D0792199

Get the most out of this book...

Use the Companion CD-ROM!

Specially developed to accompany *Kinn's The Medical Assistant: An Applied Learning Approach, 10th Edition*, the **Companion CD-ROM** offers innovative features that help you get more out of this book.

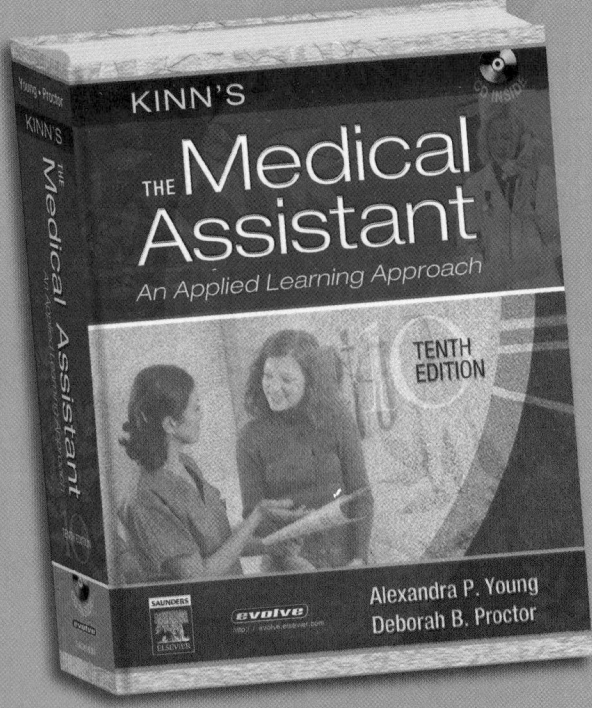

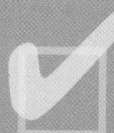 **Medical Assisting Competency Challenges**
Improve your critical thinking and decision-making skills with 35 learning activities that encourage you to apply key concepts from the textbook to realistic practice scenarios.

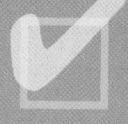 **AltaPoint's Electronic Medical Record Software**
Familiarize yourself with the technology used in today's medical office with this user-friendly software demonstration.

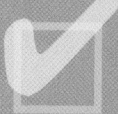 **Anatomy and Physiology Animations**
Strengthen your knowledge of the body and medical terminology with detailed anatomy and physiology animations.

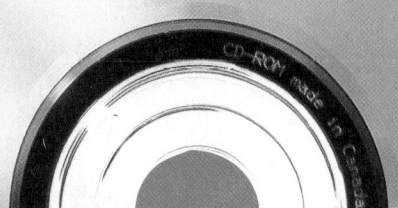

Don't wait another minute — start using the Companion CD-ROM today!

KINN'S

THE Medical Assistant

An Applied Learning Approach

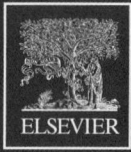

evolve

To access your Student Resources, visit:

http://evolve.elsevier.com/Kinn/

Evolve® Learning Resources for *Kinn's: The Medical Assistant: An Applied Learning Approach,* **Tenth Edition,** offer the following features:

Student Resources

- **Dosage and Calculation Exercises**
- **Altapoint Demo Exercises**
- **Study Tips**
- **Succeeding on an Externship**
- **Succeeding on the Job**
- **Weblinks**
- **Online Quizzes**
- **Medical Assisting Exam Review Practice Questions**
- **Procedure Checklists**

http://evolve.elsevier.com/Kinn/

KINN'S
THE Medical Assistant

An Applied Learning Approach

TENTH EDITION

Alexandra Patricia Young, BBA, RMA, CMA

Adjunct Instructor
Everest College, Arlington Midcities Campus
Arlington, Texas
Professional Writer
Grand Prairie, Texas

Deborah B. Proctor, EdD, RN

Professor and Medical Assisting Program Director
Butler County Community College
Butler, Pennsylvania

With over 1200 illustrations

SAUNDERS

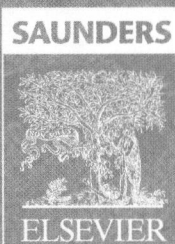

ELSEVIER

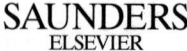

SAUNDERS
ELSEVIER

11830 Westline Industrial Drive
St. Louis, Missouri 63146

KINN'S THE MEDICAL ASSISTANT:
AN APPLIED LEARNING APPROACH

ISBN-13: 978-1-4160-2420-0
ISBN-10: 1-4160-2420-4

Copyright © 2007, 2003, 1999, 1993, 1988, 1981, 1974, 1967, 1960, 1956 by Saunders, an imprint of Elsevier Inc.

All rights reserved. No part of this publication may be reproduced or transmitted in any form or by any means, electronic or mechanical, including photocopying, recording, or any information storage and retrieval system, without permission in writing from the publisher. Permissions may be sought directly from Elsevier's Health Sciences Rights Department in Philadelphia, PA, USA: phone: (+1) 215 239 3804, fax: (+1) 215 239 3805, e-mail: healthpermissions@elsevier.com. You may also complete your request on-line via the Elsevier homepage (http://www.elsevier.com), by selecting 'Customer Support' and then 'Obtaining Permissions'.

Notice

Knowledge and best practice in this field are constantly changing. As new research and experience broaden our knowledge, changes in practice, treatment and drug therapy may become necessary or appropriate. Readers are advised to check the most current information provided (i) on procedures featured or (ii) by the manufacturer of each product to be administered, to verify the recommended dose or formula, the method and duration of administration, and contraindications. It is the responsibility of the practitioner, relying on their own experience and knowledge of the patient, to make diagnoses, to determine dosages and the best treatment for each individual patient, and to take all appropriate safety precautions. To the fullest extent of the law, neither the Publisher nor the Authors assume any liability for any injury and/or damage to persons or property arising out or related to any use of the material contained in this book.

The Publisher

ISBN-13: 978-1-4160-2420-0
ISBN-10: 1-4160-2420-4

Executive Editor: Susan Cole
Developmental Editor: Celeste Clingan
Publishing Services Manager: Patricia Tannian
Project Manager: Sarah Wunderly
Senior Book Designer: Julia Dummitt

Printed in United States of America

Last digit is the print number: 9 8 7 6 5 4 3

Working together to grow
libraries in developing countries

www.elsevier.com | www.bookaid.org | www.sabre.org

ELSEVIER   BOOK AID
            International   Sabre Foundat

DEDICATION

To my dad, J. W. Crumley, my grandmother, Lucille Saxton, and to all of the healthcare professionals who cared for them during their illnesses. Thank you for your dedication to medicine and to your patients.

To all medical assisting students who seek to improve their lives by helping others.

Alexandra Patricia Young, BBA, RMA, CMA

To my students and the students who will use this textbook to develop professional medical assistant skills. Among you are individuals who are recent high school graduates, perhaps lacking a strong academic background, worried that you will not be successful. Others are "non-traditional" students, many of you returning to school to make a better life for yourselves. Regardless of your background and your learning needs my hope is that this text, with its focus on learning principles and student achievement, will help you accomplish your goals.

To my children, Sara, Erin, Sean, and Scott, who continue to brighten my life. There are never enough moments for us to be together.

To my husband, Timothy Shields Proctor, thank you for giving me you, for patiently waiting for the endless book work to be finished, and for your unending loving support.

To my mother, Rose Conrad Beck, who lost her battle with cancer on May 26, 2006, in her home surrounded by her eight children. I miss you Mom.

Deborah B. Proctor, EdD, RN

PREFACE

Medical assisting as a profession has changed dramatically since *The Office Assistant in Medical and Dental Practice*, by Portia Frederick and Carol Towner, was first published in 1956. Each subsequent edition of this textbook has reflected the age in which it was published. Now, 50 years and ten editions later, *Kinn's The Medical Assistant: An Applied Learning Approach*, Tenth Edition, continues to represent a long-standing commitment to quality medical assisting education with its engaging, straightforward writing style and demonstrated positive outcomes. Hundreds of instructors in classrooms across the country have used this text to teach thousands of students over the years. Many of these students have gone on to teach students of their own with this very same trusted resource. To continue the use and growth of this text and its features, the tenth edition has undergone a massive revision in an effort to offer the most comprehensive, up-to-date, and innovative approach to teaching this subject today. We appreciate the opportunity to explore the exciting field of medical assisting with you!

DISTINCTIVE FEATURES OF OUR APPROACH

This textbook has endured throughout the years because it has been able to keep pace with an ever-changing profession while producing students who are well trained and qualified to enter medical practices across the country. This dependability is why the market continues to rely on this text edition after edition. Underlying this dependability is a foundation of pedagogical features that has stood the test of time and that has been expanded and improved upon yet again in this new edition. Such features include the following:

- An easy-to-read, highly interactive writing style that engages students through practical applications of medical assistant competencies.
- An emphasis on skill development with procedural steps outlining each skill, supported by rationales that provide meaning to each step.
- An organizational approach that addresses each body system with its own chapter, with additional chapters dedicated to specialty medical assistant skills.
- Each clinical chapter begins with a review of that system's anatomy and physiology, then moves to the common disorders found in that system, with the chapter concluding with patient education and legal and ethical issues.
- A pedagogical framework based on the use of learning objectives, vocabulary terms, and supportive student supplements.
- A package of supportive materials to accommodate a wide variety of student learning types and instructor teaching styles.

NEW FEATURES IN THIS EDITION

The medical field is an ever-changing one, with constant advances in diagnostic procedures and treatment protocols. Accrediting agencies, including the Committee on Accreditation of Allied Health Programs (CAAHEP) and the Accrediting Bureau of Health Education Schools (ABHES), place demands on faculty and medical assistant programs to maintain accreditation standards. The influence of current risk management practices and the potential of electronic technology as a resource for student and patient education have both complicated and expanded the opportunities available to medical assistant professionals.

To build on the long-established strengths of the Kinn textbook, the tenth edition expands and supplements the techniques used so successfully in past editions. The combined talents and backgrounds of the two primary authors and the contributors has resulted in a text that adheres to the Kinn tradition while meeting the needs of a new generation of medical assistant educators and students. The result is an innovative text that comprehensively meets the educational and accreditation needs of all types of medical assistant programs while effectively training tomorrow's medical assisting professionals.

This edition of *Kinn's The Medical Assistant* incorporates a unique approach that is reflected in the subtitle: An Applied Learning Approach. It is believed that learning takes place only when students are engaged and when the learning requires something from them in response to information that is being imparted to them.

This "applied" theme is set up-front in the first chapter, which introduces students to the concepts of critical thinking and the impact of individual learning styles on student success. This in turn transitions into time management and problem-solving skills, as well as effective study skills and test-taking strategies. The text develops from there true to the original Kinn textbook, with its distinctive Administrative and Clinical sections, and is rounded out by the last chapter that helps the student focus on preparing for and nurturing a career as a medical assistant.

This pedagogical theme and other new enhancements can be found throughout the book and its supplements in the following features:

- Each chapter opens with a scenario related to the chapter's focus. This introduces students to a medical assistant and a situation, with questions to consider, that provide a way for students to directly apply concepts they are learning. These features challenge them to think about how they would behave and the decisions they would make in certain situations.
- Each chapter also opens with national curriculum competency tables that outline current competencies for CAAHEP and ABHES, two primary accrediting associations. Within the chapters, specific CAAHEP and ABHES competencies are identified within the Procedures to ensure that students attain the necessary requirements to achieve employment in the medical assisting profession.
- Throughout the chapter, Critical Thinking Applications are designed to allow the student to use a concept that has just been learned in the context of the overall chapter scenario. These exercises help students look at the big picture and consider various angles, or approaches, to the challenges in which they will eventually find themselves in the medical office. These exercises provide a wonderful opportunity for discussion and further reflection.
- Chapters end with a Summary of Scenario that identifies concepts for student focus, as well as a discussion, where relevant, of patient education as it relates to the chapter focus and concepts within the chapter. The answers to Scenario questions provide relevant information that the student may encounter as a professional in the field.
- Well-developed Learning Objectives emphasize the cognitive and performance objectives addressed in the chapter, and are summarized at the end of each chapter for student review of learning.
- The artwork throughout has been updated and modernized, providing a more attractive textbook for student use. Many new photographs throughout better support the revised content and are more relevant to the actual medical office. Many photographs were replaced with new images that show updated equipment, provide more disease examples, and better illustrate key procedural steps.
- Chapter 8 on computers has been revised and thoroughly updated to include timely information to reflect the sophisticated computer systems found in today's busy medical practice. It provides easy-to-understand details about subjects such as the elements of microprocessors, an "inside-the-computer" section, file formats, internet connectivity, networking basics, computer security, and ergonomics. The medical records management and health information chapters also include an in-depth discussion of computer-based medical records.
- More than any previous edition, customer service is stressed throughout the chapters. As patients become more involved in their healthcare, medical assistants must realize that the healthcare field is a service industry and that patients should be treated as customers.
- New to this edition, The Office Environment and Daily Operations chapter provides information about procedures for managing an office, expenses involved in the operation of a medical office, proper waste management, and basic safety and security.
- Also new to this edition, the Privacy in the Physician's Office chapter explains how the HIPAA Privacy Rule benefits the healthcare industry and the patient, discusses rights of patients under the Privacy Rule, and what is expected of healthcare providers.
- New compliance regulations in medical billing and coding have lent a far greater emphasis on reimbursement than ever before. The billing and coding unit has been expanded and updated and includes the following: basics of diagnostic coding, basics of procedural coding, basics of health insurance, and the health insurance claim form. Chapter 20 includes an introduction to and directions for using the new CMS 1500 (08/05 version) that will be required in April of 2007.
- The clinical section includes updated protocols regarding infection control, new information about MyPyramid in the nutrition and health promotion chapter, and recommendations for IV therapy in the chapter about administering medications.
- New to this edition is the integration of administrative concepts into the discussions of the various diseases and conditions within each medical specialty, including application of telephone screening situations and related medical documentation. This innovative feature transcends the traditional separation of administrative and clinical and brings them together in the context of real-world application.
- Each clinical specialty chapter has been completely revised and has expanded its focus on medical terminology, anatomy and physiology, and pathophysiology. In addition to focusing on the diagnostic and therapeutic interventions that are most frequently used in each specialty, the equipment and pharmacology that students can expect to encounter when working in that specialty, is discussed, including drug types and dosage calculations.
- The Connections heading at the end of each chapter integrates text content with accompanying ancillaries and Internet sites. These provide students and instructors with a means to enhance their understanding of chapter concepts and to stay current on medical news, trends, and industry developments.

EVOLVE

Stay current with trends, developments, and news in the medical field, as well as access additional chapter supplemental features, advice on your externship, interviewing techniques, and more through EVOLVE, the website that is provided complimentary to this textbook. This exciting website is an interactive learning environment that adds an incredibly powerful set of instructional resources to your classroom experience. EVOLVE works in coordination with *Kinn's The Medical Assistant: An Applied Learning Approach,* Tenth Edition, by providing Internet-based course content and Internet web links to reinforce and expand your learning experience.

In addition to the Evolve Learning Resources available to students, an entire suite of tools is available to instructors that allows for communication between instructors and students, including discussion boards, e-mail, chat rooms, and more.

To access this comprehensive online resource, simply go to the EVOLVE home page at http://evolve.elsevier.com and enter your user name and password provided to you from your instructor. If your instructor has not set up a Course Management System, you can still access all the learning resources available free with this textbook by going to http://evolve.elsevier.com/Kinn/.

EXTENSIVE SUPPLEMENTAL RESOURCES

The diversity of students, instructors, programs, institutions, and teaching environments using this textbook required that we develop an integrated, comprehensive, and flexible package of supplements to support *Kinn's The Medical Assistant: An Applied Learning Approach,* Tenth Edition. Each of these innovative supplements is designed to enhance the teaching and learning experience, with the outcome of producing students well equipped to pass any certification examination, and who will go on to experience successful professional careers in medical assisting. These supplements and their unique features include the following:

Student Software Program

The free CD-ROM that comes with your textbook includes three programs designed for you to apply the key content and skills you've learned throughout the textbook. The Medical Assisting Competency Challenge provides realistic scenarios, with you making the decisions and getting feedback on each decision you make, plus a skill-building section that lets you practice both administrative and clinical competencies. All forms used throughout are included for reference in a format suitable for printing. The Anatomy and Physiology animations will help you strengthen your knowledge of the body and medical terminology. The Altapoint demo is derived from a real medical office software program and lets you practice front office skills on the computer.

Study Guide

This practical tool takes the "applied learning approach" to a whole new level, giving you the opportunity to apply the knowledge and skills you are learning in the textbook. Some of the outstanding features of this study guide include:

- Reinforcement of anatomy and physiology with extensive labeling exercises.
- Procedure checklists that serve as a valuable tool for checking your competency, as well as a tool for your instructor to gauge your skill level and proficiency for each skill in the textbook.
- A multitude of exercises to reinforce key content throughout the textbook, including vocabulary exercises that help you recall and apply medical terms.
- Coding applications, documentation scenarios, and telephone screening examples provide you with the opportunity to apply administrative concepts to clinical situations.

- Instrument identification, as well as a review of disease-specific skills, further reinforces clinical material.
- Chapter quizzes at the end of each chapter exercise set allow you to further test your knowledge.
- Study tips for all medical assisting students, as well as a section on study tips specifically designed for ESL (English-as-a-Second-Language) students, written by an ESL consultant.
- A glossary of English-Spanish terms, based on the text glossary, gives students an excellent resource for working with patients who speak English as a second language. This glossary is likewise extremely helpful for those medical assisting students who themselves speak English as a second language.

Instructor's Resource Manual

This complete instructor teaching tool includes extensive curriculum materials in both print and electronic formats. Beginning and veteran instructors alike will be able to easily prepare their lectures, presentations, labs, and assessments with an extensive course syllabus, multiple course outlines, individual chapter lesson plans, chapter Internet addresses, and ready-made tests for each chapter. Answer keys for all text and Student Study Guide questions are also included. In addition, special tips for instructors with ESL (English-as-a-Second-Language) students have been provided, written by an ESL consultant.

Test Bank

Our test bank provides an accurate and exhaustive source of test items for a wide variety of examination styles. It contains more than 1,900 questions, and is available in both printed and electronic format so you can easily prepare your quizzes and exams, tailored to your classroom format.

PowerPoint Presentation Slides

The instructor CD-ROM includes a PowerPoint viewer and a set of over 1,400 PowerPoint slides. The slides include a summary of key chapter material, and can easily be customized to support your lectures and enhance your classroom presentation. All slides have been formatted to reflect the text design, and include nearly 300 images from the text. These slides can also be easily formatted within the PowerPoint program for student note taking or as overhead transparencies.

TEACH Lesson Plan Manual

The TEACH Lesson Plan Manual includes a print version of the lesson plan manual as well as a CD containing all TEACH resources. Assets are also available via the Evolve website. The TEACH Lesson Plan Manual provides instructors with customizable lesson plans and lecture outlines based on learning objectives. With these valuable resources, instructors will save valuable preparation time and create a learning environment that fully engages students in classroom preparation. The lesson plans are linked to each chapter and are divided into 50-minute units in a three-column format. Instructors will also have lecture outlines in PowerPoint with talking points, thought-provoking questions, and unique ideas for lectures. The Instructor's

Electronic Resource on CD contains a testbank in ExamView with over 500 questions and PowerPoint slides.

KINN'S MEDICAL ASSISTING ONLINE

Today's educational environment has the potential to be more interactive than ever before. The more resources available to facilitate learning, and the more varied those resources, the greater the chances are for material to be comprehended and retained.

Kinn's Medical Assisting Online has been developed with this creative approach to education in mind. Offering a multidimensional experience that is not possible in a traditional classroom setting, these unique and innovative new products are complete courses that simulate the externship experience by creating a virtual medical practice where students have an opportunity to learn by doing.

Designed to be used together with *Kinn's The Medical Assistant: An Applied Learning Approach,* Tenth Edition, this set of two courses is divided by administrative and clinical information. Lessons draw on the text for reading assignments, then provide an opportunity for you to apply text content by entering the simulated environment, complete with an office manager who acts as your supervisor/mentor through the courses, other office personnel, physicians, and realistic patient cases. This environment is an exciting way for you to discover what it is like to work in the field of medical assisting before you ever enter your externship.

A wide range of visual, auditory, and interactive elements create this exciting environment and work together to amplify key learning objectives from the textbook, giving you the opportunity to practice key skills by first being guided through a practice of each skill, then by trying to perform that skill in a realistic application exercise. This combination of guided practice and application of skills gives you the confidence to perform these skills with competence in the laboratory or on the job.

Providing a myriad of learning opportunities, Kinn's Medical Assisting Online accommodates diverse learning styles and circumstances through the use of a sophisticated learning management system that lets your instructor tailor the program's content either to support a traditional classroom learning experience or as a true distance education course. You log on through the Evolve portal to complete lessons, take quizzes and exams online, participate in threaded discussions, post assignments to your instructor, or chat with your instructor or fellow classmates, all from any location that has an Internet connection.

Alexandra Patricia Young
Deborah B. Proctor

SPECIAL FEATURES

A **Scenario** at the beginning of each chapter is presented so that the student can think about a real-world situation when reading the chapter content.

Scenario questions provide a way for students to directly apply concepts they are learning and think about decisions they would make in certain situations.

Learning Objectives emphasize the cognitive and performance objectives presented in the chapter.

The Medical Assisting Profession

3

SCENARIO

Sandra Rameriz is a single mother who has decided on medical assisting as a career. She has always been interested in the medical field and wants a job that will allow her to spend evenings and weekends with her 3-year-old son, Roberto. The idea of working in a physician's office appeals to her, and she has applied to a school that is close to her apartment and day care provider. She plans to attend day classes and work part-time after school until it is time to pick up her son.

Sandra is very excited about her new career and has set several goals for her training. First, she hopes to attain perfect attendance, and second, she would like to graduate with honors. She has budgeted her study time and plans to ask her instructors during the first 2 weeks of school for suggestions about how she can better prepare for classes and examinations. Sandra will find medical assisting to be a rewarding career and respected profession.

While studying this chapter, think about the following questions:

- What obstacles might prevent Sandra from attending all of her classes, and how can she prepare in advance to overcome them?
- How can Sandra begin to explore the type of physician offices in which she would enjoy being employed after graduation?
- What goals might Sandra have at the commencement of her training? At the end of training?
- How can Sandra make the most of her time attending school to become a medical assistant?

LEARNING OBJECTIVES

1. Define, spell, and pronounce the terms listed in the vocabulary.
2. Briefly discuss the history of medical assisting as a profession.
3. Differentiate between administrative and clinical medical assisting duties.
4. Discuss the versatility of a career in medical assisting.
5. Explain the reasons that hiring an individual who has no formal training is often more expensive than hiring a professional medical assistant.
6. Identify several considerations to keep in mind when choosing a position as a medical assistant other than financial compensation.
7. Discuss the aspects of the medical assistant's performance on a successful externship.
8. List three unacceptable behaviors on the externship site.
9. Explain why continuing education is so important to the medical assistant.
10. Discuss the difference between a CMA and an RMA.

National Accreditation Competencies and Content

ABHES COMPETENCIES	ABHES COMPETENCIES
Professionalism	**Communication**
1.a. Project a positive attitude	2.p. Professional components
1.b. Maintain confidentiality at all times	2.q. Allied health professions and credentialing
1.c. Be a "team player"	
1.d. Be cognizant of ethical boundaries	**Legal Concepts**
1.e. Exhibit initiative	5.f. Maintain licenses and accreditation
1.f. Adapt to change	
1.g. Evidence a responsible attitude	
1.h. Be courteous and diplomatic	
1.i. Conduct work within scope of education, training, and ability	

35

National Accreditation and Competencies and Content tables outline current competencies for CAAHEP and ABHES.

Each chapter contains **Vocabulary** with definitions.

Critical Thinking Application boxes are linked to the Scenario and prompt students to apply what they have learned at the end of major sections.

Illustrated step-by-step Procedures show how to perform and document administrative and clinical procedures encountered in the health-care setting.

UNIT ONE   INTRODUCTION TO MEDICAL ASSISTING   36

VOCABULARY

allied health fields Occupational disciplines in which professionals involved with the delivery of healthcare or related services assist physicians with the diagnosis, treatment, and care of patients in many different specialty areas.

benefits Services or payments provided under a health plan, employee plan, or some other agreement, including programs such as health insurance, pensions, retirement planning, and many other options that may be offered to employees of a company or organization.

certification (ser-tuh-fuh-ka'-shun) The attesting of something as being true, as represented, or as meeting a standard; the result of having been tested, usually by a third party, and awarded a certificate based on proven knowledge.

continuing education units (CEUs) Credits for courses, classes, or seminars related to an individual's profession, designed to promote education and to keep the professional up to date on current procedures and trends in his or her field; CEUs are often required for licensing.

cross-training Training in more than one area so that a multitude of duties may be performed by one person or so that substitutions of personnel may be made in an emergency or at other necessary times.

externship or internship A training program that is part of a course of study of an educational institution and is taken in the actual business setting of that field of study; the terms are often interchanged in reference to medical assistant training.

intangibles (in-tan'-juh-buls) Qualities that are incapable of being perceived, especially by touch, or incapable of being precisely identified or realized by the mind.

invasive Involving entry into the living body as by incision or insertion of an instrument.

perks Extra advantages or benefits from working in a specific job that may or may not be commonplace in that particular profession; a shortened form of *perquisites*.

phlebotomy (fli-bah'-tuh-me) The invasive procedure used to obtain a blood specimen for testing, experimentation, or diagnosis of disease.

profit sharing Offer of a part of a company's profits to employees or other designated individuals or groups.

stock options Offers of stocks for purchase to a certain group of individuals or certain groups, such as employees of a for-profit hospital.

versatile (vur'-suh-til) Embracing a variety of subjects, fields or skills; having a wide range of abilities.

UNIT SIX   FUNDAMENTALS OF CLINICAL MEDICAL ASSISTING   626

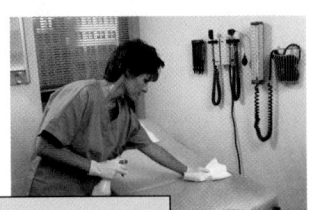

and recording vital signs. During the examination, the physician may expect the medical assistant to do the following:

- Hand instruments and equipment as requested and provide supplies as needed.
- Alter the position of a gooseneck lamp to better illuminate the area being examined, and turn lights off and on during specific phases of the examination.
- Position and drape the patient during the different phases of the examination.
- Assist in collecting and properly labeling specimens such as urine, Pap smear samplings, and throat cultures.
- Conduct follow-up diagnostic procedures as ordered including an **electrocardiogram** (ECG), eye or ear screening, urinalysis, and phlebotomy.
- Schedule postexamination diagnostic procedures such as a mammogram, x-ray examination, or **colonoscopy**.

CRITICAL THINKING APPLICATION

Felicia's first patient for the day is Harry Garcia, a 51-year-old truck driver who is scheduled for a complete physical examination. Mr. Garcia's insurance has changed since his last visit. The physician ordered an ECG to be performed and a complete blood panel to be drawn before the physical. What does Felicia need to complete before Dr. Kosto sees the patient?

Supplies and Instruments Needed for the Physical Examination

The instruments typically used during the physical examination are displayed in Figure 31-2. They enable the physician to see, feel, inspect, and listen to parts of the body. All equipment must be in good working order, properly disinfected, and readily available for the physician's use during the examination. The instruments most frequently used for the physical examination are described in the following paragraphs. Physical examinations are typically conducted from the head to the feet; the instruments are listed in the order in which the physician would typically request them.

Ophthalmoscope. An ophthalmoscope is used to inspect the inner structures of the eye. It has a stainless-steel handle containing batteries, onto which a head is attached. The head is equipped with a light and magnifying lenses and an opening through which the eye is viewed. Examination rooms are usually equipped with wall-mounted electrical units for the ophthalmoscope and otoscope, a dispenser for disposable speculums, and a wall-mounted sphygmomanometer (Figure 31-3).

Tongue Depressor. A tongue depressor is a flat, wooden blade used to hold down the tongue when examining the throat (Figure 31-4).

Otoscope. An otoscope is used to examine the external auditory canal and tympanic membrane. It has a stainless-steel handle containing batteries or is part of a wall-mounted electrical unit (see Figure 31-3). The head of the otoscope contains a light that is focused through a magnifying lens and should be covered with disposable ear speculum. The light may also be used to illuminate the nasal passages and throat.

UNIT EIGHT   ASSISTING WITH MEDICAL SPECIALTIES   896

PROCEDURE 41-4

Prepare Patient for and Assist with Routine and Specialty Examinations: Obtain Pediatric Vital Signs and Vision Screening

<u>CAAHEP COMPETENCIES:</u> 3.b.(4)(b), 3.b.(4)(e)
<u>ABHES COMPETENCIES:</u> 4.d, 4.h

GOAL: To accurately obtain vital signs for and assess vision of a pediatric patient.

EQUIPMENT and SUPPLIES

- Digital or tympanic thermometer
- Pediatric blood pressure cuff
- Wristwatch with sweep second hand
- Weight scale with height bar
- Stethoscope
- Snellen E eye chart and oculator
- Pen
- Patient's chart

PROCEDURAL STEPS

1. Gather equipment.
   PURPOSE: Efficiency.
2. Wash your hands.
   PURPOSE: Infection control.
3. Explain the procedure to the parent, and if you want the parent to help by holding the child, explain the technique you want him or her to employ.
   PURPOSE: Explanations ahead of time save time and enhance cooperation.
4. Help the child stand in the center of the scale, and weigh the child. Ask the child to turn around, and obtain the child's height. Record your findings.
5. Obtain tympanic or axillary temperature using the procedure explained in Chapter 30 (Figure 1).
6. Record the tympanic or axillary temperature. Indicate the method used: A = axillary, T = tympanic.
   PURPOSE: A procedure is not done until it is recorded in the patient's record.
7. Place the stethoscope on the child's chest at the midpoint between the sternum and the left nipple. Listen for the apical beat (Figure 2).

8. Count the apical beat for 1 full minute.
9. Record the apical pulse. Be sure to place an Ap before the rate to indicate that this is an apical pulse reading.
   PURPOSE: A procedure is not done until it is recorded on the patient's record.
10. Place your flat hand on the child's chest, and count the respirations for 1 full minute.
11. Record the respiration rate.
    PURPOSE: A procedure is not done until it is recorded on the patient's record.
12. Check to be sure that you have the correct-size blood pressure cuff, then proceed with taking the blood pressure. Follow procedure in Chapter 30 (Figure 3).
13. Record the blood pressure.
    PURPOSE: A procedure is not done until it is recorded in the patient's record.
14. If vision screening is to be done, familiarize the child with the E chart by asking him to make an E point the same way as your

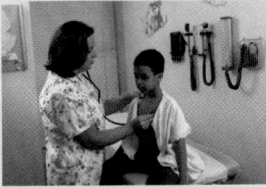

FIGURE 2

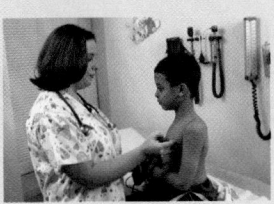

FIGURE 1

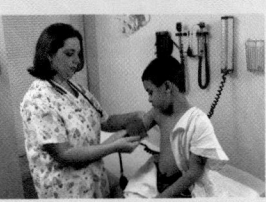

FIGURE 3

Continued

- Reinforce the instructions the physician gave the patient.
- Be sure you are comfortable performing a procedure.
- If you have any concerns about a procedure, discuss them with the physician privately before proceeding.
- Do not perform a procedure if you are uncomfortable; get someone to help you.

Always remember: You are the assistant, and this is the physician's patient. The physician is ultimately responsible for every aspect of the patient's care. If you feel uncertain or unsure of any order that the physician has written for a patient, you must get it clarified before you proceed. Always stay within the legal and ethical guidelines of the medical assisting profession in your state.

SUMMARY OF SCENARIO

Kaiwan is becoming more and more comfortable in his position as an orthopedic medical assistant at the sports medicine clinic. His enthusiasm is contagious. Patients consistently comment on his positive, upbeat manner. Kaiwan is motivated to learn new things and methods for better assisting the physicians with routine procedures. He always seeks answers to questions that occur with new patients. He has gained a great deal of confidence and now remembers to always check the paraffin bath temperature before starting a treatment. One of the most enjoyable aspects of his job continues to be assisting Dr. Alexander with treating the team members. Kaiwan has attended two sports medicine continuing education seminars with Dr. Alexander. He is now thinking about continuing his education part-time to become an athletic trainer while continuing to work at the clinic. Kaiwan recognizes the importance of continuing education in maintaining orthopedic skills.

SUMMARY of LEARNING OBJECTIVES

1. Define, spell, and pronounce the terms listed in the vocabulary.
   - Spelling and pronouncing medical terms correctly adds credibility to the medical assistant. Knowing the definition of these terms promotes confidence in communication with patients and co-workers.
2. Describe the principal structures of the musculoskeletal system and their functions.
   - The main structures of the musculoskeletal system include the skeletal muscles, which provide movement; tendons, which connect muscles to bones; bones, which provide support, protection, mineral storage, and blood cell development; and ligaments, which connect bone to bone.
3. Differentiate among tendons, bursae, and ligaments.
   - Tendons are the tough bands that connect muscles to bones; ligaments provide support by connecting bone to bone and preventing a joint from moving beyond its normal ROM. Bursae prevent friction between different tissues in the musculoskeletal system.
4. Summarize the major muscular disorders.
   - Fibromyalgia is a condition of unknown origin that causes widespread connective tissue and muscular pain with sleep disorders and extreme fatigue. Myasthenia gravis is an autoimmune disorder that affects the use of ACh at the neuromuscular junction, resulting in muscular weakness, especially in the face and eyes. A sprain is the tearing of ligaments and a strain is the overstretching or tearing of a muscle or tendon.
5. Identify and describe the common types of fractures.
   - The common types of fractures are explained in Table 42-3.

6. Explain the difference between osteomalacia and osteoporosis.
   - Osteomalacia is the softening of bone because of a problem with the metabolism or absorption of vitamin D, calcium, and phosphorus; in children the condition is called *rickets*. Osteoporosis is a decrease in bone density caused by many factors including lack of dietary calcium earlier in life; it leads to brittle bones that easily fracture.
7. Classify typical spinal column disorders.
   - Spinal column disorders are related to the shape of the spine; scoliosis is a lateral deviation, lordosis or swayback is a pronounced curve of the lower back, kyphosis is a pronounced cervical curve or hunchback.
8. Differentiate among the various joint disorders.
   - Joint disorders include dislocations when the two bones of the joint are no longer approximated; gout, which is a form of arthritis caused by a collection of uric acid crystals most commonly in the synovial membrane of the great toe; SLE, which is a widespread autoimmune disorder that can affect any organ system in the body; Lyme disease, a form of infectious arthritis that is caused by ba[...] and that can result in exten[...] if left untreated; OA, caused [...] cartilage of synovial joints; [...] causes crippling pain and d[...] and bursitis, which are infla[...] tissue that are typically caus[...]
9. Summarize the medical assista[...] procedures.
   - The medical assistant is res[...]

SUMMARY of LEARNING OBJECTIVES
Continued

rapid, weak, and thready pulse; tachypnea; and altered levels of consciousness. If the process is not reversed, the central nervous system becomes depressed and acute renal failure may occur.

10. Summarize the characteristics of common vascular disorders.
    - Varicose veins are dilated, tortuous, superficial veins in the legs that develop because the valves do not completely close, allowing blood to flow backward, thus causing the vein to distend from the increased pressure. Phlebitis is an inflammation of the veins most commonly seen in the lower legs. DVT is a thrombus with inflammatory changes that has attached to the deep venous system of the lower legs and has caused a partial or complete obstruction of the vessel. If a thrombus becomes dislodged and begins to circulate through the general circulation, it is then called an embolus. Arteriosclerosis is a general term for the thickening and loss

of elasticity of arterial walls; it can occur in arteries throughout the body and cause systemic ischemia and necrosis over time. Atherosclerosis is a form of arteriosclerosis in which the formation of an atheroma occurs. An aneurysm is a ballooning or dilation of the wall of a vessel caused by weakening of the vessel wall. Peripheral arterial disease affects the vessels outside of the heart, especially the legs and feet, in which circulation is decreased and ischemia can occur.

11. Outline typical cardiovascular diagnostic procedures.
    - Cardiovascular diagnostic procedures include Doppler studies of the patency of blood vessels; angiography to show arterial pathways; echocardiography to assess the structure and movement of the parts of the heart, especially the valves; and cardiac catheterization to show the heart chambers, valves,

CONNECTIONS

Study Guide Connection: Go to Chapter 46 Study Guide. Read the Case Study and Workplace Applications and complete the assignments. Do online research for answers to the questions in the Internet Activities associated with assisting in cardiology.

CD Connection: Go to the Medical Assisting Competency Challenge CD and do the training activities under Diagnostic Testing. For a better understanding of the function of the heart, view the animation for normal cardiopulmonary physiology.

Evolve Connection: For more information related to assisting in cardiology, go to evolve.elsevier.com/kinn and visit related weblinks for Chapter 46. Click on the Medical Assisting Exam Review and do the practice questions to sharpen your test-taking skills.

At the end of the chapter, the **Summary of Scenario** provides students with relevant information that they may encounter as a professional in the field.

Summary of Learning Objectives reviews important points of the chapter's focus, reinforcing content students must master.

Connections information at the end of the chapter presents ancillary products and resources that are available to assist students' comprehension of concepts and to enhance their learning experience

REVIEWERS

We are deeply grateful to the numerous people who have shared their comments and suggestions on this edition. Reviewing a book or supplement takes an incredible amount of energy and attention, and we are glad so many of our colleagues were able to take time out of their busy schedule to help ensure the validity and appropriateness of content in this edition. The reviewers provided us with additional viewpoints and opinions that combine to make this text an incredible learning tool. We wish to thank the following editorial reviewing team:

Michelle Buchman RN, BSN, BC
Nursing Director, St. John's Marian Center
Owner/Manager Educational Support Services, LLC
Springfield, Missouri

Amy DeVore, BA, CMA
Instructor
Butler County Community College
Butler, Pennsylvania

Monica D. Flowers, CMIS, CHI
Administrative Medical Assisting and Medical Office Specialist
Instructor
Arlington Career Institute
Grand Prairie, Texas

Deborah Holmes, RN, CMA-C
Former Medical Assisting Program Chair
Iowa Western Community College
Council Bluffs, Iowa

Maureen Messier, CMA, RMA, AS, BA
Instructor, Medical Assisting/General Education
Branford Hall Career Institute
Southington, Connecticut

Andrea Potteiger, CPC, CMAA, CBCS, CHI, NR-CAHA, NR-CMA, NR-CPT, NR-CEKG
Lead Healthcare Instructor
New Horizons
Harrisburg, Pennsylvania

Donna M. Schenkel, BA
Coding Instructor
Southeast Technical Institute
Sioux Falls, South Dakota

Janet Sesser, RMA(AMT), CMA, BSEd Admin
Director of Education for Allied Health
High-Tech Institute, Inc.
Phoenix, Arizona

Lynn Slack, CMA
Medical Programs Director
ICM School of Business and Medical Careers
Pittsburgh, Pennsylvania

CONTRIBUTORS TO THIS EDITION

The preceding section demonstrates the amount of feedback and developmental input that went into shaping the tenth edition of this book. Because the medical assisting curriculum is so broad in scope, no individual can be an expert in all areas. We therefore extend a special acknowledgment to the following people who brought their expertise to bear by contributing one or more chapters to this edition:

Robin R. Patterson, BS, MT(ASCP), MS, EdD
Professor
Department of Technology and Natural Science
Butler County Community College
Butler, Pennsylvania

Carline A. Dalgleish, MA, BS, CMA
Owner/Director
COUGAR-Ed.net LLC Department of Medicine
Arlington, Texas

AUTHOR ACKNOWLEDGMENTS

I consider it a privilege to be one of the authors of this incredible textbook. I appreciate the dedication and tireless work performed by the editorial, design, and production team that partnered with us on *Kinn's The Medical Assistant: An Applied Learning Approach*, Tenth Edition. This textbook has led countless medical assistants into a career that has allowed them to express compassion, caring, and dedication to health and wellness.

Years before I became associated with the writing of this textbook, I used it to teach my own students. Thousands of medical assistants today owe a great debt to Mary Kinn, the original author, for her innovation and dedication to the medical assisting field. I personally appreciate her vision, her past input, and her contributions that brought the text from its first edition through many subsequent editions. As we publish this tenth edition, our appreciation for Mary Kinn is heartfelt and sincere.

Susan Cole, Executive Editor, is a dedicated, sharp editor with a keen insight into the allied health profession and her professionalism is absolutely second to none. She listened to ideas, provided insight, encouragement, and endless support to Deb and me as we revised the book, determined to make the text even better than the last edition. I especially want to thank Susan for her support and her ability to help me refocus during the difficult months that my family faced while I was writing this revision.

Celeste Clingan, Developmental Editor, assisted every step of the way and her wonderful attitude made the writing process much easier. Celeste was always open to new ideas and concepts, and was complimentary to us as a writing team when those ideas worked. I know that this is a project that she will be proud of, because she did a gigantic amount of work, kept us organized, and remained supportive throughout the entire process.

I sincerely appreciate the work and contributions of Sarah Wunderly, Senior Project Manager. She was consistently cooperative and helpful during the production stages of this process. A warm thank-you goes to each one of her team members who worked on the Kinn project.

Dr. Deb Proctor is an amazing partner, always the consummate professional and a wealth of great ideas. It is a great privilege to work alongside such an outstanding leader in the medical profession. I appreciate that I can feel confident in Deb's knowledge of the clinical side of the book, knowing that she has provided medical assisting students with the exact knowledge that they need to enter this marvelous career field. Thank you, Deb, for all that you do.

Additional thanks to Amy Devore for partnering with us on the ancillary products. Amy's enthusiasm and experience is impressive and her contributions will make these products second to none. Carline Dalgleish joined our writing team and contributed four chapters in the administrative section of the text. Carline did an outstanding job and I am so grateful that she was willing to share her wealth of knowledge with today's students.

During the revision of this edition, I experienced several devastating losses and challenging times. Three individuals who inspired me and were crucial parts of my life passed away, and my son was diagnosed with a curable cancer. These events brought me into contact with the healthcare professionals that I write about in this text. As I experienced life on the other side of the thermometer, so to speak, I was reminded of the reasons that I entered the healthcare profession long ago in 1981. The dedication of the professionals who cared for my family was heartwarming and encouraging. The healthcare profession is the most rewarding career field available, and my hope is that more and more individuals choose allied health careers in the future.

And last, my family deserves so many thanks, because they allowed me to work on this textbook when they would rather have had my time to themselves. My children, Jimmie, Jonathan, Jessica, and Stacey, inspire me daily. My mother, Patricia Crumley, has been supportive ever since she held up flash cards in the wee hours of the morning while I was learning medical terminology during my own school years. Thanks also go to my sisters, Alisha Crumley and Karry Chapman, for endless encouragement and support. And last of all, tremendous thanks to my fiancé, Bentley Charles Adams. You are my rock, the man that I can always depend on, the man to whom I can release all of my concerns and know that they will be handled with care. Thank you for your belief in me and my abilities as a writer. I look forward to the rocking chairs on the front porch of our home in years to come.

Alexandra Patricia Young, BBA, RMA, CMA

Just like many of you who are starting school to learn a new profession, I have gone back to school many times since graduating from a nursing program over 30 years ago. One thing that I am absolutely sure of is that learning never ends if you have decided to pursue a career in medicine. For those of us who are lifelong learners, we have a significant ally in the Elsevier publishing team. Creating a comprehensive medical assisting text that meets the needs of accredited programs or those seeking accreditation, as well as one that fosters a user-friendly learning environment for students enrolled in those programs, is a highly complex process. From the first organizational meeting for the tenth edition to the final proofs a wide range of professionals contributed to this effort. Thank you to all of those individuals who have offered Tricia and I consistent guidance and direction, especially Sarah Wunderly, Senior Project Manager, and Celeste Clingan, Developmental Editor. As with the previous edition, I have had the pleasure of working with Tricia Young on the tenth edition of Kinn. I appreciate her contributions in the development of a text that focuses on the comprehensive coverage of material that meets national accreditation standards as well as provides students the opportunity to learn in a student-centered environment.

One of our goals with this revision was to involve the authors in the development of the ancillary package. Unfortunately, because of family concerns, I was unable to follow through with my commitment. I owe a special note of thanks to one of my former students, Amy Geibel DeVore, who has worked to create ancillaries for the clinical portion of the text that emphasize student application of learning. Amy embodies the W. B. Yeats quote, "Education is not the filling of a bucket, but the lighting of a fire." She brings energy, creativity, experience in the medical assistant profession, and a total dedication to teaching to this project which she completed shortly before giving birth to her first child

I have experienced multiple significant professional and personal events since working on the last edition of this text. Some of those include rewriting the medical assistant curriculum at Butler County Community College to better meet the needs of our students; successfully preparing for and surviving the CAAHEP continuing accreditation process at the College; my and my daughter's marriages and the challenge of helping care for my 85-year-old mother as she battled a terminal disease. So, more than anything else, I acknowledge the contribution of my mom who provided love and support, and taught me many valuable lessons...perhaps the most important is to treat all people with understanding and respect. I hope that those of you who use this text will see that message repeated over and over again as I encourage each of you to provide your patients and their families the type of care you would want for yourself or your loved ones.

Deborah B. Proctor, EdD, RN

CONTENTS

UNIT EIGHT
Assisting with Medical Specialties

List of Procedures

Becoming a Successful Student

SCENARIO

Shawna Long is a newly admitted student in a medical assistant program at your school. Shawna is anxious about starting classes and very concerned that she may not be a successful student. She had trouble with some of her classes in high school and must continue to work part time while taking medical assistant classes. Based on what you discover about the learning process in this chapter, see if you can help Shawna take steps toward success.

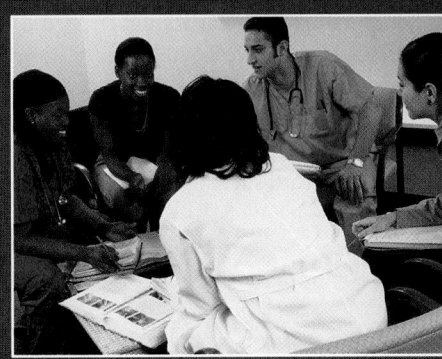

While studying this chapter, think about the following questions:

- Why is it important for Shawna to understand how she learns best?
- Time management is an important part of being a successful student as well as a successful medical assistant. What are some strategies Shawna can implement to help her manage her time as effectively as possible?
- Shawna will face many problems and conflicts while working through the MA program. How can she develop workable strategies for dealing with these issues?
- Studying may be a challenge for Shawna. What skills can she use to help her learn new material and prepare for examinations?

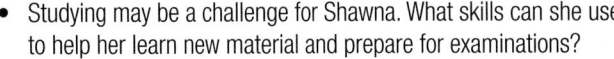

LEARNING OBJECTIVES

1. Define and spell the terms listed in the vocabulary.
2. Assess the importance of developing professional behaviors as a member of the allied health team.
3. Evaluate the concept of critical thinking and how it affects your actions.
4. Examine your learning preferences.
5. Interpret how your learning style affects your success as a student.
6. Apply time-management strategies to make the most of your learning opportunities.
7. Use problem-solving techniques to manage conflict and barriers to your success.
8. Integrate effective study skills into your daily activities.
9. Design test-taking strategies that help you take charge of your success.
10. Incorporate critical thinking and reflection to make mental connections as material is learned.

VOCABULARY

critical thinking The constant practice of considering all aspects of a situation when deciding what to believe or what to do.

empathy (em′-puh-the) Sensitivity to the individual needs and reactions of patients.

learning style The way that an individual perceives and processes information to learn new material.

perceiving (pur-sev′-ing) How an individual looks at information and sees it as real.

processing (pro′-ses-ing) How an individual internalizes new information and makes it his or her own.

professional behaviors Those actions that identify the medical assistant as a member of a healthcare profession, including being dependable, performing respectful patient care, exercising initiative, demonstrating a positive attitude, and using teamwork.

reflection (re-flek′-shun) The process of considering new information and internalizing it to create new ways of examining information.

You have taken the first step toward becoming a successful student by choosing your profession and field of study. The medical assistant profession is both challenging and rewarding. Becoming a medical assistant opens the doors to a wide variety of opportunities in both administrative and clinical practice at ambulatory or institutional healthcare settings. Medical assistants are important members of the healthcare team, and as a healthcare professional you will be expected to practice certain **professional behaviors** (Figure 1-1). These professional behaviors, which are discussed in depth in Chapter 4, include demonstrating dependability, respectful patient care, **empathy,** initiative, a positive attitude, and teamwork. In order to become a successful medical assistant you must first become a successful student. This chapter helps you discover the way that you learn best and provides multiple strategies to assist you in your journey toward success.

CRITICAL THINKING APPLICATION

Consider your history as a student. What do you think helped you to succeed? What do you think needs improvement? Create a plan for improvement that includes two or three ways you can become a more successful student.

WHO YOU ARE AS A LEARNER: HOW DO YOU LEARN BEST?

Think about what you do when you are faced with something new to learn. How do you go about understanding and learning the new material? Over time you have developed a method for **perceiving** and **processing** information. This pattern of behavior is called your **learning style.** Many different ways of examining learning styles exist, but most professionals agree that the success of students depends more on whether they can "make sense" of the information than on whether or not they are "smart." Education that is based on attention to individual learning styles is sensitive to the different ways that students learn and approaches new material with a wide variety of methods so that all students have the opportunity to learn. Determining your individual learning style and understanding

how it applies to your ability to learn new material are the first steps toward becoming a successful student (Figure 1-2).

Learning Style Inventory

For you to learn new material, two things must happen. First you must perceive the information. This is the method you have developed over time that helps you examine the material and recognize it as real. Then you must process the information. Processing the information is how you internalize it and make it your own. By investigating various learning styles, you can figure out how to combine different methods of perceiving and processing information. In his book *Becoming a Master Student,* David Ellis discusses these different methods of information perception, processing, and learning.

Information perception involves how you go about examining new material and making it real. Learners perceive new material in two ways. Some people are concrete perceivers who learn information through direct experience by doing, acting, sensing, or feeling. Concrete learners prefer to learn things that have a personal meaning or things that they feel are relevant. Other learners are abstract perceivers who take in information through analysis, observation, and **reflection.** Abstract learners like to think things through. They analyze the new material and build theories to help understand it. They prefer structured learning situations and use a step-by-step approach to problem solving.

Information processing is how you internalize the new information and make it your own. There also are two different methods for processing material. Active processors prefer to jump in and start doing things immediately. They make sense of the new material by immediately using it. They look for practical ways to apply the new material and typically do not mind taking

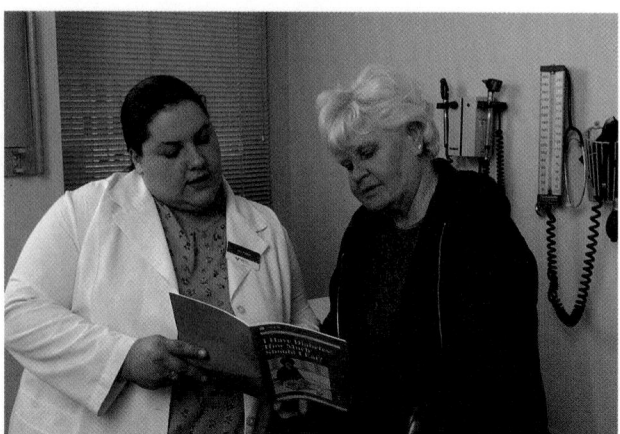

FIGURE 1-1 Professional interaction with patient.

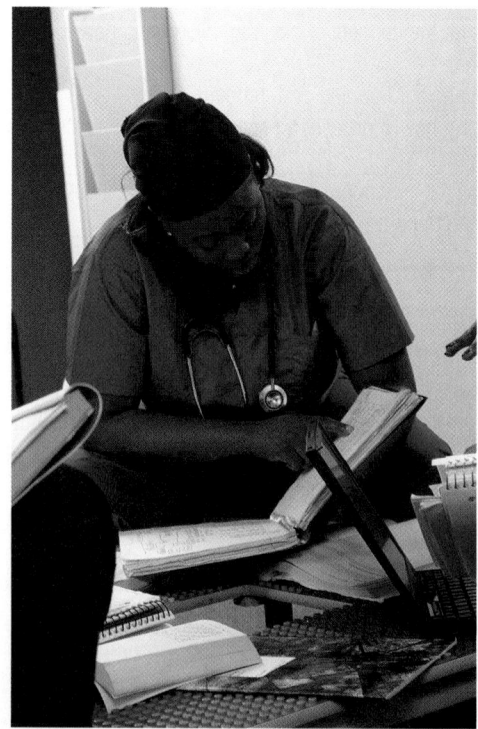

FIGURE 1-2 Student learning.

risks to get the desired results. They learn best with practice and hands-on activities. Reflective processors, however, have to think about the information before they can internalize it. They prefer to observe and consider what is going on. The only way they can make sense of new material is to spend time thinking and learning a great deal about it before acting.

CRITICAL THINKING APPLICATION

- Consider the two ways to perceive new material. Are you a concrete perceiver who ties the information to a personal experience, or do you prefer abstract perception in which you like to analyze or reflect on the meaning of the material? Choose which one you think most accurately describes your method of investigating new information.
- Then think about the way you process learning. Are you an active processor who is always looking for the practical application of what you learn, or are you a reflective processor who has to think about new material before internalizing it?
- After completing this activity write down the combination of your perceiving and processing learning styles and share it with your instructor.

Using Your Learning Profile to Be a Successful Student: Where Do I Go from Here?

No one falls completely into one or the other of these categories. However, by being aware of how we generally prefer first to perceive information and then to process it, we can be more sensitive to our learning style and can approach new learning situations with a plan for learning the material in a way that best suits our learning preferences. Your preferred perceiving and processing learning profile will fall into one of the following stages in the Learning Style Inventory created by David Kolb of Case Western Reserve University.

Learners in Stage 1 have a concrete reflective style. These students want to know the purpose of the information and have a personal connection to the content. They like to consider a situation from many different points of view, observe others, and plan before taking action. Their strengths are in understanding people, brainstorming, and recognizing and creatively solving problems. If you fall into this stage, you enjoy small group activities and learn well in study groups.

Stage 2 learners have an abstract reflective style. These students are eager to learn just for the sheer pleasure of learning rather than because the material relates to their personal lives. They like to learn lots of facts and arrange new material in a logical and clear manner. Stage 2 learners plan studying and like to create ways of thinking about the material but do not always make the connection with the practical application of the material. If you are a Stage 2 learner, you prefer organized, logical presentations of material and therefore enjoy lectures and generally dislike group work. You also need time to process and think about the new material before applying it.

Learners in Stage 3 have an abstract active style. Learners with this combination of learning style want to experiment and test the information that they are learning. If you are a Stage 3

learner, you want to know how techniques or ideas work, and you also want to practice what you are learning. Your strengths are in problem solving and decision making, but you may lack focus and may be hasty when making decisions. You learn best with hands-on practice by doing experiments, projects, and laboratory activities. You also enjoy working alone or in small groups (Figure 1-3).

Stage 4 is made up of concrete active learners. These students are concerned about how they can use what they learn to make a difference in their lives. If you fall into this stage, you like to relate new material to other areas of your life. You have leadership capabilities, can create on your feet, and are usually vocal in a group, but you may have difficulty completing your work on time. Stage 4 learners enjoy teaching others and working in groups and learn best when they can apply the new information to real-world problems (Figure 1-4).

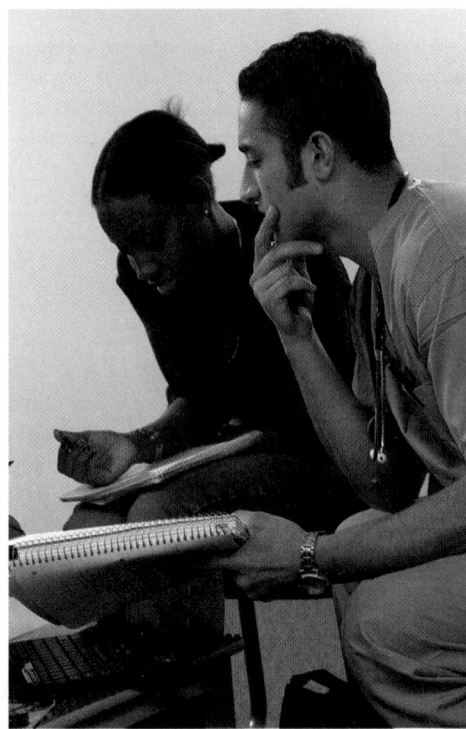

FIGURE 1-3 Learning in a small group.

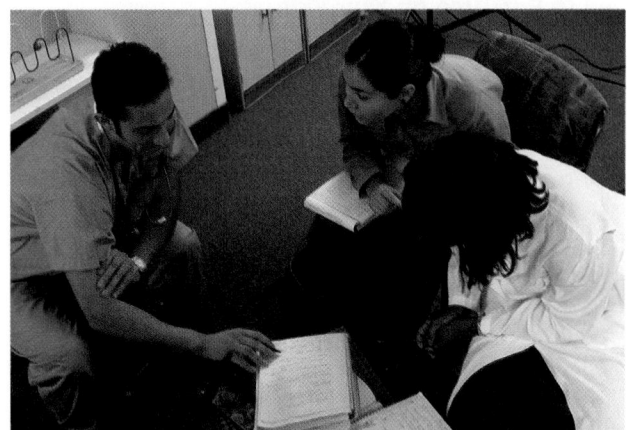

FIGURE 1-4 Teaching and working with others.

To get the most out of knowing your learning profile, you need to apply this knowledge to how you approach learning. Each of the learning stages has pluses and minuses. When faced with a learning situation that does not match your learning preference, see how you can adapt your individual learning to make the best of the information. For example, if you are bored by lectures, look for an opportunity to apply the information being presented to a real problem you are facing in the classroom or at home. If you are an abstract perceiver, take time outside of class to think about new information so that you are ready to process it into your learning system. If you benefit from learning in a group, make the effort to organize review sessions and study groups. If you learn best by teaching others, offer to assist your peers with their learning. By taking the time now to investigate your preferred method of learning, you will perceive and process information more effectively throughout your school career.

CRITICAL THINKING APPLICATION

Take a few minutes to reflect on a time when you really enjoyed learning about something new. How was the material presented, and what did you do to "make it your own"? What do you need to do to become a more effective learner?

TIME MANAGEMENT: PUTTING TIME ON YOUR SIDE

One of the most complicated tasks for a professional medical assistant is to effectively manage time. No other workplace can compete with the distractions and demands of a busy healthcare setting. Do you think that you practice effective time-management skills? Do you believe that you are in control of your time, or do you think that other people or situations control it? How frequently do you say that you just do not have enough time to do what you are supposed to do, let alone those things you would like to do? Time management gives you the opportunity to spend time in the way you choose. Effective time management is also crucial to your success as a student and as a future healthcare professional (Figure 1-5).

How to Put Time on Your Side

The following time-management skills are designed to help you effectively deal with the demands on your time. Highlight the ones that you think will be most useful in helping you deal with your situation.

1. *Determine your purpose.* What do you want to accomplish this semester, in this course, or in this unit of study? What do you want to achieve as a student? What is one thing you can do to help achieve your goals?
2. *Identify your main concern.* Besides school, what other demands do you have on your time? Based on the learning goals you have established, what do you need to do to accomplish your goals?
   - Plan time: Schedule projects in advance with notes to yourself on deadlines.

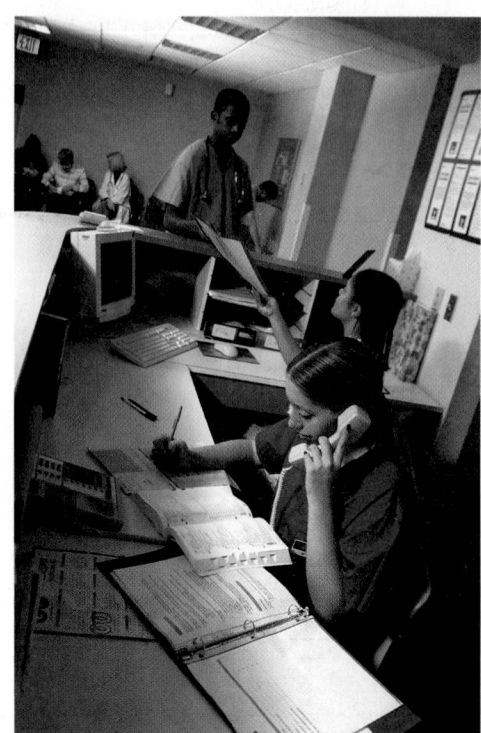

FIGURE 1-5 Time management in a busy medical practice.

   - Use down time: Take your work with you everywhere you go. Do small bits at every opportunity.
   - Guard time: Avoid distractions (e.g., television, music) that will interfere with your concentration. Notice how others abuse your time. Learn to say no to outside demands on your time.
   - Discover time: Steal time from other activities in your schedule.
   - Assign time: Ask for help when you need it from friends and family.
3. *Be organized.* What materials (e.g., books, research, supplies) do you need to have an effective study session? What preparation is needed to make the most of your time?
   - Record time: Use a day planner or calendar to write down due dates for assignments and tests. If a paper or project is due on a specific date, write yourself a reminder in your day planner to start the project on a specific date so you are sure to have it done when it is due.
   - Optimal time: Take advantage of the time of day when you study and learn the best. Schedule study time during your peak performance time—which means if you are an early riser make time for homework first thing in the day, or at night if you are a night owl. Plan on dedicating at least some of your optimal time to your school work.
4. *Stop procrastinating.* If you avoid working on your goals, you may not achieve them. Examine the following suggestions as ways to break the procrastination cycle.
   - Make the work meaningful: What is important about the work you are putting off and what are the benefits of getting it done? Reflect on your long-range goals. Is it important to do a good job on the work so you

can earn an acceptable grade, do well in the course, complete the medical assisting program, and ultimately find employment?

- Plan work deadlines: Break assignments into achievable sections that can be completed in the time slots available. Schedule those work sections in your day planner to prevent forgetting deadlines for assignments.
- Ask for help: Let your support system know you have work to get done. Ask them for encouragement to stay on track. If you have school-age children you can set an excellent example by planning "family" homework sessions. You can get some of your work done while role modeling learning behaviors for your children. Let your partner know when due dates are looming or tests are scheduled. Ask for help in meeting day-to-day demands so you can study or prepare for school.
- Prioritize: If you keep avoiding a certain task, reevaluate its priority. If it is really worth worrying about, get started now, not later. Don't waste time worrying about how you are going to get things done. Spend that time actually working on the projects that worry you the most.
- Reward yourself: Create a reward that is meaningful and something you will work for. If you want to spend time with your family or friends on the weekend, develop a plan and stick to it so you can share that special time as a reward.

5. *Remember you.* It is very easy to become overwhelmed with responsibilities both in school and at home. Part of successful time management includes setting aside time to do things you enjoy. You have chosen a profession that can be very demanding. Now is the time to remember that you have to take care of yourself as well as meet your professional and personal responsibilities. So remember to plan some time for yourself as well (Figure 1-6).

CRITICAL THINKING APPLICATION

How do you spend your time? Over 3 days this week write down the amount of time you spend on each activity. How much television do you watch? How much time do you spend talking on the phone? How about driving time, visiting time, work time, time for family and friends, and so on? At the end of the 3-day period, add up the various categories of time. Do you recognize any time you might be wasting? Can you implement any of the suggested time-management strategies to make more time available?

PROBLEM SOLVING AND CONFLICT MANAGEMENT

As a future member of the healthcare team, you will frequently face problems and conflict. Although we usually look at these situations as negative factors in our lives, problem solving and conflict management actually give us the opportunity to positively affect a potentially negative situation. Learning how to manage problems can be very useful for your practice as a medical assistant, as well as for your success as a student.

The first step in reaching an equitable solution to a problem or conflict situation is to identify the central issue. How many times have you known that you were upset about something but were not really sure why? You cannot solve a problem or resolve a negative situation unless you are sure what is at the root of your feelings. You need to understand the problem and gather as much information about the situation as possible before you decide to act. One way of doing this is to ask yourself these questions:

- When does the situation occur and under what circumstances?
- How does it make you feel?
- Is there someone else involved?
- What interferes with making a decision or resolving the conflict?

Once you understand the situation and how you feel about it, you need to decide if it is worth the effort to resolve it. Prioritize your involvement. Sometimes situations and problems may arise that you are unable to resolve or that you may decide are not important enough for you to act on. For example, if one of your co-workers refuses to take out the garbage when it is his or her turn, does that really bother you? If it does, then you need to deal with the issue. However, if the individual helps out in other ways then perhaps the garbage isn't worth the effort to resolve the conflict.

After you have gathered the details about the problem or conflict and you have decided it is important enough to act on, it is time to determine possible solutions. One way to do this is to ask for advice or brainstorm ideas with individuals you respect. Sometimes another person can give you special insight into the problem that you were unable to see on your own. After brainstorming for possible solutions, you should then get feedback regarding the workability of the suggested solutions. An alternative to brainstorming possible solutions to the problem is to list on a piece of paper the pros and cons of possible solutions. Simply looking at a list of the positive and negative aspects of the solution may clarify how you should solve the problem. Before deciding on a particular solution, make sure you critically analyze the consequences of each proposed solution: Which one best meets your needs and has the potential for providing an outcome you can live with?

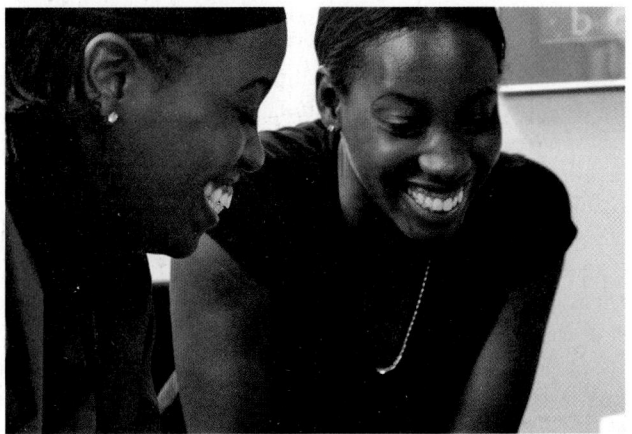

FIGURE 1-6 Making time for you.

Finally you are ready to implement the chosen solution. However, your work is not over yet. You need to evaluate the outcome of your decision and see if it truly did meet your needs. If not, it may be time to review other possible solutions and try another approach.

Conflict management requires some additional consideration. If you are in conflict with a peer, instructor, or co-worker, it is important to follow certain guidelines. You should attempt to solve the conflict in a private place at a prescheduled time. This ensures that the person will meet with you and that neither one has to worry about others overhearing the conversation. At the meeting clearly state your feelings about the conflict and how you would like it resolved. Then try to come to an agreeable solution. The best way to deal with conflict situations is through open, honest, assertive communication. However, just as with problem solving, it is important to follow up on the decided course of action to see if it effectively dealt with the source of the conflict (Figure 1-7).

CRITICAL THINKING APPLICATION

Think about a serious problem you are currently facing. Use the brainstorming and/or pros-and-cons method for creating solutions to the problem. Implement your chosen solution, and follow up on its effectiveness. Did the problem-solving process help you manage the situation more effectively?

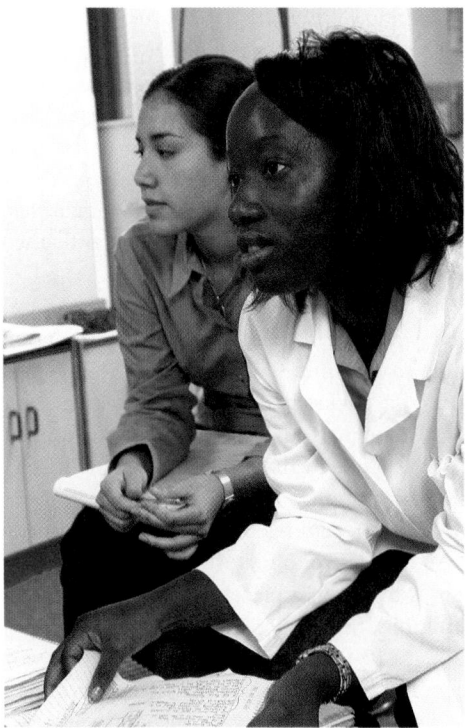

FIGURE 1-7 Dealing with conflict.

STUDY SKILLS: TRICKS TO BECOMING A SUCCESSFUL STUDENT

So far in this chapter we have looked at the influence of individual learning styles and time management on learning success. Now we will investigate some ideas that are useful in learning new material. These study skills include memory techniques, active learning, brain tricks, reading methods, and note-taking strategies.

Several techniques can help you store and remember information. The first of these involves organizing information into recognizable groups so the brain can easily find it. You can organize information by getting the big picture first before trying to learn the details. One way to implement this strategy is to skim a reading assignment before actually reading and taking notes on the material, thus getting a general impression of what you need to learn before tackling the details. Depending on your learning style, it may also help to find a way of making the new information meaningful. Think about your educational goals and how the new material will help you achieve those goals. Another way of remembering material is to create an association with something you already know. By grouping new material with already stored material, your brain will remember it much easier.

A useful study skill for some learners is to be physically active while learning. Some students learn best if they walk or talk out loud while studying. Besides encouraging learning, moving and talking while studying relieve boredom and keep you awake. Another way to be actively involved in learning is to use pictures or diagrams to represent the material you are studying. Some people are visual learners, and creating pictures of the material is the easiest method for them to retain the information. Other students find that rewriting notes or making lists of information helps them retain the material. Writing also helps those students who need to "do" something in order to learn.

Studying will go much more smoothly if you work *with* your brain rather than *against* it. If you tend to get anxious and worried while studying, you may be acting as your own worst enemy. One way of dealing with a topic that you find anxiety producing is to overlearn it. If material is overlearned, you are much less likely to experience test anxiety. Another method for remembering material is to quickly review it after class. This minireview will help the new information become part of your long-term memory system. Many students find creating songs, dances, or word associations an effective way to learn and remember new material. Putting details into a familiar song and moving to it can help trick the brain into remembering the information. This is especially helpful when trying to learn anatomy and physiology. Another excellent way of learning information is to actually teach it to someone else. Teaching requires you to have a good understanding of the material as well as the ability to describe it for others. It can be an effective reinforcer of complicated material (Figure 1-8).

A great deal of the learning process is expected to take place from assigned readings. You can use several methods to make reading assignments more meaningful. If you find a reading assignment challenging or difficult to understand, the first step

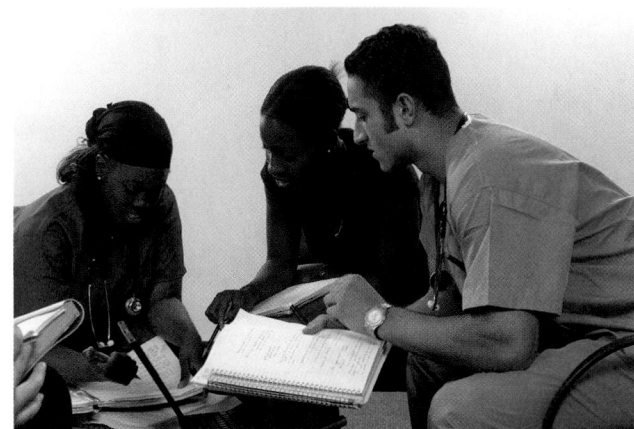

FIGURE 1-8 Effective study skills.

is to take the time to read it again. Sometimes the first time through the material is not enough to gain understanding. As you read, highlight important words or thoughts and stop periodically to summarize the material. If you get bored while reading, use your body–walk or talk your way through the assignment. Take the time to look up words or terms you do not understand, or ask your instructor or tutor for help. Outlining the material can help you create a brief overview of what you need to learn. And finally, the best way to determine if you learned anything from your reading is to try to explain it to someone else. If that is effective, you know you acquired the knowledge needed from the reading assignment.

Many students find effective note taking a challenge. The big question is, "How much of what the instructor says do I actually need to write down?" The first step in effective note taking is to come to class prepared. The more familiar you are with the material, the easier it will be to determine the important parts of the instructor's lecture. Pay attention to the instructor, and look for clues about what he or she thinks is important. Ask questions about the material if you do not understand it rather than writing down information that makes no sense to you. Think critically about what you hear before you write it down so you can start to build relationships among the things you want or need to know.

When it comes to actual note taking, some strategies can make the process of recording notes an active learning tool. Organize the information as much as possible while you are writing, in either an outline or paragraph format. Use only one side of the paper for easier reading and leave blank spaces where needed to fill in details later. Use key words to help you remember the material, and create pictures or diagrams to help visualize it. If permitted, use tape recorders when appropriate and make sure you have either handouts or notes that cover material written on the board, in an overhead, or in a PowerPoint presentation. Another helpful tool is to develop your own system of abbreviations to help simplify the writing load.

The most effective way to use your notes is to review them shortly after class. This is the time to add details, clarify information, or make notes about asking the instructor for explanations during the next class. You could even exchange

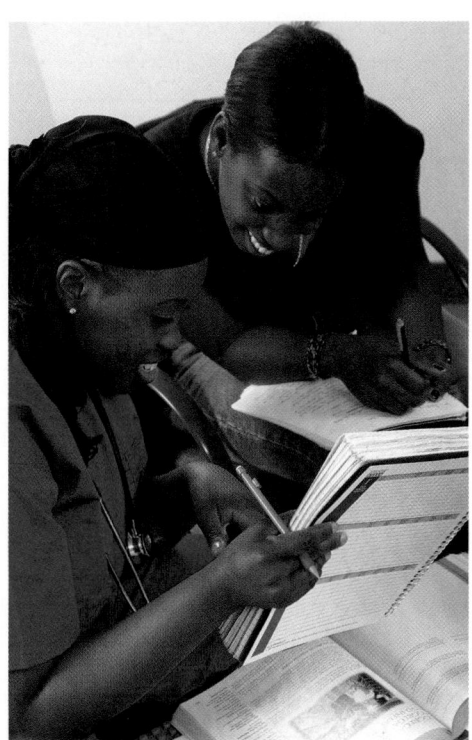

FIGURE 1-9 Sharing notes.

notes with students you trust to compare information (Figure 1-9). Some students find it beneficial to type or rewrite their notes. This can give you an opportunity to learn the material as you are transcribing it. As you are reviewing your notes you can also draw mind maps of the information or diagram outlines to help you better understand and remember the material.

Creating mind maps is a way of representing the main idea of the topic and supporting important details with a figure or picture. Healthcare textbooks are made up of complicated concepts with multiple main ideas, each with its own important details. Mind maps are a way of consolidating complex details and organizing them into a format that is easier to remember. The spider map example in Figure 1-10 presents a method for including several main ideas with details in one study guide. The fishbone map in Figure 1-11 can be used to learn complicated causes of disease. The chain-of-events map in Figure 1-12 displays the cause and effect of events such as infection control or the history of medicine. The cycle map in Figure 1-13 shows the connection between factors, such as with the chain of infection. Creating your own mind maps is a way of making the information more meaningful and easier for you to understand.

Although many techniques can help you study, perhaps the most important one is your attitude toward learning. Some students fall into the "I can't possibly learn this material" trap. That type of attitude only leads to self-defeat. The way to solve barriers is to first recognize that they exist. Once you know your weak spots, use the suggested study skills to improve in those areas. Do not be afraid to ask questions or to seek out help if you do not understand the material. Employ as many different strategies as necessary to become a successful student.

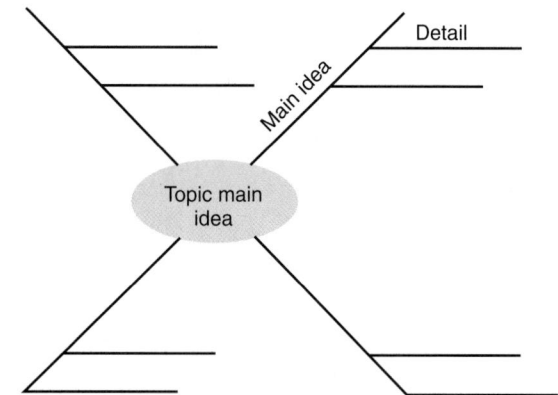

FIGURE 1-10 Spider map displays multiple main ideas with supporting details.

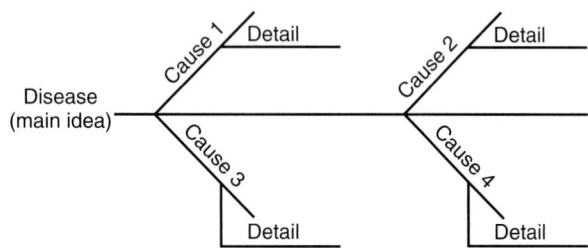

FIGURE 1-11 Fishbone map used to describe causes of disease.

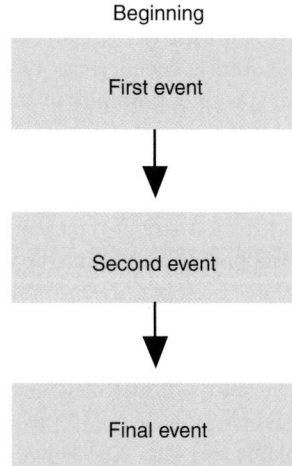

FIGURE 1-12 Chain-of-events map displays the cause and effect of events.

CRITICAL THINKING APPLICATION

Write down at least two barriers to your learning. Review the study skill suggestions discussed, and choose four you want to try out. Use them over the next week to help you when learning new material. Reflect on whether the chosen study skills helped you learn the material better.

TEST-TAKING STRATEGIES: TAKING CHARGE OF YOUR SUCCESS

What happens when you do not know the answer to the first question on a test? What if you do not know the next one? Are you able to go on without panicking? Many people find taking

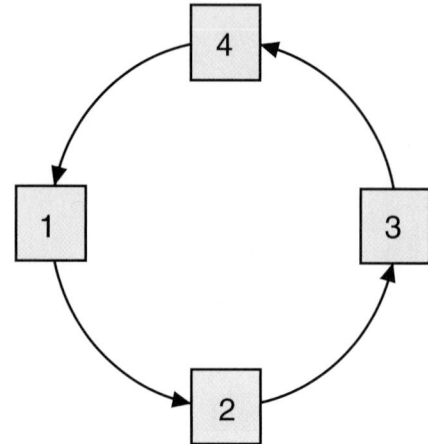

FIGURE 1-13 Cycle map shows how one action leads to another.

tests the most challenging part of being successful students. Multiple approaches are available that you can employ to take charge of your success and improve your ability to take tests. These include such strategies as adequate preparation, controlling negative thoughts during test time, and understanding how to manage various types of questions.

The first step is to go into a test adequately prepared. Use the time-management skills already outlined in this chapter to get prepared for the big day. Recognize and employ your preferred learning style to overlearn the material and increase your confidence. Use memory tools like flash cards, checklists, and mind maps to help visualize the material. Form a study group if you are the type of learner who benefits from studying in groups (Figure 1-14). Schedule and plan study time, and reward yourself for your hard work. It is also important to go into the test rested and relaxed, so eat, exercise to relieve stress, and sleep before the test so that you are as alert as possible.

Before you start the test make sure you read directions carefully and, if possible, begin with the easiest or shortest questions to build your confidence. Be aware of the amount of time allotted for the examination, and pace yourself accordingly. As you go through the test, look for clues to answers in other questions. During test time remember to use positive self-talk at the first indication of panic. Repeatedly remind yourself that you are well prepared, relax, and think about the material before you get worried. You need to stop negative thoughts as soon as they arise, and instead visualize yourself being successful. Use slow deep breathing to relax and, if helpful, close your eyes for a minute and visualize a relaxing place before you go on with the test. You may find it helpful to wear a thick rubber band on your wrist and to snap it as soon as you start to think negatively. This will provide a physical reaction to interfere with the power of your negative thoughts and serve as a reminder of what you should be concentrating on.

Some strategies can be employed when answering certain types of questions. With multiple choice questions, try to identify key words or clues in each question. Read the question carefully and answer it in your head before you review the provided answers. If you are not absolutely sure of the answer, make an educated guess or follow your instincts in choosing an

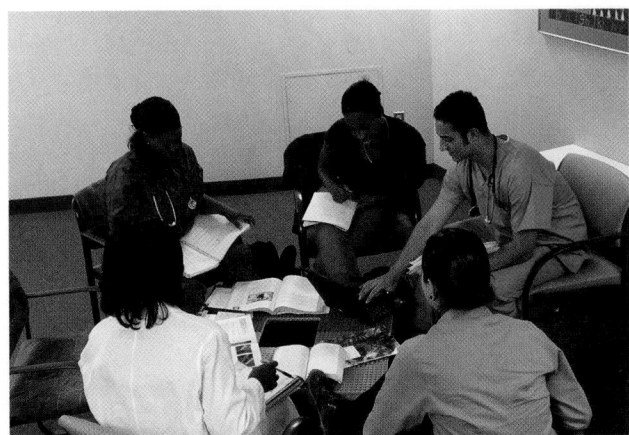

FIGURE 1-14 Study group.

answer. "True-or-false" questions give you a "50/50" chance of being correct. Remember that if any part of the question is not true, then the statement is false. Again, check the statements for key words that will help indicate the direction of the answer. Look for qualifying terms (e.g., "always," "never," "sometimes") that are key to understanding the meaning of the true-or-false statement.

CRITICAL THINKING APPLICATION

Think about a time you experienced test anxiety. Write down the details about the situation and how you felt. Choose four test-taking strategies that you think would be beneficial in handling similar situations in the future.

BECOMING A CRITICAL THINKER: MAKING MENTAL CONNECTIONS

The ability to process information and arrive at reasonable conclusions is crucial to all healthcare workers. The process of **critical thinking** involves sorting out conflicting information, weighing the knowledge you possess about that information, ignoring or letting go of personal biases, and deciding on a reasonable belief or action. Critical thinking is actually an active search for the truth. Critical thinking could be described as thorough thinking because it requires learners to be open-minded to all possibilities. Successful students are thorough thinkers because they must determine the facts about the topic being learned and come to logical conclusions about the material. Critical thinkers are also inquisitive learners who are constantly in the process of analyzing and sorting out conflicting information to reach conclusions. A crucial step in critical thinking is evaluating the results of your learning. Reflection is key to critical thinking. "How did I learn what I learned?" and "What does it mean in my life?" are questions that must be consistently asked in order to continue to learn. Becoming a successful student and ultimately a successful member of the allied health team requires the possession of critical thinking skills. Both the material presented in this chapter and the critical thinking application exercises are designed to encourage you along this lifelong learning path of critical thinking.

SUMMARY OF SCENARIO

One of the things Shawna can do to improve her learning is to determine her individual learning style. By understanding how she typically perceives and processes new information she can plan the best methods for learning the material. In addition to understanding who she is as a learner, Shawna needs to practice successful time-management skills to keep up with school and work responsibilities. Effective problem solving and developing study skills that work for her are also key to her success as a student.

SUMMARY of LEARNING OBJECTIVES

1. Define, spell, and pronounce the terms listed in the vocabulary.
   - Spelling and pronouncing medical terms correctly adds credibility to the medical assistant. Knowing the definitions of these terms promotes confidence in communication with patients and co-workers.
2. Assess the importance of developing professional behaviors as a member of the allied health team.
   - Medical assistants play a vital role in the healthcare team and are expected to display such professional behaviors as being dependable, practicing respectful patient care, having empathy,

showing initiative, having a positive attitude, and using teamwork.
3. Evaluate the concept of critical thinking and how it affects your actions.
   - Incorporate critical thinking and reflection to make mental connections as material is learned. Critical thinkers can evaluate conflicting information and make a decision to act based on their knowledge and willingness to be open-minded to all possibilities.
4. Examine your learning preferences.

Continued

SUMMARY of LEARNING OBJECTIVES

Continued

- Learning preferences are the ways that you like to learn and that have proven successful in the past.

5. Interpret how your learning style affects your success as a student.
   - Learning styles are determined by your individual method of perceiving or examining new material and the way that you process it or make it your own. People are either concrete or abstract perceivers and either active or reflective processors.

6. Apply time-management strategies to make the most of your learning opportunities.
   - Effective time-management strategies such as setting goals, prioritizing, getting organized, and avoiding procrastination will make you a more successful student as well as an effective medical assistant.

7. Use problem-solving techniques to manage conflict and barriers to your success.
   - Problem-solving and conflict-management techniques are key to your success. First, identify the central issue and how you feel about it; then consider possible solutions and their potential results, implement the chosen solution, and analyze the results.

8. Integrate effective study skills into your daily activities.
   - Study skills such as memory techniques, active learning, brain tricks, effective reading methods, note-taking strategies, and mind maps all help students to be more successful.

9. Design test-taking strategies that help you take charge of your success.
   - Test-taking strategies include preparing adequately for the examination, controlling negative thoughts during the examination, and understanding how to deal with different types of questions.

10. Incorporate critical thinking and reflection to make mental connections as material is learned.
    - Critical thinking can be described as thorough thinking because it considers all sides of the information without bias. Reflection is the process of thinking about or reviewing information before acting.

CONNECTIONS

Study Guide Connection: Go to Chapter 1 Study Guide. Read the Case Study and Workplace Applications and complete the assignments. Do online research for answers to the questions in the Internet Activities associated with becoming a successful student.

CD Connection: Go to the Medical Assisting Competency Challenge CD and review the content of the training activities. These will be referred to throughout the textbook to enhance your learning experience.

evolve   **Evolve Connection:** For more information related to becoming a successful student, go to evolve.elsevier.com/kinn and visit related weblinks for Chapter 1. Click on the Medical Assisting Exam Review and do the practice questions to sharpen your test-taking skills.

The Healthcare Industry

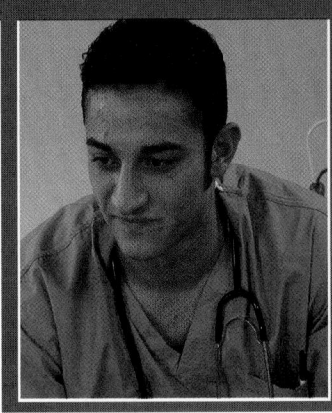

2

SCENARIO

Carlos Santos, CMA, is a medical assisting instructor with 10 years' experience in the clinical area. He worked for a group of family practitioners and for an allergist during his career as a medical assistant before becoming an instructor. Mr. Santos believes that it is very important to give his students an overview of the healthcare industry early in their training. He knows that it is exciting to show them the history and progress of medicine and introduce them to the current types of facilities available for patient care on both a national and a local level. This helps the student to understand where he or she fits into the whole picture as a medical assistant. Often Mr. Santos assigns the students a short report on one person who contributed to the progress of medicine. He finds that this is a good way to encourage the students to use the Internet and conduct research right from the start of their training; the students get a chance to grow more comfortable speaking in front of a group. The knowledge that the students will gain about the different areas of patient care will be useful once they graduate and begin working in a healthcare facility. All of these skills will make Mr. Santos's students more versatile and valuable to their eventual employers.

While studying this chapter, think about the following questions:

- Why is continuing medical research so important to the healthcare industry?
- How can the individual medical assistant contribute to the progress of medicine in today's world?
- What is the value in gaining an overview of the entire healthcare industry as one begins a career in medical assisting?

LEARNING OBJECTIVES

1. Define, spell, and pronounce the terms listed in the vocabulary.
2. Identify the ancient cultures that contributed a major portion of our medical terminology.
3. Explain the history of medicine and how it has affected today's medical industry.
4. Distinguish between and describe the two medical symbols in general use today.
5. Explain why a medical education at Johns Hopkins was considered superior, even in its early years.
6. List several medical pioneers, and discuss the importance of their contributions to the medical profession.
7. Explain the roles of the world healthcare organizations.
8. Discuss the various types of ambulatory care.
9. Distinguish among different types of doctors and medical practices.
10. Identify the medical specialties recognized by the American Board of Medical Specialties.
11. Discuss various healthcare occupations and the role these professionals play in the healthcare industry.

National Accreditation Competencies and Content

ABHES COMPETENCIES

Communication
2.g. Use appropriate medical terminology
2.q. Allied health professions and credentialing

Legal Concepts
5.f. Maintain licenses and accreditation

accreditation (u-kre-duh-ta′-shun) The process through which an organization is recognized for adherence to a group of standards that meet or exceed expectations of the accrediting agency.

advent A coming into being or use.

allopathic (al-o-pa′-thik) A word used to contrast homeopathic medicine with mainstream medicine; describes medicine supposedly characterized by an effort to counteract the symptoms of a disease by administration of treatments that produce effects that are opposite to the symptoms.

alternative medicine A variety of therapeutic or preventative health care practices that are alternatives to mainstream medicine, such as chiropractic, homeopathy, naturopathy, and herbal medicine.

ambulatory (am′-bu-la-to-re) Able to walk about and not be bedridden.

amenities Things that contribute to comfort, enjoyment, or convenience.

cardiac arrhythmias (kar′-de-ak ah-rith′-me-ahs) Irregular heartbeats resulting from a malfunction of the electrical system of the heart.

case management The process of assessing and planning patient care, including referral and follow-up, to ensure continuity of care and quality management.

chiropractic (ki′-ruh-prak-tik) A medical discipline that focuses on the nervous system and involves manual adjustment of the vertebral column to affect the nervous system to treat various disorders and to promote patient wellness.

cited Quoted by way of example, authority, or proof or mentioned formally in commendation or praise.

contamination (kun-ta-mu-na′-shun) A process by which something is made impure, unclean, or unfit for use by the introduction of unwholesome or undesirable elements.

credentialing (kri-den′-shuh-ling) The act of extending professional or medical privileges to an individual; the process of verifying and evaluating that person's credentials.

dissection (di-sek′-shun) Separation into pieces and exposure of parts for scientific examination.

encounter Any contact between a healthcare provider and a patient that results in treatment or evaluation of the patient's condition; not limited to in-person contact.

fermentation (fur-men-ta′-shun) An enzymatically controlled transformation of an organic compound.

holistic (ho-lis′-tik) Related to or concerned with all of the systems of the body, rather than breaking it down into parts.

homeopathy (ho-me-uh′-puh-the) A type of alternative medicine that attempts to stimulate the body to recover itself; a system of therapy based on the concept that disease can be treated with minute doses of drugs thought capable of producing the same symptoms in healthy people as the disease itself.

hospice (hos′-pus) A concept of care that involves health professionals and volunteers who provide medical, psychologic, and spiritual support to terminally ill patients and their loved ones.

indicators An important point or group of statistic values that, when evaluated, indicate the quality of care provided in a healthcare facility.

indicted (in-di′-ted) Charged with a crime by the finding or presentment of a jury according to due process of law.

indigent (in′-di-junt) Totally lacking in something of need.

innate Existing in, belonging to, or determined by factors present in an individual since birth.

innocuous (i′-nuh-kyu-wus) Having no effect, adverse or otherwise; harmless.

mysticism The experience of seeming to have direct communication with God or ultimate reality.

naturopathy (na-chu-ra′-puh-the) An alternative to conventional medicine in which holistic methods are used, as well as herbs and natural supplements, with the belief that the body will heal itself. Naturopathic physicians can currently be licensed in 15 states, Puerto Rico, and the Virgin Islands.

osteopathic (us-te-uh-pa′-thik) A type of medicine based on the theory that disturbances in the musculoskeletal system affect other bodily parts, causing many disorders that can be corrected by various manipulative techniques in conjunction with conventional medical, surgical, pharmacologic, and other therapeutic procedures.

pandemic (pan-de′-mik) A condition in which the majority of the people in a country, a number of countries, or a geographic area are affected.

peer review organization A group of medical reviewers contracted by the Centers for Medicare and Medicaid Services to ensure quality control and medical necessity of services provided by a facility.

philanthropist (fu-lan′-thruh-pist) An individual who makes an active effort to promote human welfare.

putrefaction (pyu-truh-fak′-shun) Decomposition of animal matter that results in a foul smell.

robotics Technology dealing with the design, construction, and operation of robots in automation.

staff privileges Allowance of a healthcare professional to practice within a specific facility.

standards Item or indicator used as a measure of quality or compliance with a statutory or accrediting body's policies and regulations.

subluxations (suh-blek-sa′-shuns) Slight misalignments of the vertebrae or a partial dislocation.

telemedicine The use of telecommunications in the practice of medicine, in which great distances can exist among healthcare professionals, colleagues, patients, and students.

teleradiology The use of telecommunications devices to enhance and improve the results of radiologic procedures.

treatises (truh-te′-ses) Systematic expositions or arguments

List continues on next page

in writing including a methodic discussion of the facts and principles involved and the conclusions reached.

triage (tre'-azh) The sorting of and allocation of treatment to patients according to a system of priorities designed to maximize the number of survivors and treat the sickest patients first.

The growth of today's healthcare industry seems unstoppable. Thanks to modern technologic advances, medicine speeds forward faster than ever in its quest to improve the health of humankind. Modern advances, such as **telemedicine,** are experiencing significant growth, and the images produced with **teleradiology** have vastly improved in their resolution. **Robotics** is assisting healthcare professionals in surgery and even delivers drugs to hospital floors using laser sensors. Education in medicine has grown exponentially: computers, the Internet, and video have enabled an instructor in New York to communicate with a student in Los Angeles. The key to this technology lies within the development and widespread use of elaborate information systems that have revolutionized the way that medicine is practiced today. Technology is advancing at an astounding rate of speed; the healthcare environment of the future is barely imaginable. This chapter looks back at the history of medicine, gazes at its present, and glances toward its future.

THE HISTORY OF MEDICINE
Medical Language and Mythology

Today's medical professional uses words with origins stemming from the romance and fantasy of classical and ancient languages. The study of anatomy reaches back to the dawn of recorded history. Today's modern terms are often similar to their original versions. Some terms are inaccurate when translated literally, because the ancients did not fully understand body functions. The word *artery,* for example, which comes from the Greek word *arteria,* literally means "a windpipe." The early Greeks believed that the arteries carried air, not blood. Greek and Roman mythology have contributed a major portion of our medical terminology, but we have also borrowed liberally from Arabic, Anglo-Saxon, and Germanic sources. Several terms originate from the Bible.

The human head rests on the first cervical vertebra, which is called the *atlas.* Atlas was the famous Greek Titan who was condemned by Zeus to bear the heavens on his shoulders. Achilles was held by the heel as his mother dipped him into the river Styx, so that he would become invulnerable. However, his heel was not immersed, and he later died from a wound in that area. "Achilles heel" is a common expression used today to show a point of weakness. Aphrodite, the Greek goddess of love and beauty, is the source of the name for drugs used to enhance sexual arousal, called *aphrodisiacs.* The equivalent Roman goddess of love, Venus, is associated with lustful desires.

A portion of the female anatomy, the mons *veneris* (mons pubis), and *venereal* diseases were named after her.

Aesculapius, the son of Apollo, was revered as the god of medicine. The early Greeks worshiped the healing powers of Aesculapius and built temples in his honor where patients were treated by trained priests. His daughters were Hygeia, goddess of health, and Panacea, goddess of all healing and restorer of health. Our modern word "hygiene" has its origin in Hygeia, and the modern meaning for panacea is "a remedy for all ills and difficulties." The staff of Aesculapius is a common medical icon. It depicts a serpent encircling a staff and signifies the art of healing. The staff of Aesculapius has been adopted by the American Medical Association as the symbol of medicine. The mythologic staff belonging to Hermes, the messenger of the gods, is the caduceus, which was thought to have magical powers. The caduceus is a staff encircled by two serpents with wings at the top. This icon is the medical insignia of the U.S. Army Medical Corps and is often misused as a symbol of the medical profession (Figure 2-1).

Medicine in Ancient Times

Although religious and mythologic beliefs were the basis of care for the sick in ancient times, evidence suggests the use of drugs, surgery, and other treatments based on theories about the body from as early as 5000 BC. In the well-developed societies of the Egyptians, Babylonians, and Assyrians, certain men acted as physicians and used the little knowledge they had to try to treat illness and injury.

Moses presented rules of health to the Hebrews at approximately 1205 BC. He was the first advocate of preventive medicine and is considered the first public health officer. Moses knew that some animal diseases could be passed to humans and that **contamination** existed, so a religious law was developed

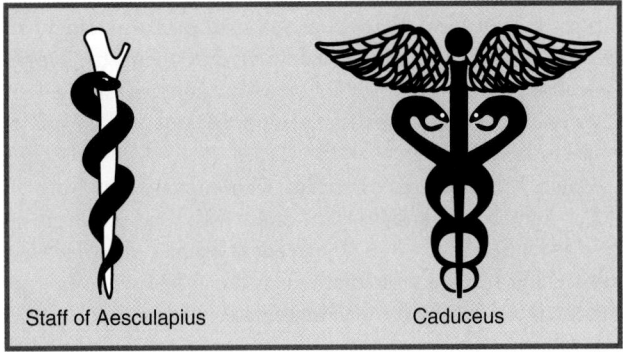

Staff of Aesculapius   Caduceus

FIGURE 2-1 Staff of Aesculapius and the caduceus.

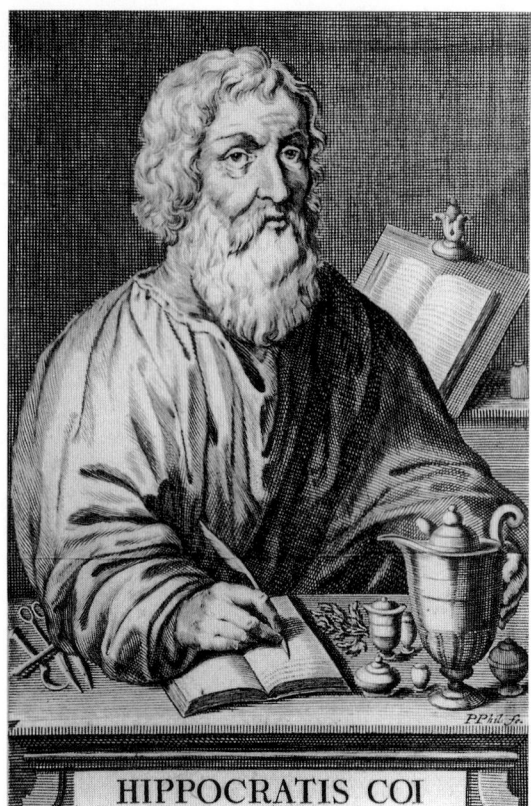

FIGURE 2-2 Hippocrates is known as the Father of Medicine. (Courtesy National Library of Medicine.)

forbidding humans to eat or drink from dirty dishes. The people of that era believed that doing so would defile their bodies and they would lose their souls.

Hippocrates, known as the Father of Medicine, is the most famous of the ancient Greek physicians (Figure 2-2). He was born in 450 BC on the island of Cos in Greece. He is best remembered for the Hippocratic Oath, which has been administered to physicians for more than 2000 years. Hippocrates is credited with taking **mysticism** out of medicine and giving it a scientific basis. During this period of history, most believed that illness was caused by demon possession; for the illness to be cured, the demon had to be removed from the body. Hippocrates' clinical descriptions of diseases and his volumes on epidemics, fevers, epilepsy, fractures, and instruments were studied for centuries. He believed that the body had the capacity to heal itself and that the physician's role was to help nature. Very little was known about anatomy, physiology, and pathology, and there was no knowledge of chemistry. Despite these limitations, many of the classifications of diseases and descriptions of symptoms that Hippocrates developed are still in use today.

Galen was a Greek physician who migrated to Rome in 162 AD and became known as the Prince of Physicians. He is said to have written more than 500 **treatises** on medicine. He wrote an excellent summary on anatomy as it was known at the time, but his work was faulty and inaccurate because it was largely based on the **dissection** of apes and swine. He is considered the Father of Experimental Physiology and the first experimental

neurologist. He was the first to describe the cranial nerves and the sympathetic nervous system, and he performed the first experimental section of the spinal cord, producing hemiplegia. Galen also produced aphonia by cutting the recurrent laryngeal nerve, and he gave the first valid explanation of the mechanism of respiration. Galen was also a champion of medical ethics: he felt that physicians "must learn to despise money," and that if a physician was interested in profit, he was not serious in his devotion to the art of medicine. Galen's beliefs about monetary profit from medicine parallel the views of many modern healthcare professionals, who understand the nature of the healthcare crisis the world faces today. Although much of what he believed about the body was incorrect, Galen's teachings remained intact until human dissections began and physicians were able to visualize exactly what was inside the human body.

Because both Hippocrates and Galen were highly respected, the authority of their observations went unquestioned. This had a negative effect on the progress of science throughout the Dark Ages and well into the sixteenth century. Their theories and descriptions were considered immutable principles, so few physicians were innovative and curious enough to challenge them. Those who did experiment in medicine were scorned by their colleagues, and physicians continued to use methods that were at best ineffectual or **innocuous** and at worst harmful to the patient. However, the establishment of universities led to a study of theories of disease rather than observation of the sick.

Early Development of Medical Education

Medical knowledge developed slowly, and distribution of such knowledge was poor. Before the printing press was invented in the mid-fifteenth century, very little exchange of scientific knowledge and ideas occurred; scientists were not well informed about the investigations of other scientists. The printing press allowed books to be distributed faster and over a widespread area. Another development important to science occurred in the seventeenth century, when European academies or societies were established, consisting of small groups of men who met to discuss subjects of mutual interest. The academies provided freedom of expression that, with the stimulus of exchanging ideas, contributed significantly to the development of scientific thought. One of the earliest of the academies was the Royal Society of London, formed in 1662. The development of communications during this era was important, and these societies contributed to the exchange of information.

Our world became more complex over the centuries, which prompted a greater need for regulation. The passage of the Medical Act of 1858 in Great Britain was considered one of the most important events in British medicine. The act established a statutory body, the General Medical Council, which controlled admission to the medical register and had regulatory power over medical education and examinations.

In the United States, medical education was greatly influenced by the Johns Hopkins University Medical School in Baltimore, Maryland, established in the early 1890s. The school admitted only college graduates with a year's training in the natural sciences. The clinical education at Johns Hopkins was superior because the school partnered with Johns Hopkins Hospital, which had been created expressly for teaching and research by members of the medical faculty. The first four professors at Johns Hopkins were Sir William Osler (Professor of Medicine), William H. Welch (Chief of Pathology), Howard A. Kelley (Chief of Gynecology and Obstetrics), and William D. Halsted (Chief of Surgery). Together these four men transformed the organization and curriculum of clinical teaching and made Johns Hopkins the most famous medical school in the world at that time.

The earliest medical school **accreditation** resulted from a report published by Abraham Flexner. He received a grant from the Carnegie Foundation Commission to study the quality of medical colleges in the United States and Canada. His report, called the Flexner Report, resulted in the closure of many low-ranking schools and the upgrading of others. These events legitimized medical education and opened new doors for many individuals to the world of medicine.

CRITICAL THINKING APPLICATION

- Mr. Santos asks his class to identify which of the individuals involved in early medicine have had the most impact on modern healthcare. Whom would you choose, and why?
- The students point out that early research was often viewed in a negative manner. How does research affect us now, and how is it viewed by the public?

Early Medical Pioneers

Andreas Vesalius (1514-1564) was a Belgian anatomist known as the Father of Modern Anatomy (Figure 2-3). At the age of 29 he published his great *De Corporis Humani Fabrica*, in which he described the structure of the human body. This work marked a turning point by breaking with past traditional beliefs in Galen's theories. Vesalius introduced many new anatomic terms, but because of his radical approach, he was subjected to persecution from his colleagues, teachers, and pupils. Despite his great

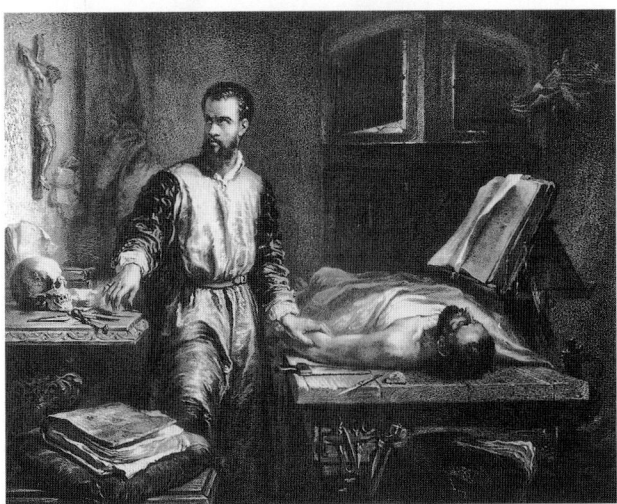

FIGURE 2-3 Andreas Vesalius is known as the Father of Modern Anatomy. (Courtesy National Library of Medicine.)

contributions to the science of anatomy, his name is not used to identify any significant anatomic structures.

Other important advances and discoveries took place throughout the world. Gabriele Fallopius (1523-1562), an Italian student of Vesalius, was also an accurate dissector. He described and named many parts of the human anatomy. He named the fallopian tubes after himself and also named the vagina and placenta. In 1628 William Harvey (1578-1657) announced his discovery that the heart acts as a muscular pump, forcing and propelling the blood throughout the body. He revealed that the blood's motion is a continuous cycle, basing his conclusion on his experimental vivisection, ligation, and perfusion as well as brilliant reasoning. Harvey's writings were recognized in Germany before the English permitted their publication at home. Modern England now considers Harvey to be its medical Shakespeare.

The unseen world of microorganisms was first revealed by Anton van Leeuwenhoek (1632-1723), a Dutch linen draper and haberdasher. Haberdashers made their living dealing in men's clothing and accessories, but it was Leeuwenhoek's hobby of grinding lenses that eventually led to his amazing discovery of the magnification process. He ground more than 400 lenses during his lifetime, some of which were no larger than a pinhead. In the grinding process, Leeuwenhoek learned how to use a simple biconvex lens to magnify the minute world of organisms and structures, never before seen. Leeuwenhoek was the first to ever observe bacteria and protozoa through a lens, and his accurate interpretations of what he saw led to the sciences of bacteriology and protozoology.

Marcello Malpighi (1628-1694) was born near Bologna, Italy, and attended the University of Bologna, where he earned a doctorate in both medicine and philosophy. He pioneered the use of the microscope in the study of plants and animals. Microscopic anatomy became a prerequisite for advances in physiology, embryology, and practical medicine. In 1661 he described the pulmonary and capillary network connecting the smallest arteries with the smallest veins. This was one of the most important discoveries in the history of science, and it validated Harvey's work. Malpighi is commonly regarded as the first histologist.

Medical Advances in the Eighteenth and Nineteenth Centuries

English scientist John Hunter (1728-1793) is known as the Founder of Scientific Surgery. An army surgeon, he became an expert on gunshot wounds and experimented with tissue transfer. His surgical procedures were soundly based on pathologic evidence. He was the first to classify teeth in a scientific manner and introduced artificial feeding by means of a flexible tube passed into the stomach. He provided a classic description of the syphilitic chancre, which is sometimes called a Hunterian chancre. During his studies of venereal diseases, he inoculated himself with what he thought was gonorrhea, but instead he acquired syphilis. His results in this study actually caused confusion in the medical community because he mistakenly thought that gonorrhea was a symptom of syphilis. This misconception was not corrected until the beginning of the twentieth century. His collection of anatomic and animal specimens formed the basis for the museum of the Royal College of Surgeons. After Hunter's death he was buried in St. Martin. His remains were later moved, however, to Westminster Abbey as a gesture of honor. A tablet was placed over his grave by the Royal College of Surgeons to "record their admiration of his genius as a gifted interpreter of the Divine Power and Wisdom at work in the laws of Organic Life and their grateful veneration for his services to mankind as the Founder of Scientific Surgery." Today in Australia the John Hunter Hospital serves more than 600 inpatients and 1000 outpatients per day.

Edward Jenner (1749-1823) was a student of John Hunter and a country physician from Dorsetshire, England. He is considered one of the immortals of preventive medicine for his development of the smallpox vaccine. While Jenner was serving as an apprentice, he assisted in treating a dairymaid. Smallpox was mentioned, and she commented, "I cannot take that disease, for I have had cowpox." Smallpox at that time was a deadly **pandemic.** Jenner observed that those who had contracted cowpox never contracted smallpox. Later, as a practicing physician, Jenner continued investigating the relationship between cowpox and smallpox almost obsessively, but the medical society members grew bored with his obsession and threatened to expel him from their ranks. On May 14, 1796 Dr. Jenner took purulent matter from a pustule on the hand of Sarah Nelmes, a dairymaid, and inserted it through two small superficial incisions into the arm of James Phipps, a healthy 8-year-old boy. This was the first vaccination. On July 1 a virulent dose of smallpox matter was given to the boy in the same arm. Phipps' vaccination kept him safe from the dreaded disease, and Jenner's method of vaccination spread throughout the world. The results of his experiments were published in 1798. He called this method of protection *vaccination*, from the Latin word *vacca*, which means "cow," and at that time, cowpox was called *vaccinia*. Today smallpox has been eradicated throughout the world as a result of a planned program of global vaccination.

Austrian physician Leopold Auenbrugger (1722-1809) developed the use of percussion in diagnosis. He became physician-in-chief to the Hospital of the Holy Trinity at Vienna in 1751, where he tested his discovery. Although scorned and ignored by his contemporaries, his techniques later made him famous and are still used today during physical examinations. René Laennec (1781-1826) was a French physician who developed the stethoscope in 1819. At first he used only a cylinder of rolled paper in his hands; later he used a wooden device because of its sound-conducting properties. With today's sophisticated stethoscopes physicians are able to hear sounds in the body, including a fetus inside the mother. Laennec's book, *Treatise on Mediate Auscultation and Diseases of the Chest*, was readily accepted and translated into many languages. It is said to be the most important treatise on diseases of the thoracic organs ever written.

Several men of the early 1800s are remembered for their fight against puerperal fever and their concern for women's health. Puerperal fever, an infectious disease that can be contracted during childbirth, was also called *puerperal sepsis* or *childbed fever*. The term *puerperal*, denoting a woman in childbed, originates from the Latin *puer*, "a child," and *pario*, "to bring forth." The word *puerperium* now designates the period from delivery to the time the uterus returns to normal size (approximately 42 days after childbirth).

The best known of these men was the Hungarian physician Ignaz Philipp Semmelweis (1818-1865); history has called him the Savior of Mothers. His fight against puerperal fever is a sad story of hardships. His theories were resisted by many professionals, including his instructors. Semmelweis noted that the fever often attacked women who were delivered by medical students coming straight from the autopsy or dissecting rooms. Semmelweis directed that in his wards the students were to wash and disinfect their hands before going to examine the women and deliver the children. This process brought about a marked reduction of cases of puerperal fever on his ward, but he still faced unrelenting opposition. As his theories were proved correct, Semmelweis felt an incredible guilt that the doctors themselves had caused so many deaths. He died at the age of 47—ironically, from the very disease he had fought. He was infected with puerperal fever from a cut on his finger during an autopsy. His grave had hardly been closed when scientists began to understand the causes of this disease, largely as a result of the investigations of two great scientists, Louis Pasteur and Joseph Lister.

Pasteur (1822-1895) was a Frenchman who did brilliant work as a chemist, but it was his studies in bacteriology that made him one of the most famous men in medical history (Figure 2-4). He was bestowed the title of Father of Bacteriology and has also been honored as the Father of Preventive Medicine. He gave unselfishly of his time outside his profession to help others solve problems. Pasteur's adventures included studying

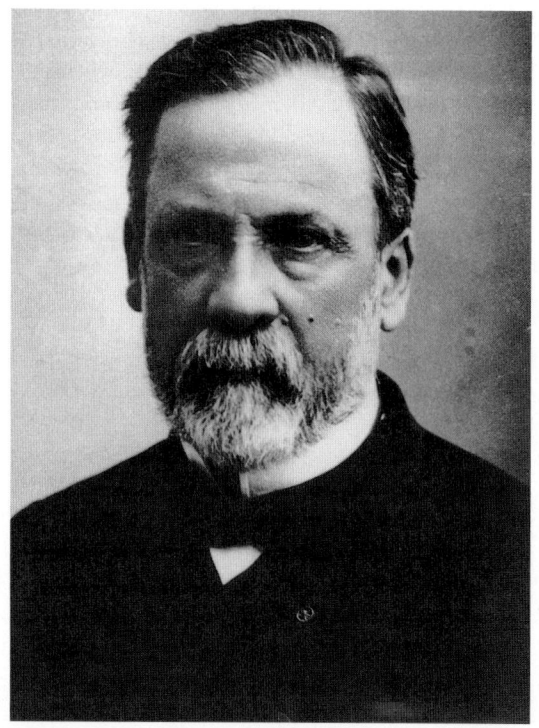

FIGURE 2-4 Louis Pasteur was a brilliant chemist who made numerous contributions to medicine. (Courtesy National Library of Medicine.)

the difficulties in the **fermentation** of wine. He averted disaster in France's critical winemaking industry by a process he developed, now called *pasteurization.* This achievement alone would have made him an immortal among the French. Through a process of supplying enough heat to destroy microorganisms, wine was prevented from turning to vinegar. The French people called on Pasteur again to help the ailing silkworm industry. He devoted years to the conquest of diseases that infected the silkworm. His efforts were impeded when he was stricken with hemiplegia, but after a long, difficult recovery, he was able to continue with a stiff hand and a limp.

Convinced that the infinite world of bacteria held the key to the secrets of contagious diseases, Pasteur left chemistry again to continue studying his theory. Many renowned scientists denied the germ theory of disease and devoted themselves to degrading Pasteur's theories and experiments. In the midst of this controversy he became involved in the prevention of anthrax, which threatened the health of cattle and sheep. Pasteur was eventually honored for his work with many other diseases, such as rabies, chicken cholera, and swine erysipelas. He devoted the last 7 years of his life to the Pasteur Institute, which was founded as a clinic for rabies treatment, a research center for infectious disease, and a teaching center. The Pasteur Institute still exists today. He died in 1895, with his family at his bedside. It is said that his last words were, "There is still a great deal to do."

Joseph Lister (1827-1912) revolutionized surgery through the application of Pasteur's discoveries. He understood the similarity between infections in postsurgical wounds and the processes of **putrefaction.** Pasteur proved that these processes were caused by microorganisms. Before this time, surgeons accepted that infections in surgical wounds were inevitable. Lister reasoned that microorganisms must be the cause of infection and should be kept out of wounds. His colleagues were indifferent to his theories, because most believed infections were God-given and natural. Lister disagreed, and he developed antiseptic methods by using carbolic acid for sterilization. By spraying the rooms with a fine mist of the acid, soaking the instruments in carbolic solutions, and washing his hands in a similar solution, he was able to prove his theories. He is honored as the Father of Sterile Surgery. Pasteur and Lister met after years of great mutual admiration. The meeting was filled with emotion, and it was written in *Pathfinders in Medicine* that "a new star should have appeared in the heavens to commemorate the event." Medicine truly owes a deep gratitude to these two pioneers for the knowledge they imparted to the art.

Robert Koch (1843-1910) is a familiar name to all bacteriologists because of his famous Koch's Postulates—his theory of rules that must be followed before an organism can be accepted as the causative agent in a given disease. Koch was a German physician who earned great honors in bacteriology and public health. He introduced many of the tools used in the laboratory, such as the culture-plate method for isolation of bacteria. He discovered the cause of cholera and demonstrated its transmission by food and water. This discovery completely transformed health departments and proved the importance of bacteriology in everyday life. Koch's greatest disappointment was his failure

to find a cure for tuberculosis, but in his attempt he isolated tuberculin, the substance produced by tubercle bacteria. Its use as a diagnostic aid was of immense value to medicine. In 1885 the University of Berlin created the Chair of Hygiene and Bacteriology in honor of Robert Koch. He became a Nobel Laureate in 1905.

One of Koch's students was a German physician named Paul Ehrlich (1854-1915). He pioneered the fields of bacteriology, immunology, and especially chemotherapy. Chemotherapy is the process of treating diseases by injecting chemicals into the body to destroy microorganisms, and this was a new science in Koch's day. Ehrlich was only 28 when he wrote his first paper on typhoid, but his greatest gift to humanity was called his "magic bullet," or formula 606, which was designed to fight syphilis. With the organism identified by scientists Bordet and Wasserman, Ehrlich set out to find a chemical that would destroy the organism but not harm the host, specifically, the human body. The six hundred–sixth drug that Ehrlich tried finally brought about healing. He called it *salvarsan* because he believed that it offered mankind salvation from the disease. This endeavor also marked the beginning of the practice of injecting chemicals into the body to destroy a specific organism. In 1908 Ehrlich shared the Nobel Prize with Eli Metchnikoff, who is remembered for his theory of phagocytosis and immunology.

Crawford Williamson Long (1815-1878) was the first to employ ether as an anesthetic agent. Early in 1842 a group of students would have a social gathering after chemistry lectures and inhale ether, a chemical commonly found in chemistry labs, as a form of amusement. Ether, an intoxicant similar to nitrous oxide, functions as a soporific or sleep-inducing agent. However, at one of these "ether frolics," as they were called, Dr. Long also observed that people under the influence of ether did not seem to feel pain. After considerable thought, he decided to use ether for a surgical operation. In March 1842 he removed a tumor from the neck of James M. Venable after placing him under the influence of ether. Dr. Horace Wells was a dentist who reported using nitrous oxide as an anesthetic in 1844. Another dentist, Dr. William T.G. Morton, reported using ether in 1846 when he extracted a tooth from a patient, and he also used the gas at Massachusetts General Hospital for a surgical procedure.

Surgeons are grateful to Wilhelm Konrad Roentgen (1845-1923), a professor of physics at the University of Wurzburg, Germany. Roentgen discovered the x-ray in 1895 while experimenting with electrical currents passed through sealed glass tubes. He was awarded the Nobel Prize in Physics in 1901. Although he called it an *x-ray,* history has honored him by calling it the *roentgen ray.* Marie and Pierre Curie discovered radium in 1898, and they were awarded the 1902 Nobel Prize in Physics for their work on radioactivity. Unfortunately, Pierre was killed 3 years later while crossing a street in a rainstorm. Marie was awarded his teaching position at the Sorbonne, a medical university in France; no woman had taught at the school in its 650-year history. In 1911 she was awarded the Nobel Prize for her discoveries of radium and polonium, the first person to receive the award twice. She died in 1934 from pernicious anemia, which was believed to have been caused by her overexposure to radiation and years of overwork.

Nineteenth Century Women in Medicine

Many other women made great contributions to medicine in the early nineteenth century. Florence Nightingale (1820-1910) is known as the founder of nursing and is fondly called the Lady with the Lamp (Figure 2-5). She was of noble birth, and somewhat late in life she sought nursing training in both England and Europe. By the dawn of the Crimean War in 1854, she had established a fine reputation for her work in hospital organization. She was invited by the British Secretary of War to visit the Crimea to help correct the terrible conditions that existed in caring for the wounded. She created the Women's Nursing Service in Scutari and Balaklava. The physicians treated her and the other 38 nurses poorly until a crisis brought thousands of wounded and sick soldiers to the army hospitals. The bravery and competence of the nurses helped the doctors realize their value to the medical profession. In 1860 she founded the Nightingale School and Home for Nurses in London, which marked the beginning of professional nursing education.

Clara Barton (1821-1912), an American, began her nursing career early in life. When she was 11 years of age her brother fell from the roof of their barn, and Clara nursed him back to health over a 2-year period. She later was a battlefield nurse and **philanthropist** whose work during the Civil War led her to recognize that very poor records were kept in Washington to aid in the search for missing men who were wounded or killed in combat. Her efforts to remedy this led to the formation of the Bureau of Records. Her organization and recruitment of supplies for the wounded led to her eventual involvement with the Red Cross in the Franco-Prussian War. In 1881 she organized a Red Cross Committee in Washington, the original formation of the American Red Cross. She served as its first president from 1881 to 1904. Her retirement came at the age of 82, just after personally leading dangerous expeditions to help victims of fires, hurricanes, and floods. The American Red Cross remains a vital organization to this day.

Elizabeth Blackwell (1821-1910) was the first woman in the United States to receive the Doctor of Medicine degree from a medical school (Figure 2-6). Blackwell's family immigrated to New York from England in 1832. She began her medical education by reading medical books and later obtained private instruction. Medical schools in New York and Pennsylvania initially refused her applications for formal study, but finally in 1847 she was accepted at the Geneva Medical College in New York. Ten years later, she established the New York Infirmary for Indigent Women and Children, the first hospital staffed entirely by women. In 1869 Blackwell returned to her native England and became a professor of gynecology at the London School of Medicine for Women, of which she was a founder.

Lillian Wald (1867-1940), a social worker and nurse, made great contributions to medical care when she founded the Henry Street Settlement in New York City. Wald operated a visiting nurse service from this establishment. When one of her nurses was assigned to the city's public schools in 1902, the New York City Municipal Board of Health established the world's first public school nursing system.

Margaret Sanger (1883-1966) was born in Corning, New York, and trained as a nurse at the White Plains Hospital. She became the American leader of the birth control movement. While working among the poor in New York City, she came to understand the public's need for information about contraception. She left nursing to devote herself to that objective. In 1873 the federal Comstock law declared it illegal to import or distribute any device, medicine, or information designed to prevent conception or induce abortion, or to mention in print the names of sexually transmitted diseases. Nurses and physicians were legally prohibited from providing this information to their patients. In 1914 Sanger was **indicted** for circulating the magazine *The Woman Rebel,* in which she attacked the legislative

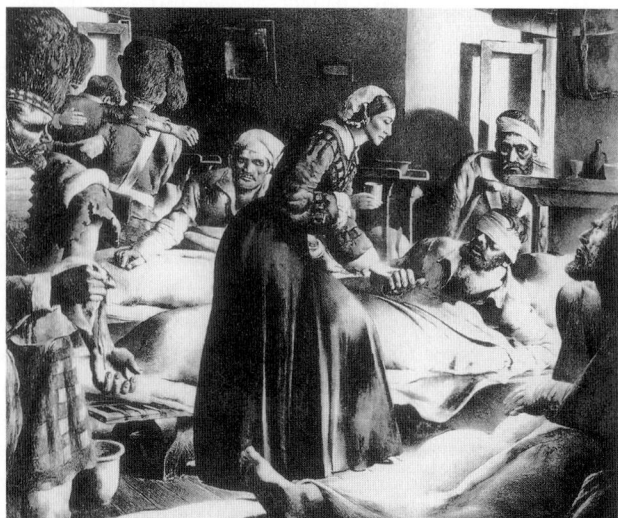

FIGURE 2-5 Considered the founder of nursing, Florence Nightingale is also known as the Lady with the Lamp. (Courtesy National Library of Medicine.)

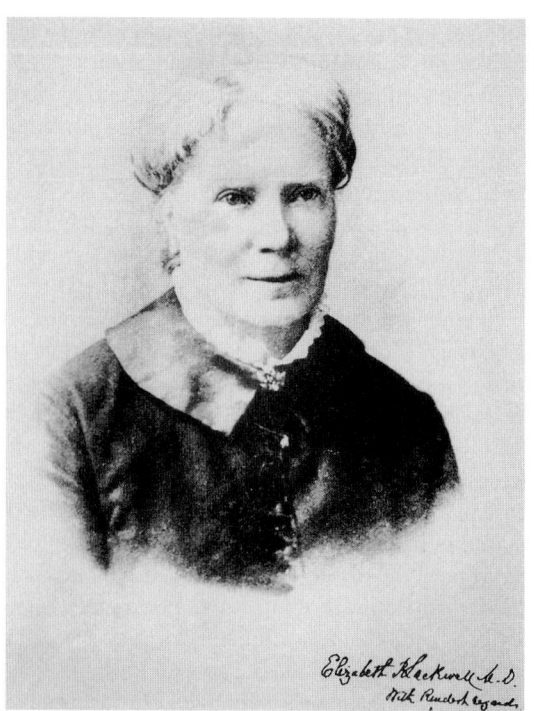

FIGURE 2-6 Elizabeth Blackwell was the first woman to receive a degree as a medical doctor in the United States. (Courtesy National Library of Medicine.)

restrictions of the Comstock law. The case was dismissed 2 years later. In the same year she established the first American birth control clinic; this led to her arrest, conviction, and time in the county jail. She continued her work, and after World War II, she successfully advocated research into hormonal contraception, because of the newfound concern about population growth. This research ultimately led to development of the birth control pill. When the Planned Parenthood Federation of America was formed in 1941, she was named honorary chairperson.

CRITICAL THINKING APPLICATION

Mr. Santos asks his students to tell him which of these early pioneers they would most like to have worked with. Whom would you choose, and why? What difficulties did they face as they worked?

MEDICAL MILESTONES

In recognition of the achievements of scientists of the past, Sir Isaac Newton spoke of our ability to discover and innovate in the medical field. He humbly said, "If I have seen a little further than others, it is because I have stood on the shoulders of giants." Great strides in medicine accompanied the twentieth century, and technology began to advance rapidly. Medical leaders continued their contributions, and knowledge, treatment, and research grew by leaps and bounds.

Walter Reed was a U.S. Army pathologist and bacteriologist who proved that yellow fever was transmitted by the bite of a mosquito. Persons with diabetes should be grateful to Sir Frederick Grant Banting, a Canadian physician who isolated insulin for treatment, along with Charles Herbert Best, a Canadian physiologist. In 1928 Sir Alexander Fleming discovered penicillin accidentally while researching influenza and working with staphylococcal bacteria. He found a substance in mold that prevented growth of bacteria even when the substance was diluted 800 times.

Cardiologist Helen Taussig and surgeon Alfred Blalock explored the health issues of children born with cyanosis resulting from a malformed heart. Dr. Taussig collaborated with Dr. Blalock to develop a lifesaving operation for these children, called "blue babies." History often omits the contributions of Vivien Thomas, an African-American who was Dr. Blalock's surgical research technician at Johns Hopkins Hospital. Thomas was a former carpenter who constructed several of the medical instruments used in the Blalock-Taussig procedure. Thomas actually created the blue-baby condition in dogs, on which he regularly practiced the surgical procedure. When Dr. Blalock and Dr. Taussig performed the first blue-baby operation at Johns Hopkins University, Thomas stood over Blalock's shoulder and advised him during the procedure, since Thomas had done the surgery several more times than Blalock. This happened at a time when African-Americans were not allowed on the main floors of the hospital, much less in the surgical suite. This surgery became known as the Blalock-Taussig procedure, and although the first blue-baby operation prolonged the patient's life by only 2 months, subsequent operations were successful

and children were able to leave the hospital with hope of a healthy life.

Jonas Edward Salk and Albert Sabin almost eradicated poliomyelitis, once the killer and crippler of thousands in the United States. Salk's injectable vaccine was developed in 1952, and after wide-scale testing in 1954 it was distributed nationally, greatly reducing the incidence of the disease. Sabin's live-virus vaccine, in a form that could be swallowed, became available less than a decade later. Werner Forssmann, a German surgeon, originated a cardiac technique called *catheterization* that is used in the diagnosis and treatment of heart disease. Christiaan Barnard, a South African surgeon, performed the first human-heart transplant in 1967. Dr. Elisabeth Kübler-Ross, a Swiss-born psychiatrist who died in 2004, was shocked at the treatment of terminally ill patients at her hospital in New York. She wrote the best-selling book *On Death and Dying*, which helped professionals and laypersons alike to understand the stages of grief.

CRITICAL THINKING APPLICATION

■ During class discussion Mr. Santos points out that the leaders in the healthcare industry had specific goals for their careers and achieved worldwide recognition for their contributions. What individuals have made contributions to medicine in recent years?
■ How can the individual medical assistant make a contribution to medicine?

MODERN MEDICINE

Many modern physicians are making important discoveries and contributions to the field of medicine. Dr. David Ho is considered by many to be one of the most brilliant minds today helping to piece together the puzzle of the human immunodeficiency virus (HIV). Ho is the scientific director and chief executive officer (CEO) of the Aaron Diamond AIDS Research Center in New York City and is also a professor at Rockefeller University. He was born in Taiwan in 1952, and his family immigrated to the United States when he was 12 years of age. He eventually entered college to study physics—medicine was actually his second choice—but once he discovered molecular biology and the concept of gene splicing, he decided to become a researcher. He still does calculations in Chinese. Ho was named *Time* magazine's "Man of the Year" in 1996 for his work in the battle against HIV and acquired immunodeficiency syndrome (AIDS).

Dr. Eve Slater served as the Assistant Secretary for Health at the U.S. Department of Health and Human Services (DHHS). Dr. Slater was former Secretary Tommy G. Thompson's primary advisor on matters regarding issues concerning the nation's public health and oversaw DHHS's U.S. Public Health Service (PHS). Before she joined DHHS, Dr. Slater served as a senior vice president of Merck Research Laboratories' external policy, and also as Vice President of Corporate Public Affairs. Dr. Slater was the first woman to hold this rank. During her time with Merck, she spearheaded the approval of major medicines used to treat the HIV infection, osteoporosis, cardiovascular disease, arthritis, chickenpox, and many others. In 1976, Dr. Slater became the first woman appointed chief resident in medicine at Massachusetts General Hospital. She served as an assistant professor at Harvard Medical School and directed laboratory research funded by the National Institutes of Health (NIH) and the American Heart Association. Currently, Dr. Slater is a board member of several prestigious medical organizations, including Theravance, Inc. and VaxGen, the company co-founded by Dr. Don Francis, who led the fight against AIDS when the disease was first discovered.

Dr. C. Everett Koop was graduated from Cornell University as a medical doctor in 1941 and spent most of his career as a pediatric surgeon. During his terms as the U.S. Surgeon General, he became a proponent of tobacco awareness, insisting that tobacco advertisements must be less attractive to the youth of today. Dr. Koop is a professor at Dartmouth Medical School. He founded the Koop Institute, an organization whose mission is to "promote the health and well-being of all people." Dr. Koop has been honored with many awards, including 41 honorary doctorates.

Dr. Marcia Angell is the former editor-in-chief of the *New England Journal of Medicine* (NEJM), one of the most prestigious medical publications in the United States. Her career with NEJM began in 1979, and her excellent articles spanned a variety of subjects, from the pharmaceutical companies' profit margins to the effects of socioeconomic status on Americans seeking healthcare services. Angell was named one of the 25 most influential Americans in 1997 by Time magazine. She has written and contributed to several books, including *Science on Trial: The Clash of Medical Evidence and the Law in the Breast Implant Case*. Angell is a board-certified pathologist and currently serves as senior lecturer in the Department of Social Medicine at Harvard Medical School.

As the director of the National Institute of Allergy and Infectious Diseases at the NIH, Dr. Anthony Fauci leads research efforts on immune–mediated disorders. His scientific leadership has resulted in major advances in several diseases, such as polyarteritis nodosa and Wegener's granulomatosis. Many of his studies now relate to HIV and the body's response to the AIDS virus, and ways to improve HIV treatment and prevention, including HIV vaccine development. Out of more than one million scientists who published during the period between 1981 and 1994, Dr. Fauci was the fifth most **cited.** He received his MD from Cornell University Medical College, and his career with the NIH has spanned more than 30 years.

Dr. Antonia Novello was the first woman, and the first Hispanic, to be honored with the post of Surgeon General. She served at the NIH and was the honorary chairperson of the National Youth Summit for Mothers Against Drunk Driving (MADD). Novello played a key role in writing the warning labels on cigarette packages. She supported and promoted the National Organ Transplant Act of 1984 and has contributed to the efforts of the United Nations Children's Fund (UNICEF). Novello was a clinical professor at Georgetown University Hospital and in 1994 was inducted into the National Women's Hall of Fame. She currently serves as New York State's health commissioner.

THE NATIONAL VIEW OF HEALTHCARE

World Health Organization

The World Health Organization (WHO), founded in 1948, is a specialized agency of the United Nations. The organization promotes cooperation among nations in their efforts to control and eliminate diseases worldwide. The purposes of WHO are as follows:

- To give worldwide guidance in the field of health
- To set global standards for health
- To cooperate with governments in strengthening national health programs
- To develop and transfer appropriate health technology, information, and standards

One of the greatest accomplishments of this agency was the eradication of smallpox. Other diseases, such as polio and leprosy, are on the verge of eradication. The agency also created and maintains the International Classification of Diseases (ICD) coding system. ICD-9 is used today to identify diseases and conditions using a specific code number. The original purpose of this system was to track worldwide morbidity and mortality statistics. WHO is committed to research and delivery of needed drugs and medical supplies to various areas of the world. In addition, WHO promotes the sharing of health information, and WHO officials meet with the leaders of the worldwide health industry to discuss various ethical and moral implications that face today's healthcare professionals.

U.S. Department of Health and Human Services

The Department of Health and Human Services (HHS) is the principal U.S. agency for providing essential human services and protecting the health of all Americans, especially those who are unable to help themselves. HHS is made up of more than 300 programs involved in the following:

- Medical and social science research
- Immunization services
- Financial assistance for low-income families
- Child support enforcement services
- Improvement of infant and maternal health
- Child and elder abuse prevention services
- Assistance programs for elderly Americans

HHS also oversees the Medicare and Medicaid programs. Medicare is the nation's largest health insurer, and HHS processes more than one billion claims every year. It is the largest grant-making agency in the federal government, providing more than 60,000 grants annually. With a budget of more than $581 billion and more than 67,000 employees, HHS works side by side with local and state governments in its effort to serve the healthcare needs of the public.

U.S. Army Medical Research Institute of Infectious Diseases

The primary focus of the U.S. Army Medical Research Institute of Infectious Diseases (USAMRIID) is protecting military service members, but the Institute conducts key research programs in national defense and infectious diseases that benefit

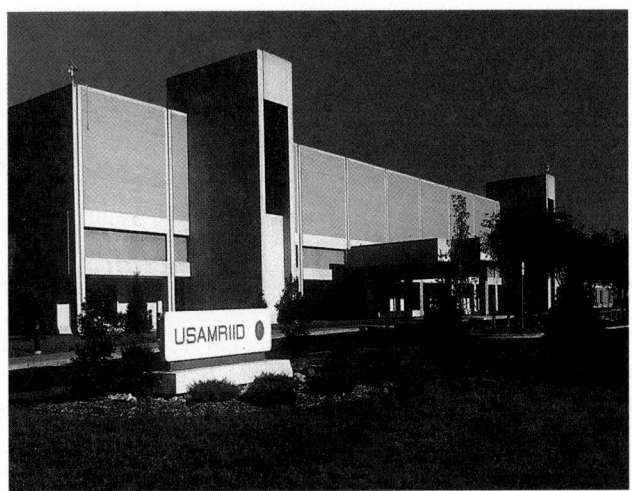

FIGURE 2-7 U.S. Army Medical Research Institute of Infectious Diseases in Fort Detrick, Maryland. (Courtesy USAMRIID, Ft. Detrick, Md.)

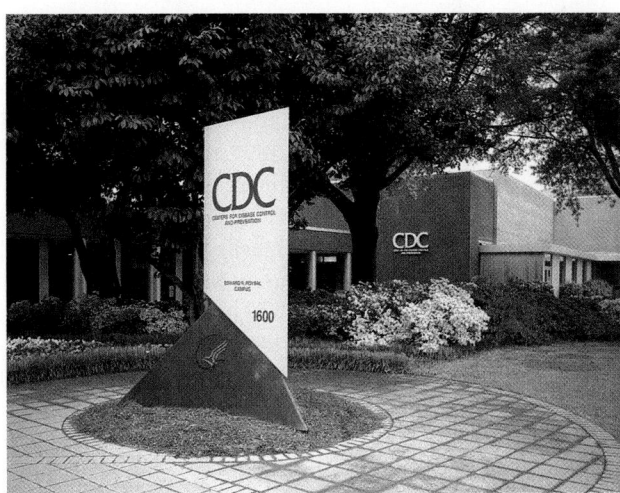

FIGURE 2-8 The headquarters of the Centers for Disease Control and Prevention (CDC) are located in Atlanta, Georgia. (Courtesy Centers for Disease Control and Prevention, Atlanta, Ga.)

everyone (Figure 2-7). USAMRIID, located at Fort Detrick in Maryland, works extensively with the Centers for Disease Control and Prevention (CDC) and WHO. USAMRIID also controls an internationally known reference laboratory with state-of-the-art facilities. This laboratory is instrumental in identifying biologic threats and the diseases those threats produce. USAMRIID is the only laboratory facility operated by the Department of Defense that is equipped to study biosafety level IV viruses and pathogens.

Four biosafety levels are commonly accepted among laboratory professionals. Biosafety level I consists of well-known agents that have a minimal or low biohazard potential to laboratory personnel and to the environment as a whole. At this level the laboratory is not necessarily separated from the regular areas of the facility. Examples of level I pathogens include *Pneumococcus* and *Salmonella*. In the biosafety level II section of the laboratory, substances with a moderate biohazard potential are studied. At levels I and II laboratory personnel have specific training in handling pathogens, and specialized equipment is used to avoid splashes and splatters. Pathogens classified as biosafety level II are hepatitis, the Lyme disease virus, and influenza virus.

Personnel working in biosafety level III have very specific training in working with the potentially deadly pathogens found at this level. All procedures performed on level III pathogens have a high biohazard risk and are done inside protective safety cabinets. Laboratory personnel are required to wear heavy personal protective equipment. Special regulations concerning exhaust air and ventilation are strictly followed, and access to the laboratory is limited when work is in progress. Human immunodeficiency virus (HIV), anthrax, and typhus are some of the pathogens classified as biosafety level III. Biosafety level IV is applied to the most deadly pathogens, which often produce incurable diseases. The biohazard risk of transmission of these agents is extreme and includes the risk of airborne transmission. Laboratory personnel are highly trained in the manipulation and handling of these dangerous pathogens. Laboratory access is strictly controlled in this section. Some of the pathogens studied at biosafety level IV include Ebola virus, Lassa virus, and hantavirus.

Centers for Disease Control and Prevention

The headquarters for the CDC are located in Atlanta, Georgia, (Figure 2-8). The CDC is the principal U.S. federal agency concerned with the health and safety of people throughout the world and is a part of HHS. It is a clearinghouse for information and statistics associated with healthcare. Several divisions within the CDC focus on specific health-related issues, such as the National Center for HIV, STD, and TB Prevention; the Public Health Practice Program Office; the National Center on Birth Defects and Developmental Disabilities; and the National Center for Health Statistics. Branch offices are located throughout the United States and in several foreign countries. The CDC has over 9000 employees who are dedicated to public health. Extensive publications and information services provide healthcare professionals all over the world with the information needed to care for patients.

The agency conducts research into the origin and occurrence of diseases and develops methods for their control and prevention. In addition, it develops immunization services and aids in the training of healthcare workers. In recent years the CDC has been intricately involved in the battle against HIV, which in its advanced form is the acquired immunodeficiency syndrome (AIDS). The agency has developed guidelines emphasizing that universal blood and body fluid precautions be used in all situations in which the risk of contamination by body fluids exists. These recommended precautions are the basis for the laws enforced by the Occupational Safety and Health Administration (OSHA) regarding blood-borne pathogens.

National Institutes of Health

The National Institutes of Health (NIH) began as a one-room laboratory in the marine hospital on New York's Staten Island in 1887. Its first major contribution to medicine was the isolation of the bacterium that causes cholera. Tuberculosis was the number one cause of death at that time. There were few drugs that could alleviate or cure diseases, and there were no vaccines, except for smallpox vaccine. There were no antibiotics, and even aspirin was not yet available. Doctors could diagnose some conditions but fell short on treatments. In 1891 the laboratory moved from Staten Island to Washington, DC. In 1930 the laboratory became the NIH, an agency of HHS. The mission of the NIH is to uncover new knowledge that will lead to better health for everyone. As a part of the public health service, it seeks to improve the health of the American people, supports and conducts biomedical research into the causes and prevention of diseases, and uses a modern communications system to furnish biomedical information to the healthcare professions.

The NIH moved from Washington, DC, to Bethesda, Maryland, in 1938 and today occupies more than 60 buildings covering 30 acres. It consists of 27 different Institutes and Centers and the National Library of Medicine. Thousands of research projects are underway in NIH laboratories and clinics at any given time. The NIH also provides support to other research projects conducted at universities, medical schools, and hospitals.

HEALTH INDUSTRY COUNCILS

Health industry councils are organizations that seek to organize and unify all of the entities providing healthcare in a certain region or community. These organizations keep statistical records about the medical trends in the area and are an important factor in drawing new businesses related to the medical field to the area that they represent. These councils are designed to function as developmental groups that promote the industry in their area and work together for the good of all those involved in healthcare. The organizations represented within the council may fiercely compete in the area market, but they work together to promote the healthcare industry in the region where they are located. The councils usually are made up of task forces and committees that study communications concepts, home health, managed care, membership and development, new business promotion, and design and construction. They are an excellent source of medical information and trends in medicine locally, statewide, and nationally. These councils are valuable assets to any region that wishes to remain on the cutting edge of healthcare.

TYPES OF HEALTHCARE FACILITIES

Hospitals

Several different types of hospitals exist. They are classified according to the type of care and services that they provide to patients, as well as by type of ownership. Acute-care hospitals offer intensive care units and emergency or trauma departments and are equipped to handle the most severely ill or injured patients. Subacute-care hospitals offer patient care for those who do not require extensive services but still need hospital super-

vision and treatment. Specialty hospitals, such as a psychiatric hospital, offer specific services. Teaching hospitals provide a learning environment and often have research departments as well. These hospitals are usually affiliated with medical schools, and interns or residents provide care supervised by licensed physician instructors. Community hospitals provide care in rural areas or in specific areas within a metropolis. Regional hospitals are usually acute-care facilities and serve a large area that may not offer intensive care in its local communities.

Private hospitals are run by a corporation or other organization and are usually designed to produce a profit for the owners or stockholders. Nonprofit hospitals exist to serve the community in which they are located and are normally run by a board of directors. The term *nonprofit* is sometimes misleading, because a difference exists between "profit" and "making money." A nonprofit hospital or organization may make money in a campaign or fund-raiser, but all of the money is returned to the organization. Nonprofit hospitals and organizations must follow strict guidelines in the area of finance and must account to the government how much money is brought in and for what purposes it is used. Sometimes the term *county hospital* is used to designate the hospital to which **indigent** patients are taken. These hospitals provide emergency care to those who cannot pay for medical expenses. Today, however, many people without insurance go to the emergency department (ER) for routine illnesses. This is one reason that ERs are busy and full. If patients have no other options, the ER physicians become primary care providers. This is a major cause of the long waiting times experienced in hospital ERs. Managed care has eased this problem somewhat by refusing to cover visits to the ER that are not true emergencies. **Triage** procedures are used to determine which patients have the most severe conditions and should be seen first.

Hospitals have various departments that are organized to provide efficient patient care. The admissions department gathers information and enters it into a computer for use by the rest of the hospital staff. Nursing service supervises all of the nursing care given to the patients and is involved in **case management.** The laboratory provides diagnostic testing on blood, body fluids, and tissues, and the radiology or nuclear medicine department offers diagnostic imaging and x-ray services. The respiratory services department offers a broad spectrum of diagnostic tests and various treatments. Most hospitals also have a physical medicine and rehabilitation department, which offers both physical and occupational therapy. The dietary department employs professionals who carefully plan menus to meet the needs of each patient served. Most modern hospitals have a surgery department, and many offer day surgery services that allow patients to have a procedure performed and go home the same day, if they recover as expected. The medical records department is responsible for the patient records related to every **encounter** that takes place in the facility. Social services works with patients to ensure continuity of care, patient education, and social intervention, all of which assist patients with emotional, economic, and social concerns.

The hospital administrators manage the hospital on a day-to-day basis, and human resource responsibilities are usually a part of the administration department. Almost every hospital has a board of directors to assist the administrators in governing the hospital, and usually a medical staff committee, led by the hospital's chief of staff, assists in the management of the facility and the **credentialing** process for the physicians that have **staff privileges.** Credentialing involves determining whether a practitioner should be allowed to practice medicine in a facility, based on his or her education, license, past performance, and other qualifications.

The National Practitioner Data Bank also gathers information that helps healthcare facilities identify physicians who are incompetent. It provides information about physicians who have had licensure problems, made malpractice settlements, had clinical privileges revoked or restricted, or had action taken against them by a professional society. This process is incredibly important, because if an incompetent physician is allowed to have staff privileges at a hospital, patients could be harmed and the facility could be held liable for the physician's actions and named as a codefendant in medical professional liability cases. Physicians' backgrounds should be carefully scrutinized by the credentialing committee and staff to avoid this threat of liability. Various types of **peer review organizations** (PROs) are also critical to good healthcare facility management.

Accreditation is considered the highest form of recognition for the quality of care that a facility or organization provides. Not only does it indicate to the public that the facility is concerned with offering high-quality care, it also provides professional liability insurance benefits and plays a role in regulatory agency relicensure and certification efforts. Hospitals and other healthcare facilities are often accredited by the Joint Commission on Accreditation of Healthcare Organizations (JCAHO), an organization that is concerned with the quality of care given in healthcare facilities. **Standards** or **indicators** have been developed that help to determine when patients are receiving high-quality care. The term *quality* refers to much more than whether the patient liked the food served or had to wait to have a procedure or test performed. Categories of compliance include the following:

- Assessment and care of patients
- Use of medication
- Plant, technology, and safety management
- Orientation, education, and training of staff
- Medical staff qualifications
- Patient rights

Ratings from 1 to 5 are given to the facility on its performance in specific areas. A "1" rating means that the facility is in full compliance with that standard, and the other ratings indicate different levels of noncompliance. HHS also regulates healthcare facilities, as does OSHA.

CRITICAL THINKING APPLICATION

- Mr. Santos has assigned his students to groups and asked them to investigate local hospitals. What types of hospitals are found in your local area, and what services do they provide? How might a hospital board decide what services are offered to the community?
- How might Mr. Santos' students find out whether a physician has staff privileges at a certain hospital?

Ambulatory Care

Many other types of healthcare facilities operate in the industry today. **Ambulatory** care centers include a wide range of facilities that offer healthcare services to patients who are able to walk around and are not bedridden. Physicians' offices, group practices, and multispecialty group practices are common types of ambulatory care facilities. Group practices may be of a single specialty, such as pediatrics, or may be multispecialty. A multispecialty practice might consist of an internal medicine specialist, an oncologist, a family practitioner, and an endocrinologist. Usually the physicians within the practice refer to each other when indicated. This is not only more convenient for the patients, but also more profitable for the physicians.

Occupational health centers are concerned with helping patients return to work and productive activity. Often, physical therapy is used in conjunction with rehabilitation services that assist the patient in regaining as much of the previous level of ability as possible. Also, freestanding rehabilitation centers can assist patients with a wide range of services. Pain management centers help patients deal with discomfort that is associated with their condition. Sleep centers diagnose and treat people who have sleep problems. Difficulty in sleeping is a symptom, like pain, and the cause of the disturbance must be found so that proper treatment can be provided. Freestanding urgent or emergency care centers provide patients with an alternative to hospital ERs. They are less expensive, have a shorter waiting time, and are conveniently located in many areas. Most have flexible hours, many are open well into the evening hours, and walk-in appointments are usually accepted.

Surgery has become more convenient because of the number of ambulatory surgical centers that exist today. Day surgery performed in hospitals has continued to provide patients with alternatives to overnight hospital care after surgery. Many insurance companies now prefer day surgery because it is more cost effective. Not many years ago, however, the only alternative to inpatient surgery was the same hospital's day-surgery department. Today more and more freestanding surgical centers are available. Patients can be treated with laser surgery, radial keratotomy, and cataract removal during the day and recover at home that same evening. Plastic surgeons are becoming very innovative in the physical structure of their offices and the types of surgery they offer on an outpatient basis. Many plastic surgeons offer breast augmentation and reduction and even abdominoplasty ("tummy tuck") and liposuction in the office setting. It was not long ago that having abdominoplasty meant staying for several days in the hospital. The new trend is becoming more accepted, partially as a result of the new "office-based surgery" accreditation offered by the Ambulatory Care Accreditation Program of the JCAHO.

Dialysis centers offer services to patients with severe kidney disorders, and many of the larger cities across the country have cancer centers for patients who need treatment by oncologists. Many other types of ambulatory care facilities exist, including centers that provide magnetic resonance imaging (MRI), student health clinics, dental clinics, endoscopy centers, community health centers, mobile health services, podiatric care centers, and women's health centers.

Geriatric and long-term patients have more options today for ambulatory care than ever before. In the past, nursing homes were the only alternative to keeping elderly patients in their own homes. These nursing homes provided care for residents who needed more than just assistance with day-to-day activities. Now there are many attractive options to traditional nursing homes or skilled nursing facilities. One of the most popular is assisted living. Most assisted living facilities provide 24-hour supervision of their residents, most meals, and a broad range of services, from the very basic, such as transportation to physician office visits and errand-running, to the extravagant, such as shopping trips and day-long outings. Most also provide exercise programs, social services, laundry and linen services, and housekeeping. The cost ranges from approximately $1000 to $3000 per month, depending on the location and the **amenities** desired by the resident. There are many new assisted-living facilities specifically designed for Alzheimer's or other memory-care patients.

Independent retirement communities offer residents the opportunity to come and go as they please. Many have a resort-like design, catering to the desire of retirees to enjoy their golden years. Usually the communities consist of apartments or duplex units, and some even offer small cottages. Activities are planned to enhance the social life of the residents, and some communities offer libraries with computer access, restaurant-style dining, beauty salons, and even gardens to grow food. The units usually have special emergency call bells and other protective devices for safety.

Other Healthcare Facilities

Several other types of healthcare facilities deserve attention in the broad overview of the healthcare industry. Diagnostic laboratories offer testing services for patients referred by their physicians. Since the enactment of the Clinical Laboratory Improvement Act (CLIA) in 1967 and its amendment in 1988, many physician offices have stopped providing laboratory tests that were performed inside their offices. These types of labs are called physician office laboratories (POLs). CLIA was enacted to ensure high-quality laboratory testing. The regulations set forth by both OSHA and CLIA rules often made it more cost effective to have the patient go to an outside laboratory to have tests done. The medical assistant should note that OSHA is an organization and division of the U.S. Department of Labor that enforces many laws related to workplace safety. CLIA is a law, not an agency. However, both influence safety and quality testing.

Home health agencies were tremendously successful in the late 1980s to the mid 1990s, but cuts in Medicare funding have caused them to suffer severe losses in recent years. This concept of care is very popular. Unfortunately, the influx of too many home health agencies and the subsequent drop in payments made to them have resulted in fewer home healthcare providers over the past several years. In addition, many hospitals began offering home healthcare, which added to the already heavy competition that smaller firms faced. Home healthcare offers its patients home care, therapy services, administration and assistance with medications, and other services so that the patient can remain at home yet still obtain the care that is needed.

Medical suppliers are retail operations that offer all types of medical devices and products. Diabetic patients can purchase glucose monitoring machines. Special hospital beds can be ordered for those who need them. All types of durable medical equipment (DME), such as bedpans, crutches, bathing assistance devices, wheelchairs, and walkers, are available, often without a physician's prescription. Most medical suppliers serve both the public and the profession.

Hospice centers play an important role in the acceptance of terminal illnesses. These facilities are designed to care for the patient with a terminal disease and provide support to family members. The goal of hospice is to provide peace, comfort, and dignity while controlling pain and promoting the best possible quality of life for the patient. Most patients involved in hospice care have a life expectancy of less than 6 months.

MEDICAL PRACTICES

Three general types of business structures exist in medical practices today: the sole proprietorship, the partnership, and the corporation. Sole proprietorships dominated medical practice until the last quarter of the twentieth century. These practices are on the decline as a result of the **advent** of managed care and its favor of the multispecialty group practice.

Sole Proprietorship

A sole proprietor is an individual who holds exclusive right and title to all aspects of the medical practice. The sole proprietor may employ other physicians to participate in the practice. The employed physician is entitled to employee benefits; however, the owner is not considered an employee and is not so entitled. In addition, the owner would be potentially liable for all of the acts of his or her professional employees and staff members. Although practicing alone has many advantages, including flexibility and independence, it also has heavy disadvantages. The drawbacks include having total responsibility for covering the practice 24 hours a day, 7 days a week. In an unincorporated solo practice, the business dies when the owner leaves it, unless it is sold to someone else. Many modern physicians do not see sole proprietorship as an avenue for a decent income as a doctor, because managed care companies often offer participation to group practices over the single-practice physician, enabling them to provide more options to the patients. Some doctors organize associate practices. In this case, physicians share office space, and often equipment and employees, but they operate their practices as sole proprietorships. Agreements such as these should always be in writing to avoid misunderstandings and legal concerns.

Partnership

When two or more physicians elect to associate in the practice of medicine, they may enter into a partnership agreement. This agreement specifies all of the rights, obligations, and responsibilities of each partner. They have more potential for profit as a partnership than they would in practice as sole proprietors, because various expenses are shared and resources are pooled. Each physician has more freedom, because the doctors rotate an "on-call" schedule so that each has some time away from the office and patients. However, one disadvantage of the partnership is the liability of each for the actions and conduct of all the others. In a partnership arrangement, the partners often pool employees, equipment, insurance, facilities, and even profits, and these resources are divided according to the specifications of the partnership agreement or contract.

A group practice is a body of at least three licensed physicians who engage in full-time practice in a formally organized and legally recognized entity. A group practice may take the form of a partnership, or it may be formed as a corporation. The group may share income and expenses, equipment, records, and personnel and may combine patient care and business management. The group practice may be an association of the same specialty or may be a multispecialty organization. Usually a group practice will take the form of a partnership or a corporation.

Corporation

A corporation may be defined as an artificial entity having a legal and business status that is independent of its shareholders or employees. Corporations are regulated by statutes of the state in which the incorporation takes place. In most cases the physician shareholders are employees of the corporation. Even one physician in a solo practice can incorporate the practice. All employees of the corporation receive income and tax advantages. Corporations are usually able to offer better benefit packages, which may include pension and profit-sharing plans, medical expense reimbursement, life insurance, disability income insurance, and many other benefits. Some offer cafeteria plans, which the employees can customize according to their specific needs, including benefits such as child care reimbursement and tuition reimbursement. Most benefits are tax deductible to both the employer and employee, and some plans offer pretax benefit packages as well. Professional employees of a corporation are liable for only their own acts, although it is always a good idea for any professional in the medical field to carry his or her own malpractice insurance. Another advantage of the corporate entity is the continuous life of the corporation. It does not dissolve with a change in shareholders.

HEALTHCARE PROFESSIONALS

Title of "Doctor"

Doctors of Medicine

Medical doctors (MDs) are considered to be **allopathic** physicians and are the most widely recognized type of physician. They diagnose illness and disease and prescribe treatment for their patients. MDs are allowed to write prescriptions and perform surgeries. They offer advice on nutrition and preventive medicine. To become an MD usually requires 4 years of undergraduate training (premed) and 4 years of medical school. Some extraordinary students are allowed entry after 3 years of undergraduate studies, but competition for entry into medical school is intense, so grades and other experience in healthcare are strongly considered. Premed students study biology, physics, organic and inorganic chemistry, mathematics, English, humanities, and social sciences. There are approximately 125 allopathic medical schools in the United States. After medical school the student faces 3 to 8 years of internship and residency programs. An intern is a medical student still in training at medical school but treating patients under the supervision of licensed doctors. A residency is a graduate medical education program, often in a specialty, and is usually a paid "on-the-job training" hospital position. Often MDs specialize in a certain field, such as cardiology or pediatrics. These doctors usually invest 3 to 6 years of training in the specialty after medical school and can obtain board certification in one or more of 24 different specialty areas recognized by the American Board of Medical Specialties (Table 2-1). An MD must have a state license to practice, and continuing education is required to maintain the license. Graduates of foreign medical schools can usually obtain a license in the United States after passing an examination and completing a residency program in this country.

Doctors of Osteopathy

Osteopathic physicians (Doctors of Osteopathy [DOs]) complete requirements similar to those of MDs to graduate and practice medicine. Osteopaths use medicine and surgery, as well as osteopathic manipulative therapy (OMT), in treating their patients. Andrew Taylor Still is considered the originator of osteopathic medicine, which he began in 1874. He believed in a more **holistic** approach to medicine, and although he was an MD, he founded the American School of Osteopathy in Kirksville, Missouri. The school was originally chartered to offer an MD degree but later focused more on the osteopathic approach. DOs stress preventive medicine and holistic patient care, as well as a special focus on the musculoskeletal system and OMT. Osteopathic medicine also promotes the **innate** ability of the body to heal itself, and many osteopaths tend to take a more conservative approach to using medications and surgical procedures than allopathic physicians. Many DOs practice **homeopathy,** believing in the body's ability to heal itself. Premed students moving toward osteopathic medicine also study biology, physics, organic and inorganic chemistry, mathematics, English, humanities, and social sciences. They also usually complete 4 years of undergraduate studies, then begin 4 years of medical studies at a school for osteopathic medicine. Most DOs participate in a 12-month rotating internship in the various specialty areas before entering a residency program lasting from 2 to 6 years, and they are eligible for board certification through either the American Board of Medical Specialists or the American Osteopathic Association. Approximately one in 20 physicians in the United States is a DO. DOs participate

TABLE 2-1 Types of Medical Specialties Recognized by the American Board of Medical Specialties

MEDICAL SPECIALTY	TITLE OF PRACTITIONER	DESCRIPTION OF SPECIALTY
Allergy and Immunology	Allergist, Immunologist	An allergist/immunologist is trained to evaluate disorders and diseases of the immune system. These include conditions such as adverse reactions to drugs and foods, anaphylaxis, problems related to autoimmune diseases, asthma, and insect stings.
Anesthesiology	Anesthesiologist	An anesthesiologist provides pain relief and management during surgical procedures and for patients with long-standing conditions accompanied by pain, such as cancer patients. Anesthesiologists also provide critical care and resuscitation for patients during cardiac or respiratory emergencies.
Colon and Rectal Surgery	Colon and Rectal Surgeon	This type of surgeon diagnoses and treats conditions affecting the intestines, rectum, and anal area, as well as organs that can cause intestinal disease. They often treat cancers that appear in these areas, as well as disorders such as hemorrhoids and fissures.
Dermatology	Dermatologist	The dermatologist works with adult and pediatric patients in treating disorders and diseases of the skin, hair, nails, and related tissues. Dermatologists are specially trained to manage conditions such as skin cancers, cosmetic disorders of the skin, scars, allergies, and other disorders, both malignant and benign.
Emergency Medicine	Emergency Physician	An emergency physician is an expert in triage and in treating patients to prevent death or serious disability. This physician gives immediate care to stabilize the patient, then refers to the appropriate professional for further care. These physicians are usually found in hospital emergency rooms or freestanding emergency centers.
Family Practice	Family Practitioner	The family practitioner offers care to the whole family, from newborns to elderly adults, and is familiar with a wide range of disorders and diseases. Preventive care is of primary concern. This is one of the more common specialties that physicians choose.
General Surgery	Surgeon	Surgery is the correction of deformities, defects, diseases, or injured parts of the body by means of operative treatment. A surgeon must be familiar with the various specialties to effectively treat patients. General surgery includes all of the aspects of surgery other than those separated into a subgroup specialty.
Internal Medicine	Internist	Internists are concerned with comprehensive care, often diagnosing and treating those with chronic, long-term conditions. They also offer treatment for common illnesses and preventative care. Internists must have a broad understanding of the body and its ailments in order to diagnose and provide treatment to the patient.
Medical Genetics	Geneticist	A geneticist is a physician trained to diagnose and treat patients who have conditions related to genetically linked diseases and may provide special genetic counseling when indicated. Often associated with research projects, this physician may participate in screening programs for defects and abnormalities, sometimes before the birth of an infant.
Neurological Surgery	Neurological Surgeon	The neurological surgeon offers nonoperative and operative care for patients with conditions of the central, autonomic, and peripheral nervous systems, including the supporting structures and vascular supplies of related organs.
Neurology, Psychiatry	Neurologist, Psychiatrist	The neurologist diagnoses and treats disorders of the brain, spinal cord, nerves, and the blood vessels that support those organs. Generally, the neurologist manages infectious, metabolic, degenerative, and systemic involvement of the nervous system. A psychiatrist is a physician whose specialty is the diagnosis and treatment of persons with mental, emotional, or behavioral disorders. The psychiatrist is qualified to conduct psychotherapy and to prescribe medications when necessary.
Nuclear Medicine	Nuclear Medicine Specialist	This specialist uses radioactive substances for the diagnosis and treatment of disease. Radiation and imaging instruments are used to detect diseases often before the affected organ is shown to be abnormal by other methods. The nuclear medicine specialist is aware of the effects of radiation on various structures, as well as the fundamentals of the principles of radiation and physics.

Continued

TABLE 2-1 Types of Medical Specialties Recognized by the American Board of Medical Specialties—*cont'd*

MEDICAL SPECIALTY	TITLE OF PRACTITIONER	DESCRIPTION OF SPECIALTY
Obstetrics and Gynecology	Obstetrician and Gynecologist	Obstetricians provide care to women of childbearing age and monitor the progress of the developing child. They deliver the baby, and care for the mother for approximately 6 weeks after birth. Gynecologists are concerned with the diagnosis and treatment of the female reproductive system.
Ophthalmology	Ophthalmologist	Ophthalmologists diagnose, treat, and provide comprehensive care to the eye and its supporting structures. These physicians also offer vision services, including corrective lenses. Screening tests are promoted as a measure of preventative care.
Otolaryngology	Otolaryngologist	These physicians treat diseases and conditions that affect the ear, nose, throat, and structures related to the head and neck. Problems that affect the voice and hearing are also referred to this specialist.
Pathology	Pathologist	Pathologists study the causes of diseases that affect the body and determine what may have caused the death of a patient. These physicians study tissues and cells, body fluids, and actual organs to assist in diagnosing the patient's ailments. Pathologists often perform autopsies.
Pediatrics	Pediatrician	Pediatricians promote preventative medicine and treat diseases that affect children and adolescents. They monitor the child's growth and development and provide a wide range of health services to keep their patients healthy.
Physical Medicine and Rehabilitation	Physiatrist	Physicians of this specialty assist patients who have physical disabilities. This may include those with musculoskeletal disorders or who are suffering from pain as a result of injury or trauma. Their primary goal is to restore the patient to the state of health the patient had before the injury or trauma as nearly as possible through rehabilitation.
Plastic Surgery	Plastic Surgeon	The plastic surgeon works with patients who have had some type of injury or condition that has left them with a physical defect. The surgeon performs reconstructive procedures, using grafts, flaps, and tissue transfer and replanting. These surgeons also perform cosmetic enhancements and procedures that are elective in nature.
Preventative Medicine	Preventative Medicine Specialist	Preventative Medicine is concerned with preventing the occurrence of both mental and physical illness and disability. Analysis of present health services and planning for future medical needs are part of this specialty. Preventative medicine consists of several components, including biostatistics, environmental studies, occupational studies, and clinical preventive medicine activities.
Radiology	Radiologist	Radiology is a specialty in which x-rays are used for diagnosis and treatment of disease. A diagnostic radiologist specializes in using x-rays, ultrasound, nuclear medicine, computed tomography, and magnetic resonance imaging for detection of abnormalities throughout the body.
Thoracic Surgery	Thoracic Surgeon	This surgical specialty is concerned with the operative treatment of the chest and chest wall, lungs, and respiratory passages. Specialists in this field are involved with heart surgery, including both valvular and coronary heart surgery.
Urology	Urologist	Urology is a medical specialty concerned with the treatment of diseases and disorders of the urinary tract. They diagnose and manage problems with the genitourinary system and practice endoscopic and percutaneous procedures related to these structures.

in continuing education programs to renew their licenses annually.

Doctors of Chiropractic

Chiropractors (Doctors of Chiropractic [DCs]) are typically thought of as "bone doctors" but actually focus on the nervous system to help patients live healthier lives. The nervous system is the master system of the body, controlling and coordinating all the other systems. Information from the environment, both internal and external, moves through the spinal cord to get to the brain, and in the same manner, information from the brain moves through the spinal cord to reach the body in a two-way flow of communication. The intention of the **chiropractic** adjustment is to remove any disruptions or distortions of this energy flow that may be caused by slight misalignments that chiropractors call **subluxations.** Chiropractors are trained to locate these subluxations and remove them, using touch as well as x-ray films, thereby restoring the normal flow of nerve energy so that the entire body functions in an optimal fashion. They believe that the same innate inner intelligence that grows the body from a single cell into a complex human being can also heal the body if it is free of disturbance to the nervous system. The philosophy is that health, not merely absence of symptoms, comes from within the body, not from the outside. Chiropractic colleges require undergraduate studies in biology, organic and inorganic chemistry, physics, English, and the humanities, and then 3 to 4 years are spent studying chiropractic. Each state offers licensing. Some chiropractors devote their practices to a specific specialty, but more often they practice general chiropractic. Continuing education is required for relicensure. Chiropractic is one of the most common fields of **alternative medicine.**

CRITICAL THINKING APPLICATION

- Mr. Santos challenges his new medical assisting students to interview several types of doctors at some point during their studies. The class discusses the different philosophies of medicine among allopathic, osteopathic, and chiropractic physicians. Discuss with your class the similarities and differences of these three aspects of medicine.
- Most of Mr. Santos' students have visited one or more of these types of doctors. What experiences have you had with medical doctors (MDs), osteopaths (DOs), or chiropractors?

Dentists

The two basic types of dentists in the United States are Doctors of Dental Medicine (DMD) and Doctors of Dental Surgery (DDS). Dentists treat and prevent problems dealing with the teeth and gums and the tissue surrounding them. They can perform oral surgery and write prescriptions for antibiotics and analgesics. Some specialist dentists perform straightening, called *orthodontics,* and some perform root canal therapy, called *endodontics.* Dental school usually lasts 4 years after completion of undergraduate studies, and state licensing is required.

Optometrists

The optometrist (OD) is trained and licensed to examine the eyes to test visual acuity and to treat vision defects by prescribing correctional lenses and other optical aids. A program of exercise may be planned for the patient's eyes. Optometrists study at accredited schools for optometry for 4 years after completing undergraduate studies in the sciences, mathematics, and English. They must be licensed in the state in which they practice. Optometrists should not be confused with ophthalmologists, who are licensed MDs.

Podiatrists

Podiatrists, or Doctors of Podiatric Medicine (DPM), are educated in caring for the feet, including surgical treatment. Normal persons spend an extraordinary amount of time on their feet, resulting in wear and tear and chronic pain. Podiatrists are trained to find pressure points and weight-distribution

problems. These doctors train for 4 years at accredited colleges after undergraduate studies in the sciences.

Other Doctorates

Other individuals may be called "doctor" based on the degree they have earned in their field. For instance, a person with a PhD has a doctoral degree in philosophy, may be addressed as "doctor," and might work as a professor at a university or in a field related to his or her discipline. A PsyD is a Doctor of Psychology, and an EdD is a Doctor of Educational Psychology. Doctors who practice **naturopathy,** called naturopathic physicians, use only natural means to help the body to heal. These medical professionals are licensed in 15 states.

Licensed Medical Professionals

Many types of licensed medical professionals assist the physician in diagnosing and treating the patient (Table 2-2). Some of the professionals that the medical assistant will commonly encounter are listed in this section. Medical assistants are usually certified professionals and are discussed in detail in Chapter 3.

Physician Assistants

Physician assistants (PAs) provide direct patient care services under the supervision of licensed physicians. They are trained to diagnose and treat patients as directed by the physician, and in 46 states and the District of Columbia they are allowed to write prescriptions. These professionals take patient histories, order and interpret tests, perform physical examinations, and even make diagnosis decisions. They can be found in physician offices, in hospitals, on military bases, and in other healthcare facilities.

Nurse Practitioners

Nurse practitioners (NPs) provide basic patient care services, including diagnosis and prescribing for common illnesses. These professionals must have advanced academic training beyond the RN degree and also have vast clinical experience. Usually the focus of nurse practitioners is on preventive care and disease prevention, and an NP is allowed to practice independently or as a part of a team of healthcare professionals.

Nurse Anesthetists

Nurse anesthetists are registered nurses (RNs) who administer anesthetics to patients during care by surgeons, physicians, dentists, or other qualified health professionals. They practice in many different settings, including offices, traditional hospitals, labor and delivery units, ophthalmology offices, plastic surgery offices, and many others. This practice is quite advanced, and they are compensated well for their skills. Nurse anesthetists can be found in both metropolitan and rural communities.

Registered Nurses

The RN has many career options available. Many nurses work in an administrative capacity within hospitals or other types of healthcare facilities as managers. They also provide direct patient care, where they are vital in assessing the patient and providing a care plan. Usually nurses find a specialty area that

TABLE 2-2 Allied Health Careers from the Health Professions Career and Education Directory

OCCUPATION	CREDENTIAL	BRIEF JOB DESCRIPTION
Anesthesiologist Assistant	AA	Functions as a specialty physician assistant under the direction of a licensed and qualified anesthesiologist; assists in developing and implementing the anesthesia care plan
Art Therapist	ATR	Uses drawings and other art or media forms to assess, treat, and rehabilitate patients with mental, emotional, physical, and/or developmental disorders
Athletic Trainer	ATC	Provides a variety of services, including injury prevention, assessment, immediate care, treatment, and rehabilitation after physical injury or trauma
Audiologist	CCC-A	Identifies individuals with symptoms of hearing loss and other auditory, balance, and related neural problems; assesses the nature of those problems and helps individuals manage them
Blindness and Visual Impairment Professions	LVT, O&M, VRT	Helps people learn to use their vision more efficiently, both with and without optical devices; provides training and offers recommendations to help patients function more successfully in their environments
Blood Bank Technology, Specialist in	SBB	Performs routine and specialized tests in blood center and transfusion services, using methods that conform to the accepted standards in the blood bank industry
Clinical Laboratory Science or Medical Technologist	MT, MLT	Performs tests in conjunction with pathologists to diagnose the causes and nature of disease; develops data on blood, tissues, and fluids of the human body using a variety of methodologies
Counseling-Related Occupations	LPC, LMHC	Deals with human development concerns through support, therapeutic approaches, consultation, evaluation, teaching, and research; practices the art of helping people to grow
Cytotechnologist	CT	Works with pathologists to evaluate cellular material from all body sites primarily using the microscope; looks for normal and abnormal cytologic changes, including malignancies
Dance Therapist	DTR, ADTR	Uses the psychotherapeutic properties of movement as a process that furthers the emotional, cognitive, social, and physical integration of the patient as a tool for healing
Dental Assistant, Dental Hygienist, Dental Laboratory Technician	CDA, RDH, CDT	Performs a wide range of tasks from assisting the dentist to instructing patients as to how they can prevent oral disease and maintain oral health
Diagnostic Cardiovascular Sonographer or Technologist	RDCS, RVT	Performs diagnostic examinations and therapeutic interventions of the heart and/or blood vessels at the request of a physician using invasive and/or noninvasive techniques.
Dietetic Technician, Dietician	DTR	Integrates and applies the principles derived from the sciences of food, nutrition, biochemistry, physiology, food management, and behavior to achieve and maintain health status
Electroneurodiagnostic Technology	REEG-T	Records and studies electrical activity in the brain and nervous system; obtains interpretable recordings of patients' nervous system function
Emergency Medical Technician, Paramedic	EMT, Paramedic	Provides medical care to people who have suffered from an injury or illness outside the hospital setting, most often in an emergency; provides basic and/or advanced life support
Genetic Counselor	IGC	Provides genetic services to individuals and families seeking information about the occurrence or risk of a genetic condition or birth defect
Health Information Management	RHIA, RHIT	Provides expert assistance in the systems and processes of health information management, including planning, engineering, administration, application, and policy making
Kinesiotherapist	RKT	Provides rehabilitation exercise and education designed to reverse or minimize debilitation and enhance the functional capacity of medically stable patients
Massage Therapist	MT	Applies manual techniques and may apply adjunctive techniques with the intention of positively affecting the health and well-being of the client
Medical Assistant	CMA, RMA	Functions as a member of the health care delivery team and performs both administrative and clinical procedures and duties; multiskilled health professional

Continued

TABLE 2-2 Allied Health Careers from the Health Professions Career and Education Directory—*cont'd*

OCCUPATION	CREDENTIAL	BRIEF JOB DESCRIPTION
Medical Illustrator	MI	Specializes in the visual display and communication of scientific information; creates visuals and designs communications to teach medical professionals as well as the public
Music Therapist	MT-BC	Uses music within a therapeutic relationship to address physical, emotional, cognitive, and social needs of individuals of all ages; assesses strengths and needs of clients
Nuclear Medicine Technologist	RT	Uses the nuclear properties of radioactive and stable nuclides to make diagnostic evaluations of the anatomic or physiologic conditions of the body and provide therapy with unsealed radioactive sources
Occupational Therapist	OTR	Uses purposeful activity and interventions to achieve functional outcomes to maximize the independence and the maintenance of health for those limited by physical injury or illness
Ophthalmic Laboratory Technician, Medical Technician or Technologist	COT, COMT	Collects data and performs clinical evaluations; performs tests and protocols required by ophthalmologists; assists the physician in treating the patient
Orthoptist	CO	Performs a series of diagnostic tests and measurements on patients with visual disorders; helps design a treatment plan to correct the disorders of vision, eye movements, and alignment
Orthotist and Prosthetist	RTO, RTP, RTPO	Designs and fits devices (orthoses) to provide care to patients who have disabling conditions of the limbs and spine and/or partial or total absence of a limb
Perfusionist	CCP	Operates extracorporeal circulation and autotransfusion equipment during any medical situation in which the patient's respiratory or circulatory function must be supported or temporarily replaced
Pharmacy Technician	CPhT	Assists pharmacists with duties that do not require the expertise or judgment of a licensed pharmacist
Physical Therapist	PT	Helps to improve patient strength and mobility, relieve pain, prevent or limit permanent physical disabilities; takes a personal, direct approach to meeting individual health goals
Physician Assistant	PA	Practices medicine with the direction and responsible supervision of a licensed doctor of medicine or osteopathy; makes clinical decisions and provides a range of services
Radiation Therapist, Radiographer	RRT	Delivers prescribed dosages of radiation to patients for therapeutic purposes; provides appropriate patient care and maintains accurate records of treatment provided
Rehabilitation Counselor	CRC	Determines and coordinates services to assist people with disabilities in moving from psychologic and economic dependence to independence
Respiratory Therapist, Respiratory Therapy Technician	RRT, CRT, RPFT, CPFT	Evaluates, treats, and manages patients of all ages with respiratory illnesses and other cardiopulmonary disorders; advanced RTs exercise considerable independent judgment
Surgical Assistant	CSA	Provides aid in exposure, hemostasis, closure, and other intraoperative technical functions that help the surgeon carry out a safe operation with optimal results for the patient
Surgical Technologist	ST, CST	Assists in preparing patients for surgery and maintaining the sterile field within the surgical suite, making certain that all members of the surgical team adhere to sterile technique
Therapeutic Recreation Specialist	CTRS	Uses treatment, education, and recreation services to help people with illnesses, disabilities, and other conditions develop and use their leisure in ways that enhance their health

they enjoy and practice within that area, although they may also "float" to different departments within the hospital. Some function as home health nurses, visiting patients and providing home care. Some work in nursing homes or in public health, and others serve in physicians' offices.

Licensed Practical and Vocational Nurses

Licensed practical nurses (LPNs) and licensed vocational nurses (LVNs) offer bedside care, assisting with the actual day-to-day personal care required by inpatients. They assess patients, chart their progress, and administer medications and intravenous fluids where allowed by law. They often work in hospitals or skilled nursing facilities and are also found in physicians' offices. They sometimes supervise nursing assistants and may also provide patient education services.

Medical Technologists

Medical technologists (MTs) perform diagnostic testing on blood, body fluids, and other types of specimens to assist the physician in arriving at a diagnosis. These professionals work with bacteria and viruses and use their technical skills combined with their knowledge of disease to perform their duties. They can make quality-control decisions and can act independently within their profession. Hospitals, teaching universities, research organizations, and laboratories employ most of the medical technologists. Usually they have a Bachelor of Science (BS) degree in addition to certification or a license.

Medical Laboratory Technicians

Medical laboratory technicians (MLTs) perform most of the same test procedures that the medical technologist performs; the difference between the two is that MLTs do not work independently. They are usually supervised by an MT and have at least an associate's degree and a certification or license. MLTs work in the same types of facilities as MTs.

Physical Therapists

Physical therapists (PTs) assist patients in regaining their mobility and improving their strength and range of motion, which may have been impaired by an accident or injury or as a result of disease. After assessing the patient, the PT devises a treatment plan in conjunction with the patient's physician. The goal of the PT is to improve how the patient functions at work and at home.

Respiratory Therapists

Most respiratory therapists (RTs) work in the hospital environment. All types of patients receive respiratory care, including newborns and geriatric patients. RTs commonly use oxygen therapy to assist with breathing, and they also perform diagnostic tests that measure lung capacity.

Occupational Therapists

Occupational therapists (OTs) work with patients who have developed conditions that disable them developmentally, emotionally, mentally, or physically. OTs assist in helping the

individual to compensate for loss of function. The goal of OTs is to bring their patients to a level of living healthy, productive lives.

Diagnostic Cardiac Sonographers

Diagnostic cardiac sonographers or technologists (DCSs or VTs) assist in the diagnosis and treatment of cardiac and vascular diseases and disorders. They perform noninvasive tests, including echocardiographs and electrocardiographs. Often ultrasonography is used by the cardiovascular technician to assist the physician in discovering the malfunction of the heart and its structures.

Diagnostic Medical Sonographers

Diagnostic medical sonographers (DMSs) assist physicians in the diagnosis of various disorders by means of ultrasound waves, which produce images of the internal structures of the body. These professionals are often called *sonographers*. Ultrasonography is used to assist the physician in many ways, including the monitoring of fetal development.

Radiology Technicians

Radiology technicians (RTs) use various machines to help the physician diagnose and treat certain diseases. These machines may include x-ray equipment, ultrasonographic machines, and MRI scanners. RTs explain procedures to patients and know correct positioning techniques, so that the images recorded are accurate and helpful for the diagnosing physician.

Paramedics

Paramedics are specially trained to provide emergency care to patients in life-threatening situations. Paramedics are highly efficient and well versed in the functions of the body. They perform advanced skills and, with more experience, are able to supervise or direct the operations of an emergency care ambulance facility.

Emergency Medical Technicians

Emergency medical technicians (EMTs) progress through several levels of training, each providing more-advanced skills. Their medical education encompasses managing respiratory, cardiac, and trauma cases and often emergency childbirth. Specialties within the EMT field also exist in certain states, such as EMT Cardiac, which includes training in **cardiac arrhythmias,** and EMT Shock Trauma, which includes starting intravenous fluids and administration of medication.

Registered Dietitians

Registered dietitians (RDs) have thorough training in nutrition and the different types of diets that patients are placed on to improve or maintain their condition. They use the advice of the physician and information about the patient to design healthy diets during hospital stays and even help to plan menus for home use. They also provide education for the patient about the diet and alternatives that will help in choosing attractive foods.

CLOSING COMMENTS

The healthcare industry is certainly one of the most exciting career fields to enter in today's world. The constant change and development of new technology and theories make medicine an attractive option for career choices. The needs of medicine extend far beyond the boundaries of the United States, and collaborative efforts among countries promote a faster move forward with new discoveries and hope for those affected by disease. Headlines grace newspapers and computer screens daily, detailing stories of human cloning, designer babies, genetic discoveries, and computer capabilities that amaze us all. Medications are being developed that bring us to the brink of eliminating certain diseases. The mapping of the human genome may lead to incredible breakthroughs in the study of colon, breast, and ovarian cancers, cystic fibrosis, neurologic degeneration, sickle cell anemia, and countless other conditions. There has never been a more thrilling time to become a part of the world of medicine and make a contribution as a healthcare professional.

SUMMARY OF SCENARIO

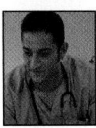

Mr. Santos is an effective instructor, and one who is concerned about providing interesting material for his students. He wishes to instill a strong respect in the students for the people who played a role in early medical advances. His classroom discussions will help the students to think about what it was like to present new ideas to the public and often be ridiculed.

While teaching them about the history of medicine and the state of healthcare today, he also provides opportunities for the students to work together in discussion groups and present information to the class. He encourages Internet research, a valuable skill that will help the medical assisting student in many areas of training. By allowing the students to speak in front of the class while giving reports on the medical forefathers, Mr. Santos teaches the students to be more at ease when speaking in public and when articulating instructions and details to patients and co-workers. All of these skills make a well-rounded medical assistant who will become a great asset to the facility in which he or she is employed.

Mr. Santos explains that continuing medical research is critical to the healthcare industry because new and more-effective drugs and treatments are necessary and because many diseases and conditions do not as yet have a cure. Medical research constantly looks for better ways to make patients well and continually strives to find cures for diseases that medicine has not yet conquered. Medical assistants may work for physicians who are involved in research projects, and this may afford them the opportunity to contribute to medical research.

By providing his students with an overview of the healthcare industry, Mr. Santos helps them to become more familiar with the professionals whom they encounter in various medical facilities and to have a better awareness of their duties and responsibilities.

SUMMARY of LEARNING OBJECTIVES

1. Define, spell, and pronounce the terms listed in the vocabulary.
   - Spelling and pronouncing medical terms correctly adds credibility to the medical assistant. Knowing the definition of these terms promotes confidence in communication with patients and co-workers.
2. Identify the ancient cultures that contributed a major portion of our medical terminology.
   - Greek and Roman mythology contributed the major portion of the medical terms we use today. Terms have also been borrowed from Anglo-Saxon, German, Arabic, and other sources, including the Bible.
3. Explain the history of medicine and how it has affected today's medical industry.
   - The history of medicine clearly influences medical practice today, because yesterday's discoveries are today's medications and treatments. Research is an ongoing necessity in the medical field. As technology becomes more and more sophisticated, medical advancements follow.
4. Distinguish between and describe the two medical symbols in general use today.
   - The American Medical Association adopted the staff of Aesculapius as the symbol of medicine. The symbol is a staff encircled by a serpent. The caduceus is often mistakenly used to represent medicine but is actually the medical insignia of the U.S. Army Medical Corps. This icon is a staff encircled by two serpents, bearing wings at the top.
5. Explain why a medical education at Johns Hopkins was considered superior, even in its early years.
   - Johns Hopkins University Medical School has been recognized as a leader in healthcare education for over a century. The university was one of the first institutions to partner with a hospital for training purposes, resulting in its superior medical education. Johns Hopkins contained a research department as well, where faculty members investigated new methods and treatments for patients. Combining the medical education with readily available patients brought the discovery of illness and disease into a new light for early medical students. Today Johns Hopkins is a multibillion-dollar organization, incorporating three acute-care hospitals and other entities in an integrated healthcare system.

Continued

SUMMARY of LEARNING OBJECTIVES
Continued

6. List several medical pioneers, and discuss the importance of their contributions to the medical profession.
   - Numerous early pioneers made tremendous contributions to the medical field. Constant growth and research have pressed the medical profession forward, and with the assistance of technology the growth speeds along today faster than ever.

7. Explain the roles of the world healthcare organizations.
   - World healthcare organizations provide information, medication, and personnel to attempt to eradicate diseases and treat those diseases for which no cure exists. Many of these organizations operate with restricted funding and rely often on volunteer donations and volunteer workers to operate. These agencies often work together in an effort to effectively solve problems of epidemics and learn more about diseases. All of the national healthcare organizations are a vital part of the medical industry today.

8. Discuss the various types of ambulatory care.
   - Physicians' offices, group practices, and multispecialty group practices are a few types of ambulatory care. This division of medicine also includes occupational health centers, dialysis centers, rehabilitation clinics, and sleep centers. Patients who are ambulatory are able to move from place to place, usually on their own or with the assistance of a wheelchair or walker.

9. Distinguish among different types of doctors and medical practices.
   - Three main provider portals of entry into the healthcare system exist today; they are medical doctors, osteopathic physicians, and chiropractic physicians. These different disciplines have some similar training, but osteopathic physicians usually use a holistic approach, and chiropractors concentrate many of their efforts on the alignment of the spine in an effort to promote a healing of the body. Most physicians work in a sole proprietorship, a group practice, or a healthcare corporation.

10. Identify the medical specialties recognized by the American Board of Medical Specialties.
    - Numerous specialties focus on particular areas of the practice of medicine. The American Board of Medical Specialties recognizes over 20 specialty groups that support various organizations designed to promote that particular branch of medicine. Although other specialties and subspecialties of medicine exist, the most common and most generally recognized are those associated with the American Board of Medical Specialties.

11. Discuss various healthcare occupations and the role these professionals play in the healthcare industry.
    - The American Medical Association recognizes more than 60 allied healthcare occupations. These allied health professionals contribute to the field of medicine, each playing a specific role in the healthcare industry.

CONNECTIONS

Study Guide Connection: Go to Chapter 2 Study Guide. Read the Case Study and Workplace Applications and complete the assignments. Do online research for answers to the questions in the Internet Activities associated with the healthcare industry.

CD Connection: Go to the Medical Assisting Competency Challenge CD and review the content of the training activities. These will be referred to throughout the textbook to enhance your learning experience.

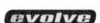

Evolve Connection: For more information related to the healthcare industry, go to evolve.elsevier.com/kinn and visit related weblinks for Chapter 2. Click on the Medical Assisting Exam Review and do the practice questions to sharpen your test-taking skills.

The Medical Assisting Profession

3

SCENARIO

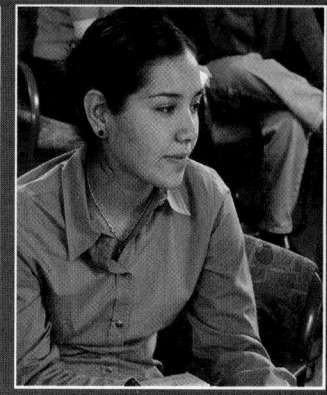

Sandra Rameriz is a single mother who has decided on medical assisting as a career. She has always been interested in the medical field and wants a job that will allow her to spend evenings and weekends with her 3-year-old son, Roberto. The idea of working in a physician's office appeals to her, and she has applied to a school that is close to her apartment and day care provider. She plans to attend day classes and work part-time after school until it is time to pick up her son.

Sandra is very excited about her new career and has set several goals for her training. First, she hopes to attain perfect attendance, and second, she would like to graduate with honors. She has budgeted her study time and plans to ask her instructors during the first 2 weeks of school for suggestions about how she can better prepare for classes and examinations. Sandra will find medical assisting to be a rewarding career and respected profession.

While studying this chapter, think about the following questions:

- What obstacles might prevent Sandra from attending all of her classes, and how can she prepare in advance to overcome them?
- How can Sandra begin to explore the type of physician offices in which she would enjoy being employed after graduation?
- What goals might Sandra have at the commencement of her training? At the end of training?
- How can Sandra make the most of her time attending school to become a medical assistant?

LEARNING OBJECTIVES

1. Define, spell, and pronounce the terms listed in the vocabulary.
2. Briefly discuss the history of medical assisting as a profession.
3. Differentiate between administrative and clinical medical assisting duties.
4. Discuss the versatility of a career in medical assisting.
5. Explain the reasons that hiring an individual who has no formal training is often more expensive than hiring a professional medical assistant.
6. Identify several considerations to keep in mind when choosing a position as a medical assistant other than financial compensation.
7. Discuss the aspects of the medical assistant's performance on a successful externship.
8. List three unacceptable behaviors on the externship site.
9. Explain why continuing education is so important to the medical assistant.
10. Discuss the difference between a CMA and an RMA.

National Accreditation Competencies and Content

ABHES COMPETENCIES

Professionalism
1.a. Project a positive attitude
1.b. Maintain confidentiality at all times
1.c. Be a "team player"
1.d. Be cognizant of ethical boundaries
1.e. Exhibit initiative
1.f. Adapt to change
1.g. Evidence a responsible attitude
1.h. Be courteous and diplomatic
1.i. Conduct work within scope of education, training, and ability

ABHES COMPETENCIES

Communication
2.p. Professional components
2.q. Allied health professions and credentialing

Legal Concepts
5.f. Maintain licenses and accreditation

VOCABULARY

allied health fields Occupational disciplines in which professionals involved with the delivery of healthcare or related services assist physicians with the diagnosis, treatment, and care of patients in many different specialty areas.

benefits Services or payments provided under a health plan, employee plan, or some other agreement, including programs such as health insurance, pensions, retirement planning, and many other options that may be offered to employees of a company or organization.

certification (ser-tuh-fuh-ka′-shun) The attesting of something as being true, as represented, or as meeting a standard; the result of having been tested, usually by a third party, and awarded a certificate based on proven knowledge.

continuing education units (CEUs) Credits for courses, classes, or seminars related to an individual's profession, designed to promote education and to keep the professional up to date on current procedures and trends in his or her field; CEUs are often required for licensing.

cross-training Training in more than one area so that a multitude of duties may be performed by one person or so that substitutions of personnel may be made in an emergency or at other necessary times.

externship or internship A training program that is part of a course of study of an educational institution and is taken in the actual business setting of that field of study; the terms are often interchanged in reference to medical assistant training.

intangibles (in-tan′-juh-buls) Qualities that are incapable of being perceived, especially by touch, or incapable of being precisely identified or realized by the mind.

invasive Involving entry into the living body as by incision or insertion of an instrument.

perks Extra advantages or benefits from working in a specific job that may or may not be commonplace in that particular profession; a shortened form of *perquisites.*

phlebotomy (fli-bah′-tuh-me) The invasive procedure used to obtain a blood specimen for testing, experimentation, or diagnosis of disease.

profit sharing Offer of a part of a company's profits to employees or other designated individuals or groups.

stock options Offers of stocks for purchase to a certain group of individuals or certain groups, such as employees of a for-profit hospital.

versatile (vur′-suh-til) Embracing a variety of subjects, fields or skills; having a wide range of abilities.

According to the U.S. Department of Labor's *Occupational Outlook Handbook,* medical assisting is projected to be one of the fastest growing occupations in the United States over the 2004-2014 period. Much of this growth is a result of the increase in the number of group practices, clinics, and other facilities that need a high number of support personnel. This makes the flexible medical assistant who can handle both clinical and administrative duties particularly valuable to the physician.

A career as a medical assistant is challenging and offers job satisfaction, opportunities for service, financial reward, and possibilities for advancement. Men and women can be equally successful as medical assistants. Individuals considering the medical assisting discipline must be dedicated and committed and must have a strong desire to become caregivers. Caregivers are people who have the ability to put the needs of the patient first and have a sincere concern for those who are not at their best. A caregiver must feel an obligation to assist the patient in whatever way possible and have patience with those who, at times, are more difficult. This strong inner desire is one of the most important qualities of the successful professional medical assistant. Through development of this "caregiving" mentality, many personal rewards will follow, as will a long and beneficial career.

THE HISTORY OF MEDICAL ASSISTING

The first medical assistant was probably a neighbor of a physician who was called on to help when an extra pair of hands was needed.

As time passed and the practice of medicine became more organized and more complicated, some physicians hired nurses to help in their office practices. Gradually, record keeping, data reporting, and an increasing number of business details became important to physicians, and they realized a need for an assistant with both administrative and clinical training. Nurses were likely to have training only in clinical skills, so many physicians began training them or other individuals to assist with all of the office duties. Community and junior colleges began offering training programs that focused on both administrative and clinical skills in the late 1940s. Medical assistant organizations at the local and state level began developing around 1950, and soon after, certifying examinations became available. Today medical assisting is one of the most respected **allied health fields** in the industry, and training is readily available through community colleges, junior colleges, and private educational institutions throughout the United States.

THE SCOPE OF PRACTICE OF A MEDICAL ASSISTANT

Versatile is an excellent descriptive term for today's medical assistant. The duties that medical assistants perform vary not only from office to office, but even within the same clinic. Medical assistants perform routine duties within the offices of many types of health professionals, including physicians, chiropractors, podiatrists, and others. Individuals with medical assisting training can accomplish many jobs in the hospital environment, and some are employed by freestanding emergency centers or surgery centers. Opportunities for medical assistants are growing because of the constant change within the medical profession and the surge of **cross-training**, which means that one individual is trained to do a variety of duties. Medical assistants work under the direct supervision of a physician in the office and perform tasks delegated by the doctor or supervisor.

The American Association of Medical Assistants (AAMA) once defined the scope of practice as the "performance of delegated clinical and administrative duties within the supervising physician's scope of practice consistent with the medical assistant's education, training, and experience." This definition remains accurate today. The duties performed by the medical assistant do not constitute the practice of medicine.

The two major categories of duties that medical assistants perform are administrative tasks and clinical tasks (Figure 3-1). On the administrative end of the spectrum, medical assistants greet patients who arrive in the office or clinic and obtain basic registration information. They may enter information into a computer and assemble the patient's medical record. They are trained to do office accounting, which may be done electronically or manually. The medical assistant is trained in filing procedures and in proper techniques for adding information to the medical record. A basic knowledge of procedure and diagnosis coding is important to today's medical assistant, and some medical assistants concentrate strictly on the billing and coding career option. They are able to complete insurance claim forms and determine insurance coverage and limitations for the patient. Medical assistants answer telephones, schedule appointments, update medical records, and handle all types of correspondence. Often the medical assistant schedules outpatient procedures and hospital admissions and may coordinate consultations with physicians. Those who enjoy the administrative side of the profession often enter into office management positions.

The clinical duties that medical assistants perform are just as broad as the administrative duties. These professionals prepare patients and the equipment needed before examinations and assist the physician during patients' office visits. They assist with or perform basic testing procedures and are usually proficient in **phlebotomy.** Medical assistants are trained in first aid skills and cardiopulmonary resuscitation. They collect and prepare laboratory specimens and know how to adhere to U.S. Occupational and Health Administration (OSHA) and Clinical Laboratory Improvement Amendment (CLIA) regulations. Often medical assistants working in the clinical area are responsible for inventorying and ordering supplies. If directed by a physician and allowed by the state, they may administer various types of medications and perform x-ray examinations. Medical assistants also perform electrocardiograms and prepare patients for x-ray evaluations. They assist in minor surgical procedures, prepare sterile trays, and perform autoclave sterilization procedures for instruments. Other clinical duties involve taking medical histories from patients, patient teaching, and obtaining and recording vital signs. Medical assistants who enjoy the clinical side of the profession may become office managers or may supervise other medical assistants.

Duties and restrictions related to medical assisting vary from state to state, but in most of the United States the medical assistant performs as an agent of the physician and is under the physician's supervision. This means that the medical assistant performs actions that he or she is told to perform by the physician and that the physician is responsible for those actions. The command may be related to the medical assistant from the physician verbally, through a supervisor, or by way of the office policy and procedure manual. *Respondeat superior* is a Latin term meaning "let the master answer." Physicians are responsible not only for their own actions, but for the actions of employees performing within the scope of their employment.

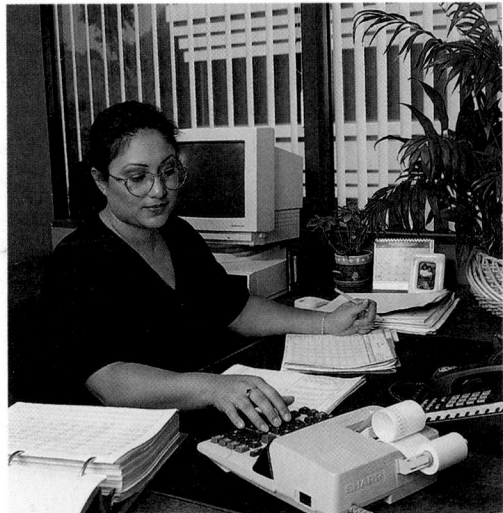
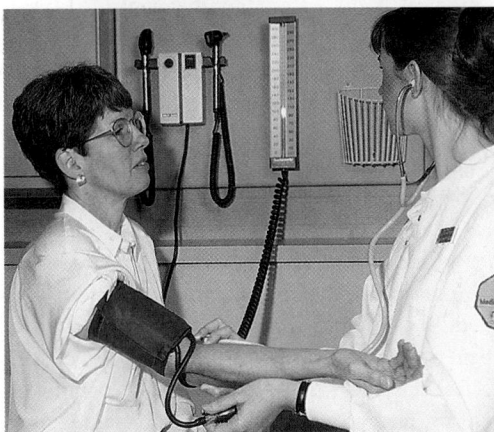

FIGURE 3-1 The responsibilities of a medical assistant include both administrative and clinical duties. (Bottom photo from Chester GA: *Modern medical assisting,* Philadelphia, 1998, Saunders.)

CRITICAL THINKING APPLICATION

- Sandra is not sure whether she will enjoy administrative or clinical assisting more. How can she begin to explore both avenues during her classroom training? During her externship or internship?
- How could Sandra explore the medical specialties and determine what areas might be of interest to her as a potential job site?

A CAREER IN MEDICAL ASSISTING

Trained medical assistants are equipped with a flexible, adaptable career in which they experience the rewards of helping other people (Figure 3-2). The skills acquired by the medical assistant are valuable, and employment is readily available anywhere in the world that medicine is practiced. Many medical assistants pursue their careers far beyond the usual retirement age, because physicians realize the value of the experienced, mature employee. This career attracts the nontraditional student who may be older than the average postsecondary student by a decade or more. Although many older students feel intimidated by the classroom, they normally have excellent experiences in school and reach the top of the class. Medical assisting is more than suitable for the student just exiting high school. Many individuals plan to work as medical assistants to earn a viable income while pursuing further academic studies.

The practice of medicine has changed dramatically in the past several decades. Increasing costs have created a trend away from hospital-based treatment and toward the delivery of care in physicians' offices and in outpatient ambulatory clinics. Although physicians have employed medical assistants in their practices for many years, computerization and technologic advances have created more opportunities for formally trained medical assistants, and their responsibilities have similarly increased. Clearly defined educational requirements have been established, and these requirements have resulted in improvement of the quality and accessibility of medical assistant training. These requirements have resulted in creating a healthy respect for medical assistants, who are considered an integral part of today's allied health field.

Employment for medical assistants is abundant. In the United States in 2004 approximately 387,000 jobs were held

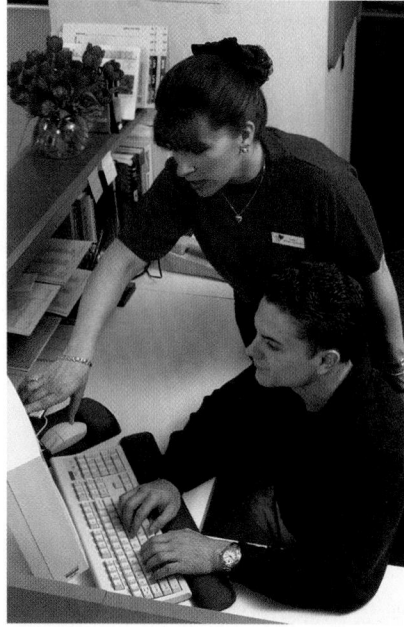

FIGURE 3-2 Medical assisting is a career with many benefits and perks, not to mention the internal rewards of assisting patients in need.

by medical assistants; approximately 60% of those were in physicians' offices, and approximately 15% were in hospitals. Career opportunities abound in public health facilities, hospitals, laboratories, medical schools, research centers, voluntary health agencies, and medical firms of all kinds. Jobs may also be available with federal agencies such as the Department of Veterans Affairs, the U.S. Public Health Service, and armed forces clinics or hospitals.

Most medical assistants derive a high degree of satisfaction from their work. Job turnover among medical assistants is surprisingly low; some begin working with a physician when the practice is opened and stay until the physician's retirement. In the past, physicians would often hire any individual to perform office and clinical duties, but these people were often untrained and unprofessional. Therefore they could be paid a minimum amount for their work. Most physicians have learned that hiring an untrained person to work in the medical office is usually more expensive in the long run. Untrained assistants often make errors that are costly to the practice, and these assistants require much more supervision. Formal training and **certification** are valuable not only to the medical assistant, but to the physician-employer.

Medical assistants are compensated in various ways, some by hourly wages and some by salary. The earnings vary from place to place. Overall, medical assistants can expect a healthy return on their investment in training, experience, and skills. Most physicians realize that a good medical assistant is worth a higher-than-average wage, and a medical assistant with formal training is almost always compensated on a higher scale than one with no training. The *Occupational Outlook Handbook,* a Department of Labor publication, reports statistics on the average salaries for many different career fields, including medical assisting. This information can be accessed at www.bls.gov/oco. More information on salaries may be obtained by monitoring the local classified advertisements and by checking online job information on sites such as Yahoo! Careers. It is important to determine a realistic entering salary. Often graduates in many fields expect to make a much higher salary than is reasonable right after graduation, with little or no experience in the medical field.

The medical field offers good **benefits** to employees. Usually, the larger the organization, the better the benefits and **perks.** Most employers offer a health insurance plan or managed care plan to their employees. Often a life insurance program is included, and dental insurance is always a valuable benefit. Some companies have **profit sharing** plans and **stock options.** Some organizations give their employees access to credit unions, and many have discount options to local businesses, such as uniform shops. Remember that benefits and perks should be considered when contemplating a job opportunity. Many medical assistants may choose to work for less money if the benefits and the opportunities for advancement are good. Consider driving time, holidays, paid parking, sick days, vacation days, and facilities when choosing a job. Do the co-workers seem to enjoy one another's company and get along? Is the physician friendly or more "aloof and cold"? All of these should be weighed carefully before making the final decision as to which position to accept. It is a truism that "money is a byproduct of services rendered." Nowhere is this more accurate than in the medical field. When the patients are served well, the medical assistant becomes more and more valuable to the employer and is compensated accordingly.

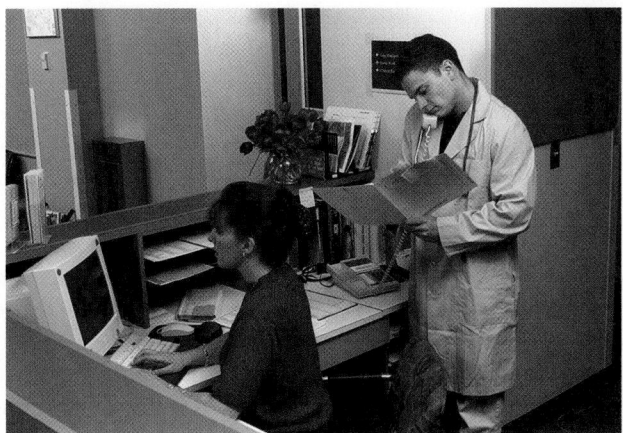

FIGURE 3-3 Medical assistants must have a professional appearance and demeanor in the medical office environment.

CRITICAL THINKING APPLICATION

■ Sandra knows that she needs certain benefits as a single mother. What might she need to look for in a potential job after her graduation?

■ What are some ways that Sandra can compare positions and opportunities?

■ What types of websites might help Sandra in learning about opportunities in her geographic location?

PROFESSIONAL APPEARANCE

A well-groomed medical assistant in appropriate attire has a positive psychologic effect on patients. The essentials of a professional appearance are good health, good grooming, and suitable dress.

Good health requires getting adequate sleep, eating balanced meals, and exercising enough to keep fit. Medical assistants can set a good example by following a sensible and healthy lifestyle that includes regular checkups of their own physical condition, both medical and dental. A radiantly healthy office staff promotes the best possible public relations image for the physician.

Good grooming is little more than attention to the details of personal appearance. Personal cleanliness, which includes taking a daily bath or shower, using deodorant, and practicing good oral hygiene, is vital. The use of perfume or aftershave cologne should be avoided or limited, because patients and co-workers may be allergic to some scents. A female medical assistant's makeup should be conservative and moderately applied. Heavy or exaggerated makeup is out of place in the professional office; subtle eye and lip makeup is best for the physician's office. Clear or muted shades of nail polish are best, and long nails are not only inappropriate but can be dangerous to the patient and the medical assistant. Nails must be kept clean and at a very conservative length. Both male and female assistants should be sure that their hair is shiny clean, neatly styled, and off the collar.

The medical assistant usually wears a uniform or lab coat, which not only presents a professional appearance but also identifies the assistant as a member of the healthcare team (Figure 3-3). Fashionable styling makes it possible for the medical assistant's uniform to be both practical and attractive. Women may choose to wear pantsuits, which are available in white or a variety of colors; a two-piece dress uniform in white or a color; an attractively styled traditional white uniform; or a scrub set. Scrubs have become increasingly popular and much more attractive over the past decade. They are now often made of pretty fabrics in rich colors and patterns and are much better suited for the professional office than the old green or blue scrubs worn in the surgical suites of hospitals. Men may also wear the newer scrubs or may choose white slacks with a white or colored shirt, jacket, or pullover top. If it is acceptable in the facility, a lab coat may be worn over street clothes, but it is important that the lab coat be buttoned when **invasive** procedures are performed. Uniforms should be laundered daily, because medical assistants are exposed to ill patients throughout their workday. Shoes should be appropriate for a uniform, spotless, and comfortable. Many attractive styles that resemble running or tennis shoes are available at uniform shops, specially conditioned for the medical professional who is on his or her feet the majority of the day. White shoes must be kept white by daily cleansing and touchups. Remember that if laced shoes are worn, the laces also need cleaning.

In some facilities the physician prefers that the staff not wear uniforms. Some psychiatrists and some pediatricians, for example, believe that the clinical appearance of a uniform may affect patients adversely. However, today's uniforms reflect so many styles and patterns that the right one for the particular office should be readily available. Some of the fabrics depict cartoon characters or drawings that will appeal to children yet still function as a durable uniform. A medical assistant who does not wear a uniform should follow the dictates of good taste and should be conservative in choosing a professional wardrobe. Jeans are rarely acceptable in the medical facility, unless the office is extremely casual or it is a special day.

The garments worn while on duty must be comfortable, allow easy movement, and still look fresh at the end of a busy day. Whatever uniform style the assistant chooses, it should be personally becoming and worn over appropriate undergarments. The lines, colors, and ornamentation of the undergarments should not be seen through the uniform; therefore it is best to wear a neutral color without a pattern. Thongs and high-cut underwear should be avoided. When a uniform is worn, jewelry should be limited to an engagement ring, wedding band, and professional pin. No more than two earrings per ear lobe should be worn, and the clothing or hairstyle should always cover tattoos. Facial and tongue piercings are unacceptable in the medical arena and must be removed during working hours. A name badge will help patients identify each staff person by name.

Be sure that the dress code that is required in the office setting is clearly understood. Adherence to that code is a demonstration of responsibility and the willingness to cooperate with office rules. Compliance with office regulations will be a factor in office promotion decisions.

EDUCATION AND TRAINING

Ideally, a medical assistant should have both administrative and clinical skills, although he or she may have a personal preference for one over the other. The physician's staff must be able to handle all responsibilities of the office except those requiring the services of the physician or another licensed professional. In an office with several assistants, each should be able and willing to substitute in an emergency for any of the others and should be cross-trained on the basics of the others' duties. Teamwork is a very important part of any occupation, and even more so in the medical environment.

Certain knowledge and skills are expected of a trained medical assistant. The skills mentioned within this chapter are not all-inclusive but suggest what may be expected on entry into employment as a professional medical assistant.

Classroom Training

Formal training is essential for today's medical assistant. Many community colleges, junior colleges, and private career institutions offer courses in medical assisting. After satisfactory completion of the program, the student usually receives a certificate or diploma. Private career institutions offer training that usually takes 7 to 10 months to complete and offer enrollment as often as monthly. Students who attend community colleges, junior colleges, and some private career institutions to study medical assisting may complete the educational requirements to obtain an associate degree in medical assisting. Courses at the community college level usually take 1 to 2 years to complete and offer enrollment from every few weeks to two or three times per year.

Currently the trend is toward offering the medical assisting program in modules, so that the student receives some clinical training, some administrative training, and some theory in each module taken. Some classes are taught in traditional classrooms, and the clinical aspect is usually taught in a laboratory at the school. Much of the equipment that the medical assistant will use in practice is found in the laboratory, such as an autoclave, medical instruments and trays, and specimen-collection equipment. Medical assisting training usually involves the study of medical terminology, anatomy and physiology, aseptic technique, clinical procedures, medical law and ethics, principals of pharmacology, insurance billing and coding, receptionist and telephone technique, patient communication, human relations, management duties, and receptionist duties, among other subjects.

Instructors are important allies as the medical assisting student pursues his or her education, and the relationship between instructor and student should be one of mutual respect (Figure 3-4). Students must realize that instructors have a strong desire to share their knowledge and that they want each student

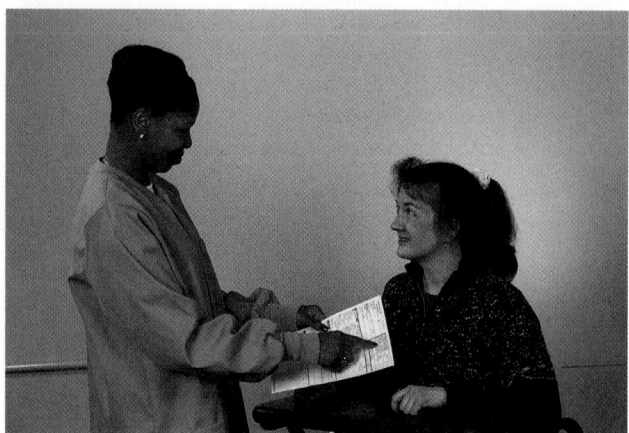

FIGURE 3-4 Get to know instructors and ask their advice on study habits and test preparation. Instructors are valuable references when the medical assistant begins the job search.

to succeed. Individual schools have certain rules and regulations that must be enforced, many of them a result of state or federal regulation or legislation. The guidelines that students must follow are not designed to hinder the education, but rather to make certain that the school graduates competent medical assistants. Complete assignments accurately, turn them in on time, and take pride in all of the work done for class. School days should be missed only when absolutely necessary. Develop good habits in school, and they will become valuable assets to future employers.

CRITICAL THINKING APPLICATION

- How can Sandra develop a positive, nurturing relationship with her instructors?
- What should she do if she has difficulty in the classroom or if her grades begin to fall?
- How can Sandra study effectively and prepare for examinations?

Externships and Internships

Most medical assisting training programs require an **externship** or **internship** before the student graduates. For the purposes of this text, the terms are interchangeable and have the same meaning. This on-the-job training allows students to put the skills they have learned in the classroom setting to use with real patients and staff members. In the majority of cases, externships and internships are unpaid positions that are a part of the medical assistant training program, not a separate entity. Most accreditation organizations do not allow student externs or interns to be paid.

The physician, probably more than any other employer, expects employees to carry out their duties independently, with little or no direct supervision. Someone at the externship site will be designated as the student's supervisor. The medical assisting student should consult frequently with the externship supervisor to determine what is expected of the student and what progress is being made (Figure 3-5).

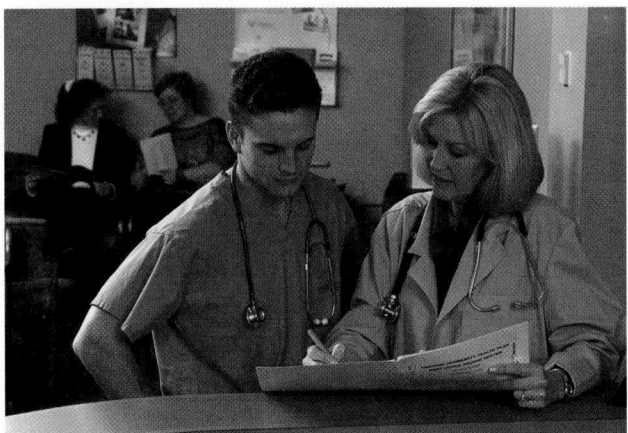

FIGURE 3-5 The externship or internship provides practical experience in the skills learned in the classroom. It is usually listed first on the resume once the medical assistant graduate prepares a resume, so it is vital to perform well and make a good impression.

The student must be open to constructive criticism and a willing learner. Techniques may be learned on the externship that were not included in the classroom training, or optional methods may be taught for various procedures. The medical assistant should never argue with the staff at the clinical site that a method taught by the school is the only correct way. Often several methods are available to obtain the same result. The medical assisting student should treat the externship experience as if it were a probationary period on an actual job. Remember, the externship is often the first medical reference that the student will be able to list on the resume.

Several general rules must be remembered on the externship site. First, the medical assistant will have to gain the trust of the employees there. This is done by eagerly performing the duties assigned in a timely manner and performing those duties to the best of the student's ability. If any questions arise at any time, the student should ask the externship supervisor instead of assuming or performing the duties the wrong way.

It is often helpful to read the job description of the medical assistant in the facility so that the student will understand what is expected of him or her. The student medical assistant must show responsibility and dependability. There should never be a time that the student is not busy while at the externship site. If all assigned duties are completed, the extern should offer to assist others in their duties or ask for additional responsibilities. Counters always need cleaning, and filing always needs to be done. The student who does these duties without being told shows initiative and a strong work ethic. In addition, all of the rules for professional appearance apply to the site and should be meticulously followed, because the medical assisting student will be working with actual patients.

The medical assistant may find it necessary to educate the patient about the definition of what a medical assistant is and does. Often, patients assume that those assisting in the offices are nurses, but medical assistants should never represent themselves in this manner. When making introductions or assisting with patients, one should state, "I am Sandra Rameriz, Dr. Patrick's medical assistant extern," or "I am Sandra, a medical assistant

intern here in Dr. Patrick's office." These words accurately portray the duties performed and help the patient to know who is caring for him or her in the physician's office.

Externs need to know a few other rules. A medical assisting student must never attempt to form a romantic relationship with patients or co-workers on the externship site. Patient confidentiality must be respected at all times, and anything that the student discovers about a patient must not be revealed or discussed under any circumstances. The student must not use any of the drug samples at the office unless specifically given permission by the physician. The student should never go to the drug storage area alone without permission or unless directed by the supervisor or physician. Externs should be extremely careful if asked to handle petty cash in the office. No student wants to be accused of any impropriety while performing their externship hours. Students must never ask the physician to treat them or any members of their family or friends. If the physician offers this as a benefit, it is acceptable, but one must not assume the physician is available for and willing to give free treatment. An extern must not ask the physician to provide prescriptions; for liability reasons, most physicians will not prescribe medications for people who are not their patients.

The externing student should bring **intangibles** to the physician's office not found in any job description. Courtesy toward others and a capacity for teamwork, a positive attitude, enthusiasm, initiative, and dedication are important personal attributes for the professional medical assistant. After becoming comfortably acquainted with what is expected on the externship, the student should concentrate on developing his or her skills and learning as much as possible during this short period. An extern becomes a valuable team player by assisting others and being reliable. By performing at peak level, the student gains the respect and trust of those on the externship site, and these people can become an excellent reference to use in beginning the search for that first paid position. Remember, the professional services of a medical assistant are extremely personal. Therefore the manner in which these services are performed can affect the health and welfare of a patient in either a positive or a negative way. When medical assisting students do their best to be sure that all contact with patients is positive in nature, they win the praise of patients, supervisors, and co-workers alike.

Benefits of Externship

- The school has a line of communication to the community and is better able to assess the needs and expectations of the public for which it is training prospective employees.
- The externship agency benefits from the new ideas and methods that the trainee may introduce. If the facility is looking for additional help, this is an ideal way to evaluate the performance of a trainee without involvement in the hiring process.
- The trainee benefits most of all by exposure to practical experience in a variety of settings. This experience in the real world removes a great deal of the anxiety that might otherwise be present in a first employment situation.

CRITICAL THINKING APPLICATION

- If Sandra has any difficulty on her externship, whom should she contact?
- What should Sandra do when she has completed her normal duties for the day at the externship and it is not yet time to leave the clinic?
- How can Sandra glean more knowledge from her co-workers on the externship?

CRITICAL THINKING APPLICATION

- When should Sandra get involved with professional organizations for medical assistants?
- How can she contribute to professional organizations in her area once she has graduated and secured a position as a medical assistant?
- Is it important that Sandra participate in volunteer organizations?

Continuing Education

Education does not end with the completion of formal training. The amount of medical knowledge gained in a given year is astounding. The practicing medical assistant must keep current with the rapid changes within the profession. Most physicians appreciate the medical assistant who asks questions about unfamiliar conditions and procedures and are willing to teach students about the function of the body and treatments that benefit the patient. Much can be learned by reading or reviewing the medical literature that arrives in the daily mail or articles that appear in newspapers, magazines, and medically related newsletters.

Continuing education classes are available to enhance the knowledge of the professional medical assistant. **Continuing education units (CEUs)** may be required to maintain the medical assistant's certification. These credits can be obtained through many sources, including the AAMA, the American Medical Technologists (AMT), and various other agencies and educational institutions. Professional seminars and workshops often offer CEUs. Notices of continuing education classes are sent in bulk to medical facilities and physicians' offices, so the staff should watch for courses that pertain to their particular job duties and take advantage of them as available.

PROFESSIONAL ORGANIZATIONS

By joining a professional organization and taking part in the activities it offers, a medical assistant can grow personally and professionally, keeping abreast of current trends. Participation in a recognized professional organization shows that the employee takes the career seriously and wants to be an asset to the employer. National organizations, state chapters of these organizations, and local groups meet to promote the profession of medical assisting. The organizations offer many benefits to members. Some offer health, disability, and malpractice insurance programs. Some offer credit card options and discount programs that are exclusive to their membership. All extend an opportunity for continuing education and learning beyond the classroom. Some schools that offer medical assistant training form local or school-based chapters of professional organizations. Both the AAMA and AMT offer discounted student memberships.

American Association of Medical Assistants and Certified Medical Assistants

AAMA was formally organized in 1955 as a federation of several state associations that had been functioning independently. Today the AAMA has 51 state societies (including Washington, DC) and more than 375 local chapters. The organization, whose national headquarters are located in Chicago, Illinois, was the driving force behind establishing a national certification program for medical assistants. AAMA has also been instrumental in the accreditation of medical assisting training programs in community colleges and private career institutes and in setting the minimum standards for entry-level medical assistants. At meetings held on national, state, and local levels, medical assistants can participate in workshops, learn about all types of advancement in the field, hear prominent speakers, and network with other medical assistants from other parts of the country. AAMA publishes a bimonthly journal called *CMA Today*, which includes articles with tests that may be submitted for CEU credit.

Since 1963 the AAMA has administered the certified medical assistant (CMA) examination. Those who pass the examination are awarded the CMA credential (Figure 3-6). Examinations are given in January, June, and October of each year at more than 200 centers throughout the United States. Certification is available to graduates of medical assisting programs accredited by the Commission on Accreditation of Allied Health Education Programs (CAAHEP) or by the Accrediting Bureau of Health Education Schools (ABHES). Recertification is required every 5 years and can be accomplished through CEUs or reexamination. More information is available at www.aama-ntl.org. CAAHEP competencies for medical assistants are located at the back of

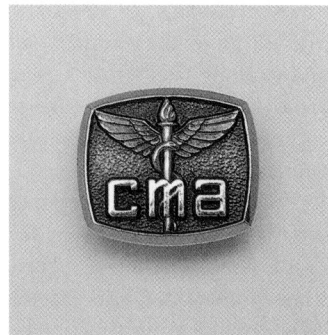

FIGURE 3-6 This pin is worn by the certified medical assistant. (Courtesy American Association of Medical Assistants, Chicago, Ill.)

this text. These competencies detail the administrative, clinical, and transdisciplinary skills required of the competent medical assistant graduate.

American Medical Technologists and Registered Medical Assistants

In the early 1970s the AMT, a national certifying body for laboratory professionals, began offering a certifying examination for medical assistants. This led to the formation of the registered medical assistant (RMA) program within the AMT organization in 1976. AMT offers this national certification to medical assistants who meet established standards and pass the examination (Figure 3-7). Several other certification examinations are offered by AMT that may be of interest to medical assistants. The certified medical laboratory assistant (CMLA) examination is available to those who have completed certain educational and work experience requirements. Most medical assistants who work in the clinical area and have at least 6 months' experience will qualify to take the examination. Medical assistants may also qualify to take the phlebotomy technician certification examination (RPT) offered by AMT after meeting specific work-related requirements. The Certified Medical Administrative Specialist (CMAS) examination is offered to those who have graduated from an accredited administrative program or who have 5 years' experience in the field. RMAs with 2 years' administrative exprience may also take the examination.

AMT also provides societal benefits, including publications such as *AMT Events*, a quarterly magazine with useful information and articles relating to the professions served by the organization. AMT also offers national, state, and local meetings to enhance the knowledge and networking opportunities of its members. CEU credits are available to assist in increasing a medical assistant's level of competence and are a requirement for those who first became certified (or will recertify) after January 1, 2006.

The national headquarters for AMT are located in Park Ridge, Illinois. More information about the RMA examination is available on the website www.amt1.com. The ABHES competencies for medical assistants are located at the back of this text. These competencies detail the administrative, clinical, and general skills required of the medical assistant graduate.

National Healthcareer Association

Some schools also offer certification through the National Healthcareer Association. These include the Certified Medical Administrative Assistant (CMAA), the Certified Clinical Medical Assistant (CCMA), as well as the Certified Billing and Coding Specialist (CBCS) and Certified Medical Transcriptionist (CMT). The costs for these certification examinations range from approximately $100 to $150. The National Healthcareer Association's website can be found at www.nhanow.com.

Taking Certification Examinations

Both the CMA and RMA certifications are national credentials. The CMA credential is offered by the AAMA, and the RMA credential is offered by the AMT. Because medical assistants are not required to be licensed, both of these examinations are voluntary. A medical assistant may practice in the United States without either certification, but most employers today require at least one certification. Both organizations have committees that develop the examinations, and they are both based on the roles that medical assistants fulfill in the workplace.

Students should take the examination soon after graduation; the intricate knowledge gained in school will be easier to recall the sooner it is taken. In addition, the fee for the CMA examination will increase 1 year after the graduation date. Although the graduate is not guaranteed more wages with certification or registration, most employers are willing to pay more for a graduate who has been through formal training and the certification or registration procedure.

The CMA examination covers three general categories, including administrative, clinical, and transdisciplinary competencies. The examination is scored by tallying correct responses, so making a guess will not count against the student. The minimum score to obtain the CMA credential is currently 425, and students are allowed 4 hours to complete the examination. AAMA offers two practice tests on its website that cover both anatomy and physiology and medical terminology review. AAMA requires either continuing education credits or reexamination to continue using the CMA credential.

The RMA examination can be scheduled nearly every day of the year other than Sundays and holidays at over 200 testing centers throughout the United States, its territories, and Canada. Applicants for the RMA examination must be graduates of a medical assisting course accredited by ABHES or by CAAHEP, or they must meet requirements related to their experience. The RMA examination covers administrative skills, clinical skills, and general skills and contains over 200 questions. Examinees are allowed 3 hours to take the paper-based test, and $2\frac{1}{2}$ hours to take the computer-based test. The scoring is based on a scale with a minimum passing score of 70. Practice examinations are available on the AMT website.

The AMT has recently mandated a point system to prove compliance with continuing education requirements. RMAs, CMASs, and CMLAs are required to earn 30 points, and RPTs are required to earn 20 points. Points can be earned through continuing education, employer evaluations, professional and formal education, and various other methods.

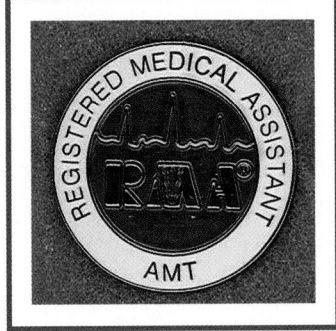

FIGURE 3-7 This pin is worn by the registered medical assistant. (Courtesy RMA/American Medical Technologists, Rosemount, Ill.)

Medical Assistant's Creed

I believe in the principles and purposes of the profession of medical assisting.

I endeavor to be more effective.

I aspire to render greater service.

I protect the confidence entrusted to me.

I am dedicated to the care and well-being of all patients.

I am loyal to my physician-employer.

I am true to the ethics of my profession.

I am strengthened by compassion, courage, and faith.

CRITICAL THINKING APPLICATION

- Why is it important for Sandra to obtain one of the medical assisting certifications after graduation?
- How might certification help her career as a medical assistant?
- When and where can the tests be taken in your area?

The Difference Between CMAs and RMAs

Two major differences between these two credentials are the examination consultant organizations and the cost. The CMA examination fee for the 2006 testing year is $95 for recent CAAHEP or ABHES graduates. The annual membership fees vary from state to state and are substantially lower if one joins while still a student. Student membership costs range from $20 to approximately $35 but must be applied for before graduating. Nonmembers must pay $170 to take the CMA examination. Annual dues thereafter are between $67 and $97, depending on the state association joined. The RMA examination cost is $90, which includes the first year's dues. Annual dues thereafter are currently $48. See Table 3-1 for a detailed comparison of the CMA and RMA.

CLOSING COMMENTS

This chapter has presented the advantages of becoming a trained medical assistant and some of the many career opportunities available. The necessary skills that must be developed and the general knowledge that must be acquired to function effectively have been presented. However, skills and knowledge alone do not ensure success. Personality traits and professional appearance are also critical. Professional societies and continuing education are vital to the professional medical assistant. The individual who accepts this career must be willing to accept the responsibilities inherent in its standards. The importance of gaining a national certification cannot be stressed enough. Whatever the career goals of the medical assistant, the ideas expressed in this chapter will be useful to all.

Medical assisting has grown into one of the most respected professions in the allied health field. When asked about the field, one should share the role a medical assistant plays in the office and the training involved. Others may be interested in a career change or have a desire to enter the medical field. A medical assistant should always be an exceptional ambassador for the profession.

TABLE 3-1 Differences between the Certified Medical Assistant and the Registered Medical Assistant

	CERTIFIED MEDICAL ASSISTANT (CMA)	REGISTERED MEDICAL ASSISTANT (RMA)
Credential awarded by	American Association of Medical Assistants (AAMA)	American Medical Technologists (AMT)
Address of certification or registration organization	American Association of Medical Assistants 20 N. Wacker Drive, Suite 1575 Chicago, IL 60606-2903 800-228-2262	American Medical Technologists 10700 West Higgins Road, Ste 150 Rosemont, IL 60018 800-275-1268
Organization website	www.aama-ntl.org	www.amt1.com/store/start.asp
Mailing address for certification applications	AAMA Certification 7999 Eagle Way Chicago, IL 60678-1079	RMA Certification/AMT 10700 West Higgins Road, Ste 150 Rosemont, IL 60018
Requirement for certification or registration	Federal licensing is not required; certification or registration is optional in most states.	Federal licensing is not required; certification or registration is optional in most states.
Qualifications to take examination	Applicants must fall into one of three categories to qualify to take the CMA examination: • Category One: Graduating student or recent graduate of a CAAHEP-accredited medical assisting program • Category Two: Nonrecent graduate of a CAAHEP-accredited medical assisting program • Category Three: Graduating student or graduate of an ABHES-accredited medical assisting program	Good moral character and at least 18 years old High school graduate or acceptable equivalent Must be a graduate of, or scheduled to graduate from: • a medical assistant program accredited by either ABHES or CAAHEP • a medical assistant program in a postsecondary school that is accredited by a regional or national organization, is recognized by the U.S. Department of Education, and includes a minimum of 720 clock hours including externship • a formal medical services training of the U.S. Armed Forces Must have 5 years of work experience unless graduated from the medical assisting program within the last 3 years
Examination approval organization	National Board of Medical Examiners (NBME) www.nbme.org	National Commission for Certifying Agencies www.noca.org/ncca/ncca.htm
Cost of examination	AAMA members pay $95 (can be a student member, which costs $25-$35, depending on the state)	$90 (membership in AMT is required as part of certification maintenance)
Length of time required to take examination	4 hours	3 hours
Content of examination	Three sections of 100 questions each, covering general or transdisciplinary skills, clinical skills, and administrative skills	More than 200 questions, covering general subject areas, clinical areas, and administrative areas
Testing sites	Over 200 centers throughout the United States, assigned when approved to take examination	Over 200 centers throughout the United States; list of sites available at www.pearsonvue.com/amt
Where to obtain practice test	www.aama-ntl.org/becomeCMA/exam_outline.aspx	www.amt1.com/site/epage/15340_315.htm
Testing dates	The application date for the January examination is October 1 of the previous year. The application date for the June examination is March 1 of the same year. The application date for the October examination is July 1 of the same year.	Testing dates are ongoing and are arranged at PearsonVue Centers throughout the United States.

SUMMARY OF SCENARIO

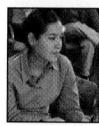

Sandra has chosen to embark on an exciting career and will find her work very rewarding. She knows that she will be proud of her efforts and looks forward to becoming a respected member of the healthcare team in a physician's office. She has set goals for her class work and attendance and is determined to meet them. Obstacles usually arise whenever one embarks on a new project, and Sandra must plan for the days that she or her child may be ill or her transportation fails. Having a backup plan in advance will help her to overcome these minor setbacks.

Many opportunities exist for the medical assistant in both administrative and clinical positions, and as Sandra progresses through her training she will find areas that appeal to her more than others. All are vitally important so that she will be a versatile medical assistant, able to perform front- and back-office duties. Exposure to various duties will be provided during the externship, and these experiences will help her to determine where she might enjoy working once she graduates. It is important that Sandra glean as much experience and knowledge as possible while in school so that she will have more options after her training.

Sandra should develop a good relationship with her instructors and go to them when she has questions or concerns. These professionals are anxious to share their knowledge and experiences with students to best prepare them for the work environment. If Sandra's grades ever drop or she is struggling, Sandra should seek the advice of the instructor to determine how to improve her performance. The externship is also critically important, because it is usually the first medical reference a new graduate will have. Any difficulties at the externship site should be brought to the attention of the externship supervisor or an instructor at her school. Learning to set goals will help her to achieve more throughout her education, and this is a habit she should carry into her career.

With so many benefits available at different facilities in the medical field, Sandra will need to carefully weigh what she needs for herself and her son before taking any position. She should look at all of her options and choose the best one after careful evaluation. Her time in school should be spent getting to know her instructors and understanding their expectations, studying hard, learning to budget time and money, and discovering as much as possible about her new career. This will result in her satisfaction with her job and new career.

SUMMARY of LEARNING OBJECTIVES

1. Define, spell, and pronounce the terms listed in the vocabulary.
   - Spelling and pronouncing medical terms correctly adds credibility to the medical assistant. Knowing the definition of these terms promotes confidence in communication with patients and co-workers.
2. Briefly discuss the history of medical assisting as a profession.
   - The first medical assistants were probably neighbors and friends of the physician. The field has grown into one of the most respected and versatile professions in allied health.
3. Differentiate between administrative and clinical medical assisting duties.
   - Administrative duties are those that involve running the office, such as scheduling appointments and filing insurance. Administrative medical assistants usually spend most of the day in the front office of the facility. Clinical duties include more patient contact and assisting the physician in the back office. Often, new graduates move toward one or the other divisions, but they should always be ready and willing to adapt to new duties or fill in at other areas when necessary.
4. Discuss the versatility of a career in medical assisting.
   - Medical assistants are versatile enough to work in many different settings. Most often they are found in physician offices, but they also work in hospitals, insurance companies, clinics, laboratories, and many other facilities. The combination of administrative and clinical training makes the medical assistant quite valuable to the employer.

5. Explain the reasons that hiring an individual who has no formal training is often more expensive than hiring a professional medical assistant.
   - Medical assistants who have been formally trained certainly deserve a fair wage, comparable to the national average for a person in whatever position they hold. When supervisors or employers attempt to find "bargain help" at a cheaper rate, often they do not hire the high-quality employee who is so necessary in the physician's office. Because medical assistants help care for the patient, they should be compensated well so that the retention of the office staff will be continuous and stable. This can only help the physician care for patients in a more effective manner and gives the patients a sense of familiarity and security as well.
6. Identify several considerations to keep in mind when choosing a position as a medical assistant other than financial compensation.
   - The medical assistant should consider many factors other than the salary when choosing a position. Location, perks, benefits, and the atmosphere of the office are all important. Many assistants are interested in growth within the organization and welcome those opportunities. Working for a friendly, caring physician and/or supervisor is invaluable. Sometimes, taking a lesser position in a well-known and reputable facility is temporarily worth a lower wage because of future opportunities. Consider all aspects of a position before accepting a job offer.

Continued

SUMMARY of LEARNING OBJECTIVES

Continued

7. Discuss the aspects of the medical assistant's performance on a successful externship.
   - The medical assisting externship offers the student an opportunity to put the skills learned in the classroom to good use. If completed successfully, this is an excellent reference for the resume. The student should perform at the optimal level and never hesitate to complete duties assigned. Offer to go above and beyond to secure the support of the externship site as the job search begins.

8. List three unacceptable behaviors on the externship site.
   - An externing medical assistant should never attempt to form relationships with patients outside the office or view the chart for personal information. Do not ask the physician to treat family members, and do not take medications without explicit permission from the physician or supervisor. Be very careful when handling cash and drugs in the office. The student should make every effort to never be late to the externship site unless a severe emergency occurs.

9. Explain why continuing education is so important to the medical assistant.
   - Continuing education is important to medical assistants so that the latest trends and information are readily available and accessible. Take advantage of local seminars and continuing education classes. Often the employer will agree to pay for classes or seminars that the medical assistant takes if they relate to his or her employment at the facility. Some will provide tuition reimbursement for college expenses, often even if the college courses are not related to the position the employee holds at the facility.

10. Discuss the difference between a CMA and an RMA.
    - The main difference between the CMA and RMA credentials is the agency that provides each certification. The CMA credential is awarded by the AAMA, and the RMA is awarded by the AMT. Both are nationally recognized certifications.

CONNECTIONS

 Study Guide Connection: Go to Chapter 3 Study Guide. Read the Case Study and Workplace Applications and complete the assignments. Do online research for answers to the questions in the Internet Activities associated with the medical assisting profession.

 CD Connection: Go to the Medical Assisting Competency Challenge CD and review the content of the training activities. These will be referred to throughout the textbook to enhance your learning experience.

 Evolve Connection: For more information related to the medical assisting profession, go to evolve.elsevier.com/kinn and visit related weblinks for Chapter 3. Click on the Medical Assisting Exam Review and do the practice questions to sharpen your test-taking skills.

Professional Behavior in the Workplace

4

SCENARIO

Karen Yon has wanted to work in the medical field for most of her adult life. She studied very hard in high school and graduated with honors. She volunteered in a local hospital, then after working for 3 years in restaurants as a server, she enrolled in medical assistant classes. After her externship, she was asked to continue as a regular employee at a family practice in her area.

Karen strives to do all of her duties professionally and compassionately in the physician's office. She maintains a professional image to patients and co-workers. However, it was difficult to learn how to be professional at all times and show compassion to patients through only the classroom experience. These are important aspects of her job, and she was able to gain valuable experience in these areas on her externship. Because this is her first job in the medical field, she wants to make a good impression on her employer and be a team player.

Throughout most of Karen's training as a medical assistant, her grandmother was confined to a rehabilitation center after a stroke. Although she has progressed well with treatment, Karen is the only relative who lives close to the rehabilitation center, and her family depends on her to check on her grandmother from time to time. Karen enjoys spending time at the center reading to her grandmother, because they are close. Still, Karen realizes that the stroke has caused permanent damage, and her grandmother's health seems to be on the decline.

While studying this chapter, think about the following questions:

- How do professional medical assistants put aside personal issues and devote themselves to the patients in the office?
- How can Karen meet her familial and work obligations equally well?

- What steps should Karen take to ensure that both her family and her supervisors understand her obligations to the other?
- How can Karen exhibit professional behavior and compassion for patients on a daily basis at the physician's office?

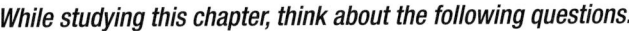

LEARNING OBJECTIVES

1. Define, spell, and pronounce the terms listed in the vocabulary.
2. Explain the meaning of the word professionalism.
3. Discuss several of the characteristics of professionalism.
4. Explain why confidentiality is so important in the medical profession.
5. Discuss the role of the medical assistant's attitude in caring for patients.
6. List some examples of office politics.
7. Identify specific ways that teamwork can be promoted in the physician's office.
8. Discuss the meaning of insubordination and why it is grounds for dismissal.
9. Identify several categories of prioritizing tasks and their meaning.
10. Talk about goal setting and how this helps in achieving career success.

National Accreditation Competencies and Content

ABHES COMPETENCIES

Professionalism

1.a. Project a positive attitude
1.b. Maintain confidentiality at all times
1.c. Be a "team player"
1.d. Be cognizant of ethical boundaries
1.e. Exhibit initiative
1.f. Adapt to change
1.g. Evidence a responsible attitude
1.h. Be courteous and diplomatic
1.i. Conduct work within scope of education, training, and ability

Communication

2.p. Professional components

Legal Concepts

5.e. Maintain liability coverage

VOCABULARY

characteristics Distinguishing traits, qualities, or properties.

commensurate (ku-men'su-rut) Corresponding in size, amount, extent, or degree; equal in measure.

competent Having adequate or requisite capabilities.

connotation (kah-nuh-ta'-shun) An implication; something suggested by a word or thing.

credibility The quality or power of inspiring belief.

demeanor (di-me'-nur) Behavior toward others; outward manner.

detrimental (de-truh-men'-til) Obviously harmful or damaging.

discretion (dis-kre'-shun) The quality of being discrete; having or showing good judgment or conduct, especially in speech.

disseminated (di-se'-muh-na-ted) To disburse; to spread around.

initiative To cause or facilitate the beginning of; to initiate something into happening.

insubordination (in-suh'-bor-din-a-shun) Disobedience to authority.

morale (mo-ral') The mental and emotional condition, enthusiasm, loyalty, or confidence of an individual or group with regard to the function or tasks at hand.

optimistic Inclined to put the most favorable construction on actions and events or to anticipate the best possible outcome.

persona (pur-so'-nuh) An individual's social facade or front that reflects the role in life the individual is playing; the personality that a person projects in public.

procrastination (pruh-kras-tuh-na'-shun) Intentionally putting off doing something that should be done.

professionalism The conduct or qualities characterized by or conforming to the technical or ethical standards of a profession; exhibiting a courteous, conscientious, and generally businesslike manner in the workplace.

reproach An expression of rebuke or disapproval; a cause or occasion of blame, discredit, or disgrace.

What is professional behavior? We tend to hold medical personnel to a higher standard of **professionalism** than those in most other career fields. The medical assistant who works to improve his or her professional approach in the workplace will be an asset to the employer and will be promoted to positions of more responsibility quickly within the healthcare industry.

THE MEANING OF PROFESSIONALISM

Professionalism is defined as exhibiting a courteous, conscientious, and generally businesslike manner in the workplace. It is characterized by or conforms to the technical or ethical

standards of a certain profession. Conducting oneself in a professional manner is essential for successful medical assistants. The attitude of those in the medical profession is generally more conservative than in other career fields. Patients expect professional behavior and will base much of their trust and confidence in those who exhibit this type of **demeanor** in the physician's office (Figure 4-1).

CHARACTERISTICS OF PROFESSIONALISM

Many **characteristics** make up the professional posture required of medical assistants. Student medical assistants should begin developing these characteristics while in school; these qualities

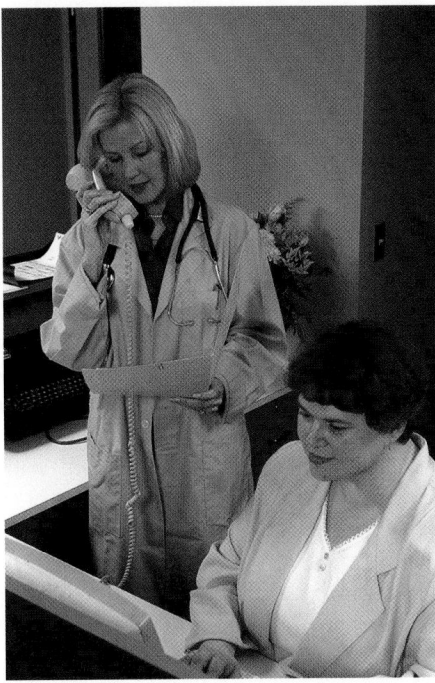

FIGURE 4-1 The professional medical assistant is an asset to the physician's office.

will not magically appear when the student begins working with actual patients. Although we might think that we would always behave appropriately during an externship or in a job setting, the habits developed in school will carry over into these experiences. If the behavior is unacceptable, it will be **detrimental** to the medical assistant's professional career. If the medical assistant wishes to advance and receive wage increases, promotions, and the trust of the employer, the following characteristics must be a part of his or her **persona.**

CRITICAL THINKING APPLICATION

- How can students practice professional behavior while still in the classroom situation?
- When students are practicing clinical skills, how can they demonstrate proficiency in professional behavior?

Loyalty

Loyalty is a faithfulness or allegiance to a cause, ideal, custom, institution, or product. Loyalty to an employer means that the employee is appreciative of the opportunity provided through the job and supports the company by giving the best effort possible. Many individuals today are interested only in what the employer can provide them. However, this is an immature approach to take toward a job. When a person is employed by a company, use of skills is exchanged for different types of compensation. Each benefits the other. Often we forget that experience alone is a great benefit from working. Loyalty to the employer is important, and the employee should feel a sense of loyalty from the company as well.

CRITICAL THINKING APPLICATION

- How can Karen demonstrate loyalty to her employer?
- What are some ways that her employer can reciprocate Karen's loyalty?

Dependability

One of the most valuable traits of a successful medical assistant is dependability. Be on time and make every attempt to be at work every day. When staff members arrive late, the schedule for the entire day can be delayed (Figure 4-2). A medical assistant must follow through when the physician or supervisor gives an order. That person will count on the medical assistant to remember and complete all assigned duties. Supervisors should be confident that once given a task to do, the medical assistant will carry it out accurately and in a timely manner.

Courtesy

Show courtesy to the patients and co-workers in the physician's office. Kind words and compassion go far in building trust between the medical assistant and patients (Figure 4-3). All

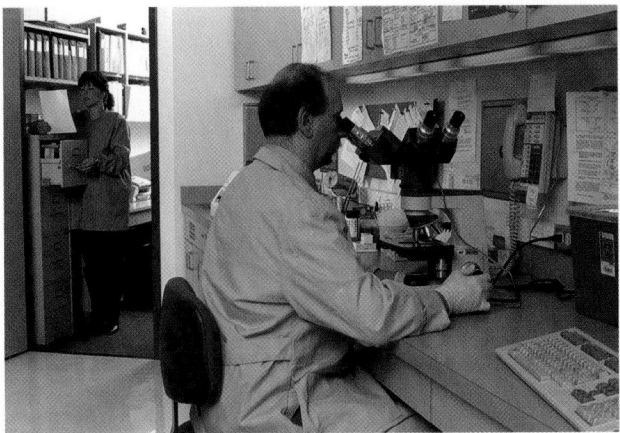

FIGURE 4-2 The physician will depend on the medical assistant to be at work on time and on each scheduled day. Absent or tardy employees cause scheduling difficulties and can greatly inconvenience the patients and remaining staff.

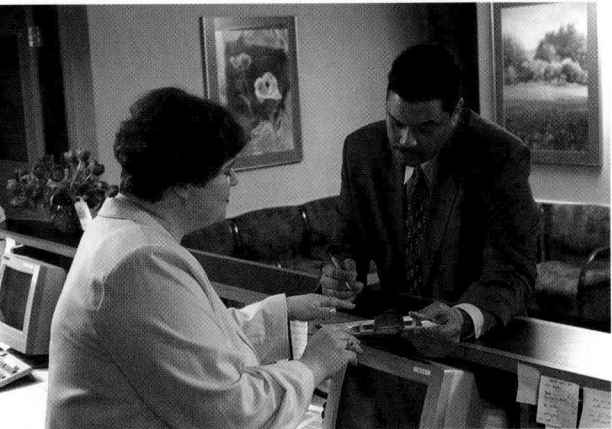

FIGURE 4-3 Taking a few moments to explain forms and bills to a patient is a courteous way to avoid misunderstandings and promote goodwill.

visitors and staff members in the office should be shown kindness and consideration. The fact that a medical assistant is having a bad day is no excuse for inflicting his or her anger or irritation on patients. Always demonstrate a good attitude and offer patients and visitors a sincere smile.

Initiative

Employee lack of **initiative** is one of the more common complaints from supervisors. Taking initiative means that the medical assistant looks for the opportunity to be of help, assisting others as the workload demands. Instead of waiting to be told to perform a task, the **competent** medical assistant looks for jobs that need to be completed; never remain idle. Some task can always be done in the medical office. Filing needs to be done on a continual basis. Inventories, supply ordering, or restocking can be performed when there is extra time. Cleaning countertops and straightening areas as work is done will help to keep the facility tidy. The medical assistant should also keep an eye on the reception area, since it may need attention several times during the day.

CRITICAL THINKING APPLICATION

■ How can Karen show her initiative on the job?
■ What types of duties can she perform when she has finished her workload for the day and there is still time left before leaving the office?

Flexibility

A medical assistant must be able to adapt to a wide variety of situations. An emergency could occur in the office, and the staff must be flexible enough to adjust the schedule and care for all patients. Being flexible also means that staff members are willing to assist one another in the performance of their duties. No one in the physician's office should ever say, "That's not my job." The patients must come first, and every staff member must be willing to lend a hand where needed. Some medical assistants trade or rotate their duties. If one assistant does not particularly enjoy doing a certain task, perhaps another assistant would be willing to trade tasks. This way, both are more satisfied with their jobs. Being able to adapt quickly and cheerfully will make the medical assistant a valuable asset to the office.

Credibility

Credibility is the perceived competence or character of a person. It leads to the belief that a person can be trusted. Because trust is a vital component of the physician-patient relationship, the credibility of the physician and those who assist in the office should be strong. The information provided to patients must be accurate. Patients expect that the physician and medical assistant will instruct them in a manner that will enhance their health and provide positive results. One must take care in giving any advice to patients, because they view the medical assistant as an agent of the physician. Patients may not distinguish between the medical assistant's comments and the physician's orders. Remember that giving anything that could be construed as medical advice is outside the scope of the duties of the medical assistant. To avoid charges of practicing medicine without a license, a medical assistant must be sure to suggest only what the physician has authorized.

Confidentiality

The importance of confidentiality cannot be stressed enough in the medical environment. Patients are entitled to privacy where their health is concerned, and they should be confident that medical professionals use information only to care for them. Never reveal any information about any patient to anyone without specific permission to do so. Always verify that the person seeking information has the right to see it and that the patient has signed a consent form. Casual conversations in hallways, elevators, and break rooms between staff members can be overheard by a family member or friend of the patient. These are a few places in the facility where confidentiality is often breached.

The rules regarding confidentiality extend beyond the medical office. While at home, medical assistants should not discuss details about patients with their families and friends. Those outside the medical profession do not understand how vital it is to keep information confidential and may pass along damaging facts to others. Medical assistants must make it a rule never to discuss a patient with anyone unless information must be shared for patient care and treatment. The Health Insurance Portability and Accountability Act (HIPAA) was created in part to assure patient confidentiality. HIPAA will be discussed more in later chapters.

Attitude

Possibly the most important asset a medical assistant brings to the office is a good attitude. A good attitude involves courtesy and kindness to others, refraining from jumping to conclusions, giving the other person the benefit of the doubt, and being **optimistic.** This trait alone can influence promotions, terminations, and the entire atmosphere of the office (Figure 4-4). Individuals are able to control their attitudes with practice. It takes skill to react calmly to people who are very upset, rather than to respond in kind, especially if being harassed or accused. Speaking in an even tone and perhaps a little softer than normal will force the listener to lower his or her voice to hear. Offer to help resolve the problem and attempt to move to a private room out of the hearing range of other patients to talk. Always display a good attitude with co-workers and be willing to assist them with their duties, especially on hectic days.

OBSTRUCTIONS TO PROFESSIONALISM

It is not always easy to be a professional. Sometimes patients, co-workers, and supervisors try our patience, and it can be hard to maintain a professional attitude in these cases. Some of the obstructions to professional behavior are discussed in this section.

Personal Problems and "Baggage"

Everyone has a life outside of the workplace, and sometimes we face challenges and difficult times that are hard to put aside.

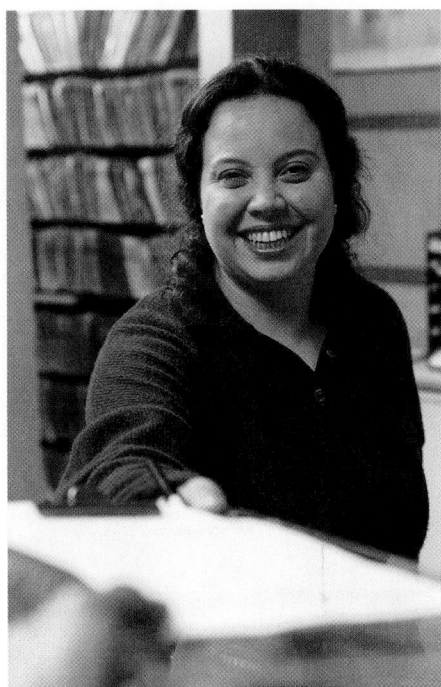

FIGURE 4-4 A good attitude goes a long way in patient and staff relationships.

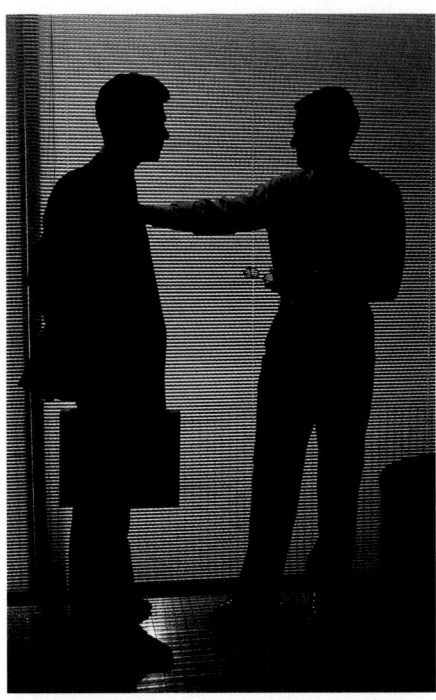

FIGURE 4-5 Gossip and rumors have no place in the medical profession. Avoid employees who participate in this type of activity.

During working hours our thoughts should be on the job at hand, especially when we are dealing with patients. However, there may be situations in our lives that are so critical or distracting that we find ourselves thinking of them constantly. This personal baggage can interfere with our ability to properly perform job duties.

When a situation intrudes on thoughts at work, it is often best to take the time to talk with a supervisor. It is not always necessary to share the intimate details, but a quick explanation that some difficulties are occurring outside of work will help the supervisor to understand any changes in habit or attitude. However, some supervisors are uncaring and are concerned only with satisfactory job performance. The medical assistant will have to use some **discretion** when discussing private affairs with the supervisor.

Never transfer personal problems and baggage to the patient. A professional medical assistant does not share personal information or problems with anyone at the medical facility, especially patients. The workday should be centered around patient care, so never allow personal business to impinge on time that should be spent assisting patients and the physician.

CRITICAL THINKING APPLICATION

It is often hard to keep from thinking about a problem while you are working. How can Karen do this if she is concerned about a grandmother who is critically ill?

Rumors and the "Grapevine"

A rumor by definition is talk or widely **disseminated** opinion with no discernible source, or a statement that is not known to be true. The definition alone suggests that spreading rumors should be avoided. Most people enjoy working in an environment in which employees cooperate and get along with each other, but rumors can cause problems with employee **morale** and are often great exaggerations or manipulations of the truth. By promoting the grapevine, rumors are passed along and become more and more outrageous with each retelling. A medical assistant should refuse to participate in the office rumor mill and should attempt to be cordial and friendly to everyone at work (Figure 4-5). Supervisors regard those who spread or discuss rumors as unprofessional and untrustworthy. Avoid passing along work-related rumors to patients, family, and friends.

Personal Phone Calls and Business

It is wise to avoid receiving unnecessary phone calls to the office from friends and family. The office phone should be considered a business line and must be used as such, except in emergencies. Using personal cell phones during working hours is not acceptable. Use breaks and lunch hours to take care of business on the phone. Never take a personal call or respond to text messages on a cell phone while working with a patient. If a phone must be carried, place it on the vibrator setting, and always step into a hall or break area if a call absolutely must be taken. This should only happen in rare cases. Visitors should not frequent the office, especially not in the area where the medical assistant is working. If someone must come to the office, always offer the reception area as a waiting room. Visitors should never be allowed to enter patient areas.

Checking personal email should also be avoided in the workplace. Any type of personal business, such as studying, looking up information on the Internet for personal use, or balancing a personal checkbook, should be done at home and not in the office setting. All of these actions distract the medical assistant from the job at hand; the focus should be on serving the patients in the office at all times.

CRITICAL THINKING APPLICATION

■ Karen has a friend who works in a video store close to her office. Her friend has begun the habit of stopping in daily during her lunch hour to chat with Karen. How can Karen politely discourage her friend from doing this?

■ Karen feels the need to check on her grandmother's condition as often as possible during the days she is ill. How might she accomplish this in a professional way?

Office Politics

Most people associate office politics with some underhanded scheme or plans to move upward in the company in whatever way possible, whether the methods used are ethical or not. The tendency is to give the word politics a negative **connotation.** *Politics* can be defined as the art or science of influencing and guiding government or some other organization. The same can be applied to medical office politics. When an individual wishes to move upward in an organization, he or she may use a positive strategy. Many people develop a specific plan regarding how they will advance and in what time period they will accomplish their goals. Medical assistants who wish to advance should be productive workers, accept responsibility, be dependable, and always conduct themselves in a professional manner. Using underhanded techniques and instigating trouble is not an effective method of career advancement.

Procrastination

Procrastination is often a symptom of the fear of failure. Some people procrastinate because this gives them an excuse for failure. Others procrastinate because they are perfectionists and feel that only they can complete a project the right way. Procrastination is the surest way to see that goals remain unfulfilled. The best way to stop this habit is to *do* something. Divide projects into small steps, and complete one at a time. When a project is divided into small segments, it is much less overwhelming. The stronger the motivation, the easier it is to fight the urge to procrastinate.

PROFESSIONAL ATTRIBUTES

Teamwork

If managers were asked what the most important attributes would be for medical professionals, teamwork would be high on the list (Figure 4-6). Staff members must work together for the good of the patients. They must be willing to perform duties outside the formal job description if they are needed in other areas of the office. Many supervisors frown on employees who state, "That's not in my job description." Any order that is given by a supervisor becomes mandatory, and an individual who refuses to perform such a task can have his or her employment terminated for **insubordination.** A medical assistant should

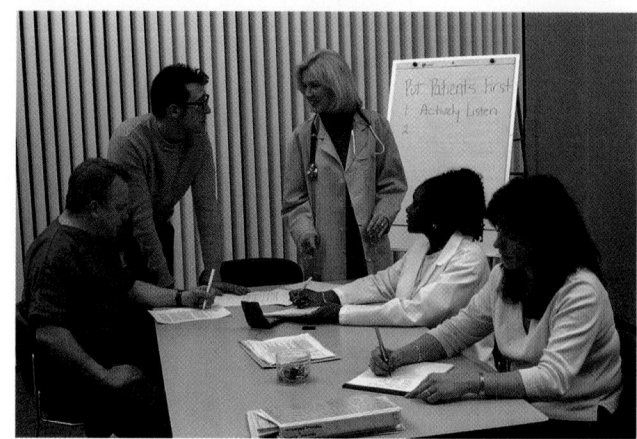

FIGURE 4-6 Teamwork is a vital part of the medical profession. All staff members must work together to care for the patient and perform required duties in the physician's office.

perform the duty and later discuss with the supervisor any valid reasons that it should have been assigned to someone else.

Although we would all enjoy working in an office in which everyone gets along and likes every other employee, this does not always happen. Personal feelings must be set aside at work, and all employees must cooperate with others to get the job done efficiently. If a medical assistant has an issue with another employee, the first move would be to discuss it privately with the other person. Then, if the situation does not improve, perhaps a supervisor should be involved for further discussions.

Time Management

We have often heard the expression "work smart." This means that we are to use our time efficiently and concentrate on the duties that are most important first. To do this we must first prioritize our duties and arrange our schedules to ensure that these duties can be performed. The first way to improve time management is to plan the tasks that need to be done that day. Taking 10 minutes to write down the tasks for the day will help to ensure that they are done. Then it is important to stay on schedule throughout the day, unless emergencies disrupt the schedule. Even then, when office days are well planned, allowances can be made for emergencies, even if they happen often, and the majority of the tasks can still be completed. The key to managing time is prioritizing.

Prioritizing

Prioritizing is simply deciding which tasks are most important. Many people make a "to do" list for the day's activities, but the secret to success is prioritizing those activities into categories that give order to the tasks.

Most tasks can be prioritized into three general categories: those that must be done that day, those that *should* be done that day, and those that could be done if time permits. Once you have a general list of tasks, review the list and further prioritize it, using a code such as M for must, S for should, and C for could (or this might be further simplified by using the letters A, B, and C). Once the tasks are divided into these categories, they can be further classified within each section. For instance, if there are six A category duties, meaning they must be done that day, these six can be numbered in the order they should be performed. The same process is completed with the B and C categories, and then as the tasks are completed, they are checked off for that day. Other categories can be added to customize the list. For example, an H category can be used for duties to perform at home, P could represent phone calls that need to be made, and E could represent errands to run. Customizing the categories will make the list more user-friendly.

Setting Goals

Those who succeed in life are planners and goal-setters. The first step in becoming a proficient goal-setter is to take the time to really think about what is to be accomplished throughout one's lifetime. These goals must be written down and reviewed often. Goals should be set for all areas in a person's life, including personal growth, career, home life, family, spiritual needs, and any others that apply to the individual. The goals should not be unreasonable. They should be measurable and specific, with written steps detailing how they will be reached. Determination and persistence in reaching the goals will help to make them happen, along with a healthy dose of hard work. The goals should be reviewed often and progress evaluated; then goals can be reset as necessary.

Remember to celebrate accomplishments and move past any goals that are missed, evaluating and restating the goals if necessary. Charles Kettering, an inventor who is most well known for his invention of the automobile self-starter, once said, "The only time you can't afford to fail is the last time you try." Never quit trying to improve and experience personal growth.

CRITICAL THINKING APPLICATION

- What are some goals that Karen might set related to her behavior on the job?
- List several goals for the new medical assistant to work toward during his or her first year in the field.

KNOWING THE FACILITY AND ITS EMPLOYEES

A much-circulated story tells of a college professor who used to end a critical test with the question, "What is the name of the woman who cleans our wing of the building?" This would perplex most students, but the question makes a good point. A professional medical assistant should attempt to get to know the people who work in the facility and should have a good idea of who handles which duties (Figure 4-7). When patients have specific problems with which they need help, they can be referred to the person who knows the most about that particular issue. It is wise to express appreciation to others whenever possible. Say "thank you" often or "I appreciate your help" when working with others. This will make co-workers more likely to assist at other times when their help is needed.

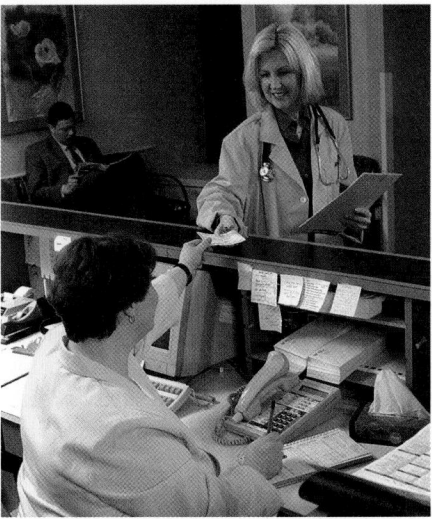

FIGURE 4-7 Knowing which employee to call when help is needed promotes goodwill among employees and often gets a task done more efficiently.

DOCUMENTATION

From the standpoint of professional behavior, documentation skills are vital to medical assistants. Charting accurately with legible, neat handwriting can make a difference in the perception of professionalism in the medical office. Be complete in any narrative regarding patients. Be sure to state facts, not opinions, and never use sarcastic remarks when charting. Phone messages must be documented carefully as well, and handled in a professional manner. Never use sarcasm when reporting messages to the physician or anyone else in the office. Use conservative speech and proper wording in all situations in the medical facility.

Note Taking

Whenever office meetings or seminars are held, be prepared by having a pad and pencil ready for note taking. A medical assistant should never be without paper and pen so that accurate information from the meeting can be jotted down for future reference. It is wise to keep a notebook or file on office meetings to refer to in case clarification of an order or a point is needed. Another good idea is to keep a small spiral notebook in a pocket with a pen, so that if an order is given in passing by the physician, the medical assistant will have a place to jot it down until he or she has access to the patient's chart. This avoids giving incorrect dosages of medication or forgetting to order a laboratory test, as well as many other errors that could be made by relying on memory.

WORK ETHICS

Work ethics can involve a whole range of activities, from individual acts to the philosophy of the entire facility. A person who has good work ethics is one who arrives on time, who is rarely absent, whose work output is **commensurate** with the pay received, and who uses his or her best abilities. Work ethics also involves other situations. If another employee is seen taking drugs from the supply cabinet or money from the cash box, the act should certainly be reported. However, if the guilty employee is also a close friend of the person who witnesses the act, an ethical dilemma is present. Ways to solve ethical problems are discussed in Chapter 6. A medical assistant must always act in such a way that his or her actions are above **reproach.**

INTERPERSONAL SKILLS

Interpersonal skills are paramount in working with patients and other health professionals. A medical assistant should work hard to perfect his or her communication techniques. Often the success of a business is directly related to the ability of its employees to communicate effectively. Interpersonal skills are discussed in detail in Chapter 5.

When speaking to patients and providing them with information, remember that most do not have any medical background and do not understand many of the phrases used by the medical community. A medical assistant must be patient and explain in a courteous manner any aspect of the instructions or details that the patient does not understand. When educating

the patient, the medical assistant should have a professional attitude of concern and helpfulness. Assure the patient that medical assistants and the rest of the staff in the facility are bound by rules of patient confidentiality if the patient seems concerned about revealing pertinent information.

CLOSING COMMENTS

Patients expect and deserve professional behavior from those who work in medical facilities. Always show compassion, caring, and consideration for a person who comes to the office, whether a patient, visitor, or co-worker. By displaying these traits, the medical assistant will earn the respect of co-workers and become indispensable to the physician-employer. Behaving in a professional manner in the medical office will help to gain the patient's trust. Trust is one of the most important factors in avoiding cases of medical professional liability. Treating patients with care and not subjecting them to poor attitudes and unnecessary information will keep the patient-physician relationship a strong one, conducive to the health and recovery of the patient.

SUMMARY OF SCENARIO

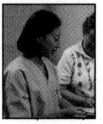

Karen is happy to be employed in a family practice in which providing quality patient care is paramount. She is learning to be careful of what she says and to remain focused on the patient instead of any difficulties she may be having. Karen knows that it is her responsibility to be a team player and to assist the other staff members as much as possible. She maintains a good attitude, even when personal issues could distract her from her duties. Karen gets a strong sense of pride in being a part of the medical profession. She insists on a neat appearance and arrives on time for each scheduled workday. She always asks others if they need help when she has any extra time throughout the day. Karen looks forward to a long relationship with her employer. The rewards she feels as a member of the health team are second to none.

Although Karen is concerned about her grandmother's health, those concerns must be minimally invasive on her work duties and her attitude toward her patients and co-workers. By making an appointment to speak with her supervisor and explaining the situation with her grandmother, Karen takes a proactive role in assuring that the supervisor understands the pressures Karen is facing. Most supervisors will be sympathetic and understanding when issues outside the practice affect employees; however, this should not happen on a regular basis. By encouraging Karen to call and check on her grandmother periodically, the supervisor helps Karen to feel more confident and less distracted during the day. By finding her supervisor a supportive ally, Karen can relax and carry out her duties professionally and competently throughout the workday. Karen puts the patients first, and this is a fine example of both professionalism and patient compassion.

SUMMARY of LEARNING OBJECTIVES

1. Define, spell, and pronounce the terms listed in the vocabulary.
   - Spelling and pronouncing medical terms correctly adds credibility to the medical assistant. Knowing the definition of these terms promotes confidence in communication with patients and co-workers.
2. Explain the meaning of the word professionalism.
   - Professionalism is the characteristic of being or conforming to the technical or ethical standards of a profession. It

involves exhibiting courtesy, being conscientious, and conducting oneself in a businesslike manner at the workplace. Professionalism is vitally important in the medical profession.
3. Discuss several of the characteristics of professionalism.
   - Some of the characteristics of professionalism include loyalty, dependability, courtesy, initiative, flexibility, credibility, confidentiality, and a good attitude.
4. Explain why confidentiality is so important in the medical profession.

SUMMARY of LEARNING OBJECTIVES
Continued

- Confidentiality is vitally important in the medical profession. Patients depend on medical personnel to keep their health information confidential and private. Breach of patient confidentiality is one reason that an employee could be immediately terminated from his or her position and can result in litigation between the patient and the physician-employer.

5. Discuss the role of the medical assistant's attitude in caring for patients.
   - Because most patients are not at their best when visiting the physician's office, the attitude of the staff plays an important role in patients' attitudes while in the office. Medical assistants need patience when working with those who are ill. A smile or a reassuring pat on the back will go a long way and be encouraging.

6. List some examples of office politics.
   - Office politics can be negative or positive. A person who uses others to be promoted in the company or takes credit for a team effort may be using office politics in a negative way; a person who strategically plans advancement through outstanding performance, dependability, and teamwork uses office politics in a positive manner. Knowing when to speak and when to listen will help the medical assistant to play the game of politics well in the medical facility.

7. Identify specific ways that teamwork can be promoted in the physician's office.
   - Teamwork makes any job easier to complete. By helping those who may be overwhelmed with duties, the medical assistant may find willing co-workers who will help when the situation is reversed in the future. If two assistants both have duties they dislike, they might trade the duties and both be satisfied. Everyone must work together for the good of the facility and the patients it serves.

8. Discuss the meaning of insubordination and why it is grounds for dismissal.
   - Insubordination can be used as grounds for immediate dismissal. Insubordination is being disobedient to any type of authority figure, usually the supervisor. When given a task to complete, the medical assistant should carry out the order unless it is unlawful or unethical. If the medical assistant does not carry out an order, the patient's life may be at risk. If the medical assistant feels that the duty should have been performed by someone else or there was some reason it should not have been performed, the supervisor should be consulted. Discuss the issue and attempt to reach an agreement about the appropriateness of performing the task in the future.

9. Identify several categories of prioritizing tasks and their meaning.
   - Prioritizing tasks can help the medical assistant to accomplish more tasks. Prioritizing can be used for work, home, and extracurricular activities. Tasks can be identified as those that must, should, or could be done that day. Then within each of these categories the tasks can be numbered in the order in which they should be completed.

10. Talk about goal setting and how this helps in achieving career success.
    - Goals should be written down and reviewed often to check progress. Taking small steps toward goals will help ensure that they are eventually reached. Individuals should set goals in each area of their lives, breaking the tasks down into manageable parts. Goals should not be unreasonable or unattainable but should provide the opportunity for small successes along the way to reaching the ultimate goal.

CONNECTIONS

Study Guide Connection: Go to Chapter 4 Study Guide. Read the Case Study and Workplace Applications and complete the assignments. Do online research for answers to the questions in the Internet Activities associated with professional behavior in the workplace.

CD Connection: Go to the Medical Assisting Competency Challenge CD and do the training activities under Communication.

Evolve Connection: For more information related to professional behavior in the workplace, go to evolve.elsevier.com/kinn and visit related weblinks for Chapter 4. Click on the Medical Assisting Exam Review and do the practice questions to sharpen your test-taking skills.

Interpersonal Skills and Human Behavior

5

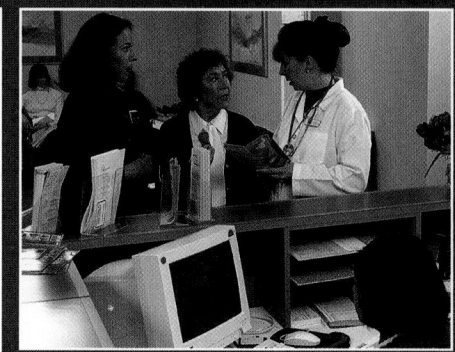

Many types of patients seek medical attention and care in the physician's office. Each has different needs and different concerns, even if the diagnoses are similar. Communication and interpersonal skills are vitally important in meeting these needs and providing optimal care to the patient. However, the patient is not the only individual to consider. Family members are often instrumental in the health and well-being of the patient.

Lucille Cloyd is an 83-year-old patient who has been diagnosed with pancreatic cancer and is seeing Dr. Neill for treatment. Her daughter, Sarah Smithson, helps to care for her; she is very close to her mother emotionally. Sarah is also Dr. Neill's patient. Although Sarah does not wish to see her mother in pain, she suffers with the knowledge that life will be very different without her. Mrs. Cloyd is widowed and visits the physician once a month in addition to receiving hospice services. She is a good-humored woman who feels she has led a fruitful life, yet she has moments of depression. She has been living with Sarah and her family for 2 months and enjoys interacting with her two grandchildren and the family's pets.

The medical assistant must consider not only Mrs. Cloyd, but also her extended family. Compassion and sensitivity will be necessary to care for this patient, as well as excellent listening skills. A good knowledge of human relations will help the medical assistant make Mrs. Cloyd's medical care as pleasant as possible under the circumstances.

While studying this chapter, think about the following questions:

- How can the medical assistant treat patients as individuals during a busy workday?
- How does the medical assistant effectively communicate with a patient's family members?

- How will developing good listening skills make the medical assistant more effective?
- How do friends and family members play a role in the health of the patient?

1. Define, spell, and pronounce the terms listed in the vocabulary.
2. Explain why first impressions are critically important.
3. Differentiate between verbal and nonverbal communication.
4. Explain the different levels of spatial separation.
5. Discuss the value of touch in the communication process.
6. Describe the elements of the transactional communication model.
7. Explain some of the barriers to effective communication.
8. List and explain the levels of Maslow's hierarchy of needs.

9. Discuss defense mechanisms, and be able to recognize commonly used defense mechanisms.
10. Describe the value of listening.
11. List several ways to deal with conflict.
12. Explain the stages that patients go through when facing death.
13. Discuss why physical and emotional needs affect our daily performance at work.

National Accreditation Competencies and Content

CAAHEP COMPETENCIES

General

3.c.(1)(b). Recognize and respond to verbal communications
3.c.(1)(c). Recognize and respond to nonverbal communications

ABHES COMPETENCIES

Communication

2.a. Be attentive, listen, and learn
2.b. Be impartial and show empathy when dealing with patients
2.c. Adapt what is said to the recipient's level of comprehension
2.d. Serve as liaison between physician and others
2.h. Receive, organize, prioritize, and transmit information expediently
2.i. Recognize and respond to verbal and nonverbal communication
2.k. Principles of verbal and nonverbal communication
2.l. Recognition and response to verbal and nonverbal communication

Instruction

7.b. Instruct patients with special needs

VOCABULARY

adage (a′-dij) A saying, often in metaphoric form, that embodies a common observation.

aggressive Forceful or intended to dominate; hostile, injurious, or destructive, especially when referring to a behavior caused by frustration.

ambiguous (am-bi′-gu-wus) Capable of being understood in two or more possible senses or ways; unclear.

animate To fill with life; to give spirit and support to expressions.

battery An offensive touching or use of force on a person without his or her consent.

caustic (kos′-tik) Marked by sarcasm.

channels Means of communication or expression; courses or directions of thought.

comfort zone A place in the mind where an individual feels safe and confident.

congruent (kun-gru′-unt) Being in agreement, harmony, or correspondence; conforming to the circumstances or requirements of a situation.

decodes Converts, as in a message, into intelligible form; recognizes and interprets.

defense mechanisms Psychologic methods of dealing with stressful situations that are encountered in day-to-day living.

encodes Converts from one system of communication to another; converts a message into code.

encroachments Actions that advance beyond the usual or proper limits.

enunciate (e-nun′-se-at) To utter articulate sounds; the act of being very distinct in speech.

external noise Sounds or factors outside the brain that interfere with the communication process.

externalization The attribution of an event or occurrence to causes outside the self.

feedback The transmission of evaluative or corrective information to the original or controlling source about an action, event, or process.

grief Reaction to an unfortunate outcome; a deep distress caused by bereavement, a loss, or a perceived loss.

internal noise Factors inside the brain that interfere with the communication process.

language barrier Any type of interference that inhibits the communication process and is related to languages spoken by the people attempting to communicate.

litigious (luh-ti′-jus) Prone to engage in lawsuits.

malediction (ma-luh-dik′-shun) Speaking evil or the calling of a curse.

media Term applied to agencies of mass communication, such as newspapers, magazines, and telecommunications.

paraphrasing To express an idea in different wording in an effort to enhance communication and clarify meaning.

perception Capacity for comprehension; an awareness of the elements of the environment.

physiologic noise Physiologic interferences with the communication process.

pitch Highness or lowness of a sound; the relative level, intensity, or extent of some quality or state.

proxemics (prok-se′-miks) The study of the nature, degree, and effect of the spatial separation individuals naturally maintain.

sarcasm A sharp and often satirical response or ironic utterance designed to cut or give pain.

stereotype Something conforming to a fixed or general pattern; a standardized mental picture that is held in common by many and represents an oversimplified opinion, prejudiced attitude, or uncritical judgment.

stressors Stimuli that cause stress.

subtle Difficult to understand or perceive; having or marked by keen insight and ability to penetrate deeply and thoroughly.

thanatology (tha-nuh-tah′-luh-je) The study of the phenomena of death and of psychologic methods of coping with death.

vehemently (ve′-uh-ment-le) In a manner marked by forceful energy; intensely emotionally.

volatile (vah′-luh-til) Easily aroused; tending to erupt in violence.

The interpersonal skills developed by the medical assistant help to set the tone of a medical office. Interpersonal skills include the communications process and how we relate to one another during that process. Human relations can be defined as the study of the problems that arise from organizational and interpersonal contact. The two entities intersect each other, and the successful medical assistant will work to enhance these attributes on a continual basis. Patients who visit the healthcare facility may not be at their best, and the way in which the medical assistant reacts to and interacts with them can make an incredible difference in their **perception** of the office, the physician, and the medical staff. These interactions may also affect the patient's treatment and recovery.

FIRST IMPRESSIONS

Our elders have stressed all of our lives that first impressions are lasting ones, and this old **adage** is still true! The opinions formed in the early moments of meeting someone remain in our thoughts long after the first words are spoken. The first impression involves much more than just physical appearance or dress; it includes attitude and compassion, and the all-important smile (Figure 5-1).

One of the primary objectives of the professional medical assistant is to care for and about the people that are being served. Patients are the reason for the existence of the facility, and they should be offered the best customer service available. They must be warmly welcomed, and it is important to call patients by their names. People enjoy hearing their names, and it gives a patient confidence that the medical staff members know for whom they are caring.

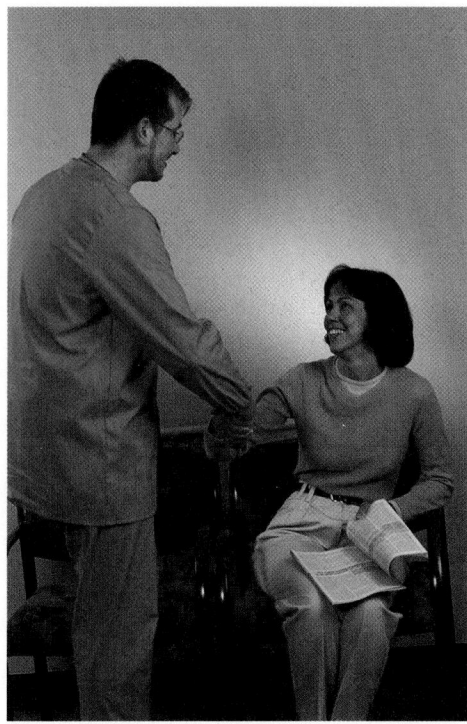

FIGURE 5-1 First impressions are critical in gaining the patient's trust.

Think for a moment about how it feels to be a new patient who is entering the unknown territory of the physician's office. Staff members of the facility are in familiar surroundings and already have some information about the new patient. However, the patient knows nothing about the staff members. One way to break that barrier is to have all staff members wear name badges, with letters large enough to be read at a distance of 3 feet. Include the staff position if several divisions of responsibility exist, for example, "medical assistant," "insurance biller," and "office manager." When the patient approaches, even when wearing a name badge, make introductions and smile. Smiles should show both facially and in the voice and eyes. Genuinely welcome the patient to the office. This small effort will help put the patient at ease in the office environment.

Some physicians make brief notes in the chart about the personal life of the patient. When the patient arrives for an appointment, the physician can ask about his or her recent trip abroad or new grandchild. This tells the patient that the doctor and the office staff see him or her as more than just an illness or a chart number. It gives the impression that they truly care, and that impression should be an accurate one. Once an impression is formed in the patient's mind, it is very difficult to change, so make the first impressions of your office positive ones.

COMMUNICATION PATHS

Verbal Communication

Messages are conveyed by the use of language, which may be written, spoken, or communicated in another way. Verbal communication depends on words and sounds. The **pitch** of the voice is a part of verbal communication. The voice lifts at the end of a question. It drops at the end of a statement. Usually when a speaker intends to continue a statement, the voice will hold the same pitch, the head will remain straight, and the eyes and hands will be unchanged. This is not an appropriate time to interrupt. If the message is interrupted, the train of thought may not be completed. Tone of voice and choice of words also affect messages.

The medical assistant should speak clearly and **enunciate** words properly. Speak loudly enough that the patients are able to hear clearly, and pay particular attention to those who wear some type of hearing assistance device. It is wise to note this information on the patient's chart to jog the memory when a patient with a hearing problem visits the office. Never assume that just because a patient is elderly, he or she has a hearing problem. When talking with patients, be sure to use the volume of speech to an advantage. Always speak at a clearly audible level, but at times it will be necessary to increase or decrease the volume of speech. When a patient is upset, for instance, it often helps to lower the volume of speech, because the patient tends to get quieter to hear the person speaking.

Eye contact is critical. Look at the person being spoken to, and do not forget a genuine smile. Many people feel that a person who speaks and cannot look another in the eyes is being deceptive. It can also mean that the speaker is very shy and has little self-confidence. Use gestures where appropriate to liven speech and **animate** the conversation.

Medical assistants must become aware of how they express themselves and how they affect the feelings of others. The tone of voice is vitally important. There is no place for **sarcasm** or **caustic** remarks. For example, saying "I hope you can manage to be on time for your next appointment" to a patient is needless and rude. The medical assistant must be conservative when speaking and not be too familiar. The patient expects professionalism and has the right to demand this in the healthcare setting. Never make an inappropriate remark and follow with "I was just kidding." This has no place in a medical facility or in any type of interpersonal communication. Take special care not to hurt anyone's feelings with words and phrases. Be very careful about what is said, especially to patients (Procedure 5-1).

Remember that patients are in the facility to be treated or cared for by the physician and staff. They are usually concerned about their illness and may have great apprehensions and fears about the future. It is completely out of place for the medical assistant to talk about his or her personal life and challenges with the patients. Allow the patient to speak, and listen instead of offering personal information. Often patients will casually mention things to the medical assistant that might influence their care. The saying that we are given "one mouth and two ears" stresses which should get more use!

Nonverbal Communication

Both verbal and nonverbal communications are important in the art of expression, and both are needed to succeed in the communication exchange. Nonverbal communications are messages conveyed without the use of words. They are transmitted by body language, gestures, and mannerisms that may or may not be in agreement with the words a person speaks. Body language is partly instinctive, partly taught, and partly imitative. It involves eye contact, facial expression, hand gestures, grooming, dress, space, tone of voice, posture, touch,

and much more. We are often unaware of our own nonverbal signals and consciously recognize only a small number of the signals sent by others. Our ability to help others increases as we hone our own skills in interpreting nonverbal communication. Nonverbal communication is almost always more accurate than verbal communication and tends to convey our true feelings and beliefs (Procedure 5-2).

Appearance is an integral part of nonverbal communication. It influences the way others view us and can present a conflicting message, or even a totally incorrect message. When we see someone who dresses or grooms in a way that is very different from our own style, we tend to assume that the personalities are also very different. This is not always true. Although we should not judge people by the way they dress, it is difficult not to form opinions based on what is seen. Visible piercings and tattoos are often looked on unfavorably in the medical profession, as are brightly painted long nails. Although these do not signify that the wearer is not professional, many patients, especially older patients, look on these trends unfavorably. For this reason alone, the medical assistant who is less conservative may be diminishing the chance for certain jobs and advancements. It is healthy to express oneself, yet in the medical profession, conservative appearance is preferred to avoid blocks in communications.

The successful medical assistant expresses self-esteem and confidence by stance, vocabulary, facial expression, and a caring attitude. The experience of speaking to someone who does not make eye contact helps one to realize the importance of greeting the patient with the eyes as well as the voice and body language. Facial expressions often convey our true feelings and are not masked by the words we use. Our eyes often tell the truth when our words are misleading or false. It is important to have an open body stance when dealing with patients. Crossed arms and legs hint that one is "closed" to the person being spoken to, and this may be construed as disinterest or disbelief.

PROCEDURE 5-1

Recognize and Respond to Verbal Communications

CAAHEP COMPETENCY: 3.c(1)(b)
ABHES COMPETENCY: 2.I

GOAL: *To be able to recognize verbal communication and respond to it in a professional manner.*

EQUIPMENT and SUPPLIES

- Cards with various patient scenarios

PROCEDURAL STEPS

1. Select a classmate as a partner for this procedure.
   PURPOSE: To practice communications with a partner whose responses will not be predictable.
2. Taking turns, draw a card and role-play the scenario described on it. Make certain that the partner understands the role on the card.
   PURPOSE: To send a clearly communicated message.

3. Allow your partner to respond to the sent message.
   PURPOSE: To make certain that your partner understood your message and allow him or her to communicate a response.
4. Restate your partner's response.
   PURPOSE: To assure understanding of the partner's message.
5. Clarify any issues that are unclear.
   PURPOSE: To make certain that the meaning of each message sent is understood.
6. Refrain from using slang or other unprofessional wording.
   PURPOSE: To maintain professional communication.
7. Continue to communicate back and forth, and be sure that each partner communicates accurately.

PROCEDURE 5-2

Recognize and Respond to Nonverbal Communications

CAAHEP COMPETENCY: 3.c(1)(c)
ABHES COMPETENCY: 2.I

GOAL: *To be able to recognize nonverbal communication and respond to it in a professional way.*

EQUIPMENT and SUPPLIES

- Cards with various statements that can be communicated in a nonverbal way

PROCEDURAL STEPS

1. Select a classmate as a partner for this procedure.
   PURPOSE: To practice nonverbal communications with a partner whose responses will not be predictable.

2. Taking turns, draw a card and communicate the thought on the card to your partner.
3. Determine if the receiver understood the message correctly.
   PURPOSE: To send a nonverbal message that is understood by the receiver.
4. Continue to communicate back and forth and be sure that each message sent is conveyed to the receiver accurately.

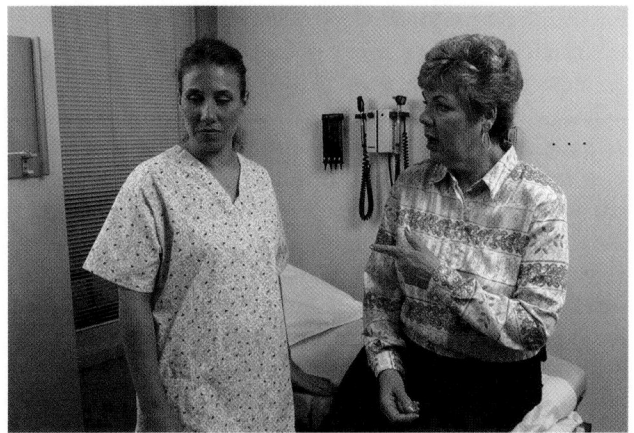 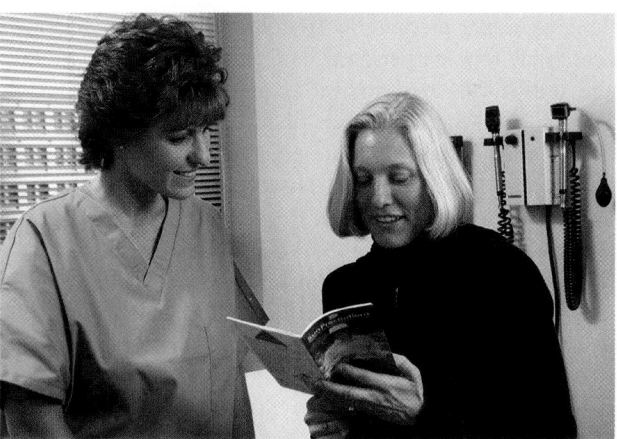

A   B

FIGURE 5-2 A, Pointing is often an accusatory gesture and causes discomfort. **B,** A bright smile helps to put the patient at ease and relax.

Nonverbal and verbal communications are dependent on each other (Figure 5-2). They must be in harmony to convey an accurate message that can be easily interpreted by the receiver. If the two are not **congruent,** the nonverbal is usually dominant and expresses the true message.

The need for personal space is demonstrated by how patients in the reception area will choose a seat. **Proxemics** is defined as the study of the nature, degree, and effect of the spatial separation individuals naturally maintain and how this separation relates to cultural and environmental factors. Seldom will a person sit in a seating space adjoining that of a stranger if there is another option. Although the need for space varies with the individual culture, some might even remain standing to satisfy the need for personal space. Public space is usually accepted as a distance of 12 to 25 feet, and social space is usually considered to be 4 to 12 feet. Personal space ranges from $1\frac{1}{2}$ to 4 feet, and intimate contact includes physical touching to approximately $1\frac{1}{2}$ feet. The medical assistant can often tell when he or she has invaded someone's personal space, because the person will tend to back up a step or two. If this happens, take a small step back and

respect the boundaries that are being set. The more familiar and comfortable patients are with the medical assistant, the closer the space they will allow.

Touch is a powerful communicator. The soft acceptance of someone's hand in yours, to the good-natured pat on the back, to the harsh slap on the face all relay different messages that need no words to accurately express. In the medical profession, as in any business, touch can be comforting or can promote a sexual harassment suit. Individuals who have experienced sexual abuse or other traumatic experiences may not want to be touched at all. Unfortunately, one must be extremely careful when using this effective communication tool. In today's **litigious** society, any nonconsensual touching may be considered **battery,** and touch should be used with great discretion and cautious care.

The medical assistant should not be afraid to touch the patient appropriately, for example, using a pat on the back or a squeeze of the hand (Figure 5-3). Some patients are receptive to a brief sideways hug, whereas others would take this as an intrusion into their personal space. Certainly patients with

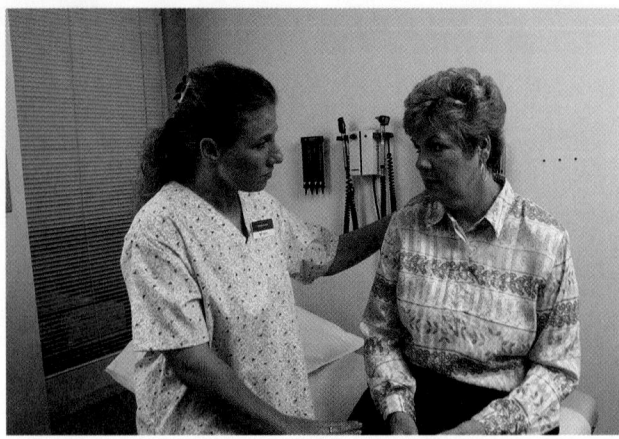

FIGURE 5-3 Touching the patient communicates care and compassion.

serious illnesses appreciate touch as an expression of empathy. Never be afraid to touch sick patients, especially those with diseases such as acquired immunodeficiency syndrome (AIDS), as long as proper precautions are followed where indicated. It is acceptable to ask a person if he or she minds being hugged. These individuals need to feel acceptance, and the attitude of the medical staff members they encounter will directly influence their adherence to keeping their appointments with the physician. If they do not feel accepted and cared for, they will not return to the physician's office. A gentle touch and a smile do wonders for showing care and concern.

Posture can signal depression, excitement, anger, or even an appeal for help. When the physician sits at the front of the chair and leans forward, he or she is giving the message of caring and interest. Positioning is important as well. Sitting behind a desk promotes an air of authority. Standing or sitting across a room may convey a negative message of denying involvement or reluctance to talk. Sitting side by side with a patient will help to initiate trust and promote open conversation. The medical assistant should practice good postural techniques as a part of projecting a positive image and for personal health reasons.

CRITICAL THINKING APPLICATION

- How might touch be an important communication tool with Mrs. Cloyd?
- How can Sarah be affected by using touch?
- Could laughter affect either of these women as they deal with death?

THE PROCESS OF COMMUNICATION

Anyone who works within the realm of public service should develop good communication skills. It is important to be able to interact with others and put them at ease, so that their comfort level increases and they develop trust. To communicate well, we must first have a general understanding of the process of communication. Once a message is sent, it cannot be retrieved and restated or expressed in a different way. Especially in the medical profession, communication must be clear and concise, and the message we intend to send must match what the receiver understands.

Although many different scientific models of communication exist, the one that best fits most types of communication is the transactional communication model. Before understanding how this model works, one must understand the elements we use to communicate.

Usually when two people interact, both people act as senders and as receivers. The sender is the person who sends a message through a variety of different **channels.** Channels can be spoken words, written messages, and body language. The sender **encodes** the message, which simply means that he or she chooses a specific way of expression using words and other channels. The receiver **decodes** the message according to his or her understanding of what is being communicated. However, sometimes the receiver incorrectly understands the message. This often is a result of noise, which is anything that interferes with the message being sent. It can be literal noise, such as a radio or a jackhammer on the street outside. This is called **external noise.** Or it can be **internal noise,** which would include the receiver's own thoughts or prejudices and opinions. **Physiologic noise** interferes with communication as well. This includes any biologic factor that would preclude the communicator from sending or receiving accurate messages, such as not feeling well or being overly tired. **Feedback** can be given through verbal expressions or body language, such as a simple nod of understanding. The perception of the receiver is very important and is discussed later in this chapter.

The transactional communication model (Figure 5-4) depicts "communicators" instead of one sender and one receiver. If two people are communicating, both are sending and receiving messages and both are encoding and decoding what is being offered. Even when two people are speaking one at a time, messages are continually sent with words, body language, facial expressions, and gestures. Various channels of communication are used, and both communicators offer feedback, even if it is done subconsciously. Noise may or may not be present, but even the best communicators experience some type of noise, even if that is only thinking of what to say next.

Listening

Listening is just as important to good communication as the spoken word. Hearing is the process, function, or power of perceiving sound, whereas *listening* is defined as paying attention to sound or hearing something with thoughtful attention. People need to know that the medical assistant is listening. This is actually true in all interpersonal relationships, including husband-wife, parent-child, supervisor-employee, and doctor-patient interactions. When listening to someone who is attempting to communicate, the first rule is to look at the speaker and pay attention. Sometimes it is important not to respond immediately, but to remain silent and offer an understanding and reassuring nod.

Sometimes it is hard to listen. We may not be able to listen effectively because we are distracted by our own thoughts. Perhaps the situations occurring in our own lives make the

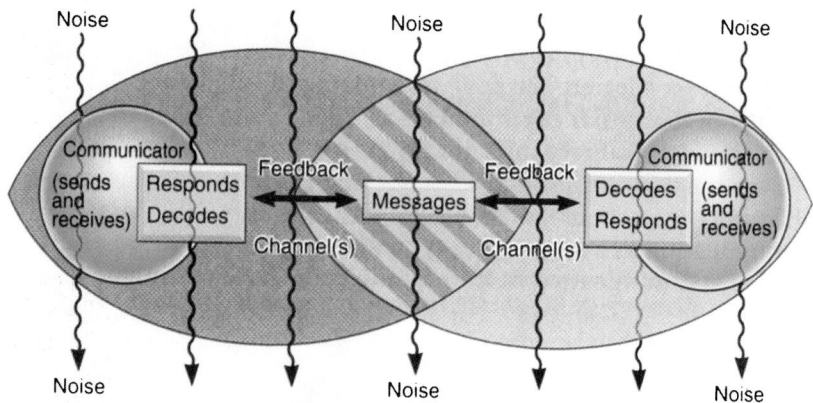

FIGURE 5-4 The transactional communication model. (From Adler RB, Towne N: *Looking out, looking in: interpersonal communication*, San Antonio, 1996, Harcourt Brace.)

conversation we are hearing seem meaningless and unimportant. Or so many messages may be attacking at once that we are unable to focus on any specific one to hear what is being communicated. At other times, such as in anger, we are so rapidly preparing our response that we cannot hear what is being said. We may simply be too tired to listen, or we may have prejudged the speaker and decided that there is no need to listen. However, while working with patients the medical assistant must be diligent in not only hearing the words being spoken, but also listening to them and to what the patient is attempting to communicate.

Active listening is the skill whereby **paraphrasing** and clarifying what the speaker has said take place. Paraphrasing is listening to what the sender is communicating, analyzing the words, and restating them to confirm that the receiver has understood the message as the sender intended it. This process clarifies the speaker's thoughts and helps to indicate that there is a common understanding of the message between both people. When communicating in this way, the receiver should reword what the sender has said and then ask a clarifying question. Consider the following example:

Patient: I have not been feeling well lately.

MA: You say you have not been feeling well. What exactly is the trouble?

This type of communicating may seem awkward at first, because most of us believe that listening involves lack of speech. Active listening means that the speaker's words are heard, and a restatement is used to verify that the message was understood correctly. This statement gives the speaker the opportunity to correct any misconceptions or misunderstandings. Consider the following example:

Patient: My back hurts.

MA: Where does it hurt?

Patient: In the middle.

MA: Can you point to exactly where it hurts?

Patient: Yes, right here. (points)

MA: Is it a sharp or dull pain?

Patient: Very sharp.

MA: How often does it occur?

Patient: Several times a day.

MA: Can you tell me on an average day how many times it bothers you?

Patient: About six times.

MA: How long does it last?

Patient: About 10 or 15 minutes.

MA: How long has this been a concern?

Patient: For about 2 weeks.

MA: So you have had a sharp pain in this part of your back, about six times a day lasting for up to 15 minutes for 2 weeks? Is that correct?

Patient: Yes.

It would have been easier if the patient had said, "I have had a sharp pain in my back that lasts up to 15 minutes, and it happens about six times a day." This example shows how the medical assistant can continue clarifying until the answer is specific enough, which is critical when obtaining information from the patient.

It is also best to ask "open" questions, as opposed to "closed" questions. An open question requires more than a "yes" or "no" answer. It forces the patient to provide more detail and expand on his or her thoughts. A closed question can be answered with "yes" or "no" and compels the medical assistant to spend more time obtaining the answers needed to accurately document the patient's needs.

CRITICAL THINKING APPLICATION

■ How can the medical assistant be sure that Mrs. Cloyd understands how she is to take her medication?

■ Often older patients do not appreciate instructions being given to their caregiver instead of directly to them. How can the medical assistant place the primary focus on communicating with Mrs. Cloyd, yet make sure that Sarah understands the instructions and care at the same time?

Often when a person or patient is talking with the medical assistant, he or she is looking for a specific type of response. Some patients want advice, some want sympathy, and others are looking for reassurance. Many patients will open up to the medical assistant more quickly and more completely than to the physician. Because it is important to build good rapport with patients, this can be a very positive aspect of the relationship the medical assistant has with the patient. However, the medical assistant should never agree to withhold information from the physician under any circumstances. If the patient asks that the assistant not reveal something to the physician, the medical assistant should politely explain that he or she has an ethical obligation to report any and all pertinent information to the physician, especially if it affects medical care. For example, if the patient asks the medical assistant not to tell the physician that the patient has been smoking against medical advice, the assistant could be jeopardizing the patient's care if the information is not reported.

This does not mean that specific details must always be aired. If, for example, the patient reveals that stress levels have been high because she has filed a sexual harassment suit against her boss, the medical assistant could report to the physician that the patient is having some legal problems that have resulted in additional stress at work. Never agree to lie to the physician! The patient must understand that if the physician questions any information given by the patient, it must be revealed so that the physician is assured that the care being provided is the right care. It is also critical to note that the physician may have worked with the patient for a long period and may have a better understanding of the patient's needs than the medical assistant. One patient may be able to handle a high degree of stress, and another may crumble at the first sign of stress. A good physician knows his or her patients and keeps accurate, complete records that will help with decision making in these situations.

If ever in doubt about telling the physician something a patient has said, the best solution is to tell. Remember, medical professionals are legally bound to confidentiality, and the patient may need to be reminded of this. Encourage him or her to talk to the physician and communicate all of his or her concerns, no matter how insignificant they may seem. Never display a judgmental attitude or express negativity about the patient's activities, thoughts, or behavior. Offer to be with the patient, if he or she desires, as the patient discusses difficult issues with the physician, or to make arrangements for a special counseling session with the physician if this is indicated. Some patients are hesitant to initiate conversation with the physician because they feel they are taking too much of his or her time. The medical assistant can help to ensure that critical issues receive the doctor's attention.

WARNINGS AGAINST ADVISING A PATIENT

The medical assistant must be extremely careful when making suggestions or comments to a patient, in order to avoid legal accusations of practicing medicine without a license. Often a patient will ask for an opinion as to which course of action to take. Medical assistants are not qualified to give any type of advice to a patient. Strict laws in most states prohibit anyone other than a licensed physician from offering medical advice. Even if the patient asks what the medical assistant would do if presented with the same options, the assistant cannot encourage

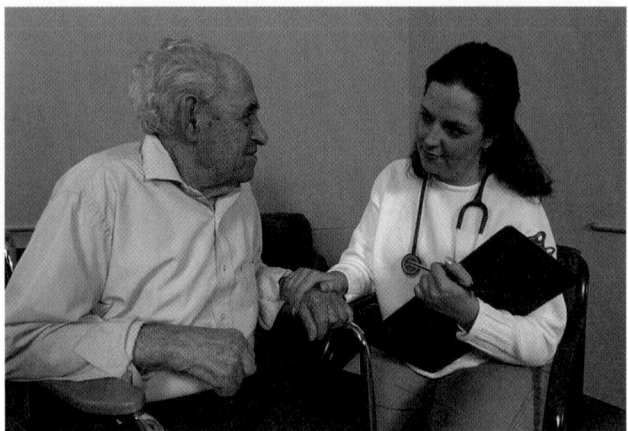

FIGURE 5-5 Careful listening and asking questions will help the patient express thoughts and feelings.

the patient to choose one option over another. The assistant can offer a listening ear, though, and help the patient process his or her own thoughts. This can be done in much the same way as using active listening techniques (Figure 5-5). When a patient expresses a concern, the medical assistant should restate the concern, then ask a clarifying question. For example:

Patient: I don't know if I should take the chemotherapy treatments the doctor suggested.

MA: You seem worried about the treatments. What are you concerned about specifically?

Patients must come to their own decisions about treatments and options that they have when faced with a medical decision. The medical assistant is often looked on not only as an authority figure, but also as an extension of the physician. Patients may mistakenly think that the medical assistant has the same opinion as the physician. It is important that all communication with the patient be professional and accurate. Always attempt to get the patient to openly discuss all of his or her concerns and fears with the physician.

The medical assistant should never agree to withhold any information from the physician, because even a small piece of information could completely change the plan of treatment. When giving instructions to patients, it is always best to have them in writing and keep a copy for the patient's chart so that a written record of what was communicated to the patient is available. Use excellent documentation technique when adding information to the patient's chart. Remember that all of the patients in the facility deserve to be treated with respect and compassion. Help the physician to establish trust with the patient. An open, trusting relationship with the patient will help to avoid legal issues in the future.

CRITICAL THINKING APPLICATION

- How should the medical assistant handle Sarah's questions about the various aspects of her mother's treatments?
- How does her mother's decision not to have chemotherapy treatments affect Sarah? What barriers to communication between them might be present?

OBSERVING CAREFULLY

In the fast-paced world of medicine, sometimes nonverbal signals sent by patients that play a critical role in their care are missed. If the patient hesitates when speaking, it may be an indication that he or she has more to say. As mentioned previously, the inability to look a person directly in the eyes sometimes, but not always, indicates deception. The medical assistant must pay close attention to what is seen as well as what is heard when communicating with the patient. Look into the patient's eyes, and watch intently for signs of trouble.

When a patient cries, the medical assistant should always question what is causing the tears. Some patients may refuse to discuss the issue or insist that nothing is wrong, but tears are always a sign of some emotion, whether it is anger, frustration, fear, pain, or some other concern. It is unwise to allow patients who are obviously emotionally upset to leave the office without reasonable assurance that they are going to be safe. The medical assistant might wish to suggest that a friend come to the office and escort the patient home. On rare occasions, it is better to be firm with the patient and insist on help getting home if he or she is in a **volatile** state. This action may save the patient from being hurt or hurting someone else. Careful observation of the patient as a whole is worth the time investment and may even save the patient's life.

DEFENSE MECHANISMS

Anxiety or stress causes the human body to react in many different ways. Some people handle **stressors** more easily than others. Most people use **defense mechanisms** when they feel pressured or attacked in some way. These are often subconscious reactions designed for emotional protection; they help us to deal with whatever difficult event has triggered such a response. Often people may not even realize that they are using these mechanisms and may **vehemently** deny that they do so. Many types of defense mechanisms exist, and the medical assistant should be familiar with them to better communicate with patients and others they come into contact with in the course of their duties.

Verbal Aggression

When a person verbally attacks another without addressing the original complaint, or disregards it, he or she is being verbally **aggressive** (Figure 5-6). Such people may attack, or they may change the subject. Some individuals get very angry at any suggestion of wrongdoing. They lash out, usually quite loudly, and attack back quickly in hopes of diminishing their role in any wrongdoing.

"When are you going to clean the drug sample closet?"

"Who are you to ask me that? You haven't finished your duties today, either!"

Sarcasm

This word has its origin in the Greek *sarkasmos*, which means "to tear flesh" or "to bite the lips in rage." This is quite an accurate definition of the nature of sarcasm. It is a biting edge added to

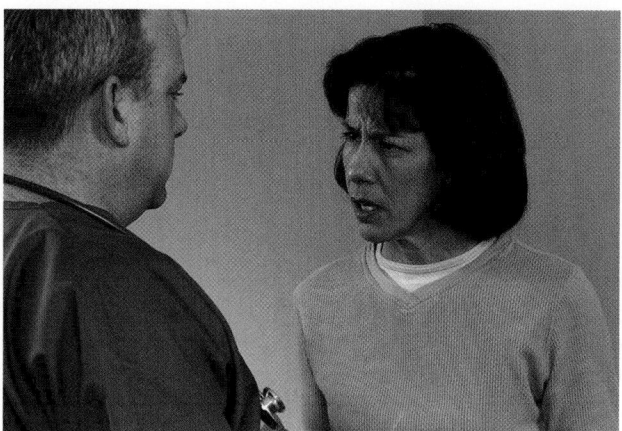

FIGURE 5-6 Remain calm even if a patient becomes verbally aggressive, and attempt to calm him or her by listening and expressing empathy whenever possible.

words that a person states with the intent to cause pain or anger. Sarcasm is hostile and cruel in most cases, and some individuals use it constantly, thinking that it is quite witty. On the contrary, it often makes bitter enemies of its victims.

"Of course it's a nice dress, if you like tents."

Rationalization

Rationalizing is attributing actions to rational and credible motives without analyzing underlying methods. When people rationalize their behavior, they are offering excuses for what has been done or said and trying to convince others that the behavior was completely justified.

"He only hits me because he is stressed at work."

Compensation

A person who compensates makes up for one behavior by stressing another. Compensation is a psychologic mechanism through which feelings of inferiority, frustration, or failure in one area are counterbalanced by achievement in another. Compensation is not always a negative response, but it is often used as an excuse for not accomplishing what should be accomplished.

"I know I gained 5 pounds, Dr. George, but I exercised three times last week."

Regression

Regression is the reversion to an earlier mental or behavioral level. Some people regress to a childlike state or period or exhibit qualities inherent to an earlier time in life. This can include making excuses for not doing a certain thing, saying that it cannot be done, instead of the truth, which is that the person does not want to do it. Replacing the word "can't" with "won't" is a good gauge of using regression.

"I'd like to get better grades, but I can't find time to study."

Repression

The process whereby unwanted desires or impulses are excluded from the consciousness and left to operate in the unconscious is called *repression*. Blocking a problem out of the mind, or changing the subject when it is mentioned, are both types of repression. The repressed urges or desires may seethe beneath the surface, absorbing energy, and force the continual repression of the desires, which takes more and more concentration to do successfully.

"I should phone my brother since we fought, but I just can't deal with that now."

Apathy

Apathy is a lack of feeling, emotion, interest, or concern. It is an indifference to what is happening or a pretense of not caring about a situation. Usually, apathy is not a true reflection of the inner feeling. It is a defense mechanism that is similar to repression, but with a more flippant attitude.

"I don't care what grade I got on the test, because I am not going to pass the class anyway."

Displacement

Displacement is the redirection of an emotion or impulse from its original object, such as an idea or person, to another object. When challenged or attacked by one person or event, displacement is used to channel negative feelings to some other area, which gives a false sense of control over issues that may not be controllable. The venting of hostile feelings is directed somewhere other than where it should be directed, but usually this is a result of a lack of confidence in addressing the true issues at hand.

"I have enough problems at work and don't need to come home to a nagging wife!"

Denial

Denial is a psychologic defense mechanism in which confrontation with a personal problem or with reality is avoided by denying the existence of the problem or reality. This is where the common expression, "He's in denial" originates. For whatever reason, the individual is unable to cope with the stress of a situation and completely pushes it or any person or thing representing it away.

"My husband can't have cancer. He is completely healthy."

Physical Avoidance

Some events are so painful for people that they completely avoid any representation of the event. This could be a person, a place, an object, or just about anything that serves as a reminder of the event that induces the negative feelings. If the problem is a person, that person may be avoided forever. If it is a place, such as a home that a couple lived in before one of them died, the other person may physically move. In some cases, such as physical abuse, the avoidance may be necessary, but it can also be quite unhealthy and may need to be explored further through therapy.

"I will never go to that restaurant again, because that is where my ex-husband told me he wanted a divorce."

Projection

Projection as a defense mechanism is the attribution of one's own ideas, feelings, or attitudes to other people or to objects. This especially includes the **externalization** of blame, guilt, or responsibility as a defense against anxiety. Some people project their feelings about a certain thing onto others, who may not be affected by the negative connotations the first person feels. Projection is a way to avoid dealing with the root issues of a problem.

"Everyone else is always late, so why am I getting reprimanded for it?"

DEALING WITH CONFLICT

Conflict is defined as the struggle resulting from incompatible or opposing needs, drives, wishes, or external or internal demands. We deal with conflict in our lives in some capacity almost daily. Knowing how to recognize the signs of conflict and what patterns people use to deal with conflict will be of great benefit to the medical assistant. This will enable the professional to be understanding and empathetic to patients, co-workers, supervisors, and others in the day-to-day work environment.

Conflict is not always negative; sometimes it is beneficial to relationships. It can be constructive and allow people to learn more about each other. This may promote a stronger understanding and deeper levels of intimacy. Unless both parties are aware that a problem exists between them, no conflict exists. The conflict begins when both realize there is a problem that needs resolution. People handle conflict in different ways. Some avoid it at all costs, and on the other end of the spectrum, some seem to thrive on conflict.

In order to understand the thought processes of others and how best to respond to them, as well as discerning how others respond, it is helpful to define some of the many types of conflict. Of itself, assertion is not conflict; assertion is stating or declaring positively, often forcefully or aggressively. Being assertive or aggressive can be very productive. Assertive people often receive job promotions and reach the goals they set for their lives. Too much aggression can make a person seem pushy, so it should be controlled and used at the appropriate times. Remember, there is a difference between assertion and aggression, which will be discussed in the following paragraphs.

Nonassertion is the inability to express needs and thoughts or the refusal to express them. Some avoid conflict and some accommodate by putting others' desires before their own. Sometimes nonassertion is justifiable. Anyone who has been involved in a long-term relationship realizes that there will be occasions when the other person's needs must come first. Many have learned the truth of the old saying, "Choose your battles wisely."

CRITICAL THINKING APPLICATION

- Why might Mrs. Cloyd and Sarah experience conflict at this stage in their lives?
- How might each deal better with disagreements, especially regarding Mrs. Cloyd's decisions about her medical care?

Aggression is defined in several ways. It can be a hostile, injurious, or destructive behavior or outlook, especially when caused by frustration. It is also the practice of making attacks or **encroachments,** especially if the acts are unprovoked. In the realm of psychologic studies, there are different types of aggression. Direct aggression occurs when a person directly attacks another, whether by criticism, **malediction,** ridiculing, or other methods. This behavior causes the victim to feel embarrassment, shame, anger, or a range of other emotions. *Passive aggression* is a familiar term, but many may not know its definition. A passive-aggressive person expresses himself or herself in an obscure, **ambiguous** way. People who experience passive aggression may have feelings of rage, inadequacy, or resentment that they cannot articulate in a direct manner. Unfortunately, this behavior usually will not provide the results that are needed or expected.

The Crazymakers: Passive-Aggressive Communications

In the book *Looking Out, Looking In: Interpersonal Communication* by Ronald B. Adler and Neil Towne, the concept of "Crazy-makers" is discussed and credited to George Bach. Bach was a psychologist who developed the theory of creative aggression; he nicknamed this passive-aggressive behavior *crazymaking*. He said that two types of aggression exist: clean fighting and dirty fighting. Crazymaking was his name for dirty fighting, which is a detrimental behavior for all involved. The term *partner* is loosely used to indicate the opposite side or victim of the crazymaker.

Following are brief descriptions of the characteristic types of passive-aggressive persons described by Bach.

The Avoider

Avoiders refuse to fight. When a conflict arises, they leave, fall asleep, pretend to be busy at work, or keep from facing the problem in some other way. This behavior makes it difficult for the partner to express feelings of anger and hurt, because the avoider will not fight back.

The Pseudoaccommodator

Pseudoaccommodators refuse to face up to a conflict either by giving in or pretending nothing is wrong. This drives the partner crazy, because the partner definitely feels there is a problem, and causes feelings of guilt and resentment toward the accommodator for bringing the situation up for discussion in the first place.

The Guiltmaker

Instead of saying straight out that they don't want or don't approve of something, guiltmakers try to make their partners feel responsible for causing pain. A guiltmaker's favorite line is, "It's OK, don't worry about me…," followed by a long sigh.

The Subject Changer

Really an avoider, the subject changer escapes facing up to aggression by shifting the conversation whenever it approaches an area of conflict. Because of their tactics, subject changers and their partners never have the chance to explore their problems and do something about them.

The Distracter

Rather than come out and express their feelings about an object of dissatisfaction, distracters attack other parts of their partners' lives. Thus they never have to share what is really on their minds and can avoid dealing with painful parts of their relationships.

The Mind Reader

Instead of allowing their partners to express feelings honestly, mind readers go into character analysis, explaining what the other person really means or what is wrong with the other person. By behaving this way, mind readers refuse to handle their own feelings and leave no room for their partners to express themselves.

The Trapper

Trappers play an especially dirty trick by setting up a desired behavior for their partners; then, when the behavior is manifested, they attack the very thing they requested. An example of this technique is for the trapper to say, "Let's be totally honest with each other," then attack the partner's words of honesty.

The Crisis Tickler

Crisis ticklers bring what is bothering them almost to the surface but never quite express their true feelings. Instead of admitting concern about the finances, they innocently ask, "Gee, how much did that cost?" dropping a rather obvious hint but never really dealing with the crisis.

The Gunnysacker

Gunnysackers do not respond immediately when angry. Instead, they put their resentment into a gunnysack, which after a while begins to bulge with both large and small gripes. Then, when the sack is about to burst, the gunnysacker pours out all the pent-up aggressions on the overwhelmed and unsuspecting partner.

The Trivial Tyrannizer

Instead of honestly sharing their resentments, trivial tyrannizers do things they know will bother their partners—leaving dirty dishes in the sink, clipping fingernails in bed, belching out loud, turning up the television too loud, and so on.

The Beltliner

Everyone has a psychologic "beltline," and below it are subjects too sensitive to be approached without damaging the relationship. Beltlines may have to do with physical characteristics, intelligence, past behavior, or deeply ingrained personality traits a person is trying to overcome. In an attempt to "get even" or hurt their partners, beltliners will use intimate knowledge to hit below the belt, where they know it will hurt.

The Joker

Because they are afraid to face conflicts squarely, jokers kid around when their partners want to be serious, thus blocking the expression of important feelings.

The Blamer

Blamers are more interested in finding fault than in resolving a conflict. Needless to say, they usually do not blame themselves. Blaming behavior almost never resolves a conflict and is an almost sure-fire way to make receivers defensive.

The Contract Tyrannizer

Contract tyrannizers will not allow their relationships to change from the way they once were. Whatever the agreements the partners had for roles and responsibilities at one time, they will remain unchanged.

The Kitchen Sink Fighter

Kitchen sink fighters are so named because in an argument they bring up things that are totally off the subject—as in everything, including the kitchen sink. Perhaps it is the way the other person behaved last New Year's Eve, or bad breath, or the unbalanced checkbook; any past imperfection is fair game for picking a fight.

The Withholder

Instead of expressing their anger honestly and directly, withholders punish their partners by holding something back—courtesy, affection, good cooking, humor, sex. Such withholding is likely to build up even greater resentments in the relationship.

The Benedict Arnold

Benedict Arnolds get back at their partners by sabotage, by failing to defend them from attackers, and even by encouraging ridicule or disregard from outside the relationship.

BARRIERS TO COMMUNICATION

Physical Impairment

Patients may have physical troubles that impair their ability to communicate effectively. This could be a vision or hearing problem, or one of many other conditions that makes communicating a bit more difficult than usual. The medical assistant should use more descriptive language when speaking with the patient who has a visual disturbance. This helps the patient to "see" what is being discussed. The person with diminished hearing may be very sensitive and in denial of the condition. Be certain that you have his or her attention and that you are face to face with the person while speaking. People who are hearing impaired are often very dependent on lip reading for comprehension. Being elderly is not an impairment at all. Many older patients are physically fit and mentally sharp and do not expect special treatment. Never increase the volume of your speech in an assumption that an older patient is hard of hearing. Some physicians make a note in the patient's medical record that indicates the patient has a hearing problem or other impairment, similar to notations about patient allergies. With such notations in an easily noticeable place, everybody that handles the record will know about the impairment and take proper measures to adapt.

CRITICAL THINKING APPLICATION

- What must be considered when communicating verbally with Mrs. Cloyd? With Sarah?
- How can the medical assistant show compassion to a terminally ill patient during her appointment when the office is extremely busy?

Language

With non–English-speaking patients the medical assistant may need to use gestures and more body language to convey messages. In such cases, be alert to the possibility of misunderstandings. Confirm that the message being sent is the message that the listener received by asking for feedback. Ask the listener to repeat the message, and if family members are present, be sure they have a good understanding of what is being communicated as well.

It is always helpful to have a bilingual staff member so that there is less chance of miscommunication with those who speak a different language (Figure 5-7). Many regions offer bilingual classes for medical professionals to assist them with basic communications with their patients. The medical assistant will find it well worth the time and financial investment to investigate such classes, because bilingual employees are quite valuable to the physician and may be able to command a higher salary.

Prejudice

Personal and social bias, or prejudice, brings about discrimination. *Discrimination* is a word that is used to describe unfair

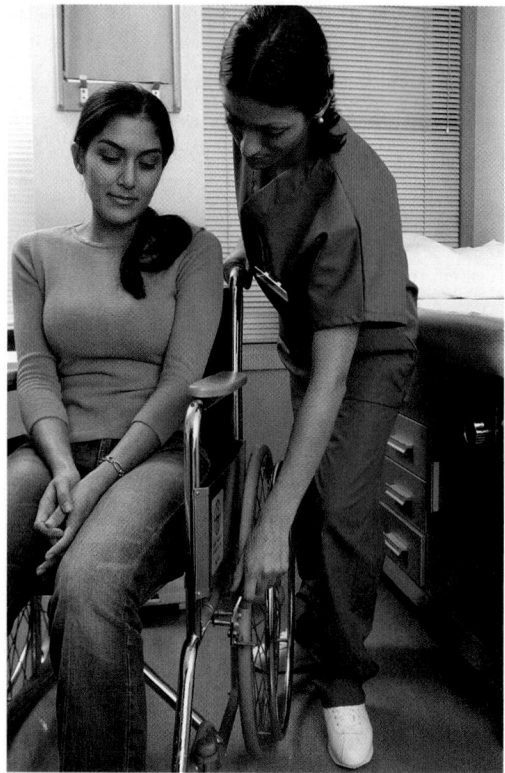

FIGURE 5-7 Bilingual staff members are valuable in ensuring accurate communications with patients who speak a different language.

treatment of a person because of race, gender, religious affiliation, or handicap, or for any other reason. Discrimination is unethical, morally and socially wrong, and in many situations illegal. It also prevents us from communicating effectively.

Some discrimination is very **subtle;** it is not expressed openly or in a blatant manner. Subtle discrimination is based on a person's appearance, values, lifestyle, or some other personal factor. Examples include discrimination against those who are obese, divorced individuals, homosexuals, welfare recipients, or those with sexually transmitted diseases. Sometimes we are not aware that our words or actions reflect subtle discrimination against others.

Personal prejudices must be recognized before one can change them. Medical professionals are exposed to a wide variety of persons who need excellent medical care. The professional cannot allow personal prejudice to affect the care of any individual. Everyone has the right to be honored as a human being and treated respectfully. This enforces the Golden Rule: treating others as you would wish to be treated. Realize the worth of each individual person, and allow that attitude to reflect in all of the actions taken with a patient.

Stereotyping

Stereotyping is defined as the application of a standardized mental picture that is held in common by members of a group and that represents an oversimplified opinion, prejudiced attitude, or uncritical judgment. It is unfair to **stereotype** anyone or categorize him or her based on preconceived, often incorrect, assumptions. Although sometimes there is a degree of truth to the assumption based on stereotypic categories, people should not be judged before there has been an opportunity to get to know them as individuals. The medical assistant should push preconceived notions aside and look at the individual when forming and building a relationship. In the medical profession, stereotypic categories should not be considered when caring for patients and developing good rapport with them.

Perception

Perhaps one of the most important issues to consider when discussing barriers to communication is the concept of perception. Perception means the capacity for comprehension, or the discernment of what is being communicated, according to the message receiver's point of reference. When we discussed the transactional communication model earlier in the chapter, it was obvious that because of different types of noise and channels, there would be times that the message sent would be distorted; the receiver would not always get the message that the sender meant to send. The receiver's perceptions could completely alter the message, no matter how clearly it was sent. If the receiver believes that all attorneys are corrupt, he or she will probably be unable to get past this perception when speaking with one and therefore may not be able to trust any attorney.

Often our perceptions stem from some experience that happened in the past with a certain group of people. This perception goes unresolved or has affected us so strongly that we group all people from that walk of life into a negative category. This is an unfair way to deal with people; everyone

should be viewed as an individual, not as a part of a stereotypic group. Remember, perception is an individual's point of view, right or wrong. The issue of interpretation also plays a role—the determination of what is meant by a certain message. There must be an attempt to understand both points of view and a willingness to discuss them calmly, even when discussing subjects that cause anger. Most people do not truly enjoy conflict. Have a healthy respect for others' opinions. The differences among individuals are part of what makes each of us unique.

COMMUNICATION DURING DIFFICULT TIMES

Communication is not an art that comes easily to everyone. It is often difficult to express feelings in an honest and open way. When a crisis occurs, it is much harder to communicate effectively and we sometimes say things that we do not mean. The medical assistant must develop communication skills that can be used in times of trouble. There must be an understanding of why a patient or co-worker is unable to communicate.

Patience is important, too, because people are not always at their best when they are concerned about their condition or that of a loved one. Always remain calm when dealing with a person who is experiencing a traumatic event or has any depressive condition. Remember that he or she may be reacting to many emotions—fear, anger, doubt, inadequacy, or many others. The key is to listen and determine the best way to help the patient out of any immediate danger and help him or her establish some type of support system.

Anger

One of the most difficult times to communicate is when we are angry. Anger is a normal emotion that all of us feel at one time or another. Usually the expression of anger is a healthy thing. Some people bottle up their emotions and do not express what they truly feel inside. If this is done repeatedly, at some point the anger will erupt, possibly over a tiny event or at an inappropriate time. Others explode over every little situation, and people who do this need anger management skills and training.

Anger, like most emotions, can cause physiologic changes. When a person feels anger, the blood pressure rises and the heart rate increases. Many things can trigger anger, from a simple traffic backup to a real or perceived betrayal, the diagnosis of a disease, or the death of a close relative. "Road rage" is one example of anger out of control and is a serious problem on our public highways today. Unexpressed anger can cause or contribute to all types of health problems, including depression and hypertension.

The medical assistant can help to calm an angry patient by speaking calmly and refusing to return the emotion. If the volume is gradually lowered with every sentence spoken, the angry person will have to lower the volume as well to hear what the assistant is saying. Suggest that the person breathe deeply and stop talking for a few minutes. Remember that the anger that is being expressed is usually not directed intentionally toward the medical assistant. Be a good listener and allow the person to speak as long as it is not abusive speech. Using logic with the angry individual may also help. Some will use words such as "never" and "always"; for example, "My wife never balances the checkbook!" or "You always make me wait for my appointment!" These statements are broad generalizations and usually untrue. Using a logical approach and maintaining a calm attitude will help the angry individual.

Address the root of the problem, and be willing to admit if the physician's office has made a mistake or contributed to a problem. Do not be afraid to say, "I'm sorry, we made an error." Arguing will never solve the situation and will only increase the intensity of the patient's feelings. Four words that will often disarm an angry person are "Let me help you." There will be times in the career of a medical professional that a patient, a co-worker, or even the physician will lash out, even though the medical assistant is not the cause of the anger. Realize that this is a part of being human, and be as caring and kind as possible. If the anger becomes abusive, either refer the situation to a supervisor or, if that is not possible, tell the patient that you can no longer discuss the situation and offer to schedule an appointment so that the matter can be discussed at a later time. By then, the patient will probably have calmed down and will be able to discuss the situation rationally.

Shock

When an event or a circumstance arises that is especially painful, an individual may experience emotional shock. This may happen when a person has just been told that a family member has been killed in an automobile accident or some other catastrophe has taken place. Many different types of shock occur, but in this chapter, the emotional aspect is discussed. Often the person cannot think or move, and other coping reactions may take place. One person may scream in agony, whereas another may calmly sit down and begin to talk about a completely unrelated subject. The person who appears calm is probably more at risk, because in addition to shock, he or she may be experiencing a denial process. We never really know in advance how we will react to events that are traumatic. Also, our reactions may differ from time to time. What else is happening in a person's life will determine how he or she will be able to cope with a traumatic event.

Never leave a person in emotional shock alone. If the healthcare professional cannot stay close by, arrangements should be made for someone to stay near, especially during the early stages, if at all possible. Because the thought processes the person is experiencing may not be under control, he or she could be a danger to himself or herself or others. People who are in shock have a strong need to get away from the situation they have found themselves in. They may try to literally run away, or they may speed off in a car, which compounds the situation. The event does not have to be a life-threatening one, but the patient may perceive it as such. For instance, a teenager who becomes pregnant may not be able to focus on anything except her perception that her life is ruined. As with anger, listening is a good disarming tool for dealing with a person in emotional shock.

The medical assistant should watch for several signs of emotional shock, including hyperactivity, disruptions in breathing patterns, a blank staring, sudden hysterics, and shaking. Humans have an innate sense of threat or danger, and this sense may initiate what psychologists call the "fight or flight" syndrome. When a person feels a threat of some kind, the hormone adrenaline is released in the body quickly, and this hormone promotes an increased heart rate and blood pressure. The oxygen level in the body increases, which prepares the muscles to help the body flee. Awareness is increased, as are energy and performance. The individual either runs, avoiding the danger, which is the "flight" aspect, or stays to "fight," facing the stressors or threat. With either choice, the body must have this increased energy level and awareness to deal with the situation. When the immediate period of shock abates, the individual may feel a debilitating, drained sensation as the hormonal levels return to normal.

CRITICAL THINKING APPLICATION

■ Is it possible that Sarah might experience shock months after her mother's death?

■ How can the medical assistant help Sarah to deal with these emotions?

Death and Dying

Years ago patients who were considered terminally ill were placed in hospital wards and left to their demise. The medical community did not focus on understanding the fears and concerns of the dying, and very few measures that preserved their dignity were offered to them. However, in 1969 a groundbreaking book, *On Death and Dying,* was published by Dr. Elisabeth Kübler-Ross, who studied **thanatology.** Kübler-Ross (Figure 5-8), a Swiss psychiatrist, realized that terminally ill patients were somewhat ignored, even by medical professionals, and she spent many hours interviewing these patients, discovering their fears and concerns. Kübler-Ross listened to them and realized that there were certain stages that patients passed through as they dealt with their impending death. She held seminars during which she interviewed dying patients as medical students listened. When the book was published, she was recognized internationally as an authority on the subject of death. She wrote more than 20 books about the process of dying. In *Life Lessons,* she shares many of the truths she learned from the dying to encourage us to live. Dr. Kübler-Ross died in August 2004.

Kübler-Ross believed that the process of dealing with death or loss has five specific stages. These stages include denial, bargaining, anger, depression, and acceptance. She believed that all people go through each stage in the grieving process, but they may not go through the stages in the same order. A stage could take days to work through or several months. Although she related these stages to dying patients, they are not exclusively limited to those who are dying. Anyone experiencing **grief** may progress through these five stages, and having a good understanding of them will help the medical assistant to better care for the patient.

Denial is the first stage, during which the patient or grieving person denies the issue that is causing the grief and thinks,

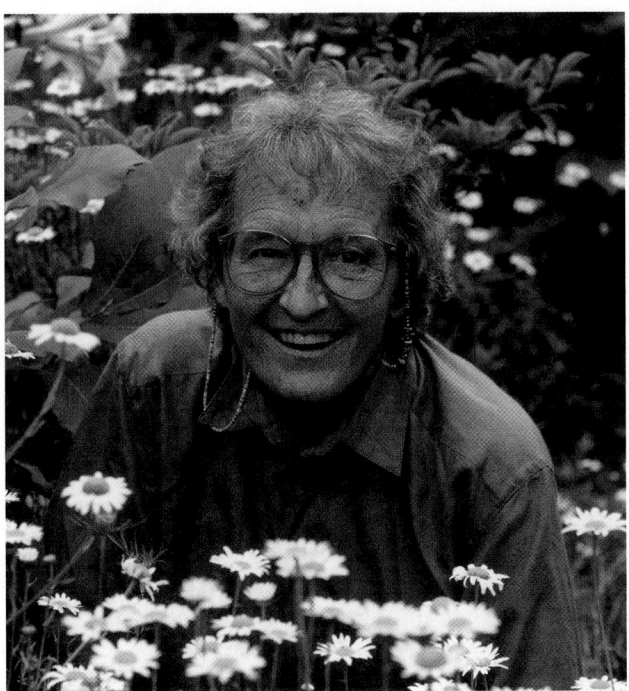

FIGURE 5-8 Dr. Elisabeth Kübler-Ross is the author of more than 20 books, many of which deal with the subject of death and dying, and is considered an international authority on the stages of grief. Dr. Kübler-Ross died in 2004. (Photograph copyright Kenneth Ross, 1985.)

"No, not me." The person is shocked and rejects the facts. The denial is a defense mechanism that helps the individual to deal with the news. The second stage is anger, when the dying patient begins to ask, "Why me?" The anger is often directed at others, and that may include the people in the family taking care of the patient, or it may include healthcare workers who cannot present a cure. In the third stage the patient begins to bargain in an attempt to postpone death or eliminate it altogether. This bargaining is usually with God, and the patient may pray to see a child marry or to witness some other upcoming event. The event is not the true hope of the patient, but life itself is. These patients say, "Yes, me, but..." in the attempt to postpone death. The fourth stage is depression, and during this stage patients realize that they are going to die and may feel regret for the goals they did not accomplish or for not taking better care of themselves. These patients say, "Yes, it's me..." and they must be allowed this period of grieving. However, family and friends should watch the patient carefully for signs of deep depression. The final stage of grief is acceptance, during which the patient is able to say, "Yes, me, and I'm ready." The reality of the impending death or distressing situation is accepted, and although the patient may continue to experience some depression, he or she is better equipped to deal with the arrangements that have to be made and may even demonstrate good humor during this time.

Patients who are dying must be treated with dignity and respect. This does not mean that they are unable to laugh and enjoy the life they are still living. Gentle touch and kind words will help patients to know the medical assistant cares for them. It is important to be careful with words and phrases around dying patients, but be natural in your conversations with them and do not be afraid to laugh. Never suggest to such patients that you "know how they feel." This phrase belittles their situation, and we never really know how another person feels. Asking questions is a good method of communication when you are not sure what to say. Use questions such as, "How do you feel about that?" or "What does your family think about your plans to discontinue treatment?" Then listen to the patient and make eye contact with him or her as you listen. You may also ask, "How can I help you?" as opposed to "Is there anything I can do?" There will be a natural tendency for the patient to say "No" to the second question. However, if you ask specifically how to help, they may open up and allow you or the office staff to be of help. They may simply need suggestions about who could cut their grass or how to contact Meals on Wheels. Hospice services provide terminally ill patients and their families with care and support, often from the point of diagnosis to bereavement. Many have found hospice services invaluable in the process of coping with a loved one close to death. The medical office should have listings of community resources to assist in these types of situations.

CRITICAL THINKING APPLICATION

- Often people put off writing a will. Could this be procrastination or a fear of death?
- When is it important to have a will?
- How can the medical assistant help Sarah to deal with her mother's impending death?
- What stage of grief might Mrs. Cloyd currently be experiencing? What stage might Sarah be experiencing?

MULTICULTURAL ISSUES

Cultural differences influence the way we deal with those from various parts of the world. We often become isolated in our thinking and incorrectly assume that people all over the world think and do things the same way that we do. However, there are vast differences in cultures from country to country, and even from areas within the same country. In the United States we see a difference between northerners and southerners. The speech of people in New York is significantly different from that of people in south Texas, and the dialect changes again from Texas to the West Coast. We picture Texans with cowboy boots and hats, but that is not how most Texans dress. Some of us still associate Alaska with Eskimos and igloos. Perhaps this stems from the books we read in elementary school, but cultures today are much more widely mixed in the United States, and because many people immigrate to our country for various reasons and opportunities, it is wise to learn a bit more about the cultures and the variety of people who inhabit the world.

We sometimes stereotype people of other cultures and think that we understand what they are like and how they live. Often, some type of **media** has influenced our thinking. There is much to learn from other cultures, and sharing is a way to gain an understanding of the experiences in other places. This helps us to be more well-rounded individuals and to enjoy and appreciate our own cultural differences. Remember that those people who have come to the United States from other countries have to deal with their ideas of both their own homeland and this country as well. There may be significant misconceptions, so in the medical facility, patience will be necessary as explanations are provided. Take extra time and care with patients of other cultures, without assuming they know or understand local culture. Also understand that culture is something that is passed from generation to generation, so many of the ideas people hold dear have been handed down for centuries.

Some people who enter a new country go through a period of what is called "culture shock"—a state of being in unfamiliar surroundings and being away from the things that were present in everyday life in the homeland. Street signs are different; in some cases, people drive on the opposite side of the street. Affected people quickly realize that their "normal" ways of doing things no longer work, and they must make some type of adaptation to survive. This adaptation may mean changing the habits and customs of a lifetime. This can be a very exciting prospect for some, but a very frightening prospect for others. Simple processes, such as enrolling in school, become extremely difficult tasks. Patience is a critical tool to help others adjust to the American way of life.

Examples of Cultural Traditions

- A husband speaks for his wife. The wife does not speak to the physician.
- The palm of the hand, facing down, is used to beckon someone. The hand motion signaling one to come or follow, performed with the back of the hand toward the patient, is used only when calling an animal. An open hand is used to point, rather than one finger.
- A female's clothing is not removed without the presence of another female family member.
- Emotional crying and sobbing denote femininity.
- Going to the doctor is a sign of weakness.
- The female medical assistant never touches the male patient.
- Acquaintances are not permitted to stand within 3 feet of the patient; only immediate family members are permitted to stand within this space.
- The Chinese do not like to be touched by people they do not know.
- The Laotian's "yes" response may not mean "yes," because it is considered rude to say "no" to others or to cause conflict.
- A native of Cambodia, as well as a Laotian, will not look into the eyes of the person being addressed because long eye contact means disrespect and is impolite.
- Cambodians do not like to have their blood drawn because they believe it will weaken them.
- Afghans and Mexicans have a concept of time that is less precise than in the United States.
- Vietnamese consider the head to be a sacred part of the body and are offended by being touched on the head or shoulders. Only the elderly may touch the head of a child without giving offense.

Communicating with People of Other Cultures

People from other cultures want to be treated just as you would like to be treated if you were visiting another country; they wish to be respected and treated fairly. Much can be learned about the background of others, and much can be shared about the culture we know, too. Cultural differences are responsible for many misunderstandings. We must make an attempt to understand people of other walks of life.

When speaking with those from a foreign country, there may be a **language barrier.** Even if the person knows some English, there will be words and phrases that do not make sense in the way that we use them in the United States. A period of time must pass during which the words are heard frequently before they will take on meaning to a person who is unfamiliar with them. It is important to speak a little more slowly than usual to a person whose primary language is not English—not to insinuate they are less intelligent but to give them a chance to absorb the words and mentally translate them into their own language, then prepare a response. There is no need to increase the volume of speech; people from other cultures are not hard of hearing. They merely need a little more time to process the words that are said.

Medical assistants should have an awareness of the nonverbal messages being sent by the persons who are interacting. In our society a simple up-and-down nod of the head means "yes" and a side-to-side shake means "no." However, in Bulgaria and some other countries, these signals have the opposite meaning. It is important to be sensitive to and aware of the beliefs of the many cultures that will be represented in the patient population. If you work in a practice that predominantly serves a distinct ethnic group, discuss possible cultural differences with the physician and with influential people within the cultural group. Learning to understand cultural differences helps you to gain the confidence and respect of patients.

EMOTIONAL AND PHYSICAL NEEDS

Human beings have certain emotional and physical needs that must be met for us to live balanced lives and a healthy existence. Many of us take these needs for granted until they become an absolute necessity; then our focus becomes directed toward meeting them. Few in the United States have faced hunger as those in some Third World countries have, and when hunger is our need, it suddenly becomes our prime concern. This section provides some insight into the needs we have as humans and their role in the total health of the body, mind, and spirit.

Maslow's Hierarchy of Needs

Psychologist Abraham Maslow created what he called the hierarchy of needs (Figure 5-9). A hierarchy is defined as "things arranged in order, rank, or a graded series." Maslow believed that our human needs can be categorized into five levels and that the needs on each level must be satisfied before we can move to the next level. These levels are often depicted as a triangle, with the most basic needs at the bottom and the highest potential for growth as a human being at the top.

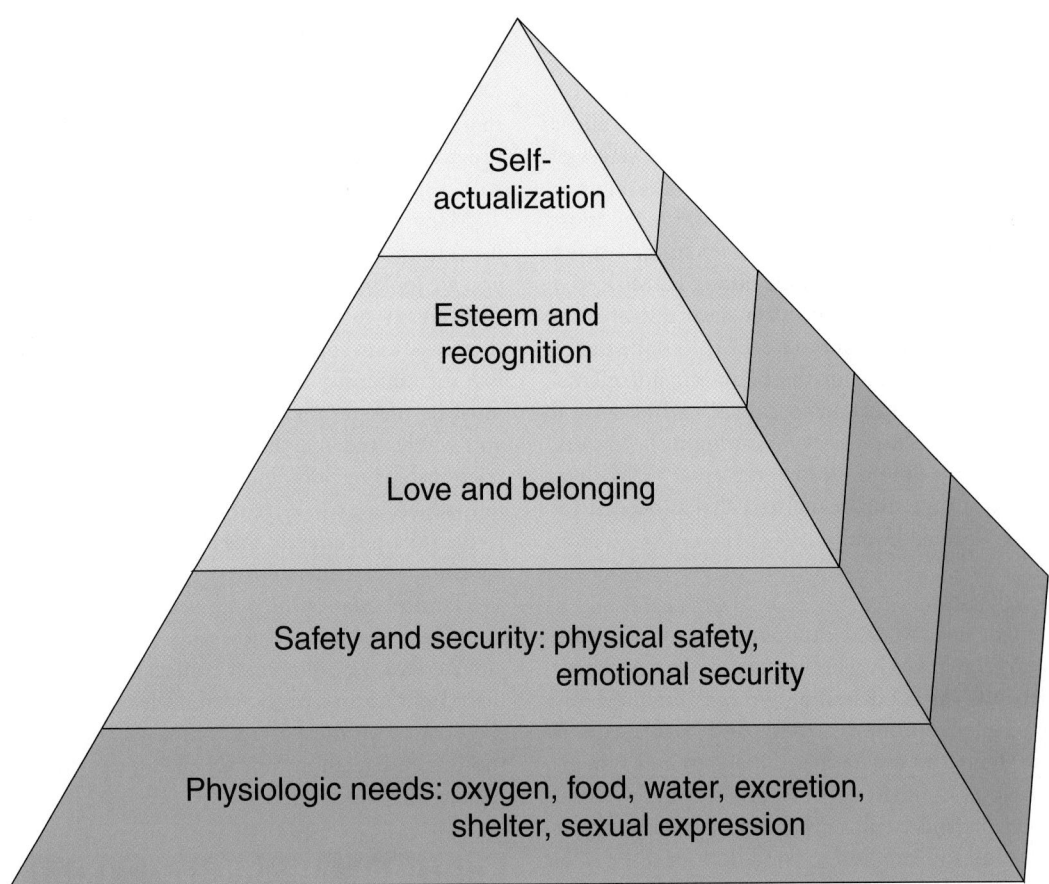

FIGURE 5-9 Maslow's hierarchy of needs. (From Adler RB, Towne N: *Looking out, looking in: interpersonal communication*, San Antonio, 1996, Harcourt Brace.)

The needs we have as humans, at the most basic level, are those that involve our physical well-being. These include food, rest, sleep, water, air, and sex. The second level includes issues related to our safety. We need to feel safe and secure in our homes and our environments, as well as the places where we work. The third level involves our social needs for love, a sense of belonging, and interaction with others. The fourth level relates to our self-esteem. We have an inner need to feel good about ourselves and to know that others view us in a positive manner. The last level is the self-actualization stage, in which we maximize our potential. In this level, we attempt to be at our best and to live our lives to the fullest extent possible.

Approval, Acceptance, and Achievement

Three specific needs that we have, apart from Maslow's hierarchy of needs, are critical to our happiness. These three needs are approval, acceptance, and achievement. Although most would agree that we do not need everyone's approval at all times, there exist specific people whose approval we do seek. Children usually wish to please their parents, even when the child is an adult. We seek to please our supervisors, and even our own children. However, this need to please can be taken too far. Various books address personalities called *pleasers*, who often place their own needs second to the needs of those they feel they must please in order to feel of worth.

We have a healthier self-esteem if we feel accepted by others. This resembles the sense of belonging discussed earlier but is a bit more extensive in nature. A feeling of acceptance includes the belief that our actions, words, dress, mannerisms, and other personality traits are acceptable to others we wish to impress.

Last, we have an inner need for achievement. Most humans want to do something great and contribute to their world in some way. A great thing to one person may be winning an Olympic race, but to another it may be reading to an elderly grandmother at a nursing home. We all enjoy praise for a job well done, or for losing weight, or for passing a difficult examination. It is beneficial to all when legitimate praise is shared freely and appreciated. This is especially true in our close relationships but is just as important in the workplace. It is much easier to work for a supervisor who praises for work well done than for one who never offers a pat on the back.

A Good Night's Sleep

Many of us do not realize the value of our sleep time. Sleep is one of the most important physical needs that we have and is the one most often sacrificed during busy, stressful periods of life. This is called *sleep deprivation*. Human beings need approximately 8 hours of sleep each night, although many can function for a period of time with less sleep. Eventually this lack of sleep will take a physical and emotional toll on the body.

The two main phases of sleep are non–rapid eye movement (NREM) and rapid eye movement (REM). During NREM sleep the eyes are fairly still and the body relaxes and slows down. There are four stages of NREM, which progress into a deeper sleep. After the body moves through the four stages of NREM, it enters REM sleep. During REM sleep the brain is highly active and the eyes move rapidly. Breathing is more irregular, and most people experience REM sleep in the last few hours of the sleep cycle. Dreaming occurs during REM sleep.

Many professionals who study and treat sleep disturbances agree that if an individual does not reach REM sleep, he or she will have provided physical rest for the body but not mental rest. This rest is critical in stress management, and because it occurs at the end of most sleep cycles, or during its last hours, those who cut their sleep time short may not enter REM sleep often. Thus they do not get the mental rest that is needed for them to perform at optimal levels.

Healthy Nutrition

We have been taught since we were children that good nutrition is vital to healthy bodies. Our bodies are machines whose performance depends on good health. We care for the body with a balance of good nutrition, activity, and health care. A balanced diet is essential to ensure that the organs and systems within us function at optimal levels. When the body is not receiving the nutrients and vitamins that it needs, various parts may malfunction, and this can lead to conditions or diseases or a worsening of the problems already present.

In today's diet-conscious society, some people attempt to lose weight by eating less food or cutting out meals altogether. This is a dangerous practice. Losing weight quickly through fad diets and "miracle" supplements is usually a guarantee that the weight will eventually return.

One should always begin weight loss programs under the advice and care of a physician. Do not skip meals in an effort to lose weight, and do choose foods from the four basic food groups. Avoid unhealthy snacks and sodas, and drink at least 8 to 10 glasses of water every day. Exercise regularly and take walks to provide cardiovascular benefits to the body. If you take good care of your body, the chances are increased that it will function properly for a longer period of time, resulting in a longer, healthier lifetime to enjoy to the fullest.

CRITICAL THINKING APPLICATION

- Could Sarah's sleep and nutrition habits affect her ability to care for her mother?
- How might these affect Sarah's personal stress levels, and how can she ensure that she is caring for herself, when her thoughts are primarily on her mother?

Positive Relationships

As mentioned earlier in this chapter, all of us need to feel approval, acceptance, and achievement. This is a vital component within our relationships as well. When we are involved in a relationship that is not going well, it will naturally reflect in our attitude, our opinions, and our sense of self-esteem. This can greatly influence our performance at work. Often, because of infatuation, we find ourselves in a situation that might not be a positive one. Once the relationship is in progress, it is sometimes hard to end it and find a connection with a supportive, caring individual.

Many individuals really have not determined what they need from a relationship. It is helpful to make a list of what you are looking for in a partner and commit not to compromise with regard to the critical points on the list. The sparks and fireworks that appear in the beginning of a relationship may lose their intensity as time goes on, and a firm foundational base must be present after the newness wears off. Choose carefully and wisely, and the chances of becoming involved in healthy relationships greatly increase. In addition, more and more individuals are choosing to remain single and are enjoying life to the fullest. Certainly this choice is better than being a part of a destructive partnership.

Harmful relationships are not always just between partners. Often we experience stress and strain with relatives, friends, and co-workers. Sometimes contact with the person causing the discontent cannot be avoided, at least for a period of time. In these cases we must learn coping techniques for dealing with the difficult relationship. Open, honest communication is of paramount importance.

CRITICAL THINKING APPLICATION

- Often survivors feel a sense of "unfinished business" with a person who has died, and have a more difficult time bringing closure to the relationship. How might Sarah spend high-quality time with her mother and come to terms with her death in a positive way?
- Is there anything that should not be discussed with a terminally ill patient?

Healthy Self-Esteem

Self-esteem is a confidence and satisfaction in oneself. To have high self-esteem, an individual must also be self-aware, and that takes some honesty. It means taking a look at your strengths and your weaknesses and knowing what you have to offer as a person. To feel well and accomplish goals in life, you must develop positive attitudes and positive responses to the pressures in life. It can sometimes be difficult to keep a positive attitude when others are being negative. Some people believe that if they inflict their bad feelings on others, they will feel better about themselves. It is important to remember, though, that no one can make you feel a certain way; it is a choice that you make. Blaming others for one's situation in life or negative emotions is self-defeating.

We are able to control two things in life—our attitude and our actions. Even when faced with a potentially volatile situation, our attitude and reactions are decisions that we make. These decisions should be made with careful thought, even if the reaction must be a swift one. Think before speaking. Pause a moment if needed, before reacting. Take a time out. Choose your battles wisely. All of these suggestions will help you to react in a more positive, constructive way when faced with a difficult situation.

Improving Yourself

No matter how great the training or how many opportunities are placed in front of a person, fear and doubt can sabotage efforts to improve the self-image, confidence, and potential of an individual. Almost every failure or mistake experienced can be traced to fear or doubt; either we are afraid to take a specific action or we doubt our own abilities. Blaming the circumstances around us is no excuse for a poor performance. It is also important to remember that small, daily decisions make a huge impact on our lives, sometimes even more than what we consider critical life decisions. For example, a student decides not to study for 30 minutes daily for an upcoming major examination, then fails it. This small decision to do something other than study results in failing an examination, which may force course repetition and delay the graduation date.

Self-esteem will improve if a person is able to adapt to situations well. To be human is to be a changing, growing, imperfect, but amazing living creation. Adapting means being flexible and open to the actions of others. Although we should have empathy for others, we cannot allow others to ruin our day or lower our confidence level. Inventor-philanthropist Charles Kettering once said, "The only time you can't afford to fail is the last time you try." Our failures often teach us much more than our successes. The important thing is to get up, evaluate why the failure occurred, then move forward armed with the new knowledge gained from mistakes.

Procrastination is often a symptom of the fear of failure and the fear of success. Many people procrastinate because they feel it will give them an excuse for their failure. They say, "There is no way I could pass that test—I only had 2 days to study!" Others are perfectionists and put off doing a job or delegating because they feel no one can do it as well as they can. The best way to stop procrastinating is to do something! Divide projects into small steps and complete one at a time. This makes tasks much less overwhelming.

The self-improvement process is ongoing. Periodically stop and evaluate where you stand in relation to the goals you have set for your life. Set goals—short- and long-term goals—for all of the areas of life, including career, relationships, and personal growth. Write the goals down; make them specific and measurable. Be sure that the goals are reasonable. Start with smaller, short-term goals and work toward long-term goals. Be persistent and never give up. Post a list of them on the refrigerator, and note progress. Do not count on having a whole lifetime to pursue goals; instead, move toward them consistently and enthusiastically.

Comfort Zones

We all have comfort zones. When faced with new ideas or changes, many of us tend to be a bit unsure of ourselves. Think back to the first day at school, the first day on a new job, the first time going to a fancy restaurant, a first date—these events often make us feel a bit uncomfortable. New experiences may be outside of our **comfort zone.** Psychologists often speak about a comfort zone, which is a place in the mind where we feel safe and comfortable, where we can perform comfortably and confidently. Most goals, however, require movement outside the comfort zone to reach them. Striving to reach a goal means trying new things, and this can be quite stressful. Because we do not want to become so stressed that we give up on our goals, we should take slow, small steps that are challenging, then move to the next step. Procrastination is a failure concept, but it can be overcome through dedication and consistent planning. Remember, too, that patients are usually outside of their comfort zones while visiting the physician's office. Do everything possible to make them feel at home and comfortable.

CLOSING COMMENTS

Interpersonal skills are critically important to the successful medical assistant. Communication will be a part of all interactions throughout the day, and the better developed these skills are, the better the medical assistant will be able to serve the patients in the facility. Every attempt should be made to enhance the interpersonal and human relations skills that the medical assistant currently has and to strive to better these skills continually. This will ensure that effective communication will be a part of the relationship with patients as well as others with whom the medical assistant interacts.

SUMMARY OF SCENARIO

Mrs. Cloyd and her daughter are facing a difficult time. Death is inevitable for everyone, but when a loved one is diagnosed with a terminal illness, it is particularly distressing. Both of these women need compassion and caring from the medical team. They will need to feel as if they are being heard and that their opinions are important. Some of their needs are similar, but they have differing needs as well. A gentle touch and laughter will brighten their day, and these expressions are critical to a person experiencing the stress of a devastating illness.

The medical assistant must ensure that Mrs. Cloyd understands her medications and treatments. The office should assist her and her daughter in finding community resources for which she might be eligible. Be sure to instruct Mrs. Cloyd primarily, and make certain that Sarah also understands any directions her mother should follow. Sarah will need compassion as she deals with her mother's illness and impending death. Because she is also a patient of the clinic, she should be given care and attention and may have emotional needs or periods of great stress also. Even on the busiest of days, these two women deserve warmth from the staff and should be made as comfortable as possible as they seek medical care.

Although the medical office is always a busy place, the medical assistant can take a moment to individualize the care that they provide to patients. Looking into the patients' eyes and genuinely asking how they have been getting along demonstrates interest in them. Call patients by their name and ask about their families. These techniques allow the medical assistant to develop rapport, which will result in a more pleasant office visit for the patient.

Often, the patient will be accompanied by a relative or friend, and the medical assistant may find it necessary to interact with these individuals. Remember that all information about the patient must be kept in strict confidence. Friends and family play a role in the overall health of the patient. When relations are strained, patients may feel depressed and stressed. This can affect their health in a negative way. The patient with strong family support will often heal faster and have a better outlook toward their health issues.

Listening is a skill that must be practiced and refined. The patient needs to know that the medical assistant is focusing attention on him or her, hearing their concerns and paraphrasing to make certain that the patient is understood correctly. Listening is one of the most important skills that the medical assistant can develop.

SUMMARY of LEARNING OBJECTIVES

1. Define, spell, and pronounce the terms listed in the vocabulary.
   - Spelling and pronouncing medical terms correctly adds credibility to the medical assistant. Knowing the definition of these terms promotes confidence in communication with patients and co-workers.

2. Explain why first impressions are critically important.
   - First impressions are critical in the medical profession. Dress, attitude, and appearance all influence the credibility of the medical assistant. The medical assistant should always treat patients and visitors to the office as individuals who deserve the best in customer service.

3. Differentiate between verbal and nonverbal communication.
   - Verbal communication depends on words and sound, whereas nonverbal communication consists of messages that are conveyed to another without the use of words. Body language, eye contact, facial expressions, and hand gestures are some of the many ways we use body language. Sometimes our body language conflicts with verbal communication, and a mixed signal is sent to the receiver. Often we are unaware of nonverbal signals and notice only a small number of the signals that other people send.

4. Explain the different levels of spatial separation.
   - Spatial separation can be defined as the space of comfort between individuals. Public space is usually considered to be

12 to 25 feet, whereas social space is approximately 4 to 12 feet. Personal space is the range of $1\frac{1}{2}$ to 4 feet, and intimate space would include touching up to approximately $1\frac{1}{2}$ feet.

5. Discuss the value of touch in the communication process.
   - Touch is important in the process of communication because it projects an air of care and compassion to the receiver. The medical assistant should never be afraid to touch patients, as long as precautions are taken with those who are contagious. Touching the patient shows empathy and often can be more eloquent than the spoken word.

6. Describe the elements of the transactional communication model.
   - The transactional communication model includes a sender and a receiver who both offer messages to each other using various channels. The sender encodes a message, then the receiver decodes it, to the best of his or her ability. Often some type of noise interferes as well, such as internal, external, and physiologic noise. Perception is important when communicating because messages are sometimes easily misinterpreted.

7. Explain some of the barriers to effective communication.
   - Some of the barriers to communication include physical impairment, language differences, prejudice, stereotyping, and perception. Barriers may also be present during difficult times, such as when a crisis occurs, when a person is angry or

Continued

SUMMARY of LEARNING OBJECTIVES
Continued

in shock, or when a patient or family member is experiencing an impending death or illness or has experienced a serious accident.

8. List and explain the levels of Maslow's hierarchy of needs.
   - Maslow's hierarchy of needs includes five levels, beginning with our most basic needs, such as food, rest, sleep, water, and anything that involves our physical well-being. The second level is related to safety issues, and the third, our social needs, such as love and interaction with others. The fourth level deals with our self-esteem, and the fifth is self-actualization, where our potential is maximized.

9. Discuss defense mechanisms, and be able to recognize commonly used defense mechanisms.
   - Defense mechanisms are psychologic methods of dealing with stressful situations and include sarcasm, denial, repression, compensation, and several others. Often these mechanisms are our only way of dealing with circumstances that are difficult to cope with.

10. Describe the value of listening.
   - Listening is one of the most important skills the medical assistant can possess. Listening involves not only silence, but active feedback as well. Open-ended questions help the medical assistant to restate what the patient is saying, to be sure that the patient is understood clearly.

11. List several ways to deal with conflict.
   - Everyone experiences conflict in daily living, so it is necessary to develop skills in dealing with conflict in as positive a way as possible. Conflict is not always negative and can be quite beneficial to relationships. Knowing the different types of conflict, as well as how people attempt to process conflict, will help the medical assistant to recognize patterns and respond appropriately. Some individuals deal with conflict by being aggressive, assertive, or nonassertive. There are also many passive-aggressive methods of dealing with conflict, such as avoidance, changing the subject, distraction, blaming, and several others.

12. Explain the stages that patients go through when facing death.
   - Elisabeth Kübler-Ross suggests that there are five stages to the process of grief: denial, bargaining, anger, depression, and acceptance. She believes that all stages are experienced while grieving, but not necessarily in the same order. The medical assistant can better care for the patient and the patient's loved ones when a good understanding of the grieving process is present.

13. Discuss why physical and emotional needs affect our daily performance at work.
   - Everyone needs physical and emotional rest to function throughout the day. A good night's sleep, consisting of at least 8 hours, regular exercise, and healthy nutrition will help to keep the medical assistant fit for duty. When these needs are not being met, work performance may suffer and the medical assistant may not be able to give proper attention and care to the patients. Exhaustion will affect the ability to perform, as will pressing concerns that linger in the mind. Make every effort to clear all negative thoughts and completely focus on the patients.

CONNECTIONS

Study Guide Connection: Go to Chapter 5 Study Guide. Read the Case Study and Workplace Applications and complete the assignments. Do online research for answers to the questions in the Internet Activities associated with interpersonal skills and human behavior.

CD Connection: Go to the Medical Assisting Competency Challenge CD and do the training activities under Communication.

Evolve Connection: For more information related to interpersonal skills and human behavior, go to evolve.elsevier.com/kinn and visit related weblinks for Chapter 5. Click on the Medical Assisting Exam Review and do the practice questions to sharpen your test-taking skills.

Medicine and Ethics

6

SCENARIO

Monica Johnson has been employed for 6 months as a medical assistant in a family practice. She works as the clinical medical assistant for Dr. Richard Wray. One of Dr. Wray's patients, Anna Walsh, recently adopted a baby after 8 years of trying to conceive a child. The baby, Delaney Gracelia, was born to a single mother, Susan, who participated in an open adoption in which she and the Walshes met and got to know each other during her pregnancy. Susan dated the baby's father for about 6 months before discovering that she was pregnant, and they are no longer dating. Susan wanted to make a good decision for the baby and decided to place her for adoption.

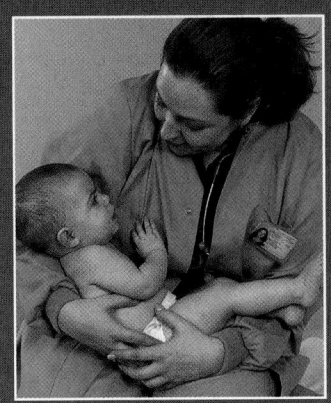

Dr. Wray performed some genetic testing on Delaney, and the adoptive parents were involved throughout the pregnancy, even meeting Delaney's birth mother for physician appointments from time to time. Monica observed both Susan and the Walshes and saw many benefits from the arrangement, noticing that everyone was primarily concerned with Delaney and her happiness and well-being. However, there were periods that were difficult, as well, for both sides. This prompted Monica to give some thought to her own feelings and ideas about many different ethical situations and issues and how she would react in the face of having to make ethical decisions.

While studying this chapter, think about the following questions:

- What difficulties do patients who are placing their babies for adoption face?
- What difficulties do adoptive parents face when participating in an open adoption?
- How can the medical assistant be supportive of both the adoptive parents and the birth mother?
- Should the medical assistant discuss personal beliefs about ethical situations with patients?

LEARNING OBJECTIVES

1. Define, spell, and pronounce the terms listed in the vocabulary.
2. Explain rights and duties as related to ethics.
3. List and define the four types of ethical problems.
4. Discuss the process used for making an ethical decision.
5. Detail the impact that the CEJA has on the ethical decisions made by healthcare professionals.
6. Describe the way unique identifiers help HIV-positive patients to avoid some discrimination.
7. Note some of the concerns regarding ethics that surround genetic information.
8. Explain why confidentiality is an ethical issue.
9. Discuss several of the CEJA opinions and how they might differ from the views of the class as a whole.

National Accreditation Competencies and Content

CAAHEP COMPETENCIES	ABHES COMPETENCIES
General	**Professionalism**
3.c.(2)(b). Perform within legal and ethical boundaries	1.d. Be cognizant of ethical boundaries

VOCABULARY

advocate (ad'-vuh-kat) One who pleads the cause of another; one who defends or maintains a cause or proposal.

allocating (a'-luh-ka-ting) Apportioning for a specific purpose or to particular persons or things.

annotations (a-nuh-ta'-shun) Notes added by way of comment or explanation.

beneficence (buh-ne'-fuh-sens) The act of doing or producing good, especially performing acts of charity or kindness.

clinical trials Research studies that test how well new medical treatments or other interventions work in the subjects, usually human beings.

disparities (di-spar'-uh-tes) Marked differences or distinctions.

disposition (dis-puh-zi'-shun) The tendency of something or someone to act in a certain manner under given circumstances.

duty Obligatory tasks, conduct, service, or functions that arise from one's position, as in life or in a group.

euthanasia (yu-thuh-na'-zhe-uh) The act or practice of killing or permitting the death of hopelessly sick or injured individuals in a relatively painless way for reasons of mercy.

fidelity (fuh-de'-luh-te) Faithfulness to something to which one is bound by pledge or duty.

gametes (ga'-mets) Mature male or female germ cells, usually possessing a haploid chromosome set and capable of initiating formation of a new diploid individual; a sex cell, whether sperm or ovum.

genome (jeh'-nom) The genetic material of an organism.

idealism The practice of forming ideas or living under the influence of ideas.

impaired Being in a less-than-perfect or less-than-whole condition; includes having handicaps or functional defects and

being under the influence of drugs, alcohol, and/or controlled substances.

infertile Not fertile or productive; not capable of reproducing.

introspection (in-truh-spek'-shun) An inward, reflective examination of one's own thoughts and feelings.

nonmaleficence (non-mal-fe'-zens) Refraining from the act of harming or committing evil.

opinions Formal expressions of judgment or advice by an expert; formal expressions of the legal reasons and principles on which a legal decision is based.

philosopher A person who seeks wisdom or enlightenment; an expounder of a theory in a certain area of experience.

postmortem Done, collected, or occurring after death.

procurement (pro-kuhr'-ment) To get possession of, to obtain by particular care and effort.

public domain The realm embracing property rights that belong to the community at large, are unprotected by copyright or patent, and are subject to use or appropriation by anyone.

ramifications (ra-muh-fuh-ka'-shuns) Consequences produced by a cause or following from a set of conditions.

reparations (re-puh-ra'-shuns) Amends, acts of atonement, or satisfaction given as a result of a wrong or injury.

sociologic Oriented or directed toward social needs and problems.

surrogate (suhr'-uh-gat) A substitute; to put in place of another.

unique identifiers Codes used instead of names to protect the confidentiality of the patient in a method of anonymous HIV testing.

veracity (vuh-ra'-suh-te) A devotion to or conformity with the truth.

---

*E*thics is defined as the thoughts, judgments, and actions on issues that have implications of moral right and wrong. The concept of ethics concerns itself with the philosophies underlying ideal relationships between human beings, as well as the promotion of the highest good for humanity as a whole. Various beliefs exist about what is and is not ethical in everyday life and in the medical profession. The decisions that people make based on ethical beliefs can quite possibly alter the course of human existence.

A medical assistant not only must have a strong knowledge base about ethical issues that might be faced throughout the profession, but also must come to terms with some of the deeply rooted value systems that have been a part of his or her life since youth. The trials and tribulations we have experienced, as well as the joys, will all influence our thought patterns when we are faced with an opportunity to make a good ethical decision.

HISTORY OF ETHICS IN MEDICINE

From earliest recorded history, humans have pondered ethics— the judgment of right and wrong. Ethics should not be confused with etiquette. *Etiquette* refers to courtesy, customs, and manners, whereas ethics explores the moral right or wrong of an issue. It is not surprising that for centuries the field of medicine has set for itself a rigid standard of ethical conduct toward patients and professional colleagues.

The earliest written code of ethical conduct for medical practice was conceived in approximately 2250 BC by the Babylonians and was called the *Code of Hammurabi*. It elaborated on the conduct expected of a physician and even set the fees that a physician could charge. The Code was quite lengthy and detailed, which is the probable reason it did not survive the ages. In approximately 400 BC Hippocrates, the Greek physician known as the Father of Medicine, developed a brief statement

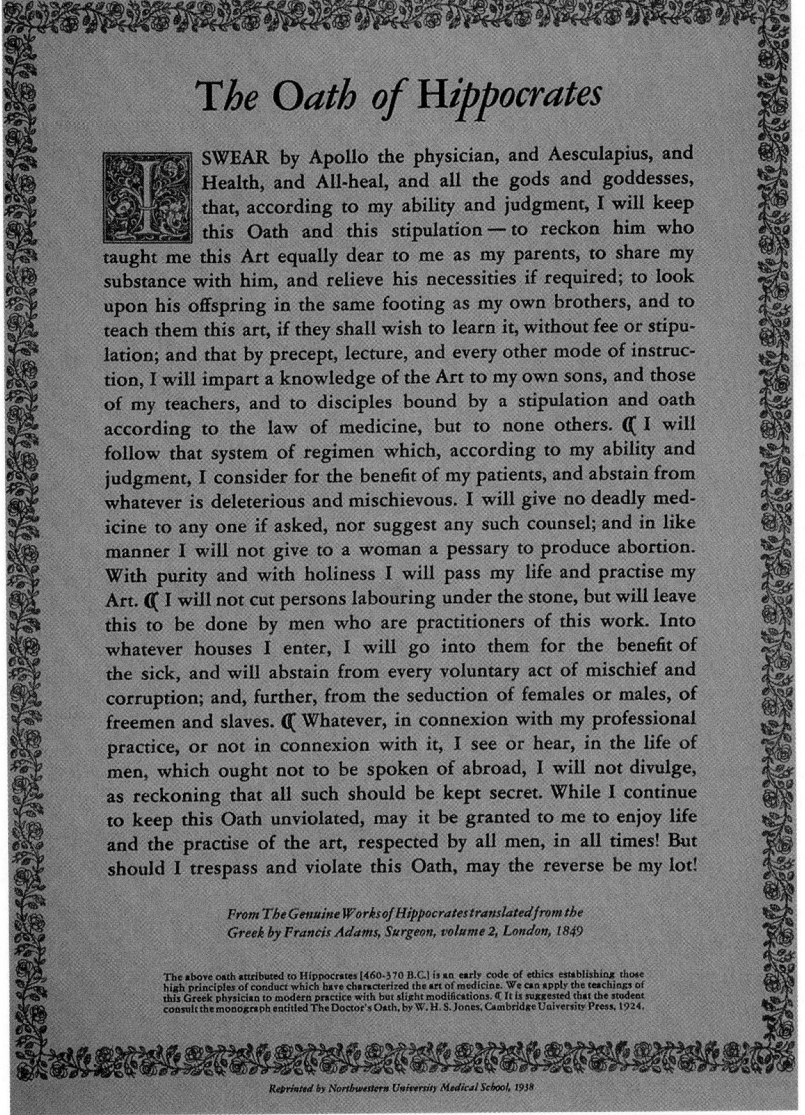

FIGURE 6-1 The Oath of Hippocrates. (Courtesy National Library of Medicine.)

of principles that remains an inspiration to the physicians of today. The Oath of Hippocrates has been administered to many medical graduates (Figure 6-1). The most significant contribution to medical ethics after the time of Hippocrates was that of Thomas Percival. Percival was a physician, **philosopher,** and writer from Manchester, England. In 1803 he published his Code of Medical Ethics. Percival was very interested in **sociologic** matters and took a great interest in the study of ethical concepts as related to the medical profession.

In 1846, as the American Medical Association (AMA) was being organized in New York City, medical education and medical ethics were already considered important aspects of the profession. At the first annual AMA meeting in 1847, a Code of Ethics was formulated and adopted. It specifically acknowledged Percival's code as its foundation, and this document became a part of the fundamental standards of the AMA and its component parts. Even today sections of the AMA Code of Ethics stem from Percival's writings.

WHO DECIDES WHAT IS ETHICAL?

When we weigh the question of who decides what is ethical, the answer is evident: you do. Every day medical professionals face the task of making ethical decisions. Although many different groups of people meet to discuss the ethics of a procedure or decision from the local level to national and worldwide levels, fundamentally, each individual decides what is ethical and what is not for him or her and the individuals these decisions will affect. As with any important choice, one must consider the short- and long-term effects and consequences. Although it is a completely acceptable practice to depend on groups and committees to guide ethical decisions, the responsibility for making these decisions ultimately rests with the individual (Figure 6-2).

Organizations that study ethical dilemmas may decide that a concept such as abortion is an ethical medical practice. But if an individual does not find abortion to be an acceptable

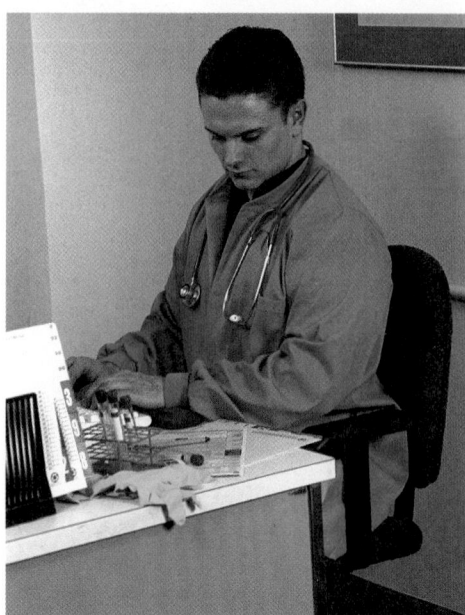

FIGURE 6-2 Medical assistants may find themselves making ethical decisions on a daily basis.

practice for religious or other reasons, abortion is not ethical for that individual. A great freedom that Americans often take for granted is that we can exercise free will in decisions related to individual conscience in this country, that we can choose from a variety of options—but we must exercise this responsibility carefully.

CRITICAL THINKING APPLICATION

■ Monica knows that she has deep-rooted thoughts and ideas about many ethical matters. However, she has never really thought about where she formed her ideas. Where do we get most of our opinions on ethical or moral issues?

■ What is the difference between an opinion's being personal and its being someone else's?

THE ROLE OF THE AMERICAN MEDICAL ASSOCIATION AND THE COUNCIL ON ETHICAL AND JUDICIAL AFFAIRS WITH REGARD TO ETHICS

The AMA serves physicians as a national organization providing various types of information and support. One of the most important facets of the AMA is its Council on Ethical and Judicial Affairs (CEJA). The CEJA consists of nine active members of the AMA, including one resident physician member and one medical student member, and is responsible for interpreting the *AMA Principles of Medical Ethics* as adopted by the House of Delegates of the AMA. The AMA's Code of Ethics has four components:

• Principles of medical ethics
• The fundamental elements of the patient-physician relationship

• Current opinions of the CEJA with **annotations**
• Reports of the CEJA

The *Code of Medical Ethics: Current Opinions with Annotations* is a publication that contains the first three components, with discussion of more than 135 ethical issues encountered in medicine. A separate publication, *Reports of the Council on Ethical and Judicial Affairs,* discusses the rationale of the Council's **opinions** (Figure 6-3).

The *AMA Principles of Medical Ethics* has been revised several times to follow current trends in medicine, but there has never been a change in the moral intent or overall **idealism** of the statements. In 1957 the *AMA Principles of Medical Ethics* was condensed to a preamble and 10 sections. In 1980 the principles were reduced to seven sections to clarify and update the language, eliminate reference to gender, and seek a proper and reasonable balance between professional standards and contemporary legal standards in our changing society. The most recently adopted changes, presented at the 2001 Annual Meeting of the AMA House of Delegates, reflect wording consistent with today's privacy issues and stress the importance of informed consent in deoxyribonucleic acid (DNA) database information in genomic research. Opinions are issued on a variety of subjects at the annual and interim meetings, and often older opinions are updated or changed based on current societal trends.

MAKING ETHICAL DECISIONS

Before discussing the opinions of AMA's CEJA, it is best to understand a few of the elements of ethics, the different types of ethical problems, and how a good ethical decision is made. Then, as some of the opinions are presented in this text, students can begin to evaluate their own positions regarding each issue. This section will enable the medical assistant to recognize the type of ethical problems that might arise in the physician's office and will provide a pattern to follow when making an ethical decision.

Elements of Ethics

Ruth Purtilo, in her book *Ethical Dimensions in the Health Professions,* presents three general elements of ethics: duties, rights, and character traits. A **duty** is an obligation that a person has or perceives himself or herself to have. A daughter may feel the obligation to care for her elderly parents, or a husband who has hurt his spouse may feel an obligation to somehow make up for his act.

Purtilo mentions several types of duties that relate to the medical profession. **Nonmaleficence** refers to refraining from harming the self or another person. **Beneficence** refers to bringing about good. **Fidelity** is the concept of promise-keeping, and **veracity** refers to the duty of telling the truth. Justice, in relation to medical ethics, deals with the fair distribution of benefits and burdens among individuals or groups in society having legitimate claims on those benefits. When a person has wronged another, he or she has a duty to make **reparations,** or right the wrong. Last, a person should feel grateful after being

---

FUNDAMENTAL ELEMENTS OF THE PATIENT-PHYSICIAN RELATIONSHIP

From ancient times, physicians have recognized that the health and well-being of patients depend on a collaborative effort between physician and patient. Patients share with physicians the responsibility for their own healthcare. The patient-physician relationship is of greatest benefit to patients when they bring medical problems to the attention of their physicians in a timely fashion, provide information about their medical condition to the best of their ability, and work with their physicians in a mutually respectful alliance. Physicians can best contribute to this alliance by serving as their patients' advocates and by fostering these rights:

1. The patient has the right to receive information from physicians and to discuss the benefits, risks, and costs of appropriate treatment alternatives. Patients should receive guidance from their physicians as to the optimal course of action. Patients are also entitled to obtain copies or summaries of their medical records, to have their questions answered, to be advised of potential conflicts of interest that their physicians might have, and to receive independent professional opinions.
2. The patient has the right to make decisions regarding the healthcare that is recommended by his or her physician. Accordingly, patients may accept or refuse any recommended medical treatment.
3. The patient has the right to courtesy, respect, dignity, responsiveness, and timely attention to his or her needs.
4. The patient has the right to confidentiality. The physician should not reveal confidential communications or information without the consent of the patient, unless provided for by law or by the need to protect the welfare of the individual or the public interest.
5. The patient has the right to continuity of healthcare. The physician has an obligation to cooperate in the coordination of medically indicated care with other healthcare providers treating the patient. The physician may not discontinue treatment of a patient as long as further treatment is medically indicated, without giving the patient reasonable assistance and sufficient opportunity to make alternative arrangements for care.
6. The patient has a basic right to have available adequate healthcare. Physicians, along with the rest of society, should continue to work toward this goal. Fulfillment of this right is dependent on society providing resources so that no patient is deprived of necessary care because of an inability to pay for the care. Physicians should continue their traditional assumption of a part of the responsibility for the medical care of those who cannot afford essential healthcare. Physicians should advocate for patients in dealing with third parties when appropriate.

FIGURE 6-3 Fundamental elements of the patient-physician relationship. (From Report of the Council on Ethical and Judicial Affairs of the American Medical Association. Originally adopted June 1990; last updated August 2001. Report 26, 1990. Available at: www.ama-assn.org/ama/pub/category/8313.html.Accessed June 26, 2006.)

the beneficiary of someone else's goodness. This is also a type of duty.

Rights are defined as claims that a person or group makes on society, a group, or an individual. The Bill of Rights appended to the U.S. Constitution guarantees certain liberties that we enjoy as American citizens. However, some individuals think that they have rights that are really privileges. For instance, Americans do not have the "right" to healthcare services. Individuals may "expect" to be cared for when sick, but this is not a right that is guaranteed to anyone in America. Some countries provide medical care to all their citizens, but the United States is not one of those countries. A right applies to all people within a group, without prejudice. One of the most intense ethical arguments faced today is the right-to-life concept. If our Constitution states that we all have the right to life, liberty, and the pursuit of happiness, how can abortion be considered ethical? Or if an individual is trying to end his or her suffering from a terminal illness, could the "pursuit of happiness" be interpreted to include seeking a physician's help in committing suicide? These are the types of ethical questions that arise in the healthcare field.

Character traits are defined in Purtilo's book as a **disposition** to act in a certain way. A person who feels honesty is an important character trait can usually be trusted to speak the truth. One who feels that it is acceptable to take small items from work for use at home may not be able to resist an opportunity to take something more valuable. Character traits will certainly not always provide an indication of how a person will react in all situations. No human being is perfect, and we are sometimes unpredictable. Stress can also interfere with our normal reactions, and other factors, such as depression or anger, influence how we act as well. The phrase that someone is acting "out of character" usually means that he or she is deviating from his or her normal behavior patterns.

With an understanding of these basic elements of ethics, we have a good foundation that will help us to look more objectively at ethical problems and solve them to the best of our ability.

Types of Ethical Problems

Purtilo presents four basic types of ethical problems (Figure 6-4). They are:

- Ethical distress
- Ethical dilemmas
- Dilemmas of justice
- Locus of authority issues

Ethical distress is the type of problem faced when a certain course of action is indicated, but some type of hindrance or

WHAT SHOULD BE DONE?

1. **Ethical Distress**
   I know which course of action I (the "agent") should take for the patient's benefit, but there is a structural barrier to my being able to do it.

   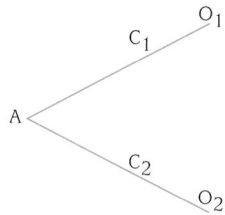

   $$A \underset{C}{\rule{3cm}{0.4pt}} \|\ O$$

   A = Agent
   C = Course of Action
   O = Outcome

2. **Ethical Dilemma**
   There are two (or more) courses of action, each of which is right (or wrong). No matter which one I (the "agent") choose, something of value will be compromised.

   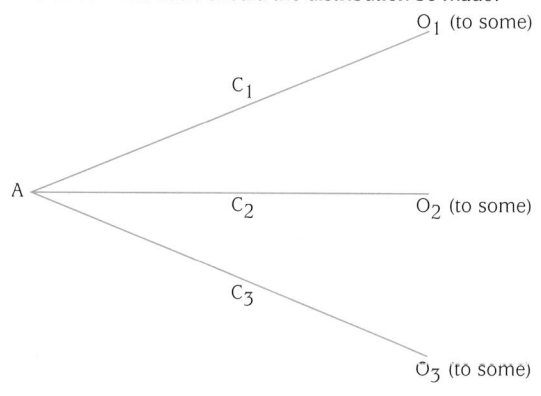

3. **Distributive Justice**
   There are benefits to be distributed among several potential beneficiaries. Not everyone can receive a full measure of the benefit. On what basis should the distribution be made?

WHO SHOULD DO IT?

4. **Locus of Authority**
   There are 2 (or more) agents or "authorities" in this situation. Each believes he or she knows what outcome will benefit the patient the most, but only one authority will prevail.

   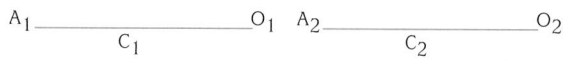

   $$A_1 \underset{C_1}{\rule{2.5cm}{0.4pt}} O_1 \quad A_2 \underset{C_2}{\rule{2.5cm}{0.4pt}} O_2$$

FIGURE 6-4 Summary of types of ethical problems. (From Purtilo R: *Ethical dimensions in the health professions*, ed 4, Philadelphia, 2005, Saunders.)

barrier prevents that action. A professional knows the right thing to do but for some reason cannot do it.

An ethical dilemma is a situation in which an individual is faced with two or more choices that are acceptable and correct, but doing one precludes doing another. A choice must be made, and something of value may be lost if a second choice is eliminated. This could be viewed as the proverbial "being caught between a rock and a hard place," whereby a choice must be made that has more of an effect than what may be seen on the surface.

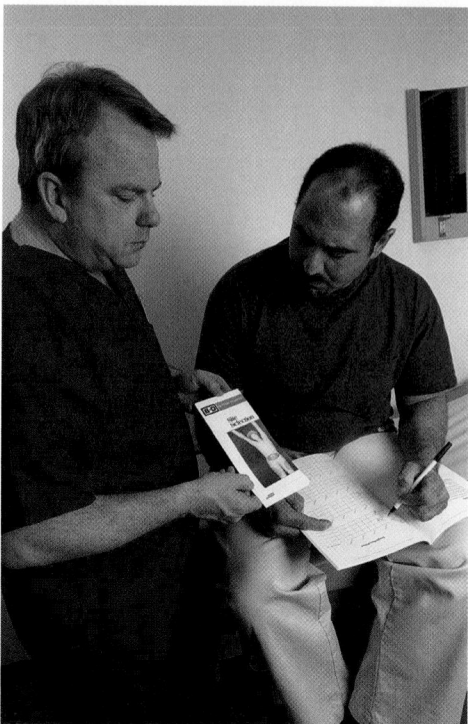

FIGURE 6-5 One of the duties of a medical assistant is to ensure that the patient understands the instructions given. Only when the patient fully understands the choices available can he or she make sound decisions.

The third type of ethical problem is the dilemma of justice. This problem focuses on the fair distribution of benefits to those who are entitled to them. Choices must be made regarding who receives these benefits and in what portion. A few examples of the dilemma of justice would include organ donations and distribution of scarce or costly medications.

In locus of authority issues, two or more authority figures have their own ideas about how a situation should be handled, but only one of those authorities will prevail. If one physician feels a patient should have surgery and another does not, how does the patient decide (Figure 6-5)?

Recognizing the type of ethical problem is not always easy. Sometimes a medical professional is faced with an issue that is a mixture of one or more types of ethical problems. When possible, it is wise to take some time in weighing the right course of action to take before making an important decision. Unfortunately, this is not always possible in the fast pace of the medical profession. Some decisions must be made in a split second, so it is wise to have a thorough grasp of ethical decision-making before the need arises.

The Ethical Decision-Making Process

In her book Purtilo presents a five-step process for ethical decision making. The steps include:

- Gathering relevant information
- Identifying the type of ethical problem
- Determining the ethics approach to use
- Exploring the practical alternatives
- Completing the action

To gather information a medical professional should ask questions, review charts, talk to the patient and other professionals, and search for other data so that the full view of the situation is available for scrutiny. Once the information is gathered, the medical professional must decide which ethical problem or problems are being presented. In determining the ethical approach to use, we must consider duties, rights, and character traits of all the individuals involved with this issue, paying close attention to the **ramifications** of all possible decisions. All of the alternatives must be considered and evaluated, and then an action should be taken (Procedure 6-1).

Although it is best to have time to give these areas some thought, this may not always be possible. It is a good practice for those entering the medical profession to take stock of what their core beliefs are. Scan the newspapers and search professional journals for ethical situations, think about the facts, then decide how you would react to each one. This is excellent preparation for the day that you will be faced with making a quick ethical decision.

CURRENT OPINIONS OF THE COUNCIL ON ETHICAL AND JUDICIAL AFFAIRS AND MEDICINE'S ETHICAL ISSUES

Now, armed with a basic knowledge about the types of ethical problems and the process used to solve them, we will take a look at some of the Council opinions. Remember, physicians and other medical professionals are not bound to abide by the CEJA opinions. They have the freedom to make their own decisions, but many of the medical professionals in our country tend to agree with the decisions made by the committee.

Abortion

In 1973 the U.S. Supreme Court heard the case of *Roe v. Wade*. Norma McCorvey (using the name Jane Roe) petitioned the court for permission to have an elective abortion when at age 21 she found herself pregnant with her third child. The class action suit she filed against Henry Wade, then the District Attorney in Dallas, Texas, eventually was appealed to the United States Supreme Court. Although she won her case, it was too late for her to have an abortion, and her child was born and placed for adoption. McCorvey went public with her true identity in the early 1980s and later became a staunch opponent of abortion and has spent many years promoting the overturn of *Roe v. Wade* (Figure 6-6).

Since the ruling was handed down in 1973, abortion has been one of the most volatile issues in medical ethics. According to

---

CRITICAL THINKING APPLICATION

- What are the ramifications of an open adoption such as Delaney's? What problems might occur during the first year of her life?
- How might these problems be avoided?
- What are the positive aspects of the adoption?

PROCEDURE 6-1

Perform Within Ethical Boundaries

CAAHEP COMPETENCIES: 3.c(2)(b)
ABHES COMPETENCIES: 1.d

GOAL: *To enable the medical assistant to perform in an ethical manner in all situations.*

EQUIPMENT and SUPPLIES

- Copy of the AAMA Code of Ethics
- Copy of the Medical Assistant Creed
- Copy of the Oath of Hippocrates

PROCEDURAL STEPS

1. Become familiar with the AAMA Code of Ethics and the Medical Assistant Creed.
   PURPOSE: To understand the purpose of medical assisting and the ethical boundaries that surround the profession.
2. Study the Oath of Hippocrates.
   PURPOSE: To gain knowledge of the roots of ethical behavior.
3. Consider the ethical problem at hand.
4. Gather relevant information about the problem.
   PURPOSE: To make certain that all of the facts are considered when solving the problem.

5. Identify the type of ethical problem.
   PURPOSE: By accumulating information about the problem and determining the type of ethical problem, the medical assistant will be better able to solve the problem.
6. Determine the ethical approach to use.
   PURPOSE: Knowing the type of problem helps the medical assistant to determine which ethical approach to use to solve the issue.
7. Explore practical alternatives.
   PURPOSE: Considering all practical alternatives helps the medical assistant to make the best ethical decisions.
8. Make the best ethical decision.
   PURPOSE: By gathering information, identifying the problem and the best ethical approach to use, and considering all practical alternatives, the medical assistant can arrive at a sound ethical decision.

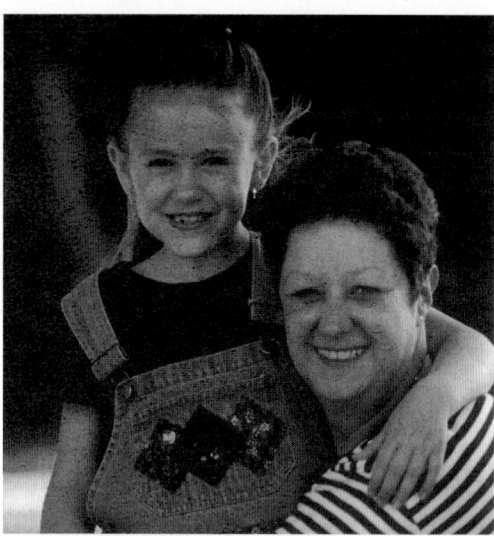

FIGURE 6-6 Norma McCorvey was "Jane Roe" in *Roe v. Wade*, the Supreme Court decision that legalized abortion. More than 20 years later, she became one of the pro-life movement's biggest advocates and has worked to get *Roe v. Wade* overturned.

the *AMA Principles of Medical Ethics,* the AMA does not prohibit a physician from performing an abortion in accordance with good medical practice and under circumstances that do not violate the law. In recent years laws have been passed in some states requiring mandatory parental notification of a minor's intent to have an abortion. In some cases this means that the minor must have parental consent, and in others, parents only must be notified of their daughter's intent to have an abortion. Some states also require a 24-hour or more waiting period after the notification has been made. However, CEJA states that the patient, even if an adolescent, should ultimately be in control of the decision as to whether parents should be involved in the abortion decision.

The AMA strongly encourages physicians to persuade the minor toward seeking counseling with someone she trusts, such as a school counselor, teacher, or relative, if the minor's parent is not to be involved in the abortion decision. However, the AMA agrees that the physician should not feel compelled to require minors to involve the parent in the decision. Medical professionals must be aware of the laws in their respective states that deal with the mandatory notification requirements and should contact the medical societies in their region to determine what constitutes proper notification.

Case to Discuss

Should a woman who has been raped and become pregnant seek an abortion?

Abuse

The AMA requires that a physician be familiar with the signs of physical, psychologic, and sexual abuse of spouses, children, mentally incompetent persons, and the elderly. Discovery of abuse creates a difficult situation for a medical professional. The patient may be the object of abuse but may deny its existence because of fear of further attacks. The law requires that abuse

be reported, and if the physician does not report abuse, ethical standards have been breached. In addition, the abuse may continue. Any medical assistant who suspects abuse must report this information to the physician first, who must determine whether the incident is reportable by law and take action. If action is not taken, the medical assistant is responsible for making a report to the proper authority in the city or state.

Case to Discuss

What harm can come to a patient's family if the medical professionals are incorrect about their assessment of abuse?

Allocation of Health Resources

Sometimes society must decide who will receive care when serving all who need care is not possible. Decisions must be made fairly and should be weighed carefully. The criteria to consider when **allocating** health resources include urgency of need, likelihood of benefit, duration of benefit, amount of resources required for successful treatment, and potential for change in quality of life. Nonmedical criteria, such as ability to pay, social worth of the individual, age, obstacles to treatment, and the patient's contribution to the illness, should not be considered. The physician who is treating the patient must remain the **advocate** of the patient and should not be involved in making allocation decisions for that patient. Procedures for such allocations are determined in an objective manner by the institutions involved in the patient care.

Case to Discuss

If the chief executive officer (CEO) of American Airlines, the winner of last year's Academy Award for Best Actor, and a drug-abusing mother of three all were equally ill and needed a liver transplant, which should receive the organ, and on what would you base the decision?

Artificial Insemination

Any individual or couple considering artificial insemination must be thoroughly counseled and endure lengthy screening procedures for communicable and genetic diseases that the donor and/or recipient may have. Informed consent must be provided, and further regulations are based on the marital status of the people involved. If the recipient is married to the donor, the resultant child will have all of the rights of a child naturally conceived. If the donor is anonymous, the husband must sign consent if he is to become the legal father of the resultant child. If the donor and recipient are not married, the recipient is considered the sole parent, unless both parties agree to recognize a right to paternity. It is not considered unethical to provide artificial insemination to a single woman or a woman who is a part of a homosexual couple. It is usually considered unethical to offer compensation to donors other than reimbursement of actual expenses and/or compensation for the donor's time.

Physicians should keep permanent records regarding donors so that:

- Individuals who test positive for communicable diseases can be excluded from the donor pool

- The number of pregnancies resulting from a single donor source can be limited
- Donors can be notified about screenings that demonstrate the presence of a communicable disease
- Donors can be notified about a disease or disorder found in a child born through artificial insemination that may have been transmitted by the donor

Much discussion is ongoing about the use of extra embryos that are harvested for reproductive purposes. The control and use of these **gametes** should logically be left to the man and woman who produced them, but the AMA agrees that both must give their consent regarding how they are used. In vitro fertilization is considered an ethical procedure.

Case to Discuss

A man fertilized eggs that were frozen for later use, but he died without having made provision for the use of those eggs after his death. Should the man's wife be able to use those eggs after her marriage to a second man?

Stem Cell Research

Many organizations feel that using human embryos for stem cell research destroys the most vulnerable of beings, and laws are designed to protect them. Others want to explore the possibility of developing cures from this research for diseases such as Alzheimer's disease, diabetes, Parkinson's disease, and heart disease. Stem cell research continues to be an area of disagreement because of the controversy regarding the point at which life begins. Those who believe that life begins at conception usually oppose stem cell research, because it involves experimentation and testing on a "viable human being." Many physicians believe that their commitment is first to "living persons" as opposed to embryos, and therefore support stem cell research. One of the strongest proponents of stem cell research was actor Christopher Reeve, who played Superman in several movies and was later paralyzed in an equestrian accident (Figure 6-7).

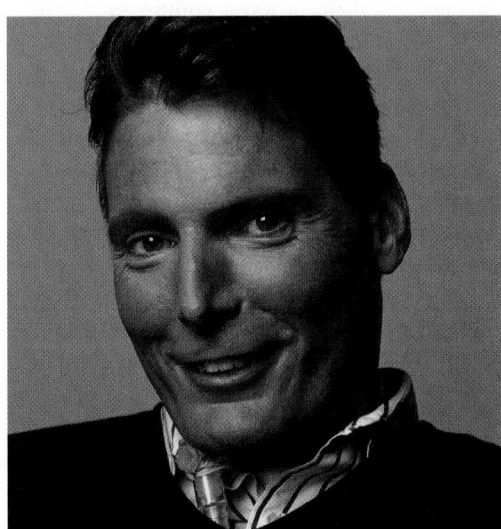

FIGURE 6-7 Christopher Reeve played the role of Superman in movies but was more admired for his untiring efforts toward medical research after the equestrian accident that left him paralyzed. Reeve died in 2004. (Courtesy Corbis.)

Case to Discuss

A medical student is recruited to work with a physician who is researching paralysis. Once the project is underway, the student discovers that the physician is using embryos that have been questionably obtained in the experimentation. What should the medical assistant do?

Surrogate Motherhood

Surrogate motherhood introduces many different ethical, legal, and social problems to the individuals involved. However, this could be the only opportunity for **infertile** couples to have a child. The benefits of surrogacy must be heavily weighed against the possible risks and psychologic problems that might arise. The AMA feels that the birth mother must be given a period of time during which she can reverse her decision to give up the child she has delivered and void the contract. However, in cases of gestational surrogacy, the legality and ethical implications are more complicated. In gestational surrogacy the child is not genetically linked to the birth mother. Usually the couple engaging the surrogate mother would be the genetic parents of the resultant child. One must also consider what will happen if the child were to be born with a deformity or handicap. This is a contract that should never be entered into without strong forethought and counseling.

Case to Discuss

What is a fair length of time to give a surrogate mother to petition to void a surrogacy contract?

Human Cloning

The AMA agrees that physicians should not at this time participate in human cloning, or somatic cell nuclear transfer, because of the numerous legal and moral issues that must be explored. Most agree that our current ethical and moral standards would interpret that a "cloned human" be granted the same rights as "normal humans," much in the same way as an adopted child is accepted legally and socially as part of a family. The AMA does not feel there has been nearly enough research into the long-term effects of cloning and therefore does not advocate the practice today.

Case to Discuss

If a couple loses a child through death but it were possible to clone the child, what concerns would be present for the family?

Genetic Counseling

Genetic counseling is also an area in which the AMA recommends caution. Through genetic counseling, parents of tomorrow may be able to choose eye color, talents, and intellect levels for their children (Figure 6-8). There are already humans who were conceived as "designer babies" in the world today. In 1980 the Repository for Germinal Choice (more commonly known as the "Genius Sperm Bank") was founded. Although it was not established to create a perfect "master race," it did attempt to produce leaders and creators. As with cloning, the AMA

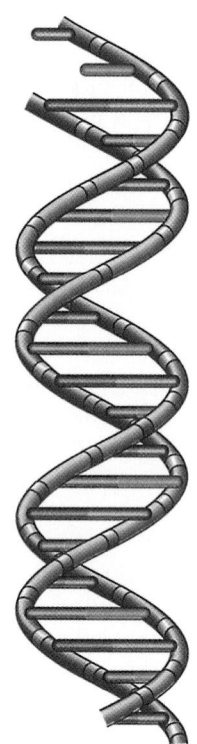

FIGURE 6-8 DNA, known as the "blueprint of the body," contains all the genes and chromosomes that make each human a unique creation, unlike any other human. (From Chester GA: *Modern medical assisting*, Philadelphia, 1998, Saunders.)

recommends that much more research be done before instituting genetic counseling on a global scale.

Case to Discuss

What could happen if parents were to "design" a baby, but it arrived flawed in some way or did not meet their expectations?

CRITICAL THINKING APPLICATION

- How might the genetic testing done in Delaney's case have caused an ethical dilemma?
- Discuss whether genetic testing can be counted on to predict disease.
- How many in your class would have genetic testing done on their own child before birth?

Physician-Assisted Suicide

The AMA believes that physician-assisted suicide interferes with the fundamental purpose of being a physician—being a healer. The CEJA advocates that physicians aggressively provide care and alternatives in treatment for those who are near the end of life but not promote or provide the means with which the patient could end his or her own life. This includes not only assisting the patient to inject chemicals that will induce death, but also prescribing drugs and information about lethal doses or administering a lethal dose of a drug to a patient to promote death (Figure 6-9). This is sometimes called **euthanasia,** or mercy-killing.

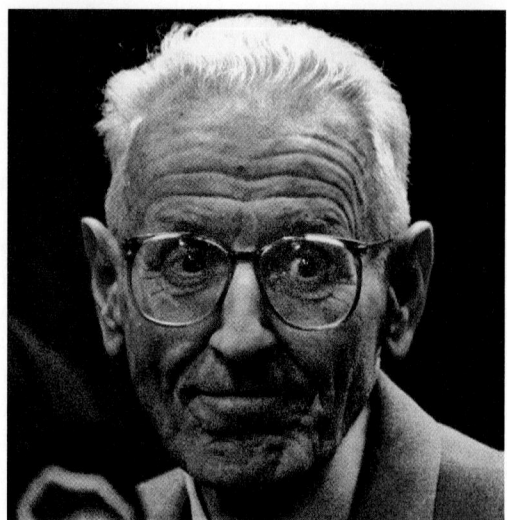

FIGURE 6-9 Dr. Jack Kevorkian, after being acquitted for numerous assisted suicides, was convicted in 1999 of second-degree murder and delivery of a controlled substance in the death of Thomas Youk, 52, who had amyotrophic lateral sclerosis (ALS or Lou Gehrig's disease). (© AFB/CORBIS.)

Case to Discuss

If a parent mentioned in passing that he or she would want the right to commit suicide in the event of a terminal illness, would you support that decision if the situation did in fact arise?

Surrogate Decision Making

According to CEJA, physicians should encourage patients to document their preferences regarding advance directives through a living will or durable power of attorney. However, many patients do not have any type of documentation of their wishes available when tragedy strikes. In these cases a surrogate may be asked to make decisions for the patient with regard to his or her medical treatment. Even when such provisions have been made, the documents are sometimes unavailable in an emergency, so patients should discuss treatment options in advance with those who may be called on to be a surrogate decision maker. If patients cannot make medical decisions for themselves and documented advance directives are unavailable or nonexistent, absent any state regulation to the contrary the physician should approach the patient's family, domestic partner, or a close friend as the surrogate decision maker. There may be cases in which family members disagree about the decisions that are necessary for the health and well-being of the patient. In these instances the physician should work to resolve the conflict through mediation or should consult the facility's ethics committee. The ultimate goal of the physician is to act in the best interests of the patient, and in the absence of any other basis for interpreting how a patient would wish to proceed with treatment, the physician should make the decision that would, in the physician's professional opinion, most benefit the patient.

Case to Discuss

A physician recommends that a patient be taken off life support. The patient lives with his homosexual partner and has not had contact with his parents in more than 10 years. Both the partner and the parents discuss the situation with the physician. The partner does not wish to remove life support, stating that the patient would want to have every opportunity to live. The parents insist that they know what is best for their son and demand that he be taken off life support. Who should prevail?

Withholding or Withdrawing Life-Prolonging Treatment

A physician is committed to saving life and relieving suffering. Sometimes these two goals are incompatible, and a choice between them must be made. If possible the patient should decide what treatment is given. Often the patient makes his or her wishes known to a responsible relative or other representative, in case the patient becomes incapacitated. Some patients wish to have a "do not resuscitate" (DNR) or "no code" order added to their charts. Usually such an order is desired so that no heroic measures are taken in a situation in which a patient would be unable or incompetent to make a decision. In any case, the decision to withdraw life support should be made before any mention of organ donation is made by the medical professionals tending the patient. In the best situation the patient has formally completed advance directives. Two types of advance directives are usually used in the United States. These documents are written instructions for healthcare and usually are in the form of a living will or a durable power of attorney. This documentation is strongly recommended by the AMA.

Patients are urged to create a living will. This is a document that states the wishes of the patient in case of terminal illness or an accident after which the patient cannot express his or her wishes. A durable power of attorney is a legal document that allows the patient to appoint someone who is trusted to make medical decisions for the patient in the event that the patient cannot make those decisions. This person is sometimes called a *patient advocate* or *healthcare proxy*. Federal law requires that patients be given information about advance directives by all facilities that participate in the Medicare and Medicaid programs.

Case to Discuss

How would a medical assistant handle the family of a patient who asks for advice about withdrawing life-prolonging treatment? To whom should the medical assistant defer the question?

Quality of Life

Physicians must sometimes participate in or advise on decisions affecting the fate of a person whose prognosis is poor, such as a deformed newborn or a person of advanced age with many physical problems. The first thought may be the burden that the patient's care will place on the family or society. However, the AMA insists that the physician's primary consideration be what is best for the patient.

Case to Discuss

A mentally ill single woman who is institutionalized becomes pregnant and refuses to give up her maternal rights so that the child can be adopted. Even if she were to reconsider, what complications result if the child is born deaf and has a severe liver disorder? Should the child be fed and cared for by the hospital staff?

Clinical Trials and Investigation

Without **clinical trials** and investigation, no new drugs or procedures would be developed. However, all such investigation must follow a competently designed systematic program with due concern for the welfare, safety, and comfort of patients. The physician-patient relationship does exist in clinical investigation, and when treatment of the patient is involved, voluntary written consent must be obtained from the patient or the patient's legally authorized representative. Additional restrictions apply to minors or mentally incompetent adults. Physicians must show the same concern for the welfare and safety of the person involved in the clinical trials as they would if the person were a private patient.

Case to Discuss

If your brother were homosexual and wanted to participate in clinical trials for a vaccination against human immunodeficiency virus (HIV), would you support his decision?

Cost of Healthcare Services

Concern for the quality of patient care should be the physician's first consideration. However, the physician should be conscious of costs and should not provide or prescribe unnecessary services. Access to an adequate level of healthcare for all members of our society is now a moral expectation, but certainly not a right. Cost must be considered when providing these services, as well as the degree of benefit to the patient, the duration of the benefit, and the number of people who will benefit.

Case to Discuss

Should an 87-year-old patient with cardiovascular disease and stomach cancer undergo expensive breast reconstruction surgery?

Organ Donation

Organ donation is not only considered ethical by the AMA, it is encouraged. However, it is considered unethical to participate in proceedings in which the donor receives payment, except reimbursement of expenses directly incurred in the removal of the donated organ. The rights of both the patient and the donor must be equally protected. In cases in which the donor has lost his or her life, the death must be certified by a physician other than the recipient's physician.

Because the need for donated organs is so extreme, protocols have been established by healthcare facilities to determine when it is proper to harvest organs. Organ **procurement** may occur immediately after a person has died, or it may happen after a patient has been kept alive artificially for a period of time. Hospitals also have specific guidelines for donation of organs from living donors, such as a kidney donation. When donations are made from one living person to another, both patients must have an advocate team that includes a physician, so that the interests and well-being of each patient are addressed. Payment to a living donor other than legitimate expenses incurred in connection with removal of the organ is also considered unethical.

Blood donations are probably the most common form of organ donation. Some religions do not believe in transfusing blood, and cases in which such beliefs come to bear must be dealt with carefully. If the patient is a minor and the parents refuse the child a blood transfusion, or any other medical care, some states would hold the parents liable for danger to or abuse of a child. However, the court system is reluctant to fight the parents over their religious beliefs and would intervene only in extreme circumstances.

CEJA has recommended that two proposals related to organ donation be considered; these are aimed at increasing organ donations and would change the approach to consent for deceased donations. The two proposed models include the mandated choice model and the presumed consent model. The mandated choice model would require individuals to express their preferences regarding organ donation at the time of performing some state-regulated task, such as renewal of a driver's license. This method would be ethically appropriate only if the individual's choice was made in accordance with the principles of informed consent. The presumed consent model would mean that deceased individuals were presumed to be organ donors unless they indicated their refusal to donate. It is unknown at this time whether the implementation of such models would affect the number of organs transplanted in a positive way, but CEJA encourages physicians to support policies that would increase the number of organ donors in the United States.

Case to Discuss
A woman dies with a living will that states that she wishes her organs to be donated. Her mother, still living, disagrees with the decision and does not want her daughter's organs donated. What should health professionals do in this situation?

CRITICAL THINKING APPLICATION
- Monica has often thought about being an organ donor. She is very much in favor of organ donation because of her interest in the medical field. Her parents are very opposed to this because of their religious beliefs. How can Monica deal with this conflict within her family?
- If Monica dies before her parents do, how can she ensure that her wishes are carried out?

Capital Punishment
The CEJA does not consider participation in the act of capital punishment by a physician to be ethical. The physician may certify the death of the person but should not administer a lethal injection or induce death in any way. This conflicts with the physician's role as a healer, much in the same manner as physician-assisted suicide does.

Case to Discuss
A very emotional patient, the parent of a child who was raped and killed, has been given the opportunity to attend the execution of the murderer. During a visit to her family physician, she expresses concerns about being able to cope with the memory of her daughter during the execution and asks you if you would attend in the same situation. How do you handle this situation?

ETHICAL ISSUES SURROUNDING HIV

Being HIV positive creates a whole new world of ethical concerns for patients as well as those who support and care for them. When the HIV crisis first came to public attention, many variables about the virus were unknown and this created a wealth of misinformation. Those infected with the virus were often forced to leave their homes and lost their jobs, were shunned in society, and faced rejection seemingly everywhere they turned, all because of fear of the illness (Figure 6-10).

Today clinical trials are underway for vaccinations against HIV, but clinical trials need volunteers for testing. Because vaccinations are often made of an attenuated or weakened strain of a virus, serious concerns exist about who will receive the vaccination. Researchers have considered testing the vaccination in several Third World countries that have a high number of prostitutes and a thriving sex industry. These people, with no intentions of changing their lifestyle no matter the risks, may see vaccination trials as their chance of not contracting HIV. However, the situation raises the question of the ethics of not submitting our own citizens to testing instead of those from disadvantaged countries.

Because of the discrimination practiced even today against people who are infected with HIV, problems occur with testing in some states that report the names of HIV-positive patients to various health departments and agencies. Although the stated intention is to ensure that these patients receive care, the accompanying effect is the risk of discriminatory practices. Some states use code systems called **unique identifiers** to assist in helping maintain the confidentiality of those getting tested for HIV. However, other states insist by statute that the names

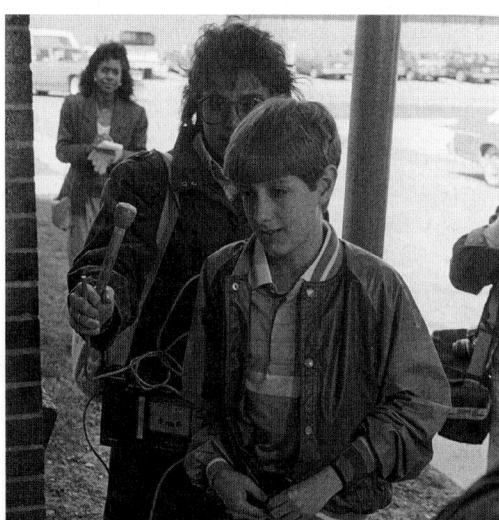

FIGURE 6-10 After a long court battle, Ryan White won the right to attend public school, despite his HIV status. (© Bettmann/CORBIS.)

be reported. Some states require mandatory HIV testing for prisoners and those who have committed sex crimes. Insurance is a difficult issue when a person is infected with HIV, and some policies can be cancelled if HIV infection is discovered. This may prompt providers who want to treat patients infected with HIV to delay reporting the infection as long as possible, using other diagnoses regarding symptoms as opposed to the underlying cause of the patient's problems. Many details are involved when HIV is a factor, even the reporting of HIV-positive status on the **postmortem** report. All of these ethical issues are difficult to resolve, and great care should be taken when making decisions surrounding a patient who is HIV positive.

ETHICS AND THE HUMAN GENOME

The mapping of the human **genome** has been in the news for several years. The genome project formally began in 1990 with the goals of identifying all of the 20,000 to 25,000 genes present in the human body, determining the sequences of the three billion chemical base pairs that make up human DNA, and finding ways to catalog this information in databases to make it readily available to those who need it. The project was completed in 2003, but the data discovered during the 13 years of the project will be studied for years to come.

Highlights of the project included the completion of the sequence mapping of chromosome 19, which is the most "gene-rich" of all of the human chromosomes. Chromosome 13 sequence mapping provided information about the genes that carry breast cancer type 2, as well as information about bipolar disorder and schizophrenia. The medical potential of the analysis of information provided by the Human Genome Project is mind boggling and will surely provoke advances in various medical fields and new technology and procedures.

Access to genetic information prompts many concerns and presents ethical, legal, and moral questions. Most of the major healthcare agencies and organizations in the United States and worldwide will be involved in the decisions made about this type of information, including the Centers for Disease Control and Prevention (CDC), National Institutes of Health (NIH), Department of Health and Human Services (DHHS), Food and Drug Administration (FDA), Centers for Medicare and Medicaid Services (CMS), and many others. Experts will be needed to educate Congress, federal agencies, and state and local governments, because laws must be passed regarding the use of genetic information. The rapid pace of science surpasses the ability of lawmakers to keep up, so the challenge ahead with regulation of the use of genetic information is a mammoth one.

The mapping of the human genome and the information provided have raised concerns about privacy and confidentiality issues. Who actually owns genetic information, and who will be allowed to control it? Logically, it would seem that the patient owns his or her own genetic information, but if that is so, then the patient should be able to control access to it. Also, decisions must be made regarding the fair use of genetic information. Employers, schools, courts, insurance companies, adoption agencies, and the military are just a few examples of organizations that could potentially misuse genetic information and discriminate against those whom they may wish to target for inclusion or exclusion. Reproductive issues arise, as well, along with questions about the reliability of genetic testing.

Patients will have to be counseled thoroughly about the risks and limitations of genetic technology. The answers to many questions are uncertain. Should a parent be allowed to test a minor child for adult-onset diseases? Should testing be performed for diseases that have no cure? All of these issues need resolution before the use of genetic information is widespread.

OTHER ETHICAL ISSUES

Interprofessional Relationships

If a medical assistant recognizes or suspects an error in a physician's orders, he or she has an ethical obligation to report this to the physician. Questioning a possible error is necessary, even if it means risking the displeasure of the physician or supervisor. It could save a life or prevent a lawsuit if an error has been made.

Physicians often refer a patient to another physician for diagnosis and treatment when it is necessary. A physician should make these referrals only when confident that the patient will receive competent treatment. It is considered unethical to offer a financial incentive or other valuable consideration to patients in exchange for recruitment of other patients.

Unless the state imposes legal restrictions, a physician in private practice is free to choose whom he or she will treat. Although private practitioners may refuse certain patients, they must treat those who have already been accepted in the practice or face possible charges of neglect. This does not include referring a patient to another physician for a condition that is not within the scope of the original physician's practice.

A sports medicine physician must keep in mind that the professional responsibility at a sporting event is to protect the health and safety of the participants, with personal judgments being governed only by medical considerations. Players should not be allowed to play and risk injury to ensure winning games.

In years past it was considered unethical for a physician to have any type of romantic relationship with nurses or assistants in the office or hospital. Although this is not as stringent a rule today, it is wise to not fraternize with co-workers, especially subordinates, at the workplace.

Confidentiality and Patient Privacy

Confidentiality is one of the cardinal rules of the medical profession. It is completely unethical and unacceptable to divulge any information about a patient to any other person not directly related to the patient's care. The places where confidentiality is often breached include elevators, hallways, waiting or reception areas, break rooms, and lunch rooms. One never knows whose relative is standing behind the medical assistant, listening to conversations that would be inappropriate for those not personally involved in the patient's care to hear. Breach of patient confidentiality is grounds for immediate termination from a healthcare facility or physician's office.

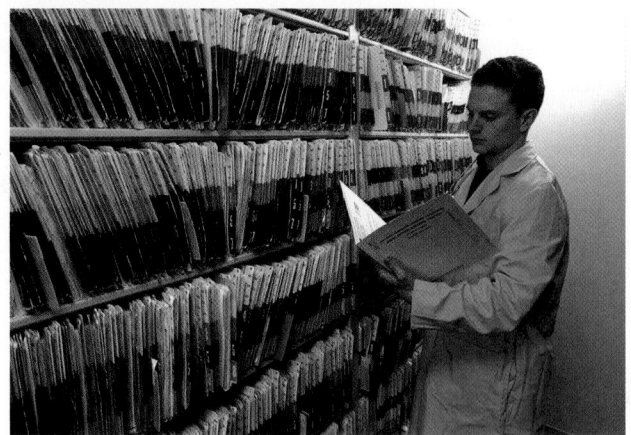

FIGURE 6-11 Confidentiality issues apply to all information about the patient, including what is charted and what is spoken between the patient and the medical assistant.

Confidentiality restrictions apply to information in patient records and charts, as well as what the medical assistant is told by the patient or patient's family (Figure 6-11). Never investigate a patient record strictly for curiosity. All information in the record must be kept in confidence. If records are computer based, accessing records of patients who do not fall directly under the medical assistant's realm of duty is also considered unethical. Never share information about patients with anyone outside the medical facility or office, including your own immediate family.

The prime objective of the medical profession is to render service to humanity, and this must be a medical assistant's first concern as well. The importance of respecting the confidentiality of information learned from or about patients in the course of employment cannot be overemphasized. It is unethical to reveal patient confidences to anyone, and this includes family, spouse, best friends, and other medical assistants. A medical assistant must never mention the names of patients outside the place of employment, because sometimes the doctor's specialty reveals the patient's reason for consultation. Confidential papers, case histories, and even the appointment book should be kept out of sight of curious eyes. In addition, outside observers should be present during the patient encounters with the physician only with the patient's explicit permission. Outside observers may include a friend who drove the patient to the physician's office or a medical student or intern who is observing in the clinic. It is advisable to document this permission in the patient's chart.

Never discuss one patient's case with another patient. If curious patients ask questions about others, simply explain that medical assistants are obligated to keep all patient information confidential. This can be done in a tactful and kind manner. Patients who ask questions of a medical nature about their own case should be referred to the physician for information and instructions, unless the physician has authorized the medical assistant to provide this information. When minors request confidential services, physicians should encourage them to include their parents. However, if the minor does not wish to involve them and the law does not require otherwise, physicians

should allow competent minors to consent to medical care and should not notify the parents without the minor patient's consent.

Remember that the Health Insurance Portability and Accountability Act (HIPAA) provides strict regulations for patient confidentiality and disclosure of private health information. Make certain that the physician's office is abiding by its own privacy policy and that all patients have been given the opportunity to review that policy. A document stating that the patient has read and understands the privacy policy or that he or she has refused to sign should be a part of the patient's medical record.

Patients may not always understand the ethical standards to which physicians and medical assistants adhere. They may ask questions about their own health or the health of a fellow patient. Medical assistants must educate patients regarding the issues of confidentiality in such a way that the patients are not offended, explaining that all patients deserve to have their medical and personal information kept private. Now more than ever the obligation of the medical assistant to keep information private is not only an ethical responsibility but also a legal responsibility. All patients should understand they are entitled to confidential treatment of their records and that the facility is dedicated to that principle.

CRITICAL THINKING APPLICATION

- Susan, Delaney's birth mother, comes to the office for a checkup 6 weeks after the baby was born. Susan looks a little sad, and when Monica questions her, she asks how Delaney is doing. What should Monica tell her?
- How can the office protect itself from issues involving confidentiality in this unusual adoption scenario?

Advertising

The only restrictions on advertising by physicians are those that specifically protect the public from deceptive practices. Standards regarding advertising and publicity have been liberalized over the years, but any advertisement or publicity must be true and not misleading. Testimonials of patients, for instance, should not be used in advertising, because they are difficult to verify or measure by objective standards. Statements regarding the quality of medial services are highly subjective and difficult to verify.

Communications with the Media

Although information regarding some patients such as celebrities and politicians may be considered news, the physician cannot discuss any patient's condition with the press without authorization from the patient or the patient's legal representative. The physician may release only authorized information or that which is public knowledge. Certain kinds of news are a part of public records. This is known as news in the **public domain** and includes births, deaths, accident reports, and police cases.

A medical assistant must be aware that only the physician is authorized to release information, and under no circumstances should the medical assistant violate the confidential nature of the physician-patient relationship. It is unethical even to certify or verify that the patient is under the physician's care without the patient's permission. Policy must be in place for every medical office regarding how media inquiries should be handled and to whom they should be referred. Never voluntarily speak to the press without authorization from the physician. Communications with the media fall within the HIPAA guidelines. Do not release a patient's health information without written permission.

Physician Obligations in Disaster Preparedness and Response

Physicians are ethically obligated to provide urgent medical care during disasters. Because extensive physician involvement is required during national, state, regional, and local disasters, physicians are expected to contribute both their time and their skills to assist in such emergencies. Examples of instances when the physician would be obligated to act include natural disasters, epidemics, and terrorist attacks.

Malevolent Use of Biomedical Research

Because biomedical research may produce information that has potential for both harmful and beneficial applications, the physician must assess the possible ramifications of participation in such research before engaging in projects. One of the most harmful uses of biomedical research involves biologic weapons. Physicians are expected to hold public trust as sacred and consider the welfare of society as a whole as well as the welfare of individual patients.

Racial and Ethnic Healthcare Disparities

Patients are entitled to the same quality of care regardless of their race or ethnic background. CEJA demands that physicians strive to eliminate biased behavior toward patients. Discrimination toward any patient or patient group cannot be tolerated. In addition, physicians must take into account any language barriers that might hinder effective treatment of the patient. Every effort must be made to make certain that the patient understands the physician and that the physician understands the patient. Physicians should also participate in efforts to encourage diversity in the profession.

Diagnostic Imaging on Request

Patients may request diagnostic imaging services for reasons such as determination of a baby's sex. Physicians should perform diagnostic imaging only when they believe that the benefits of the imaging service outweigh the risks involved.

Computers

The expanding uses of computer technology permit the accumulation of an unlimited amount of medical information. With the use of computers in the physician's office and the employment of computer service organizations, confidentiality becomes even more difficult to maintain. In general, all

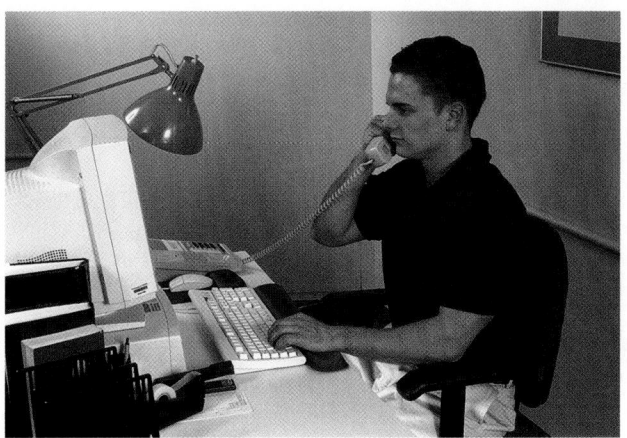

FIGURE 6-12 With the advent of advanced computer technology, a medical assistant must be particularly careful about using information about patients on the computer.

information must be entered and accessed only by authorized personnel, and a tracking system should be used to identify which employees access information. Breaches in computer policies should be considered a breach of patient confidentiality, and the consequences should be stringent enough to deter employees from accessing information to which they are not entitled (Figure 6-12). Information from the computer should be disseminated only to those who have a legitimate reason for needing the information.

Fees and Charges

Charging or collecting an illegal or excessive fee is unethical. The medical assistant is responsible for keeping informed about current billing regulations and to see that they are conscientiously followed.

Requesting that payment be made at the time of treatment is entirely appropriate and very common in today's medical offices. Often, managed care patients are asked to remit their co-payment before seeing the physician on the day of the visit. If the patient is notified in advance, adding interest or other reasonable charges to delinquent accounts is also considered ethical. Most offices use a patient information booklet that provides a written reference of all policies and that is given to new patients on their first visit. A reasonable charge may be made for the cost of duplicating patient records.

Fee Splitting and Contingent Fees

If a physician accepts payment from another physician solely for the referral of a patient, both are guilty of an unethical practice called *fee splitting*. This practice, whether with another physician, a clinic, a laboratory, or a drug company, is unethical.

Although attorneys often accept a case on a contingent fee basis, it is unethical for a physician to engage in this practice. The fee in this case is contingent on a successful outcome, but a physician should never set his or her fee on the successful outcome of medical treatment. A physician's fee must always be based on the value of service provided to the patient.

Insurance Forms

Although physicians' offices in times past would willingly file the claim on all insurance policies for their patients, some have changed their policies to a payment up-front system and give patients the information needed to file the claim themselves. Many offices will still file at least one insurance claim for established patients but may charge for multiple or complex insurance filing. This practice is entirely ethical if in conformity with local custom.

Waiver of Insurance Copayments

Physicians may opt to write off or waive copayments to facilitate patient access to medical care. If access to care is directly threatened because the patient cannot make the copayment, the physician may forgive the payment. However, routine waiver of copayments may violate the policies of some insurers, both public and private. Physicians should ensure that their policies on copayments are consistent with applicable law and within legal boundaries of their contracts with insurers.

Professional Courtesy

Professional courtesy is defined as the provision of medical care to physician colleagues or their families and staff free of charge or at a reduced fee. This is a long-standing tradition but certainly not an ethical requirement. Physicians make the decision as to who will receive professional courtesy in their offices, and this should be written into the office policy manual. In some cases, extending professional courtesy is contrary to insurance and/or managed care contracts. In addition, some physicians have stopped offering professional courtesy because of the rising costs of healthcare and shrinking reimbursements.

Appointment Charges

It is ethical for a physician to charge for a missed appointment or one that was not cancelled within a stated time if the patient has been fully advised in advance that such a charge may be made. Discretion should be used in applying such charges, however, since the patient may have encountered an emergency. Often, adding a missed appointment charge to the bill of a patient who never cancels in advance will prompt a call in the future when the appointment cannot be kept.

Prescribing Drugs and Devices

The physician should not be influenced in the prescribing of drugs, devices, or appliances by a direct or indirect financial interest in the supplier. A physician may own or operate a pharmacy but generally may not ethically refer his or her patients to that pharmacy. Patients should enjoy the same freedom of choice in deciding who will fill their prescriptions as they do in choosing a physician.

Professional and Contractual Relationships

Physicians often enter into contractual relationships, which may be as simple as monthly pest control services for the office. However, contracts can be quite complicated and contain numerous provisions, necessitating the assistance of an attorney. Physicians should negotiate the wording of contracts such that there is no question of financial incentives for the physician that would in any way compromise professional judgment or integrity.

Health Facility Ownership by a Physician

A physician may ethically own or have a financial interest in a for-profit or other health care facility, such as a freestanding clinic or health club. However, before admitting or referring a patient to that facility, the physician has an ethical obligation to reveal such ownership to the patient. In general, physicians should not refer patients to a health facility that is outside their office practice and at which they do not directly provide care or services.

Ghost Surgery

The substitution of another surgeon without the patient's consent is called *ghost surgery.* The patient has a right to choose his or her own physician or surgeon. Ghost surgery may happen when the patient has already received anesthesia and has no idea that a substitution has been made. To make a substitution without consulting the patient is deceitful and unethical.

Discipline within Medicine

A physician should expose incompetent, corrupt, dishonest, or unethical conduct on the part of members of the profession without fear of loss of favor. A physician may be subject to civil or criminal liability, including loss of license to practice medicine, for violation of government laws. Expulsion from membership is the maximum penalty that may be imposed by a medical society for violation of ethical standards.

Physician Health and Wellness

Physicians are responsible to maintain their own good health and be well enough to treat their patients. When the physician is not well, both physically and mentally, his or her health can interfere with the ability to provide good care to patients and engage in the safe execution of professional medical activities and decision making. When a physician is not in such good health, he or she is said to be **impaired.**

CEJA recommends that all physicians have their own personal doctor who will use uncompromised objectivity in caring for the physician's health. Healthcare providers are expected to intervene promptly when the health or wellness of a colleague appears to have become compromised. CEJA suggests types of intervention such as the offer of encouragement as well as referrals to physician health programs or other programs that will restore and maintain the physician's health and wellness.

A physician who knows that he or she has an infectious disease should not engage in any activity that creates an identified risk of transmission to the patient. Simple colds and other minor illnesses will arise occasionally, but illnesses that would cause a significant risk to the patient should not be given a chance to cause infection.

Substance Abuse

It is unethical for a physician to practice medicine while under the influence of a controlled substance, alcohol, or other chemical agents that could impair the ability to properly care for the patient or perform procedures. Healthcare providers who are aware of other providers with substance abuse problems must take action to ensure patient safety, which may include reporting the physician to the appropriate authority in the city or state in which he or she practices medicine.

Unethical Conduct by Members of the Health Profession

In rare instances a medical assistant is faced with a situation in which the physician-employer's conduct appears to violate established ethical standards. Before making any judgments, the medical assistant must be absolutely sure of all the information and circumstances. If unethical conduct occurs, the medical assistant must then make his or her own decision about continued employment in the facility and whether the unethical behavior should be reported to a law enforcement agency, the local medical society, or the hospital where the physician has been granted privileges. Would it be wise to remain in the office under the circumstances? Would it be better to seek other employment? Would remaining adversely affect future opportunities for employment with another physician?

These decisions are difficult, especially if the relationship and employment conditions have been favorable and congenial. An ethical medical assistant will not wish to participate in known substandard or unlawful practices, especially those that might be harmful to patients. In addition, the medical assistant must never make inaccurate reports regarding unethical behavior and should realize that some states can prosecute individuals who file a false report. Be absolutely certain of the facts before making such accusations against any health professional.

CLOSING COMMENTS

Medical assistants have an ethical obligation to keep abreast of current developments that affect the practice of medicine and care of the patients. Membership in a professional organization provides access to continuing education for maintaining knowledge and skills pertaining to the performance of medical assisting.

The study of ethics requires much thought and honest appraisal of what the medical assistant believes. Sometimes **introspection** of this type is difficult. Often our beliefs are a result of our environment, upbringing, and other factors that have influenced our thinking and actions from the time we were small children to our current age. It is important that our belief system be one that we have created personally, not just a set of beliefs accepted from another source. Medical assistants should take a serious look at the thoughts and concepts that make up their own concepts of ethics. It is important to approach ethical decisions calmly, logically, and without haste.

SUMMARY OF SCENARIO

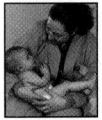

Pregnancy is usually a joyous time, but Monica has learned that even such an anticipated event can bring ethical issues to light. She has realized that there are two or more sides to every situation and that she must be open and willing to look at all sides when making an ethical decision.

Medical assisting is a rewarding career, but sometimes the decisions that face medical professionals are quite difficult. Monica must learn to be nonjudgmental and not to inflict her opinions on her patients. They must make their own decisions regarding their health and emotional well-being, and the medical assistant should not influence their thinking unfairly.

Monica will continue to evaluate her own ideas and beliefs throughout her career as a medical assistant. Periodic self-evaluation is good for everyone, and she will grow emotionally from the experiences that patients bring about where ethical issues are concerned.

Patients who place their babies for adoption often feel the same type of grief experienced on the death of a loved one. Sometimes this loss does not register with the patient for many years after the event. Adoptive parents face many fears as well, such as the concern that the adoptive mother will change her mind about the proceedings and want the child back. Some families find the adjustment to having an adopted child in the family a difficult one. Siblings may be less than accepting of the new child, and later in life other children may tease the adopted child. However, adoption is most often a positive event in the life of a family.

The medical assistant should be supportive to both adoptive parents and birth mothers. Personal beliefs should be set aside as the patient and others involved make the best decisions they are able to make for their own lives.

SUMMARY of LEARNING OBJECTIVES

1. Define, spell, and pronounce the terms listed in the vocabulary.
   - Spelling and pronouncing medical terms correctly adds credibility to the medical assistant. Knowing the definition of these terms promotes confidence in communication with patients and co-workers.

2. Explain rights and duties as related to ethics.
   - Ethics are judgments of right and wrong or actions on issues that have implications of a moral right and wrong. Etiquette deals with courtesy, customs, and manners. A duty is an obligation that a person has or perceives himself or herself to have. Rights are claims that are made by a person or group on society, a group, or an individual. Although these terms have different definitions, the concepts are interrelated, and often all are involved in ethical questions.

3. List and define the four types of ethical problems.
   - Ethical distress is caused when a problem has an obvious solution but some type of barrier hinders the action that needs to be taken. An ethical dilemma is a situation that has two or more solutions, but if one is chosen, something of value is lost in not choosing the other. A dilemma of justice involves allocation of benefits and how they are to be fairly distributed. Two or more authority figures, each with his or her idea of how to handle a certain situation, are the center of the locus of authority ethical problem. Only one of the authority figures can prevail. Often an ethical problem has several aspects and more than one type of problem is presented.

4. Discuss the process used for making an ethical decision.
   - Making an ethical decision is easier when the situation is approached logically and considered using a five-step process. First, one gathers relevant information; then the type of problem is identified. After determining the ethical approach to use, one should explore alternatives. Finally, all that is left is to complete the action and make the decision.

5. Detail the impact that the CEJA has on the ethical decisions made by healthcare professionals.
   - Although healthcare professionals do not have to abide by the opinions of the CEJA, the Council's opinions are highly regarded, and many professionals practice in accordance with these opinions. Often providers will abide by the opinions to avoid controversy, but many still openly oppose the decisions of the CEJA.

6. Describe the way unique identifiers help HIV-positive patients to avoid some discrimination.
   - Unique identifiers maintain the confidentiality of patients who are tested for HIV. Some individuals might hesitate to be tested if they were concerned that their names would be reported to various agencies. Using the unique identifiers, patients may have much more confidence that the chances of discrimination resulting from HIV status are lessened.

7. Note some of the concerns regarding ethics that surround genetic information.
   - Many ethical concerns exist regarding genetic testing. Many patients are concerned about how the information gained will be used and who will have access to the information. Questions arise regarding the ownership of the information. When negative information is found, other ethical problems arise that will need to be addressed. Knowledge of a person's genetic blueprint could lead to discrimination. Countless issues must be examined before the use of genetic information becomes widespread.

8. Explain why confidentiality is an ethical issue.
   - Confidentiality is of major importance in the medical profession. The patient's privacy should be of prime concern to a medical assistant. It is a serious enough issue that a breach of patient confidentiality is sufficient reason for immediate termination of an employee. Because it is such a critical aspect of patient care, it is considered highly unethical to reveal any information about a patient to anyone else. All medical assistants are required and expected to uphold the confidentiality of the information with which they come into contact.

9. Discuss several of the CEJA opinions and how they might differ from the views of the class as a whole.
   - The opinions put forth by CEJA are just one group of opinions. Class members may share very differing views based on culture, past experience, or serious consideration of the issues. Each individual is entitled to have an opinion, and these opinions should be discussed and shared calmly and respectfully.

CONNECTIONS

 Study Guide Connection: Go to Chapter 6 Study Guide. Read the Case Study and Workplace Applications and complete the assignments. Do online research for answers to the questions in the Internet Activities associated with medicine and ethics.

 CD Connection: Go to the Medical Assisting Competency Challenge CD and do the training activities under Legal Concepts.

evolve **Evolve Connection:** For more information related to medicine and ethics, go to evolve.elsevier.com/kinn and visit related weblinks for Chapter 6. Click on the Medical Assisting Exam Review and do the practice questions to sharpen your test-taking skills.

Medicine and Law

7

SCENARIO

Barbara Johnson is the new office manager for two neurologists in an urban area. Recently she was subpoenaed to appear in court with medical records to testify about a patient. This particular patient was referred to one of the physicians in the clinic, Dr. Rebecca Patrick. Dr. Patrick saw the patient several years ago, and the patient has brought a medical professional liability case against a surgeon in another city. Barbara is considered the custodian of medical records and will take them to court and answer questions about the information contained within them.

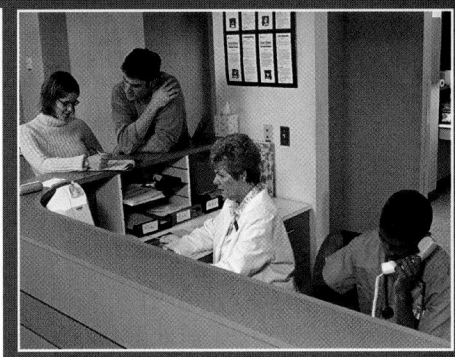

One of Barbara's first priorities at her new job is to make certain that the office is operating in compliance with the legal regulations that affect the facility. She is knowledgeable about OSHA requirements, and because her father was an attorney, she is very familiar with legal issues.

Two of the employees Barbara supervises, Samantha and Lynda, are newly graduated from medical assisting school and are anxious to learn more about the statutes and laws that affect the physicians' office. Barbara is more than happy to share what she has learned with them. She is excited about her new job and eager to be a great success.

While studying this chapter, think about the following questions:

- How can the medical assistant help to comply with legal regulations in the medical office?
- How can new graduates learn about the laws that affect them in their state?
- What are some ways that medical professional liability suits can be avoided?
- What should the medical assistant do if the employer is not in compliance with legal regulations?

LEARNING OBJECTIVES

1. Define, spell, and pronounce the terms listed in the vocabulary.
2. Distinguish among an act, a statute, and an ordinance.
3. Know the two types of law.
4. Explain the three basic categories of criminal law.
5. Distinguish which type of civil law deals with medical professional liability.
6. Explain the four essential elements needed for a valid contract.
7. Distinguish between interrogatories and depositions.
8. List three things to remember when testifying in court.
9. Discuss the advantages of arbitration.
10. Differentiate among malfeasance, misfeasance, and nonfeasance.
11. Explain the "four D's" of negligence.
12. Define the types of damages.
13. Explain the importance of informed consent.
14. List several legal disclosures the physician must make.
15. Explain the importance of the Health Insurance Portability and Accountability Act.
16. Distinguish between OSHA and CLIA, explaining which of the two is an actual agency.
17. Discuss the three ways in which a physician can obtain a license to practice medicine.
18. Discuss the ways that a physician might lose a license to practice medicine.

National Accreditation Competencies and Content

CAAHEP COMPETENCIES

General

3.c.(2)(a). Identify and respond to issues of confidentiality
3.c.(2)(b). Perform within legal and ethical boundaries
3.c.(2)(d). Document accurately
3.c.(2)(e). Demonstrate knowledge of federal and state health care legislation and regulations

ABHES COMPETENCIES

Legal Concepts

5.a. Determine needs for documentation and reporting
5.b. Document accurately
5.c. Use appropriate guidelines when releasing records or information
5.d. Follow established policy in initiating or terminating medical treatment
5.e. Dispose of controlled substances in compliance with government regulations
5.f. Maintain licenses and accreditation
5.g. Monitor legislation related to current healthcare issues and practices

Office Management

6.e. Maintain liability coverage

VOCABULARY

abandonment To withdraw protection or support; in medicine, to discontinue medical care without proper notice after accepting a patient.

act The formal action of a legislative body; a decision or determination of a sovereign state, a legislative council, or a court of justice.

allegation (a-li-ga′-shun) A statement by a party to a legal action of what the party undertakes to prove; an assertion made without proof.

appeal A legal proceeding by which a case is brought before a higher court for review of the decision of a lower court.

appellate (uh-pe′-lut) Having the power to review the judgment of another tribunal or body of jurisdiction, such as an appellate court.

arbitration (ar-buh-tra′-shun) The hearing and determination of a cause in controversy by a person or persons either chosen by the parties involved or appointed under statutory authority.

arbitrator (ar-buh-tra′-ter) A neutral person chosen to settle differences between two parties in a controversy.

assault An intentional, unlawful attempt of bodily injury to another by force.

assent To agree to something, especially after thoughtful consideration.

bailiff An officer of some U.S. courts usually serving as a messenger or usher, who keeps order at the request of the judge.

battery A willful and unlawful use of force or violence on the person of another.

Code of Federal Regulations (CFR) A coded delineation of the rules and regulations published in the *Federal Register* by the various departments and agencies of the federal government. The CFR is divided into 50 titles that represent broad subject areas, and then chapters that provide specific detail.

concurrently Occurring at the same time.

contributory negligence Statutes in some states that may prevent a party from recovering some damages if he or she contributed in any way to the injury or condition.

damages Loss or harm resulting from injury to person, property, or reputation; compensation in money imposed by law for losses or injuries.

decedent (di-se′-dent) A legal term for a deceased person.

defendant A person required to make answer in a legal action or suit; in criminal cases, the person accused of a crime.

docket A formal record of judicial proceedings; a list of legal cases to be tried.

due process A fundamental constitutional guarantee that all legal proceedings will be fair; that one will be given notice of the proceedings and given an opportunity to be heard before the government acts to take away life, liberty, or property; a constitutional guarantee that a law will not be unreasonable or arbitrary.

emancipated minor A person under legal age who is self-supporting and living apart from parents or guardian; a mature minor considered by the courts to possess a sufficient understanding of self-care and responsibility.

expert witnesses People who provide testimony to a court as experts in certain fields or subjects to verify facts presented by one or both sides in a lawsuit, often compensated and used to refute or disprove the claims of one party.

felony A major crime, such as murder, rape, or burglary; punishable by a more stringent sentence than that given for a misdemeanor.

fine A sum imposed as punishment for an offense; a forfeiture or penalty paid to an injured party or the government in a civil or criminal action.

guardian ad litem Legal representative for a minor.

implied consent Presumed consent, such as when a patient offers an arm for a phlebotomy procedure.

informed consent A consent, usually written, which states understanding of what treatment is to be undertaken and of the risks involved, why it should be done, and alternative methods of treatment available (including no treatment) and their attendant risks.

List continues on next page

List continued from previous page

infractions (in-frak'-shuns) Breaking the law; minor offenses against the rules, usually punishable by fines.

judicial (ju-di'-shuhl) Of or relating to a judgment, the function of judging, the administration of justice, or the judiciary.

jurisdiction (jur-uhs-dik'-shun) A power constitutionally conferred on a judge or magistrate to decide cases according to law and to carry sentence into execution; jurisdiction is original when it is conferred on the court in the first instance, called *original jurisdiction;* or it is appellate when an appeal is given from the judgment of another court.

jurisprudence (jur-uhs-proo'-dens) The science or philosophy of law; a system or body of law or the course of court decisions.

law A binding custom or practice of a community; a rule of conduct or action prescribed or formally recognized as binding or enforceable by a controlling authority.

liable (li'-uh-buhl) Obligated according to law or equity; responsible for an act or circumstance.

libel A written defamatory statement or representation that conveys an unjustly unfavorable impression.

litigious (luh-ti'-juhs) Prone to engage in lawsuits.

manifestation (ma-nuh-fuh-sta'-shun) Something that is easily understood or recognized by the mind.

misdemeanor (mis-duh-me'-nuhr) A minor crime, as opposed to a felony, punishable by fine or imprisonment in a city or county jail rather than in a penitentiary.

municipal (myu-ni'-suh-puhl) **courts** Courts that sit in some cities and larger towns and that usually have civil and criminal jurisdiction over cases arising within the municipality.

negligence (ne'-gli-jents) Failure to exercise the care that a prudent person usually exercises; implies inattention to one's duty or business; implies want of due or necessary diligence or care.

ordinance (or'-di-nens) Authoritative decree or direction; law set forth by a governmental authority–specifically, municipal regulation.

other potentially infectious materials (OPIM) Substances or materials other than blood that have the potential to carry infectious pathogens, such as body fluid, urine, semen, and others.

paraphrased Restated; applies to restatement of text, passage, or work to convey the meaning in another form.

perjured testimony The voluntary violation of an oath or vow either by swearing to what is untrue or by omission to do what has been promised under oath; false testimony.

physician office laboratories (POLs) Laboratories owned by a private physician or corporation, such as the laboratory inside a physician's office or a freestanding laboratory.

plaintiff The person or group bringing a case or legal action to court.

precedence (pre-sed'-ens) To surpass in rank, dignity, or importance; to be, go, or come ahead or in front of.

precedents (pre'-suh-dens) A person or thing that serves as a model; something done or said that may serve as an example or rule to authorize or justify a subsequent act of the same kind.

preponderance of the evidence Evidence that is of greater weight or more convincing than the evidence offered in opposition to it; evidence that as a whole shows that the fact sought to be proven is more probable than not.

prudent Marked by wisdom or judiciousness; shrewd in the management of practical affairs.

quackery The pretense of curing disease.

reasonable doubt Doubt based on reason and arising from evidence or lack of evidence; it is not doubt that is imagined or conjured up, but doubt that would cause reasonable persons to hesitate before acting.

recourse A turning to something or someone for help or protection.

relevant Having significant and demonstrable bearing on the matter at hand.

respondent (ri-spahn'-dunt) The person required to make answer in a civil legal action or suit; similar to a defendant in a criminal trial.

slander Oral defamation; a harmful, false statement made about another person.

statutes (sta'-choots) Laws enacted by the legislative branch of a government.

stipulate To specify as a condition or requirement of an agreement or offer; to make an agreement or covenant to do or forbear from doing something.

subpoena (suh-pe'-nuh) A writ or document commanding a person to appear in court under a penalty for failure to appear.

subpoena duces tecum A legally binding request to appear in court and provide records or documents that pertain to a particular case.

testimony A solemn declaration usually made orally by a witness under oath in response to interrogation by a lawyer or authorized public official.

Uniform Commercial Code (UCC) A unified set of rules covering many business transactions; it has been adopted in all 50 states, the District of Columbia, and most U.S. territories. It regulates the fields of sales of goods; commercial paper, such as checks; secured transactions in personal property; and particular aspects of banking, letters of credit, warehouse receipts, bills of lading, and investment securities.

verdict The finding or decision of a jury on a matter submitted to it in trial.

Law is a fascinating subject. When law is applied to medicine, it can provoke interesting case studies and complex decisions. In today's **litigious** society, medical assistants, as well as physicians and other staff members, must take steps to protect themselves from lawsuits. Legal issues underlie many aspects of the provision of healthcare in a physician's office. Although the wording of **statutes** and regulations is often long and complicated, medical assistants must stay abreast of the rules governing medical facilities and do everything possible to remain in compliance with the standards and regulations for all organizations that oversee the medical industry.

Generally, the law holds that every person is **liable** for the consequences of his or her own **negligence** when another person is injured as a result. In some situations this liability also extends to the employer. Physicians may be held responsible for the mistakes of those who work in their healthcare facility, and sometimes they must pay **damages** for the negligent acts of their employees.

Under the doctrine of respondeat superior, physicians are legally responsible for the acts of their employees when the employees are acting within the scope of their duties or employment. Physicians are also responsible for the acts of assistants who are not their own employees if the assistant commits acts of negligence in the presence of the physician while under the physician's immediate supervision. *Respondeat superior* is a Latin term meaning "let the master answer." When physicians practice as partners, they are liable not only for their own acts and those of their partners, but also for the negligent acts of any agent or employee of the partnership. A medical assistant acting within the scope of the employment contract is considered an agent of the employer.

Medical assistants who are guilty of negligence are liable for their own actions, but the injured party generally sues the physician, because the chance of collecting damages is greater. However, even an assistant who has no money can still be liable for any negligent action. This fact illustrates the continuing importance of exercising extreme care in performing all duties in the professional office.

JURISPRUDENCE AND THE CLASSIFICATIONS OF LAW

Jurisprudence, the science and philosophy of law, comes from the Latin words *juris*, which means "law, right, equity, or justice," and *prudentia*, which means "skill or good judgment."

Law is a custom or practice of a community. It is a rule of conduct or action prescribed or formally recognized as binding or enforceable by a controlling authority. Law is the system by which society gives order to our lives. The U.S. Constitution is the supreme law of the land, which takes **precedence** over federal statutes, court opinions, and state constitutions. However, within the states the state constitution is the supreme law within the boundaries of that state, unless it conflicts with the U.S. Constitution. States cannot pass laws that conflict with the U.S. Constitution, nor can local governments pass laws that conflict with the state constitution.

A law enacted at the federal level, which must be passed by Congress, is called an **act.** Statutes are laws that have been enacted by state legislatures. Local governments create and enact **ordinances.** Much of our law is based on previous **judicial** and jury decisions, which are called **precedents.** Often judges and juries follow precedents when making a decision on a case before them. The two basic categories of jurisprudence are criminal law and civil law.

Criminal Law

Criminal law governs violations of the law that are punishable as offenses against the state or the government. Such offenses involve the welfare and safety of the public as a whole rather than of one individual. Criminal offenses are classified into three basic categories: misdemeanors, felonies, and treason. In order to ensure fair treatment under the law, all physicians are entitled to **due process,** which guarantees that the accused will have an opportunity to defend himself or herself against any charges brought in opposition.

Misdemeanors

A minor crime, as opposed to a **felony,** is called a **misdemeanor.** Such a crime is punishable by **fine** or imprisonment in a city or county jail rather than in a penitentiary. Misdemeanors vary from state to state and are often divided into subgroups or classes, such as class A, class B, or class C misdemeanors. In most states the subgroups are divided from most serious offenses to lesser offenses. Some states have created a subcategory of misdemeanors for **infractions,** which are often called *violations.* Infractions are minor offenses, such as traffic tickets, which are punishable only by a fine.

Felonies

A felony is a major crime, such as murder, rape, or burglary, and is punishable by a more stringent sentence than that given for a misdemeanor. Federal law and most state statutes classify felonies as crimes punishable by imprisonment for more than 1 year, whereas misdemeanors are punishable by imprisonment for 1 year or less. Usually a convicted felon cannot vote, hold public office, or possess a firearm. Felonies are often divided into subgroups or degrees, such as first degree, second degree, and third degree. The first-degree offense is normally the most serious.

Treason

Treason, the most serious crime, is the offense of attempting to overthrow the government. High treason constitutes a serious threat to the stability or continuity of the government, such as an attempt to kill the president. The President of the United States has the right to declare an action against the United States to be an act of war, as opposed to an act of treason, which is considered a crime. For instance, although the terrorist attacks of September 11, 2001, were certainly a threat against the United States, they were declared acts of war.

Civil Law

Civil law is concerned with acts that are not criminal in nature but involve relationships of individuals with other individuals, organizations, or government agencies. Many types of civil law address numerous issues. The three that most directly affect the medical profession include tort law, contract law, and administrative law.

Tort Law

Tort law provides a remedy for a person or group that has suffered harm from the wrongful acts of others. Four elements must be established in every tort action. First, the **plaintiff** must establish that the **respondent** or **defendant** was under a legal duty to act in a particular fashion. Second, the plaintiff must demonstrate that the defendant breached this duty by failing to conform his or her behavior accordingly. Third, the plaintiff must prove that the breach of the legal duty proximately caused some injury or damage. Fourth, the plaintiff must prove damages, the injury or loss suffered. Medical professional liability, or medical malpractice, falls into the category of tort law. **Libel** and **slander** are common complaints that fall into the category of tort law.

Contract Law

A contract is an agreement creating an obligation. Contract law touches our lives in many ways practically every day, but we usually do not give much thought to its influences. If a person parks a car in a parking garage for a monthly fee and signs a contract for a year, then begins parking elsewhere and refuses to pay the fee, the person may be liable for the fees for the duration of the entire contract. If damage occurs to the person's vehicle while it is parked in the garage, the garage may be responsible for reimbursement, if the contract does not **stipulate** otherwise. A contract does not have to be formalized in writing to be binding on the parties involved. Oral contracts are also valid in many states in most situations. The **Uniform Commercial Code** is a long, elaborate act that attempts to harmonize the law of sales and other commercial transactions in all 50 states. This code directly affects contract law.

Administrative Law

Administrative law involves regulations set forth by governmental agencies. For example, the Internal Revenue Service (IRS) has thousands of regulations and codes, and the typical American does not understand all of them, which may result in errors when filing taxes. The laws that allow the IRS to collect taxes and pursue restitution are administrative laws. Other agencies that are involved with administrative law include the Social Security Administration (SSA), Citizenship and Immigration Services (USCIS), and the Centers for Medicare and Medicaid Services (CMS).

ANATOMY OF A MEDICAL PROFESSIONAL LIABILITY LAWSUIT

A medical liability case often stems from a breach of trust or miscommunication between the physician and the patient. These cases fall into the category of tort law. Even when the physician has made an error, often the level of trust between the physician and patient will determine whether a lawsuit will be pursued. First, the physician-patient relationship must be formed. Before discussing this relationship, it is important to understand what is necessary for a contract to be valid and enforceable.

What Constitutes a Valid Contract?

A valid legal contract has four essential elements. First, there must be **manifestation** of **assent** or a "meeting of the minds." This element is proven by an "offer" and the "acceptance" of that offer. The parties to the contract must understand and agree on the intent of the contract. Second, the contract must involve legal subject matter. An obligation that requires an illegal action, such as a gambling contract, is not an enforceable contract. Third, both parties must have the legal capacity to enter into a contract. This means that each party must be an adult of sound mind or an **emancipated minor.** Fourth, some type of consideration must be present. Consideration is an exchange of something of value, for example, money for the physician's time.

CRITICAL THINKING APPLICATION

Barbara works for Dr. Rebecca Patrick, who saw the patient bringing the lawsuit against the surgeon as a referral patient. Does Dr. Patrick have a contract with the patient, based on a physician-patient relationship? Why or why not?

The physician-patient relationship is generally held by courts to be a contractual relationship that is the result of three steps:
- The physician invites an offer by establishing availability.
- The patient accepts the invitation and makes an offer by arriving for or requesting treatment.
- The physician accepts the offer by accepting the patient and undertaking treatment. The physician may explicitly accept the patient's offer or implicitly accept the offer by exercising their independent medical judgment on behalf of the patient.

Before accepting a patient, the physician is under no obligation, and no contract exists. However, once the physician has accepted the patient, an implied contract does exist (Figure 7-1). This implied contract assumes that the physician will

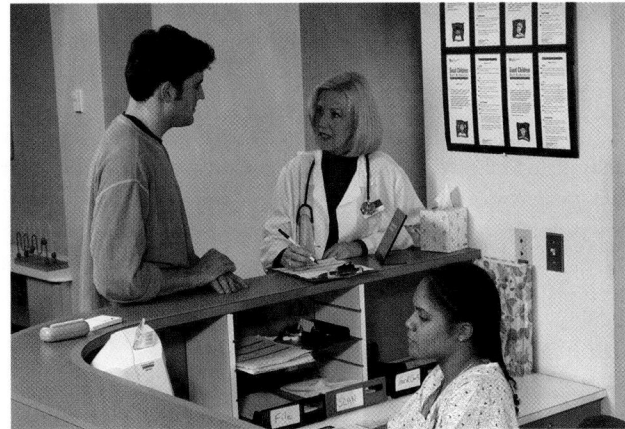

FIGURE 7-1 The physician-patient relationship is built on a strong foundation of trust, but it is also a contractual relationship.

treat the patient using reasonable care and that the physician possesses a degree of knowledge, skill, and judgment that might be expected of any other physician in the same locality and under similar circumstances. It is extremely important that no express promise of a cure be made by anyone in the office, including the physician, because this would become a part of the contract.

The patient's responsibility in this agreement includes the liability of payment for services and a willingness to follow the advice of the physician. Most physician-patient contracts are implied contracts. Although many forms may be completed by the patient before he or she is accepted by the physician, they do not in most cases constitute a formal contract for each specific visit to the physician.

CRITICAL THINKING APPLICATION

- If the patient does not pay for the services rendered by the physician, does this negate the physician-patient contract?
- How might Barbara, Samantha, and Lynda ensure that patients understand that they are expected to follow the advice of the physician?

After the physician-patient relationship has been established, the physician is obligated to attend the patient as long as attention is required, unless the physician or patient terminates the contract. When a physician terminates the contract, the patient must be given notice of the physician's intentions so that the patient has sufficient time to secure another physician. The physician may write a letter of withdrawal from medical care of the patient, and it should be delivered by certified mail, return receipt requested. A copy of the letter and the return receipt should be attached to the patient's chart and permanently retained. Reasonable time should be allowed for the patient to secure other medical care.

To protect the physician against a lawsuit for **abandonment,** the details of the circumstances under which the physician is withdrawing from the case should be included in the patient's medical chart. The letter of withdrawal does not have to specify a reason for withdrawal unless the physician so chooses, but it should state the following:

- That professional care is being discontinued
- That the physician will provide copies of the patient's records to another physician on request
- That the patient should seek the attention of another physician as soon as possible

A patient who wishes to terminate the physician-patient relationship simply no longer seeks the physician for treatment. The patient does not have to inform the office; however, if this is done, the office manager or physician should follow up with a letter confirming notice that the patient has ended the relationship.

The Statute of Frauds

In 1677 a statute was adopted in England that was designed to reduce the occurrence of **perjured testimony** by providing that certain contracts could not be enforced if they depended on the **testimony** of witnesses alone and were not evidenced in writing.

The provisions of this English statute have been closely followed by statutes adopted in all 50 states in the United States.

The promise to pay the debts of another person is an example of a contract that usually must be made in writing. If a third party who is not otherwise legally responsible for a patient's medical bills agrees to pay them, the agreement cannot be enforced unless it is in writing. If a physician were to enter into an agreement to perform a series of treatments for a given sum, and this series covered a time span of more than 1 year, the contract would have to be in writing to be enforceable.

Preliminaries of Litigation

Once a patient has decided to file a lawsuit against a physician, the first step is usually to find an attorney who will accept the case. This may be a frustration to many patients: attorneys may not wish to initiate litigation against a physician. Like physicians, attorneys do not have to accept cases they do not wish to pursue; this often occurs because the attorney does not see enough of a financial benefit from the time it would take to work on the case. Although this sounds a bit harsh, the attorney runs a business, as does a physician, and must make good business decisions as to how his or her time is spent and invested.

CRITICAL THINKING APPLICATION

- For what reasons might a physician not wish to accept a patient?
- Must the physician treat every patient who attempts to make an appointment?
- How might Barbara tactfully explain that the physician will not accept the patient into treatment?

Lawsuits are filed in a variety of different courts, and different states have different types of courts at various levels. The state judiciary has several branches. At the local level are usually **municipal courts.** These are courts in a city or town that usually deal with ordinance violations. Municipal judges may issue search and arrest warrants. Some states also have justice of the peace courts, which have **jurisdiction** over many misdemeanors and some civil matters, as well as concurrent jurisdiction over some matters along with the municipal courts. The judges that preside over justice of the peace courts may also issue search warrants and arrest warrants. They often function as small claims courts, with which the medical assistant may have contact in cases of patients who do not pay their bills. Both municipal and justice of the peace courts are local trial courts with limited jurisdiction.

County courts are higher than municipal and justice of the peace courts. These courts handle misdemeanors and civil matters up to a certain monetary limit. District courts have unlimited jurisdiction in criminal and civil matters. They are the highest state courts, other than **appellate** courts. When one party of a lawsuit is dissatisfied with a lower court's decision, it has the right to **appeal** to a higher court for review and possible reversal of the decision. Most states have an appellate court for both criminal and civil matters. The U.S. District Court handles federal matters of both a criminal and a civil nature. States

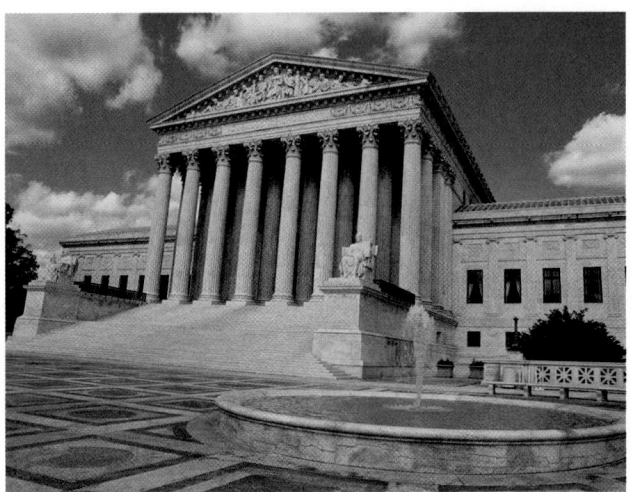

FIGURE 7-2 The U.S. Supreme Court. The Supreme Court decides cases that involve interpretation of the Constitution of the United States.

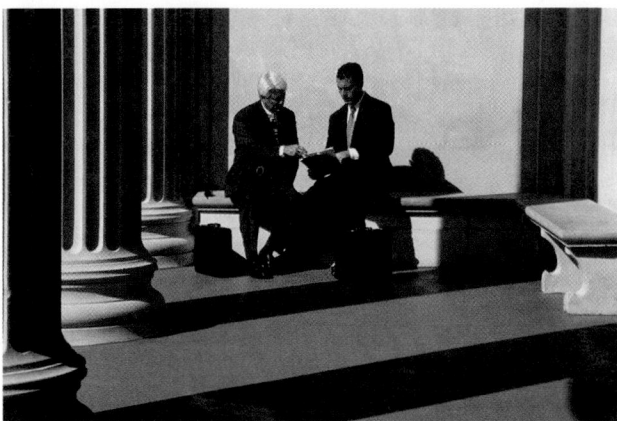

FIGURE 7-3 Preparation is of primary importance to the physician facing a medical professional liability case. A competent and experienced attorney is necessary to provide an adequate defense and present the physician's views to the court. Always be completely honest with the representing attorney.

also have Supreme Courts that handle a limited number of appellate cases.

The U.S. Supreme Court has authority given by Article III, Section One of the Constitution to ensure equal justice under the law (Figure 7-2). The Supreme Court interprets and guards the Constitution. The Court's one Chief Justice and eight Associate Justices are appointed by the President and confirmed by the Congress. The current Chief Justice of the Supreme Court is the Honorable John G. Roberts, Jr., who was appointed by President George W. Bush and confirmed by the U.S. Senate in 2005. The other Justices include Justice John Paul Stevens, Justice Antonin Scalia, Justice Anthony M. Kennedy, Justice David H. Souter, Justice Clarence Thomas, Justice Ruth Bader Ginsburg, Justice Stephen G. Breyer, and Justice Samuel Anthony Alito, Jr. Justice Sandra Day O'Connor, the first woman appointed to be a Supreme Court Justice, retired in 2005. Approximately 8000 cases are on the **docket** per term, which runs from the first Monday in October to the first Monday of October in the next year. Only 80 to 90 cases are chosen each year for full oral argument in front of the Justices.

CRITICAL THINKING APPLICATION

Samantha and Lynda are curious as to how Supreme Court decisions affect the individual physician's office. What Supreme Court decisions have affected the medical profession?

Preparing for Court

Medical professional liability suits are far from rare, and every physician faces the probability of being sued at least once during his or her career. When a suit is filed, preparation for court should start expeditiously. A medical assistant may be involved in preparing materials for court and scheduling or participating in depositions. The best advice for a medical assistant in this position is to remember to tell the truth. Attorneys will help to prepare the defense of the physician and the staff, but everyone should be truthful in the answers that are

given to the court to avoid losing his or her credibility in the trial and to avoid charges of perjury. Be especially careful to present a true and complete statement to the representing attorney. Unless he or she knows the whole truth, an appropriate defense cannot be prepared (Figure 7-3).

Interrogatories

Before the trial, the physician may be requested to complete an interrogatory, which is a list of questions from each party to the other in the lawsuit. Answers to the interrogatory must be provided within a specified time, and the answers are considered to be given under oath. Only the parties named in the lawsuit may be questioned through interrogatories.

Depositions

A deposition is testimony taken from a party or witness to the litigation and is not limited to the parties named in the lawsuit. A witness who is not a party to the lawsuit may be summoned by **subpoena** for the deposition. The deposition is usually taken in an attorney's office in the presence of a court reporter and is taken under oath. The person giving the deposition is called the *deponent*. The transcribed deposition, once finished, is sent to the deponent for review, and the deponent is at liberty to request any necessary changes or corrections in the document.

CRITICAL THINKING APPLICATION

- Samantha and Lynda are anxious to hear about Barbara's experiences in testifying in court. She mentions that attorneys often advise witnesses to "answer the question, then be quiet." What might be meant by this advice?
- Discuss the phrase, "the truth, the whole truth, and nothing but the truth."

Subpoenas

A subpoena is a document issued by a court requiring a person to be in court at a specific time and place to testify as a witness in a lawsuit, either in a court proceeding or in a deposition. A **subpoena duces tecum** is a legally binding request to provide records or documents to appear in court and is usually issued to the person considered the custodian of the records. This may be the medical assistant or office manager. A fee may be demanded for the time spent in compiling the records and for photocopying charges, but this fee must be requested at the time the subpoena duces tecum is served, or it is considered to be waived. Physician approval must be obtained to release or copy any patient records. Original records should never be released under any circumstances. Release only the information requested in the subpoena.

Before responding to a subpoena, make certain that it is valid. Although some variances may occur from state to state, some general rules can be used to judge the validity of a subpoena:

- A subpoena issued in one state court is generally not valid in another state. Always verify the state in which the subpoena was issued.
- A subpoena issued by a federal court in one state is generally not valid in another state unless a federal statute authorizes nationwide service of process.
- Any duly authorized law officer may execute a valid subpoena anywhere in the same state. The officer will notify the issuing court once the subpoena has been served.
- Generally, the person or entity who is issued a subpoena has 21 days to respond to the subpoena, but this time period can differ from place to place.
- A subpoena duces tecum should be filed no less than 15 days before a trial. One served less than 15 days before a trial should not be honored.

Read the subpoena carefully to determine exactly what records are being requested. The physician should always be notified of subpoenas served to the medical facility. Never copy records required in a subpoena without bringing the matter to the attention of the physician and/or office manager. It is also advisable to keep a log of subpoenas served to the office, what records were involved, and the disposition of the request, including when the records were presented to the court.

Discovery

Discovery is the pretrial disclosure of pertinent facts or documents by one or both parties to a legal action or proceeding. Many states have extensive discovery statutes that require each side to reveal to the other the facts that they "discover" while investigating the case. Discovery is also considered the process of uncovering facts in a lawsuit before the court proceedings.

Presentation of evidence may be by testimony. A witness is called who has some information about an aspect of the case and is asked questions by one or both attorneys. The witness will not know about every part of the case, but something that the person knows will be **relevant** to the case.

Another type of evidence may be documentary evidence. This is any type of evidence brought before the court by document or display. It could be a patient's chart, or a letter, a laboratory result, or a photograph. All of these are usually entered into evidence and numbered for easy reference.

CRITICAL THINKING APPLICATION

Samantha wonders what she should do if she ever finds negative information during a medical professional malpractice case that might harm her employer's defense. What advice would you offer? Would it be considered an obligation or a choice to report the employer of wrongdoing?

Preparing Witnesses and Testifying

Attorneys will prepare witnesses who may be called to testify during the court proceedings. They will review the questions that will be asked and potential questions that the opposite side may present. The attorney will help the witness to clarify the answers that he or she gives so that they are sharp and succinct. One of the first rules that attorneys learn in law school is to never ask a question to which they do not already know the answer.

Witnesses should be certain that they know the exact location of the courthouse and to which floor and courtroom they are to report. They should always be on time for a court appearance, because the judge and jury may frown on those appearing late. That frown may also include a fine or confinement in jail for contempt of court! When called to testify, it is critical that the witness dress conservatively and in a manner that shows respect for the court. Normal business attire should be adequate, but if any doubt is present, consult the attorney.

If any documents are to be referenced while testifying, the witness should review the documents before the court appearance if possible, so that the needed information will be easy to locate and discuss. The witness should speak clearly and at a volume audible to the attorneys and parties to the suit, the judge, the jury, and the court reporter. The witness should always answer each question aloud, because the court reporter must record those answers and cannot specify that the witness "nodded yes" as a response to a question.

If a question is confusing, the witness should ask the attorney to restate or repeat it. Attorneys may ask the witness to speak up, but this should not be intimidating to the witness. If the witness does not know the answer to a question or does not recall, that should be stated clearly and confidently. Above all, the parties involved are expected to tell the truth and must be seen as credible witnesses (Figure 7-4). Lying under oath constitutes perjury, which carries stiff penalties. Listening is as important as speaking, so the witness should be sure to listen to the question, and answer it, elaborating only if the attorney asks for more details.

If an attorney lodges an objection to a question, the witness should be silent until the judge rules on the objection. The objection may be sustained or overruled. Sustaining the objection means that the judge agrees with the objection and will not allow the question stated in that manner. If the judge allows the question, he or she will overrule the objection. Then the witness will be allowed to answer. The witness should never display a combative or hostile attitude and should not make sarcastic remarks while testifying in court. This is the fastest way to show disrespect for the judge, the jurors, and the court itself. No

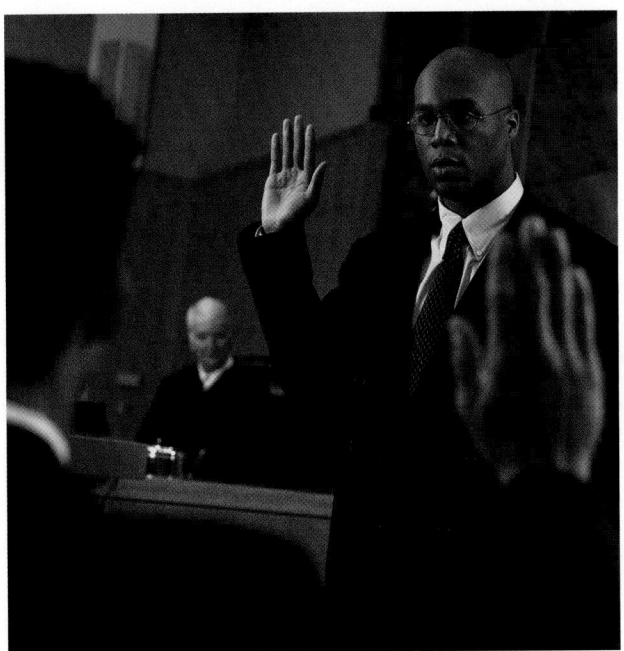

FIGURE 7-4 Witnesses must be credible and tell the truth on the stand in court to avoid charges of perjury.

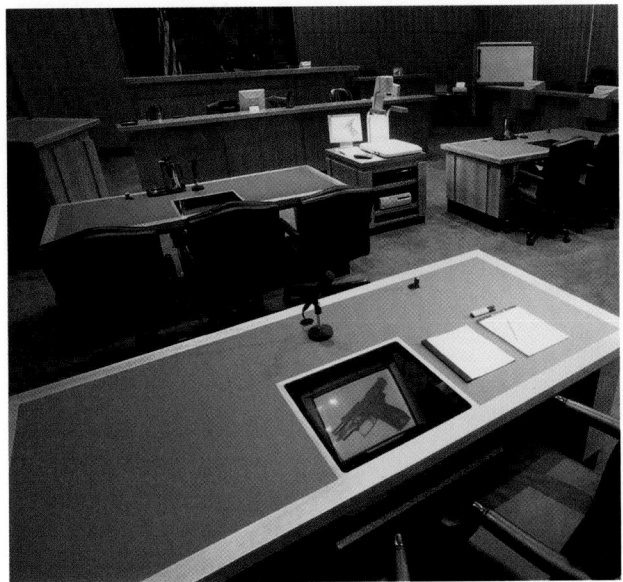

FIGURE 7-5 The inside of a typical U.S. courtroom.

matter the circumstances, the court is no place to express discontent. The witness should be professional at all times and restrain inappropriate comments and belligerent behavior. Using "yes, sir" and "no, ma'am" is appropriate in the courtroom. Always address the judge as "Your Honor."

Inside the Courtroom

Today's courtrooms are a far cry from the ones depicted on television shows representing the old west. Modern courtrooms are equipped with computer and video equipment, and elaborate security systems often monitor those who enter the building (Figure 7-5). The advent of Court TV has changed the

way Americans see the justice system. By simply turning on our televisions, we can watch justice at work.

It is beneficial to know the role of each person in a court of law. The person or body bringing the lawsuit to court is referred to by different terms, depending on what type of case is to be presented. In a criminal court, the government brings the case and is represented by a prosecutor. Legal documents will read, for example, "The State of Texas v. Robert Smith" in criminal cases. In this case, the fictitious Robert Smith is the defendant. In civil court, the person or group bringing the case to court is called the *plaintiff* (or *complainant* in some court systems), and the opposite party is called the *defendant* or *respondent*. A judge will preside over the case, providing instructions concerning the law to the jury, if a jury is present. If no jury is present, the judge decides the case. This is called a "bench trial." A witness is a person who gives testimony, knowing some pertinent information about the case (Figure 7-6). Often a court reporter takes notes of the proceedings, and a **bailiff** may be present, who assists in keeping order. All of these individuals should be treated with respect and courtesy.

Burden of Proof

In a criminal case the burden of proof is on the prosecution, which must prove guilt beyond any **reasonable doubt.** Reasonable doubt is defined as the level of certainty a juror must have to find a defendant guilty of a crime. It is real doubt, based on reason and common sense after careful and impartial consideration of all the evidence, or lack of evidence, in a case.

Civil cases must be proven by a **preponderance of the evidence.** This means that there must be a greater weight of evidence that points to the defendant or respondent as being responsible for the act involved in the case.

To understand the difference between reasonable doubt and preponderance of the evidence, think of the scales of justice (Figure 7-7). For a case to be proven beyond a reasonable doubt, the scales should tip heavily toward either guilt or innocence. However, for a case to be proven by preponderance of the evidence, the scales need only tip slightly one way or the other.

To illustrate the difference in the burden of proof in criminal and civil cases, consider "The People of the State of California v. Orenthal James Simpson." In O.J. Simpson's criminal trial, although there was much circumstantial evidence, there was also enough doubt that the scales could not tip heavily toward a **verdict** of guilty, and Mr. Simpson was acquitted. But in the civil trial brought by family members of Nicole Brown Simpson and Ron Goldman after the criminal trial had ended, there was just enough evidence to tip the scales in favor of the families' claim that Mr. Simpson was somehow responsible for the deaths of the two victims. This is the equivalent of a preponderance of the evidence.

CRITICAL THINKING APPLICATION

A discussion of the burden of proof prompts Barbara, Samantha, and Lynda to discuss the case of O.J. Simpson. Discuss whether reasonable doubt existed in his criminal trial.

HUMOR IN THE COURTROOM

Mary Louise Gilman has very possibly heard it all. As the editor of the *National Shorthand Reporter*, she collected enough courtroom bloopers to fill two books: "*Humor in the Court*" and "*More Humor in the Court.*" Here are a few examples!

Q: Were you acquainted with the deceased?
A: *Yes, Sir.*
Q: Before or after he died?

Q: What happened then?
A: *He told me, he says, "I have to kill you because you can identify me."*
Q: Did he kill you?
A: *No.*

Q: When he went, had you gone and had she, if she wanted to and were able, for the time being excluding all the restraints on her not to go, gone also, would he have brought you, meaning you and she, with him to the station?
A: *Objection. That question should be taken out and shot.*

Q: And lastly, Gary, all your responses must be oral. O.K.? What school do you go to?
A: *Oral.*
Q: How old are you?
A: *Oral.*

Q: ...and what did he do then?
A: *He came home, and next morning he was dead.*
Q: So when he woke up the next morning he was dead?

Q: ...any suggestions as to what prevented this from being a murder trial instead of an attempted murder trial?
A: *The victim lived.*

Q: What is your date of birth?
A: *July fifteenth.*
Q: What year?
A: *Every year.*

Q: This myasthenia gravis–does it affect your memory at all?
A: *Yes.*
Q: And in what ways does it affect your memory?
A: *I forget.*
Q: Can you give me an example of something you've forgotten?

Q: What was the first thing your husband said to you when he woke that morning?
A: *He said, "Where am I, Cathy?"*
Q: And why did that upset you?
A: *My name is Susan.*

Q: She had three children, correct?
A: *Yes.*
Q: How many were boys?
A: *None.*
Q: Were there any girls?

Q: Doctor, before you performed the autopsy, did you check for a pulse?
A: *No.*
Q: Did you check for a blood pressure?
A: *No.*
Q: Did you check for breathing?
A: *No.*
Q: So, then it is possible that the patient was alive when you began the autopsy?
A: *No.*
Q: How can you be sure, Doctor?
A: *Because his brain was sitting on my desk in a jar.*
Q: But could the patient have still been alive nevertheless?
A: *Yes, it is possible that he could have been alive and practicing law somewhere.*

FIGURE 7-6 Humor in the courtroom. (From Gilman M, editor: *More humor in the court*, Vienna, Va, 1985, National Shorthand Reporters Association.)

Outcome of the Case

Once both sides have presented their case to the judge or jury, they are usually given the opportunity to present a final summation of their case. After this is done, the jury retires to consider the verdict. This can take minutes, hours, days, or weeks. After the jury reaches a decision, the judge may enter it as a final verdict or may disregard it if the evidence does not support the jury's decision. The judge may also revise the verdict to comply with statutes, such as statutory limits on the amount of punitive damages. The final decision of the trial court is reflected in the judgment, signed by the judge.

Either side normally has the right to appeal the decision to a higher court. However, not all appellate courts are required to hear all cases. For instance, the U.S. Supreme Court chooses the cases that it hears each year, and it is restricted to cases that involve interpretation of the Constitution and how that interpretation affects the people it governs.

In criminal cases when a person is found guilty of the crime with which he or she is charged, a sentencing date will be set, usually a few weeks to a few months after the verdict is announced, at which time the punishment will be announced.

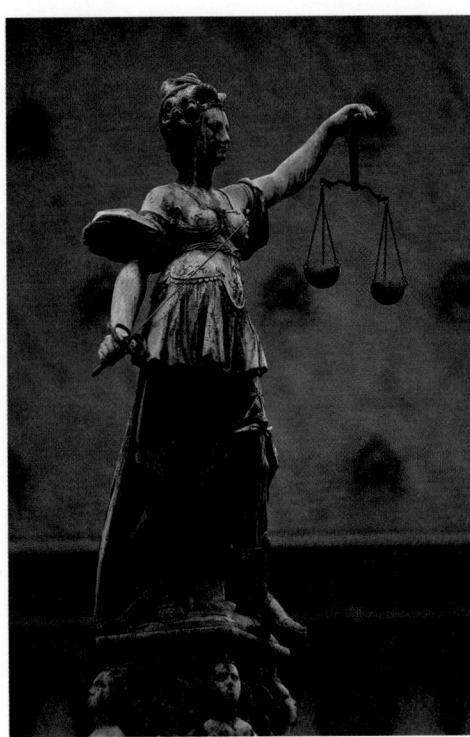

FIGURE 7-7 "Lady Justice." Justitia was the Roman goddess of justice and is the figure depicted in statues across the world, often holding both scales and a sword. Her scales imply the weighing of justice, and the blindfold represents the impartiality of justice.

ARBITRATION

Arbitration is an alternative to trial that uses a third party who has been selected because of the party's familiarity with or knowledge of the law or the issues involved to hear evidence and make a decision. Arbitration is common in modern business life. It is recognized by statute in the majority of the states and is usually available to the medical profession, affording an alternative method for resolving legal disputes between physician and patient. Many physicians and attorneys see arbitration as one way to solve the crisis of litigation in this country. Court battles can take years and can be extremely expensive, and much of the money will revert to the attorneys involved in the case instead of the victors of the lawsuit.

In arbitration the patient and the physician agree to submit the dispute to an **arbitrator** in an informal hearing. The arbitrator will render a legally binding decision based on very specific rules of arbitration. Arbitration applies essentially the same rights and the same measure of damages as a court. It is fair, less expensive, faster, and more confidential than court litigation.

The staff of each medical office should know whether arbitration statutes exist in the state where the office conducts business. The state medical board or local medical society should be able to provide this information. An arbitration agreement is a contract and is subject to the judgment of the courts only as to the fairness of the agreement. The agreement is precisely worded by an attorney and should not be **paraphrased** when explaining it to a patient. Signing the agreement is a voluntary act by the patient, who has a grace period in which to revoke the agreement if he or she later decides against it. Likewise, a physician always has the option to decide not to care for a patient but must formally notify a patient if the decision is made to no longer render care.

If a physician elects to implement an arbitration agreement procedure with patients, every member of the physician's staff should know the details of the agreement, how and when the patient should sign up, and how to answer the patient's questions. The way that the program is presented to the patient and the willingness with which the office personnel answer the patient's questions will play a large part in whether courts will uphold the arbitration agreement as being fair and legal.

Both the patient and the physician have the opportunity to agree on who will arbitrate the case, so that it does not favor one side over the other. By prior agreement the arbitrator (or arbitrators) may be appointed by or from the American Arbitration Association, which is a neutral, private, nonprofit association dedicated to the advancement of out-of-court remedies. Its panels of arbitrators are made up of persons from business, the professions, and public interest groups.

MEDICAL PROFESSIONAL LIABILITY AND NEGLIGENCE

When injury results to a patient as a result of a physician's negligence, the patient may initiate a malpractice lawsuit to recover financial damages. However, experience has shown that the incidence of malpractice claims is directly related to the personal relationship and trust that exist between the physician and the patient. A deterioration of the physician-patient relationship is a common reason for the patient's decision to sue the physician for malpractice, even in situations in which no real injury has been sustained by the patient.

Medical professional liability, commonly called *medical malpractice,* is governed by the law of torts. The term *medical professional liability* encompasses all possible civil liability that can be incurred during the delivery of medical care. Medical professional liability is much more easily prevented than defended.

To understand medical malpractice, one must first understand the term *negligence.* Negligence, in general, implies inattention to one's duty or business, or the implication of a lack of necessary diligence or care. In medicine, negligence is defined as the performance of an act that a reasonable and **prudent** physician would not do or the failure to do an act that a reasonable and prudent physician would do. This, of course, also applies to any other healthcare professional. The standard of prudent care and conduct is not defined by law but would be left to the determination of a judge or jury, usually with the help of **expert witnesses** (Figure 7-8). Expert witnesses are members of the profession involved—in this case, medicine. To be considered an expert witness, a person usually belongs to a certifying or qualifying organization against which the qualities of the defendant may be compared.

Professional negligence in medicine falls into one of three general classifications:

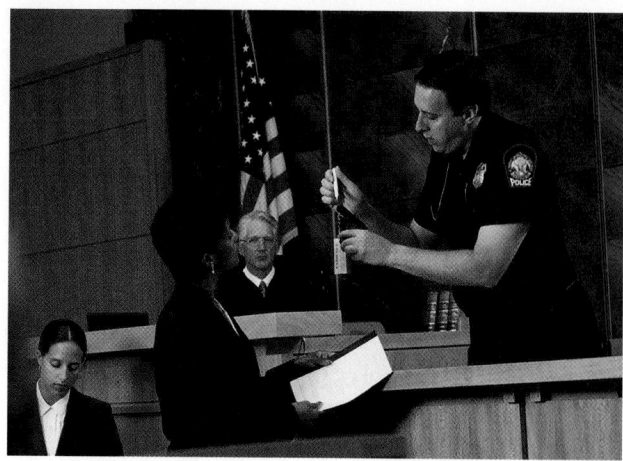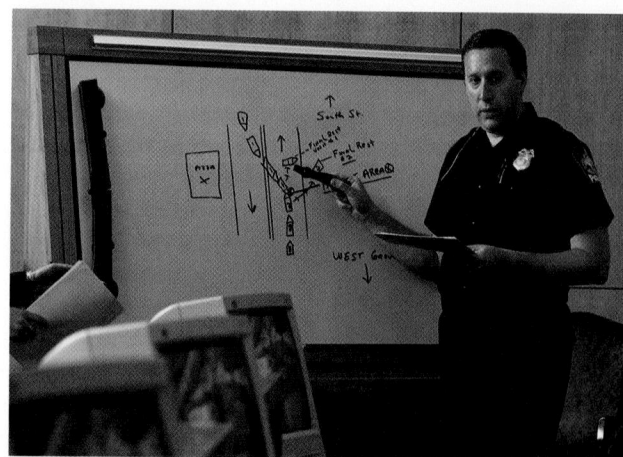

FIGURE 7-8 Expert witnesses help attorneys to prove or disprove the case in question by drawing on their experience with a given subject.

- Malfeasance: The performance of an act that is wholly wrongful and unlawful
- Misfeasance: The improper performance of a lawful act
- Nonfeasance: The failure to perform an act that should have been performed

A physician who performs an operation carelessly or fails to render care that should have been given may be found to have been negligent. Although a medical assistant acts as an agent of the physician in carrying out the majority of his or her duties, it is possible for the medical assistant to perform an act that can result in litigation.

For instance, if the medical assistant gives a patient the wrong medication or the wrong dose of medication, both the physician and the medical assistant can be held liable for the error. Some states limit the scope of practice of medical assistants where medications are involved; however, if medical assistants are performing within the realm of duties for which they have received training and the physician is accepting responsibility for the actions of those in the medical office, they are usually allowed to dispense and administer medications unless prohibited by state law. The medical assistant should always perform within the legal boundaries of his or her state (Procedure 7-1).

CRITICAL THINKING APPLICATION

Lynda is curious as to whether a physician is guilty of medical professional liability if he or she makes a mistake in diagnosing a patient. When might this be considered malpractice, and when might it not be considered malpractice?

What if the patient makes his or her condition worse? Is the physician then fully responsible? **Contributory negligence** exists when the patient contributes to his or her own condition and can lessen the damages that can be collected or even prevent them from being collected altogether.

The Four D's of Negligence

Negligence is not presumed; it must be proven. The Committee on Medicolegal Problems of the American Medical Association (AMA) has determined that patients must present evidence of four elements before negligence has been proven. These elements have become known as the "four D's of negligence":

- Duty: Duty exists when the physician-patient relationship has been established. The patient has sought the assistance of the physician, and the physician has knowingly undertaken to provide the needed medical service.
- Dereliction: Dereliction, or failure to perform a duty, is the second element required. There must be proof that the physician somehow neglected the duty to the patient.
- Direct cause: There must be proof that the harm to the patient was directly caused by the physician's actions or failure to act and that the harm would not otherwise have occurred.
- Damages: The patient must prove that a loss or harm has resulted from the actions of the physician.

If all four of these elements exist, then the patient may obtain a judgment against the physician in a medical professional liability case.

Types of Damages

Several types of damages are commonly seen in tort cases. They are nominal, punitive, compensatory, general, and special damages.

Nominal damages are small awards that are token compensations for the invasion of a legal right in which no actual injury was suffered. For instance, if an unauthorized medical facility employee accesses a patient's medical record and is discovered but has not revealed any of the information in the record, the patient has not actually been harmed but may be awarded nominal damages in a lawsuit for the invasion of the patient's privacy.

Punitive damages are designed to punish the party who committed the wrong in such a way so as to deter the repetition of the act and are sometimes called *exemplary damages*. These damages were historically set so that the amounts would discourage intentional wrongdoings, misconduct, and outrageous behaviors. The amount of damages awarded would coincide in some percentage with the wealth of the defendant. Today there is much discussion of tort reform, which would place a cap on

PROCEDURE 7-1

Perform Within Legal Boundaries

CAAHEP COMPETENCY: 3.c.(2)(b)
ABHES COMPETENCY: 5.g

GOAL: *To perform duties within legal boundaries in the state where employed as a medical assistant.*

EQUIPMENT and SUPPLIES

- Computer
- Access to text of various laws and regulations affecting the practice

PROCEDURAL STEPS

1. Become familiar with the laws that affect medical practices in your state.
   PURPOSE: To understand which laws apply to the employer's facility.
2. Read the laws and regulations thoroughly.
   PURPOSE: To understand the concept and intent of the laws and regulations.
3. Obtain additional training on compliance with the laws and regulations, if necessary.
   PURPOSE: To make certain that all actions and procedures in the office are in compliance with applicable, current laws.
4. Read journals and any information available about the laws.

PURPOSE: To remain current in compliance activities.

5. Stay aware of licensure issues that affect the physician, including:
   - Licensure
   - Registration
   - Certification
   - Suspension
   - Revocation
   PURPOSE: To ensure that the physician is always practicing legally.
6. Know the scope of practice for a medical assistant.
   PURPOSE: To ensure that the medical assistant is always practicing legally.
7. Make certain that information is available on current laws and regulations at all times.
8. Perform all activities in accordance with applicable laws and regulations.
   PURPOSE: To insure compliance with applicable laws and regulations.

---

the amount of money that could be collected during personal injury litigation, including medical malpractice cases. Some have suggested a specific monetary figure, such as $500,000, as a limit on punitive damages, and others have suggested that plaintiffs be allowed to collect only up to three times the amount of compensatory damages.

CRITICAL THINKING APPLICATION

Samantha and Lynda disagree as to whether punitive damages should be awarded in medical professional liability cases. Samantha feels that nothing will compensate for certain losses, but Lynda feels that monetary compensation is reasonable when a loss has been suffered. Discuss both sides of the issue.

Compensatory damages are designed to compensate for any actual damages that are caused by the negligent person. They are intended to make the injured person "whole." Of course, nothing can substitute for the loss of an arm or a leg, for example, but compensatory damages help the patient or the patient's family recover from the loss.

General damages include compensation for pain and suffering, for loss of a bodily member or faculty, for disfigurement, or for other similar direct losses or injuries. The fact of the losses must be proven, but the monetary value does not.

Special damages are those injuries or losses that are not a necessary consequence of the physician's negligent act or omission. These may include the loss of earnings or costs of travel. Both the fact of these losses and the monetary value must be proven.

Standard of Care

If a physician were to be held legally responsible for every unsuccessful result occurring in the treatment of a patient, no person would undertake the responsibility of practicing medicine. The courts hold that a physician must do the following:

- Use reasonable care, attention, and diligence in the performance of professional services
- Follow his or her best judgment in treating patients
- Possess and exercise reasonable skill and care that are commonly possessed and exercised by other reputable physicians in the same type practice in the same or a similar locality

Physicians who represent themselves as specialists must meet the standards of practice of their specialty. Whether or not they have met these requirements in treating a particular patient is generally a matter for the court to decide on the basis of testimony provided by an expert witness. Physicians are not required to possess extraordinary learning and skill, but they must keep abreast of medical developments and techniques, and they cannot experiment. They are also bound to advise their patients if they discover that the condition to be treated is one beyond their knowledge or technical skill.

In the worst of cases, a physician or medical facility may be faced with wrongful death litigation. A wrongful death **allegation** is one in which the physician or medical facility is being blamed for the death of a patient as a result of error or inappropriate treatment. A wrongful death suit is usually brought by the family of the **decedent** against the physician or others involved with the patient.

A medical assistant should treat every chart touched as if it will end up in a court of law. Handwriting must be implicitly clear and legible, information must be detailed, and absolutely no room must be left for errors. Never mark out, cross out, erase, or white-out a mistake. Always draw one line through the error, then initial and date it. Nothing should be committed to memory. Remember, if it is not in the chart, it did not happen!

Consent

A physician must have consent to treat a patient, even though this consent is usually implied by virtue of the patient's appearance at the office for treatment. This **implied consent** is sufficient for common or simple procedures that are generally understood to involve little risk. Phlebotomy and taking vital signs are examples of procedures that usually involve implied consent. When more-complex procedures are anticipated, the physician must obtain the patient's **informed consent.** A physician who fails to secure some formal expression of consent could be charged with the crime of **battery.**

The Health Insurance Portability and Accountability Act (HIPAA) was designed for two major purposes. First, a standardization of electronic data exchange was sought in hopes that the efficiency of the healthcare system would be improved. Second, HIPAA was developed to protect health information and secure the contents of patient medical records. In the past a section of the Health Insurance Claim Form (CMS-1500) was reserved for the patient to authorize the release of medical information to the insurance company so that the claim could be evaluated and paid. Today, because of the influence of HIPAA, many medical offices are moving toward the use of a general consent form that is signed before the physician sees the patient. This form allows the physician to not only treat the patient, but also to use and submit health information to third parties for reimbursement.

Informed consent involves a deeper understanding of the patient's condition and a full explanation of the plan for treatment. Informed consent is not satisfied merely by having the patient sign a form. A discussion must occur during which the physician provides the patient or the patient's legal representative with enough information to decide whether the patient will undergo the treatment or seek an alternative. After such discussion, the patient either consents to the proposed therapy and signs a consent form or refuses to consent. According to the AMA's standards for informed consent, the discussion should contain the following elements, at a minimum:

- The patient's diagnosis, if known
- The nature and purpose of a proposed treatment or procedure
- The risks and benefits of a proposed treatment or procedure

- Alternative treatments or procedures, regardless of the cost or the extent to which the treatment options are covered by health insurance
- The risks and benefits of the alternative treatment or procedure
- The risks and benefits of not receiving or undergoing a treatment or procedure

The discussion should be fully documented in the patient's medical record, and a copy of the signed form should be placed in the record. Treatment may not exceed the scope of the consent that the patient has given. Often the consent forms will be lengthy and mention excessive possibilities and complications. There may be language that attempts to be all-inclusive, such as "included, but not limited to" when risks are listed. It is wise to have an attorney review the forms that are used for informed consent, because those that are too broad or too specific can be detrimental to the physician in a medical professional liability case.

Patients cannot be forced to undergo any type of medical treatment or care. The ultimate decision regarding care must be left to the patient, and although medical professionals should disclose information to help the patient make a good, informed decision, the patient should never be persuaded to act in any manner or accept any treatment with which he or she does not agree. Should the patient decide not to undergo treatment that the physician feels is necessary, an informed refusal of treatment or care should be signed. This should be a statement similar to the informed consent but will indicate that the patient has elected not to undergo treatment. Some physicians will discontinue all treatment if a patient does not participate in the care that the physician recommends. This document, once signed, should be added to the patient's medical record.

CRITICAL THINKING APPLICATION

Barbara stresses to Samantha and Lynda that there may be times in their professional career when a patient asks for their advice as to whether he or she should undergo a certain procedure or treatment. Barbara explains that patients often consider advice from the medical assistants in the office to be an extension of the physician's opinions. How might they handle such questions from patients? Should a medical assistant offer any type of advice?

Giving Consent to Medical Procedures

Mentally competent adults are certainly able to consent to medical procedures. However, if an act is unlawful, then the consent is invalid. For instance, if an abortion is performed in a state where abortion is illegal, then the consent to that procedure is null. Consent is also invalid if it is given by a person who is unauthorized to do so or if it is obtained by misrepresentation or fraud.

In an emergency, one may render aid or care to prevent loss of life or serious illness or injury. However, implied consent in this circumstance lasts only as long as the emergency exists, and formal consent must be obtained for further treatment as soon as the emergency has passed.

Physicians are sometimes reluctant to render aid in an emergency to someone who is not their patient for fear that they will later be charged with negligence or abandonment. In 1959 California passed the first Good Samaritan Act, which provides immunity from liability to volunteers at the scene of an accident for any civil damages as a result of rendering emergency care. Today, the majority of states have either Good Samaritan or Volunteer Protection statutes. As long as the emergency care is given in good faith and without gross negligence, and the healthcare worker provides only emergency care that he or she has been trained to provide, the likelihood of a successful lawsuit against that individual is very slim.

Adults who have been found by a court to be insane or incompetent usually cannot consent to medical treatment. Consent must be obtained from the guardian except in emergency situations.

Generally, when the patient is a minor, consent for surgery or treatment must be obtained from a parent, guardian, or **guardian ad litem,** except in an emergency requiring immediate treatment. If the parents are legally divorced or separated, consent should be obtained from the custodial parent, but if the child is visiting the second parent, consent may be obtained from that parent, because in such a situation that parent has temporary custody.

Consent is not required for minors in the following circumstances:

- When consent may be assumed, such as in a life-threatening situation
- When a certain treatment is required by law, such as a vaccination or x-ray evaluation for school entry or safety
- When a court order has been issued, as in a situation in which parents withhold consent for a necessary treatment because of religious reasons

In many states, treatment of sexually transmitted diseases, drug abuse, alcohol dependency, or pregnancy or providing birth control measures does not require parental consent.

Emancipation is defined by statute and varies from state to state. An emancipated minor is a person younger than the age of majority (usually 18 to 21 years) who meets one or more of the following conditions:

- Is married
- Is in the armed forces
- Is living separate and apart from parents or a legal guardian
- Is self-supporting

Some states include a minimum age for emancipation. Unless a statute declares otherwise, a minor who has the right to consent to treatment is entitled to the protection of his or her confidences, even from parents.

Statute of Limitations

A statute of limitations is a period of time after which a lawsuit cannot be filed. The statute of limitations varies from state to state and differs for various types of litigation. Many states have a 2-year statute of limitations for medical malpractice issues. However, in some instances, the statute of limitations may be extended because of a delay in the discovery of an

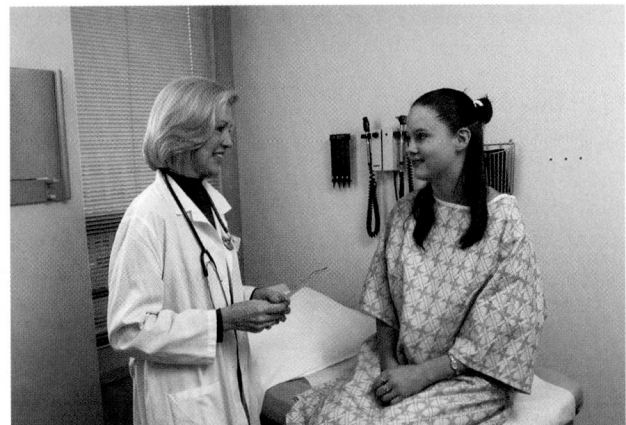

FIGURE 7-9 Patient confidentiality is the most important trust that exists between the physician and the patient.

injury. For example, a patient has surgery to replace a valve in the heart, and the surgery seems successful. Two years later, the patient undergoes a routine echocardiogram and the physician discovers that the surgeon mistakenly replaced the aortic valve when the surgery was intended for the pulmonary valve. Although 2 years have already passed, the statute of limitations begins at the point of discovery of the injury, so the patient could now bring suit against the surgeon for the error.

Confidentiality

Confidentiality is one of the most sacred trusts that the patient places in the hands of the physician and his or her staff (Figure 7-9). Breach of patient confidentiality is grounds for immediate dismissal of a healthcare professional. The strictest care must be taken when handling patient records and discussing information about patients.

In many special cases patient confidentiality plays a vital role. A patient who is human immunodeficiency virus (HIV) positive may face discrimination if the information about his or her medical condition surfaces. Physicians who treat such patients may wish to take extra care when leaving phone messages or sending mail. Instead of leaving a message for a patient from "Dr. Watson's office," the medical assistant could say that the message is from "Terry Watson's office." This could indicate an attorney, accountant, or real estate broker. Curious co-workers or relatives may not grow as suspicious as they might if they were to encounter a message from a physician's office.

Patients who are receiving treatment for substance abuse are protected by federal statutes. Confidentiality is also of utmost importance to patients receiving treatment for mental health issues, sexually transmitted diseases, sexual **assault,** and any type of abuse.

LAW AND MEDICAL PRACTICE

Law affects the day-to-day practice of the physician. Some of the ways in which the medical assistant will encounter legal issues in the physician's offices are discussed in this section. The medical assistant must comply with both state and federal laws and regulations while performing the duties associated with his or her job (Procedure 7-2).

Legal Disclosure

The physician is charged with safeguarding patient confidences within the constraints of the law, but according to state laws, which vary somewhat throughout the nation, certain disclosures must be made. Frequently the medical assistant is involved with the responsibility for reporting these events.

Births and deaths must be reported. In some states, detailed information about stillbirths is required. Physicians must also report cases that may have been a result of violence, such as gunshot wounds, knife injuries, or poisonings. Any death from accidental, suspicious, or unexplained causes must also be reported. In some states, occupational diseases and injuries must be reported within specific time limits.

Sexually transmitted diseases are reportable in every state. All 50 states require that patients who have confirmed cases of acquired immunodeficiency syndrome (AIDS) be reported by name to the local health department. However, just over 30 states require that patients who are HIV positive be reported. Individuals are reported either by name or by unique identifiers. A continuing controversy exists as to whether the reporting prompts patients to receive care or deters patients in high-risk groups from seeking care.

Child abuse is a leading cause of death among children younger than 5 years of age, and healthcare professionals are required by law to report any suspected cases of child abuse. The report should be made as soon as evidence is discovered that gives the physician "cause to believe" that abuse or neglect has occurred. Even if the evidence is uncertain, the physician should report the evidence and allow the government to investigate and determine what action to take to protect the child. However, it is essential to make every attempt to ensure that the report is legitimate, because it could lead to the child's being removed from the home and placed in foster care. Cases of spousal and elder abuse are difficult, because the person being abused is often reluctant to report the situation for fear of further mistreatment. The law requires that suspected cases of abuse of children, elderly persons, or any others at risk be reported to the authorities.

Local health departments publish lists of diseases that are reportable as well as the method that should be used in reporting. Often this can be done by telephone or mail. Appropriate forms must be used for mail reporting and are supplied by the health department or available on their websites. County and state health departments periodically issue bulletins that are sent to healthcare providers and provide information about disease outbreaks and various statistics. Local health departments should be consulted for specific procedures and reporting protocols.

PROCEDURE 7-2

Demonstrate Knowledge of Federal and State Health Care Legislation and Regulations

CAAHEP COMPETENCY: 3.c(2)(e)
ABHES COMPETENCY: 5.g

GOAL: *To be aware of federal and state legislation and regulations that apply to the employer's facility.*

EQUIPMENT and SUPPLIES

- Computer
- Access to organizational websites that have established legislation and regulations that pertain to medical facilities
- Information about changes to and new federal and state legislation and regulations

PROCEDURAL STEPS

1. Consistently review applicable legislation and regulations that apply to the facility.
   PURPOSE: To ensure compliance with the law.
2. Discover the federal and state ramifications of issues related to healthcare workers, such as:
   - Regulatory bodies
   - Education and credentials
   - Scope of practice
   - Job qualifications
   - CEU requirements
   - Loss of credentials
   PURPOSE: To ensure full compliance in the medical facility.

3. Review and understand federal and state legislation and regulations related to:
   - Americans with Disabilities Act
   - Controlled Substance Schedules
   - OSHA
   - Centers for Disease Control
   - Local Public Health Departments
   - Materials Safety Data Sheets (MSDS)
   PURPOSE: To ensure full compliance in the medical facility.
4. Review and understand accrediting agency requirements that affect the facility.
   PURPOSE: To ensure full compliance in the medical facility.
5. Stay aware of new state and federal legislation and regulations.
   PURPOSE: To ensure full compliance in the medical facility.
6. Always follow office policy when performing any action at the facility.
   PURPOSE: To ensure full compliance in the medical facility.

Patient Self-Determination Act

The Patient Self-Determination Act of 1990 brought the term *advance directives* to the forefront of medical care. This act requires healthcare facilities to develop and maintain written procedures that ensure that all adult patients receive information about living wills, durable powers of attorney for healthcare, and advance directives. These documents place the decision-making power into the hands of the patient and the patient's family, providing them with written notification of their right to consent to or refuse medical treatment.

Patients' Bill of Rights

In March of 1998, President Bill Clinton received the final report from the President's Advisory Commission on Consumer Protection and Quality in the Healthcare Industry. The Commission was created to advise the President on the current issues facing the healthcare industry and make recommendations that would assure that patients would receive high-quality healthcare services. The report, entitled *"Quality First: Better Healthcare for All Americans,"* led to the development of a Consumer Bill of Rights and Responsibilities for the healthcare industry. This is usually called the Patients' Bill of Rights. The document lists three specific goals:

- To strengthen consumer confidence by assuring the healthcare system is fair and responsive to consumer's needs, provides consumers with credible and effective mechanisms to address their concerns, and encourages consumers to take an active role in improving and assuring their health
- To reaffirm the importance of a strong relationship between patients and their healthcare professionals
- To reaffirm the critical role consumers play in safeguarding their health by establishing rights and responsibilities for all participants in improving their health

Most healthcare facilities have adopted a Patient Bill of Rights that provides a condensed version of the entire report, which contains eight sections. Often this information is presented to patients when they are admitted to healthcare facilities, or one might see it posted in a prominent place within the facility.

Because it is a patient's right to understand his or her diagnosis, prognosis, and all aspects of care, one must take special care when dealing with a patient with whom there may be a language barrier. If the patient's ability to understand is limited, an interpreter may be needed to ensure that communication from physician to patient is adequate.

Controlled Substances Act

On May 1, 1971, the Controlled Substances Act of 1970 became effective. In October 1973 a regulatory agency known as the Drug Enforcement Administration (DEA) became a part of the U.S. Department of Justice. The DEA works with local, state, federal, and international agencies and organizations to address and regulate the serious issues of drug use and abuse in the United States.

Before administering, prescribing, or dispensing any drugs, a physician is required to register with the regional office of the DEA. This registration is renewable every 3 years. If a physician

---

Patients' Bill of Rights

I. Information Disclosure
You have a right to receive accurate and easily understood information about your health plan, healthcare professionals, and healthcare facilities. If you speak another language, have a physical or mental disability, or just don't understand something, assistance will be provided so you can make informed healthcare decisions.

II. Choice of Providers and Plans
You have the right to a choice of healthcare providers that is sufficient to provide you with access to appropriate high-quality healthcare.

III. Access to Emergency Services
If you have severe pain, an injury, or sudden illness that convinces you that your health is in serious jeopardy, you have the right to receive screening and stabilization emergency services whenever and wherever needed, without prior authorization or financial penalty.

IV. Participation in Treatment Decisions
You have the right to know all your treatment options and to participate in decisions about your care. Parents, guardians, family members, or other individuals that you designate can represent you if you cannot make your own decisions.

V. Respect and Nondiscrimination
You have a right to considerate, respectful, and nondiscriminatory care from your doctors, health plan representatives, and other healthcare providers.

VI. Confidentiality of Health Information
You have the right to talk in confidence with healthcare providers and to have your healthcare information protected. You also have the right to review and copy your own medical record and request that your physician amend your record if it is not accurate, relevant, or complete.

VII. Complaints and Appeals
You have the right to a fair, fast, and objective review of any complaint you have against your health plan, doctors, hospitals, or other healthcare personnel. This includes complaints about waiting times, operating hours, the conduct of healthcare personnel, and the adequacy of healthcare facilities.

---

works from more than one office, he or she must register each individual office. Regulations regarding the writing, telephoning, and refilling of prescriptions vary according to which schedule is involved.

Under the Controlled Substances Act, drugs are categorized into Schedules I, II, III, IV, and V. Drugs in Schedule I have the highest potential for abuse and addiction, and those in Schedule V have the lowest abuse potential.

Schedule I substances are those that have no accepted medical use in the United States. Examples include heroin and lysergic acid diethylamide (LSD). Only the physician who is involved in conducting research with such drugs is concerned with Schedule I substances.

Schedule II drugs have a high abuse potential, with severe risk of mental and physical dependence. They include certain narcotic, stimulant, and depressant drugs, such as opium, morphine, codeine, and methylphenidate (Ritalin). Controlled substances in Schedule II can be obtained only with a federal triplicate order form obtained from the DEA. A special inventory must be maintained on controlled substances and retained for 2 to 3 years, depending on state requirements. When a controlled substance is removed from inventory, it must be recorded. The record must show the date, the name of the drug, the dosage, and the name of the patient, physician, and employee involved. Schedule III, IV, and V substances do not require triplicate forms.

Schedule III substances have an abuse potential that is lower than that of the first two schedules. They include compounds that contain limited quantities of certain narcotic drugs combined with nonnarcotic substances. Examples include acetaminophen (Tylenol) with codeine, hydrocodone, butalbital with aspirin and caffeine (Fiorinal), and several steroids.

Schedule IV substances have still lower potential for abuse. Phenobarbital, diazepam (Valium), propoxyphene (Darvon and Darvocet), alprazolam (Xanax), chlordiazepoxide (Librium), and pentazocine lactate (Talwin) are examples.

Schedule V substances have lower abuse potential than those in Schedule IV but still warrant control. They include preparations that contain moderate quantities of certain narcotics as may be found in cough medicines and antidiarrheal products.

The physician may call a prescription to the pharmacist, but the pharmacist must transcribe it in writing before filling it. With permission from the physician, the medical assistant may orally transmit a prescription for controlled substances only in Schedules III, IV, or V, and the dispensing pharmacist must put the prescription into writing before filling it. The medical assistant cannot under any circumstances orally transmit a prescription for a Schedule II drug. These prescriptions must be presented in writing to the pharmacist on the appropriate form.

Stored controlled substances must be kept in a locked cabinet or safe. Any loss of controlled drugs by theft must be reported to the regional office of the DEA at the time the theft is discovered. If a physician discovers that his or her DEA number is being used in the unauthorized prescribing of controlled substances, he or she should report the incident to the DEA, to the state regulatory agency, and to the local police authorities. This is especially important in the case of employees whose employment has been terminated and who are suspected of drug theft in the office. There have been numerous cases of retaliation by fired employees who report to the DEA exactly what they have actually taken, yet accuse the physician or other staff members of taking the controlled substances. This results in messy investigations and months of follow-up, so any suspected employee drug use or abuse should be documented and reported to the local authorities. Periodic drug testing of employees is one way to help prevent office drug abuse. Many states now have laws to prevent the filing of false reports, so if

the physician is wrongly accused by a disgruntled employee, the physician often has some **recourse.**

A physician who discontinues medical practice must return the registration certificate and any unused order forms and triplicate prescription pads to the nearest office of the DEA. The regional DEA office will advise the physician on the disposition of any controlled drugs still on hand.

CRITICAL THINKING APPLICATION

Barbara explains the importance of reporting any employee who is suspected of using drugs or taking drugs from the office. This may be difficult, because co-workers are often friendly with one another and may hesitate to report such acts. Discuss ways to handle this situation.

Uniform Anatomical Gift Act

The Uniform Anatomical Gift Act was approved by the National Conference of Commissioners on Uniform State Laws in 1968. Although many states had passed laws before this time that permitted living persons to make a gift of their body or portions of it after death, the laws were so different from state to state that arrangements for a donation in one state might not be recognized in another. All states have adopted the Uniform Anatomical Gift Act or similar legislation.

Essentially, the model law for donation states the following:

- Any person of sound mind and 18 years of age or older may give all or any part of his or her body after death for research, transplantation, or placement in a tissue bank.
- A donor's valid statement of gift is paramount to the rights of others except when a state autopsy law may prevail.
- If a donor has not indicated an intent to donate during his or her lifetime, his or her survivors, in a specified order of priority, may do so.
- Physicians who accept organs or tissues, relying in good faith on the documents, are protected from lawsuits. The physician attending at the time of death, if acquainted with the donor's wishes, may dispose of the body under the Uniform Anatomical Gift Act.
- The time of death must be determined by a physician who is not involved in the transplantation, and the attending physician cannot be a member of the transplant team.
- The donor may revoke the gift, or the gift may be rejected by the proposed recipient.

The most important clause of the act permits the donation to be made by a will (without waiting for probate) or by other written or witnessed documents, such as a card designed to be carried by the person or a Uniform Donor Card (Figure 7-10). The Uniform Donor Card is considered a legal document in all 50 states. Many states now list donor preference on the driver's license as well.

The provisions of the Uniform Anatomical Gift Act are so designed that the offer is exercised only after death. Therefore

```
 _____
|  ┌─────────┐                                |
|  │ DONOR   │              DONOR CARD        |
|  └─────────┘                                |
|  I _____, have spoken to my family about |
|  organ and tissue donation. I wish to donate: |
|  __ any needed organs and tissue            |
|  __ only the following organs and tissue: _____ |
|  The following people have witnessed my     |
|  commitment to be a donor.                  |
|  donor signature _____ date _____ |
|  witness_____ |
|  witness_____ |
|  next of kin _____ ph _____ |
 _____
```

FIGURE 7-10 Organ donation card.

donors should reveal their intentions to as many of their relatives and friends as possible and to their physician. Because the human body and its parts are not commodities in commerce, no money can be exchanged in making an anatomic donation itself. Fees are charged for performing the transplant and various procedures, but organs cannot be bought and sold. It is also important to note that family members should be prepared to receive the body of the person who has donated his or her entire body to research once the research facility has completed its study. This can often be a traumatic experience, rekindling the grief process once again, so the procedures and final disposition of the body should be decided at the time of the donation to avoid this difficult situation.

Health Insurance Portability and Accountability Act

HIPAA was signed into law on August 21, 1996, and all healthcare providers were required to comply with HIPAA's privacy standards by April 2003. Its history began in the Clinton healthcare reform proposals. HIPAA was designed for several purposes, with many goals in mind. Limiting administrative costs of healthcare and privacy issues, as well as prevention of fraud and abuse, are of primary importance within the HIPAA regulations. The law has two provisions, which include Title I (Insurance Reform) and Title II (Administration Simplification). The use of electronic transmissions ideally lowers the administrative costs of providing healthcare, but this led to problems with privacy regarding health information. The law also had to provide security and confidentiality guarantees for the individual patient. Extensive privacy rules, including the use of unique identifiers, have shaped the law.

The final regulations regarding the privacy legislation sections of HIPAA were published in December 2000, after HCFA reviewed more than 50,000 comments on and concerns about this important subject. All healthcare organizations that transmit any health information electronically must comply with HIPAA; fines as well as prison terms can be imposed on those who do not comply with the regulations.

HIPAA has had a tremendous effect on the healthcare industry. All healthcare providers, clearinghouses, and health plans that use electronic information must comply with HIPAA regulations. The benefits of HIPAA compliance include the following:

- Lower administrative costs
- Increased accuracy of data
- Increased patient and consumer satisfaction
- Reduced revenue cycle time
- Improved financial management

HIPAA's Title I, which deals with insurance reform, includes several provisions that protect individuals and their insured dependents in the event that they change jobs or lose a job. Preexisting condition clauses are limited, and an individual cannot be discriminated against for a poor health history when changing insurance coverage. HIPAA also ensures that an individual can renew health insurance coverage even if he or she has a health condition that is covered under the policy. In many cases, individuals are guaranteed the right to purchase health insurance coverage after the loss or change of a job.

Title II details the process of administrative simplification. The standardization of the exchange of healthcare data is one way in which HIPAA promotes computer-to-computer transactions. This standardization process helps to reduce the number of forms and methods used in the claims processing cycle, including electronic transactions, standard code sets (such as diagnosis, procedure, and supply codes), and the provision for unique identifiers for providers, employers, health plans, and patients. These unique identifiers use alphanumeric systems to ensure privacy. Title II also details the implementation of privacy and security procedures designed to prevent the misuse of health information by ensuring confidentiality. Security standards were required to be in place by April 2005. Medical professionals who access medical information must use log-in and password systems that prevent unauthorized individuals from accessing protected health information.

Occupational Safety and Health Act and the Bloodborne Pathogens Standard

In 1970 President Nixon signed the Occupational Safety and Health Act, which created what we know today as the Occupational Safety and Health Administration (OSHA). OSHA is a division of the U.S. Department of Labor, and since its creation workplace injuries, illnesses, and fatalities have been significantly reduced. OSHA's mission is to ensure workplace safety and a healthy environment within the workplace.

Although OSHA is commonly thought of as the regulatory agency that requires steel-toed boots and hard hats, the medical industry moved into the OSHA spotlight in the late 1980s, when the threat of HIV infection extended to healthcare workers. Hepatitis and other pathogens were already of concern to healthcare workers, but when HIV, the virus that causes AIDS, was identified, action was needed to better protect the individuals who cared for patients with these infectious diseases. OSHA's Final Ruling on Bloodborne Pathogens became fully effective in July 1992, and since that time various additions have been made to update the regulations in light of new information learned about blood-borne pathogens.

The law requires medical facilities to comply with the Bloodborne Pathogens standard and to be able to prove that compliance to OSHA inspectors if necessary. The actual standard can be found in the 29 **Code of Federal Regulations**

(CFR) 1910.1030. The following information details the legal requirements of the OSHA Standard as it pertains to the physician's office.

General Duty Clause

No law can cover every single situation that may arise in the course of daily living. Because of this, OSHA's general duty clause is a catch-all regulation that fits almost any situation not specified in any other section of the law. The general duty clause simply states that a workplace must be free of any hazard that might cause serious harm or death. For example, one breach of the general duty clause is the "failure of a facility to provide reasonable security procedures at a retail store." Although not a specific breach of any regulation, this fits nicely into the general duty clause.

Occupational Safety and Health Administration Regulations as Performance-Based Standards

OSHA regulations are considered performance-based standards. This means that adequate compliance depends largely on what happens in the facility. For instance, the same regulations may not apply to two offices located right next to each other. Would it be possible that a family practitioner could be fined for not having sharps containers, whereas a surgeon in the office next door, inspected by the same OSHA inspector, does not receive a fine for not having sharps containers? It is possible if the surgeon does not perform any invasive, surgical, or any other procedures that involve blood in the office! Some surgeons perform all procedures at facilities other than the office.

This is one reason that employees must be trained in their individual facilities. Even if training was done 1 month before a job change, the employee must be trained again in the new facility. Offices and procedures are different from place to place, and the employee must have adequate training to function successfully in the medical office.

OSHA inspectors can recommend fines when a facility is found to be out of compliance with an OSHA standard. One of the most common infractions is that the facility has an Exposure Control Plan in the facility but is not using it or following the procedures and policies set forth within it. This could lead to an inspector's declaring the facility to be willfully negligent. Willful negligence exists when "an employer representative was aware of the requirements of the [OSHA] Act, or the existence of an applicable standard or regulation, and was also aware that the condition or practice was in violation of those requirements, and did not abate the hazard." Fines for noncompliance can quadruple for willful negligence.

Exposure Control Plan

The Exposure Control Plan can be a part of the regular safety plan written for the medical facility or may be a stand-alone document, but it must cover all of the elements required by OSHA. This plan must be in writing and be reviewed annually, and there must be written documentation that the plan was reviewed and updated or revised, if needed. A hard copy must be provided to employees on their request within 15 working

---

Common Occupational Safety and Health Administration Violations

- No eyewash facilities available
- No labeling or improper labeling of hazardous chemicals
- No MSDS for each hazardous chemical
- Storage of contaminated laboratory coats with clean ones
- Not communicating hazards to employees
- No documentation of initial employee training
- No documentation of annual employee training
- No annual hazard assessment performed
- Having an Exposure Control Plan but not following it
- No proof of destruction of hazardous waste
- No Emergency Action Plan in the facility
- No written Exposure Control Plan
- OSHA Form 300A not posted during required period
- No records of hepatitis B vaccinations or declination forms

MSDS, Material Safety Data Sheets; *OSHA*, Occupational Safety and Health Administration.

---

days, and the plan must be available at all times in the workplace.

The plan must delineate the tasks that employees perform where risk of blood exposure is present. It must also classify jobs within the facility according to the likelihood of exposures. For instance, some job duties would always expose the employee to blood or **other potentially infectious materials (OPIM)**, often on a daily basis. Some duties would only occasionally expose the employee, and other duties would never expose the employee to blood or OPIM. Employees must be told which category they are a part of and what duties they will perform that could lead to exposures. In addition, there must be a clear follow-up procedure in place that details how the medical facility will track employee exposures. The employee cannot be abandoned after an exposure incident. Periodic counseling must take place in which the facility determines and documents the progress of the employee who has had an exposure, including laboratory tests and medical treatment received.

The Exposure Control Plan must contain a Waste Management section that details how waste is removed from the facility and destroyed. Most medical offices contract with companies that specialize in removing and destroying medical waste. The office must keep the receipts given by the company that prove that the waste was taken away from the facility and then incinerated or otherwise destroyed.

The plan must also contain a section on Hazardous Materials Communication, which explains what substances in the facility are hazardous and how to handle a spill or exposure to those products. Only the manufacturer of a chemical can determine whether it is hazardous, and Material Safety Data Sheets (MSDS) must be kept on almost all chemicals and reagents in the facility. Recent rulings have exempted some chemicals, but without the MSDS information, a medical assistant could not determine what type of health, reactivity, flammability, or other risks the chemical could have.

If the facility has equipment for x-ray studies, a Radiation Safety Plan must also be written and followed. All facilities should have an Emergency Action Plan in place, which provides procedures in case of tornadoes, fires, floods, or any other type of emergency that might occur in the office. This plan should contain floor plans of the facility, diagrams depicting the most efficient exits from the building, and the chain of command in an emergency. Diagrams with exit routes should be posted in every room of the medical office. At least annually, a hazard assessment must be performed on the entire facility. The hazard assessment is an inspection for problem areas in which the facility might be out of compliance. The facility must have documentation that the hazard assessment was done.

Occupational Safety and Health Administration Record Keeping Regulations.

An injury or illness is considered to be work related when an event or exposure in the work environment contributed to or caused the condition or significantly aggravated a preexisting condition. OSHA made several changes in the regulations concerning work-related injury record keeping to simplify forms, protect employee privacy, encourage employee involvement, and enable computer usage for meeting OSHA requirements. The revised rules took effect on January 1, 2002. Three basic forms are now used to keep records regarding injuries, accidents, and illnesses related to the workplace. The forms are as follows:

- OSHA Form 300–Log of Work-Related Injuries and Illnesses (Figure 7-11): Information is posted on form 300 regarding work-related deaths and every work-related injury or illness that involves loss of consciousness, restricted work activity or job transfer, days away from work, or medical treatment beyond first aid. An OSHA Form 301 (Injury and Illness Incident Report) should be completed for each entry on the log.
- OSHA Form 300A–Summary of Work-Related Injuries and Illnesses (Figure 7-12): Form 300A must be completed even if no injuries or illnesses occurred during the year that were work related. It must be posted in a common area for viewing by all employees, and provides the total number of accidents, illnesses, and injuries in the facility for the previous year. The length of time that this information must be posted has increased from 1 month to 3 months, specifically from February 1 to April 30 each year. An additional change is the certification of the form. A company executive must examine the document and certify that it is accurate.
- OSHA Form 301–Injury and Illness Incident Report (Figure 7-13): Form 301 is used to report what actually happened when an employee suffers a work-related injury or illness. This form, or an acceptable substitute, such as a state worker's compensation form, must be completed within 7 calendar days after notification of the illness or injury. The form should be completed as quickly as possible so that an exact recollection of events can be documented. Now that the new record-keeping regulations have become effective, employees are

guaranteed access to their OSHA 301 forms for the first time.

The log and summary forms must be kept on file for a minimum of 5 years. Only the Summary should be posted during the specified time period from February 1 to April 30 each year, reflecting information from the previous calendar year. The forms are not sent to OSHA unless specifically requested.

CRITICAL THINKING APPLICATION

Barbara quickly realizes that the office is using older versions of OSHA Forms 300 and 301. Where might she look or go to find updated information and forms?

It is wise to keep a communication log of calls to OSHA in which questions were asked or information verified. Note the day and time called, the first and last name of the person spoken to, the person's title, and the question asked and response given. Take detailed notes while discussing the issue on the phone. This log could be invaluable if a question ever arises about a subject discussed with a local OSHA official. It may make the difference when an OSHA inspector suggests a hefty fine. If the medical facility can show documentation that a certain procedure was discussed with an OSHA official and decisions were made based on that discussion, the facility may have sufficient evidence that the law was considered and the facility did its best to comply.

Needlestick Safety and Prevention Act

An estimated 600,000 to 800,000 injuries occur annually among healthcare workers. One third of these injuries happen during the disposal process. In an effort to reduce these injuries, which can lead to exposure to HIV, hepatitis B virus (HBV), or other blood-borne pathogens, OSHA revised its Bloodborne Pathogens standard to comply with the Needlestick Safety and Prevention Act, which became law on November 6, 2000. The regulations became effective on April 18, 2001.

Employers are now required to involve employees in the selection of needle safety devices. The facility must be able to prove that consideration was given to various types of devices that promote needle safety, what led to the decision to choose the device currently in use, and which employees were involved in these decisions. A list should be kept of which employees contributed to the selection decisions. Minutes from meetings, copies of employee response forms, and the forms used to solicit input are good methods of proving that employees were involved in the selection process.

CRITICAL THINKING APPLICATION

Barbara needs input about the needle safety devices being used in the facility. Should she call a meeting of the entire office, or are there specific employees who should be present? If so, discuss who should have input in these decisions.

A needlestick and sharps injury log must also be kept in the medical facility. At a minimum, the log must include the following information:

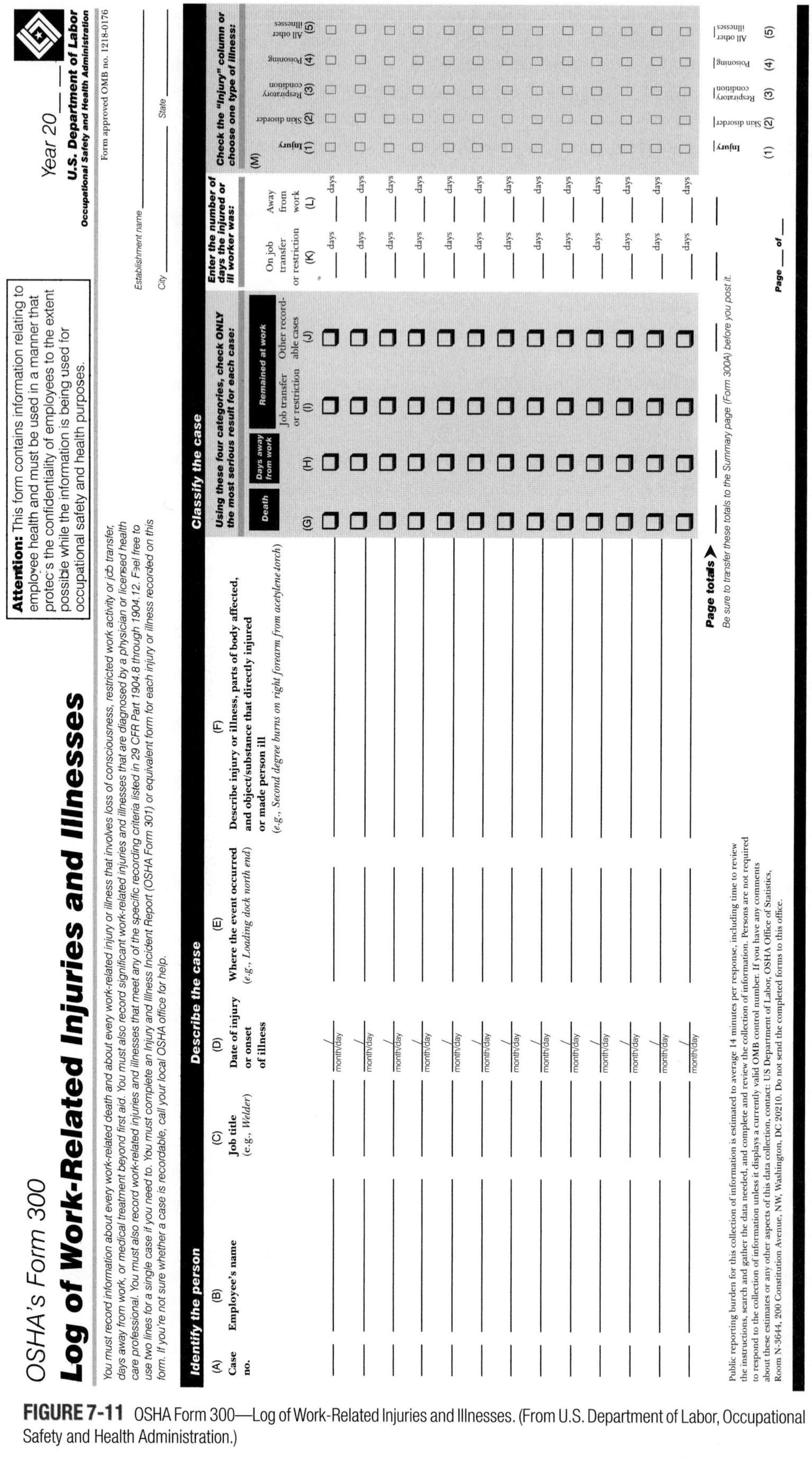

FIGURE 7-11 OSHA Form 300—Log of Work-Related Injuries and Illnesses. (From U.S. Department of Labor, Occupational Safety and Health Administration.)

FIGURE 7-12 OSHA Form 300A—Summary of Work-Related Injuries and Illnesses. (From U.S. Department of Labor, Occupational Safety and Health Administration.)

OSHA's Form 301
Injury and Illness Incident Report

U.S. Department of Labor
Occupational Safety and Health Administration

Form approved OMB no. 1218-0176

This *Injury and Illness Incident Report* is one of the first forms you must fill out when a recordable work-related injury or illness has occurred. Together with the *Log of Work-Related Injuries and Illnesses* and the accompanying *Summary*, these forms help the employer and OSHA develop a picture of the extent and severity of work-related incidents.

Within 7 calendar days after you receive information that a recordable work-related injury or illness has occurred, you must fill out this form or an equivalent. Some state workers' compensation, insurance, or other reports may be acceptable substitutes. To be considered an equivalent form, any substitute must contain all the information asked for on this form.

According to Public Law 91-596 and 29 CFR 1904, OSHA's recordkeeping rule, you must keep this form on file for 5 years following the year to which it pertains.

If you need additional copies of this form, you may photocopy and use as many as you need.

Attention: This form contains information relating to employee health and must be used in a manner that protects the confidentiality of employees to the extent possible while the information is being used for occupational safety and health purposes.

Information about the employee

1) Full name _____

2) Street _____

City _____ State _____ ZIP _____

3) Date of birth ___ / ___ / ___

4) Date hired ___ / ___ / ___

5) ☐ Male
☐ Female

Information about the physician or other health care professional

6) Name of physician or other health care professional _____

7) If treatment was given away from the worksite, where was it given?

Facility _____

Street _____

City _____ State _____ ZIP _____

8) Was employee treated in an emergency room?
☐ Yes
☐ No

9) Was employee hospitalized overnight as an in-patient?
☐ Yes
☐ No

Information about the case

10) Case number from the Log _____ *(Transfer the case number from the Log after you record the case.)*

11) Date of injury or illness ___ / ___ / ___

12) Time employee began work _____ AM / PM

13) Time of event _____ AM / PM   ☐ Check if time cannot be determined

14) *What was the employee doing just before the incident occurred?* Describe the activity, as well as the tools, equipment, or material the employee was using. Be specific. *Examples:* "climbing a ladder while carrying roofing materials"; "spraying chlorine from hand sprayer"; "daily computer key-entry."

15) *What happened?* Tell us how the injury occurred. *Examples:* "When ladder slipped on wet floor, worker fell 20 feet"; "Worker was sprayed with chlorine when gasket broke during replacement"; "Worker developed soreness in wrist over time."

16) *What was the injury or illness?* Tell us the part of the body that was affected and how it was affected; be more specific than "hurt," "pain," or sore." *Examples:* "strained back"; "chemical burn, hand"; "carpal tunnel syndrome."

17) *What object or substance directly harmed the employee? Examples:* "concrete floor"; "chlorine"; "radial arm saw." *If this question does not apply to the incident, leave it blank.*

18) *If the employee died, when did death occur?* Date of death ___ / ___ / ___

Completed by _____

Title _____

Phone (___) ___ - ___   Date ___ / ___ / ___

Public reporting burden for this collection of information is estimated to average 22 minutes per response, including time for reviewing instructions, searching existing data sources, gathering and maintaining the data needed, and completing and reviewing the collection of information. Persons are not required to respond to the collection of information unless it displays a current valid OMB control number. If you have any comments about this estimate or any other aspects of this data collection, including suggestions for reducing this burden, contact: US Department of Labor, OSHA Office of Statistics, Room N-3644, 200 Constitution Avenue, NW, Washington, DC 20210. Do not send the completed forms to this office.

FIGURE 7-13 OSHA Form 301—Injury and Illness Incident Report. (From U.S. Department of Labor, Occupational Safety and Health Administration.)

- Description of the incident
- The type and brand of device used when the incident took place
- Location of the incident

The regulations that took effect in 2001 require all needlestick and sharps injuries to be reported and documented, not just the ones that result in injury or illness.

Occupational Safety and Health Administration Training Requirements

All employees, including full-time, part-time, and temporary employees with a risk of occupational exposure, must receive training within the facility in which they are employed at two very specific times. Initial training must be conducted before commencement of any work-related duties by a new employee. In addition, training must be conducted on an annual basis to update and inform employees about new regulations and procedures related to OSHA compliance. The initial training requirement is one of the most frequently breached regulations, yet it is critical for the safety of the employee.

Training must include the following:

- Making accessible a copy of the regulatory text of the standard and explanation of its contents
- General discussion of blood-borne diseases and their transmission
- Universal precautions and body substance isolation
- The Exposure Control Plan
- Engineering and work practice controls, including handling of needles and sharps
- Personal protective equipment
- Hepatitis B vaccine
- Response to emergencies involving blood
- Potential sources of infection and tasks that might preempt exposure
- Written schedules for cleaning
- Handling of contaminated laundry
- How to handle exposure incidents and spills
- The postexposure evaluation and follow-up program
- Reading of MSDS, signs, labels, and color-coding (Figure 7-14), and locations of these items

There must be an opportunity for questions and answers, and the trainer must be knowledgeable about the subject matter. Documentation of the training sessions should be kept in each employee's personnel file or a special file for OSHA-related information.

CRITICAL THINKING APPLICATION

Barbara reviews the employee files and finds that neither Samantha nor Lynda received OSHA training when they were initially hired. How might Barbara rectify this, and what documentation would be helpful?

Hepatitis B Vaccination

The hepatitis B vaccination series must be offered to employees at risk of occupational exposures at no cost to the employee. The employee cannot be asked to pay in advance for the vaccination and be reimbursed, nor can the employee be asked to put the vaccination series on his or her personal health insurance policy. It must be made available to the employee within 10 working days of initial hire or assignment. The vaccination series can be declined by the employee, who must sign a declination form. If at any time the employee decides to receive the vaccination series, this must still be offered at no cost. The employee does not have to offer a reason for the declination. Prescreening or postvaccination serologic tests cannot be required.

The vaccination series is completed within a 6-month period. The second vaccination is given 1 month after the first, and the third 5 months after the second. Documentation should be provided to the employee for each vaccination received. Currently a booster dose of the hepatitis B vaccination is not required. However, if a routine booster is recommended by the U.S. Public Health Service in the future, it must be made available at no cost to employees.

CRITICAL THINKING APPLICATION

Lynda has not disclosed to anyone at the facility that she has had a case of hepatitis. Should she discuss this matter with Barbara? Is Lynda required to discuss this matter with Barbara? Is Lynda placing her patients at risk? If Lynda declines the hepatitis vaccination, must she explain why on the declination form?

Clinical Laboratory Improvement Amendments

The Clinical Laboratory Improvement Amendments (CLIA) was a result of the Congressional investigation of **physician office laboratories (POLs)** and the deficiencies in the quality of the services and results provided by these laboratories. A set of minimum standards for laboratories was established and involved quality improvement in test procedures. Quality control and assurance, as well as personnel and proficiency testing, are of utmost importance to the facility complying with CLIA.

CLIA regulations set the minimum standard for laboratory practice and quality. Remember that CLIA is not a governmental agency, but a law. CLIA is enforced by the Department of Health and Human Services (HHS). OSHA is a law (Occupational Safety and Health Act), but also an agency (Occupational Safety and Health Administration). This is an important difference between the two.

Some tests conducted in the laboratory are exempt from CLIA standards. These tests include the following:

- Nonautomated dipstick or tablet urinalysis
- Fecal occult blood
- Ovulation using visual color comparison
- Urine pregnancy using visual color comparison
- Erythrocyte sedimentation rate
- Hemoglobin by copper sulfate method
- Spun microhematocrit
- Blood glucose using certain devices cleared by the FDA for home use
- Specialized self-contained hemoglobin tests

Offices that perform only these tests may obtain a certificate of waiver and will not be routinely inspected for CLIA compliance. Tests of moderate or high complexity must be performed by trained personnel with education and experience

Material Safety Data Sheets communicate hazards to employees about the products and chemicals used in the medical office. They also inform the employee as to what to do in case of an exposure. OSHA requires that MSDS sheets are kept on all hazardous chemicals, unless exempted. Only the manufacturer can determine if a product is hazardous. MSDS sheets can be obtained from either the manufacturer or the medical supply company from which the product was ordered. They must be provided after requested from the manufacturer within 30 days. Keep copies of requests to prove that an attempt has been made to obtain the MSDS information.

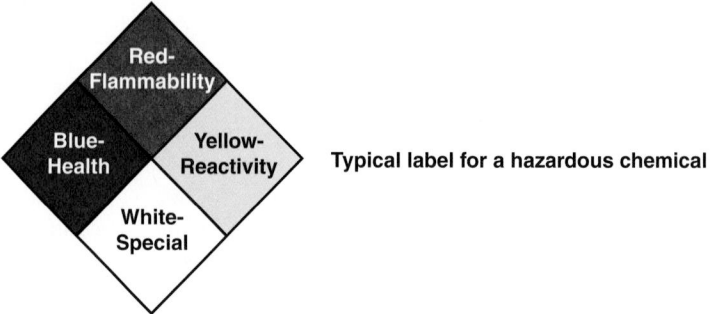

Typical label for a hazardous chemical

The appropriate number should be placed inside each box that applies in the figure above. Most offices use the National Fire Protection Association Rating System. Many MSDS sheets provide the labeling information on the sheet. Others must be read thoroughly to determine how the labels should be completed. If the MSDS says that a chemical has a "moderate to high" hazard, label it high. If it says "low to moderate," label it moderate.

Never guess at the numbers used for the label—always consult the MSDS. If individual containers are labeled, the facility is said to always be out of compliance, because it is easy to miss a container that may have just arrived in a shipment. Many medical facilities place labels on a permanent fixture next to where the product is stored, but it must be permanently stored in that area.

Simple Rating Guide
0—no hazard
1—slight hazard
2—moderate hazard
3—high hazard
4—extreme hazard

NFPA Rating Summary

Health (Blue)			Reactivity (Yellow)		
4	Danger	May be fatal on short exposure. Specialized protective equipment required.	4	Danger	Explosive material at room temperature.
3	Warning	Corrosive or toxic. Avoid skin contact or inhalation.	3	Danger	May be explosive if shocked, heated under confinement, or mixed with water.
2	Warning	May be harmful if inhaled or absorbed.	2	Warning	Unstable or may react violently if mixed with water.
1	Caution	May be irritating.	1	Caution	May react if heated or mixed with water but not violently.
0		No unusual hazard.	0	Stable	Not reactive when mixed with water.
Flammability (Red)			**Special Notice Key (White)**		
4	Danger	Flammable gas or extremely flammable liquid.	W		Water reactive.
3	Warning	Flammable liquid flash point below 100° F.	Oxy		Oxidizing agent.
2	Caution	Combustible liquid flash point of 100° to 200° F.			
1		Combustible if heated.			
0		Not combustible.			

FIGURE 7-14 Labeling and the National Fire Protection Association (NFPA) Rating System. (Courtesy the National Fire Protection Association.)

in the test areas in which they are working. A list of the moderate- and high-complexity procedures can be found in the July 26, 1993, issue of the *Federal Register,* and updates are periodically published that detail any changes in the list or regulations regarding testing procedures. Laboratories apply for a CLIA certificate through their local health departments and will be periodically inspected for compliance.

Americans with Disabilities Act

In 1990, the Americans with Disabilities Act (ADA) was signed into law with the intent of eliminating discrimination against individuals with disabilities. The act is comprehensive legislation that addresses many areas in which a person might experience discrimination, including telecommunications, housing, public transportation, air carrier access, voting accessibility, education, and rehabilitation. Physician offices fall under the category of public accommodations, which is defined as a private entity that owns, lease, lease to, or operates public facilities.

Public accommodations must comply with basic nondiscrimination requirements that prohibit exclusion, segregation, and unequal treatment. They also must comply with specific requirements related to architectural standards for new and altered buildings; reasonable modifications to policies, practices, and procedures; effective communication with people with hearing, vision, or speech disabilities; and other access requirements. Additionally, public accommodations must remove barriers in existing buildings where it is easy to do so without much difficulty or expense, given the public accommodation's resources.

These regulations affect the physician office because those individuals with disabilities must be able to enter and exit the facility without difficulty. This means that a person in a wheelchair would need a ramp to enter and exit the building. They must also be able to navigate throughout the office without major barriers. Any facility with 15 or more employees must comply with the Americans with Disabilities Act. To be protected by the ADA, one must have a disability or have a relationship or association with an individual with a disability. An individual with a disability is defined by the ADA as a person who has a physical or mental impairment that substantially limits one or more major life activities, a person who has a history or record of an impairment, or a person who is perceived by others as having an impairment. The ADA does not specifically name all of the impairments that are covered. Every medical facility must comply with the Americans with Disabilities Act (1990). This law requires that public medical facilities must allow persons with disabilities to easily and safely do the following

- Reach door handles for opening and closing
- Enter and exit buildings
- Move through doors and hallways
- Use drinking fountains, phones, and restrooms
- Move from floor to floor (elevators are required for multilevel buildings)
- Do everything that the general public is able to do in a public place

PHYSICIAN LICENSURE AND REGISTRATION

A graduate of a medical school must be licensed before beginning the practice of medicine. Licensure is regulated by state statutes through the Medical Practice Acts. It is important for a medical assistant to understand licensing and other laws and regulations that are intended to protect patients, physicians, medical assistants, and other healthcare workers.

Medical Practice Acts

Medical practice acts existed as early as colonial days. However, these acts were later repealed, and in the mid-nineteenth century practically none of the states had laws governing the practice of medicine. As one might expect, a rapid decline in professional standards followed. The general welfare of the people was endangered by medical **quackery** and inadequate care. By the beginning of the twentieth century, medical practice acts were established by statute and were again in effect in every state. The purpose of the medical practice acts is as follows:

- To define what is included in the practice of medicine within that state
- To govern the methods and requirements of licensure
- To establish the grounds for suspension or revocation of license

Licensure

A Doctor of Medicine (MD), Doctor of Osteopathy (DO), or Doctor of Chiropractic (DC) degree is conferred on graduation from medical or chiropractic school. The license to practice medicine or chiropractic is granted by a state board, frequently known as the State Board of Medical Examiners or Board of Registration. Licensure may be accomplished by examination, reciprocity, or endorsement.

Examination

Every state requires medical doctors to pass a written examination. The Federation of State Medical Boards and the National Board of Medical Examiners agreed in 1990 to establish a single licensing examination—the Federation Licensing Examination (FLEX)—for graduates of accredited medical schools. Medical graduates in the United States must pass either the FLEX examination, the U.S. Medical Licensing Examination (USMLE), or the National Board of Medical Examiners' Examination (NBME). Osteopathic physicians pass the National Board of Osteopathic Medical Examiners' Comprehensive Osteopathic Medical Licensing Examination (COMLEX).

Reciprocity

Some states grant the license to practice medicine by reciprocity; that is, they automatically recognize that the requirements of the state in which the license was granted meet the standards required by the second state.

Endorsement

Most graduates of medical schools in the United States have been licensed by endorsement of the National Board certificate. To explain in simpler terms, a state will offer a license to a physician based on the examinations taken to grant the license, not by virtue of the license granted from another state. Licensure by endorsement is granted on a case-by-case basis. Graduates who have not been licensed by endorsement are required to pass a state board examination.

In all states, graduates of foreign medical schools who are seeking licensure by endorsement must meet the same requirements as graduates of medical schools in the United States, in addition to various other qualifying factors.

Exemptions

Some graduates may not wish to engage in the practice of medicine; their interests may lie in research or administration, or even in the practice of law with a special interest in medical liability. In such instances licensure is not required. Licensed physicians in the Armed Forces, Public Health Service, or

Veterans Administration facilities need not be licensed in the state in which they are employed. However, the Department of Defense is encouraging states to require full licensure of military personnel.

Registration and Reregistration

After a license is granted, periodic reregistration is necessary annually or biennially. A physician can be **concurrently** registered in more than one state. The issuing body notifies the physician when reregistration is due. A medical assistant can aid the physician by being aware of when the registration fees are due, thereby preventing a possible lapsing of the registration.

Many states require proof of continuing education in addition to payment of a registration fee. Continuing education units (CEUs) are granted to physicians for attending approved seminars, lectures, scientific meetings, and formal courses in accredited colleges and universities. A total of 50 hours per year is the average requirement for a license renewal. A medical assistant may be expected to help the physician arrange for completing the required units for license renewal.

Revocation or Suspension

Under certain conditions, the license to practice medicine may be revoked or suspended. Grounds for revocation or suspension of the license to practice medicine fall within one of three categories:

- Conviction of a crime: This may include felonies such as murder, rape, larceny, and narcotic violations.
- Unprofessional conduct: Failure to uphold the ethical standards of the medical profession may be indicated by betrayal of patient confidence, giving or receiving rebates, and excessive use of narcotics or alcohol.
- Personal or professional incapacity: Such incapacity is difficult to label or prove. For example, advanced age or an injury may reduce the apparent capacity of some physicians. Certain illnesses can affect the memory or judgment necessary to practice medicine.

A physician studies many years to learn the profession before becoming licensed by the state to practice medicine. A medical assistant is not licensed to practice medicine and must never prescribe or attempt to diagnose a patient's ailment. This is the illegal practice of medicine. For this reason a medical assistant must use great care in discussing the patient's complaints and treatment with them because patients identify the medical assistant's remarks as being the opinion of the physician.

CLOSING COMMENTS

The majority of patients never entertain the thought of taking legal action against their physicians, and a medical assistant should not develop an attitude of skepticism. However, a medical assistant can play an important role in preventing medical claims.

Give scrupulous attention to the needs of each patient and avoid leaving them alone for long periods. This especially applies to young children and elderly patients. Always avoid criticism of other physicians or healthcare facilities. Never give out any information about the patient without written consent, and verify the identity of anyone asking for information about a patient.

Use discretion in phone and office conversations. One never knows who is standing just around the corner. Be aware of tone of voice and attitude during spoken conversations. Communicate office policies and procedures to patients clearly in advance of treatment whenever possible.

Keep accurate records that show exactly what was done to the patient and when it was done. The medical assistant must never make any promises as to the outcome of treatment. Record cancelled and no-show appointments and record the facts if a patient discontinues treatment.

Check office equipment often to ensure that it is working properly. Keep drug samples and prescription pads out of sight. Never diagnose, prescribe, or offer a prognosis. Perform only the tasks for which you are trained and keep abreast of new findings and procedures in healthcare. Correctly follow all federal and state regulations.

Play a positive part in the prevention of medical liability claims. Take care of the patient in a compassionate and competent way, and malpractice will not be a frequent issue in the medical facility.

SUMMARY OF SCENARIO

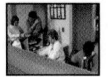

Barbara is enthusiastic about her new job and duties. She is confident about appearing in court to represent Dr. Patrick and discuss the contents of the medical record of the patient suing his surgeon. Dr. Patrick is not a party to the lawsuit but has a physician-patient relationship with the patient just the same. An offer existed, as well as the acceptance of that offer. The relationship was based on legal subject matter, and the physician and the patient had the legal capacity to enter into a contract. Consideration existed as well, because the patient paid for services and the physician treated the patient. Both received something of value. Samantha and Lynda would like to accompany Barbara to the court proceedings to watch and learn.

Even if a patient does not pay for treatment, a contract still exists. The physician may elect to terminate the physician-patient relationship if the patient does not pay, but the trust that the patient places in the physician can be considered a thing of value. Patients should understand their role in their treatment, and their responsibilities to the physician. Often this information is communicated in the patient policy brochure or may be verbally discussed with the patient. Physicians are not required to accept all patients; for instance, not all

SUMMARY OF SCENARIO—*cont'd*

physicians deliver babies. Some physicians do not treat patients with worker's compensation claims. The physician does have the right to see the types of patients he or she wishes and is competent to treat but should never discriminate on the basis of race, sex, or any other protected status. A physician may not always be correct in his or her diagnoses, but this does not mean that the physician has committed malpractice. However, if expert witnesses feel that the physician should have made a different diagnosis based on the case, then the physician might be held liable for negligence. If an employee has information about a case that is damaging to the physician, he or she is ethically obligated to report the information, but rarely legally liable to speak up unless a law has been broken.

Samantha and Lynda have learned many new concepts about law from Barbara and are anxious to follow the court proceedings. They will learn more by seeing the actual process of law at work. Barbara looks forward to sharing more knowledge with the employees as they continue to work together.

Medical assistants can help the physician comply with legal regulations in the office by making certain that they understand the policies and procedures that are required by the facility. Rules are set in place in order to assure compliance so that both patients and employees are kept safe and risks in the office are at a minimum. Patient confidentiality is one of the most important

rules to remember. New graduates can learn about the laws that affect medical facilities in their area by discussing them with their supervisors and by attending seminars and training. Much information is available on the Internet regarding legal issues. Trust is a critical factor in avoiding medical professional liability lawsuits. When the patient trusts the physician, he or she is much more likely to work through issues that might otherwise lead to legal action against the physician. Keeping accurate patient records and documenting all information required in the patient chart will help to prove that the physician adequately cared for the patient. Clearly legible handwriting is vital in this process.

The medical assistant may find that the physician is not in compliance with certain rules and regulations. Never jump to conclusions and assume that the physician has no intention of complying. There are various reasons for noncompliance, and any issues should be brought to the attention of the office manager or the physician for clarification. It is the medical assistant's responsibility to question noncompliance and make every effort to bring the facility into compliance with the cooperation of supervisors, co-workers, and the physician. As a team, medical professionals can remain in compliance and deliver excellent care to all patients.

SUMMARY of LEARNING OBJECTIVES

1. Define, spell, and pronounce the terms listed in the vocabulary.
   - Spelling and pronouncing medical terms correctly adds credibility to the medical assistant. Knowing the definition of these terms promotes confidence in communication with patients and co-workers.
2. Distinguish among an act, a statute, and an ordinance.
   - Different types of laws and regulations affect us, depending on the origination of the law. Acts are introduced at the federal level and must be passed by Congress. State legislative bodies develop statutes, and local governments create ordinances.
3. Know the two types of law.
   - Criminal law governs violations that are punishable as offenses against the state or government. Civil law is concerned with acts that are not criminal in nature but involve relationships between individuals and other individuals, groups, or government agencies.
4. Explain the three basic categories of criminal law.
   - Misdemeanors are minor crimes punishable by a fine or imprisonment in a city or county jail. Felonies are major crimes, such as rape, murder, or burglary. Most felonies carry punishment of imprisonment for at least 1 year, and they are divided into subgroups, usually first-, second-, and

third-degree felonies. Treason is an attempt to overthrow the government. High treason constitutes a serious threat to the stability of the government—for example, an attempt on the life of the president.

5. Distinguish which type of civil law deals with medical professional liability.
   - Tort law is the division of civil law that deals with medical professional liability. Tort law provides relief for those who have suffered harm from the actions of others. The plaintiff must establish duty, breach of duty, damages as a result of the breach of duty, and the extent of the damages suffered.
6. Explain the four essential elements needed for a valid contract.
   - Four elements are essential to a valid, legal contract: (1) there must be a "meeting of the minds" or manifestation of assent; (2) the contract must involve legal subject matter; (3) the parties to the contract must have the legal capacity to enter into a contract; and (4) some type of consideration must be offered.
7. Distinguish between interrogatories and depositions.
   - Interrogatories are lists of questions directed from each party of a lawsuit to the other. Interrogatories are answered under oath and directed only to the parties actually named in the

Continued

SUMMARY of LEARNING OBJECTIVES

Continued

lawsuit. Depositions, however, can be taken from any witness or party to the lawsuit. They are also taken under oath, and often witnesses are subpoenaed to offer a deposition.

8. List three things to remember when testifying in court.
   - Testifying in court can sometimes be an intimidating experience, but good preparation beforehand will alleviate many anxieties. Discussing potential questions with the attorney will help prepare the witness for giving testimony. Always tell the truth to avoid charges of perjury. Speak clearly and distinctly, and do not hesitate to ask the attorney to repeat a question. A brief pause to think about an answer causes no harm. Dress conservatively, know the location and room of the court in advance, and always arrive on time. Credibility is critical in a medical professional liability trial.

9. Discuss the advantages of arbitration.
   - Arbitration is a popular alternative to court trials. It involves the use of a third party familiar with law or the issues at hand. It is recognized by statute in most states and provides a faster, confidential, fair, and less expensive resolution to a dispute.

10. Differentiate among malfeasance, misfeasance, and nonfeasance.
    - Malfeasance, misfeasance, and nonfeasance are types of negligence often involved in medical professional liability cases. Malfeasance is performing an act that is completely wrong or unlawful. Misfeasance, comparable to a mistake, is the improper performance of a lawful act. Nonfeasance is the failure to perform some act that should have been performed.

11. Explain the "four D's" of negligence.
    - The four D's of negligence include the duty to care for the patient; dereliction or failure to perform that duty; proof that this failure was the direct cause of a patient's injury; and proof that the patient suffered damages from the injury.

12. Define the types of damages.
    - Nominal damages are token compensations for invasion of a legal right. Punitive damages are designed to punish an offender and discourage repetition of an act. Compensatory damages are designed to compensate for the actual damages suffered, whereas general damages include compensation for pain and suffering, loss of a body member, disfigurement, and other similar losses. Special damages can include such losses as earnings or travel costs.

13. Explain the importance of informed consent.
    - Informed consent gives the patient a full understanding of the condition that has been diagnosed, including what could happen if the patient undergoes treatment, refuses treatment, or delays treatment. It provides the patient with information on the advantages and risks of a medical procedure and alternative treatments that the patient may wish to consider. Informed consent places the control in the hands of the patient, who is given the opportunity to make the decisions about his or her healthcare. Patients can never be forced to undergo any type of procedure or treatment.

14. List several legal disclosures the physician must make.
    - Several disclosures must be made by the physician with regard to a patient's health that do not require patient consent. Information about births and deaths, injuries or illnesses as a result of violence, accidental or suspicious deaths, sexually transmitted diseases, and any type of abuse are examples of legal disclosures that must be made by healthcare professionals.

15. Explain the importance of the Health Insurance Portability and Accountability Act.
    - Passage of HIPAA in 1996 offered the healthcare profession extensive privacy rules and regulations concerning the electronic transfer of information. The act also limited administrative costs by supporting the use of electronic transfer of information and presented fraud and abuse prevention guidelines. The privacy issues that surround HIPAA, however, have been the most discussed and debated topics related to this law.

16. Distinguish between OSHA and CLIA, explaining which of the two is an actual agency.
    - OSHA is an agency and a division of the U.S. Department of Labor. More than 2300 employees work for OSHA, and the agency runs on an annual budget of approximately $443 million as of 2002. Twenty-six states have their own OSHA programs, which adds an additional 3100 employees. The Occupational Safety and Health Act of 1970 created this agency to ensure safety in the workplace. CLIA is a law that regulates the quality of services provided by laboratories. CLIA is enforced by the HHS.

17. Discuss the three ways in which a physician can obtain a license to practice medicine.
    - Physicians may receive a license to practice medicine through examination, reciprocity, or endorsement. FLEX, USMLE, and NBME are all designed for graduates of accredited medical schools. Some states recognize the requirements of another state in which a license was granted, and through reciprocity will give a physician a license to practice medicine. Endorsement is the method of obtaining a license by recognition of the passed examinations, instead of by virtue of the license obtained in another state. Most physicians in the United States are licensed by endorsement, because they take the examination after graduating from medical school and this prompts the receipt of the license, after proper application and providing all required documentation. Practicing medicine without a license is illegal.

18. Discuss the ways that a physician might lose a license to practice medicine.
    - A physician may lose his or her license to practice medicine if convicted of a crime, if found guilty of unprofessional conduct, or as a result of personal or professional incapacity. An arrest will not cause the physician to lose the license, because this is an allegation not yet proven in court. Unprofessional conduct is usually determined by local medical societies or other organizations, such as a hospital, with which the physician is affiliated.

CONNECTIONS

 Study Guide Connection: Go to Chapter 7 Study Guide. Read the Case Study and Workplace Applications and complete the assignments. Do online research for answers to the questions in the Internet Activities associated with medicine and the law.

 CD Connection: Go to the Medical Assisting Competency Challenge CD and do the training activities under Legal Concepts.

Evolve Connection: For more information related to medicine and the law, go to evolve.elsevier.com/kinn and visit related weblinks for Chapter 7. Click on the Medical Assisting Exam Review and do the practice questions to sharpen your test-taking skills.

Computer Concepts

8

SCENARIO

Dr. Michael Bouchard is aware of the advantages of networking his office computers and having Internet access to meet the needs of his facility. Every day he sends and receives many important email messages to and from patients and colleagues. His staff members use the computer for communications and to access sources of online information. Patient tracking, accounting functions, and health information retrieval are immensely faster on a computer than with the use of a paper-based system. One other distinct advantage to Dr. Bouchard is the scheduling features of his software. Because the schedule is shared, everyone in the office knows the doctor's schedule and avoids double-booking and miscommunications. Dr. Bouchard sends his staff members for regular computer training so that all of them can use the computers in the best and most efficient ways possible.

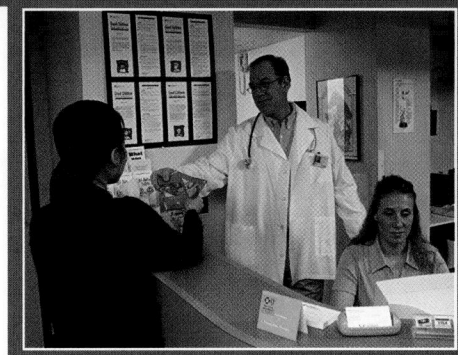

HIPAA requirements have altered the methods in which information may be used in medical facilities. No employee is allowed to access information in the clinic that is not necessary to that employee for patient care and assistance. Dr. Bouchard takes the HIPAA guidelines seriously and makes certain that all of his staff members understand the importance of keeping health information secure.

While studying this chapter, think about the following questions:

- How do computers help the physician's office to run more efficiently?
- Can an employee in the physician's office invade a patient's right to privacy by accessing medical records?
- How can information on the computer be kept secure from curious employees who do not need to access the information for the purpose of patient care?

- How does logging in and logging out of the office network help to ensure proper access to medical records?
- How could the computer be considered a co-worker in the medical office?

LEARNING OBJECTIVES

1. Define, spell, and pronounce the terms listed in the vocabulary.
2. List several ways that the computer can be effective in a medical office.
3. Explain the basic functions that a computer performs.
4. Explain the basic parts of a computer.
5. List the three elements that differentiate microprocessors.
6. Discuss the differences among various types of printers.
7. Explain the importance of a motherboard.
8. Explain and give examples of peripheral devices.
9. List and discuss several types of file formats.
10. Explain the concept of computer networking.
11. Define the function of browsers.
12. Discuss the importance of computer security.

National Accreditation Competencies and Content

CAAHEP COMPETENCIES

General

3.c.(4)(c). Utilize computer software to maintain office systems

ABHES COMPETENCIES

Communication

2.n. Application of electronic technology

Administrative Duties

3.d. Apply computer concepts for office procedures

Office Management

6.d. Evaluate and recommend equipment and supplies for practice

Financial Management

8.a. Use manual and computerized bookkeeping systems

VOCABULARY

application software Computer programs designed to perform specific tasks.

artificial intelligence The aspect of computer science that deals with computers taking on the attributes of humans, such as mimicking human thought. One example is expert systems, which are capable of making decisions, such as software that is designed to help a physician diagnose a patient, given a set of symptoms.

ASCII codes Acronym for American Standard Code for Information Interchange; a code representing English characters as numbers, where each is given a number from 0 to 255.

backup Any type of storage of files to prevent their loss in the event of hard disk failure.

banners Advertisements often found on a Web page that can be animated to attract the user's attention in hopes that he or she will click on the ad, be redirected to the advertiser's home page, and purchase from the site or gain information from the site.

bits The smallest units of information inside the computer, each represented by either the digit "0" or "1"; 8 bits equal 1 byte.

byte A unit of data that contains 8 binary digits, or bits.

cache (kash) A special high-speed storage that can either be a part of the computer's main memory or can be a separate storage device. One function of a cache is to store websites visited in the computer memory for faster recall the next time the website is requested.

CD burner A device that is capable of "writing" data onto a blank compact disk (CD) or copying data from one CD to a blank CD.

computer A machine that is designed to accept, store, process, and give out information.

cookies Messages sent to a Web browser from a Web server that identify users and can prepare custom Web pages for them, possibly displaying their name on return to the site.

cursor A symbol appearing on the monitor that shows where the next character to be typed will appear.

cyberspace The nonphysical space of the online world of computer networks in which communication takes place.

database A collection of related files that serves as a foundation for retrieving information.

device driver The program or commands given to a device connected to a computer that enable the device to function. For instance, a printer may come equipped with software that must be loaded onto the computer first, so that the printer will work.

digital subscriber line (DSL) High-speed, sophisticated modulation scheme that operates over existing copper telephone wiring systems; often referred to as "last-mile technologies," because DSL is used for connections from a telephone switching station to a home or office, and not between switching stations.

Digital video disk (DVD) An optical disk that holds approximately 28 times more information than a CD; a DVD is most commonly used to hold full-length movies. Compared with a CD, which holds approximately 600 megabytes, a DVD has the capacity to hold approximately 4.7 gigabytes. Also called a digital versatile disk.

disk A removable device shaped like a hard plastic square with a magnetic surface that is capable of storing computer programs; also called *diskettes*, and early versions were called *floppy disks*.

disk drives Devices that load a program or data stored on a disk into the computer.

ecommerce An abbreviation for electronic commerce; used to describe the sale and purchase of goods and services over the Internet; doing business over the Internet.

email Communications transmitted via computer or computer network.

environment The state of a computer, usually determined by the programs that are running as well as hardware and software characteristics.

fax Abbreviation for facsimile; also, a document sent using a facsimile (fax) machine.

flash Animation technology often used on the opening page of a website to draw attention, excite, and impress the user.

flash drive A small portable device that connects into the USB port that can carry 2 to 8 or more gigabytes of information.

List continues on next page

List continued from previous page

font   A design for a set of type characters; a combination of typeface, spacing, pitch, and other qualities. Fonts are named; examples include Times Roman, Arial, and Garamond.

format   To magnetically create tracks on a disk where information will be stored, usually done by the manufacturer of the disk.

gigabyte   Approximately 1 billion bytes; abbreviated GB.

hard copy   The readable paper copy or printout of information.

hardware   The physical components of the computer system, such as the CPU, monitor, and printer.

HTML   Acronym for HyperText Markup Language, which is the language used to create documents for use on the Internet.

HTTP   Acronym for HyperText Transfer Protocol, which defines how messages are formatted and transmitted over the Internet. When a URL is entered into the computer, an HTTP command tells the Web server to retrieve the requested Web page.

hub   A common connection point for devices in a network containing multiple ports, often used to connect segments of a LAN.

icons   Pictures, often on the desktop of a computer, that represent programs or objects. By clicking on an icon, the user is directed to the program.

input   Information entered into and used by the computer.

Java   A commonly used object-oriented high-level programming language that is well suited for the Internet.

kilobyte   Approximately 1024 bytes, abbreviated KB.

megabyte   Approximately 1 million bytes; abbreviated MB.

megahertz   The measuring device for microprocessors, abbreviated MHz. A megahertz is 1 million cycles of electromagnetic currency alternation per second and is used as a unit of measure for the clock speed of computer microprocessors. The hertz is a unit of measure named after Heinrich Hertz, a German physicist.

MIDI   Acronym for Musical Instrument Digital Interface; a MIDI interface allows computers to record and manipulate sound.

modem   A device that allows information to be transmitted over telephone lines, at speeds measured in bits per second (bps); short for modulator-demodulator. Modem speed is generally listed somewhere on the actual unit.

monochromatic   Having or consisting of one color or hue.

multimedia   The presentation of graphics, animation, video, sound, and text on a computer in an integrated way, or all at once. CD-ROMs are efficient multimedia devices.

output   Information that is processed by the computer and transmitted to a monitor, printer, or other device.

queries   Requests for information from a database.

router (rau'-ter)   A device used to connect any number of LANs, which communicate with other routers and determine the best route between any two hosts.

scanner   Device that reads text or illustrations on a printed page and can translate the information on that page into a form that the computer can understand.

search engines   Programs that search documents for keywords and return a list of documents containing those words.

server   A computer or device on a network that manages shared network resources.

sound card   Device that allows a computer to output sound through speakers that are connected to the main circuitry board, or motherboard.

switch   In networks, a device that filters information between LAN segments and decreases overall network traffic and increases speed and bandwidth usage efficiency.

system software   The operating system and all utility programs that allow the computer to function and perform operations.

TCP/IP   Acronym for Transmission Control Protocol/Internet Protocol; a suite of communications protocols used to connect users or hosts to the Internet.

telecommunications   The science and technology of communication by transmission of information from one location to another via telephone, television, telegraph, or satellite.

terabyte   Approximately 1 trillion bytes, abbreviated TB.

URL   Acronym for Uniform Resource Locator; specifies the global address of documents or information on the Internet. The URL provides the IP address and the domain name for the Web page, such as microsoft.com.

virtual reality   An artificial environment presented to a computer user that feels as if it were a real environment, often involving use of special gloves, earphones, and goggles to enhance the experience.

zip drive   A small, portable disk drive that is primarily used for backing up information and archiving computer files. A 100-megabyte Zip disk will hold the equivalent of approximately 70 floppy disks.

COMPUTERS TODAY

Nearly 60 years ago, in 1946, the first electronic **computer** (ENIAC) was completed after $2^1/_2$ years in the making. It weighed 30 tons, required a space of 15,000 square feet, and cost more than $1 million. Since that time, a computer explosion has taken place, and today our lives are affected by computers on a daily basis. Personal computers (PCs), laptop or notebook computers, and even cell phones that send and receive **email** are commonplace. Our world is now one of enhanced **telecommunications**, where faster processing of information is both needed and expected. Advances in technology happen daily; as soon as one "new and improved" device is on the market, its "better and faster" competitor is released. Most people venture into **cyberspace** on a daily basis, where a world of information is waiting with the simple click of a mouse!

For many years computers have been used in medical facilities, including physicians' offices. The development of software, the decrease in the cost of computer **hardware,** and the time savings that the computer brings to the office make it well worth the investment. Computers are now standard equipment in healthcare facilities (Figure 8-1). A medical assistant must have more than computer literacy; a good understanding of the way computers work and their capabilities is essential in a medical office.

Getting Started

Even with some basic knowledge of computer components and of what computers can do, without hands-on knowledge, the beginner may have some initial fear of the unknown. However, the computer is only a machine that takes its direction from the person operating it. It will perform the tasks that it is told to do. A computer can simulate the thought process and make decisions, but most computers found in medical facilities will wait for commands that prompt it to act. Dialog boxes appear that ask for **input** from the user. This is how the computer communicates with the person using it. Computers assist workers in medical offices in some of the following ways:

- Performing repetitive tasks
- Reducing errors
- Speeding up production
- Recalling information on command
- Saving time
- Reducing paperwork and storage space
- Allowing for more creative and productive use of workers' time

The more familiar a medical assistant becomes with the computer, the better skilled he or she will become in its use. Occasionally errors will be made, and the computer may respond with an error message. However, the monitor screen normally indicates what to do next. The computer will usually allow the operator the opportunity to figure out the correct information and input that information into the computer. A help menu can always be accessed, or the instruction manual can be consulted; help lines and technical support are available as well when problems occur. The problem may be with the software or with the computer itself. Usually it is fairly easy to determine which is causing the problem.

Rarely will the computer "break," although this is a common fear among new users. It is unlikely that records will be destroyed by accident; usually very specific commands are needed to delete stored information. However, a medical assistant must take care not to shut off the computer without saving the information that has been entered. By using a computer in the classroom and practicing at home or at a library, if possible, the medical assistant will gain familiarity with computer operation and confidence that it can be mastered. Mastery is accomplished only through practice.

With knowledge of computer terms, the ability to follow step-by-step instructions, and reasonable expertise with a keyboard, a medical assistant can rapidly learn and use almost any computer system. Although the computers and the software may vary from facility to facility, basic computer operation is similar, and if the instructions given by the computer are carried out, the user should be successful in the tasks attempted.

Although it seems elementary, the first step to computer use is to turn the system on. If nothing happens when the power button is pushed, the primary troubleshooting protocol is to make certain that the system is plugged into the power outlet. If it is, then check all of the cords that attach the hardware to determine if they are securely fastened. Once the power is on, the computer goes through a process called *booting*. The boot sequence is a set of operations that the computer performs that loads the operating system and prepares it for use.

Once the computer is on, the desktop will appear and the user will see several **icons.** To open a certain program, double-click on its icon. Once a program has been opened, many functions can be performed, such as creating a document, a spreadsheet, or a presentation or maintaining a **database.** Some of the basic computer functions include the following:

- *Formatting a* **disk**. Most of today's diskettes are purchased preformatted, but that formatting can be erased if the user desires. Formatting a disk prepares it for use on the system and divides it into sectors and tracks where information can be written by the computer.
- *Opening a document.* A document stored on the computer can be opened by clicking on its icon, if it is stored on the desktop. If the document is stored in a folder, open the folder and click on the document icon.
- *Saving a document.* Most toolbars have a button that allows a document to be saved to a folder or to the desktop. Click the button, then name the file so that it can be easily found when it is needed. Word processing programs usually have a "save as" option as well, so that a document can be saved and edited without changing the original file.
- *Creating a folder.* Folders in which documents can be stored are easily created. For instance, in a Windows **environment,** one can create a folder called "Study Guides" on the desktop. To do this, right-click on the desktop away from other files, folders, and icons, then select the command "new." When the second dialog box appears, select "folder." Click "folder" and a folder titled "new

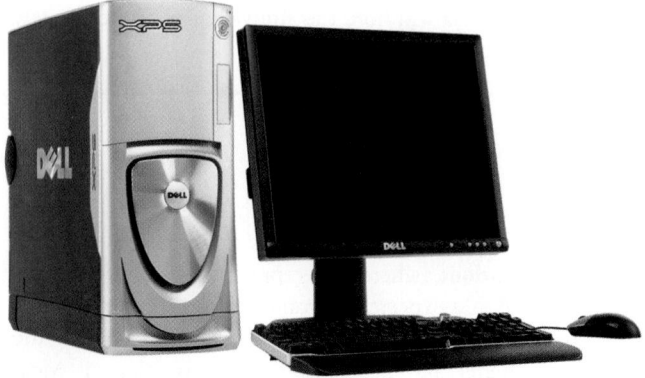

FIGURE 8-1 Computers are an invaluable tool for today's medical office. (Photo courtesy of Dell Corporation.)

folder" will appear on the desktop. To rename it, click twice on the words "new folder" and type in the words "Study Guides" or whatever title is to be used. The folder is now ready for use. To move documents into the folder, click on the document icon and hold the left mouse button down while dragging the document on top of the folder. This is called "drag and drop" or sometimes, "click and drag." To place documents that are not on the desktop into the folder, use the "save as" feature and save the document to the desired folder. Or the document can be saved to the desktop, after which the "drag-and-drop" feature can be used to place it in the desired folder.

- *Copying, moving, deleting, and renaming files.* Most word processing programs allow the user to copy, move, delete, and rename files. In Windows, a file may be copied easily by right-clicking on the document icon and then clicking "copy." Then, open the folder to which the file is to be copied, right-click inside the folder, and click "paste." A copy of the file will appear in the folder. Moving files from one place to another can be accomplished by using the drag-and-drop method. To delete a file, right-click on the document icon and click "delete." A dialog box will open that will confirm the user's choice to delete the file. The file will remain in the recycle bin on the desktop for a brief period of time once deleted, so if a mistake has been made and the file is needed, the user should look to see if it is still available. Renaming files is as simple as clicking twice on the filename and typing in the new one. The user can also right-click on the document icon and select "rename," which will allow the user to change the name of the document.

- *Cutting, copying, and pasting text.* Text can be moved from one place to another by cutting and pasting. First, highlight the text that is to be moved, then press the "cut" button. This function can also be accomplished by right-clicking the mouse and selecting "cut." Next, place the **cursor** at the point where the text should be inserted, then click the "paste" key or right-click the mouse and select "paste." Copying text is done in the same manner. Instead of clicking the "cut" button, press the "copy" button. These functions allow the user to be more efficient when creating documents.

- *Finding files.* Computers have a "search" mechanism that will allow the user to search for a file with certain keywords or extensions. In the Windows environment, click the "start" button, then click on "search." The dialog box that appears will ask the user what to search for, whether it be a picture, audio file, document, or other file type. An option to search all files and folders is also available. Enter keywords that pertain to the desired file, and click "search."

- *Copying an entire disk.* It is possible to copy an entire diskette or compact disk (CD). First, click on "start" and then click on "my computer." Find the drive that contains the diskette or CD and right-click on that icon. Then, click on "copy." Open the folder to which the contents should be copied, then click "paste." The actual diskette or CD could also be opened, then under the "edit" drop-down menu, the user can choose "select all." This also allows all of the files on the diskette or CD to be copied or permanently moved to another location.

- *Exiting a program.* Press the "x" key on the upper right corner of the document to exit a program. If the work has not yet been saved, the user will be prompted to either save the document or cancel the action. The user can also exit the program by clicking on "file" then "exit."

Once the user is finished with the computer for the day, it should always be shut down properly. To accomplish this, click the "start" icon, then click "turn off computer." The dialog box that appears will allow the user to turn the computer off, restart the computer, stand by, or cancel the action. The restart function is helpful when the computer "freezes" or fails to function as it should. This takes the computer back through the booting sequence and will often correct problems and allow the user to continue working. Never attempt to fix problems on the computer that are beyond the medical assistant's scope of knowledge. Often a technical assistance desk will be able to walk the user through various steps to correct basic issues. Always report computer malfunctions to the proper person or department.

Computer systems have user manuals that can be consulted when functions do not perform as they should or when a user is working with an unfamiliar system. Tutorials may be available that will help the new user to learn the system or to refresh the skills of the experienced user.

COMPUTER BASICS

A computer is a machine that is designed to accept, store, process, and provide information (Figure 8-2). Computers serve the following basic functions:

- *Input:* Input includes any information that enters the computer. It can take a variety of forms, from commands that are entered from the keyboard to data from another computer or device, such as a **scanner.** The device that feeds data into a computer, such as a mouse, scanner, keyboard, or voice recognition system, is called an *input device.*

- *Processing:* Processing is the act of manipulating the data that are currently inside the computer to carry out a certain task.

- *Output:* **Output** is anything that exits the computer. Output can appear in many forms, such as binary numbers, characters, pictures, printed pages, or a simple image on the computer screen. Output devices include monitors, speakers, printers, scanners, and modems.

- *Storage:* The act of retaining data or applications is called *storage.* Data can be stored on disks, on CDs, or on separate drives, such as a **zip drive** or a **flash drive.** The type of storage device used depends on the amount of information that needs to be saved and where it needs to be used. CDs and flash drives are common portable storage devices used in the business world.

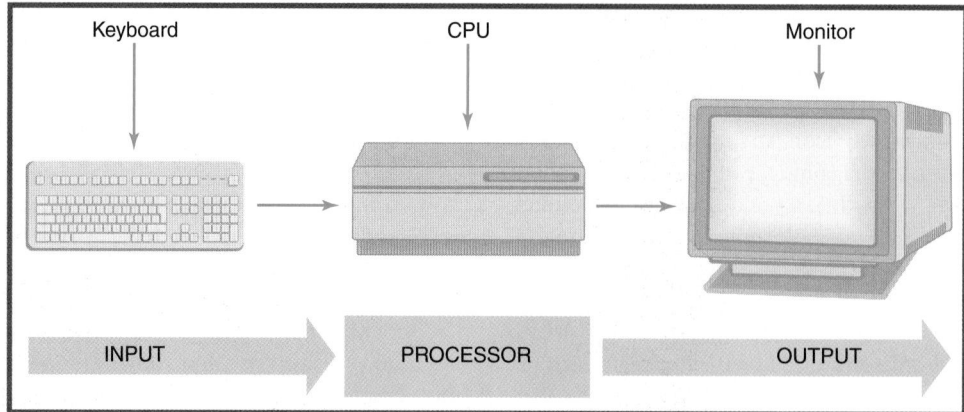

Keyboard   CPU   Monitor

INPUT → PROCESSOR → OUTPUT

FIGURE 8-2 Input devices allow data to be entered into the computer, where they are processed; output is available in several different forms.

CRITICAL THINKING APPLICATION

■ Dr. Bouchard plans to send two of his employees to a training class on using a new software program designed to perform all computer functions needed for his practice. Although he can send only two employees, how can the others learn the system?

■ Would it be beneficial or detrimental to close the office for a day to educate the other employees about the system? What should the physician consider before losing a day of patient visits?

TYPES OF COMPUTERS

Various types of computers meet the needs of staff in today's physician office. The most common type is the desktop computer, which consists of a central processing unit (CPU), monitor, mouse, and keyboard, in most cases. The laptop, notebook, and personal digital assistant (PDA) have grown in popularity because they are compact and portable (Figures 8-3 and 8-4). Some physicians and office employees carry the computer from room to room while treating patients. Information can be entered directly into the computer, which saves time and is much more efficient than handwritten or transcribed notes. The PDA is small enough to carry in a pocket or purse. Physicians may use this device when treating patients or making hospital rounds, as it is lighter and even more convenient than a laptop. The PDA also organizes personal information, such as addresses and phone numbers, and most models allow the user to access the Internet and read email messages. The user can also use the PDA as a day planner, keeping track of appointments, meetings, and other important events.

Embedded computers are those that are inside another device, such as an ultrasound unit or electrocardiograph (ECG). These computers allow for data input and output and usually analyze information. A mainframe is a large, expensive computer that is capable of processing huge amounts of information. These computers are usually found in large companies and government institutions.

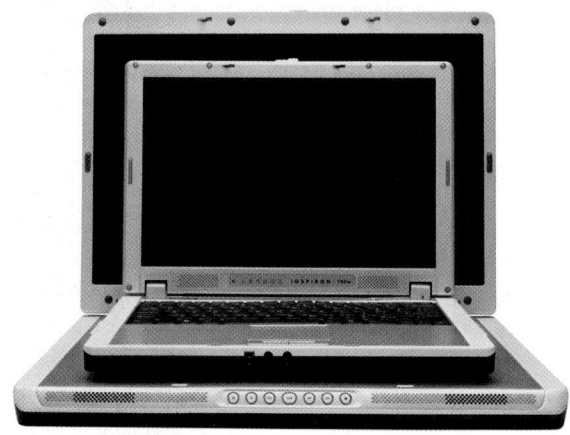

FIGURE 8-3 Laptop computers vary in size and weight and are easily portable. (Photo courtesy of Dell Corporation.)

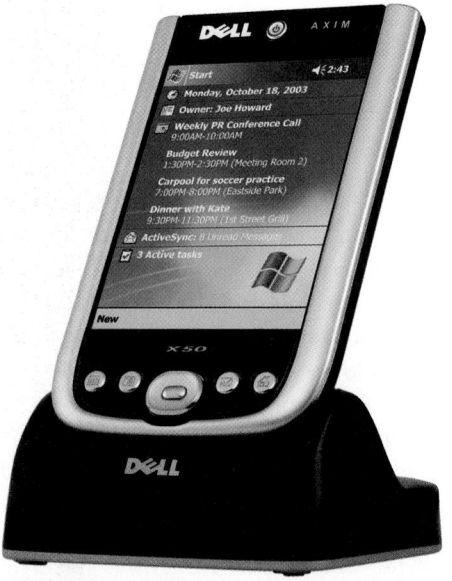

FIGURE 8-4 The PDA is a hand-held device that usually contains an address and phone book and a personal organizer and allows the user to access the Internet. (Photo courtesy of Dell Corporation.)

PARTS OF THE COMPUTER

A medical assistant must understand the function of the different parts of a computer. The physical pieces that can be touched and seen are called *hardware*. Computers using Windows software have an option in the control panel for adding hardware. This shortcut makes adding new equipment easy and provides instruction all along the way. Hardware provides the medium on which software can be used. Most PCs have a microprocessor, monitor, keyboard, and mouse and many are connected to a printer.

Microprocessor

Inside the casing of the main computer hardware, the microprocessor is housed. The microprocessor is the central unit of the computer that contains the logic circuitry, which carries out the instructions of a computer's programs. It is considered the most important piece of hardware in a computer system. Microprocessors act as the brain of the computer and interpret instructions from a program. Microprocessors, sometimes called CPUs, are differentiated by three basic elements:

- *Bandwidth:* Bandwidth describes how much information can be sent over a connection at one time, or how many **bits** can be processed in one single instruction. Bits, short for binary digits, are the smallest pieces of information on the computer. Eight bits make up 1 **byte.** A **kilobyte** is approximately 1024 bytes, and a **megabyte** is approximately 1 million bytes. A **gigabyte** consists of approximately 1 billion bytes. A **terabyte** provides a huge amount of storage, consisting of approximately 1 trillion bytes.
- *Clock speed:* Clock speed determines how many instructions per second that the processor can handle. Clock speed is measured in **megahertz** (MHz). One megahertz equals 1 million cycles per second, so a processor that operates at 300 MHz executes 300 million cycles per second.
- *Instruction set:* The instruction set is the set of instructions that the microprocessor can execute.

The higher the bandwidth and clock speed, the faster and more powerful the microprocessor. For instance, a 32-bit microprocessor that runs at 50 MHz is more powerful than a 16-bit microprocessor that runs at 25 MHz.

A microprocessor contains memory consisting of electronic and magnetic cells, each of which contains information. Two kinds of memory exist: read-only memory (ROM) and random-access memory (RAM). ROM is internal memory that contains a portion of the operating system and computer language. This is sometimes known as *main memory.* Data that have been "burned" onto a ROM chip cannot be removed and can only be read, similar to a CD-ROM, unless the CD is a "rewriteable" type. With this permanent memory, much less information has to be transferred from a disk to start the computing process. ROM cannot be overwritten and is not erased when the power is shut off. RAM can be thought of as an internal scratch pad for the computer. It contains the program instructions and the data that are currently processing. RAM is normally erased when the power is shut off.

CRITICAL THINKING APPLICATION

A colleague of Dr. Bouchard's has mentioned that he knows about a website that has several computer programs online that can be downloaded free of charge. Dr. Bouchard investigates the site and realizes the software has been pirated. What concerns could this cause if he uses the software in his office? What would happen if any of this software were to malfunction?

Monitor

A monitor, which looks very much like a television (TV) screen, is a device used to display computer-generated information. A few are **monochromatic,** but most monitors today are color, capable of being adjusted for brightness, sharpness, and other settings of the user's choice. Many are high-definition monitors that rival the best plasma TV screens. Color monitors allow for a high-quality display, and the more advanced models have resolutions capable of reproducing high-quality pictures good enough for viewing a **digital video disk (DVD).** By viewing the monitor, the user receives instant feedback on entries into the computer. Monitors are sometimes referred to as *displays* and are considered output devices.

Keyboard

For most computers the keyboard is the primary text input device. Keyboards contain special function keys, such as the escape key, tab key, cursor movement keys, numeric keys, shift keys, and control keys. Additional function keys, numbered F1 to F12, are used to perform specific word processing or other computer-related operations. Used alone, a function key may create bold print, underline, indent, or call up a help screen. Used in conjunction with the Ctrl, Alt, or Shift key, the function keys can produce other desired results, such as activating the printer, inserting the current date into a document, retrieving a file, or moving a designated block of text. Wireless keyboards are a popular alternative that allow the user to move around more freely while operating the computer. Wave keyboards, and others designed with ergonomics in mind, are also popular.

Mouse

The mouse first became a widely used computer tool when Apple Computers made it a standard part of the Apple Macintosh computer. It resembles a mouse because of its shape and the cord, which attaches it to the microprocessor. A wireless mouse allows the user to manipulate the cursor without a cord attached. The mouse is a pointing device with a ball on the bottom that is moved by rolling it on a flat tabletop or mouse pad. The optical mouse has a photosensor instead of the rolling ball device. Some computers, especially laptops, have a built-in device called a *trackball* that is moved with the finger or thumb and serves the same function as a mouse. Other computers have a touchpad or a track-point that is manipulated to control the cursor. The cursor is a pointer or flat bar appearing on the monitor that shows where the next character will appear, which is the insertion point. The mouse allows the user to navigate around the screen quickly and click on links to access websites.

Printer

Printers are output devices. Documents appearing on the monitor may be directed to a printer to produce a printout or **hard copy** of a document. Many printers are bidirectional, which means they print both from left to right and from right to left. The type of printer used should depend on the job being performed.

Dot matrix printers are inexpensive and produce a moderate-quality hard copy. They form letters or shapes that they are directed to print by arranging patterns of dots on the paper. They operate faster than letter-quality machines, but the print lacks the clarity generally desired for a professional look.

Inkjet printers use an ink cartridge that feeds an array of nearly microscopic tubes, each of which has a heating element that is energized during the printing process. The ink cartridge may be black and white or color. Inkjet printers cost less than laser printers, but the ink cartridges they use are fairly expensive and increase the operating cost.

Laser printers use xerographic technology similar to that in photocopiers, so the laser printer is able to produce an almost limitless variety of forms and sizes as well as complex graphics. One disadvantage of inkjet and laser printers is that they are incapable of producing multiple copies with carbon sets or multicopy forms, which are often used by insurance companies for their filing forms.

Some printers today are multifunctional, serving as printers, **fax** machines, scanners, and copiers. Although these are excellent for home offices, they may not be the best investment for offices that will use these machines often during the day.

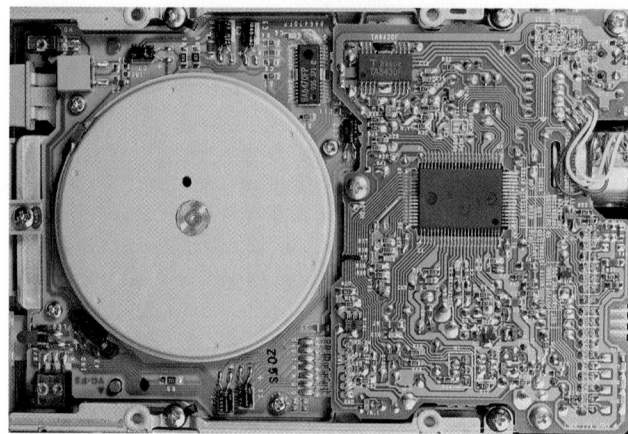

FIGURE 8-5 Hard drives store data and applications for fast and effective access and retrieval. Although a program installed on a hard drive can be removed, most programs are placed there for permanent use, such as Microsoft Office or Peachtree Accounting.

to the hard disk and stored there on the computer for use when needed. This is commonly called the *C drive.*

Floppy disks or diskettes are normally used in the computer's A drive, although the drives can have different names or labels, depending on the brand of computer. Floppy disks were so named because the original $5^1/_4$-inch variety was housed in a soft plastic cover that would "flop" if waved up and down. The $3^1/_2$-inch diskettes are less frequently used now because CDs have a higher capacity for holding information. Flash drives make transporting information from one computer to another quick and easy and are used more often today than diskettes.

CRITICAL THINKING APPLICATION

Dr. Bouchard has asked his office manager to perform a cost comparison on a printer for three of the office computers. He prefers that they have scanning and fax capability. What are some of the features that the office manager will be interested in knowing about these machines?

CRITICAL THINKING APPLICATION

Dr. Bouchard mentions that he noticed CD-R disks on sale over the weekend. The price that he saw was $30 for 100 CD-Rs. One of the medical assistants noticed a 30-pack of CD-Rs for $9.99. Which is the better buy?

INSIDE THE COMPUTER

Basic knowledge of the parts of a computer and their function will help a medical assistant to deal with minor technical issues and easily communicate with technical support personnel.

Motherboard

A motherboard is the main circuit board for the computer, to which other devices can be attached. Usually it contains the processor, the memory, and other controllers and devices that allow the system to operate and function.

Disk Drives

Today's computers have various **disk drives** on which information can be stored or accessed. The hard disk or hard drive is a magnetic disk inside the computer that holds from approximately 10 megabytes to several hundred gigabytes of information (Figure 8-5). Application software is normally saved

CD-ROM

Most of today's PCs are equipped with CD-ROM drives, which allow the storage of data on a CD. CDs hold much more information than floppy disks. A single CD can store as much information as approximately 700 floppy disks, which is the equivalent of about 300,000 text pages (Figure 8-6). A CD-RW is one on which data can be written, erased, and rewritten. Computers that have a **CD burner,** or CD-R drive, can take information from one CD or another source and write it to another CD. The computer must also have software that enables the burner to work. Software that is installed on a computer to allow a hardware device to function is called a **device driver.**

Expansion Boards

Expansion boards are devices that are inserted into a computer that give the computer added capabilities. For example, a **sound card** may be installed so that music or **MIDI** files can be heard from the unit. Other expansion boards are video adapters, internal modems, and graphics accelerators.

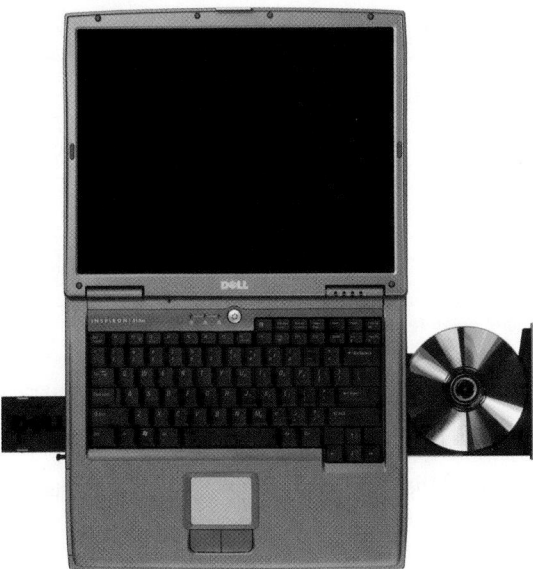

FIGURE 8-6 CD-ROMs allow the user to store and retrieve large amounts of information. Many computers are now equipped with CD-ROM burners, which allow copying of information from one CD to another, or from Internet files to CD-ROMs. (Photo courtesy of Dell Corporation.)

Software

Software is the programs and utilities that are loaded onto or inside the computer and used to carry out the work performed by the machine. There are two types of software: systems software and applications software. **System software** serves as the operating system of the computer and allows it to run and carry out the functions that the computer performs. For instance, Windows XP, Linux, and the now somewhat antiquated DOS are all types of operating system software. **Application software** refers to the programs loaded onto the computer that carry out the work for the actual users of the computer. Examples of application software are Microsoft Office, MediSoft, and Medical Manager. Applications (programs) are designed to perform specific tasks, such as word processing, billing, accounting, appointment setting, insurance form preparation, payroll, and **database** management. Many software applications are available for complete medical practice management (Procedure 8-1).

Modems

A **modem,** short for modulator-demodulator, is a device over which data can be transmitted via telephone lines and other media, such as a coaxial cable. Modems can be internal or external. An internal modem is built into or added to the inside of the computer casing. A cable modem operates over cable TV lines and uses the coaxial cable to provide faster Internet access. **Digital subscriber line (DSL)** modems operate over phone lines like normal modems, but they use a different frequency; therefore the telephone can be used while the computer is accessing the Internet. Often a filter is attached to the phone that removes other frequencies wherein the DSL is working, avoiding interference with the telephone line operation.

Speakers and Microphones

Some computers have external speakers to provide a higher quality sound from the computer. Many computers also have built-in speakers that provide a fair quality of sound. Microphones can be built in or attached so that the user can speak directly into the computer, even to someone on the other side of the world!

PERIPHERAL DEVICES

Peripheral devices are those that are not essential to the operation of the computer. For instance, the computer will operate without a modem, although a modem is necessary to access the Internet. A mouse is even considered a peripheral device, because everything that the mouse can access can also be reached by certain buttons on the keyboard, although often multiple keys have to be pressed at once. This section discusses some of the peripheral devices in use today.

Scanners

Scanners read text, illustrations, or photographs printed on paper and put them into a **format** that the computer can understand. Photographs can be placed into the scanner, saved on the computer, then used in a document. Some advanced scanners are used like highlighters and can collect notes from printed text.

Digital Cameras

Digital cameras use a charge-coupled device (CCD) to convert light into electrical charges. Digital cameras do not use film. Light strikes the surface of a photosite inside the camera, then filters add color and create the digital image. Many digital cameras can be attached directly to a computer or printer, and photos can be downloaded directly from the camera. Other cameras use a disk to load the pictures onto the computer.

CRITICAL THINKING APPLICATION

How might a digital camera be of use to a physician in his or her medical practice? What care should be taken when using the camera with a patient?

Zip Drives

A zip drive is a disk drive that has a very high storage capacity and is attached externally to a computer. It is usually used as a **backup** device for important data that should not be lost. Zip drives can hold between 100 and 250 megabytes of data and can even be stored somewhere other than the facility so that they are safe in case of fire or other destructive event.

ADDING A PROGRAM TO A COMPUTER

Adding or loading a program onto a computer is relatively easy. Most programs today come on a CD-ROM. The program will come with instructions as to how it should be loaded onto

PROCEDURE 8-1

Utilize Computer Software to Maintain Office Systems

CAAHEP COMPETENCY: 3.c(4)(c)
ABHES COMPETENCIES: 2.n, 3.d

GOAL: *To use the office computer system at maximum capacity to run the various aspects of the physician's office.*

EQUIPMENT and SUPPLIES

- Computer
- Computer software applications
- Software manuals
- Description of office systems
- Patient data
- Business data

PROCEDURAL STEPS

1. Determine the types of data that the physician's office needs to computerize.
   PURPOSE: To effectively plan the needs of the physician's office.
2. Discuss these needs with the physician and office manager.
3. Compile a budget for computer systems and/or upgrades.
   PURPOSE: Any large or capital purchases must be budgeted.

4. Research computer systems that can handle the tasks designated by the physician.
5. Invite sales representatives to present their options during a staff meeting.
   PURPOSE: The staff members may have significant questions that pertain to their particular area of concern.
6. Compare benefits and drawbacks of each system.
   PURPOSE: The comparison process will help in the decision as to which system should be used.
7. Ask sales representatives any questions that arise in the comparison process.
8. Discuss the final few choices with the physician and office manager.
9. Decide on a computer system or upgrade that best fits the needs of the office.
10. Purchase or lease the computer system.

---

the computer. Watch the monitor for steps to complete and information concerning the user's preferences, then follow all of the directions given.

In a Windows environment, the control panel provides an option to "add/remove programs." Once clicked, this will allow the program in the CD disk drive to be loaded onto the computer. At several points the computer may ask the user questions about his or her preferences for the program. Often the computer needs to be restarted after installation.

To remove a program from the computer, the "add/remove programs" **icon** should be accessed and the directions followed for removal of the program. This may be the only way to completely remove the program from the computer system.

FILE FORMATS

A file is a collection of data. Many types of files are related to computers. A text file, for example, contains some type of text, which is the main body of printed words or written matter on a page. Often an extension exists at the end of the filename that designates what type of file the document is. A file named manual.com might indicate that the file is some type of command file. A few of the common file extensions include the following:

- jpg: *JPEG* stands for Joint Photographic Experts Group and is a format often used for photographs.
- gif: *GIF* stands for Graphics Interchange Format, which supports color and is often used for scanned images and illustrations rather than photographs.

- doc: A file that includes the extension .doc is usually a file created by a word processor or word processing software; *doc* stands for document.
- txt: A text file usually has the extension .txt after its name. Characters in a text file are represented by their **ASCII codes.**
- rtf: *RTF* stands for Rich Text Format. This type of file combines ASCII codes with special commands that distinguish variations, such as a certain **font.**
- bmp: Bit-mapped graphics are indicated by the extension .bmp. These are compiled by a graphics image that is set in rows or columns of dots.

A medical assistant who is familiar with these types of files will be able to save and open them correctly and use the computer to the fullest advantage in the medical office.

COMPUTER NETWORKING

A network is a group of two or more computer systems that are linked together. Several types of networks exist:

- LAN: A LAN is a Local Area Network, or a computer network spanning a relatively small area. Most LANs are contained in a single building or group of buildings and are connected by a **router,** but LANs can be connected to other LANs even at a distance. A **hub** is a device that connects several computers or networks together, and a **switch** is designed to help the LAN run more efficiently by controlling local network traffic.
- MAN: A MAN is a Metropolitan Area Network. A MAN

spans an area that does not exceed a metropolitan area or city and connects several LANs.

- WAN: A WAN is a Wide Area Network, which spans a relatively large geographic area. Typically, a WAN consists of two or more LANs or MANs. These networks can be connected through public networks, such as a telephone system, or through leased lines or satellites. The largest WAN that exists is the Internet.
- HAN: A HAN is a Home Area Network, which connects computers inside a user's home.
- CAN: A CAN is a Campus Area Network, often used on college campuses and sometimes on military bases.

SERVERS

A **server** is important to the network, because it is the computer that manages the shared network resources. Several types of servers exist. When many computers are connected to one printer, often a print server manages these printers. File servers are used for file storage, and database servers are used to process database **queries.** Some servers are considered to be dedicated servers, meaning they perform tasks only as a server, although a server may also operate as a normal computer.

CLIENTS

A client is a computer that is configured to request access to resources from a server. Server applications, like access to the Internet, network printing, or email access, can run on a server and are accessed by the clients so that they can accomplish these tasks.

THE INTERNET

The Internet is a global network that connects millions of computers together. This fascinating structure has made the world a smaller place (Figure 8-7). Through chat programs one can talk with individuals literally on the other side of the world and be introduced to cultures that 20 years ago would never have been understood. Through Web pages we

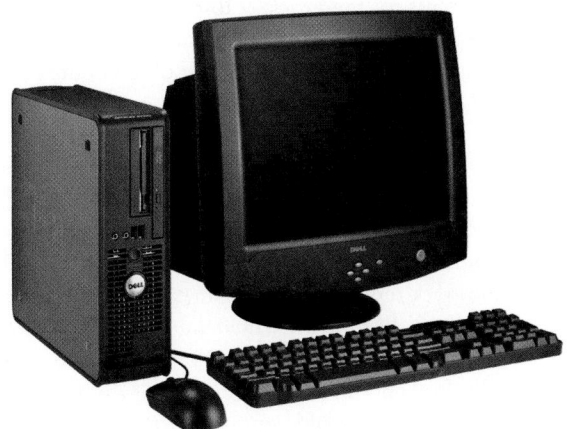

FIGURE 8-7 Computers in today's businesses can speak to one another from across the room or across the world. (Photo courtesy of Dell Corporation.)

can visit different parts of the world and learn and see many things that previously were impossible for the average person to experience. **Ecommerce** allows us to shop on the net, from the most exclusive shops in Beverly Hills to the corner grocery store. The Internet has changed the way we learn, do business, communicate, and entertain ourselves.

Each computer connected to the Internet is called a *host* and is independent of all the others. The users of each computer determine which services to make available to other users on the Internet. Often a company or organization also has an Intranet, which is a local network that uses Internet technology within a company or single location but does not have access to the Internet directly.

Internet service providers (ISPs) are companies that provide access to the Internet. Examples include America Online, Mindspring, Verizon, Earthlink, and Yahoo. ISPs issue each user an IP (Internet Protocol) address, which is a unique identifier for that user's particular computer on a Transmission Control Protocol/ Internet Protocol **(TCP/IP)** network. An IP address is a 32-bit number written as four numbers separated by a period. Each number can be zero to 255, so a valid IP address could be 10.145.32.254. Messages are defined and transmitted over the Internet when a Uniform Resource Locator **(URL)** is entered into the browser and a HyperText Transfer Protocol **(HTTP)** command tells the Web server to retrieve the requested Web page.

Domain names identify one or more IP addresses, such as microsoft.com or ama-assn.org. A limited number of top-level domains are available to which a domain name can be attached. Some of these top-level domains include .com (familiarly called *dot-com)* for commercial businesses; .org for organizations, usually nonprofit; .edu for educational institutions; .gov for government agencies; and .net for network organizations. Most Internet sites use a language called HyperText Markup Language **(HTML),** which was one of the first and is still one of the most popular languages used to create Web pages. **Java** is another popular language used in website creation.

Hotspots are locations that offer an access point providing public wireless broadband network services and are found in places such as airports, libraries, convention centers, and hotels. Users may be able to connect to the network for no charge or may be required to place a credit card number on file or make a deposit. This service is convenient for the medical professional who is traveling or attending events away from the office.

Many physicians and health organizations offer a website with information about their services. In today's data-driven society, this is an excellent way to educate the public about the services the organization offers and to provide all types of information to the audience that the organization wishes to reach. To obtain a domain name, one must pay a small fee to have the name registered and added to a central database, if the desired name is available. Companies such as register.com or verisign.com offer domain name registration services.

Websites often contain **banners,** which attract the eye of the user and tempt a click of the mouse, taking the user to a new website. They are similar to Internet commercials. These sites usually contain advertisements or surveys and can track the number of times a user views the site. These views are called "hits." Banners and website home pages sometimes use **Flash**, which is designed to grab the interest of the user with **multimedia** and encourage further exploration of a website.

A word of caution: Because most medical offices have some type of connection to the Internet, the medical assistant may be tempted to check personal email, "surf" the Web, or participate in instant messaging during working hours. Remember, personal business should not be conducted while at work. Supervisors appreciate the medical assistant who is honest with his or her time and spends it in productive, work-related activities.

BROWSERS

Web browsers are software applications that allow the user to locate and display Web pages. Two commonly used browsers are Netscape Navigator and Microsoft Internet Explorer. These browsers are able to display graphics as well as text and can also present multimedia information, the quality of which is dependent on the computer system in use and the Internet connection speed. Browsers also have a bookmark capability that allows the user to mark a certain Web page then easily return to it by clicking on its link in a drop-down box in the browser's menu. The **cache** allows quick retrieval of previously viewed sites because the computer remembers and saves the information on the hard drive. **Cookies** are stored information about individual users, like screen names and passwords.

Browsers and other websites also contain **search engines.** These are programs in which a topic, word, or group of words can be entered, and the engine will search the Internet for matches. A listing of those matches will appear, and the user can click on each match to reference information and complete research. Information on just about any subject can be found through using search engines.

CRITICAL THINKING APPLICATION

Dr. Bouchard wants all employees to have Internet access at his office but is still concerned that there will be occasional misuse of the computer. He does not want the staff to use the computer for personal business but does not mind if they check their personal email on a break or at lunch. What are some reasonable policies for office Internet use?

Popular Search Engines

www.alltheweb.com	www.lycos.com
www.altavista.com	www.metacrawler.com
www.ask.com	www.netscape.com
www.dogpile.com	www.search.aol.com
www.excite.com	www.search.msn.com
www.google.com	www.webcrawler.com
www.hotbot.com	www.yahoo.com

THE COMPUTER AS A CO-WORKER

The computer is a valuable tool in the medical office. It can assist in filing insurance claims by sending information from the computer in the office to the computers at the insurance company using a modem. Electronic processing of insurance claims not only saves time but also provides immediate information as to whether a claim will be accepted. Errors in coding or procedure are immediately evident, and many rejections can be avoided even before the claim is transmitted. Most insurance companies require that providers file claims electronically.

The demographics about a patient will appear on computerized patient ledgers, listing name, address, telephone number, and insurance information. As services are rendered, charges are entered into the computer, and payments will be displayed as well. This helps the medical facility to maintain an accurate balance of all patient accounts.

At the appropriate time each month, the computer can print a patient's billing statement, which shows a detail of charges, payments, adjustments, and the current balance. In addition, the computer can be programmed to age the accounts according to any criteria selected and to include this information on the billing statement. A series of collection letters can be developed and personalized for individual patients as they are needed.

Database software makes it possible to organize a large volume of information that can be used in a number of ways. One of the most practical uses is the organization of identifying information on each patient. The computer can also store clinical information about patients using much less space and with greater security than papers in a patient's chart. Access to records can be limited with passwords.

The computer has virtually replaced the appointment book in many medical offices today. Software for appointment-setting ranges from relatively simple programs to very sophisticated systems. An advantage to computer scheduling is that more than one person can access the system at one time, and the same information is available to all users.

Computers are even being used as marketing tools and virtual secretaries in some modern medical offices (Figures 8-8 and 8-9). Computers can be programmed to call all patients with appointments for the next day to remind them to visit the doctor, or perhaps to call all patients due for a 6-month eye or dental examination. As a marketing tool, computers can be programmed to call all phone numbers in a certain area code with a prerecorded message about a new procedure available at the office or a new physician in the area. Although many individuals are annoyed by the telemarketing concept and being called by a computer, the success rate is good. Computers can call thousands on thousands of phone numbers, relay a message, and track replies within a matter of hours. This could never be accomplished in the same time period by humans. These methods of using the computer open all kinds of doors for the medical practice of the future.

The medical office should routinely perform a file backup to be sure that valuable data can be retrieved in the event of a system failure. Many medical office computer programs have an

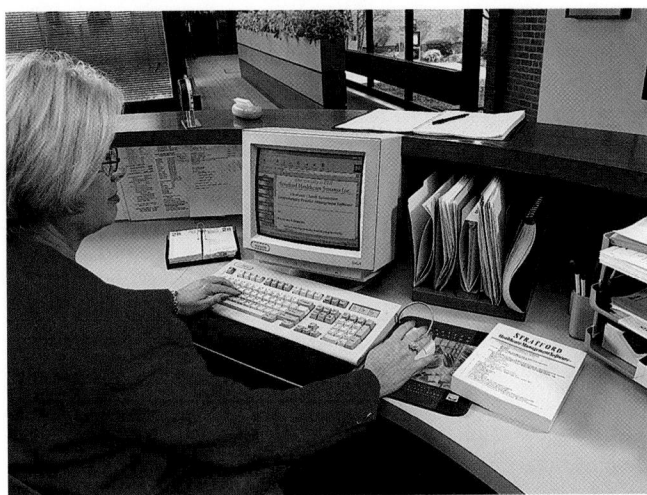

FIGURE 8-8 Computers assist the staff members and physicians of the medical office in numerous ways, making the office run in a more efficient manner.

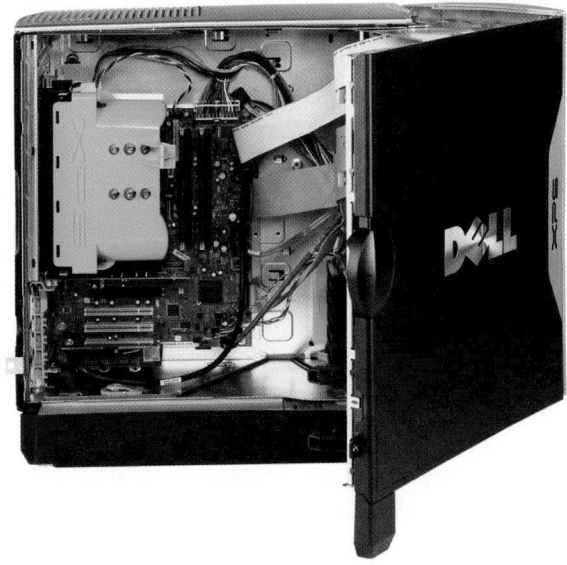

FIGURE 8-9 Inside a computer. Today's microprocessors are designed so that memory, additional drives, and other hardware can be easily added to the system. (Photo courtesy of Dell Corporation.)

automatic backup function, but some must be done manually. It is wise to keep backup copies of the database and other critical documents off the premises in case of fire or other tragedy.

COMPUTER SECURITY

Patients are entitled to the utmost confidentiality with respect to their medical records and the release of any information of a personal nature. Computer technology allows the accumulation and storage of a vast amount of data that may be accessible to a variety of individuals, making it imperative that guidelines be set up for the protection of such data.

Encryption is the translation of data into a code that is not readily understood by most users. It is one effective way to achieve data security. To access or read an encrypted file, the user must have a password that enables the code to be decrypted.

Once the code is decrypted, the file is then useable by the application. Encrypted data are called *cipher text*.

Some individuals attempt to access information in a computer without the owner's consent. These people may intend to use the information just for fun or may have a malicious intent, such as to steal or corrupt the data. Although these people are commonly called *hackers*, computer enthusiasts insist that the correct term for individuals who break into computers with dishonorable intent is *crackers*. The term *hacker* originally simply described a person who enjoyed learning about using computers and becoming proficient in that use.

Various ways may be used to protect computers and data from unauthorized access. Firewalls are systems designed for just such a purpose and can be implemented into both the hardware and the software of the computer. Firewalls are often used to prevent individuals from accessing private networks. Each message sent and received is examined, and the firewall blocks those that do not meet specific security criteria. Passwords, frequent password changes, and user logs also help protect data and the integrity of the database.

Viruses are programs or pieces of code that are loaded onto a computer, usually without the owner's knowledge, and can act like a physical virus in that they can make the computer "sick." Viruses can replicate themselves, copying themselves over and over again, and can be passed to other computers through emails, usually without the sender's knowing that a virus was passed along. Even simple viruses can quickly use all available memory and bring the system to a standstill; some can completely corrupt the computer's hard drive. More dangerous types of viruses can transmit over networks, bypassing security systems and destroying valuable data. This is why antivirus software is an important part of any computer system. Check for updates to the antivirus program at least weekly.

COMPUTERS AND THE HEALTH INSURANCE PORTABILITY AND ACCOUNTABILITY ACT

The Health Insurance Portability and Accountability Act (HIPAA) was developed in part to make certain that patient health information would be kept private and confidential. The wide use of computers in healthcare facilities sometimes makes this a difficult goal. The law limits who can look at and/or receive a patient's health information. Health information may be used and shared as follows:

- For patient care and treatment coordination
- To pay physicians and facilities for healthcare
- With family, friends, and relatives whom the patient has identified as being involved in the patient's healthcare
- To make certain that good care is provided in clean facilities
- To protect public health
- To make required reports to law enforcement officials

Health information cannot be shared or used without patient permission in most cases. Specifically, the provider cannot do the following:

- Give health information to a patient's employer
- Use or share health information for marketing purposes

- Share mental health information obtained in counseling sessions

The healthcare facility must take action to train those who use computer systems as to what information can and cannot be shared. Individual computer users should have their own log-in names and passwords that are not provided to anyone else. All users should be required to use the log-in name and password every time they use the computer system. Patient information must not be accessed unless the user needs to know the contents of the patient's file in order to provide patient care. Be careful when releasing any type of medical information to anyone. Questions should be directed to the office manager or to the physician. HIPAA will be discussed in more detail in Chapter 15, which covers Health Information Management.

ELECTRONIC SIGNATURES

A recently introduced convenience option is the electronic signature. Electronic signature programs are offered both as stand-alone products and as part of computerized medical record systems. After dictated reports are transcribed, a physician can use a password and personal identification number (PIN) to electronically "sign" the document by clicking on an icon after the document has been reviewed for accuracy. Once the document has been signed, it cannot be altered—only addenda are allowed.

COMPUTERS AND ERGONOMICS

The increased use of computers in the workplace has underscored the need to choose comfortable, safe furniture and equipment. Repetitive strain injury (RSI) accounts for the majority of work-related injury claims. This includes a number of conditions that are caused by repeatedly straining certain nerves, muscles, or tendons. Carpal tunnel syndrome is one example of RSI.

To avoid such injuries, office staff should use posture chairs that support the lumbar section of the back, with a correct angle of the knee and the feet resting on the floor. Of the many designs for keyboards available, one should be chosen that allows the correct angle at the elbow and the wrist to be held in a neutral position.

Eyestrain is another danger arising from continuous use of a computer. The monitor should be just below eye level and at an arm's length away. At least once each hour, the user should take a break from looking at the monitor.

CLOSING COMMENTS

Computers should be thought of as additional workers in the office. A medical assistant who learns how best to use the computer and discovers as many of its capabilities as possible will be a valuable employee.

Read the manuals that accompany equipment and programs and try new applications for old procedures. Computers are designed to save time, so look for ways to make the day's workload lighter by taking full advantage of the computer.

The future promises more rapid technologic advances; computer equipment can become archaic in as short a time as 6 months after purchase. **Artificial intelligence,** voice recognition, **virtual reality,** and retinal scanning, seen mostly in the movies, will become commonplace in our homes and businesses. These tools will make the work environment even faster and more efficient as the world becomes a smaller place.

The evolution of computers will continue to bring about changes in medical facilities of the future. Medical staffs will find themselves educating their patients about computer use, because numerous programs in development will allow patients to "check in" once they arrive at the office and verify their identity. A medical assistant will need patience to instruct these procedures and assure the patients that these new methods will increase their security as well as the protection of their medical records.

With the growing number of medical databases online, physicians can now use information on the Internet to help educate their patients about the illnesses that they are facing. While consulting with the patient, with a few clicks of the mouse the physician can print out excellent information, which often will assist the patient with referrals to help agencies and suggestions for better healthcare.

SUMMARY OF SCENARIO

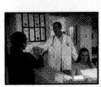

Dr. Bouchard is a progressive physician who believes that the use of technology will assist him in the care of his patients and help his office to run more efficiently. The computer assists the staff to complete tasks in a timely manner and provides records of business transactions. Staff members are able to function much faster than when records were kept by hand. He understands the need to train his staff and keep them up to date on the latest versions of their computer software. His willingness to close his office for staff-wide training demonstrates his commitment. He is cost conscious and looks for the best available equipment for the investment he is willing to make.

Dr. Bouchard often uses digital camera equipment to take "before" and "after" pictures of his patients, but only with their special written consent. He also uses the computer to send his patients a monthly email newsletter with health information and special news about the practice.

He monitors his staff's Internet use but is reasonable about allowing them a small degree of personal access on breaks and at lunch. The doctor cautions his staff about accessing medical records that they are not actively involved with in patient care to avoid invading the patient's privacy. The computer system prints a daily log of all employees and what information they accessed throughout the day, so he stresses the importance of logging on and off the computer using their individual passwords and log-on IDs. Dr. Bouchard's employees realize the importance of keeping medical information private. Unless a staff member needs to know the information in the chart to care for the patient, he or she may be accused of invading the patient's privacy when accessing medical information.

He is very interested in new developments for healthcare facilities, such as those that will allow his patients to check themselves in and gain access to limited information about their own medical record. He has a vision that one day his patients will be able to download their statements or perhaps their child's immunization records from their home computers, reducing the staff's workload and providing instant access to some information for his patients. Insightful physicians like Dr. Bouchard see the computer as a co-worker in the medical facility.

SUMMARY of LEARNING OBJECTIVES

1. Define, spell, and pronounce the terms listed in the vocabulary.
   - Spelling and pronouncing medical terms correctly adds credibility to the medical assistant. Knowing the definition of these terms promotes confidence in communication with patients and co-workers.
2. List several ways that the computer can be effective in a medical office.
   - The computer can be an effective tool in the medical office. It performs repetitive tasks, reduces errors, speeds up production, recalls information on command, saves time, reduces paperwork, and allows for more creative and productive use of workers' time.
3. Explain the basic functions that a computer performs.
   - The computer performs four basic functions: input, processing, output, and storage. Input includes information that is put into the computer, and output is information that comes out of the computer. Processing is in-between, and is the actual manipulation of data. Storage is the retention of data inside the computer or on storage media.
4. Explain the basic parts of a computer.
   - Several basic parts make up a computer system. The microprocessor is the brains of the system that interprets the instructions given to it by an application program. The monitor allows the user to see immediate output on a screen, and printers allow the output to be printed to a hard copy. The keyboard and mouse serve as input devices.
5. List the three elements that differentiate microprocessors.
   - Three elements differentiate microprocessors. The bandwidth describes the amount of information that can be sent over a connection at one time, and the clock speed determines the number of instructions per second that the processor can handle. The instruction set is the instructions that the microprocessor can execute.
6. Discuss the differences among various types of printers.
   - Three main types of printers are in use in today's medical offices. Dot matrix printers produce output of moderate quality but are inexpensive. Inkjet printers use a cartridge and a heating element to produce an image on a page. A laser printer uses technology similar to a photocopier.
7. Explain the importance of a motherboard.
   - The motherboard is the main connection board to which all other devices are connected inside the computer. It contains all of the essential wiring and expansion devices needed to operate the computer, as well as the battery that keeps the clock and calendar running when the computer is turned off.
8. Explain and give examples of peripheral devices.
   - Peripheral devices, such as scanners, Zip drives, and other devices, are not necessary to the function of the computer but perform special functions.
9. List and discuss several types of file formats.
   - File format refers to the extension just after the filename and describes the method used to save the file. This also helps to

Continued

SUMMARY of LEARNING OBJECTIVES

Continued

identify the type of file on the computer. For example, a JPEG file is often used for photographs, a GIF file is used for scanned illustrations or images, and a TXT file is usually specifically for text for a printed page.

10. Explain the concept of computer networking.
    - Computer networks are groups of two or more computers linked together. These networks can be local or can cover a city or wide geographic area. Some are limited to a few buildings. Networks often share resources, such as printers.
11. Define the function of browsers.
    - Browsers are software applications that allow a user to find information on the Internet. They are able to show graphics, and often multimedia, such as videos. Commonly used browsers include Internet Explorer and Netscape Navigator.
12. Discuss the importance of computer security.
    - Computer security is critical, especially because confidential patient information is stored on computers in medical facilities. Several methods may be used to enhance computer security, such as the use of firewalls and antivirus programs. Restrictions on who may log in and the use of passwords also will assist the facility to ensure that only authorized individuals have access to confidential information.

CONNECTIONS

 Study Guide Connection: Go to Chapter 8 Study Guide. Read the Case Study and Workplace Applications and complete the assignments. Do online research for answers to the questions in the Internet Activities associated with computers in the medical office.

 CD Connection: Go to the Medical Assisting Competency Challenge CD and review the content of the training activities. These will be referred to throughout the textbook to enhance your learning experience.

 Evolve Connection: For more information related to computers in the medical office, go to evolve.elsevier.com/kinn and visit related weblinks for Chapter 8. Click on the Medical Assisting Exam Review and do the practice questions to sharpen your test-taking skills.

Telephone Techniques

9

Ashlynn McDowell is a recent graduate of a medical assisting program and has begun her first position as a receptionist in an obstetrician's office. It has been Ashlynn's lifelong goal to work in obstetrics, and she is determined to perform to the best of her abilities. However, Ashlynn has never held a job in a professional office. She knows that she will need to practice all of the skills she learned in school with regard to being an effective receptionist.

Ashlynn works for Dr. Stella Frank, who is customer service oriented and wants her patients to feel special and cared for. She insists that all of their concerns be taken seriously. Ashlynn is anxious to build trust with the patients and offer them help with the problems they encounter that fall into her realm of responsibility.

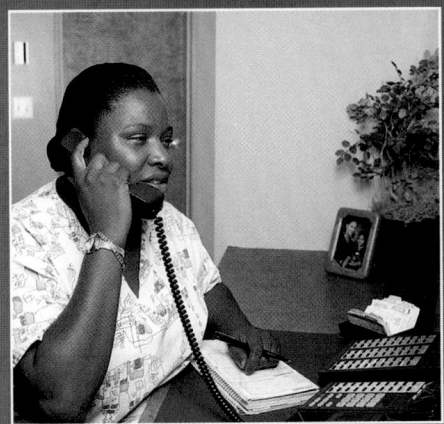

She knows that she will be required to speak clearly and distinctly and be adept at follow-up skills. She plans to dress professionally each day so that she projects the right image to the patients with whom she comes in contact. Ashlynn will strive to be the type of employee who presents a willingness to learn, an ability to adapt, and a heart full of compassion for the patient. She is a team player who sincerely wishes to cooperate with other staff members that might need her help.

Dr. Frank is pleased that she has found such an eager person to add to her staff and will provide assistance and guidance to Ashlynn as she learns how to make her patients feel a part of her clinic family. Ashlynn's self-esteem has increased because she feels she is making a great contribution to healthcare.

While studying this chapter, think about the following questions:

- How can Ashlynn's telephone demeanor convince patients that she wants to help them?
- Why does the tone of voice play an important role in patient perception?

- How does the medical assistant speaking to patients on the telephone strike a balance between too much and too little time?
- How can the medical assistant reduce patient frustration with telephone issues?

LEARNING OBJECTIVES

1. Define, spell, and pronounce the terms listed in the vocabulary.
2. Determine and discuss the source of incoming and outgoing calls to a physician's office.
3. Describe how one develops a pleasing telephone voice.
4. Demonstrate the correct way to hold a telephone handset.
5. Explain why courtesy is so important when speaking on the telephone.
6. Discuss different ways to handle callers who wish to speak to the physician.
7. List the seven items needed to take a telephone message correctly.
8. Explain how angry callers might be handled.

9. Discuss how the medical assistant should handle callers who have a complaint.
10. List several questions to ask when handling an emergency call.
11. Discuss several useful sections of the introductory pages of the phone directory.
12. Demonstrate the correct way to answer the telephone in the office.
13. Demonstrate the correct way to accurately record a message and take a request for action.
14. Demonstrate the most efficient way to call in a prescription or a prescription refill to a pharmacy.

National Accreditation Competencies and Content

CAAHEP COMPETENCIES

General
3.c.(1)(b). Recognize and respond to verbal communication
3.c.(1)(d). Demonstrate telephone techniques
3.c.(2)(a). Identify and respond to issues of confidentiality
3.c.(3)(a). Explain general office policies
3.c.(3)(d). Identify community resources

ABHES COMPETENCIES

Professionalism
1.h. Be courteous and diplomatic

Communication
2.a. Be attentive, listen, and learn
2.b. Be impartial and show empathy when dealing with patients
2.c. Adapt what is said to the recipient's level of comprehension
2.d. Serve as liaison between physician and others
2.e. Use proper telephone techniques
2.h. Receive, organize, prioritize, and transmit information expediently
2.k. Principles of verbal and nonverbal communication
2.l. Recognition and response to verbal and nonverbal communication
2.m. Adaptation for individualized needs
2.n. Application of electronic technology

Administrative Duties
3.a. Perform basic secretarial skills

VOCABULARY

clarity The quality or state of being clear.

competent Having adequate abilities or qualities; having the capacity to function or perform in a certain way.

cultivate To foster the growth of; to improve by labor, care, or study.

diction The choice of words especially with regard to clearness, correctness, or effectiveness.

enunciation (e-nun-se-a′-shun) Utterance of articulate, clear sounds.

inflection (in-flek′-shun) A change in pitch or loudness of the voice.

invariably (in-var′-e-uh-buh-le) Consistently; not changing or capable of change.

jargon The technical terminology or characteristic idiom of a particular group or special activity.

monotone A succession of syllables, words, or sentences in one unvaried key or pitch.

multitasking Performing multiple tasks at the same time.

pitch The property of a sound, especially a musical tone, which is determined by the frequency of the waves producing it; the highness or lowness of sound.

provider Individual or company that provides medical care and services to a patient or the public.

salutation (sal-yu-ta′-shun) An expression of greeting, goodwill, or courtesy by words or gestures.

screen Something that shields, protects, or hides; to select or eliminate through a screening process.

STAT Medical abbreviation for immediately; at this moment.

tactful Having a keen sense of what to do or say to maintain good relations with others or to avoid offense.

tedious (te′-de-yus) Tiresome because of length or dullness.

The telephone is the lifeline of a medical practice as well as a powerful public relations tool. The majority of patients who are seen in a medical facility make their initial appointments by telephone. When used appropriately, the telephone can help build a medical practice from its beginning and throughout its life (Figure 9-1). If used inappropriately, it can destroy a flourishing practice. Always remember that the voice on the other end of the line is that of the patient, and telephone calls can never be considered an interruption of the work day.

Most incoming calls are from the following sources:
- Established patients calling for appointments or to ask questions
- New patients making a first contact with the physician's office
- Patients and medical workers reporting treatment results or emergencies
- Other physicians who are making referrals or discussing a patient
- Laboratories reporting vital patient information

EFFECTIVE USE OF THE TELEPHONE

Active Listening

Although great emphasis is placed on rules for speaking, the importance of active listening is often overlooked. The same

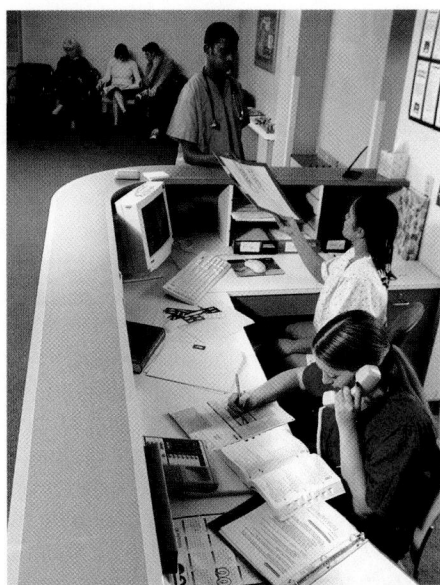

FIGURE 9-1 The telephone plays a vital role in the success of a medical practice.

attention should be given to a telephone conversation that would be given to a face-to-face conversation. Concentration is not always easy for a medical assistant who is juggling several duties at once in the medical office, so he or she must practice focusing on the call at hand. Effective active listening also provides vital information about the nature of the call—whether the caller is distressed, is agitated, or has a concern that needs to be addressed immediately.

Developing a Pleasing Telephone Voice

Individuals who call a physician's office should hear a pleasant, friendly voice when they are greeted. It is a common sales technique to be sure that the caller "hears a smile." Customer service is critical in today's medical offices, and this technique is quite useful for medical assistants because they are likely to be the caller's first point of contact with the practice. Be sure to enunciate words clearly, pronouncing them separately and distinctly. **Diction, pitch,** and **clarity** are important as well. Avoid speaking in a **monotone;** instead, use **inflection,** or a change in the pitch and loudness of the voice when speaking. This helps the speaker to emphasize certain points during the conversation.

When a telephone call is received from a stranger, one usually tries to visualize that person's appearance and perhaps will form an opinion of his or her personality. The caller may sound mature, somewhat worried, well educated, or frantic. As discussed in Chapter 5, communication is a two-way street, so the caller will be forming an impression of the person answering the phone at the same time. Sometimes these impressions are incorrect, but much can be inferred from what is heard on the telephone.

The tone of voice used by the medical assistant, as well as other medical staff members, plays a role in the attitude of the patient. A study conducted by Harvard University claims that the tone of voice used by surgeons has a direct link to medical professional liability claims. How something is said to a patient

is just as important as what is said. Always use a friendly and warm tone of voice and project confidence when speaking with patients. Be courteous and **tactful** and choose words carefully. Every caller should be made to feel that the medical assistant has time to attend to his or her wishes. A small mirror placed near the telephone will serve as a reminder to smile. If the medical assistant is rushed to pick up the telephone, he or she should wait a few seconds until able to answer graciously without seeming breathless or impatient.

Be alert and interested in the person who is calling. Always give full attention to the caller, and do not allow distractions to interfere with the conversation. Build a pleasant, friendly image for the office. Talk naturally and avoid repetition of mechanical words or phrases, such as "uh huh" and "you know." Avoid the use of professional **jargon,** such as referring to *otalgia* when the patient is reporting an earache. Using correct grammar adds to the caller's favorable impression. Speak distinctly; clear pronunciation and **enunciation** are vital. Move the lips, tongue, and jaw freely. Talk directly into the mouthpiece. Never answer the telephone when eating, drinking, or chewing gum. A well-modulated voice carries best. Use a normal tone of voice, neither too loud nor too soft. Talk at a moderate rate, neither too quickly nor too slowly. Be expressive, and vary the tone of voice. This will bring out the meaning of sentences and add color and vitality to what is said.

CRITICAL THINKING APPLICATION

Ashlynn has a tendency to speak a little fast in her normal conversations. How will she need to adjust as she is answering phones in the medical office? She is also a friendly person and enjoys talking on the phone. What precautions should she take so that this does not become an issue on the job?

Holding the Telephone Handset Correctly

A medical assistant must develop professional telephone habits and correct the more casual ones that are used at home. Consider how the handset is held. It should be placed so that the medical assistant's voice is relayed distinctly and accurately. Practice holding the handset around the middle, with the mouthpiece approximately 1 inch from the lips and directly in front of the teeth (Figure 9-2). Never hold it under the chin. Check the proper distance by taking the first two fingers and passing them through sideways in the space between the lips and the mouthpiece. If the fingers just squeeze through, then the lips are the correct distance from the telephone and the voice will go over the line in as close to its natural tone as possible. When using a headset, speak directly into its mouthpiece, positioning it the same distance from the mouth as a regular telephone.

Speak directly into the telephone immediately after removing it from its cradle. When turning to face another part of the room, make sure the handset moves, too; otherwise, the voice will be lost. A medical assistant who speaks too fast, enunciates poorly, or fails to speak directly into the transmitter may not be easily understood by the person on the other end of the receiver.

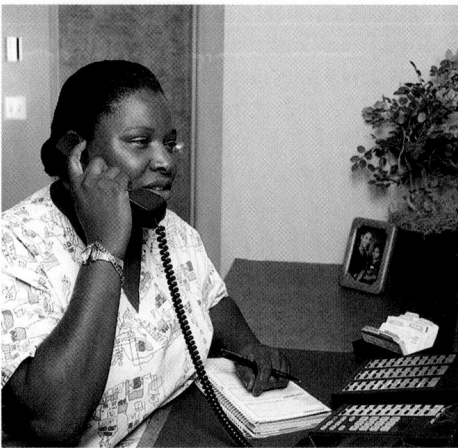

FIGURE 9-2 The handset should be held in the center, with the mouthpiece approximately 1 inch in front of the lips.

Maintaining Confidentiality

Keep in mind that all communications in a healthcare facility are confidential. If others are nearby, use discretion when mentioning the name of the caller. Be careful about being overheard when repeating any symptoms or other information received by telephone. Never use a speaker phone to listen to voicemail or to hold a phone conversation within the hearing range of others. Do not place patients on speakerphone at any time. Another individual may hear private medical information, which is a violation of HIPAA regulations.

CRITICAL THINKING APPLICATION

Ashlynn hears two employees speaking on the intercom in a derogatory manner about a patient who just left the office. How should she handle this situation? To whom should Ashlynn report this activity, if anyone, and why? What problems could be caused when staff members are overheard talking in this manner?

Thinking Ahead

It is always helpful to think ahead when an important call must be made. Have the patient's chart or the bill in question at hand before dialing the phone. Write down a list of questions to ask or goals for the conversation. Keep the call short and simple, then free the line for other calls.

Most offices keep a list of frequently called phone numbers both for staff use and to offer to patients. A list of local pharmacies, hospitals, and their departments is helpful. All of these are time-savers that will help the medical assistant to better serve patients.

TECHNIQUES FOR INCOMING TELEPHONE CALLS

Many incoming calls will be received in the medical office during the course of a single day. Each one deserves the medical assistant's complete and **competent** attention.

Answering Promptly

Whenever possible, answer the telephone on the first ring, and always by the third ring. If the facility has several incoming lines or more than one telephone, it will sometimes be necessary to interrupt a conversation to answer another call. It is courteous to say, "Excuse me just a moment; the other line is ringing." Answer the second call and determine who is calling. If it is not an emergency, ask that person to hold while the first call is completed. If possible, get the phone number of the second caller, but do not allow that request to turn into a lengthy conversation. Do not make the mistake of continuing with the second call while the first caller waits. Return to the first call as soon as possible and apologize briefly for the interruption. Think of what would happen during a face-to-face conversation. A second person who approaches people involved in a conversation should not expect to interrupt and be heard at length. However, if the second call is an emergency, take a moment to return to the first line and alert the caller that he or she will have to be kept waiting or be called back.

Never answer a call by saying, "Please hold" without first finding out who is calling. The call could be an emergency, and this type of greeting is extremely discourteous. It takes only a moment to be polite. If the call is an emergency, prompt attention to it could save a life.

Keep the focus on the call. Do not attempt to multitask while answering the telephone because this practice takes attention away from the patient. Callers can hear keyboard strokes and other office activity; therefore a caller might assume that the medical assistant is not giving full attention to the person on the phone. Treat the phone call just as if the patient were standing in the office face to face (Procedure 9-1).

Identifying the Facility

The medical assistant should identify the facility first, then state his or her name to the caller. Numerous telephone greetings can be used. Discuss which are best with the physician or office manager. Examples of telephone greetings include the following:

- "This is Dr. Frank's office, Miss McDowell speaking. How may I help you?"
- "Frank Maternal Health Clinic, this is Miss McDowell. How may I help you?"
- "Stella Frank's office, this is Miss McDowell. How may I help you?"

Some physicians avoid using the title "Doctor" so that they may protect their patient's confidentiality. For instance, if a physician needs to call a work number and leave a message for a patient, curious co-workers might attempt to investigate what type of physician is being seen. Dropping the "Doctor" when leaving messages and when answering the telephone can be an effective means of protecting patient privacy. However, merely saying "Hello" is unsatisfactory. The caller will **invariably** ask if he or she has reached the physician's office, so time is wasted, and the opportunity to create a favorable impression of your facility has been lost.

The use of a **salutation** in telephone identification is optional. Sometimes the addition of "Good morning" or

PROCEDURE 9-1

Demonstrate Telephone Techniques: Answer the Telephone

<u>CAAHEP COMPETENCY:</u> 3.c.(1)(d)
<u>ABHES COMPETENCY:</u> 2.e

GOAL: *To answer the telephone in a physician's office in a professional manner and respond to a request for action.*

EQUIPMENT and SUPPLIES

- Telephone
- Message pad
- Pen or pencil
- Appointment book
- Notepad

PROCEDURAL STEPS

1. Answer the telephone by the third ring, speaking directly into the mouthpiece, which should be positioned 1 inch from the mouth.
   <u>PURPOSE:</u> Answering promptly conveys interest in the caller. Proper positioning of the handset allows for audible tone and carries the voice well.
2. Speak distinctly with a pleasant tone and expression, at a moderate rate, and with sufficient volume for the calling party to understand every word.
3. Identify the office and/or physician and yourself.
   <u>PURPOSE:</u> The caller will know that the correct number has been reached and the identity of the staff member.
4. Verify the identity of the caller.
   <u>PURPOSE:</u> To confirm the origin of the call.

5. Triage the call, if necessary.
   <u>PURPOSE:</u> To determine if the caller has an emergency and needs immediate attention or a referral to the emergency department of a hospital.
6. Determine the needs of the caller, and provide the requested information or service, if possible. Provide the caller with excellent customer service. Be as helpful as possible.
   <u>PURPOSE:</u> The medical assistant can handle many calls and conserve the time and energy of the physician or other staff members.
7. If unable to assist the caller, transfer the call to the appropriate person. Before transferring the call, provide the person to whom the call is being transferred with as much information as possible about the caller and his or her needs.
   <u>PURPOSE:</u> To provide good customer service and be as helpful to the caller as possible.
8. Take a proper message for further action, if required.
   <u>PURPOSE:</u> Not all calls can be responded to immediately.
9. Terminate the call in a pleasant manner, and replace the receiver gently. Always allow the caller to hang up first.
   <u>PURPOSE:</u> To promote good public relations, provide excellent customer service, and ensure that the caller has no further questions.

"Good afternoon" to the identification is awkward. A rising inflection or a questioning tone of voice indicates interest and a willingness to assist and eliminates the need for an additional greeting. When the type of greeting to use has been decided, practice until it can be said easily and smoothly. It is critical that the greeting not be rushed so that all callers can clearly understand exactly what is being communicated.

CRITICAL THINKING APPLICATION

Most offices dictate how the phone is to be answered. What should Ashlynn do if she is very uncomfortable with the way she is being asked to answer the phone? Who should ultimately make the decision as to how the phone is answered?

Identifying the Caller

If the caller does not identify himself or herself, ask who is calling. It is helpful to write the name down immediately on a pad of paper or phone message form. Repeat the caller's name by using it in the conversation as soon as possible. Individuals like to hear their own names, and name repetition assures the

patient that he or she has been correctly identified. Try to use the person's name at least three times during the call, and remember other courteous expressions, such as "thank you," "please," and "you're welcome" as often as possible. However, if other patients are within the range of your voice, remember that the caller's privacy must be respected.

Occasionally a caller will refuse to identify himself or herself to the medical assistant and may be quite insistent on speaking with the physician. The individual could be a patient, so every attempt to identify the patient and assist him or her should be made. Such callers may also be salespersons who are fully aware that if their identity is revealed, they will never get the opportunity to speak to the physician. These people may be firmly told, "Dr. Frank is busy with a patient and has asked that we take messages for her. If you will not leave a message, you may wish to write a letter to her and mark it 'personal.'"

Screening Incoming Calls

Most physicians expect the medical assistant to **screen** all telephone calls. The physician and office manager will provide guidance as to the type of calls that should be routed to the physician and those that he or she will want to return at a later

STAYING IN CONTROL OF CALLS

The Dartnell Corporation publishes a newsletter entitled "Effective Telephone Techniques" that is an excellent tool for building good customer relations while using the phone. One issue suggests ways to control calls and keep them from becoming too lengthy. Try the tips below to keep callers on track and make all phone time productive.

- Ask the caller, "How may I help you today?"
- If the caller becomes sidetracked, say "You were describing the pain in your side?"
- When making a call, get right to the purpose of it after the initial greeting by saying "I was calling you about…"
- Keep explanations short and direct.
- Type information directly into the database, if used, while speaking on the phone.
- Keep personal and friendly comments to a minimum, or only one per call.
- Once the business is concluded, say "If there are no other questions…" and bring the conversation to a close.

FIGURE 9-3 Several tips to stay in control of the telephone calls in the medical office.

time. The medical assistant should become familiar with their preferences and also use good judgment, much of which comes with experience, in deciding whether to put a call through to the physician (Figure 9-3).

If it is the policy of the office, put calls from other physicians through at once. If the physician is busy and cannot possibly come to the telephone, explain this briefly and politely, then say that the physician will return the call as soon as possible.

Many callers will ask, "Is the doctor in?" or "May I speak to the doctor?" Avoid answering this question with a simple "Yes" or "No" or by responding with the question, "Who is calling, please?" If the physician is not in, say so before asking the identity of the caller. Otherwise, the impression may be created that the physician is just not willing to talk with this person.

If the physician is away from the office, the rule of offering assistance still holds. The medical assistant may say, "No, I am sorry, Dr. Frank is not in. May I take a message?" or "No, I am sorry, but Dr. Frank will be at the hospital most of the morning. May I ask her to return your call after 1 o'clock?"

If the physician is in and is available for telephone calls, a typical response would be, "Yes, Dr. Frank is in; may I say who is calling, please?"

When physicians prefer to keep telephone calls to a minimum, say, "Yes, Dr. Frank is in the office, but she is not free to come to the phone. May I take a message, please?" By responding in this way, the physician is not committed to taking the call.

During the time that a physician is examining a patient, he or she will not wish to be interrupted with a routine call. In such cases you might say, "Yes, Dr. Frank is in but is with a patient right now. May I help you?" or "Yes, Dr. Frank is in but is with a patient right now. Is there anything you would like me to ask her?"

Try to guard against being overprotective. A patient should be able to talk with the physician when necessary; but unless it is an emergency, the patient is probably willing to do so at the convenience of the physician. The medical assistant who answers the telephone acts as a screen, not a roadblock.

Find out exactly how calls are to be handled when the physician is out of the office and under what circumstances he or she can be interrupted when the physician is on the premises. **Cultivate** a reputation for being helpful and reliable. A medical assistant will save the physician many interruptions if patients develop confidence in the medical assistant's ability to help them and have faith in his or her promises to take messages and deliver them properly.

CRITICAL THINKING APPLICATION

Ashlynn answers the phone and a male pharmaceutical representative who has been visiting the clinic for several months is on the phone. She cheerfully greets him and asks if he is calling to make an appointment. He states that he wants to make an appointment with Ashlynn—for a date. How should she handle this call? What problems could arise if this were a patient and Ashlynn were to accept the date?

Minimizing Wait Time

When a call cannot be put through immediately, ask, "Would you prefer to wait, or should I call you back when Dr. Frank is free?"

If the caller elects to wait, remember that waiting with a silent telephone can be irritating and **tedious.** The waiting time always seems long, no matter how brief it really is. Many of today's phones are equipped with timers that tell the caller exactly how long they have been waiting on hold. The longer they wait, the more irritated they may become. Let no more than 1 minute pass without breaking in with some reassuring comment. For instance: "I'm sorry, Dr. Frank is still busy. Would you like to continue to hold?" or "I'm sorry to keep you waiting so long, Ms. Hughes. Would you prefer to have me return your call when Dr. Frank is free?" If the wait is longer than expected, the caller may wish to reconsider and call back at another time or have the call returned. By going back on the line at frequent intervals, the medical assistant allows the caller an opportunity to express such concerns.

Try to give the caller some estimate of when he or she may expect the return call. In any event, be considerate and remember that irritation can be lessened each time the medical assistant returns to the call by saying, "Thank you for waiting, Ms. Hughes."

When it is necessary to leave the telephone and obtain information, ask the caller, "Will you please wait while I get the information?" Listen for a reply. If it will take longer than a few seconds to get the information, give some estimate of the time required and offer to call back. When returning to the telephone, always thank the caller for waiting. Requests that might require pulling the patient's chart from the files are best handled with a call back to the patient.

Remember that leaving a person on hold ties up one of the physician's telephone lines, and an emergency call could be coming through, or new patients might be attempting to call. The majority of phone calls that come in to a physician's office during the day are important, so the lines should be kept clear as much as possible.

Transferring a Call

Always ask the patient's permission to place him or her on hold and to transfer the call. Identify the person on the phone when a call is transferred to the physician or another person in the facility. It is considered poor customer service to transfer the call to a co-worker's voicemail without warning the caller that the person is not available. Any person who refuses to give a name should not be put through unless the medical assistant has been specifically instructed to do so. If the person is not immediately available, ask the caller whether he or she would prefer to be put through to voicemail. Some callers simply believe their call will receive more attention if a human takes the message. If the caller insists, take a written message and deliver it to the proper person as soon as possible.

All medical assistants should learn "who does what" in the medical facility. Knowing about the functions of the office and which person is responsible for which areas will make a significant difference in the customer service provided to the patient. For example, suppose that the medical office employs one insurance receptionist, named Sarah, and three insurance billers. Opel handles names that begin with A through G, David handles names that begin with H through P, and Andrea handles names that begin with Q through Z. If a call comes to the office and the patient has an insurance question, the medical assistant could put the call through to Sarah. However, better customer service dictates that the medical assistant ask the name of the patient and put the call through to the person who handles that patient's particular claims. If the patient's name is Rebecca Whitehead, the medical assistant should call Andrea and ask if she may transfer Ms. Whitehead's call to her. The fewer times the caller is transferred, the happier the caller.

When the caller is a patient, the physician or clinical medical assistant will probably need his or her medical record at hand during the conversation. Remember that it is vital to protect the patient's right to privacy. If others are within hearing range, take the chart to the person responsible for the call and say, "This patient is waiting on the telephone." Because physician offices are often hectic, most require that a message be taken so that the medical record can be reviewed, the patient's request considered, and the patient called back with questions or instructions from the doctor.

Taking a Telephone Message

Always have a pen or pencil in hand and a message pad nearby when answering the telephone. Several calls may be answered before an opportunity arises to relay a message or carry out a promise of action. The written message is a vital part of competent patient care (Procedure 9-2).

Many types of message pads are available today (Figure 9-4). Ordinary spiral-bound notebooks are inexpensive, sturdy, and well proportioned. These usually lie flat on a desk and can be filed for future reference. Never use small scraps of paper for messages; they are too easily lost. Message books should be kept indefinitely in the medical office, because they could be used as evidence in a court of law. A copy of a phone message could be added to the patient's chart once acted on, or at a minimum the information could be noted in the chart if it concerns the patient's medical care.

A minimum of seven items are needed to take a telephone message correctly:

- The name of the person to whom the call is directed
- The name of the person calling
- The caller's daytime, evening, and/or cellular telephone number
- The reason for the call
- The action to be taken
- The date and time of the call
- The initials of the person taking the call

Impression-sensitive message pads that provide a copy of each page ensure that no message will be forgotten and are the best way to keep track of messages. This also provides a copy of the message in the event that one is somehow lost, and will help to assure that all messages are acted on. The nature of the message will determine whether it should be reported immediately. The person who completes the call must sign and date the message. If the call is from a patient and relates in any way to the medical history, or if any instructions were given or queries answered, this information should be placed in the patient's chart. Message forms are available that have a self-adhesive backing and can be placed permanently in the patient's case history.

Taking Action on Telephone Messages

The message procedure is not complete until the necessary action has been taken. Notations on the memo pad should be carried over to the following day if they have not been completed, but this should be a rare occurrence. Do not trust to memory messages that were not attended to from previous days; always carry them forward in writing.

Make brief notations of patients' reactions while talking to them on the telephone. The physician does not require a character study, but it is helpful to know when a patient appears fearful, apprehensive, or nervous. If a patient shows such symptoms, it may be wise to consult with or transfer the call to the physician or clinical medical assistant.

Ending a Call

When a caller's requests have been satisfied, do not encourage inappropriate chatting or permit the call to monopolize your time unnecessarily. The telephone lines should be cleared for other calls. Allow the person who placed the call to hang up first, and be sure to thank him or her for calling. Close the conversation with some form of "good-bye," and replace the telephone on its cradle gently.

PROCEDURE 9-2

Demonstrate Telephone Techniques: Take a Telephone Message

CAAHEP COMPETENCY: 3.c(1)(d)
ABHES COMPETENCY: 2.e

GOAL: *To take an accurate telephone message and follow up on the requests made by the caller.*

EQUIPMENT and SUPPLIES

- Telephone
- Message pad
- Pen or pencil
- Notepad

PROCEDURAL STEPS

1. Answer the telephone using the guidelines in Procedure 9-1.
   PURPOSE: Answering promptly and courteously conveys interest in the caller and promotes good customer service.

2. Using a message pad or notepad, take the phone message, obtaining the following information:
   - The name of the person to whom the call is directed
   - The name of the person calling
   - The caller's telephone number
   - The reason for the call
   - The action to be taken
   - The date and time of the call
   - The initials of the person taking the call
   PURPOSE: Accurate information allows the staff member to address the caller's issues quickly and efficiently.

3. Repeat the information back to the caller after the message is recorded on the message pad.
   PURPOSE: To verify that all information taken has been recorded accurately.

4. Provide the caller with an approximation of the time and date that he or she will be called back, if possible.
   PURPOSE: To be considerate of the patient's time and to keep him or her from sitting next to the phone awaiting a call.

5. End the call and wait for the caller to hang up first.

6. Deliver the phone message to the appropriate person. Separate trays or slots for each staff member are helpful.

7. Follow up on important messages.
   PURPOSE: To make certain that important issues are addressed in a timely manner.

8. Keep old message books for future reference. Carbonless copies will allow the facility to keep a permanent record of phone messages.
   PURPOSE: To have a permanent source of messages in case a number is needed after the paper message has been discarded.

9. File pertinent phone messages in the patient's chart.
   PURPOSE: To keep a permanent record of important information in the patient's chart.

Retaining Records of Telephone Messages

Each office must develop a policy regarding retention of telephone message records. Many offices elect to keep message pads for the same period that the statute of limitations exists for medical professional liability cases. Remember, phone records would include telephone bills, especially those that detail long-distance charges. Keeping message records can be of assistance in proving any number of claims, including the number of times that patients called the office and the fact that calls to the patient were returned. Be sure that accurate telephone records are kept to ensure good patient care and customer service.

TYPICAL INCOMING CALLS

One reason for having a medical assistant answer incoming calls is to spare the physician unnecessary interruptions during visits with patients. Many calls relate to the administrative aspects of the office and can actually be better handled by the medical assistant. The policy regarding how calls are to be handled should be clearly set forth in the office procedures manual.

New Patients and Return Appointments

Procedures for handling appointments for new patients and scheduling return appointments are discussed in the chapter on appointment scheduling. Always provide excellent customer service to the caller. Remember that the routine questions that may be asked should be answered in a polite and cheerful manner. Health matters are important to the individual patients whom the practice serves. Follow the designated office procedure as to what information should be gathered and recorded when appointments are made.

Directions

Each office should have a clear set of directions written out that can be read to the caller who requests directions. Prepare them from various points in the area; for instance, one set would guide a patient who is coming from the north, and another set would be for a patient coming from the south. Place these directions close to the telephone so that all employees can access them easily. Not all employees live close to the clinic or are familiar with the area, so the written set of directions will be helpful to all staff members and those who call the facility. Place a map on the office website and direct patients there for printable instructions.

Inquiries about Bills

A patient may ask to speak with the physician about a recent bill. Ask the caller to hold for a moment while the ledger is obtained. If nothing irregular is found on the ledger, return to the telephone and say, "I have your account in front of me now.

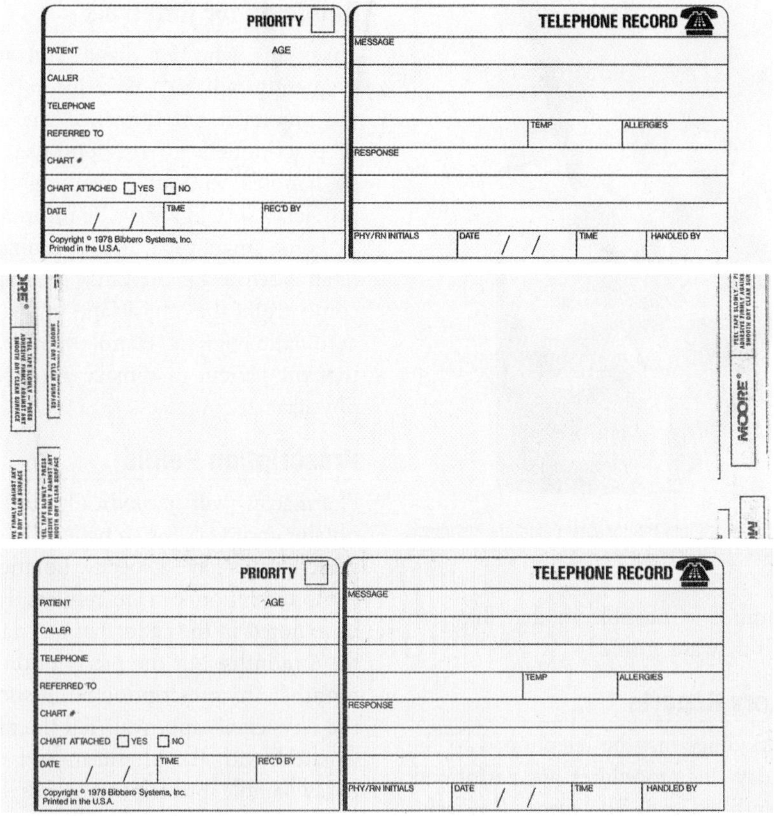

PRIORITY
PATIENT AGE
CALLER
TELEPHONE
REFERRED TO
CHART #
CHART ATTACHED ☐ YES ☐ NO
DATE / / TIME REC'D BY
Copyright © 1978 Bibbero Systems, Inc. Printed in the U.S.A.

TELEPHONE RECORD
MESSAGE
TEMP ALLERGIES
RESPONSE
PHY/RN INITIALS DATE / / TIME HANDLED BY

PRIORITY
PATIENT AGE
CALLER
TELEPHONE
REFERRED TO
CHART #
CHART ATTACHED ☐ YES ☐ NO
DATE / / TIME REC'D BY
Copyright © 1978 Bibbero Systems, Inc. Printed in the U.S.A.

TELEPHONE RECORD
MESSAGE
TEMP ALLERGIES
RESPONSE
PHY/RN INITIALS DATE / / TIME HANDLED BY

FIGURE 9-4 Phone message forms with self-adhesive backing make charting the call easier and more time efficient. (Courtesy Bibbero Systems, Inc., Petaluma, Calif.)

Perhaps I can answer your question." Most likely the caller will have some simple inquiry, such as whether the insurance has paid, or he or she may wish to delay making a payment until the next month. Not all patients realize that the medical assistant usually makes such decisions and is the best person with whom to discuss these matters.

A patient may have a question about a statement that was received in the mail. If billing matters are handled by another employee, tell the patient that the call will be transferred to the billing office. If you are responsible for billing, politely ask the patient to hold the line while you obtain the patient ledger. On returning to the line, thank the patient for waiting and explain the charges carefully. If an error has occurred, apologize and say that a corrected statement will be sent out at once. Always remember to thank the patient for calling. If patients are properly advised about charges at the time that services are rendered, the number of these calls will be considerably reduced.

Inquiries about Fees

Fees vary widely in each medical office, and it is very difficult to quote an exact fee before the patient is seen by the physician. However, a good estimate should be given to the patient as to what they should expect to pay, especially on the first visit. Asking a patient to just appear at the office without having any idea of the cost is unreasonable. Discuss with the physician or office manager what range should be quoted to the patient, then follow your quotes with the statement that the fees will vary, depending on the patient's condition and tests that the physician orders. If fees are regularly discussed on the telephone, write a suggested script in the policy manual. Do not be evasive. Have a schedule of fees available.

Participating Provider

Patients may call the office to inquire as to whether the physician is a participating **provider** with their particular insurance plan or managed care organization. The physician should keep a carefully updated list of which plans are valid. This is important, because insurance benefits vary for participating and nonparticipating providers.

Requests for Assistance with Insurance

In today's environment of managed care, copays, Medicaid, and Medicare, insurance claims will more than likely be completed and filed by the healthcare facility. Nevertheless, patients may call to inquire about their coverage or ask whether there has been any response to claims. A medical assistant or member of the staff who is responsible for insurance filing will have the knowledge to answer these inquiries (Figure 9-5). Be patient with these inquiries; insurance is a difficult subject to understand, even for those who are trained and familiar with the various forms and procedures to use. Some patients, especially elderly ones, are quite confused when dealing with insurance

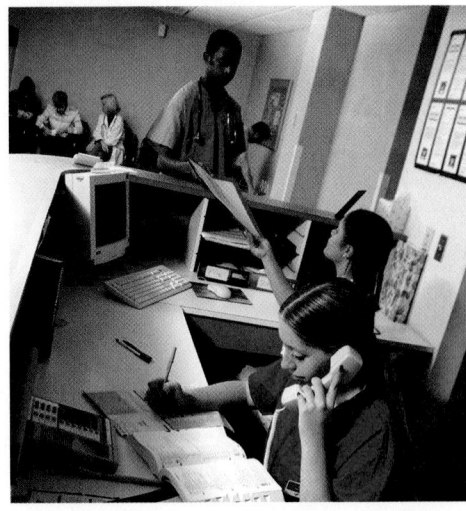

FIGURE 9-5 Many of the calls that come into the medical office are insurance questions, with which the medical assistant will assist the caller.

companies. Help them as much as possible so that they can collect the benefits to which they are entitled.

Radiology and Laboratory Reports

Laboratory and radiologic findings may be telephoned to the physician's office on the day the procedures are performed, when their results are urgently needed. The medical assistant should take these reports and relay them to the physician. Reports may also be faxed to the physician's office, especially if the test has been marked **"STAT,"** which means that the physician wants the results immediately. Original reports will usually be delivered by mail for the permanent record. Some facilities are equipped to receive laboratory results directly from the laboratory by computer.

Satisfactory Progress Reports from Patients

Physicians sometimes ask patients to phone the office to report on their condition a few days after the office visit. The medical assistant can take such calls and relay the information to the physician if the report is satisfactory. Assure the patient that you will inform the physician about the call. The physician should always be immediately informed about unsatisfactory progress reports. The doctor should provide instructions for the patient to follow in such situations.

Routine Reports from Hospitals and Other Sources

Routine calls may be received from hospitals and other sources reporting a patient's progress. Take the message carefully and make sure that the physician sees it. The message should then be placed in the patient's medical record.

Office Administration Matters

Not all calls concern patients. Calls may come from the accountant or the auditor or about banking procedures, office supplies, or office maintenance, most of which the medical assistant can handle or refer to the appropriate person. For some of these calls the medical assistant may need to gather additional information and return the call.

Requests for Referrals

Physicians who are liked and respected by their patients frequently will be called for referrals to other specialists. If the physician has furnished the medical assistant with a list of practitioners for this purpose, these inquiries can usually be handled without consulting the physician. However, the physician should always be informed of such requests.

Some managed care organizations require a physician referral before a patient may see a specialist. This referral should come from the physician, unless he or she has authorized automatic referrals. Handle these calls as quickly as possible so that the patient may make an appointment to see the referral physician.

Prescription Refills

Pharmacies will periodically call the physician's office to obtain approval for a patient to refill a prescription. Most prescriptions have a specific notation as to the number of times the prescription can be refilled. However, the physician may have noted in the chart that a certain medication is to be taken for 6 months, but the prescription was only written for 1 to 2 months. Any prescription refills should be authorized only with the physician's approval. Tell the pharmacist that you will have to check with the physician and call back. Many pharmacies today handle prescription refills by fax so that they have a written record that the refill was authorized. Be sure that state regulations and procedures are followed any time the medical assistant deals with prescription refills or calls (Procedure 9-3). Some medications cannot be called to the pharmacy and require a written prescription.

SPECIAL INCOMING CALLS

Patients Refusing to Discuss Symptoms

Occasionally patients will call and wish to talk with the physician about symptoms that they are reluctant to discuss with a medical assistant. Patients do have a right to privacy, but the physician cannot be expected to take numerous calls from patients who do not wish to speak to the medical assistant. If the patient refuses to discuss any symptoms, suggest that he or she make an appointment with the physician to discuss the problem in person.

Unsatisfactory Progress Reports

If a patient under treatment reports that he or she is still not feeling well or that the prescription the doctor provided is not helping, do not try to practice medicine by giving the patient medical advice. Make detailed notes about the patient's comments, then present them to the physician. He or she will make the decision as to whether the patient should return to the office or may make a medication change. Follow up with the patient, and convey the physician's instructions.

Requests for Test Results

When the physician orders special tests for the patient, the patient may be told to call the office in a couple of days for

PROCEDURE 9-3

Demonstrate Telephone Techniques: Call the Pharmacy with New or Refill Prescriptions

CAAHEP COMPETENCY: 3.c.(1)(d)
ABHES COMPETENCY: 2.h

GOAL: *To call in an accurate prescription to the pharmacy for a patient in the most efficient manner.*

EQUIPMENT and SUPPLIES

- Prescription
- Notepad
- Patient chart
- Telephone

PROCEDURAL STEPS

1. Receive the call from the patient requesting a prescription; use appropriate telephone technique.
   PURPOSE: To provide consistently good customer service when speaking with callers.

2. Obtain the following information from the patient:
   - Patient's name
   - Telephone number where he or she can be reached
   - Patient's symptoms and current condition
   - History of this condition
   - Treatments the patient has tried
   - Pharmacy name and telephone number
   PURPOSE: To have the information the physician will need to make a determination as to whether a prescription will be called in for the patient or whether he or she needs to come to the office to be seen by the doctor.

3. Write in the patient's chart the prescription that the physician wishes the patient to have. Be very careful to transcribe the information correctly. Read it back to the physician.
   PURPOSE: To have a permanent record of the prescription in the chart and to make certain that the prescription is exactly what the physician wants the patient to take, eliminating errors in medication name and dosage.

4. If the prescription is a refill, give the physician the patient's chart with the message requesting a refill attached, along with the information in procedure step 2.
   PURPOSE: To have the patient's chart as a reference and to provide the physician with the information needed to determine if the medication requested should be refilled.

5. Note the comments that the physician writes in the chart. If the prescription is written or a refill is approved, call the patient's pharmacy and ask to speak to a member of the pharmacy staff.

6. Ask the pharmacy staff member to repeat the prescription back to you.
   PURPOSE: To verify that the pharmacy staff member took the prescription down accurately.

7. Note in the chart the date and time that the prescription was called to the pharmacy.
   PURPOSE: To provide a permanent record of the medication being called to the pharmacy, along with the correct dose amounts and frequency of doses.

8. Call the patient to notify him or her that the prescription has been called in. Provide any information regarding the prescription doses, frequency, etc, that is requested by the physician. Tell the patient when to return to the office, if necessary. Ask the patient to write this information down.
   PURPOSE: To inform the patient as to the dosage and frequency, so that if an error is made by the pharmacy, the patient will notice a discrepancy and the error can be corrected before the patient takes any doses of the medication.

---

the results. Never assume that the patient will call for results. It is ultimately the responsibility of the physician to notify the patient of test results, especially if they are abnormal. Be certain that the physician has seen the results and has given permission before sharing the results with the patient. Patients do not always understand that the medical assistant does not have the privilege of giving out information without the permission of the physician. If the result is unfavorable, the physician should be the one to inform the patient and give further instructions. This call must be handled tactfully; otherwise, the patient may feel as if the staff is concealing information.

Most physicians prefer that medical assistants provide only normal test results to the patients. However, the medical assistant may provide abnormal test results to the patient if authorized by the physician. For example, when a patient has a questionable Pap smear, the medical assistant is usually the person who calls the patient with the results and further instructions from the physician. If the patient then has any questions about the test results, he or she must be referred to the physician. The medical assistant will need good communication skills to relay information such as this without crossing the lines of practicing medicine without a license. Human immunodeficiency virus (HIV) test results should never be given on the telephone, and the physician should always inform the patient when an HIV test returns a positive result.

Patients who call the office for results of tests must be appropriately identified before the results are given. Some offices use a special code that is written in the chart, and knowledge of this code or password gives the person access to the information. Make sure the right individual is on the line before offering test results. Especially be careful in situations in which the family includes a "Senior" and "Junior." If the medical assistant calls and asks for Robert Smith, the elder Mr. Smith may answer, whereas the younger Mr. Smith is the one who came to the office for tests. Awkward situations can be created when the office staff does not accurately identify the patient.

Requests for Information from Third Parties

The patient must give written permission before any member of the physician's staff can give information to third-party callers. This includes insurance companies, attorneys, relatives, neighbors, employers, and any other third party. Releases of information will be discussed in more detail in Chapter 14.

Complaints about Care or Fees

A medical assistant may be able to offer a satisfactory explanation to a patient who complains about the care he or she received or the fee charged. If a patient seems angry, offer to pull the chart, research the problem, and if needed, discuss it with the physician. Four magic words often calm the angry patient: "Let me help you." This reassures the patient that someone is willing to talk about the problem. However, if you are unable to appease the patient easily, the physician or office manager may prefer to talk directly to the patient.

Calls from the Physician's Family and Friends

Personal calls to the physician from family members or friends are handled in accordance with instructions from the physician. If the physician does not wish to take the calls, the medical assistant must tactfully tell the caller that the physician cannot be disturbed at that time.

Calls from Staff Members' Family and Friends

The telephone lines should never be burdened with an excess of personal calls to the staff. A call is necessary in emergencies, but staff members should never monopolize the telephone for personal business and conversations. Emergency calls could be coming through, and the lines must be clear. Keep personal calls to an absolute minimum.

HANDLING DIFFICULT CALLS

Angry Callers

No matter how efficient you are on the telephone or how well liked your employer may be, sooner or later an angry caller will be on the line. There may be a legitimate reason for the anger, or the caller's irritation may have resulted from a misunderstanding. It is a real challenge to handle such calls. First, take the required action—even if it is to say that the matter will be discussed with the physician as soon as possible and the patient will be called back later. If answers are not readily available, a friendly assurance that the situation is important and that every attempt will be made to find the answer quickly will usually calm the angry feelings.

The medical assistant may find that lowering the tone of voice and volume of speech may force the angry caller to do the same in order to hear. This method does not always work, but it is usually true that when dealing with an angry person, calm promotes calm. There are always those who will misread

this method and become even angrier, thinking that their complaint is not being taken seriously. Interpersonal skills are critical when dealing with other individuals, because the more skilled the medical assistant becomes, the better able he or she is to deal with multiple types of personalities.

Always avoid getting angry in response, and try to get to the root of the real problem. Express interest and understanding, take careful notes, and follow through with the problem to the most appropriate resolution. Never "pass the buck" by saying, "That isn't my job," or "I am not the person who filed that insurance claim." No matter whose fault the problem is, it is best to deal with it and find a solution instead of placing blame.

CRITICAL THINKING APPLICATION

An angry caller raises his voice at Ashlynn over an issue that happened before she began to work at the facility. She suggests that he speak with the office manager, but he refuses and continues to berate Ashlynn. What choices does she have in this situation, and should she simply hang up on the patient?

Aggressive Callers

Aggressive callers insist that they receive whatever action they feel is necessary, and they usually insist on action immediately. Treat these callers with a calm, poised attitude, but do not allow the caller's aggression to initiate inappropriate action. Reassure the caller that the concern being shared is valid and will receive the full attention of the right person. Explain when the caller can expect a response from the office, and be sure to follow up that the appropriate action was taken on the call.

Unauthorized Inquiry Calls

Some individuals call the physician's office requesting information to which they are not entitled. These callers must be told politely but firmly that such information cannot be provided to them because of privacy laws. Insistent callers should be referred to the office manager or physician.

Sales Calls

Sales calls are often thought of as an interruption to the physician's busy day, but some salespersons may have important information on products, equipment, or services that the office uses regularly. Do not completely disregard salespersons, but do not allow them to monopolize time or telephone lines, either. Keep these calls quick and to the point. Most professional salespersons realize that the physician's and the staff's time is extremely valuable and will respect this. Developing a good rapport with representatives ("reps") from the companies whose products are frequently used in the practice may result in discounted prices and first news of sales and promotions. In turn, these people rarely waste the time of office personnel.

Physician Shopping

Some calls will be from prospective patients seeking information about the office and the types of illnesses or conditions that the physician treats. Consider these callers to be future patients, or as those who may refer patients to the office. Always be polite and answer questions respectfully. Remember, even if the caller does not become a patient, he or she may share his or her impressions of the practice with another prospective patient.

Complaints

When callers complain, use an approach similar to the one used with angry callers. Do not make an attempt to blame, and never argue with the patient. Find the source of the problem, then present the options to the caller as to how the situation can be resolved. Remember to treat callers in the same manner that you would wish to be treated. A complaint may seem small and insignificant to the office staff, but to the patient it could be paramount. Provide good customer service to patients, and complaints will be few and far between.

EMERGENCY CALLS

Many emergency calls require judgment on the part of the person answering the phone in the medical practice. Good judgment comes from experience and proper training by the physician with regard to what constitutes a real emergency in each type of practice and how such calls should be handled. If the physician is not immediately available, what should the staff do? The person answering the telephone should first determine whether the call is truly urgent. Emergency calls could include such conditions and/or symptoms as chest pain, profuse bleeding, severe allergic reactions, cessation of breathing, injuries resulting in loss of consciousness, and broken bones. Often, the physician will instruct the patient to go straight to the closest hospital emergency room or to call an ambulance. Office policy and procedure manuals should dictate the action to take in such emergency situations.

If the physician is in, the call should be transferred immediately. All offices should have a written plan of action for the times that the physician is not physically present in the office to handle the call. The physician and medical assistant may also jointly develop typical questions to ask the caller to determine the validity and disposition of an emergency. Some examples of questions to ask would include the following:

- At what telephone number can you be reached?
- Where are you located?
- What are the chief symptoms?
- When did they start?
- Has this happened before?
- Are you alone?
- Do you have transportation?

If the call is such that an ambulance is dispatched, the policy in most offices is to stay on the line until the paramedics or police arrive on the scene.

Triage Guidelines

In the facility with multiple employees, the physician may designate one individual as the triage nurse or assistant. Within the environment of managed care, every physician would be wise to have a written telephone protocol for handling urgent

situations and emergencies. The protocol should state that the employees are bound by the written guidelines and that any giving of advice by unauthorized personnel may be grounds for dismissal.

A special sheet of instructions listing specific medical emergencies such as chest pain, heavy bleeding, fainting, seizure, and poisoning should be posted by each telephone. The phone numbers for the nearest poison control center, hospital, and ambulance should be listed. Such calls should be routed to a physician immediately. Additional instructions should include what action to take if no physician is available, such as sending the patient to an emergency department or calling an ambulance. Most offices have some means of constant contact with the physician, whether by pager, cell phone, or another method.

Getting the Information the Physician Needs

As the medical assistant gains experience and knows the physician better, he or she will begin to have a sense of the questions that the physician will have for patients that call the facility. For instance, the physician will be interested in how long the patient has had symptoms, what makes the symptoms better or worsens them, what remedies have been tried, what has worked and not worked, and other specifics about the condition the patient is experiencing. If the patient complains of painful urination, the medical assistant will learn to ask about pain in the back, blood in the urine and/or stool, and cramping. One way to learn about questions to ask is to listen to the physician carefully as he or she questions patients about their symptoms. This will help the medical assistant to learn more about signs and symptoms and will enable him or her to be a better assistant to the physician.

Remember to always be "patient with your patients." Those who call the medical office for help are almost never at their best. When feeling ill, people are often short-tempered and even display poor manners. Some can be verbally abusive. Care for patients as if they were family members, and they will feel care and compassion in the medical facility.

OUTGOING CALLS

The majority of the outgoing calls in a physician's office are responses to the incoming calls. The same rules regarding courtesy and diction apply to the calls being made from the office to patients, other individuals, or businesses.

It is helpful to plan outgoing calls in advance. For instance, if the medical assistant is placing an order for office supplies, a list should be made that includes the product, the price, the quantity needed, and a catalog page number, if applicable. Questions about the various products ordered should be noted so that they can be asked while the sales representative is on the phone.

Some medical assistants find it helpful to make all outgoing calls at once, when possible. This way the calls can be made one after another, and if a call back is necessary, it is likely that the medical assistant may still be by the phone. Organizing calls will help to increase office efficiency.

Never be rude to an individual on the phone. Remember to treat those on the other end of the phone as you would wish to be treated. Do not forget that the medical assistant is a representative of the physician and should behave in a professional manner at all times (Procedure 9-4).

TELEPHONES IN THE MILLENNIUM

Voicemail

Voicemail is widely used in today's business offices because it affords an around-the-clock method for receiving patient messages. Unfortunately, it can prove frustrating to those who find themselves speaking to an electronic device more often than with a human being. Voicemail allows the caller to hear a recorded message that may also provide information about what to do in case of an emergency. Similar to an answering machine, voicemail will record a caller's message that can later be retrieved. It often allows special temporary greetings when the user is away from the office. Keep patients happy by answering voicemail messages promptly.

Answering Machines

Answering machines do the same job as voicemail, but a machine is attached to the telephone rather than being an integral part of the office phone system. With the inexpensive cost of voicemail, most businesses have retired their answering machines and have chosen more modern methods of message-taking.

Answering Services

Because a physician's telephone is an all-important tool of the practice, there must be someone to answer it at all times—day and night, weekends and holidays. This presents no problem during weekdays, but nights and weekends require special attention. Most physicians subscribe to telephone answering services that provide round-the-clock coverage. Answering services normally provide an operator (rather than a recording device) to answer the phones, and this is often preferred over standard voicemail. Two types of operator-answered services exist. With the first type, physician-subscribers leave messages with, or obtain patients' messages from, a service whose number appears in the local telephone directory after the physician's

---

PROCEDURE 9-4

Demonstrate Telephone Techniques

CAAHEP COMPETENCY: 3.c.(1)(d)
ABHES COMPETENCY: 2.e

GOAL: *To project a professional image while handling telephone calls.*

EQUIPMENT and SUPPLIES

- Telephone
- Message Pad

PROCEDURAL STEPS

1. Answer incoming calls quickly and always by the third ring.
   PURPOSE: Individuals prefer prompt responses to their calls.
2. Greet the caller professionally, using words that identify the office.
   PURPOSE: To assure the caller that he or she has reached the right number.
3. Identify the caller and determine to whom the caller wishes to speak or what the caller needs from the office.
   PURPOSE: To be able to assist the caller and to direct the call to the right person.
4. Ask if you may put the caller on hold before transferring the call.
   PURPOSE: To show consideration for the caller's time.
5. Call the person to whom the call will be transferred, and explain that you will be transferring a call to him or her.
   PURPOSE: To make certain that the staff member is available to take the call to avoid wasting the patient's time and to prepare the staff member for the call, in case a file or other information is needed.
6. Go back to the caller, and tell him or her that you are prepared to transfer the call.
   PURPOSE: This process lets the caller know that you value his

or her time and have found the staff member who will be of assistance.
7. Transfer the call immediately.
   PURPOSE: To quickly and efficiently route the caller to the person to whom he or she wishes to speak.
8. If a second call comes in while you are speaking to the first caller, ask permission to place the first caller on hold.
   PURPOSE: Asking permission to place a caller on hold is polite and shows consideration for the caller's time.
9. Answer the second call and ask permission to place the call on hold. Listen for a response to make certain that the caller does not have an emergency.
   PURPOSE: Always listen for a response to make sure that the second caller does not need immediate attention.
10. Place the second caller on hold, and return to the first caller.
    PURPOSE: The first caller's needs should be addressed before moving to the second caller.
11. Address the first caller's needs, complete the call, and go back to the second caller.
    PURPOSE: Callers should be assisted in the order that the calls come to the office, barring any emergency.
12. Take a message if necessary, following the guidelines in Procedure 9-2.
13. Always allow the caller to hang up first.
    PURPOSE: To remain on the line in case the caller has a last comment or question.

number, with a notation to call the second number after hours. This form of service is somewhat inconvenient for the patient but is far better than no coverage at all. With the second type the answering service has a direct connection with the office telephone. When the telephone rings in the physician's office or at home, it also signals on the switchboard of the answering service. As long as the telephone is ringing, it will continue to signal at the answering service. If no one answers within a certain agreed-on number of rings (or immediately in some cases), the answering service operator takes the call. This method provides continuous live telephone coverage.

Even during the day, such an answering service can function effectively. There may be times when the staff members are assisting the physician and not available to answer the telephone. Not answering the telephone is extremely poor policy, so if the office has an agreement with the answering service, its operators will accept calls in such situations. With this direct-wire answering method, the operator answers the telephone in the same manner as the regular staff.

The answering service will greatly appreciate receiving a call every day from a member of the physician's staff before leaving the office with information as to where the physician will be during the evening or other special messages. The next morning, a staff member should call the service and ask for any messages that may have been taken. Usually there will be messages from patients who called after office hours but whose calls were not urgent enough to merit an emergency call to the physician. An answering service can act as a buffer for the physician and help eliminate too frequent, unnecessary calls during the late evening or night hours.

Automatic Call Routing

In automatic call routing, a call is answered by an automated operator's message that presents a list of options, such as "If you are calling about your account, press 1; to make an appointment, press 2; and so forth. The impersonal nature of automation does not lend itself well to answering the telephone in a private physician's office, but the medical assistant will encounter it frequently when placing outgoing calls. Some larger clinics and hospitals may use automatic call routing on a daily basis.

CRITICAL THINKING APPLICATION

Ashlynn has had many complaints from patients about the new call-routing system, because it takes so long to "get to a human being." How can she get her patients to be more accepting of modern call-routing systems? What methods might help elderly patients in dealing with automated call routing more easily?

Call Forwarding

Call forwarding allows the user to forward calls to another designated number, such as a cellular phone. Usually a code is entered, then the phone number to which the calls should be forwarded. This keeps the user from missing important calls when away from the main telephone.

Caller ID

Caller ID allows the user to see who is calling before picking up the handset to answer the phone. The caller's phone number and name appear on a screen, and the user can decide whether to take the call. If the user subscribes to call-waiting services, another benefit called *call-waiting caller ID* is often available. Call-waiting caller ID allows the user to see who is calling even when the user is already on the phone.

Cellular Phones

Considered a luxury item only 10 years ago, cellular (or cell) phones have become commonplace in today's world (Figure 9-6). Many people no longer have a home phone because of the expense of having two phones, and the cell phone is usually the better buy for the money. Several of the more popular cell phone companies offer free long-distance calls in the United States and may provide users free night and weekend minutes as a bonus. Some of today's advanced cell phones will even allow the user to access the Internet through the telephone, and the user can check email. Cell phone companies usually offer a text messaging service, which allows the user to type a message using the cell phone keys which is then sent directly to a cell phone number.

Pagers

The popularity of pagers has dwindled somewhat with the growth of cell phones. However, pagers are quite useful for reaching individuals to notify them that they are needed

---

CELL PHONE RULES OF ETIQUETTE

1. *Hang Up and Drive:* Take care when using the phone and driving. It is best to pull over and talk on the phone instead of trying to manipulate the car and carry on a conversation.
2. *Turn Off the Phone at the Right Time:* Never leave the phone on during meetings or at public events like movies and formal dinners.
3. *Respect Personal Space:* Most people do not want to hear personal or business conversations while they are in line for a movie or eating dinner. Step away when speaking on the cell phone in public.
4. *The Phone Is Not a Human:* Nothing is more rude than having dinner with a friend and taking a casual call on the cell phone. Pay attention to the human and turn the phone off until later.
5. *Keep it Charged:* It is very frustrating to speak to someone on a cell phone who cannot hear. Keeping the phone charged will cause less periods of static and more clarity when in use.

FIGURE 9-6 Etiquette rules for cellular phones.

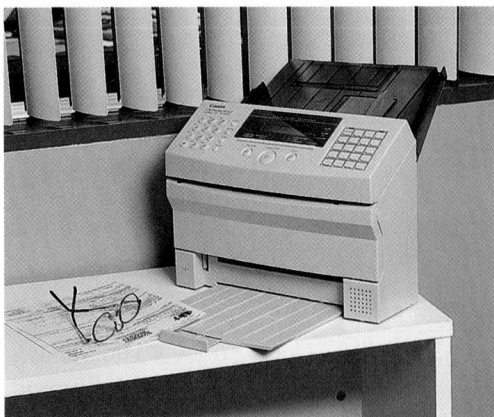

FIGURE 9-7 Fax machines allow the transfer of written data from one place to another with the simple dial of a telephone number.

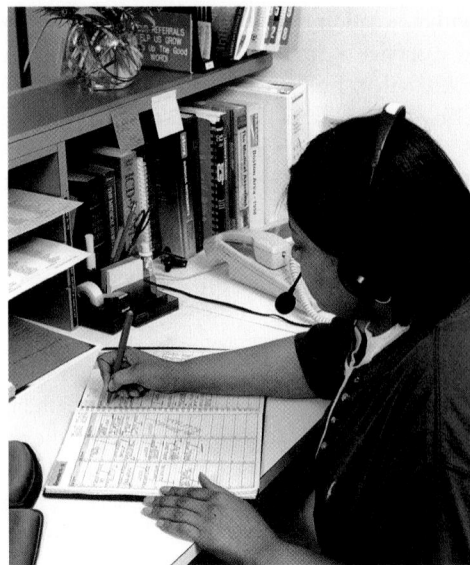

FIGURE 9-8 Using a headset helps the medical assistant keep hands free while using the telephone and is better ergonomically.

quickly. Physicians often carry pagers with them at all times. Many models allow the user to type into the pager a text message that is sent to the receiver electronically.

Fax Machines

A fax machine can be a great time and labor saver in conveying patient information from physician to physician or from physician to hospital. It allows its user to send and receive copies of printed documents over telephone lines to other facilities that have fax machines (Figure 9-7). Most offices find this machine indispensable. Unless precautions are taken to ensure security of information arriving by fax, the danger of loss of confidentiality is present. When sensitive material is sent, it is wise to telephone ahead to alert the receiver that this information will be arriving so that the appropriate person will be on hand to receive it. A fax cover sheet should be used that instructs individuals who receive faxes in error to destroy them and states that the information contained in the fax is strictly confidential.

Headsets

In today's world of **multitasking,** the headset helps a medical assistant to keep hands free while speaking on the phone. A popular headset is a very lightweight plastic earphone and microphone combination that allows the wearer to move about the room and to have the hands free (Figure 9-8). Some units weigh less than 1 ounce and are worn behind the ear or clipped to the wearer's glasses. Some headsets can be equipped with a cord that allows for easy mobility. Some also have a quick-disconnect feature that allows the user to separate the headset even during a call without breaking the connection.

USING LONG DISTANCE AND SPECIAL SERVICES

Long-distance calls are simple to place, usually inexpensive, and efficient. When information is needed in a hurry, it is much more expedient to telephone rather than wait for an exchange of letters. Before placing a long-distance call, have the correct number ready. This number often may be obtained from a letterhead or from other records. If you do not have the number,

you may obtain directory assistance by dialing the area code of the party you are calling, followed by 555-1212. In some areas you must dial 1 before the area code. Directory assistance is now an automated service in many regions, and you will be asked for the name of the city and the person you are calling. There is often a charge for using directory assistance.

One alternative to directory assistance is using the Internet to find phone numbers. A search for the business or physician the medical assistant is looking for may yield the information needed. There are also Internet services that allow the user to call long distance, and sometimes even internationally, through the computer with absolutely no long-distance charges.

Time Zones

The continental United States is divided into four standard time zones: Pacific, Mountain, Central, and Eastern (Figure 9-9). When it is noon Pacific time, it is 3 PM Eastern time. When calling from San Francisco to New York, plan to make the call no later than 2 PM if the call is to a business or professional office. When it is 2 PM on the West Coast, it is 5 PM on the East Coast.

International Service

International Direct Distance Dialing (IDDD) is available in many areas. International dialing codes are the same for all companies offering IDDD. Depending on the long-distance company, additional numbers or codes may preface the international access, country, and city codes. IDDD is still not available in all areas. If it is available, you may place international station-to-station calls by dialing the following in sequence:

1. International code 011
2. Country code
3. City code
4. Local telephone number
5. The pound sign (#) button if the telephone is touch-tone

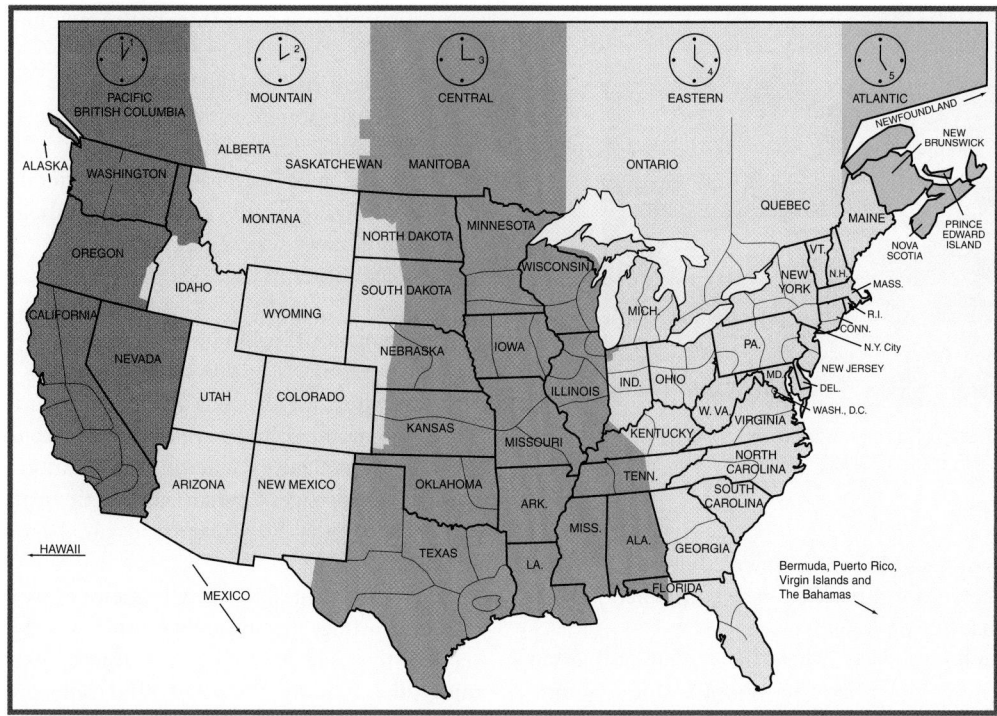

FIGURE 9-9 Time zones across the United States.

After dialing any international code, allow at least 45 seconds for the ringing to start. Consult the Internet for updates on international call procedures and country or city codes.

Wrong Numbers

One slip in direct distance dialing can mean a call to Los Angeles or New York instead of Dallas. If you reach a wrong long-distance number, be sure to obtain the name of the city and state that was called. Report this information promptly to the local operator, so the facility will not be charged for the call. If you are cut off before terminating a call, report this as well. The operator will either reconnect the call or make an adjustment of the charge.

Conference Calls

Conference telephone service is of great value to the medical profession in notifying and explaining to a family how a patient is progressing. It has exceptional value in family conferences, at which a quick decision by the entire family regarding a patient's condition is required.

This service can connect numerous points for a conference in which each person can hear or talk to all others participating. Conference calls may be local or long distance. Charges are added for the number of places connected, the distance between parties, and the length of the conversation.

Conference calls can be set up by a normal long-distance operator or through conference call services. To schedule a call, contact either an operator or the calling service and relay the pertinent information about time, date, and the individuals who are to be included in the call. Many businesses have conference call capabilities on their phone or computer systems. Notify everyone participating in the call of the time, date, number to

call, and subjects to discuss. If prior arrangements are made with all parties, there is a better chance of reaching everyone and having a successful conference.

Operator-Assisted Calls and Services

Operator-assisted calls include the following:
- Person-to-person
- Billing to a third party
- Collect calls
- Requests for time and charges
- Certain calls placed from hotels
- Credit for wrong numbers
- Conference calls
- Some international calls

There is an initial charge and a service charge for operator-assisted calls provided through most phone service providers. Fewer and fewer calls are operator-assisted in today's business world, because the cost for these calls is often high. Try other alternatives before making an operator-assisted call.

OFFICE TELEPHONE EQUIPMENT NEEDS

Number and Placement of Telephones

Familiarity with a multiple-line telephone system is a must for medical assistants. Few healthcare facilities can get along with just one telephone line. Two incoming lines along with a private outgoing line with a separate number for the physician's exclusive use is the minimum recommended number of lines.

One medical assistant can handle no more than two incoming lines, so the addition of more lines may also involve additional staffing (Figure 9-10). If a staff member is assigned solely to

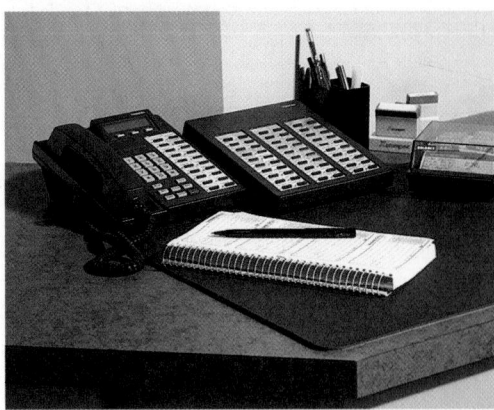

FIGURE 9-10 Multiline telephones allow numerous calls to come into the office at once. Each call deserves the same kind of attention and care from the medical assistant.

dealing with insurance and billing, a separate line and listing in the telephone directory for this service may considerably lessen the load on the main incoming lines.

Telephones should be placed where they are accessible but private. Some facilities also place a telephone in the reception room for the convenience of patients and to prevent their asking to use the facility's phones. However, recent trends suggest that a separate telephone line with a limited calling area for the convenience of patients who need to call out may be preferable. This telephone should not be in the reception room but in an area available to patients on request. It should be placed low enough for use by patients in wheelchairs. Wherever possible, other telephones should be placed on the wall to conserve desk space.

Equipment Selection

Selection of telephone equipment and services offers many options that differ from region to region. As with any major equipment purchase, research the availability and cost before making a purchase.

USING A TELEPHONE DIRECTORY

The primary purpose of the telephone directory is to provide lists of those who have telephones, their telephone numbers, and in most cases their addresses. In addition, the directory is an aid in checking the spelling of names and in locating certain types of businesses through the yellow pages. Some directories are color coded, with residence listings on white pages, business numbers on pink pages, and business by categories and advertisements on yellow pages. Often, federal, state, county, and city government listings are included as blue pages. Directories are usually organized into three sections:

- Introductory pages
- Alphabetic pages (white pages)
- Yellow pages

The introductory pages are sometimes entirely overlooked by subscribers. This section precedes the white alphabetic pages and provides basic information concerning the telephone services in the area, including the following:

- Emergency services (fire, police, ambulance, and highway patrol)
- Service calls
- Dialing instructions for local and long-distance calls
- Area codes for some cities

The introductory pages may also include the following:

- A survival guide for newcomers to the community
- Community service numbers
- Prefix locations
- Rates
- International calling information
- Time zones

Some directories include ZIP code maps for the local area. Take a few moments to become familiar with the local directory, then use it frequently for getting information fast.

The white pages are an alphabetic listing of telephone subscribers with their telephone numbers and often their addresses.

The yellow pages directory, sometimes published separately, contains listings for businesses arranged by the product or services they sell. Physicians are listed alphabetically, usually under the heading Physicians and Surgeons, and have the option of another listing by type of practice.

In some metropolitan areas, a street address and telephone directory is published that is arranged by street address, followed by the name and telephone number of the person or business at that address.

Organizing a Personal Phone Directory

Organize telephone numbers in a tabbed 3- × 5-inch desktop file or a rotary file. Binders with clear sheet protectors also work well as personal phone directories. Emergency numbers might be typed on a colored card or flagged with a color tab. A personal directory of telephone numbers should include all the numbers that are frequently called.

Identifying Community Resources

Patients will often call the physician's office looking for information on various community resources. Those who are fighting cancer may be interested in programs offered by the American Red Cross. Those who are diabetic may wish to know the options for ordering blood glucose testing supplies through online services. Some patients may benefit from Meals on Wheels. The medical assistant should be concerned with providing good customer service to patients and visitors with whom they come into contact. Therefore it is helpful to keep a list of the community resources that might be of assistance to patients. Often, information can be found in the first few sections of the telephone book. The physician may wish to keep a list of those services that are most often used by the patients of the clinic. Patients will appreciate staff members who try to offer assistance and resources outside the physician's office.

Using the Telephone to Educate Patients

Today's telephone systems allow physicians to educate patients while they are on hold; recordings may be played that offer health information on subjects from A to Z. These messages can be professionally recorded or custom designed by the physician and staff. Special events may be announced, with the option to press a certain number for more information about the event.

Some phone directories offer listings of health information in the introductory pages. A patient may call a main number, then press a second number to reach the subject of his or her choice. Such features help to address the needs of today's more information-oriented consumers of healthcare, who have an interest in healthy lifestyles and in gaining useful information immediately.

CLOSING COMMENTS

A telephone can be a tool to build a physician's practice, or one to break it apart. Medical assistants must become proficient in good telephone technique and must ensure that the caller hears compassion and patience in the voice of the medical assistant, even over the phone. A medical assistant must convey a genuine sense of caring for the patients who call the facility, just as if they were standing in the office face-to-face. By keeping this in mind, the medical assistant will play a major role in patient satisfaction, and the patients will find their medical care a pleasant process.

SUMMARY OF SCENARIO

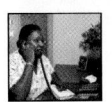

Ashlynn is quickly becoming a part of the team at Dr. Frank's office and is developing into a well-liked asset to the staff. She has learned to slow down when speaking on the phone and to adjust her volume and pitch, depending on the patient with whom she is speaking. Although she tends to be quite talkative, she is balancing just the right amount of friendly chat with the business at hand. She does this by offering a friendly greeting to callers, getting to the business at hand, then being affable before ending the call. By expressing her concern and asking how she can be of help to the patients, Ashlynn shows them that she sincerely cares about their problems. She is careful about her tone of voice, realizing that patients may take her comments the wrong way if she does not treat them in a cordial manner. Dr. Frank is very pleased with her performance.

Ashlynn takes care when she speaks to patients and others on the phone so that she does not breach confidentiality in any way. She has become comfortable with the way she is to answer the telephone. The pace of her speech and the wording are now a habit. Ashlynn is determined to maintain a professional relationship with all of the people related to her work environment. She is adept now at handling calls from angry patients and can maintain control with even the most aggressive callers. She leaves callers on hold for a minimum amount of time and reassures them frequently that she is attending to their situation. By treating callers as she would want to be treated, Ashlynn reduces frustration, and she feels that the office is more efficient in handling the large volume of calls that come into the office each day. She shows much promise for a long and rewarding career in the medical field and is satisfied with the track her career is on at the present time. As she continues to settle into her position, she looks forward to learning more about efficiency and time management. Her good attitude and desire to learn will only enhance her performance at work and make her an employee worth promoting and of great value in the facility.

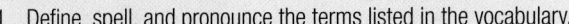

SUMMARY of LEARNING OBJECTIVES

1. Define, spell, and pronounce the terms listed in the vocabulary.
   - Spelling and pronouncing medical terms correctly adds credibility to the medical assistant. Knowing the definition of these terms promotes confidence in communication with patients and co-workers.
2. Determine and discuss the source of incoming and outgoing calls to a physician's office.
   - Incoming calls to a physician's office come from a wide variety of sources. Established or new patients may be calling to set appointments. Insurance companies may be seeking information about a claim. Hospitals, nursing facilities, or other healthcare units may need to report the progress of a patient. Laboratory results may be coming in for a patient who is very ill. Routine sales calls and telemarketing calls also come to the

office, in addition to personal calls to the physician and staff members.
3. Describe how one develops a pleasing telephone voice.
   - A pleasing telephone voice is one that is friendly and conveys a favorable impression of the physician's practice. Enunciate words and pronounce them clearly and distinctly. Vary the pitch of your voice, avoiding a monotonous or droning manner. Always be courteous and use tact. Both incoming and outgoing calls should be businesslike and handled in a professional manner.
4. Demonstrate the correct way to hold a telephone handset.
   - The telephone handset should be held around the middle of the shaft, with the mouthpiece situated approximately 1 inch from the lips, in front of the teeth. Talk directly into the handset

Continued

SUMMARY of LEARNING OBJECTIVES
Continued

so the caller can clearly hear what is being said. Do not hold the mouthpiece beneath the chin, because the voice may not be heard clearly. Do not lean the head downward to hold the phone between the ear and the shoulder, to avoid sore muscles and neck problems.

5. Explain why courtesy is so important when speaking on the telephone.
   - It is vital to be courteous to patients and other callers. First impressions are important, and a medical assistant's phone manner sets the tone for the caller's perception of the physician's practice. Customer service is important to today's physician, because many patients have choices among their healthcare providers as to which physician provides their care, and the attitude of staff members may play a large part in such a decision. Good customer care to patients means that they will not only continue to see the provider, but they will also refer other patients to the physician. This is one of the best ways to help a practice grow.

6. Discuss different ways to handle callers who wish to speak to the physician.
   - The physician's time is valuable but is also centered around his or her patients. It would be physically impossible for the physician to take all of the calls from those who wish to talk each day. Therefore the medical assistant must screen the physician's calls and make decisions about which ones should be put through to the physician. The medical assistant should offer to take a message and attempt to find out exactly what the caller's needs are and how they can be resolved. The patient should not feel that the physician is totally inaccessible but must also understand that the patient in the office must have the physician's full attention.

7. List the seven items needed to take a telephone message correctly.
   - Seven distinct items are needed when taking a phone message, including the name of the person to whom the call should be directed and the name of the person calling. The caller's telephone number must be noted as well as the reason for the call. The medical assistant should describe the action to be taken. The date and time of the call should always be noted, as well as the initials of the person taking the call, so that if any question arises, that person can be identified and asked.

8. Explain how angry callers might be handled.
   - Never return anger when a caller is angry. Remain calm and speak in tones that are perhaps slightly quieter than those of the caller. This often prompts the caller to lower his or her tone of voice. Offer to help the angry person, and ask questions to gain control of the conversation, moving it toward resolution. Do not argue with angry callers.

9. Discuss how the medical assistant should handle callers who have a complaint.

- Callers who have a complaint should be handled in a similar way as angry callers. Remain calm and offer to help. Take a serious interest in what the caller has to say. Let the caller know that his or her concerns are important to the staff and the physician. Find the source of the problem, and determine exactly what the caller wants or expects with regard to its resolution. Always follow up with complaints, and be sure that they were resolved as much to the caller's satisfaction as possible.

10. List several questions to ask when handling an emergency call.
    - Several questions should be asked when an emergency call comes to the medical office. First, obtain a phone number at which the caller can be reached in case of a sudden disconnection. Ask about the chief symptoms and when they started. Find out if the patient has had similar symptoms in the past and what happened in that situation. Determine whether the patient is alone, has transportation, or needs an ambulance dispatched to the location. In cases of severe emergencies, do not hang up the phone until the ambulance or police arrive.

11. Discuss several useful sections of the introductory pages of the phone directory.
    - The introductory pages of the telephone book contain several sections of useful information, such as area codes, emergency service information, long-distance calling information, time zones, government listings, and community service numbers. It may be helpful to tear these pages out, place them in clear sheet protectors, then add them to a binder for easy reference.

12. Demonstrate the correct way to answer the telephone in the office.
    - Medical assistants should answer the telephone promptly and professionally. The physician's image is affected by the way that telephone calls are handled. Be courteous and polite to all callers. The correct way to answer the telephone is addressed in Procedure 9-1.

13. Demonstrate the correct way to accurately record a message and take a request for action.
    - When taking a telephone message, strive for accuracy. Be sure to get all of the information that the physician will need to act. Repeat any words or numbers that are not heard clearly. The steps in taking an accurate telephone message are detailed in Procedure 9-2.

14. Demonstrate the most efficient way to call in a prescription or a prescription refill to a pharmacy.
    - The medical assistant should follow the office policy and procedure manual when calling new prescriptions or refills to a pharmacy. If a question ever arises as to what the physician meant, ask—do not guess. Mistakes with medication can cost a patient his or her life. Calling the pharmacy with new or refill prescriptions is explained in Procedure 9-3.

CONNECTIONS

 Study Guide Connection: Go to Chapter 9 Study Guide. Read the Case Study and Workplace Applications and complete the assignments. Do online research for answers to the questions in the Internet Activities associated with telephone techniques.

 CD Connection: Go to the Medical Assisting Competency Challenge CD and do the training activities under General Office Duties and Communication.

Evolve Connection: For more information related to telephone techniques, go to evolve.elsevier.com/kinn and visit related weblinks for Chapter 9. Click on the Medical Assisting Exam Review and do the practice questions to sharpen your test-taking skills.

Scheduling Appointments

10

SCENARIO

Ramona West is the medical assistant in charge of scheduling appointments for Dr. Charlotte Brown. Ramona is an extremely organized person who thinks quickly and creatively. One of her professional goals is to ensure that the office remains on schedule throughout each day and that patient wait time is kept to an absolute minimum. She is fortunate that Dr. Brown is cooperative and time oriented, so they work well together to reach this common goal.

Ramona usually arrives at work at least 15 minutes early to begin her preparations for the day. She pulls patient charts each evening for the next day so that they will be easily accessible the next morning. She pays particular attention to the patients who arrive in the office as she completes her daily tasks. Ramona greets each patient by name and carries on a brief but cordial conversation. Patients appreciate that she goes the extra mile to remember something about them, and this promotes excellent patient relations.

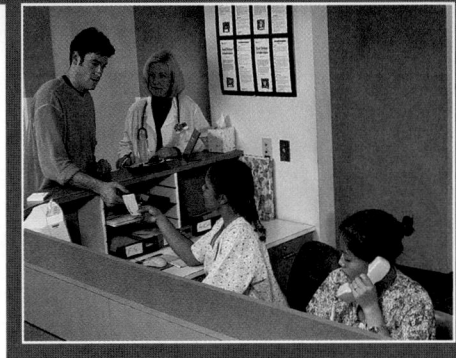

Ramona leaves a little time in the morning and afternoon for emergency appointments. She calls or emails patients to confirm appointments in advance, and this increases her show rate. Her friendly, caring attitude makes her a favorite among the patients, and Dr. Brown is pleased with the relationship-building skills that Ramona has developed.

While studying this chapter, think about the following questions:

- How can the medical assistant contribute to an efficient daily routine?
- How does the medical assistant keep the daily schedule on track?
- How can the schedule be put back on track when emergencies disrupt the day?
- How does the flexibility of the medical assistant contribute to office efficiency?

LEARNING OBJECTIVES

1. Define, spell, and pronounce the terms listed in the vocabulary.
2. Discuss three items that must be considered when scheduling appointments.
3. Explain the features that should be considered when choosing an appointment book.
4. Discuss the advantages of computerized appointment scheduling.
5. Explain how self-scheduling would reduce calls to the medical office.
6. List and explain at least three methods of appointment scheduling.
7. Explain the basic procedure to follow when the office is behind schedule.
8. Discuss offering choices to patients when scheduling appointments.
9. Explain the importance of legible writing in the appointment book.
10. Discuss several methods of dealing with patients who consistently arrive late.
11. Name several reasons for failed appointments.

National Accreditation Competencies and Content

CAAHEP COMPETENCIES

Administrative
3.a.(1)(a). Schedule and manage appointments
3.a.(1)(b). Schedule inpatient and outpatient admissions and procedures

General
3.c.(1)(b). Recognize and respond to verbal communication
3.c.(1)(d). Demonstrate telephone techniques
3.c.(2)(a). Identify and respond to issues of confidentiality
3.c.(2)(d). Document appropriately
3.c.(3)(a). Explain general office policies
3.c.(3)(b). Instruct individuals according to their needs
3.c.(4)(a). Utilize computer software to maintain office systems

ABHES COMPETENCIES

Professionalism
1.h. Be courteous and diplomatic

Communication
2.e. Use proper telephone techniques
2.h. Receive, organize, prioritize, and transmit information expediently
2.k. Principles of verbal and nonverbal communication
2.l. Recognition and response to verbal and nonverbal communication
2.m. Adaptation for individualized needs
2.n. Application of electronic technology
2.p. Professional components

Administrative Duties
3.a. Perform basic secretarial skills
3.c. Schedule and monitor appointments
3.f. Manage physician's professional schedule and travel
3.g. Schedule inpatient and outpatient admissions

Legal Concepts
5.b. Document accurately

VOCABULARY

disruption An unexpected event that throws a plan into disorder; an interruption that prevents a system or process from continuing as usual or as expected.

established patients Patients who are returning to the office who have previously been seen by the physician.

expediency (ik-spe'-de-un-se) A means of achieving a particular end, as in a situation requiring haste or caution.

integral (in'-ti-grul) Essential; being an indispensable part of a whole.

interaction A two-way communication; mutual or reciprocal action or influence.

intermittent Coming and going at intervals; not continuous.

interval Space of time between events.

matrix Something in which a thing originates, develops, takes shape, or is contained; a base on which to build.

no-show A person who fails to keep an appointment without giving advance notice.

prerequisite (pre-re'-kwe-zut) Something that is necessary to an end or to carry out a function.

proficiency (pruh-fi'-shun-se) Competency as a result of training or practice.

socioeconomic Relating to a combination of social and economic factors.

triage (tre'-awzh) Process of evaluating the urgency of medical need and prioritizing treatment.

The physician's time is the most valuable asset of a medical practice. The person responsible for scheduling this time must understand the practice, be familiar with the working habits and preferences of the physicians, and have clear guidelines for time management within the practice.

Appointment scheduling is the process that determines which patients will be seen by the physician, the dates and times of appointments, and how much time will be allotted to each patient based on his or her complaint, as well as the physician's availability. Time management involves the realization that unforeseen interruptions and delays will always occur. Most providers of medical care find that efficient scheduling of appointments is one of the most important factors in the success of the practice. Many approaches to scheduling are available, and each facility must find what suits it best.

GUIDELINES FOR APPOINTMENT SCHEDULING

One of the most common complaints that patients make is the amount of money they pay for such short visits with the physician. A patient may say, "I only saw the doctor for 5 minutes and could not even remember all the questions I wanted to ask!" The patient must feel confident that the physician will take enough time to understand his or her concerns. Well-planned scheduling and adherence to that schedule will allow the physician to do more than run in and out of examination rooms, leaving little time for the patient to talk with the physician.

Some medical offices stick to a strict schedule, with little room for maneuvering, whereas many are more flexible in scheduling to meet the needs of the patients and the providers.

The key to good scheduling is organization and teamwork in the office. Without these, even the best-planned schedule will not succeed.

The person who is scheduling appointments must learn the physician's habits and desires. If the physician suggests scheduling patients every 15 minutes but always spends 20 to 25 minutes with a patient, the schedule must be adjusted. Talk with the physician and/or office manager and compromise so that the schedule is a workable one. Some physicians need prompting to end the patient visit and move to the next patient. The medical assistant who is assisting in the examination room can help the physician remain on schedule, because he or she teams with the scheduler and both work together for the efficient flow of patients through the office.

The scheduling system must be individualized to each specific practice. The following guidelines are general and can be applied to any practice, whether paper-based or computer-based. Three items must be considered when scheduling: patient need, physician preference and habits, and available facilities.

Patient Need

A major consideration in determining office hours and appointment times is the **socioeconomic** status of the area being served. The office staff should answer the following questions:

- Is the office located in a busy metropolitan area or a rural agricultural community?
- Are the patients young, middle-aged, or retirement age?
- Is the area more industrial or residential?
- What type of patients are seen? Are they of a specific age or gender? Do they have common diagnoses? Is the physician a general practitioner?
- Are evening and weekend appointments essential for most of the patients served?

After these items are considered, the scheduler must allot time based on the patient needs for each individual office visit. These needs can be assessed by determining the following:

- What is the purpose of this visit?
- What is the age of the patient?
- Will the patient require the physician's time for the entire visit, or will another staff member perform all or part of the service?
- Is the patient a parent who prefers to schedule appointments while the children are at school?
- Does the patient object to traveling after dark?
- Is the patient a day worker who cannot take time off from a job?
- Is the patient a child whose parents are both working during the day?

The office should make every attempt to meet the patient's needs while balancing the physician's preferences and available facilities.

Physician Preferences and Habits

The preferences and habits of the physicians in the practice must be considered before a scheduling plan can be established and followed. Consider the following:

- Does the physician become restless if the reception room is not packed with waiting patients?
- Does the physician worry if even one patient is kept waiting?
- Is the physician methodic and careful about being in the facility when patient appointments are scheduled to begin?
- Is the physician habitually late?
- Does the physician move easily from one patient to another?
- Does the physician require a "break time" after a few patients?
- Would the physician rather see fewer patients and spend more time with each one, or schedule more patients each day?

All of these preferences and habits become an **integral** part of the scheduling process (Figure 10-1). Keep in mind that the physician cannot spend every moment of the day with patients. The physician also has telephone calls to make and receive, reports to examine and dictate, meetings to attend, mail to answer, and many other business responsibilities that require his or her attention. An experienced staff can handle many—but not all—of these tasks.

CRITICAL THINKING APPLICATION

■ Ramona has noticed that Dr. Brown is taking a little longer with patients than normal and that she is running consistently behind schedule by approximately 5 to 15 minutes. How can Ramona help to rectify this situation?

■ Discuss ways of approaching the physician when he or she is the cause of the delays in the schedule. What opening remarks can the medical assistant use to start the discussion in a positive way?

Available Facilities

It is pointless to get a patient into the office at a time when no facilities are available for the services needed. For example, suppose that a two-physician office has only one room that can be used for minor surgery. You would not schedule two patients requiring minor surgery for the same time block even if both

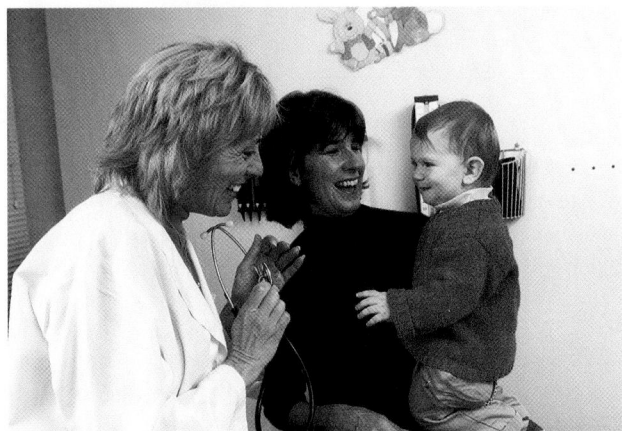

FIGURE 10-1 The habits and preferences of the physician must be considered when scheduling appointments for patients.

doctors could be available. If the office has only one electrocardiograph, you would not book two electrocardiographic procedures at the same time. As the medical assistant gains **proficiency** in scheduling, patient needs will be paired with the available facilities, according to the physician's preference. Major equipment that is frequently used or a certain room containing such equipment may need its own scheduling column in the appointment book or software system.

SELECTING THE METHOD OF APPOINTMENT SCHEDULING

The two most common methods of appointment scheduling are using an appointment book and computer-based scheduling. Each has advantages and disadvantages, and the physician's office should weigh the benefits and choose the method that best suits the physician and the staff.

Appointment Books

Office suppliers carry a variety of appointment book styles. Certain basic features should be considered when choosing an appointment book:

- The size should conform to the desk space available.
- It should be large enough to accommodate the practice.
- It should open flat for easy writing and reference.
- It should allow space for writing when, who, and why.

Some appointment books show an entire week at a glance, and many are color-coded, with a special color for each day of the week (Figure 10-2). This is very helpful when the physician asks the patient to return, for instance, in 2 weeks. If Wednesdays are colored yellow, the medical assistant can flip quickly to the correct day 2 weeks later and schedule the appointment. Multiple columns may be available to correspond with the number of doctors in a group practice, and the time can be divided according to their preferences.

Computer Scheduling

The computer has replaced the appointment book in many practices. Software for appointment scheduling ranges from relatively simple programs that merely display available and scheduled times to more sophisticated systems that perform several other functions. Many programs can display such information as the length and type of appointment required and day or time preferences. The computer can then select the best appointment time based on the information entered into the computer.

The computer can also be used to keep track of future appointments. For example, when a patient calls and inquires about an appointment, the system can search by his or her name to find the time and date. Printouts can also run to show the physician's daily schedule, including the patients' names and telephone numbers and the reason for the visit. Multiple copies of these schedules can be made, according to the needs of the practice.

One advantage of computer scheduling is that more than one person can access the system at one time, and the information is available to all operators. The medical assistant can generate a hard copy of the next day's appointments before leaving each evening. In some facilities, employees still maintain an appointment book as a backup to computer scheduling.

Self-Scheduling

The future of appointment scheduling includes self-scheduling, which is a method by which a patient can log on to the Internet and view a facility's schedule, then select his or her own appointment time and make the appointment right then. The system should allow for patient confidentiality by showing only available times. Other patients' names should never be visible on an online system.

Software is available that will allow the patient to self-schedule through secure links to the physician's appointment book. The software or Internet site for the physician's office should give the patient guidelines as to the amount of time needed for certain appointments or should allow only a certain length of time to be self-scheduled, such as 15 minutes. These systems will reduce calls to the office and are available to the patient 24 hours a day. Some of these systems will also send an automatic email reminder to the patient the day before the appointment, requesting a reply to confirm. These systems are less frustrating to patients, who do not have to wait on hold to speak to the person who does scheduling for the office. Appointments that are more lengthy or complicated should be scheduled through the office staff.

Although this type of appointment-setting system will appeal to most technologically savvy people, some patients will stringently reject online scheduling because it requires at least minimal computer skills that the patient may not be capable of or comfortable with performing. If this method is used, some allowance must be made for those who are computer illiterate. Other patients may object to online scheduling because they do

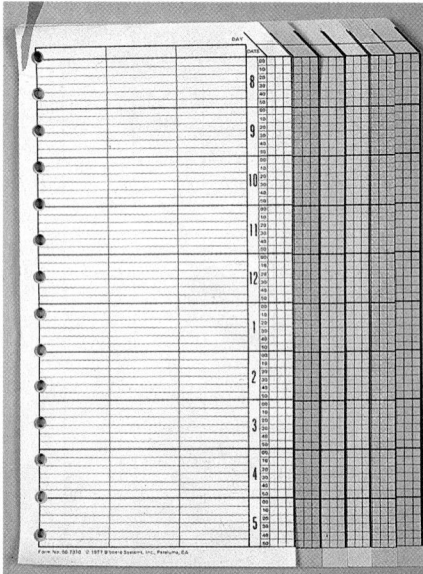

FIGURE 10-2 Color-coded appointment book pages help a medical assistant to flip to the right day of the right week quickly. Appointments for multiple physicians can be color-coded in the book.

not wish their name to be anywhere on the Internet. This is a valid issue and the office should allow these patients to schedule over the phone.

CRITICAL THINKING APPLICATION

Ramona has heard about patient self-scheduling and would like to try this method in her office, but Dr. Brown is concerned that her patients enjoy personal contact and is not sold on the idea. What can Ramona say to convince Dr. Brown to try this new, time-saving method of scheduling?

ADVANCE PREPARATION

Having chosen an appropriate method of appointment setting, some advance preparation should be done. This is sometimes called establishing the **matrix** (Procedure 10-1). Block off time slots when the physician is routinely not available to see patients, such as days off, holidays, lunch or dinner breaks, time for hospital rounds, and meetings. In the space in which a patient's name would normally be placed, note the reason the time is blocked off. Always try to account for every time period in each day. The medical assistant should also make a note of social or family engagements to help the physician remember these obligations. Because time is a valuable commodity for the physician and the office staff, the schedule is the tool that assists in making certain that the day runs smoothly.

TYPES OF APPOINTMENT SCHEDULING

Different types of appointment scheduling are used to meet the various needs of the medical facility, the providers, and the patients served. Some offices use a combination of methods to create the right mix of activity during the day and to ensure that the day runs smoothly and efficiently. The medical assistant should become proficient at managing appointments (Procedure 10-2).

Open Office Hours

When using the open office hours method, the facility is open at given hours of the day or evening, and the patients are "scheduled" by the physician by mentioning to the patient that he or she should return "in a couple of weeks" for follow-up. At **intermittent** times the patients come in, knowing in advance that they will be seen in the order of their arrival. Physicians who use this method say that it eliminates the annoyance of broken appointments and of the office running behind schedule. The open office hours method has also been referred

---

PROCEDURE 10-1

Schedule and Manage Appointments: Prepare Appointment Pages by Matrixing

<u>CAAHEP COMPETENCY:</u> 3.a.(1)(a)
<u>ABHES COMPETENCY:</u> 3.c

GOAL: *To establish the matrix of the appointment page and enter information according to office policy.*

EQUIPMENT and SUPPLIES

- Appointment book or computer
- Office procedure manual
- Information regarding physician office hours and availability
- Clerical supplies
- Calendar

PROCEDURAL STEPS

1. Determine the proper methods to use when scheduling an appointment by consulting the office procedure manual.
   <u>PURPOSE:</u> To follow prescribed office policy for appointment scheduling.
2. Become familiar with any software that is used for scheduling appointments.
   <u>PURPOSE:</u> To become proficient with the scheduling software used in the office.
3. Determine the hours that the physician(s) will not be available.
   <u>PURPOSE:</u> To make certain that patients are not scheduled when the physician is unavailable and to avoid rescheduling issues.
4. Make a column in the appointment book for each provider.
   <u>PURPOSE:</u> Some medical facilities have multiple providers who will maintain a schedule of patients—for example, many physicians employ physician assistants or nurse practitioners who also see patients.
5. Establish the matrix of the appointment book by blocking out the times that the physician(s) will be unavailable or the office will be closed.
   <u>PURPOSE:</u> To leave available only those time slots that can be used for patient appointments.
6. Allow buffer time in the morning and afternoon.
   <u>PURPOSE:</u> To allow for emergencies and short rest or catch-up times for the staff and providers.
7. Determine the number of available rooms for patient examinations, treatments, and procedures.
   <u>PURPOSE:</u> The number of available rooms affects the number of patients that can be seen during a day.
8. Establish a list of procedures that details the amount of time needed for an appointment.
   <u>PURPOSE:</u> To better gauge the amount of time that the physician will spend with patients.
9. Place the book in a convenient place for all employees who will schedule appointments.
   <u>PURPOSE:</u> To make certain that the appointment book is always readily available.

PROCEDURE 10-2

Schedule and Manage Appointments: Manage Appointments

CAAHEP COMPETENCY: 3.a.(1)(a)
ABHES COMPETENCY: 3.c

GOAL: *To manage appointments as they are cancelled, no showed, or rescheduled throughout the business day.*

EQUIPMENT and SUPPLIES

- Appointment book or computer
- Office procedure manual
- Appointment cards
- Clerical supplies
- Telephone

PROCEDURAL STEPS

1. Determine the names of patients who have appointments either the day before or the morning of the appointment.
   PURPOSE: To prepare the medical records for the patients who have appointments.
2. Confirm the appointments if required.
   PURPOSE: To make certain that the patient plans to keep the appointment and provide an opportunity to reschedule or call in a patient on the waiting list.
3. Make note of any patient arriving late in the appointment book. If this behavior has become a pattern, note it in the medical record as well.
   PURPOSE: Repeated behavior that disrupts the clinic schedule should be documented.

4. Document failure to arrive for an appointment in the appointment book or scheduling program and in the patient's medical record.
5. Call the patient to attempt to reschedule the appointment and obtain a reason for the no-show.
   PURPOSE: To document failure to comply with physician's recommendation to return.
6. Reschedule missed appointments if possible after talking with the patient.
   PURPOSE: To keep the patient on schedule for medical care.
7. Write the new appointment time, date, and day on an appointment card, or give the information to the patient over the telephone.
   PURPOSE: To ensure that the patient is aware of the new appointment time.
8. If the physician is running more than 15 minutes late, inform patients of the delay.
   PURPOSE: To offer the patients the opportunity to reschedule if necessary.
9. As patients arrive, place a check next to the name in the appointment book.
10. Offer the sign-in sheet to the patient for his or her signature.
    PURPOSE: To verify that the patient arrived in the clinic.

to as *tidal wave scheduling.* Some of these facilities allow online or telephone check-in, and patients are notified when it is close to their turn with the provider.

Few healthcare facilities in metropolitan areas have open office hours with no scheduled appointments, but this system is still found in some rural areas, where the way of life is governed not so much by the clock as by the needs of the people in the area. Many freestanding emergency clinics also offer open office hours, as do many laboratories and imaging facilities.

There can be many disadvantages to open office hours. The office may already be crowded when the physician arrives, resulting in an extremely long wait for some patients. Patients may arrive in waves throughout the day, which causes parts of the day to be very busy and parts to be slow. This makes it difficult to get other office duties accomplished. Without planning, the facilities and staff can be overburdened.

Other types of practices that have open office hours include emergency departments, many of which are open 24 hours a day. Although called *emergency departments,* many of these facilities deal with general practice cases.

Scheduled Appointments

Studies have shown that practitioners are able to see more patients with less pressure when their appointments are scheduled.

Unfortunately, the skill required for scheduling appointments is often not fully appreciated by the practitioner or office manager, resulting in the responsibility being delegated to the least-qualified medical assistant. An efficient, bright individual proficient at multitasking should be assigned to scheduling duties. Although the skill and attitude of the assistant who manages the appointment schedule is very important, the ultimate success of the system lies in the cooperation of the physicians.

Different procedures take varying amounts of time; the scheduler must understand how long it takes to draw blood, fill out new patient paperwork, weigh and check the patient in—all procedures, even the simplest ones, must have an associated amount of time that is necessary to complete the task. If the patient needs an average of 15 minutes to do new patient paperwork, then this time must be included in the schedule. (This is why many offices ask new patients to arrive 15 minutes early for their appointment.) If an allergy shot takes only 20 minutes from check-in to checkout and does not require the patient to see the physician, the scheduler knows that other patients can see the physician while the medical assistant gives the allergy shot. The scheduler cannot accurately set appointments without skill in knowing how long it takes to complete office procedures.

Remember, people other than patients will want to make appointments to see the physician or office staff members, such as pharmaceutical reps or office salespersons. They must make appointments and adjust to the physician's schedule. Patients should not be moved around to accommodate salespersons.

Flexible Office Hours

Most scheduling practices are carryovers from the days when expectant mothers of families with young children relied on one wage earner. Today families commonly have two working parents. As a result, many healthcare providers are turning to extended-day and flexible office hours. Staff hours are affected by these schedules, but this flexibility works to the advantage of the employee and the employer. For instance, if a medical assistant has decided to continue his or her education, morning class hours become available if he or she agrees to work evening hours. Scheduling evening and weekend hours may increase the size of the practice because of the convenience offered to patients.

CRITICAL THINKING APPLICATION

Dr. Brown would like to implement evening appointments 1 night each week and open the office every other Saturday morning. She feels this will better serve her patients with children who have difficulty making daytime appointments. If this is her primary goal, should other types of patients be seen during these time slots? Why or why not?

Wave Scheduling

Wave scheduling is an attempt to create short-term flexibility within each hour. Wave scheduling assumes that the actual time needed for all of the patients seen will average out over the course of the day. Instead of scheduling patients at each 20-minute **interval,** wave scheduling places three patients in the office at the same time, and they are seen in the order of their arrival. Therefore one person's late arrival will not disrupt the entire schedule.

Modified Wave Scheduling

The wave schedule can be modified in several ways. One method is to have two patients scheduled to come in at, for example, 10:00 AM, and a third at 10:30 AM. This hourly cycle is repeated throughout the day. Another application would have patients scheduled to arrive at given intervals during the first half of the hour, and none scheduled to arrive during the second half of the hour. Physicians can modify wave scheduling to best suit the clinic's needs. If a patient complains that more than one patient was scheduled for the same time, explain the method of scheduling used and its efficiency. Patients are usually more cooperative when they understand why tasks are completed a certain way in the office.

Double Booking

Booking two patients to come in at the same time, both of whom are to be seen by the physician, is poor practice. Of course, if each appointment is expected to take only 5 minutes, there is no harm in telling both to come at the same time and reserving a 15-minute period for the two. This is simply one method of wave scheduling. However, if each patient requires 15 minutes, two will require 30 minutes. This must be reflected in the scheduling. It is not considered double booking if a patient comes to the office to receive a treatment by someone other than the physician, such as a patient receiving a physical therapy modality or an allergy injection.

Grouping Procedures

Grouping or categorizing of procedures is another method of scheduling that appeals to many practitioners. For instance, an internist might reserve all morning appointments for complete physical examinations or a pediatrician for well-baby visits. A surgeon might devote one day each week to seeing only referral patients. Obstetricians often schedule pregnant patients on different days than gynecology patients. The physician and staff can experiment with different groupings until the plan that works best for the practice eventually becomes evident. In applying a grouping system of appointments, the medical assistant may find it helpful to color-code the sections of the appointment book being reserved for designated procedures.

Advance Booking

Often appointments are made months in advance. When any appointment is made, an appointment card should be completed and given to the patient. All appointment cards should mention that patients must give 24 hours' notice if they are unable to keep the time reserved for them. Most offices have some type of confirmation procedure by which patients are called the day before to verify that they will keep the appointment.

TIME PATTERNS

When booking appointments, a medical assistant should make it a policy to leave some open time during each day's schedule, so that if a patient calls with a special problem that is not an immediate emergency, there will be some time available to book the patient for at least a brief visit. It is also wise to keep one time slot available in the morning and afternoon specifically for emergencies. A busy physician will always be able to fill these open slots of time, and having them in the schedule will cause the least amount of **disruption** during the day. If possible, time should be set aside in the morning and afternoon for a break. Even 15 minutes will give the physician time to return calls from patients, verify prescription calls, or answer questions.

In the average medical practice, Mondays and Fridays are the most hectic days of the week. Patients may have been waiting the whole weekend to call for an appointment and expect to be seen immediately on Monday. Similarly, toward the end of the week, small problems that could magnify if left unattended over the weekend may prompt the patient to be anxious to see the physician on Friday. Incorporating more buffer time on these 2 days may be worthwhile.

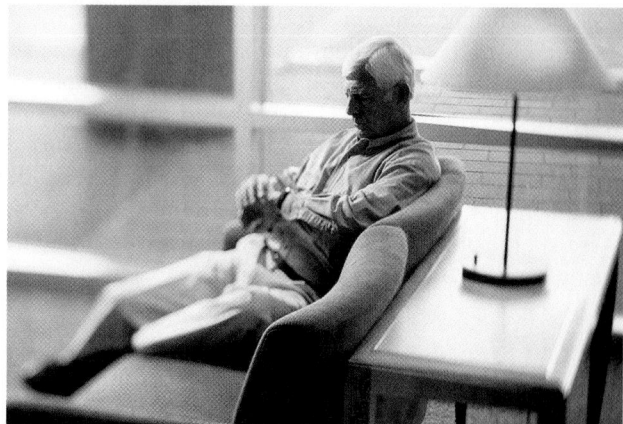

FIGURE 10-3 One of the most common patient complaints is the time spent in the reception area.

PATIENT WAIT TIME

Be conscious about the amount of time that the patient sits in the reception area. Ideally the patient's name will be called to go to the examination room precisely at the scheduled appointment time (Figure 10-3). However, the scheduling has failed if the patient then waits in the back office for 30 minutes to see the physician. Make it clear to the patient whether he or she is free to leave the office after the physician has finished the examination. Some patients mistakenly wait in the examination room until actually told that they are free to leave. Always make certain that the patient knows when to go where.

If a patient has waited more than 15 minutes in the reception area, the medical assistant should briefly explain the delay and offer to reschedule the appointment. The longer patients sit and wait, the more anxious and frustrated they become. Remember, some patients are there to see the physician for test results or may be expecting a negative diagnosis. Do not make their visit more stressful by forcing them to wait for a long time.

Of course, some delays are unavoidable. The physician may be delayed as a result of unforeseen circumstances, or there could be a patient with an emergency. Occasionally a physician becomes ill or must be unexpectedly absent from the office. Briefly explain the situation to the patient and allow him or her to decide whether to wait or reschedule. If a delay is forthcoming, attempt to call patients who may be en route to the office and inform them that there will be a delay. Again, offer to reschedule, or allow the patient to come in and wait to see the physician. Always ask for the patient's cell phone number for just such events.

CRITICAL THINKING APPLICATION

Ramona offers to reschedule patient appointments if the schedule ever falls more than 15 minutes behind. If a patient becomes belligerent about the delays, how can Ramona handle the situation in a professional manner?

TELEPHONE SCHEDULING

It is just as important for a medical assistant to be pleasant and express a desire to be helpful on the telephone as it is when meeting face to face. This is especially true when making appointments, because the telephone contact may be the patient's first impression of the facility. Often the manner in which the booking is made makes more of an impact than the convenience of the appointment time.

Be especially considerate if the time requested for an appointment must be refused. Briefly explain why the time is not available and offer a substitute date and time. Comply with the patient's desires as much as possible, and do not show any annoyance if the patient does not understand the scheduling process. Most people, however, understand the need for a well-managed office and are willing to cooperate.

Many offices offer the patient a choice when scheduling the appointment and let the patient decide which option is best for him or her. For example, the following dialog might take place during the scheduling call:

MA: Mrs. Thomas, Dr. Stern is available to see you in the office next Tuesday or Wednesday, January 6 or 7. Which day is better for you?
Patient: I will be working on Wednesday, so I would like to come on Tuesday.
MA: Do you prefer a morning or afternoon appointment?
Patient: The afternoon is best for me.
MA: Great. Would 1:30 or 3:30 be a better time?
Patient: I can be there at 1:30.
MA: Then Dr. Stern will see you at 1:30 next Tuesday, January 6. Thank you for calling, Mrs. Thomas. We'll see you then!

These small courtesies will give patients the feeling that they are in control of their time. Always repeat the time to reinforce the appointment, and do not hesitate to ask the patient if he or she has a pen with which to jot down the time and date. While repeating the information to the patient, check the appointment book or computer screen to ensure that it was posted correctly.

Write legibly when using an appointment book. These records could be called to court, and the medical assistant must be able to read his or her own writing if asked to testify. Form the habit of entering the patient's daytime telephone number after every entry. It may become necessary to cancel or rearrange the schedule in a hurry, and many precious minutes can be saved if the telephone number is handy. Cell phone numbers are also quite useful for tracking down a patient quickly.

SCHEDULING APPOINTMENTS FOR NEW PATIENTS

Arranging the first appointment for a new patient requires time and attention to detail (Procedure 10-3). This first encounter provides the first impression of the office and may set the tone for all subsequent visits. Tact, courtesy, and professionalism are extremely important. During the conversation with the new patient, request preliminary information to assist in deciding

PROCEDURE 10-3

Schedule and Manage Appointments: Schedule New Patients

CAAHEP COMPETENCY: 3.a.(1)(a)
ABHES COMPETENCY: 3.c

GOAL: *To schedule a new patient for a first office visit.*

EQUIPMENT and SUPPLIES

- Appointment book
- Scheduling guidelines
- Appointment card
- Telephone

PROCEDURAL STEPS

1. Obtain the patient's full name, birth date, address, and telephone number.
   NOTE: Verify the spelling of the name.
2. Determine whether the patient was referred by another physician.
   PURPOSE: You may need to request additional information from the referring physician, and your physician will want to send a consultation report.
3. Determine the patient's chief complaint and when the first symptoms occurred.
   PURPOSE: To assist in determining the length of time needed for the appointment and the degree of urgency.
4. Search the appointment book for the first suitable appointment time and an alternate time.
5. Offer the patient a choice of these dates and times.
   PURPOSE: Patients are better satisfied if they are given a choice.
6. Enter the mutually agreeable time in the appointment book, followed by the patient's telephone number.
   NOTE: Indicate that the patient is new by adding the letters NP.
7. If new patients are expected to pay at the time of the visit, explain this financial arrangement when the appointment is made.
   PURPOSE: The patient will be aware of the payment policy and can come prepared to pay at the time of the visit.
8. Offer travel directions for reaching the office as well as parking instructions.
   PURPOSE: To relieve any anxiety about being able to find the medical facility.
9. Repeat the day, date, and time of the appointment before saying goodbye to the patient.
   PURPOSE: To verify the patient understands the date and time of the appointment.

how much time to allot for the visit on the appointment schedule. The physician may also expect the medical assistant to give general instructions to patients seeking care for specific complaints. For example, the patient may be required to bring a urine specimen or to make certain that laboratory tests are completed before the appointment. Some offices obtain enough information to build a patient chart before the office visit; others wait until the patient actually arrives to construct the chart.

After the necessary information has been recorded, offer the first available appointment to the patient. Whenever possible, offer the patient choices between two dates and times. Ask the patient if he or she knows the directions to the office, or offer the physical address for those who wish to obtain exact directions from one of the many Internet sites, such as Mapquest. Tell the patient whether there are any special parking conveniences and whether the office will provide a token or parking validation. The options that the patient will have for the first payment should also be discussed. If payment is expected immediately, inform the patient. The office staff should expect patient concerns about the amount of the first bill and should address this issue in advance of the appointment so that there are no surprises or misunderstandings. Before ending the conversation, repeat the appointment date and time, then thank the patient for calling.

Some medical offices mail an information packet about their facility to new patients, especially if the appointment is several days away. With today's technology and the patient's email address, such information can also be sent via the Internet. This information should tell the patient about the nature of the practice, should introduce the medical staff, and should explain appointment policies and financial arrangements.

If another physician has referred the patient, the medical assistant may need to call the referring physician's office to obtain additional information before the patient's appointment. This information should be printed out and given to the attending physician in advance of the patient's arrival. Remember to send a thank-you note to anyone who refers a patient to the facility.

Many offices call each patient the day before the appointment as a reminder and a courtesy. This can be a time-consuming procedure, but most patients appreciate this service, and it may open appointments for others if the original patient cannot keep the scheduled time slot. Email and automatic dialers can also be programmed to call or send electronic reminders to patients about their appointments. This procedure can run automatically if the office has access to the proper equipment, which takes no time away from the medical assistant's other duties.

SCHEDULING APPOINTMENTS FOR ESTABLISHED PATIENTS

In Person

Most return appointments for **established patients** are arranged when the patient is leaving the office. It is a good policy for all patients to stop by the front desk before leaving, in case any information is needed from the patient or any outside scheduling must be done. The patient's chart can be reviewed to see whether the physician ordered any laboratory tests or procedures, and these can be scheduled and discussed with the patient. When making a return appointment, follow the same procedures as scheduling any appointment by phone, offering the patient choices in the day and time slots (Procedure 10-4). If a certain time is not available that the patient specifically requests, offer two alternatives. Always give the patient an appointment card and any necessary instructions at this time, along with a bright smile (Procedure 10-5). Never forget to provide excellent customer service to the patient.

By Telephone

Usually it is necessary only to determine when the patient is required to return and to find a suitable time on the schedule. Established patients do not usually need directions and parking information, unless the office has recently moved. If there has been a lengthy interval since the patient's last visit, the medical assistant should recheck certain information and enter any changes on the patient's chart. Be sure to ask whether insurance companies or benefits have changed, and it is always a good idea to verify the address and phone numbers of the patient. If an email address is not on file, obtain one for quick and easy notification of appointments and other events.

PROCEDURE 10-4

Schedule and Manage Appointments: Schedule Appointments with Established Patients or Visitors

CAAHEP COMPETENCY: 3.a.(1)(a)
ABHES COMPETENCY: 3.c

GOAL: To schedule a general appointment either by telephone or in person.

EQUIPMENT and SUPPLIES

- Appointment book or computer
- Office procedure manual
- Clerical supplies
- Appointment cards
- Telephone

PROCEDURAL STEPS

1. Know the proper methods to use when scheduling an appointment by consulting the office procedure manual.
   PURPOSE: To follow prescribed office policy for appointment scheduling.

2. Ask the name of the person wishing to make the appointment and obtain his or her phone number.
   PURPOSE: To be able to speak professionally with the individual and to identify the person in the patient database, if applicable. Ask for the phone number in case the line is disconnected or the appointment needs to be changed.
   Say: "To whom am I speaking, please?"

3. Ask the reason for making the appointment.
   PURPOSE: To determine the length of time needed for the appointment.
   Say: "What is the reason for making this appointment?"

4. Determine who the appointment is for, if necessary.
   PURPOSE: To schedule the individual with the right provider or person.
   Say: "Mr. Adams, would you like to see Dr. Blake, or would you like to see our office manager, Mrs. Jackson?"

5. Give the person a choice between 2 days of the week.
   PURPOSE: To allow the individual to choose a convenient time; this decreases missed appointments. If the suggested days are not satisfactory, allow the person to suggest an alternate day.
   Say: "Would you prefer to come on Monday or Tuesday, Mr. Adams?"

6. Give the person a choice between a morning or an afternoon appointment.
   PURPOSE: To allow the individual to choose a convenient time of day.
   Say: "Would morning or afternoon be better for you?"

7. Give the person a choice between two specific times.
   PURPOSE: To allow the individual to choose the best time for his or her needs.
   Say: "Mr. Adams, would you prefer 9 am or 11 am?"

8. Write the name of the individual and the phone number on the appropriate line of the appointment book, or enter this information into the scheduling system.
   PURPOSE: To document the appointment and assure that the time is reserved.

9. Repeat the appointment day, date, and time back to the person being scheduled.
   PURPOSE: Repeating the appointment time reduces errors and misunderstandings.
   Say: "I have you scheduled for 9 am on Tuesday, March 14, Mr. Adams. If you are not able to keep your appointment, please let us know."

10. If the person scheduling the appointment is in the office instead of on the phone, give an appointment card to him or her.
    PURPOSE: Providing appointment cards reduces missed appointments.

PROCEDURE 10-5

Schedule and Manage Appointments: Prepare an Appointment Card

CAAHEP COMPETENCY: 3.a.(1)(a)
ABHES COMPETENCY: 3.c

GOAL: *To provide a written notation of the appointment for the convenience of the patient (or other individual making the appointment) and to reduce missed appointments.*

EQUIPMENT and SUPPLIES

- Appointment book or computer
- Office procedure manual
- Appointment cards
- Clerical supplies
- Telephone

PROCEDURAL STEPS

1. Make an appointment following the steps listed in Procedure 10-2.
   PURPOSE: The information about the appointment is necessary to complete the appointment card.

2. Copy the appointment information onto the appointment card directly from the appointment book or the computer, including the day, date, and time.
   PURPOSE: To provide a written record of the scheduled appointment.

3. Mention that a 24-hour notice is appreciated when canceling an appointment.
   PURPOSE: To allow others to fill the empty slot that a missed appointment creates.

4. Give the individual the appointment card.

SCHEDULING OTHER TYPES OF APPOINTMENTS

There are other appointments that a medical assistant will make and that will appear on the appointment schedule, such as surgeries the physician will be performing at a hospital or other facility, hospital rounds and consultations, appointments and meetings, and even house calls if the physician performs them. The physician must also have time to get from one location to another, so driving time must be considered when arranging all appointments.

Inpatient Surgeries

When scheduling a surgery, call the facility where the procedure will be performed as soon as the operation is planned. Most surgical departments and centers have a surgical secretary who makes these arrangements. Provide all necessary information as well as any special requests that the physician may have, such as the amount of blood to have available for the patient. The secretary may want all of the patient's insurance information and will certainly want a phone number so that the patient can be contacted before the surgery if necessary. Be sure that all of this information is handy before placing the call.

Some hospitals request that the patient complete a pre-admission form so that all records can be processed before the patient is admitted. In such cases it may be the medical assistant's responsibility to see that this is done. These are general guidelines only, because procedures vary in different areas and hospitals.

Outpatient and Inpatient Procedure Appointments

A medical assistant is often requested to arrange laboratory or radiography appointments for patients. Before calling the facility to schedule the appointment, be sure all necessary information is handy. When the patient is informed of the time and place for the appointment, relay any special instructions that may be necessary, then note these arrangements in the patient's chart. Some offices will make a reminder call to the patient, or a reminder email message can be sent.

Outpatient testing is common, because most physicians do not have extensive x-ray or laboratory equipment in their offices. Magnetic resonance imaging (MRI), computed tomography (CT) scans, numerous x-ray evaluations, ultrasonography, and simple blood tests all may need to be scheduled (Procedure 10-6). Provide the patient with the name, address, and phone number of the facility where the tests will be performed.

Some patients may require a series of appointments, such as at weekly intervals. Try to set up these appointments on the same day of each week at the same time of day. This considerably reduces the risk that the patient will forget an appointment.

In some cases the medical assistant may be responsible for scheduling inpatient admissions or inpatient surgical procedures (Procedures 10-7 and 10-8). This is similar to scheduling outpatient testing, but the medical assistant must coordinate with the hospital instead of with an outside facility.

Outside Visits

If the physician regularly makes house calls or visits patients in skilled nursing facilities, a special block of time will need to be reserved in the appointment schedule. The physician will need demographic information, such as addresses, room numbers, and the best route to each home or facility. Remember to allow for travel time. Although most physicians never make house calls because of the ease of seeing patients in the office, they may be necessary in certain situations. The physician's medical bag should always be prepared and well stocked before he or she has to make any outside visits.

PROCEDURE 10-6

Schedule Outpatient Admissions and Procedures

CAAHEP COMPETENCY: 3.a.(1)(b)
ABHES COMETENCY: 3.c

GOAL: *To schedule a patient for outpatient admission or procedure within the time frame needed by the physician, confirm with the patient, and issue all required instructions.*

EQUIPMENT and SUPPLIES

- Diagnostic test order from physician
- Name, address, and telephone number of diagnostic facility
- Patient demographic information
- Patient chart
- Test preparation instructions
- Telephone
- Consent form

PROCEDURAL STEPS

1. Obtain an oral or written order from the physician for the exact procedure to be performed.
   PURPOSE: To have a documented order for the procedure to be performed

2. Precertify the procedure with the patient's insurance company, if necessary.
   PURPOSE: To make certain that expected insurance benefits are valid and the procedure will be covered by the patient's insurance policy.

3. Determine the physician and patient availability.
   PURPOSE: To be certain that the patient will be able to comply with the arrangements for the test and that the physician is available, if he or she must be present for the procedure. The urgency of the needed test results affects the time and date of the appointment needed.

4. Telephone the diagnostic facility and schedule the procedure or test.
   - Order the specific test needed.
   - Provide the patient's diagnosis.
   - Establish the date and time.
   - Give the name, age, address, and telephone number of the patient.
   - Provide the demographic information for the patient, including insurance policy numbers and addresses for filing claims.
   - Determine any special instructions for the patient or special anesthesia requirements.
   - Notify the facility of any urgency for test results..
   PURPOSE: To schedule the procedure or admission and provide needed information.

5. Notify the patient of the arrangements, including:
   - Giving the name, address, and telephone number of the diagnostic facility
   - Conveying the date and time to report for the test
   - Giving instructions concerning preparation for the test (e.g., eating restrictions, fluids, medications, enemas).
   - Telling what preadmission testing will be necessary, if any
   - Asking the patient to repeat the instructions.
   PURPOSE: To be certain that the patient understands the preparation necessary and the importance of keeping the appointment. If time permits, issue written instructions to the patient.

6. Have the physician review the consent form with the patient. The patient should sign the consent form, and a copy should be placed in the chart. Note arrangements on the patient's chart.
   PURPOSE: To make certain that the patient understands the risks, benefits, and alternatives to the procedure. To ensure follow-up on diagnosis and/or treatment.

7. Place reminder on the physician's tickler or desk calendar, if needed. Be sure the information is listed on the office schedule. Check the postsurgical status of the patient. Follow up if results are not received in a timely manner.
   PURPOSE: To check whether the appointment was kept and a report was received from the testing facility.

SPECIAL CIRCUMSTANCES

Late Patients

Probably every medical practice has a few patients who are habitually late for appointments. This seems to be a problem for which no cure has been found. Emergencies and small delays can happen to anyone, but a patient who constantly arrives late can place a strain on the practice. Such patients can be booked as the last appointment of the day. Then, if closing time arrives before the patient does, the staff has no obligation to wait. Some medical assistants tell the patient to come in 30 minutes before the appointment time that is actually scheduled. Make an attempt to work with patients who have occasional difficulties arriving on time, but do not allow the schedule to be constantly disrupted by late patients.

CRITICAL THINKING APPLICATION

Seth Jones is always late for his appointments. How might Ramona approach him about this? What can Ramona do to assist Mr. Jones in arriving for appointments on time?

PROCEDURE 10-7

Schedule Inpatient Admissions

CAAHEP COMPETENCY: 3.a.(1)(b)
ABHES COMPETENCY: 3.c

GOAL: *To schedule a patient for inpatient admission within the time frame needed by the physician, confirm with the patient, and issue all required instructions.*

EQUIPMENT and SUPPLIES

- Admission orders from physician
- Name, address, and telephone number of inpatient facility
- Patient demographic information
- Patient chart
- Any preparation instructions for the patient
- Telephone
- Admission packet for the patient

PROCEDURAL STEPS

1. Obtain an oral or written order from the physician for the admission.
   PURPOSE: To have a documented order for the admission.
2. Precertify the admission with the patient's insurance company, if necessary.
   PURPOSE: To make certain that expected insurance benefits are valid and the admission will be covered by the patient's insurance policy.
3. Determine the physician and patient availability if the admission is not an emergency.
   PURPOSE: To be certain that the patient will be able to comply with the arrangements for the admission and that the physician is available to care for the patient during the admission. The urgency of the admission affects the time and date of the appointment needed.
4. Telephone the diagnostic facility and schedule the admission.
   - Order any specific tests needed.
   - Provide the patient's admitting diagnosis.
   - Establish the date and time.
   - Convey the patient's room preferences.
   - Give the name, age, address, and telephone number of the patient.
   - Provide the demographic information for the patient, including insurance policy numbers and addresses for filing claims.
   - Determine any special instructions for the patient.
   - Notify the facility of any urgency for test results.
   PURPOSE: To schedule the admission and provide needed information.
5. Notify the patient of the arrangements, including:
   - Giving name, address, and telephone number of the facility
   - Conveying date and time to report for admission
   - Giving instructions concerning preparation for any procedures, if necessary (e.g., eating restrictions, fluids, medications, enemas)
   - Outlining preadmission testing that will be necessary, if any
   - Asking the patient to repeat the instructions
   PURPOSE: To be certain that the patient understands the preparation necessary and the importance of admittance. If it is your office policy to do so, give an admission packet to the patient that contains the orders and basic instructions for the admission.
6. Note arrangements and the admission on the patient's chart.
   PURPOSE: To ensure follow-up on diagnosis and/or treatment.
7. Place reminder on the physician's tickler or desk calendar, if needed. Be sure the information is listed on the office schedule. If the physician keeps a list of all inpatients, add the patient's name to that list.
   PURPOSE: To keep a record of the number of days the patient was seen in the hospital by the physician during rounds for insurance billing purposes.

Rescheduling Canceled Appointments

Changes sometimes must be made in the appointment schedule. Unexpected conflicts might arise that force a patient to change the appointment time. When rescheduling an appointment, be sure that the first appointment day and time is removed from the appointment book or database, then set the new appointment. Otherwise, the patient will be expected in the office on 2 days, and time will be wasted with calls and follow-up, only to find out that the appointment was rescheduled.

Emergency Calls

Periodically, emergency or urgent calls will come to the office and an appointment will need to be scheduled. To some extent, all calls that come to the office go through a **triage** process, and emergencies are prioritized to evaluate the urgency of the need to see the physician. Triage is an extremely important function that requires experience and knowledge of signs and symptoms, as well as tact.

Emergencies may include emotional crises as well as the more obvious physical problems. Patients with emergencies should be seen the same day. The urgency of the call can be initially determined by having a list of questions prepared for reference with the help of the physician. The physician should determine what is considered urgent. The patient may need to be referred directly to the emergency department of a hospital, or the physician may want to see the patient that day in the office. In many cases, the caller will consider the situation more urgent than his or her responses to the medical questions may indicate. Skillful handling of such situations requires

PROCEDURE 10-8

Schedule Inpatient Procedures

CAAHEP COMPETENCY: 3.a.(1)(b)
ABHES COMPETENCY: 3.c

GOAL: *To schedule a patient for inpatient surgery within the time frame needed by the physician, confirm with the patient, and issue all required instructions.*

EQUIPMENT and SUPPLIES

- Orders from physician
- Name, address, and telephone number of inpatient facility
- Patient demographic information
- Patient chart
- Any preparation instructions for the patient
- Telephone
- Consent form

PROCEDURAL STEPS

1. Obtain an oral or written order from the physician for the admission.
   PURPOSE: To have a documented order for the admission.
2. Precertify the admission with the patient's insurance company, if necessary.
   PURPOSE: To make certain that expected insurance benefits are valid and the admission will be covered by the patient's insurance policy.
3. Determine the physician availability if the surgery is not an emergency. Another physician may be the surgeon. If this is the case, the surgery will need to be coordinated with his or her office as well.
   PURPOSE: To be certain that the physician is available to care for the patient during the admission and the surgery. The urgency of the surgery affects the time and date of the appointment needed.
4. Telephone the hospital surgical department and schedule the procedure.
   - Order any specific tests needed.
   - Provide the patient's admitting diagnosis.
   - Establish the date and time.
   - Give the name, age, address, and telephone number of the patient.
   - Provide the demographic information for the patient, including insurance policy numbers and addresses for filing claims.
   - Determine any special instructions for the patient.
   - Notify the facility of any urgency for the surgery.
   PURPOSE: To schedule the surgery and provide needed information to the facility.
5. Notify the patient of the arrangements, if the patient is not already admitted to the hospital. Include:
   - Name, address, and telephone number of the facility.
   - Date and time to report for admission.
   - Instructions concerning preparation for any procedures, if necessary (e.g., eating restrictions, fluids, medications, enemas).
   - Tell what preadmission testing will be necessary, if any.
   - Ask the patient to repeat the instructions.
   PURPOSE: To be certain that the patient understands the preparation necessary and the importance of surgery. If it is your office policy to do so, give an admission packet to the patient that contains the orders and basic instructions for the surgery.
6. The physician should review the consent form with the patient. Have the patient sign a consent for the surgical procedure. Keep the original consent in the patient's chart and give a copy to the patient.
   PURPOSE: To ensure that the patient understands the risks, benefits, and alternatives to the surgical procedure.
7. Note arrangements on the patient's chart.
   PURPOSE: To ensure follow-up on diagnosis and/or treatment.
8. Place reminder on the physician's tickler or desk calendar, if needed. Be sure the information is listed on the office schedule. If the physician keeps a list of all inpatients, add the patient's name to that list. Follow up with the hospital after the procedure regarding the patient's condition as required by the physician.
   PURPOSE: To check on the patient's status and keep a record of the number of days the patient was seen in the hospital by the physician during rounds for insurance billing purposes.

---

considerable tact. Maintaining a caring and reassuring response will frequently alleviate the fear evidenced by the caller.

Acutely Ill Patients

There is sometimes a fine line between an emergency patient and an acutely ill patient, but the latter should be seen as soon as possible. At the very least, let the physician decide whether an appointment should be made for another day. For example, a patient may report having had flu symptoms for several days and now having an elevated temperature. The physician will probably want more information before deciding whether the patient should be seen immediately or whether some other course of action is appropriate. The 15- to 20-minute breather time saved in the middle of the morning may rescue the schedule and provide the needed time for the patient. Escort these patients to the examination room on their arrival if possible. Patients with symptoms of infection should be placed so as to prevent cross-contamination.

Physician Referrals

If another physician telephones and requests that a patient be seen today, most offices will honor that request if at all possible. It is important to keep a schedule that will not be intolerant of this type of request.

Patients Without Appointments

There must be a policy agreed to by the physician and carried out by medical assistants for patients without appointments. A patient who requires immediate attention will most likely be accommodated into the schedule somehow. If the patient does not need immediate care, a brief visit with the physician and a scheduled appointment at a later time may be the answer. The medical assistant may simply have to turn down the request. Follow established office policy.

The medical assistant should always make it clear, even when accommodating patients without appointments, that the office runs on an appointment basis. Try to convey the message that appointments save not only the physician's time but also the patient's time. Emphasize that the physician is able to give the patient full attention and more time if an advance appointment is made.

FAILED APPOINTMENTS

Why do patients fail to keep appointments? Some are simply forgetful. Once this tendency is detected in a patient, form the habit of telephoning or emailing a reminder the day before the appointment, or send a postcard timed to arrive 1 or 2 days in advance.

A patient who has been pressed for a payment may stay away because of his or her inability to pay for medical services. Do not make the mistake of classifying all such patients as "deadbeats." Many have every desire to pay, but they cannot afford to and feel embarrassed about their situation, so they avoid their appointments.

If the office consistently runs behind schedule, some patients may not be willing to waste any time waiting to see the physician. Time is a valuable commodity for patients as well, and every effort must be made to get patients in at their appointment time and out quickly.

One other reason for failed appointments that is often overlooked is a patient's state of denial regarding his or her condition. For instance, if a patient has been recently diagnosed as human immunodeficiency virus (HIV) positive, he or she may avoid doctor appointments, because going to see the physician forces the patient to face the reality of the disease. Take special care with such patients, and if denial is suspected, discuss this with the physician, who may wish to refer the patient for counseling.

It is important to determine the reason for failed appointments and do whatever is possible to remedy the situation. Telephone the patient to be sure no misunderstanding has occurred. If the patient's health is such that medical care must continue, write a letter and explain this to the patient. Send the letter by certified mail, with return receipt requested. Keep the letter in the patient's chart for legal protection.

No-Show Policy

Some patients may not realize the importance of keeping their appointments. The patient who does not arrive for a scheduled appointment or reschedule it is called a **no-show.** A busy practice must have a very specific policy on appointment no-shows and must enforce it effectively. The first time a patient fails to show, note the fact on the medical chart and/or ledger card. The second time, warn the patient, and if a third no-show occurs, consider dropping the patient by using the customary methods that provide legal protection for the physician.

The physician may wish to charge patients for not showing up or for rescheduling the appointment. Be understanding whenever possible, but do not let a patient take advantage of the physician's time. The office policy manual must state that patients may be charged for missed appointments, especially if the time slot could not be filled with another patient. Many physicians do not press this issue, but it is an available tool if needed.

Recording the Failed Appointment

When a patient fails to keep an appointment, a notation should be made in the patient's chart as well as in the appointment book or database. If the patient is seriously ill, the physician should also be told about the failure to show. In some cases it may be necessary to call or write the patient to remind that a missed appointment may have serious effects on the patient's health.

INCREASING APPOINTMENT SHOW RATES

Everyone benefits from a full schedule of appointments that are kept. Appointment show rates may be increased in several ways.

Appointment Cards

Most healthcare facilities use appointment cards to remind patients of scheduled appointments, as well as to eliminate misunderstandings about dates and times (Figure 10-4). Make a habit of reaching for an appointment card while writing an entry in the appointment book. After the date and time have been written on the card, double-check with the book to see that the entries agree.

Confirmation Calls

Patients who have made appointments in advance may appreciate a confirmation call to remind them that they have a time set aside to see the physician. Always note the phone number that the patient prefers the office to use for such calls. Many individuals now have home phone, cell phone, and work phone numbers; however, they may wish calls from the physician to go only to their home phone. The preferred phone number can be highlighted in the chart or on the computer. The office must use caution in making calls to patients because of the significance of privacy guidelines and standards. Some offices may wish to prepare a release form in which the patient grants the office staff permission to contact the patient. Many physicians insist

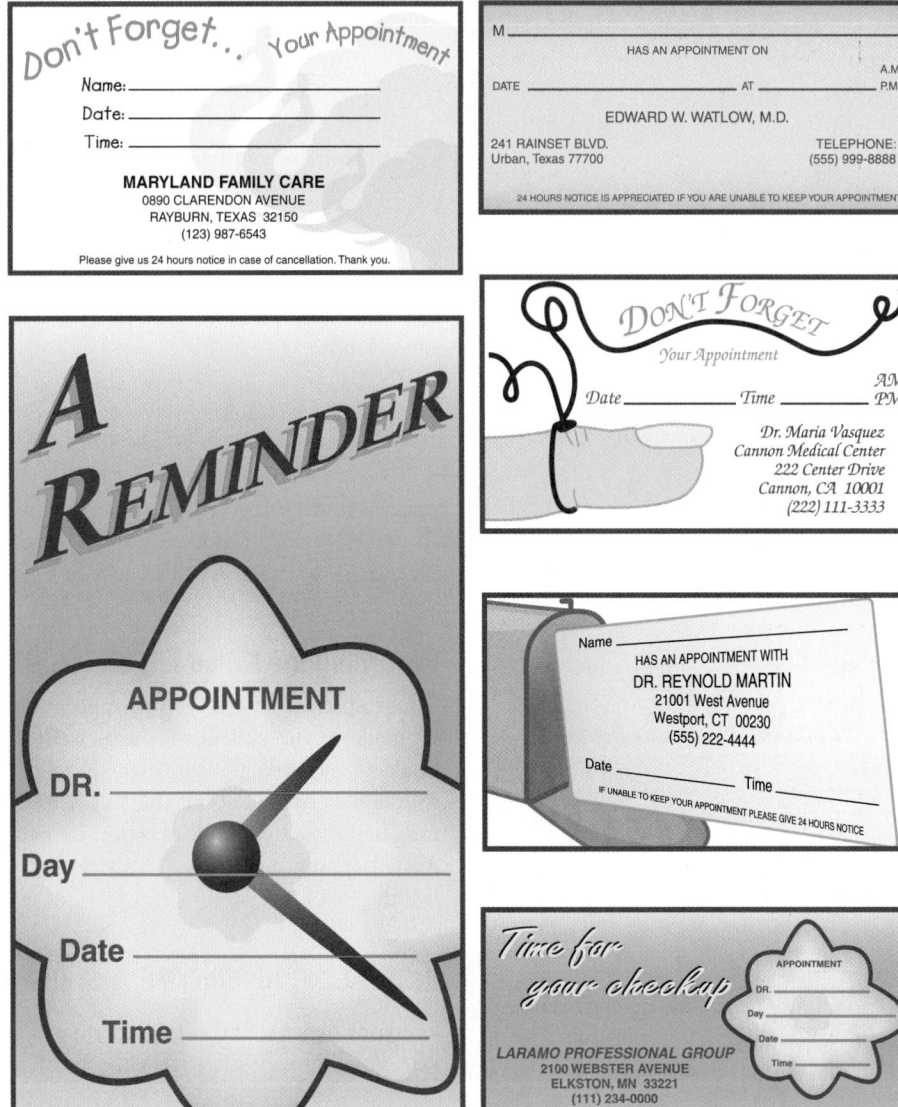

FIGURE 10-4 Examples of appointment cards.

that messages left on voicemail not mention the term "doctor" or "doctor's office" for confidentiality reasons. The medical assistant might say, "This is Pam at Robert Welch's office confirming your appointment tomorrow at 2:00 PM. Please call us if you cannot make the appointment. Our number is 555-212-0909. Thank you!"

If the patient has signed the privacy policy, and the policy states that messages may be left at certain numbers from the physician's office, then the office can certainly leave messages at that number and mention that the call is from the physician's office. Still, it is a good idea to have an established policy regarding leaving messages that does not breach any patient's confidentiality.

Email Reminders

Many computer scheduling programs have the capacity to send an email to patients to remind them of appointments the day before. This is a great timesaver for the office staff, because no time is taken to perform this duty, other than the original scheduling of the appointment.

Mailed Reminders

Mailed reminder cards may be sent to patients by the office staff. This method is a bit time consuming, but worth the effort if the patients show up for their appointments.

A patient who is due for an appointment but has not yet arranged a date and time may be sent a reminder. A simple way of handing this is to have a supply of postcards on hand, and while patients are still in the office, have them write their name and address on the postcard. Then place the card in a tickler file box under the date it is to be mailed.

Innovative Ideas

Knowing that time is valuable to patients as well as to the physician, many of today's offices try to make the time spent at the office as productive as possible for the patient. Some reception areas are equipped with computers, televisions, and even video games and movies for children. Often a small desk with a phone will allow the patient to do a limited amount of work, if needed, while waiting to see the physician. Keeping the patient's needs in mind makes the patient less likely to break an appointment.

HANDLING CANCELLATIONS AND DELAYS

When the Patient Cancels

Inevitably, some cancellations will occur. If a list is kept of patients with advance appointments who would like to come in sooner, the medical assistant can begin calling to try to get one of them in to fill the available opening. By keeping a list of patients willing to take the first cancelled appointment, the medical assistant can readily identify which patients to call to fill the vacancy. Each patient cancellation should be noted in the medical record, along with a note regarding why the appointment was cancelled, if that information is available. If the patient simply reschedules an appointment, it is not necessary to make a notation in the medical record, unless a pattern develops that might be significant to his or her medical treatment.

When the Physician Is Delayed

There will be days when the physician is delayed in reaching the office. If there is advance notice of the delay, start calling patients with early appointments and suggest that they come later. If some patients have already arrived before the office learns of the delay, explain that an emergency has detained the physician.

Show concern for the patient but avoid being overly apologetic, which might imply some degree of guilt. Most patients realize that a physician has certain priorities. The patient who is in the office may be inconvenienced, but it is not a life-or-death matter. If this kind of situation occurs frequently, however, consider devising a different scheduling system.

When the Physician Is Called for Emergencies

Physicians are conscious of their responsibilities for responding to medical emergencies, and most patients will be sympathetic to such occurrences if the medical assistant takes the time to explain what has happened. The medical assistant may say:

"Dr. Wright has been called away to answer an emergency. She asked me to tell you she is very sorry to keep you waiting. There will be at least a 1-hour delay."

Ask the patient:

"Do you wish to wait? If it is inconvenient, I'll be glad to give you the first available appointment on another day. Or perhaps you'd like to have some coffee or do some shopping and return in an hour."

As quickly as possible, call the patients who are scheduled for a later hour. In many offices, especially those of obstetricians, surgeons, and general practitioners, it sometimes is necessary to cancel a whole day's appointments. For this reason, it is particularly important to have the daytime telephone number of each patient available so that the appointment can be rescheduled.

If it is at all possible, cancel appointments before the patient arrives in the office to find that the physician is not available. The **expediency** of the office staff in contacting the patients who will be affected by an emergency will be most appreciated.

When the Physician is Ill or Out of Town

Physicians get ill, too, and the patients who are scheduled to be seen during the course of the physician's expected recovery period must be informed of this. They need not be told the nature of the illness. When the physician is called out of town for personal or professional reasons, the appointments will have to be canceled or rescheduled. It is customary to give the patient the name of another physician, or possibly a choice of several, who will be providing care during such absences. For security reasons, it is best to merely state that the doctor is unavailable. Stating over the telephone that the physician is out of town could lead to attempted burglary or other unauthorized intrusion of the premises.

OTHER TYPES OF APPOINTMENTS

There will be a wide range of other unscheduled callers with whom the physician will need to meet. Handle all of these individuals with care and courtesy.

Physicians

Another physician dropping into the facility should be ushered in to see the physician as soon as possible, regardless of the appointment schedule. If the physician is seeing a patient, explain the situation and, if possible, take the visiting physician into a private room to wait. Then notify the physician as soon as possible. Visits from other physicians are usually brief and do not appreciably affect the schedule.

Pharmaceutical Representatives

Also known as *detail persons* or *reps,* representatives from pharmaceutical companies are frequent visitors to physicians' offices and are generally welcomed when the schedule permits. They are well trained and bring valuable information on new drugs to the physician. The medical assistant is often expected to screen such visitors and turn away those whose products would not be used in that practice. If the representative or the pharmaceutical company is unknown to the office, ask for a business card, then check with the physician, who will decide whether to see the caller.

Specialists usually limit their conferences with pharmaceutical representatives to their line of practice. The medical assistant, together with the physician, can prepare a list of the representatives with whom the physician is willing to spend time, then let the list be the determining factor in future conferences. The medical assistant can say whether the physician will be available that day and give an estimate of the waiting time or suggest a later time at which the caller may return. The caller can then make a decision regarding whether to wait or return later. The pharmaceutical representative is usually quite understanding and cooperative and is willing to wait patiently a long while for just a brief visit with the physician. The medical assistant should in turn treat the representative with courtesy, showing as much cooperation as possible.

In some cases the representative will just leave literature or materials for the physician with the medical assistant. The detail person who is not on the calling list for a particular physician will also appreciate the time saved by knowing this in advance. Most representatives say they would rather be told outright if the physician does not wish to see them than to be given some evasive reply.

Salespersons

Salespersons from medical, surgical, and office supply houses call regularly at physicians' offices. Sometimes they will want to see the physician, but the office manager or the medical assistant who is in charge of ordering supplies usually is able to handle these calls.

Unsolicited salespersons can sometimes present a problem in the professional office. If the physician does not wish to see such callers, the medical assistant must firmly but tactfully send them away. Suggest that they leave their literature and cards for the physician to study and say that the physician will contact them if further information is desired.

Miscellaneous Callers

From time to time other callers appear in the medical office. Some are civic leaders seeking the physician's aid in community projects. Others may be church leaders, insurance representatives, solicitors for fund drives, and so forth. A general policy regarding seeing such callers should be established so that each incident does not require a separate discussion and decision.

Civic leaders should be treated with courtesy and consideration when they telephone or come into the office. Most physicians feel a responsibility to take an active part in community affairs, but no one can participate in all activities. The responsibility for accepting or refusing such community appointments is sometimes delegated to the office manager or medical assistant. In this event, one should use discretion and exercise great tact and courtesy. Turning away community leaders with a blunt refusal does not create good medical public relations.

When it is necessary to refuse requests for community projects, the medical assistant can explain that the physician is already participating in such community projects as, for example, the Boy Scouts, Girl Scouts, Kiwanis, and the Health Council and cannot accept additional responsibilities at this time. The practice of tact, courtesy, and consideration applies to every caller in the healthcare facility.

PLANNING FOR THE NEXT DAY

Before leaving at the end of the day, look over the appointments scheduled for the next day. Review the charts for scheduled patients. If laboratory tests or other procedures were scheduled on the patient's last visit, determine that the reports are available in the chart. If the patient is scheduled for specific procedures on this visit, make certain that everything that will be needed for the procedure is on hand and available. Planning can save many precious moments at the time of the patient visit.

CLOSING COMMENTS

The person charged with the responsibility for scheduling appointments will have a huge impact on the efficiency of the medical office. A friendly and helpful attitude is a **prerequisite** for cordial **interaction** with patients and the ability to make compromises that will benefit both the physician and the patient. The office that runs smoothly and stays on schedule indicates professionalism and competence and will be greatly appreciated by all who come into contact with the medical office.

Providing patients with an information booklet about the office will familiarize them with the policies and procedures of the office. Many physicians compile an extensive booklet that even provides tips as to when the physician should be called immediately, listing symptoms and signs of emergencies.

Educating the patient regarding office policies will help the facility to run smoothly from day to day. All patients should be familiar with the policies about appointments. This leads to fewer misunderstandings and conflicts over bills that might include a charge for a missed appointment.

If the facility offers Internet-based appointment scheduling, patients will have to be taught how to use the system. A printed pamphlet or information sheet will be helpful in providing instruction to the patient. It would be wise to have a special phone number that patients can call if they have problems with the scheduling system. For best results choose a program that is simple to use and easy to understand and one that does not breach patient confidentiality.

The appointment schedule may be used as a legal record and could be brought by subpoena into a court of law. Be sure that all handwriting in the book is completely legible and that information is routinely collected in a consistent manner for each entry. Do not fail to note a no-show in the patient's chart as well as the appointment schedule. This is often helpful when a physician must prove that the patient did not follow medical advice or that the patient contributed to his or her poor condition by missing appointments. Old appointment schedules should be kept for a time equal to the statute of limitations in the state in which the practice exists.

SUMMARY OF SCENARIO

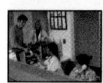

Ramona is an asset to the medical office because her dedication and customer service skills help her to interact with patients in a positive way. She genuinely cares about the patients and makes every effort to meet their needs while following the preferences of her physician. She has found that her bright smile is a valuable tool to use when patients have been waiting and are growing restless.

Ramona cooperates with other staff members to get the patients seen as quickly as possible and to minimize wait time. She is flexible and can change the order of the patients seen, if needed, to maximize the use of time and facilities in the office. Because she is so cheerful and friendly, patients do not seem to mind when she asks for their cooperation. She keeps current phone numbers and cell phone information so that she can notify a patient quickly if Dr. Brown is running behind schedule. Ramona's proficiency on the computer also is an asset, and she makes frequent use of email to take care of patient problems or rescheduling desires.

Because of the cooperation she receives from staff and patients alike, Ramona successfully runs an efficient office. She contributes to that efficiency by constantly refining her knowledge about her job. She pays attention to the times during the day that don't run as smoothly as others, evaluates the problems at those times, and then corrects them. Ramona also keeps the schedule moving by communicating with the clinical medical assistants and keeping them informed about arriving patients, and those who have come early or are running late. She is able to quickly adjust and substitute a patient who has already arrived. Ramona has learned how to manipulate the schedule to accommodate an emergency. She knows that by making minor adjustments and keeping the waiting patients informed, the staff can handle any emergency. All medical assistants need to develop skills in flexibility. Through the establishment of a system that works and through correct use of it, patients and staff will be more content with their experience in the physician's office.

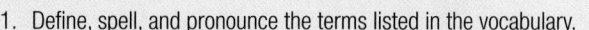

SUMMARY of LEARNING OBJECTIVES

1. Define, spell, and pronounce the terms listed in the vocabulary.
   - Spelling and pronouncing medical terms correctly adds credibility to the medical assistant. Knowing the definition of these terms promotes confidence in communication with patients and co-workers.
2. Discuss three items that must be considered when scheduling appointments.
   - When scheduling appointments, a medical assistant must consider the patients' needs, the physician's preferences, and the available facilities. Make every attempt to schedule a patient at his or her most convenient time. This will help to avoid no-shows. The physician will outline preferences, which should be of high priority to the medical assistant. However, most physicians are flexible and will make adjustments according to the needs of the office. The availability of facilities within the office is perhaps the most inflexible factor. If a certain room or piece of equipment is being used for one patient, it usually cannot be used for another.
3. Explain the features that should be considered when choosing an appointment book.
   - When choosing an appointment book, all of the needs of the office should be considered. If there are multiple physicians, the book should be arranged so that each physician is readily identified. Books that open flat on the surface of the desk are much easier to handle, but if not enough space is available to open the book entirely, another style might be better. The book should also provide enough space to write all of the patient information needed in the various time slots, such as the name, phone number, and reason for the visit.

4. Discuss the advantages of computerized appointment scheduling.
   - Computerized scheduling programs are in demand today because they are easy to operate, simplifying scheduling appointments and making changes to the schedule. The computer can find the first available time much more quickly than a person scanning through an appointment book. Most programs can prepare reports and even notify patients automatically by email of the impending appointment. Web-based self-scheduling programs are becoming popular; these allow a patient to see the physician's available appointments and book his or her own date and time.
5. Explain how self-scheduling would reduce calls to the medical office.
   - Self-scheduling would vastly reduce calls to the office, because a high number of everyday calls are requests to schedule appointments. Patients could make an appointment at midnight, if they desired.
6. List and explain at least three methods of appointment scheduling.
   - Open office hours allow patients to come to the physician's office when it is convenient and wait in turn to see the physician. Scheduling specific appointments is the most popular method for seeing patients. Flexible office hours allow patients to see the physician during the evening and often on weekends. Many of today's medical offices have some flexible scheduling, because most families now consist of two working parents. Wave scheduling brings two or three patients to the office at the same time, and they are seen in the order of their arrival. This type of scheduling can be modified in many ways to suit the needs of the facility. Other scheduling methods include double booking and grouping of like procedures.

Continued

SUMMARY of LEARNING OBJECTIVES

Continued

7. Explain the basic procedure to follow when the office is behind schedule.
   - When the office is running 15 minutes behind schedule, the medical assistant should briefly explain the delay to the waiting patients, then offer to reschedule their appointments. Keep the patients informed of wait times until the schedule resumes.

8. Discuss offering choices to patients when scheduling appointments.
   - Giving a patient a choice in appointment times to better meet his or her needs is a part of good customer service. Offering the patient a choice of 2 days, morning or afternoon, and two times helps to ensure that the patient will keep the appointment.

9. Explain the importance of legible writing in the appointment book.
   - Because the appointment schedule might be called into a court of law, it is vital that the handwriting in the book be completely legible. Even if the book is 5 years old, the person charged with testifying in court should be able to clearly read all entries. Scribbled, messy handwriting implies incompetence and reflects on the practice.

10. Discuss several methods of dealing with patients who consistently arrive late.
    - Patients who are habitually late for appointments might be told to arrive 15 minutes before the time written in the book. Some offices book these patients as the last appointment of the day, so that if they do not arrive promptly, they do not see the physician. Usually talking with the patient and gaining an understanding of why the patient arrives late will improve the situation. The office can work with the patient to choose the best times that will result in a show appointment.

11. Name several reasons for failed appointments.
    - Some patients forget the appointment with the physician, and some are habitually careless about remembering their scheduled time. Small emergencies often come up, and in today's busy business world, some patients just cannot get away from their own offices or other obligations to visit the physician. In some cases patients do not keep appointments because they do not want to deal with a health issue confronting them.

CONNECTIONS

 Study Guide Connection: Go to Chapter 10 Study Guide. Read the Case Study and Workplace Applications and complete the assignments. Do online research for answers to the questions in the Internet Activities associated with scheduling appointments.

 CD Connection: Go to the Medical Assisting Competency Challenge CD and do the training activities under General Office Duties.

evolve **Evolve Connection:** For more information related to scheduling appointments, go to evolve.elsevier.com/kinn and visit related weblinks for Chapter 10. Click on the Medical Assisting Exam Review and do the practice questions to sharpen your test-taking skills. To learn more about office software, do the exercises for the Altapoint demo that is on the CD.

Patient Reception and Processing

SCENARIO

Most people enter the healthcare field for very specific reasons. Georgina Robertson recalls being in a serious car accident when she was 6 years old. As a result, her vision was temporarily impaired. She remembers seeing a woman in a white uniform who offered words of comfort. The woman seemed to have a haze around her that, when combined with the hospital lights, made her look as if she had wings. The vision of an angel never left Georgina's thoughts and led her into the medical field.

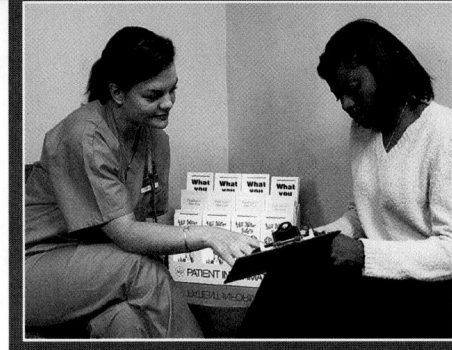

Today Georgina works for Dr. Stuart Wade, a cardiologist in a metropolitan city. Georgina is an experienced medical assistant, and she enjoys getting to know her patients. She makes notes on the chart that remind her of special events in the lives of the patients who visit Dr. Wade's office. The patients feel that she truly cares about them, aside from her duties at the clinic. Although she is efficient and time conscious, she always has a moment to share a warm smile or hear about a new grandchild. Georgina is a valued member of the medical team in her office. She is currently attending a state college in the evening hours, gaining credits toward her bachelor's degree. She plans to continue her education and apply to medical school in the future.

While studying this chapter, think about the following questions:

- What are some ways to develop good rapport with patients?
- Why is the sign-in register a potential breach of patient confidentiality?

- What is the value in knowing some information about patients' personal lives?

LEARNING OBJECTIVES

1. Define, spell, and pronounce the terms listed in the vocabulary.
2. Explain the purpose of the office mission statement.
3. List several patient amenities and why these are important additions to the medical office.
4. Describe how to prepare for patient arrivals.
5. Explain why it is important to use the patient's name as often as possible.

6. Discuss how the medical assistant may help the patient prepare for an examination.
7. List and explain two methods of chart placement.
8. Discuss how the medical assistant might deal with talkative patients.
9. Discuss ways to make the patient feel at ease and comfortable in the medical office.

National Accreditation Competencies and Content

CAAHEP COMPETENCIES

Administrative
3.a(1)(c). Organize a patient's medical record

General
3.c(1)(b). Recognize and respond to verbal communication
3.c(2)(a). Identify and respond to issues of confidentiality
3.c(2)(c). Establish and maintain the medical record
3.c(2)(d). Document appropriately
3.c(3)(a). Explain general office policies
3.c(3)(b). Instruct individuals according to their needs

ABHES COMPETENCIES

Communication
2.l. Recognition and response to verbal and nonverbal communication

Administrative
3.a. Perform basic secretarial skills
3.b. Prepare and maintain medical records

Legal Concepts
5.a. Determine needs for documentation and reporting
5.b. Document accurately
5.c. Use appropriate guidelines when releasing records or information

Instruction
7.a. Orient patients to office policies and procedures
7.b. Instruct patients with special needs

VOCABULARY

amenity (uh-me'-nuh-te) Something conducive to comfort, convenience, or enjoyment.

demographic (de-muh-gra'-fik) The statistical characteristics of human populations (as in age or income) used especially to identify markets.

depleted Lessened markedly in quantity, content, power, or value.

fervent Exhibiting or marked by great intensity of feeling.

flagged Marked in some way as to remind or remember that specific action needs to be taken.

harmonious Marked by accord in sentiment or action; having the parts agreeably related.

immigrant A person who comes to a country to take up permanent residence.

intercom A two-way communication system with a microphone and loudspeaker at each station for localized use.

perception A quick, acute, and intuitive cognition; a capacity for comprehension.

phonetic (fuh-ne'-tik) Constituting an alteration of ordinary spelling that better represents the spoken language, that employs only characters of the regular alphabet, and that is used in a context of conventional spelling.

progress notes Notes used in the patient chart to track the progress and condition of the patient.

sequentially (si-kwen'-shuh-le) Of, relating to, or arranged in a sequence.

The patient reception area should be an inviting place in which patients feel comfortable. Visits to the physician can be times of great stress, so the office staff must do everything possible to make the experience pleasant for patients. A patient usually has a choice of healthcare providers and should be given excellent customer service. Good patient relations will result in referrals to the physician, and this helps the practice grow. When patients have a good experience with a physician, they are likely to tell others. When the office staff is committed to making the patient feel welcome and the focus is on care of the patient, the success of the practice is inevitable.

THE OFFICE MISSION STATEMENT

Healthcare providers often have a **fervent** reason for entering the medical field. One physician remembers the heritage his **immigrant** grandfather left in his heart. The physician has fond memories of his grandfather's pride and thankfulness for the opportunities he found in America, after coming to the United States with nothing but the clothes on his back. The grandfather's dream was to see his grandson become a physician, and that is exactly what he did. Even on the most trying days, he can step into his office and see a picture of his grandfather. His memories helped him to find the strength and determination to care for his patients.

The office mission statement reflects this deep-seated desire by expressing the reasons for the existence of the practice (Figure 11-1). The physician develops the mission statement alone or may consult the office staff for input. Many offices display the mission statement prominently in the reception area and on printed material, such as patient information booklets. Whatever the contents, each employee of the facility should be

WADE CARDIAC CLINIC MISSION STATEMENT

The mission of the Wade Cardiac Clinic is fourfold:

- The staff of the clinic promotes the highest standards of ethical medical practice.
- The physician and staff members commit to serving their patients with respect and courtesy.
- All staff members shall promote a healthy lifestyle and preventative measures for the patients that present to the clinic.
- The clinic will support medical patient education, scientific research and development, community service, and community health promotion.

It is our desire to give the best customer service to our patients and care for them as if they were members of our own families.

FIGURE 11-1 The mission statement should be presented to all employees early in their tenure, and the staff should strive to meet the mission every day.

familiar with the statement and have a personal commitment to promoting the mission statement in everyday practice.

THE RECEPTION AREA

A first impression is lasting. Nowhere is this more important than in the healthcare facility, where the environment must appear orderly and faultlessly clean. The facility may be a physician's office, a hospital, a health maintenance organization, an insurance company, or one of the many other healthcare establishments. No matter what type of facility is involved, the appearance of the reception room and the front desk as well as a cordial greeting by the receptionist influence a patient's **perception** of the entire facility and the care that he or she will receive.

The reception room is just that—a place to receive patients and visitors. The area should be planned for the patients' comfort, made as attractive and cheerful as possible, and kept clean and uncluttered. Often a medical assistant has the opportunity to assist in the design and decoration of this very important area. Consider traffic flow; the movement of patients from place to place within the reception room—as well as in the rest of the office—should be unhindered and logical (Figure 11-2).

CRITICAL THINKING APPLICATION

Georgina feels that her patients enjoy a homelike atmosphere, which is less intimidating than the sterile, clinical feel of some medical offices. How might she accomplish giving her office a homelike feeling?

Fresh, **harmonious** colors and cleanliness are the foundation of an attractive room (Figure 11-3). Select comfortable furniture

that is adequate to accommodate the peak load of patients seen each day, and arrange it in conversational groups. Individual chairs are best (Figure 11-4); people usually prefer to stand rather than sit next to a stranger on a sofa. Provide good lighting, ventilation, and regulated temperature, and the essentials are in place for an attractive, comfortable reception area. Reduce room clutter by providing a place to hang coats, rainwear, and umbrellas. Professional designers can be consulted regarding reception room décor and improvements or to solve a problem area that inhibits office traffic.

Most physicians' offices are well supplied with recent magazines, and some have various books. Publications with short items of popular interest are favorites, like *Reader's Digest*. Any reading material placed in the reception room should be of interest to the general public; *Good Housekeeping*, *U.S. News and World Report*, *Real Simple*, *Oprah*, and *People* are examples of interesting magazines that most people would enjoy reading. The reception room, incidentally, is not the place for the physician's professional journals.

A writing desk with writing paper in the reception area for the convenience of patients is a nice touch, as is restful music from a concealed speaker. A lighted aquarium or an educational display of some sort enhances the attractiveness and individuality of the reception area in the professional practice. Patients are often interested in health-related brochures. The physician may also have a videotape or healthcare book library that allows patients to check out items of interest to them. A telephone in the reception area is an asset and can be programmed by the phone company not to allow long-distance calls.

A television VCR or DVD player will help the time pass much faster, especially in pediatric offices. Children enjoy Disney movies and cartoon programs, and these hold their interest until it is time to see the physician. Young patients would be thrilled to find a video game system in the waiting area, although this may make them more uncooperative when called back to see the physician—they may want to continue playing the game! A children's corner equipped with small-scale furniture and some playthings works well (Figure 11-5). Youngsters who might otherwise get into mischief are kept pleasantly occupied. Toys should be easily cleanable; plastic washable items are especially good. Take extra care to ensure that no toy has sharp corners that could cause injury or small parts that could be swallowed. In selecting toys, make certain that they will not stimulate the child toward noisy activity. And no rubber balls, unless there is time to chase them around the room!

CRITICAL THINKING APPLICATION

Georgina has a few patients who bring young children to their appointments. Sometimes the children are a bit disruptive and make other patients feel uncomfortable. How might Georgina handle this problem in the medical office? Some children misbehave in public, and the parents do not respond or correct them. How might Georgina deal with this situation if it happens in her office?

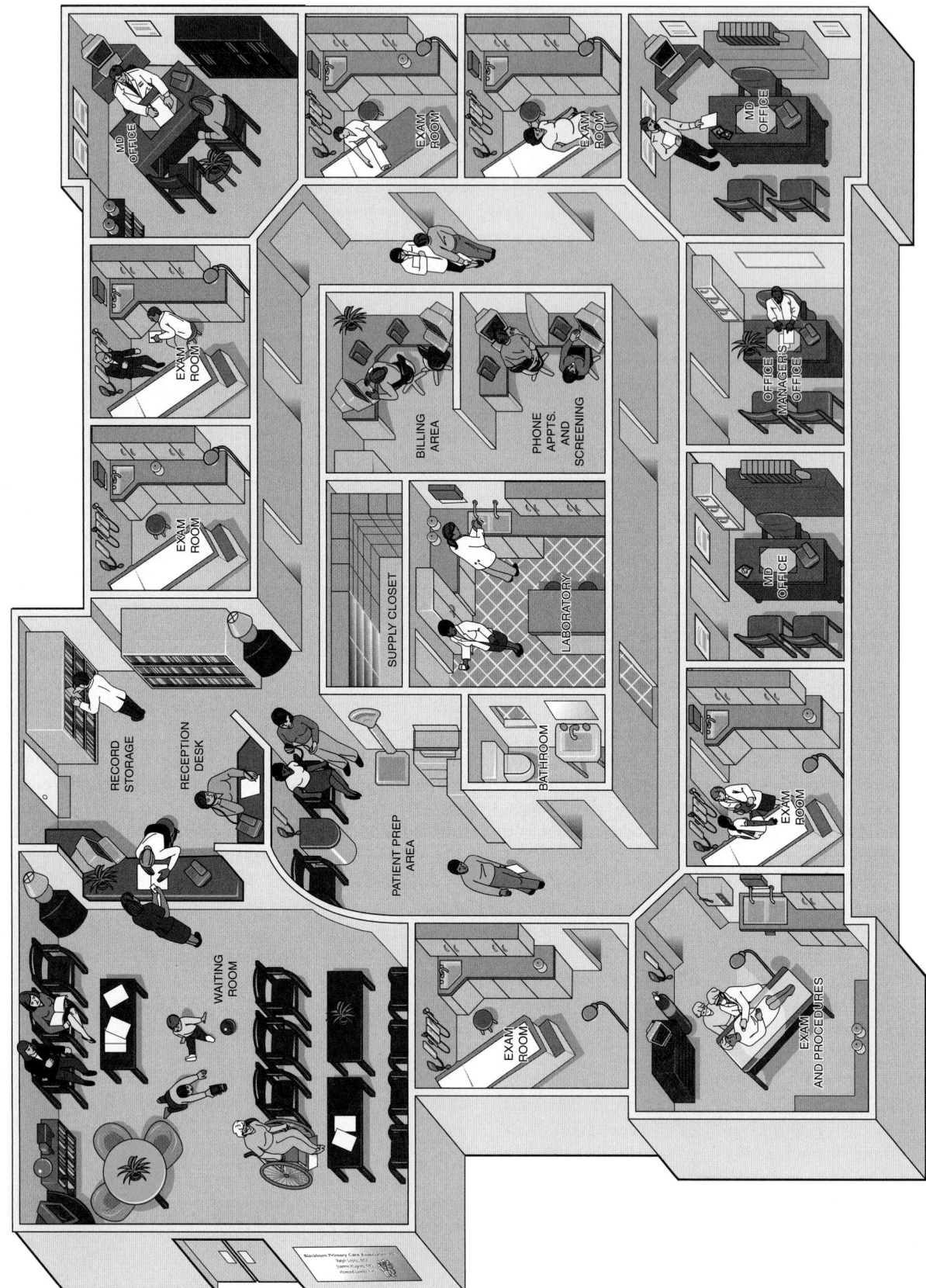

FIGURE 11-2 The medical office should be arranged so that the flow of traffic is conducive to the movement of patients throughout the office.

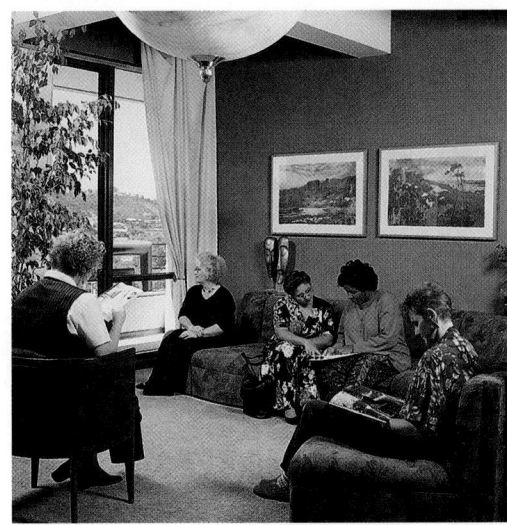

FIGURE 11-3 Patients appreciate cleanliness, restful colors, good ventilation, and light to read by when waiting in the reception area.

Many of today's modern offices offer a computer for patient use while waiting to see the physician. This is a wonderful **amenity** because the patient can make good use of his or her time while in the reception area. Some patients may bring their personal laptop computers and use their time in the waiting room to complete projects. An amazing amount of work can be done just by checking office email, so providing Internet access to patients is also helpful, whether it is wired or wireless. If patients are allowed to connect to the office wireless network, it is wise to provide one specific log-on name and password just for them, to maintain control over access to private health information.

Periodically, take an objective look around the reception room. Could it use a little brightening or freshening up? Try to look at the room as if seeing it for the first time. The receptionist is partly responsible for the appearance of the area by making certain that the room remains neat and orderly throughout the day. Check the temperature and lighting for comfort. Scan the room at various intervals during the day to ensure that the room is in good order.

If the medical assistant's desk is in the reception area or in open view of the patients, it should be free of clutter. In particular, patients' medical and financial records should not be in sight. Keep computer monitors out of view to protect patient confidentiality. Some offices use privacy screens that allow only the user to see the monitor. Personal articles, coffee cups, and other personal items should not be on the receptionist's desk.

PREPARING FOR PATIENT ARRIVAL

Advance preparation helps to make the day go smoothly and contributes toward a more relaxed atmosphere for all concerned. Some offices prepare for the next day on the evening before, whereas others prepare each morning. The office should be consistent and should always perform the same routine so that important preparations are not left undone. More information about opening the office, closing the office, and its daily operation can be found in Chapter 12.

CRITICAL THINKING APPLICATION

There will always be housekeeping chores associated with preparing for each day in the physician's office. What are some ways that Georgina can divide these tasks fairly among the staff members? How should Georgina handle the employee who feels that general housekeeping duties are not a part of the job description?

Preparing Medical Records

Pull the medical records for the day (or the next day if this is done in the evenings), and check off the patient's name on a copy of the appointment schedule to be sure that all of the records have been located and are ready (Figure 11-6).

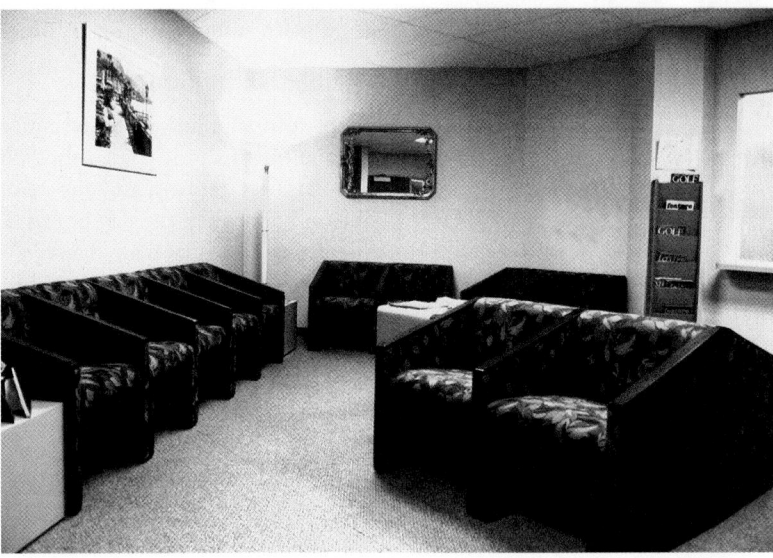

FIGURE 11-4 Patients tend to prefer individual seating. Comfortable seating helps patients relax and be at ease while waiting to see the physician. (Courtesy August Incorporated, Centerville, Ohio.)

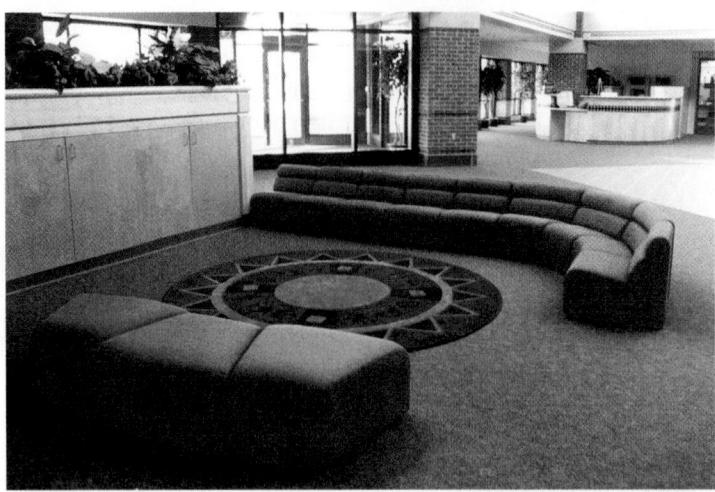

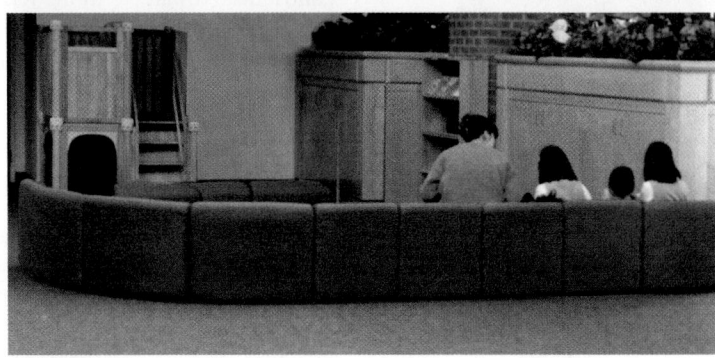

FIGURE 11-5 Furniture in a pediatrician's office should be durable and fun, child sized, and able to withstand the most active children. (Courtesy August Incorporated, Centerville, Ohio.)

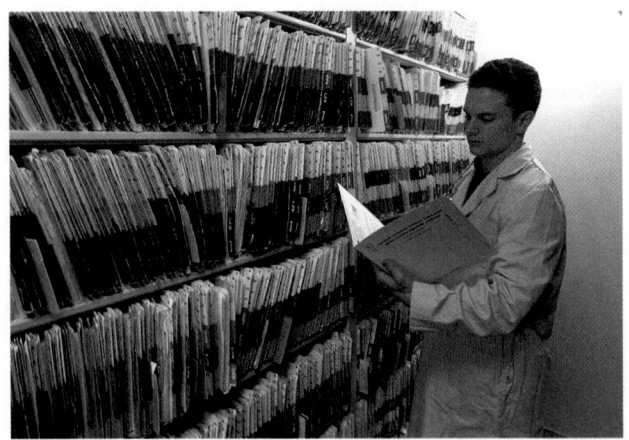

FIGURE 11-6 Charts should be pulled in advance for the patients arriving for appointments. Each chart should be checked to see whether it has adequate forms and is in good order for the physician's use.

Occasionally more than one patient may have the same or a similar name. Check the patient's social security number, date of birth, or other pertinent information to ascertain that the right medical record has been pulled. Review each record to verify that any recently received information, such as laboratory reports and radiograph readings, has been correctly entered into and permanently attached to the record (Procedure 11-1).

Arrange the medical records **sequentially** in the order in which the patients are scheduled to be seen. The medical assistant may be expected to place the records of all the patients to be seen that day on the physician's desk, but it is more likely that the physician will prefer to review each record just before entering the examination room. Be sure that there is enough space on the **progress notes** for the physician to write in the record. If not, place additional progress notes in the record.

Replenishing Supplies

Replenish supplies at the reception desk regularly. Stationery, appointment cards, charge slips, sharpened pencils, pens, telephone message pads, and any items likely to be needed should be on hand when the day begins. Discovering that supplies are **depleted** during a busy day can seriously interrupt the flow of patient care. One person should be in charge of checking the inventory of supplies on a regular basis and ordering as necessary. Inventories and supply ordering will be discussed in Chapter 12.

In a multiple-employee practice, a clinical assistant usually has the responsibility of checking clinical supplies and preparing the patient rooms; however, in a small practice there may be only one assistant available for all duties. Before patients begin to arrive, everything should be ready for the day so that the physician and medical assistant can give undivided attention to the patients' needs.

PROCEDURE 11-1

Establish and Maintain the Medical Record: Organize a Patient's Medical Record

CAAHEP COMPETENCY: 3.c(2)(c)
ABHES COMPETENCY: 3.b

GOAL: *To prepare patient charts for the daily appointment schedule and have them ready for the physician before the patients' arrival.*

EQUIPMENT and SUPPLIES

- Appointment schedule for current date
- Patient files
- Clerical supplies (e.g., pen, tape, stapler)

PROCEDURAL STEPS

1. Review the appointment schedule.
2. Identify full name of each scheduled patient.
3. Pull patients' charts for files, checking each patient's name on your list as each is pulled.
   PURPOSE: To determine that the correct charts have been pulled and that no charts have been omitted.
4. Review each chart.
   PURPOSE: To reaffirm that:

- The correct patient chart has been pulled
- Any previously ordered tests have been performed
- The results of the tests have been mounted or entered in the chart
- Forms have been replenished inside the chart, such as progress notes, and so forth

5. Annotate the appointment list with any special concerns.
   PURPOSE: To alert the physician regarding matters that should be checked or discussed with the patient.
6. Arrange the charts sequentially according to each patient's appointment.
7. Place the charts in the appropriate examination room or other specified location.

GREETING THE PATIENT

Every patient has the right to expect courteous treatment in a physician's office. No matter what the patient's economic or social status may be, each individual who enters the reception room should receive a cordial, friendly greeting (Figure 11-7). Using a personal touch, such as greeting the patient by name, is an easy way to develop patient rapport. Use the patient's last name and title unless the patient insists on using his or her first name.

"How are you today, Mr. Roberts?"

"Ms. Nelson, the doctor will be in to see you shortly."

If the office creates a policy of obtaining a copy of all patients' photo identification cards, such as the driver's license,

it can be used to identify patients and greet them by name, even if they do not visit the office often.

Patient Check-In

The reception desk should be in clear view of all visitors who come into the office. If only one medical assistant is present, it is sometimes impossible for each new visitor to be welcomed personally. Develop an announcement system that alerts staff when people enter the office. The patient who enters an empty reception room does not know whether to sit down, knock on the glass partition, or try to announce his or her presence in some other way. One solution would be a bell that the patient can ring on arrival. A sign placed in the reception room that reads, "Please sit comfortably. The receptionist will be with you shortly," will assure patients that their presence will be acknowledged.

The receptionist should check the reception room each time he or she has been away from the desk to see if additional patients have arrived. Greet these patients by name; if the staff member is unaware who has entered the reception area, ask the person his or her name. Use a sign-in register that promotes patient privacy. Patient confidentiality is violated when others can read the names on the register. The best registers allow the staff to remove the patient's name and information after he or she signs the document. Pressure-sensitive labels, printed with lines for the patient name, appointment time, and changes in insurance coverage, are a practical, inexpensive solution for confidential patient registers. The signed label can then be placed in a separate log book or even inside the patient's medical record. The office can order custom registers that work like a pegboard, making the identifying information invisible to

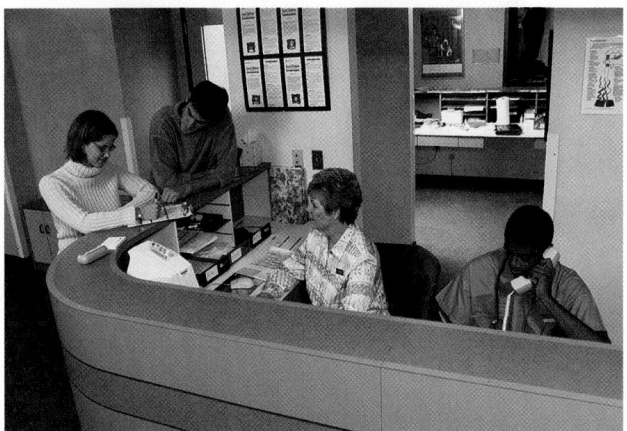

FIGURE 11-7 Greet all patients with a warm smile, and assist them with forms they need to complete for the chart.

subsequent patients. Patients should not be expected to provide details of the reason for their visit in a public area.

CRITICAL THINKING APPLICATION

Everyone forgets someone's name on occasion. How might Georgina and her staff members remember names? What special tips or techniques assist in remembering names? Eventually a patient will come to the clinic whose name just cannot be recalled. How can the staff determine who the patient is without offending him or her?

Knowing the Patients

Cultivate the habit of greeting each patient immediately in a friendly, self-assured manner. Establish eye contact and smile while introducing yourself to the patient. For example, "Good morning, I'm Elizabeth Parr, Dr. Wade's medical assistant." Remember to ask about the patient before asking about insurance coverage; no patient wants to feel that the physician's main interest in him or her is the collection of an insurance check.

Patients like to be acknowledged when they arrive. All staff members should review the day's schedule in the morning to be prepared to greet patients by name and to know whether the patient is new or established (Figure 11-8). Learn how to pronounce each patient's name correctly; incorrect pronunciations may offend or irritate some people. If the name is unusual, write the **phonetic** spelling on the record for reference. By using the patient's name often, the medical assistant ensures that he or she is treating the correct patient.

Make brief notes in the medical record about the current events in the patient's life. With this information, the medical assistant and the physician can read those notes before entering the examination room and share a short dialog with patients at the beginning of their visits. An example follows:

Georgina: Hello, Mrs. Williams, how are you today?

Mrs. Williams: I am doing very well, Georgina, how are you?

Georgina: I'm fine. How was the cruise you took with your husband last month?

Mrs. Williams: It was wonderful! The water was the bluest I have seen!

Georgina: You went to Cozumel, didn't you?

Mrs. Williams: Yes, we did! I'm surprised you remember, as many patients as you see each day!

This brief chat will confirm that the staff members care about the individual patients because they take an interest in their personal lives (Figure 11-9). Because the patient does not see the medical assistant or physician look at the notes before entering the patient room, the patient assumes that the information is being recalled from memory. This is an impressive customer service technique. Most patients appreciate the interest of the physician and the staff in their families, hobbies, and work.

Some state regulations prohibit information other than health details being placed in the medical record; however, most health professionals agree that the mental and emotional health of a patient is connected to his or her physical health. Details about what is happening in patients' lives provide clues to physical problems they are experiencing. As a simple example, a patient going through a divorce may experience depression that needs to be treated with medication. Without knowledge of the divorce, the physician would not have all of the information needed to make a sound medical decision. Physicians can treat patients more effectively when such information is available in the medical record.

REGISTRATION PROCEDURES

On a patient's first visit to the physician's office, the staff performs certain registration procedures (Procedure 11-2). Most physicians use a patient information form to gather **demographic** information about the patient. The form may

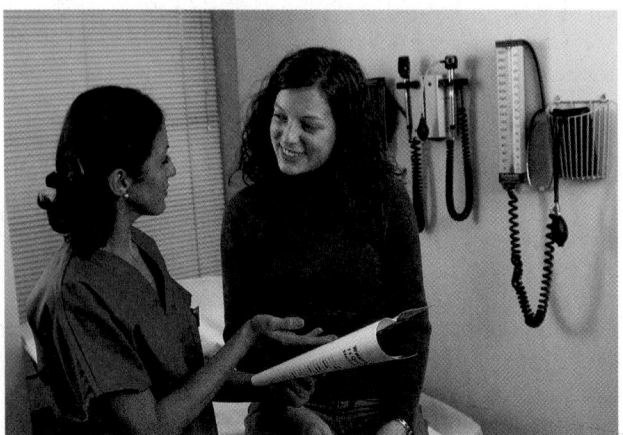

FIGURE 11-8 The medical assistant should develop a good relationship with the patient and be a caring advocate.

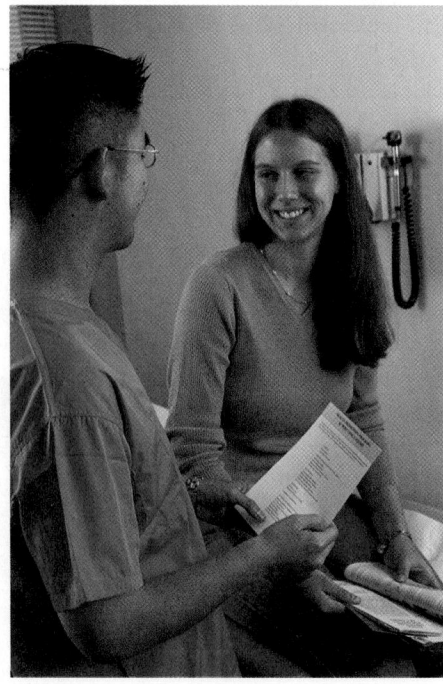

FIGURE 11-9 Patients appreciate being called by name and remembered from visit to visit.

PROCEDURE 11-2

Establish and Maintain the Medical Record: Register a New Patient

CAAHEP COMPETENCY: 3.c.(2)(c)
ABHES COMPETENCY: 3.b

GOAL: *To complete a registration form for a new patient with information for credit and insurance claims, and to inform and orient the patient to the facility.*

EQUIPMENT and SUPPLIES

- Registration form
- Clerical supplies (pen, clipboard)
- Private conference area

PROCEDURAL STEPS

1. Determine whether the patient is new to the practice.
2. Obtain and record the necessary information:
   - Full name, birth date, name of spouse (if married)
   - Home address, telephone number (include ZIP and area codes)
   - Occupation, name of employer, business address, telephone number
   - Social Security number and driver's license number, if any
   - Name of referring physician, if any
   - Name and address of person responsible for payment
   - Method of payment
   - Health insurance information (photocopy both sides of insurance ID card)
   - Name of primary carrier

- Type of coverage
- Group policy number
- Subscriber number
- Assignment of benefits, if required

   PURPOSE: This information is necessary for credit and insurance claims.
3. Review the entire form and confirm patient eligibility for insurance coverage.
   PURPOSE: To verify that the given information is complete and legible.
4. Determine that required referrals have been received, if applicable.
   PURPOSE: Insurance coverage may not be valid without referral.
5. Explain medical and financial procedures to patients.
   PURPOSE: The patient develops a comfort level and knows what to expect.
6. Collect co-payments or balance payment charges.
   PURPOSE: Keeps accounts current and prevents the necessity of mailing statements.

---

be attached to a clipboard and handed to the patient with instructions to complete sections. The medical assistant must be ready and willing to answer any questions (Figure 11-10). The patient's name should appear prominently at the top of the form, followed by other pertinent facts in logical order. Most information sheets contain the following:

- Patient's full name and date of birth
- Responsible person's name and relationship to the patient

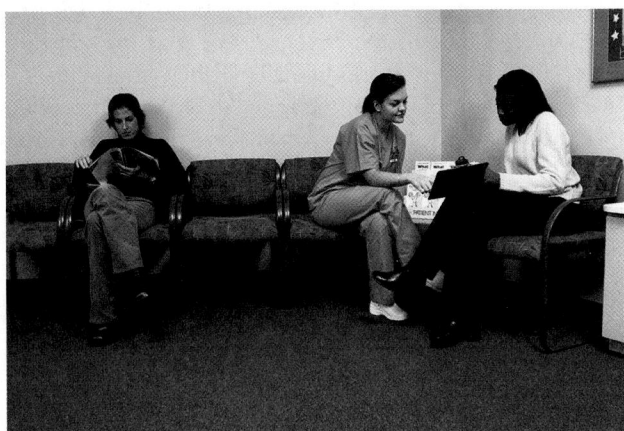

FIGURE 11-10 The medical assistant should take the time to explain forms that the patient does not understand and always be willing to answer questions.

- Address and telephone number
- Name, address, and telephone number of spouse
- Occupation
- Place of employment
- Social Security number
- Driver's license number
- Nearest relative not living with patient, and his or her relationship
- Source of referral, if any

When the completed form is returned, check carefully to verify that all the necessary information has been provided.

CRITICAL THINKING APPLICATION

Often some time is needed to complete patient forms when a new patient arrives in the office. How might Georgina keep the office on schedule when new patients arrive, necessitating chart construction and form completion? What are some ways to trim time from these activities?

Obtaining a Patient History

The personal and medical history and the patient's family history may be obtained by asking the patient to complete a questionnaire; the physician can augment this information during the patient interview. Some experienced medical assistants conduct the interview to obtain the patient's personal and medical history, family history, and chief complaint. This is a specialized procedure, and the medical assistant should be specifically trained to perform it for the individual practice.

CONSIDERATION FOR PATIENTS' TIME

The patient expects to see the physician or practitioner at the appointed time. The medical assistant should get the patient into the examination room for treatment or consultation as near the appointment time as possible or explain delays. All patients want to be kept informed about how long they should expect to wait to see the physician. They will usually respond positively when the physician or the assistant comes to the reception area to apologize for any delay. Always consider the patient's time and make every effort to streamline the office visit.

In a solo or small practice there should seldom be more than three to five patients in the reception room. Patients complain that the wait time in medical facilities is one of the most frustrating aspects of the medical profession. The patient who complains about medical fees or the care received may have first become agitated during a long wait to see the physician. Many patients are fearful and tense; long wait times intensify these feelings. The medical assistant can often put patients in a better frame of mind with just a friendly smile and a show of concern.

A crowded reception room is not always an indication of a physician's popularity. It may simply mean that the physician or the assistant is inefficient in scheduling patients. Business people, for example, who are in the habit of making the most of their time, are particularly displeased at what may appear to them to be inefficient scheduling of appointments. Any delay of longer than 10 to 15 minutes should be explained to the person waiting. Some personal attention, such as offering a drink of water, a cup of coffee, or a new magazine, may help to calm a patient who appears irritated with the delay. However, be sure that the patient is allowed caffeine before offering coffee. Be careful that the refreshment offered does not go against the physician's orders or would interfere with scheduled blood testing or other procedures.

Patients with Special Needs

Some patients will be physically challenged, some very ill, and some severely uncomfortable. There may be language or cultural barriers. Observe the patient's appearance and behavior. Is the patient pale? Do the eyes or voice reflect pain or discomfort? Find out how the patient is feeling before suggesting that he or she be seated to wait for the physician. The patient may need to lie down in a cool room or perhaps be seen as an emergency case.

Patients with disabilities, such as those in a wheelchair or using a cane, walker, or crutches, may need extra attention. Some patients may need help in disrobing even when a disability is not obvious. Ask if the patient needs assistance.

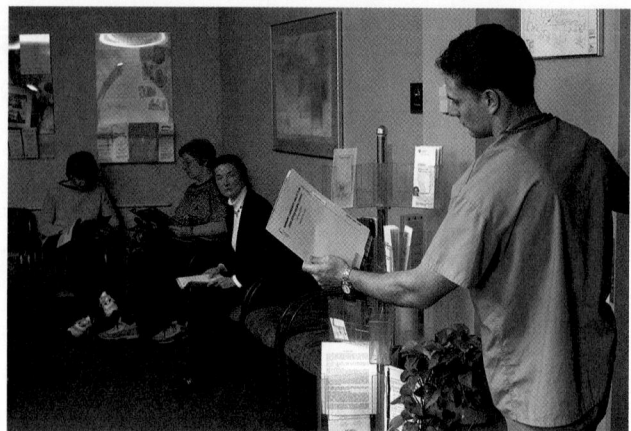

FIGURE 11-11 Pronounce the patient's name correctly, and use it often. This promotes good customer service and pleases the patient.

ESCORTING AND INSTRUCTING THE PATIENT

Patients prefer to be escorted while inside the physician's office rather than simply told where to go. This is usually the responsibility of the clinical medical assistant, but the task could be assigned to administrative staff, including the receptionist. Pronounce the patient's name correctly when he or she is called to the clinical area (Figure 11-11). If unsure of the pronunciation, ask the patient. Write the name phonetically on the medical record for quick retrieval at the next appointment.

Remember that to an employee of the practice the office surroundings may become as familiar as home. A stranger to the practice's environment may be confused or disoriented by all the hallways, doors, and rooms. Uncertainty creates anxiety. Take the time to personally escort the patient to the appropriate examination or treatment room; do not point to the room and expect the patient to find the way. If a urine specimen is needed, direct the patient to the restroom and always explain what to do with the specimen.

On arrival in the examination room, tell the patient if he or she needs to disrobe. Explain what garments, if any, can be left on, whether shoes are to be removed, whether jewelry needs to be removed, and any other necessary instructions. If a gown is to be worn, specify whether the opening should be in the front or back and tell the patient where he or she can hang up clothes if this is not obvious. An examination table should never be placed in such a position that the patient is exposed to passersby in the hallway if the door is opened. Imagine a patient ready for a Pap smear, facing the door as the physician enters! Allow patients a sense of modesty at all times, and make all instructions completely clear. Be equally clear when the examination has been completed. Do not assume that patients will know what is expected of them. Tell the patient whether he or she should go to the physician's office for consultation, or return to the reception area to wait, or whether he or she is free to check out with the front office and leave.

The medical assistant helps keep the schedule operating smoothly by immediately tidying each examination room and escorting the next patient in so that the physician has no idle moments waiting for a patient to be prepared. Try not to place a patient in an examination room just to clear out the reception area. It is especially inconsiderate to keep the patient waiting after being gowned, draped, and positioned on the examining table. Medical offices are often chilly or even cold, which will make a draped patient quite uncomfortable. A magazine rack on the wall of the treatment room is a welcome addition in some practices.

Remember that in today's litigious society, physicians prefer a second person in the room during examinations to avoid claims of sexual assault or harassment. The office may be equipped with a buzzer that alerts the medical assistant to enter the examination room after the physician has initially consulted with the patient. Be prompt in answering the buzzer, and provide assistance during the examination. Patients may be uncomfortable and uneasy, so it is appropriate to offer words of encouragement, a smile, and a pat on the shoulder.

MEDICAL RECORD PLACEMENT

Medical records should never be left in the examination room to be picked up and read by a patient. This can cause misunderstandings because patients rarely know medical terms and abbreviations. A number of different methods are used to signal that a patient is ready to be seen. Often there are file holders on the doors of the examination rooms, where the medical record can be placed horizontally when the patient is ready to be seen. Then the physician can signal the medical assistant that he or she is finished examining the patient by placing the chart in an upright position on leaving the examination room. Some offices have call systems, by which a physician can press a button to call the medical assistant for help with the examination. Others have a visual item outside the door that signals what that particular patient needs next.

Other offices place patients in examination rooms in a certain order, and the physician knows, for instance, that when he or she has finished with the patient in room one, the next patient will be waiting in room two. The office should develop a method that allows the most efficient use of time while providing high-quality care to the patients.

PROBLEM SITUATIONS

Talkative Patients

Problem patients exist in any professional office. Talkative patients, for example, take up far more of the physician's time than is justified. An alert medical assistant can usually spot this tendency during the initial interview. The patient's history can be **flagged** with a symbol to alert the physician. The medical assistant can buzz the physician's **intercom** and remind him that the next patient is ready. Once the medical assistant has learned which patients take extra time, they can be booked for the end of the day or more time can be allowed for them.

CRITICAL THINKING APPLICATION

Georgina has one patient who insists on sitting close to her desk and attempting to chat the entire time she is waiting to see the physician. What is worse, she comes to her appointments at least an hour early. How might Georgina subtly deal with this patient?

Children

Children frequently present special management problems, whether they are patients or they accompany a patient. Sometimes younger patients are escorted into the treatment room without the parent. Of course, this should be at the discretion of the physician and must be with the permission of the parent. The physician cannot force the parent to leave the examination room by any means. Although this practice of separating children from their parents to treat their needs is not always feasible, it sometimes can be applied with great success. In some offices a token of the physician's friendship, such as a trinket or toy, is given to the child at the completion of the visit.

Angry Patients in the Reception Area

Every medical assistant will eventually be confronted by an angry patient. The anger may simply be a reflection of the patient's pain or fear of what the physician may discover during the examination. If possible, invite the patient into another room out of the reception area. Usually it is best to let the patient talk out his or her anger. Pacify the patient using a calm attitude, and speak using a low tone of voice. Under no circumstances should the assistant return the anger or become argumentative.

Patient's Relatives and Friends

Patients are sometimes accompanied by a relative or well-meaning friend who may become restless while waiting for the patient and attempt to discuss the patient's illness. The medical assistant should sidestep any discussion of a patient's medical care, except by direction of the physician. Avoid a too-casual attitude, such as, "I'm sure there's nothing to worry about." A show of moderate concern and reassurance that "the patient is in good hands" usually takes care of the situation. Remember that health information cannot be released to anyone, including concerned friends and relatives, without patient consent.

PATIENT CHECKOUT

When the patient returns to the front office for checkout, greet him or her with a friendly smile and call the patient by name. Form the habit of asking patients if they have any questions. Check the medical record to determine when the physician wishes the patient to return to the office. Most physicians will note this information on the encounter form. Make the return appointment, remembering the technique of giving the patient choices as to which day they wish to come, morning or afternoon, and specific time. Then ask the patient for payment, using phrases such as, "Your co-pay today is $15, Mrs. Williams.

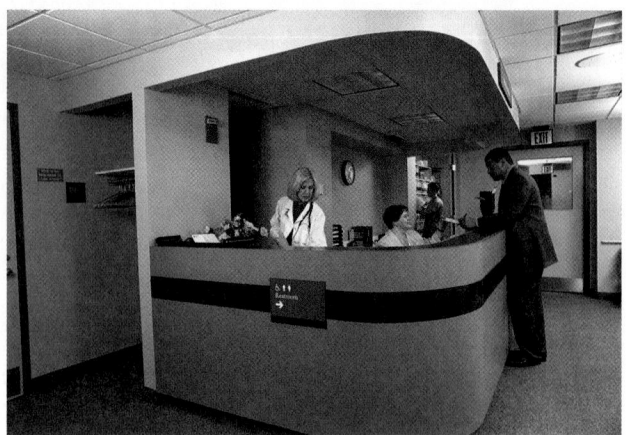

FIGURE 11-12 Always thank the patient for coming and wish him or her well.

Will you be writing a check or would you like to charge this visit to your Visa?"

Be sure to thank the patient for coming, and wish him or her well as they leave the office (Figure 11-12).

THE FRIENDLY FAREWELL

As soon as the visit with the physician has been completed, the medical assistant should be ready to assist the patient in dressing, if necessary, and make certain that any questions the patient may have are answered. Answer questions if they can be addressed ethically and legally; otherwise, direct the patient to the physician. Some questions can be answered only by the physician; in such cases the assistant can offer to get answers for the patient or bring the physician back to the examination room to answer the questions. Remember, patients view the medical assistant as an extension of the physician and the medical assistant must be very careful to avoid accusations of practicing medicine without a license.

The assistant can help convey a sense of caring by terminating the patient's visit cordially. If the patient is returning for another visit, the assistant can say something like, "We'll see you next week." If it is the patient's last visit, a pleasant "I certainly hope you'll be feeling fine from now on" is appropriate. The assistant may wish to tell a patient on a last visit that it has been a pleasure to make his or her acquaintance. Whatever words of goodbye are chosen, all patients should leave the facility with the feeling that they have received top-quality care and were treated with friendliness, respect, and courtesy.

CLOSING COMMENTS

A medical assistant must never offer medical advice to a patient unless specifically instructed to do so by the physician. The patient sees the medical assistant as an extension of the physician and tends to weigh advice and comments by the medical assistant with the same validity as if they came from the physician. Provide only information that the physician has approved or is included in the office policy and procedure manuals.

When a patient complains, listen carefully and attempt to resolve the problem or assure the patient that the issue will be discussed with the appropriate staff member to find a solution. If someone other than the patient asks for information about the patient, refrain from discussion unless the patient or physician has authorized the release of information.

A personal touch is vital to projecting a sense of care to the patients seen in the physician's office. Many medical offices are not concerned enough about the customer service aspect of the business. Patients talk about their experiences with their friends and relatives and may be an excellent source of referrals if they are treated with dignity and courtesy. If they have had a good experience, they will tell several people. If they have a poor experience, they tend to tell everyone they know! Be sure to have a part in each patient feeling a sense of satisfaction as they leave the office. All patients should feel that their time and money were well spent.

SUMMARY OF SCENARIO

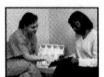 Georgina is a person who truly makes a difference in the healthcare profession. She takes her role as a patient advocate seriously and strives to make her patients feel comfortable in her physician's office. She keeps the mission statement posted close to her desk and rereads it often to keep her focus clear. She shares the vision with the other staff members, who are supportive and in agreement with the purpose for which the office exists.

Dr. Wade promotes continuing medical education and encourages his staff members to participate in courses and seminars that will assist them in being more effective patient advocates. The office sends birthday and Christmas cards to the patients in the database, and at the annual holiday party the staff hand-signs each Christmas card. Georgina sends a monthly newsletter to the patients, some by mail and some by email, to keep the patients up to date on office policies and interesting health information. All of these activities indicate a strong caring attitude toward the patients. Georgina considers each one a customer of the clinic, and she is determined that they receive excellent customer service.

Wait times are at a minimum in Dr. Wade's office. Cell phone numbers and email addresses are gathered at registration and updated frequently so that the staff can quickly contact patients. Georgina offers new patients a form for evaluation of

SUMMARY OF SCENARIO—cont'd

the office so that they can provide input about the experience they had as a new patient. All of these efforts promote a trusting, caring relationship among physician, staff, and patients.

By treating patients as one would wish to be treated, the medical assistant will develop a strong rapport. Patients enjoy hearing their own names and being recognized by medical staff members. Georgina remembers to greet each patient on his or her arrival to the clinic and always asks the names of patients she does not know. She knows that having a bit of personal

knowledge about the patients will be of benefit to Dr. Wade, so the entire staff is cordial and friendly to all patients.

Georgina knows that she must keep the sign-in register confidential and uses a form that is HIPAA compliant. This prevents patients from obtaining private health information during check-in procedures. By protecting patient confidentiality, the office not only remains in compliance with federal regulations but also puts the patients' interests first, assuring that they can enter the office with confidence and trust.

SUMMARY of LEARNING OBJECTIVES

1. Define, spell, and pronounce the terms listed in the vocabulary.
   - Spelling and pronouncing medical terms correctly adds credibility to the medical assistant. Knowing the definition of these terms promotes confidence in communication with patients and co-workers.

2. Explain the purpose of the office mission statement.
   - The office mission statement is the philosophy of why the office exists. Often physicians themselves develop the mission statement, which outlines their vision and reasons for entering medical practice. Some physicians allow the office staff to assist in its development. All employees should become familiar with the mission statement and promote its ideas to all patients and visitors.

3. List several patient amenities and why these are important additions to the medical office.
   - Patient amenities include such things as a VCR, television, computer, telephone, and a desk where patients can sit and balance a checkbook or review work while away from the office. These features turn the time spent in the physician's office into productive minutes instead of wasteful ones.

4. Describe how to prepare for patient arrivals.
   - Some offices prepare for patient arrivals the evening before, and some in the morning. Patient charts must be pulled and should be reviewed, checking for completed laboratory tests and posting of results, and to ensure that progress notes for this visit are ample. Rooms should be checked and inventoried to make certain that sufficient supplies are on hand and that they present a clean, neat appearance.

5. Explain why it is important to use the patient's name as often as possible.
   - People like hearing their own names; a better relationship is built between the staff and patients when the names are used often. Patients feel that the office staff cares enough about them to acknowledge them, and this custom adds a personal touch.

6. Discuss how the medical assistant may help the patient prepare for an examination.
   - The medical assistant should escort the patient to the examination rooms and other areas of the office. Always tell the patient when to disrobe and exactly what should be removed. Offer to assist with disrobing if the patient needs extra help. Take care that the patient's purse or wallet is in a secure place. Be sure that doors do not open and expose the disrobed patient. Instruct the patient as to whether he or she may leave or should wait after seeing the physician. Ask whether the patient has any questions.

7. List and explain two methods of chart placement.
   - Some medical offices place patient charts in a door file, which alerts the physician that the patient is ready to be seen. The chart may be placed horizontally or vertically, one placement meaning that the patient is ready for the physician, and the other meaning that the doctor is finished with the patient. Other offices place the charts in door files in a certain order. For example, if examination rooms one, two, and three are available, patients are seen in that order by the physician.

8. Discuss how the medical assistant might deal with talkative patients.
   - Patients who are talkative may be lonely and enjoy the social interaction of their visits to the physician's office. Be as courteous as possible with talkative patients, expressing to them when necessary that another patient is waiting or that the physician needs assistance. When this is said with a smile, most patients understand.

9. Discuss ways to make the patient feel at ease and comfortable in the medical office.
   - The personal touch will help the patient to feel at home and comfortable in the office. An attractive reception area with various patient amenities will provide a warm atmosphere. Using the patient's name often and a gentle touch will impart a sense of caring as well.

CONNECTIONS

 Study Guide Connection: Go to Chapter 11 Study Guide. Read the Case Study and Workplace Applications and complete the assignments. Do online research for answers to the questions in the Internet Activities associated with patient reception and processing.

 CD Connection: Go to the Medical Assisting Competency Challenge CD and do the training activities under General Office Duties.

Evolve Connection: For more information related to patient reception and processing, go to evolve.elsevier.com/kinn and visit related weblinks for Chapter 11. Click on the Medical Assisting Exam Review and do the practice questions to sharpen your test-taking skills. To learn more about office software, do the exercises for the Altapoint demo that is on the CD.

Office Environment and Daily Operations

12

SCENARIO

Kayla Kemper performed her externship at Dr. Richard Tarago's office, a general practice clinic located downtown that serves patients who do not have medical insurance. Some patients must pay a copayment of $5 to $25, and others pay no copayment, depending on their income level. Kayla's family is quite wealthy, and it was an eye-opening experience for her to see patients who live a very different life than she does. There were many days that she wanted to leave the clinic because she realized that many of the patients were unable to seek medical care when the illness first began, and when they finally came to the clinic they were in worse condition. Kayla is a caring person, and she saw the suffering that many of the patients experienced on a daily basis. She found it hard to see people who had difficulty obtaining healthcare, yet she realized that a large number of Americans have no insurance coverage at all. Kayla discussed her feelings with the clinic manager, Elaine Mays, and expressed her concern for the patients in the clinic. Elaine asked if Kayla would like to continue working with the patients, and Kayla admitted that she would, although it was not easy for her. Elaine then suggested that because Kayla's background was so different from the patients, she might wish to stay at the clinic as a volunteer for a few months to add to her learning experience. She accepted the offer, and after Kayla worked for 3 months as a volunteer, Elaine hired Kayla to work in the clinical area full-time. The patients consistently commented on Kayla's compassion and considerate treatment while they were at the clinic. Kayla truly learned the meaning of giving as it relates to the medical profession, and her externship was the start of her full-time career.

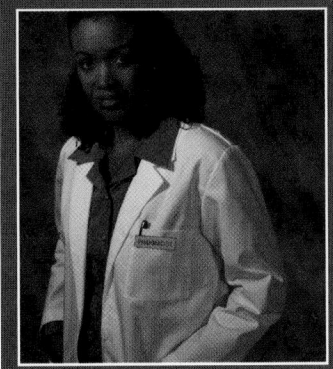

While studying this chapter, think about the following questions:

- What are some of the issues that might prevent a medical assistant from showing compassion to all patients? How can these issues be resolved?
- Why is it a good practice to allow the person who uses a certain supply to order it?
- Why might outsourcing be less expensive than doing testing or procedures in the office?
- How might an extensive list of community resources be helpful to patients?

LEARNING OBJECTIVES

1. Define, spell, and pronounce the terms listed in the vocabulary.
2. List five actions that need to be taken before the office opens in the morning.
3. Explain why patient traffic flow is an important consideration in office design.
4. List some of the expenses involved in the operation of a medical practice.
5. Describe how prices can be compared for medical office supplies.
6. Describe the purpose of white noise.
7. List several ways to save money in the medical office.
8. Explain the difference between medical waste and regular waste.
9. Explain why keys and alarm codes should be shared with only a few people.

National Accreditation Competencies and Content

CAAHEP COMPETENCIES

General

3.c.(3)(a). Explain general office policies
3.c.(3)(b). Instruct individuals according to their needs
3.c.(3)(d). Identify community resources
3.c.(4)(a). Perform an inventory of supplies and equipment
3.c.(4)(b). Perform routine maintenance of administrative and clinical equipment

ABHES COMPETENCIES

Communication

2.m. Adaptation for individualized needs

Administrative Duties

3.a. Perform basic secretarial skills
3.e. Locate resources and information for patients and employers
3.f. Manage physician's professional schedule and travel

Office Management

6.a. Maintain physical plant
6.b. Operate and maintain facilities and perform routine maintenance of administrative and clinical equipment safely
6.c. Inventory equipment and supplies
6.d Evaluate and recommend equipment and supplies for practice

Instruction

7.a. Orient patients to office policies and procedures
7.b. Instruct patients with special needs

VOCABULARY

backorder An ordered item that has not been delivered when promised or demanded but will be supplied at a later date.

bookmarking Marking a document or a specific place within a document for later retrieval; a feature supported by most browsers that allows the user to save the address (or URL) so that the document can be located when it is needed again.

budget A plan for the coordination of resources and expenditures; the amount of money that is available or required for a particular purpose.

circumvent To manage to get around, especially by ingenuity or strategy.

discrepancies Differences among conflicting facts, claims, or opinions.

fiscal year An accounting period of 12 months during which a company determines earnings and profit; the fiscal year does not necessarily begin in January—instead, the beginning of the fiscal year is determined by the business.

incur To become liable or subject to; to bring down on oneself.

outsourcing The practice of subcontracting work to an outside company.

packing slip A list of items that are included in a shipment.

proactive Acting in anticipation of future problems, needs, or changes.

The physician's office is a busy environment where the medical assistant encounters new challenges each day. The more flexible the medical assistant is, the more valuable he or she becomes to the physician. By learning and refining adaptation skills, office efficiency increases and the schedule can handle interruptions and emergencies.

Chapter 11 covered patient reception and processing. Remember that the patient is the reason the office exists and is of primary importance to the office staff. However, various tasks demand attention in the daily operation of the medical office. This chapter explores many of the duties that the medical assistant performs throughout a typical day at work.

OPENING THE OFFICE

The employees arrive earlier than the patients so that the office can be prepared for the day ahead. Some office policies dictate that the office be readied for the next day on the evening before, but for the purposes of this chapter, assume that the policy requires that preparation be done in the mornings.

Although the physician may trust the employees, office policy should demand that supervisors be **proactive** in avoiding the risk of theft. Depending on the size of the clinic, a certain number of employees will have keys and will know the alarm codes to the facility. The best policy is to strictly monitor this access and information. When numerous keys are distributed, more employees will have after-hours access to the office. By limiting this access, the physician may **circumvent** losses by theft. Two items in particular make the physician's office a target—money and drugs. Usually only limited cash is found in the office, but some medications are narcotics, and many, even those that are not narcotics, can be addictive. These items must be protected, not only for safety but also to remain in compliance with the law.

PREPARING FOR THE DAY AHEAD

Once the employees have arrived for work, all of them will begin to prepare for patients and visitors. Each employee is responsible for his or her own work space, and employees may work as a team to prepare common areas of the office, such as the reception area. When each person understands the required duties and they are divided among the staff, work can be completed quickly and efficiently.

Several duties are completed before patient arrival. The answering service should be called to collect any messages that were left since the last time the staff was in the office (Figure 12-1). Make certain that the phone message book is handy when calling the answering service; write each message into the message book, and include all information necessary to properly respond to the message. This action ensures that copies of the messages are available if one happens to get lost. Patient records may need to be pulled so that the medical assistant can take action and follow up on the messages.

Make two copies of the day's appointments, and place one copy on the physician's desk. Use the other copy to pull medical records for the patients who will visit the office during the day. In multiphysician practices, a copy of the day's appointments should be made for each physician. Keep the medical records in a convenient, central area so that staff members can find them easily once the patients begin to arrive. Make certain that there is enough room in the progress notes section of the medical record for the physician to write the details of the office

visit. If not, add a new sheet of progress notes. Glance over the notes from the last visit to ascertain whether laboratory work or treatments were ordered, then verify that the results are available to the physician.

Patient examination rooms should be restocked with all of the regular supplies used in the individual rooms. Items such as cotton balls, adhesive bandages, gauze pads, patient gowns, and drapes need to be replenished daily. The medical assistant should never force the physician and patient to wait in the examination room while the medical assistant searches for supplies. Check the restrooms as well, to make sure that toilet paper, soap, and hand towels are available. If urine specimen cups are kept in patient restrooms, there should be enough available to last throughout the day.

Be sure that prescription pads are available for the physician, although they should not be left in open areas or on counters (Figure 12-2). Patients should never have access to the prescription pads, because an unscrupulous patient might try to forge a prescription. Take extra care that the pads are out of the patient's' sight.

Certain equipment may need to be turned on, such as computers, laboratory equipment, and copy machines. Lights should be turned on in all of the examination rooms. If quality-assurance tests need to be performed on any of the laboratory machines, run the tests and record the results.

Some specimens from previous days may need to be checked for results or additional testing; for example, a blood culture may be ready to view for growth after 1 or 2 days. Always record test results in the patient's medical record. Make certain that the physician sees all test results as dictated in the office policy manual, especially if they fall outside normal ranges. The physician may need to perform follow-up work or see the patient again if the results are not normal.

CRITICAL THINKING APPLICATION

Kayla realizes that there is no set method through which the medical assistants know that laboratory results are ready to be filed. How might she handle this, and what suggestions can Kayla make to Elaine?

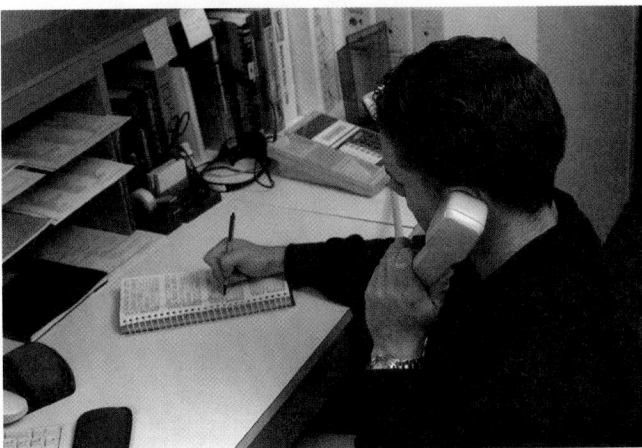

FIGURE 12-1 The telephone is the lifeline of a medical practice. The medical assistant will take several phone messages throughout the course of the day. (From Hunt SA: *Saunders fundamentals of medical assisting,* Philadelphia, 2002, Saunders.)

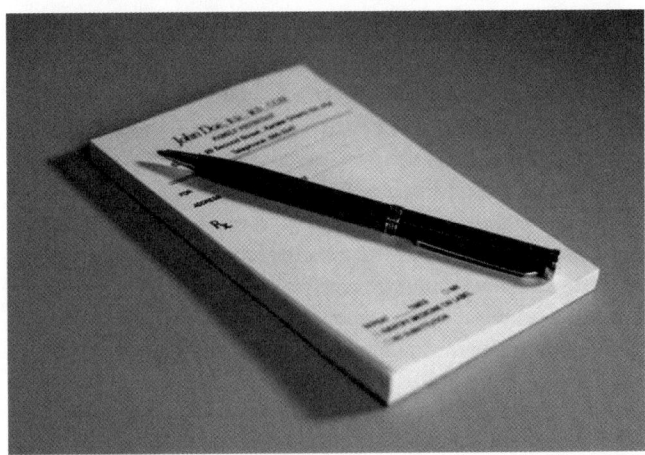

FIGURE 12-2 Keep a close watch on prescription pads so that patients do not have access to them.

The patient accounting software or day sheets should be prepared for the day. Secure enough encounter forms for each patient on the appointment book. Stock the patient checkout area with plenty of appointment cards. If the office gives small gifts to patients, like refrigerator magnets or coffee mugs, be sure that they are available for use. Many offices place the physician's business card just outside the receptionist's window or in the patient reception area. Because patients often take a card, this supply should also be checked.

Various specialty offices may need to prepare additional equipment, so make certain that everything necessary is available for the physician and staff members. Some offices use a checklist to ensure that all of the opening duties are completed. In others the staff knows each person's responsibilities by memorization and carries them out successfully each day. Whichever method is used, the day will go much more smoothly when the office is completely prepared for the patients. Once all of these duties are completed, the last task is to unlock the front door and begin welcoming patients to the practice.

PATIENT TRAFFIC FLOW

The design of the medical office is usually outside the realm of the medical assistant's control; however, the employees of the office can adapt to the physical design and determine the best room layout for efficient patient traffic flow. The reception area is the first room that most patients enter. Some physicians allow patients who are very ill to enter a back doorway or maintain a room separate from the reception area for these patients. This accommodation helps to prevent well patients from contracting a communicable disease.

CRITICAL THINKING APPLICATION

One of the older patients expresses concern that an ill child is coughing so much in the waiting area. How can Kayla help to alleviate the patient's concern? What can Kayla do to resolve the issue?

The fewer steps that patients have to walk as they work their way through the medical office, the better the traffic flow. Avoid making the patient backtrack over their previous steps, if possible. Many offices perform all procedures or treatments in the examination room. If the patient needs blood drawn, the medical assistant brings the equipment to the examination room where the patient is waiting. Some procedures, such as x-ray procedures, require that the patient go to another room. Move the patient from one room to another only when no other options exist.

When moving through hallways, the medical assistant should walk on the right side, leaving the left side for those traveling in the opposite direction—similar to the way people drive in the United States. The same principle applies to patients in wheelchairs or using some other form of walking assistance. Push or direct them along the right side of the hallway.

VISITORS TO THE OFFICE

Many people who are not patients visit the physician's office. Some of these people have appointments, and others stop by at random. The office policy manual should detail the procedure to follow when dealing with such individuals. Most physicians prefer that a specific time be set aside for pharmaceutical representatives (also called *detail persons*). Some will see one representative in the morning and one in the afternoon. Others will speak briefly to representatives in the hallway, then allow them to replenish the supply of drug samples in the storage area. Sometimes the representative will not need to speak to the physician; other times he or she will make an appointment to supply the entire office with lunch so that he or she can spend some time with the physician to explain new drugs. These professionals are usually quite competent in their knowledge of various drugs, and they should be treated with respect (Figure 12-3). Often, they leave giveaways for the staff and patients, such as pens, pencils, notepads, coffee mugs, videos relating to their products, pamphlets, and other novelty items. All of their efforts go toward convincing the physician to prescribe their drugs more often or to begin prescribing a new drug.

CRITICAL THINKING APPLICATION

One of the pharmaceutical representatives is extremely pushy. How can Kayla express that the physician cannot meet with the representative? What can Kayla do if the representative continues to be insistent about seeing the physician?

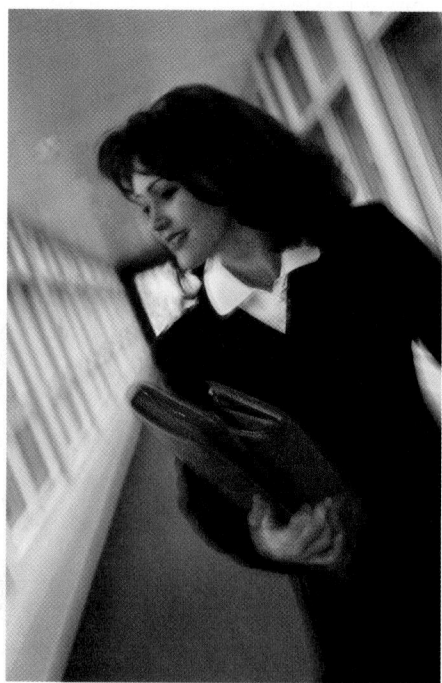

FIGURE 12-3 Pharmaceutical representatives are highly trained, knowledgeable professionals who can help the office staff understand the medications that patients are taking.

PROCEDURE 12-1

Explain General Office Policies

CAAHEP COMPETENCY: 3.c(3)(a)
ABHES COMPETENCY: 7.a

GOAL: *To effectively communicate office policies and procedures to employees, patients, and visitors in the office.*

EQUIPMENT and SUPPLIES

- Office policy manual
- Office procedure manual (if not included in policy manual)
- Patient information sheets (if needed)
- Patient information brochure

PROCEDURAL STEPS

1. Design an office policy manual and patient information brochure that contains general information for employees and patients. At a minimum the following information should be included:
   - Philosophy statement
   - Goals
   - Description of the medical practice
   - Location and/or map
   - Phone numbers
   - Pager numbers
   - Email and website addresses
   - Staff names and credentials
   - Services offered
   - Hours of operation
   - Appointment system
   For employees:
   - Vacation, sick leave
   - Confidentiality
   - Grievances
   - Benefits
   - Payroll information
   - Other employee information
   PURPOSE: To give the employees and patients a written document that details general information that can be used as a reference when needed.
2. Offer the brochure to new employees and patients or to any other employees and patients who do not have a current brochure.
3. Briefly discuss each section of the brochure with new employees and patients.
   PURPOSE: To acclimate the employees and patients to the contents of the policy manual and answer questions that might arise about each section.
4. Watch for verification of understanding from the employee or patient, both verbally and nonverbally.
   PURPOSE: By watching a patient's body language and listening to his or her questions, the medical assistant can determine whether the patient truly understands the information presented.
5. Ask the employee or patient if he or she has any questions.
   PURPOSE: To ensure understanding of the information presented.
6. Document that the employee or patient received the information in the medical record, if required.
   PURPOSE: This action is helpful in proving that an employee or patient was given certain information about policies and procedures.

Pharmaceutical representatives are not the only salespersons that may visit the physician's office. Sales people from office supply stores, medical equipment sellers, and others may stop by the office to make appointments or to take orders for various items. Usually the office manager can address the needs of salespeople and is authorized to place orders.

At times other physicians will stop by the office to see the doctor. They may not have an appointment, but the physician should be notified at once when another doctor is waiting in the reception area. If office policy allows, take the visiting physician to the doctor's office instead of forcing him or her to wait in the patient reception area. Usually the physician will agree to see the visiting doctor, if only for a few moments. Because doctors understand busy schedules, most will not stop by another doctor's office without having important information to share.

The physician's family members or friends may stop by the medical office, but they have usually been given restrictions by the physician as to when they can stop by and for what reasons. Never send family members or friends away without notifying the physician of their presence and asking whether he or she has time to speak to them.

USING THE OFFICE POLICY MANUAL

All employees should read the office policy manual when they begin to work in the physician's office. By reading the manual the medical assistant will become informed about the expectations of supervisors. However, the office policy manual is not used only for new employees (Procedures 12-1 and 12-2). The manual should be a daily source of information for all employees to reference whenever needed. The policy manual should be reviewed at least annually to make certain that all of the information contained within it is accurate and up to date. Whenever revisions are made, insert a page in the manual that tells the date that revisions became effective.

After review and acceptance of the revised manual, it is helpful to distribute a memo detailing what changes were made and where to look for the changes.

PROCEDURE 12-2

Instruct Individuals According to Their Needs

CAAHEP COMPETENCY: 3.c(3)(b)
ABHES COMPETENCY: 2.m

GOAL: To effectively communicate office policies and procedures to employees, patients, and visitors in the office so that they understand instructions from the physician.

EQUIPMENT and SUPPLIES

- Office policy manual
- Office procedure manual (if not included in policy manual)
- Patient information sheets (if needed)
- Physician orders, if applicable
- Patient information brochure

PROCEDURAL STEPS

1. Determine the communication needs of the employee, patient, or visitor.
   PURPOSE: To discover the best way to communicate information to an employee, patient, or visitor who may have special needs.
2. Arrange for an interpreter, if needed.
   PURPOSE: To make certain that information is communicated and received accurately.
3. Provide instructions to the employee, patient, or visitor.
4. Watch for verification of understanding from the patient, both verbally and nonverbally.
   PURPOSE: By watching body language and listening to questions, the medical assistant can determine whether the employee, patient, or visitor truly understands the information presented
5. Ask if there are any questions.
   PURPOSE: To ensure understanding of the information presented.
6. Document that the employee, patient, or visitor (if necessary) received the instructions in the medical record, if required.
   PURPOSE: This action is helpful in proving that an employee or patient was given certain instructions about policies, procedures, and expectations or directions regarding treatment.

The office policy manual should include sections that deal with several topics:

- Expected performance of the employee
- Tardiness and absenteeism
- Sexual harassment
- Confidentiality
- Vacations, sick time, paid time off
- Employee evaluation
- Continuing education
- Chain of command
- How to deal with certain patients and visitors

Some offices require that employees sign a document that states they have read and understand the policy in its entirety. The manual should be written in clear, concise language that is easily understood and should be used whenever a question about policy matters arises or the employee is unsure about why or how to proceed when completing a task. Often a procedure manual is combined with policy manuals. There should be no office tasks that are not detailed in either the policy manual or the procedure manual.

DAILY, WEEKLY, AND MONTHLY DUTIES

Develop a list of duties that are done daily, weekly, and monthly. Checklists are helpful when staff members want to make certain that all duties are completed. The lists help the supervisors divide chores evenly among staff members. Be specific on the checklist, and include every task that needs to be done, even the smallest ones. Staff members should cheerfully accept assignments they are given and should complete them quickly and efficiently. If one staff member is struggling with finishing her daily duties, other staff members should assist so that all required jobs are finished for the day. Usually, that employee will later help others complete their own duties when help is needed.

Constant Cleaning

Patients expect the physician's office to be immaculate. Nothing should be or appear dirty in any part of the facility. If the office is truly clean, it is less likely that germs and communicable diseases will spread, though not impossible. Effective cleaning products should be used on a daily basis, especially in high-traffic areas. There will never be a lack of equipment or furniture that could use a wipe down with a disinfectant or a light dusting. Countertops, sinks, door handles, and restrooms should be checked frequently and cleaned whenever needed. During slow periods between patients or during lengthy office visits, take a cloth and use a disinfectant on nearby counters and on the areas on doors near the handle. Look for things to clean in the office. By being conscientious about these things, the medical assistant will become more valuable to the physician. Supervisors and physicians will notice this productivity; good cleaning habits reflect positively on the medical assistant and will be important factors during employee evaluations.

Cleaning Services

Many offices employ a cleaning service that performs more intensive chores for the office. These professionals usually come

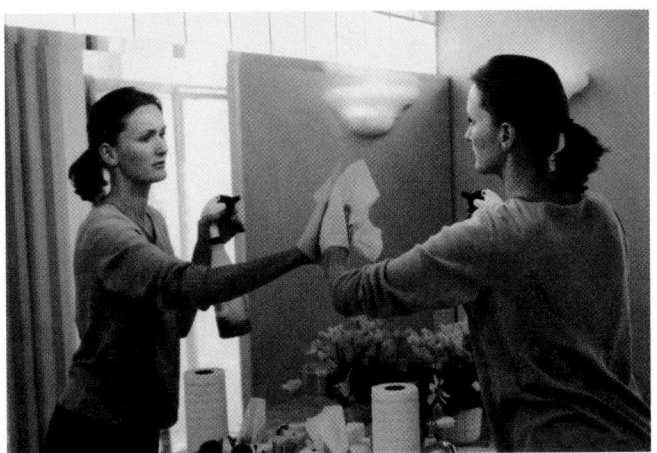

FIGURE 12-4 Cleaning services usually work in the evenings and keep the office looking professional and attractive.

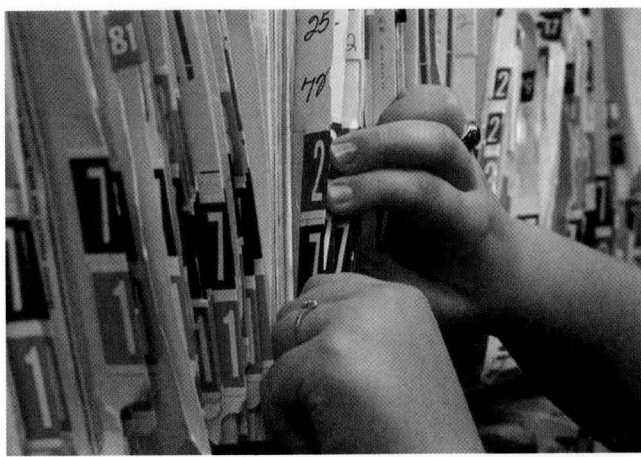

FIGURE 12-5 Filing is a critical job that must be done on a daily basis.

to the facility during the evening when patients and staff are not present. They clean and disinfect the bathrooms, vacuum, dust, empty trash, and may perform other specific tasks as required by the office staff (Figure 12-4). Some form of communication should exist between the office manager and the person who heads the cleaning team. Many offices leave a notebook for the cleaning crew that will detail what specific cleaning tasks should be performed in addition to the regular cleaning tasks. The office manager should delegate a staff member to be the contact person for the service. If any task is not completed in a satisfactory manner, the contact person should immediately contact the cleaning supervisor and resolve the problem. Make certain that a log is kept so that tasks are listed and a notation is made regarding whether they were completed or why they were not completed. Always inspect; the cleaning service must perform the jobs that they are being paid to do. Do not allow situations to go unresolved. Be open and frank with services that do not meet expectations.

CRITICAL THINKING APPLICATION

Kayla has noticed that on the days after the cleaning crew has come, sodas, plastic tableware, and other small items seem to be missing from the kitchen area. Today, she notices that an entire box of toilet paper is gone from the office. Kayla knows the box was there the day before, because she personally checked in the shipment. How can Kayla handle this situation? How is the situation complicated if one of the people who cleans the office at night is a co-worker's sister?

Filing

The medical assistant will rarely find a shortage of documents that are ready to file in the physician's office. Although this task is sometimes monotonous, filing is a critical job that must be completed accurately and in a timely manner (Figure 12-5). If a laboratory result is not placed in the right medical record, important information that may affect the patient's health could be lost. Chapter 14 explains rules that apply to the filing process and describes the equipment and supplies needed to perform this task.

SUPPLIES AND EQUIPMENT IN THE PHYSICIAN'S OFFICE

Physicians become frustrated when they reach for an item in an examination room and do not find it in its proper place. The medical assistant is responsible for stocking examination rooms and making certain that all supplies and equipment are available and in good working order. The following section describes the process of ordering and receiving medical supplies and equipment.

Identifying the Need for Specific Supplies

The medical assistant orders supplies periodically to ensure that the physician has everything he or she needs to treat patients. The office policy and procedure manual details the way that employees should identify the need for certain supplies, order them, check them in, and place them into the office inventory for use. Communication is the key to keeping supplies in stock. Once a method for ordering is established, all employees must adhere to the plan so that employees and patients are not affected by an item or product being out of stock.

Budgeting

Most offices operate using an annual **budget** to determine the amount of money that is to be spent on various categories of expenses (Figure 12-6). Some of the expenses that are involved in the operation of a medical practice include the following:

- Salaries
- Medical supplies
- Business equipment
- Medical equipment
- Utilities
- Rent or mortgage
- Insurance
- Maintenance
- Taxes
- Laboratory fees
- Office supplies

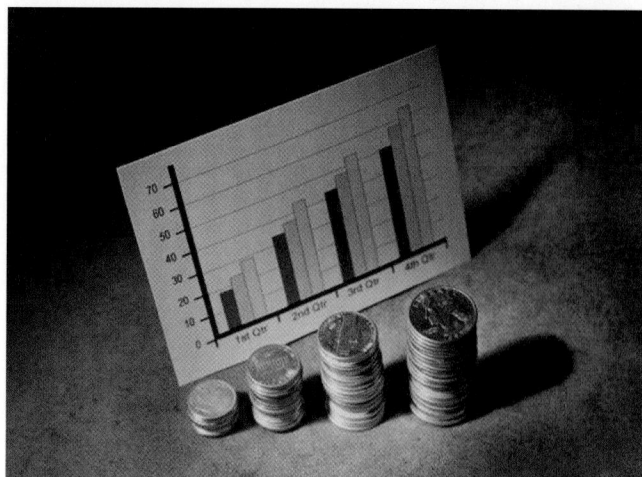

FIGURE 12-6 Smart budgeting is important to every physician.

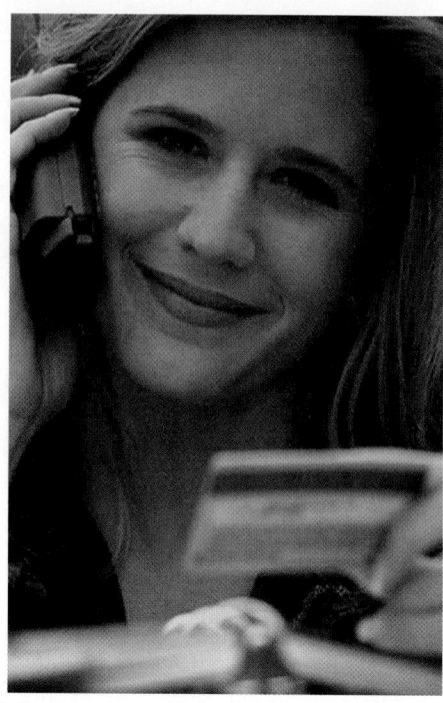

FIGURE 12-7 Compare prices before deciding on suppliers, then make a confident purchase.

Expense categories may be very specific and detailed or may constitute a more general list, such as the one above. A specific category listing would separate expenses for electricity, gas, and water, as opposed to grouping these expenses together as "utilities." These categories are important because most business expenses can be deducted on tax returns. Always keep receipts when shopping for items that will be used in the medical office and submit them in a timely manner to the office manager or other designated individual.

CRITICAL THINKING APPLICATION

Elaine has asked Kayla to prepare a budget for next year for her department. Kayla has never done this before. How can she get through her first challenging task?

The majority of people operate their households using some type of budget. The process of planning the coordination of resources and expenditures defines budgeting. Businesses usually plan expenses for the year in advance, allocating expected income into various categories of expenses. Then, on at least a monthly basis, expenses are logged onto a ledger or spreadsheet and separated into specific categories. This process allows tracking of expenses to make certain that a category is not over budget. If a specific category of expenses is over budget, adjustments may need to be logged to allow more funds in that category, or spending may need to be stopped in that category until the next year. It is not necessarily uncommon for budgets to exceed allowed amounts, but good business practice dictates that budgets be very close to estimations made at the beginning of the budget year. When a category goes over budget, money must often be taken from another budget category to cover the amount. This reduces the money available in the second category. Employees should not be allowed to spend money needlessly or wastefully. The physician should designate a minimum of persons authorized to make purchases on behalf of the facility.

Comparing Prices

A good shopper is an asset to the physician's office. Compare prices when shopping for supplies and equipment. Make it clear to salespersons that comparisons will be conducted and that price will be a strong consideration when the time comes to make a purchase (Figure 12-7). However, price may not be the only consideration. Warranties, bulk purchase opportunities, maintenance agreements, and other factors may influence the best deal available on a certain item. Quality is another important factor; the physician may be willing to pay more for an item based on its quality and durability. Personal preference also influences purchasing decisions. The clinical medical assistant may prefer one brand of needles over another even though they are the same price. In most circumstances, the person or persons who regularly use a certain item should be allowed to make decisions as to the brand, model, or other specifics before the item is purchased.

Most companies use a catalog, whether it is a paper catalog or one that is available online. Once a need is identified, compare the prices from at least three sources before placing an order. For instance, if 70% isopropyl alcohol is the product, and a stock is needed to last for 6 months, first determine how much is needed. Suppose that approximately one 16-ounce bottle of the alcohol is used per month in each of five treatment rooms. Further suppose that the following prices are listed:

Smith's Medical Supply	1 dozen bottles	$10.53
Argosy Medical and Dental Supply	2 dozen bottles	$17.44
Walgreen's	1 bottle	$0.53
Gibson's Pharmacy	1 gallon	$6.12

By comparing these prices, assuming that all other aspects of the products are equal, it is clear that buying bottles of alcohol at Walgreen's is a better deal than buying one or two dozen at either Smith's Medical Supply or Argosy Medical and Dental Supply. The alcohol at Smith's costs approximately $0.87 per bottle, and at Argosy a bottle costs approximately $0.72. Is the gallon a better buy? The alcohol can always be poured into containers from the gallon bottle. However, because there are 128 ounces in a gallon, only eight bottles with 16 ounces each could be divided from the gallon container. This means that the cost of the eight bottles is approximately $0.76 each. Walgreen's offers the best price. Still, if the only Walgreen's location is 35 miles away, the gas used in getting the product may make the overall cost to obtain the alcohol higher than driving 2 miles to Argosy. In addition, consider delivery, shipping, and handling charges that might be added to the total cost of the order. Some suppliers may cut the cost on certain items to get the order, either meeting or beating the deal offered by another supplier. Examine all costs before awarding the order to a supplier.

Ordering Supplies

The responsibility for ordering supplies in the medical office should be assigned to one person. The medical assistant who assumes this task can use various methods to track the supplies that are needed and place orders to replenish them. The simplest method is to develop a spreadsheet listing all of the products and supplies that need to be ordered periodically. Post the sheets in areas where supplies are stored. When staff members take supplies from storage, they should make a note on the spreadsheet. When it is time to place an order, the sheets are gathered and used to determine which supplies need to be replenished. Some offices use software to prepare orders, and others use a computer system to enter products that are taken from the supply area. Still others may use a sticker system, whereby a coded sticker is removed when a product is used and placed on a card or form, then that amount is charged to the patient. Others use a notecard system, wherein a notecard is prepared for each supply item and after inventory is performed; orders are completed based on the needs reflected on the note cards (Procedure 12-3). The physician should use the system that works best in that particular office. After determining the items that need to be ordered, browse medical or office supply catalogs to shop for the best prices. The order may need to be divided and offered to two different suppliers if certain items can be obtained at a better rate (Procedure 12-4).

Remember that the Internet is a source for shopping for supplies, too. Often businesses can find excellent prices by ordering online. Some physicians and office managers may be hesitant to use credit card accounts online; however, if an account is established with an online supply company, they will hold payment information or perhaps extend credit, and the company credit card need not be used. Investigate this helpful source, and use it to lower costs wherever possible.

Ordering Equipment

Ordering equipment is more involved than ordering simple supplies. Much of the equipment acquired for the physician's office is considered a capital purchase. Before purchasing this type of equipment, compare price, features, and benefits.

The physician is almost always involved in the purchase of capital equipment. Different businesses use different monetary amounts to classify capital purchases; some use $1000, whereas others may consider a capital purchase to be one that is over $5000. Physicians consult with accountants to determine limits on capital purchase amounts. At least three estimates should be obtained before making a major equipment purchase.

The physician and staff members who will use the equipment will have questions about the features and benefits, as well as the cost to purchase and the cost to use in the facility. Sometimes, the cost to use certain equipment may exceed the cost of **outsourcing.** For instance, the cost to perform a complete blood count (CBC) in the office may be $10. If the test can be outsourced and sent to an outpatient lab, resulting in a cost of $8, the physician could avoid equipment and maintenance costs. In addition, if the physician continues to charge $10, he will make a profit of $2 on every CBC performed. Physicians should not order unnecessary testing, but it is certainly ethical to make a profit on procedures and treatments performed. Remember, the physician's office is a business, and there is nothing unethical about making a profit.

CRITICAL THINKING APPLICATION

Kayla is talking with a patient who tells her husband that she doesn't know how they will afford the laboratory tests the doctor wants run. When Kayla walks by them, they stop talking. How can Kayla help the patient in this situation?

The medical assistant has numerous options when looking for equipment to purchase. Local suppliers offer catalogs detailing the products and equipment available, and the suppliers' sales representatives will be able to answer questions. Investigate whether used equipment might be for sale from the supplier. Physicians who are selling their practice or retiring might have equipment for sale. Research the Internet, even eBay, to find bargains on quality equipment (Figure 12-8). Obviously,

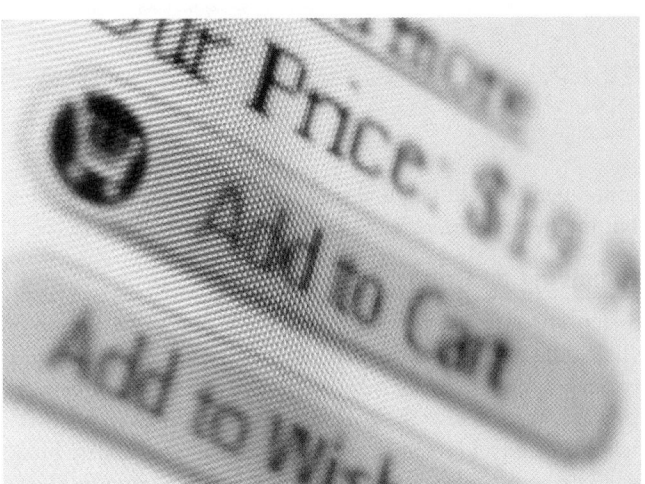

FIGURE 12-8 Check prices on the Internet and compare with those of local suppliers.

PROCEDURE 12-3

Perform an Inventory of Supplies and Equipment

CAAHEP COMPETENCY: 3.c.(4)(a)
ABHES COMPETENCY: 6.c

GOAL: *To establish an inventory of all expendable supplies in the physician's office and follow an efficient plan or order control using a card system.*

EQUIPMENT and SUPPLIES

- File box
- Inventory and order control cards
- List of supplies on hand
- Metal tabs
- Pen or pencil

PROCEDURAL STEPS

1. Write the name of each item on a separate card (Figure 1*).
   PURPOSE: To establish a record of all items in inventory.
2. Write the amount of each item on hand in the space provided.
   PURPOSE: To establish beginning inventory.
3. Place a reorder tag at the point where the supply should be replenished (Figure 2*).
   PURPOSE: The tag will serve as an alert that supply is low.
4. Place a metal tab over the *order* section of the card.
   PURPOSE: The metal tab will be a reminder to include this item in the next order.
5. When the order has been placed, note the date and quantity ordered and move the tab to the *on order* section of the card.
6. When the order is received, note the date and quantity in the appropriate column, remove the tab, and refile the card.
   NOTE: If the order is only partially filled, let the tab remain until the order is complete.

*Courtesy of Colwell Systems, Champaign, Illinois.

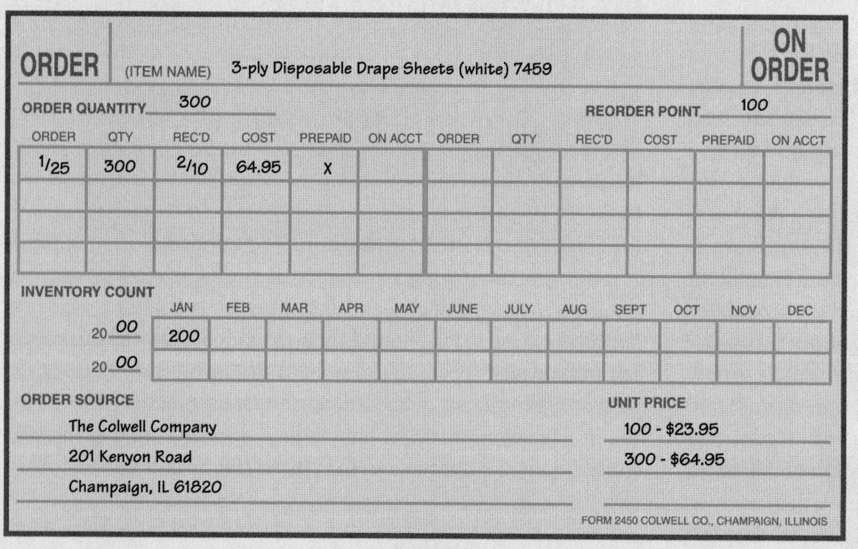

ORDER (ITEM NAME) 3-ply Disposable Drape Sheets (white) 7459 — ON ORDER

ORDER QUANTITY 300 — REORDER POINT 100

ORDER	QTY	REC'D	COST	PREPAID	ON ACCT	ORDER	QTY	REC'D	COST	PREPAID	ON ACCT
1/25	300	2/10	64.95	X							

INVENTORY COUNT

	JAN	FEB	MAR	APR	MAY	JUNE	JULY	AUG	SEPT	OCT	NOV	DEC
20 00	200											
20 00												

ORDER SOURCE
The Colwell Company
201 Kenyon Road
Champaign, IL 61820

UNIT PRICE
100 - $23.95
300 - $64.95

FORM 2450 COLWELL CO., CHAMPAIGN, ILLINOIS

FIGURE 1

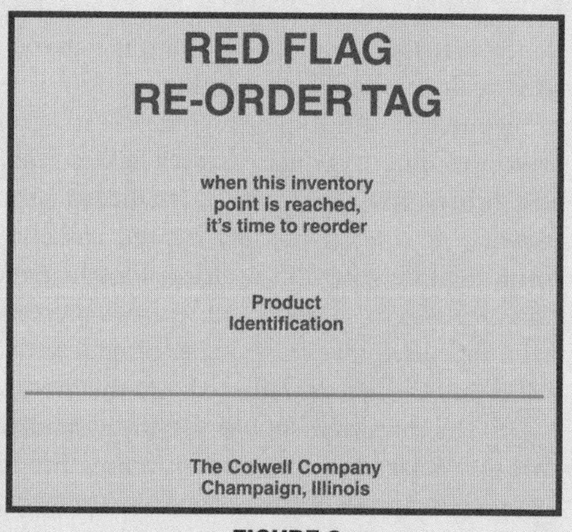

FIGURE 2

some items should be purchased only from a medical supplier, but many great deals are available from various sources.

Receiving an Order

When an order arrives from a supplier, notify the person in charge of inventory. Boxes should be opened only if there is enough time to check them in properly. Carefully open the package, and look for the **packing slip.** A packing slip is a list of items ordered and items shipped. Occasionally, an ordered item will not be included in the package because it has been placed on **backorder.** The item may be out of stock but will be sent to the physician as soon as it becomes available. Compare the items listed on the packing slip with the items found inside the box. If any **discrepancies** are found, bring them to the attention of the supplier immediately. Discourage other employees from taking items from the package before they are checked against the packing slip. Once the order is checked in, make a note on the packing slip that the package was received as expected, then place new stock in the proper place.

Warranty Information

Many purchased items include a warranty. The medical assistant should always mail warranty information to the manufacturer. Warranty cards usually resemble a postcard and contain several

PROCEDURE 12-4

Prepare a Purchase Order

<u>CAAHEP COMPETENCY:</u> 3.c(4)(a)
<u>ABHES COMPETENCY:</u> 6.c

GOAL: *To prepare an accurate purchase order for supplies or equipment.*

EQUIPMENT and SUPPLIES

- List of current inventory
- Purchase order
- Pen
- Phone
- Fax machine

PROCEDURAL STEPS

1. Review the current inventory and determine what items need to be ordered.
   <u>PURPOSE:</u> To determine what is needed so that the office will not be overstocked or understocked.
2. Complete the purchase order accurately, filling in all applicable spaces and blanks with the information requested.
   <u>PURPOSE:</u> An accurately completed purchase order helps to eliminate mistakes in the order and in shipments.
3. List the items to be ordered, including quantity, item numbers, size, color, price, and extended price. Be sure that all applicable information is included.
   <u>PURPOSE:</u> To help ensure accurate orders.
4. Provide the physician's signature, DEA certificate, and medical license when needed.
   <u>PURPOSE:</u> Some items require these documents to verify that the physician is eligible to order them.
5. Call in, fax, mail, or electronically submit the order to the vendor. Keep a copy for your records. Keep any verification provided that the order was received.
   <u>PURPOSE:</u> To document exactly what was ordered on what date and provide proof that the order was received.
6. Note on the inventory which items are on order.
   <u>PURPOSE:</u> To keep other staff members from preparing duplicate orders.
7. Keep a copy of the order in the appropriate place in the office filing system.
   <u>PURPOSE:</u> To reference the order if needed and have a copy of the items ordered to compare with the packing list once the items arrive at the office.

---

questions about the purchaser. By completing the warranty card and mailing it, the manufacturer will be able to contact those who have purchased a certain product if defects are discovered. The warranty period begins on the date of purchase and usually lasts 1 year but can be lengthier, depending on the item purchased. Keep a copy of the completed warranty in a file that contains other information on the specific product or piece of equipment, such as the receipt of purchase, expense records, owner's manuals, and maintenance records.

Invoices and Statements

An invoice is an itemized list of goods shipped that specifies price and the terms of a sale. A statement is a summary of a financial account that shows the balance due, as well as transactions that affect the account. Invoices precede statements. A medical supplier may send an invoice when a sale has been completed, and statements are mailed whenever a balance exists on an account. Some invoices request payment on receipt, and some allow a certain period of time to make a payment (Figure 12-9). Read invoices and statements carefully and make certain that there are no errors before making payment.

Troubleshooting Equipment Failure

When equipment fails to function properly, consult the owner's manual to determine the steps for troubleshooting. The owner's manual is usually found in the package that the product was in when purchased. Many are published on the Internet, which allows

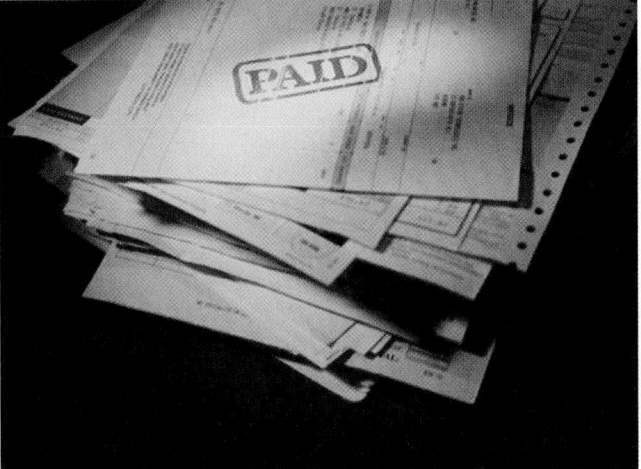

FIGURE 12-9 Invoices and statements must be compared carefully with orders actually received at the physician's office.

for quick access to details about the item. The owner's manual includes contact information so that the purchaser can reach the manufacturer if necessary. Today, purchasers have additional contact options, such as email and chat rooms; both offer fast access for problems that need to be quickly solved. Remember to consider the reasonable, simplest solutions first—is the equipment plugged in? Does the computer need to be rebooted? Often, the solution is a straightforward one that can be easily deduced.

Perform Routine Maintenance of Administrative and Clinical Equipment

CAAHEP COMPETENCY: 3.c.(4)(b)
ABHES COMPETENCY: 6.b

GOAL: *To ensure that all office equipment is in good working order at all times.*

EQUIPMENT and SUPPLIES

- Notecard or spreadsheet containing information on each piece of office equipment, including serial number and periods that the equipment needs servicing
- Pen or pencil
- Computer
- Access to all office equipment

PROCEDURAL STEPS

1. Gather information about each piece of equipment. The following information is needed at a minimum:
   - Name of equipment
   - Type of equipment
   - Manufacturer or maker's name
   - Address of manufacturer
   - Contact phone numbers for technical support
   - Contact phone numbers for main office
   - Date purchased
   - Cost of product
   - Original receipt showing where the item was purchased
   - Date warranty begins and ends
   - Addresses to send equipment if under warranty
   - Number of times the equipment needs service in a year
   - Last date of service
   - Explanation of what was done during last servicing
   - A number assigned by the office manager to identify the equipment

PURPOSE: To give the medical assistant all of the information needed for maintenance and service for the equipment.

2. Place all of the information about each piece of equipment into a document or spreadsheet.
   PURPOSE: This provides a written recording of all information about each piece of equipment.

3. Make a list containing each month of the year. Note which equipment needs servicing in which months.
   PURPOSE: To provide a calendar for servicing equipment.

4. On the first of each month, check the spreadsheet and list to determine which equipment needs servicing that month.

5. Schedule servicing and maintenance for equipment during the current month.
   PURPOSE: To provide a specific time that the equipment will be available for servicing.

6. Check with co-workers to make certain that servicing dates work with all schedules, especially if a piece of equipment will be out of service for any length of time.
   PURPOSE: To prevent scheduling conflicts during times when the equipment is needed by the staff.

7. Oversee scheduling appointments to make certain they are kept.

8. Record new information on the document or spreadsheet to reflect new times for servicing and any additional information.
   PURPOSE: To ensure that the most accurate information is on file about every piece of equipment in the physician's office.

Equipment Maintenance

Medical office equipment must be maintained regularly, especially machines that perform testing procedures. The Clinical Laboratory Improvement Act (CLIA) requires that controls and calibrations be performed, and all of these requirements are designed to ensure that patient testing is accurate and that the results are reliable. The maintenance process is similar to maintaining a car in good working condition. Periodically, oil, filters, and tires must be changed, brake pads must be removed and replaced, and engines must be kept clean. Similarly, medical office machines must be kept in good repair and working condition (Procedure 12-5).

Maintenance guidelines are found in most owners' manuals, and they should be the basis of any maintenance plan. The medical assistant can develop a maintenance schedule to ensure that all office equipment receives proper, timely attention. Keep all information about each equipment item in a separate file, and add maintenance records to it as they are produced.

PREVENTING WASTE

Waste prevention reduces or eliminates waste before it is generated. Companies can reduce the cost of waste management, reduce long-term liability for disposal of hazardous waste materials, and become more efficient to enhance profit margins. The key to successful waste management is the cooperation of employees–unless they are willing to participate in waste management efforts, the efforts will be unsuccessful.

Physician office employees can reduce waste while saving money in the following ways:

- Use solar powered calculators and battery rechargers
- Use refillable pens, pencils, and tape dispensers
- Use refillable calendars
- Use two-way envelopes
- Reuse file folders and binders
- Refurbish office equipment
- Use bulletin boards

- Change to cloth towel dispensers
- Reuse printer toner and ribbon cartridges
- Retrofit exit sign bulbs
- Convert to high efficiency fluorescent lighting
- Reuse dishware
- Use reusable forced air filters
- Eliminate single-use cups
- Reuse paper printed on only one side

Avoiding waste and being conservative with products at the office will save money and may result in an increase in employee wages and benefits. Always participate in efforts to preserve products and be open to trying new conservation methods.

LUNCH AND BREAK ETIQUETTE

Even though the physician's office is a busy place and often hectic, all staff members should take a morning and afternoon break, as well as a lunch period. Many offices close between noon and 2:00 PM so that the staff can have lunch and use the moments to rest, refocus, and catch up (Figure 12-10). Try to alternate lunch times so that some assistants go to lunch during the first hour and some during the second hour. Be respectful of lunch hours and break times by leaving and returning at the appropriate time. Remember to clean any dishes used and put them away, as well as food items that should be returned to the refrigerator. Medical supplies that need to be refrigerated cannot be stored with food. Leftovers should be removed at least once a week. All employees should have a hand in keeping the lunch or break area clean.

SENDING AND RECEIVING EMAIL

Electronic communications are sent and received frequently throughout the business day. Email messages are similar to memos, and when used in the professional office they should

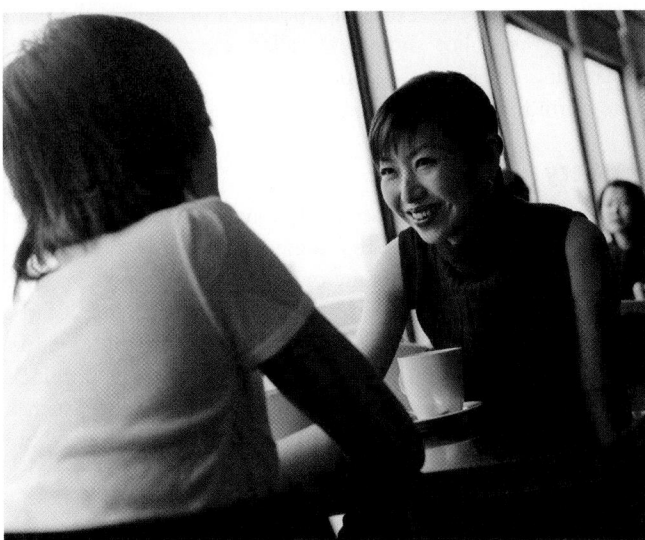

FIGURE 12-10 Use lunch periods and breaks to relax. Don't skip lunch or breaks, because this practice can lead to burnout.

project a professional tone. More information about the format of emails is available in Chapter 13. Use the office email system for work-related messages only. Never forward comic email or messages that are sexual in nature using the office email system. A good general rule to follow is to refrain from sending any email at the workplace that supervisors should not read. Remember that the information services staff of a facility can often find emails and other improper files on computers even if they have been deleted. A file is not completely gone from a computer until another file is written over it. In addition, computers can be monitored in real time, with every keystroke recorded and every website visited logged. Several free email sites allow the user to create an email account with substantial storage space. Use the separate, personal email address for non–business-related information. The medical assistant should treat email information as confidential if it relates to a patient.

INTERNET RESEARCH

The medical assistant may be asked to research various types of information using the Internet. If a word or phrase is entered into a search engine, it produces a results screen containing links to various websites that contain the word or phrase in the search. The medical assistant can then enter the websites and look for the required information. Not all of the articles found on the Internet are reliable; some are completely false and others are simply one person or group's opinion. Look for information from sites that can be trusted, such as the American Heart Association or the American Medical Association. Once a good, informative site is found, read through it carefully, because it may lead to more sites that will provide additional information. **Bookmarking** the site allows it to be easily referenced at a later time. In the Internet Explorer environment, a site is bookmarked by clicking on "Favorites" then clicking on "Add to favorites."

Various types of information can be found on the Internet, such as the following:

- Company reports
- Financial information
- Company profiles
- Conference proceedings
- Seminar announcements
- Law, government announcements, and parliamentary debates
- News and current affairs
- Databases of reference material
- Places to discuss topics and ask for help

Before beginning a search online for information, jot down several keywords that are relevant to the research topic. For instance, consider the subject "medical office management." A search for those three words on www.yahoo.com reveals over 37,000,000 sites with information on the topic. Once a listing has been obtained, the medical assistant can begin to research the sites and determine which ones contain pertinent information. When writing a paper using information contained on websites, be sure to cite the website in the proper place at the end of the paper.

TRAVELING FOR BUSINESS PURPOSES

Throughout the course of a **fiscal year,** employees may attend seminars or workshops to gain additional information, learn new techniques or procedures, and obtain continuing education units (CEUs), which may be needed to maintain certification (Figure 12-11). There is more to these workshops than registering and attending. Shifts must be covered for employees attending the seminar, and travel arrangements must be secured.

Seminars and Workshops

Both physicians and office staff members will periodically attend seminars or workshops to participate in continuing education events or learn new skills. Physicians are required to accumulate a certain number of continuing education credits each year, and medical assistants may need continuing education credits as well, depending on the type of certification that he or she has earned. When planning to attend a seminar, consider not only the cost of the sessions, but also the cost of travel to and from the seminar and hotel, gas, and food costs. Invitations to attend seminars often arrive in the mail, although some arrive by email. Watch for enrollment deadlines, and make certain that registration is done before the deadline date. Some seminars offer great discounts if registration is completed early.

Scheduling Travel, Hotel Rooms, and Car Rentals

The location of the event will often dictate the type of travel arrangements that should be made (Procedure 12-6). Distant locations usually require an airline flight. A travel agent is sometimes used to book flights and hotel rooms, but companies are booking their own flights using the Internet more than ever

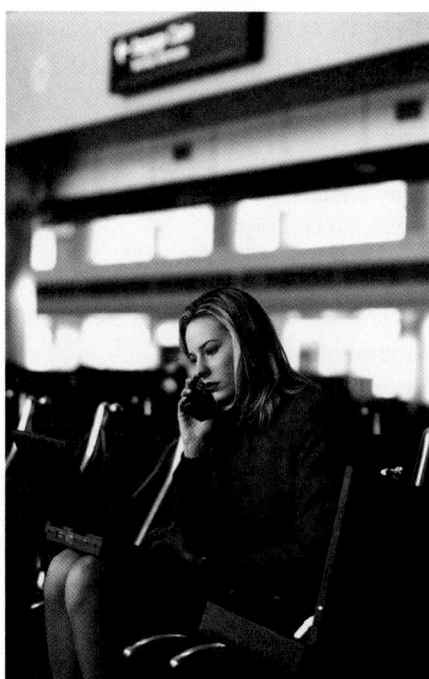

FIGURE 12-11 The medical assistant may need to travel to attend seminars or workshops.

before. Other trips involve car travel. Staff members who travel by car are entitled to reimbursement for mileage expenses. In fact, if staff members **incur** any reasonable business expense, they should be reimbursed by the company.

The brochures for many events that the physician and staff will attend list suggested hotels. If the physician has a preference for a certain hotel, reservations should be made at that location if possible. However, do not hesitate to suggest a different hotel if one is closer to the event or offers a better price for the same amenities.

A car rental may be necessary so that staff members can travel from place to place while attending the seminar. Take care when using a debit card to pay for rentals or deposits. Many establishments will place a hold on the estimated total balance due, even when the balance is paid in cash. This process could place a hold on available funds until the payment actually clears.

BASIC SAFETY AND SECURITY IN THE MEDICAL OFFICE

No one knows when our safety and the security we enjoy will be jeopardized. The saying "Better safe than sorry" has never been truer than today. Don't think that any place of business is immune to crime.

Suspicious Persons

If a suspicious person enters the office, make every effort to keep a distance. Staff members should stay behind the counter or desk so that the person cannot grab or gain control of one of the employees. When feeling serious concern about a suspicious individual, attempt to notify another employee early in the conversation. Pick up the telephone and dial the office manager's extension. Plan a code in advance for different emergency situations. For instance, use the phrase "Norman is here to see you," which relates to Norman Bates of the *Psycho* films, an individual who was at least frightening. This will alert the office manager that there is a potential problem at the front desk and the police should be called. Even if it isn't a life-threatening emergency, the police would rather respond to a false alarm than arrive to find a situation that is out of control.

Robbery

Although physician's offices rarely have an excess of cash on hand, thieves may assume that there is money to steal or, more likely, narcotics. Do not argue or fight with such people. Give them what they want—the object is to get them out of the office as quickly as possible. Once they are out, lock the doors and call the police. Do not touch any items that the criminals touched so that the crime scene is preserved. When such a situation occurs, the employees will clearly be under stress, but make every effort to remember basic identifying markers, such as the following:

- Height
- Weight
- Hair color and length

PROCEDURE 12-6

Locate Resources and Information for Patients and Employers:
Make Travel Arrangements

ABHES COMPETENCY: 3.f

GOAL: *To make travel arrangements for the physician or another staff member.*

EQUIPMENT and SUPPLIES

- Travel plan
- Telephone
- Telephone directory
- Typewriter or computer
- Typing paper

PROCEDURAL STEPS

1. Verify the dates of the planned trip. Consider the following:
   - Desired date and time of departure
   - Desired date and time of return
   - Preferred mode of transportation
   - Number in party
   - Preferred lodging and price range
   - Preferred ticketing method (electronic or paper).
2. Telephone a trusted travel agency to arrange for transportation and lodging reservations, or book the trip using Internet resources.
   PURPOSE: A travel agent might be better suited to answer questions involving regulations for international travel. The Internet is an easy way to book trips on your own.
3. Arrange for traveler's checks, if desired.
   PURPOSE: Traveler's checks are a better alternative than carrying large sums of cash and can be easily replaced if lost or stolen.
4. Pick up tickets or e-receipts or arrange for their delivery.
5. Check tickets to confirm conformance with the travel plan.
   PURPOSE: To avoid any error resulting from misunderstanding and to verify compliance with requests.
6. Check to see that hotel and air reservations are confirmed.
7. Prepare an itinerary, including all the necessary information:
   - Date and time of departure
   - Flight numbers or identifying information for other modes of travel
   - Mode of transportation to hotel(s)
   - Name, address, and telephone number of hotel(s), with confirmation numbers if available
   - Name, address, and telephone number of travel agency
   - Date and time of return.
   PURPOSE: The itinerary provides the details of the entire trip at a glance and is a more organized way to keep up with times, dates, confirmation numbers, and other details all on one document.
8. Place one copy of itinerary in the office file, and give one to the office manager.
   PURPOSE: It may be necessary to contact the traveler or to forward mail.
9. Give several copies of the itinerary to the traveler.
   PURPOSE: The traveler may wish to have extra copies for family or friends.

- Clothing, especially the color
- Race
- Distinctive marks (scars, tattoos, etc.)

Make the observations as subtly as possible; criminals who think they are being sized up for later identification may not react well!

If the criminals don't leave the office and the situation escalates, make every effort to find out what they want that will prompt them to leave. Remain as calm as possible throughout the ordeal. If the employee remains calm, a criminal will usually remain calm as well. Unfortunately, this is not always the case, but most criminals want to leave the crime scene as opposed to being present when the authorities arrive. Review the general safety tips for employees in Figure 12-12.

Office Security

Various items of value can be found in the medical office. Narcotic medications are stored in a locked cabinet, and cash and checks are kept in the office as well. For these reasons the office must always be secure.

Alarm systems are often used to protect the medical office; such systems either are monitored or simply sound an alarm when tripped. Monitored alarms go off when a door or window is opened and the security code is not entered into the unit. When the alarm is tripped, an employee of the alarm company will attempt to call the office to determine if there is a true emergency. If no one answers, the alarm company will send police to the facility. An alarm that sounds will also be active until a code is entered, but these systems allow a short period of time for the alarm code to be entered before the main alarm begins to ring. Occasionally a false alarm will sound and prompt the police to investigate; however, many alarm companies charge the business a fee when the alarm is not a valid emergency.

Only a few staff members need to know the alarm code. The office manager and those who open and close the facility need to know the code, as does the physician. The fewer people who know the code, the better. A combination of letters and numbers is best for alarm codes, instead of a strictly numeric or alphabetic code.

General Safety Tips for Employees

- Be sure to always lock the car when leaving it, no matter how short a visit to the destination.
- Park in a well-lighted area and have the car key in hand when approaching the vehicle.
- Attempt to walk out of the office with another person. If there is no choice but to walk alone, walk confidently and with determined stride.
- Be aware of the surroundings. Walk in the middle of parking lanes, not too close to cars on the left or right to avoid being pulled in between two vans or SUVs.
- Take a good look at the vehicle on approach, including underneath, if possible. Once the door is open, glance around the vehicle. If parked in a well-lit area, it is easier to see into the back seat.
- Once inside the vehicle, immediately lock the doors, start the car, and leave. Don't perform menial tasks, such as balancing a checkbook, applying makeup, or talking on the phone, while sitting in a parking lot.
- Never leave valuable items lying in the car in plain sight, such as iPods, cell phones, CD players, laptop computers, etc.
- Don't be afraid to ask security personnel to provide an escort when leaving for the day, if security is available.
- Report all suspicious activity immediately; don't wait until the next day.

FIGURE 12-12 General safety tips for employees.

Smoke Alarms and Fire Extinguishers

Smoke alarms should be installed in every physician's office. The two basic types of smoke alarms are photoelectric and ionization alarms. If nuisance alarms continually sound (for instance, from cooking popcorn in the lounge area), changing alarm types may solve the problem. Smoke alarm batteries must be changed twice a year; the best time to do this is when daylight savings time begins and ends. Although the old batteries may not be dead, new ones will be fresh and will certainly last for 6 months.

Fire extinguishers must be readily available in the office and must be prominently mounted in a visible, convenient place. The extinguishers must be serviced annually by a fire professional who holds a valid certificate to perform inspections. In addition, staff members should be trained in the use of fire extinguishers; most fire departments offer this training either free or for a nominal charge. A multipurpose ABC fire extinguisher is appropriate for a small business. Staff members can remember the basic use of the fire extinguisher by memorizing the mnemonic device PASS:

  P–pull the pin
  A–aim the hose
  S–squeeze
  S–sweep the nozzle

To determine whether a physician's office is safe, answer the following questions:

- Are all exit ways accessible and unobstructed?
- Are all of the fire extinguishers operational and properly locatable?

- Are all of the emergency lighting units and exit signs operational?
- Are any extension cords or multiplug adaptors in use?
- Is there an escape plan with two ways out, and do employees know how to use it?
- Are the fire alarms and sprinkler system functioning correctly and easily accessible?
- Is all storage neat and orderly and not obstructing sprinkler heads?
- Are all flammable liquids and materials stored away from heat sources?
- Are all plumbing, mechanical, and electrical systems functioning properly?

Fire Exits and Exit Routes

At least two exits must be designated as fire exits in the medical facility. These exits must be clearly marked and easily accessible. The exit doors must remain unlocked during business hours so that people can get out in case of a fire or other emergency. For security reasons, doors can be locked on the outside, yet have an exit bar on the inside that allows exit by pushing on the exit bar.

An escape plan must be posted in several areas of the facility, and employees should have regular drills that allow them to practice evacuating the building. If escape plans are posted in every room, then the escape from that particular room can be diagrammed. Two escape routes should be posted from each room—a primary route and a secondary route. Before exiting through a door, touch it and determine whether it feels warm. If it does, then use another route. If the facility is two stories tall, have ladders ready that attach to a window and unfold to allow escape. Buildings with two or more stories should have stairwells that can also be used in case of fire.

Locked Storage Areas

Several items in the medical office must be kept in locked cabinets or storage areas. Narcotic drugs and other prescription medications should be secured, and employees should have limited access to them. Because some over-the-counter medications are readily available, such as pseudoephedrine (an ingredient in common cold medication), most pharmacies and discount stores have begun limiting the number of packages of the medicine that one person can purchase.

Narcotics must be logged when a dose is used. More details about the requirements when administering a dose of medication can be found in Chapter 32. Prescription pads should also be kept under lock and key unless the physician is using the pad. Most doctors are protective of prescription pads because they realize that patients, or even employees, sometimes steal them.

WASTE STORAGE AND DESTRUCTION

Two basic types of waste are found in physicians' offices: medical waste and regular waste. Medical waste includes anything that was once a part of the human body. Most offices use a trash service to remove regular waste, whether it is contracted or a service provided by the city. Removing medical waste is

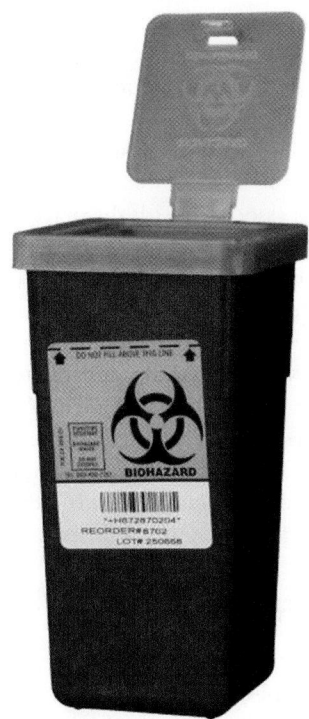

FIGURE 12-13 OSHA requires that medical waste be disposed of properly and that the office keep records of waste removal and incineration.

somewhat more complicated (Figure 12-13). The Occupational Safety and Health Administration (OSHA) requires records that prove that (1) medical waste was collected by the removal waste service, and (2) the same waste was destroyed by the waste service. The medical waste service usually comes every few days; the waste is picked up, then destroyed by incineration.

Regular trash is usually collected twice a week. Holiday weeks may result in additional trash, and that may mean additional fees. Trash pickup will occur two or three times per week; make certain that all trash is brought to the predetermined location for disposal outside. Do not place trash outside early, as it may attract animals and insects.

ERGONOMICS

Ergonomics is the applied science concerned with designing and arranging things people use so that the people and the things interact efficiently and safely. OSHA developed a four-pronged approach to quickly and efficiently address musculoskeletal disorders in the workplace. The approach includes a combination of industry-specific and task-specific guidelines, outreach, enforcement, and research. Since these measures have been implemented, OSHA has seen significant improvement in these areas. A plethora of information on ergonomics is available online, both through a general search and on the OSHA website.

ACOUSTICS AND WHITE NOISE

Acoustics is defined as the science that deals with the production, control, transmission, reception, and effects of sound. Acoustics

differ from room to room. When acoustics are good, sound reception is sharp and clear. In a room that has poor acoustics, the sound seems to be more muffled.

Acoustics are important in the medical office because they can affect confidentiality. Most people have visited a medical office in which a patient sitting in an examination room could hear every word spoken in the next room. If the diagnosis is revealed and overheard by another patient, then patient confidentiality has been broken. Medical professionals must be aware of the acoustics in the office and attempt to work with them, guarding patients' right to confidentiality.

Although the technical definition of *white noise* is long and complicated, for the purposes of this text, the shortened definition will help students understand the term. White noise is commonly used with architectural acoustics, where it "masks" undesirable noises, such as multiple conversations in interior spaces, by generating a low level of background noise that is used as background sound. It is also used on some sirens for emergency vehicle use because of its ability to cut through background noise; one benefit of this ability is that the siren is easier to distinguish as a separate sound and it does not create an echo, so it is easier to determine the direction from which the siren sound is coming.

White noise is often used in medical offices because the stark quiet of the facility can be unnerving for patients. Most people have no idea that white noise is being generated. Even if soft music is playing in the office, white noise can be in the background. Sometimes white noise sounds like a soft static. Some businesses use a CD of white noise, and they can contain the sounds of waterfalls, thunderstorms, rushing water, jungle sounds, and many others, all designed to make the office visit less frightening and more relaxing and to absorb distracting noise.

IDENTIFYING AND SHARING COMMUNITY RESOURCES

The medical assistant must be able to identify community resources so that he or she can assist patients with needs that are not office related, and possibly not medically related. At various times, patients need help with meals, rehabilitation, Medicare issues, exercise groups, and other services. Grocery stores that deliver are a great convenience resource for the older patient. Get to know the people in the community, trade information, and refer patients when they need help with a particular issue. Figure 12-14 includes some of the more common community resources in which patients may be interested. This can be used to create a phone directory for a local community resource list (Procedure 12-7). To expand the knowledge base as to what resources are available in the community, get involved in various organizations, especially health industry councils and organizations for medical assistants or other office staff members. Make introductions, and be prepared to talk about the services that the clinic offers. Ask questions about other facilities. Exchange business cards, if they are available. Stay in touch with community resource contacts to make certain that information being provided to patients is accurate. Patients

---

Community Resources

Check with these organizations for services available in the local area.

Alcoholics Anonymous
Alzheimer Support Organizations
American Cancer Society
American Heart Association
American Red Cross
Child Protective Services
Civic Organizations
Council on Aging
Family Services
Homeless Organizations
Hospice Services
Legal Aid Societies
Mental Health and Mental Retardation Services
Public Health Department
United Way

FIGURE 12-14 Examples of community resources.

appreciate that the office staff can refer them to local resources and can assist them in gathering information.

Emergency Phone Numbers

Every medical facility should keep a list of emergency and frequently called numbers close to each telephone in the office.

The list should include 911, which summons police and fire departments in most areas in the country. Other numbers on the list might include those for the following:

- Local hospitals
- Local pharmacies, including extensions to the emergency room
- All physicians associated with the practice
- All employees
- Nonemergency police services
- Physicians who are periodically on call

Each office will have different numbers on the emergency phone numbers list. The physician and office manager often provide input about the numbers that are included. Periodically the numbers will need to be updated. If the list is kept on a computer, a new one can be printed and distributed each time a phone number changes. Because the list is used in emergencies, it must be current and accurate at all times.

CLOSING THE OFFICE

When the day comes to an end, several duties must be completed before the doors are locked and the office is closed. First, check to see that all patients have left the facility. Walk through all examination rooms and treatment areas to make certain that they are empty. At the same time, straighten the examination rooms so that they are ready for the next day's patients. Because the rooms are tidied in between patients, they should be easy

---

PROCEDURE 12-7

Identify Community Resources

CAAHEP COMPETENCY: 3.c.(3)(d)
ABHES COMPETENCY: 3.e

GOAL: *To help patients find organizations that can assist with their needs beyond the physician's office and to establish a listing of community resources that can be used for referral purposes.*

EQUIPMENT and SUPPLIES

- Phone book
- Internet access
- Library access
- Newspapers
- Local volunteer guides
- Computer
- Pen or pencil
- Notepad

PROCEDURAL STEPS

1. Research the resources available in the local community using the Internet, phone book, newspapers, and other guides.
   PURPOSE: To become familiar with various agencies that provide services in the local area.

2. Open a document on the computer, either using a word-processing program or a spreadsheet. Create a list of the resources within the document. Include the following information on the list:
   - Name of agency
   - Purpose or mission of agency
   - Physical address
   - Mailing address, if different
   - Phone numbers
   - Contact name
   - Hours of operation
   - Services offered or performed
   PURPOSE: To make information readily available.

3. Update the information whenever a change is needed.
   PURPOSE: To provide the most accurate information possible.

4. Provide referrals to agencies when patients, their friends, or their families ask for it or when the physician recommends referral.
   PURPOSE: To get patients the help that they need.

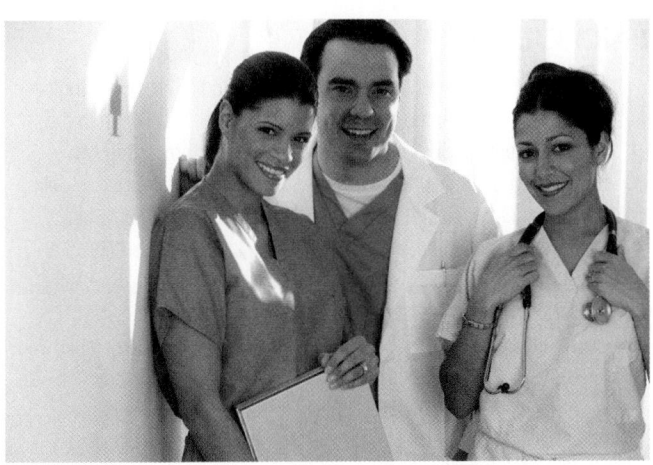

FIGURE 12-15 Teamwork is vital to ensure successful completion of the workday in the physician's office.

to clean at day's end. Work with fellow employees as a team to accomplish all of the tasks that are required each day (Figure 12-15).

Other duties include locking patient file cabinets, placing laboratory specimens in the outside lockbox for pickup, performing general housekeeping duties, running accounting reports, balancing the day sheet, and preparing the bank deposit. The phones will need to be turned over to the answering service or voicemail. Using a mnemonic device, as discussed in the last chapter, helps the medical assistant to remember closing duties. Remember the safety tips for leaving offices and returning to vehicles. The saying bears repeating: "Better safe than sorry."

CLOSING COMMENTS

Although the tasks discussed in this chapter include duties that are done on a daily basis, the medical assistant should not be lazy about completing them. When the physician sees that employees are competent about completing small duties, he or she will consider the medical assistant to be competent in completing more difficult tasks. By consistently proving to be a skilled, dependable worker, the medical assistant will be promoted to higher levels of responsibility.

Always keep in mind that the patient is of primary concern in the physician's office. The medical assistant's efforts should be directed at making the patients feel more at ease and encouraging them to follow the treatment plan devised by the physician. Therefore even the smallest of office duties plays a part in the health and well-being of the patient.

SUMMARY OF SCENARIO

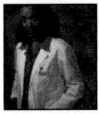

Kayla learned much more on her externship than she thought she would. She saw patients who had few belongings and no health insurance coverage. Her experience helped her to realize just how difficult it is to obtain medical care without insurance. Kayla is happy that her clinic sees these patients and allows the patients to pay what they can to obtain medical care. She feels slightly guilty that she has had such an easy life as she listens to her patients' stories and their problems.

Kayla has developed a sense of caring for the people she helps in the clinic. She does not treat the patients disrespectfully; on the contrary, she treats them as individuals who deserve dignity. She understands that although she might not connect with all patients, she can make a difference to the ones who enter the clinic by expressing an emotion that she truly feels—compassion.

Elaine allowed Kayla to order many of the supplies that she needs, because Kayla is the primary user of those items. This allows Kayla to use the items she has found perform the best and with which she is most comfortable. Kayla suggested that the clinic outsource some of their laboratory tests because of the expense of buying the supplies to run the tests. This has allowed the clinic to keep their prices lower, a great help to the patients.

Kayla found that most of the patients who come to the clinic are in need of referrals, whether it be for food, clothing, other medical services, child care, or other issues. She designed a lengthy list of community resources, and she can tell patients where to go to receive help with various problems. The patients appreciate Kayla's willingness to help them. Even though Kayla comes from a completely different background, the patients have accepted her as a medical assistant who truly cares.

SUMMARY of LEARNING OBJECTIVES

1. Define, spell and pronounce the terms listed in the vocabulary.
   - Spelling and pronouncing medical terms correctly adds credibility to the medical assistant. Knowing the definition of these terms promotes confidence in communication with patients and co-workers.
2. List five actions that need to be taken before the office opens in the morning.
   - Before the medical office is opened in the morning, several tasks must be completed. The office should be clean, whether it is done the evening before or as one of the morning duties. Examination rooms should be checked for supplies and replenished, if necessary. The phone should be taken off of voicemail or the answering service called to inform them that the office staff has arrived for the day. Make two copies of the appointment book, placing one on the physician's desk and using the other to pull the medical records of the patients who have appointments. Individual offices may assign additional duties to the medical assistants who work in the office.
3. Explain why patient traffic flow is an important consideration in office design.
   - Patient traffic flow is important because patients should not have to repeatedly retrace their steps as they move throughout the clinic. Furnishings should be arranged so that it is easy to get from one place to another without having to dodge objects in the room.
4. List some of the expenses involved in the operation of a medical practice.
   - Many types of expenses affect the operation of a physician's office. Lease or mortgage payments are one of the largest expenses. Utilities, payroll, equipment and supplies, professional organization dues, insurance, maintenance, and taxes are all examples of items that must be worked into the annual budget.
5. Describe how prices can be compared for medical office supplies.
   - Compare unit prices by determining what each individual item costs. If a bulk package of eight containers of correction fluid costs $9.99, then each individual bottle costs $1.25. If another company offers the same product at 10 for $12.00, then the individual cost is $1.20, which is the better buy of the two. However, the cost to buy the product, meaning the gas to get to the store, or the shipping and handling costs, if any, may increase the price. Be aware of these situations and figure all costs possible before placing an order.
6. Describe the purpose of white noise.
   - White noise is used to absorb sound and mask undesirable noises. It creates a low-level noise so that a conversation in one room won't be heard in the next room. White noise can also be in the form of CDs that play sounds of waterfalls, thunderstorms, rain, and other nature sounds.
7. List several ways to save money in the medical office.
   - Physicians can save money in several ways when purchasing items for the office. Make sure that trash bags are completely full before taking trash out. Use refillable print cartridges and solar-powered calculators and adding machines. Print on both sides of paper when possible. Monitor ordering to determine where budget cuts could be made. Watch carefully for areas where money could be saved or items could be bought in bulk.
8. Explain the difference between medical waste and regular waste.
   - Medical waste includes any disposed-of item that was once a part of the human body or used to clean up blood or body fluids. Regular waste is any other trash that does not have to go into a biohazard waste container.
9. Explain why keys and alarm codes should be shared with only a few people.
   - The fewer people who know alarm codes and have keys, the easier it is to keep track of them. In addition, if fewer people have the codes and keys, there is less chance that someone will use them to enter the office and steal equipment and supplies.

CONNECTIONS

Study Guide Connection: Go to Chapter 12 Study Guide. Read the Case Study and Workplace Applications and complete the assignments. Do online research for answers to the questions in the Internet Activities associated with the office environment and daily operations.

CD Connection: Go to the Medical Assisting Competency Challenge CD and do the training activities under General Office Duties.

Evolve Connection: For more information related to the office environment and daily operations, go to evolve.elsevier.com/kinn and visit related weblinks for Chapter 12. Click on the Medical Assisting Exam Review and do the practice questions to sharpen your test-taking skills. To learn more about office software, do the exercises for the Altapoint demo that is on the CD.

Written Communications and Mail Processing

13

SCENARIO

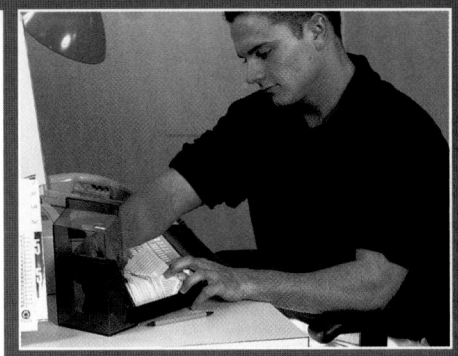

Brandon Tipps is a medical assistant working with his father, Dr. Rick Tipps. Brandon has considered continuing his education to become a doctor, but he is not sure whether he would like to be a medical doctor, an osteopathic physician, or a chiropractor. He decided to spend his summer off from college working in his father's family practice so that he could get a closer look at the inner workings of a physician's office.

Brandon has assisted with every procedure in the clinic, including the administrative skills required in the front office. The staff has been impressed with Brandon's ability to do any task, no matter how small, as if it were the most important task in the office. He continuously moves from employee to employee to ask what he can do to help. When the administrative medical assistant working in the front office, Darla Grover, was injured in a car accident and had to be off work for a while, Brandon stepped right in to do her job and quickly learned her duties. His help enabled the office to continue to run smoothly even with one employee absent for several weeks.

Brandon has an excellent command of the English language and types about 60 words per minute. He is organized and efficient, so he is able to handle the enormous amount of incoming and outgoing mail with very little assistance from the office manager. He is also able to answer phones and schedule appointments. He speaks clearly and is an expert at customer service. Many of Dr. Tipps' patients have known Brandon since he was a small child, and they enjoy seeing him helping in his father's office. The patients and staff alike will certainly miss him once he returns to college.

While studying this chapter, think about the following questions:

- What types of difficulties are faced when a physician's family member works at the office?
- How do proofreader's marks help the medical assistant to save time?
- What types of impressions could be formed by the receiver of mail from a physician's office?
- Explain why any written communication discussed in this chapter should be worded in a professional manner.

LEARNING OBJECTIVES

1. Define, spell, and pronounce the terms listed in the vocabulary.
2. Discuss the responsibility of the medical assistant with respect to equipment and supplies.
3. List the four common sizes of letterhead stationery.
4. Explain the various parts of speech.
5. Name some of the essential references for the medical assistant's library.
6. List several steps to complete before answering a business letter.
7. Discuss the process of developing and the value of keeping a communications portfolio.
8. Discuss the differences in the four letter styles.
9. Explain the four standard parts of a business letter.
10. List several ways to save money when mailing.
11. Open, sort, and annotate incoming mail.
12. Compose, proofread, and mail a business letter.
13. Properly send a fax.
14. Process incoming mail.
15. Address an envelope according to Postal Service optical character reader guidelines.

National Accreditation Competencies and Content

CAAHEP COMPETENCIES

General

3.c.(1)(a). Respond to and initiate written communications
3.c.(1)(b). Recognize and respond to verbal communications
3.c.(1)(c). Recognize and respond to nonverbal communications
3.c.(2)(d). Document appropriately

ABHES COMPETENCIES

Communication

2.g. Use appropriate medical terminology
2.h. Receive, organize, prioritize, and transmit information expediently
2.i. Recognize and respond to verbal and nonverbal communication
2.j. Use correct grammar, spelling, and formatting techniques in written works
2.k. Principles of verbal and nonverbal communication
2.l. Recognition and response to verbal and nonverbal communication
2.o. Fundamental writing skills

Administrative Duties

3.a. Perform basic secretarial skills
3.d. Apply computer concepts for office procedures

Legal Concepts

5b. Document accurately

VOCABULARY

academic degree A title conferred by a college, university, or professional school on completion of a program of study.

amiable (a'-me-uh-buhl) Having qualities that make one liked and easy to deal with.

annotating Furnishing with notes that are usually critical or explanatory.

archaic (ar-ka'-ik) Of, relating to, or characteristic of an earlier or more primitive time.

archived To have filed or collected records or documents.

bond A durable, formal paper used for documents.

categorically Placed in a specific division of a system of classification.

clauses Groups of words containing a subject and predicate and functioning as a member of a complex or compound sentence.

collect on delivery (COD) Method of payment used when an article or item is delivered and payment is expected before it is released.

concise (kun-sis') Expressing much in brief form.

condescending Assuming an air of superiority.

continuation pages The second and following pages of a letter.

curt Marked by rude or peremptory shortness.

disseminate (di-se'-muh-nat) To disperse throughout.

domestic mail Mail that is sent within the boundaries of the United States and its territories.

flush Directly abutting or immediately adjacent, as set even with an edge of a type page or column; having no indention.

girth A measure around a body or item.

grammar The study of the classes of words, their inflections, and their functions and relations in the sentence; a study of what is to be preferred and what avoided in inflection and syntax.

international mail Mail that is sent outside the boundaries of the United States and its territories.

intrinsic (in-tri'-zik) Belonging to the essential nature or constitution of a thing; indwelling, inward.

mailpiece A piece of mail.

microfiche (mi'-kro-fish) A sheet of microfilm containing rows of microimages of pages of printed matter.

portfolio A set of pictures, drawings, documents, or photographs either bound in book form or loose in a folder.

ream A quantity of paper weighing 20 lb or consisting of, variously, 480, 500, or 516 sheets.

recipient The receiver of some thing or item.

stationers (sta'-shuh-nerz) Sellers of stationery.

substance number A number based on the weight of a ream of paper containing 500 sheets.

superfluous (suh-puhr'-flu-uhs) Exceeding what is sufficient or necessary.

watermark A marking in paper resulting from differences in thickness usually produced by the pressure of a projecting design in the mold or on a processing roll and visible when the paper is held up to the light.

Entrepreneur and co-founder of the Amway Corporation, Rich de Vos, believed in a simple principle regarding the many business papers that crossed his desk on a daily basis. He believed that each paper should be handled only once. Whatever the news, information, or action required, the paper should be dealt with immediately, and this resulted in the most efficient use of his time. This excellent idea is beneficial for any business, including the medical office.

Written correspondence and mail processing consumes a large part of the administrative medical assistant's day. Many physicians, when queried about the skills they most desire in an administrative assistant, say that a person who can spell accurately and write a good letter is a valuable addition to the medical office. When a physician delegates the responsibility of composing letters or reports that have the potential to reflect positively or negatively on the practice, he or she is expressing confidence in that medical assistant's abilities.

IMPORTANCE OF WRITTEN COMMUNICATIONS

Written communications offer the perfect opportunity for making a good impression on others, but they do not just happen. They require thought, preparation, skill, and a positive attitude. Written communications take many forms in the medical office. The medical assistant needs skills in creating various forms of communication.

Written communications include original letters, memorandums, replies to inquiries, responses to requests for information, telephone messages, email, transcriptions, orders for supplies, instructions for patients, and a variety of other forms. Communications that are courteous to the reader, correct in content, and **concise** without being **curt** are most appreciated. Communication is truly an art as well as a skill. The ability to communicate effectively is extremely important to the administrative medical assistant who wishes to succeed and advance his or her career.

CRITICAL THINKING APPLICATION

Brandon has just found a small backlog of correspondence that accumulated during the first 3 days that Darla was out of the office. A large amount of mail comes to the office each day. How can Brandon manage the daily mail and clear the pile of communications that accumulated over those 3 days?

WRITTEN COMMUNICATION AS A PUBLIC RELATIONS TOOL

Public relations involves "telling the organization's story." The public relations department or director of any organization exists to present a business in the best possible light and to communicate to the public and other interested parties all of the positive aspects of a business. With this understanding, it is easy to see why written communications are so important. These documents can present a professional image or a very poor image to the receiver. Individual medical offices rarely employ public relations professionals, so each member of the staff must be conscientious about the documents and materials that are present within and that leave the office. An envelope addressed carelessly or a patient information sheet that has been photocopied over and over insinuates that the office personnel are not concerned about the appearance of documents that leave the office. If the staff is careless in this respect, many patients will assume that the staff is careless with everything, including patient care.

REFLECTION ON THE PHYSICIAN

Everything that happens in the medical office is a reflection on the physician or physicians who practice there. Letters with misspelled words or errors will give the reader a negative impression of the physician and the practice itself. Great care must be taken to ensure that each document in the office and sent from the office is well written and grammatically correct. Table 13-1 lists proofreader's marks. Although these marks are usually used in copyediting, medical assistants who take the time to learn them will be able to process written communications twice as fast as those who make lengthy notes on documents that need revision or need an answer. Tables 13-2 and 13-3 list frequently misspelled and misused words.

WRITING SKILLS AND COMPOSING TIPS

Business letters are much different from the social letters that the medical assistant may have written. Social letters tend to be long and chatty and do not necessarily follow any organized plan. Most business letters should be less than one page in length and carefully organized (Procedure 13-1, p. 229). This takes practice and preparation. Every person who writes letters develops his or her own personal style.

The medical assistant should carefully read the letter to be answered. Make note of or underline any questions asked or materials requested. Then decide on the answers to the questions and verify the information. This is called **annotating.** Draft a reply, proofread it, then rewrite for clarity (Procedure 13-2, p. 230). Keep most of the sentences short. Put only one idea in each sentence, and eliminate **superfluous** words. Be careful about using medical terms in correspondence with patients. Instead, use language that the reader will easily understand.

Most physicians conform to a highly professional and formal style in their dictation. The medical assistant who is given the responsibility of composing correspondence for the medical office should strive for the same degree of formality used by the physician. It would be inappropriate for the assistant to write in a breezy, informal style when acting as the representative of an employer who has a more formal approach. The principal point to remember is that every letter produced in your office should project the image of the physician regardless of who composes or signs the letter.

Grammar Review

Good **grammar** is essential to writing effective, professional business letters. Medical assistants need an understanding of the elements of acceptable grammar and writing skills.

TABLE 13-1 Proofreader's Marks

Symbol or Margin Notation	Meaning	Example
ϑ or Ϭ or ϒ	Delete	take it out
⌒	Close up	print as o ne word
ϑ	Delete and close up	close up
∧ or ⟩ or ⋏	Insert	insert here ⟨ something
#	Insert a space	put onehere
eq#	Space evenly	space evenly ∧ where indicated
stet	Let stand	let marked text stand as set
tr	Transpose	change order the
[	Set farther to left	∟ too far to the right
]	Set farther to right	too∣ far to the left
¶	Begin a new paragraph	the same is true. ¶ In conclusion
⑤ⓟ	Spell out	set 5 lbs as five pounds
cap	Set in CAPITALS	set nato as NATO
lc	Set in lowercase	set South as south
ital	Set in italic	set oeuvre as oeuvre
bf	Set in boldface	set important as **important**
∨	Superscript or superior	∨ as in πr^2
∧	Subscript or inferior	∧ as in H_2O
⅋	Comma	red blue, and yellow
⅋	Apostrophe	Calvin's lizard was green.
⊙	Period	The end is near ⊙
; or ⅉ/	Semicolon	1, this 2, that
: or ⊙	Colon	is the following :
⅋⅋ or ⌣⌣	Quotation marks	He said, I did it.
( )	Parentheses	Run fast now.

Parts of Speech

Nouns. A noun is a person, place, or thing. Nouns can also be thoughts, ideas, or concepts, as in *freedom* or *courage*. Common nouns name general persons, places, or things, such as *teacher* and *city*. Proper nouns are specific, such as *Mrs. Adams* and *New York City*.

Pronouns. Pronouns replace nouns and provide the writer with shortcuts so that proper nouns do not have to be constantly repeated. Pronouns include words such as *it, you, he, she, her, his, them, mine, you, yours, its, ours,* and *theirs.*

Verbs. Verbs are action words that express movement, such as *runs, drove,* or *typed.* Linking verbs express a condition or state of being and include *is, am, are, was, be,* and *been.* Linking verbs also express the senses, as in *smell, hear, taste, touch, feel,* and *look.*

Adjectives. Adjectives are words that describe nouns and pronouns or may show which one, how many, and what kind

TABLE 13-2   One Hundred and Fifty Frequently Misspelled or Misused English Words

absence	corroborate	inimitable	persistent	ridiculous
accede	definitely	inoculate	personal	sacrilegious
accessible	description	insistent	personnel	seize
accommodate	desirable	irrelevant	possession	separate
achieve	despair	irresistible	precede	siege
affect	development	irritable	precedent	similar
agglutinate	dilemma	judgment	predictable	sizable
all right	disappear	labeled	predominant	stationary
altogether	disappoint	led	predominate	stationery
analyses (pl.)	disastrous	leisure	prerogative	subpoena
analysis (s.)	discreet	license	prevalent	succeed
analyze	discrete	liquefy	principal	suddenness
anoint	discriminate	maintenance	principle	superintendent
argument	dissatisfaction	maneuver	privilege	supersede
assistant	dissipate	miscellaneous	procedure	surprise
auxiliary	drunkenness	mischievous	proceed	tariff
balloon	ecstasy	misspell	professor	technique
believe	effect	necessary	pronunciation	thorough
benefited	eligible	newsstand	psychiatry	tranquility
brochure	embarrass	noticeable	psychology	transferred
bulletin	exceed	occasion	pursue	truly
category	exhilaration	occurrence	questionnaire	tyrannize
changeable	existence	oscillate	rearrange	unnecessary
clientele	February	paid	recede	until
committee	forty	pamphlet	receive	vacillate
comparative	grammar	panicky	recommend	vacuum
concede	grievous	parallel	referring	vicious
conscientious	height	paralyze	repetition	warrant
conscious	incidentally	pastime	rheumatism	Wednesday
coolly	indispensable	perseverance	rhythmical	weird

of. *A*, *an*, and *the* are special types of adjectives called articles. Examples of adjectives include a *golden* sunset, a *mangy* dog, and a *crooked* nose.

Adverbs. Just as adjectives describe nouns, adverbs describe verbs, adjectives, or other adverbs. Adverbs specify when, where, to what extent, or how. Examples include *unusually* warm, *never* won, and *quite* cold.

Prepositions. Connecting words that show a relationship between nouns, pronouns, or other words in a sentence are called prepositions. Examples of prepositions include *by, from, of, to, in, at, with, into,* and *on.*

Conjunctions. Conjunctions join words or phrases. These helpful words include *and, or, nor,* and *but.*

Interjections. Interjections show strong feeling. They are often followed by an exclamation point and sometimes by a comma. *"Ouch! That really hurt!"* is a sentence that uses an interjection.

Making Sense of Sentences

Sentence structure is important when writing a professional letter or document. The medical assistant should know the basics of good sentence structure so that written documents will make sense and represent the medical facility and staff in a positive way.

Types of Sentences. The four basic sentence types are as follows: declarative, interrogatory, imperative, and exclamatory. Declarative sentences make a statement, whereas interrogatory sentences ask a question. Imperative sentences state a command or request. Exclamatory sentences express strong feeling. An example of each type follows:

TABLE 13-3 Frequently Misspelled Medical Words

abscess	defibrillator	intussusception	parietal	pruritus
additive	desiccate	ischemia	paroxysmal	psoriasis
aerosol	ecchymosis	ischium	pemphigus	pyrexia
agglutination	effusion	larynx	percussion	respiratory
albumin	epididymis	leukemia	perforation	rheumatic
anastomosis	epistaxis	malaise	pericardium	roentgenology
aneurysm	eustachian	malleus	perineum	sagittal
anteflexion	fissure	melena	peristalsis	sciatic
arrhythmia	flexure	mellitus	peritoneum	scirrhous
bilirubin	glaucoma	menstruation	petit mal	serous
bronchial	gonorrhea	metastasis	pharynx	sessile
cachexia	graafian	neurilemma	pituitary	sphincter
calcaneus	hemorrhage	neuron	plantar	sphygmomanometer
capillary	hemorrhoids	occlusion	pleura	squamous
cervical	homeostasis	optic chiasm	pleurisy	staphylococcus
chromosome	humerus	oscilloscope	pneumonia	suppuration
cirrhosis	idiosyncrasy	osseous	polyp	trochanter
clavicle	ileum	palliative	prophylaxis	venous
curettage	ilium	parasite	prostate	wheal
cyanosis	infarction	parenteral	prosthesis	xiphoid

Declarative   *She was the last person here.*
Interrogatory   *Are we going to the fair today?*
Imperative   *Clean your room before dinner.*
Exclamatory   *I am so excited for you!*

Sentence Structure. Sentences, when written correctly, follow certain patterns. Three very basic patterns are used in constructing sentences. These patterns are as follows:

- Subject-predicate
- Subject-object
- Subject-complement

The subject of a sentence is usually a noun and is the word or group of words in a sentence that acts, is acted on, or is described by the verb. The predicate is the part of the sentence that contains the verb and tells what the subject is doing or experiencing or what is being done to the subject. The object is a noun, pronoun, or group of words functioning as a noun or pronoun that receives the action of the verb. The complement is a word or group of words in the predicate of a sentence that renames or describes a subject or object in that sentence.

Sentence Errors. Three main sentence errors plague most writers. These include the sentence fragment, the run-on sentence, and the comma splice.

A sentence fragment is an incomplete thought or a portion of a sentence that is punctuated as though it were a complete sentence. An example follows:

Although the doctor had seen the patient.

A run-on sentence contains independent **clauses** without a semicolon, comma, or conjunction between them. These sentences are also called *run-together* or *fused* sentences. An example follows:

The office was clean when the staff left on Friday the doors were locked.

A comma splice is a sentence in which a comma alone joins independent clauses. An example follows:

The storm grew worse, it began to snow.

Personal Tools

Competent handling of written communications requires a basic knowledge of composition. A personal reference library that includes an up-to-date standard dictionary, a medical dictionary, a composition handbook, an English-language reference manual, and a thesaurus will be a tremendous help. The book *English Grammar for Dummies* by Geraldine Woods is actually used in many masters-level English courses and is extremely easy to understand. This helpful book would be a good addition to a personal tools list.

For those who have difficulty with spelling, keep a small loose-leaf indexed notebook or card index of words that are troublesome. When it is necessary to look up a word in the dictionary for spelling, record the word in the notebook or card index for quick reference. The physician or a medical assistant who is familiar with the practice might compile a basic list of frequently used medical terms and abbreviations as a reference.

PROCEDURE 13-1

Respond to and Initiate Written Communications: Compose Business Correspondence

<u>CAAHEP COMPETENCY:</u> 3.c.(1)(a)
<u>ABHES COMPETENCY:</u> 2.j

GOAL: *To compose a letter that will convey information in an accurate and concise manner and that is easy for the reader to comprehend.*

EQUIPMENT and SUPPLIES

- Computer or word processor
- Word processing software
- Draft paper
- Letterhead
- Printer
- Pen or pencil
- Highlighter
- Envelope
- Correspondence to be answered
- Other pertinent information needed to compose a letter
- Electronic or paper dictionary and thesaurus
- Writer's handbook
- Portfolio

PROCEDURAL STEPS

1. Determine the purpose of initiating correspondence or read through any correspondence to be answered, and highlight the specific questions that should be addressed.
   <u>PURPOSE:</u> To make certain that all of the issues raised in the correspondence are addressed or answered.
2. Make any necessary notes on the letter or a copy of the letter. A scrap sheet of paper may be used.

3. Prepare a draft of the letter using good grammar, and save it in the computer or word processor.
   <u>PURPOSE:</u> To put the thoughts on paper for later revision and make the letter easy to understand for the reader.
4. Proofread a printed copy of the letter, using proofreader's marks to make corrections.
   <u>PURPOSE:</u> To see the document as it will look once printed and to speed the process by using proofreader's marks.
5. Make any necessary corrections.
6. Allow the physician or other interested parties to proofread the letter, if the medical assistant is not the person whose signature will appear at the bottom.
   <u>PURPOSE:</u> To give the physician an opportunity to correct the letter and add additional thoughts, if desired.
7. Make any final changes, then print the letter on stationery. Allow the person whose name appears at the bottom to sign the letter.
8. Address the envelope using OCR guidelines, and place the letter and any supporting documents inside. (See Procedure 13-5 for using postal OCR guidelines.)
9. Mail the letter using correct postage.
   <u>PURPOSE:</u> Using incorrect postage or guessing can delay the arrival time of the document.

EQUIPMENT AND SUPPLIES

To create a favorable impression with letters, the medical assistant must use good equipment and high-quality supplies. Whatever kind of equipment is available, it is the medical assistant's responsibility to know how to use it to the best advantage and to keep it in good working condition. If the equipment manual is available, study it and keep it handy for reference when problems occur. Know how to maintain equipment so that the effort made in composing the correspondence results in a high-quality appearance.

Equipment

Computers

Computers have made composing correspondence simple. Various letters and documents may be saved and reused time after time by changing the name and basic information contained within the text. Computers can add graphics to text, compute figures, and use multimedia in communications—all of which enhance the appearance and effectiveness of the document.

Word Processors

Word processors are used mainly for letter writing and simple documents. The word processor has taken a backseat to today's desktop and notebook computers.

Typewriters

Typewriters, too, are becoming **archaic,** given the versatility of the computer. Most typewriters use correctable film ribbons that pass through the spool only one time. However, if the typewriter uses a cotton or silk ribbon that becomes lighter with use, be sure to change the ribbon before the resulting type impression becomes too light. The typewriter keys need to be cleaned frequently in typewriters that use a cotton ribbon.

Copiers

Maintain the copier so that copies are crisp and clear. The toner cartridge must be changed when necessary and can be expensive. Multiple copies of documents are usually made on a copier rather than printed from the computer.

PROCEDURE 13-2

Respond to and Initiate Written Communications: Proofread Documents for Accuracy

CAAHEP COMPETENCY: 3.c.(1)(a)
ABHES COMPETENCY: 2.j

GOAL: *To compose a clearly written, grammatically correct business letter that is easily understood by the reader, and to eliminate spelling and grammatic errors.*

EQUIPMENT and SUPPLIES

- Stationery
- Computer or typewriter
- Correspondence to be answered or notes
- Proofreader's marks guide

PROCEDURAL STEPS

1. Scan through the letter to be answered or the notes about the correspondence to be written and highlight any questions that should be answered or points to be made.
   PURPOSE: To ensure that the goals of the correspondence are fulfilled and no important points are omitted.
2. Write the letter using good grammar.
3. Print a draft copy of the letter. Read it carefully and highlight changes to be made or note any additions to be made. Use proofreader's marks.

PURPOSE: Seeing a hard copy of a letter is more conducive to finding errors and grammatic mistakes.

4. Revise the letter using the notes and proofreader's marks.
5. Read the letter once again on the screen. Complete spelling and grammar checks if those tools are available on the computer.
   PURPOSE: To locate any missed errors or misspelled words.
6. Print a final draft. Read the letter word for word, and check once again for errors.
7. Have another person proofread correspondence that is especially important.
   PURPOSE: Often another person can locate missed errors quickly.
8. Complete the final preparations for mailing the letter. Address the letter using guidelines for OCR and fast processing at the post office.

Scanners

Occasionally documents are scanned and sent by email. Scanners provide high resolution and can produce images of written text and photos. Scanners are often used to create images so that older documents can be stored, much like the **microfiche** systems of the past.

Supplies

Stationery

The quality of paper unquestionably affects the reader's total impression of the communication. **Stationers** or printing companies are qualified to advise on the selection of paper, which can range from all-sulfite (a wood pulp) to all-cotton fiber (sometimes called *rag).* Letterhead paper is usually on **bond** with a 25% or higher cotton fiber content.

The weight of paper is described by a **substance number.** This number is based on the weight of a **ream** consisting of 500 sheets of 17- × 22-inch paper. The larger the substance number, the heavier the paper. If the ream weighs 24 lb, the paper is referred to as *Sub 24* or *24-lb weight).* Letterhead stationery and matching envelopes are usually 16-, 20-, or 24-lb weight. This is often abbreviated as 16#, 20#, or 24#.

Sizes and Types of Letterhead Paper. Letterhead paper is available in four basic sizes:

Standard or letter	$8^{1}/_{2} \times 11$ inches
Monarch or executive	$8^{1}/_{2} \times 10^{1}/_{2}$ inches
Baronial	$5^{1}/_{2} \times 8^{1}/_{2}$ inches
Legal	$8^{1}/_{2} \times 14$ inches

Standard letterhead is used for general business and professional correspondence. Monarch is often used by professional people for informal business and social correspondence. Baronial, which is a half-sheet of standard, is used for very short letters or memoranda. Legal, as its name indicates, is used for the lengthy documents presented in court or of a legal nature. Each size of letterhead should have its matching envelope.

Letterhead should be well designed and of a high-quality paper. The letter represents the sender, and the letterhead paper should be carefully chosen to promote the image that the sender wishes to convey. The paper itself makes a strong statement about the business or person it represents and can help the receiver form an impression of the professionalism of the business.

Bond paper has a felt side and a wire side. When a sheet of letterhead is picked up and held to the light, a design or letters can be read from the printed side. This design is called a **watermark** and is an indication of quality. The side from which the watermark can be read is the felt side of the paper and is the side on which printing or typing should be done. The watermark should always read across the page in the same direction as the typing.

Paper with a linen finish is so named because it is similar to fine cloth, with finely spaced lines crossing each other at right angles. Wove is a smooth paper that is normally inexpensive. Antique finish has a semismooth texture, and laid has a finish similar to that of corduroy. All of these paper finishes can make a very professional, impressive letterhead.

CRITICAL THINKING APPLICATION

Brandon realizes that his father's office does not have a method of logging letters sent by certified mail. This forces the receptionist to dig through a patient's file to determine if a certified mail was actually sent and the notice of delivery received. How can this issue be resolved?

Continuation Pages. The second and continuing pages of a letter are placed on plain bond that matches the letterhead in weight and fiber content and are called **continuation pages.** The stationery used for continuation pages should be an exact match to the letterhead, only without the letterhead printing. It is considered unprofessional to use different paper for the continuation pages.

Envelopes. Envelopes are usually made of the same paper as the letterhead stationery. Just as the continuation pages should be the same type of paper as the letterhead, so should the envelopes.

Envelopes also come in the following basic sizes or types:

*   No. 10
*   No. $6^3/_4$
*   Window

No. 10 envelopes are the general business size used for letter and legal stationery. No. $6^3/_4$ envelopes and window envelopes are often used for statements.

LETTER STYLES

A business letter is usually arranged in one of three styles: block, modified block or standard, or modified block indented. A fourth style, called *simplified,* is occasionally used. The block and modified block styles are most commonly used in the physician's office.

Block Letter Style

When block letter style is used, all lines start **flush** with the left margin (Figure 13-1). This style is considered the most efficient but is less attractive on the page.

Modified Block Letter Style

The dateline, the complimentary closing, and the typewritten signature all begin at the center when typing in modified block letter style. All other lines begin at the left margin (Figure 13-2).

Modified Block Letter Style with Indented Paragraphs

The modified block letter style with indented paragraphs is identical to the block style except that the first line of each paragraph is indented five spaces (Figure 13-3).

Simplified Letter Style

With the simplified letter style, all lines begin flush with the left margin (Figure 13-4). The salutation is replaced with an

---

Elizabeth Blackwell, M.D.
223 Orange Avenue, N.W.
Cottonwood, UT 84121

January 26, 20—

Mr. Richard Fluege
3678 North Willow Avenue
Palm Beach, FL 33480

Dear Mr. Fluege:

Please send me full particulars on the professional suites you expect to offer for sale or rent in the Medical Arts Professional Annex.

In about six months, I will be ready to open my practice, and I am interested in locating in Florida. My preference is a street-level suite of approximately 2,000 square feet.

After I have had an opportunity to study the information you send me, I will write or telephone you if I have further questions.

Very truly yours,

Elizabeth Blackwell, M.D.

EB:mek

FIGURE 13-1 Block letter style.

MEDICAL ARTS PROFESSIONAL ANNEX
3678 North Willow Avenue
Palm Beach FL 33480

January 29, 20—

Elizabeth Blackwell, M.D.
223 Orange Avenue, N.W.
Cottonwood, UT 84121

Dear Doctor Blackwell:

We have two remaining street-level suites available for occupancy about July 1. These are marked on pages 3 and 4 of the enclosed descriptive brochure. If one of these suites appeals to you, we will be pleased to customize it for your practice.

Please feel free to call me collect at the number on the brochure for further discussion of your needs.

Sincerely yours,

Richard Fluege
Business Manager

RF:ab
Enclosure

FIGURE 13-2 Modified block letter style.

WILLIAM OSLER, M.D.
1000 South West Street
Park Ridge, NJ 07656

January 26, 20—

Robert Koch, M.D.
398 Main Street
Park Ridge, NJ 07656

Dear Doctor Koch:

Mrs. Elaine Norris

Thank you for referring your patient, Mrs. Elaine Norris, for consultation and care. She was examined in my office today.

FINDINGS: The patient complained of pain in the left lower quadrant and some abdominal tenderness. She had a temperature of 100.2 degrees.

RECOMMENDATIONS: The patient was placed on a soft, low-residue, bland diet, antibiotics, and bed rest for a few days. Upper and lower gastrointestinal x-rays will be performed next week.

TENTATIVE DIAGNOSIS: Diverticulitis of large bowel.

Mrs. Norris has been asked to return here for reevaluation in about ten days.

Sincerely yours,

William Osler, M.D.

WO:gm

FIGURE 13-3 Modified block letter style with indented paragraphs.

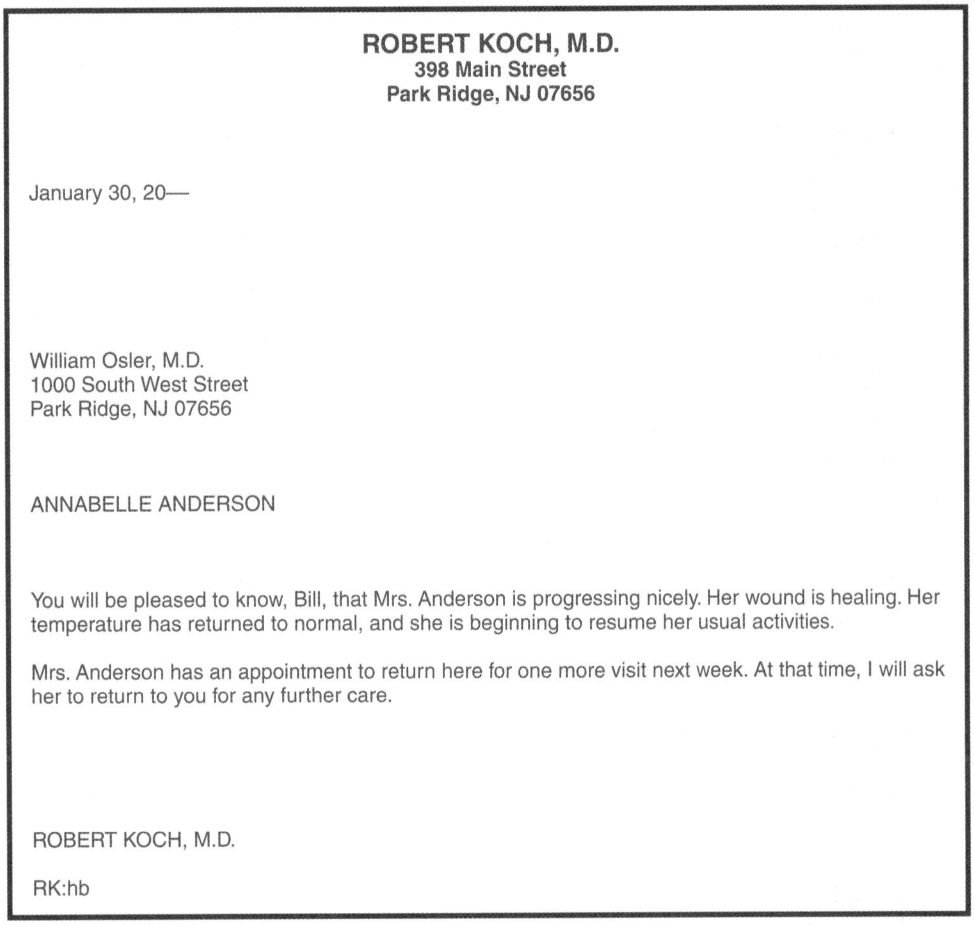

ROBERT KOCH, M.D.
398 Main Street
Park Ridge, NJ 07656

January 30, 20—

William Osler, M.D.
1000 South West Street
Park Ridge, NJ 07656

ANNABELLE ANDERSON

You will be pleased to know, Bill, that Mrs. Anderson is progressing nicely. Her wound is healing. Her temperature has returned to normal, and she is beginning to resume her usual activities.

Mrs. Anderson has an appointment to return here for one more visit next week. At that time, I will ask her to return to you for any further care.

ROBERT KOCH, M.D.

RK:hb

FIGURE 13-4 Simplified letter style.

all-capital subject line on the third line below the inside address. The body of the letter begins on the third line below the subject line. The complimentary closing is omitted. An all-capital typewritten signature is entered on the fifth line below the body of the letter.

Types of Punctuation for Letter Styles

Traditionally the punctuation pattern is selected on the basis of letter style. Normal punctuation is always used within the body of a business letter. The other parts use either standard or open punctuation.

When standard punctuation is used, a colon is placed after the salutation, and a comma is placed after the complimentary closing. This is the punctuation pattern most commonly used. It is appropriate with the block or modified block letter styles. When open punctuation is used, no punctuation is used at the end of any line outside the body of the letter unless that line ends with an abbreviation. This pattern is always used with the simplified letter style.

SPACING AND MARGINS

Generally a letter centered on a page is the most attractive. Accomplishing this is easy with today's computer programs, such as Microsoft Word or WordPerfect. Business letters are almost always single-spaced. If a letter consists of only a few lines, double-space both the inside address and the message and indent the first line of each paragraph five spaces.

The first typed entry, which is the date on the first page of the letter, is usually placed on the third line below the letterhead or on line 13 if there is no letterhead. The typing on continuation pages begins 1 inch from the top.

On standard letterhead, the side margins are usually $1\frac{1}{2}$ inches to 1 inch on each side. The appearance of a very short letter is improved by increasing the width of all margins.

A 1-inch bottom margin is the minimum. This can be increased if the letter is to be carried over to a second page. Never use a second page to type only the complimentary closing and signature. Carry over a minimum of two lines of the body of the letter onto a continuation page.

PARTS OF LETTERS

The structure of a letter and its placement on a page have been fairly well standardized into the following four main parts:
- Heading
- Opening
- Body
- Closing

Heading

The heading includes the letterhead and the dateline. The printed letterhead is usually centered at the top of the page and includes the name of the physician or group and the address. It may include the telephone number and the medical specialty or specialties. In a group or corporate practice, the names of the physicians may also be listed. Occasionally, the heading also includes the name of an office manager.

The dateline consists of the name of the month written in full, followed by the day and year. The date should not be abbreviated, nor should ordinal numbers (e.g., 1st, 2nd, and 3rd) be used after the name of the month.

Opening

The opening consists of the inside address, the salutation, and the attention line, if there is one. The inside address has two or more lines, starts flush with the left margin, and contains at least the name of the individual or firm to whom the letter is addressed and the mailing address. When the letter is addressed to an individual, the name is preceded by a courtesy title, such as Dr., Mr., Mrs., Miss, or Ms. When addressing a letter to a physician, omit the courtesy title and type the physician's name followed by his or her **academic degree,** such as *Rick P. Tipps, MD.* The name could also be written as *Dr. Rick P. Tipps.* Do not use both a courtesy title and a degree that means the same thing, as in *Dr. Rick P. Tipps, MD.* Although this construction is often seen, even on the sign in front of physician's' offices, it is wrong to write a doctor's name in this manner.

CRITICAL THINKING APPLICATION

Brandon has noticed that some of the correspondence leaving the office is signed incorrectly, with "Dr. Rick P. Tipps, MD" in the typed signature line. This is an uncomfortable situation because Brandon realizes that the person who is typing the signature this way is the office manager.

- How might he approach her so that the mistake can be corrected?
- Is it wise to approach the office manager, or should Brandon go to his father? Why or why not?

The salutation is the letter writer's introductory greeting to the person being addressed; it is typed flush with the left margin on the second line below the last line of the address and is followed by a colon unless open punctuation is used. The words in the salutation vary depending on the degree of formality of the letter.

The attention line, if used, is placed on the second line below the inside address. If the name of the person for whom the letter is intended is known, that person's name is used in the inside address and he or she is addressed personally. If the letter is being addressed to a company or organization and directed to a division or department within the company, the division or department name is placed on the attention line.

Body

The body of a letter includes the subject line, if one is used, and the message. In medical office correspondence, the subject of a letter is frequently a patient; in that instance, the patient's name is used as the subject line. Because the subject line is considered to be a part of the body of the letter, it is placed on the second line below the salutation. It may start flush with the left margin or at the point of indentation of indented paragraphs, or it may be centered. The word subject, followed by a colon, may be used or omitted entirely.

Begin typing the message on the second line below the subject line or on the second line below the salutation if there is no subject line. The first line of each paragraph may be indented five spaces or may start flush with the left margin, depending on the chosen letter style.

Closing

The closing includes the complimentary closing, the typed signature, the reference initials, and any special notations.

The complimentary closing is the writer's way of saying goodbye. This closing is placed on the second line below the last line of the body of the letter and is followed by a comma unless open punctuation is used. Only the first word is capitalized. The words used are determined by the degree of formality in the salutation. For example, if the salutation is *Dear Herb,* the closing might be *Cordially, Very truly yours,* or *Sincerely yours* with consistent punctuation. If the letter is addressed to a business, the complimentary closing most used is *Sincerely.*

A typewritten signature is a courtesy to the reader, especially if the name does not appear on the printed letterhead or if the personal signature is difficult or impossible to decipher. The typewritten signature is placed on the fourth line directly below the complimentary closing.

Reference initials that identify the typist are placed flush with the left margin on the second line below the typewritten signature. If the writer's name is included on the signature line, the writer's initials need not be included in the reference block unless desired. The writer's initials, if used, should precede the typist's initials and are separated by a colon or diagonal line. Examples include *mek, GB:mek,* and *GB/mek.*

Special notations are sometimes needed to indicate that enclosures are included with the letter or that copies of the letter are being distributed to others. If the letter indicates an enclosure, type the word *Enclosure* or *Enc.* on the first line below the reference initials. If there is more than one enclosure, specify the number (e.g., *Enclosures 3*). If copies are to be sent to others, type this notation in the same manner as the enclosure notation or after it if both notations are needed. The copy notation is usually written as *cc:* or *copy to:* followed by the name or names of those to whom a copy will be sent. If the person to whom the letter is addressed is not to know that copies are being distributed to others, use the notation *bc:* for "blind copy" on all copies except the original. Place this notation either in the upper left of the letter at the margin or below the last notation at the lower left margin.

Postscripts

Although a postscript may sometimes be used to express an afterthought, it is often used to place emphasis on an idea or statement. Begin the postscript on the second line below the last special notation. Follow the style of the letter, indenting the first line if paragraphs were indented in the body of the letter or starting at the margin if indentation was not used in the letter.

Continuation Pages

If the letter requires one or more continuation pages, the heading of the second and subsequent pages must contain the following three items of information:

- The name of the addressee
- The page number
- The date

The heading should begin on the seventh line from the top of the page. Continuation of the body of the letter begins on the tenth line or the third line below the heading. The three accepted forms for the continuation page heading are as follows:

RICK P. TIPPS, M.D.
Page 2
July 5, 2003

Rick P. Tipps, M.D.
Page 2
July 5, 2003
Subject: Susan Clemmons

Rick P. Tipps, M.D.   -2-   July 5, 2003

Signing the Letter

Some physicians prefer to compose and sign all letters that leave their offices. The majority are more than pleased to delegate to a competent assistant the responsibility of composing and signing letters of a business nature. Although not all authorities agree on the form to be followed, most recommend that a woman's typewritten signature includes a courtesy title (Miss, Mrs., or Ms.) and that the title not be enclosed in parentheses. It is not necessary to include the courtesy title in the handwritten signature.

In general, the physician signs all of the following:

- Letters that deal with medical advice to patients
- Letters to officers or committees of the medical society
- Referral and consultation reports to colleagues
- Medical reports to insurance companies
- Personal letters

The medical assistant usually composes and signs letters dealing with the following matters:

- Routine matters such as arranging or rescheduling appointments
- Orders for office supplies
- Notification to patients about surgery or hospital arrangements
- Collection of delinquent accounts
- Letters of solicitation

CRITICAL THINKING APPLICATION

One of the employees has brought an urgent letter to Brandon that Brandon's father neglected to sign before leaving the office for the day. The letter is to another physician reporting his findings on a referred patient. The employee asks Brandon to sign the letter. What should he do? What are some ways to resolve this situation, if the letter must leave in the mail today?

Continued

MORE TYPES OF WRITTEN COMMUNICATIONS

There are many types of written communications other than a business letter. Remember, every piece of written communication that leaves the office is a reflection on the office. Make certain to follow the rules of grammar even when sending a simple business email.

Telephone Messages

One of the most common types of written communications in the medical office is the telephone message. Seven items must be recorded when taking a phone message, including the following:

- The name of the person to whom the call is directed
- The name of the person calling
- The caller's daytime and/or cell phone number
- The reason for the call
- The action to be taken
- The date and time of the call
- The initials of the person taking the call

Email Messages

Email is a very popular way to send written communications in today's computer-literate society. Email messages can be saved, printed for the patient's chart, and **archived** for storage. Emails that are pertinent to the patient's care or a conflict situation should be printed, and a copy placed in the patient's medical record. Emails that show a pattern of cancelled appointments should also be added to the patient's medical record. Any email sent in a professional capacity from the physician's office or by a physician's representative should adhere to proper rules of grammar and should use accurate spelling. People tend to classify email as casual communication, but because it is so frequently used in business, it should be considered just as professional as a mailed letter. Use of the proper letter format, including the inside addresses and date, is not necessary. However, the rest of the email should read similarly to a letter. Some emails are only one-line responses, but they can still be grammatically correct.

The medical assistant should also avoid the tendency to immediately answer an email that is derogatory, accusatory, or negative in some other way. Print the email and go through it calmly, marking what needs to be addressed. Because attitude is often easily detectable in an email, avoid any hint of negativity in the response. Once a professional response has been crafted, then type and send it. In this situation, it is often best to cc: the office manager, either openly or blindly, depending on the situation. By doing this the medical assistant is including the supervisor in the conflict and keeping him or her aware of the brewing situation. If necessary the office manager will get involved, or he or she may just monitor the situation and how it is handled by the medical assistant.

Faxed Messages

Faxes are another form of written communication. All faxes should have a cover sheet that states that the information contained within it is of a confidential nature and is intended only for the person to whom the fax was sent (Procedure 13-3). Use correct grammar in all faxed messages. Use a fax only when absolutely necessary or when the information sent would not breach patient confidentiality. This helps to avoid other individuals on the receiving end from reading faxed information.

Memorandums

Most offices **disseminate** various memorandums throughout the business week (Figure 13-5). These written documents must also be clear, concise, and grammatically correct. Remember that people reading memos, emails, faxes, and letters can often detect attitudes in written communications, so make the document sound professional, even if the subject matter is frustrating or difficult.

When sending emails to employees, make certain that the important points are all included and presented in a way that does not sound **condescending.** Sometimes, it is wise to include a supervisor's initials on memos that might not receive a positive response, so that employees realize that the writer's supervisor is aware of and supports the information in the memo. This action sometimes avoids a rush to the boss's office to complain about the contents of a memo.

CRITICAL THINKING APPLICATION

- Email is used more and more often to communicate with employees. Brandon has noticed that very few printed memos circulate throughout the office. What are the advantages and disadvantages of communicating through email with employees?
- The office manager has given Brandon information to disseminate to all of the employees of the clinic. She did not specify whether to give out the memo by hand or by email but did state that the information was very important. Which would be the best method?

DEVELOPING A PORTFOLIO

Letter composition can be sped up by developing a **portfolio** of sample letters to suit the various situations that frequently arise. As the physician approves letters, add them to the office portfolio. Suppose, for instance, a letter is needed for a patient who wishes to change an appointment. Compose a letter that is clear, concise, and courteous—and make an extra copy to place in the portfolio of letters. Alternatively, if using a computer, store the letter on a disk or on the computer's hard drive. If letters and other documents are stored on the hard drive, be sure to back the files up on disk or a zip drive. Do this each time a new kind of letter is written. Soon the medical assistant will be able to select a letter from the portfolio and change it slightly to suit the current situation. This will make letter writing in the medical office quick and easy.

PROCEDURE 13-3

Respond to and Initiate Written Communications: Prepare a Fax for Transmission

CAAHEP COMPETENCY: 3.c.(1)(a)

GOAL: *To send a fax from the medical office and ensure that it arrives at its destination in a confidential manner.*

EQUIPMENT and SUPPLIES

- Fax machine
- Fax cover sheet
- Correspondence to be sent

PROCEDURAL STEPS

1. Fill out a fax cover sheet. Include the name of the person sending the fax and that person's phone number. List the name of the person to receive the fax and the fax number to which the document is being sent. Use cover sheets that contain a confidentiality statement.
   PURPOSE: To identify a fax that has been misdirected and to ensure that it goes to the right person when it arrives.
2. Note the number of pages that are being sent, including the cover page.
   PURPOSE: To ensure that all pages are received.

3. Turn the last page upside down, and write the fax number on the top of the document. Many machines require the documents to be in place before the fax is started. This allows the user to see the number without having to memorize it and make an error.
   PURPOSE: To see the fax number clearly once the pages have been placed in the fax machine.
4. Follow the instructions for individual fax machines.
5. Be sure the machine is set to provide a verification that the fax went through. Print the verification and attach it to the fax. Verify the arrival of critical fax documents by phone.
   PURPOSE: To document that the fax arrived at its destination.
6. File the fax and verification sheet in the appropriate location.
   PURPOSE: To maintain a record of information sent via fax.

INTEROFFICE MEMORANDUM

TO   All Staff

FROM   Office Manager

DATE   December 1

SUBJECT   Holiday Schedule

Our entire facility will be closed on December 24, December 25, December 31, and January 1. The office will be on reduced staff during the days of December 26, 27, 28, 29, and 30. Assignments will be based on seniority of staff members. Please submit your preferences as soon as possible.

A

MEMO TO: George Walker

FROM: Stanley Barr

DATE: February 8

SUBJECT: Office rental

We are experiencing unexpectedly rapid growth in our business office and will soon need additional space for our increased number of employees. Do you have a larger facility available in this building? If so, I would like to hear from you regarding the location, square footage, and anticipated rental costs.

B

FIGURE 13-5 Examples of memorandums. Memos are intended to be short, specific, and to the point.

U.S. POSTAL SERVICE

The U.S. Postal Service (USPS) is an independent establishment of the executive branch of the U.S. government. The organization is not a part of the government but was established by the government and operates independently. Established on July 26, 1775, by the Second Continental Congress, the organization we know as the USPS is the second oldest federally established department or agency in the United States.

The Postal Service has transformed from messages sent to neighbors in colonial times to a service dedicated to providing mail service to every single home and business in the United States. Today, many operations can be done online at www.usps.com.

MAIL PROCESSING

Incoming Mail

Each day, a great variety of mail comes into the professional office and must be processed. Common items in the daily mail include the following:

- General correspondence
- Payments for services
- Bills for office purchases
- Insurance claim forms to be completed
- Laboratory reports
- Hospital reports
- Medical society mailings
- Professional journals
- Promotional literature and samples from pharmaceutical houses
- Advertisements

In large clinics and medical centers the mail is opened by specially designated people in a central department to speed up this daily task. In the average medical office, however, a medical assistant, often the receptionist, opens the mail using the ordinary letter-opener method.

Opening the Mail

Before opening any mail the medical assistant should have an agreement with the physician as to what procedure to follow regarding incoming mail—in other words, what letters should be opened and what pieces, if any, the physician prefers to open personally. For example, the physician may prefer to open any communications from an attorney or accountant, even when they are not marked personal. If there is any doubt with regard to opening an envelope, do not open the item and forward it to the person to whom it is addressed. Even a simple procedure such as opening the daily mail can be done with more efficiency if a good system is followed (Procedure 13-4).

Annotating

Annotating the mail is an additional service the medical assistant can perform. Reading each letter through, underlining the significant words and phrases, and noting in the margin any action required make taking action on the mail much easier. If the letter needs no reply, code it for filing at this

PROCEDURE 13-4

Respond to and Initiate Written Communications: Process Incoming Mail

CAAHEP COMPETENCY: 3.c.(1)(a)
ABHES COMPETENCY: 2.h

GOAL: *To efficiently sort through the mail that arrives in the medical office on a daily basis.*

EQUIPMENT and SUPPLIES

- Computer or word processor
- Draft paper
- Letterhead stationery
- Pen or pencil
- Highlighter
- Staple remover
- Paper clips
- Letter opener
- Stapler
- Transparent tape
- Date stamp

PROCEDURAL STEPS

1. Clear a working space on the desk or countertop.
2. Sort the mail according to importance and urgency:
   - Physician's personal mail
   - Ordinary first-class mail
   - Checks from insurance companies and patients
   - Periodicals and newspapers
   - All other pieces, including drug samples.

   PURPOSE: To prioritize the mail for the physician so that the most important issues can be addressed first.

3. Open the mail neatly and in an organized manner.
4. Stack the envelopes so that they are all facing in the same direction.
5. Pick up the top one and tap the envelope so that when you open it you will not cut the contents.
   PURPOSE: To avoid damaging any of the contents inside the envelope.
6. Open all envelopes along the top edge for easiest removal of contents.
7. Remove the contents of each envelope, and hold the envelope to the light to see that nothing remains inside.
8. Make a note of the postmark when this is important.
9. Discard the envelope after you have checked to see that there is a return address on the message contained inside. Some offices make it a policy to attach the envelope to each piece of correspondence until it has received attention.
10. Date-stamp the letter, and attach any enclosures.
    PURPOSE: The date stamp identifies when the envelope and its contents was received at the office.
11. If there is an enclosure notation at the bottom of the letter, ensure that the enclosure was included. If it is missing, indicate this on the notation by writing the word *no* and circling it. This may be as far as your employer will want you to proceed with handling the correspondence.

---

time. A highlighter that does not photocopy may be used for annotating. When mail refers to previous correspondence, obtain this from the file and attach it or a copy. If the patient's chart is needed when replying to an inquiry, pull the chart and place it with the letter.

There should be a specific place for the opened and annotated mail in the medical office. This will probably be some area on the physician's or office manager's desk. After sorting, opening, and annotating the mail, place those items that the physician will wish to see in the established place, with the most important mail on top. Personal mail, of course, is to remain unopened. If a piece of personal mail addressed to the employer is opened in error, fold and replace it inside the envelope, and write across the outside *opened in error,* followed by the initials of the person who opened the mail. Use the same procedure with a piece of mail addressed to another office that may have been opened in error. In such cases reseal the envelope with transparent tape and hand it to the mail carrier.

Responding to the Mail

In some offices, the physician and the medical assistant go over the mail together. Once the medical assistant gains

confidence, he or she will find it easy to draft a reply to most inquiries. Usually, the physician is very pleased to delegate this responsibility, especially for matters that do not relate to patient care.

Letters of referral from other physicians should be carefully noted so that an answer can be sent after the patient has been seen and the physician can give a report. If considerable time may pass before such information can be sent, it is a courteous gesture to write a letter to the referring physician advising that a detailed report will follow. Some physicians send printed cards expressing thanks for referrals; others prefer to write thank-you letters to professional colleagues.

Mail Requiring Special Handling

Payment Receipts

Payments from patients and insurance companies will come to the office on a daily basis. All payments should be separated and recorded immediately in the day's receipts. A payment received on Monday should be recorded on Monday. Most patients consider their cancelled check as a receipt; if the patient requests a receipt, one should be mailed. Otherwise, the receipt may be placed in the patient's chart for delivery on a future office visit.

CRITICAL THINKING APPLICATION

Brandon notices that Mrs. Attaway, a widow and long-time patient of his father's, sent in a check for $125 for a bill. However, her insurance company had already paid $112 toward the bill. Brandon knows that Mrs. Attaway must be very careful with her money and has always paid her bills quickly. The policy of the office is to route the overpayment through the system, but refund checks are cut only once per month. What should Brandon do in this situation?

Insurance Information

Insurance information should be put in a predetermined place for handling by the billers. Documents relating to insurance should be passed to the appropriate person immediately to avoid delays and time limitations that might cause the claim to go unpaid.

Drug Samples

Sample drugs and related literature are usually delivered by pharmaceutical representatives and may occasionally arrive in the mail. Determine from the physician what types of literature and samples should be saved. Most physicians keep pertinent new samples in a locked sample storage area, along with the accompanying literature for immediate reference. Other drug samples are **categorically** stored. Drugs should never be tossed into the trash.

Vacation Mail

When the physician is away from the office, it is generally the responsibility of a medical assistant to handle all mail. In this event, all pieces should be examined carefully. The medical assistant can then decide how to handle each piece based on the following questions:

- Is this important enough that I should phone or fax the physician?
- Shall I forward this for immediate attention?
- Shall I answer this myself or send a brief note to the correspondent, explaining that there will be a slight delay because the physician is out of the office?
- Can this wait for attention until the physician returns, or would that give the appearance of negligence?

If the medical assistant is unable to contact the physician or to forward important mail, he or she should always answer the sender immediately, explaining the delay and requesting cooperation. Instead of forwarding an original piece of mail and risking possible loss, make a copy for forwarding. Then, if the physician wishes the letter answered, notations can be made on the copy and then the copy may be returned to the office staff for answering and returned without defacing the original letter.

When the physician is traveling from place to place, the envelopes for all communications sent to him or her should be numbered consecutively. Doing this enables the physician to easily determine whether any mail has been lost or delayed. By keeping a record of each piece of mail sent out, with its corresponding number, anything that might be lost can be identified and remailed if necessary.

Correspondence not requiring immediate action that the medical assistant is unable to answer until the physician returns should be placed in a special folder marked *Requires Attention* and placed on top of other accumulated mail. Mail that the medical assistant can compose but that requires the physician's approval before mailing should be put into another special folder marked *For Approval*. When the physician returns, these letters can be rapidly checked and signed.

Any letters marked *Personal* may be acknowledged to the return address on the envelope. The brief acknowledgment should state that the physician is out of town for a certain length of time and will attend to the letter immediately on returning. This acknowledgment should also offer help in any way possible in the meantime.

Discard any mail that would ordinarily not be brought to the physician's attention. Some promotional literature falls into this category. Make certain that mailings from professional organizations are saved.

There may be rare periods during which the entire facility is closed. In such cases the post office can be contacted to hold mail until the facility reopens. The postal carrier cannot accept an oral request, so a formal written request must be made. Never leave mail unattended to gather outside a mailbox or clutter up a doorway in a hall. Even mail slots may become filled, or magazines may become stuck in them, causing important mail to pile up outside the slot. Far too much money and mail of a confidential nature are sent to physicians' offices to take chances on mail theft or destruction.

Outgoing Mail

Folding and Inserting Letters

Standard ways of folding and inserting letters are used so that the letter fits properly into the envelope and so that it can be easily removed without damage (Figure 13-6).

No. 10 Envelope. Bring the bottom third of the standard-sized letter up and make a crease. Fold the top of the letter down to within about $3/_8$ inch of the creased edge, and make a second crease. The second crease goes into the envelope first.

No. 6³/₄ Envelope. For a standard-sized letter, bring the bottom edge up to within about $3/_8$ inch of the top edge and make a crease. Then, folding from the right edge, make a fold a little less than one third of the width of the sheet and crease it. Folding from the left edge, bring the edge to within about $3/_8$ inch of the previous crease. Insert the left creased edge into the envelope first.

Window Envelope. To fold a letter for insertion into a window envelope, bring the bottom third of the letter up and make a crease, then fold the top of the letter back to the crease you made before. The inside address should now be facing forward. This method is often followed for mailing statements.

Addressing the Envelope

Delivery Addresses. The USPS attempts to have all mail in standard-sized envelopes read, coded, sorted, and canceled automatically at regional sorting stations where mail can be

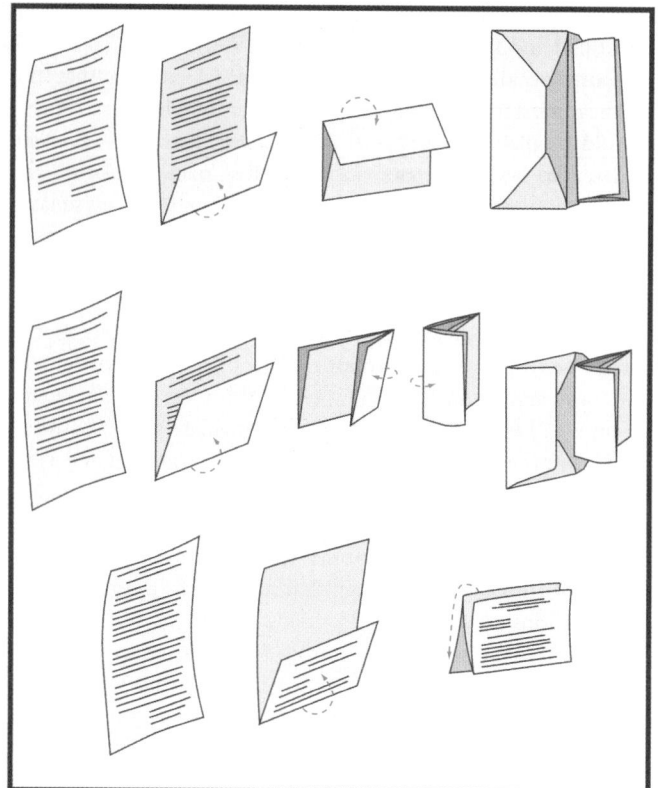

FIGURE 13-6 Correct methods of folding letters.

processed at a rate of over 30,000 letters per hour. The success of automatic sorting depends on the cooperation of mailers in preparing envelopes in a format that can be read by automatic equipment (Procedure 13-5).

Many regulations affect delivery addresses, because this is the most important information on the envelope. The goal of the **mailpiece** is to get delivered.

The Postal Service provides three special sets of abbreviations: (1) state names; (2) long names of cities, towns, and places; and (3) names of streets and roads and general terms, such as University or Institute. The information can be obtained from the Postal Service, or a program can be purchased for the computer. When these abbreviations are used, it is possible to limit the last line of any **domestic mail** address to 27 strokes. The next-to-last line in the address block should contain a street address or post office box number.

The address block should start no higher than $2^{3}/_{4}$ inches from the bottom. Leave a bottom margin of at least $^{3}/_{8}$ inch and left and right margins of at least 1 inch. Nothing should be written or printed below the address block or to the right of it.

The regulations for addressing envelopes were developed mainly for volume mailers with computerized mailing lists (Figure 13-7, p. 243). Some exceptions are acceptable to the Postal Service and its scanning equipment. For example, the traditional style of typing an address in lower case with initial capital letters is readable by the optical scanners. Also, if the ZIP code cannot fit on the line with the city and state, it can be placed on the line immediately below. When using a suite number, most people place it after the delivery address, which is fine. However, if it does not fit in that space, it should be placed *above* the delivery address, not below it.

Return Addresses. Always place a complete return address on the envelope. If there is no stamp on the envelope or if the stamp falls off and there is no return address, it will go to the dead letter office. There, the postal employees will open the mail in an attempt to identify the sender, but huge time delays may make the mail useless on delivery. If an address is found for the sender, the mail will be returned in an official envelope with a notice of postage due. If an address is not found for the sender, the mail is destroyed.

Notations. Any notations on the envelope directed toward the addressee, such as Personal or Confidential, should be typed and underlined on line 9 or on the third line below the return address, whichever is lower. Align it with the return address on the left edge of the envelope.

Any notations directed toward the Postal Service, such as special delivery or Certified Mail, should be typed in all capital letters on the upper right side of the envelope immediately below the stamp area. If an address contains an attention line, it should be typed above the organization line or on the line immediately above the street address or post office box number.

Sealing and Stamping Hints

Here is a suggestion for speeding up the sealing of a number of envelopes—at statement time, for example, when many envelopes go into the mail at one time:

- Fan out unsealed envelopes, address side down, in groups of six to 10.
- Draw a damp sponge over the flaps, and starting with the lower piece, turn down the flaps and seal each one.

Do not use too much moisture because this may cause the glue to spread and several envelopes to stick together. A similar process simplifies stamping several letters at one time if not using a postage meter. If possible, purchase stamps by the roll. Tear off about ten stamps from the roll. Fanfold the stamps on the perforations so that they separate easily. Fan the envelopes address side up. Wet a strip of stamps with the sponge and, starting at one end of the fanned envelopes, attach the stamp at the end of the strip, tear it off, and proceed to the next envelope. Automated sealers and stampers are also available to make this procedure easier and more efficient.

Cost-Saving Mailing Procedures

Using ZIP Codes. The ZIP code is a very important part of an address, just as the area code is a very important part of a telephone number. ZIP codes start with the number 0 on the East Coast and gradually increase to number 9 on the West Coast and in Hawaii.

The five-digit ZIP code was introduced in 1961. The first three digits identify a major city or distribution point, and all five digits identify an individual post office, zone of a city, or other delivery unit. The Postal Service later developed the nine-digit ZIP code, consisting of the original five digits followed by a hyphen and four additional digits that further identify the addressee's street location. The ZIP code is electronically transformed into a bar code. The office computer may have this

Basic U.S. Postal Service Delivery Address Guidelines

- Always put the address and the postage on the same side of your mailpiece.
- On a letter the address should be parallel to the longest side.
- Use the following:
  - All capital letters
  - No punctuation
  - At least 10-point type
  - One space between city and state
  - Two spaces between state and ZIP code
  - Simple type fonts
  - Left-justified format
  - Black ink on white or light paper
  - No reverse type (white printing on a black background)
- If your address appears inside a window, make sure there is at least 1/8 inch clearance around the address. Sometimes parts of the address slip out of view behind the window, and mail processing machines can't read the address.
- If you are using address labels, make sure you don't cut off any important information. Also make sure your labels are on straight. Mail processing machines have trouble reading crooked or slanted information.

More Tips

- Always put the attention line on top—never below the city and state or in the bottom corner of your mailpiece.
- If you can't fit the suite or apartment number on the same line as the delivery address, put it on the line *above* the delivery address, *not* on the line below.

From the U.S. Postal Service website.

- Words like "east" and "west" are called *directionals* and they are *very* important. A missing or a bad directional can prevent your mail from being delivered correctly.
- Use the free ZIP code Lookup and the ZIP+4 code lookup on the Postal Service website to find the correct ZIP codes and ZIP+4 codes for your addresses.
- Almost 25% of all mailpieces have something wrong with the address—for instance, a missing apartment number or a wrong ZIP code. Can some of those mailpieces be delivered in spite of the incorrect address? Yes. But it costs the Postal Service time and money to do that.
- When a first-class-mail letter weighs 1 oz or less and the address is parallel to the shortest side, the piece may be nonmailable or will be charged the nonmachineable surcharge.
- Sometimes it is not important that your mailpiece reach a specific customer, just that it reach an address. One way to do this is to use a generic title such as "Postal Customer" or "Occupant" or "Resident," rather than a name, plus the complete address.
- Fancy fonts such as those used on wedding invitations do not read well on mail processing equipment. Fancy fonts look great on your envelopes but also may slow down your mail.
- Use common sense. If you can't read the address, then automated mail processing equipment can't read the address.
- Some types of paper interfere with the machines that read addresses. The paper on the address side should be white or light in color. No patterns or prominent flecks, please! Also, the envelope shouldn't be too glossy—avoid shiny, coated paper stock.

capability. The Postal Code claims that the ZIP-plus-4, when used with the automated letter-sorting machinery, can eliminate 20 mail-handling steps and result in considerable savings. This saving is passed on to bulk mailers on mailings of 250 or more pieces that have typewritten addresses in machine-readable format along with the nine-digit ZIP code.

Presorting. Bulk mailers can get a discount on postage for presorting their mail. A discounted presort rate is charged on each piece that is part of a group of 10 or more pieces sorted to the same five-digit code or a group of 50 or more pieces sorted to ZIP codes with the same first three digits. The USPS uses the words "presorting" and "bulk" interchangeably.

Using Correct Postage. Although mailing fees are still one of our better bargains, the mailing costs for even a small office are a sizable item in the annual budget, and carelessness can cause them to soar. If the facility does not have a postage meter that dispenses postage exactly, then be sure that you are not putting too many stamps on your outgoing mail. Use an accurate postage scale and remember that only the first ounce requires the base rate; additional ounces are at a lower rate. Remember, the USPS will not deliver mail without postage.

Getting Faster Mail Service

Postage Meters. The postage meter is the most efficient way of stamping the mail in a large business office (Figure 13-8, p. 244). It can print postage onto adhesive strips that are then placed onto the envelopes or packages, or it can print the postage directly onto an envelope. Metered mail does not have to be canceled or postmarked when it reaches the post office. This means that it can move on to its destination faster. Meters vary in size and capabilities. Consult an office-equipment dealer for information on postage meters.

CRITICAL THINKING APPLICATION

- Brandon knows that the mail processing would go much faster if the office invested in a postage meter. The office manager states that she has mentioned this to Brandon's father several times, but he did not purchase a meter. How might Brandon approach his father about this issue?
- What should Brandon do before discussing the postage meter with his father?

PROCEDURE 13-5

Respond to and Initiate Written Communications: Address an Envelope According to Postal Service Optical Character Reader Guidelines

CAAHEP COMPETENCY: 3.c(1)(a)
ABHES COMPETENCY: 2.j

GOAL: *To correctly address business correspondence so that the mail arrives at and is processed by the U.S. Postal Service as efficiently as possible.*

EQUIPMENT and SUPPLIES

- Envelopes
- Computer or typewriter
- Correspondence

PROCEDURAL STEPS

1. Place the envelope into the printer or typewriter.
2. Enter the word processing program, such as Microsoft Word, and check the "Tools" section for envelopes. If this is not available in the word processing program or if a typewriter is being used, judge the area on the envelope that can be read by the optical character reader (OCR). The address block should start no higher than 2¾ inches from the bottom. Leave a bottom margin of at least ⅝ inch and left and right margins of at least 1 inch. Nothing should be written or printed below the address block or to the right of it.
   PURPOSE: To ensure the correct placement of the address for accurate reading by the OCR.
3. Use dark type on a light background and no script or italics, and capitalize everything in the address.
   PURPOSE: To ensure that the OCR can read the address.
4. Type the address in block format, using only approved abbreviations and eliminating all punctuation. If a suite number is to be included, type it above the delivery address on a separate line.
5. Type the city, state, and ZIP code on the last line of the address.
6. No line should have more than 27 total characters, including spaces.
7. Leave a ⅝-inch by 4¾-inch space blank in the bottom right corner of the envelope.
   PURPOSE: To allow for bar code scanning (BCS).
8. Mail addressed to other countries includes the city and postal code on the third line, and the name of the country on a fourth line.

Mailing Practices. For large mailings, local letters should be separated from out-of-town letters. Letters or packages that need to be rushed should be taken directly to the post office for mailing. Others can be placed in street boxes or the building's mail chute for pickup. Packages should always be taken to a post office and weighed for proper postage. Place a letter tray on the desk or some other convenient place so that all outgoing mail is kept together until it is ready to leave the office.

Classifications of Mail

Mail is classified according to type, weight, and destination. The ounce and pound are the units of measurement. Domestic mail is sent to a destination within the United States and its territories, and **international mail** is sent to a destination outside the United States. Letters to distant points of the globe are in almost all cases sent by air and can be expected to reach their destination within a few days. The rates for international mail are based on increments of ½ to 1 ounce. A table of rates can be obtained from the post office.

Express Mail. Express Mail is available 7 days per week, 365 days per year for items weighing up to 70 lb and measuring 108 inches in combined length and **girth.** This includes delivery on Sundays and holidays. It is the fastest mail service offered by the USPS. Service features include the following:

- Noon delivery between major business markets
- Merchandise and document reconstruction insurance
- Express mail shipping containers
- Shipment receipt
- Optional return receipt service
- Optional **collect-on-delivery (COD)** service
- Waiver of signature option
- Collection boxes
- Optional pickup service

First-Class Mail. First-class mail includes sealed or unsealed handwritten or typed material, such as letters, postal cards, postcards, and business reply mail. Postage for letters weighing 13 ounces or less is based on weight, in 1-ounce increments. Envelopes larger than the standard No. 10 business envelope should have the green diamond border to expedite first-class delivery. The minimum quantity to mail at discount prices is 500 mailpieces. First-class mail over 13 ounces automatically becomes Priority Mail. At the time of this publishing, first-class stamps cost $0.39 cents.

Priority Mail. First-class mail weighing over 13 ounces is classified as Priority Mail, and the postage is calculated on the basis of weight and destination, with the maximum weight being 70 lb. A few tips about Priority Mail include the following:

- If using an envelope or box not purchased from the USPS, make certain to mark it *Priority Mail.*
- Priority mail drop shipment is a special way to get mail delivered sooner. Sacks or trays of standard mail are sent to the post office nearest the zip code for delivery, then sent via standard mail.

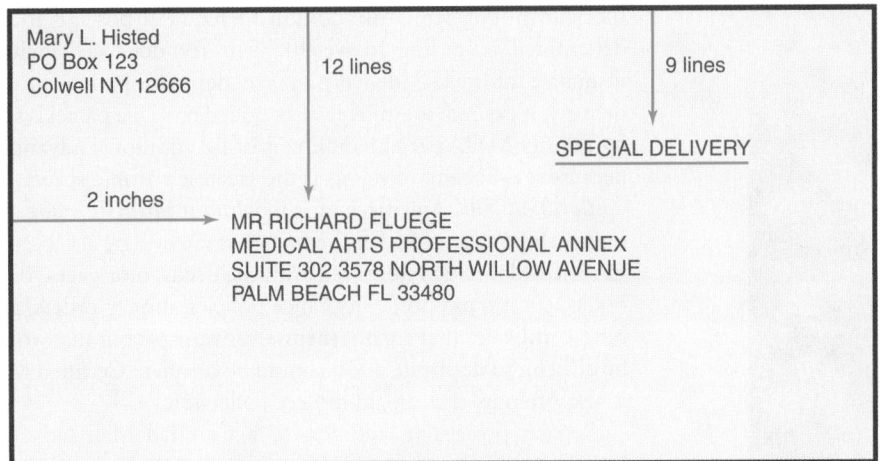

Placement of return address, mailing address, and mailing notation on 6³/₄ envelope

Placement of mailing address and personal notation on No. 10 envelope

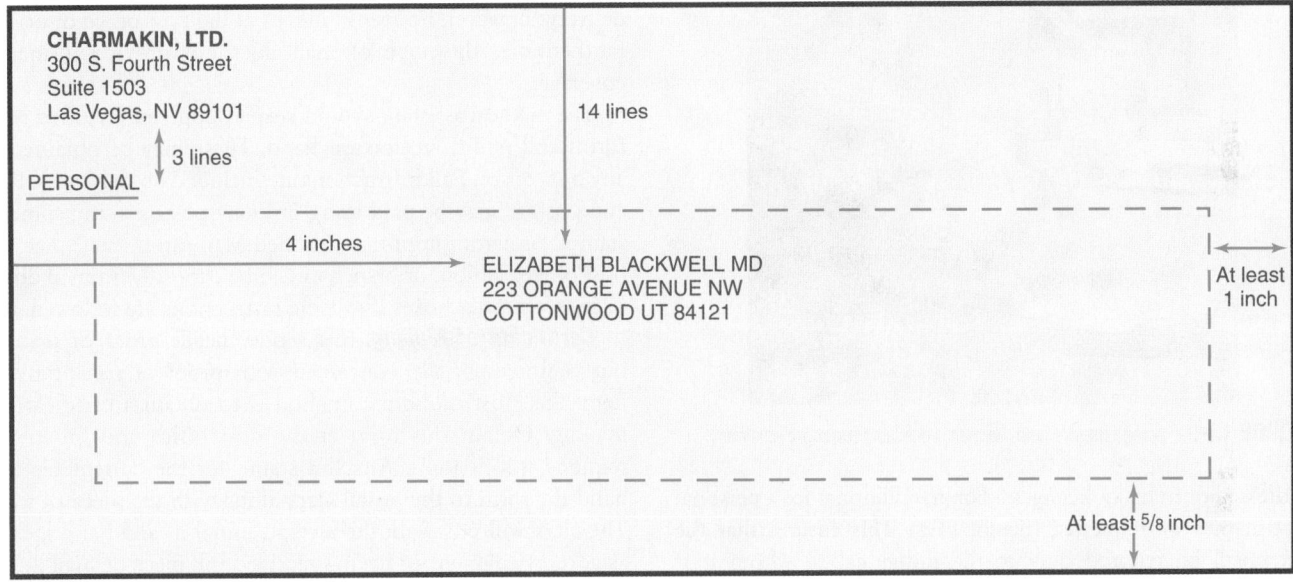

FIGURE 13-7 Addressing envelopes.

- Priority mail parcels that weigh more than 15 lb and are larger than 84 inches in combined length and girth are charged a balloon rate.

Bound Printed Matter. Bound printed matter consists of advertising, promotional, directory, or editorial material (or any combination of such material). It must be securely bound by permanent fastenings such as staples, spiral binding, glue, or stitching, and cannot have the nature of personal correspondence. Loose-leaf binders and similar fastenings are not considered permanent. Mail in this class cannot weigh over 15 lb.

Media Mail. Media mail is used for books, film, manuscripts, printed music, printed test materials, sound recordings, play scripts, printed educational charts, loose-leaf pages and binders consisting of medical information, videotapes, and computer recorded media such as CD-ROMs and diskettes. Media mail cannot contain advertising, and it cannot weigh over 70 lb.

Special Services

Insured Mail. Insurance for coverage against loss or damage is available for Priority Mail, first-class mail, and parcel post.

Registered Mail. Mail of all classes, particularly that of unusually high value, can be additionally protected by registering it. The sender may request evidence of its delivery. Registering a piece of mail also helps to trace delivery, if necessary. The Hope Diamond, worth an estimate of up to $250,000,000, was sent via Registered Mail from New York City to the Smithsonian Institute in Washington, D.C. when Harry Winston donated it to the museum.

When sending a registered letter, it is necessary to go to the post office and fill in the required forms. All articles to be registered must be thoroughly sealed with USPS tape. Cellophane tape is not permitted. On receipt of the item, the **recipient** is required to sign a form that acknowledges delivery. A registered letter may be released to the person to whom it is

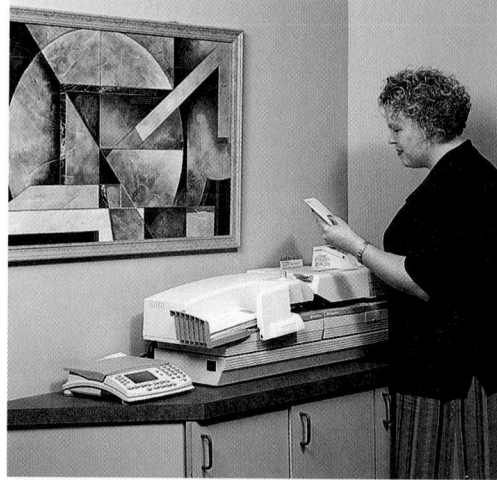

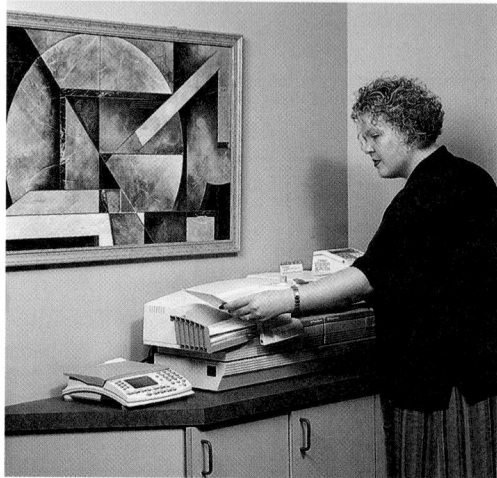

FIGURE 13-8 Postage meters help the mail processing run more efficiently.

addressed or to his or her agent. For an additional fee a personal receipt may be requested (Figure 13-9). This ensures that the letter will be released only to the individual to whom it is addressed. Such pieces bear the label *To Addressee Only*.

Registered Mail is accounted for by number from the time of mailing until the time of delivery and is transported separately from other mail under a special lock. In case of loss or damage, the customer may be reimbursed up to certain limits, provided that the value of the registered article has been declared at the time of mailing and that the appropriate fee has been paid.

Postal Money Orders. Postal money orders are a convenient way of mailing money, especially for the individual who does not have a personal checking account. They may be purchased in amounts as high as $700.

Special Delivery. Mail of any class that has been marked *special delivery* is charged at the special-delivery rate. Such pieces may be regular first- or second-class, registered, insured, or COD pieces. The special-delivery designation generally does not speed up the normal travel time between two cities but does ensure immediate delivery of the item when it arrives at the designated post office.

Special Handling. Third- and fourth-class mail sent by special handling receives the fastest service and ground transportation practicable—about the same as that for first-class mail. The special-handling fee is in addition to required postage and is determined according to weight. This fee does not include insurance or special delivery at the destination, but special delivery, if desired, is available at an added cost. If a parcel is sent by Priority Mail, special handling is of no additional advantage because it is already traveling at the greatest possible speed.

Certified Mail. Any piece of mail without **intrinsic** value and on which postage is paid at the first-class rate will be accepted as Certified Mail. Such items as contracts, deeds, mortgages, bank books, checks, passports, insurance policies, money orders, and birth certificates that are not themselves valuable but that would be difficult to duplicate if lost should be certified. Certified Mail is also often used as an aid in debt collection.

Regular postage in addition to a Certified Mail fee must be affixed. For an additional fee a receipt verifying delivery can be requested (Figure 13-10). Certified Mail can be sent special delivery if the prescribed fees are paid. A record of delivery of Certified Mail is kept for 2 years at the post office of delivery; however, no record is kept at the post office of origin. Furthermore, this type of mail does not provide insurance coverage.

The medical assistant should keep a supply of Certified Mail forms and return receipts on hand. These may be obtained at any post office. Full instructions are included on the forms. Fees and postage may be paid using ordinary postage stamps, meter stamps, or permit imprints. Certified Mail can be mailed at any post office, station, or branch or can be deposited in mail drops or in street letter boxes if specific instructions are followed.

Certificate of Mailing. If a sender needs proof of mailing but is not especially concerned with proof of receipt of an item, the most economic method is to obtain a certificate of mailing. Obtain this form at the post office and fill in the required information. Attach a stamp for the current fee and hand the form to the postal clerk along with the piece of mail. The clerk will postmark the receipt, initial it, and hand it back as acknowledgment of having received the piece of mail at the post office. This is sometimes used when mailing tax reports or other items that must be postmarked by a certain date.

Private Delivery Services

Not all mail is delivered by the USPS. Actually, the USPS delivers only about 44% of the mail in the United States. Many private services pick up and deliver mail overnight. Among these are Federal Express, United Parcel Service, Emery, Airborne Express, and DHL. These services are highly advertised and competitive. All large cities and many smaller communities have centralized points where packages can be dropped off for the service of the sender's choice. Pickup service is also available in many communities.

CRITICAL THINKING APPLICATION

- The office has always used FedEx for sending packages. However, Brandon is curious as to whether FedEx offers the best rates. How might he gather this information?
- What should be considered when choosing a private delivery service?

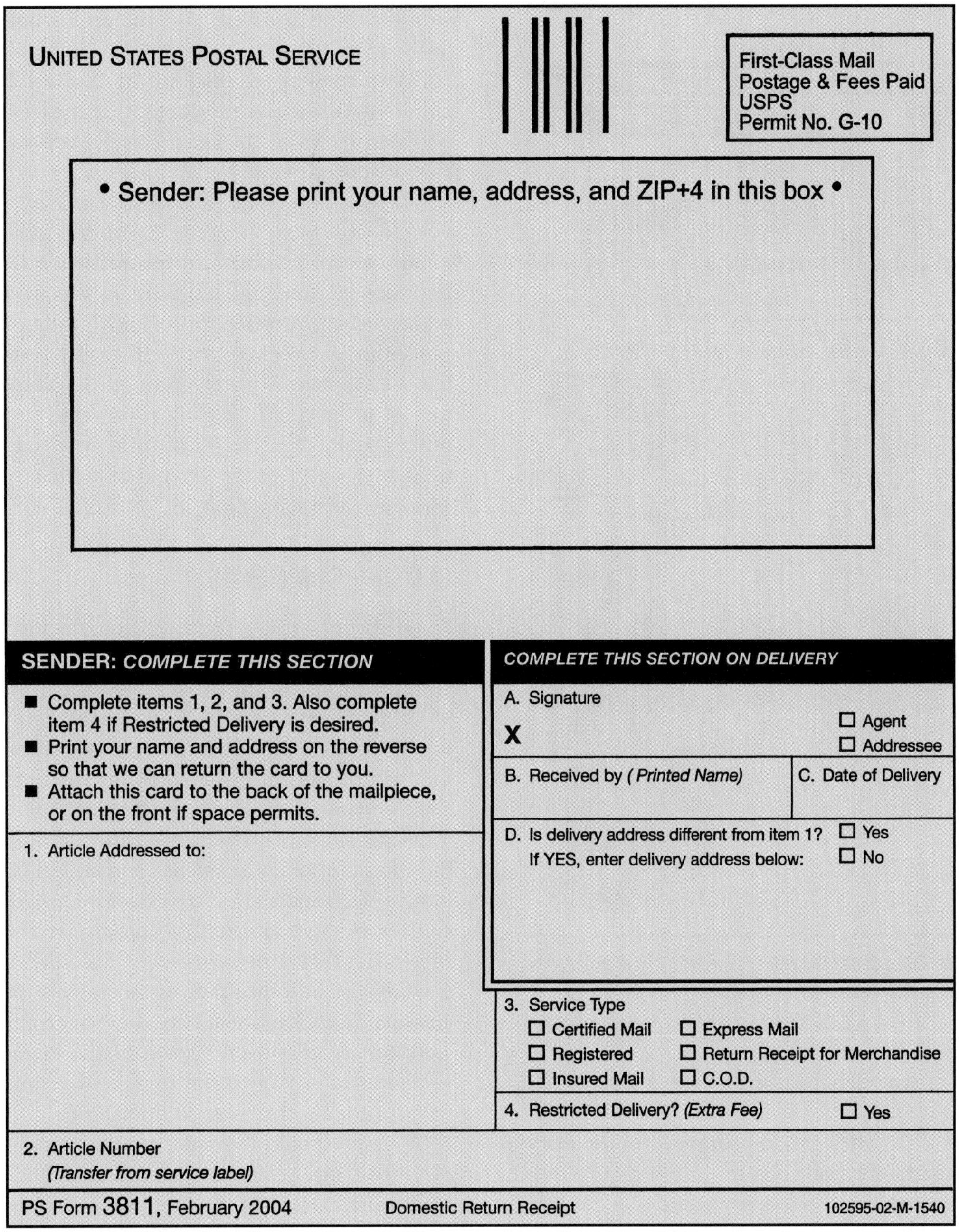

UNITED STATES POSTAL SERVICE

First-Class Mail
Postage & Fees Paid
USPS
Permit No. G-10

• Sender: Please print your name, address, and ZIP+4 in this box •

SENDER: COMPLETE THIS SECTION

- Complete items 1, 2, and 3. Also complete item 4 if Restricted Delivery is desired.
- Print your name and address on the reverse so that we can return the card to you.
- Attach this card to the back of the mailpiece, or on the front if space permits.

1. Article Addressed to:

COMPLETE THIS SECTION ON DELIVERY

A. Signature

X
☐ Agent
☐ Addressee

B. Received by (*Printed Name*) | C. Date of Delivery

D. Is delivery address different from item 1? ☐ Yes
   If YES, enter delivery address below: ☐ No

3. Service Type
   ☐ Certified Mail ☐ Express Mail
   ☐ Registered ☐ Return Receipt for Merchandise
   ☐ Insured Mail ☐ C.O.D.

4. Restricted Delivery? *(Extra Fee)* ☐ Yes

2. Article Number
   (Transfer from service label)

PS Form 3811, February 2004   Domestic Return Receipt   102595-02-M-1540

FIGURE 13-9 Delivery receipts for Certified Mail, Registered Mail, and insured mail. Attach to the back of the article, and endorse the front with the phrase *return receipt requested* adjacent to the article number.

Handling Special Situations

Forwarding and Obtaining a Changed Address. By marking a piece of mail with the notation *Forwarding Service Requested,* the U.S. Post Office will forward mail to the new address if it is sent within 12 months of the change or if the receiver has left a forwarding order with the post office. At that time the forwarding order is expired unless the receiver requests that it be continued. Between 12 and 18 months, the piece will be returned to the sender with the new address noted. After 18 months, mail is usually returned with the reason for nondelivery noted. There is no charge for forwarding when priority or first-class mail is used.

If the mailer wants to know an addressee's new address, this service can be obtained from the post office by placing the words *Address Correction Requested* beneath the return address on the envelope. This can be handwritten, stamped, typewritten, or printed. The new address will be noted on a sticker and returned to the sender, and there is no charge for this if the item is sent priority or first-class mail. The post office charges a weighted fee for this service for standard mail and packages. If the envelope is marked *Change Service Requested,* the post office will dispose of the piece of mail and return a card to the sender showing the forwarding address of the addressee. If the piece was sent priority or first class, no charge is incurred for the service unless

FIGURE 13-10 Receipt for Certified Mail. Attach the bottom portion of the receipt to the top of the envelope, just to the right of the return address.

the notification is sent electronically, in which case there is a small charge.

Recalling Mail. If a letter has been dropped in the mailbox by mistake, do not ask the mail collector to give it to you; he or she is not permitted to do so. However, mail can be recalled by making written application at the post office, together with an envelope addressed identically to the one being recalled. If the letter has already left the local post office, the postmaster, at the sender's expense, can notify the postmaster at the destination post office to return the letter. However, there is no guarantee that the letter will be retrieved.

Returned Mail. If a letter is returned to the sender after an attempt has been made to deliver it, it cannot be mailed again without new postage. It is best simply to prepare a new envelope with the correct address, affix the proper postage, and place it in the mail.

When mail is returned to the medical office, be sure to correct the database, indicating that mail to a certain patient has been returned, so that postage is not wasted sending mail to that address again.

Tracing Lost Mail. Receipts issued by the post office, whether for money orders, Registered Mail, Certified Mail, or insured mail, should be retained until receipt of the item has been acknowledged. If after an adequate time elapses no acknowledgment of receipt for such mailing arrives, notify the post office to trace the letter or package. Regular first-class mail is not easily traced, but the post office will make every attempt to find it for you. In tracing a lost letter or package, the post office requires that a special form be filled out; information from any original receipt should be written on this form, along with any other identifying information.

CLOSING COMMENTS

Remember that every letter sent from the medical office should project a professional image. Use neat handwriting when correspondence is not typed or generated on a computer. All of the office staff must be able to read items written years ago. It is worth the time and effort to brush up on English skills so that writing documents becomes as comfortable as setting an appointment or assisting in a procedure.

Medical offices often use brochures and printed material for the education of their patients. It is critical that these materials look professional and reflect a positive image for the physician and the facility. Be sure that copied material is clean without streaks and that it looks attractive to the eye. If the information is written by an office staff member, make certain that correct grammar is used and that several office members proofread the work for errors and proper use of the English language. It is wonderful to make a good first impression, but every impression in the medical office is an important one.

A copy should be kept of all communications leaving the office that relate to patient care. If any information is handwritten, it must be completely legible to the patient. Certainly, everyone should be able to read his or her own handwriting, even years later.

Because the appointment book is also considered a communications tool, the information entered by hand in the book must also be clear and easy to read. Take enough time to write legibly so that there is no confusion when the document is referred to at a later date. In legal battles, all written documentation must be concise and must not promote questions about the content.

SUMMARY OF SCENARIO

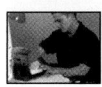

Brandon has been a tremendous help to the office staff over the summer months. He has learned about every area of the medical clinic and has mastered several of the office procedures, both clinical and administrative. He has a greater understanding now of the business aspect of the medical office.

His duties as a temporary administrative medical assistant have opened his eyes to the value and importance of the administrative personnel. He can easily see that everyone–from the receptionist to the scheduler to the insurance billers–plays a vital role in the smooth operation of the facility.

Toward the end of the summer, the office staff honored Brandon with a going-away party. He announced with a smile that he had decided that he wished to become a pediatrician, based on his experience in his father's family practice. He expressed to the staff that he planned to hire them all away from his father! Then on a serious note, he thanked all the employees for their patience and for their willingness to let him learn from them. Everyone expects Brandon to be a complete success.

Sometimes it is difficult to work with a member of the physician's family. Employees should understand that family members often have as much at stake on the success of the practice as the employee. Make every attempt to get along with family members, even when they are less than **amiable.**

By learning proofreader's marks the medical assistant will find that it is much easier and faster to work through a document that needs revision or simple grammatic corrections. The marks are simple to use, once learned, and will be helpful throughout the medical assistant's career.

All documents make an impression, and that impression may be negative or positive. Each document that is generated by the medical assistant needs to make a positive impression. Proofread everything, including emails and memos, and look for ways in which the wording can be made more accurate or more fitting for the message that is being communicated. Because of the reflection on the physician, all documents must be professional–each one, each day, every single time.

SUMMARY of LEARNING OBJECTIVES

1. Define, spell, and pronounce the terms listed in the vocabulary.
   - Spelling and pronouncing medical terms correctly adds credibility to the medical assistant. Knowing the definition of these terms promotes confidence in communication with patients and co-workers.
2. Discuss the responsibility of the medical assistant with respect to equipment and supplies.
   - The medical assistant is responsible for making certain that equipment is in good working order. Warranties should always be mailed when new equipment is purchased, and the correct maintenance procedures should be followed to keep machines working at an optimal level. Supplies should be ordered before they run out, and prices should be compared to find the best quality for the best price available.
3. List the four common sizes of letterhead stationery.
   - Letterhead stationery comes in four basic sizes. Standard or letter stationery, which is most commonly used for business purposes, is 8½ × 11 inches. Monarch or executive stationery is 8¼ × 10½ inches and is used for informal business correspondence. Baronial stationery is 5½ × 8½ inches, whereas legal stationery is 8½ × 14 inches.
4. Explain the various parts of speech.
   - The medical assistant should be familiar with the various parts of speech and the way to use them correctly in a sentence. Nouns name something, such as a person, place, or thing; pronouns are substitutes for nouns. Verbs are action words and express movement, a condition, or a state of being. Adjectives usually describe nouns, whereas adverbs usually describe

verbs. Prepositions are connecting words, as are conjunctions. Interjections show strong feelings and are often followed by an exclamation point.
5. Name some of the essential references for the medical assistant's library.
   - It is quite helpful to develop a personal tool collection that will assist the medical assistant with written communications in the medical office. An up-to-date dictionary, a medical dictionary, a composition handbook, an English-language reference manual, and a thesaurus will be valuable additions to the tool library.
6. List several steps to complete before answering a business letter.
   - Before any type of correspondence is answered, the piece should be read carefully. Often a highlighter is used for marking questions that must be answered, or notes may be written on the correspondence in pencil. A draft of the reply should be written first, then the correspondence should be rewritten in its final draft.
7. Discuss the process of developing and the value of keeping a communications portfolio.
   - Subsequent letters will be much easier to draft if the medical assistant develops a portfolio that contains sample letters and other types of communications. Once a letter is written, it can be saved on the computer hard drive or on a disk, or it can be printed and placed in a binder for easy viewing. If the letter is printed in a binder, it is wise to note on each example the file name as it is saved on the computer so that the document can be easily found again when needed. This is an excellent way to save time in the busy medical office.

Continued

SUMMARY of LEARNING OBJECTIVES

Continued

8. Discuss the differences in the four letter styles.
   - Block is an efficient but less attractive letter style wherein all lines begin flush with the left margin of the paper. Modified block is similar, but some lines begin at the center of the page instead of the left margin. Modified block with indented paragraphs is identical to block style, with the exception of the indention of the paragraphs. Simplified letter style contains lines that begin flush at the left margin, but other items, such as the salutation and complimentary closing, are omitted.

9. Explain the four standard parts of a business letter.
   - The four standard parts of a business letter include the heading, the opening, the body, and the closing. The heading includes the letterhead and dateline, whereas the opening includes the inside address and any attention or salutation line. The body is the message of the document, and the closing includes the signature, complimentary closing, reference initials, and special notations.

10. List several ways to save money when mailing.
    - Money can be saved by consulting the post office when mailing, checking for better rates, and using ZIP codes. Consult a local post office when mailing in bulk to obtain the best rates.

11. Open, sort, and annotate incoming mail.
    - Mail is one of the most common types of communication used in the physician's office. The process for responding to and initiating written correspondence is outlined in Procedure 13-1.

12. Compose, proofread, and mail a business letter.
    - Business letters must look professional and contain sentences that are grammatically correct. The process for proofreading a business letter or publication for accuracy is outlined in Procedure 13-2.

13. Properly send a fax.
    - Transmissions sent by fax must arrive at their destination in a confidential manner. The process for preparing a fax for transmission is outlined in Procedure 13-3.

14. Process incoming mail.
    - Most physician offices have a process for dealing with mail that arrives at the facility. The method for processing incoming mail is outlined in Procedure 13-4.

15. Address an envelope according to postal service optical character reader guidelines.
    - Addresses should be written in such a way that they are quickly and efficiently read by postal service machines. The process for addressing an envelope according to Postal Service optical character reader guidelines is outlined in Procedure 13-5.

CONNECTIONS

 Study Guide Connection: Go to Chapter 13 Study Guide. Read the Case Study and Workplace Applications and complete the assignments. Do online research for answers to the questions in the Internet Activities associated with written communications and mail processing.

 CD Connection: Go to the Medical Assisting Competency Challenge CD and do the training activities under Communication.

 Evolve Connection: For more information related to written communications and mail processing, go to evolve.elsevier.com/kinn and visit related weblinks for Chapter 13. Click on the Medical Assisting Exam Review and do the practice questions to sharpen your test-taking skills.

Medical Records Management

14

SCENARIO

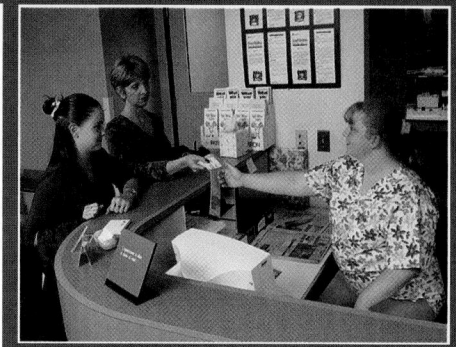

Susan Beezler has just begun her career in the medical assisting profession. She is attending medical assisting school in the morning hours and works part-time for a family practitioner in the afternoons as a clerical record assistant. Susan is eager to learn about medicine and looks forward to taking on more responsibility at the office.

The practice is growing swiftly and recently added a new physician, Dr. Alex Thomas. Dr. Thomas has enjoyed working with Susan and feels that her energy will be just what his patients need. He has taken a special interest in Susan and often lets her assist him with patients when her other duties allow.

Susan knows that although she is a beginner in the office, she will gain trust from her supervisors and patients as long as she projects a teachable attitude. She cheerfully performs filing and often does transcription for Dr. Thomas. The other staff members are pleased with her willingness to perform the most mundane tasks. Her warm personality and caring way with patients ensure that she has a great chance at a long career in this medical office.

Susan enjoys sharing her experiences with the other students in her class. She is the only person who is currently working in the medical field, so the other students ask many questions about what Susan has experienced in the real world of medicine. She is very careful not to breach patient confidentiality as she discusses situations in general, never mentioning any patient names.

Susan feels a great sense of pride that she is already a member of the healthcare team and able to make a positive contribution to the lives of her patients.

While studying this chapter, think about the following questions:

- How can the medical assistant help to alleviate patient concerns about electronic medical records?
- How can the medical assistant earn the patient's trust so that he or she is comfortable revealing the very private information contained in health histories?

- Why is the simple task of filing such a critical action in the physician's office?

LEARNING OBJECTIVES

1. Define, spell, and pronounce the terms listed in the vocabulary.
2. State several important reasons for keeping accurate medical records.
3. Discuss the ownership of records.
4. Explain the difference between a traditional medical record and a problem-oriented medical record.
5. Illustrate the difference between subjective and objective information.
6. Discuss changing an entry in the patient record and the importance of following correct procedures.
7. List and discuss the basic equipment used in a filing system.
8. Describe the steps in filing a document.
9. List and discuss application of the basic filing systems.

10. Explain how color-coding of files can be useful in a medical facility.
11. Establish a patient's medical record.
12. Prepare an informed consent for treatment form.
13. Add supplementary items to an established patient record.
14. Prepare a record release form.
15. Transcribe a machine-dictated letter using a computer or word processor.
16. File medical records and documents using an alphabetic system.
17. File medical records and documents using a numeric system.
18. Color-code medical records.
19. Document appropriately and accurately.

National Accreditation Competencies and Content

CAAHEP COMPETENCIES

Administrative
3.a.(1)(c). Organize a patient's medical record
3.a.(1)(d). File medical records

General
3.c.(2)(c). Establish and maintain the medical record
3.c.(2)(d). Document appropriately

ABHES COMPETENCIES

Communication
2.j. Use correct grammar, spelling, and formatting techniques in written works
2.n. Application of electronic technology
2.o. Fundamental writing skills

Administrative Duties
3.b. Prepare and maintain medical records
3.h. File medical records

Legal Concepts
5.a. Determine needs for documentation and reporting
5.b. Document accurately
5.c. Use appropriate guidelines when releasing records or information
5.d. Follow established policy in initiating or terminating medical treatment

VOCABULARY

alphabetic filing Any system that arranges names or topics according to the sequence of the letters in the alphabet.

alphanumeric Of or relating to systems made up of combinations of letters and numbers.

audit A formal examination of an organization's or individual's accounts or financial situation; a methodic examination and review.

augment To make greater, more numerous, larger, or more intense.

caption A heading, title, or subtitle under which records are filed.

chronologic order Of, relating to, or arranged in or according to the order of time.

continuity of care Continuation of care smoothly from one provider to another, so that the patient receives the most benefit and no interruption in care.

dictation (dik-tay′-shun) The act or manner of uttering words to be transcribed.

direct filing system A filing system in which materials can be located without consulting an intermediary source of reference.

gleaned Gathered bit by bit (e.g., information or material); picked over in search of relevant material.

indirect filing system A filing system in which an intermediary source of reference, such as a card file, must be consulted to locate specific files.

microfilm A film bearing a photographic record on a reduced scale of printed or other graphic matter.

numeric filing The filing of records, correspondence, or cards by number.

objective information Information that is gathered by watching or observation of a patient.

obliteration (uh-bli-tuh-ra′-shun) Act of making undecipherable or imperceptible by obscuring or wearing away.

OUTfolder A folder used to provide space for the temporary filing of materials.

OUTguide A heavy guide that is used to replace a folder that has been temporarily moved from the filing space.

power of attorney A legal instrument authorizing one to act as the attorney or agent of the grantor.

pressboard A strong, highly glazed composition board resembling vulcanized fiber; heavy card stock.

procrastination (pruh-kras-tuh-na′-shun) The intentional postponement of doing something that should be done.

provisional diagnosis A temporary diagnosis made before all test results have been received.

quality control An aggregate of activities designed to ensure adequate quality, especially in manufactured products or in the service industries.

requisites (re′-kwuh-zuhts) Entities considered essential or necessary.

retention schedule A method or plan for retaining or keeping medical records, and their movement from active, to inactive, to closed filing.

shelf filing A system that uses open shelves rather than cabinets for storing records.

shingling A method of filing whereby one report is laid on top of the older report, resembling the shingles of a roof.

subjective information Information that is gained by questioning the patient or taken from a form.

tickler file A chronologic file used as a reminder that something must be taken care of on a certain date.

transcription To make a written copy of, either in longhand or by machine.

vested Granted or endowed with a particular authority, right, or property; to have a special interest in.

A medical records management system is only as good as the ease of retrieval of the data in the files. Because the pace of the medical office is usually quite rapid, patient medical records must be found quickly and also be functional, so that the information inside is easily obtainable.

Few phrases are more frustrating to the patient than "we cannot locate your records." Patients have every right to question the competence of the medical care they are receiving if the office has problems simply finding a chart. Organization and adherence to set routines will help to ensure that medical records are accessible when they are needed.

WHY MEDICAL RECORDS ARE IMPORTANT

Medical records exist for four basic reasons. First, the medical record assists the physician in providing the best possible medical care for the patient. The physician examines the patient and enters the findings on the patient's medical record. These findings are the clues to diagnosis. The physician may order many types of tests to confirm or **augment** the clinical findings. As the reports of these tests come in, the findings fall into place like the pieces of a jigsaw puzzle. Then, with the confirmation data to support the diagnosis, the physician can prescribe treatment and form an opinion about the patient's chances for recovery, assured that every resource has been used to arrive at a correct judgment. The medical record provides a complete history of all of the care given to the patient.

The medical record also provides critical information for others. By reading through the record and discovering the methods used to treat the patient, healthcare professionals can provide a **continuity of care.** Each person knows what the patient has experienced and can provide continued care, even from one facility to another. For example, when a patient is transferred from a hospital to a skilled nursing facility, the information from the patient's hospital record will help the nursing facility staff to better care for the patient. When patients move from place to place or caregivers change, copies of the pertinent information should move with the patient to provide this continuity of care.

The second reason for keeping medical records is to offer legal protection for those who provided care to the patient. A documented medical record is excellent proof that certain procedures were performed or medical advice was given. An accurate record is the foundation for legal defense in cases of medical professional liability. This is one reason that it is critical to write legibly in the record and document exactly what happens to the patient. Remember: *If it isn't charted, it didn't happen.*

Third, medical records provide statistical information that is helpful to researchers. The patient's record provides information about medications taken and the reactions to them. Medical records may be used to evaluate the effectiveness of certain kinds of treatment or to determine the incidence of a given disease. Often, physicians take part in drug studies that track adverse reactions and side effects. The effects of various treatments and procedures can also be tracked and statistics **gleaned** from the information gathered from patient records.

Correlation of such statistical information may result in a new outlook on some phases of medicine and can lead to revised techniques and treatments. The statistical data from medical records are also valuable in the preparation of scientific papers, books, and lectures.

Fourth, medical records are vital for financial reimbursement. The information in the medical record supports claims for reimbursement and is required by most third-party payors.

OWNERSHIP OF THE MEDICAL RECORD

Who actually owns the medical record? Patients often assume that because the information contained in the medical record is about them, the ownership of the record rightfully belongs to the patient. However, the owner of the physical medical record is the physician or medical facility, often called the "maker," that initiated and developed the record. The patient has the right of access to the information within but does not own the physical chart or other documents pertaining to the record. The patient has a **vested** interest and therefore has the right to demand confidentiality of all of the information placed in the chart.

The actual medical record should never leave the medical facility from which it originated. Even the physician should refrain from taking the record from the office to the hospital or nursing facility. If information from the record is needed, copies can be placed in a file, and progress notes written on-site and returned to the original record later. Patient records should be kept in a locked room or locked filing cabinets when the office is closed.

CRITICAL THINKING APPLICATION

On Susan's third day at work, a man comes into the office and demands to see his mother's medical chart. Susan pulls the chart and sees an entry stating that the mother does not wish the son to have any information about her. What should Susan do in this situation? Are there any viable reasons why the son should have access to the mother's medical information?

CREATING AN EFFICIENT MEDICAL RECORD MANAGEMENT SYSTEM

The medical record management system used in the medical office should provide an easy method for retrieving information. The files should be organized in an orderly fashion, and all of the information within the record must be completely legible to the average reader. The information must also be accurate, and corrections should be made and documented properly. The wording in the record should be easily understood and grammatically correct. An efficient method of adding documents to the chart must be in place so that the physician or other provider always has the most up-to-date information.

Above all, the medical record management system must be one that works for the individual facility. Attempting to adopt a method used by another facility may not always be best. The system should be adapted to the needs of the facility and the provider.

Types of Records

The two major types of patient records include the paper-based medical record and the computer-based medical record. As computer technology advances, the paper-based medical record seems more and more inefficient. It is difficult to use a paper-based record for multiple purposes. In most cases, only one person can use the paper-based record at any given time, and the record is not available to others who need it when it is in use by a single person. Misfiled information is common, and the entire record can be misfiled as well. Data cannot be accessed easily for research and **quality control,** and in facilities with multiple departments the information is difficult to share. The paper-based record is a good evidence of patient care, but it not nearly as useful in other capacities.

The computer-based medical record (also called the *electronic health record)* is much more efficient than the paper-based record. The book *Electronic Health Records: Changing the Vision* offers the following definition:

An electronic health record is any information relating to the past, present, or future physical/mental health, or condition of an individual which resides in electronic systems used to capture, transmit, receive, store, retrieve, link, and manipulate multimedia data for the primary purpose of providing healthcare and health related services.

Some healthcare professionals distinguish between a computer-based medical record and an electronic health record. To simplify a difficult definition, consider the computer-based medical record as one in which the bulk of information is entered via computer but there are still paper aspects to the record. For instance, an x-ray film may not be included in a patient's computer-based record. The x-ray film may still be filed in a room among all other patient x-ray films. However, using an electronic health record, all healthcare information is stored in one format. This means that x-ray studies, bone scans, magnetic resonance imaging (MRI) studies, and so on would be scanned into the electronic health record and become a permanent part of the record.

Granted, not all physicians today have the means or desire to convert to a total electronic health record. The cost of such a conversion would be tremendous. However, physicians who are just opening and establishing their practices may look more toward the future and plan for an electronic medical practice. Even today, many physicians use laptop computers, or smaller electronic units, to record patient information during office visits.

Be aware that for a medical assistant, learning never stops. As facilities grow, medical assistants will be asked to make changes and learn new ways of completing tasks. Be willing to move into the future and embrace new ideas. Those who balk and complain about change will find themselves left behind as technology advances.

The computer-based medical record is a great improvement over the paper-based record, but it is not without its disadvantages. Patient confidentiality is critical and sometimes difficult to maintain with computer-based records. Many providers worry about computer malfunctions that would inhibit access to the record in an emergency.

Still, the advantages of the computer-based record seem to far outweigh the disadvantages. Information can be accessed in a variety of physical locations, and more than one person can see the record at any given time. The patient database usually allows various types of statistical information to be recalled, which is a valuable tool. Patient information is available quickly in an emergency, even when the patient is not in his or her hometown. All of these advantages mean that the computer-based record will continue to be a key tool in the future.

CRITICAL THINKING APPLICATION

Some of the patients who visit Dr. Thomas have expressed concern that computer-based medical records may not be private enough. They are worried that unauthorized individuals could somehow access their information on the computer and somehow cause the patients harm. How might Susan alleviate the patients' fears? What disadvantages regarding confidentiality are associated with the computer-based patient record? Should a patient be allowed to decide whether his or her records will be kept on computer or on paper?

ORGANIZATION OF THE MEDICAL RECORD

Source-Oriented Records

The traditional patient record is source oriented; that is, observations and data are cataloged according to their source—physician, laboratory, radiology department, nurse, technician—with no recording of a logical relationship among them. Forms and progress notes are filed in reverse **chronologic order** (most recent on top) and filed in separate sections of the record by the type of form or service rendered—all laboratory reports together, all x-ray reports together, and so on.

Problem-Oriented Medical Records

The problem-oriented medical record (POMR) is a radical departure from the traditional system of keeping patient records. It is sometimes referred to as the *Weed system,* because it was originated by Dr. Lawrence L. Weed, a professor of medicine at the University of Vermont's College of Medicine. The POMR is a record of clinical practice that divides medical action into four bases:

- The database includes chief complaint, present illness, patient profile, review of systems, physical examination, and laboratory reports.
- The problem list is a numbered and titled list of every problem the patient has that requires management or workup. This may include social and demographic troubles as well as strictly medical or surgical ones.
- The treatment plan includes management, additional workups needed, and therapy. Each plan is titled and numbered with respect to the problem.
- The progress notes include structured notes that are numbered to correspond with each problem number.

Several companies have developed file folders for the organization of patient data consistent with the POMR (Figure 14-1). The problem list is entered on the divider cover for

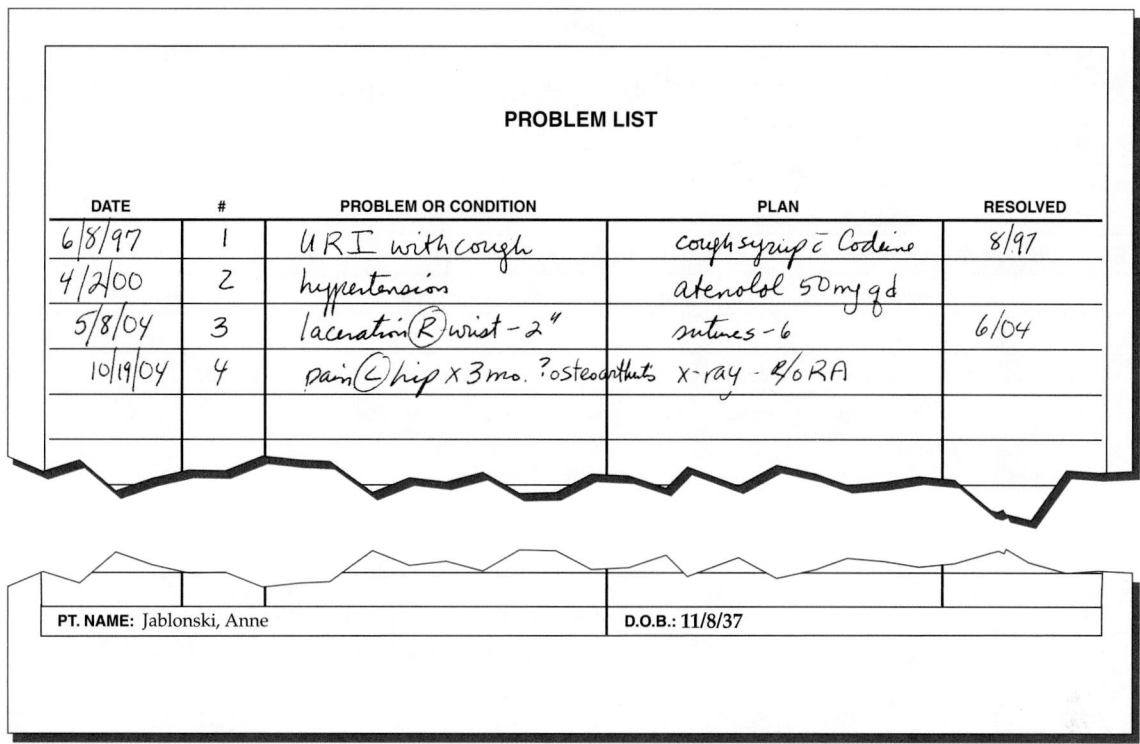

PROBLEM LIST

DATE	#	PROBLEM OR CONDITION	PLAN	RESOLVED
6/8/97	1	URI with cough	cough syrup c̄ Codeine	8/97
4/2/00	2	hypertension	atenolol 50mg qd	
5/8/04	3	laceration (R) wrist – 2"	sutures – 6	6/04
10/19/04	4	pain (L) hip X 3 mo. ?osteoarthritis	x-ray - R/o RA	

PT. NAME: Jablonski, Anne   D.O.B.: 11/8/37

FIGURE 14-1 A chart designed for a problem-oriented medical record (POMR). Some charts are specifically adapted to the POMR. (Courtesy Bibbero Systems, Inc., Petaluma, Calif. 94954, (800) 242-2376, www.bibbero.com.)

laboratory reports. Special sections are provided for current major and chronic problems and for inactive major or chronic problems. The divider cover for progress notes is a chart for listing medications and other therapeutic modalities. Progress notes follow the SOAP approach. SOAP is an acronym for the following:

- *S*ubjective impressions
- *O*bjective clinical evidence
- *A*ssessment or diagnosis
- *P*lans for further studies, treatment, or management

Some medical offices also used an "E" in the record, to represent "Evaluation." This section is used to record an assessment of the patient's understanding of and possible compliance with the treatment plan. As this is not used in every practice, the medical assistant may never see or use it to complete a patient record.

The POMR has the advantage of imposing order and organization on the information added to a patient's medical record. The records are more easily reviewed, and the likelihood of overlooking a problem is greatly reduced. The SOAP method essentially forces a rational approach to patient problems and assists in formulating a logical and orderly plan of patient care (Figure 14-2).

CRITICAL THINKING APPLICATION

Dr. Thomas wants Susan to thoroughly understand the SOAP method of charting. How would Susan explain each aspect of this method to a classmate? Distinct differences exist between the SOAP method and the POMR. Help Susan distinguish between the two. Which method seems easier and more efficient to you?

Popularity of the POMR has continued to grow since its introduction in the 1960s, and it is especially advantageous in clinics, group practices, and hospitals, where more than one person must be able to find essential information in the chart.

CONTENTS OF THE COMPLETE CASE HISTORY

The medical case history is the most important record in a physician's practice. For completeness, each patient's record should contain **subjective information** provided by the patient and **objective information** provided by the physician. If all entries are completed, the case history will stand the test of time. No branch of medicine is exempt from the necessity of keeping patient history records.

Subjective Information

Personal Demographics

The patient's case history begins with routine personal data, which the patient usually supplies on the first visit (Procedure 14-1). Most patients are required to complete a patient information form (Figure 14-3). The basic facts needed are the following:

- Patient's full name, spelled correctly
- Names of parents if patient is a child
- Patient's sex
- Date of birth
- Marital status
- Name of spouse, if married
- Number of children, if any
- Home address, telephone number, and email

OUTLINE FORMAT PROGRESS NOTES

Patient Name _____Fletcher, LeRoy_____

Page_____1_____

Prob. No. or Letter	DATE	**S** Subjective	**O** Objective	**A** Assess	**P** Plans
2	01/26/06	Patient complains of two days of severe high epigastric pain and burning, radiating through to the back. Pain accentuated after eating.			
			On examination there is extreme guarding and tenderness, high epigastric region. No rebound. Bowel sounds normal. BP 110/70		
				R/O gastric ulcer, pylorospasm.	
					To have upper gastrointestinal series. Start on Cimetidine, 300 mg. q.i.d. Eliminate coffee, alcohol, and aspirin. Return in two days.

Start each Progress Note (Subjective, Objective, through the intervening columns to the right   Assessment and Plans) at the appropriate margin of the page.   shaded column to create an outline form. Write

ANDRUS/CLINI-REC® PRIMARY CARE CHARTING SYSTEM FORM NO. 26-7115, ©1976 BIBBERO SYSTEMS, INC., PETALUMA, CA.

FIGURE 14-2 SOAP progress notes. The SOAP method keeps information organized and in a logical sequence. An actual progress note would include the physician's signature or initials after this entry. (Courtesy Bibbero Systems, Inc., Petaluma, Calif. 94954, (800) 242-2376, www.bibbero.com.)

PROCEDURE 14-1

Establish the Medical Record

<u>CAAHEP COMPETENCY:</u> 3.a(1)(c), 3.c.(2)(c)
<u>ABHES COMPETENCY:</u> 3.b

GOAL: *To initiate a medical file for a new patient that will contain all the personal data necessary for a complete record and any other information required by the facility.*

EQUIPMENT and SUPPLIES

- Computer or typewriter
- Clerical supplies (pen, clipboard)
- Information on the agency's filing system
- Registration form
- File folder
- Label for folder
- Identification (ID) card if using numeric system
- Cross-reference card
- Financial card
- Routing slip
- Private conference area

PROCEDURAL STEPS

1. Determine that the patient is new to the office.
2. Obtain and record the required personal data.
   <u>PURPOSE:</u> Complete information is necessary for credit and insurance claim processing.
3. Type the information onto the patient history form.

4. Review the entire form.
   <u>PURPOSE:</u> To confirm that the information is complete and correct.
5. Select a label and folder for the record.
   <u>EXPLANATION:</u> If color-coding is used, a decision must be made regarding the appropriate color for the patient name.
6. Type the caption on the label and apply it to the folder.
   <u>EXPLANATION:</u> Use the patient's name for alphabetic filing or appropriate number for numeric filing.
7. For a numeric filing system, prepare a cross-reference card and a patient ID number.
   <u>PURPOSE:</u> Numeric filing is an indirect system and requires a cross-reference to a patient's name for locating the chart. The patient will use the number of the ID card when arranging appointments or making inquiries.
8. Prepare the financial card, or place that patient's name in the computerized ledger.
9. Place the patient's history form and all other forms required by the agency into the prepared folder.
10. Clip an encounter form on the outside of the patient's folder.

- Occupation
- Name of employer
- Business address and telephone number
- Employment information for spouse
- Healthcare insurance information
- Source of referral
- Social Security number

Personal and Medical History

The personal and medical history, which is often obtained by having the patient complete a questionnaire, provides information about any past illnesses or surgical operations that the patient may have had and includes data about injuries or physical defects, whether congenital or acquired (Figure 14-4). It also includes information about the patient's daily health habits. The presence of allergies, advance directives, and other information can be easily indicated on the front of the medical record by the use of stickers (Figure 14-5). These are useful when important facts about the patient need to be on the forefront of the health professional's mind while treating the patient.

Patient's Family History

The family history is composed of the physical condition of the various members of the patient's family, any illnesses or diseases that individual members may have experienced in the past, and a record of the causes of death. This information is

important, because a hereditary pattern may be present in the case of certain diseases.

Patient's Social History

The patient's social history includes information about the lifestyle the patient lives. If the patient drinks, how many drinks per day or per week are consumed? If the patient uses cigarettes, how many packs a day are smoked? Drug use and even marital information can be considered part of the social history.

CRITICAL THINKING APPLICATION

While taking a medical history from a patient, Susan asks about the social history. She questions the patient as to whether he drinks alcohol. The patient immediately becomes defensive and accuses Susan of getting too personal about his affairs. How might Susan explain her reasons for asking these questions? What options are available if the patient refuses to discuss the social history with Susan? Could this opposition to questions about the social history raise suspicion in Susan's mind? What might she suspect?

Patient's Chief Complaint

The patient's chief complaint is a concise account of the patient's symptoms, explained in the patient's own words. It should include the following:

Thank you for selecting our health care team!
To help us meet all your health care needs, please
fill out this form completely in ink. If you have any questions
or need assistance, please ask us - we will be happy to help.

Welcome

Patient # _____

Soc. Sec. # _____

Date _____

Patient Information (CONFIDENTIAL)

Name _____ Birth date _____ Home phone _____

Address _____ City _____ State _____ Zip _____

Check appropriate box: ☐ Minor ☐ Single ☐ Married ☐ Divorced ☐ Widowed ☐ Separated

☐ Full time ☐ Part time

If student, name of school/college _____ City _____ State _____

Patient's or parent's employer _____ Work phone _____

Business address _____ City _____ State _____ Zip _____

Spouse or parent's name _____ Employer _____ Work phone _____

Whom may we thank for referring you? _____

Person to contact in case of emergency _____ Phone _____

Responsible Party

Name of person responsible for this account _____ Relationship to patient _____

Address _____ Home phone _____

Driver's license # _____ Birth date _____ Financial institution _____

Employer _____ Work phone _____ SSN# _____

Is this person currently a patient in our office? ☐ Yes ☐ No

Insurance Information

Name of insured _____ Relationship to patient _____

Birth date _____ Social Security # _____ Date employed _____

Name of employer _____ Union or local # _____ Work phone _____

Address of employer _____ City _____ State _____ Zip _____

Insurance company _____ Group # _____ Policy/ID # _____

Ins. co. address _____ City _____ State _____ Zip _____

How much is your deductible? _____ How much have you used? _____ Max. annual benefit _____

DO YOU HAVE ANY ADDITIONAL INSURANCE? ☐ Yes ☐ No   IF YES, COMPLETE THE FOLLOWING:

Name of insured _____ Relationship to patient _____

Birth date _____ Social Security # _____ Date employed _____

Name of employer _____ Union or local # _____ Work phone _____

Address of employer _____ City _____ State _____ Zip _____

Insurance company _____ Group # _____ Policy/ID # _____

Ins. co. address _____ City _____ State _____ Zip _____

How much is your deductible? _____ How much have you used? _____ Max. annual benefit _____

I authorize release of any information concerning my (or my child's) health care, advice and treatment provided for the purpose of evaluating and administering claims for insurance benefits. I also hereby authorize payment of insurance benefits otherwise payable to me directly to the doctor.

X _____

Signature of patient or parent if minor   Date

FIGURE 14-3 The patient information form provides all of the information that the medical assistant needs to construct a patient chart.

PART A — PRESENT HEALTH HISTORY (continued)

IV. GENERAL HEALTH, ATTITUDE AND HABITS (continued)

Have you recently had any changes in your: If yes, please explain:
Marital status?   No ___ Yes ___
Job or work?   No ___ Yes ___
Residence?   No ___ Yes ___
Financial status?   No ___ Yes ___
Are you having any legal problems
or trouble with the law?   No ___ Yes ___

PART B — PAST HISTORY

I. FAMILY HEALTH
Please give the following information about your immediate family:

Relationship	Age, If Living	Age At Death	State of Health Or Cause of Death
Father			
Mother			
Brothers and Sisters			
Spouse			
Children			

Have any **blood relatives** had any of the following illnesses?
If so, indicate relationship (mother, brother, etc.)

Illness	Family Members
Asthma	
Diabetes	
Cancer	
Blood Disease	
Glaucoma	
Epilepsy	
Rheumatoid Arthritis	
Tuberculosis	
Gout	
High Blood Pressure	
Heart Disease	
Mental Problems	
Suicide	

II. HOSPITALIZATIONS, SURGERIES
Please list all times you have been hospitalized.

Year	Operation

III. ILLNESS AND MEDICAL PROBLEMS
Please mark with an (X) any of the following
If you are not certain when an illness started,

Illness	(X)
Eye or eye lid infection	
Glaucoma	
Other eye problems	
Ear Trouble	
Deafness or decreased hearing	
Thyroid trouble	
Strep throat	
Bronchitis	
Emphysema	
Pneumonia	
Allergies, asthma or hay fever	
Tuberculosis	
Other lung problems	
High blood pressure	
Heart attack	
High cholesterol	
Arteriosclerosis	
(Hardening of arteries)	
Heart murmur	
Other heart condition	
Stomach/duodenal ulcer	
Diverticulosis	
Colitis	
Other bowel problem	
Hepatitis	
Liver trouble	
Gallbladder trouble	

Page 2   © 1979, 1983 Bibbero Systems Int'l
(REV. 6/92)

ANDRUS/CLINI-REC® HEALTH HISTORY QUESTIONNAIRE

Identification Information   Today's Date _____
Name _____   Date of Birth _____
Occupation _____   Marital Status _____

Chart No. _____

PART A — PRESENT HEALTH HISTORY

I. CURRENT MEDICAL PROBLEMS
Please list the medical problems for which you came to see the doctor. About when did they begin?

Problems	Date Began

What concerns you most about these problems?

If you are being treated for any other illnesses or medical problems by another physician, please describe the problems and write the name of the physician or medical facility treating you.

Illness or Medical Problem	Physician or Medical Facility	City

II. MEDICATIONS
Please list all medications you are now taking, including those you buy without a doctor's prescription (such as aspirin, cold tablets or vitamin supplements)

III. ALLERGIES AND SENSITIVITIES
List anything that you are allergic to such as certain foods, medications, dust, chemicals, or soaps, household items, pollens, bee stings, etc., and indicate how each affects you.

Allergic To:	Effect	Allergic To:	Effect

IV. GENERAL HEALTH, ATTITUDE AND HABITS

How is your overall health now?   Health now: Poor ___ Fair ___ Good ___ Excellent ___
How has it been most of your life?   Health has been: Poor ___ Fair ___ Good ___ Excellent ___
In the past year:
  Has your appetite changed?   Appetite: Decreased ___ Increased ___ Stayed same ___
  Has your weight changed?   Weight: Lost ___ lbs. Gained ___ lbs. No change ___
  Are you thirsty much of the time?   Thirsty: No ___ Yes ___
  Has your overall 'pep' changed?   Pep: Decreased ___ Increased ___ Stayed same ___
Do you usually have trouble sleeping?   Trouble sleeping: No ___ Yes ___
How much do you exercise?   Exercise: Little or none ___ Less than I need ___ All I need ___
Do you smoke?   Smokes: No ___ Yes ___ If yes, how many years? ___
How many each day?   ___ Cigarettes ___ Cigars ___ Pipesfull
Have you ever smoked?   Smoked: No ___ Yes ___ If yes, how many years? ___
How many each day?   ___ Cigarettes ___ Cigars ___ Pipesfull
Do you drink alcoholic beverages?   Alcohol: No ___ Yes ___ I drink ___ Beers ___ Glasses of Wine
                                                       ___ Drinks of hard liquor - per day
Have you ever had a problem with alcohol? Prior problem: No ___ Yes ___
How much coffee or tea do you usually drink? Coffee/Tea: ___ cups of coffee or tea a day.
Do you regularly wear seatbelts?   Seatbelts: No ___ Yes ___

DO YOU:	Rarely/Never	Occasionally	Frequently	DO YOU:	Rarely/Never	Occasionally	Frequently
Feel nervous?				Ever feel like committing suicide?			
Feel depressed?				Feel bored with your life?			
Find it hard to make decisions?				Use marijuana?			
Lose your temper?				Use "hard drugs"?			
Worry a lot?				Do you want to talk to the doctor about a personal matter? No ___ Yes ___			
Tire easily?							
Have trouble relaxing?							
Have any sexual problems?							

Created and Developed by "Medical Economics" Professional Systems
Copyright © 1979, 1983 Bibbero Systems International, Inc.
STOCK NO. 19-711-4 5/83   Page 1

PART C — BODY SYSTEMS REVIEW

MEN: Please answer questions 1 through 12, then skip to question 18.
WOMEN: Please start on question 6.

N ONLY
Have you had or do you have
prostate trouble   No ___ Yes ___
Do you have any sexual problems or with impotency? No ___ Yes ___
Have you ever had sores or lesions on your penis?   No ___ Yes ___
Have you ever had any discharge from your penis?   No ___ Yes ___
Do you ever have pain, lumps or swelling in your testicles? No ___ Yes ___
ck here if you wish to discuss any special problems with the doctor.

	Rarely/Never	Occasionally	Frequently
Is it sometimes hard to start your urine flow?			

19-711-4   5/83   Page 3

CONFIDENTIAL

FIGURE 14-4 Database self-administered general health history questionnaire. Lengthy questionnaires should be completed by the patient before he or she is seen by the physician. Either mail the information to the patient in advance or ask the patient to come in early to complete the paperwork. (Courtesy Bibbero Systems, Inc., Petaluma, Calif. 94954, (800) 242-2376, www.bibbero.com.)

- Nature and duration of pain, if any
- Time when the patient first noticed symptoms
- Patient's opinion as to the possible causes for the difficulties
- Remedies that the patient may have applied before seeing the physician
- Other medical treatment received for the same condition in the past

Objective Information

Objective findings, sometimes referred to as *signs,* become evident from the physician's examination of the patient.

Physical Examination and Findings and Laboratory and Radiology Reports

This section of the case history varies greatly with the specialty of the physician and the complaint of the patient. After the

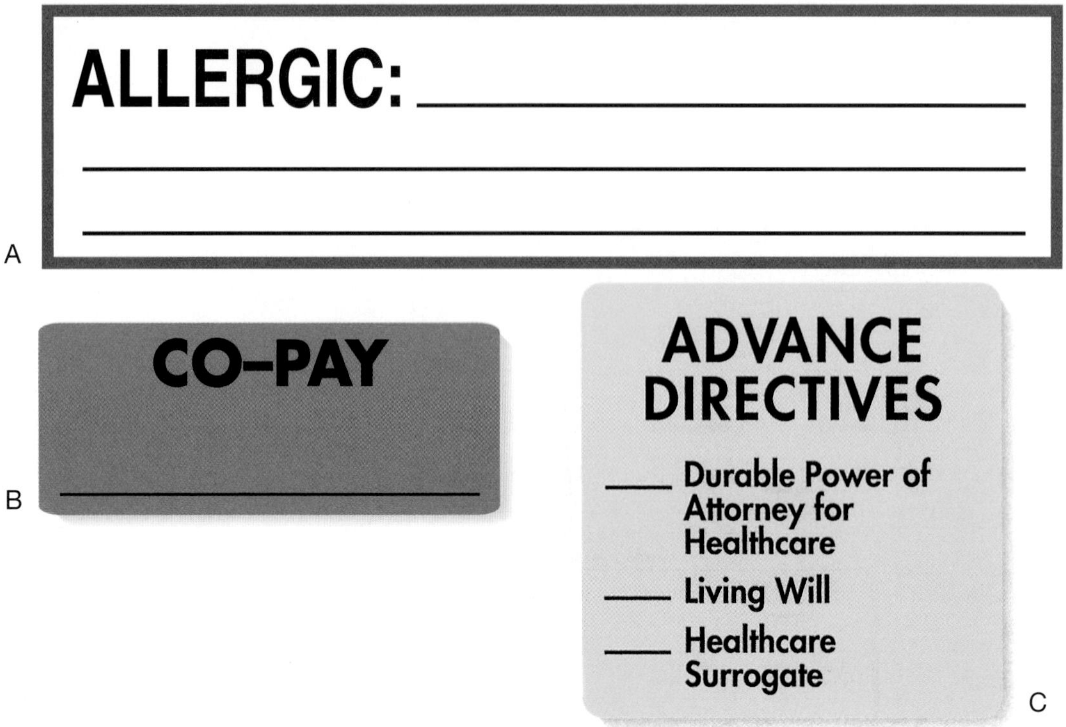

A   **ALLERGIC:** _____

B   **CO-PAY** _____

C   **ADVANCE DIRECTIVES**
_____ **Durable Power of Attorney for Healthcare**
_____ **Living Will**
_____ **Healthcare Surrogate**

FIGURE 14-5 Chart stickers. Information on stickers on the outside of the chart allows the physician and medical staff to quickly see important information about the patient. (Courtesy Bibbero Systems, Inc., Petaluma, Calif. 94954, (800) 242-2376, www.bibbero.com.)

physician has examined the patient, the physical findings are recorded in the history. Results of other tests or requests for these tests are then recorded or, if they appear on separate sheets, are attached to the history.

Diagnosis

The physician, on the basis of all evidence provided in the patient's past history, the physician's examination, and any supplementary tests, places the diagnosis of the patient's condition on the medical record. If some doubt remains, this may be termed a **provisional diagnosis.**

Treatment Prescribed and Progress Notes

The physician's suggested treatment is listed after the diagnosis. Generally, instructions to the patient to return for follow-up treatment in a specific period of time are noted here as well. If surgery or other treatment is needed, the patient must sign a consent form (Procedure 14-2).

On each subsequent visit the date must be entered on the chart and information about the patient's condition and the results of treatment added to the history, on the basis of the physician's observations. Notations of all medications prescribed or instructions given, as well as the patient's own progress report, should be placed in the record. Any home visits are noted. If the patient is hospitalized, the name of the hospital, the reason for the admission, and the dates of admission and discharge are recorded. Much of this information may be obtained from the hospital discharge summary.

Condition at the Time of Termination of Treatment

When the treatment is terminated, the physician will record that information. For example:

August 18, 2006. Wound completely healed. Patient discharged.

Obtaining the History

The medical assistant usually secures the routine personal data. The personal and medical history and the patient's family history may be secured by asking the patient to complete a questionnaire, with the physician augmenting the information provided during the patient interview (see Procedure 27-1).

The Medical Assistant's Role

When the medical assistant is responsible for recording the patient's history, care must be exercised to ensure that the patient's answers are not heard by others in the reception room. If privacy is not possible, it is better to give the patient a form to fill out, then to transfer this information to permanent records later. When privacy is available, the medical assistant may ask the patient questions and at the same time write or type the answers directly on the record. This method offers an opportunity to become better acquainted with the patient while completing the necessary records. In facilities where lengthy questionnaires are to be completed by the new patient, the questionnaire may be mailed to the patient with a request that it be completed and returned to the physician before the appointment. If the record

PROCEDURE 14-2

Establish and Maintain the Medical Record: Prepare an Informed Consent for Treatment Form

CAAHEP COMPETENCY: 3.c.(2)(d)
ABHES COMPETENCY: 3.b., 5.a

GOAL: *To adequately and completely inform the patient regarding the treatment or procedure that he or she is to receive, and to provide legal protection for the facility and the provider.*

EQUIPMENT and SUPPLIES

- Pen
- Consent form

PROCEDURAL STEPS

1. After the physician provides the details of the procedure to be done, prepare the consent form. Be sure that the form addresses the following:
   - The nature of the procedure or treatment
   - The risks and/or benefits of the procedure or treatment
   - Any reasonable alternatives to the procedure or treatment
   - The risks and/or benefits of each alternative
   - The risks and/or benefits of not performing the procedure or treatment

   PURPOSE: To make certain that the patient is fully informed about the procedure or treatment and the risks and/or benefits of having or not having it performed.

2. Personalize the form with the patient's name and any other demographic information that the form lists.
   PURPOSE: To correctly identify the patient and the procedure.

3. Deliver the form to the physician for use as the patient is counseled about the procedure.

PURPOSE: To avoid charges of practicing medicine without a license. The physician should explain procedures, risks, benefits, and alternatives and answer all of the patient's questions.

4. Witness the signature of the patient on the form, if necessary. The physician will usually sign the form as well.

5. Provide a copy of the consent form to the patient.
   PURPOSE: To make certain that the patient is fully informed regarding the procedure and has a copy of the information for his or her personal records.

6. Place the consent form in the patient's chart. The facility where the procedure is to be performed may require a copy.
   PURPOSE: To maintain a permanent copy of the signed consent form.

7. Ask the patient if he or she has any questions about the procedure. Refer questions that the medical assistant cannot or should not answer to the physician. Be sure that all of the questions expressed by the patient are answered.
   PURPOSE: To make certain that the patient is fully informed.

8. Provide information regarding the date and time for the procedure to the patient.

---

is to be computerized, requesting the information ahead of time gives the office staff the opportunity to transfer information to the computer before the new patient's visit.

The patient's chief complaint may have been indicated to the medical assistant, but the physician will question the patient in more detail. Many practitioners write their own entries on the chart in longhand. Some may key the findings directly into the computer. Others may dictate the material, either directly to the medical assistant or by using a recording device. If the material is dictated and typed, the physician should check each entry then initial the entry to verify accuracy. For a chart to be admissible as evidence in court, the person dictating or writing the entries must be able to attest that they were true and correct at the time they were written. The best indication of that is the physician's signature or initials on the typed entry.

MAKING ADDITIONS TO THE PATIENT RECORD

As long as the patient is under the physician's care, the medical history is building. Each laboratory report, radiology report, and progress note is added to the record, with the latest information

always on top (Procedure 14-3). Although each item is important, the most recent is usually of greatest significance to the patient's care. Again, the physician should read and initial each of these reports before it is placed in the record.

Laboratory Reports

Different colors of paper are often used for reporting different procedures. For example, urinalysis report forms may be yellow, blood count forms pink, and so on. When laboratory slips are smaller than the history form, they should be placed on a standard $8^{1}/_{2}$- × 11-inch sheet of colored paper. Type or print the patient's name in the upper right corner; then, with transparent tape, fasten the first report even with the bottom of the page. The second laboratory report will be taped or glued in place on top of and approximately $^{1}/_{2}$ inch above the first slip, allowing the date to show on the first report. By this method, called **shingling,** the latest report always appears on top (Figure 14-6). When checking previous reports, it is necessary only to run a finger down the slips until the desired date is found; then flip up the slips above. Laboratory report carrier forms with adhesive strips may be purchased.

PROCEDURE 14-3

Establish and Maintain the Medical Record: Add Supplementary Items to Established Patient Records

<u>CAAHEP COMPETENCY:</u> 3.c.(2)(c)
<u>ABHES COMPETENCY:</u> 3.b

GOAL: *To add supplementary documents and progress notes to patient histories, observing standard steps in filing, while creating an orderly file that will facilitate ready reference to any item of information.*

EQUIPMENT and SUPPLIES

- Assorted correspondence, diagnostic reports, and progress notes
- Patient files
- Computer or typewriter
- Mending tape
- FILE stamp or pen
- Sorter
- Stapler

PROCEDURAL STEPS

1. Group all papers according to patients' names.
   PURPOSE: To expedite the filing process.
2. Remove any staples or paper clips.
   PURPOSE: Staples in the file folders are hazardous; paper clips are bulky and may become inadvertently attached to other materials.
3. Mend any damaged or torn records.
4. Attach any small items to standard-size paper.
   PURPOSE: Small items are easily lost or misplaced in files.
5. Group any related papers together.
6. Place your initials or FILE stamp in the upper left corner.
   PURPOSE: To indicate that the document is released for filing.
7. Code the document by underlining or writing the patient's name in the upper right corner.
   PURPOSE: To indicate where the document is to be filed.
8. Continue steps 2 through 7 until all documents have been conditioned, released, indexed, and coded.
9. Place all documents in the sorter in filing sequence.
   EXPLANATION: Sorter can be taken to file cabinet or shelf for placing documents in patient folders.

Radiology Reports

Radiology reports are usually typed on standard letter-size stationery. They are placed in the patient's history folder, with the most recent report on top. All radiology reports may be stapled together or kept behind a special divider in the chart.

Progress Notes

Reports on the patient's progress are continually being added to the medical record. Each visit of the patient should be entered on the chart, with the date preceding any notations about the visit. The medical assistant can type or stamp the date on the chart when readying the charts for the patient's visits. Every instruction, prescription, or telephone call for advice should be entered with the correct date. It is always advisable to initial each entry, especially when several persons are handling and making entries on a patient's record. This aids in tracing entries about which there may be some question.

MAKING CORRECTIONS AND ALTERATIONS TO MEDICAL RECORDS

Sometimes it is necessary to make corrections to medical records. Erasing, using correction fluid, or any other type of **obliteration** is never acceptable. To correct a handwritten entry, follow these three steps:

1. Draw a line through the error.
2. Insert the correction above or immediately after the error.
3. In the margin, write *correction* or *Corr.*, the initial of the person correcting the entry, and the date.

Errors made while typing are corrected in the usual way. However, an error discovered in a typed entry at a later date is corrected in the same manner as described for a handwritten entry. Never attempt to alter medical records without using this specific correction procedure, because this alteration of records may indicate a fraudulent attempt to cover up a mistake made by a staff member or the physician. Do not hide errors. If the error could in any way affect the health and well-being of the patient, it must immediately be brought to the attention of the physician.

Additions to electronic health records must be made by making an additional entry. Never delete a previous entry or change it, unless it was entered seconds ago. A good rule of thumb is to avoid changing any electronic entry after the initials of the maker have been added. This, of course, should happen immediately after the note is placed into the record. Once this has happened, a new entry must be made to correct information in a previous entry.

CRITICAL THINKING APPLICATION

Susan has been using an incorrect abbreviation for several weeks and is having a difficult time remembering the right abbreviation. After taking a call from Mrs. Johnston, she remembers that she used the incorrect abbreviation in her chart last week. When Susan pulls the

Continued

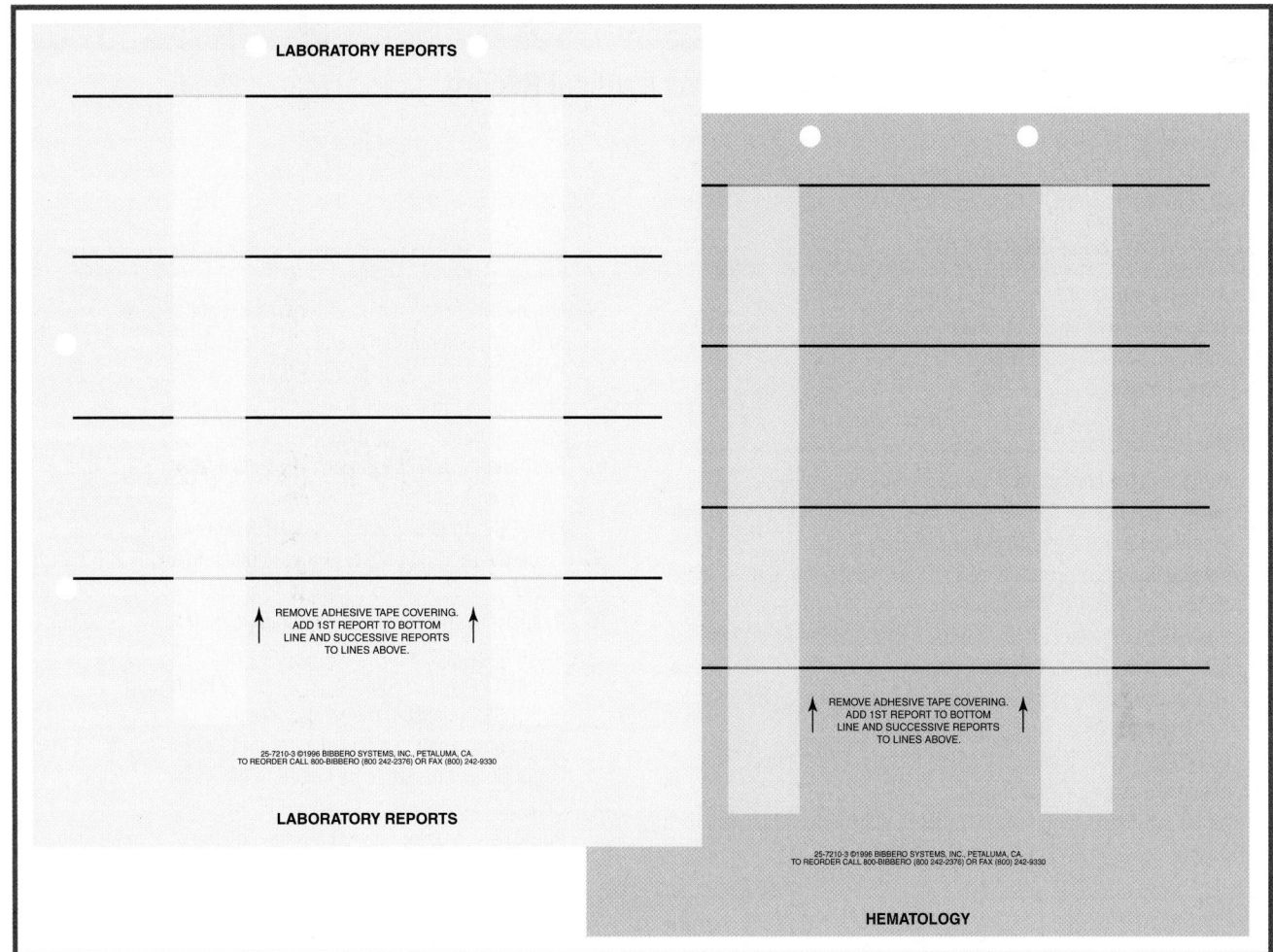

FIGURE 14-6 Shingled laboratory report forms. These forms make filing laboratory reports easy and provide a good adhesive so that the reports will not fall out of the chart if they are not standard size. (Courtesy Bibbero Systems, Inc., Petaluma, Calif. 94954, (800) 242-2376, www.bibbero.com.)

chart, she notices that entries have been made after the ones that Susan made on Mrs. Johnston's last visit. How does Susan correct her error?

KEEPING RECORDS CURRENT

One of the greatest dangers to good record keeping is **procrastination.** The record must be methodically kept current (Procedure 14-4). The medical assistant is responsible for seeing that this is done.

Case histories and reports may accumulate on the physician's or the medical assistant's desk during the day. After the last patient has gone, check each history to make certain that all necessary information has been recorded and that each entry is sufficiently clear for future understanding. Give the physician all abnormal reports to read and initial so that action can be taken and they may be filed in the patient's case history folder. Some physicians will want to see every laboratory report, whether it is normal or abnormal. Follow the requirements as set forth in the office policy and procedure manual.

While the physician is reviewing these reports, pull the histories of any patients seen outside the office that day, as well as those of patients who have been given special instructions by telephone or for whom prescriptions were ordered. These entries are made in the same manner as for an office visit, but the type of call is explained in parentheses after the date.

A prescription pad, printed on no-smear, carbonless paper, is available for a timesaving, write-it-once system. By placing the prescription blank over the patient's record, the prescription is automatically copied on the record as it is written. Prescription carriers with adhesive strips are also available for the physician who uses duplicate prescription blanks (Figure 14-7).

The patient record should not leave the office. A physician's pocket call record can be used for outside calls, and the information can be transferred to the chart in the office (Figure 14-8). Notations should be made of any missed appointments or of refusals to cooperate with instructions as they occur.

After all records have been reviewed for the day, they should be placed in a file tray and locked away for the night if there is insufficient time to file them. Do not leave histories out in view at night, especially if the facility has a cleaning service. On

PROCEDURE 14-4

Maintain the Medical Record

<u>CAAHEP COMPETENCY:</u> 3.c(2)(c)
<u>ABHES COMPETENCY:</u> 3.b

GOAL: *To make certain that the medical record is maintained and usable by all parties involved in patient care.*

EQUIPMENT and SUPPLIES

- Patient medical record
- Various forms used inside the medical record
- Results and reports, if applicable
- Clerical supplies

PROCEDURAL STEPS

1. Verify that the correct medical record has been pulled.
   <u>PURPOSE:</u> To make certain that all items placed into the medical record pertain to the right patient.
2. Inspect the medical record to determine which forms need to be added.
   <u>PURPOSE:</u> To make certain that the forms that the physician needs are available at all times.
3. Add all necessary forms to the record to enable the physician to document the office visit properly.
   <u>PURPOSE:</u> To make certain that the forms that the physician needs are available at all times.
4. Attach the forms to the record permanently or according to office policy.

<u>PURPOSE:</u> To keep information from falling out of the chart and getting lost or misplaced.

5. Make certain that all laboratory results and reports are available to the physician in the medical record.
   <u>PURPOSE:</u> All results and reports must be available to the physician so that he or she can make an accurate diagnosis and treat the patient accordingly.
6. Permanently attach laboratory results and/or reports in the record, with the most recent on top.
   <u>PURPOSE:</u> To easily access the most recent patient data.
7. Place the record in the designated place to await arrival of the patient.
8. If other documents are to be added to the record, condition each document.
9. Release each document to be added to the record.
   <u>PURPOSE:</u> Releasing the record means to place a mark on the document to indicate that the information is ready to be filed.
10. Index all documents to be added to the medical record.
11. Code all documents to be added to the medical record.
    <u>PURPOSE:</u> To determine where the document is to be filed.

---

arrival the next morning the medical assistant can index the histories for filing. Attach extra reports and information sheets. Always attach material to the chart permanently—do not simply drop forms into the folders. When this has been done, the records are ready for filing.

The physician may prefer to dictate progress notes rather than write them in longhand. At appropriate times during the day, everything is dictated: patient histories, physical examination findings, medications prescribed, follow-up findings, and summaries of telephone conversations. At the end of the day, the recorded information is given to the medical assistant for transcribing onto the records.

A great deal of time may be saved in transcribing these notes by using a continuous roll or pages of self-adhesive strips. When the **transcription** has been completed, the physician may wish to check the notes, underline important points, and initial each entry before returning the notes to the medical assistant for insertion into the charts to verify that they are correct in the event of **audit** or litigation. The use of self-adhesive strips saves removing the sheet from a chart that may be bound with metal fasteners, inserting the sheet into the typewriter, and putting the sheet back into the folder (Figure 14-9). It also simplifies the physician's part in checking and initialing the notes, because only the transcribed material is handled, not the bulky charts.

TRANSFER, DESTRUCTION, AND RETENTION OF MEDICAL RECORDS

Regular Transfer of Files

In most medical offices, records are filed according to three classifications:

- Active files are those of patients currently receiving treatment.
- Inactive files generally are those of patients whom the doctor has not seen for 6 months or longer. When such individuals return for care, their folders are replaced in the active file.
- Closed files are records of patients who have died, moved away, or otherwise terminated their relationship with the physician.

Some system must be established for regular transfer of files from active to inactive status or possibly destruction. The yearly expansion of charts and the file space available can influence the transfer period. Charts for patients who are currently hospitalized may be kept in a special section for quick reference, then placed in the regular active file when the patient is discharged from the hospital. In a surgical practice there frequently is a specific date on which the patient is discharged from the physician's care, and

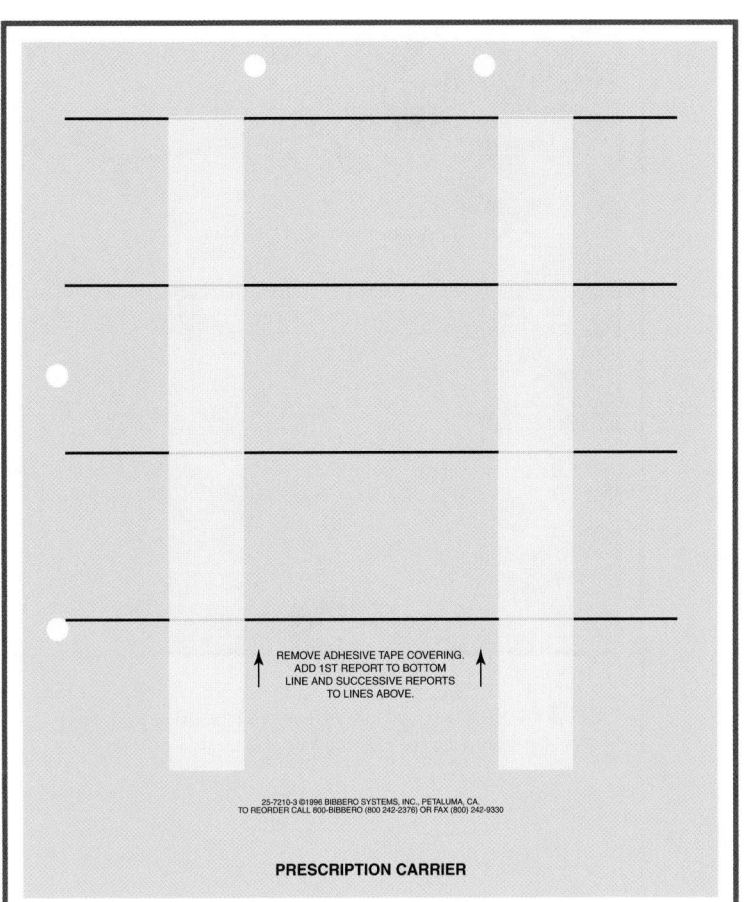

FIGURE 14-7 Filing copies of prescriptions. The self-adhesive on this form allows a copy of the prescription to be filed inside the patient's chart, and saves time over handwriting the information a second time. (Courtesy Bibbero Systems, Inc., Petaluma, Calif. 94954, (800) 242-2376, www. bibbero.com.)

PHYSICIANS POCKET CALL RECORD		DATE _____			
NAME	ADDRESS OR REMARKS	SYMBOL	MONEY RECEIVED	HOME CHARGES	HOSPITAL CHARGES
	Post these TOTALS to office book daily. ☞				

FIGURE 14-8 Physician pocket call record. The pocket call record may be used to record information about patients seen away from the clinic, such as skilled nursing facility patients or hospital patients.

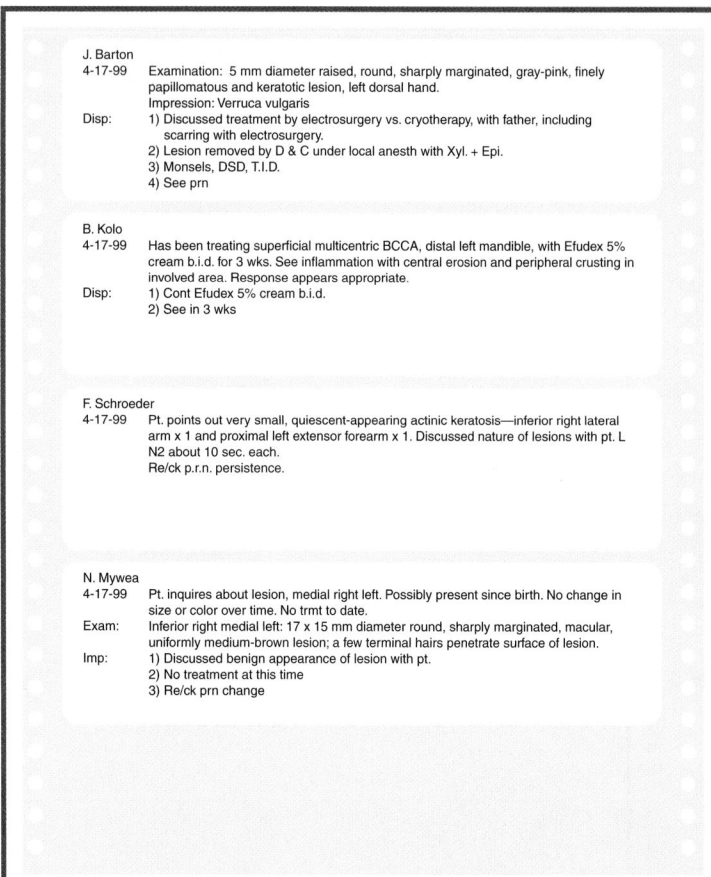

J. Barton
4-17-99   Examination: 5 mm diameter raised, round, sharply marginated, gray-pink, finely
           papillomatous and keratotic lesion, left dorsal hand.
           Impression: Verruca vulgaris
Disp: 1) Discussed treatment by electrosurgery vs. cryotherapy, with father, including
              scarring with electrosurgery.
           2) Lesion removed by D & C under local anesth with Xyl. + Epi.
           3) Monsels, DSD, T.I.D.
           4) See prn

B. Kolo
4-17-99   Has been treating superficial multicentric BCCA, distal left mandible, with Efudex 5%
           cream b.i.d. for 3 wks. See inflammation with central erosion and peripheral crusting in
           involved area. Response appears appropriate.
Disp: 1) Cont Efudex 5% cream b.i.d.
           2) See in 3 wks

F. Schroeder
4-17-99   Pt. points out very small, quiescent-appearing actinic keratosis—inferior right lateral
           arm x 1 and proximal left extensor forearm x 1. Discussed nature of lesions with pt. L
           N2 about 10 sec. each.
           Re/ck p.r.n. persistence.

N. Mywea
4-17-99   Pt. inquires about lesion, medial right left. Possibly present since birth. No change in
           size or color over time. No trmt to date.
Exam: Inferior right medial left: 17 x 15 mm diameter round, sharply marginated, macular,
           uniformly medium-brown lesion; a few terminal hairs penetrate surface of lesion.
Imp: 1) Discussed benign appearance of lesion with pt.
           2) No treatment at this time
           3) Re/ck prn change

A

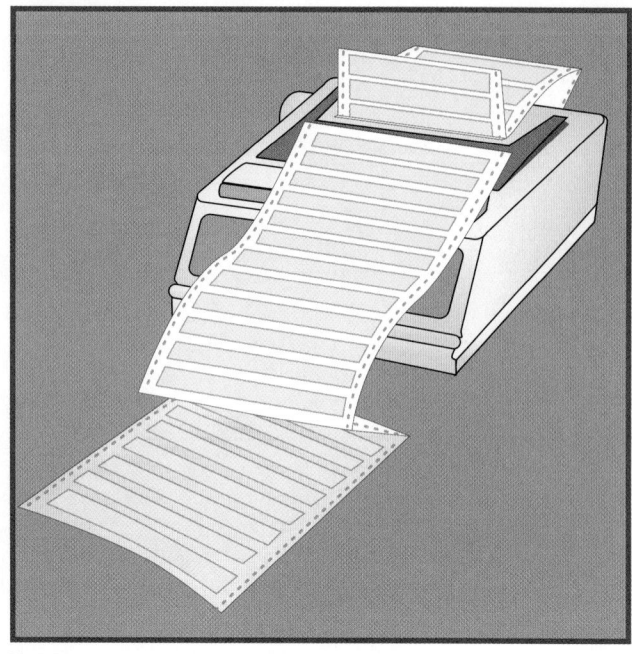

B

FIGURE 14-9 Self-adhesive progress notes. Progress notes can be quickly filed into the chart when self-adhesive forms are used.

the notation made on the chart "Return prn" (for the Latin pro re nata, "as the occasion arises" or "when needed"). This record may safely be placed in the inactive file. In a general practice office, the outside of the folder may be stamped with the date of the visit each time the patient is seen. It will then be a simple matter to determine when the chart should be transferred to the inactive status. This is called the *perpetual transfer method*.

Retention and Destruction

Physicians have an obligation to retain patient records that may reasonably be of value to a patient, according to the American Medical Association (AMA) Council on Ethical and Judicial Affairs. There is no standard, nationwide rule to follow in establishing a records **retention schedule** at this time.

Medical considerations are the primary basis for deciding how long to retain medical records. For example, operative notes and chemotherapy records should always be part of the patient's chart. The laws regarding the retention of medical records vary from state to state, and many governmental programs, such as Medicare and Medicaid, have their own guidelines for records retention. These guidelines range anywhere from 3 years to permanent retention. When no restriction exists for the retention of medical records, it is best to keep the records for a 10-year period. However, when retaining the records of a minor, the facility should keep the records until the minor reaches the age of majority, plus an additional 3 years.

If a particular record no longer needs to be kept for medical reasons, the physician should check state law to see whether there is a requirement that records be kept for a minimum length of time (most states do not have such a provision). The time is measured from the last professional contact with the patient.

In all cases, medical records should be kept for at least as long as the length of time of the statute of limitations for medical malpractice claims, which may be 3 or more years, depending on state law. In the case of a minor the statute of limitations may not apply until the patient reaches the age of majority.

The records of any patient covered by Medicare or Medicaid must be kept at least 6 years. The Health Insurance Portability and Accountability Act (HIPAA) recommends that records for patients who have died should be kept for at least 2 years.

Before old records are discarded, patients should be given an opportunity to claim a copy of the records or have them sent to another physician, if it is feasible to give the patient that opportunity. To preserve confidentiality when discarding old records, the documents should be destroyed by shredding or through a professional document destruction service.

Protection of Records

Releasing original case histories to anyone outside the healthcare facility should be avoided. Instead, prepare a summary or photocopy the materials needed for reference and retain the original in the physician's office. With the facsimile machine becoming standard equipment in business facilities, as well as in many of our homes, the transfer of information is simplified and the records remain in safekeeping. Often only certain aspects of the record are requested by colleagues or others, and these can easily be supplied by faxing the required pages, observing precautions for confidentiality.

Occasions may arise when records are temporarily out of the office, although this should be an extremely rare occurrence. Some physicians release case histories to their colleagues, or an original record may be subpoenaed by the court. In such instances, a colored **OUTfolder** should be inserted in the file in place of the regular folder and a notation made of the name, date, and to whom the record was released. Interim papers may be placed in the OUTfolder until the original is returned.

Long-Term Storage

Large healthcare facilities may find it advisable to **microfilm** records for storage. Another option is the transfer of paper records by laser beam onto optical disks. Microfilm and optical disk technology are both expensive and probably are not practical for any but a very large group practice or health maintenance organization.

Facilities that have computerized the patient records will be able to keep those records indefinitely on disk. Scanners can convert a paper record into an image on the computer screen, resulting in an electronic medical record. Records can be scanned and stored in electronic format on writeable CD-ROM or DVD-ROM. The bulky paper files can then be put in storage or eliminated. There is no longer a need to fill hundreds of square feet of storage space or search through stacks of storage file boxes for an inactive or closed file.

RELEASING MEDICAL RECORD INFORMATION

The medical facility must be extremely careful when releasing any type of medical information. The patient must sign a release for information to be given to any third party (Procedure 14-5).

Often a family member will call to inquire about a patient, but without the patient's specific request or release, no information may be given. Some offices have a "code" system whereby the patient gives the facility a code word that must be used by a family member to receive medical information about the patient.

Requests for medical information should be made in writing (Figure 14-10). It is unwise to accept a faxed request for medical information or a faxed release of information from a patient. Even requests from the patient's attorney or third-party payors must be cleared by the patient to receive information. Some attorneys may present a legal document called a **power of attorney**, which authorizes them to see the records. Still, this document is signed by the patient, so it is a release in itself.

PROCEDURE 14-5

Establish and Maintain the Medical Record: Prepare a Record Release Form

<u>CAAHEP COMPETENCY:</u> 3.c.(2)(c)
<u>ABHES COMPETENCY:</u> 5.c

GOAL: *To provide a legal document that indicates the patient's consent to the release of his or her medical records to another provider or healthcare facility.*

EQUIPMENT and SUPPLIES

- Medical record release form
- Pen
- Envelope

PROCEDURAL STEPS

1. Explain to the patient that a medical record release form will be necessary to obtain records from another provider. If the patient is having records sent to another provider, a release for that will also be required.
   <u>PURPOSE:</u> To ensure the patient's understanding of the record release procedure and purposes.

2. Review the record release form with the patient and ask if the form is understood or if the patient has any questions about the form.
   <u>PURPOSE:</u> To provide the opportunity for questions and to ensure the patient's understanding of the form.

3. Have the patient sign the form in the space indicated. If other demographic information is required, such as a social security number or other names used, complete that information as well.
   <u>PURPOSE:</u> The patient must sign the form for records to be released by any medical facility.

4. Make a copy of the form for the file, then mail it to the appropriate facility. Note the date that the form was sent. Provide a copy to the patient if requested.
   <u>PURPOSE:</u> To provide a record that the information or documents were actually requested on a certain date

5. Follow up to ensure that the requested records actually arrived.
   <u>PURPOSE:</u> To make certain that the records needed by the physician to accurately and competently treat the patient are available in a timely manner.

6. Check the patient's medical record to determine if a signed, current privacy policy document is on file. If not, have the patient sign one, and place it in the record.
   <u>PURPOSE:</u> To ensure that all patients are notified of the office privacy policy.

RECORDS RELEASE AUTHORIZATION

TO _____
Doctor or Hospital

_____
Address

I HEREBY AUTHORIZE AND REQUEST YOU TO RELEASE TO:

ALL RECORDS IN YOUR POSSESION CONCERNING _____

_____ ILLNESS AND/OR

TREATMENT DURING THE PERIOD FROM _____ TO _____.

NAME _____ TEL. _____

ADDRESS_____

SIGNATURE _____ DATE _____
(If relative, state relationship)

WITNESS_____ DATE _____

25-8104 © 1973 BIBBERO SYSTEMS, INC., PETALUMA,, CA.

FIGURE 14-10 Authorization to release medical records. All requests for medical records should be in writing, and the request should be kept in the patient chart. (Courtesy Bibbero Systems, Inc., Petaluma, Calif. 94954, (800) 242-2376, www.bibbero.com.)

CRITICAL THINKING APPLICATION

Susan has never seen a power of attorney and is curious about this type of document. How might she investigate and learn more about them? Whom should Susan approach first for this information? The physician has an attorney that Susan has met once. Should she call him and ask about the document without notifying the physician? Why or why not?

The time may come when a patient decides that he or she no longer agrees to the release of medical information. In this case the patient should sign a revocation form, and it must be made a part of the medical record (Figure 14-11).

Sometimes the patient will want to view his or her own record. They certainly have a right to see this information, but some patients may not understand the terminology used in the record. A staff member should always remain with the patient who is viewing his or her medical record. Remember, the original medical record should never leave the medical facility.

When a release is presented to the office, copy only the records requested in the release. Do not provide additional information that is not requested. It is acceptable to charge reasonable copying fees to the person requesting the information.

DICTATION AND TRANSCRIPTION

Administrative medical assistants may find that transcribing **dictation** is one of the job requirements they perform periodically. Transcription can be performed from handwritten notes, such as those in shorthand, or from machine dictation. In a healthcare facility, the medical transcriptionist is a part of the team. Smooth operation of the facility may depend on the timely and accurate performance of assigned responsibilities, such as record documentation and the preparation of special reports.

The transcriptionist will find that accuracy and speed are primary **requisites,** as well as a strong grasp of medical knowledge, especially anatomy and physiology (Figure 14-12). Income depends on the transcriptionist's productivity, which may be measured by the number of pages, characters, or lines typed. The person who intends to do transcribing exclusively should take a special course in transcription techniques. Certification is available through the American Association for Medical Transcriptionists.

Machine Transcription

Three stages of activity are involved in the process of dictation and transcription:

REVOCATION OF AUTHORIZATION TO RELEASE MEDICAL RECORDS

_____ , who resides at _____
Name   Street Address

_____ , hereby revokes authorization to the physician, hospital, clinic,
City/State/Zip

lab, radiology center or other healthcare provider listed below:

_____
Name

_____
Street Address

_____
City/State/Zip

to disclose information from the medical records of:

_____
Name

_____
Street Address

_____
City/State/Zip

My revocation extends to the data or documents I have initialed below:
_____ Records of visits (all visits)
_____ Record of visit for a specific date or dates, including or limited to _____
_____ Copies of records or reports provided to the above named (i.e. hospital, lab, etc.)
_____ Statements of charges or payments
_____ Mental health, alcohol and/or drug abuse treatment _____
_____ HIV information
_____ Hepatitis information
_____ Other (specific) _____

This revocation is given freely with the understanding that:

1. Disclosures made in good faith may have already occured based upon my previously issued authorization and that this renovation cannot apply retroactively to such disclosures. I also understand that the disclosure of health information may be required by law in some instances, such as for the reporting of communicable diseases.
2. The facility, it's employees, officers, and physicians are hereby released from any legal responsibility or liability for disclosure of the information I authorized previously.

_____   _____   _____
Patient's Printed Name   Social Security # (for identification purposes only)   Date

_____   _____
Patient's Signature (Or Guardian, if for a minor)   Revocation Date (if other than 60 days from date above)

_____   _____
Witness   Date

#25-8402 • 12/02 • BIBBERO SYSTEMS, INC • PETALUMA, CA   TO REORDER FORMS: (800) BIBBERO (800 242-2376) OR FAX: (800) 242-9330 MFG IN U.S.A.

FIGURE 14-11 Revocation of release of medical records. (Courtesy Bibbero Systems, Inc., Petaluma, Calif 94954, (800) 242-2376, www.bibbero.com.)

- Dictating into a dictation unit
- Listening to what has been dictated
- Keyboarding the dictated text to a printed document using correct format and required punctuation

Dictation Unit

A dictation unit is used by the physician to record material to be typed. Dictation units vary in design and capabilities. A desktop dictation unit is common in an office setting. This may be a combination unit used for both dictation and transcription. Alternatively, a machine used only for dictation may remain at the physician's desk; a separate transcription unit, including headphones and a foot pedal, remains at the transcriptionist's station. A lightweight, portable, handheld dictation unit may be used for times when the physician wishes to dictate while traveling or attending meetings away from the office. Digital dictation machines are now available; these are lightweight and portable and hold more information than standard dictation recorders. Physicians in a larger setting may install transcribing

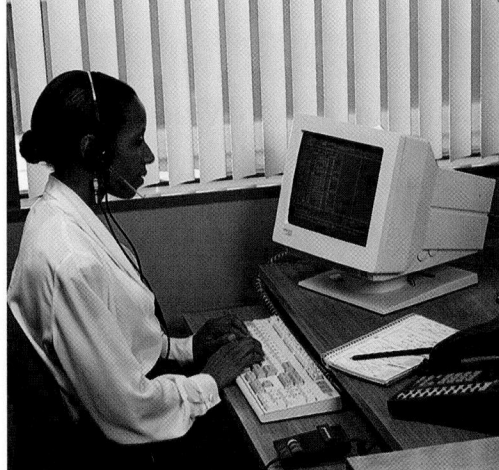

FIGURE 14-12 Medical transcriptionists must have excellent typing skills and good hearing. They must be accurate and use good grammar while completing transcription duties.

equipment that they can access by telephone wherever they may be. Many hospitals have this arrangement. All produce a recording that the transcriptionist listens to while keyboarding the text.

CRITICAL THINKING APPLICATION

Susan would like to practice transcription skills at home, but she does not have a transcription unit. How could she do this without the proper equipment? Medical terminology is important to the medical assistant who does transcription. What are some ways Susan can improve her medical terminology skills?

Transcriber Unit

The unit operated by the transcriptionist may use magnetic tape, a cassette, or a disk. A desktop unit using minicassettes, microcassettes, or standard cassettes is typical in the physician's office.

There are many types and manufacturers of transcribing equipment, but most units contain certain standard features. Before using any equipment, the medical assistant should study the manufacturer's instruction manual. Most transcription units have at least the following features:

- Stop and start control, with backup and fast-forward ability
- Speed control
- Volume control
- Tone control
- Indicator for locating special instructions and determining the document length

A beginning transcriptionist tends to listen to a few words, stop the machine, type those words, then restart the transcriber unit. Through practice, the transcriptionist learns to coordinate keyboarding activity with listening skills and listen ahead, thereby retaining in memory more and more of the dictated material so that it becomes unnecessary to stop and start the machine for this purpose.

Keyboarding Unit

The most important piece of equipment for the transcriptionist is the typewriter or computer on which the printed text will be produced (Procedure 14-6). Many improvements have occurred within the past few years. Computers have attachable foot pedals and headphones that allow the medical assistant to perform transcription directly onto the unit. A variety of computer programs are available to assist with transcription duties.

FILING EQUIPMENT

The vertical four-drawer steel filing cabinet, used with manila folders with the patient's name on the tab, was the traditional system of choice for years. The most popular system today is color-coding on open shelves. Rotary, lateral, compactable, and automated files are also available. Some records are kept in card or tray files. Regardless of the type or style of equipment, the best quality is always an economy. Some of the considerations in selecting filing equipment are as follows:

- Office space availability
- Structural considerations
- Cost of space and equipment
- Size, type, and volume of records
- Confidentiality requirements
- Retrieval speed
- Fire protection

Drawer Files

Drawer files should be full suspension; they should roll easily, close securely, and be equipped with a locking device. The best cabinets have a center trough at the bottom of each drawer with a rod for holding divider guides. Floor space of twice the depth of the drawer must be allowed so that the drawer can be pulled out to its full extent. A drawback of the vertical four-drawer files is that only one person can use a file cabinet at any given time. Filing is also slower because the drawer must be opened and closed each time a file is pulled or filed. Drawer files are

---

PROCEDURE 14-6

Transcribe a Machine-Dictated Letter Using a Computer or Word Processor

CAAHEP COMPETENCY: 3.c.(1)(a)
ABHES COMPETENCIES: 2.j, 2.n, 2.o

GOAL: *To transcribe a machine-dictated letter into a mailable document without error or corrections, using a computer or word processor.*

EQUIPMENT and SUPPLIES

- Transcribing machine
- Word processor or computer with appropriate software
- Stationery
- Reference manual

PROCEDURAL STEPS

1. Assemble supplies.
2. Set up format for selected letter style.
3. Keyboard the text while listening to the dictated letter.
4. Edit the letter on the monitor.
   PURPOSE: The letter should be in mailable form before printing.
5. Execute a spell check.
6. Direct the letter to the printer.

relatively easy to move, but for safety reasons they should be bolted to the wall or to one another.

File cabinets are heavy and can tip over, causing serious damage or injury unless reasonable care is observed. Open only one file drawer at a time, and close it when the filing has been completed. A drawer left even slightly open can cause injury to a passerby.

Shelf Files

Shelf files should have doors to protect the contents. A popular type of shelf file has doors that slide back into the cabinet; the door from a lower shelf may be pulled out and used for work space. Approximately 50% more material per square foot of floor space may be filed in shelf files when compared with the four-drawer file. Open shelf units hold files sideways and can go higher on the wall because there is no drawer to pull out (Figure 14-13). File retrieval is faster because several individuals can work simultaneously.

Open shelf units without doors are the most economic but offer little protection or confidentiality to the records. They are susceptible to water and fire damage. Shelf files are available in many attractive colors and can add a decorative note to the business office. Special storage or shelf space should be provided for x-ray films, if many films are stored.

Rotary Circular Files

Rotary circular files can hold a large volume of records. They save space and clerical motion. The files revolve easily; some come with push-button controls. Several persons can work at one rotary file and use records at the same time. One disadvantage is that they afford less privacy and protection than files that can be closed and locked.

Lateral Files

Lateral files are good for personal files and are especially attractive for the physician's private office. They use more wall space than the vertical file but do not extend out into the room

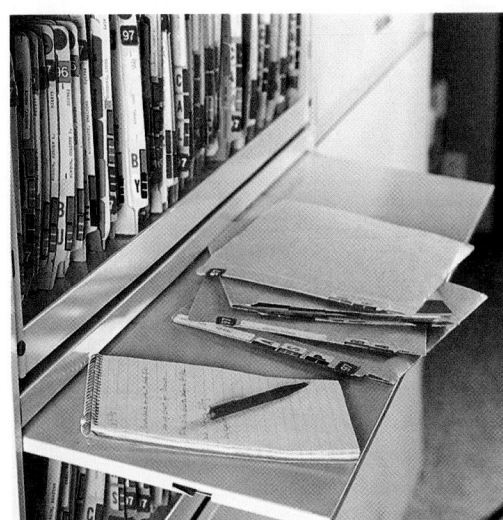

FIGURE 14-13 Open shelf filing is an efficient method, especially for color-coded filing systems. The shelf doors can often be used as workspace.

so far. The folders are filed sideways in the lateral file, left to right, instead of front to back as in a vertical file. Some have a pull-out drawer, as the vertical file does; others have doors that slide into the cabinet, exposing the filing space.

Compactable Files

The office with little space and a great volume of records might use compactable files, which are a variation of open shelf files. The files are mounted on tracks in the floor, and the units slide along the tracks so that access is gained to the needed records. The rolling may be either automated or manual. One drawback is that not all records are available at the same time.

Automated Files

Automated files are very expensive initially and require more maintenance than do the other types of filing equipment. They will probably be found only in very large installations such as clinics or hospitals. These files bring the record to the operator instead of the operator going to the record. When the operator presses a button indicating the appropriate shelf, the shelf automatically moves into position in front of the operator for record retrieval. The automated or power file is fast and can store large numbers of records in a small amount of space. Only one person can use the unit at one time.

Card Files

Almost every office has some occasion to use a card file. This may be for patient ledgers, a patient index, a library index, an index of surgical tray setups, telephone numbers, or numerous other records. A good-quality steel box or tray is a sound investment.

Special Items

Metal framework is available that can convert a regular drawer file into suspension-folder equipment. The assistant with a great deal of filing may wish to purchase a portable filing shelf that fits on the side of an opened drawer and can be moved from place to place as needed. Another special filing item is a sorting file, which can be a great time saver. A portable file cart for the temporary filing of unbilled insurance claims may be quite useful. It may also be used for the preliminary sorting of charts to be refiled. This is sometimes called a *suspense file*.

SUPPLIES

Divider Guides

Each file drawer or shelf should be equipped with plenty of dividers or guides. Some authorities recommend one guide for approximately each $1^{1}/_{2}$ inches of material, or every eight to ten folders. Guides should be of good-quality **pressboard** or strong plastic. Economy guides will soon become bent and frayed and have to be replaced. Divider guides have a protruding tab, which either may be an integral part of the card or may be made of metal or plastic. The guides reduce the area of search and serve as supports for the folders. They are available in single, third, or fifth cut (one, three, or five different positions). The guide may have a projection at the bottom edge with a ring or hole through which a rod may go. This type of guide card is used in drawers that have a trough for the projection and a rod to hold the guides in place.

OUTguides

An **OUTguide** is a heavy guide that is used to replace a folder that has been temporarily removed (Figure 14-14). It should be of a distinctive color for quick detection. This makes refiling simpler and alerts the file clerk that a file is missing. Several colors may be used, each color designating the temporary location of the file. The OUTguide may have lines for recording information, or it may have a plastic pocket for inserting an information card.

Chart Covers of Folders

Most records to be filed are placed in covers or tabbed folders. The most commonly used is a general-purpose third-cut manila folder that may be expanded to 3/4 inch. These are available with a double-thickness reinforced tab that will greatly lengthen the life of the folder. Folders kept in drawers have tabs at the top; those kept on shelves have tabs at the side. Many variations of folder styles are available for special purposes.

The vertical pocket, which is of heavier weight than the general-purpose folder, has a front that folds down for easy access to contents and is available with up to a 3 1/2-inch expansion. These are used for bulky histories or correspondence.

Hanging or suspension folders are made of heavy stock and hang on metal rods from side to side in a drawer. They can be used only with files equipped with suspension equipment.

Binder folders have fasteners with which to bind papers within the folder. These offer some security for the papers, but filing the materials is time consuming.

The number of papers that will fit in one folder depends on the thickness of the papers. Near the bottom edge of most folders are one or more score marks, which should be used as the contents of the folders expand. If folders are refolded at these score marks, the danger of their bending and sliding under other folders is reduced, and a neater file results. Papers should never protrude from the folder edges, and they should always be inserted with their tops to the left. When papers start to ride up in any folder, the folder is overloaded.

Labels

The label is a necessary filing and finding device. Use labels to identify each shelf, drawer, divider guide, and folder. A label on

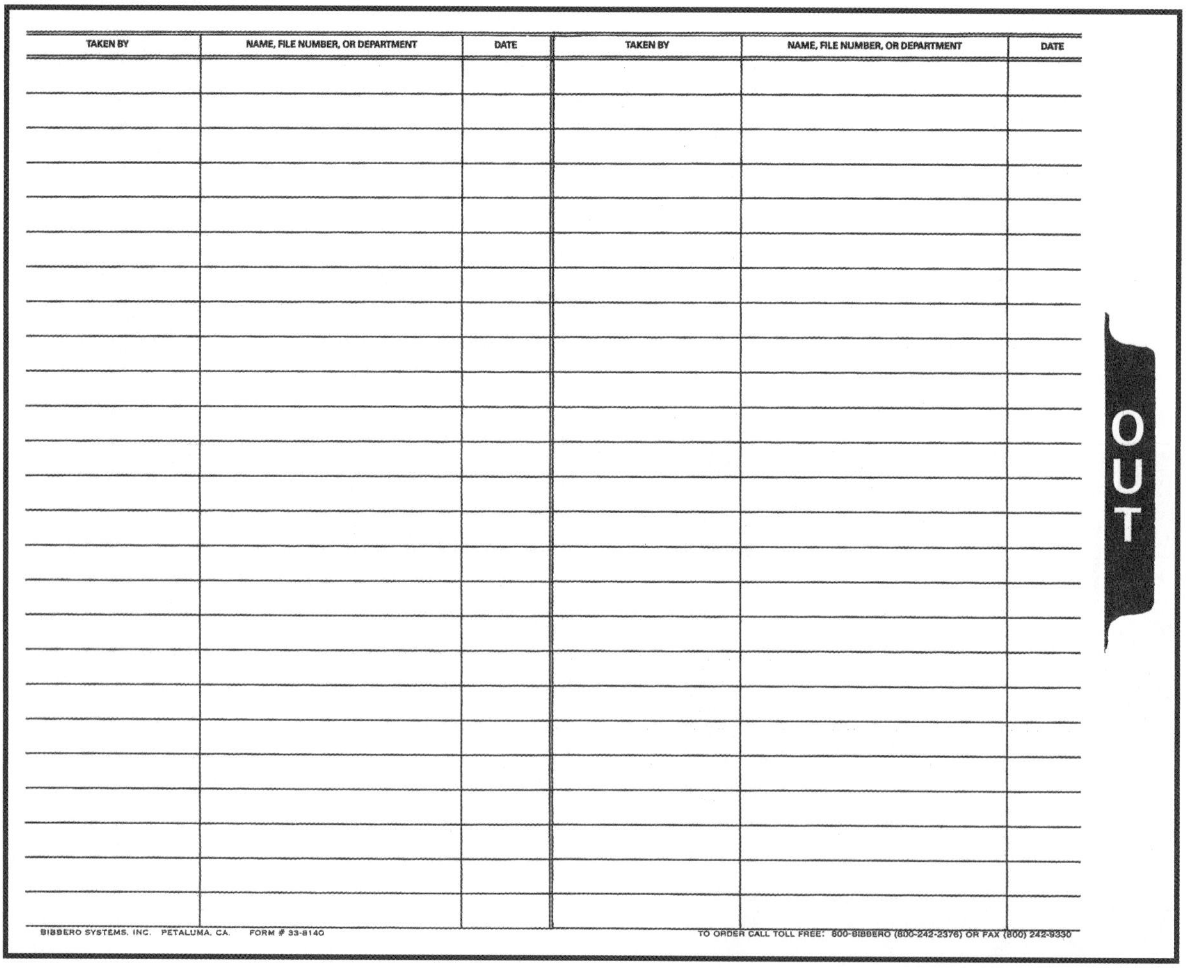

FIGURE 14-14 OUTguides provide tracking for files that are not in their proper location. The guide gives information as to where the file can be located. (Courtesy Bibbero Systems, Inc., Petaluma, Calif. 94954, (800) 242-2376, www.bibbero.com.)

the drawer or shelf identifies the nature of its contents. It should also indicate the range (alphabetic, numeric, or chronologic) of the material filed in that space.

The label on the divider guide identifies the range of folder headings following that divider guide up to the next divider; for example, BaBo. The label on the folder identifies the contents of that folder only. This may be the name of the patient, subject matter of correspondence, a business topic, or anything at all that needs to be filed. Label a folder when a new patient is seen or existing folders are full or when materials need to be transferred within the filing system.

Paper labels may be purchased on rolls of gummed tape; another type has adhesive backs that are peeled from a protective sheet. Labels are available in almost any size, shape, or color to meet the individual needs of any facility. Visit a stationer and study the catalogs to find the best product to meet the needs of the facility.

A narrow label applied to the front of the folder tab is the easiest to use and is satisfactory for folders kept in a drawer file. Labels for **shelf filing** should be identifiable from both front and back. Always type the label before separating it from the roll or protective sheet. Type the **caption** on the label in indexing order.

FILING PROCEDURES

Filing of all materials involves five basic steps: conditioning, releasing, indexing and coding, sorting, and storing and filing.

Conditioning

Conditioning of papers involves removing all pins, brads, and paper clips; stapling related papers together; attaching clippings or items smaller than page-size to a regular sheet of paper with rubber cement or tape; and mending damaged records.

Releasing

The term *releasing* simply means that some mark is placed on the paper indicating that it is now ready for filing. This will usually be either the medical assistant's initials or a FILE stamp placed in the upper left corner.

Indexing and Coding

Indexing means deciding where to file the letter or paper, and coding means placing some indication of this decision on the paper (Table 14-1). This may be done by underlining the name or subject, if it appears on the paper, or writing the indexing subject or name in some conspicuous place. If there is more than one logical place to file the paper, the original is coded for the main location and a cross-reference sheet prepared, indicating this location and coded for the second location. Every paper placed in a patient's chart should have the date and name of the patient on it, usually in the upper right corner.

Sorting

Sorting is arranging the papers in filing sequence. Sort papers before going to the file cabinet or shelf. Do any necessary

TABLE 14-1 Application of Indexing Rules				
INDEXING RULE	NAME	UNIT 1	UNIT 2	UNIT 3
1	Robert F. Grinch	Grinch	Robert	F.
	R. Frank Grumman	Grumman	R.	Frank
2	J. Orville Smith	Smith	J.	Orville
	Jason O. Smith	Smith	Jason	O.
3	M. L. Saint-Vickery	Saint-Vickery	M.	L.
	Marie-Louise Taylor	Taylor	Marielouise	
4	Charles S. Anderson	Anderson	Charles	S.
	Anderson's Surgical Supply	Andersons	Surgical	Supply
5	Ah Hop Akee	Akee	Ah	Hop
6	Alice Delaney	Delaney	Alice	
	Chester K. DeLong	Delong	Chester	K.
7	Michael St. John	Stjohn	Michael	
8	Helen M. Maag	Maag	Helen	M.
	Frederick Mabry	Mabry	Frederick	
	James E. MacDonald	Macdonald	James	E.
9	Mrs. John L. Doe (Mary Jones)	Doe	Mary	Jones (Mrs John L.)
10	Prof. John J. Breck	Breck	John	J. (Prof.)
	Madame Sylvia	Madame	Sylvia	
	Sister Mary Catherine	Sister	Mary	Catherine
	Theodore Wilson, M.D.	Wilson	Theodore (M.D.)	
11	Lawrence W. Sloan, Jr.	Sloan	Lawrence	W. (Jr.)
	Lawrence W. Sloan, Sr.	Sloan	Lawrence	W. (Sr.)
12	The Moore Clinic	Moore	Clinic (The)	

stapling of papers at the desk or filing table. Invest in a desktop sorter with a series of dividers, between which papers are placed in filing sequence. One general-purpose sorter has six means of classification: alphabetic sections, numbers 1 to 31, days of the week, months of the year, numbers in groups of five, and space on the tabs for special captions to be taped when desired. In the preliminary sorting, place the papers in the appropriate division in the sorter. Then it is comparatively simple to arrange these groups into the proper sequence for filing.

Storing and Filing

In storing or filing papers in the folder, items should be placed face up, top edge to the left, with the most recent date at the front of the folder. Lift the folder 1 or 2 inches out of the drawer before inserting new material, so that the sheets can drop down completely into the folder. It is best to permanently attach items to the file folder. When refiling completed folders, arrange them in indexing order before going to the file cabinets.

Locating Misplaced Files

Unless files are promptly replaced after use, they may become lost. Papers may be misfiled, requiring a thorough search to find them, which wastes valuable time. After a methodic and complete search through the proper folder, there are several places one may look for a misplaced paper: (1) in the folder in front of and behind the correct folder; (2) between the folders; (3) at the bottom of the file under all the folders; (4) in a folder of a patient with a similar name; or (5) in the sorter.

Indexing Rules

Indexing rules are fairly well standardized, based on current business practices. The Association of Records Managers and Administrators takes an active part in updating the rules. Some establishments adopt variations of these basic rules to accommodate their needs. In any case the practices need to be consistent within the system.

1. Last names of persons are considered first in filing; given name (first name), second; and middle name or initial, third. Compare the names beginning with the first letter of the name. When a letter is different in the two names, that letter determines the order of filing. For example:

> ab*e*
> ab*i*
> ab*m*
> ab*x*
> ac*l*
> ac*m*
> ad*a*
> ad*e*
> ad*i*

2. Initials precede a name beginning with the same letter. This illustrates the librarian's rule, "Nothing comes before something." For example:

> Smith, J.
> Smith, Jason

3. Hyphenated personal names. The hyphenated elements of a name, whether first name, middle name, or surname, are considered to be one unit. For example:

> Carlotta Freeman-Duque is filed as
> Freemanduque, Carlotta
> Cindy-Jean Green is filed as Green, Cindyjean

4. The apostrophe is disregarded in filing. For example:

> Andersons' Surgical Supply
> Andersons Surgical Supply

5. When indexing a foreign name when you cannot distinguish the first and last name, index each part of the name in the order in which it is written:

> Cau Liu
> Talluri Devi

If you can make the distinction, you should use the last name as the first indexing unit:

> Liu, Jason

6. Names with prefixes are filed in the usual alphabetic order, with the prefix being considered as part of the name. For example:

> von Schmidt is filed as Vonschmidt
> DeLong is filed as Delong
> LaFrance is filed as Lafrance

7. Abbreviated parts of a name are indexed as written if that is the form generally used by that person. For example:

> Ste. Marie is filed as Stemarie
> St. John is filed as Stjohn
> Wm. is filed as Wm
> Edw. is filed as Edw
> Jas. is filed as Jas

8. Mac and Mc are filed in their regular place in the alphabet:

> Maag
> Mabry
> MacDonald
> Machado
> MacHale
> Maville
> McAulay
> McWilliams
> Meacham

If the files contain a great many names beginning with Mac or Mc, some offices file them as a separate letter of the alphabet for convenience.

9. The name of a married woman is indexed by her legal name (her husband's surname, her given name, and her middle name or maiden surname). For example:

> Doe, Mary Jones (Mrs. John L.)
> not Doe, Mrs. John L. (unless first name is unknown)

10. Titles, when followed by a complete name, may be used as the last filing unit if needed to distinguish from another identical name. For example:

> Mr. James D. Conley
> Conley James D Mr.
> Dr. James D. Conley
> Conley James D Dr.

Titles without complete names are considered the first indexing unit:

> Madame Sylvia
> Sister Theresa

11. Terms of seniority, or professional or academic degree, are used only to distinguish from an identical name. For example:

> Theodore Wilson, PhD
> Theodore Wilson, Sr.
> Theodore Wilson, Jr.
> Theodore Wilson, MD
> These examples would be filed in the following order:
> Theodore Wilson, Jr.
> Theodore Wilson, MD
> Theodore Wilson, PhD
> Theodore Wilson, Sr.

12. Articles such as The and A are disregarded in indexing:

> Moore Clinic (The)

FILING METHODS

The three basic methods of filing used in healthcare facilities are these:
- Alphabetic by name
- Numeric
- Subject

Patient charts are filed either alphabetically by name or by one of several numeric methods. Subject filing is used for business records, correspondence, and topical materials.

Alphabetic Filing

Alphabetic filing by name is the oldest, simplest, and most commonly used system. It is the system of choice for filing patient records in the majority of physicians' offices. If the medical assistant can find a word in the dictionary or a name in the telephone directory, then he or she already knows some of the rules.

The alphabetic system of filing is traditional and simple to set up, requiring only a file cabinet or shelf, folders, and some divider guides (Procedure 14-7). It is a **direct filing system,** in that the person filing need know only the name in order to find the desired file. Alphabetic filing does have some drawbacks:
- The correct spelling of the name must be known.
- As the number of files increases, more space is needed for each section of the alphabet. This results in periodic shifting of folders from drawer to drawer or shelf to shelf to allow for expansion.
- As the files expand, more time is required for filing or retrieving each folder because of the greater number of folders involved in the search. The time can be greatly reduced by color-coding.

Numeric Filing

Some form of **numeric filing** combined with color and shelf filing is used by practically every large clinic or hospital. Management consultants differ in their recommendations; some recommend numeric filing only if there are more than 5000 charts, more than 10,000 charts, or in some cases more than 15,000 charts. Others recommend nothing but numeric filing. Numeric filing is an **indirect filing system,** requiring the use of an alphabetic cross-reference to find a given file. Some people object to this added step and overlook the advantages, which are as follows:
- It allows unlimited expansion without periodic shifting of folders, and shelves are usually filled evenly.
- It provides additional confidentiality to the chart.
- It saves time in retrieving and refiling records quickly. One knows immediately that the number 978 falls between 977 and 979. By contrast, an alphabetic system, even with color-coding, requires a longer search for the exact spot.

There are several types of numeric filing systems. In the straight or consecutive numeric system, patients are given consecutive numbers as they visit the practice. This is the simplest of the numeric systems and works well for files of up to 10,000 records. It is time consuming, and the chance for error is greater when filing documents with five or more digits. Filing activity is greatest at the end of the numeric series.

In the terminal digit system, patients are also assigned consecutive numbers, but the digits in the number are usually separated into groups of twos or threes and are read in groups from right to left instead of from left to right. The records are filed backward in groups. For example, all files ending in 00 are grouped together first, then those ending in 01, etc. Next the files are grouped by their middle digits so that the 00 22s come before the 01 22s. Finally the files are arranged by their first digits, so that 01 00 22 precedes 02 00 22.

Middle-digit filing begins with the middle digits, followed by the first digit and finally by the terminal digits.

Some practices use the last four digits of each patient's Social Security number to file patient records. However, there is no

PROCEDURE 14-7

File Medical Records and Documents Using the Alphabetic System

CAAHEP COMPETENCY: 3.a.(1)(d)
ABHES COMPETENCY: 3.h

GOAL: *To file records efficiently using an alphabetic system and ensure that the records can be easily and quickly retrieved.*

EQUIPMENT and SUPPLIES

- Medical records
- Physical filing equipment
- Cart to carry records, if needed
- Alphabetic file guide
- Staple remover
- Stapler

PROCEDURAL STEPS

1. Using alphabetic guidelines, place the records to be filed in alphabetic order. If a stack of documents is to be filed, place them in alphabetic order inside an alphabetic file guide or sorter. Use rules for filing documents alphabetically.
   PURPOSE: To organize the filing process and file the record or document quickly without retracing steps and skipping from letter to letter.

2. Go to the filing storage equipment (shelves, cabinets, or drawers), and locate the correct spot in the alphabet for the first file.

3. Place the file in the cabinet or drawer in correct alphabetic order.

4. If adding a document to a file, place it on top so that the most recent information is seen first. This puts the information in the file in reverse chronologic order.
   PURPOSE: To provide access to the most pertinent and recent information.

5. Securely fasten documents to the chart. Do not just drop the documents inside the chart.
   PURPOSE: To keep vital information from falling out of the chart and being lost.

6. Refile the chart in its proper place.

---

legal requirement that every U.S. resident have a Social Security number; if a patient does not, a "pseudo number" would have to be issued.

Numeric filing requires more training, but once the system is mastered, fewer errors occur than with alphabetic filing (Procedure 14-8).

CRITICAL THINKING APPLICATION

Susan is unsure whether alphabetic or numeric filing is best in the medical office. What are some advantages and disadvantages of each method?

Subject Filing

Subject filing can be either alphabetic or **alphanumeric** (A 1-3, B 1-1, B 1-2, and so on) and is used for general correspondence. The main difficulty with subject filing is indexing, or classifying—deciding where to file a document. Many papers require cross-referencing. All correspondence dealing with a particular subject is filed together. The papers within the folders are filed chronologically, the most recent on top. The subject headings are placed on the tabs of the folders and filed alphabetically.

Color-Coding

When a color-coding system is used, both filing and finding are easier, and misfiled folders are kept to a minimum (Procedure 14-9). The use of color visually restricts the area of search for a specific record. A misfiled chart is easily spotted even from a distance of several feet. In color-coding, a specific color is selected to identify each letter of the alphabet. The application of the principle may be through using colored folders, adhesive colored identification labels, or various combinations of these. Any selection of colors may be used, and the division of the alphabet is determined by one's own needs. However, studies have shown that there is wide variation in the frequency with which different letters occur.

Alphabetic Color-Coding

There are several ways of color-coding files. One alphabetic system uses five different colored folders, with each color representing a segment of the alphabet. The second letter of the patient's last name determines the color.

As medicine continues to consolidate into larger facilities, with more patients under one management, the filing of patient charts becomes more complicated and color-coding becomes more useful. Several color-coding systems use two sets of 13 colors—one set for letters A-M, and a second set of the same colors on a different background for the letters N-Z.

Many ready-made systems are available (e.g., Bibbero, Colwell, Kardex, Remington Rand, Smead, TAB, VisiRecord). Self-adhesive colored letter blocks with either two or three letters in the specific colors are supplied in rolls. The color blocks with the appropriate letter are placed on the index tab of the folder, along with the patient's full name. The letters are in pairs so that they can be seen from either side of the chart.

PROCEDURE 14-8

File Medical Records and Documents Using the Numeric System

CAAHEP COMPETENCY: 3.a.(1)(d)
ABHES COMPETENCY: 3.h

GOAL: *To file records efficiently using a numeric system and ensure that the records can be easily and quickly retrieved.*

EQUIPMENT and SUPPLIES

- Medical records
- Physical filing equipment
- Cart to carry records, if needed
- Numeric file guide
- Staple remover
- Stapler
- Paper clips

PROCEDURAL STEPS

1. Using numeric guidelines, place the records to be filed in numeric order. If a stack of documents is to be filed, write the chart number on the document. Use rules for filing documents alphabetically.
   PURPOSE: To organize the filing process and file the records or documents quickly without retracing steps and skipping from letter to letter.
2. Go to the filing storage equipment (shelves, cabinets, or drawers) and locate the numeric spot for the first file.
3. Place the file in the cabinet or drawer in correct numeric order.
4. If adding a document to a file, place it on top so that the most recent information is seen first. This puts the information in the file in reverse chronologic order.
   PURPOSE: To provide access to the most pertinent and recent information.
5. Securely fasten documents to the chart. Do not just drop the documents inside the chart.
   PURPOSE: To keep vital information from falling out of the chart and being lost.
6. Refile the chart in its proper place.

PROCEDURE 14-9

Establish and Maintain the Medical Record: Color-Code Medical Records

CAAHEP COMPETENCY: 3.a.(1)(d)
ABHES COMPETENCY: 3.h

GOAL: *To color-code patient records using the agency's established coding system to effectively facilitate filing and finding.*

EQUIPMENT and SUPPLIES

- List of patient medical records to code
- File folders
- Information on agency's coding system
- Full range of color tabs

PROCEDURAL STEPS

1. Assemble patient records.
2. Arrange records in indexing order.
   PURPOSE: When records have been color-coded, they will be in filing order.
3. Pick up the first record, and note the second letter of the patient's surname.

EXPLANATION: For the purpose of this activity, the color-coding system described in the text will be used.

4. Choose a tab of the appropriate color.
5. Type the patient's name on the label in indexing order, and apply tab to the folder tab.
   PURPOSE: To identify the sequence of folders in the filing system.
6. Repeat steps 4 and 5 until all records have been coded.
7. Check the entire group for any isolated color.
   PURPOSE: If the order and color of the folders are correct, all charts of the same color within each letter of the alphabet will be grouped together.

Strong, easily differentiated colors are used, creating a band of color in the files that makes it easy to spot out-of-place folders (Figure 14-15).

Numeric Color-Coding

Color-coding is also used in numeric filing. Numbers 0 through 9 are each assigned a different color. In a terminal digit filing system, the colors for the last two numbers would be affixed to the tab. If the number 1 is red and 5 is yellow, all files with numbers ending in 15 form a red and yellow band. Usually a predetermined section of the number is color-coded.

Other Color-Coding Applications

There are many other ways to make color work for the efficient medical office. Small pressure-sensitive tabs in a variety of colors may be used to identify certain types of insured patients and

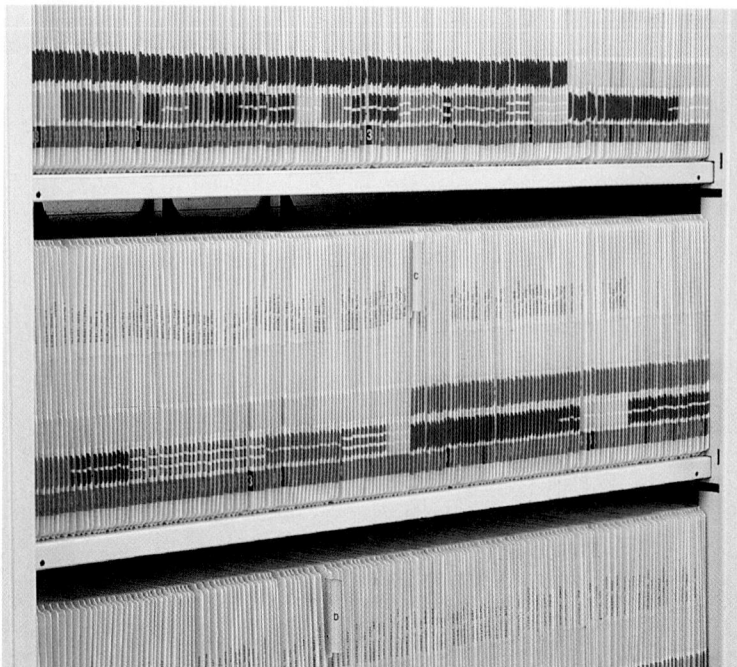

FIGURE 14-15 Color-coding patient charts makes it easy to see a file that is misplaced. (Courtesy Bibbero Systems, Inc., Petaluma, Calif. 94954, (800) 242-2376, www.bibbero.com.)

other specific information. For example, a red tab over the edge of the folder may identify a patient on Medicaid; a blue tab may identify a CHAMPUS patient; a green tab may identify a workers' compensation patient; matching tabs may be attached to the insured's ledger card; research cases may be identified by a special color tab; and brightly colored labels on the outside of a patient chart can indicate certain health conditions, such as drug allergies. In a partnership practice, a different color folder or label may identify each physician's patients. Color can also be used to differentiate dates—one color for each month or year.

Business records may also use color-coding. Main divider guide headings may be in one color, subheadings in a second color, and subdivisions in a third color. A fourth color might be used for personal items.

The use of color in filing is limited only by the imagination. One word of caution: Every person in the facility who uses the files must know the key to the coding, and the key should also be written in the facility's procedures manual.

ORGANIZATION OF FILES

It is very difficult for a physician to study a disorganized history. Some systematic method must be followed in placing items in the patient folder. The content of the patient record has already been discussed. From the filing standpoint, it should be emphasized that when a patient record is not in actual use, it should be in only one place—in the filing cabinet or on the shelf. Many precious hours can be lost in searching for misplaced or lost records that were carelessly left unfiled.

The patient's full name, in indexing order, should be typed on a label, and the label attached to the folder tab. A strip of transparent tape can be placed on the label to prevent smudging if this is a problem. The patient's full name should also be typed on each sheet within the folder.

Health-Related Correspondence

Correspondence pertaining to patients' medical records should be filed with the case history. Other medical correspondence should probably be filed in a subject file.

General Correspondence

The physician's office operates as a business as well as a professional service. There will be correspondence of a general nature pertaining to the operation of the office. In all likelihood, a special drawer or shelf will be set aside for the general correspondence. The correspondence is indexed according to subject matter or names of correspondents. The guides in a subject file may appear in one, two, or three positions, depending on the number of headings, subheadings, and subdivisions.

Practice Management Files

The most active financial record is, of course, the patient ledger. In facilities that still use a manual system, this will be a card or vertical tray file, and the accounts will be arranged alphabetically by name. There will be at least two divisions:
- Active accounts
- Paid accounts

Miscellaneous Folder

Papers that do not warrant an individual folder are placed in a miscellaneous folder. Within the folder, all papers relating to one subject, or with one correspondent, are kept together in chronologic order, with the most recent on top, then filed alphabetically with other miscellaneous material. Related materials may be stapled together. Never use paper clips for this purpose. When as many as five papers accumulate with one correspondent or subject, a separate folder should be prepared.

Other business files include records of income and expenses, financial statements, income and payroll tax records, canceled checks, and insurance policies. These papers may be filed chronologically.

Tickler or Follow-Up Files

The most frequently used follow-up method is that of a **tickler file,** so called because it tickles the memory that something needs to be done or followed up on a particular date. The tickler file is always a chronologic arrangement. In its simplest form, it consists of notations on the daily calendar. If information, such as an x-ray report or laboratory report, is expected concerning a patient who has an appointment to come in, the medical assistant might make a note on the calendar or tickler file a day ahead to check on whether the report has arrived.

The tickler file is often a card file with 12 guides for the names of the months and 31 guides printed with numbers 1 through 31 for the days of the month. The guide for the current month, followed by the 31-day guides, is placed at the front of the file. Notations of actions to be taken are placed behind the guides for specific days of the current month. Notations for future months are placed behind the guide for that month. To be effective, the tickler file must be checked the first thing each day.

CRITICAL THINKING APPLICATION

Susan is responsible for checking the tickler file on a daily basis. What types of documents and duties might she find inside these files?

The tickler file can be used in many ways. It is a useful reminder for recurring events such as payments, meetings, and so forth. On the last day of each month, all the notations from behind the next month's guide are distributed among the daily numbered guides, and the guide for the month just completed is placed at the back of the file.

Transitory or Temporary File

Many papers are kept longer than necessary because no provision is made for segregating those that have a limited usefulness. This situation is avoided by having a transitory or temporary file. For example, if a medical assistant writes a letter requesting a reprint, the file copy is placed in the transitory folder. When the reprint is received, the file copy is destroyed. The transitory file is used for materials that have no permanent value. The paper may be marked with a T and destroyed when the action is completed.

CLOSING COMMENTS

Just as in every aspect of the medical profession, advances in medical records management are occurring rapidly, allowing physicians and other caregivers to perform their duties in a more efficient and accurate way. A medical assistant must constantly be willing to learn and to adapt to changes that result from legislation and technologic strides. Because patients are fast becoming more computer literate, computers will become more generally accepted as a viable means of recording medical information. This is a positive change, because many patients and providers were not in favor of computer-based medical records when the concept was first presented to the general public.

The medical assistant should always explain to the patient any paperwork that he or she may be required to complete. Patients do not like to be told to simply "sign here." Take the time to explain any form that needs completion or a signature, so that the patient will understand the reason for collecting the information and the necessity for the information to be available to the medical facility.

Many forms are similar, and patients may complain about answering the same questions on multiple forms. It can be frustrating for patients when they must list their address and phone numbers on each of several forms. Review and revise the forms used in the office often so that they are user-friendly for the office and patient alike.

Patients may need reassurance that each staff member in the physician's office is committed to complete patient confidentiality. Always be open to answering questions regarding the patient medical record.

The authority to release information from the medical record lies solely with the patient unless required by law by subpoena. Ownership of the record is often a subject of controversy. The record belongs to the physician; the information belongs to the patient.

When a medical record is used as evidence in a court case, the person who entered information in the chart must be able to read it, no matter how much time has elapsed since the entry was created. When a chart is corrected, the proper method must be followed, and the record should never be obliterated.

Be sure to understand the laws concerning records retention. Records should be kept through the period of the statute of limitations, and possibly longer in certain situations. Take care with the medical chart, as it is the lifeline of patient care in the medical facility. When a chart is corrected, the proper method must be followed, and the record should never be obliterated (Procedure 14-10).

PROCEDURE 14-10

Document Appropriately and Accurately

CAAHEP COMPETENCY: 3.c(2)(d)
ABHES COMPETENCY: 5.b.

GOAL: *To document appropriately and accurately on all patient medical records and other office paperwork that concerns the patient.*

EQUIPMENT and SUPPLIES

- Any medical document
- Clerical supplies
- Computer or word processor
- Office policy and procedure manual

PROCEDURAL STEPS

1. Determine the information that needs to be added to the patient's medical record, appointment book, telephone message, or other office paperwork that concerns the patient.
   PURPOSE: To place pertinent, accurate information into the document.
2. Make certain that the information is factual, timely, and accurate.
   PURPOSE: To ensure that the information is usable.
3. Write or type the information into the document.
4. Re-read the information to make certain that it is legible.
   PURPOSE: To be sure that the information can be read even after several years by anyone who needs to access the information.
5. Date and sign the entry, if necessary.
   PURPOSE: To authenticate the entry.

6. Make certain that the entry meets any local, state, or federal guidelines that may apply to the information contained in the document.
   PURPOSE: To remain in compliance with local, state, and federal rules and regulations.
7. Make certain that the entry is written in compliance with office policies and procedures.
   PURPOSE: To comply with office policy.
8. If the entry needs to be corrected, draw one line through the entry, and make the new entry below or in the required place within the document.
   PURPOSE: To correct the document according to office policy and procedure guidelines.
9. Place the date and initial the corrected entry.
   PURPOSE: To authenticate the correction.
10. Make certain that the correction has not obliterated any part of the medical record or documentation that affects the patient.
    PURPOSE: TNo obliteration is acceptable in any part of the medical record.

SUMMARY OF SCENARIO

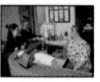 Susan looks forward to attending her medical assisting classes each day and works diligently to perform to the best of her ability in the classroom. She strives to do well on each procedure check-off and each examination that she completes. Her instructors provide excellent feedback and appreciate her contributions to the classroom experience.

Susan has the attitude that everything she is allowed to do in the medical office is a learning tool. She regularly asks for additional responsibilities and is always ready to assist a co-worker. Dr. Thomas has recognized that she has the desire to learn, and he gives her many opportunities to glean more knowledge through the everyday activities in the office.

Although she is new to the medical profession, Susan learns quickly and thinks logically. She knows the rules and regulations regarding patient confidentiality and is always careful about the information she provides to those who request it. She is never hesitant about asking her office manager for guidance if she is unsure about any aspect of her duties. Susan is understanding and respectful when patients are concerned about their privacy. Her confidence and warm personality play a role in the trust that she earns from the patients at the clinic.

Susan is willing to admit when she has made an error and has sought advice from Dr. Thomas and her office manager when an error needed correction. Although filing is not one of her favorite duties, she can be counted on to do her best while completing this important task. She realizes that filing is a critical task, because the documents contained in the patient's medical record direct the care provided to the patient. An abnormal laboratory report that is missing may make a crucial difference in the patient's care. She takes pride in her work and is efficient and accurate where medical records are concerned. When she is faced with a task that is new to her, she considers it a learning experience and seeks help when she is not completely certain about the way to handle a given situation.

Susan's co-workers are supportive and always willing to assist her as she learns to be the best medical assistant that she can possibly be. Her future as a professional medical assistant will certainly be laden with opportunity and advancement. Just as important, the patients extend their trust to Susan. She has alleviated patient concerns about electronic medical records by taking the time to explain privacy policies and exactly what information will be accessible to third parties. This trust also gives patients the confidence to reveal personal information and know that it will be held in the strictest confidence, not just by Susan, but by each employee at the physician's office.

SUMMARY of LEARNING OBJECTIVES

1. Define, spell, and pronounce the terms listed in the vocabulary.
   - Spelling and pronouncing medical terms correctly adds credibility to the medical assistant. Knowing the definition of these terms promotes confidence in communication with patients and co-workers.

2. State several important reasons for keeping accurate medical records.
   - Medical records must be accurate primarily so that the right care can be given to the patient. The record also helps to provide continuity of care between providers so that there is no lapse in treatment of the patient. The record serves as indication and proof in court that certain treatments and procedures were performed on the patient, so it can be excellent legal support if it is well maintained and accurate. Medical records also aid researchers with statistical information.

3. Discuss the ownership of records.
   - The physician owns the physical medical record, whereas the patient owns the information contained within it.

4. Explain the difference between a traditional medical record and a problem-oriented medical record.
   - The POMR categorizes each problem that a patient has and elaborates on the findings and treatment plan for all concerns. Detailed progress notes are kept for every individual problem. This method separates each of the patient's concerns and addresses them separately, whereas a traditional record may address all problems and concerns at one time. The POMR helps to assure that all individual problems are addressed.

5. Illustrate the difference between subjective and objective information.
   - Very simply, subjective information is provided by the patient, whereas objective information is provided by the physician or provider. Subjective information includes items such as the patient address, social security number, insurance information, and the patient's explanation of the condition he or she is experiencing. Objective information is obtained through the questions the physician asks and the observations made during the examination.

6. Discuss changing an entry in the patient record and the importance of following correct procedures.
   - Correct procedures must be followed when making corrections to a patient chart. A single line should be drawn through the incorrect information, then initialed and dated. Some offices require a notation of "Corr." or "correction" on the chart as well. A medical assistant should never try to alter the medical record or cover up an error in charting.

7. List and discuss the basic equipment used in a filing system.
   - Several types of equipment and supplies are necessary when managing patient records. A variety of shelving units and filing containers is available. Open shelving allows the maximized use of color-coded charts, which make finding misfiles quick and easy. Many file folder styles are available, and several types of forms can be used within the patient charts. The preference of the physician and staff members who use these tools is important, as well as concerns such as cost and availability. A medical assistant should be conservative when ordering supplies and purchasing equipment, ordering only the number needed to save on office supply costs.

8. Describe the steps in filing a document.
   - Five basic steps are involved in filing documents. The papers are conditioned, which is the preparatory stage for filing. Releasing the documents means that they are ready to be filed because they have been reviewed or read, and some type of mark is placed on the document to indicate this. Indexing involves the decision as to where the document should be filed, and coding is placing some type of mark on the paper relative to that decision. Sorting is placing the files in filing sequence. The last step is the actual filing and storing of the document.

9. List and discuss application of the basic filing systems.
   - Alphabetic filing is a simple and traditional filing system whereby documents are filed in alphabetic order. Numeric filing systems use a number code to give order to the files. An alphanumeric system is a combination of the two.

10. Explain how color-coding of files can be useful in a medical facility.
    - Color-coding is an excellent way to keep patient charts in order and swiftly locate those charts that have been misfiled. The medical assistant can tell at a glance when a chart is out of place. Color-coding also makes retrieval and refiling of files quick and easy.

11. Establish a patient's medical record.
    - The patient's chart must be organized so that the components are easy to find. The process for establishing the medical record is outlined in Procedure 14-1.

12. Prepare an informed consent for treatment form.
    - Patients must sign an informed consent for treatment form so that the physician can perform specific treatments and/or procedures. The process for preparing an informed consent for treatment form is outlined in Procedure 14-2.

13. Add supplementary items to an established patient record.
    - Items must be periodically added to patient records when test results arrive or new information becomes available. The process for adding supplementary items to an established medical record is outlined in Procedure 14-3.

14. Prepare a record release form.
    - Records cannot be released without the express permission of the patient. The process for preparing a record release form is outlined in Procedure 14-5.

15. Transcribe a machine-dictated letter using a computer or word processor.
    - At times, the medical assistant will be required to transcribe information from a recorder or other device into a medical record. The process for transcribing a machine-dictated letter using a computer or word processor is outlined in Procedure 14-6.

Continued

SUMMARY of LEARNING OBJECTIVES
Continued

16. File medical records and documents using an alphabetic system.
    - Some offices use an alphabetic filing system. The process for filing records and documents using an alphabetic filing system is outlined in Procedure 14-7.
17. File medical records and documents using a numeric system.
    - Some offices use a numeric filing system. The process for filing records and documents using a numeric filing system is outlined in Procedure 14-8.

18. Color-code medical records.
    - Color coding records is a great help in filing accurately. The process for color coding records is outlined in Procedure 14-9.
19. Document appropriately and accurately.
    - All medical documentation must be correct and complete. The process for documenting appropriately and accurately is outlined in Procedure 14-10.

CONNECTIONS

Study Guide Connection: Go to Chapter 14 Study Guide. Read the Case Study and Workplace Applications and complete the assignments. Do online research for answers to the questions in the Internet Activities associated with documentation and medical records management.

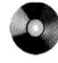

CD Connection: Go to the Medical Assisting Competency Challenge CD and do the training activities under General Office Duties: The Medical Record.

Evolve Connection: For more information related to documentation and medical records management, go to evolve. elsevier.com/kinn and visit related weblinks for Chapter 14. Click on the Medical Assisting Exam Review and do the practice questions to sharpen your test-taking skills. To learn more about office software, do the exercises for the Altapoint demo that is on the CD.

Health Information Management

15

SCENARIO

Laura Kelly graduated from her medical assistant training 1 year ago and is now employed at a regional hospital in the quality-assurance department as an administrative assistant. She enjoys working with statistics, is very detail oriented, has excellent computer skills, and is able to comprehend the lengthy regulatory text, such as that set forth in the Health Insurance Portability and Accountability Act (HIPAA) rules and guidelines. She has proven to be a valuable employee and her efforts help the hospital to comply with privacy laws.

Laura thought that quality assurance involved only patient satisfaction when she began working for the hospital. She has learned that this is just a small part of the total quality picture of the facility. The hospital has developed a patient questionnaire to solicit input from patients, and she enjoys talking with them about their experiences. Laura rarely encounters complaints, and she is proud to work for a medical facility that employs individuals who are concerned about giving exceptional care to patients. She understands that there are many aspects to providing quality in a healthcare facility.

Laura also realizes that health information encompasses much more than the patient's medical record. She knows that health statistics are vital to research and that physicians rely on statistical information when prescribing drugs, giving treatments, and performing other services. Providers frequently contact Laura to determine how many cases of a certain disease or disorder occurred at the hospital during a given period. The hospital database is very sophisticated and allows her to access many types of statistics quickly. Her office also monitors who enters the database and what information is accessed. This is one method of ensuring that privacy is maintained.

Laura has attended continuing education workshops that allow her to gain information and help the staff stay in compliance with the numerous regulations that govern the facility. She is eager to learn and assist her employers in keeping the hospital safe for all patients and visitors.

While studying this chapter, think about the following questions:

- How is health information used in today's medical facilities?
- What can the individual medical assistant do to improve the quality of care given in his or her employer's facility?
- Why is quality management an important aspect of today's healthcare industry?
- How do statistics impact healthcare?

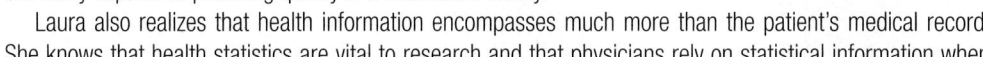

LEARNING OBJECTIVES

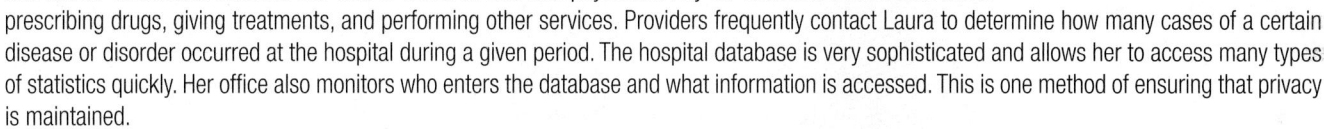

1. Define, spell, and pronounce the terms listed in the vocabulary.
2. Describe several ways that health information is used.
3. Contrast the nine characteristics of quality health data.
4. Explain the four concerns of quality assurance.
5. Discuss the importance of the Health Insurance Portability and Accountability Act (HIPAA).
6. Explain the functions of the National Center for Health Statistics (NCHS).
7. Discuss the types of statistics kept by the NCHS.
8. Define total quality management.
9. Explain the function of the Joint Commission on Accreditation of Healthcare Organizations (JCAHO).
10. Discuss the importance of healthcare standards in medical facilities.

National Accreditation Competencies and Content

CAAHEP COMPETENCIES

General

3.c.(2)(a). Identify and respond to issues of confidentiality
3.c.(2)(b). Perform within legal and ethical boundaries
3.c.(2)(d). Document appropriately
3.c.(2)(e). Demonstrate knowledge of federal and state health care legislation and regulations

ABHES COMPETENCIES

Professionalism

1.b. Maintain confidentiality at all times
1.d. Be cognizant of ethical boundaries

Legal Concepts

5.a. Determine needs for documentation and reporting
5.b. Document accurately
5.c. Use appropriate guidelines when releasing records or information
5.g. Monitor legislation related to current healthcare issues and practices
5.h. Perform risk management procedures

VOCABULARY

authenticated Proved; with regard to medical records, it applies to a signature, initials, or computer keystroke by the maker of the record to verify that the record is correct.

circumvent (suhr-kuhm-vent′) To manage to get around, especially by ingenuity or stratagem.

contraindications (kahn-truh-in-duh-ka′-shuns) Factors, such as symptoms or conditions, that make a particular treatment or procedure inadvisable.

disparities (di-spar′-uh-tez) Fundamentally different and often incongruous elements; elements that are markedly distinct in quality or character.

encrypted (in-kript′-ed) Encoded; converted from one system of communication to another.

erroneous (eh-ro′-ne-uhs) Containing or characterized by error or assumption.

gradients Changes in response with distance from a stimulus.

nosocomial (no-suh-ko′-me-uhl) Originating or taking place in a hospital.

quality assurance Activities designed to increase the quality of a product or service through process or system changes that increase efficiency or effectiveness.

sentinel events Unexpected occurrences involving death or serious physical or psychologic injury, or the risk thereof.

standards Models or examples established by authority, custom, or general consent; something set up and established by authority as a rule for the measure of quantity, weight, extent, value, or quality.

transposed Altered in sequence; interchanged.

Before the 1990s, practitioners in the healthcare field were barely familiar with the term *health information management*. Today, this well-respected profession employs thousands of individuals across the United States. As more medical facilities move toward computer-based medical records, more trained health information management professionals are needed. The medical assistant may wish to pursue employment in this growing field.

The health information management profession is supported by a national organization called the *American Health Information Management Association*. This association's House of Delegates developed a statement in 1994 that defines the profession. The statement reads:

"Health information management is the profession that focuses on healthcare data and the management of healthcare information resources. The profession addresses the nature, structure, and translation of data into usable forms of information for the advancement of health and healthcare of individuals and populations. Health information professionals collect, integrate, and analyze primary and secondary healthcare data; disseminate information; and manage information resources related to research, planning, provision, and evaluation of healthcare services."

EVOLUTION OF THE PROFESSION

In 1928 the American College of Surgeons realized that accurate medical records promoted good medical care. This desire for quality led to the establishment of the Association of Record Librarians of North America. Years later in 1970 the organization changed its name to the American Medical Record Association. Medical records professionals found employment in hospitals, health clinics, insurance companies, and other organizations that used medical records.

In 1991 the organization became known as the *American Health Information Management Association*. Advances in technology have brought the health information management profession from a paper-based environment into a highly sophisticated computer age, where physicians can access patient and statistical data in seconds.

In 2005, nearly a quarter of U.S. physicians used some form of electronic patient record, according to the CDC. Most experts agree that electronic records can reduce medical errors by keeping prescriptions, allergies, and other information organized, as well as reduce costs by avoiding duplicate tests. Electronic records may also reduce staffing needs, since fewer personnel are needed to manage them. The CDC agrees that progress has been made toward a presidential goal of having digital health data for every American by 2014, but states that there is still a long way to go toward meeting that goal.

CRITICAL THINKING APPLICATION

■ Laura is eligible to join the American Health Information Management Association, and her employer will pay her dues. How might joining this professional organization benefit Laura?

■ How would the hospital benefit from Laura's membership in the organization?

THE USE OF HEALTHCARE DATA

Many people and various organizations use healthcare data in a multitude of ways (Figure 15-1). Primarily, healthcare data are used to plan care for patients and ensure that they receive continuity of care from one healthcare provider to another. However, the information provided through healthcare records is useful in other capacities.

For example, when a drug is being evaluated, statistics must be kept to help the manufacturers of the product determine its effectiveness. Information on side effects and other **contraindications** is reviewed and used to make the product safer and more marketable. Sometimes the drug must be changed then returned to clinical trials.

Healthcare organizations gather information on the number of patients who enter the facility with the same diagnosis. This and other information helps them to plan what types of equipment will be needed to meet the needs of the patient population. For instance, if the geographic area where the facility is located contains a large number of patients with cardiac disease, a hospital may need to add a cardiac intensive care unit. If the facility is located in a neighborhood where there are many young families, the obstetrics and pediatrics departments may be expanded. Healthcare data and statistics guide planning for the needs of next week and for the next decade.

CRITICAL THINKING APPLICATION

■ Laura has noticed that the hospital keeps extensive records on the admitting diagnosis and the discharge diagnosis. Why is this information important?

■ If a certain physician is admitting numerous patients with the same diagnosis and is a family practitioner, what concerns might this raise for the facility?

Third-party payors use healthcare information to determine whether claims should be paid. The data provide proof that a certain procedure or treatment was medically necessary and therefore its cost should be reimbursed (Figure 15-2). Government and regulatory agencies use data to make certain that healthcare facilities are in compliance with the various statutes and **standards** that govern them. Data also are used by facilities in determining whether high-quality healthcare is being provided to patients.

WHAT ARE HIGH-QUALITY DATA?

The information that is contained in a database is only as reliable as the person who entered it into the computer. Most database systems require information to be saved after it is entered by clicking an additional button. Unless the data information is saved, the time and effort spent in entering the data have been wasted.

Health Information: Management of a Strategic Resource* identifies nine characteristics of quality health data. These characteristics are validity, reliability, completeness, recognizability, timeliness, relevance, accessibility, security, and legality.

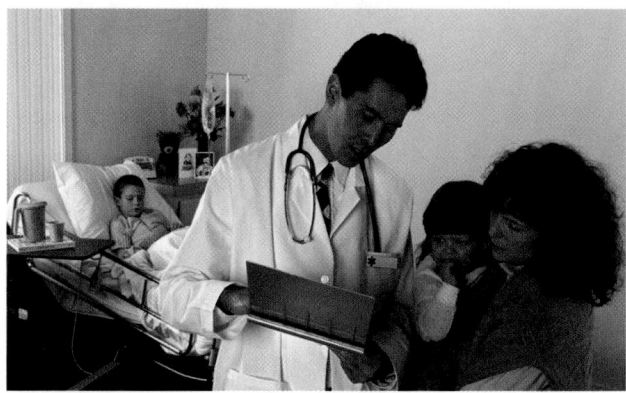

FIGURE 15-1 Physicians rely on health information to provide high-quality care to their patients.

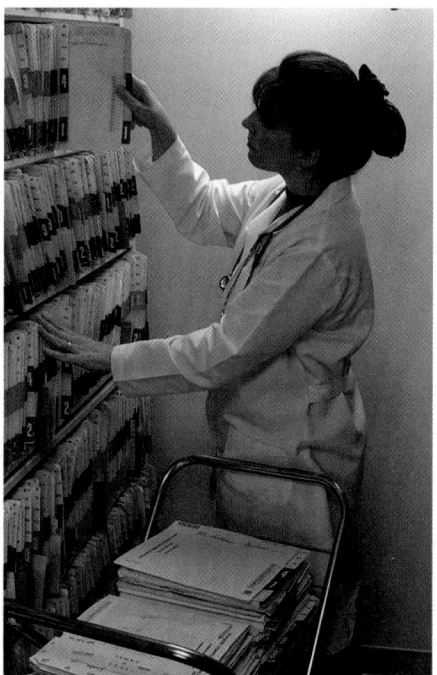

FIGURE 15-2 Healthcare providers often rely on statistics when treating their patients. Most statistical information is gleaned from patient charts.

Validity

The validity of health data is synonymous with accuracy. Accuracy is one of the most important characteristics of data, whether in paper-based or computer-based records. Great care must be taken when characters are typed on the keyboard, so that letters or numbers are not **transposed.**

Reliability

The healthcare professional must be able to rely on the data presented. If a patient's medical chart is marked to indicate that he or she has no allergies, the medical assistant must be able to trust that information and give an injection with the confidence that the patient is not allergic to the medication. Reliability also pertains to the degree to which the information in the database can be trusted.

Completeness

The information not only must be accurate; it also must be complete. If the medical assistant gives an injection yet fails to document it in the patient's chart, then the record is incomplete. If a computer system is designed to upload new information into the database every night and the system malfunctions, there is a strong possibility that the records contained within the system are incomplete, possibly lacking vital information needed to care for the patient.

Recognizability

All users of health information must be able to interpret the data that are presented in the health record. The facility should have a consistent use of abbreviations so that no misunderstandings occur when reviewing a patient's chart.

Timeliness

Health information must be entered into the chart or database as soon as it is available. The medical assistant should never commit information to memory intending to enter it later. Reports from laboratories or medical tests also should be placed in the chart as soon as the information is reviewed by the physician, so that decisions made are supported by the latest information about the patient's condition.

Relevance

The information contained in the database must be relevant to be useful. Needless and meaningless statistics about patient treatments or drug interactions do not benefit providers and users of health information.

Accessibility

One of the advantages of a computer-based patient record is that it is accessible to multiple users at the same time. The facility must take care to provide access only to individuals who are authorized to view the records. The computer should have a login system that prompts for a password. In addition, the computer system should keep records of who accesses information by time and date. Paper-based patient records should be returned to their proper place when they are not in use so that they will be accessible to all staff members.

Security

Although only certain employees are allowed to access health information, precautions must be taken to prohibit access to intruders. Firewalls are similar to filters that allow only certain types of data to enter or exit. Information can be **encrypted,** which means that it is changed into a code that can be read only after it has been unencrypted. These precautions are necessary because of the sensitivity of patient information. Also, care must be taken to ensure that no one can change the information already contained in the record.

Legality

Many statutes govern medical records. The laws concerning record retention vary from state to state. Medical records cannot be altered but should be corrected according to accepted guidelines. The record must be completely legible and **authenticated** properly (Figure 15-3).

CRITICAL THINKING APPLICATION

- One of Laura's duties involves making sure that medical records have been authenticated. Why is the authentication of records important?
- One physician, Dr. Anthony, is consistently careless about record authentication. How can the hospital encourage him to complete this critical duty?

THE CHALLENGES OF QUALITY-ASSURANCE PROBLEMS

Many of the larger medical facilities today have entire departments that are devoted to **quality assurance.** *Quality*

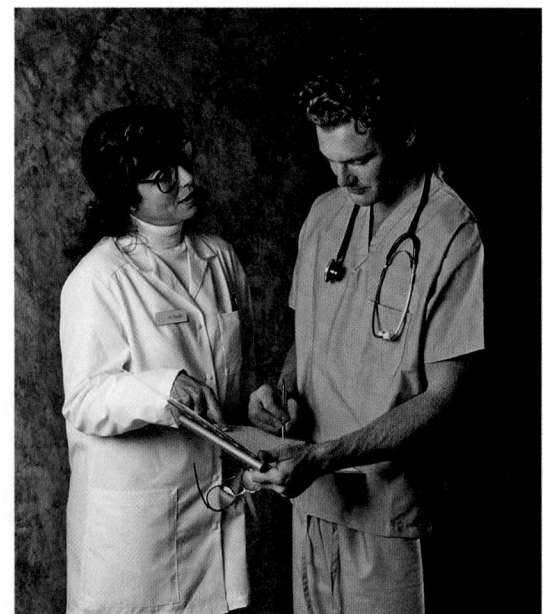

FIGURE 15-3 Physicians must authenticate medical records by initialing or signing their entries. Some computer systems automatically authenticate records.

assurance is defined as the activities designed to increase the quality of a product or service through process or system changes that increase efficiency or effectiveness. Although many people assume that quality is determined solely by the patient, much more is involved in quality assurance than just the patient's satisfaction with services rendered. Quality assurance also is concerned with the overuse, underuse, misuse, and variations in use of different healthcare services.

Healthcare services that are excessive and unnecessary cause costs to rise. Treatments and services that are overused include hysterectomies, tympanostomy tubes, and antibiotics. Medical studies have shown that up to 16% of all hysterectomies performed in 1993 were unnecessary and up to 23% of tympanostomy tube operations performed between 1991 and 1992 were unnecessary. Antibiotics are prescribed widely for common colds and acute bronchitis, but the drugs do not benefit patients with these illnesses.

The underuse of services and treatments can be equally costly. Mammograms and cervical cancer screening tests can detect medical problems yet are not taken advantage of by enough at-risk patients (Figure 15-4). The use of beta-blockers has been proven to reduce mortality in patients who have had heart attacks by as much as 43%, but often they are not prescribed for these patients. Diabetic patients should have their eyes checked regularly, but many do not. All of these are examples of the underuse of services that can affect the quality of healthcare.

CRITICAL THINKING APPLICATION

■ How might a hospital employee encourage patients to have screening tests done, such as mammograms and for cervical cancer?

■ What marketing strategies could Laura assist in developing that will result in more patients taking advantage of health screening opportunities?

■ How do these services benefit the health facility?

Some healthcare services are misused. These errors can cause death, delay of correct diagnosis, unnecessary injuries,

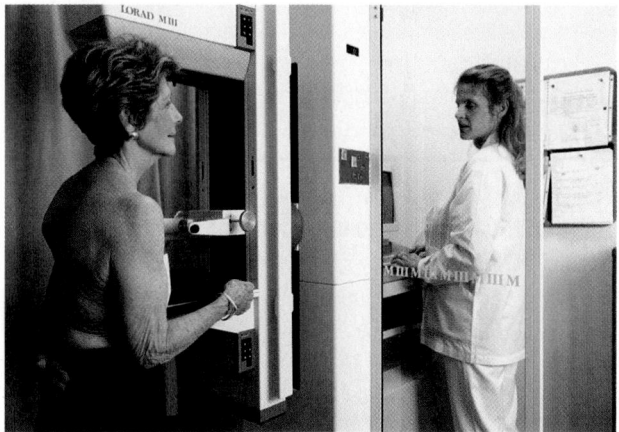

FIGURE 15-4 Healthcare professionals must encourage at-risk patients to have screening tests done, such as those for breast and cervical cancer.

and increased healthcare costs. Examples of misuse can include laboratory tests that provide **erroneous** results. Medication errors can be fatal to patients or can cause complications to illnesses that are already present. Hospital injuries and **nosocomial** infections promote further complications. A study at the Harvard School of Public Health published in 1994 estimated that up to 180,000 needless deaths occurred each year as a result of preventable errors.

Wide variations exist in services in different parts of the country. Discharge rates (which indicate that the patient left the hospital without expiring) are higher in some areas of the United States than others. Individuals who seek medical care are more conscientious and likely to seek health services in different geographic areas. All of these issues contribute to the concept of high-quality healthcare.

Health Insurance Portability and Accountability Act

As technology advanced and more health records became computerized, legislation dealing with privacy became imperative. The Health Insurance Portability and Accountability Act (HIPAA) 1996 was developed, in part, to help ensure the confidentiality of medical records. The statute, which became law in August 1996, applies to those records that are created or maintained by healthcare providers, health plans, and healthcare clearinghouses that engage in certain electronic transactions. The Office for Civil Rights, a division of the Health and Human Services Department, regulates HIPAA.

In August 2002, the Department of Health and Human Services Secretary Tommy Thompson announced the final ruling relating to HIPAA's privacy act, which became effective April 14, 2003. Under the privacy rule the following apply:

• Patients must give specific authorization before entities covered by the regulation could use or disclose protected information in most nonroutine circumstances—such as releasing information to an employer or for use in marketing activities. Doctors, health plans, and other covered entities would be required to follow the rule's standards for the use and disclosure of personal health information.

• Covered entities generally will need to provide patients with written notice of their privacy practices and patients' privacy rights. The notice will contain information that could be useful to patients choosing a health plan, doctor, or other provider. Patients would generally be asked to sign or otherwise acknowledge receipt of the privacy notice from direct treatment providers.

• Pharmacies, health plans, and other covered entities must first obtain an individual's specific authorization before sending marketing materials. At the same time, the rule permits doctors and other covered entities to communicate freely with patients about treatment options and other health-related information, including disease management programs.

• Specifically, improvements to the final rule strengthen the marketing language to make clear that covered entities cannot use business associate agreements to **circumvent** the rule's marketing prohibition. The improvement explicitly prohibits pharmacies and other covered entities from selling personal medical information to a business that would market its products or services under a business associate agreement.

- Patients generally will be able to access their personal medical records and request changes to correct any errors. In addition, patients generally could request an accounting of nonroutine uses and disclosures of their health information.

Many healthcare organizations have concern about the costs of implementing and maintaining measures that will comply with the privacy regulations. However, the benefits of the act far outweigh the inconveniences of remaining in compliance. Patients have the right to expect complete confidentiality with regard to their health records (Figure 15-5).

CRITICAL THINKING APPLICATION

- Laura is concerned about the number of employees in her facility who are allowed to access patient information. For instance, all nurses have access to health information on all patients. Is this a good policy? Why or why not?
- Should all physicians have access to all patient records? Why or why not?

National Center for Health Statistics

The National Center for Health Statistics (NCHS) is a division of the Centers for Disease Control and Prevention. The agency is the primary provider of health information statistics used to guide the actions and policies that relate to the health of the American public. The functions of the NCHS include the following:

- Documentation of the health status of the population and of important subgroups
- Identification of **disparities** in health status and use of healthcare by race, ethnicity, socioeconomic status (SES), region, and other population **gradients**
- Description of experiences with the healthcare system

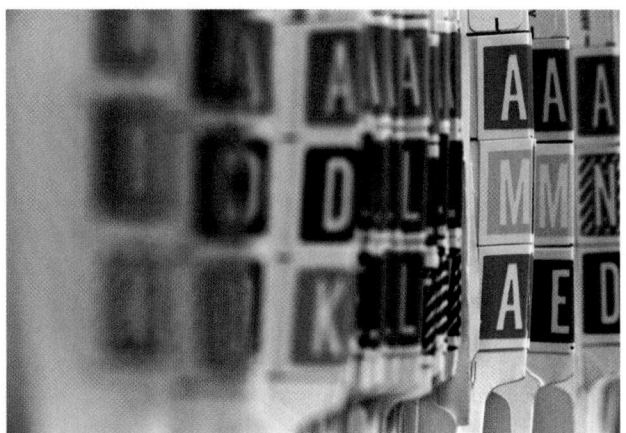

FIGURE 15-5 Patients must have the assurance that their medical records are accessed only by authorized individuals.

- Monitoring of trends in health status and healthcare delivery
- Identification of health problems
- Support for biomedical and health services research
- Provision of information for making changes in public policies and programs
- Evaluation of the impact of health policies and programs

Statistics are of vital importance to many entities that are interested in the healthcare industry. Some of the statistics available through the NCHS are related to the following:

- Teenage pregnancy
- Incidence of human immunodeficiency virus (HIV) infection
- Alcohol and drug use
- Births
- Deaths
- Communicable diseases
- Infant health and mortality
- Leading causes of death
- Life expectancy
- Sexually transmitted diseases
- Suicide

Total Quality Management

Total quality management is management and control activities based on the leadership of top-level management, supported by the involvement of all employees and departments from planning and development to sales and service. These management and control activities focus on quality assurance. Ideally, qualities that satisfy the customer are built into products and services as they receive care or services from providers.

For total quality management practices to be effective, all employees must make a commitment to provide patients with the best care possible. This includes top-level management as well as the staff members who work directly with the patients.

CRITICAL THINKING APPLICATION

- Laura has noticed that many employees are frustrated when confronted with quality-assurance regulations. Often employees complain that the policies are a waste of time. How can Laura convince these employees that the regulations are important, and how can she foster cooperation from these people?
- Should adherence to quality-assurance policies be a mandatory part of the employee's job description?

The Total Quality Management Concept

Much of the thrust of today's interest in total quality management originated from the teachings of W. Edwards Deming. Deming obtained a doctorate in mathematical physics from Yale University in 1928. He is perhaps best known for the work he did with Japanese managers and engineers regarding quality management. Deming compiled 14 points for managers to institute that were designed to place the emphasis on quality rather than quantity.

The following is an excerpt from Deming's book *Out of the Crisis* and briefly describes the Fourteen Points for Management.

- Create constancy of purpose toward improvement of product and service, with the aim to become competitive, to stay in business, and to provide jobs.
- Adopt the new philosophy. Western management must awaken to the challenge, must learn their responsibilities, and take on leadership for change.
- Cease dependence on inspection to achieve quality. Eliminate the need for inspection on a mass basis by building quality into the product or service in the first place.
- End the practice of awarding business on the basis of price tag. Instead, minimize total cost. Move toward a single supplier for any one item, on a long-term relationship of loyalty and trust.
- Constantly improve the system of production and service, to improve quality and productivity, and thus constantly decrease costs.
- Institute training on the job.
- Institute leadership. The aim of supervision should be to help people and machines and gadgets to do a better job. Supervision of management is in need of overhaul as well as supervision of production workers.
- Drive out fear, so that everyone may work effectively for the company.
- Break down barriers between departments. People must work as a team, to foresee problems of production and in use that may be encountered with the product or service.
- Eliminate slogans, exhortations, and targets for the work force asking for zero defects and new levels of productivity. Such exhortations only create adversarial relationships. Eliminate quotas and substitute leadership. Eliminate management by objective. Eliminate management by numbers and numerical goals. Substitute leadership.
- Remove barriers that rob the hourly worker of his right to pride of workmanship. The responsibility of supervisors must be changed from sheer numbers to quality.
- Remove barriers that rob people in management and in engineering of their right to pride of workmanship. This means the abolishment of the annual merit rating and of management by objective.
- Institute a vigorous program of education and self-improvement.
- Put everybody in the company to work to accomplish the transformation. The transformation is everybody's job.

Deming believed that these points would assist managers in bringing quality to the facility or business in which they were used (Figure 15-6). They are widely used in countless business and service organizations today.

Joint Commission on Accreditation of Healthcare Organizations

The Joint Commission on Accreditation of Healthcare Organizations (JCAHO) is a nonprofit organization that assists healthcare facilities by providing accreditation services. The

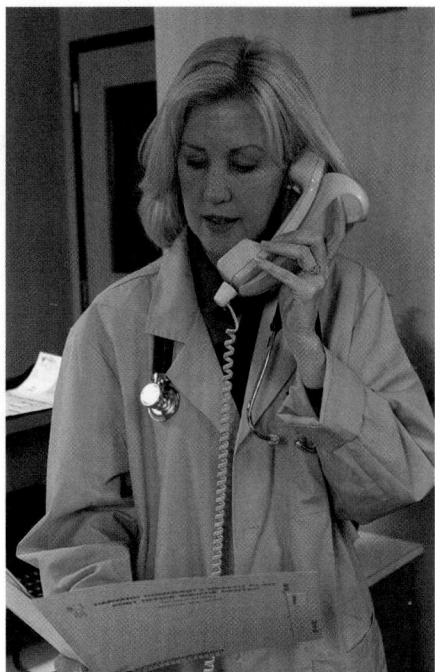

FIGURE 15-6 Quality management is a vital part of accreditation of healthcare organizations, and all physicians should be dedicated to providing optimal, high-quality care to patients.

facilities participate in obtaining accreditation voluntarily, but over 17,000 healthcare facilities in the United States are accredited by JCAHO and comply with its standards.

For many years, healthcare facilities were interested in meeting the minimum standards that would reflect quality healthcare. Recently, there has been a shift from simply meeting minimum standards to exceeding standards and providing optimal healthcare to patients (Figure 15-7). Standards are a set of criteria that the facility must adhere to, and the facility must be able to prove such compliance.

Risk Management

A risk is any occurrence that could result in patient injury or any type of financial loss to the healthcare facility. The policies and procedures that facilities develop are designed to manage risk and prevent situations that can cause harm to persons or property for which the healthcare facility could be held liable.

Risk management programs in healthcare facilities should focus on financial loss prevention and reduce the possibility of negative publicity resulting from **sentinel events.** JCAHO defines a sentinel event as an "unexpected occurrence involving death or serious physical or psychological injury, or the risk thereof." Sentinel events must be investigated thoroughly and their contributing factors rectified so that they are avoided in the future. Records are kept of the sentinel events that happen in a facility, especially those that involve injury to patients.

CLOSING COMMENTS

Health information management is a critical aspect of today's healthcare facility. Although regulations may seem stringent,

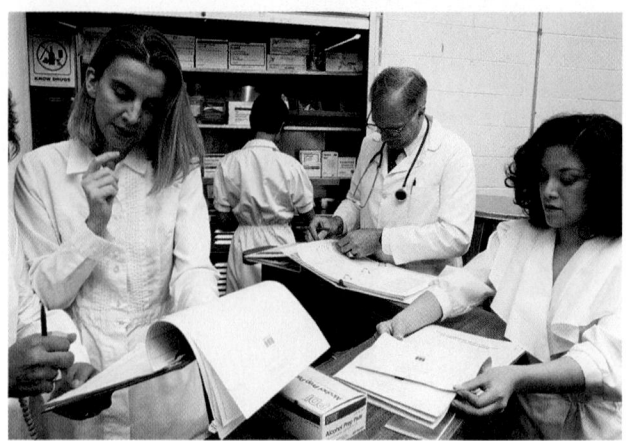

FIGURE 15-7 Accreditation of a healthcare facility takes teamwork and a commitment to quality assurance.

the value of protecting the patient's privacy is immeasurable. Patients have the right to expect their health information to be kept confidential. The medical assistant should focus on meeting privacy guidelines and should take great care when working with medical records and information.

Many patients may have questions about HIPAA and the extent of their rights to limit access to their records. Be prepared to answer these questions or guide such patients to the right source for information.

The medical assistant must be familiar with the laws surrounding privacy issues and be able to guide patients as concerns arise. Seminars that will target the compliance issues that affect the physician's office often are available to the medical assistant. Most employers are willing to pay for such seminars so that the office can remain in strict compliance with legal issues. Remember that the medical profession is one of constant change. The medical assistant must have a positive attitude about the learning process, especially when new rules and regulations take effect.

SUMMARY OF SCENARIO

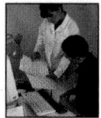

Laura is learning more about health information management each day that she goes to work. She has earned the respect of her supervisors, who often give her a lengthy, complicated document concerning regulations and ask her to read and summarize it for the staff. She has a knack for weeding out the actual requirements amid the excess of legalese.

Laura has developed good relationships with many of the staff physicians at the hospital. She has approached several of them about record authentication, and her bright personality helps to foster a sense of cooperation between the medical staff and the hospital staff. She has even begun to give coupons good for one lunch in the cafeteria when physicians form the habit of authenticating their records in a timely manner. The physicians appreciate the recognition for completing their duties on schedule.

Laura has given thought to continuing her education in the health management field and possibly gaining certification in this area. She knows that this will lend credibility to the knowledge that she has gained on the job. Her supervisors are pleased with her performance, and know they can count on Laura to complete any task she is assigned on time with accurate results. Laura looks forward to a long career at the hospital and being of service to the patients and staff alike in the years to come.

Health information is used on a daily basis in medical facilities. The patient record is probably the most common source of health information that healthcare professionals use, but they also access databases that provide statistical and other information that impacts patient care. Laura knows that she can contribute to quality healthcare by making certain that records are accurate, complete, and reliable for the medical professionals who use them. Providing quality healthcare is mandatory in today's society, because physicians are susceptible to lawsuits and complaints when patients feel that they did not receive optimal care. Additionally, patients have the right to choose their healthcare providers and they deserve and insist upon quality healthcare.

Laura has noticed that today's patients are more sophisticated and knowledgeable about health-related issues, primarily because of the ease of looking up their health issues on the Internet. Patients often tell the doctor what they think their diagnosis is, based upon their own Internet research. This is proof that even patients are using healthcare information. Statistical information helps Laura's employer determine the diseases and disorders that are most likely to affect patients in their hospital. Computers are an invaluable tool that allows healthcare providers and facilities to share information that will result in quality patient care.

SUMMARY of LEARNING OBJECTIVES

1. Define, spell, and pronounce the terms listed in the vocabulary.
   - Spelling and pronouncing medical terms correctly adds credibility to the medical assistant. Knowing the definition of these terms promotes confidence in communication with patients and co-workers.

2. Describe several ways that health information is used.
   - Both physicians and employees of medical facilities use health information in many ways. The information helps to ensure continuity of care from provider to provider. It assists manufacturers in determining side effects of drugs. It provides statistical information regarding primary and secondary diagnoses. Health information also helps the medical facility plan for future needs and capital equipment.

3. Contrast the nine characteristics of quality health data.
   - High-quality health data have nine characteristics. Validity refers to the accuracy of the information, and reliability means that the information can be counted on to be accurate and that medical decisions can be made based on the information. Completeness simply means that the information is available in its entirety, and recognizability refers to the data being understood by the users. Timely information allows the provider to make decisions based on the latest data about a patient or a treatment. Relevance refers to the usefulness of the health information, and accessibility means that the information is easily available to the provider when it is needed. Security encompasses the effort to keep unauthorized people from accessing health information. Legality refers to the correctness of the information and its authentication by the healthcare provider.

4. Explain the four concerns of quality assurance.
   - Four concerns that surround quality assurance include the overuse, underuse, misuse, and variations in use of healthcare services. Overused services are excessive and cause cost increases. An example includes using the emergency room for nonemergencies. Underuse means that patients do not take advantage of many services they should be using, especially if they are at-risk patients. Misuse of services often reflects errors, such as laboratory errors or misdiagnoses. Variations in services simply means that in various parts of the country, individuals use services in different ways, which can influence the quality of care overall in the United States.

5. Discuss the importance of the Health Insurance Portability and Accountability Act (HIPAA).

   - HIPAA is a milestone in support of patient privacy issues. The act has several facets, but the most widely publicized sections deal with the right to patient privacy. The act will give a degree of control to patients and allow them information about who accesses their records. Patients must also give specific authorization for the use and dissemination of the information contained in the medical record.

6. Explain the functions of the National Center for Health Statistics (NCHS).
   - The NCHS is a part of the Centers for Disease Control and Prevention. Health statistics are important, because they enable providers to better treat their patients. For instance, if a certain area has a high number of outbreaks of a particular disease, the physician may be better prepared to cope with patients with the symptoms of that disease, treating them faster and promoting a full recovery. Health statistics provide information about these types of issues. The NCHS helps to compile information such as the number of HIV infections, the number of teen pregnancies, and other vital health data that are useful to medical professionals.

7. Discuss the types of statistics kept by the NCHS.
   - Some of the statistics kept by the NCHS include alcohol and drug use information, births, deaths, communicable diseases, infant health and mortality, and life expectancy.

8. Define total quality management.
   - Total quality management is management and control activities based on the leadership of top-level management, supported by the involvement of all employees and departments in an effort to provide quality assurance.

9. Explain the function of the Joint Commission on Accreditation of Healthcare Organizations (JCAHO).
   - JCAHO is a nonprofit organization that offers accreditation services to healthcare facilities that wish to excel in healthcare services. Accreditation is voluntary; however, more than 17,000 healthcare facilities in the United States are accredited by this agency.

10. Discuss the importance of healthcare standards in medical facilities.
    - Without strong healthcare standards, quality cannot exist. The focus of quality assurance has shifted in recent years from just meeting the minimum standards to providing optimal quality. People expect high-quality healthcare when they get treatment. Today's organizations that seek accreditation or focus their efforts on quality will exceed standards, not just meet them.

CONNECTIONS

 Study Guide Connection: Go to Chapter 15 Study Guide. Read the Case Study and Workplace Applications and complete the assignments. Do online research for answers to the questions in the Internet Activities associated with health information management.

 CD Connection: Go to the Medical Assisting Competency Challenge CD and do the training activities under Patient Care and General Office Duties.

Evolve Connection: For more information related to health information management, go to evolve.elsevier.com/kinn and visit related weblinks for Chapter 15. Click on the Medical Assisting Exam Review and do the practice questions to sharpen your test-taking skills.

Privacy in the Physician's Office

16

SCENARIO

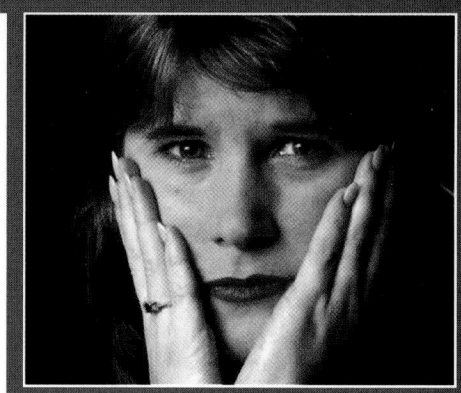

Sabrina Ragland, a medical assistant with 12 years' experience, works for a gastroenterologist, Dr. Tim Taylor. She comes from a family heavily involved in the medical field. Her father was a surgeon and her mother was his office assistant. Two of Sabrina's sisters are nurses, and her brother is a respiratory therapist. Her husband, Joe, is a biomedical technician, and his mother, Elsa Ragland, has been an RN for 40 years. For more than half of her career, Elsa has worked for a local internist, Dr. Royce Berry. A casual comment at the Ragland family picnic resulted in a medical professional liability lawsuit based on violation of patient privacy. Sabrina and Elsa's careers were jeopardized by a simple exchange of what seemed to be innocent information.

Vivian Adams, a 42-year-old hospital insurance biller, saw Dr. Berry in his office for pain located in her lower left quadrant. Ms. Adams was not a new patient but had not visited the office in approximately 2 years. When she arrived for her visit, she was presented with the office privacy policy and was asked to sign the document. Vivian glanced through it, signed it, and saw the doctor. He performed an examination and found that Vivian was likely suffering from irritable bowel syndrome and prescribed medication. Ms. Adams called the physician 1 week later complaining that she was no better. Dr. Berry changed her medication without seeing her and did not hear from her again, other than her requests for refills of the medication. After 6 months with no improvement, Ms. Adams went to Dr. Taylor; after several diagnostic tests, she was told that she had colon cancer and was given a bleak prognosis. She told Dr. Taylor that she blamed Dr. Berry for not being more thorough in his testing. Sabrina was in the room and heard the comment.

That weekend at the picnic, Sabrina mentioned Ms. Adams to her mother-in-law and stated that the patient might sue Dr. Berry, although the patient never said those words. Elsa defended Dr. Berry and proclaimed that he was a good doctor, then expressed her hope that Ms. Adams would not sue her employer. One week later, Elsa was in a grocery store and saw Ms. Adams. Elsa immediately expressed her sympathy about her diagnosis, and then asked if there was anything she could do. Her intent was to be kind and try to avert litigation against Dr. Berry. Her gesture might have been well received had Ms. Adams' daughter, Terri, not been standing with her. Terri was not yet aware that her mother had been diagnosed with cancer. Ms. Adams had told no one about her illness at that point. After the incident at the grocery store the first person Ms. Adams told was her attorney.

While studying this chapter, think about the following questions:

- When can the medical assistant discuss a patient, and with whom, and under what circumstances?
- What has HIPAA done for the medical industry and the patients it serves?

- When new policies and procedures are implemented, how can the staff embrace the changes and make the transitions easier?
- What happens if the patient refuses to sign the privacy policy?

LEARNING OBJECTIVES

1. Define, spell, and pronounce the terms listed in the vocabulary.
2. Explain how the HIPAA Privacy Rule benefits the healthcare industry and patients.
3. List what must be included on a Notice of Privacy Practices.
4. Explain the difference between Title I and Title II of the HIPAA Privacy Rule.
5. List the rights that patients have under the Privacy Rule.
6. Briefly explain what is expected of healthcare providers in relation to the Privacy Rule.

7. Describe an incidental disclosure.
8. List the three instances when a parent is not considered the child's representative.
9. Explain why a provider can discuss protected health information with a patient's friends and family.
10. Discuss the role of the Notice of Privacy Practices in emergencies.

National Accreditation Competencies and Content

CAAHEP COMPETENCIES

General

3.c.(2)(a). Identify and respond to issues of confidentiality
3.c.(2)(b). Perform within legal and ethical boundaries
3.c.(2)(d). Document accurately

ABHES COMPETENCIES

Professionalism

1.b. Maintain confidentiality at all times
1.d. Be cognizant of ethical boundaries

Legal Concepts

5.a. Determine needs for documentation and reporting
5.b. Document accurately
5.c. Use appropriate guidelines when releasing records or information
5.g. Monitor legislation related to current healthcare issues and practices
5.h. Perform risk management procedures

VOCABULARY

business associates Individuals or organizations that perform or assist a covered entity in the performance of a function or activity that involves the use or disclosure of individually identifiable health information.

complainant (kuhm-pla'-nuhnt) Person making a complaint against a person or organization.

covered entity An organization that transmits information in an electronic form during a transaction, as defined by HIPAA.

divulge (duh-vuhlj') To make known, as a confidence or secret.

due diligence Also known as *due care;* the effort made by an ordinarily prudent or reasonable party to avoid harm to another party or himself; doing everything possible to prevent something from happening.

electronic media Means of electronic transmission, including the Internet, private networks, dial-up phone lines, and fax modems; includes information moved from one place to another while stored on an electronic device.

healthcare providers Providers of medical or health services, individually or as organizations, that furnish, bill for, or are paid for services or products.

individually identifiable health information Any part of a patient's health record that is created or received by a covered entity.

infer To derive as a conclusion from facts and premises.

Office for Civil Rights (OCR) The division of the federal government that enforces privacy standards.

Office of Inspector General (OIG) Established to protect the integrity of the Department of Health and Human Services (HHS), the office conducts audits, investigations, and inspections involving the laws that pertain to HHS.

personal health information The patient's own information that pertains to his or her health.

preclude To rule out in advance.

prevalent Generally or widely accepted, practiced, or favored.

privacy officer A person designated to ensure compliance with privacy standards for a covered entity.

protected health information (PHI) Any individually identifiable health information that is transmitted and/or maintained in electronic form.

transactions As defined by HIPAA, transmissions of information between two parties to carry out financial or administrative activities related to healthcare.

verbiage A manner of expressing oneself in words.

One of the most valuable character traits that the medical assistant develops is the ability to adjust to change and be flexible. The medical profession evolves rapidly, and advances in technology allow medicine to progress. Think of how few computers were found in physician's offices 40 years ago. Today, computers adorn almost every desk. Change is a concept that many individuals resist.

The creation of privacy and security laws was a huge step toward more efficient healthcare and faster reimbursements. Technology often forces organizations to move forward somewhat quickly. Healthcare facilities with already strapped budgets sometimes view such innovations as a hindrance. Compliance officers at larger facilities may wonder if additional federal regulations are necessary.

Many healthcare workers feel that they can say nothing to anyone, about any patient, at any time. By understanding the compliance that HIPAA requires, the employees of the physician's office can feel secure about their dealings with the patients and other individuals who frequent the facility.

THE HEALTH INSURANCE PORTABILITY AND ACCOUNTABILITY ACT

The Health Insurance Portability and Accountability Act (HIPAA) was introduced in Chapter 7. HIPAA, enacted in 1996, is a group of laws that affect both employees of a healthcare facility, insurance company, or other **covered entity** and the patients the organizations serve. The federal government required all covered entities to be in compliance with HIPAA by April 14, 2003 (small healthcare plans received an extra year to comply, extending their deadline to April 14, 2004).

Effect of the HIPAA Privacy Rule

The HIPAA Privacy Rule creates national standards to protect individuals' medical records and other personal health information. This is the first time that such a group of laws has been enacted to protect patient privacy. The creation of the HIPAA Privacy Rule provides benefits to both patients and their **healthcare providers:**

- Patients have more control over their medical records.
- Patients are able to make informed choices regarding how their personal health information is used.
- Boundaries are set on the use and release of health records.
- Safeguards are established that healthcare providers must achieve to protect the privacy of health information.
- Violators are held accountable and face both civil and criminal penalties if patient privacy rights are compromised.
- The Privacy Rule protects public health by striking a balance when public responsibility supports disclosure of personal health information.

Under the few laws that existed before the HIPAA Privacy Rule, personal health information could be distributed to others without either notice or authorization from the patient, even if the reason for the exchange of information had nothing to do with the patient's medical treatment or healthcare reimbursement. A health plan could pass patient information to a financial lender, who might then deny the patient a home mortgage or credit card based on his or her health history. Employers could obtain health information and use it in personnel decisions. Because computers make information exchange so much easier, laws had to be enacted to protect patient privacy (Figure 16-1).

Title I and Title II Provisions

HIPAA contains two provisions, Title I and Title II. Title I regulates insurance reform, and Title II deals with administrative simplification. Title I limits the use of preexisting health

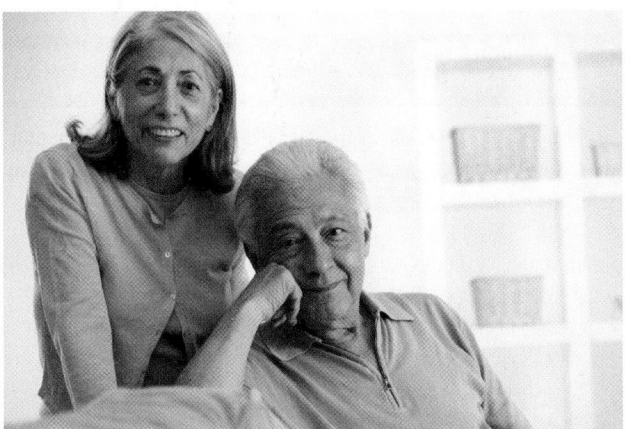

FIGURE 16-1 The HIPAA Privacy Rule was created in part to give patients more control over their personal health information.

conditions that in the past prevented or limited an employee from obtaining health insurance coverage. If an individual left a job with insurance coverage and attempted to secure new coverage, a preexisting health condition would often **preclude** that person from obtaining coverage for that illness. Many individuals were refused any coverage at all, especially if the condition was a serious one, such as a heart condition or high blood pressure. Today, because of HIPAA laws, discrimination against individuals who are in poor health now or were in the past is prohibited. The regulations limit the use of preexisting condition exclusions and guarantee that certain individuals can purchase healthcare insurance after leaving or losing a job.

The goal of Title II is to reduce administrative costs in the healthcare industry. Often goals sound simple, but to reach a goal, many actions are necessary. The medical assistant who enters school sets graduation as his or her goal. However, in order to graduate, he or she must study, pass tests, arrange for childcare, sacrifice sleep, adjust working hours, readjust to the school environment, and make any number of other adjustments to reach the goal. Likewise, to simplify the administrative costs involved in patient care, many different objectives must be met.

Provisions of Administrative Simplification

If given a choice to use a computer or an electric typewriter to write a report, most individuals would likely choose the computer. Because computers can perform so many duties much more rapidly than those that were performed manually, they have become indispensable to the healthcare profession. **Electronic media** is used daily in modern physician offices and healthcare facilities. However, as computers have become **prevalent,** patients have begun to express concerns about who sees **protected health information (PHI)** and what is done with that information. Title II contains two parts:

- Development and implementation of standardized electronic **transactions** using Standard Code Sets
- Implementation of privacy and security procedures to prevent the misuse of health information by ensuring confidentiality

The second part of the administrative simplification provision deals with privacy, confidentiality, and security of PHI and is the focus of this chapter.

Patient Rights

Separate from the Patients' Bill of Rights, HIPAA provides for several patient rights. These include the following:

- The right to notice of a facility's privacy practices
- The right to have access to, view, and obtain a copy of their PHI
- The right to restrict certain parts or uses of their PHI
- The right to request that communications from the facility be kept confidential
- The right to request the facility to amend the PHI
- The right to receive notice of all disclosures of their PHI

These patient rights are the heart of the HIPAA Privacy Rule. These rights must be protected by those involved in the healthcare profession and are explained in more detail in the following section.

Right to Notice of Privacy Practices

Patients have the right to a copy of the Notice of Privacy Practices used in the physician's office (Figure 16-2). A copy of the Notice of Privacy Practices must also be prominently displayed in the office. This policy is developed by the individual facility and must be written in terminology that the patient will understand. Patients should be given a copy of the Notice of Privacy Practices and sign an acknowledgement that they received the copy. If a patient refuses to sign the acknowledgement, the medical assistant can note that the document was offered to the patient and he or she refused to sign. This proves **due diligence** on the part of the office and that a good faith effort was made to provide the patient with privacy information. Most patients will sign the document. Be prepared to explain the Notice of Privacy Practices to the patients.

The Notice of Privacy Practices must include the following:
- How PHI is used and disclosed by the facility
- The duties of the provider to protect health information
- Patient rights regarding PHI
- How complaints can be filed if patients believe their privacy has been violated
- Whom to contact at the facility for more information
- The effective date of the Notice of Privacy Practices

Right to Access Protected Health Information

Patients must be allowed access to their personal health information. The maker, not the patient, owns the record; however, the HIPAA Privacy Rule grants patients the right to access, inspect, and obtain a copy of their health information. Most physicians' offices require patients to request access in writing and act on that request within 30 days (Figure 16-3). HIPAA does restrict access to psychotherapy notes, information compiled for use in legal proceedings, and information exempted from disclosure by the Clinical Laboratory Improvement Amendment (CLIA).

Right to Request Restrictions on Certain Uses and Disclosures of Protected Health Information

Patients can request restrictions on the use of their PHI. For instance, if a patient had an abortion many years ago and does not want that information released, she has the right to ask a provider not to **divulge** that information. The provider does not have to agree to the request but must review it and give a good reason for the restriction not to be honored. An appeal process should be in place for instances when the provider does not agree with the restriction.

Right to Request Confidential Communications

Patients have the right to express where they wish to receive communications from the provider. The patient may prefer to be contacted on a cell phone instead of a home phone, or through email. Providers must accommodate reasonable requests. Suppose a married female patient comes to the clinic for a pregnancy test. Further suppose that her husband has had

a vasectomy. Clearly, a call to her home phone number with test results could initiate personal and private difficulties for the patient. Make certain that the preferred method of communication is used when contacting any patient (Procedure 16-1).

Right to Request Amendment of Protected Health Information

Patients can request that changes be made to their medical record, if they inspect it and find an error. This request should be made in writing. Providers must review the request and act on it in a timely manner, generally within 60 days. The request may be denied if the provider was not the creator of the record, as in the case of records provided by a consulting physician. Or, the provider may believe that the information is correct and complete. A review process must be in place by which such requests can be considered.

Right to Receive an Accounting of Disclosures of Protected Health Information

Patients may request that the physician provide an accounting of all disclosures of the patient's PHI that are nonroutine (as defined in the facility's Notice of Privacy Practices). Patients are entitled to receive this accounting annually without charge, but the provider can charge patients for additional accountings.

Responsibilities of Providers or Health Plans

The responsibilities placed on providers and health plans seems extensive when one reads the actual **verbiage** of the law. Do not be intimidated when reading a publication written by the federal government. These documents are rarely written for ease of understanding and may need to be reread several times before the reader grasps the meaning of a regulation.

In general, the HIPAA Privacy Rule requires activities such as the following.
- Notifying patients of their privacy rights
- Explaining how their health information might be used
- Development of privacy procedures in the facility
- Implementation of those privacy procedures
- Training employees so that they understand the procedures in place

---

Seven Components of HIPAA Compliance Offered by the Office of Inspector General

To simplify compliance with HIPAA regulations, the **Office of Inspector General (OIG)** has developed seven components of an effective compliance program. These components are as follows:
- Conducting internal monitoring and auditing
- Implementing compliance and practice standards
- Designating a compliance officer or contact
- Conducting appropriate training and education
- Responding appropriately to detected offenses, and developing corrective action
- Developing open lines of communication
- Enforcing disciplinary standards through well-publicized guidelines

WALNUT HILL FAMILY AND PREVENTIVE MEDICINE CLINIC, PA
1701 W. Walnut Hill Lane, Suite 200
Dallas, Texas 75229
214-549-1111   214-549-1222 (FAX)
info@walnuthillclinic.com

NOTICE OF PRIVACY PRACTICES

THIS NOTICE DESCRIBES HOW MEDICAL INFORMATION ABOUT YOU MAY BE USED AND DISCLOSED
AND HOW YOU CAN GET ACCESS TO THIS INFORMATION.
PLEASE REVIEW IT CAREFULLY.

YOUR MEDICAL RECORD (CHART) contains your symptoms, examination, and test results, diagnoses, treatment, and plan for follow-up. This is protected health information (PHI), and is used for many reasons. Your medical record serves as a

- basis for planning your care and treatment (this includes scheduling and appointment reminders)
- means of communication among the many health professionals who contribute to your care
- legal document describing the care you received
- means by which you or a third-party payer can verify services billed
- tool in educating health professionals
- source of data for quality control programs and medical research
- source of information for public health officials (by law, certain illnesses must be reported)

YOUR HEALTH INFORMATION RIGHTS
Although your medical record (chart) is the physical property of the clinic, the information contained within the record belongs to you. You have the right to:

- request a restriction on certain uses and disclosures of your information
- obtain a paper copy of this notice
- inspect and obtain a copy of your medical record as provided in our office policy manual
- amend your health record (requests must be made in writing)
- request communications of your health information by alternative means or at alternative locations
- revoke your authorization to use or disclose health information except to the extent that action has already been taken
- obtain an accounting of any non-routine disclosures of your health information

OUR RESPONSIBILITIES
The Walnut Hill Family and Preventative Medicine Clinic is required to:

- maintain the privacy of your medical record (chart)
- abide by the terms of this notice
- notify you if we are unable to agree to a requested restriction
- accommodate reasonable requests you may have to communicate health information by alternative means or at alternative locations or phone numbers

We reserve the right to change our practices and to make new provisions effective for all protected health information we maintain. We will post a copy of our current notice in a visible location at all times. We will not use or disclose your protected health information without your authorization, except as described in this notice.

FOR MORE INFORMATION OR TO REPORT A PROBLEM
Please contact Sue Singer or Ron Rachels during regular office hours at 214-549-1111 or you can email or mail questions or complaints to Dr. Robbie Speasak at the above address. If you believe that your privacy rights have been violated, you can file a complaint with the Secretary of the Department of Health and Human Services. You will not be penalized in any way for filing a complaint.

FIGURE 16-2 Notice of Privacy Practices.

REQUEST TO ACCESS MEDICAL RECORD

Patients have the right to access their personal health information. We will be happy to accommodate any patient who wishes to exercise this access to inspect or obtain a copy of the record. Please provide the information requested on this form. This request will be acted upon within thirty (30) days. Standard copy charges will apply.

Patient Name _____

Date of Birth _____ Phone _____

Address _____

City _____ State _____ Zip _____

Email Address _____

Date of Last Office Visit _____

Please note below what information should be copied or provided:

_____

_____

_____

Please note below the following change(s) that need to be addressed:

_____

_____

I wish to receive a regular accounting of non-routine disclosures of my protected health information.

❏ Yes   ❏ No

_____   _____
Patient Signature   Date

FOR OFFICE USE ONLY

Date Copied _____ Date Mailed _____

Certified Mail # _____

FIGURE 16-3 Request to access a medical record.

PROCEDURE 16-1

Identify and Respond to Issues of Confidentiality

CAAHEP COMPETENCY: 3.c(2)(a)
ABHES COMPETENCY: 1.b

GOAL: *To become proficient at identifying issues involving confidentiality and respond to them in the manner prescribed by office policy.*

EQUIPMENT and SUPPLIES

- Office policy manual
- Office procedure manual, if separate
- Release of information forms
- Notice of Privacy Practices
- Clerical supplies
- Patient medical records

PROCEDURAL STEPS

1. Review office policy regarding release of patient information and confidentiality in the facility.
   PURPOSE: To make certain that office policy is stringently followed and that the office remains in HIPAA compliance.

2. Review the Notice of Privacy Practices for the facility.
   PURPOSE: To be sure that the office's privacy policies are followed.

3. Review the facility's Authorization to Release Medical Records form.

4. Thoroughly read the request for information that is presented to the facility.
   PURPOSE: To determine what information is being requested.

5. Determine if the document is valid.
   PURPOSE: No information should be released if the requesting documents are not valid.

6. Determine the exact information that is being requested.
   PURPOSE: Only the exact information being requested should be released.

7. Make certain that the release of information form either is one designed by the facility or contains all of the same information.

8. Make the requestor complete one of the facility's request forms, if necessary.

9. Forward only the information requested to the person or organization that presented the authorization for release of information.
   PURPOSE: No information that has not been requested can be released without additional consent by the patient.

10. Release the information by mail or to the agent of the requestor.

- Designating an individual to be responsible for implementation
- Securing medical records so that they are not available to those who do not need them

PERMISSION TO DISCLOSE PROTECTED HEALTH INFORMATION

Once the patient has signed the Notice of Privacy Practices, the physician may disclose PHI in the manner that is described on the policy. Virtually all of the daily operations that involve PHI are covered under the Notice of Privacy Practices.

Some offices ask patients to sign a receipt of privacy practices annually. Others simply post the current policy prominently in the office, and state where it can be found on the original notice that the patient signs. Using either method, every current medical record should contain a signed Notice of Privacy Practices, an acknowledgement that the patient received the Notice of Privacy Practices, or a statement that the patient refused to sign the notice. Physicians also use separate release of information forms that detail exactly where to call a patient, whether the patient prefers email communications, and/or specific releases for human immunodeficiency virus (HIV)–related and psychotherapy information (Figures 16-4 and 16-5).

At times, conflicting permissions may be an issue when disclosing PHI. Suppose that a patient requests that a copy of his or her medical record be sent to a third party, such as an attorney. The patient signs the release at an office visit. Before the medical record is copied and sent, the attorney forwards a signed release for just the progress notes. Call the patient first and attempt to verify what he or she wishes sent. Another option is to adhere to the most restrictive request; in this case, send only the progress notes. Always document any form of communication about the patient's preference in writing. The medical assistant may find it necessary to ask the patient to sign a new permission form. Do not hesitate to contact the patient if any question arises about what he or she wishes to be released.

Identifying the Patient

Providers see numerous patients each day and the medical assistant may not know each one by sight. Always insist on identification when releasing any type of health information to anyone. A state-issued drivers license or identification card is the best method of identification, but alternates may be necessary for those who do not have that particular document. The office policy manual should list acceptable forms of identification. When making any type of disclosure, make certain to note why the person has the authority to request and receive the PHI.

Patient Names and Sign-In Sheets

A staff member in a physician's office may call out a patient's name when it is time to see the physician. Sign-in sheets that list patient names may also be used. Covered entities are permitted to make such incidental disclosures if they comply with the

Patient Consent to the Use and Disclosure of Health Information for Treatment, Payment, or Health Care Operations

I understand that as part of my health care, the practice originates and maintains paper and/or electronic records describing my health history, symptoms, examination and test results, diagnoses, treatment, and any plans for future care or treatment. I understand that this information serves as:

- A basis for planning my care and treatment,
- A means of communication among professionals who contribute to my care,
- A source of information for applying my diagnosis and treatment information to my bill,
- A means by which a third-party payer can verify that services billed were actually provided,
- A tool for routine health care operations, such as assessing quality and reviewing the competence of staff.

I have been provided the opportunity to review the *"Notice of Patient Privacy Information Practices"* **that provides a more complete description of information uses and disclosures. I understand that I have the following rights:**

- The right to review the *"Notice"* prior to acknowledging this consent,
- The right to restrict or revoke the use or disclosure of my health information for other uses or purposes, and
- The right to request restrictions as to how my health information may be used or disclosed to carry out treatment, payment, or health care operations.

Restrictions:

I request the following restrictions to the use or disclosure of my health information:

_____

_____

May discuss treatment, payment, or health care operation with the following persons:

(Please check all that apply)   Spouse [   ]   Your Children [   ]   Relatives [   ]   Others [   ]   Parents [   ]

Please list the names and relationship, if you checked "Relatives" or "Others" above

_____

_____

Messages or Appointment Reminders: (Please check all that apply)

May we leave a message on your answering machine at home [   ] or at work [   ]. **Do not leave a message** [   ]
May we leave a message with someone at your **home** using the doctor's name or the practice name: Yes [   ]   No [   ]
May we leave a message with someone at your **work** using the doctor's name or the practice name: Yes [   ]   No [   ]
Messages will be of a nonsensitive nature, such as appointment reminders.

I understand that as part of treatment, payment, or health care operations, it may become necessary to disclose health information to another entity, i.e., referrals to other health care providers, labs, and/or other individuals or agencies as permitted or required by state or federal law.

I fully understand and accept the information provided by this consent.

_____   _____   _____
Signature   Print name of person signing   Date

*If other than patient is signing, are you the parent, legal guardian, custodian, or have Power of Attorney for this patient for treatment, payment, or health care operations? Yes [   ]   No [   ]

FOR OFFICE USE ONLY
[   ] Patient refused to sign the consent form.
[   ] Restrictions were added by the patient (see restrictions listed above)
[   ] "Consent form" received and reviewed by _____ on (date) _____
[   ] "Consent form" placed in the patient's medical record on (date) _____

FIGURE 16-4 Example of HIPAA-compliant patient disclosure form. (From Klieger DM: *Saunders textbook of medical assisting*, St Louis, 2005, Saunders.)

GENERAL MEDICAL HEALTH CARE

AUTHORIZATION FOR RELEASE OF MEDICAL INFORMATION

I, _____ ____/____/____ _____ hereby authorize
    Print Patient's Name   Date of Birth   Social Security Number

General Medical Health Care 1234 Riverview Road, Anytown, FL 33333

to release medical, including HIV Antibody Testing, Psychiatric/Psychological, Alcohol and/or Drug Abuse, information records to:

To: _____

Address _____
        (Street)   (City)   (State)   (Zip)

For the purpose of: 1. Drs. appointment on: _____

                       2. Other: _____

                       _____
                              Please Specify Reason for Disclosure

I understand that if I consent to the release of any of my medical records, the results of any HIV Antibody Testing, Psychiatric/Psychological, Alcohol and/or Drug Abuse information will be released.

I understand this consent may be cancelled upon written notice to the hospital, except that action by the hospital has been taken in reliance on this authorization, and that this authorization shall remain in force for a 90-day period in order to effect the purpose for which it is given. Alcohol and drug abuse information, if present, has been disclosed from records whose confidentiality is protected by Federal Law.
FEDERAL REGULATIONS (42CFR, part II) prohibit making any further disclosure of records without the specific written authorization of the undersigned, or as otherwise permitted by such regulations.
The confidentiality of HIV antibody test results is protected by Florida Law [Fla. Stat.ANN. 381.609 (2) (F)], which prohibits any further disclosure by a person to whom this information has been disclosed, without specific written consent of the undersigned or as otherwise permitted by state law.

_____   From: _____ To: _____
    (Date of Authorization)   (Dates to be Released)

_____
    Patient's Signature

_____
Parent, Legal Guardian, or Authorized
Representative Signature

_____
    Relationship to Patient

_____
    Witness

FIGURE 16-5 Example of HIPAA-compliant patient disclosure form containing HIV and psychologic information release. (From Klieger DM: *Saunders textbook of medical assisting*, St Louis, 2005, Saunders.)

HIPAA MINIMUM NECESSARY STANDARD
[45 CFR 164.502(b), 164.514(d)]

Background

The minimum necessary standard, a key protection of the HIPAA Privacy Rule, is derived from confidentiality codes and practices in common use today. It is based on sound current practice that protected health information should not be used or disclosed when it is not necessary to satisfy a particular purpose or carry out a function. The minimum necessary standard requires covered entities to evaluate their practices and enhance safeguards as needed to limit unnecessary or inappropriate access to and disclosure of protected health information. The Privacy Rule's requirements for minimum necessary standards are designed to be sufficiently flexible to accommodate the various circumstances of any covered entity.

How the Rule Works

The Privacy Rule generally requires covered entities to take reasonable steps to limit the use or disclosure of, and requests for, protected health information to the minimum necessary to accomplish the intended purpose. The minimum necessary standard does not apply to the following:

- Disclosures to or requests by a health care provider for treatment purposes.
- Disclosures to the individual who is the subject of the information.
- Uses or disclosures made pursuant to an individual's authorization.
- Uses or disclosures required for compliance with the Health Insurance Portability and Accountability Act (HIPAA) Administrative Simplification Rules.
- Disclosures to the Department of Health and Human Services (HHS) when disclosure of information is required under the Privacy Rule for enforcement purposes.
- Uses or disclosures that are required by other law.

The implementation specifications for this provision require a covered entity to develop and implement policies and procedures appropriate for its own organization, reflecting the entity's business practices and workforce. While guidance cannot anticipate every question or factual application of the minimum necessary standard to each specific industry context, where it would be generally helpful we will seek to provide additional clarification on this issue in the future. In addition, the Department will continue to monitor the workability of the minimum necessary standard and consider proposing revisions, where appropriate, to ensure that the Rule does not hinder timely access to quality health care.

http://www.hhs.gov/ocr/hipaa/

FIGURE 16-6 HIPAA's Minimum Necessary Standard Overview.

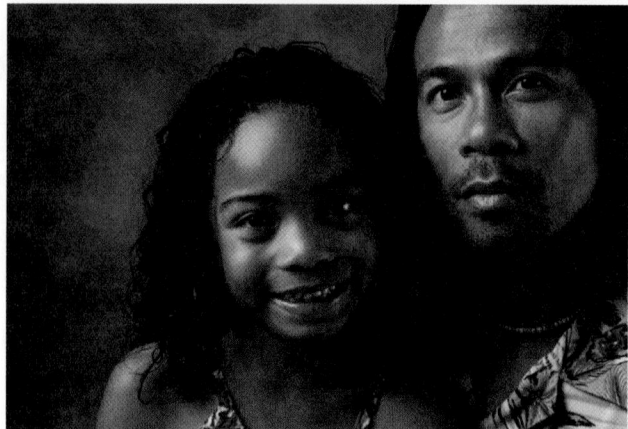

FIGURE 16-7 In most cases the parent is considered the child's representative and is allowed to view 'the child's medical records.

Privacy Rule is not intended to impede customary and necessary healthcare communications or practices or to require that all risk of incidental use or disclosure be eliminated to satisfy the Privacy standards. Disclosures that could occur as a byproduct of engaging in healthcare communications or practices may be considered acceptable under the Privacy Rule.

Incidental disclosures could include the following:
- Confidential conversations between providers or with patients, if a possibility exists that they may be heard (e.g., by hearing the patient and physician talking through the wall when in an adjacent examination room)
- Seeing other patient names when signing in
- A person not authorized to see PHI walks by medical equipment and sees material containing **individually identifiable health information** (e.g., seeing a patient's name on an ultrasound screen)
- Physicians speaking with patients in semiprivate hospital rooms
- Healthcare staff orally coordinating patient care services at a nurse's station or central location within an office
- A pharmacist discussing a patient with a physician on the phone when another person is standing nearby

Most physician offices have implemented sign-in sheets that ideally allow only one patient to sign in at a time and prevent them from seeing other patient names. Sign-in sheets that use pressure-sensitive stickers are a good example. The patient signs in on the form, then the sticker is removed and placed either in the patient's medical record or on a log sheet. Some offices are more technologically advanced and have a computer sign-in system. The patient arrives and goes to the computer screen, sees his or her name, and then presses "enter" to signify that he or she has arrived for the appointment. The patient name appears only for 15 minutes or so before the appointment and for 15 minutes after. If the name is not on the screen, the patient is directed to see the office staff. This subtly teaches the patient to be on time for appointments. These devices save time, although the patient must receive brief training on how to use the system. The short time that the patient's name is viewable on the screen is an incidental exposure but is acceptable through HIPAA guidelines as explained previously.

minimum necessary requirements of HIPAA (Figure 16-6). An incidental use or disclosure is a secondary use or disclosure that cannot reasonably be prevented, is limited in nature, and occurs as a result of another use or disclosure that is permitted. The

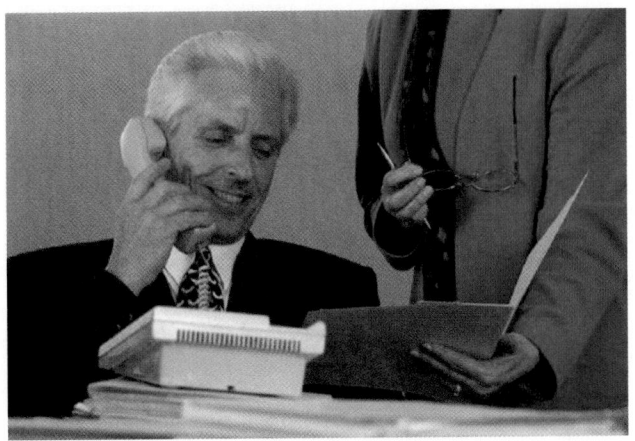

FIGURE 16-8 The telephone remains one of the most vital tools for communication with patients.

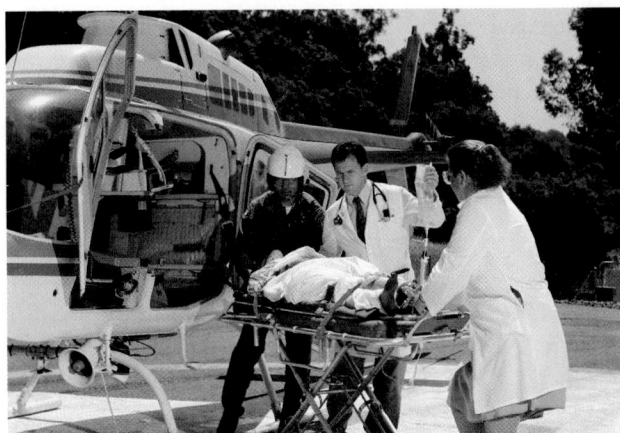

FIGURE 16-9 In emergencies the Notice of Privacy Practices does not have to be offered until it is practical to do so.

Placement of Patient Medical Records

Many physician offices place medical records inside a wall folder just outside of the examination room. By turning the record so that the name cannot be seen by someone passing through the hallway, the facility meets the minimum necessary requirement in protecting patient privacy. The hallway area should be supervised, and nonemployees should be escorted when in the clinical area of the office.

Children's Health Records

The Privacy Rule does allow parents to see the medical records of their children as long as this is not inconsistent with state law. In most cases the parent is the child's personal representative under the Privacy Rule (Figure 16-7). However, several instances exist in which the parent is not considered the child's personal representative. These instances include the following:

- When the minor is the one who consents to care and the consent of the parent is not required under state or other applicable law (for example, in the case of an emancipated minor)
- When the minor obtains care at the direction of a court or a person appointed by the court
- When the parent agrees that the minor and healthcare provider can have a confidential relationship

Discussing Information with Friends and Family

The Privacy Rule specifically permits covered entities to share information that is directly relevant to the patient's care with a spouse, family members, friends, or other persons identified by a patient. The covered entity may also share relevant information with the family and these other persons if it can reasonably **infer,** based on professional judgment, that the patient does not object or that the action is in the best interest of the patient. Remember that if the patient has requested that such information not be shared with others, the provider must honor that request unless it is deemed unreasonable.

Both covered entities and **business associates** can discuss a patient's bill with a person other than the patient to obtain reimbursement. No limit is placed on to whom such a disclosure may be made. However, the Privacy Rule does require a covered entity or business associate to reasonably limit the amount of information disclosed for such purposes to the minimum necessary and to abide by reasonable requests for confidential communications and restrictions that the patient has requested.

Telephone Messages and Faxes

Medical assistants must communicate with patients, and that communication is often initiated with a telephone call (Figure 16-8). At times the patient is not at home or available and the medical assistant must use professional judgment about leaving a message, as well as about how much information to disclose to the person who answers the telephone. Even leaving a message on an answering machine can be questionable, because no one is sure who will hear a message containing PHI.

If the patient has requested that the provider or provider's employees communicate only in a confidential manner, such as by alternative means or at an alternative location, the provider must honor that request if it is reasonable. For instance, requests to receive calls at work instead of at home are reasonable requests, unless there are extenuating circumstances.

A fax can be sent containing PHI to another healthcare provider for treatment purposes or to another individual as requested by the patient. Use reasonable care in sending a fax, such as verifying the correct numbers, directing the fax to a certain person, and using cover sheets that stress confidentiality. All fax machines should be located in secure areas to prevent unauthorized access to PHI. Information used for treatment purposes can be shared by fax, email, or telephone with other healthcare providers.

Emergencies

Healthcare providers and facilities, such as hospitals, with a direct treatment relationship with individuals are not required to provide their Notices of Privacy Practices to patients at the time they are providing emergency treatment (Figure 16-9). In such situations the HIPAA Privacy Rule requires only that providers give patients a notice when it is practical to do so after the emergency situation has ended. In addition, the Privacy Rule does not require that providers make a good faith effort to obtain the patient's written acknowledgement of receipt of the notice.

Complaints about Privacy Violations

When a patient has a complaint regarding his or her privacy information, the first person he or she should seek out is the **privacy officer** at the facility where the incident took place. If the complaint is not resolved, patients should be directed to the office manager or physician. In the event that the patient's issue has still not been resolved, he or she has the option to file a written complaint either on paper or electronically with the **Office for Civil Rights (OCR).** The complaint must be filed within 180 days of when the **complainant** knew or should have known that the act had occurred (Figure 16-10). The OCR may waive the 180-day time limit if good cause is shown.

Complaints must meet the following criteria:
- They must be filed in writing, either on paper or electronically.
- They must name the entity that is the subject of the complaint.
- They must describe the acts or omissions believed to be in violation of the Privacy Rule.
- They must be filed within 180 days of the incident.
- They must apply to an incident that occurred after April 14, 2003 (2004 for small health plans).

OCR has 10 regional offices, and each one covers certain states. Complaints must be filed with the correct regional office that has jurisdiction over the state in which the incident occurred. A complaint form is available on the OCR website. The **Office of the Inspector General (OIG)** conducts investigations and audits when there is a question regarding privacy laws.

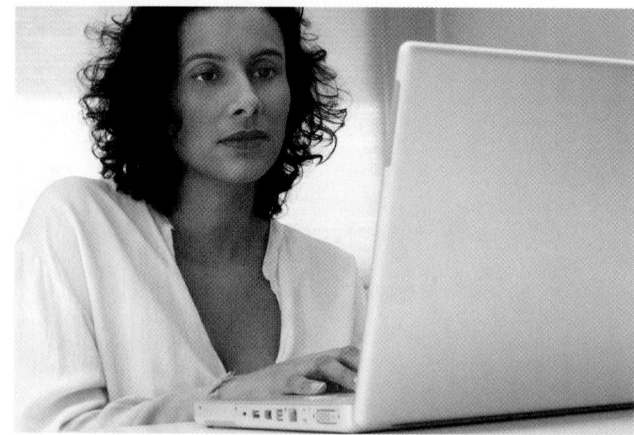

FIGURE 16-10 The time may come when a patient files a complaint against a provider for a violation of privacy practices.

CLOSING COMMENTS

Every employee of the physician's office must read the policy and procedure manual to make certain that he or she has a firm understanding of the HIPAA Privacy Rule and how it relates to the individual office (Figure 16-11). The medical assistant is responsible for learning and following the guidelines set forth by HIPAA. If uncertain about any situation, contact the privacy officer in the organization for direction or research the question on the HIPAA website. Never assume that a patient will not mind if certain information is disclosed. Always check the medical record to determine patient preferences. Keep current on changes to HIPAA regulations and continue to function in a state of constant learning. Embrace changes designed to improve patient care and treatment.

Guidelines for HIPAA Privacy Compliance

1. Consider that conversations occurring throughout the office could be overheard. The reception area and waiting room are often linked, and it is easy to hear the scheduling of appointments and exchange of confidential information. It is necessary to observe areas and maximize efforts to avoid unauthorized disclosures. Simple and affordable precautions include using privacy glass at the front desk and having conversations away from settings where other patients or visitors are present. Health care providers can move their dictation stations away from patient areas or wait until no patients are present before dictating. Phone conversations by providers in front of patients, even in emergency situations, should be avoided. Providers and staff must use their best professional judgment.

2. Be sure to check in the patient medical record and in the computer system to see if there are any special instructions for contacting the patient regarding scheduling or reporting test results. Follow these requests as agreed by the office.

3. Patient sign-in sheets are permissible, but limit the information requested when a patient signs in, and change it periodically during the day. A sign-in sheet must not contain information such as reason for visit because some providers specialize in treating patients with sensitive issues. Showing that a particular individual has an appointment with the physician may pose a breach of confidentiality.

4. Make sure patients sign a form acknowledging receipt of the NPP. The NPP allows the physician to release the patient's confidential information for billing and other purposes. If the practice has other confidentiality statements and policies besides HIPAA mandates, these must be reviewed to ensure they meet HIPAA requirements.

5. Format policies for transferring and accepting outside PHI must address how the office keeps this information confidential. When using courier services, billing services, transcription services, or email, ensure that transferring PHI is done in a secure and compliant manner.

6. Computers are used for a variety of administrative functions, including scheduling, billing, and managing medical records. Computers typically are present at the reception area. Keep the computer screen turned so that viewing is restricted to authorized staff. Screensavers should be used to prevent unauthorized viewing or access. The computer should automatically log off the user after a period of being idle, requiring the staff member to reenter their password.

7. Keep usernames and passwords confidential, and change them often. Do not share this information. An authorized staff member such as the PO will have administrative access to reset passwords if they are lost or if someone discovers the password. Also, practice management software can track users and follow their activity. Do not ever give out a password. Safeguards include password protection for electronic data and storing paper records securely.

8. Safeguard the work area; do not place notes with confidential information in areas that are easy to view by nonstaff. Cleaningservices will access the building, usually after business hours; ensure that PHI is protected.

9. Place medical record charts face down at reception areas so the patient's name is not exposed to other patients or visitors to the office. Also, when placing medical records on the door of an examination room, turn the chart so that the identifying information faces the door. If medical record are kept on countertops or in receptacles, ensure that non-staff persons will not access the records. Handling and storing medical records will certainly change because of HIPAA guidelines.

10. Do not post the health care provider's schedule in areas viewable by non-staff individuals. The schedules are often posted for professional staff convenience, but this may be a breach in patient confidentiality.

11. Fax machines should not be placed in patient examination rooms or in any reception area where non-staff persons may view incoming or sent documents. Only staff members should have access to the faxes.

12. Direct mail and phone calls only to the appropriate staff members.

13. Recognize, learn, and use HIPAA TCS if involved in coding and billing.

14. Send all privacy-related questions or concerns to the appropriate staff member.

15. Immediately report any suspected or known improper behavior to supervisors or the PO so that the issue may be documented and investigated.

16. Direct all questions to the supervisors or PO.

FIGURE 16-11 Guidelines for HIPAA Privacy Compliance. (From *Quick Guide to HIPAA for the physician's office*, St Louis, 2004, Saunders.)

SUMMARY OF SCENARIO

Sabrina and Elsa will experience many challenges as a result of the information exchange they shared at the family picnic. Their conversation probably began like any other, but once Sabrina told Elsa the details of Ms. Adams' visit, they violated patient privacy laws. Their future in the medical field is now uncertain.

Ms. Adams suffered emotionally after the breach of privacy. Her daughter, Terri, does not understand why her mother did not tell her about the illness. The relationship between the mother and daughter is now stressful, an interference with their normal bond during this critical time. The family questions whether to pursue the matter legally or spend the time they have left together in more productive ways. They have many decisions to make.

Dr. Taylor placed Sabrina on probation for 3 months. Before this incident, she had never received any type of disciplinary action. Elsa was not formally disciplined, largely because of her long-standing relationship with Dr. Berry. Still, there is sharp tension between them in the office now, as he faces a possible medical professional liability lawsuit, as well as complaints

about the privacy of Ms. Adams' PHI. Neither Sabrina nor Elsa will look at their jobs the same way as before the incident—for them, everything is different. They both feel that they have disappointed their employers, their patients, and themselves.

The medical assistant must remember that patients should be discussed only with others who are directly involved in the patient's medical care. The HIPAA Privacy Rule has made great strides in protecting patient privacy and in simplifying administrative processes. However, the rule is effective only if office policies are established and practiced. New policies may be difficult to implement, but gaining an understanding of the reason for the policy and its major goals will help the medical assistant embrace changes more readily.

Patients may not agree with the privacy practices or may not understand them. Make an effort to help the patient see the benefit in the policies that the office has established, reminding the patient that such policies are designed for their protection. The patient does not have to agree with the policy or sign it as long as the staff members make a good faith effort toward this end.

SUMMARY of LEARNING OBJECTIVES

1. Define, spell, and pronounce the terms listed in the vocabulary.
   - Spelling and pronouncing medical terms correctly adds credibility to the medical assistant. Knowing the definition of these terms promotes confidence in communication with patients and co-workers.

2. Explain how the HIPAA Privacy Rule benefits the healthcare industry and patients.
   - As a result of the HIPAA Privacy Rule, patients have more control over their medical records. They are able to make informed choices as to how their personal health information is used, and boundaries are set on the use and release of health records. Safeguards are established that healthcare providers must achieve to protect the privacy of health information. Violators are held accountable and face both civil and criminal penalties if patient privacy rights are compromised. The HIPAA Privacy Rule also protects public health by striking a balance when public responsibility supports disclosure of personal health information.

3. List what must be included on a Notice of Privacy Practices.
   - A Notice of Privacy Practices must include details as to how PHI is used and disclosed by the facility; the duties of the provider to protect health information; patient rights regarding PHI; how complaints can be filed if patients believe their privacy has been violated; whom to contact at the facility for more information; and the effective date of the Notice of Privacy Practices.

4. Explain the difference between Title I and Title II of the HIPAA Privacy Rule.
   - Title I of the HIPAA Privacy Rule regulates insurance reform. It limits the use of preexisting health conditions that in the past would have prevented or limited an employee from obtaining health insurance coverage. If an individual left a job with insurance coverage and attempted to secure new coverage, a preexisting health condition would often preclude that person from obtaining coverage for that illness. Title II deals with administrative simplification. This section is the source of privacy and security laws that affect the patient. The goal of Title II is to reduce administrative costs in the healthcare industry.

5. List the rights that patients have under the Privacy Rule.
   - Patients have several rights under the Privacy Rule, including the right to notice of a facility's privacy practices; the right to have access to, view, and obtain a copy of their PHI; the right to restrict certain parts or uses of their PHI; the right to request that communications from the facility be kept confidential; the right to request the facility to amend the PHI; and the right to receive notice of all disclosures of their PHI.

6. Briefly explain what is expected of healthcare providers in relation to the Privacy Rule.
   - Healthcare providers are expected to notify patients of their privacy rights; explain how their health information might be used; develop privacy procedures in the facility; implement

Continued

SUMMARY of LEARNING OBJECTIVES

Continued

those privacy procedures; train employees so that they understand the procedures in place; designate an individual to be responsible for implementation; and secure medical records so that they are not available to those who do not need them.

7. Describe an incidental disclosure.
    - An incidental disclosure is a secondary use or disclosure that cannot reasonably be prevented, is limited in nature, and occurs as a result of another use or disclosure that is permitted.

8. List the three instances when a parent is not considered the child's representative.
    - A parent is not considered the child's representative in any of three instances: when the minor is the one who consents to care and the consent of the parent is not required under state or other applicable law (e.g., in the case of an emancipated minor); when the minor obtains care at the direction of a court or a person appointed by the court; or when the parent agrees that the minor and healthcare provider can have a confidential relationship.

9. Explain why a provider can discuss protected health information with a patient's friends and family.
    - A provider can discuss PHI with a patient's friends and family unless the patient has limited disclosure and requested that he or she receive only confidential communication with the provider. Unless the patient makes this request, which should be in writing, the provider is able to discuss the patient with others as long as good judgment is used and the communication is related to the patient's treatment.

10. Discuss the role of the Notice of Privacy Practices in emergencies.
    - Healthcare providers and facilities, such as hospitals, with a direct treatment relationship with individuals are not required to provide their Notices of Privacy Practices to patients at the time they are providing emergency treatment (Figure 16-9). In such situations the HIPAA Privacy Rule requires only that providers give patients a notice when it is practical to do so after the emergency situation has ended.

CONNECTIONS

 Study Guide Connection: Go to Chapter 16 Study Guide. Read the Case Study and Workplace Applications and complete the assignments. Do online research for answers to the questions in the Internet Activities associated with privacy in the physician's office.

 CD Connection: Go to the Medical Assisting Competency Challenge CD and do the training activities under Legal Concepts.

 Evolve Connection: For more information related to privacy in the physician's office, go to evolve.elsevier.com/kinn and visit related weblinks for Chapter 16. Click on the Medical Assisting Exam Review and do the practice questions to sharpen your test-taking skills.

Basics of Diagnostic Coding

17

Carline A. Dalgleish
Alexandra Patricia Young

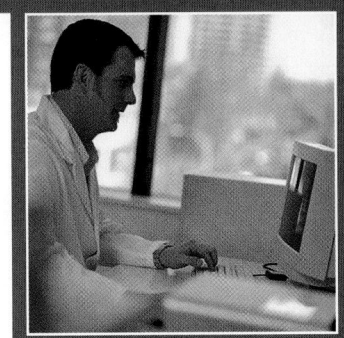

SCENARIO

Mike Simeone has been employed with Drs. Shuman and Taylor in their gastroenterology practice for the last 2 years. He works as an administrative assistant in medical records and simultaneously has been enrolled in the medical assistant program at his local college. Since he has become more knowledgeable, Mike has been given more responsibility in both diagnostic and procedural coding tasks. Diagnostic coding is a system of numeric codes used in insurance claims processing and for statistical purposes. To perform diagnostic coding, Mike uses a manual called the International Classification of Diseases, Ninth Revision, Clinical Modification, or ICD-9-CM.

Mike's experience from working in medical records gives him an understanding of the importance of correct and thorough documentation. His strong skills in reading and understanding physician's orders, treatment plans, chart notes, and diagnostic statements will prove invaluable as Mike learns more about diagnostic coding and refines his coding skills.

Mike is aware of the legalities and importance of proper billing as it affects reimbursement. Now he will use his experience and hopes to advance his position within the office. He knows that the practice is committed to compliance with all of the regulations affecting the operation of the facility and he knows that the patient charts are well documented, making his new tasks easier to accomplish. Mike is a conscientious worker and looks forward to success in his new role and the exposure to more aspects of the medical assisting profession.

While studying this chapter, think about the following questions:

- How do the format, layout, and conventions of the ICD-9-CM manual help the medical assistant search for the most accurate and specific diagnostic code?
- Why is medical record documentation so critical in relationship to diagnostic coding?

- Why does the medical assistant need to know the steps for performing diagnostic coding?
- What are the benefits of using diagnostic codes found in the ICD-9-CM?

LEARNING OBJECTIVES

1. Define, spell, and pronounce the terms listed in the vocabulary.
2. Identify three purposes of the ICD-9-CM.
3. Explain the proper use of the ICD-9-CM.
4. Understand and apply the basic coding rules in the use of the ICD-9-CM.
5. Understand the importance of the Tabular Index, which contains the most specific coding information.

6. Comprehend and use instructional terms and symbols as defined in the ICD-9-CM.
7. Explain the use of V and E codes.
8. Properly perform basic diagnostic coding.

National Accreditation Competencies and Content

CAAHEP COMPETENCIES

Administrative

3.a.(3)(d). Perform diagnostic coding

General

3.c.(2)(d). Document appropriately

ABHES COMPETENCIES

Administrative Duties

3.v. Perform diagnostic coding

Legal Concepts

5.a. Determine needs for documentation and reporting
5.b. Document accurately

Financial Management

8.b. Implement current procedural terminology and ICD-9 coding

VOCABULARY

ancillary diagnostic services Services that support patient diagnoses (e.g., laboratory or radiology services).

ancillary therapeutic services Services that support patient treatment (specialists or surgery).

"and" In the context of ICD-9-CM, the word *and* should be interpreted as *and/or.*

chapters Broad sections of the ICD-9-CM coding manual grouped by disease or illness, (e.g., Chapter 10 contains diagnostic codes for diseases of the genitourinary system).

"code also" Used when more than one code is necessary to fully identify a given condition, "code also" or "use additional code" is used.

coding Converting verbal or written descriptions into numeric and alphanumeric designations.

diagnosis The determination of the nature of a disease, injury, or congenital defect.

etiology The cause of the disorder; a claim may be classified according to etiology.

"excludes" Exclusion terms are always written in italics, and the word "excludes" is often enclosed in a box to draw particular attention to these instructions. Exclusion terms may apply to a chapter, a section, a category, or a subcategory. The applicable code number usually follows the exclusion term.

"includes" This term appearing under a subdivision, such as a category (three-digit code) or two-digit procedure code, indicates that the code and title include these terms. Other terms also classified to that particular code and title are listed in the Alphabetic Indexes.

International Classification of Diseases, Ninth Revision, Clinical Modification (ICD-9-CM) System for classifying disease to facilitate collection of uniform and comparable health information, for statistical purposes and indexing medical records for data storage and retrieval.

International Statistical Classifications of Diseases and Related Health Problems, Tenth Revision, Clinical Modifi-

cation (ICD-10-CM) System containing the greatest number of changes in ICD history. To allow more specific reporting of disease and newly recognized conditions, the ICD-10-CM contains approximately 5500 more codes than ICD-9.

manifestation The signs and symptoms of a disease.

notations Notations, also known as instructional notations, are found in both the Alphabetic Index and the Tabular Index as instructions or guides in classification assignments, defining category content or the use of subdivision codes.

primary diagnosis Initial identification of the condition or complaint that the patient expresses in the outpatient medical setting.

"see" A direction given to the coder to look in another place. This term must always be followed and is found in the Alphabetic Index, Volumes 2 and 3.

"see also" A direction given to the coder to look elsewhere if the main term or subterm (or subterms) for that entry are not sufficient for coding the information. If a code number follows, "see also" is enclosed in parentheses. If there is no code number, "see also" is preceded by a dash.

"see category" A direction given to the coder to see a specific category (three-digit code). This must always be followed.

"use additional code" This term appears only in Volume 1 in those subdivisions in which the user should add further information by means of an additional code to give a more complete picture of the diagnosis. In some cases you will find "if desired" following the term. For the purpose of coding, the "if desired" phrase will not be used. When the term "use additional code...if desired" appears, disregard "if desired" and assign the appropriate additional code.

"with" In the context of ICD-9-CM, the terms "with," "with mention of," and "associated with" in a title dictate that both parts of the title be present in the statement of the diagnosis order to assign the particular code.

To facilitate accurate medical record keeping and the processing of claims, it is essential to identify appropriate services and descriptions of diseases, injuries, and procedures. The **International Classification of Diseases, Ninth Revision, Clinical Modification** (ICD-9-CM) statistically classifies elements of a subject according to diseases, injuries, and operations. The ICD-9-CM is used by healthcare providers for **coding** and reporting clinical information, as required for participation in Medicare and Medicaid programs. In addition, the ICD-9-CM is used for tracking healthcare statistics. Practice management software and third-party payors recognize these codes, which simplify the reimbursement process and speed payment to healthcare providers.

GETTING TO KNOW ICD-9-CM

What Is Diagnostic Coding?

Diagnostic coding is described as the translation or transformation of written descriptions of diseases, illnesses, and injuries into numeric codes. Accurate use of the ICD-9-CM manual is essential for accuracy in translating the medical record's diagnostic statement(s) into numeric codes. The medical assistant facilitates accurate medical record keeping and the efficient processing of claims by using the ICD-9-CM, which identifies the disease or injury for which a patient was treated by code. ICD-9-CM codes are used in the claims submission process to request reimbursement from payors, to track the diagnoses treated by the physician, and to provide statistical data for research and other purposes.

Why Use ICD Codes?

There are several pertinent reasons for the use of ICD-9-CM codes, including:

- Standardizing a system of diagnostic coding accepted and understood by all parties in the reimbursement cycle
- Creating a more convenient method of data storage and retrieval
- Assisting in the maximization of reimbursement
- Shortening the claims-processing time
- Facilitating and measuring guideline and usage compliance
- Assisting in measuring the appropriateness and timeliness of medical care

The Evolution of ICD Coding

Classification systems are used by healthcare organizations to organize health care data and make retrieval meaningful. The early Greeks were the first to group data by disease processes. Captain John Graunt of London was the first to publish mortality and morbidity statistics in his publication, *London Bills of Mortality (1662)*, which was the first real attempt at studying disease processes from a statistical viewpoint. Later, in the 1830s, William Farr introduced uniformity in the use of statistics. His work helped classify diseases by anatomic site. He published the *International List of Causes of Death* and provided the foundation for current vital statistics.

In 1893 Dr. Jacques Bertillon developed the Bertillon Classification of Causes of Death. The American Public Health Association (APHA) recommended adoption of this classification system for Canada, Mexico, and the United States, and further recommended that the system be revised every 10 years. Subsequent revisions were called the *International Classification System of Causes of Death*. Revisions were completed in 1900, 1910, 1920, 1929, and 1938.

In the 1950s the U.S. Public Health Service published the *International Classification of Diseases*, which was adapted for indexing hospital records by diseases and operations *(International Classification of Diseases, Adapted* [ICDA]). Subsequent modifications made in 1962 provided greater detail and introduced a classification for surgical operations. In 1968, because of a need for even greater detail and specificity, the Eighth Revision of ICDA was adapted for use in the United States (ICDA-8). ICDA-8 provided a basis for coding morbidity and mortality statistics in the United States and served as a method of indexing all diagnoses and operative procedures in hospital records.

The ninth revision of ICD was published in 1975 and was renamed the *International Classification of Diseases, Ninth Revision* (ICD-9). In 1979 the National Center for Health Statistics (NCHS) developed a modification of ICD-9 for use in the United States. The modification is ICD-9-CM, which has been in use in the United States since that time.

At present, legislation is being written to formally adopt the Tenth Revision of the diagnostic coding manual for use within the United States. ICD-10 is a significant upgrade and improvement to the current Revision currently in use. See Appendix B for more information about the **International Statistical Classifications of Diseases and Related Health Problems, Tenth Revision, Clinical Modification,** also known as ICD-10-CM.

The ICD-9-CM Code

The ICD-9-CM code consists of a three-digit category code that represents a specific disease within a general disease category—for example, 250 is the disease classification for diabetes mellitus. Up to two additional digits can be used, which add further definition and specificity. These two additional digits are called the *fourth digit* or *subcategory* and the *fifth digit* or *subclassification*, respectively. The ICD-9-CM manual is used to assign a standardized numeric or alpha-numeric code to the diagnostic statement written by the provider of service, including those diagnostic statements found in operative reports, discharge summaries, history and physical (H&P) reports, **ancillary diagnostic services** and **therapeutic services**, or services that support the patient's diagnoses—for example, radiology, laboratory and pathology reports, as well as physical therapy or chemotherapy reports.

Using the diabetes classification code 250 example in Figure 17-1, a fourth digit can be added that describes any disease manifestation caused by the diabetes (e.g., renal, ophthalmic), and a fifth digit can be added that describes the type of diabetes (juvenile or adult, insulin-dependent diabetes mellitus [IDDM] or non–insulin-dependent diabetes mellitus [NIDDM]).

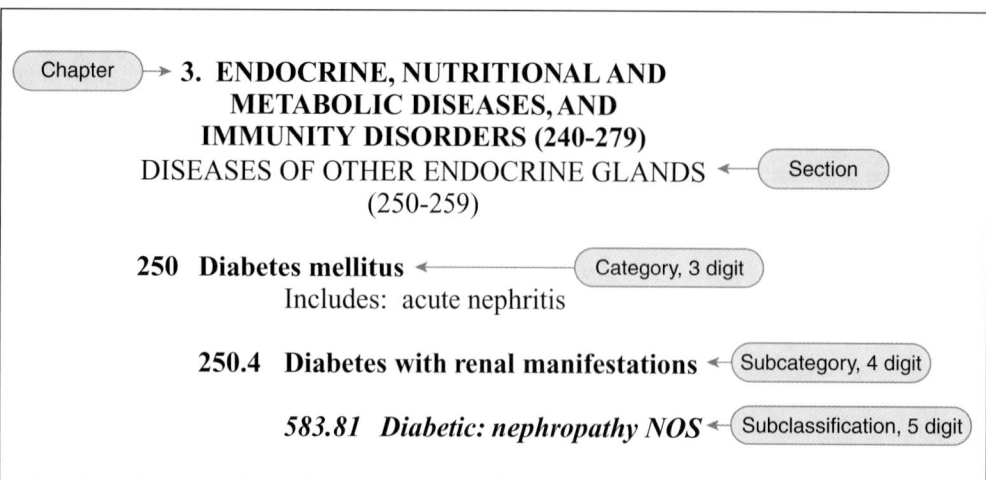

Figure 17-1 Example of Category, Sub-category, and Subclassification.

STRUCTURE OF THE ICD-9-CM

The ICD-9-CM is published in various media, including book, CD, and downloadable file. Depending on the publisher, the layout, symbols, color-coding, and some other features vary somewhat; however, the format, conventions, tables, appendixes, content, and basic structure remain the same. The basic ICD-9-CM manual contains three volumes. Volumes 1 and 2 are used for diagnostic coding by hospitals, physicians, and all other providers of service. Volume 1, also known as the *Tabular Index*, contains all of the diagnostic codes grouped into 17 classifications of disease and injury. Volume 2 is called the *Alphabetic Index* and is used in the same way an alphabetic index in any textbook is used except that it refers the user back to the category codes in the Tabular Index, rather than specific page numbers. Volume 3 is used by hospitals to code procedures and services performed within the hospital environment. Volume 3 is not used by most physician-providers.

Volume 1—Tabular Index

Volume 1, the Tabular Index, is a numeric listing of **diagnosis** codes and descriptions. A diagnosis is the determination of the nature of a disease, injury, or congenital defect. Volume 1 consists of 17 **chapters** that classify diseases and injuries; two sections containing supplementary classification codes (V and E), and five appendixes.

Each of the 17 chapters of the Tabular Index is further subdivided into four levels: section, category, subcategory, and subclassification. Refer back to Figure 17-1 for an example from the ICD-9-CM manual.

- Section: A group of three-digit code numbers describing a general disease category–e.g., 250-259 is the section for Endocrine, Nutritional and Metabolic Diseases. The section is also known as a chapter. This section, which includes codes 250 through 259, is also called Chapter 3.
- Category: A three-digit code representing a specific disease within the section–e.g., category 250 represents diabetes mellitus.
- Subcategory: A further breakdown of the category, assigning a fourth digit–e.g., in category 250, the fourth digit

describes whether any disease process or manifestation exists as a result of the diabetes mellitus.
- Subclassification: Five-digit code giving the highest level of specificity to the disease state. In this category the fifth digit specifies the type of diabetes mellitus–e.g., IDDM or NIDDM, controlled or uncontrolled.

Supplemental Classifications

The two supplementary classifications included in the Tabular Index are V codes, which describe factors influencing health status and which describe contact with health services that cannot be classified elsewhere, and E codes, which describe external causes of injury and poisoning.

V Codes. The V code is used on occasions when the patient is not currently ill or to explain problems that influence his or her current illness or injury. The *Supplementary Classification of Factors Influencing Health Status and Contact with Health Service* (V Code, V01-V85.4) is used in cases such as preventive vaccination or chronic disease states such as dialysis for renal disease.

E Codes. The E code classification, named the *Supplemental Classification of External Causes of Injuries and Poisoning*, is used to classify environmental causes of injury, poisoning, or other adverse effects on the body.

Appendixes

The five appendixes contained in Volume 1, Tabular Index, of the ICD-9-CM are as follows:
- Appendix A–Morphology (the form or structure) of Neoplasms. Morphology code numbers consist of five digits. The first four digits identify the histological type of neoplasm, and the fifth digit indicates its behavior. M codes are used for statistical data only and are not used in physician billing. This section of the appendix is used primarily by inpatient coders.
- Appendix B–Glossary of Mental Disorders. This glossary is an alphabetic listing of the psychiatric terminology that appears in Chapter 5 of Volume 1 (Tabular Index), entitled "Mental Disorders."
- Appendix C–Classification of Drugs. The adverse effects of drugs are coded according to the American Hospital

Formulary Service (AHFS) list. This section is used almost exclusively by pharmacies.

- Appendix D—Classification of Industrial Accidents. This appendix concerns the Statistics of Employment Injuries categorized by the type of industry where the accident occurred. This section is usually used by government organizations, such as the Occupational Safety and Health Administration (OSHA). It is seldom used by physician-providers.
- Appendix E—List of Three-Digit Categories. All of the three-digit category codes from the Tabular Index are listed in order, by chapter.

Conventions Used in Volume 1—the Tabular Index

Conventions refer to abbreviations, punctuation, symbols, instructional notations, and related entities that provide guidance to the medical coder in selection of an accurate and specific code. These conventions are found in Volume 1, the Tabular Index, of the ICD-9-CM. Understanding their meaning and using their guidance is crucial to accurate coding. Many different publishers offer the ICD-9-CM, and there may be some differences in the symbols, notations, colors, or other reference marks used for convenience or to convey specific meaning, depending on the publisher; however, the most common conventions are described here.

Abbreviations. There are two primary abbreviations used in the Tabular Index of the ICD-9-CM, NEC and NOS (Figure 17-2).

NOS—Not otherwise specified. This abbreviation is the equivalent of "unspecified" and means that the diagnostic statement does not provide more specificity or definition.

NEC—Not elsewhere classifiable. The category number for the term including NEC is to be used only when the coder lacks the information necessary to code the term to a more specific category. NEC means that the diagnostic statement contains specific wording but no specific classification exists to match the wording.

Punctuation. Four basic forms of punctuation are used in the Tabular Index: brackets, parentheses, colon, and braces (Figure 17-3). Each form serves a different purpose in the reading and understanding of code descriptions.

Symbols. Symbols are used to designate the requirement of a fourth and/or fifth digit, new entries, and revised text or codes. Other symbols may be found, depending on the publisher. Added symbols or other changes will be described completely in the Introduction to the ICD-9-CM, regardless of the publisher. The most common symbols are shown in Figure 17-4.

Other Conventions. Two other conventions used in both the Alphabetic Index and the Tabular Index are the use of bold and italic fonts.

Bold: Bold type is used for all codes and titles in the Tabular Index.

Italics: Italic type is used for exclusion notes and to identify any diagnosis that cannot be used as the **primary diagnosis.**

Instructional Notations. **Instructional notations** are notes included in the Tabular Index to provide additional guidance

---

NEC

Diagnosis: Pneumonia due to gram-negative bacteria

Index: **Pneumonia**
        gram-negative bacteria NEC 482.83

Tabular: **482.8 Pneumonia due to other specified bacteria**
         482.83 Other gram-negative bacteria

Code: 482.83 Pneumonia due to gram-negative bacteria

Code 482.83 identifies gram-negative bacterial pneumonia that cannot be classified more specifically into the other subclassifications. The other subclassifications within 482.8 are for anaerobes, *Escherichia coli [E. coli]*, "other than gram-negative" bacteria, Legionnaire's disease, and other specified bacteria. None of these other subclassifications can be assigned to the diagnostic statement; therefore, 482.83 is the most appropriate choice.

NOS

Diagnosis: Bronchitis

Index: **Bronchitis** 490

Tabular: **490 Bronchitis, not specified as acute or chronic Bronchitis NOS**

Code: 490 Bronchitis

The diagnosis was not specified by the physician as acute or chronic; therefore, the "not otherwise specified" code 490 must be assigned. In this situation, it would be appropriate for the coder to request specificity from the practitioner.

Figure 17-2 Example of NEC and NOS Abbreviations. (Modified from Buck CJ: *Step by step medical coding,* St Louis, 2006, Saunders.)

[ ]	Brackets enclose synonyms, alternative wording, or explanatory phrases.
( )	Parentheses are used to enclose supplementary words, which may be present or absent in the statement of a disease or procedure. These supplementary words do not usually affect the code number selected, but instead provide further definition or specificity to the code description.
:	Colons are used in the Tabular Index after an incomplete term that needs one or more of the modifiers or adjectives that follow to make it assignable to a given category.
{ }	Braces enclose a series of terms, each of which is modified by the statement appearing to the right of the brace.

Figure 17-3 Example of punctuation usage in ICD-9-CM

when selecting a specific diagnosis code (Figure 17-5). The most common instructional notations include:

INCLUDES: A notation indicating that under a category or other subdivision separate terms can be found that will serve to further define, give examples of, or provide modifying adjectives, and sites or conditions.

□ or ○	The lozenge or circle symbol is found to the left of a disease code. The symbol will contain the number 4 or 5 and indicates that use of a fourth or fifth digit is required.
§	The section mark symbol is only used in the Tabular Index of Diseases and precedes a code denoting a footnote on the page.
•	The bullet symbol indicates a new entry.
△	The triangle symbol indicates a revision in the Tabular Index and a code change in the Alphabetic Index.

Figure 17-4 Symbols in the ICD-9-CM.

TUBERCULOSIS (010-018)

INCLUDES   Infection by *Mycobacterium turberculosis*
                    (human) (bovine)

EXCLUDES   *Congenital tuberculosis (771.2)*
                    Late effects of tuberculosis (137.0-137.4)

006   Amebiasis

INCLUDES   infection due to *Entamoeba histolytica*

EXCLUDES   *amebiasis due to organisms other than*
                   Entamoeba histolytica (007.8)

006.0 Acute amebic dysentery without mention of
               abscess
               Acute amebiasis

Figure 17-5 Example of instructional notations. (Modified from Buck CJ: *Step by step medical coding*, St Louis, 2006, Saunders.)

EXCLUDES: Exclusion terms are enclosed within a box and are printed in italics. The excludes notation indicates that there are some code classifications that cannot be used with the code being selected.

NOTES: Notes are used to define terms and give coding instructions. They are often used to list the fifth-digit subclassification(s) for certain categories.

SEE: The SEE instruction follows a main term and indicates that a different term should be referenced.

SEE CATEGORY: This notation is a variation of the SEE instruction.

SEE ALSO: The SEE ALSO instruction is generally found following a main term in the Alphabetic Index and directs the coder to another area with additional index entries that may be useful.

CODE FIRST: This note directs the use of codes that are not normally intended to be used as a principal diagnosis or are not to be sequenced before the underlying disease.

USE ADDITIONAL CODE: This note indicates that a supplemental code should be used in addition to the one being selected. Using an additional code will help to give a more complete picture of the diagnosis.
Related Terms.

AND: The word *and* should be interpreted to mean either *and* or *or*.

WITH: The word *with* in the Alphabetic Index is sequenced immediately following a main term. It provides additional definition or specificity to the code description.

Volume 2—Alphabetic Index

The Alphabetic Index, Volume 2, consists of an alphabetic list of diagnostic terms and related codes; three supplementary sections (the Hypertension Table, Neoplasm Table, and Table of Drugs and Chemicals); and a separate Alphabetic Index for E Codes (Index to External Causes). In most published versions of Volumes 1 and 2, a Summary of the Additions, Deletions, and Revisions to the Tabular Index for the current year is included and is typically found at the end of the main Alphabetic Index. The Alphabetic Index structure includes main terms, subterms and carry-over lines.

- Main terms—appear in bold type
- Subterms—indented two spaces to the right under the main term
- Carryover lines—always indented two additional spaces from the level of the preceding line

A diagnostic statement from the physician may contain many medical terms, but there is typically only one main term that describes the patient's illness or injury. All accompanying words that further describe the main term are called modifiers. Modifiers are found in the Alphabetic Index indented below main terms. There are two types of modifiers: essential and non-essential. An essential modifier is indented under the main term. Essential modifiers affect code selection, and are used in the coding process only if they are specified in the diagnostic statement. A non-essential modifier is shown in parentheses after the term it modifies. These do not affect code selection.

Supplementary Sections of the Alphabetic Index

Three tables and one supplementary index are in the Alphabetic Index, the Hypertension Table, the Neoplasm Table, the Table of Drugs and Chemicals, and the Index to External Causes of Injuries and Poisoning (E codes). These tables and the index are discussed at length later in this chapter.

- Hypertension Table—The Hypertension Table lists types of hypertension and the manifestations and causes. The types of hypertension are further subdivided into three categories: malignant (a clinical course that progresses rapidly to death), benign (does not threaten health status significantly), and unspecified. Unspecified hypertension is used only when there is no documentation in the clinical record that the hypertension is malignant or benign.
- Neoplasm Table—The Neoplasm Table lists neoplasms by anatomic location. The neoplasms are further categorized into categories:

- Malignant Neoplasm—The malignant neoplasm category is broken down into three subclassifications: primary, secondary, and Ca (carcinoma) in situ.
  - Benign Neoplasm—Non-cancerous growth.
  - Unspecified Behavior
  - Uncertain Behavior
- Table of Drugs and Chemicals—This table contains a classification of drugs and other chemical substances to identify poisoning states and external causes of adverse effects.
- Index to External Causes of Injuries and Poisoning (E Codes)—E codes classify environmental events, circumstances, and other conditions as the cause of injury and other adverse effects.

Volume 3—Procedures: Tabular Index and Alphabetic Index

Volume 3 contains a Tabular Index and Alphabetic Index of procedures. Unlike Volumes 1 and 2, it is not used in a physician's office but is primarily used in hospitals and other facilities to code the procedures performed in those settings. The procedure codes are two digits, followed by a decimal and one or two additional digits. The Tabular Index of Volume 3 includes 16 chapters containing codes and descriptions for surgical, diagnostic, and therapeutic procedures performed in a hospital setting. The Alphabetic Index of Volume 3 is an alphabetic listing of the surgical, diagnostic, and therapeutic procedure codes used as a guide to finding a specific code or codes in Volume 3 of the ICD-9-CM.

BEGINNING THE CODING PROCESS

Medical Documentation

The steps for using the ICD-9-CM manual actually begin with interpretation and abstracting of the medical documentation. Information pertinent to code selection is culled from a variety of medical documents. Sources of diagnostic statements can include the following:

- Encounter form, also known as a *superbill, fee slip,* or *charge ticket*
- History and physical report (H&P)
- Discharge summary
- Treatment or progress notes
- Operative report
- Radiology, laboratory, or pathology report

The basic steps in diagnostic coding are to analyze and abstract the diagnosis or assessment documented in the medical record. To *abstract* means to create an outline or summary of information from a text or record. In diagnostic coding, an abstract is created to find all of the diagnostic statements performed during a patient encounter, and ensure nothing has been omitted or added to the encounter form or charge ticket that is not documented in the patient's medical record. When comparing the diagnosis, diagnostic statement, or even signs and symptoms, against any code description, all of the elements of that code must match, with nothing added or missing. These

abstracted data are then broken down into main term(s) and any modifying or subterms, as described earlier in this chapter.

Main and Modifying Terms

The Alphabetic Index is organized by main terms—usually the condition, illness, or injury. Subterms, also known as modifying terms as described earlier, are terms that modify or act as adjectives. Subterms are below the main term and indented two spaces. These modifying terms further describe or add additional information or definition needed to narrow the search for an appropriate diagnostic code. Modifying terms affect the selection of appropriate codes; therefore it is important to review the list of modifying terms when selecting a code or code range.

A main term is typically the primary condition, disease, or injury, with any modifying terms providing further specificity, such as the anatomic site or additional manifestations of the condition. For example, in the diagnostic statement "atherosclerotic heart disease," the condition, and thus the main term, is "disease." The modifying term "heart" adds the anatomic location, and "atherosclerotic" adds the type of heart disease. Main terms can also be found by eponym, synonym, or acronym. An eponym describes a disease, condition or injury named after a person, such as Hodgkin's disease. Acronyms are abbreviations of words—for example, the acronym for an upper respiratory infection is URI. Synonyms are words that are similar in meaning and can be used interchangeably. It is important for the medical coder to have reference books on hand, including a medical dictionary that includes abbreviations, to assist in thoroughly understanding the diagnostic statement.

CRITICAL THINKING APPLICATION

Mike is sometimes confused as to which term is the main term and which are modifying terms. What documents can help him determine the main term? Who can he consult within the office to make certain he understands the main term?

Using the Alphabetic Index

Once the diagnostic statement has been abstracted from the medical record, and the main terms identified, the medical coder will begin the search for the best code in Volume 2, the Alphabetic Index, of the ICD-9-CM manual. The Alphabetic Index is a comprehensive, alphabetic listing of all procedures and services contained within the ICD-9-CM manual. The most important thing to remember about the Alphabetic Index is that it should be used only as an aid to finding the section, category, subcategory, or subclassification within the Tabular Index of the ICD-9-CM to evaluate and select the proper code. The Alphabetic Index is not a substitute for the main text, so the medical assistant must never code directly from the Alphabetic Index. Even if only one code is found in the Alphabetic Index, the code can be used only if a thorough review of the conventions and instructional notations in the Tabular Index, Volume 1, do not contraindicate the use of the code.

STEPS IN ICD CODING

Nine basic steps are required for accurate ICD-9-CM coding.

1. Abstract the diagnostic statement or statements from the encounter form and/or the patient's medical record.
2. Determine the main terms in the diagnostic statement describing the patient's condition.
3. Determine what modifying words describe the main term in the diagnostic statement.
4. Locate the main terms taken from the diagnostic statement in the Alphabetic Index of the ICD-9-CM manual.
5. Locate the modifying words listed under the main term in the ICD-9-CM manual.
6. Review any notes or cross-references (e.g., See and See Also) found with the main or modifying terms in the Alphabetic Index.
7. Choose a tentative code or codes found in the Alphabetic Index; and write them on a sheet of paper.
8. Verify the tentative code's accuracy in the Tabular Index. Carry the codes to their highest level of specificity (fourth and fifth digits if they are available).
   a. Review instructional notations
      i. Includes or Excludes statements
      ii. Code First, Code Also, Code Additional statements
      iii. "and", "or," and/or "with" statements
   b. Review conventions and punctuation
   c. Determine if a fourth or fifth digit is required
9. Assign the code selected from the Tabular Index as the appropriate code for the patient's condition. Document the code on the encounter form and/or the medical record.

Diagnostic Coding Decision Tree

A series of questions called a *decision tree* assists in navigating the Alphabetic and Tabular Index while the steps for diagnostic coding are performed. The decision tree for the main text is designed to guide the selection of the appropriate ICD-9-CM diagnostic code (Figure 17-6). Consider the following example for using the decision tree:

The medical documentation narrative describes the following disease: "ruptured abdominal cyst." Begin the search in the Alphabetic Index using the main term "Aneurysm" and the modifying terms "abdominal" and "ruptured" Through use of the decision tree and code selection steps, the code found in the Alphabetic Index should be 441.3.

In the Tabular List, code 441.3 is found in Chapter 7 of the ICD-9-CM, Diseases of the Circulatory System, in Category 441, aortic aneurysm and dissection, and subcategory 441.3. The code description for 441.3 is "aortic aneurysm, ruptured."

Decision Tree Question 1: Does the medical documentation entirely match the code description?

Answer: Yes. If the answer to Question 1 had been no, a new search in the Alphabetic Index using a different or synonymous main term would have been required.

Decision Tree Question 2: Does the code description add anything that is not documented in the medical record?

Examples of Steps in Diagnostic Coding

1. The diagnostic statement is "cholecystitis." There is only one main term: "Cholecystitis." In the Alphabetic Index, the main term "Cholecystitis" has a single code, 575.10. Turning to the Tabular Index, 575.10 states "Cholecystitis, unspecified." The surrounding codes all add information that is not contained in the diagnostic statement—for example: 575.1 does state "Cholecystitis," but a symbol convention to the left of the code contains the number 5, which means a fifth digit must be used for this diagnosis. Code 575.0 states "Acute cholecystitis." The diagnostic statement does not specify acute, therefore 575.0 adds inaccurate information. In the same way, codes 575.11, 575.12 and 575.2 add information that is not contained in the diagnostic statement. The final and most accurate code for the diagnostic statement "Cholecystitis," therefore, is 575.10.

2. Changing the diagnostic statement "cholecystitis" only slightly, by adding "with calculus (cholelithiasis)," changes the Alphabetic Index search, and the code as well. The main term remains "Cholecystitis," although "Cholelithiasis" could also be used as the main term. Choice of either as a main term guides the coder to the same place in the Tabular Index. Using "Cholecystitis" again as a main term guides the coder to 575.10; however, indented below the main term is the subterm "with calculus," followed by "See Cholelithiasis." The code for cholelithiasis is 574.2, but again indented below cholelithiasis is the subterm with cholecystitis and the code 574.1. In the Tabular Index, code 574.2 refers only to the cholelithiasis, code 574.1; however, it is a combination code that includes cholelithiasis with cholecystitis. There is one more step according to the symbol convention to the left of the code, which indicates a fifth digit must be added. At the beginning of the subcategory for cholelithiasis (574) an instructional note provides the fifth digit definitions: 0 means "without mention of obstruction," 1 means "with obstruction." Because the diagnostic statement did not mention an obstruction, the most specific and accurate code to choose from the Tabular Index is 574.11.

Answer: No. Had the answer to this question been yes, more evaluation would have been required–either returning to the Alphabetic Index to search further, or proceeding through the next questions to evaluate the instructional notations, punctuation, and other conventions in the Tabular Index.

Decision Tree Question 3: Read all the instructional notations for the section (chapter), category, subcategory, and, if necessary, subclassification. Are there any "includes," "excludes," "code first," or "code also" instructions?

Answer: In this case there are no instructional notations that affect the selection of code 441.3 for the diagnostic statement. If the answer had been yes, the medical assistant would have followed the instructions in the notes. Since the answer was no, the assistant would proceed to the next question.

Decision Tree Question 4: Evaluate the conventions and symbols. Is a fourth and/or fifth digit required?

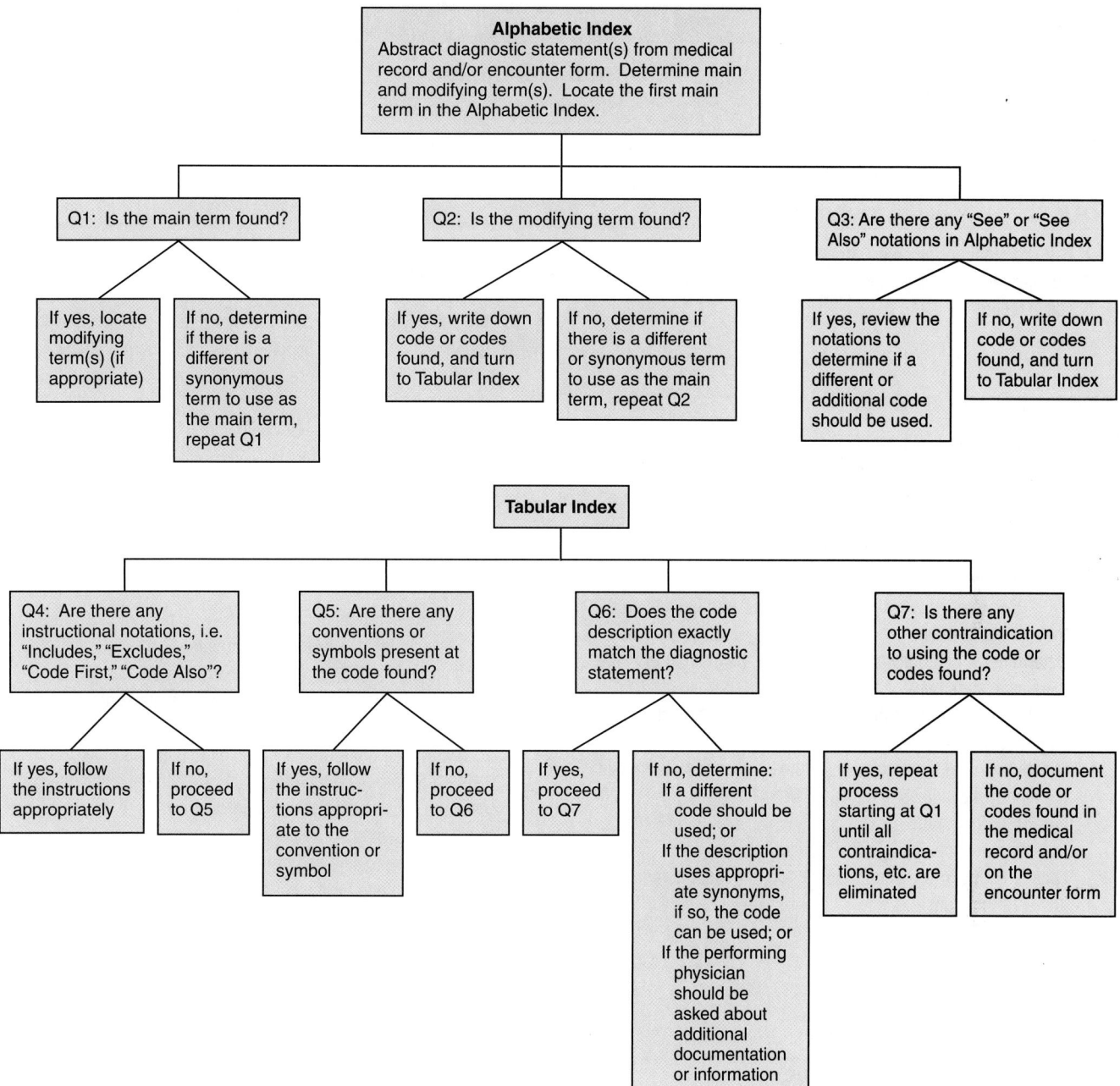

Figure 17-6 Decision Tree for ICD-9-CM Diagnostic Coding

Answer: No. In this case, 441.3 already has a fourth digit and there is no symbol showing a fifth digit is required. If the answer had been yes, the medical assistant should determine which additional digit is appropriate. Since the answer was no, proceed to next question.

Based on the answers to these questions, code 441.3 is the most accurate and specific code to use with the diagnostic statement "*ruptured abdominal aneurysm.*" At this point, the diagnosis code should be documented on the encounter form and on the medical record next to the diagnostic statement.

Abstracting the diagnosis from the patient medical record or encounter form is only the first step in the coding decision process. Procedure 17-1 describes the steps for using the Alphabetic and Tabular Index of the ICD-9-CM to guide the medical assistant in the selection of the most specific and accurate diagnosis code or codes.

CRITICAL THINKING APPLICATION

Mike is working with a medical record that contains the terms "cholelithiasis" and "acute cholecystitis with calculus." How will the coding steps and decision tree questions affect or change the selection of a diagnosis code?

PROCEDURE 17-1

Perform ICD-9 Coding

<u>CAAHEP COMPETENCY:</u> 3.a.(3)(d)
<u>ABHES COMPETENCY:</u> 3.v.

GOAL: *To perform accurate diagnosis coding using the ICD-9-CM manual*

EQUIPMENT and SUPPLIES

- ICD-9-CM manual, Volumes 1 and 2, current year
- Encounter form or charge ticket
- Medical record
- Paper
- Pen or pencil

PROCEDURAL STEPS

1. Abstract the diagnostic statement or statements from the encounter form and/or the patient's medical record.
   <u>PURPOSE:</u> To ensure all parts of the diagnostic statement are included on the encounter form, with nothing missing or added.

2. Determine the main terms in the diagnostic statement describing the patient's condition.
   <u>PURPOSE:</u> To provide a starting point for performing a search in the Alphabetic Index.

3. Determine what modifying words exist of the main term in the diagnostic statement.
   <u>PURPOSE:</u> To ensure further specificity of the codes found in the Alphabetic Index.

4. Locate the main terms taken from the diagnostic statement in the Alphabetic Index of the ICD-9-CM manual.
   <u>PURPOSE:</u> To find the code or codes which will be reviewed for accuracy and specificity in the Tabular Index.

5. Locate the modifying words listed under the main term in the ICD-9-CM manual.

   <u>PURPOSE:</u> To ensure further specificity of the codes found in the Alphabetic Index.

6. Review any notes or cross-references (e.g., See and See Also) found with the main or modifying terms in the Alphabetic Index.
   <u>PURPOSE:</u> To ensure there are no additional searches needed in the Alphabetic Index.

7. Choose a tentative code or codes found in the Alphabetic Index; and write them on a sheet of paper.
   <u>PURPOSE:</u> To prevent backtracking and repeated searches in the Alphabetic Index.

8. Verify the tentative code's accuracy in the Tabular Index. Carry the codes to their highest level of specificity (fourth or fifth digits if they are available).
   a. Review Instructional Notes:
      i. Includes or Excludes statements
      ii. Code First, Code Also, Code Additional statements
      iii. Review "and," "or," and/or "with" statements
   b. Review conventions and punctuation.
   c. Determine if a fourth or fifth digit is required.
   <u>PURPOSE:</u> To ensure the most accurate and specific code is selected, and that there is no contraindication to use of the code or codes selected.

9. Assign the code selected from the Tabular Index as the appropriate code for the patient's condition. Document the code on the encounter form and/or the medical record.

SPECIAL CODING INSTRUCTIONS

Remember that all ICD-9-CM coding manuals, regardless of the publisher, will contain comprehensive instructional notes and conventions to aid the coder in selection of the most accurate diagnostic code or codes. When any discrepancy occurs between reference sources, including this text, the current year's ICD-9-CM coding manual is the final authority. This fact cannot be overemphasized. The medical assistant must always thoroughly review and refer to the conventions, instructional notations, code definitions, and other guidelines in the Tabular Index when coding. The following instructions are designed to provide some additional guidance in selecting diagnosis codes from various chapters within the ICD-9-CM; however, they are not to be considered a replacement for the ICD-9-CM manual, nor do they provide all the coding information, definitions, or explanations found in the manual. The steps for diagnosis coding found in Procedure 17-1 are the same for all chapters of

the ICD-9-CM, but there are special rules and considerations for some chapters that must be considered during the coding selection process.

Signs and Symptoms

Signs and symptoms are coded only when the physician has not yet reached a determination of the final diagnosis. If the physician's notes contain terminology such as *"rule out"* or *"suspected,"* for example, the medical coder should use the patient's documented signs and symptoms, including subjective and objective findings. Subjective findings include the patient's chief complaint (CC) or statements regarding why the patient is seeing the physician. Objective findings are any measurable indicators found during the physical examination. Ill-defined conditions, signs, and symptoms are found in the ICD-9-CM manual in Chapter 16, of Volume 1, the Tabular Index. See Figure 17-7 for an illustration of Chapter 16's Signs and Symptoms Section.

- Use only if there is no final or determining diagnosis
- Use if "rule out" or "suspected" are included in the assessment or diagnostic statement.
- Signs and symptoms can be subjective and/or objective findings
  - Subjective: Chief complaint (CC) or patient's verbal statements
  - Objective: Any measurable indicators found during the physical examination
- Signs and Symptoms are found in Chapter 16, Ill-Defined Conditions, Signs and Symptoms, Volume 1 of the ICD-9-CM.

Figure 17-7 Rules for Coding Signs and Symptoms.

Suspected Conditions

When a diagnosis is stated as "questionable, probable, likely, or rule out," code the documented symptoms, signs, or chief complaint(s) of the patient. Do not code the suspected condition if there is no final assessment or diagnosis. If a patient is asymptomatic or has a family or personal history of a condition, a screening code from the Supplementary Classification of V Codes should be used.

Multiple Coding

Some single conditions require the use of more than one code. "Use additional code" means to use another code in conjunction with one selected; and "Code first" means that if more than one code is used, the code with the notation "Code first" should be the first or **primary diagnosis.** Multiple codes may be needed for late effects, complication codes, and obstetric codes, to more fully describe a condition. Always review the ICD-9-CM manual guidelines, instructional notes, and conventions to determine when it is appropriate to use multiple codes. A patient who is diagnosed with diabetic retinopathy with type I diabetes would require multiple codes. The first code, 362.01, represents the diabetic retinopathy, while 250.51 represents diabetes with ophthalmic manifestations. The subclassification of 1 designates Type I diabetes. Figure 17-8 shows an example of multiple coding.

Combination Codes

A combination code is used to fully identify when two diagnoses or a diagnosis with a secondary process (manifestation) or complication is included in the description of a single code number. Combination codes are identified by referring to the subterms in the Alphabetic Index (Volume 2) or the "inclusion" and "exclusion" terms in the Tabular Index (Volume 1). An example of a combination code from the ICD-9-CM is shown in Figure 17-9.

Late Effects

A late effect is a residual problem remaining after the acute phase of an illness or injury has terminated. There is no time limit on when a late effect code can be used. Coding of late effects generally requires two codes; the condition or nature of the late effect, such as hemiplegia, is coded first, and the code designating that the condition or nature is a late effect is coded second. A late effect will sometimes be described in the medical

---

Multiple Coding

Diagnosis: Diabetic retinopathy with type I diabetes

(Note: Retinopathy is the manifestation and diabetes is the etiology, or cause, of the retinopathy or retinal hemorrhage.)

Diagnosis: Index: **Retinopathy**, diabetic 250.5 [362.01]

The Index subterm "diabetic" identifies the code for the etiology as 250.5 and directs you to the code for the manifestation of [362.01] retinopathy. The italicized code is never sequenced first as the principal diagnosis but is used to identify a manifestation.

Tabular: **250 Diabetes mellitus**

   250.5 Diabetes with ophthalmic manifestations

   Use additional code to identify manifestation

   250.51 Type I, not stated as uncontrolled

Note that the diagnosis of diabetes mellitus will always be reported with a five-digit code because the fifth digit indicates the type of diabetes. See the fifth-digit codes listed after code 250 in the Tabular Index of your ICD-9-CM.

   Code 250.51 is the correct code to describe the diabetes (etiology). The statement "Use additional code to identify manifestation…" directs you to assign a code that identifies the manifestation (retinopathy).

Tabular: **362. Other retinal disorders**

   362.0 Diabetic retinopathy
   Code first diabetes (250.5)
   362.01 Background diabetic retinopathy

Note that the *"Code first diabetes"* directs you to the etiology code.

   Code: 250.51, 362.01 Diabetic retinopathy with type I diabetes.

The multiple codes fully describe the diagnostic statement. The guideline directs you to place the etiology code first, followed by the manifestation code.

Figure 17-8 Example of Multiple Coding. (Modified from Buck CJ: *Step by step medical coding,* St Louis, 2006, Saunders.)

documentation as old, residual, a sequela, or some other phrase that indicates the passage of time since the onset of the original condition. Be sure to distinguish between a late effect and a historical statement in a diagnosis. Whenever the statement uses the term "effects of old…," "sequela of…," or "residuals of…," then code as a late effect. If the diagnosis is expressed in terms of "history of…," then code using V codes to indicate a personal history of an illness or injury.

Impending or Threatened Conditions

When a condition is stated as "impending" or "threatened," it is coded only if there is a code specifically describing the condition in this way.

Combination Codes

Diagnosis: Acute cholecystitis with cholelithiasis

Index: **Cholecystitis** with calculus (stone in the gallbladder) directs you to *See* Cholelithiasis

Index: **Cholelithiasis** with, cholecystitis, acute 574.0

Tabular: **574 Cholelithiasis**

574.0 Calculus of gallbladder with acute cholecystis

A fifth-digit subclassification is indicated as 0 for a case without mention of obstruction and as 1 when there is obstruction; since there was no mention of obstruction, use the fifth digit 0.

Code: 574.00 Acute cholecystitis with cholelithiasis

The single code 574.00 fully describes the diagnosis of acute cholecystitis with cholelithiasis

---

Figure 17-9 Example of Combination Codes. (Modified from Buck CJ: *Step by step medical coding*, St Louis, 2006, Saunders.)

Infectious and Parasitic Diseases

Most often, multiple codes will be needed for coding infectious or parasitic diseases. The first code will identify the disease or condition, such as bacterial infection, and the second code will identify the organism causing the disease—for example, streptococcal bacteria. The basic coding principles regarding the use of either combination or multiple codes will apply throughout this section of the ICD-9-CM.

Coding Organism-Caused Diseases

Two categories for identifying the organism that is causing disease are found in other sections or categories. These codes, 041 and 079, may be used as either additional codes or as solo codes depending on the diagnostic statement. For example, for a urinary tract infection (UTI) caused by *Escherichia coli*, the UTI is coded first (599.0) and the *E. coli* is coded second (041.4).

Human Immunodeficiency Disease and Acquired Immune Deficiency Syndrome

It is essential first to understand the descriptions of the codes available. For coding, the key is whether or not the patient has symptoms.

- Human immunodeficiency virus (HIV)—This indicates only that the virus is present.
- Acquired immunodeficiency syndrome (AIDS)—A syndrome is defined as a "group of symptoms occurring together." AIDS is the manifestation(s) and/or symptoms that can occur as a result of having HIV.

Never code a patient as having HIV unless it is clearly documented as confirmed. Probable and suspected cases are never coded; instead, the signs and symptoms present should be coded. The code for a confirmed diagnosis of HIV is 042. The codes for illnesses and symptoms associated with Acquired Immune Deficiency Syndrome are primarily found in Chapter 3

Rules for Coding Impending or Threatened Conditions

1. If it did occur, code as a confirmed diagnosis.
2. If it did not occur, reference the Alphabetic Index to determine if the condition has a subentry term for "impending" or "threatened," and also reference main term entries for "impending" and for "threatened."
3. If the subterm "threatened" or "impending" is found, assign the given code.
4. If the subterm "threatened" or "impending" is not found, code the existing underlying condition(s), signs, or symptoms, and not the condition described as "threatened" or "impending."

---

of the ICD-9-CM manual. Remember that stringent restrictions are placed on the disclosure of medical information regarding patients with HIV infection and/or AIDS. Make certain that the patient has signed the appropriate release of medical information form before any disclosures are made to third parties.

Complications of Care

A complication of medical or surgical care generally results in additional procedures or services being ordered for a patient, but often the complication is not mentioned as part of the diagnostic statement, which results in reduced reimbursement. It is important to review the medical documentation to determine if a complication exists, and to code the complication in addition to the diagnostic statement.

- Postoperative complications that affect a specific anatomic site or body system are classified according to the appropriate ICD-9-CM chapter (1 through 16) of the Tabular Index.
- Postoperative complications that affect more than one anatomic site or body system are classified according to ICD-9-CM, Volume 1, Tabular Index, Chapter 17, Injury and Poisoning.
- If the Alphabetic Index does not provide a specific main term and/or subterm to identify a postoperative complication, classify the complication to categories 996 through 999, Complications of Surgical and Medical Care, Not Elsewhere Classified.

Etiology and Manifestation

Etiology refers to the underlying cause or origin of a disease. **Manifestation** describes the signs and symptoms of the disease. In the Alphabetic Index, the etiology and manifestation codes are listed together. The etiology code is listed first, with the manifestation listed beside it in italicized brackets. These italicized codes are always listed secondary to the etiology code.

Neoplasms

Neoplasm, or new growth, is coded by the site or location of the neoplasm and its behavior. The Table of Neoplasms (Figure 17-10) is located in the ICD-9-CM, Volume 2, or Alphabetic Index under the main term "Neoplasms." This table gives the

	Malignant					
	Primary	Secondary	Ca in situ	Benign	Uncertain Behavior	Unspecified
Neoplasm *(continued)*						
bone (periosteum)	170.9	198.5	—	213.9	238.0	239.2
Note—Carcinomas and adenocarcinomas, of any type other than intraosseous or odontogenic, of the sites listed under "Neoplasm, bone," should be considered as constituting metastatic spread from an unspecified primary site and coded to 198.5 for morbidity coding and to 199.1 for underlying cause of death coding.						
acetabulum	170.6	198.5	—	213.6	238.0	239.2
acromion (process)	170.4	198.5	—	213.4	238.0	239.2
ankle	170.8	198.5	—	213.8	238.0	239.2
arm NEC	170.4	198.5	—	213.4	238.0	239.2
astragalus	170.8	198.5	—	213.8	238.0	239.2
atlas	170.2	198.5	—	213.2	238.0	239.2
axis	170.2	198.5	—	213.2	238.0	239.2
back NEC	170.2	198.5	—	213.2	238.0	239.2
calcaneus	170.8	198.5	—	213.8	238.0	239.2

Figure 17-10 Neoplasm Table. (Modified from Diamond MS: *Mastering medical coding,* St Louis, 2006, Saunders.)

code numbers for neoplasms by anatomic site in alphabetic order. Six possible code numbers exist for each anatomic site, depending upon whether the neoplasm is malignant or benign, exhibits uncertain behavior, or is of an unspecified nature. Malignant neoplasms are separated into three separate subclassifications: primary, secondary, and in situ.

Malignant Neoplasm Site and Behavior Definitions
- Primary: Identifies the originating anatomic site of the neoplasm. A primary malignancy is defined as the original site(s) of the cancer.
- Secondary: Identifies sites to which the primary neoplasm has metastasized (spread). A secondary malignancy defines a second location to which the cancer has spread from the primary location.
- In situ: Carcinoma in situ is defined as the absence of invasion of surrounding tissues. Tumor cells are undergoing malignant changes but are still confined to the point of origin without invasion of surrounding normal tissue. The In Situ column is used only if the physician uses that precise terminology.

Benign, Uncertain Behavior, and Unspecified Nature
- Benign: The growth is non-cancerous, nonmalignant, and does not invade adjacent structures or spread to distant sites.
- Of Uncertain Behavior: The pathologist is unable to determine whether the neoplasm is benign or malignant.

- Unspecified Nature: Neither the behavior nor the histologic type of neoplasm is specified in the diagnostic statement.

The ICD-9-CM instructional notes state that the behavior of the neoplasm should be determined first when coding. Most coding decisions for malignant neoplasms are between primary and secondary; in situ is used only when the diagnostic statement contains that exact phrase. Unspecified is used only when no pathology study has been done and the neoplasm is still described with a term such as *tumor* or *growth*. Uncertain is used only when the neoplasm's behavior is not malignant, the tumor is not in situ, or the behavior is unpredictable. Note that there is also a code beginning with M that is called the *morphology code*. The morphology code is not typically used by physicians or providers when coding diagnoses.

Five Steps for Coding Neoplasms
When coding for neoplasms, the additional steps shown below will assist in determining the most specific and accurate neoplasm diagnostic code. These should be considered in addition to the basic diagnostic steps.
1. Using the Neoplasm Table in the Alphabetic Index, determine the site (anatomic location) of the neoplasm, and select the row in the Neoplasm Table in which it appears.
2. Determine the neoplasm behavior, and select the Neoplasm Table column that best defines the behavior: Malignant, Benign, Of Uncertain Behavior, or Of Unspecified Nature.

3. If the neoplasm is malignant, determine whether the malignancy is primary, secondary, or in situ.
4. Link the appropriate Neoplasm Table column to the appropriate row to find the code.
5. Check the code in the Tabular Index to ensure the code complies with the guidelines, conventions, and instructional notations in the Tabular Index.

The ICD-9-CM manual also always provides additional information, definitions, and guidelines for coding neoplasms, just as it does for all other diseases, illnesses, and injuries.

Circulatory System

Physicians use a large variety of terms and phrases to identify components of the circulatory system. To accurately code disorders of the circulatory system, the coder must carefully review all inclusions, exclusions, conventions, guidelines, and instructional notations associated with each potential code selected. The major sections concerning the circulatory system are as follows:

Acute Rheumatic Fever	Category 390 to 392
Chronic Rheumatic Heart Disease	Category 393 to 398
Hypertensive Disease	Category 415 to 417
Ischemic Heart Disease	Category 410 to 414
Diseases of Pulmonary Circulation	Category 415 to 417
Other Forms of Heart Disease	Category 420 to 429
Cerebrovascular Disease	Category 430 to 438
Diseases of Arteries and Lesser Vessels	Category 440 to 448
Diseases of Veins and Lymphatics	Category 451 to 459

Ischemic Heart Disease

Ischemic heart disease is usually caused by a lesion on one of the coronary arteries that causes a lack of blood flow to the heart. The most common cause of heart disease is atherosclerosis, which is one type of arteriosclerosis. Both atherosclerosis and arteriosclerosis are coded to category 440, with the exception of certain specified arteries including, but not limited to, coronary, carotid, cerebral, pulmonary, and vertebral; coronary atherosclerosis, for example, is found at category 414.0.

Myocardial Infarction

A myocardial infarction (MI) is coded as acute if it is documented as such in the diagnostic statement or has a stated duration of 8 weeks or less. The MI is considered chronic if it is so stated in the diagnostic statement or if symptoms still are present after 8 weeks. If an MI is specified as "old" or "healed" without any current or presenting symptoms, it should be coded using category 412.

History of an MI uses code 412, which describes an "Old Myocardial Infarct." This code is used only if the patient has no symptoms and only if the old MI was diagnosed via an electrocardiogram. When the patient is symptomatic, code the underlying condition or symptoms only if the underlying condition is not known. Acute MIs are coded to category 410 for the first 8 weeks. If symptoms persist beyond 8 weeks, the chronic MI category code is used.

Arteriosclerotic Cardiovascular Disease

Arteriosclerotic cardiovascular disease (ASCVD) is classified to subcategory 429.2, with an additional code added to identify whether or not arteriosclerosis is present. For example, the diagnostic statement "generalized arteriosclerotic cardiovascular disease" should be coded using 429.2 followed by 440.9, "generalized and unspecified atherosclerosis."

Cerebrovascular Accident

The terms *stroke* and *cerebrovascular accident* (CVA) are often used interchangeably to refer to a cerebral infarction. When the patient is initially treated for CVA or stroke, use the code for the underlying condition that caused the stroke, and an additional code for any condition or deficit it caused if that condition or deficit is still present at discharge. These conditions or deficits may eventually resolve; sometimes they do not. When they persist they are considered residuals of the CVA. For coding purposes, this means there is now a late effect to take into consideration.

Hypertensive Disease

A distinction is made in the ICD-9-CM coding system between "elevated" and "high" blood pressure. High blood pressure is defined as hypertension. If a diagnostic statement does not contain the word *hypertension* or the phrase *high blood pressure*, it is coded as elevated blood pressure, not hypertension.

The Alphabetic Index contains a Hypertension Table (Figure 17-11) under the main term "Hypertension." Within the table are subterms that identify different types of hypertension and any complications caused by the hypertension. Hypertension is classified three ways: malignant, benign, and unspecified. Malignant hypertension is usually considered acute and life-threatening; benign hypertension, although considered dangerous, is not. Unless the diagnostic statement specifically states malignant or benign hypertension, hypertension should be classified as unspecified.

Hypertension is frequently the cause of various forms of heart and vascular disease; however, the mention of hypertension in the diagnostic statement does not mean that a combination code for hypertensive heart disease should be used. If there is a cause-and-effect relationship between the hypertension and the heart disease it should be clearly documented in the clinical record or diagnostic statement.

Coding for Complications of Pregnancy, Childbirth, and the Puerperium

Coding for the obstetric patient is like using a specialty codebook within the main codebook. This is challenging for those who do not code obstetrics often. Some important terminology regarding pregnancy includes the following: *antepartum* = pregnancy (as soon as there is a positive pregnancy test); *childbirth* = delivery; and *postpartum* = puerperium (6 weeks after delivery).

Obstetric Coding Guidelines

To begin searching for obstetric codes, start at either of the main terms "Pregnancy" or "Delivery." Look for a subterm regarding the condition, or start at the main term for the condition and

	Malignant	Benign	Unspecified
Hypertension, hypertensive (arterial) (arteriolar) (disease) (essential) (fluctuating) (idiopathic) (intermittent) (labile) (low rennin) (orthostatic) (paroxysmal) (primary) (systemic) (uncontrolled) (vascular)	401.0	401.1	401.9
with			
heart involvement (conditions classifiable to 428, 429.0-429.3, 429.8, 429.9 due to hypertension) (*see also* Hypertension, heart)	402.00	402.10	401.90
with kidney involvement – *see* Hypertension, cardiorenal			
renal involvement (only conditions classifiable to 585, 586, 587) (excludes conditions classifiable as 584) (*see also* Hypertension, kidney)	403.00	403.10	403.90
with heart involvement – *see* Hypertension, cardiorenal			
failure (and sclerosis) (*see also* Hypertension, kidney)	403.01	403.11	403.91
sclerosis without failure (*see also* Hypertension, kidney)	403.00	403.10	403.90
accelerated (*see also* Hypertension, by type, malignant)	401.0	—	—
antepartum – *see* Hypertension, complicating pregnancy, childbirth, or the puerperium			

Figure 17-11 Hypertension Table. (Modified from Diamond MS: *Mastering medical coding,* St Louis, 2006, Saunders.)

Benign, Malignant, and Unspecified Hypertension

- **Malignant** hypertension - acute and life-threatening;
- **Benign** hypertension - dangerous, but not life threatening
- **Unspecified** hypertension—use only if the diagnostic statement does not specify malignant or benign.

Use of Category 650 and V-Codes in Pregnancy Coding

- Use codes from Volume 1, Tabular Index, Chapter 11, of the ICD-9-CM in the range of 630 to 677. If the pregnancy is documented as a normal pregnancy or is unrelated to the reason for the physician encounter, use a V code, V22.2, in place of any Chapter 11 code.
- Chapter 11 codes are to be used only on the maternal record, not on the newborn record.
- Categories 640 to 648 and 651 to 676 require a fifth digit. These fifth digits indicate whether the encounter is antepartum or postpartum, or whether the delivery occurred.

look for a subterm that states "affecting pregnancy" or "during pregnancy." Normal, uncomplicated prenatal and postpartum care for the mother as well as routine visits for the baby are coded with V codes as long as there is no current problem. Some mothers have conditions that put them at high risk; these situations are also coded with V codes unless a problem manifests itself during the pregnancy.

Normal, uncomplicated delivery for the mother is coded using category 650. A normal, uncomplicated delivery is described as one in which no problem or complication occurred during the entire encounter and no procedures were performed other than those deemed "normal." The normal, uncomplicated procedures are episiotomy, amniotomy, administration of analgesia, fetal monitoring, and sterilization. The use of forceps or suction-assisted delivery is not considered normal for the purposes of ICD-9-CM coding.

Normal routine obstetric care does not use fifth digits; fifth digits are used only for obstetric patients with complications. The fifth digits divide the pregnancy into three different "time zones": before delivery (antepartum), delivery (the episode of care when the delivery occurs), and after delivery (postpartum). In addition, the delivery "time zone" is divided into two subclassifications. The fifth digit 1 describes delivery (birth) without postpartum complication; and the fifth digit 2 describes a delivery (birth) with postpartum complication(s).

If the baby has a problem while the mother is still pregnant, code it only if there is an impact on the mother's condition or management. Code the baby's problem on the mother's chart only if it creates a medical concern or a medical need for the mother to undergo testing or treatment. When it is appropriate to code a fetal condition that affects the mother's management, use codes for pregnant patients, not codes for babies.

Cesarean Delivery

Cesarean codes only define the reasons why a cesarean delivery was performed; they do not describe cesarean deliveries as separate from vaginal births. A cesarean delivery is considered the treatment for a problem or condition that exists at the time of delivery.

Outcome of Delivery and Liveborn Infant Codes

Other sets of V codes that must be discussed are the Outcome of Delivery codes and Liveborn Infant codes. The Outcome of Delivery codes (V27) are reported on the mother's health record after the delivery; the Liveborn infant code(s) (V30-V39) describe the condition of the baby at delivery (e.g., live or stillborn), and are reported on the newborn record.

Late Effects of Complication of Pregnancy

The Late Effect of Complication of Pregnancy code can be used any time after the 6-week postpartum period. Use this code following the code to represent the current problem to indicate that it is a residual effect of pregnancy complications.

Abortions

All of the codes for abortion require a fifth digit to indicate whether or not the abortion was complete before the admission. Remember that the term *abortion* applies to the termination of a pregnancy before 22 weeks, regardless of whether it was spontaneous or induced.

Newborn Coding

Babies are considered newborn or perinatal for the first 28 days. The codes used for these patients range from 760 to 779 in Volume 1, Tabular Index, Chapter 15 of the ICD-9-CM manual. After the twenty-eighth day of life, do not use codes that are specific to perinatal patients. Newborn codes are found in Chapter 15 of the ICD-9-CM. Codes from Chapter 15 should never be used on the maternal record. If a newborn is healthy, a code from the V code category 30 should be used in addition to any Chapter 15 code.

Liveborn Infant Category

The only time to use a fifth digit from the Liveborn Infant category is when the fourth digit of 0 is assigned. The fourth digit of 0 means that the baby was born in the hospital; the fifth digit then specifies whether the birth was cesarean. The other fourth digits, 1 and 2, represent births that occurred outside of the hospital. It is assumed no cesarean is performed outside of the hospital, and so no fifth digit is provided.

Injury

Injuries constitute a major section of ICD-9-CM. Injuries are classified first according to the type of injury, then by anatomic site. When coding injuries, separate codes should be assigned for each individual injury unless a combination code is provided. In cases in which a patient has multiple injuries, the most severe injury should be coded first. Superficial injuries such as abrasions or contusions are not coded when associated with more severe injuries of the same site. If an injury results in minor or major damage to peripheral nerves or blood vessels, the injury is coded first, with additional codes from categories 950 to 957, Injury to Nerves and Spinal Cord, and/or 900 to 904, Injury to Blood Vessels.

Coding Fractures

Fractures are coded first by anatomic site, then by type of fracture. The code category range for fractures is 800 to 829, in Volume 1, Tabular Index, Chapter 17, Injury and Poisoning. Fractures can be classified as either "open" or "closed." A fracture is said to be "open" when the skin has been broken and the bone protrudes outside the skin surface or when a wound, such as a puncture, enables the bone to be seen. In a "closed" fracture the bone does not have contact with the outside of the body. At any time if there is no indication as to whether the fracture is open or closed, it should be coded as if it were closed.

Burns

The same principles for combination and multiple coding apply here; code each burn separately unless specific combination codes are given in Volume 1, the Tabular Index. There are many combination codes. Because burns are coded by site and degree and by extent of body surface involvement, all burn cases should have at least two codes, and a third if they are infected. Other types of wounds, lacerations, punctures, and so on, use a different fifth digit to show that they are infected and therefore complicated. Burn codes use their fifth digits for other information, so an additional code is necessary to indicate infection.

Steps for Coding Burns

* Code the burn to the site by degree. Under the main term "Burn" find the subterm for the site, then the subterm for the degree. If the burn is stated to be at the same site but of a different degree, code to the highest degree. Omit the code for the lower level burn at the same site.
* Determine the percentage of body burned, using category 948 in the Tabular Index, Chapter 17, Injury and Poisoning. The fourth digit describes the total burned surface; the fifth digit describes the percent of only third-degree burns—for example, 50% of total body surface burned with 15% third-degree burns.
* If the burn is said to be infected, use code 958.3 as a third code to identify the infection.

E Codes

To describe the circumstances of an accident or injury, the ICD-9-CM manual provides E codes, which are listed in a separate Tabular Index and Alphabetic Index (Figure 17-12). E codes describe the following:

* Nature of an event (fire, fall, collision, abuse, etc.)
* Place of occurrence
* Late effect of an injury

Lund-Browder Chart for Determining Burn Percentages in Children

	0 yr	1 yr	5 yr	10 yr	15 yr
a—1/2 of head	9$\frac{1}{2}$	8$\frac{1}{2}$	6$\frac{1}{2}$	5$\frac{1}{2}$	4$\frac{1}{2}$
b—1/2 of 1 thigh	2$\frac{3}{4}$	3$\frac{1}{4}$	4	4$\frac{1}{4}$	4$\frac{1}{4}$
c—1/2 of lower leg	2$\frac{1}{2}$	2$\frac{1}{2}$	2$\frac{3}{4}$	3	3$\frac{1}{4}$

E CODE INDEX

Railway Accidents	E800-E807
Motor Vehicle Traffic Accidents	E810-E819
Motor Vehicle Nontraffic Accidents	E820-E825
Other Road Vehicle Accidents	E826-E829
Water Transport Accidents	E830-E838
Air and Space Accidents	E840-E845
Vehicle Accidents Not Classified Elsewhere	E846-E848
Place of Occurrence	E849
Accidental Poisoning by Drugs, Medicinal Substances, Biologicals	E850-E858
Accidental Poisoning by Other Solid and Liquid Substances, Gases, Vapors	E860-E869
Misadventure to Patients During Surgical/Medical Care	E870-E876
Surgical/Medical Procedures Cause of Abnormal Reaction of Patient or Later Complication, Without Mention of Misadventure at Time of Procedure	E878-E879
Accidental Falls	E880-E888
Accidents by Fire and Flames	E890-E898
Accidents Due to Natural/Environmental Factors	E900-E909
Accidents Caused by Submersion, Suffocation and Foreign Bodies	E910-E915
Other Accidents	E916-E928
Late Effects of Accidental Injury	E929
Drugs, Medicinal and Biological Substances Causing Adverse Effects in Therapeutic Use	E930-E949
Suicide and Self-Inflicted Injury	E950-E959
Homicide and Injury Purposely Inflicted by Other Persons	E960-E969
Legal Intervention	E970-E978
Injury Undetermined Whether Accidentally or Purposely Inflicted	E980-E989
Injury Resulting from Operations of War	E990-E999

Figure 17-12 Example of E Codes. (Modified from Diamond MS: *Mastering medical coding,* St Louis, 2006, Saunders.)

- Intent (self-inflicted, assault, accident, etc.)
- Drugs and chemicals that caused the injury or disease

E codes are never principal or listed first, because they are only supplementary information. They are most often used with injury codes but may be used with any condition that is the result of an external cause, such as a respiratory problem caused by smoke inhalation. The E code describing the initial incident is only used once, the first time the patient is treated for the condition. Some major categories of E codes include the following:

- Transport accidents
- Poisoning and adverse effects of drugs, medicinal substances, and biologicals
- Accidents and falls
- Accidents caused by fire and flames
- Accidents caused by natural and environmental factors
- Late effects of accidents, assaults, or self-injury
- Assaults or purposely inflicted injury
- Suicide or self-inflicted injury

It is correct to use as many E codes as necessary to describe all of the information provided by the record. It is acceptable to use non-physician documentation to support these codes, if they do not conflict with the physician documentation.

Table of Drugs and Chemicals

The Table of Drugs and Chemicals contains a classification of drugs and other chemicals. It is used to identify poisoning states and external causes of adverse effects. Each of the substances is assigned a code which is used based on the type of poisoning—for example, overdose, wrong substance given or taken, or intoxication. The table also contains a listing of external causes of adverse effects caused by the ingestion or exposure to a drug or chemical. The poisoning codes in the first column of the Table of Drugs and Chemicals should be determined and coded first, followed by the external cause (E-Code). There are five E-code headings in the Table of Drugs and Chemicals: accidental poisoning, therapeutic use, suicide attempt, assault, and undetermined cause.

E Codes Used with the Table of Drugs and Chemicals

An E code to identify a drug or chemical may be added to clarify the patient's circumstance whenever a drug or chemical is identified in the medical record as a causative substance. In addition to the E codes that identify the causative substances, the table includes a column for poisoning associated with each substance. These codes can be used with an E code from the other columns with one exception: a Poisoning code cannot be used with a Therapeutic Use code. Problems caused by correct substances properly used are considered "adverse effects," not poisoning.

V Codes: Classification of Factors Influencing Health Status and Contact with Health Service

V codes are used to describe circumstances or encounters with a physician or healthcare provider when no current illness or injury exists. V codes may stand alone or may be principal or secondary. Some codes have notation that they cannot be principal or stand-alone.

V Code Index for History Codes

Under the main term "History" in the Alphabetic Index, the subterm "personal" follows the main term. This means that

External Cause Codes (E-Codes) Used with Table of Drugs and Chemicals

- Accidental Poisoning (E850-E869). Accidental overdose of drug, wrong substance given or taken, taken inadvertently, accidents in the usage of drugs in medical and surgical procedures, and to show external causes of poisonings coded using Volume 1, Tabular Index, Chapter 17, Injury and Poisoning, category codes 980-989.
- Therapeutic Use (E930-E949). A correct substance properly administered in the proper dosage caused an adverse effect.
- Suicide attempt (E962). Self-inflicted injury or poisoning.
- Assault (E961-E962). Injury or poisoning inflicted by another person with the intent to injure or kill.
- Undetermined (E980-E982). To be used only when either accidental or intentional circumstances can not be determined.

Use of Fourth and Fifth Digit with Diabetes Mellitus

Fourth Digit Subcategories for Diabetes Mellitus
- 250.0 Diabetes mellitus without mention of complication
- 250.1 Diabetes mellitus with ketoacidosis (defined as a life-threatening condition in which ketones, which result from the breakdown of fat for energy, accumulate in the blood stream and the pH of the blood decreases)
- 250.2 Diabetes with hyperosmolarity (defined as a concentration of the body fluids that is abnormally increased)
- 250.3 Diabetes with other coma
- 250.4 Diabetes with renal manifestations
- 250.5 Diabetes with ophthalmic manifestations
- 250.6 Diabetes with neurological manifestations.
- 250.7 Diabetes with peripheral circulatory disorders
- 250.8 Diabetes with other specified manifestations
- 250.9 Diabetes with unspecified complication

Fifth Digit Subclassifications for Diabetes Mellitus
- 250.x0 = type II Adult onset (even if using insulin). Unspecified. Not stated as uncontrolled.
- 250.x1 = type I Juvenile type not stated as uncontrolled.
- 250.x2 = type II Adult onset (even if using insulin). Unspecified as to whether it is uncontrolled.
- 250.x3 = type I Juvenile type, uncontrolled.

the subterms are considered the patient's personal history. The subterm "family" indented two spaces under the "History" main term describes family history rather than personal history. Watch the subterm indentations closely to ensure that the code selected is for the proper history code.

Diabetes Mellitus

Diabetes mellitus codes always require use of a fourth and a fifth digit. The fourth digit describes any manifestations of the diabetes that may be present; and the fifth digit describes the type of diabetes. The fourth digit subcategories in Volume 1, Tabular Index, Chapter 3, Blood and Blood-Forming Organs, category 250, diabetes mellitus are divided by the presence or absence of complications and the nature of the complication. In the case of DM (diabetes mellitus) the word "with" is used rather than the words "due to." Words such as "with," "with mention of," "associated with," and "in" indicate that both elements in the title (of the code) must be present in the diagnostic statement. There are ten fourth digit subclassifications for manifestations of diabetes mellitus.

A fifth digit is also required for coding the type of diabetes mellitus. Determining the type of diabetes is critical to proper code assignment. There are two types of DM. Type I includes both juvenile-onset DM and IDDM (insulin-dependent diabetes mellitus). Type II DM is sometimes called *adult-onset diabetes mellitus*. Type II DM is not always treated with insulin, and is therefore also called *non–insulin-dependent DM*. When selecting the fifth digit it is important to remember that a patient has insulin-dependent diabetes only if he or she has type I diabetes.

There are four fifth digits to use, specifying the type of diabetes and whether it is under control.

MAXIMIZING THIRD-PARTY REIMBURSEMENT

The most important aspect to remember with ICD-9-CM is to code the diagnosis to the highest level of specificity, linking the ICD-9-CM code to the *Current Procedural Terminology, 4th Edition*

(CPT-4) code. CPT-4, or procedure and service coding, is further explained in the next chapter of this text, Chapter 18, Basics of Procedural Coding, and Chapter 20, The Health Insurance Claim Form.

Obtaining the correct reimbursement is important to the practice cash flow and depends on proper coding and billing techniques. Some other crucial points to remember when submitting diagnostic codes for claims are as follows:

- Use the current year ICD-9-CM manual, staying informed of all changes, revisions, and additions published for that year.
- Code accurately from documented information.
- Be sure the diagnosis corresponds to symptoms and treatment.
- Review data entry to ensure that no transposition of digits has occurred.
- Know the insurance carrier's rules and requirements for completion and submission of claims.
- Incomplete or inaccurate codes may result in delay or denial of reimbursement.

CLOSING COMMENTS

Medical assistants are entrusted by the physician and practice that employs them. To this extent, a medical assistant must be responsible and knowledgeable to ensure that no fraud takes place in the coding and claims submission process. Medical assistants are expected to adhere to ethical standards, assigning and reporting only codes that are clearly supported by concise documentation in the patient chart. When in doubt, a medical assistant should consult the attending healthcare provider for clarification. Maintaining and continually enhancing coding skills and keeping informed of changes in codes, guidelines, and regulations are necessary responsibilities for a coding professional.

SUMMARY OF SCENARIO

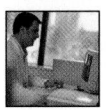

Mike is enthusiastic about his position and enjoys learning more about the coding process. He knows that as he gains experience and earns his certificate, he will be even more valuable as an employee. As Mike progresses with diagnostic coding, he will also be able to help the physicians and nursing staff to be attentive to details in documentation of the patient chart.

Although using the superbill to enter the codes for billing is an easy tool, Mike has learned that knowing how to use the ICD-9-CM volumes is a necessary asset to ensure accurate coding. He also knows it is important when coding a diagnosis to ensure the medical documentation matches the encounter form, and

that all elements of the diagnostic statement are included, and to ensure that the diagnosis listed on the encounter form is fully documented in the patient's medical record. In addition, Mike has learned that the layout and structure of Volumes 1 and 2 of the ICD-9-CM manual are designed to aid in the selection of the most specific and accurate diagnosis code. Every feature of the manual provides guidance in choosing and confirming a diagnostic code that matches the diagnostic statement on the encounter form, and in the medical record. The steps and decision tree for diagnostic coding ensure that Mike will be coding to the highest level of specificity and accuracy.

SUMMARY of LEARNING OBJECTIVES

1. Define, spell, and pronounce the terms listed in the vocabulary.
   - Spelling and pronouncing medical terms correctly adds credibility to the medical assistant. Knowing the definition of these terms promotes confidence in communication with patients and co-workers.
2. Identify three purposes of the ICD-9-CM.
   - The ICD-9-CM is used to track healthcare statistics, as well as to facilitate accurate medical record keeping and ease in processing claims. Use of the ICD-9-CM is mandatory for participation in many federal, state, and private insurance programs.
3. Explain the proper use of the ICD-9-CM.
   - Each of the three volumes of the ICD-9-CM has a specific use. Using Volume 2, the Alphabetic Index, look for the disease(s) documented in the clinical record. Proceed to the Tabular Index, Volume 1, to find and assign a code. Follow guidelines that are provided in the specific manual used for coding in the medical facility.
4. Understand and apply the basic coding rules in the use of the ICD-9-CM.
   - Several basic coding rules exist that will assist the medical assistant in coding. Be sure that the most recent ICD-9-CM manual is being used, and keep a medical dictionary handy. Proofread the claim, and be sure that it makes good sense. Avoid nonspecific codes, and use care when coding preexisting conditions.
5. Understand the importance of the Tabular Index, which contains the most specific coding information.

- Never code directly from the index. The Tabular Index contains the most specific information. Check and recheck the codes, making certain that the documentation supports the codes that are used on the claim.
6. Comprehend and use instructional terms and symbols as defined in the ICD-9-CM.
   - The medical assistant should become familiar with all of the symbols used in the ICD-9-CM. Instructional notations should be read thoroughly and all directions followed while coding a claim.
7. Explain the use of V and E codes.
   - V or E codes may help to clarify a code or further explain the code. V codes are used when the patient is not currently ill but is being seen by health service professionals. E codes are used to explain that some external cause contributed to an adverse effect within the body.
8. Properly perform basic diagnostic coding.
   - The medical assistant's knowledge of accurate diagnostic coding contributes to the legal and financial health of the practice. In most cases ICD-9-CM codes are found on the provider's encounter form (or superbill) and/or in the practice management software. However, with literally thousands of current diagnostic codes, it may be necessary to code from the ICD-9-CM manual. Because these codes are updated yearly, they are an asset in coding compliance. The process for diagnosis coding is outlined in Procedure 17-1.

CONNECTIONS

 Study Guide Connection: Go to Chapter 17 Study Guide. Read the Case Study and Workplace Applications and complete the assignments. Do online research for answers to the questions in the Internet Activities associated with basics of diagnostic coding.

 CD Connection: Go to the Medical Assisting Competency Challenge CD and do the training activities under Health Insurance Activities.

 Evolve Connection: For more information related to basics of diagnostic coding, go to evolve.elsevier.com/kinn and visit related weblinks for Chapter 17. Click on the Medical Assisting Exam Review and do the practice questions to sharpen your test-taking skills. To learn more about office software, do the exercises for the Altapoint demo that are on the CD.

Basics of Procedural Coding

Carline A. Dalgleish
Alexandra Patricia Young

18

SCENARIO

Kay James has excelled on her diagnostic coding examinations, and she now looks forward to learning procedural coding. The process for coding procedures and services will prove to be similar to that of ICD-9-CM and diagnostic coding, except she will use a different coding manual called *Current Procedural Terminology* (CPT-4) for most procedural coding. She will also use a manual called the *Healthcare Common Procedural Coding System*, or HCPCS (pronounced "*hixpix*"). As with the ICD-9-CM, accurate coding begins with the proper analysis of clinical information to abstract the correct data and accurately assign a procedure or service code. In the ICD-9-CM, she learned about coding conventions and guidelines. In the CPT-4, there are new conventions, symbols, guidelines, and formal steps specific to procedural coding that Kay will use to correctly assign procedure codes. Kay is beginning to fully understand the impact diagnostic and procedural coding has on reimbursement, and her responsibility to uphold ethical standards when coding to keep her employer in compliance with federal and state guidelines. She is excited to begin this new phase of her education and to have the opportunity to learn more skills in her goal of becoming an even more valuable asset to the practice.

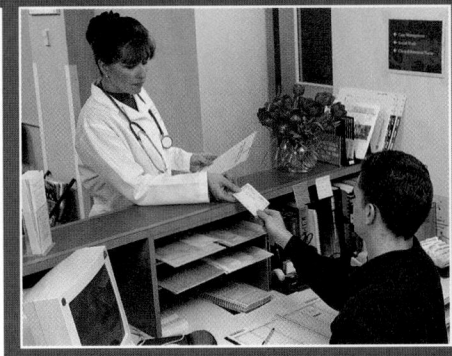

While studying this chapter, think about the following questions:

- What will Kay find similar to what she learned with the ICD-9-CM as she performs procedural coding?
- What will help Kay in selecting the most specific and accurate CPT-4 code?
- What are the differences between coding for the CPT-4 and coding for HCPCS?
- What will Kay learn about the legal and compliance implications of improper coding?

LEARNING OBJECTIVES

1. Define, spell, and pronounce the terms listed in the vocabulary.
2. Describe the steps for abstracting procedural data from clinical documentation.
3. Identify four purposes of the CPT-4.
4. List the main sections of the CPT-4, and describe their content.
5. Describe the coding conventions, guidelines, and layout of the CPT-4 manual and their importance.
6. Describe the process and steps for selecting the most accurate code based on clinical documentation.
7. Explain the importance of correctly assigning evaluation and management codes.
8. Discuss the importance of modifiers.
9. Define *upcoding*, and explain why it must be avoided.
10. Demonstrate an understanding of the process and procedures for code selection.
11. Demonstrate an understanding of main and modifying term selection.
12. Find codes in the Alphabetic Index of the CPT-4 manual.
13. Analyze and select codes using the CPT-4 main text.

National Accreditation Competencies and Content

CAAHEP COMPETENCIES

Administrative
3.a.(3)(c). Perform procedural coding

General
3.c.(2)(d). Document appropriately

ABHES COMPETENCIES

Administrative Duties
3.v. Perform procedural coding

Legal Concepts
5.a. Determine needs for documentation and reporting
5.b. Document accurately

Financial Management
8.b. Implement current procedural terminology and ICD-9 coding

VOCABULARY

abstract An outline or summary of the diagnostic statement and/or procedures and services performed. In procedural coding, the outline or summary assists in ensuring that all procedures and services are included in an insurance claim submission, and that nothing was omitted or added to the encounter form or charge ticket; to abstract also means to compile this outline or summary for use in procedural coding.

acronyms Abbreviations, such as ECG for electrocardiography.

add-on code A code that indicates additional or supplemental procedures carried out in addition to the primary procedure.

Alphabetic Index The reference section of the CPT-4 manual that is used to help find a code or code range.

bundled codes Codes designating procedures or services that are grouped together and paid for as one procedure or service.

categories Indented one level below a subsection in the CPT-4 coding manual, usually refers to a specific anatomic site or procedures and/or services.

category I code The primary procedure or service code selected when performing insurance billing or statistical research.

category II codes Special codes that can help providers track revenue and reimbursement.

category III codes Codes for a new or experimental procedure or service.

downcoding A change in code submitted for reimbursement, usually performed by the insurance company. This change generally occurs because the code submitted does not match in some way to the specifications of the insurance company.

eponyms Procedures, services, or diagnoses named after people, such as Mohs' micrographic surgery or Crohn's disease.

established patient (EP) A patient who has been seen by the same physician or same group of physicians over time. An established patient becomes a new patient if not seen by the physician or group in 3 years.

guidelines Found at the beginning of each of the six sections of the CPT-4. The guidelines define items that are necessary to appropriately interpret and report the procedures and services found in the section.

HCPCS Health Care Common Procedural Coding System; level II codes created to supplement procedures and services not covered in the CPT-4.

modifiers Code additions that explain circumstances that alter a provided service, or provide additional clarification or detail about a procedure or service.

new patient (NP) A patient who has his or her first encounter (visit) with a physician or physician group or who was an established patient with a physician or provider but has not been seen in 3 years.

patient status (PS) The state of a patient as either new or established; appears in the Evaluation and Management section of the CPT-4.

physical status The physical condition of the patient.

place-of-service (POS) codes Codes that indicate where a procedure or service was performed.

providers People who perform a medical procedure or service.

section The main divisions of the CPT-4 manual.

subsection Indented one level below a section, a subsection usually describes an anatomic site or organ system—e.g., integumentary system or cardiology.

subcategory Indented one level below a category, usually a procedure or service unique to a specific category.

unbundled codes Codes in which the components of a procedure are separated and reported separately.

upcoding A deliberate increase in a CPT-4 code, despite the lack of documentation, to the next highest reimbursable code in order to receive higher reimbursements.

*P*rocedural coding is defined as the transformation of verbal descriptions of medical services and procedures into numeric or alphanumeric designations. As with diagnostic coding and use of the ICD-9-CM coding manual, accurate use of the American Medical Association's (AMA's) *Current Procedural Terminology* (CPT-4) and the *Healthcare Common Procedural Coding System* **(HCPCS)** is essential. The medical assistant facilitates accurate medical record keeping and the efficient processing of insurance claims by using the CPT-4 and HCPCS, which identify appropriate procedures and services common to the physician's office. CPT-4 and HCPCS are used in the claims submission process to receive reimbursement from payors as well as to track physician productivity, and provide statistical data for research and other purposes.

GETTING TO KNOW THE CPT-4

The Evolution of CPT-4 Coding

The CPT-4 manual is a listing of descriptive terms and identifying codes for reporting medical services and procedures performed by physicians in order to provide a uniform or standard language that will accurately describe medical, surgical, and diagnostic services and enhance reliable communication among physicians, patients, and third parties. The manual was developed after the AMA recognized a need for a standardized description of services that would be universally understood by physicians, hospitals, insurance companies, and everyone involved in the reimbursement or statistical data collection process.

The second edition of the CPT-4, published in 1970, presented an expanded system of terms and codes to designate diagnostic and therapeutic procedures in surgery, medicine, radiology, laboratory, pathology, and medical specialties. At that time the four-digit classification was replaced with the current five-digit coding system. The fourth edition was published in 1977 and represented significant updates in medical technology. At the same time a system of periodic annual updating was introduced to keep pace with the rapidly changing environment. The fourth edition is still in use today; however, at this writing, the AMA is in the process of developing the fifth edition of the CPT-4–the first major revision since 1977.

Purpose of CPT-4 Procedural Coding

According to the AMA, the CPT-4 contains a five-digit classification system that is designed to do the following:

- Encourage the use of standard terms and descriptors to document procedures in the medical record
- Help communicate accurate information on procedures and services to agencies concerned with insurance claims
- Provide the basis for a computer-oriented system to evaluate operative procedures
- Contribute basic information for actuarial and statistical purposes

Before continuing, keep this important fact in mind. There are roughly 150,000 procedure and service codes in the CPT-4 manual, and thousands more in the HCPCS manual. Memorizing the codes for each specific procedure and service would be impractical, if not impossible. Instead, learning how to use the coding manuals to find the most specific and accurate code based on interpretation of the medical record is the key to success. This requires a solid understanding of medical terminology, anatomy, and physiology and knowledge of how to use the CPT-4 manual and its symbols, conventions, **guidelines,** and notes. The goal of this chapter is to teach the skills, processes, and decisions required to use the CPT-4 and HCPCS manuals. The final authorities are always the CPT-4 and HCPCS manuals for the current year. The symbols, guidelines, conventions, and other instructions found in the CPT-4 manual contain all the information needed to select the correct code for the procedure or service documented in the medical record.

FORMAT OF THE CPT-4 CODING MANUAL

Each procedure or service is represented by a five-digit numeric code (Figure 18-1)–a type of medical shorthand that saves enormous amounts of time and effort and helps to ensure accuracy of information. Just imagine, for example, if a billing department had to describe, in writing, every single one of the medical procedures and services represented by the codes in the CPT-4 manual. Preparing one bill for one patient could take an hour or more and still affect reimbursement negatively when the health insurance or third-party payor has additional questions or, worse, reduces or even denies payment based on their interpretation of the written narrative. Using the five-digit CPT-4 codes eliminates the need, in most instances, for written descriptions, thus assuring clear communication, and the standardization of codes ensures that everyone in the reimbursement cycle understands exactly what procedure or service was provided to the patient. These codes also enable

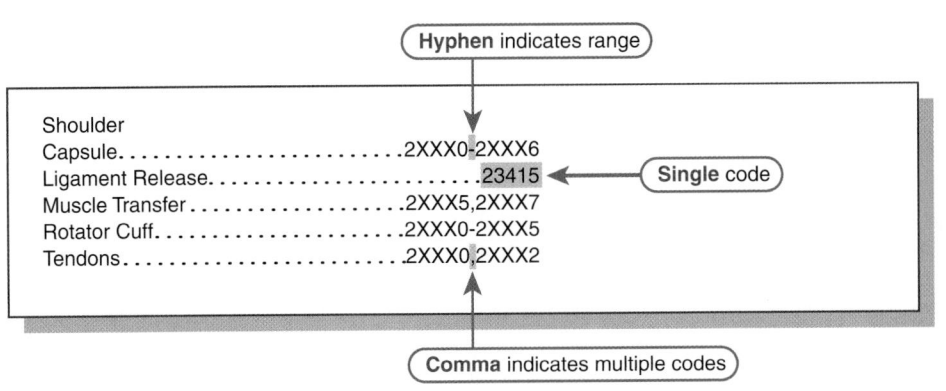

Figure 18-1 CPT code example. (From Buck CJ: *Step-by-Step medical coding,* 2006, St Louis, 2006, Saunders.)

automated computer processing of claims, which saves time and effort.

Modifiers

Modifiers provide a way for **providers** of service to indicate that a service or procedure performed has been altered by some specific circumstance but not changed in its definition. Two-digit alphanumeric modifiers, used in conjunction with a five-digit CPT-4 code, can also be used to add additional information or describe extenuating circumstances that affect the rendered procedure or service. Modifiers can be used, for example, to show that a procedure was performed bilaterally (on both sides of the body); in such a case, the modifier is -50. To describe a situation in which an assistant surgeon is needed for a surgical procedure, modifier -80 can be used to allow the assistant surgeon to submit charges for his or her time and services. Table 18-1 illustrates some commonly used modifiers.

CPT-4 Content

The CPT-4 manual includes the following content:
- Comprehensive instructions for use of the manual, including steps for coding
- A complete Alphabetic Index
- Main text (Tabular Index)
- Six **sections**
- Guidelines and notes
- Conventions
- Twelve appendixes
- Two addenda

CPT-4 Manual Structure

The CPT-4 contains two main divisions, the **Alphabetic Index** and the main text, also called the *Tabular Index*. The Alphabetic Index is like any other index within a textbook; it is simply a guide to finding data in the body of the textbook, however, instead of providing the page numbers where the information is located, as a typical index does, the CPT-4 Alphabetic Index lists the code or code ranges, which are then found in numeric order within each section of the main text.

The structure of the main text of the CPT-4 is as follows:
- Six sections divided into Evaluation and Management, Anesthesia, Surgery, Radiology, Pathology and Laboratory, and Medicine.

- Conventions, also called symbols
- Guidelines and notes
- Appendixes and other addenda

Sections of the CPT-4 Main Text

A **section** is a broad category in the main text of the CPT-4 manual, and each of the six sections is divided by the general type of service. The six sections of the CPT-4 main text are Evaluation and Management, Anesthesia, Surgery, Radiology, Pathology and Laboratory, and Medicine. Sections are subdivided into **subsections**, subsections are further divided into **categories**, and categories can be further subdivided into **subcategories**. Each level of a section provides more specificity regarding the procedure or service being performed, and the anatomical site or organ system involved. In most instances all four levels are found within a section, although this is not a hard and fast rule. See Table 18-2 for an illustration of a section, subsection, category, and subcategory.

The subsection of the CPT-4 manual is indented two spaces below a section, and typically describes an anatomical site or an organ system—for example, the heart, femur, or skull (anatomic site), or gastrointestinal, integumentary, or cardiology (organ system). Categories are indented two additional spaces below the subsection, and generally refer to a specific procedure or service, but can also be a more specific anatomical site—for example, esophagoscopy, incision and drainage, or cardiac catheterization (procedures); or mitral valve, distal femur, or occipital bone (specific anatomic site). Subcategories are the lowest level of code description and specificity. The subcategory is indented two spaces below a category, and provides even more specificity about an anatomical site, or procedure.

Evaluation and Management Section

The Evaluation and Management (E&M) section contains codes for the different types of encounters or visits patients have with providers, including office, hospital, and emergency room visits; consultations; and physician contact with patients in intensive care units, skilled nursing facilities, nursing homes, and other facilities. The code range within the E&M section is 99201 to 99499. The E&M section is further divided into subsections that include different types of services (e.g., office visits, hospital visits). The subsections, categories, and subcategories are written to further modify or describe the service or procedure performed.

Anesthesia Section

The Anesthesia section includes codes for anesthesia services rendered by anesthesiologists and anesthetists before, during, and after surgery. The code ranges within the Anesthesia section are 00100 to 01999 and 99100 to 99140. Codes are included for the types of anesthesia administered—for example, general, local, and sedation anesthesia administration; other support services, including preoperative and postoperative anesthesiologist encounters with the patient, evaluation of the **patient status,** the administration of anesthesia, fluids, and/or blood; and monitoring services, such as blood pressure, temperature, or electrocardiography (ECG).

TABLE 18-1 Example of CPT Code Modifiers	
MODIFIER	**DESCRIPTION**
-50	Bilateral procedure. If procedure was performed on both sides of the body (e.g., both knees, both eyes) and the code description does not indicate procedure or service was performed bilaterally, modifier -50 is used.
-62	Two surgeons. When two surgeons work together as primary surgeons performing distinct parts of a procedure, each surgeon should report the procedure he or she performed to the insurance carrier and use modifier -62. (This prevents the insurance carrier from possibly rejecting a surgical charge as a duplicate)

TABLE 18-2 Section, Subsection, Category, and Subcategory Illustration			
SECTION	**SUBSECTION**	**CATEGORY**	**SUBCATEGORY**
Surgery	Musculoskeletal System	Application of Casts and Strapping	Body and Upper Extremity
Surgery	Cardiovascular System	Arteries and Veins	Embolectomy/Thrombectomy
Medicine	Physical Medicine and Rehabilitation	Modalities	
Medicine	Neurology and Neuromuscular Procedures	Sleep Testing	
Radiology	Diagnostic Radiology	Head and Neck	
Radiology	Vascular Procedures	Aorta and Arteries	

Surgery Section

The Surgery section, which is the largest section in the CPT-4, includes standardized codes for all invasive surgical procedures performed by physicians. Invasive procedures are defined as any medical procedure in which a bodily orifice or the skin must be penetrated by cutting, puncture, or other method. This section is divided into subsections typically identifying specific body systems, beginning with the integumentary (skin) system and ending with ophthalmologic (eyes) and otologic (ears) systems; in most instances each subsection is further divided into categories and subcategories, which describe procedures and services unique to that anatomic subsection.

Radiology Section

The Radiology section includes codes for diagnostic imaging, including x-ray studies and scans, as well as radiation therapy used in the treatment of cancer. The codes used in the Radiology section are in the range of 70000 to 79999.

Pathology and Laboratory Section

Codes are included for all diagnostic tests performed on bodily fluids and tissue, including urine, blood, sputum, and feces, as well as excised or biopsied cells, tissue, or body organs; and evaluation of those fluids and tissues to identify any pathology or disease present in those fluids or tissue. The code ranges for the Pathology and Laboratory section are 80010 to 89999.

Medicine Section

The codes for the Medicine section range from 90281 to 99199 and 99500 to 99602 (excluding anesthesia code ranges). The Medicine section includes many and varied subsections, categories, and subcategories. This section can be called a "catch-all" section, in that it includes codes for services and procedures that do not fit in any of the other sections of the CPT-4 manual. Medical specialties, such as ophthalmology, otolaryngology, and allergy, whose procedures and services vary greatly from the traditional office encounter, are grouped in the Medicine rather than the E&M section. In addition, noninvasive diagnostic tests are included here rather than in the Surgery section, which typically includes only invasive procedures.

Conventions of the CPT-4 Main Text

Conventions are special symbols used to provide additional information about certain codes. Seven conventions are used in the current CPT-4 manual. The most common conventions are shown in Figure 18-2.

Unlisted Procedure or Service Code

Occasionally, even with the best documentation and the coder's best efforts, an accurate, specific code will not be found in the CPT-4 manual that matches the procedure or service performed. In each section, and sometimes subsection, **category,** and/ or **subcategory** of the CPT-4, nonspecific codes have been provided. These codes are called *unlisted procedures and services.*

Special Reports

When bills are submitted for services rendered or procedures performed, in most instances most insurance carriers or third-party payors require no additional information except for the procedure or service CPT-4 code. When a bill is submitted for a service that is unlisted, unusual, or newly adopted, the third-party carrier, in order to determine whether providing that service or procedure was medically appropriate, will require a special report.

Bundled and Unbundled Codes

Bundled codes are procedure codes designating procedures or services that are grouped together and paid for as one procedure or service. A good example of bundled codes are the Organ Panels found in the Laboratory and Pathology section. Each panel contains several different diagnostic tests that are "bundled" together under one code. **Unbundled codes** are codes which are separated into several components of a procedure. One procedure is separated into several different codes and reported separately.

Guidelines

Guidelines, found at the beginning of each section as well as some subsections of the CPT-4 manual, define items necessary to appropriately interpret and report the procedures and services contained in that section or subsection. For example, in the Medicine section specific instructions are provided for handling unlisted services or procedures, special reports, and supplies and materials provided to the insurance company or the patient (Figure 18-3). Guidelines are written specifically to assist in understanding when and under what circumstances codes may be used. It is important to thoroughly read and understand the guidelines provided throughout the main text. This is especially

⊘   **Modifier -51 exempt.** This symbol is used to specify when a code is exempt from use of the modifier -51. Modifier -51 allows coders to specify that one procedure was performed multiple times. Normally, in the instance when the same procedure has been performed more than once, reporting of modifier -51 would be required to indicate that the same procedure (with the same definition and code) was performed two or more times; however, when this symbol appears in front of the code, the code description already indicates the procedure was performed more than once, and therefore modifier -51 is not required.

✚   **Add-on code.** An add-on code is used when more than one code must be used to completely describe a specific procedure or service. Some medical procedures are commonly carried out at the same time a primary procedure is being performed and are described as procedures performed by the same physician to include an additional treatment or procedure done at the same time or in conjunction with the main procedure being performed. Add-on codes can be readily identified by specific words used in the code description, such as additional digit(s), lesions(s), neurorrhaphy, etc. Add-on codes are always used in addition to the primary service or procedure and must never be reported as a standalone code.

•   **New code.** In healthcare, scientific research results in new emerging technology procedures and services. Once a new procedure or service is approved for use or judged to be effective, a temporary **category III** code is assigned. If the procedure or service is then adopted, and statistics bear out the integration of the new procedure with the more mainstream or traditional codes, then a permanent CPT-4 code is assigned, and the code is added to the main text of the CPT-4 manual.

▲   **Revised code.** In addition to the new codes added to the CPT-4 each year, many code descriptions are revised as well. The change may be only to clarify or improve the wording of the description, or, as is the case in most instances, it may be revised to add or remove terminology or information.

►◄   **New or revised text.** Text within the guidelines is often revised to add or remove information, correct grammar, or further clarify the content.

⊙   **Conscious sedation.** This is a new convention, added in 2005, to describe CPT-4 codes that include conscious sedation use. Codes with this convention do not require the use of separate Conscious Sedation codes from the Medicine Section of the CPT-4.

⟋   **FDA approval pending.** A symbol indicating that a CPT-4 category I code has been assigned to a vaccine product in anticipation of approval for use from the Food and Drug Administration (FDA)

Figure 18-2 CPT-4 main text conventions.

important when first learning to code, or working in a section of the CPT-4 that is rarely used. It is also important to reread the guidelines after the CPT-4 annual revisions, additions, and deletions are released in October of each year. Selecting a code without reading the guidelines will usually lead to selection of the wrong code; not only will this result in the potential for delayed or denied reimbursement, but continued inappropriate code selection can be considered fraud or abuse and can result in serious civil or criminal penalties.

Notes

Notes are typically found only in the category, subcategory, or code description area of the CPT-4. Notes apply only to the designated group of codes following the note, and not the whole section as guidelines do. Like guidelines, notes provide additional information to assist in the selection of specific codes.

Appendixes

Appendixes found in the CPT-4 are as follows:
- Appendix A: Modifiers. Lists all of the two-digit numeric or alphanumeric codes used to increase specificity and provide additional information about certain procedures and services.
- Appendix B: Summary of Additions, Deletions, and Revisions. At each annual update of the CPT-4, this appendix lists, for easy reference, all changes made to the CPT-4 from the previous year.

- Appendix C: Clinical Examples. Clinical examples are helpful narrative examples that aid in selection of the correct and most specific level of E&M codes.
- Appendix D: Summary of CPT-4 Add-on Codes. Services and procedures that require more than one code to fully describe the service or procedure rendered, or to identify a procedure that is performed concurrently with another procedure, are called *add-on codes*.
- Appendix E: Summary of CPT-4 Codes Exempt from Modifier -51. Lists all procedures and services exempt from the use of modifier -51.
- Appendix F: Summary of CPT-4 Codes Exempt from Modifier -63. Lists all procedures exempt from use of modifier 63. Modifier -63 is used to report procedures performed on infants less than 4 kg to identify the significantly increased complexity common to these patients. **Category I codes** that state specifically "Exempt from modifier -63" do not require use of this modifier.
- Appendix G: Summary of CPT-4 Codes that Include Moderate (Conscious) Sedation. Lists all procedure codes that include conscious sedation as part of the code description, thus eliminating the need to code the sedation separately.
- Appendix H: Alphabetic Index of Performance Measures by Clinical Condition or Topic. Used by providers in determining appropriate uses of optional **category II codes** (performance measurement codes).

99000—99116 Medicine

Miscellaneous Services

99000 Handling and/or conveyance of specimen for transfer from the physician's office to a laboratory

99001 Handling and/or conveyance of specimen for transfer from the patient in other than a physician's office to a laboratory (distance may be indicated)

99002 Handling, conveyance, and/or any other service in connection with the implementation of an order involving devices (e.g. designing, fitting, packaging, handling, delivery or mailing) when devices such as orthotics, protectives, prosthetics are fabricated by an outside laboratory or shop but which items have been designed, and are to be fitted and adjusted by the attending physician

(For routine collection of venous blood, use 36415)

99024 Postoperative follow-up visit, normally included in the surgical package, to indicate that an evaluation and management service was performed during a postoperative period for a reason(s) related to the original procedure

(As a component of a surgical "package," see **Surgery Guidelines**)

(99025 has been deleted)

Figure 18-3 Example of Miscellaneous Services in Medicine section.

- Appendix I: Genetic Testing Code Modifiers. Lists all modifiers, and their descriptions, unique to genetic testing.
- Appendix J: Electrodiagnostic Medicine Listing of Sensory, Motor, and Mixed Nerves. A listing of each sensory, motor, and mixed nerve conduction study code which can be used to assist in accurate use of codes 95900, 95903, and 95904.
- Appendix K: Product Pending FDA Approval. A list of vaccine products for which FDA approval is pending and that have already been assigned category I codes before approval.
- Appendix L: Vascular Families. A listing of the vascular system, grouped by families, starting from the aorta and branching from there. This appendix is designed to assist in coding for the Cardiology subsection of the Surgery and Medicine sections.

Other Addenda

Category II Codes

Category II codes are a relatively new addition to the CPT-4 manual. The AMA, in preparation for the release of the fifth edition of the CPT-4, added category II codes to the CPT-4 manual in 2004 in an effort to assist healthcare providers in development of automated statistical and reimbursement procedural tracking tools. Category II codes are optional "tracking" codes designed to help facilitate quality-of-care data collection, which can be used by the provider for practice performance measurement. They are not used for billing or reimbursement.

Category III Codes

Category III codes are temporary codes used to identify emerging technology, services, and procedures that have not been globally accepted or adopted as medically appropriate treatment or diagnostic procedures. They are to be used only when a category I code description does not match all the elements listed in the medical documentation but does match the category III code description.

BEGINNING THE CODING PROCESS

Medical Documentation

The steps for using the CPT-4 manual actually begin not in the CPT-4 coding manual but in the medical documentation. Information pertinent to code selection is taken from a variety of medical documents. Sources of information include the following:

- Encounter form, also known as a *superbill, fee slip,* or *charge ticket*
- History and physical report (H&P)
- Discharge summary
- Operative report
- Pathology report

Many physician offices have CPT-4 and even ICD-9-CM codes preprinted on the encounter forms or charge ticket; however it is important to review the medical record, and compile an **abstract**, which is a complete list of all the procedures and services performed. For instance, if, on the encounter form, the physician checked off the procedure for an EGD (esophagogastroduodenoscopy), but in the medical record the operative report states an EGD with biopsy was performed, the code selected, had the medical record not been reviewed, would have resulted in a loss of revenue because a code with a lower reimbursement amount was submitted to the insurance carrier. Update encounter forms annually to ensure that new code additions, changes, and revisions are documented on the preprinted forms.

When comparing the medical documentation against any code description, all of the elements of that code must match, with nothing added or missing. If a code is selected that doesn't fully describe the documented procedure or service, the procedure is "downcoded," and it can, and will, affect reimbursement. Consistent **downcoding** results in a loss of revenue, and it can also trigger an audit by the health insurance carrier, especially if the downcoding occurs in the Evaluation and Management section. If a code is selected that not only matches the procedure or service performed but also adds modifying information that is not in the medical documentation, the information is considered **"upcoded."** Consistent upcoding can result in legal charges of fraud or abuse as discussed earlier.

The steps and process outlined later in this chapter, including use of the Alphabetic Index and the main text of the CPT-4 are applicable to all of the text's sections. Some special considerations and differences apply to the E&M and Anesthesia sections and are also discussed later in this chapter.

Hint: Health Insurance Portability and Accountability Act

When abstracting medical records in preparation for coding, remember that patient-identifiable information must be safeguarded. Any handwritten notes that are not to be placed in the confidential patient record and that could identify the patient must be shredded.

The basic steps in medical coding are to read, analyze, and abstract the procedure or service documented in the medical record, and compare it with the encounter form or charge ticket to ensure all services and procedures have been recorded. The term abstract, used as a verb in this context, means to create an outline or summary of information from a text or record. In procedural coding, an abstract is created to find all of the procedures and services performed during a patient encounter, and ensure that nothing has been omitted or added to the encounter form or charge ticket that is not documented in the patient's medical record. The abstracted data are then broken down into main terms and modifying terms. A main term is defined usually as the primary procedure or service performed, with a modifying term further defining, or adding information to, a main term. Next, the main and modifying terms are used to find the code or code ranges in the Alphabetic Index, and last, the code selected is confirmed by reviewing the guidelines and conventions in the CPT-4 main text to verify that the most specific and accurate code was chosen.

USING THE ALPHABETIC INDEX

The Alphabetic Index is a comprehensive, alphabetic listing of all procedures and services contained within the CPT-4 manual. The most important thing to remember about the Alphabetic Index is that it should be used only as an aid to finding the area in the main text of the CPT-4 to evaluate for selection of the proper code. The Alphabetic Index is not a substitute for the main text. Even if only one code is assigned, the main text must be used to ensure that the code selection is accurate.

The Alphabetic Index of the CPT-4 is used as a guide to search for code(s) or code ranges. The index is similar to the index found in any textbook. It is an alphabetic list of major terms or concepts found within the main text of the book. Each term or concept found in the index then references a page or pages where detailed information can be found in the main text. The Alphabetic Index in the CPT-4 is used in the same way, except that the CPT-4 Alphabetic Index references code or code ranges, rather than pages. As discussed earlier, the main text of the CPT-4 is divided into sections, and the procedures and services are then listed in numeric order by the category I code.

The Alphabetic Index is organized by *main terms* that can stand alone or be further modified by up to four *modifying terms* indented under the main term. Do not confuse the two-digit modifiers discussed earlier in the chapter with modifying terms.

Modifiers are numeric supplements to a category I CPT-4 code, whereas modifying terms are words that add to or modify the meaning of the main term.

Modifying terms are indented below the main term. These modifying terms further describe or add additional information or definition needed to narrow down the search for an appropriate procedure or service code. A main term might be a procedure such as an *excision,* and each modifying term could provide further information about the anatomic location or organ being excised, the type of instrument used, or a special technique or whether other procedures were performed at the same time as the excision, such as the taking of biopsy tissue for examination. Modifying terms affect the selection of appropriate codes; therefore it is important to review the list of modifying terms when selecting a code or code range.

For example, look at Table 18-3. If the medical documentation contains the narrative description of a procedure as a diagnostic cystoscopy, the main term is "Cystoscopy" and the modifying term is "diagnostic," because it describes the type of cystoscopy performed. Another example is "esophagogastroscopy with biopsy and fulguration of lesions." In this example, the main term would be "Gastroscopy" (the procedure being performed), with the modifying terms being "esophago-" (it adds another anatomic site scoped at the same time as the gastroscopy was performed); "with biopsy" and "fulguration" (biopsy and fulguration are two additional procedures performed during the gastroscopy); and "lesions" (describes the object of the biopsy and fulguration).

Two rules should be followed when coding any procedure or service:

- Be as specific as possible in code selection, and use all pertinent words within the description given in your documentation.
- Never add any words, modifying terms, or descriptors to the procedure or service code description that are not documented.

Once the medical documentation has been abstracted to determine the procedures and services performed, and the main and modifying term or terms have been identified, the next step is to look for the terms in the Alphabetic Index. Use the Alphabetic Index to search for a code, code(s), or code range that best describes the procedure or service documented in the medical record. Using the code or codes found in the Alphabetic Index search, locate each in the appropriate section, subsection, category, or subcategory of the CPT-4's main text, and select the most specific code that best matches the medical record documentation. The steps for using the Alphabetic Index are as follows. Further steps for use of the main text are added later in the chapter.

Using the Alphabetic Index to Search

Begin the search by using one or all of the four primary classifications (or types) of main and modifying term entries:
- Procedure or service
- Organ or anatomic site
- Condition, illness, or injury
- Eponym, synonym, or acronym

TABLE 18-3   Main and Modifying Terms Identification in the Alphabetic Index

CODE	MAIN TERM(S)	FIRST MODIFYING TERM	SECOND MODIFYING TERM	THIRD MODIFYING TERM	FOURTH MODIFYING TERM
	Cystoscopy	Diagnostic			
	Gastroscopy	Esophago-	With biopsy	With fulguration	Of lesions
492000	**Cyst**	Abdomen Ankle Bartholin's gland Bile duct			
21030	**Excision**	Cheekbone			
23140		**Clavicle**			
23146				**With allograft**	
23147				With autograft	
27355-27758		Femur			
Cyst excision: 49200					
Cyst excision of clavicle: 23140					
Cyst excision of clavicle with allograft: 23146					

Acronyms are abbreviations of words—for example, the acronym for an electrocardiogram is either ECG or EKG; the acronym for a transurethral resection of the prostate is TURP; and the acronym for gastroesophageal reflux disease is GERD. **Eponyms** are procedures or services named after their inventor or developer. Examples of eponyms are *Mohs' micrographic surgery* and *Dupuy-Dutemps' operation.* Synonyms are words that are similar in meaning and can be used interchangeably.

Earlier in the chapter it was explained that the CPT-4 is divided into sections (E&M, Surgery, Radiology, and so on). The sections could first list the procedure (e.g., excision, incision, repair), the organ or anatomic site (e.g., clavicle, liver), or a condition (e.g., a fracture or laceration). Select a main term that is the procedure, anatomic site, or condition, or, if an acronym or eponym is used, search by the synonym, acronym, or eponym first.

Start the search by using the name of the performed procedure or service (anastomosis, splint, repair, stress test, therapy, vaccination); by the organ or other anatomic site of the procedure (tibia, colon, salivary gland, aorta); by the condition, illness, or injury (abscess, fracture, cholelithiasis, strabismus); or, if applicable, by the synonyms, eponyms, or abbreviations (ECG, Stookey-Scarff procedure, Mohs' micrographic surgery). Usually, but not always, it is helpful to begin by searching for the procedure.

Using "See" and "See Also" in the Alphabetic Index
The "See" statement in the Alphabetic Index points to another location in the Alphabetic Index to find the code or code range. The "See Also" statement points to additional code or code ranges in the Alphabetic Index that may be useful in addition to the code found in the original search.

Stand Alone Code and Code Ranges
When searching the Alphabetic Index, a procedure or service may list a single code—called a *stand alone code*—or may list a range of possible codes that will match the medical documentation. Remember that the Alphabetic Index is an index—it is designed as a guide to the most suitable codes that match the documentation. It does not provide specificity; that is the purpose of the main text. At this point the search is only looking for the closest match or matches to the medical documentation.

Because some medical procedures and diagnostic tests can be quite complex, there may be a single code (standalone) or a code range that may include one main term but several variations—or modifying terms—of the main procedure or service. For example, the code for "Craterization, phalanges, toe" is 28124—a standalone code; however, using the same main term, "Craterization," this time of any of the phalanges (toes or fingers), yields a range of codes: 26235 to 29236. The range of codes is separated by a hyphen to indicate that all codes within that range could be appropriate. There will sometimes also be a standalone code and range of codes listed for the same service or procedure—for example, "Craterization, femur" lists both the range of codes 27070 to 27071 and the standalone code 27360. Once a standalone code or code range is found in the Alphabetic Index, the next step is to look up each code or code range found in the main text of the CPT-4 and select which code or codes most closely match the medical documentation (Table 18-4).

Steps for Using the Alphabetic Index
1. Using the Alphabetic Index, analyze the medical documentation to determine what procedures or services were provided.
2. Select main term classification to begin search in the Alphabetic Index.
3. Select modifying term(s), if needed, once main term is located, to narrow down search.
4. If no modifying term produces an appropriate code or code range, repeat steps 2 and 3 using a different main term classification.

TABLE 18-4 Comparing Codes in the Range of 52234 to 52250

CODE	MAIN TERM(S)	FIRST MODIFYING TERM	SECOND MODIFYING TERM	THIRD MODIFYING TERM	FOURTH MODIFYING TERM
52234	Cystourethroscopy	Treatment or fulgurations	Of a lesion or lesions	Using either cryosurgery or laser surgery	With or without a biopsy
52235/52240	Same	Same	Same except for size of lesions	Same	Same
52204	Cystourethroscopy	with biopsy			
52214	Cystourethroscopy	with fulguration	Of bladder, urethra or glands		
52224	Cystourethroscopy	with fulguration	No mention of specific urinary system structure or organ		

5. Find code or code ranges that include all or most of the medical record procedure or service description.

6. Disregard any code or code range containing additional descriptions or modifying terms not found in the medical record.

7. Write down the code or code ranges that best match the medical documentation.

CRITICAL THINKING APPLICATION

Kay is having trouble finding a procedure in the Alphabetic Index. What are some options and alternative ways Kay can perform an Alphabetic Index search?

Use of the Semicolon

If a main description is followed by a semicolon, this indicates that there are modifying terms and descriptions following it. Every indented description following a standalone code is related to that standalone code. Once there are no additional modifying terms for a main term, a new standalone description of a different procedure begins and is positioned flush left, without indentation.

Coding Decision Tree

A series of questions, sometimes called a decision tree, assists in navigating the Alphabetic Index and main text of the CPT-4. The decision tree for the main text is designed to guide the selection of the appropriate CPT-4 category I code or code range (Figure 18-4).

Following is an example of how to use the decision tree. The medical documentation narrative describes the following procedure: "excision of clavicular cyst." Begin the search in the Alphabetic Index using the main term "Excision" (procedure) and the modifying terms "clavicle" (anatomic site) and "cyst" (condition). Through use of the decision tree and code selection steps for the Alphabetic Index, the code found should be 23140.

In the main text, code 23410 is found in the Surgery section, the "musculoskeletal" subsection, the "excision" category, and finally the "shoulder" subcategory. The description of code 23410 is: "Excision or curettage of bone cyst or benign tumor of the clavicle or scapula."

Question 1: Does the medical documentation match the code description? Answer: Yes.

- The use of the word *or* between excision and curettage allows us to select "excision."
- The cyst is also included in the description.
- It states a bone cyst is acceptable; the clavicle is a bone.
- The use of the word *or* between clavicle and scapula allows us to select "clavicle."

Question 2: Does the code description add anything that is not documented in the medical record? Answer: No.

- Look above or below 23410, and read the descriptions. Notice that information is either missing or added to the documentation of "excision of clavicular cyst."
- Code 23145 is related to excision of a clavicular cyst but adds the description "with allograft," which is not in the documentation.
- The description for code 23130 directly above 23140 is "acromioplasty or acromionectomy, partial, with or without coracoacromial ligament release"—which certainly does not match the documentation in any way.

Question 3: Read the guidelines at the beginning of the Surgery section and before and after the subsection "musculo-skeletal system," the category "shoulder," and subcategory "excision." Is there anything in the guidelines that would prevent using code 23140 as the final code? Answer: No.

Question 4: Evaluate the conventions.

- Is there any indication that this is a revised or new code that might require a special report be sent with the insurance claim form? Answer: No.
- Is there an add-on code symbol, indicating that another procedure code should be used in addition to code 23140? Answer: No.
- Are any of the following conventions associated with code

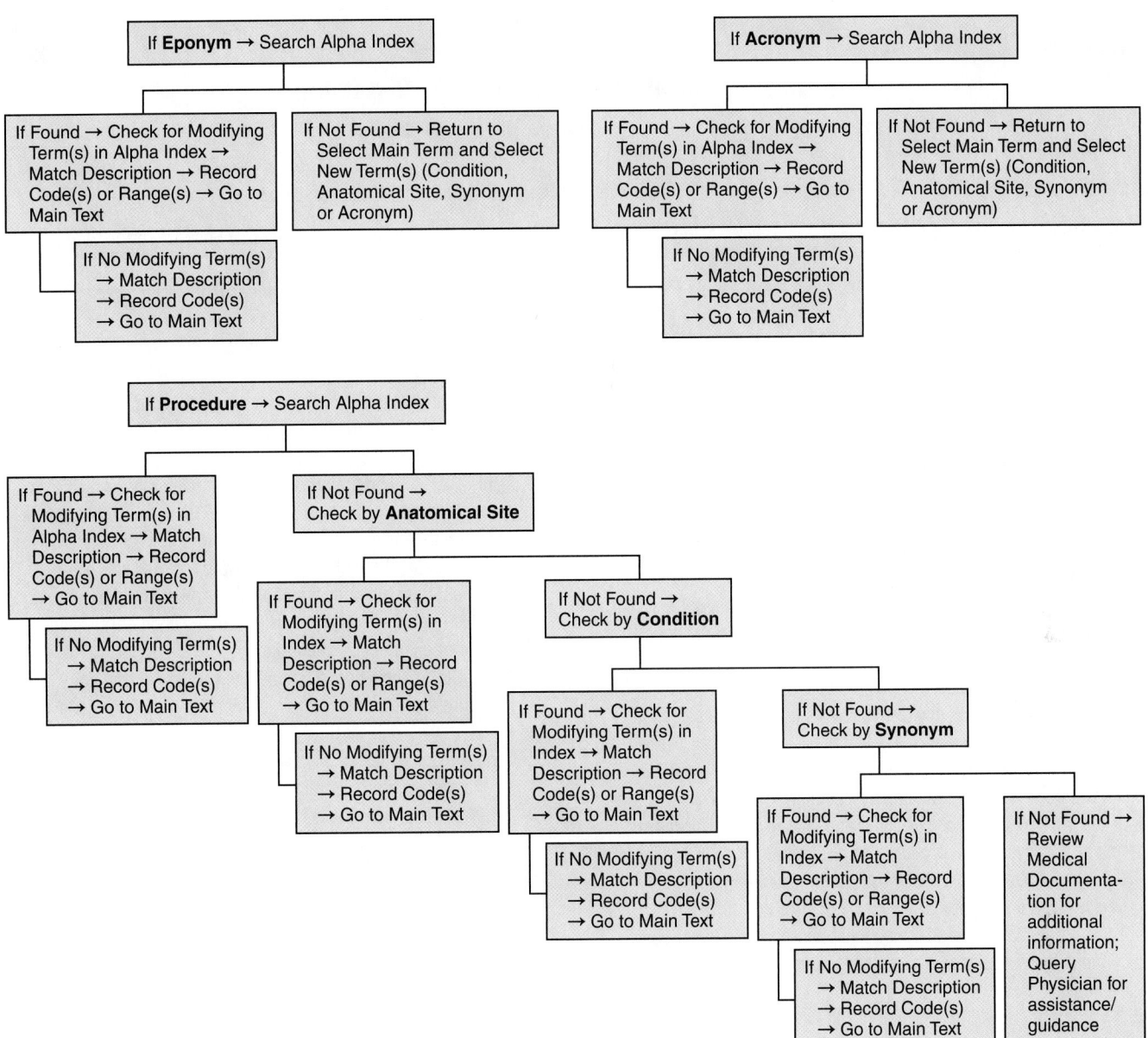

Figure 18-4 Decision tree for the CPT-4 main text.

23140: conscious sedation, exemption from modifier -63, or FDA approval pending? Answer: No.
- Code 23140 is not associated with any of the conventions or symbols that might require further action.

Question 5: Is there any indication in the medical documentation that a modifier might be required? Answer: No.

Based on these answers, 23140 is the most accurate and specific code to use with the medical narrative "excision of clavicular cyst."

Abstracting the procedure and service information from the patient medical record or encounter form is only the first step in the coding decision process. Procedure 18-1 illustrates the steps for using the Alphabetic Index and main text to guide the medical assistant to the selection of the most specific and accurate procedure or service code from the CPT-4 coding manual.

CRITICAL THINKING APPLICATION

If a patient was referred for epigastric pain and Dr. Shuman performed an ultrasound examination of the gallbladder, what would Kay need to consider to properly code this encounter for the ultrasound examination?

UNDERSTANDING EVALUATION AND MANAGEMENT

In order to properly code E&M services, it is important to understand how E&M services are classified. The E&M section is divided into broad subsections (Figure 18-5), such as "office visit," "emergency room visit," "hospital visit," and "consultation." These subsections are further divided into subcategories that include the place where the services were rendered—for example,

PROCEDURE 18-1

Perform Procedural Coding: Perform CPT-4 Coding

CAAHEP COMPETENCY: 3.a.(3)(c)
ABHES COMPETENCY: 3.v

GOAL: *Use the steps for procedure and service coding to find the most accurate and specific CPT-4 category I code.*

EQUIPMENT and SUPPLIES

- CPT-4 Coding Manual (current year)
- Encounter form (charge ticket)
- Medical record
- Paper
- Pen or pencil
- Medical dictionary or medical terminology reference book

PROCEDURAL STEPS

1. Read medical documentation to determine what procedures or services were provided.
   PURPOSE: To ensure all procedures and/or services are listed in the encounter form; that all procedures and services on the encounter form match the medical record; and that nothing documented in the medical record is missing from the encounter form.

2. Select main term classification to begin search.
   PURPOSE: To identify the term or terms to begin the search in the Alphabetic Index.

3. Select modifying term(s) if needed once main term is located.
   PURPOSE: To provide additional specificity and help narrow down the search for the code or code range in the Alphabetic Index.

4. If no modifying term produces an appropriate code or code range, repeat steps 2 and 3 using a different main term classification.
   PURPOSE: To aid in finding the most appropriate code or code range by using alternative methods of searching the Alphabetic Index.

5. Find code or code ranges that include all or most of the medical record procedure or service description.
   PURPOSE: To assist in directing the medical assistant to the proper section, subsection, category or subcategory of the main text of the CPT-4.

6. Disregard any code or code range containing additional descriptions or modifying terms not found in the medical record.

   PURPOSE: To prevent upcoding or downcoding errors and other compliance issues.

7. Write down the code or code ranges that best match medical documentation.
   PURPOSE: To prevent repeated references to the Alphabetic Index by recording all possible matches to the code or code range being sought. It saves both time and redundant effort.

8. Turn to the main text, and find the first code or code range found while searching the Alphabetic Index.
   PURPOSE: To begin the process of finding the most specific and accurate code.

9. Compare the description of the code with the medical documentation. Verify that all or most of the medical record documentation matches the code description and that there is no additional element or information in the code description that is not found in the documentation.
   PURPOSE: To avoid upcoding and downcoding errors, and to ensure there are no contraindications to use of the code selected.

10. Read the guidelines for the section, subsection, and code to ensure there are no contraindications to the use of the code.
    PURPOSE: To ensure there are no instructions that would prevent use of the code selected.

11. Evaluate the conventions, especially add-on codes (+) and exemption from modifier -51.
    PURPOSE: To ensure there are no instructions that would prevent use of the code selected.

12. Determine if there are special circumstances that require the use of a modifier.
    PURPOSE: To select, if appropriate, modifiers that provide additional information for the code selected to explain certain circumstances or provide additional detail.

13. Record the CPT-4 code selected in the medical record documentation next to the procedure or service performed and in the appropriate block of the insurance claim form.

---

the provider's office, the emergency room, a skilled nursing facility, or the patient's home—and the patient status—that is, whether the patient is new or established.

The first two steps in choosing an E&M code are identifying the **place of service** (POS) and the patient status. The two most common place of service are "office" and "hospital." Table 18-5 provides a more complete list of POS locations and their two-digit identifying numbers. The patient status choices are new or established patient. A **new patient** (NP) is new to the practice or has not been seen by the physician or any of the physicians in

a group practice for more than 3 years. An **established patient** (EP) is one who has a continuing relationship with the practice and has been seen within the last 3 years.

Once the place of service and patient status are established, the next step in selection of an E&M code is determining the level of service provided. Three key components affect code selection: history, examination, and medical decision making. The findings of the history and physical examination, the complexity of the history and examination, and the complexity of medical decision making all factor into the level of E&M

►Initial Nursing Facility Care◄

New or Established Patient

When the patient is admitted to the nursing facility in the course of an encounter in another site of service (eg, hospital emergency department, physician's office), all evaluation and management services provided by that physician in conjunction with that admission are considered part of the initial nursing facility care when performed on the same date as the admission or readmission. The nursing facility care level of service reported by the admitting physician should include the services related to the admission he/she provided in the other sites of service as well as in the nursing facility setting.

Hospital discharge or observation discharge services performed on the same date of nursing facility admission or readmission may be reported separately. For a patient discharged from inpatient status on the same date of nursing facility admission or readmission, the hospital discharge services should be reported with codes 99238, 99239 as appropriate. For a patient discharged from observation status on the same date of nursing facility admission or readmission, the observation care discharge services should be reported with code 99217. For a patient admitted and discharged from observation or inpatient status on the same date, see codes 99234-99236.

(For nursing facility care discharge, see 99315, 99316)

►Typical unit times have not been established for 99304-99306.◄

►(99301-99303 have been deleted)◄

● **99304** Initial nursing facility care, per day, for the evaluation and management of a patient which requires these three key components:

■ **a detailed or comprehensive history;**

■ **a detailed or comprehensive examination; and**

■ **medical decision making that is straightforward or of low complexity.**

Counseling and/or coordination of care with other providers or agencies are provided consistent with the nature of the problem(s) and the patient's and/or family's needs.

Usually, the problem(s) requiring admission are of low severity.

Subsequent Nursing Facility Care

►All levels of subsequent nursing facility care include reviewing the medical record and reviewing the results of diagnostic studies and changes in the patient's status (ie, changes in history, physical condition, and response to management) since the last assessment by the physician.◄

● **99307** Subsequent nursing facility care, per day, for the evaluation and management of a patient, which requires at least two of these three key components:

■ **a problem focused interval history;**

■ **a problem focused examination;**

■ **straightforward medical decision making.**

Counseling and/or coordination of care with other providers or agencies are provided consistent with the nature of the problem(s) and the patient's and/or family's needs.

Usually, the patient is stable, recovering, or improving.

● **99308** Subsequent nursing facility care, per day, for the evaluation and management of a patient, which requires at least two of these three key components:

■ **an expanded problem focused interval history;**

■ **an expanded problem focused examination;**

■ **medical decision making of low complexity.**

Counseling and/or coordination of care with other providers or agencies are provided consistent with the nature of the problem(s) and the patient's and/or family's needs.

Usually, the patient is responding inadequately to therapy or has developed a minor complication.

● **99309** Subsequent nursing facility care, per day, for the evaluation and management of a patient, which requires at least two of these three key components:

■ **a detailed interval history;**

■ **a detailed examination;**

■ **medical decision making of moderate complexity.**

Counseling and/or coordination of care with other providers or agencies are provided consistent with the nature of the problem(s) and the patient's and/or family's needs.

Usually, the patient has developed a significant complication or a significant new problem.

Figure 18-5 Example of Evaluation and Management: new or established patient and place of service.

TABLE 18-5 Place-of-Service List

CODE	PLACE OF SERVICE	CODE	PLACE OF SERVICE
01	Pharmacy	41	Ambulance—land
03	School	42	Ambulance—air
04	Homeless shelter	49	Independence clinic
11	Office	50	Federally qualified health center
12	Patient's home	51	Inpatient psychiatric facility
13	Assisted-living facility	52	Partial hospitalization, psychiatric facility
14	Group home	53	Community mental health center
15	Mobile unit	54	Intermediate care facility/mentally retarded
20	Urgent care facility	55	Residential substance abuse treatment facility
21	Inpatient hospital	56	Psychiatric residential treatment center
22	Outpatient hospital	57	Nonresidential substance abuse treatment facility
23	Emergency department (ED) hospital	60	Mass immunization facility
24	Ambulatory surgery center (ASC)	61	Comprehensive inpatient rehabilitation facility
25	Birthing center	62	Comprehensive outpatient rehabilitation facility
26	Military treatment facility	65	End-stage renal disease treatment facility
31	Skilled nursing facility (SNF)	71	State or local public health clinic
32	Nursing facility	72	Rural health clinic
33	Custodial care facility	81	Independent laboratory
34	Hospice	99	Other unlisted facility

code selected. There are also contributing factors that aid in level of service determination: counseling, coordination of care, nature of presenting problem, and time.

The steps for finding a category I code for E&M services are quite different from those discussed earlier in this chapter (Procedure 18-2). The instructions include identifying the section, subsection, category, and subcategory of the procedure or service; reviewing the reporting instructions and guidelines for the code chosen; reviewing the level of E&M service; determining the extent of history obtained and examination performed; and determining the complexity of medical decision making.

Considerations for Evaluation and Management (E&M) Coding

Evaluation and Management Level of Service Components

There are seven components for determining the level of service for E&M: history, examination, medical decision making, counseling, nature of presenting problem, coordination of care, and time. The history, examination, and medical decision-making components are considered key. In other words, they are typically the three most important components for deciding the level of service. Counseling, coordination of care, nature of presenting problem, and time are secondary considerations and are called *contributing factors.*

Key Components

History. To understand the levels of history it is important to know the definition and components of the patient's history. The history relates to the patient's clinical picture and depends on the patient for answers to specific questions. The history is a subjective narrative account in the patient's own words. The history is composed of the following:

- Chief complaint (CC), or reason the patient is being seen: This is usually in the patient's own words.
- History of present illness (HPI): Identifies the location, severity, timing, modifying factors, quality, duration, context, and associated signs and symptoms relating to the chief complaint.
- Review of systems (ROS): The patient answers questions about the following systems and organs: constitutional; eyes; ear, nose, and throat (ENT), and mouth; cardiac; gastrointestinal; musculoskeletal; endocrine; neurologic; integumentary; psychiatric; genitourinary; allergic or immunologic; respiratory; and hematologic or lymphatic.
- Past medical, family, and social history (PMFSH): Patient's experiences with illness and surgery; whether they smoke or use illicit drugs and/or alcohol; whether the patient is married or has children; where the patient lives; and what diseases the patient's blood relatives have had play an extremely important part in determining risk factors for illness.

Levels of history.
- Problem-focused history: A problem-focused history concentrates on the chief complaint; it looks at the symptoms,

PROCEDURE 18-2

Perform Procedural Coding: Perform Evaluation and Management Coding

CAAHEP COMPETENCY: 3.a.(3)(c)
ABHES COMPETENCY: 3.v

GOAL: *Use the steps for Evaluation and Management (E&M) coding to find the most accurate and specific CPT-4 category I E&M section code.*

EQUIPMENT and SUPPLIES

- CPT-4 Coding Manual (current year)
- Encounter form (charge ticket)
- Medical Record
- Paper
- Pen or pencil
- Medical dictionary or medical terminology reference book

PROCEDURAL STEPS

1. Identify the place of service.
   PURPOSE: To determine where the procedure or service was performed.
2. Identify the patient status.
   PURPOSE: To determine if the patient is new or established.
3. Identify the subsection, category, or subcategory of service in the Evaluation and Management section.
   PURPOSE: To ensure that the correct place of service and patient status are used, as well as the appropriate level of service is selected.
4. Review the guidelines and notes for the selected subsection, category, or subcategory.

PURPOSE: To determine if there are any contraindications for use of the code selected.

5. Review the level of E&M service descriptions for each code in the subsection, category, or subcategory chosen.
   PURPOSE: To assist in selection of the appropriate level of service.
6. If needed, compare medical documentation against examples in Appendix C, Clinical Examples, of the CPT-4 manual.
   PURPOSE: To compare the medical documentation to the examples in Appendix C for assistance in selection of the appropriate level of service.
7. Determine the extent of history obtained.
   PURPOSE: To ensure the correct level of history is chosen.
8. Determine the extent of examination performed.
   PURPOSE: To ensure the correct level of examination is chosen.
9. Determine the complexity of medical decision making.
   PURPOSE: To ensure the correct level of medical decision making is chosen.
10. Select the appropriate level of E&M service code, and document it on the medical record or encounter form.

---

severity, and duration of the problem. It usually does not include an ROS or family and social history.

- Expanded problem-focused history: The physician proceeds as in the problem-focused history but includes a review of the systems that relate to the chief complaint. Usually past, family, and social histories are not included.
- Detailed history: The physician will document a more extensive history, ROS, and pertinent past, family, and social histories.
- Comprehensive history: The physician will document responses to all of the components listed previously. A comprehensive history is usually taken during an initial visit with patients who have a significant history of illness.

Examination. The examination is the objective part of the patient's visit. The physician examines the patient, obtains measurable findings, and makes notes referring to body areas and/or organ systems, as follows:

- Body areas: Head including face and neck; chest including breasts and axillas; abdomen; genitourinary (GU) system; back, including spine and extremities
- Organs and organ systems: Constitutional; eyes; ENT and mouth; cardiovascular; respiratory; gastrointestinal (GI); GU; musculoskeletal; skin; neurologic; psychiatric; and hematologic, lymphatic, and immunologic

The examination is divided into the following levels:
- Problem-focused examination: The examination is limited to the single body area or single system mentioned in the chief complaint.
- Expanded problem-focused examination: In addition to the limited body area or system, related body areas or organ systems are examined.
- Detailed examination: An extended examination is performed on the related body areas or organ systems.
- Comprehensive examination: A complete multisystem examination is performed.

Medical Decision Making. When a physician makes medical decisions, the decisions are based on many years of education and experience. Three elements comprise the medical decision-making process: number of diagnoses and management options; amount and complexity of data reviewed; and risk of complications and/or morbidity or mortality.

- Number of diagnoses and management options: The physician's notes during the history and examination should help identify whether the patient's problem is minor, acute, stable, or worsening. The medical documentation should also identify whether a new problem exists or whether the physician plans to order any diagnostic tests to further investigate the patient's illness or injury.

TABLE 18-6 Complexity of Medical Decision Making

NUMBER OF DIAGNOSES OR MANAGEMENT OPTIONS	AMOUNT AND/OR COMPLEXITY OF DATA TO BE REVIEWED	RISK OF COMPLICATIONS AND/OR MORBIDITY OR MORTALITY	TYPE OF MEDICAL DECISION MAKING
Minimal	Minimal or none	Minimal	Straightforward
Limited	Limited	Low	Low complexity
Multiple	Moderate	Moderate	Moderate complexity
Extensive	Extensive	High	High complexity

- Amount and complexity of data reviewed: The medical documentation should also identify what laboratory tests, x-ray diagnostic procedures, and other tests have been ordered or reviewed.
- Risk of complications and morbidity or mortality: Risk is often involved in medical care, either from the treatment given to the patient or from the lack of treatment and professional care. Morbidity, the relative incidence of disease, and mortality, which relates to the number of deaths from a given disease, is an integral part of the assessment of risks made by the physician.

Medical decision-making complexity levels. There are four levels of complexity in medical decision making: straightforward and low, moderate, and high complexity. See Table 18-6 for a description of each of the four levels.

- Straightforward: Minimal diagnosis and management options, minimal to no complex data to be reviewed, and minimal risk to the patient of complications or death if untreated
- Low complexity: Limited number of diagnoses or management options, limited data to be reviewed, and low risk to the patient of complications or death if untreated
- Moderate complexity: Multiple diagnoses or management options, moderate amount and complexity of data to be reviewed, and moderate risk to the patient of complications or death if untreated
- High complexity: Extensive diagnoses or management options, extensive amount and complexity of data to be reviewed, and high risk to the patient for complications and/or death if the problem is untreated

Contributing Factors

Counseling. Counseling is a discussion with a patient and/or family regarding diagnostic results, impressions, recommended diagnostic studies, prognosis, risks and benefits of management or treatment options, and instructions for management, treatment, and/or follow-up. Almost all E&M services contain a degree of counseling with the patient and/or the family. This is factored into the E&M code, and as long as this factor does not exceed 50% of the time spent with the patient, it is included in the E&M code. It can be considered a contributing factor when the counseling exceeds 50% of the encounter.

Coordination of care. Some patients need assistance in arranging for care beyond the visit or hospitalization. Some will need care in a skilled nursing facility or home health care. Others will need hospice care. The primary physician usually coordinates this care. Coordination of care is also factored into the E&M code and is a consideration for determining level of service only when it exceeds 50% of the patient encounter.

Nature of presenting problem. The presenting problem is usually explained in the chief complaint. It can range from something as simple as a cold in an otherwise healthy patient to a life-threatening problem. Unless the nature of the presenting problem exceeds half of the patient encounter, it is included in the E&M code description and is not a factor in selecting the level of service.

Time. Time is included in the E&M code descriptions only to assist physicians in selecting the most appropriate level of E&M service. The times expressed in the code descriptions are averages, and time is not a determining factor in code selection unless counseling exceeds more than 50% of the encounter. Only then can time be used as a determining component to code level selection.

Selecting a Level of E&M Service

1. Identify the category and subcategory of service.
2. Review the guidelines and reporting instructions for the selected category or subcategory.
3. Review the level of E&M service descriptions and examples.
4. If needed, compare medical documentation against examples in Appendix C: Clinical Examples to assist in selection of service level.
5. Determine the extent of history obtained.
6. Determine the extent of examination performed.
7. Determine the complexity of medical decision making.
8. Select the appropriate level of E&M service based on the following:
   a. All of the key components—history, examination, and medical decision making—must meet or exceed the stated requirements to qualify for the level selected if service is in the following category or subcategory:
      i. Office, new patient
      ii. Hospital observation service
      iii. Initial hospital care
      iv. Office consultations
      v. Emergency department services
      vi. Initial nursing facility care
      vii. Domiciliary care
      viii. New patient
      ix. Home, new patient
   b. Two of the three key components must meet or exceed

the stated requirements to qualify for the level selected if service is in the following category or subcategory:

  i. Office, established patient
  ii. Subsequent hospital care
  iii. Subsequent nursing facility care
  iv. Domiciliary care
  v. Established patient
  vi. Home, established patient

c. Time may be considered one of the key components if counseling and/or coordination of care dominates more than 50% of the encounter.

Evaluation and Management (E&M) coding is difficult at first to understand and put into practice. The steps for E&M coding will act as a guide in determining the place of service, patient status, and the level of care provided in order to select the most accurate E&M code. Using Appendix C's clinical examples and comparing them to the medical documentation will also help provide a better understanding of E&M coding.

CRITICAL THINKING APPLICATION

Dr. Shuman performed a colonoscopy at the hospital on a patient, Cecil Matthews, who has been Dr. Shuman's patient for several years. Mr. Matthews came to the office with left lower quadrant pain and a history of colon cancer. What other factors or information would Kay need to know to properly code Mr. Matthews' office visit (encounter)?

ANESTHESIA CODING

The codes for anesthesia are listed in the Anesthesia section of the CPT-4 primarily, although codes for conscious sedation are found in the Medicine section. The codes are selected based primarily on the anatomic location of the surgery being performed—for example, code 00402 is for anesthesia during a reconstructive procedure on the breast in the integumentary system. In addition, there are categories and subcategories for radiologic procedures, burns, excisions, debridement, obstetric procedures, physiologic support during the harvesting of organs, and anesthesia delivered during nerve block procedures. The anesthesia codes include preoperative and postoperative visits, anesthesia care during the procedure, the administration of fluids and/or blood, and the usual monitoring services performed during anesthesia. The provider of anesthesia cannot bill separately for any of these services unless unusual circumstances exist. What makes anesthesia coding different from any other coding is the way in which anesthesia services are billed. There is a standard formula for payment of anesthesia services: basic units + time units + modifying units (B + T + M). This formula is also affected by two factors: the patient's **physical status** (PS), and any qualifying circumstances (QC). The steps for anesthesia coding are shown in Procedure 18-3.

Anesthesia Formula

Basic Unit Value (B)

The Anesthesia Society of America (ASA) publishes a *Relative Value Guide* (RVG), which lists the codes for anesthesia services.

The RVG compares anesthesia services with one another and assigns a numeric value to each service based on the level of complexity. This numeric value is called the *basic unit value.*

Time Unit (T)

Anesthesia services are provided based on the time during which the anesthesia was administered, in hours and minutes. Typically 15 minutes equals one time unit, although this can vary because insurance carriers make that determination independently. The time starts when the anesthesiologist begins preparing the patient to receive anesthesia, continues though the procedure, and ends when the patient is no longer under the personal care of the anesthesiologist. The hours and minutes during which anesthesia was administered are recorded in the patient record.

Modifying Unit (M)

Modifying units reflect circumstances or conditions that change or modify the environment in which the anesthesia service is provided. There are two modifying characteristics for anesthesia services: qualifying circumstances and physical status modifiers. A list and the descriptions of these modifiers are located in the Anesthesia section of the CPT-4. They are also shown in Table 18-7.

Qualifying Circumstances (QC)

Sometimes anesthesia is provided in situations that make the administration of the anesthesia more difficult. These types of cases include those performed in emergency situations, to patients of extreme age, during the use of controlled hypotension, and with hypothermia. There are four qualifying circumstances (QC) codes. Each of the five-digit codes is preceded by a + symbol, indicating that it is an add-on code, and is used in addition to the category I anesthesia code.

Physical Status Modifiers (PS)

The second type of modifying unit used in anesthesia coding is the physical status modifier. These modifiers are used to indicate the patient's physical condition at the time anesthesia was administered. There are five physical status modifiers, composed of two characters: first the letter P, followed by a ranking of 1 to 5 (e.g., P1, P2, P3). P1 represents a normal healthy patient, and P5 represents a brain-dead patient whose organs are being harvested.

Conversion Factors

A conversion factor is the dollar value of each basic unit value. Each third-party payor issues a list of conversion factors. The conversion factor for any given geographic location is multiplied by the number of basic unit values assigned to each procedure. See Figure 18-6 for a sample list of geographic conversion factors.

Calculating Anesthesia Services

Calculation of the fee for anesthesia services is performed using the anesthesia billing formula, B + M + T multiplied times the conversion factor (Figure 18-7).

PROCEDURE 18-3

Perform Procedural Coding: Perform Anesthesia Coding

<u>CAAHEP COMPETENCY:</u> 3.a.(3)(c)
<u>ABHES COMPETENCY:</u> 3.v

GOAL: *Use the steps to select the most accurate and specific anesthesia code, and perform the anesthesia formula calculation to determine the charge for the service.*

EQUIPMENT and SUPPLIES

- CPT-4 Coding Manual (current year)
- Encounter form (charge ticket)
- Medical record
- Conversion factor list (issued by an insurance carrier: for the purposes of this exercise, use the example in Figure 18-5).
- Paper
- Pen or pencil
- Calculator

PROCEDURAL STEPS

1. Read the medical documentation to determine what procedure or service was provided.
   PURPOSE: To ensure all procedures and/or services are listed on the encounter form; that all procedures and services on the encounter form are documented in the medical record; and that nothing documented in the medical record was omitted from the charge ticket.
2. Determine the anatomic site or organ system involved.
   PURPOSE: Anesthesia service codes use the anatomical site and organ system as a category.
3. In the Alphabetic Index, go to the heading "Anesthesia" and find the code or code range that includes all or most of the medical record procedure or service.
   PURPOSE: To avoid selecting a surgery or other type of procedure or service code other than anesthesia-related codes.
4. Write down the code or code range found in the Alphabetic Index, under the Anesthesia heading, that best matches the medical documentation.
   PURPOSE: To prevent repeated references to the Alphabetic Index by recording all possible matches to the code or code range being sought. It saves both time and redundant effort.
5. Turn to the main text, Anesthesia section, and find the code or code range found while searching the Alphabetic Index.

PURPOSE: To verify and select the most specific anesthesia code.

6. Read the guidelines and notes for the section, subsection, category, or subcategory.
   PURPOSE: To ensure the correct code is chosen and there are no instructions that prevent use of the code selected.
7. Evaluate the conventions, especially add-on codes (+) and exemptions from modifier -51.
   PURPOSE: To ensure the correct code is chosen and there are no contraindications to use of the code.
8. Document the code selected.
   PURPOSE: To determine the basic unit value and perform the anesthesia calculation to determine the charge.
9. Determine the Basic Unit Value from the Relative Value Guide.
   PURPOSE: Use to perform the anesthesia calculation to determine the charge for the anesthesia service.
10. Determine the patient's physical status, and document the appropriate modifier.
    PURPOSE: Used to perform the anesthesia calculation to determine the charge for the anesthesia service.
11. Determine if any qualifying circumstance modifier should be used. If yes, document the modifier.
    PURPOSE: Used to perform the anesthesia calculation to determine the charge for the anesthesia service.
12. Determine the total anesthesia time, divide by 15 (minutes) and document the time.
    PURPOSE: Used to perform the anesthesia calculation to determine the charge for the anesthesia service.
13. Select the appropriate geographic conversion factor.
    PURPOSE: Used to perform the anesthesia calculation to determine the charge for the anesthesia service.
14. Calculate the charge for the anesthesia service using the anesthesia formula.
    PURPOSE: To determine the charge for the anesthesia service or procedure.
15. Document the anesthesia charge and the code in the medical record and on the encounter form or charge ticket.

RADIOLOGY CODING

The Radiology section contains all diagnostic imaging codes, including not just x-ray studies, but also ultrasound, magnetic resonance imaging (MRI), and nuclear medicine procedures, as well as radiation oncology and several other types of diagnostic imaging procedures, services, and therapies. See Figure 18-8 for an illustration of the Radiology section from the CPT-4. The Radiology section is further subdivided into subsections, such as head and neck, then chest, spine, and pelvis, upper and lower extremities, abdomen, gastrointestinal and urinary tracts, gynecologic, obstetric and vascular procedures. The next subdivision, categories, define the types or function of various procedures—e.g., diagnostic ultrasound, radiation oncology, hypothermia, and so on—that are unique to the anatomic site subsection. In addition to the radiology procedure codes, codes are included for physician supervision and interpretation of diagnostic imaging data; clinical and radiation treatment

TABLE 18-7 Anesthesia Physical Status and Qualifying Circumstances Modifiers

MODIFIER	DESCRIPTION
Physical Status Modifiers*	
P1	A normal healthy patient
P2	A patient with mild systemic disease
P3	A patient with severe systemic disease
P4	A person with severe systemic disease that is a constant threat to life
P5	A moribund patient who is not expected to survive without the procedure
P6	A declared brain-dead patient whose organs are being removed for donor purposes
Qualifying Circumstances Modifiers†	
99100	Anesthesia for patient of extreme age, under 1 year or over 70
99116	Anesthesia complicated by utilization of total body hypothermia
99135	Anesthesia complicated by utilization of total body hypothermia

*A physical status modifier is required for use in performing anesthesia calculations.
†Use a qualifying circumstances modifier code, if appropriate, in addition to the primary CPT category I Anesthesia code.

Locality Name	Anesthesia Conversion Factor
Manhattan, NY	19.49
NYC suburbs/Long I., NY	19.25
Queens, NY	18.97
Rest of state	16.16
North Carolina	15.56
North Dakota	15.25

Figure 18-6 Anesthesia conversion factors. (From Buck CJ: *Step-by-step medical coding,* 2006, St Louis, 2006, Saunders.)

Medical Narrative

A 25-year-old female patient in good physical condition has anesthesia services while undergoing laparoscopy (CPT-4 Code 00840). The time for the anesthesia administration was 2 hours. For the purposes of this example the RBV basic unit value will be 4.

Basic Unit Value = 4
+ Modifying Units: PS = 0
+ QC = 0
+ Time Units = 8
= 12 Total Units

The total units value of 12 is then multiplied by the conversion factor for the geographic location of the anesthesiologist's office. For the purposes of this exercise, the conversion factor for Manhattan, NY, will be $20.48, and for North Carolina, $15.77. For the office located in Manhattan, NY, multiply $20.48 by 12. The fee for the anesthesia services would be $245.76. For the office located in North Carolina, multiply 12 times $15.77, for a fee of $189.24.

Figure 18-7 Anesthesia formula and calculation example.

planning, and administration of contrast materials during radiologic procedures.

The coding steps for radiologic procedures are the same as those for other category I codes. When searching by main term in the Alphabetic Index, using "Radiology" as the main term, a "See" note directs the codes to the more specific subcategories of nuclear medicine, ultrasound, radiation therapy, and x-ray studies. As always, a thorough review of the conventions, guidelines, and notes in the CPT-4 main text is essential to accurate coding.

PATHOLOGY AND LABORATORY SECTION

The subcategories for the Pathology and Laboratory section include organ and disease panels, drug testing, therapeutic drug assays, evocative or suppression testing, consultations, urinalysis, chemistry, molecular diagnostics, infectious agents, microbiology, anatomic pathology, cytopathology, cytogenetic studies, and surgical pathology. Figure 18-9 is an illustration of the organ panels subsection of the Pathology and Laboratory section.

Organ or disease panels are groupings of numerous tests performed to diagnose the health or disease status of specific

Radiology

Diagnostic Radiology (Diagnostic Imaging)

Head and Neck

70010   Myelography, posterior fossa, radiological supervision and interpretation

70015   Cisternography, positive contrast, radiological supervision and interpretation

70030   Radiologic examination, eye, for detection of foreign body

70100   Radiologic examination, mandible; partial, less than four views

70110   complete, minimum of four views

70120   Radiologic examination, mastoids; less than three views per side

70130   complete, minimum of three views per side

70134   Radiologic examination, internal auditory meati, complete

70140   Radiologic examination, facial bones; less than three views

Figure 18-8 Radiology section of CPT-4.

organ systems. In order to use a panel code, all of the tests listed under the code selected must have been performed. Otherwise, the individual tests should be billed using a separate code for each. The codes for drug testing are qualitative—they are based on which *type* of drug is found. Quantitative assays on the other hand, are performed to determine the *amount* of drug found.

MEDICINE SUBSECTIONS

Immune Globulins

When coding immune globulins administration, identify the immune globulin product being administered and the method of administration using the codes in the "hydration, therapeutic, prophylactic, and diagnostic injections and infusions" subsection (Figure 18-10).

Immunization Administration for Vaccines or Toxoids

These codes are for the administration of vaccines and toxoids only and should be reported in conjunction with the appropriate codes in the "immunization administration for vaccine/toxoids" subsection (Figure 18-11).

Pathology and Laboratory

Organ or Disease Oriented Panels

These panels were developed for coding purposes only and should not be interpreted as clinical parameters. The tests listed with each panel identify the defined components of that panel.

These panel components are not intended to limit the performance of other tests. If one performs tests in addition to those specifically indicated for a particular panel, those tests should be reported separately in addition to the panel code.

80048   Basic metabolic panel

This panel must include the following:

Calcium (82310)

Carbon dioxide (82374)

Chloride (82435)

Creatinine (82565)

Glucose (82947)

Potassium (84132)

Sodium (84295)

Urea nitrogen (BUN) (84520)

(Do not use 80048 in addition to 80053)

80050   General health panel

This panel must include the following:

Comprehensive metabolic panel (80053)

Blood count, complete (CBC), automated and automated differential WBC count (85025 or 85027 and 85004)

Figure 18-9 Pathology and laboratory section of CPT-4.

Vaccines, Toxoids

These codes identify the vaccine product only. Codes in the Immunization Administration for Vaccines/Toxoids subsection must be used in addition to the vaccine or toxoid product codes. To meet the reporting requirements of immunization registries, vaccine distribution programs, and reporting systems the exact vaccine product administered needs to be reported on the insurance claim form.

Medicine

Immune Globulins

►Codes 90281-90399 identify the immune globulin product only and must be reported in addition to the administration codes 90765-90768, 90772, 90774, 90775 as appropriate. Immune globulin products listed here include broad-spectrum and anti-infective immune globulins, antitoxins, and various isoantibodies.◄

⊘ **90281**   Immune globulin (Ig), human, for intramuscular use

⊘ **90283**   Immune globulin (IgIV), human, for intravenous use

⊘ **90287**   Botulinum antitoxin, equine, any route

⊘ **90288**   Botulism immune globulin, human, for intravenous use

⊘ **90291**   Cytomegalovirus immune globulin (CMV-IgIV), human, for intravenous use

⊘ **90296**   Diphtheria antitoxin, equine, any route

⊘ **90371**   Hepatitis B immune globulin (HBIg), human, for intramuscular use

⊘ **90375**   Rabies immune globulin (RIg), human, for intramuscular and/or subcutaneous use

⊘ **90376**   Rabies immune globulin, heat-treated (RIg-HT), human, for intramuscular and/or subcutaneous use

Figure 18-10 Relationship of immune globulins and infusions in CPT-4.

Hydration, Therapeutic, Prophylactic, and Diagnostic Injections and Infusion

Hydration codes are intended to report a hydration intravenous (IV) infusion to consist of a prepackaged fluid and electrolytes but are not used to report infusion of drugs or other substances. When multiple drugs are administered, report the service(s) and the specific materials or drugs for each.

Psychiatric Diagnostic or Evaluative Interview Procedures

Psychiatric diagnostic interview examination includes a history, mental status, and a disposition and may include communication with family or other sources and ordering of and medical interpretation of laboratory or other medical diagnostic studies.

Psychiatric Therapeutic Procedures

Psychotherapy is the treatment for mental illness and behavioral disturbances in which the clinician attempts to alleviate the emotional disturbances, reverse or change maladaptive patterns of behavior, and encourage personality growth and development.

Dialysis

These codes are reported once per month to distinguish age-specific service related to the patient's end-stage renal disease

Immunization Administration for Vaccines/Toxoids

Codes 90465-90474 must be reported in addition to the vaccine and toxoid code(s) 90476-90749.

Report codes 90465-90468 only when the physician provides face-to-face counseling of the patient and family during the administration of a vaccine. For immunization administration of any vaccine that is not accompanied by face-to-face physician counseling to the patient/family, report codes 90471-90474.

If a significant separately identifiable Evaluation and Management service (e.g., office or other outpatient services, preventive medicine services) is performed, the appropriate E/M service code should be reported in addition to the vaccine and toxoid administration codes.

(For allergy testing, see 95004 et seq)

(For skin testing of bacterial, viral, fungal extracts, see 86485-86586)

►(For therapeutic or diagnostic injections, see 90772-90779)◄

90465   Immunization administration under 8 years of age (includes percutaneous, intradermal, subcutaneous, or intramuscular injections) when the physician counsels the patient/family; first injection (single or combination vaccine/toxoid), per day

(Do not report 90465 in conjunction with 90467)

+ 90466   each additional injection (single or combination vaccine/toxoid), per day (List separately in addition to code for primary procedure)

(Use 90466 in conjunction with 90465 or 90467)

Figure 18-11 Relationship of immune vaccines/toxoids and administration codes in CPT-4.

(ESRD) performed in an outpatient setting. Dialysis codes describe a full month of ESRD-related service provided in an outpatient setting.

Cardiology

Echocardiography

Echocardiography is an ultrasound examination of the cardiac chambers and valves, the adjacent great vessels, and the pericardium.

Cardiac Catheterization

Cardiac catheterization is a diagnostic medical procedure that includes introduction, positioning and repositioning of catheter(s), recording of intracardiac and intravascular pressure, obtaining blood samples for measurement purposes, cardiac output measurements with or without electrode catheter placement, and final evaluation and reporting of the procedure.

Intracardiac Electrophysiologic Procedures and Studies

Intracardiac electrophysiologic studies (EPS) are invasive diagnostic medical procedures that include the procedure itself, insertion and repositioning of electrode catheters, recording of electrograms before and during pacing or programmed stimulation of multiple locations in the heart, analysis of recorded information, and reporting of the procedure.

Peripheral Arterial Disease Rehabilitation

Peripheral arterial disease (PAD) rehabilitative physical exercise consists of a series of sessions, lasting 45 to 60 minutes per session, involving use of either a motorized treadmill or a track.

Noninvasive Vascular Diagnostic Studies

Vascular studies include patient care required to perform the studies, supervision of the studies, and interpretation of study results, with copies for patient records of hard copy output with analysis of all data.

Sleep Testing

Sleep studies and *polysomnography* refer to the continuous and simultaneous monitoring and recording of various physiologic parameters of sleep for 6 or more hours with physician review, interpretation, and report. The studies are performed to diagnose a variety of sleep disorders and to evaluate a patient's response to therapies such as nasal continuous positive airway pressure (NCPAP).

Nervous System

Central Nervous System Assessments and Tests

Codes for central nervous system assessments and tests are used to report the services provided during testing of the cognitive function of the central nervous system.

Health and Behavior Assessment and Intervention

Health and behavior assessment procedures are used to identify the psychologic, behavioral, emotional, cognitive, and social factors important to the prevention, treatment, or management of physical health problems.

Chemotherapy Administration

Chemotherapy administration codes apply to parenteral administration of specific drugs and agents that are provided for treatment of cancer and noncancer diagnoses.

Injection and Intravenous Infusion Chemotherapy

IV or intraarterial push is defined as an injection in which the healthcare professional who administers the substance or drug is continuously present to administer the injection and observe the patient, or as an infusion of 15 minutes or less.

Modalities

Modality codes apply to any physical agent applied to produce therapeutic changes to biologic tissue; this includes but not is limited to thermal, acoustic, light, mechanical, or electric energy.

Active Wound Care Management

Active wound care procedures are performed to remove devitalized and/or necrotic tissue and promote healing. The provider is required to have direct (one-on-one) patient contact to use these codes.

Acupuncture

Acupuncture is reported based on 15-minute increments of personal (face-to-face) contact with the patient, not the duration of acupuncture needle(s) placement. Only one code may be reported for each 15-minute increment.

Osteopathic Manipulative Treatment

Osteopathic manipulative treatment (OMT) is a form of manual treatment applied by a physician to eliminate or alleviate somatic dysfunction and related disorders.

Chiropractic Manipulative Treatment

Chiropractic manipulative treatment (CMT) is a form of manual treatment to influence joint and neurophysiologic function. The CMT codes include a premanipulation patient assessment. For purposes of CMT, the five spinal regions referred to are the cervical region, thoracic region, lumbar region, sacral region, and pelvic region.

Education and Training for Patient Self-Management

These codes are used to report education and training services prescribed by a physician and provided by a qualified, non-physician healthcare professional using a standardized curriculum to an individual or a group of patients for the treatment of established illness(s) or disease(s).

Home Health Procedures and Services

These codes are used by nonphysician health care professionals only. They are used to report services provided in a patient's residence (including assisted living apartments, group homes, nontraditional private homes, custodial care facilities, and schools).

HEALTHCARE COMMON PROCEDURE CODING SYSTEM (HCPCS)

HCPCS (pronounced *"hixpix"*), developed by CMS, is a collection of codes and descriptions that represent procedures, supplies, products, and services that are not covered by or included in the CPT-4. HCPCS codes, like CPT-4 codes, are updated annually. They are designed to promote standardized reporting and statistical data collection of medical supplies, products, services, and procedures. Figure 18-12 is an excerpt from the HCPCS that illustrates HCPCS codes and the HCPCS manual format.

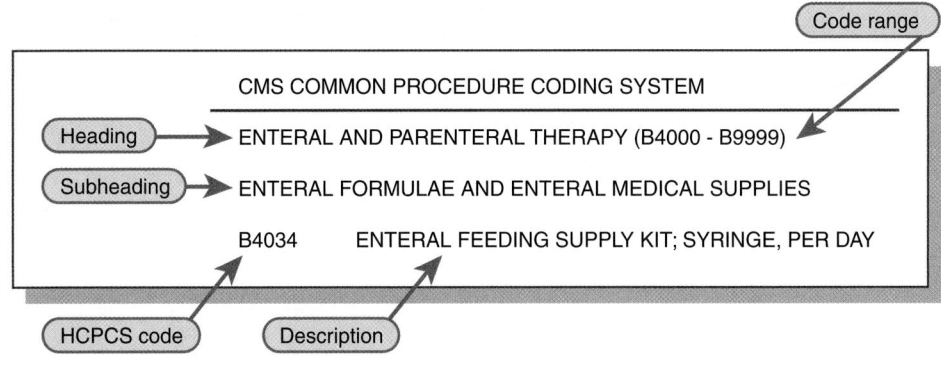

Figure 18-12 CMS's Healthcare Common Procedure Coding System (HCPCS), national codes. (Courtesy U.S. Department of Health and Human Services, Centers for Medicare and Medicaid Services.)

CODING LEVELS: CPT-4 VERSUS HCPCS

There are currently two levels of procedure codes:
- Level I: Developed by the AMA and contained in the current CPT-4 manual
- Level II: HCPCS codes developed by the Center for Medicare and Medicaid Services (CMS) to describe medical services and supplies not covered in the CPT-4

HCPCS Codes

The HCPCS Level II codes are five alphanumeric digits, beginning with one letter followed by four numerals. HCPCS also uses two alphabetic or alphanumeric character modifiers to add information or supplement the Level II Codes.

Conventions

HCPCS uses five conventions as shown in Figure 18-13.

HCPCS Manual

The HCPCS manual is divided into two parts; the Alphabetic Index and the Tabular Index. Procedures and services can be looked up in the Alphabetic Index as with CPT-4, then confirmed as the most accurate and appropriate code by using the Tabular Index. There are no subsections, categories, or subcategories in the HCPCS, only sections as outlined earlier. There is also an appendix of all the HCPCS modifiers and their descriptions for use.

The coding steps are almost identical to the steps for category I CPT-4 codes. A main term is determined, which is used to help find the procedure or service in the Alphabetic Index. The Alphabetic Index will list a code, codes, or code range. These codes or code ranges are then reviewed in the Tabular Index for specificity and accuracy. As with the CPT-4 codes, the clinical documentation is the starting point, and the final code selected should add nothing to nor omit any part of the medical documentation description. The final step is determining whether the code selected can stand alone or requires a modifier to further define or add needed information. Procedure 18-4 shows the coding steps in their entirety.

Coding using the HCPCS manual is essentially the same as coding for a CPT-4 procedure or service. The conventions,

⊗ **Special coverage instructions.**
Indicates that there are instructions provided regarding circumstances in which the code might be included for reimbursement.

◆ **Not covered by or valid for Medicare.**
These codes might result in reimbursement by private health insurance payors but not by Medicare. Their value may be only for statistical data collection but not for reimbursement.

✳ **Carrier discretion.** These codes may or may not be paid by health insurance carrier including Medicare.

▶ **New.**

➡ **Revised.** The revised symbol is placed in front of codes with any data, payment, or miscellaneous change from the prior year.

Figure 18-13 Healthcare Common Procedure Coding System (HCPCS) conventions.

Upcoding and Downcoding "Penalties"

There are no legal consequences for undercoding procedures for reimbursement; however, not selecting the most accurate and complete code(s) will result in, at a minimum, a reduction in reimbursement to the performing provider. Always attempt to choose the most appropriate code using the available medical documentation, and to check the medical record to ensure that no primary or secondary procedures were accidentally omitted.

Upcoding is much more serious from a legal standpoint. Using higher-reimbursed codes without having the medical documentation can result in civil or criminal charges of fraud or abuse. The penalties for fraud or abuse can be monetary (fines), jail time, a loss of privilege to use Medicare, Medicaid, and other governmental insurance programs, and in some cases revocation of a provider's license to practice medicine.

layout, and format of the HCPCS manual are different, and there are only sections and subsections found in the HCPCS manual. The HCPCS codes can be used when a specific procedure or service is not found in the CPT-4 coding manual.

PROCEDURE 18-4

Perform Procedural Coding: Perform HCPCS Coding

CAAHEP COMPETENCY: 3.a.(3)(c)
ABHES COMPETENCY: 3.v

GOAL: *Use the steps for procedure and service coding to find the most accurate and specific HCPCS code.*

EQUIPMENT and SUPPLIES

- HCPCS Coding Manual (current year)
- Medical Record
- Encounter form (charge ticket)
- Paper
- Pen or Pencil

PROCEDURAL STEPS

1. Read medical documentation to determine what procedures or services were provided.
   PURPOSE: To ensure all procedures and/or services are listed in the encounter form; that all procedures and services on the encounter form match the medical record; and that nothing documented in the medical record is missing from the encounter form.
2. Select main term classification to begin search.
   PURPOSE: To identify the term or terms to begin the search in the Alphabetic Index.
3. Select modifying term(s) if needed once main term is located.
   PURPOSE: To provide additional specificity and help narrow the search for the code or code range in the Alphabetic Index.
4. If no modifying term produces an appropriate code or code range, repeat steps 2 and 3 using a different main term classification.
   PURPOSE: To aid in finding the most appropriate code or code range by using alternative methods of searching the Alphabetic Index.
5. Find code or code ranges that include all or most of the medical record procedure or service description.
   PURPOSE: To assist in directing the medical assistant to the proper section, subsection, category, or subcategory of the main text of the HCPCS manual.
6. Disregard any code or code range containing additional descriptions or modifying terms not found in the medical record.

PURPOSE: To prevent upcoding or downcoding errors and other compliance issues.

7. Write down the code or code ranges that best match medical documentation.
   PURPOSE: To prevent repeated references to the Alphabetic Index by recording all possible matches to the code or code range being sought. It saves both time and redundant effort.
8. Turn to the main text, and find the first code or code range found while searching the Alphabetic Index.
   PURPOSE: To begin the process of finding the most specific and accurate code.
9. Compare the description of the code with the medical documentation. Verify that all or most of the medical record documentation matches the code description and that there is no additional element or information in the code description that is not found in the documentation.
   PURPOSE: To avoid upcoding and downcoding errors, and to ensure there are no contraindications to use of the code selected.
10. Read the guidelines for the section, subsection, and code to ensure there are no contraindications to the use of the code.
    PURPOSE: To ensure there are no instructions that would prevent use of the code selected.
11. Evaluate the HCPCS manual conventions.
    PURPOSE: To ensure there are no instructions that would prevent use of the code selected.
12. Determine if there are special circumstances that require the use of a modifier.
    PURPOSE: To select, if appropriate, modifiers that provide additional information for the code selected to explain certain circumstances or provide additional detail.
13. Record the HCPCS code selected in the medical record documentation next to the procedure or service performed and in the appropriate block of the insurance claim form.

CLOSING COMMENTS

Medical assistants must be responsible and remain knowledgeable about CPT-4 to ensure that no fraud takes place in the coding and claims submission process. Medical assistants should also ensure that proper precautions are taken to avoid incorrect coding, data entry errors, and false claims submissions.

Codes or narratives should not be altered in patient chart documentation to increase insurance reimbursement or to accommodate policy coverage requirements. Deliberate misrepresentation may carry criminal and/or civil penalties.

Downcoding, in which lower level codes are used even when the diagnostic statement indicates a higher level procedure or service, usually affects reimbursement only by lowering the amount received, but may have civil and criminal penalty implications if it is done to skirt insurance policy restrictions or preexisting condition clauses. **Upcoding,** on the other hand, in which a higher level procedure or service code is used than is supported by the medical documentation, can result in civil and criminal penalties, including fines, loss of privileges as a participating provider, and even prison time.

SUMMARY OF SCENARIO

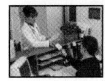 Kay has learned that procedural coding using the CPT-4 is similar in many ways to ICD-9-CM diagnostic coding. Both coding manuals have unique but similar steps, conventions, and guidelines. She has also learned that proper abstracting of procedural data from the medical record is just as important in both the ICD-9-CM and the CPT-4. Kay also discovered that HCPCS codes describe procedures and services not found in the CPT-4, such as medicines, ambulance services, and durable medical equipment. Kay now knows the legal implications of coding compliance errors, such as upcoding and downcoding.

Kay enjoys working toward becoming a medical assistant. As Kay progresses with learning procedural coding, she envisions herself as becoming more well rounded in her knowledge of the practice's administrative operations. The encounter form is a common document used to enter the procedure when a patient checks out, but knowing how to use the CPT-4 manual is essential when notes must be coded from procedures or services performed by Dr. Shuman or Dr. Taylor. As with diagnostic coding, Kay can pull the patient chart for research and documentation if any questions arise about a claim. Kay knows that coding to the highest level of specificity will help in accuracy and in obtaining maximum reimbursement. Kay continues to use the Internet to network and research. She stays informed of the changes in procedural coding by ordering the updated CPT-4 manual each year.

SUMMARY of LEARNING OBJECTIVES

1. Define, spell, and pronounce the terms listed in the vocabulary.
   - Spelling and pronouncing medical terms correctly adds credibility to the medical assistant. Knowing the definition of these terms promotes confidence in communication with patients and co-workers.
2. Describe the steps for abstracting procedural data from clinical documentation.
   - The medical assistant must thoroughly read clinical documentation and look for all of the procedures that were performed and should be charged to the patient. Most physician offices use the encounter form to document procedures and services, but there are instances when the medical assistant will need to read through the medical record to determine what was done to the patient and what charges should be made.
3. Identify four purposes of the CPT-4.
   - The CPT-4 is designed to encourage the use of standard terms and descriptors to document procedures in the medical record; to communicate accurate information on procedures and services to agencies concerned with insurance claims; to provide the basis for a computer-oriented system to evaluate operative procedures, and to contribute basic information for statistical purposes.
4. List the main sections of the CPT-4 and describe their content.
   - There are six sections in the main text: E&M, Anesthesia, Surgery, Radiology, Pathology and Laboratory, and Medicine. Each section contains subsections, categories, and subcategories that further define, modify, and describe the procedure or service codes.
5. Describe the coding conventions, guidelines, and layout of the CPT-4 manual and their importance.
   - The CPT-4 guidelines, symbols, conventions, notes, and steps are designed to guide a medical coder through the process of analyzing and translating clinical documentation and selecting the most accurate code for the procedure performed or the services rendered.
   - The CPT-4 contains a comprehensive Alphabetic Index, a main text listing of the category I CPT-4 codes, and several appendixes and addenda. The Alphabetic Index is composed of main and modifying terms that help provide specificity in selecting code or code ranges to evaluate in the main text.
   - The main text numerically lists all of the CPT-4 procedure and service codes and provides guidelines and conventions in selecting the most specific and most accurate code for insurance billing, reimbursement, and statistical data collection. Several appendixes and addenda provide lists of deletions, additions, and changes to the previous year's CPT-4, modifiers, category II and III codes, clinical examples for use of the E&M codes, add-on codes, exempt codes, codes that include conscious sedation, and drugs pending FDA approval.
6. Describe the process and steps for selecting the most accurate code based on clinical documentation.
   - To use the CPT-4 properly, the coder begins by reading and abstracting the medical documentation, then follows several specific steps using the CPT-4 Alphabetic Index to find a numeric, category I, CPT-4 procedure or service code, codes, or range of codes. The steps for using the Alphabetic Index include the following: (1) Read medical documentation; (2) Select main term classification to begin search; (3) Select modifying term(s) once main term is located; (4) If no modifying term produces an appropriate code or code range, repeat steps 2 and 3 using a different main term classification; (5) Find code or code ranges that include all or most of the medical record procedure or service description; (6) Disregard any code or code range containing additional descriptions or modifying terms not found in the medical record; (7) Write down the code or code ranges that best match medical documentation. Once the code, codes, or code range is found in the Alphabetic Index,

Continued

SUMMARY of LEARNING OBJECTIVES
Continued

the coder moves to the CPT-4 main text to further refine the search and find the appropriate code.

7. Explain the importance of correctly assigning evaluation and management codes.

- The physician can only bill for services that are actually rendered to patients and must use the evaluation and management guidelines to determine the correct codes for each patient. The amount of time spent with the patient and the level of medical decision making, as well as the length and complexity of the history and examination process all affect the code choice that applies to that particular encounter with the patient.

8. Discuss the importance of modifiers.

- Modifiers provide a way for the physician to indicate that a service or procedure was altered in some way but not changed in definition. Modifiers also allow the provider to add additional information or describe extenuating circumstances that affect the rendered procedure or service.

9. Define upcoding and explain why it must be avoided.

- If a code is selected that not only matches the procedure or service performed but also adds modifying information that is not in the medical documentation, then the information is considered "upcoded." Consistent upcoding can result in legal charges of fraud or abuse.

10. Demonstrate an understanding of the process and procedures for code selection.

- The medical assistant must understand the process for selecting the correct procedure codes that are used for billing

purposes. The selection directly influences the physician's total reimbursements. The process for code selection is outlined in Procedure 18-1.

11. Demonstrate an understanding of main and modifying term selection.

- The Alphabetic Index is organized by main terms that can stand alone or be further modified by using modifying terms that are indented under the main terms. The medical assistant should be as specific as possible in code selections, using all pertinent words within the description as found in the medical documentation.

12. Find codes in the Alphabetic Index of the CPT-4 manual.

- First, analyze the medical documentation to determine what services or procedures were performed. Select the main term from the documentation and search for it in the Alphabetic Index. Modifying terms will assist in finding the accurate code, which should then be located in the main text. Determine which code is the most accurate description for the procedure or service provided.

13. Analyze and select codes using the CPT-4 main text.

- After the Alphabetic Index has been searched, turn to the appropriate codes in the main text to perform final coding steps. Read the section thoroughly to determine the most accurate code to assign to the procedure or service rendered to the patient. Code the procedure or service. The process for using the Alphabetic and main texts of the CPT-4 manual are detailed in Procedures 18-2, 18-3, and 18-4.

CONNECTIONS

Study Guide Connection: Go to Chapter 18 Study Guide. Read the Case Study and Workplace Applications and complete the assignments. Do online research for answers to the questions in the Internet Activities associated with basics of procedural coding.

CD Connection: Go to the Medical Assisting Competency Challenge CD and do the training activities under Health Insurance Activities.

Evolve Connection: For more information related to basics of procedural coding, go to evolve.elsevier.com/kinn and visit related weblinks for Chapter 18. Click on the Medical Assisting Exam Review and do the practice questions to sharpen your test-taking skills. To learn more about office software, do the exercises for the Altapoint demo that is on the CD.

Basics of Health Insurance

Carline A. Dalgleish
Alexandra Patricia Young

19

SCENARIO

The instructor in Ann Grant's administrative medical assistant class, June Anderson, knows that working with medical insurance can be quite rewarding, and experienced billers find the field financially rewarding as well. Ms. Anderson works with Ann and her classmates, answering their questions and helping them to see that medical insurance is not as complicated as it seems.

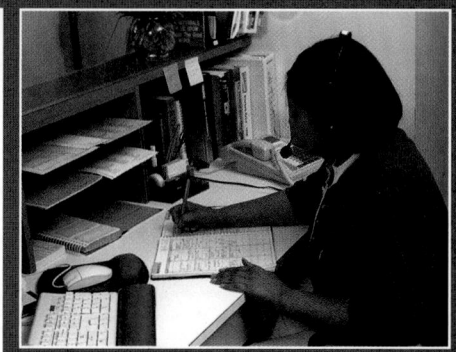

The medical assistant who is able to pay attention to detail and likes paperwork will usually enjoy billing and coding activities. The person who performs these duties in the physician's office is a critical staff member, because the tasks that are done related to billing influence the physician's income. That income is used to pay clinic expenses and payroll, so all of the employees of the facility indirectly count on accurate and timely billing. The individual who contributes billing and coding skills, as well as an understanding of health insurance and reimbursement guidelines, will be an asset to the practice and can look forward to a long and rewarding career.

Ann will learn that when insurance billing is broken down into manageable segments of information and applied to real-life situations, it becomes an interesting task. She will learn about the importance of verifying insurance eligibility and the steps for obtaining authorization for referrals and procedures; and that those benefits differ among insurance carriers, whether a private, commercial, federal or state insurance payor.

While studying this chapter, think about the following questions:

- How will the medical assistant be able to remember all the benefits, exclusions, authorizations, and other required information for the multiple insurance carriers and third party administrators?
- Why is it important to verify insurance eligibility and benefits before the patient is seen in a provider's office?

- Why is it important to understand the procedures for obtaining referrals and authorizations?
- How does the medical assistant perform insurance deductible and co-insurance calculations?

LEARNING OBJECTIVES

1. Define, spell, and pronounce the terms listed in the vocabulary.
2. Discuss the purpose of health insurance.
3. Differentiate among the various types of insurance policies.
4. Explain the numerous classifications of insurance benefits available.
5. Explain how insurance benefits are determined.
6. Differentiate among the different types of managed care options.
7. List and discuss other major third-party payors.

8. Interpret the procedure for verifying insurance benefits.
9. Discuss the different types of fee schedules.
10. Obtain managed care referrals and precertifications.
11. Perform eligibility and verification of benefits procedures.
12. Perform a preauthorization procedure.
13. Demonstrate how insurance benefits are determined by calculating deductible and co-insurance payments.

National Accreditation Competencies and Content

CAAHEP COMPETENCIES

Administrative
3.a.(3)(a). Apply managed care policies and procedures
3.a.(3)(b). Apply third-party guidelines

General
3.c.(2)(b). Perform within legal and ethical boundaries
3.c.(2)(d). Document appropriately
3.c.(3)(a). Explain general office policies

ABHES COMPETENCIES

Administrative Duties
3.t. Apply managed care policies and procedures
3.u. Obtain managed care referrals and precertification
3.x. Use physician fee schedule

Legal Concepts
5.a. Determine needs for documentation and reporting
5.b. Document accurately

Instruction
7.a. Orient patients to office policies and procedures

Financial Management
8.c. Analyze and use current third-party guidelines for reimbursement

VOCABULARY

allowed charge (allowable amount) The maximum amount of money that many third-party payors allow for a specific procedure or service.

authorization A term used in managed care for an approved referral.

beneficiary Individual entitled to receive benefits from an insurance policy or program or a governmental entitlement program offering healthcare benefits. Also called a *participant, subscriber, dependent, enrollee,* or *member.*

benefits The amount payable by an insurance company for a monetary loss to an individual insured by that company, under each coverage.

birthday rule Under law, the rule stating that when an individual is covered under two insurance policies, the insurance plan of the policyholder whose birthday comes first in the calendar year (month and day, not year) becomes the primary insurance. This rule applies when there is a question as to whose insurance should be determined as primary, such as for a dependent child, and not used when the individual is the owner of one of the two policies, which would make that the primary policy.

capitation Payment method used by many managed care organizations wherein a fixed amount of money is reimbursed to the provider for patients enrolled during a specific period of time, no matter what services were received or how many visits were made.

carriers As related to insurance, companies that assume the risk of an insurance policy.

Civilian Health and Medical Program of the Uniformed Services (CHAMPUS) See TRICARE.

Civilian Health and Medical Program of the Veterans Administration (CHAMPVA) A health benefits program run by the Department of Veterans Affairs (VA) that helps eligible beneficiaries pay the cost of specific healthcare services and supplies.

co-insurance A policy provision frequently found in medical insurance whereby the policyholder and the insurance company share the cost of covered losses in a specified ratio (e.g., 80/20 means 80% is covered by the insurer and 20% by the insured).

commercial insurance Plans that reimburse the insured for expenses resulting from illness or injury according to a specific fee schedule as outlined in the insurance policy and on a fee-for-service basis. Sometimes called *private insurance.*

copayment A sum of money that is paid at the time of medical service; a form of co-insurance.

deductibles Specific amounts of money a patient must pay out of pocket before the insurance carrier begins paying. Usually this amount ranges from $100 to $500. This deductible amount is met on a yearly or per-incident basis.

dependents The spouse, children, and sometimes domestic partner or other individuals designated by the insured who are covered under a healthcare plan.

disability income insurance Insurance that provides periodic payments to replace income when an insured person is unable to work as a result of illness, injury, or disease.

effective date The date on which an insurance policy or plan takes effect so that benefits are payable.

eligibility A term which describes whether a patient's insurance coverage is in effect, and eligible for payment of insurance benefits.

exclusions Limitations on an insurance contract for which benefits are not payable.

explanation of benefits (EOB) A letter or statement from the insurance carrier describing what was paid, denied, or reduced in payment. It also contains information about amounts applied to the deductible, the patient's co-insurance, and the allowed amounts.

explanation of Medicare benefits (EOMB) The EOMB is the name for an explanation of benefits from Medicare. See explanation of benefits above for the definition.

VOCABULARY

fee for service An established schedule of fees set for services performed by providers and paid by the patient.

fiscal intermediary An organization that contracts with the government to handle and mediate insurance claims from medical facilities, home health agencies, or providers of medical services or supplies.

government plans Entitlement programs or healthcare plans that are sponsored and/or subsidized by the state or federal government, such as **Medicaid** and **Medicare**.

group policy Insurance written under a policy that covers a number of people under a single master contract issued to their employer or to an association with which they are affiliated.

guarantor The person who is responsible for paying a medical bill.

health insurance Protection in return for periodic premium payments that provides reimbursement of expenses resulting from illness or injury. Includes the following forms of insurance: accident, disability income, medical expense, and accidental death and dismemberment. Also known as *accident and health insurance* or *disability income insurance*.

Health Insurance Portability and Accountability Act (HIPAA) The Kassebaum-Kennedy Act, designed to improve portability and continuity of health insurance coverage; to combat waste, fraud, and abuse in health insurance and healthcare delivery; to promote the use of medical savings accounts; to improve access to long-term care services and coverage; to simplify the administration of health insurance; and to serve other purposes.

health maintenance organization (HMO) An organization that provides a wide range of comprehensive healthcare services for a specified group at a fixed periodic payment. HMOs can be sponsored by the government, medical schools, hospitals, employers, labor unions, consumer groups, insurance companies, and hospital-medical plans.

indemnity plans Traditional health insurance plans that pay for all or a share of the cost of covered services, regardless of which physician, hospital, or other licensed healthcare provider is used. Policyholders of indemnity plans and their **dependents** choose when and where to get healthcare services.

individual policy An insurance policy designed specifically for the use of one person (and his or her dependents), not associated with the amenities of a group policy, namely higher premiums. Often called *personal insurance.*

insured An individual or organization covered by an insurance policy according to the policy terms, usually the individual or group that pays the premiums. Blue Cross/Blue Shield refers to this person or group as the *subscriber.*

managed care plans An umbrella term for all healthcare plans that provide healthcare in return for preset monthly payments and coordinated care through a defined network of primary care physicians and hospitals.

medical savings accounts Tax-deferred bank or savings accounts that are combined with a low-premium, high-deductible insu-rance policy, designed for individuals or families who choose to fund their own healthcare expenses and medical insurance.

Medicaid A federal and state sponsored health insurance program for the medically indigent.

Medicare A federally sponsored health insurance program for those over 65 or individuals under 65 but disabled.

Medigap A term sometimes applied to private insurance products that supplement Medicare insurance benefits.

participating provider (PAR) A physician or other healthcare provider who enters into a contract with a specific insurance company or program, and by doing so agrees to abide by certain rules and regulations set forth by that particular third-party payor.

policyholder A person who pays a premium to an insurance company and in whose name the policy is written in exchange for the insurance protection provided by a policy of insurance.

preauthorization A process required by some insurance carriers where the provider obtains permission to perform certain procedures or services, or refer a patient to a specialist.

premium The periodic (monthly, quarterly, or annual) payment of a specific sum of money to an insurance company for which the insurer, in return, agrees to provide certain benefits.

primary care provider (PCP) A general practice, or non-specialist provider or physician responsible for the care of a patient for some health maintenance organizations. Also called a gatekeeper.

referral An insurance term used when a primary care provider wants to send a patient to a specialist. Typically, the provider must obtain authorization from the insurance carrier in advance to refer a patient.

remittance advice (RA) An explanation of benefits which comes from Medicaid. See explanation of benefits above for the definition.

resource-based relative value scale (RBRVS) A fee schedule designed to provide national uniform payment of Medicare benefits after being adjusted to reflect the differences in practice costs across geographic areas.

rider A special provision or group of provisions that may be added to a policy to expand or limit the benefits otherwise payable. It may increase or decrease benefits, waive a condition or coverage, or in any other way amend the original contract.

self-insured plan An insurance plan funded by an organization having a large enough employee base that it can afford to fund its own insurance program.

self-referral The act of a patient or insured individual who refers himself or herself to a specialist without requesting the referral from the primary provider, such as a woman seeking an annual gynecologic examination. Managed care guidelines may require the patient to report the self-referral.

service benefit plans Plans that provide benefits in the form of certain surgical and medical services rendered, rather than cash. A service benefit plan is not restricted to a fee schedule.

VOCABULARY

third-party administrator An organization that processes claims and performs other business-related functions for a health plan.

third-party payors Entities that make payment on an obligation or debt but are not parties of the contract that created the debt.

TRICARE A government-sponsored program wherein authorized dependents of military personnel receive medical care. This program was originally called *CHAMPUS*.

utilization review A review of individual cases by a committee to make sure that services are medically necessary and to study how providers use medical care resources.

workers' compensation Insurance against liability imposed on certain employers to pay **benefits** and furnish care to employees who are injured and to pay benefits to dependents of employees killed in the course of or arising out of their employment.

THE PURPOSE OF HEALTH INSURANCE

The purpose of **health insurance** is to help individuals and families offset the costs of medical care. Health insurance is defined as protection against financial losses resulting from illness or injury. This protection provides payment of monetary benefits for covered sickness or injury depending on the insurance policy purchased. There are various types of health insurance, such as accident insurance, **disability income insurance,** hospitalization, medical expense insurance, and accidental death and dismemberment insurance.

More and more of today's health insurance policies cover "preventative" care, which includes services provided to help prevent certain illnesses or lead to an early diagnosis. Health insurance typically covers services and procedures considered medically necessary. Most insurance policies do not cover "elective" procedures, such as certain cosmetic surgeries that are not considered medically necessary.

CRITICAL THINKING APPLICATION

There is so much to learn in the medical insurance field, and it seems that rules and regulations change on a daily basis. How can Ann keep current on healthcare issues that affect insurance? How can Ann advise patients to keep abreast of the changes in their own personal coverage, such as Medicare?

CYCLE OF HEALTH INSURANCE

The information that follows describes common types of insurance coverage and insurance carriers, the steps for obtaining insurance coverage information, and some of the terminology associated with obtaining insurance coverage and insurance billing. The **insured** or **policyholder,** defined as an individual, group, or employer, pays a set amount called a **premium.** A premium is the periodic (monthly, quarterly, or annual) payment of a specific sum of money to an insurance company for which the insurer agrees to provide certain benefits. This premium, in return, pays for an insurance policy that covers the insured for a specific type(s) of coverage, such as basic and major medical coverage, accidental death or disability, and so on. When an insured or a covered **beneficiary** or **dependent** of the insurance policy becomes ill or suffers an injury, treatment is provided by a physician or other provider of service in a doctor's office, emergency room, or hospital.

Tasks Related to the Cycle of Health Insurance

The medical assistant's tasks related to health insurance processing are described in this section. These tasks are initiated when the patient encounters the provider, either by appointment, as a walk-in or in the emergency room or hospital. Each task will be discussed in more detail later in this chapter. Tasks completed by the medical assistant include:

- Obtain information from the patient and insured, including demographic, employment, and insurance data.
- Verify the patient's **eligibility** for insurance payment with the insurance carrier(s), as well as benefits available, exclusions, and whether special **authorization**s are needed to refer patients to specialists or perform certain services or procedures—for example, surgery or diagnostic tests.
- Perform diagnostic and procedural coding and review the encounter form or charge ticket for completeness once the patient is seen by the provider.
- Calculate insurance deductibles and co-insurance amounts and provide the patient with a statement showing the out-of-pocket expense amount owed by the patient.
- Obtain preauthorization for referral of the patient to a specialist or for special services or procedures that require advance permission. This information may be obtained verbally, but should also be documented in writing and should be obtained in advance of commencing any procedures or treatments.
- Complete an insurance claim form and submit it to the insurance company for reimbursement for services and procedures performed. In Chapter 20, detailed instructions are provided for completing a health insurance claim form.
- Post payments and adjustments on the patient ledger or account, and examine the **explanation of benefits (EOB), explanation of Medicare benefits (EOMB) or the remittance**

advice (RA) from the insurance company to identify what was paid, reduced, or denied, and includes deductible, co-insurance, and allowable amounts. Adjustments are made to the account, and the **allowable amount** is either written-off (adjusted) or passed on to the patient for payment.

- Bill the patient for any outstanding balance, or, if there is a secondary insurance, complete the secondary insurance claim form and submit it to the insurance company.
- Follow-up on any rejected or unpaid claims, and any requests from the insurance carrier for more information about specific claims are answered as soon as possible. Chapter 20 includes more information regarding insurance follow-up, as well as tips to help minimize claims rejections, reduce the number of requests for additional data, and maximize reimbursement.

Cost of Coverage

In this age of rising health care costs, most insurance **carriers** do not reimburse the full amount for services and procedures rendered. A carrier is an insurance company or third-party that pays for medical care. The insured, or beneficiary, in most instances will be required to pay certain "out-of-pocket" expenses such as **deductibles, copayment** or **co-insurance** charges, and costs for noncovered services.

A deductible is an amount a **policyholder** agrees to pay per claim or per accident toward the total amount of an insured loss before the insurance company will begin payment of benefits. A deductible amount is stated in the insurance contract and normally ranges from $100 to $500. Under most circumstances the deductible must be paid only one time per calendar year; however, some policies have a deductible per occurrence. The medical assistant should always verify the **effective date,** or date the insurance coverage began, on the patient's insurance card. An excellent policy for any provider's office is to call the insurance company to verify insurance eligibility, benefits, and **exclusions** before the patient's appointment or encounter with the provider. This verification is done by phone or fax and ensures that the insurance is in effect, and the patient is eligible for benefits. More about verification of benefits will be covered later in the chapter. Co-insurance is a policy provision frequently found in medical insurance whereby the policyholder and the insurance company share the cost of covered losses in a specified ratio, such as 80/20 (i.e., 80% of services are paid by the insurance carrier and 20% by the insured). Many plans now require a copayment, which is a type of co-insurance that is collected at the time of service. Copayments usually range from $10 to $25 for office visits but can vary according to the services rendered. Most **managed care plans** require a copayment. In addition, any services or procedures that are not covered under the terms of an insurance policy are the responsibility of the policyholder or insured.

TYPES OF HEALTH INSURANCE

Health insurance is available to the majority of persons in this country through group or individual plans. In addition, many people are covered by **government plans** or entitlement programs. However, although health insurance might be available, it is not always affordable. A recent survey revealed that more than 56 million Americans–roughly 21% of the population–have no regular source for obtaining medical care, and lack of health insurance was a major obstacle.

The types of health insurance available include group insurance, individual insurance, government-sponsored insurance, **self-insured plans,** and medical savings accounts. Government plans can be federal and/or state sponsored and include **Medicare, Medicaid, TRICARE, the Civilian Health and Medical Program of the Veterans Administration (CHAMPVA),** and **worker's compensation**.

Group Policies

Insurance written under a **group policy** covers a number of people under a single master contract issued to their employer or to an association with which they are affiliated. Group coverage usually provides greater benefits at lower premiums because of the large pool of people from whom premiums are collected. Physical examinations are normally not required, and preexisting conditions are often waived. Often the employee shares the cost of coverage through payroll deductions.

Individual Policies

Individuals who do not qualify for inclusion in a group or government-sponsored plan may apply to companies that offer individual policies, often called *personal insurance* or **individual policies.** The applicant is normally required to fill out an extended health questionnaire and undergo a physical examination before acceptance. Unlike with group policies, with personal insurance there is a risk that coverage may be denied, or the individual may have to accept a **rider,** or limitation, on benefits the policy will cover. Premiums are almost always higher with individual policies, and often the benefits are less.

Government Plans

Many large groups of people are covered by government plans or entitlement programs. A patient who is older than age 65 is covered by Part B of Medicare. A medically indigent patient may be eligible for Medicaid with or without Medicare. **Dependents** of military personnel are covered by **TRICARE** (formerly known as the **Civilian Health and Medical Program of the Uniformed Services** *(CHAMPUS);* surviving spouses and dependent children of veterans who died as a result of service-related disabilities are covered by CHAMPVA.

Some wage earners are protected against the loss of wages and the cost of medical care resulting from an occupational accident, disease, or disability through **workers' compensation** insurance. An individual may collect benefits for health expenses from an automobile policy if the injury is related to a car accident or other such loss.

TRICARE

The federal government first became responsible for insuring a large group of people in 1956 with passage of Public Law 569. This law authorized dependents of military personnel to receive treatment from civilian physicians at the expense of the government. The program administering these benefits became CHAMPUS, which today is known as *TRICARE* (discussed in detail later in this chapter).

Medicaid

In 1965 the federal government provided for another group—the medically indigent—through a program that is known as *Medicaid*. Title XIX of Public Law 89-97, under the Social Security Amendments of 1965, provided for agreements with states for assistance from the federal government to provide medical care for people meeting specific eligibility criteria.

Medicare

Established in 1965, Medicare is a federal health insurance program that provides health care coverage for individuals age 65 and older. The program also covers certain persons under age 65 with disabilities. The Medicare program was developed by the Healthcare Financing Administration (HCFA), now called the Centers for Medicare and Medical Services (CMS), as part of Title XVIII of the Social Security Act.

Workers' Compensation

All state legislatures have passed workers' compensation laws to protect wage earners against the loss of wages and the cost of medical care resulting from occupational accident or disease. State laws differ as to the classes of employees included and the benefits provided.

Self-Insured Plans

Many large companies or organizations have a big enough employee base that they choose to fund their own insurance program. This is called a **self-insured plan.** Technically, a self-funded plan is not insurance by true definition. The employer pays employee healthcare costs from the firm's own funds. Recent surveys indicate that about 40% of workers with employment-based health insurance are enrolled in plans that their employers self-insure. Usually benefits and premium costs under self-insured plans are similar to those under group plans. Self-funded plans tend to work best for companies that are large enough to offer good coverage and reasonable premium rates and are able to pay large claims for expensive medical services. Often a **third-party administrator** (TPA) or **fiscal intermediary** handles paperwork and claim payments for a self-insured group.

Medical Savings Account

In 1996 Congress made tax-free **medical savings accounts** (MSAs) available to 750,000 American workers and their families. This is a type of self-insurance. Under a provision of the Kassebaum-Kennedy health insurance reform bill, small companies (with 50 or fewer employees), self-employed persons, and the uninsured can purchase health insurance policies and make tax-free deposits to an MSA. They can use their MSA money to pay small and routine healthcare expenses, reserving a high-deductible medical insurance policy to pay large, catastrophic expenses. Money that remains in the account at year's end earns tax-free interest. People can also elect to use MSA money to pay their health insurance premiums during a job change,

which should reduce job lock, a situation in which people do not change jobs for fear of losing their health insurance.

There are both advantages and disadvantages to having an MSA, and it is wise to investigate them thoroughly to learn the values and limitations of these accounts.

CRITICAL THINKING APPLICATION

Ann understands how medical assistants can easily become intimidated by all of the regulations that affect insurance coverage. Discuss differences and similarities between the different types of insurance companies and insurance coverage. How can the medical assistant effectively keep up with all of the rules pertaining to policies that frequently are presented in the office?

TYPES OF INSURANCE BENEFITS

An insurance package is tailored to the needs of each individual or group policy, and the combinations of benefits are limitless. A policy may contain one or any combination of the following benefits as described here and in Table 19-1.

Hospitalization

Hospital coverage pays the cost of all or part of the insured person's hospital room and board and specific hospital services, such as the costs involved in having surgery in a hospital. Hospital insurance policies frequently set a maximum amount payable per day and a maximum number of days of hospital care. Some insurance companies require that the hospital be an accredited or a licensed hospital.

Surgical

Surgical coverage pays all or part of a surgeon's fee; some plans also pay for an assistant surgeon. Surgery includes any incision or excision, removal of foreign bodies, aspiration, suturing, and reduction of fractures. Surgery may be accomplished in a hospital, physician's office, or elsewhere. The insurer frequently provides the subscriber with a surgical fee schedule that establishes the amount the insurer will pay for commonly performed procedures.

Basic Medical

Basic medical coverage pays all or part of a physician's fee for nonsurgical services, including hospital, home, and office visits. Usually there is a deductible amount payable by the patient as well as a copayment or co-insurance payment each time service is received. The insurance plan may include a provision for diagnostic laboratory, radiology, and pathology fees. Some medical plans do not cover routine physical examinations or preventative health checkups such as mammograms or prostate examinations if the patient does not have a specific complaint or illness.

Major Medical

Major medical insurance (formerly called *catastrophic coverage*) provides protection against especially large medical bills

TABLE 19-1 Types of Health Insurance, Plan Benefits

BENEFIT	COVERED	PAYS
Hospitalization	Cost of all or part of the hospital room and board; and, specific hospital services, i.e., costs involved in having surgery in a hospital	Maximum amount per day and maximum number of days
Surgical	Any surgical procedure, including but not limited to: incision or excision; removal of foreign bodies; aspiration; suturing; reduction of fractures	Surgeon's fee Assistant surgeon's fee
Basic medical	Outpatient and/or physician office procedures and services	Physician's fees diagnostic, radiologic, laboratory, and pathology fees
Major medical (catastrophic)	Catastrophic or prolonged illness or injury	Takes over when basic medical, hospitalization and surgical benefits end
Disability	Accident or illness resulting in an inability for patient to work; can be paid whether work-related or non-work related.	Cash benefits paid in lieu of salary while patient is unable earn an income
Dental care	Preventative care and/or teeth and gum treatment and repair	Typically pays 100% for preventative care, 50% for repair and treatment
Vision care	Eye exam and glasses	Set benefit amount depending on vision care policy for examination and/or glasses
Medicare supplement	Deductible and co-insurance amounts unpaid by Medicare	Deductible and co-insurance amounts unpaid by Medicare
Special risk	Certain specific illnesses (cancer, heart failure) or accidents (automobile, airplane)	Typically pays a maximum benefit
Life insurance	Loss of life	Usually lump sum payment of life insurance benefit
Long-term care	Long-term skilled nursing or rehabilitation care	Set amount determined by policy benefits

resulting from catastrophic or prolonged illnesses. It may be a supplement to basic medical coverage or a comprehensive integrated program providing both basic and major medical protection.

Disability (Loss of Income) Protection

Weekly or monthly cash benefits are provided to employed policyholders who become unable to work as a result of an accident or illness. Many disability policies do not start payment until after a specified number of days or until a certain number of sick leave days have been used. Payment is made directly to the individual and is intended to replace lost income resulting from an illness or other disability. It is not intended for payment of specific medical bills, and it should not be confused with a regular insurance plan, entitlement program, or workers' compensation, in which compensation is provided for an employee who is injured on the job or cannot work as a result of a job-related illness or other disability.

Dental Care

Dental coverage is included in many fringe benefit packages. Some policies are based on a copayment and incentive program, in which preventive dental care (such as cleaning and x-ray films) is covered 100%, with most other coverage paid at 50%.

Vision Care

Vision care insurance may include reimbursement for all or a percentage of the cost for refraction, lenses, and frames.

Medicare Supplement

Many Medicare beneficiaries purchase a supplemental health insurance policy to help defray medical costs not covered, or only partially covered, by Medicare. Federal regulations now require that Medicare supplement contracts must be uniform in benefits to avoid confusion for the purchaser. Medicare supplements that cover Medicare recipients' out-of-pocket expenses, including the deductible and co-insurance payments, are called **Medigap** policies.

Special Risk Insurance

Special risk insurance protects a person in the event of a certain type of accident, such as an automobile or airplane crash, or for certain diseases, such as tuberculosis or cancer. There is usually a maximum benefit.

Liability Insurance

There are many types of liability insurance, including automobile, business, and homeowners' policies. Liability policies often include benefits for medical expenses payable to individuals who are injured in the insured person's home or car, without regard to the insured person's actual legal liability for the accident.

Life Insurance

Life insurance provides payment of a specified amount on an insured's death, either to his or her estate or to a designated beneficiary, or in the case of an endowment policy, to the policyholder at a specified date. Life insurance policies sometimes provide monthly cash benefits if the policyholder becomes permanently and totally disabled. Sometimes the proceeds from life insurance are used to meet the expenses of the insured person's last illness.

Long-Term Care Insurance

Long-term care insurance is a relatively new type that covers a continuum of broad-ranged maintenance and health services to chronically ill, disabled, or mentally retarded persons. Services may be provided on an inpatient basis (at a rehabilitation facility, nursing home, or mental hospital), on an outpatient basis, or at home. The **Health Insurance Portability and Accountability Act (HIPAA)** of 1996 gives some federal income tax advantages to people who buy certain long-term care insurance policies.

HOW BENEFITS ARE DETERMINED

Insurance benefits may be determined and paid in one of several ways:

- By indemnity schedules
- By **service benefit plans**
- By determination of the usual, customary, and reasonable (UCR) fee
- By relative value studies

Indemnity Schedules

Indemnity plans are traditional health insurance plans that pay for all or a share of the cost of covered services, regardless of which physician, hospital, or other licensed healthcare provider is used. Because physicians and other providers are paid for each office visit, test, procedure, or other service they deliver, indemnity plans are often called *fee-for-service plans*.

Policyholders of indemnity plans and their dependents choose when and where to get healthcare services. In exchange for premiums that members pay, the indemnity plan reimburses members or the provider when claims are filed. The subscriber is often given a schedule of indemnities (fee schedule), which explains the benefit payment amounts of the policy, when the policy is purchased. Indemnity benefits are usually paid to the person insured unless that person has authorized payment directly to the provider, which is a common practice.

Service Benefit Plans

In a **service benefit** plan the insuring company agrees to pay for certain surgical or medical services without additional cost to the person insured. There is no set fee schedule. In a service benefit plan, surgery with complications would warrant a higher fee than an uncomplicated procedure would. Premiums are sometimes higher for this type of coverage, but often payments are larger. Frequently payment of benefits is sent directly to the physician and is considered full payment for services rendered.

For example, the service benefit plan states it will pay $900 for a cholecystectomy. If Dr. Jones charges $1500 for this procedure, he has the right to either accept the $900 as payment in full and write off the balance due or to request payment for the remaining $600 balance from the patient or **guarantor**—the individual or group responsible for payment.

Usual, Customary, and Reasonable Fee

Some insurance companies agree to pay on the basis of all or a percentage of the physician's UCR fee. Charges for a specific service are compared with a database of charges for the same service to other patients by the same type of physician, and to patients by other physicians performing the same or similar services in the same geographic area. The insurance company determines whether the charge is UCR, and any amount over this **allowed charge** will not be paid.

Resource-Based Relative Value Scale

The **resource-based relative value scale (RBRVS)** is one of the outcomes of the Medicare Physician Payment Reform that was enacted in the Omnibus Budget Reconciliation Act of 1989 (usually called *OBRA '89*). Since the beginning of Medicare, Part B of the program has paid physicians using a fee-for-service system based on customary, prevailing, and reasonable charges that was similar in structure to the UCR fees described in the previous paragraph; however, implementation of the RBRVS, which came into effect in 1992, changed this system to a fee scale consisting of three parts: physician work, charge-based professional liability expenses, and charge-based overhead.

The physician work component includes the degree of effort invested by a physician in a particular service or procedure and the time it consumed. The professional liability and overhead components are computed by the Centers for Medicare and Medicaid Services (CMS). The fee schedule is designed to provide national uniform payments after being adjusted to reflect the differences in practice costs across geographic areas. The fee schedule includes a conversion factor, which is a single national number applied to all services paid under the fee schedule. Conversion factors are changed, usually annually, by Congress at the request of the CMS.

HEALTH INSURANCE PROVIDERS

Health insurance providers include managed care plans, Blue Cross/Blue Shield (BC/BS), **commercial insurance** companies, and federal and state government programs including Medicare, Medicaid, TRICARE, workers' compensation, and disability insurance.

Managed Care

Managed care is an umbrella term for all healthcare plans that provide healthcare in return for preset scheduled payments and coordinated care through a defined network of physicians and hospitals. Managed care refers to healthcare plans that provide healthcare in return for scheduled payments and coordinate healthcare through a defined network of **primary care providers** (PCPs), hospitals, and other providers.

The passage of the Health Maintenance Organization Act in 1973 provided for federal aid to health insurance prepayment plans that met certain criteria. This brought about a rapid growth of the **health maintenance organization** (HMO), which is an organization that provides comprehensive healthcare to an enrolled group for a fixed periodic payment. Some of these plans pay by **capitation,** which means that the provider is paid a fixed amount for each individual enrolled in the plan during a specified time period, regardless of the number of services provided to the patient. The provider still collects only the contracted rate, even if expenses cost much more than that rate for the time period (Procedure 19-1).

Managed care has been met with considerable controversy and has pros and cons that must be considered. It is important that medical assistants be well versed in the various types of managed care plans to fully understand their impact on healthcare costs.

Advantages of managed care include the following:

- Healthcare costs are usually contained.
- There are established fee schedules.
- Authorized services are usually paid for.
- Most preventive medical treatment is covered.
- Patients' out-of-pocket expenses tend to be less than with traditional insurance.

Disadvantages of managed care include the following:

- Access to specialized care and referrals can be limited.
- Physician choices in treatment of patients can be limited.
- The amount of paperwork may be increased.
- Treatment may be delayed because of preauthorization requirements.
- Reimbursement is historically less than that through traditional insurance.

Models of Managed Care

There are two basic models of managed care: the health maintenance organization (HMO) and the preferred provider organization (PPO). The HMO can be structured as an independent practice association (IPA), staff, or group model, or as an exclusive provider organization (EPO). Table 19-2 illustrates these HMO models.

Health Maintenance Organization. An HMO is a plan that contracts with a medical center or group of physicians to provide preventative as well as acute care for the insured. HMOs are state-licensed health plans that are regulated by HMO laws, which require them to include preventative care such as routine physical examinations and other services as part of their benefits package. HMOs always require referrals to specialists, precertification, and preauthorization for hospital admissions, outpatient procedures and treatments.

An HMO member is typically enrolled for a specified period of time (month, quarter, or year). The HMO receives a "per member per month" (pmpm) fee for each enrollee if they are on a capitation plan.

Providers receive payment in various structures. The two most common structures are **capitation** and **fee for service**. Capitation is payment in advance to the provider by the HMO for a contracted group of patients, regardless how often the patients are seen, and even if the patients are never seen by the provider. Fees charged for services to group members may be billed directly to the IPA rather than to the patient. Fees for services to nonmember patients are handled in the same manner as any other fee for service. The payment structure is based on the type of HMO model and the contract negotiated between the HMO and the provider(s). The most common models include the examples that follow.

Independent Practice Association. An independent practice association (IPA) consists of physicians with separately owned practices who formally organize a physician association and continue to practice in their own offices. The physician may be contracted with several IPAs. Payments to providers by an IPA can be structured either as a capitation or fee for service.

Staff model. A staff model HMO hires physicians and pays a salary to its physicians. Rather than contracting with physicians to create a network, the HMO owns the network. Medical care is given by, or authorized by, the patient's PCP. No capitation or fee for service payment structure is used with the staff model; however, the physicians may receive bonuses biannually or annually based on the number of patients treated and/or the cost savings.

Group model. A group model HMO contracts with a multispecialty medical group to deliver care to its members. It is similar to an IPA in that the multispecialty group may organize a physician association, but they typically practice together in one facility. The payment structure to the providers can be either capitation or fee for service.

Exclusive Provider Organization. An Exclusive Provider Organization (EPO) combines features of HMOs (e.g., an enrolled group or population, primary care providers, and an **authorization** system) and Preferred Provider Organizations (PPOs; e.g., flexible benefit design, and fee-for-service payments). It is referred to as "exclusive" because employers agree not to contract with any other plan. Members must choose medical care from network providers, with certain exceptions for emergency or out-of-area services. If a patient decides to seek care outside the network, he or she generally will not be reimbursed for the cost of treatment. Technically, many HMOs can be considered EPOs; however, EPOs are regulated under insurance statutes rather than federal and state HMO regulations.

Preferred Provider Organizations. The PPO model of managed healthcare preserves the fee-for-service concept that many physicians prefer. An insurer representing its clients contracts

TABLE 19-2 Comparison of HMO Models		
MODEL	**STRUCTURE**	**BILLING MODEL**
IPA	General or family practice physician or physician group that practices independently and may contract with several IPAs	Capitation or fee for service
Staff	Physician(s) hired by HMO	Salaried
Group	Multispecialty group with or without PCP (gatekeeper); may contract with several IPAs	Capitation or fee for service

PROCEDURE 19-1

Apply Managed Care Policies and Procedures

<u>CAAHEP COMPETENCY:</u> 3.a(3)(a)
<u>ABHES COMPETENCY:</u> 3.t

GOAL: *To act within the guidelines of the managed care contracts that the physician and/or medical facility has partnered.*

EQUIPMENT and SUPPLIES

- Managed care contracts
- Managed care handbooks
- Clerical supplies
- Forms from managed care organizations

PROCEDURAL STEPS

1. Determine which managed care organization the patient belongs to.
   <u>PURPOSE:</u> To make certain that the right information is applied to the right patient.
2. Read and study the policies and procedures that are set forth by the managed care organization.
   <u>PURPOSE:</u> To understand regulations and abide by them when working with patients that the regulations affect.
3. Obtain any forms that are needed to process patient claims.

<u>PURPOSE:</u> To submit the correct forms to the managed care organization.
4. Become familiar with the information in managed care policy manuals and handbooks.
   <u>PURPOSE:</u> By becoming familiar with handbooks and guidelines, the medical assistant will be able to assist patients in finding needed information.
5. Determine whom to contact in case of questions about the various managed care organizations.
   <u>PURPOSE:</u> To be able to refer patients to the best source of information when they have questions or concerns.
6. Attend seminars and workshops when offered by the managed care organizations.
   <u>PURPOSE:</u> To stay up-to-date on information and policies.
7. Use information gained on a daily basis when working with managed care organizations.

---

with a group of providers who agree on a predetermined list of charges for all services including those for both normal and complex procedures. Unlike HMOs, PPOs have no capitation or prepaid care. Typically there are deductibles or co-insurance payments of 20% to 25% of the predetermined charge that the patient pays, and the insurer pays the balance. A provider who joins a PPO does not need to alter the manner of providing care and continues to treat and bill the patients on a fee-for-service basis. When a patient covered under a PPO plan comes for treatment, the physician treats the patient and bills the PPO.

Technically PPOs are not HMOs, but they do have more patient care management than regular indemnity insurance plans. PPOs furnish their subscribers with a list of member-providers from which subscribers can receive healthcare at PPO rates. Rates are quite often lower than those charged to non-PPO patients. If a patient goes to a physician who is not in the PPO network, the out-of-pocket cost is higher.

CRITICAL THINKING APPLICATION

The physicians in the practice where Ann works are not members of a PPO that is often used in their geographic area. Many patients are confused when they have to pay a larger out-of-pocket fee for their medical services. How can Ann explain the reason for these higher fees to patients?

Blue Cross/Blue Shield

BC/BS is America's oldest and largest system of independent health insurers. It began in 1929 when an executive at Baylor University in Dallas came up with a plan for teachers to budget for their future hospital bills. The teachers paid $6 a year into a fund and were, in turn, guaranteed 21 days of free hospital care. Within 10 years the American Hospital Association officially embraced the concept of prepaid hospital care and symbolized their new program with a blue cross.

At the same time, workers in lumber camps in the Northwest developed a similar approach to deal with frequent logging accidents. Camp owners provided medical care for workers by paying physicians monthly fees, for which a physician would provide all the care the workers needed. Physicians formed groups, or medical service bureaus, which were linked to specific employers. The bureaus were identified with a blue shield, and they too quickly expanded in popularity.

BC/BS offers incentive contracts to healthcare providers. If the provider chooses to sign a member contract, he or she becomes a **participating provider (PAR).** The healthcare provider then agrees to accept BC/BS reimbursement as payment in full for covered services. In turn, BC/BS agrees to reimburse providers directly and in a shorter time.

BC/BS identification (ID) cards (Figure 19-1) carry the subscriber's name and ID number with a three-character alphabetic prefix. The letters are an important part of the number and must be included on the claim form.

Medicaid

Title XIX of Public Law 89-97 under the Social Security Amendments of 1965 provides for agreements with states for assistance from the federal government in providing healthcare for the medically indigent. All states and the District of Columbia

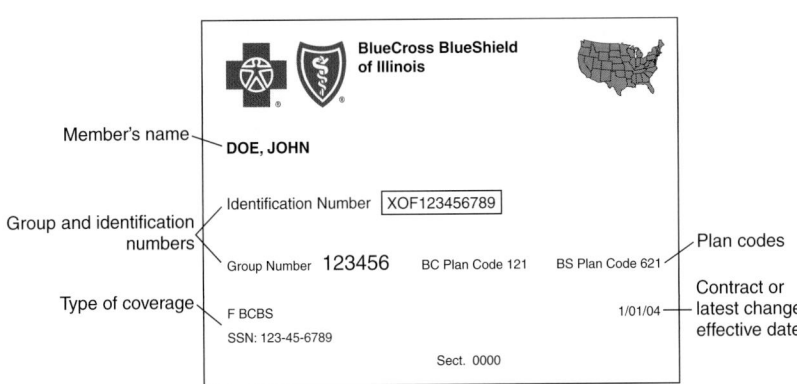

Figure 19-1 Blue Cross/Blue Shield identification card.

have Medicaid programs, but wide variations exist among these programs.

The federal government provides basic funding to the state, after which the states individually elect whether to provide funds for extension of benefits. The state determines the type and extent of medical care that will be covered within the minimum requirements established by the federal government. Some local areas and states are developing HMOs that serve only patients who qualify for Medicaid.

A physician may accept or decline to treat Medicaid patients. The physician who does accept Medicaid patients automatically agrees to accept Medicaid payment as payment in full for covered services. The patient cannot be billed for the difference between the Medicaid fee and the physician's normal fee. The patient can be billed for any services that are not covered by Medicaid. Eligibility for benefits is determined by the respective states.

Examples of individuals who qualify for benefits include the following:

- Persons who are medically needy
- Recipients of Aid to Families with Dependent Children (AFDC)
- Persons who receive Supplemental Security Income (SSI)
- Persons receiving certain types of federal and state aid
- For Qualified Medicare Beneficiaries (QMBs), Medicaid pays for Medicare Part B premiums, deductibles, and co-insurance for qualified low-income elderly
- Persons in institutions or receiving long-term care in nursing facilities and intermediate care facilities

Depending on the state in which the Medicaid is being administered, Medicaid recipients are identified with a benefits ID card (BIC), a monthly sticker, a label, or a letter, showing proof of eligibility. A BIC looks like a white credit card (Figure 19-2) and is verified by a point-of-service (POS) device similar to a credit card verification machine. The medical assistant must verify coverage each time the patient comes into the office regardless of the type of ID the recipient is issued.

Medicare

Medicare is a federal health insurance program for the following people:

- People 65 years of age and older
- People who are permanently disabled or blind

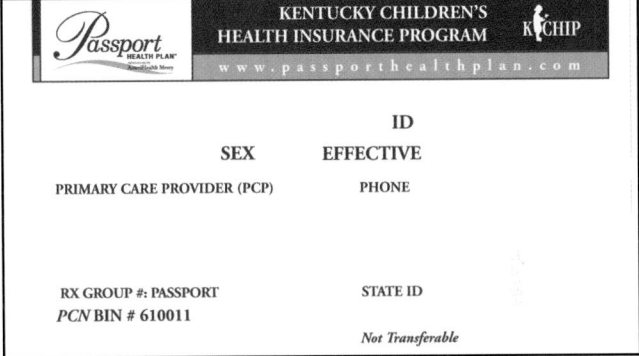

Figure 19-2 Medicaid benefits identification card.

- People receiving dialysis for permanent kidney failure or who have had a kidney transplant

On July 1, 1966, Medicare was established under the Social Security Administration as a national health insurance program for persons age 65 and older. Before Medicare only 50% of the nation's elderly had any health insurance. Today Medicare is the world's largest insurance program. It serves more than 38 million older and disabled Americans. The scope of coverage increased in 1973 to include disabled persons younger than age 65 receiving Social Security benefits, railroad retirees, and civil service retirees. This also included disabled workers of any age, disabled widows, disabled dependent widowers, adults disabled before age 18 whose parents are eligible or are retired on Social Security benefits, children and adults with end-stage renal disease, and living kidney donors (including all expenses related to the kidney transplant).

Medicare is administered by the Centers for Medicare and Medicaid Services (CMS), which was formerly known as the *Health Care Financing Administration (HCFA)*. CMS is a division of the Department of Health and Human Services (DHHS), and the Medicare program is regulated by laws enacted by Congress. Medicare has two parts that cover healthcare services: Part A and Part B.

Part A is hospital insurance. Retired people 65 years of age and older and people who receive monthly Social Security or railroad retirement checks are automatically enrolled for hospital insurance benefits and pay no premiums for this insurance. Part A covers the following:

- Inpatient hospital care
- Skilled nursing facilities
- Home healthcare
- Hospice services

Part A is financed with special contributions deducted from employed individuals' salaries, with matching contributions from their employers. These sums are collected, along with regular Social Security contributions, from wages and self-employment income earned during a person's working years. There is a deductible that a hospitalized patient must pay toward hospital expenses. Typically the deductible amount changes annually by congressional enactment.

Part B is medical insurance. Persons who are eligible for Part A are also eligible for Part B, but they must apply for this coverage and pay a monthly premium. Some federal employees and former federal employees who are not eligible for Social Security benefits and Part A may still enroll in Part B. Certain disabled persons younger than age 65 years are also eligible. Part B covers the following:

- Outpatient hospital care
- Durable medical equipment
- Physicians' services
- Other medical services

A patient with Medicare Part B must meet an annual deductible before benefits become available, after which Medicare pays 80% of the covered, or allowed, benefits. Usually the physician accepts assignment of benefits for Medicare patients and is paid directly. In these cases the physician must accept the payment that Medicare allows and bills the patient for 20% of the charge allowed by Medicare. If the physician does not accept assignment, the patient must pay the entire bill (which cannot be greater than the limit set by Medicare for nonparticipating physicians), and the patient will receive a reimbursement check directly from Medicare.

Medicare health insurance cards (Figure 19-3) typically show nine numbers with a suffix of one or two alphabetic characters that denote the patient's status, such as wage earner (A), spouse of a wage earner (B), widow (D), or other designations. The health insurance claim number (HICN or HIC#) also identifies whether a person has Part A alone or has both Part A and Part B insurance. A patient who is issued a Medicare card with a claim number ending with the letter A will have the same HICN as his or her Social Security number. A person whose Social Security number is different from his or her issued HICN will have a suffix of B or D.

Many Medicare enrollees also carry private supplemental insurance that pays the deductible and the 20% copayment not covered by Medicare. If the supplemental policy pays the deductible and the 20% copayment, it is called a *Medigap policy.*

In 1997 a new option was added, called Medicare+Choice. This program is commonly referred to as *Part C,* although the Medicare administration does not label it as such. Medicare+Choice offers expanded benefits for a fee through private health insurance programs such as HMOs and PPOs that have contracts with Medicare. In 2004, as a result of congressional action to reform Medicare, Medicare+Choice was renamed Medicare Advantage.

In 2006, drug and prescription benefits were added, which are Part D of Medicare. In Medicare Part D, the Medicare recipient has the option to choose, at a reduced cost, a prescription drug plan that pays for prescription drugs with just a small copayment by the patient. Everyone with Medicare can get this coverage that may help lower prescription drug costs and help protect against higher costs in the future. Medicare Prescription Drug Coverage is insurance that is provided by private companies. Beneficiaries choose the drug plan and pay a monthly premium. Like other insurance, if a beneficiary decides not to enroll in a drug plan when they are first eligible, they may pay a penalty if they choose to join later.

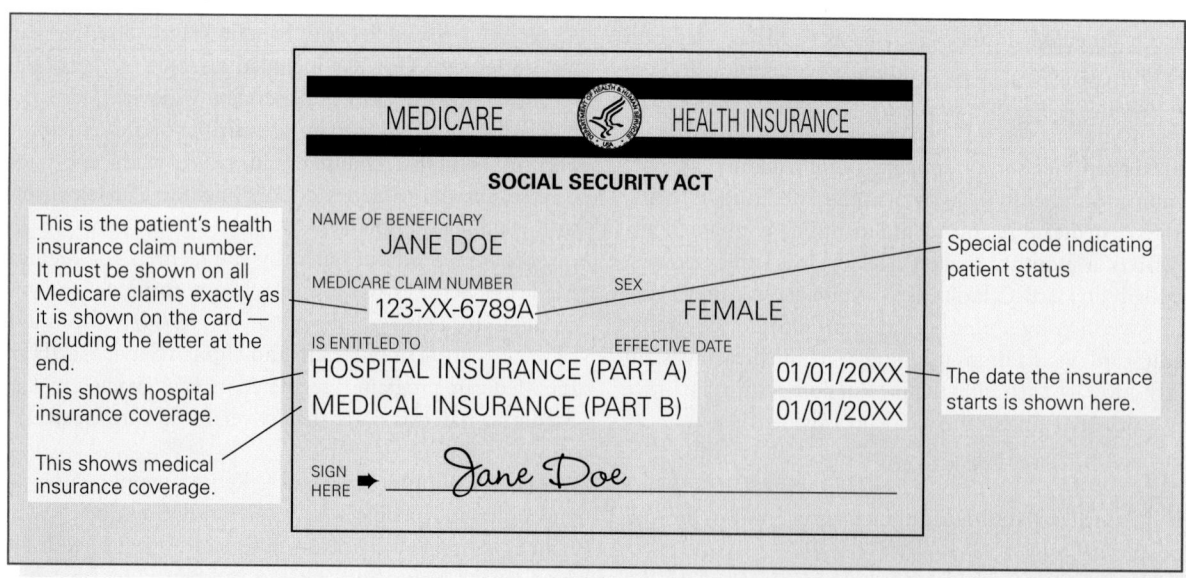

Figure 19-3 Medicare health identification card. (From Fordney MT: Insurance handbook for the medical office, ed 8, St Louis, 2004, Saunders.)

TRICARE (Formerly CHAMPUS)

TRICARE is the Department of Defense and the military's comprehensive healthcare program for family members of active duty personnel, military retirees and their eligible family members under the age of 65, and survivors of all uniformed services. Before January 1994, this program was known as *CHAMPUS*, created in 1966 under Public Law 89-614.

The TRICARE program is managed by the military in partnership with civilian hospitals and clinics. It is designed to expand access to healthcare, ensure high-quality care, and promote medical readiness. All military hospitals and clinics are part of the TRICARE program and offer high-quality healthcare at low costs to plan users.

To be eligible for TRICARE, an individual must be a TRICARE or CHAMPVA (covered later in this chapter) recipient, be entitled to retired, retainer, or equivalent pay, and be listed in the Defense Department's Defense Enrollment Eligible Reporting System (DEERS), which is a computerized database that lists all active and retired service members. Coverage is also available for a TRICARE-eligible spouse under age 65, and dependent, unmarried children under age 21, or age 23 if in college full-time. Eligible spouses and children of active-duty service members may enroll, as may TRICARE-eligible widows, widowers, and certain ex-spouses (who have not remarried).

There are three choices under TRICARE:
- TRICARE Prime: The Department of Defense's managed care option, similar to a civilian HMO
- TRICARE Extra: A preferred provider network option
- TRICARE Standard: A traditional fee-for-service option formerly known as *CHAMPUS*

Figure 19-4 illustrates the eligibility requirements and benefits of the three plans.

CHAMPVA

In 1973 a program similar to TRICARE was established for the spouses and dependent children of veterans suffering total, permanent, service-connected disabilities and for surviving spouses and dependent children of veterans who had died as a result of service-related disabilities. This program, CHAMPVA, is a health benefits program in which the Department of Veterans Affairs (VA) shares with eligible beneficiaries the cost of certain healthcare services and supplies. After eligibility for CHAMPVA has been determined and ID cards issued, the insured persons may obtain covered services and supplies from any provider who is appropriately licensed or certified to perform the services offered. Exceptions include certain mental health categories and freestanding ambulatory surgical centers.

Workers' Compensation

All state legislatures have passed workers' compensation laws to protect wage earners against the loss of wages and the cost of medical care resulting from occupational accident or disease. State laws differ as to the classes of employees included and the benefits provided.

No state's workers' compensation laws cover all employees. However, if a patient says that he or she was injured in the workplace or is suffering from a work-associated illness, the medical assistant should check with the patient's employer to verify the insurance coverage.

Compensation benefits include medical care benefits, weekly income replacement benefits for temporary disability, permanent disability settlements, and survivor benefits when applicable. The provider of service (e.g., doctor, hospital, therapist) accepts the workers' compensation payment as payment in full and does not bill the patient. Time limitations are set for the prompt reporting of workers' compensation cases. The employee is obligated to promptly notify the employer; the employer, in turn, must notify the insurance company and must refer the employee to a source of medical care.

In some states the employer and insurance company have the right to select the physician treating the patient. In essence, the purpose of workers' compensation laws is to provide prompt medical care to an injured or ill worker so that the person may be restored to health and return to full earning capacity in as short a time as possible.

Disability Programs

Disability income insurance is a form of health insurance that provides periodic payments to an individual to replace income (actual or presumed) when a sickness, injury, or disability that is not a work-related condition results in the insured being unable to work. A disability insurance policy can be obtained through employer-sponsored and/or government-funded programs, or private policies can be purchased through a commercial insurance company.

COMMERCIAL INSURANCE

Many people are covered by health insurance issued by private (commercial) insurance companies, such as Aetna, Connecticut General, Metropolitan, and Prudential. Physicians and medical societies control neither the premiums paid nor the benefits received from such policies. For traditional types of policies, payment is normally made to the subscriber unless the subscriber or insured has authorized that payment be made directly to the physician.

VERIFICATION OF INSURANCE BENEFITS

It is important to verify insurance benefits before providing services to patients. To verify benefits, the following steps should be taken (Procedure 19-2):
- When a patient calls for an appointment, identify what type of insurance the patient has or what managed care organization the patient belongs to.
- When the patient arrives for the appointment, photocopy both sides of the patient's ID card (because copayments or amounts to be paid may appear on the back for hospital, office, and the emergency department).
- Contact the insurance carrier to verify that the patient is eligible for benefits, and determine the basic benefits,

ADFM = active duty family members
RFMS = retirees, family members and survivors

Benefit and Coverage Chart

Outpatient Services	Programs and Beneficiary Costs					
Program and Classification	**Tricare Prime**		**Tricare Extra**		**Tricare Standard**	
	ADFM	**RFMS**	**ADFM**	**RFMS**	**ADFM**	**RFMS**
Annual Enrollment Fee* (per fiscal year)	None	$230/person $460/family	None ⟶		None ⟶	
Annual Deductible (per fiscal year 10/1 to 9/30) (applied to outpatient services before cost-share is determined)	None (except when using Point-of-Service option)		E-4 and below $50/person $100/family E-5 and above $150/person $300/family	$150/person $300/family	E-4 and below $50/person $100/family E-5 and above $150/person $300/family	$150/person $300/family
Physician Services	None	$12	15% of contracted fee	20% of contracted fee	20% of maximum allowable charge	25% of maximum allowable charge
Ancillary Services (certain radiology, laboratory, & cardiac services)	None ⟶	(RFMS may have $12 copay if test provided independent of office visit)				
Ambulance Services	None	$20				
Home Health Services	None	$12				
Family Health Services	None	$12				
Durable Medical Equipment (greater than $100)	None	20% cost-share				
Emergency Services (network and non-network)	None	$30 copayment				
Outpatient Behavioral Health (limitations apply)	None	$25 copayment $17 group visits				
Immunizations (for required overseas travel)	None	Not covered		Not covered		Not covered
Ambulatory Surgery (same day)	None	$25 copayment (applied to facility charges only)	$25 copayment for hospital charges	20% of contracted fee	$25 copayment for hospital charges	*Professional:* 25% of maximum allowable charge *Facility:* 25% of maximum allowable charge OR billed charges, whichever is less
Eye Examinations (limitations apply)	None	Clinical Preventive Service	15% of contracted fee	Not covered	20% of maximum allowable charge	Not covered
Prescription Drugs– Network Pharmacy	$3 copayment for each 30-day supply of **generic** medication $9 copayment for each 30-day supply of **brand name** medication					
Prescription Drugs– National Mail Order Pharmacy	$3 copayment for each 90-day supply of **generic** medication $9 copayment for each 90-day supply of **brand name** medication (Note: if the beneficiary has primary insurance that covers presciption medication, the beneficiary is not eligible for the mail order pharmacy benefit)					
Prescription Drugs– Non-network Pharmacy	$9 or 20% of total cost (whichever is greater) plus deductible					

*No enrollment fee for those who are eligible for Medicare (enrolled in Part B) on the basis of disability or end-stage renal disease

NOTE: TRICARE Prime Remote–benefits are similar to TRICARE Prime program; however, ADSMs have no copayment costs-share or deductible

Program for Persons with Disabilities–no deductible; monthly cost-share varies from $25 to $250, depending on sponsor's rank

Figure 19-4 TRICARE plans: eligibility and benefits. (From Fordney MT: *Insurance handbook for the medical office*, ed 8, St Louis, 2004, Saunders.)

PROCEDURE 19-2

Apply Managed Care Policies and Procedures: Perform Verification of Eligibility and Benefits

<u>CAAHEP COMPETENCY:</u> 3.a.(3)(a)
<u>ABHES COMPETENCY:</u> 3.t

GOAL: *Confirm patient's insurance is in effect and determine what benefit and exclusions are covered.*

EQUIPMENT and SUPPLIES

- Patient record
- Precertification form
- Patient's insurance information
- Telephone and fax machine
- Pen

PROCEDURAL STEPS

1. When a patient calls for an appointment, identify the patient's insurance plan or managed care organization.
   <u>PURPOSE:</u> To prepare for and begin gathering required information to perform both insurance verification and insurance claim completion procedures.

2. At the time of the appointment, obtain and photocopy both sides of the patient's insurance ID card(s).
   <u>PURPOSE:</u> To ensure the correct ID, group, and policy numbers are obtained, as well as the name, address, and phone number of the insurance carrier(s).

3. Complete the patient portion of the Verification of Eligibility and Benefit form, including demographic and insurance information for the patient, and the contact information for the insurance plan. Complete one form for each of the patient's insurances.

PURPOSE: To document the information needed to perform the verification of eligibility and benefits. This form will later be filed in the patient's insurance record.

4. Contact the insurance carrier(s) by phone to a) verify that the patient is eligible for benefits and the insurance is in effect; b) determine the basic benefits, exclusions, or non-covered services of the insurance plan; c) determine if there are deductibles, co-payments or any other out-of-pocket expenses the patient is responsible for paying; d) determine if preauthorization is required for referrals to specialists or for any procedures and/or services.
   <u>PURPOSE:</u> To confirm the insurance is in effect, and to determine what benefits, preauthoritizations, deductibles and/or out-of pocket expenses the patient is responsible for.

5. Obtain the name, title, and phone number of the person contacted.
   <u>PURPOSE:</u> To identify and document the name of the individual providing the benefits and eligibility information, and to have as a reference if additional questions arise.

6. Document the information collected in the patient's medical record and on the Verification of Eligibility and Benefits form.

---

exclusions or non-covered services, and whether pre-authorization is required for referrals to specialists or for any procedures and/or services. Obtain the name, title, and phone number of the person contacted.

- Document the information collected in the patient's medical record and on a Verification of Benefits form.
- Give the patient a letter to read and sign, outlining the plan requirements and possible restrictions or non-covered items.
- When referrals are required, explain the procedure to the patient so it is understood that without the referral, it is the patient's responsibility to pay for the physician's services.
- Collect any copayments or deductibles.

PRECERTIFICATION AND PREAUTHORIZATION

Most insurance companies require precertification or preauthorization, usually within 24 hours, when a patient is going to be hospitalized or undergo certain procedures. In addition, most managed care systems require preauthorization for a patient to be referred to a specialist or even for certain laboratory tests or other procedures. Insurance claims for payment will be denied if proper authorization is not obtained.

It is standard when a new patient makes an appointment to ask what type of insurance the patient has and to collect the patient and insured's personal, employment, and insurance information on a patient registration form. The patient registration form will be discussed further in Chapter 20. If the patient belongs to an HMO, the medical assistant should check that plan contract for precertification or preauthorization requirements. Typically, only HMOs require preauthorization (precertification); however, it is recommended that the need for preauthorization be obtained during the verification of eligibility and benefits for all insurance carriers. The following lists the information that should be obtained and recorded on the preauthorization form (Figure 19-5) before the contact with the insurance carrier is made.

- Patient name, address, phone number and identification number(s)
- Provider name, address, phone number, and provider identification number (PIN)
- Plan name, address, and contact person
- Telephone number (or numbers) of contact person and fax number
- Preliminary diagnosis
- Planned surgery, diagnostic test or reason for referring patient to a specialist

Mary Jo Smith
College Clinic
4567 Broad Avenue, WH
Telephone No.: (555) 486-9002
Fax No.:(555) 487-8976

MANAGED CARE PLAN AUTHORIZATION REQUEST

☐ Health Net   ☐ Met Life
☐ Pacificare   ☐ Travelers
☐ Secure Horizons ☐ Pru Care
☐ Other

Member/Group No.: 54098XX

**TO BE COMPLETED BY PRIMARY CARE PHYSICIAN
OR OUTSIDE PROVIDER**

Patient Name: Louann Campbell   Date: 7-14-20XX

☐ Male   ☐ Female   Birthdate: 4-7-1952   Home Telephone Number: (555) 450-1666

Address: 2516 Encina Avenue, Woodland Hills, XY 12345-0439

Primary Care Physician: Gerald Practon, MD   Provider ID #:   TC 14021

Referring Physician: Gerald Practon, MD   Provider ID #:   TC 14021

Referred to: Raymond Skeleton, MD   Office Telephone Number: (555) 486-9002

Address: 4567 Broad Avenue, Woodland Hills, XY 12345

Diagnosis Code: 724.2   Diagnosis   Low back pain

Diagnosis Code: 722.10   Diagnosis   Sciatica

Treatment Plan: Orthopedic consultation and evaluation of lumbar spine; R/O herniated disc L4-5

Authorization requested for: ☐ Consult Only   ☐ Treatment Only   ☐ Consult/Treatment
                               ☐ Consult/Procedure/Surgery   ☐ Diagnostic Tests

Procedure Code: 99244   Description: New patient consultation

Procedure Code: Description:

Place of service: ☒ Office ☐ Outpatient ☐ Inpatient ☐ Other   Number of Visits: 1

Facility: Length of Stay:

List of potential future consultants (i.e., anesthetists, surgical assistants or medical/surgical):

Physician's Signature: *Gerald Practon, MD*

TO BE COMPLETED BY PRIMARY CARE PHYSICIAN

PCP Recommendations: See above   PCP Initials: *GP*

Date eligibility checked: 7-14-20XX   Effective Date: 1-15-20XX

TO BE COMPLETED BY UTILIZATION MANAGEMENT

Authorized: Auth. No.   Not Authorized

Deferred: Modified:

Comments:

Figure 19-5 Sample preauthorization (referral) form.

- Name, address, phone number of facility or specialist
- Copayment amount or deductible
- Hospital benefits for inpatient and outpatient surgery
- Participating hospitals, radiology service providers, laboratories, and physicians

Once the information is collected it should be faxed to the insurance company. In case of an emergency, the authorization may be obtained by phone; however, the form should be faxed as soon as possible afterward. The form will be faxed back to the provider from the insurance carrier with the authorization number and other vital information as described in the next section. The **birthday rule** determines the primary insurance for those who are covered by more than one policy.

Obtaining preauthorization for referrals or certain procedures and services is required. Typically, the PCP or "gatekeeper" is responsible for obtaining the authorization. A gatekeeper

PROCEDURE 19-3

Apply Managed Care Policies and Procedures: Perform Preauthorization (Precertification) and/or Referral

<u>CAAHEP COMPETENCY:</u> 3.a.(3)(a)
<u>ABHES COMPETENCY:</u> 3.u

GOAL: *Using the information in the case study, obtain precertification from a patient's HMO for requested services or procedures.*

EQUIPMENT and SUPPLIES

- Patient record
- Precertification form
- Patient's insurance information
- Telephone and fax machine
- Pen

PROCEDURAL STEPS

1. Assemble the necessary documents and equipment.
2. Examine the patient record, and determine the service or procedure for which preauthorization is being requested, including, if applicable, the specialist's name and phone number and the reason for the request.
   <u>PURPOSE:</u> To correctly complete the required form for gaining authorization from the patient's insurance carrier for the specified treatment.
3. Complete the referral form, providing all pertinent information requested.

<u>PURPOSE:</u> To document for the insurance carrier the patient demographic and insurance information, the physician's identification information, and either the diagnosis and planned procedure or treatment, or the name and contact information of the physician to whom the patient is being referred.

4. Proofread the completed form.
   <u>PURPOSE:</u> To ensure the accuracy of the information.
5. Fax the completed form to the patient's insurance carrier.
   <u>PURPOSE:</u> To inform the insurance carrier of the patient's medical condition; to request preauthorization for the requested treatment; to request a verification number; and to confirm the specific number of physical therapy sessions, or to obtain authorization for referral of the patient to a specialist.
6. Place a copy of the returned, completed approval form in the patient's medical record.

---

can be a PCP, a general or family practitioner, an internist, a pediatrician, and in some instances an obstetrician or a gynecologist.

Referral is a term used in managed care when a patient is referred from a PCP to a specialist. When completing a referral form, it is imperative that all necessary information be included (Procedure 19-3). A referral can take from a few minutes to a few days to be reviewed and approved or denied. The three types of referral are as follows:

- A regular referral usually takes 3 to 10 working days for review and approval. This type of referral is used when a patient has not responded to a PCP's treatment and/or medication and the physician believes that the patient must see a specialist to continue treatment.
- An urgent referral will usually take about 24 hours for approval. This type of referral is used when an urgent situation occurs but is not life-threatening.
- A STAT referral can be approved by telephone immediately after faxing it to the utilization review department. A STAT referral is used in an emergency situation as indicated by the physician, such as life-or-death situations, miscarriage, loss of limb, or other conditions of similar magnitude. Usually the physician will refer the patient by telephone and will fax the information with the referral afterward.

A regular referral is the most common and can be inconvenient for the patient. Most managed care plans require contacting the member services department to check the status

of a referral. A cardinal rule is to never tell the patient that the referral has been approved unless you have a hard copy of the authorization. *Authorization* is a term used in managed care for an approved referral. A referral becomes an authorization after it is reviewed by utilization management and/or the medical director and has been approved. When a referral is approved, the PCP's office will receive a copy of the authorization by mail or fax. Always review the authorization thoroughly. The patient will receive a letter with an authorization number and the approved services. The patient must present the authorization to the specialist's office receptionist on the day the services will be provided. An authorization provides the following information to both the referring PCP and the specialist:

1. An authorization code, which may be alphabetic, numeric, or alphanumeric.
2. The date on which it was received by utilization management, the date on which it was approved, and the expiration date.
   a. An authorization is good for 60 days.
   b. If services are provided after the expiration date, the services will be denied. If this happens, you need to contact utilization management or member services, ask for an extension, and answer a few questions. Sometimes it is necessary to involve the patient and/or the specialist's office.
   c. If the authorization expires and services have not been provided, an extension may be requested. Utilization

management will change the expiration date and will fax a copy to the PCP and specialist or will generate a new authorization with a new number.

3. A diagnosis code.

4. The name, address, and telephone number of the contracted specialist where services will be provided. Sometimes the PCP will refer the patient to a specialist but will not receive approval for that specialist and must get approval for another. Always be sure that any specialist to whom the physician refers a patient is contracted with the same managed care plan as the PCP.

5. The comments section is the most critical area of a referral, because this area will designate what services are approved.

   a. It includes the specified number of authorized visits to the specialist.

   b. An authorization may be issued for (1) evaluation only, (2) evaluation and treatment plan, (3) evaluation and biopsy, (4) evaluation and one injection, etc.

   c. When authorization for only an evaluation and/or treatment plan is given, the medical assistant must inform the patient that there will not be any treatment—only an evaluation and/or a treatment plan.

If a referral is denied because of insufficient information or no medical necessity, the PCP's office will be notified. Some medical groups will notify both the PCP and the patient. When the PCP's office provides the utilization management committee with the necessary information, the referral will be reviewed again for approval.

Managed care changes on a day-to-day basis. To compete within this market, some insurance companies have added a benefit that will allow a member or patient to self-refer (meaning an authorization is not required to see a specialist). Many plans for senior citizens now have a **self-referral** and a copayment as well as some other insurance coverage. The procedure for obtaining a self-referral is essentially the same as for a provider of service. An authorization form is completed by the patient or with the assistance of the referred provider and faxed to the insurance company for approval.

CRITICAL THINKING APPLICATION

Many private carriers and managed health plans have precertification or preauthorization requirements. How can Ann explain the rationale of preapproval to inquiring patients?

FEE SCHEDULES

A healthcare practitioner has three commodities to sell—time, judgment, and services. In every case the healthcare practitioner must place an estimate on the value of these services. Fees for medical procedures and services differ from office to office based on the type of practice and the needs of the facility. The physician or physicians establishing the practice normally set the fees for procedures and services. In the past most physicians worked on a fee-for-service basis (e.g., patients were charged for the provider's service based on each individual service performed).

In recent years **third-party payors** (particularly government and managed healthcare organizations) have greatly influenced what healthcare providers can charge by establishing what is referred to as the *allowable charge*. The allowable charge is the maximum that third-party payors will pay for a particular procedure or service (Procedure 19-4).

When healthcare providers establish a fee schedule, other factors influence what the charge for a particular procedure or service can be; these factors include the relative value scale (RVS) and the RBRVS.

Relative Value Scale

The RVS was pioneered by the California Medical Association in 1956 to help physicians establish rational, relative fees. Other states soon followed suit. Hundreds of the most commonly performed procedures were compiled, given procedure numbers similar to those in the AMA's Current Procedural Terminology (CPT) code list, and assigned a unit value. The assigned unit value represented the value of that procedure in relation to other procedures commonly performed. Although no monetary value was placed on the units, many insurance companies used the RVS to determine benefits by applying a conversion factor to assign a monetary value to the unit value. In 1978 the Federal Trade Commission (FTC) interpreted the California RVS as a fee-setting instrument and prohibited its publication and distribution. The FTC was attempting to make medical practice more competitive by ruling against the setting of fees and by encouraging physicians to advertise.

Resource-Based Relative Value Scale

As discussed earlier in this chapter, CMS developed the first comprehensive RBRVS-based fee schedule, which was adopted by Medicare in 1992. The RBRVS-based fee schedule adjusts fees for differences in resources used to provide each service. The amount of resources required to perform a service is determined through the use of relative value units (RVUs) assigned to the CPT codes developed by the AMA. This system was implemented to standardize payment with an adjustment for overhead costs in different geographic areas. Since Medicare's introduction of RBRVS, most third-party payors have adopted similar approaches in developing their fees.

DEDUCTIBLES AND CO-INSURANCE

Many types of health insurance plans, such as indemnity, managed care, and Medicare, require a deductible and co-insurance amount that the patient must pay out of pocket. These plans typically have an annual deductible amount the patient must pay before the plan pays anything. In addition, members usually must also pay a percentage of each charge, which is called *co-insurance*. Most indemnity plans have an annual "out-of-pocket limit" on the amount members must pay for co-insurance payments. This type of plan takes the major expense out of medical bills and helps keep premium costs down.

PROCEDURE 19-4

Apply Third-Party Guidelines

<u>CAAHEP COMPETENCY:</u> 3.a(3)(b)
<u>ABHES COMPETENCY:</u> 8.c

GOAL: *To ensure that claims are processed quickly and result in the highest allowable reimbursement.*

EQUIPMENT and SUPPLIES

- Managed care contracts
- Managed care handbooks
- Clerical supplies
- Forms from managed care organizations
- Claim forms

PROCEDURAL STEPS

1. Determine the patient's health insurance plan.
   <u>PURPOSE:</u> To bill the correct health insurance plan for services rendered.

2. Review the rules and regulations that govern that particular organization.
   <u>PURPOSE:</u> To be sure that the claim is accurate according to the guidelines in place for the patient's policy.

3. Make certain that a signature is on file for the patient.
   <u>PURPOSE:</u> The signature authorizes the provider to release medical information to the insurance carrier and authorizes the carrier to pay the provider directly.

4. Determine the procedures and services that are to be billed on the claim.

5. Determine if all procedures and services to be billed are covered by the health insurance plan.
   <u>PURPOSE:</u> Procedures and services that are not covered should not be billed on the health insurance claim form; the patient must pay for those services.

6. Make sure that the patient is aware of any procedures that will not be covered by the health insurance plan.

7. Pay close attention to the blocks on the insurance claim form that are designated "for local use.".
   <u>PURPOSE:</u> These blocks are designed to include information particular to certain policies.

8. Determine that all procedures and services that are billed on the claim pertain to one or more of the diagnoses listed.
   <u>PURPOSE:</u> All of the procedures and services must relate to one or more diagnoses to be deemed medically necessary.

9. Submit the claim to the correct address or clearinghouse.

	Column A	Column B
Total charge	$10,000	$20,000
Deductible (paid by Mrs. Jones)	(500)	(500)
5% (Mrs. Jones' portion)	(500)	(500)
Total amount paid by Mrs. Jones	$900	$1000
Total amount paid by insurance	$9000	$19,000

Figure 19-6 Calculation of deductible and co-insurance.

For example, Mrs. Jones' plan has a $500 deductible, after which the insurance company pays 95% of all charges, which leaves Mrs. Jones with a 5% co-insurance expense in addition to the deductible. In addition, she has a $1000 out-of-pocket expense maximum for which she is responsible, which means that once Mrs. Jones has paid $1000 total, the insurance company then pays 100% of any balance remaining. She has incurred a $10,000 charge for a cardiac surgery performed by her physician. Column A in Figure 19-6 shows that Mrs. Jones' total out-of-pocket expense is $1000. She paid the $500 deductible, and 5% of 10,000, or an additional $500. The insurance company then paid the remaining balance of $9000. Column B in Figure 19-6 shows that the cardiac surgery in this instance was $20,000. Mrs. Jones' total out-of-pocket expense remains $1000, therefore, in this instance the insurance company is responsible for payment of the balance of $19,000. Because her maximum

out-of-pocket expense according to the plan described is $1000, even though the charges were doubled, she still only pays the $1000 total out-of-pocket expense.

With Medicare and some other plans, a limit is placed on the amount that will be reimbursed for any procedure or service. This limit is called an *allowable amount*. The allowable amount can be all or part of a charge for a service or procedure. For example, for a level I office visit if the provider typically charges $80, the insurance company benefit allowable amount might only be $60. Depending on the contract between the provider and insurance carrier, the provider will either write-off the $20 difference or pass the non-allowed portion of the charge on to the guarantor for payment. The contracts between the physician and provider vary greatly, it is important for the medical assistant to examine the explanation of benefits from the insurance carrier closely, and to be knowledgeable about the contract provisions between the provider of service and all insurance carriers the provider uses.

CRITICAL THINKING APPLICATION

An elderly patient comes to the office complaining that Medicare did not pay her bill in full. "Medicare is supposed to pay 80% of all of my bills and I have already paid my portion," she insists.

■ What information does Ann need to get to the bottom of this problem?

■ How can she explain situations like this to patients?

PROCEDURE 19-5

Apply Managed Care Policies and Procedures: Perform Deductible, Co-Insurance, and Allowable Amount Calculations

<u>CAAHEP COMPETENCY:</u> 3.a.(3)(a)
<u>ABHES COMPETENCY:</u> 3.t

GOAL: *To calculate the patient's out-of-pocket expense or amount to be billed to a secondary insurance carrier, and to determine what amounts are to be written off and/or passed on to the patient for payment.*

EQUIPMENT and SUPPLIES

- Explanation of benefits (EOB) form (or explanation of Medicare benefits (EOMB) form or remittance advice (RA) form OR Verification of eligibility and benefits form
- Patient accounts receivable ledger
- Calculator
- Pen
- Paper

PROCEDURAL STEPS

1. Assemble the required materials and equipment.
   <u>REMEMBER:</u> Deductibles and co-insurance are generally deducted from the total charge for services rendered; however, depending on the policies and procedures of the provider they can be calculated for each individual charge. Allowable amounts are almost always deducted from an individual charge.

2. Using the EOB, EOMB, and/or the RA and/or the Verification of Eligibility and Benefits form; and the patient accounts receivable ledger:
   - Write down the total charge from the EOB and/or the patient accounts receivable ledger.
   - Subtract the deductible amount from the total charge. If the deductible exceeds the total amount, subtract only that amount of the deductible that equals the total charge, and stop—do not continue with the other steps. Proceed to the other steps only after all of the patient's deductible has been paid.
   <u>PURPOSE:</u> To calculate and record the appropriate amount of deductible that must be met (and paid) by the patient according to the terms of his or her insurance policy.

3. If it is determined that all of the patient's deductible has been met, proceed by then identifying the co-insurance amount that the patient must pay (e.g., 20%).
   - Multiply this amount (e.g., 20%) by the total charge.
   - Subtract the sum from the total charge balance.

<u>PURPOSE:</u> To calculate and record the appropriate amount of co-insurance that must be met (and paid) by the patient according to the terms of his or her insurance policy.

4. Record the deductible and, if applicable, co-insurance amount(s) on separate lines in the patient balance due column of the patient's account receivable ledger. The sum becomes the patient's responsibility, or if the patient has a secondary insurance carrier, the sum can be billed to the secondary insurance carrier.
   <u>PURPOSE:</u> To maintain a current balance and audit trail on the patient accounts receivable ledger and, when appropriate, to submit a statement to the patient for payment and/or submit a claim to a secondary insurance company.
   <u>NOTE:</u> If there is an allowable amount shown on the EOB, EOMB, or RA which is less than the amount of either the total charge or the individual charge for the date of service, proceed to steps 5 and 6. Otherwise, stop here.

5. Subtract the allowable amount of each individual charge from the actual (billed) charge.

6. Record the difference either in the adjustments or patient balance column.
   - If the provider of service writes off the difference either as a courtesy, hardship adjustment, or as part of the contract the provider has with the insurance company, the amount is recorded in the adjustments column.
   - If the patient is responsible for paying the difference between the actual charge and the allowable amount, the amount is recorded in the patient balance column.
   <u>PURPOSE:</u> To adjust and reconcile the patient accounts receivable ledger and deduct the appropriate allowable amounts from the patient ledger; or, pass those amounts on to the patient for payment.

The steps for calculating deductible, co-insurance, and allowable amounts are illustrated in Procedure 19-5. Calculating deductibles, co-insurance, and allowable amounts is relatively simple. The deductible and co-insurance are subtracted from the total charge for the services and procedures. The sum becomes the patient's responsibility, or if the patient has a secondary insurance, it can be billed to the secondary insurance carrier. Deductibles and co-insurance are generally deducted from the total charge for services rendered; however, depending on the policies and procedures of the provider they can be calculated for each individual charge. Allowable amounts are almost always deducted from an individual charge. Using the example in Figure 19-7, if the allowable amount for Mrs. Jones' $10,000 cardiac surgery is $8500, the $1500 difference between the physician's charge and the allowed amount would either be written off or passed on to the patient as an out-of-pocket expense. In Figure 19-7, Column A, a line has been added to show the $8500 allowable amount and that $1500 has been

	Column A	Column B
Total charge	$10,000	$20,000
Deductible (paid by Mrs. Jones)	(500)	(500)
5% (Mrs. Jones' portion)	(500)	(500)
Allowable amount $8500	(1500)	
Allowable amount $8500 with write off		(1500)
Total amount paid by Mrs. Jones	$2500	$1000
Total amount paid by insurance	$7500	$17,500

Figure 19-7 Calculation of allowable amount.

billed to the patient. In Column B, the amount has been written off, or absorbed as a cost, by the provider. Notice, too, that the insurance carrier pays $1500 less for the cardiac surgery charge in Figure 19-7 than in Figure 19-6.

CRITICAL THINKING APPLICATION

Ann has been working with Max Carter, who is having coronary bypass surgery in one week. Discuss the possible differences in Max's coverage if he has Medicare, Medicaid, or commercial insurance.

UTILIZATION MANAGEMENT

Patient care review by healthcare professionals who do not provide the care is a necessary component of managed care to control costs. A **utilization review** committee reviews individual cases to make certain that medical care services are medically necessary and to study how providers use medical care resources. This committee reviews all physician referrals and cases of emergency department visits and urgent care. After review this department will either approve or deny the referral, so it is important to submit exact documentation and precise statements. The medical assistant should contact this department directly; it should never be left to the patient or covered member to contact this department.

THE *FEDERAL REGISTER*

The *Federal Register* is the official daily publication for rules, proposed rules, and notices of federal agencies and organizations, as well as Executive Orders and other presidential documents. Publications are sponsored by the Office of the *Federal Register* (OFR) and produced by the Government Printing Office (GPO). The system was established to regulate complex social and economic issues after it was decided that agencies and the general public needed a centralized filing and publication system to keep track of rules and regulations.

Medical assistants can use the *Federal Register* for researching rules and regulations governing health insurance and coding. The *Federal Register* website is user-friendly and can be accessed by typing http://fr.cos.com into the computer's browser (such as Internet Explorer or Netscape) address line and pressing Enter. The *Federal Register* search page will be accessed, and from

that point a search can be launched by topic, issue, or agency. Medical assistants may want to take a few minutes to browse this interesting website.

CRITICAL THINKING APPLICATION

- Ann has obtained precertification and knows the benefits that will be paid toward Max's bill. Discuss how to best explain insurance benefits, exclusions, co-insurance, deductibles, and allowable amounts to Max. Should the medical assistant explain other bills, such as those to the hospital and anesthesiologist?
- Suppose that Max has two different insurance policies in effect. Discuss the tasks and procedures associated with collecting information about his insurance. How does the medical assistant determine the primary carrier?

CLOSING COMMENTS

Understanding how insurance plans handle reimbursement of benefits is challenging for a patient as well as a medical assistant. However, it is important that patients understand how their insurance works. Many, especially elderly persons, believe that if they have health insurance, all charges for their healthcare will be covered, and they do not always understand the intricacies of deductibles, copayments, medical necessity, and allowable charges.

The responsibilities of a medical assistant include keeping the patient informed and answering questions as they arise. Often medical facilities will provide informational brochures to their patients that explain how health insurance and reimbursement works, giving definitions of some of the more common terms used in the insurance claims process. If patients are well advised and comfortable with insurance facts before treatment begins, the medical experience will go more smoothly, and collection of fees not covered by the carrier will be easier. The medical assistant must use good communication skills, patience, and tact when discussing third-party reimbursement issues with patients.

Throughout their careers, medical assistants must remember that an individual's medical record is personal and private. Conversations between patients and their healthcare providers (and staff) are considered privileged communication. Nearly every day a medical assistant is in a position to read and hear information of a private medical nature, and both the caregiver and the patient expect that this information will not leave the medical office.

Unauthorized release of medical information carries over into the insurance claims processing area. Even though the patient expects the insurance form to be filled out and submitted for payment, this cannot be done without proper written release. This medical release form should be kept in the patient's chart, and it should be updated on a regular basis.

Managed care has often been criticized by the news media. Some types of managed care can create a physician-patient barrier that did not exist during the fee-for-service era. An extra effort in human relations by the medical assistant can help to overcome this barrier and put the patient at ease.

SUMMARY OF SCENARIO

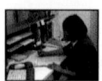

There is still a lot of information on health insurance to digest, but Ann is now much more comfortable with its concepts and no longer feels that understanding the various topics is impossible. Ann understands that there are many different types of insurance carriers, including federal and state programs, commercial carriers, health maintenance organizations, and preferred provider organizations, and that each of these programs offers different benefits, and has different requirements. Ann understands that the best way to remember all of the carriers and benefits offered is to keep an up-to-date manual or computer record that keeps track of addresses, phone numbers, and benefits information for each carrier. In addition, she's learned that failure to verify benefits

and eligibility, or authorization for referrals, treatments, or procedures, can result in a denial of payment for services rendered.

In addition, understanding how to calculate the deductibles, co-insurance, and allowed amounts for procedures and services benefits both the provider and patient. The provider's productivity, income, and losses can be easily tracked, and the patient can be educated as to the exact amounts he or she is responsible for paying.

Now that Ann understands the basics about health insurance, she can look forward to learning the procedure for completing insurance claim forms for various insurance carriers for reimbursement.

SUMMARY of LEARNING OBJECTIVES

1. Define, spell, and pronounce the terms listed in the vocabulary.
   * Spelling and pronouncing medical terms correctly adds credibility to the medical assistant. Knowing the definition of these terms promotes confidence in communication with patients and co-workers.
2. Discuss the purpose of health insurance.
   * Medical assistants should have an understanding of the purpose of health insurance. This will help in the workplace not only by facilitating their knowledge of the subject, but also in helping them educate patients. The trend for insurance policies to encourage preventive medicine can be appreciated.
3. Differentiate among the various types of insurance policies.
   * Insurance policies fall into many different categories and are available in many different forms. The ability to differentiate among the various types of insurance policies gives medical assistants a solid background in what is available on the market, what is included in each policy category, and the function of each. It is also important for medical assistants to understand and appreciate that there are still many people in this country who cannot afford and do not receive high-quality healthcare.
4. Explain the numerous classifications of insurance benefits available.
   * Insurance packages are often tailored to the needs of each individual or group, and the ways to combine benefits are limitless. Health insurance policies normally contain a combination of the different benefits discussed in this chapter (e.g., surgical, basic medical, and major medical).
5. Explain how insurance benefits are determined.
   * Benefits are determined and paid in one of several ways: indemnity schedules, service benefit plans, UCR fees, and relative value studies and scales. Medical assistants should become familiar with each of these methods and understand the ramifications of all.

6. Differentiate among the different types of managed care options.
   * *Managed care* is a broad term used to describe a variety of health plans developed to provide healthcare services at lower costs. When the medical assistant is employed in a medical facility, he or she will undoubtedly be working with many types of managed care plans. Therefore it is important to know the various types (e.g., HMO, IPA, and PPO) and understand how each one functions. Managed care has had both positive and negative effects on modern medicine. The medical assistant should be well informed about the managed care policies most frequently seen in the practice.
7. List and discuss other major third-party payors.
   * Other major third-party payors the medical assistant should become familiar with are BC/BS, Medicaid, Medicare, CHAMPVA, TRICARE, and workers' compensation. Medicare is the largest third-party insurer in the country, making high-quality healthcare affordable for the elderly and select other groups. Medicaid is another government-sponsored healthcare plan for individuals who qualify for these benefits. Workers' compensation covers employees who are injured or who become ill as a result of accidents or adverse conditions in the workplace. Disability programs reimburse individuals for monetary losses incurred as a result of an inability to work for reasons other than those covered under workers' compensation. The medical assistant should be familiar with the major plans that are presented in the practice.
8. Interpret the procedure for verifying insurance benefits.
   * Many problems can be prevented for both the patient and the medical office if the medical assistant develops and follows a procedure for verifying insurance benefits before services are rendered. This procedure includes gathering as much information as possible about the demographics of the patient and his or her insurance coverage. A pragmatic and tactful discussion with all new patients explaining the established

Continued

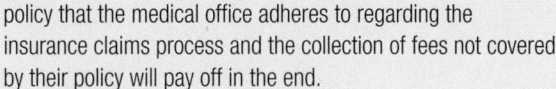

SUMMARY of LEARNING OBJECTIVES
Continued

policy that the medical office adheres to regarding the insurance claims process and the collection of fees not covered by their policy will pay off in the end.

9. Discuss the different types of fee schedules.
   - It is important for both the medical assistant and patients to realize that fees for medical procedures and services differ from office to office based on the type of practice and the needs of the facility. Until the advent of managed care, most physicians operated on a fee-for-service basis in which the provider would render his or her services and charge accordingly. In recent years, government and managed care organizations have greatly influenced what healthcare providers can charge. Many third-party payors base reimbursements on what is referred to as the allowable charge. Other fee schedule types include the RVS and the RBRVS.

10. Obtain managed care referrals and precertifications.
    - Obtaining precertifications and making referrals is a process that must be done according to the guidelines of the individual insurance companies. If uncertain about the procedure, always refer to the company's insurance manual or check the process online, if possible.

11. Perform eligibility and verification of benefits procedures.
    - Verification of insurance benefits is done to make certain that the physician will be reimbursed for his or her services performed on the patient. The process for verifying insurance benefits is outlined in Procedure 19-1.

12. Perform a preauthorization procedure.
    - Preauthorization helps the medical assistant to ensure that the physician will be paid for the services provided to the patient. The process for obtaining preauthorization or precertification is outlined in Procedure 19-2.

13. Demonstrate how insurance benefits are determined by calculating deductible and co-insurance payments.
    - Medical assistants should become proficient at calculating the amounts due to the physician, considering deductibles, copayments, and coinsurance amounts. The process for calculating insurance payments is outlined in Procedure 19-3.

CONNECTIONS

 Study Guide Connection: Go to Chapter 19 Study Guide. Read the Case Study and Workplace Applications and complete the assignments. Do online research for answers to the questions in the Internet Activities associated with third-party reimbursement.

 CD Connection: Go to the Medical Assisting Competency Challenge CD and do the training activities under Health Insurance Activities.

 Evolve Connection: For more information related to third-party reimbursement, go to evolve.elsevier.com/kinn and visit related weblinks for Chapter 19. Click on the Medical Assisting Exam Review and do the practice questions to sharpen your test-taking skills. To learn more about office software, do the exercises for the Altapoint demo that is on the CD.

The Health Insurance Claim Form 20

Carline A. Dalgleish
Alexandra Patricia Young

SCENARIO

The school where Machelle Van Cleve receives her medical assistant training offers an optional job-shadowing module. For her assignment she chose a nearby health center, where she observed the administrative responsibilities of the medical assistants employed in this multi-specialty practice. Machelle found that some of the offices were organized and efficient, whereas others lacked a structured routine, especially in the insurance department. Machelle, a detail-oriented person who enjoyed her studies related to billing and coding, heard numerous comments from employees in the administrative area related to the volumes of work in the billing offices. Her office manager explained that the mountainous paperwork was created as a result of managed care requirements, rejected claims needing further research, and inconsistencies in the demands of the various insurance companies. Machelle agreed that keeping up with the requirements and regulations of the many third-party payors and government entitlement programs must be an overwhelming task. She concluded that billing and reimbursement are at the heart of the medical facility, and the correct completion of insurance claim forms is central to the success of the practice. She realized that becoming familiar with the complexities of the insurance claims process would be challenging, but she was convinced that through education, organization, and dedication she could become a valuable employee and an advocate for the patients who needed her assistance in resolving issues related to their claims for reimbursement.

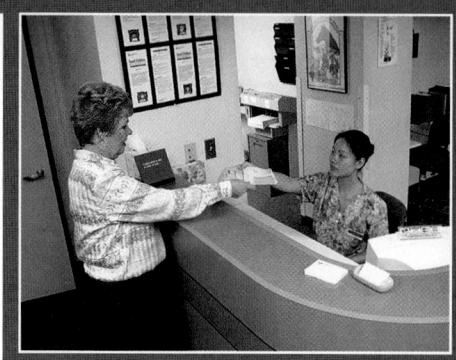

While studying this chapter, think about the following questions:

- What will Machelle find is one of the most important, and basic, tasks that must be done properly before even beginning the insurance claim preparation?
- Why was it important for Machelle to learn the specific insurance billing requirements of different insurance companies and third party payers?

- What has Machelle learned about the importance of auditing claims before they're sent to the insurance carrier for reimbursement?
- What does Machelle know about reimbursement and insurance claims followup?

LEARNING OBJECTIVES

1. Define, spell, and pronounce the terms listed in the vocabulary.
2. Discuss the differences between paper claims and electronic claims.
3. Understand the guidelines for completing the CMS-1500 claim form.
4. Explain how to complete each of the 33 blocks of the CMS-1500 claim form.
5. Differentiate between "clean" and "dirty" claims.
6. Discuss methods of preventing claim rejections.
7. Describe ways of checking the status of claims.
8. Gather information for use on insurance claim forms.
9. Complete a CMS 1500 insurance claim form appropriately for various federal, state and commercial third-party payors.

National Accreditation Competencies and Content

CAAHEP COMPETENCIES

Administrative
3.a.(3)(a). Apply managed care policies and procedures
3.a.(3)(b). Apply third-party guidelines
3.a.(3)(e). Complete insurance claim forms

General
3.c.(2)(a). Identify and respond to issues of confidentiality
3.c.(2)(b). Perform within legal and ethical boundaries
3.c.(2)(d). Document appropriately
3.c.(3)(a). Explain general office policies
3.c.(4)(c). Utilize computer software to maintain office systems

ABHES COMPETENCIES

Professionalism
1.b. Maintain confidentiality at all times
1.d. Be cognizant of ethical boundaries

Administrative Duties
3.d. Apply computer concepts for office procedures
3.t. Apply managed care policies and procedures
3.u. Obtain managed care referrals and pre-certification
3.w. Complete insurance claim forms
3.x. Use physician fee schedule

Legal Concepts
5.a. Determine needs for documentation and reporting
5.b. Document accurately

Instruction
7.a. Orient patients to office policies and procedures

VOCABULARY

assignment of benefits The transfer of the patient's legal right to collect benefits for medical expenses to the provider of those services, authorizing the payment to be sent directly to the provider.

audit A process done prior to claims submission to examine claims for accuracy and completeness. An audit can be performed manually or, if computer billing software is used, electronically.

audit trail The path left by a transaction when it has been completed; often referred to when tracking medical services used by patients or researching claims.

clean claims Insurance claim forms that have been completed correctly (no errors or omissions) and can be processed and paid promptly if they meets the restrictions on covered services and items.

clearinghouse A centralized facility to which insurance claims are transmitted. Clearinghouses separate, check, and redistribute claims electronically to various insurance carriers and may offer additional services to the physician.

direct billing A method of electronic claims submission where computer software allows a provider to submit an insurance claim directly to an insurance carrier for payment.

dirty claims Claims that contain errors or omissions which must be corrected and resubmitted to an insurance carrier in order to obtain reimbursement.

electronic claims Claims that are submitted to insurance processing facilities using a computerized medium, such as direct data entry, direct wire, dial-in telephone digital fax, or personal computer download or upload.

Electronic Data Interchange (EDI) The transfer of data back and forth between two or more entities using an electronic medium.

electronic (or digital) signature A scanned signature or other such mark that is accepted as proof of approval of and/or responsibility for the content of an electronic document.

employer identification number (EIN) The number used by the Internal Revenue Service that identifies a business or individual functioning as a business entity for income tax reporting.

incomplete claim A claim that is missing information and is returned to the provider for correction and resubmission. This is sometimes also called an invalid claim.

Intelligent Character Recognition (ICR) The electronic scanning of printed items as images and use of special software to recognize these images (or characters) as ASCII text for upload into a computer database.

National Provider Identifier (NPI) A lifetime number consisting of 10 digits that Medicare will use to replace the Provider Identification Number (PIN) and the Unique Physician Identification Number (UPIN).

paper claims Hard copies of insurance claims that have been completed and sent by surface mail.

provider Any company, individual, or group that provides medical, diagnostic, or treatment services to a patient.

Provider Identification Numbers (PINs) Numbers assigned to providers by a carrier for use in submission of claims.

rejected claims Claims returned unpaid to the provider for clarification of any question and that must be corrected before resubmission.

Unique Provider Identification Number (UPIN) A number

List continues on next page

List continued from previous page

assigned by fiscal intermediaries to identify providers on claims for services.

universal claim form The form developed by the Health Care Financing Administration (HCFA) (now known as the Centers for Medicare and Medicaid Services [CMS]) and approved by the AMA for use in submitting all government-sponsored claims. Also known as the CMS-1500 form.

Medical insurance means many things to many people. To some, it is a mound of paperwork. To others, it is a mass of confusion and regulations that seem to constantly change. To a patient with an illness or injury, health insurance helps defray the high costs associated with health care.

The **universal claim form,** originally called the *HCFA-1500,* was first developed in 1988 by the Health Care Financing Administration (HCFA) and approved for use by physicians and **providers** of outpatient services when submitting Medicare Part B claims for reimbursement. A provider is any health care worker who performs any diagnostic assessment or treatment in relation to a patient's illness or injury. In July 2001, HCFA was renamed the Centers for Medicare and Medicaid Services (CMS) and the claim form was renamed the CMS-1500. The form was subsequently adopted by almost all health insurance companies and third-party payors for use in submitting physician claims for reimbursement.

TYPES OF CLAIMS

A medical assistant may submit insurance claims to a third-party payor or an insurance carrier either on **hard copy** (paper) or electronically. Hard copy claims are insurance claims submitted manually, on paper, by surface mail (i.e., the U.S. postal service). **Electronic claims** are insurance claims that are submitted to an insurance carrier via electronic media, such as the internet. Most of today's computer programs generate claims internally from the information that is entered into the database. There are advantages and disadvantages associated with hard-copy or **paper claims** creation. The advantages include minimal start-up costs, because the forms are readily available through many vendors, and the ability to attach documentation explaining unusual circumstances that might affect reimbursement. The cost in time, labor, and postage is higher with paper claim submission, and reimbursement is much slower. Paper claims also require a lot of storage space.

Electronic Claims

Electronic claims are insurance claims that are transmitted over the Internet from the **provider** to the health insurance company. Most claims-processing software is designed to permit electronic claims generation, and with the standardization of the process that was mandated by the Health Insurance Portability and Accountability Act (HIPAA) security and privacy rules, it is far less complicated to send claims electronically. One of the mandates coming out of HIPAA includes the development of "transaction and code sets" for all insurance-related information sent electronically, including claim form submissions, claims status requests, and remittance (payment) processing. The transaction and code sets for the CMS-1500 electronic claims submission is called the **837P (HIPAA Health Care Claim: Professional).**

Electronic claims can be submitted in several ways. Claims can be transmitted directly to the insurance carrier, also known as **direct billing,** or to a claims **clearinghouse,** which then submits the claims to the insurance carrier. Direct billing occurs when an insurance carrier allows a provider to submit insurance claims directly to the carrier electronically. Most major insurance carriers, including Medicare and Medicaid, provide small computer programs that assist providers in the transmission of the claims. A clearinghouse is a vendor which, for a small fee per claim, provides a service which allows a provider to submit all of the insurance claims generated by the provider to the clearinghouse using special software. The clearinghouse then audits and sorts the claims, and sends them in batches electronically to each of the different insurance carriers. A clearinghouse charges the healthcare provider a small fee for the service of receiving claim transmissions, checking and preparing the claims for processing, consolidating claims so that one transmission can be sent to each carrier, and submitting claims in correct data format to the applicable insurance payor. Clearinghouses typically also provide the following additional services:

- Audit claims to make sure all required fields are completed and data are correct
- Report the number of claims submitted and the number of errors and their specifics
- Forward claims to insurance carriers that accept electronic claims (Medicare, Medicaid, Blue Cross/Blue Shield, and others) or to another clearinghouse that may hold the contracts with specific payors
- Keep provider offices updated as new carriers are added to the database
- Generate informative statistical reports

Typically, with electronic claims processing, payments are received in less than half the time required for turnaround of paper claims. Very soon after claims are transmitted, tracking reports will be sent from the clearinghouse that describe which claims were received, audited, and forwarded to the insurance carrier. These tracking reports also provide information regarding **rejected claims** and those needing additional information.

HIPAA 837 Health Care Claim: Professional (837P) Overview

In Chapter 16 information about HIPAA was introduced that discussed the privacy and security of patient information. As part of HIPAA, standards were developed to protect patient health information being transmitted electronically. These standards, known also as *Transaction and Code Sets,* mandate the format of insurance claims, remittance information, claims attachments, and claims status submitted electronically. The insurance claim form for physician and provider services is called the *HIPAA 837 Health Care Claim: Professional,* or *837P.* This standard contains the format and establishes the data contents of the Health Care Claim Transaction Set (837) for use within the context of an **Electronic Data Interchange (EDI)**—data that are transmitted electronically via the Internet. This transaction set can be used to submit healthcare claim billing information, encounter information, or both from providers of healthcare services to payors, either directly or via intermediary billers and claims clearinghouses.

After 2003 all insurance claims submitted electronically, whether the claim was submitted directly to the payor or a clearinghouse, must be submitted using the 837P standard, in order to comply with the HIPAA mandates. Any provider, payor, employer, or other entity found not

using these standards can be removed from participation in federal programs such as Medicaid, Medicare, and TRICARE and could also face stiff civil and/or criminal fines and imprisonment. All vendors, providers, clearinghouses, employers, and health insurance carriers that transmit protected health information electronically must have updated software that conforms to the HIPAA standards, including but not limited to the 837P. These software upgrades will be transparent to the medical assistant entering data into the computer for insurance claims processing—in other words, the format, screens, steps, and processes for entering data into the computer for the purpose of generating insurance claim forms, whether on paper to be mailed, or to be transmitted electronically, should look and feel the same as before the transaction and code sets were implemented.

For more information about the Transaction and Code Sets for the HIPAA 837 Health Care Claim: Professional, and the standards for other electronically submitted data, such as the Claims Payment and Remittance Advice (835), Healthcare Claims Status (276/277), Coordination of Benefits (837), and Referral Certification and Authorization (278), log on to the CMS website

Advantages and Disadvantages: Electronic vs. Paper Billing

Electronic Claims

Advantages
- Cost savings from shorter preparation time
- Cost savings in postage
- Quicker payment turnaround time
- Generation of claim status reports
- New HIPAA rules make claims submission, attachments, and claims status follow-up quicker and easier

Disadvantages
- Computer hardware/software glitches and/or power outages can delay preparation or transmission
- Creating electronic attachments can be problematic
- Initial start-up is expensive

Paper Claims

Advantages
- Minimal start-up costs
- Can attach documentation explaining unusual circumstances

Disadvantages
- The cost in time, labor, and postage is higher
- Reimbursement is much slower
- Require much more storage space

Electronic claims processing reduces payment turnaround time by shortening the payment cycle and can reduce average error rates to less than 1% or 2%. Some insurance companies even waive the attachment requirements for many procedures when claims are submitted electronically.

CRITICAL THINKING APPLICATION

Machelle is interested in learning more about filing claims electronically. In the medical facility where she is doing her externship, she has asked to work with Mrs. Leonard, who performs this procedure in the office. How can working closely with Mrs. Leonard benefit Machelle with regard to this subject?

National Provider Identifier

In the past, each insurance carrier, including government programs, assigned an identifier to each provider of service. Now, also as part of HIPAA, all allied healthcare providers of service will be assigned one individual **National Provider Identifier (NPI)** that the provider can use regardless which insurance carrier is being billed for reimbursement. The NPI is a uniform, national identification number providers will use in lieu of the many provider identification numbers currently used. The NPI, which should be issued in 2007, will replace Medicare's **Unique Provider Identification Number (UPIN)** and almost all other federal, state, and private insurance carriers' **Physician Identification Numbers (PINs).** When following the steps for preparing a health insurance claim form, use the UPIN and PIN numbers where indicated, unless and until the provider's NPI has been issued. At that time, use the NPI in lieu of any references to a UPIN or PIN. This NPI does not replace the Social Security number (SSN), employer identification number (EIN), or federal tax identification number (TIN) used by a provider of service. The SSN, EIN, and TIN are used for income and tax purposes and for reporting to the Internal Revenue Service.

DATA GATHERING GUIDELINES

When the first appointment is made for a patient, it is routine to ask the patient for all pertinent insurance information. Much of this information is on the patient information form that is completed when the patient comes to the medical office for the initial visit and is inserted into the medical chart as well as entered into the computer's patient database. This information should always be collected from every new patient seen by the provider. Returning or established patients should be asked during each visit whether their insurance information is complete and current. Many offices use a form that allows the patient to provide address and phone updates, as well as new insurance information.

The information required to properly complete an insurance claim form includes a patient registration form, verification of eligibility and benefits, referral and authorization information (when required by the insurance carrier), the patient's medical record and/or encounter form or charge ticket, and a CMS-1500 insurance claim form.

The patient registration form (Figure 20-1) is generally divided into several sections. The first section includes the patient information, including the full name, address, phone number, date of birth, gender, and insurance information.

The information needed to complete an insurance claim form includes patient and guarantor demographic and insurance information, the name, address, and phone number of the insurance company, the diagnostic, treatment, and procedures and services information, and the provider's billing information, including name, address, phone number, place of service, and the tax and provider identification numbers.

A medical assistant can use the following general guidelines for collecting information in preparation for insurance claim preparation. More information about the importance of collecting this information and its use in completing an insurance claim form will be discussed later in this chapter.

- Photocopy the back and front of the patient's insurance card, and place the photocopy in the medical record and/ or patient insurance file.
- Obtain the patient's full name, address, phone number, date of birth, gender, and employer or, if a student, school information.
- If a patient has more than one insurance policy, it is important to get the name, address, group, and policy number for each company.
- Record the name of the subscriber or guarantor if it is someone other than the patient, and obtain the guarantor's address, date of birth, employer information, and the guarantors relationship to the patient (i.e., spouse, parent, self, or other)
- Signatures to authorize insurance billing, supplying of information to insurance companies, and acceptance of assignments of benefits (if appropriate) should be obtained from all new patients.

Verification of Eligibility and Benefits

Once this information has been collected, the next step is to verify the patient's eligibility and benefits. This is done, usually by phone, by calling the insurance carrier(s) for the patient and confirming that the patient is covered by the insurance, and to obtain a general overview of the benefits available for the patient from the insurance policy. Figure 20-2 is an example of a basic form to use as a guide when completing the eligibility and benefits verification.

THE CMS-1500 HEALTH INSURANCE CLAIM FORM

The CMS-1500 Health Insurance Claim Form (Figure 20-3) is used for most health payors for claims submitted by physicians and suppliers. In the 1960s, there were a number of different claim forms used by third-party payors, but no standardized form for physicians to use in reporting health care services. In the 1980s, the American Medical Association and the Centers for Medicare and Medicaid Services (then known as the Health Care Financing Administration or HCFA) formed a group called the Uniform Claim Form Task Force. The group was charged with creating a standardized claim form and promoting its use among the insurance entities.

In the mid 1990s, the Uniform Claim Form Task Force was replaced by the National Uniform Claim Committee (NUCC). The goal of NUCC was to develop a standardized data set for use in an electronic environment, but still be applicable to and consistent with evolving paper claim form standards.

The CMS-1500 claim form has been revised slightly to accommodate the National Provider Identifier (NPI) and current identifiers until the NPI is fully implemented. An instruction manual is available on the NUCC website for completion of the claim form. The date of the new form is 08-05, replacing the old CMS-1500 form, dated 12-90. Physicians can use either form during the time period between October 1, 2006 and March 31, 2007. On April 1, 2007, the CMS-1500 (12-90 version) will be discontinued and all claims must be submitted on the CMS-1500 (08-05 version). NUCC will provide a data set crosswalk between the 837P and the CMS-1500. The data set is currently being revised to reflect the changes in the CMS-1500 and updated information will be available on the NUCC website when available.

Each item number, or box, in the guidelines below contains the box title, instructions, description, field specifications, and an example. Examples are only for completion of the information required in the box and are not indicative of billing methods. Punctuation is noted in the instructions for each box.

Insurance cards copied   ☒
Date: Jan. 20, 20XX

Patient Registration Information

Account #: 84516
Insurance #: H-550-64-5172-02
Co-Payment : $ OV $10 ER $50

Please PRINT AND complete ALL sections below!

Is your condition the result of a work injury? YES (NO)   An auto accident? YES (NO)
Date of injury: _____

PATIENT'S PERSONAL INFORMATION Marital status ☐ Single ☒ Married ☐ Divorced ☐ Widowed
Sex: ☐ Male ☒ Female
Name: _____ FUHR _____   LINDA   L.
         last name   first name   initial
Street Address: 3070 Tipper Street   (Apt # 4) City: Oxnard   State: CA Zip: 93030
Home phone:(555)276-0101   Work phone:(555)372-1151   Social Security # 550-XX-5172
Date of Birth: 11/05/65   Driver's License: (State & Number) G0075012
Employer/Name of School Electronic Data Systems   ☒ Full Time ☐ Part Time
Spouse's Name: FUHR   GERALD   T.   Spouse's Work phone: (555)921-0075
                     last name   first name initial
How do you wish to be addressed? LINDA   Social Security # 545-XX-2771

PATIENT'S/ RESPONSIBLE PARTY INFORMATION
Responsible party: GERALD T. FUHR   Date of Birth: 06-15-64
Relationship to patient: ☐ Self ☒ Spouse ☐ Other   Social Security # 545-XX-2771
Responsible party's home phone:(555) 276-0101   Work phone:(555)921-0075
  Address: 3070 Tipper Street   (Apt # 4) City: Oxnard   State: CA Zip: 93030
Employer's Name: General Electric   Phone number: (555) 485-0121
  Address: 317 East Main   City: Oxnard   State: CA Zip: 93030
  Your occupation: Technician
Spouse's Employer's Name: Electronic Data Systems   Spouse's Work phone: (555)372-1151
  Address: 2700 West 5th Street   City: Oxnard   State: CA Zip: 93030

PATIENT'S INSURANCE INFORMATION Please present insurance cards to receptionist.
PRIMARY insurance company's name: ABC Insurance Company
Insurance address: P.O. Box 12340   City: Fresno   State: CA Zip: 93765
Name of insured: Linda L. Fuhr   Date of Birth: 11/05/65 Relationship to insured: ☒ Self ☐ Spouse / ☐ Other ☐ Child
Insurance ID number: H-550-XX-5172-02   Group number: 17098-020-00004
SECONDARY insurance company's name: None
Insurance address: _____ City: _____ State: ___ Zip: ___
Name of insured: _____ Date of Birth: _____ Relationship to insured: ☐ Self ☐ Spouse / ☐ Other ☐ Child
Insurance ID number: _____ Group number: _____
Check if appropriate: ☐ Medigap policy ☐ Retiree coverage

PATIENT'S REFERRAL INFORMATION
                                                          (Please circle one)
Referred by: Margaret Taylor (Mrs. W. T.) If referred by a friend, may we thank her or him? (Yes) No
Name(s) of other physician(s) who care for you: Jason Smythe, MD

EMERGENCY CONTACT
Name of person not living with you: Hannah Gildea   Relationship: Aunt
Address: 4621 Lucretia Avenue   City: Oxnard   State: CA Zip: 93030
Phone number (home):(555) 274-0132   Phone number (work):(___)_____

Assignment of Benefits • Financial Agreement

I hereby give lifetime authorization for payment of insurance benefits be made directly to Gerald Practon, MD, and any assisting physicians, for services rendered. I understand that I am financially responsible for all charges whether or not they are covered by insurance. In the event of default, I agree to pay all costs of collection, and reasonable attorney's fees. I hereby authorize this healthcare provider to release all information necessary to secure the payment of benefits.
I further agree that a photocopy of this agreement shall be as valid as the original.
Date: Jan 20, 20XX   Your signature: *Linda L Fuhr*
Method of payment: ☐ Cash ☒ Check ☐ Credit Card

Figure 20-1 Patient registration form. (Courtesy Bibbero Systems, Inc., Petaluma, Calif.)

ASSIGNMENT OF INSURANCE BENEFITS

I, the undersigned, represent that I have insurance coverage with and do hereby authorize
_____ to pay and assign directly to _____
(NAME OF COMPANY)   (NAME OF DOCTOR)

all surgical and/or medical benefits, if any, otherwise payable to me for services as described on the attached forms hereof, but not to exceed the charges for those services. I understand that I am financially responsible for all charges whether or not paid by said insurance. I hereby authorize said assignee to release all information necessary to secure the payment of said benefits.

Date _____   Signed _____

Figure 20-2 Insurance Eligibility/ Preauthorization form.

CARRIER

1500

HEALTH INSURANCE CLAIM FORM

APPROVED BY NATIONAL UNIFORM CLAIM COMMITTEE 08/05

☐☐☐ PICA | | PICA ☐☐☐

| 1. MEDICARE ☐ (Medicare #) MEDICAID ☐ (Medicaid #) TRICARE CHAMPUS ☐ (Sponsor's SSN) CHAMPVA ☐ (Member ID#) GROUP HEALTH PLAN ☐ (SSN or ID) FECA BLK LUNG ☐ (SSN) OTHER ☐ (ID) | 1a. INSURED'S I.D. NUMBER (For Program in Item 1) |

2. PATIENT'S NAME (Last Name, First Name, Middle Initial)

3. PATIENT'S BIRTH DATE MM DD YY   SEX M☐ F☐

4. INSURED'S NAME (Last Name, First Name, Middle Initial)

5. PATIENT'S ADDRESS (No., Street)

6. PATIENT RELATIONSHIP TO INSURED Self☐ Spouse☐ Child☐ Other☐

7. INSURED'S ADDRESS (No., Street)

CITY | STATE

8. PATIENT STATUS Single☐ Married☐ Other☐ Employed☐ Full-Time Student☐ Part-Time Student☐

CITY | STATE

ZIP CODE | TELEPHONE (Include Area Code) ( )

ZIP CODE | TELEPHONE (Include Area Code) ( )

9. OTHER INSURED'S NAME (Last Name, First Name, Middle Initial)

10. IS PATIENT'S CONDITION RELATED TO:

11. INSURED'S POLICY GROUP OR FECA NUMBER

a. OTHER INSURED'S POLICY OR GROUP NUMBER

a. EMPLOYMENT? (Current or Previous) YES☐ NO☐

a. INSURED'S DATE OF BIRTH MM DD YY SEX M☐ F☐

b. OTHER INSURED'S DATE OF BIRTH MM DD YY SEX M☐ F☐

b. AUTO ACCIDENT? PLACE (State) YES☐ NO☐

b. EMPLOYER'S NAME OR SCHOOL NAME

c. EMPLOYER'S NAME OR SCHOOL NAME

c. OTHER ACCIDENT? YES☐ NO☐

c. INSURANCE PLAN NAME OR PROGRAM NAME

d. INSURANCE PLAN NAME OR PROGRAM NAME

10d. RESERVED FOR LOCAL USE

d. IS THERE ANOTHER HEALTH BENEFIT PLAN? YES☐ NO☐ If yes, return to and complete item 9 a-d.

READ BACK OF FORM BEFORE COMPLETING & SIGNING THIS FORM.
12. PATIENT'S OR AUTHORIZED PERSON'S SIGNATURE I authorize the release of any medical or other information necessary to process this claim. I also request payment of government benefits either to myself or to the party who accepts assignment below.

SIGNED _____ DATE _____

13. INSURED'S OR AUTHORIZED PERSON'S SIGNATURE I authorize payment of medical benefits to the undersigned physician or supplier for services described below.

SIGNED _____

14. DATE OF CURRENT: MM DD YY ► ILLNESS (First symptom) OR INJURY (Accident) OR PREGNANCY(LMP)

15. IF PATIENT HAS HAD SAME OR SIMILAR ILLNESS. GIVE FIRST DATE MM DD YY

16. DATES PATIENT UNABLE TO WORK IN CURRENT OCCUPATION MM DD YY FROM   TO MM DD YY

17. NAME OF REFERRING PROVIDER OR OTHER SOURCE 17a. 17b. NPI

18. HOSPITALIZATION DATES RELATED TO CURRENT SERVICES MM DD YY FROM   TO MM DD YY

19. RESERVED FOR LOCAL USE

20. OUTSIDE LAB? YES☐ NO☐ $ CHARGES

21. DIAGNOSIS OR NATURE OF ILLNESS OR INJURY (Relate Items 1, 2, 3 or 4 to Item 24E by Line)
1. ⌊___.___⌋   3. ⌊___.___⌋
2. ⌊___.___⌋   4. ⌊___.___⌋

22. MEDICAID RESUBMISSION CODE   ORIGINAL REF. NO.

23. PRIOR AUTHORIZATION NUMBER

24. A. DATE(S) OF SERVICE From MM DD YY To MM DD YY	B. PLACE OF SERVICE	C. EMG	D. PROCEDURES, SERVICES, OR SUPPLIES (Explain Unusual Circumstances) CPT/HCPCS MODIFIER	E. DIAGNOSIS POINTER	F. $ CHARGES	G. DAYS OR UNITS	H. EPSDT Family Plan	I. ID. QUAL.	J. RENDERING PROVIDER ID. #
1									NPI
2									NPI
3									NPI
4									NPI
5									NPI
6									NPI

25. FEDERAL TAX I.D. NUMBER SSN☐ EIN☐

26. PATIENT'S ACCOUNT NO.

27. ACCEPT ASSIGNMENT? (For govt. claims, see back) YES☐ NO☐

28. TOTAL CHARGE $

29. AMOUNT PAID $

30. BALANCE DUE $

31. SIGNATURE OF PHYSICIAN OR SUPPLIER INCLUDING DEGREES OR CREDENTIALS (I certify that the statements on the reverse apply to this bill and are made a part thereof.)

SIGNED _____ DATE _____

32. SERVICE FACILITY LOCATION INFORMATION a. NPI b.

33. BILLING PROVIDER INFO & PH # ( ) a. NPI b.

PATIENT AND INSURED INFORMATION

PHYSICIAN OR SUPPLIER INFORMATION

Figure 20-3 CMS-1500 Insurance Claim form.

Completing the CMS-1500 (08-05)

The CMS-1500 Claim Form is divided into three sections. The first contains the address of the insurance carrier and is located at the top of the form (Figure 20-4). The second section contains information about the patient and insured person, and contains Boxes 1 through 13. The third section contains Boxes 14 through 33 and details physician or supplier information. The following text provides a brief description of each of the blocks on the form. Procedure 20-1 outlines detailed instructions on how to complete each block.

CARRIER BLOCK   The name and address of the payor is entered in this block. The payor is the carrier, health plan, third-party administrator, or other payor who will handle the claim. Use the format shown in Figure 20-4.

Suggestions for Claims Submission Planning

Medical assistants might consider the following items when creating a work-friendly routine for completing insurance claims:

- If possible, set aside a definite time for completing insurance claims.
- Have a central location for all insurance forms.
- Have readily available the necessary manuals, code books, and other references needed.
- Create a master list of codes most often used by the practice, including fourth and fifth digits, if appropriate. The list should be updated annually and should never be considered a replacement for the coding manuals.
- Make it a practice to complete the forms as soon as possible after service is rendered, usually at the end of the day.
- Complete the forms by type of insurance category (e.g., all Blue Cross, all Medicare).
- Transmit claims electronically whenever possible.

Patient/Insured Section—Blocks 1 to 8 (Figure 20-5)

Block 1   **Type of Insurance.** This block indicates the type of insurance that the patient has. The "other" block is used when the insurance type is HMO, commercial insurance, automobile accidents, liability, or workers compensation. This information directs the claim to the correct payor and may establish primary liability. EXAMPLE: If the claim is primary for Medicare, check the Medicare box. If Medicare is secondary, check the "Other" box.

Block 1a   **Insured's ID Number.** The ID number identifies the patient to the payer. The patient may not be the insured, but the ID number should identify that the patient is covered for benefits.

Block 2   **Patient's Name.** The name of the patient is the person who received treatment or supplies.

Block 3   **Patient's Birth Date and Sex.** The patient's birth date and sex help to identify the patient and distinguishe patients with similar names.

Block 4   **Insured's Name.** The insured's name identifies the person who owns the policy. For employee-sponsored plans, the insured would be the employee.

Block 5   **Patient's Address.** The patient's address and telephone number are entered here. Use the patient's permanent address; do not use a temporary or school address.

Block 6   **Patient Relationship to Insured.** "Self" indicates that the patient is the insured. "Spouse" indicates that the patient is married to the insured. "Child" means that the patient is the insured's minor

---

1500

HEALTH INSURANCE CLAIM FORM

APPROVED BY NATIONAL UNIFORM CLAIM COMMITTEE 08/05

☐☐☐☐ PICA

XYZ INSURANCE COMPANY
102 MAIN STREET
ANYTOWN, MO 63030

← CARRIER →

PICA ☐☐☐

Figure 20-4 CMS-1500 insurance claim form: carrier information.

Figure 20-5 CMS-1500 insurance claim form: patient and insured information, blocks 1 to 8.

PROCEDURE 20-1

Complete an Insurance Claim Form

CAAHEP COMPETENCY: 3.a.(3)(e)
ABHES COMPETENCY: 3.x

GOAL: *Accurately complete a CMS-1500 (formerly HCFA-1500) claim form.*

EQUIPMENT and SUPPLIES

- Patient registration form
- Photocopy of patient's insurance ID card
- Encounter form
- Patient record
- Patient's ledger
- CMS-1500 form
- Typewriter or computer

PROCEDURAL STEPS

Carrier Section

Enter the name and address of the payer to whom this claim is being sent in the following format:
1st Line: Name of carrier
2nd Line: First line of address
3rd Line: Second line of address, if needed
4th Line: City, State, and Zip code

Patient/Insured Section

Block 1   Place an "X" in the appropriate box to indicate the type of healthcare coverage that applies to this claim. Mark only one box. **NOTE:** One (1) character may be entered in any box within the field. Only one box can be marked.

Block 1a   Enter the insured's ID number as shown on the health insurance ID card for the specific payor that this claim addresses. **NOTE:** A total of twenty-nine (29) characters may be entered in this block.

Block 2   The patient's full last name, first name, and middle initial should be entered into Block 2. Suffixes should be entered after the last name. Do not include titles or professional suffixes. Use commas to separate each name. Do not use periods. Use a hyphen for hyphenated names. **NOTE:** A total of twenty-eight (28) characters may be entered in this block.

Block 3   Use an 8-digit birth date (MM/DD/YYYY). Enter an "X" in the correct box to indicate the sex of the patient. Only one box can be marked. Leave blank if the gender is for some reason unknown. **NOTE:** Two (2) characters may be entered for month and date, and four (4) characters may be entered for the year. One (1) character may be entered in the box denoting sex.

Block 4   Enter the insured's full last name, first name, and middle initial. Suffixes should be entered after the last name. Do not include titles or professional suffixes. Use commas to separate each name. Do not use periods. Use a hyphen for hyphenated names. **NOTE:** Twenty-nine (29) characters may be entered in this box.

Block 5   Enter the patient's mailing address and phone number. The first line is for the number and street, the second line is for the city and state, while the third line is for the zip code and phone number. Do not use punctuation in the address, other than a hyphen in a nine digit zip code. Do not use a hyphen in the phone number. **NOTE:** Twenty-eight (28) characters are allowed for the street address, twenty-four (24) characters are allowed for the city, and three (3) for the state. Twelve (12) characters are allowed for the zip code, three (3) for the area code, and ten (10) for the phone number.

Block 6   Place an "X" in the correct box that indicates the relationship of the patient to the insured. Mark only one box. **NOTE:** One (1) character may be entered in any box. Only one box should be marked.

Block 7   Enter the insured's address in this block. The first line is for the number and street, the second line is for the city and state, while the third line is for the zip code and phone number. Do not use punctuation in the address, other than a hyphen in a nine digit zip code. Do not use a hyphen in the phone number. **NOTE:** Twenty-nine (29) characters are allowed for the street address, twenty-three (23) characters are allowed for the city, and four (4) for the state. Twelve (12) characters are allowed for the zip code, three (3) for the area code, and ten (10) for the phone number.

Block 8   Place an "X" in the appropriate box indicating marital status and employment status. Mark only one box on each line. **NOTE:** Only one (1) character may be marked in the boxes and only one box per line should be marked.

Block 9   Complete blocks 9 and 9 a-d only if block 11d is marked. Use this block when other group health coverage exists. Enter the last name, first name, and middle initial of the other insured if it is different from block 2. Suffixes should be entered after the last name. Do not include titles or professional suffixes. Use commas to separate each name. Do not use periods. Use a hyphen for hyphenated names. **NOTE:** Twenty-eight (28) characters may be entered in this block.

Block 9a   Enter the group number or policy of the other insured. **NOTE:** Twenty-eight (28) characters can be entered in this field.

Block 9b   Use an 8-digit birth date (MM/DD/YYYY). Enter an "X" in the correct box to indicate the sex of the other insured. Only one box can be marked. Leave blank if the gender is for some reason unknown. **NOTE:** Two (2) characters may be entered for month and date, and four (4)

Continued

PROCEDURE 20-1—cont'd

characters may be entered for the year. One (1) character may be entered in the box denoting sex.

Block 9c Enter the name of the other insured's employer or school. <u>NOTE</u>: Twenty-eight (28) characters may be entered in this field.

Block 9d Enter the other insured's insurance plan or program name. <u>NOTE</u>: Twenty-eight (28) characters may be entered in this field.

Block 10a-c Enter an "X" in the correct box to indicate whether one or more of the services described in block 24 are for a condition or injury that occurred on the job or as a result of an automobile or other accident. Only one box on each line can be marked. Place the state postal code in the blank next to auto accident if the "yes" box is marked in that line. <u>NOTE</u>: One (1) character may be entered per line in either box, and two (2) characters may be entered in the place/state field.

Block 10d Refer to the most recent instructions from the applicable public or private payor regarding the use of this field. <u>NOTE</u>: Nineteen (19) characters may be entered in this field.

Block 11 The policy, group, or FECA number should be entered as it appears on the health care identification card. If block 4 was completed, then this block must be completed. <u>NOTE</u>: Twenty-nine (29) characters may be entered in this field.

Block 11a Enter an 8-digit date of birth, in the MM/DD/YYYY format. Place an "X" in the box that indicates the sex of the patient. <u>NOTE</u>: Two characters are allowed in the month and day spaces, and four in the year space. One entry is allowed in the block to indicate sex.

Block 11b Enter the name of the insured's employer or school. <u>NOTE</u>: Twenty-nine (29) characters are allowed in this block.

Block 11c The insurance plan or program name should be placed in this block. Some payors prefer an identification number of the primary insurer instead of a name in this block. <u>NOTE</u>: Twenty-nine (29) characters are allowed in this field.

Block 11d Mark the appropriate box. If there is another health plan, blocks 9 and 9a-d must be completed. <u>NOTE</u>: One (1) character may be entered in either box.

Block 12 Enter either "signature on file," "SOF," or an actual legal signature. When using a legal signature, enter the date signed in 6-digit format (MMDDYY) or 8-digit format (MMDDYYYY). <u>NOTE</u>: Use the space available to enter the signature and date.

Block 13 Enter either "signature on file," "SOF," or an actual legal signature. When using a legal signature, enter the date signed in 6-digit format (MMDDYY) or 8-digit format (MMDDYYYY). <u>NOTE</u>: Use the space available to enter the signature.

Block 14 Enter the 6-digit (MMDDYY) or 8-digit (MMDDYYYY) date of the first time the present illness, injury, or pregnancy began. In the case of pregnancy, use the date of the last menstrual period (LMP). <u>NOTE</u>: Two (2) characters may be entered under MM and DD, and four (4) characters may be entered under the YYYY.

Block 15 Enter the first date that the patient experienced the same or a similar illness in either 6-digit (MMDDYY) or 8-digit (MMDDYYYY) format. Do not indicate previous pregnancies. Leave blank if unknown. <u>NOTE</u>: Two (2) characters may be entered under MM and DD, and four (4) characters may be entered under the YYYY.

Block 16 If the patient is employed and is unable to work in the current occupation, use the 6-digit (MMDDYY) or 8-digit (MMDDYYYY) date in the "from" and "to" spaces that explain the time period that the patient was unable to work in his or her current occupation. <u>NOTE</u>: Two (2) characters may be entered under MM and DD, and four (4) characters may be entered under the YYYY.

Block 17 Enter the name (first name, middle initial, last name) and credentials of the professional who referred or ordered the service(s) or supply(ies) on the claim. Do not use period or commas within the name. A hyphen can be used for hyphenated names. <u>NOTE</u>: Twenty-six (26) characters may be entered in this field.

Block 17a The other ID number is the referring provider, ordering provider, or other source and is reported in 17a in the shaded area. The qualifier indicating what the number represents is reported in the qualifier field to the immediate right of 17a. The NUCC defines the qualifiers (see Table 20-1), since they are the same as those used in the electronic 837P. <u>NOTE</u>: Two (2) characters may be entered in the qualifier field and seventeen (17) characters may be entered in the other ID# field.

Block 17b Enter the NPI number of the referring provider, ordering provider, or other source in block 17b. <u>NOTE</u>: This field allows for the entry of a ten (10) digit NPI number.

Block 18 Enter the date that the patient was in the hospital, beginning with the admission date and ending with the discharge date in 6-digit (MMDDYY) or 8-digit (MMDDYYYY) format. If the patient is not yet discharged, leave the discharge date blank. This block is used only when the hospitalization is related to the current illness or injury. <u>NOTE</u>: This field allows for the entry of the following in each of the date fields: Two (2) characters may be entered under MM and DD, and four (4) characters may be entered under the YYYY.

Block 19 Please refer to the most current instructions from the applicable public or private payor regarding the use of this field. Some payors ask for certain identifiers in this field. If identifiers are reported in this field, enter the appropriate qualifiers describing the identifier. Do not

Continued

PROCEDURE 20-1—cont'd

enter a space, hyphen, or other separator between the qualifier code and the number. Refer to Table 20-1 for the qualifiers, which are the same as those used on the 837P. <u>NOTE</u>: Eighty-three (83) characters are allowed in this field.

Block 20   Use this field when billing for purchased services. Enter an "X" in "yes" if the reported services were performed by an entity other than the billing provider. Then enter the purchase price of those services. A "yes" mark indicates that an entity other than the one billing for the services performed the purchased services. A "no" mark indicates that no purchased services are included on the claim. When "yes" is marked, Block 32 must be completed. When billing for multiple purchased services, each service should be submitted on a separate claim form. Only one box can be marked. When entering the charge amount, enter the amount in the field to the left of the vertical line. Enter the number right justified to the left of the vertical line. Do not use commas or a decimal point when reporting amounts. Negative dollar amounts are not allowed. Dollar signs should not be entered. Use "00" for the cents if the amount is a whole number. Leave the righthand field blank. <u>NOTE</u>: One (1) character may be entered in either box in the Outside Lab area and eight (8) characters to the left of the vertical line and in the charges area.

Block 21   Enter the patient's diagnosis/condition. List up to four ICD-9-CM diagnosis codes. Relate lines 1, 2, 3, and 4 to the lines of service in 24E by line number. Use the highest level of specificity. Do not provide narrative descriptions in this field. When entering the number include a space (accommodated by the period) between the two sets of numbers. If entering a code with more than three beginning digits, (e.g., E codes), enter the fourth digit on top of the period. <u>NOTE</u>: The field allows for the entry of three (3) characters prior to the period, one (1) character above or on the period, and four (4) characters after the period in each of the four line areas.

Block 22   List the original reference number for resubmitted claims. Please refer to the most current instructions from the applicable public or private payor regarding the use of this field. <u>NOTE</u>: This field allows for the entry of eleven (11) characters in the code area and eighteen (18) characters in the original reference number area.

Block 23   Enter any of the following: prior authorization number, referral number, mammography precertification number, or Clinical Laboratory Improvement Amendments number, as assigned by the payor for the current service. Do not enter hyphens or spaces within the number. <u>NOTE</u>: Twenty-nine (29) characters are allowed in this field.

Block 24   The six service lines in block 24 have been divided horizontally to accommodate submission of both the NPI and to accommodate the submission of supplemental information to support the billed service. The top area of the six service lines is shaded and is the location for reporting supplemental information. It is NOT intended to allow billing for twelve items. <u>NOTE</u>: The shaded area of lines 1 through 6 allow for the entry of sixty-one (61) characters from the beginning of 24A to the end of 24G.

Block 24A   Enter the dates of service, both from and to. If there is one date of service only, enter that date under "from" and leave the "to" blank or re-enter the date placed in "from." <u>NOTE</u>: Two (2) characters are allowed for each section of month, day, and year.

Block 24B   Enter the appropriate 2-digit code from the Place of Service code list for each item used or service performed. <u>NOTE</u>: Two (2) characters are allowed in the unshaded area.

Block 24C   Determine if the services provided were an emergency. If required, place a "Y" for "yes" and an "N" for "no" in the bottom, unshaded section of the field. The definition of emergency would be either defined by federal or state regulations or programs, payor contracts, or as defined in the electronic 837P implementation guide. <u>NOTE</u>: Two (2) characters may be entered in the unshaded area.

Block 24D   Enter the CPT or HCPCS code(s) and modifiers (if applicable) from the appropriate code set in effect on the date of service. This field accommodates the entry of up to four 2-digit modifiers. The procedure code must be shown without a narrative description. <u>NOTE</u>: Six (6) characters may be entered in the unshaded area of the CPT/HCPCS field and four sets of two (2) characters in the modifier area.

Block 24E   In 24E, enter the diagnosis code reference number (pointer) as shown in Block 21 to relate the date of service and the procedures performed to the primary diagnosis. When multiple services are performed, the primary reference number for each service should be listed first, other applicable services show follow. The reference numbers should be 1, 2, 3, or 4, or multiple numbers as explained. ICD-9-CM diagnosis codes should be entered in Block 21 only. Do NOT enter them in 24E. Enter the numbers justified to the left. Do not use commas between the numbers. <u>NOTE</u>: Four (4) characters may be entered in the unshaded area.

Block 24F   Enter the charge for the listed service or procedure. Enter the number right justified in the dollar area of the field. Do not use commas when reporting dollar amounts. Negative dollar amounts are not allowed. Dollar signs should not be entered. Enter 00 in the cents column area if the amount is a whole number. <u>NOTE</u>: Six (6) characters may be entered to the left of the vertical line and two (2)

Continued

PROCEDURE 20-1—cont'd

characters to the right of the vertical line in the unshaded area.

Block 24G   Enter the number of days or units. This is usually used for multiple visits, units of supplies, anesthesia units or minutes, or oxygen volume. If only one service is performed, enter "1." Enter numbers right justified in the field. No leading zeros are required. If reporting a fraction of a unit, use the decimal point. Refer to Table 20-3 for a description of qualifiers. <u>NOTE</u>: This field allows for the entry of three (3) characters in the unshaded area.

Block 24H   If the claim is Early & Periodic Screening, Diagnosis, and Treatment related, enter "Y" for "yes" or "N" for "no" in the unshaded area of the field. If the claim is family planning, enter "Y," or leave blank if "N" is in the unshaded area of the field. <u>NOTE</u>: One (1) character is allowed in this field.

Block 24I   Enter in the shaded area of 24I the qualifier identifying if the number is a non-NPI. The Other ID# of the rendering provider is reported in 24J in the shaded area. The NUCC qualifiers are defined in Table 20-1, which are used in the 837P. <u>NOTE</u>: This field allows for entering two (2) characters in the shaded area.

Block 24J   The individual rendering the service is reported in 24J. Enter the non-NPI ID number in the shaded area of the field. Enter the NPI number in the unshaded area of the field. <u>NOTE</u>: Eleven (11) characters can be entered in the shaded area and ten (10) characters for the NPI number are allowed in the unshaded area.

Block 25   Enter the federal tax ID number or social security number. Place an "X" in the appropriate box to show which was provided. Do not enter hyphens with numbers. Enter numbers left justified in the field. <u>NOTE</u>: Fifteen (15) characters may be entered for the federal tax ID number or social security number and one (1) character for the description of which number is being provided.

Block 26   Enter the patient account number, if desired. <u>NOTE</u>: This field allows for fourteen (14) characters.

Block 27   Enter an "X" in the correct box. Only one box can be marked. <u>NOTE</u>: One (1) character is allowed per box.

Block 28   Enter the total charges for the services in 24F. <u>NOTE</u>: Seven (7) characters may be entered to the left of the vertical line and two (2) characters may be entered to the right of the vertical line.

Block 29   Enter the total amount that was paid toward this claim by the patient or guarantor. <u>NOTE</u>: Six (6) characters may be entered to the left of the vertical line and two (2) characters may be entered to the right of the vertical line.

Block 30   Enter the total amount due. This information does not exist in the 837P. <u>NOTE</u>: Six (6) characters may be entered to the left of the vertical line and two (2) characters may be entered to the right of the vertical line.

Block 31   Enter the legal signature of the practitioner or supplier, "signature on file," or "SOF." Enter a 6-digit (MMDDYY) date or 8-digit (MMDDYYYY) date reflecting the day that the claim was signed.

Block 32   Enter the name, address, city, state, and zip code of the location where the services were rendered. Enter the name and address in the following format:
>   1st line: Name
>   2nd line: Address
>   3rd line: City, State, and Zip code

<u>NOTE</u>: Seventy-eight (78) characters may be used in this block.

Block 32a   Enter the NPI number of the service facility location in 32a. <u>NOTE</u>: Ten (10) characters may be entered in this space.

Block 32b   Enter the 2-digit qualifier identifying the non-NPI number followed by the ID number. Do not enter a space, hyphen, or other separator between the qualifier and number. Refer to Table 20-1 for qualifiers. <u>NOTE</u>: Fourteen (14) characters may be entered in 32b.

Block 33   Enter the provider's or supplier's billing name, address, and use the following format:
>   1st line: Name
>   2nd line: Address
>   3rd line: City, State, and Zip Code

Block 33 identifies the provider that is requesting to be paid and should always be entered. <u>NOTE</u>: Three (3) characters are available for area code, nine (9) for phone number, and eighty-seven (87) for billing provider information.

Block 33a   Enter the NPI number of the billing provider. <u>NOTE</u>: Ten (10) characters are allowed.

Block 33b   Enter the two digit qualifier as shown in Table 20-1. <u>NOTE</u>: Thirty-three (33) characters may be entered in this space.

Final Steps

1. Review the claim for accuracy and completeness.
   <u>PURPOSE</u>: To double-check that no blocks or fields are inaccurate or missing required information.

2. Run or prepare an insurance claims log for all claims completed. For paper claims, make copy of claim and place in tickler file.
   <u>PURPOSE</u>: To provide an audit trail of claims submitted.

3. For paper claims:
   a. Paperclip any attachments to be sent with the claim.
   b. Group all claims going to the same carrier and mail together in one large envelope.
   c. Address the envelope, weigh the contents, attach postage, and mail.

4. For claims to be submitted electronically, follow the computer software instructions for the software being used.
   <u>PURPOSE</u>: To submit all claims electronically or by surface mail to the appropriate insurance carrier.

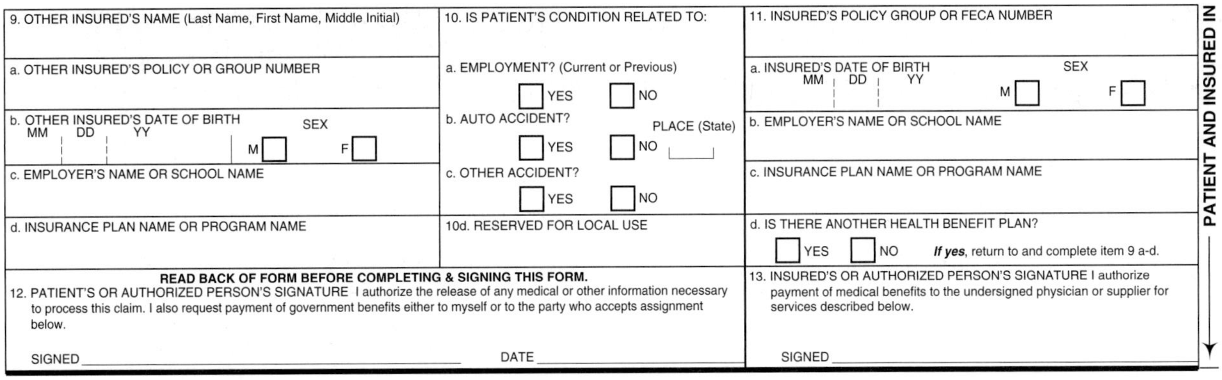
9. OTHER INSURED'S NAME (Last Name, First Name, Middle Initial)
a. OTHER INSURED'S POLICY OR GROUP NUMBER
b. OTHER INSURED'S DATE OF BIRTH MM DD YY SEX M F
c. EMPLOYER'S NAME OR SCHOOL NAME
d. INSURANCE PLAN NAME OR PROGRAM NAME
10. IS PATIENT'S CONDITION RELATED TO:
a. EMPLOYMENT? (Current or Previous) YES NO
b. AUTO ACCIDENT? PLACE (State) YES NO
c. OTHER ACCIDENT? YES NO
10d. RESERVED FOR LOCAL USE
11. INSURED'S POLICY GROUP OR FECA NUMBER
a. INSURED'S DATE OF BIRTH MM DD YY SEX M F
b. EMPLOYER'S NAME OR SCHOOL NAME
c. INSURANCE PLAN NAME OR PROGRAM NAME
d. IS THERE ANOTHER HEALTH BENEFIT PLAN? YES NO *If yes*, return to and complete item 9 a-d.
READ BACK OF FORM BEFORE COMPLETING & SIGNING THIS FORM.
12. PATIENT'S OR AUTHORIZED PERSON'S SIGNATURE I authorize the release of any medical or other information necessary to process this claim. I also request payment of government benefits either to myself or to the party who accepts assignment below.
SIGNED DATE
13. INSURED'S OR AUTHORIZED PERSON'S SIGNATURE I authorize payment of medical benefits to the undersigned physician or supplier for services described below.
SIGNED
PATIENT AND INSURED IN

Figure 20-6 CMS-1500 Insurance Claim form: patient and insured information, blocks 9 to 13.

dependent. "Other" could mean that the patient is an employee, ward, or other dependent as defined by the insured's plan.

Block 7 **Insured's Address.** The insured's address and telephone number are entered here. Use the insured's permanent address, which may be different from the patient's address in block 5.

Block 8 **Patient Status.** These boxes are important in determining liability and for coordinating benefits. Mark the employment box if the patient has a job. Full- or part-time student would be marked depending on the school's definition of full- and part-time status.

Patient/Insured Section—Blocks 9 to 13 (Figure 20-6)

Block 9 **Other Insured's Name.** The other insured's name indicates that there is a holder of another policy that may cover the patient.

Block 9a **Other Insured's Policy or Group Number.** The other insured's group number or policy number identifies coverage for the insured as indicated in block 9.

Block 9b **Other Insured's Date of Birth and Sex.** The other insured's birth date and sex help to identify the birth date and gender of the insured as indicated in block 9.

Block 9c **Employer's Name or School Name.** This block identifies the other insured's employer or school name as indicated in block 9.

Block 9d **Insurance Plan or Program Name.** The insurance plan name or program name identifies the name of the plan or program of the other insured as indicated in block 9.

Blocks 10a to 10c **Is Patient's Condition Related to.** This block indicates whether the patient's condition is the result of an employment injury or illness, auto accident, or other accident.

Block 10d **Reserved for Local Use.** Some third-party payors require that this boxed be used. Refer to the applicable third-party payor instructions.

Block 11 **Insured's Policy, Group, or FECA Number.** The policy, group, or FECA number is the alphanumeric identifier for the insurance plan coverage. Workers' compensation claims use the carrier's alphanumeric identifier. FECA numbers are the 9-digit alphanumeric identifier assigned to the patient claiming a work-related condition under the Federal Employees Compensation Act.

Block 11a **Insured's Date of Birth, Sex.** This information applies to the person identified in block 1a.

Block 11b **Insured's Employer's Name or School Name.** This refers to the name of the employer or school attended by the insured as indicated in Box 1a.

Block 11c **Insurance Plan Name or Program Name.** The insurance plan name or program name refers to the name of the plan or program of the insured as indicated in Block 1a.

Block 11d **Is There another Health Benefit Plan.** This block indicates whether the patient has insurance coverage other than that indicated in Block 1.

Block 12 **Patient's or Authorized Person's Signature.** The signature is an authorization for the release of any medical or other information necessary to process or adjudicate the claim.

Block 13 **Insured or Authorized Person's Signature.** The insured's or authorized person's signature indicates that there is a signature on file authorizing payment of medical benefits.

CRITICAL THINKING APPLICATION

It is office policy to request that patients assign benefits when the patient does not pay for services immediately. One of the patients, Mr. Jones, seems hesitant to sign block 13 of the CMS-1500 form. How should Machelle explain the office policy to Mr. Jones?

Physician/Supplier Section—Blocks 14 to 23 (Figure 20-7)

Block 14 — **Date of Current Illness, Injury, or Pregnancy.** The date should be the first date of the onset of the illness, the date the injury happened, or the LMP in case of pregnancy.

Block 15 — **Same or Similar Illness.** A patient having had same or similar illnesses would indicate that the patient had a previously related condition.

Block 16 — **Dates Patient Unable to Work in Current Occupation.** This section refers to the time span that the patient was unable to work in his or her current occupation.

Block 17 — **Name of Referring Provider or Other Source.** The name of the referring provider, ordering provider, or other source that referred or ordered the service or supply on the claim.

Block 17a — **Other ID.** The non-NPI number of the referring provider, ordering provider, or other source refers to the payor assigned unique identifier number of the professional. The qualifier indicating what the number represents is reported in the qualifier field to the immediate right of 17a. Table 20-1 shows the two-character qualifiers used in this block.

Block 17b — **NPI Number.** The NPI number refers to the HIPAA National Provider Identifier Number.

Block 18 — **Hospitalization Dates Related to Current Services.** The hospitalization dates related to current services would refer to an inpatient stay and indicates the admission and discharge dates associated with the service on the claim.

TABLE 20-1 Qualifiers Used in Blocks 17a, 19, 24I, 32b, and 33b

QUALIFIER	DESCRIPTION
0B	State License Number
1B	Blue Shield Provider Number
1C	Medicare Provider Number
1D	Medicaid Provider Number
1G	Provider UPIN Number
1H	TRICARE CHAMPUS Identification Number
E1	Employer's Identification Number
G2	Provider Commercial Number
LU	Location Number
N5	Provider Plan Network Identification Number
SY	Social Security Number (cannot be used for Medicare)
X5	State Industrial Accident Provider Number
ZZ	Provider Taxonomy

Block 19 — **Reserved for Local Use.** Some payors ask for certain identifiers in this field. Refer to the applicable third-party payor instructions. (See Table 20-1 for a list of the identifiers used in this block.)

Block 20 — **Outside Lab and Charges.** This field refers to services that have been rendered by an independent provider as indicated in Block 32 and the related costs.

Block 21 — **Diagnosis or Nature of Illness or Injury.** The diagnosis or nature of illness or injury refers to the signs, symptoms, complaint, or condition of the patient relating to the services on the claim. It should be coded to the highest level of specificity.

Block 22 — **Medicaid Resubmission.** Medicaid resubmission means the code and original reference number assigned by the destination payor or receiver to indicate a previously submitted claim or encounter.

Block 23 — **Prior Authorization Number.** The prior authorization number refers to the

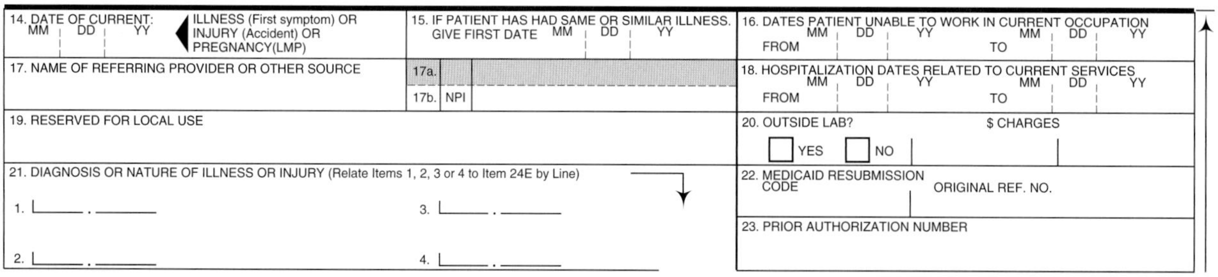
14. DATE OF CURRENT: MM DD YY — ILLNESS (First symptom) OR INJURY (Accident) OR PREGNANCY(LMP)
15. IF PATIENT HAS HAD SAME OR SIMILAR ILLNESS. GIVE FIRST DATE MM DD YY
16. DATES PATIENT UNABLE TO WORK IN CURRENT OCCUPATION MM DD YY FROM MM DD YY TO
17. NAME OF REFERRING PROVIDER OR OTHER SOURCE
17a.
17b. NPI
18. HOSPITALIZATION DATES RELATED TO CURRENT SERVICES MM DD YY FROM MM DD YY TO
19. RESERVED FOR LOCAL USE
20. OUTSIDE LAB? YES NO $ CHARGES
21. DIAGNOSIS OR NATURE OF ILLNESS OR INJURY (Relate Items 1, 2, 3 or 4 to Item 24E by Line)
1. 2. 3. 4.
22. MEDICAID RESUBMISSION CODE ORIGINAL REF. NO.
23. PRIOR AUTHORIZATION NUMBER

Figure 20-7 CMS-1500 Insurance Claim form: physician or supplier information, blocks 14 to 23.

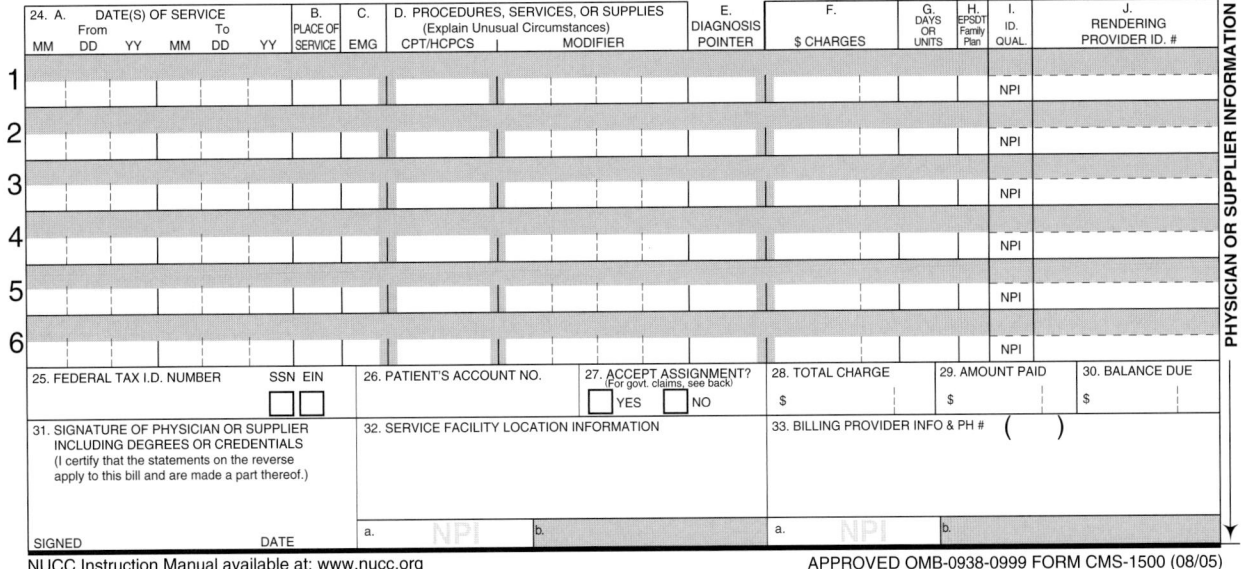

Figure 20-8 CMS-1500 Insurance Claim form: physician or supplier information, blocks 24 to 33.

TABLE 20-2 Place of Service Codes

CODE	DESCRIPTION	CODE	DESCRIPTION
11	Doctor's office	51	Inpatient psychiatry facility
12	Patient's home	52	Psychiatric facility-partial hospitalization
21	Inpatient hospital	53	Community mental health care (outpatient, twenty-four-hours-a-day services, admission screening, consultation, and educational services)
22	Outpatient hospital		
23	Emergency department—hospital		
24	Ambulatory surgical center	54	Intermediate care facility/mentally retarded
25	Birthing center	55	Residential substance abuse treatment facility
26	Military treatment facility/uniformed service treatment facility	56	Psychiatric residential treatment center
31	Skilled nursing facility (swing bed visits)	60	Mass immunization center
32	Nursing facility (intermediate/long-term care facilities)	61	Comprehensive inpatient rehabilitation facility
33	Custodial care facility (domiciliary or rest home services)	62	Comprehensive outpatient rehabilitation facility
34	Hospice (domiciliary or rest home services)	65	End-stage renal disease treatment facility
35	Adult living care facilities (residential care facility)	71	State or local public health clinic
41	Ambulance-land	72	Rural health clinic
42	Ambulance-air or water	81	Independent laboratory
50	Federally qualified health center	99	Other unlisted facility

payor-assigned number authorizing the service(s).

Physician/Supplier Section—Blocks 24 to 33 (Figure 20-8)

Block 24A   **Date(s) of Service (lines 1-6).** Date(s) of service indicate the actual month, day, and year that the service was provided.

Block 24B   **Place of Service (lines 1-6).** This section identifies where the services were provided. Table 20-2 shows the two-digit place of service codes.

Block 24C   **EMG (lines 1-6).** This field is used to indicate whether or not the services provided involved an emergency.

Block 24D   **Procedures, Services, or Supplies (lines 1-6).** The procedures, services, or supplies refer to a listing of identifying codes for reporting medical services and procedures.

Block 24E   **Diagnosis Pointer (lines 1-6).** The diagnosis pointer refers to the line number from Block 21 that relates to the reason the services were performed.

TABLE 20-3 Qualifiers Used to Report NDC Units

QUALIFIER	DESCRIPTION
F2	International unit
GR	fram
ML	milliliter
UN	unit

Block 24F **$ Charges (lines 1-6).** $ charges refers to the total billed amount for each service line.

Block 24G **Days or Units (lines 1-6).** Days or units refer to the number of days that correspond to the dates entered in 24A or units as defined in CPT or HCPCS coding manual(s). Table 20-3 shows the qualifiers to be used in this block.

Block 24H **EPSDT/Family Plan (lines 1-6).** The EPSDT/Family Plan identifies certain services covered under state plans.

Block 24I **Rendering Provider ID Qualifier (lines 1-6).** The Rendering Provider is the person or company who rendered or supervised the care. If the provider does not have an NPI number, enter the appropriate qualifier and identifying number in the shaded area. There will always be providers who do not have an NPI and will need to report non-NPI identifiers on their claim forms. The qualifiers will indicate the non-NPI number being reported. See Table 20-1 for the two-character qualifiers used in this block.

Block 24J **Rendering Provider ID Number (lines 1-6).** The individual performing/rendering the service is reported in 24J and the qualifier indicating if the number is a non-NPI goes into 24I. The non-NPI ID number of the rendering provider refers to the payor assigned unique identifier of the professional.

Block 25 **Federal Tax ID Number.** The federal tax ID number refers to the unique identifier assigned by a federal or state agency.

Block 26 **Patient's Account Number.** The patient's account number is that which is assigned by the provider and leads to the patient's financial information.

Block 27 **Accept Assignment.** The accept assignment indicates that the provider agrees to accept assignment under the terms of the Medicare program.

Block 28 **Total Charge.** The total charges indicate the amount billed on this claim form for all services rendered.

Block 29 **Amount Paid.** The amount paid refers to the payment received from the patient or other payors.

Block 30 **Balance Due.** The amount left after the patient has paid a copay or coinsurance is placed in this block.

Block 31 **Signature of Physician or Supplier (include degrees or credentials).** The signature is the verification from the provider that the claim is correct.

Block 32 **Service Facility Location Information.** The name, address, city, state, and ZIP code identify the site where services were rendered.

Block 32a **NPI Number.** The NPI number refers to the HIPAA National Provider Identifier Number of the service facility.

Block 32b The non-NPI number of the service facility refers to the payor-assigned unique identifier of the facility. The qualifier for the non–NPI number is entered here (see Table 20-1 for the two-character qualifiers used in this block.).

Block 33 **Billing Provider Info and Phone Number.** This block refers to the address and phone number of the provider that wishes to be paid on this claim.

Block 33a **NPI Number.** The NPI number of the billing provider is entered here. The NPI number refers to the HIPAA National Provider Identifier Number.

Box 33b **Other ID Number.** The non–NPI number of the billing provider refers to the payor-assigned unique identifier of the professional. The two-character qualifier of the non–NPI number is also entered here (see Table 20-1).

PREVENTING CLAIM REJECTION

It is important for the medical assistant to understand and comply with the guidelines specific to completion of a CMS-1500 form for each third-party payor and insurance company to prevent delays in reimbursement—or worse, denial of payment. The guidelines for Medicare, Medicaid, TRICARE, and worker's compensation can be found online at any of the fiscal intermediaries—e.g., Medicare billing guidelines are on the CMS website. Most computer software billing systems have built-in "claim scrubbers" that help in the process, and if claims are sent electronically through a clearinghouse, claims auditing is done before the clearinghouse submits the claim to the third-party payor. Claims without significant errors of any type are called **clean claims.** Claims with incorrect, missing, or insufficient data are called **dirty claims.**

Guidelines for Claims Review Before Submission

- Proofread the form carefully for accuracy and completeness.
- Make certain any necessary attachments are included with the completed form.
- Follow office policies and guidelines for claim review and signatures.
- Forward the original claim to the proper insurance carrier either by mail or electronically.
- If creating a paper claim, make a copy of the completed and signed claim form for the office records.
- Enter the appropriate information in the insurance log, and record the insurance submission information on the patient's ledger.
- The patient's and/or insured's name, address, and ID, group, and/or policy number should be identical to the information printed on the insurance card.
- Patient's birth date and sex should correspond with the medical record.
- The word "NONE" should appear in block 11 if Medicare is the primary payor.
- The referring, consulting, or ordering provider's name and identification number should be entered in blocks 17 and 17a, if applicable.
- Accept assignment should be checked "yes" if the physician is a participating provider (PAR).
- Be sure the diagnosis is not missing or incomplete.
- The diagnosis must be coded accurately and must correspond with the treatment.
- The patient must have authorized the release of information, and block 12 should contain a handwritten signature, the words "Signature on File," or the acronym SOF.
- The patient section (blocks 1-13) should be completed accurately according to the guidelines of the insurance carrier.
- Fees for each charge must be listed individually.
- All required fields of the diagnosis and procedure section of the claim form (blocks 14-24K) should be accurate and completed according to the guidelines of the third-party payor or insurance company.
- The physician signature must be on the form in an accepted manner.
- The federal **Employer Identification Number (EIN)** or Social Security number (SSN) should be double-checked to identify potential number transposition.
- The physician's correct billing or provider identification number corresponding to the insurance carrier being billed should be entered in block 24k and again to the right of "PIN #" in block 33, when required

Intelligent Character Recognition

Only claims which are completed on hard copy (paper) and submitted via surface mail such as the postal service are affected by the **Intelligent Character Recognition (ICR)** system and the guidelines given below. ICR is a system used to scan documents and capture claims information directly from the CMS-1500 form. Medicare, Medicaid, TRICARE (formerly CHAMPUS), and many other insurance carriers have adopted the ICR system.

The ICR system replaces the more antiquated optical character recognition (OCR) process, which had been in use until the early twenty-first century. The ICR scanners transfer the information on claim forms to their carrier's computer memories using a red bulb scanner, which causes the red preprinted portion of the CMS-1500 form to disappear or "drop out," and "transfers" to the computer only those characters printed in black ink. The resulting image allows for "clean" recognition of the data inserted without the characters being obstructed by the lines and text of the form. The benefits of ICR scanning include greater efficiency in processing claims, improved accuracy, more control over the data input, and reduced data entry cost for the insurance carrier.

There are rules for completing the CMS-1500 form in order for the insurance carriers to scan the claims; these rules include the following:

- Entries should be clear and sharp; carbon copies are not acceptable.
- A proportionally spaced 12-point font such as Courier works best.
- All uppercase letters should be used.
- All punctuation should be omitted.
- The MM DD CCYY format (with a space between each set of digits) should be used for all birth dates.
- All entries should be kept within their respective boxes. Xs must fall completely within the designated box.
- For the following, a blank space should be substituted:
  - Dollar signs and decimal points in charges and ICD codes
  - Dashes preceding procedure code modifiers
  - Parentheses around telephone area codes
  - Hyphens in Social Security numbers
- Titles and other designations, such as Sr., Jr., II, or III, should be omitted unless they appear on the identification (ID) card.
- When the charge is expressed in whole dollars, two zeros should be used in the "cents" column.
- If a typewriter is used, do not use lift-off tape, correction tape, or correction fluid.
- Because photocopies of claims cannot be scanned, all resubmissions must be prepared using the original (red print) claim form.
- No handwritten data (other than signatures) may be included on the forms.
- Nothing should be stapled to the form.
- The name and address of the insurance company should be inserted in the proper area in the top margin of the claim form.

Denied or Rejected Claims

The two main reasons for denial of payment are technical errors and insurance policy coverage issues. Technical errors include incorrect or incomplete information or typographic or mathematic errors. A common reason for insurance coverage rejections is that a procedure listed on the claim is not a covered service or is involved with a preexisting condition. The reason for a claim denial or reduction in reimbursement is listed on

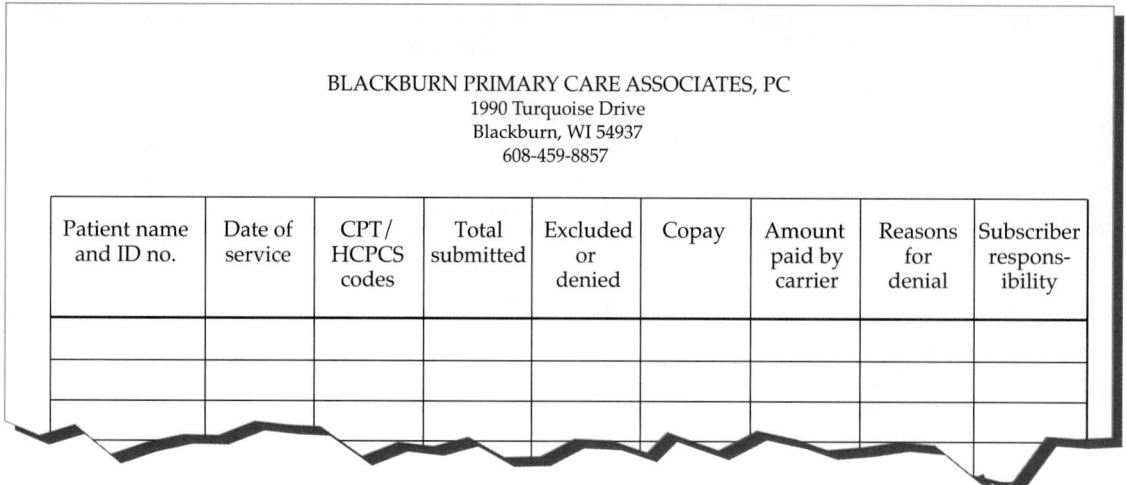

Figure 20-9 Example of explanation of benefits form. (From Hunt SA: *Saunders fundamentals of medical assisting*, Philadelphia, 2002, Saunders.)

the explanation of benefits (EOB) of commercial carriers, the remittance advice (RA) for commercial carriers and on Medicaid claims, and the explanation of Medicare benefits (EOMB) on Medicare claims. The EOMB, EOB and RA are hard copy or electronic forms that list the amount paid by the insurance company, as well as information about any non-covered services, denied claims (and the reason), deductible and/or co-insurance amounts, and other information about the claim or claims submitted. Figure 20-9 is an example of an insurance carrier benefits explanation.

A complete, accurate claim is called a **clean claim.** Claims returned unpaid by the third-party payor can be called "dingy," (also known as "incomplete,") or "rejected."

- **Dingy claims.** An inaccurate or incomplete insurance claim returned for more information or correction.
- *Rejected claims.* A claim for which payment has been denied for any reason (e.g., non-covered service, pre-existing condition, or ineligibility) is called an incomplete claim.

At times, a denied claim may involve policy issues beyond the control of the medical assistant. When this happens, he or she should contact the patient and discuss the problem. Normally, it is the patient's responsibility to resolve disputes regarding payment with the payor. The insurance policy is a contract between the company and the insured. However, the provider and those involved with the billing process in the medical facility should have a good understanding of the guidelines and requirements for the types of claims and various insurers handled most often in the facility.

CRITICAL THINKING APPLICATION

In her externship at the women's health center, Machelle sees a file containing a number of rejected claims. On closer examination she notices that similar errors in certain blocks are repeatedly the cause for rejection. Discuss common errors on the CMS-1500 claim form and what can be done to prevent these mistakes and/or omissions.

CHECKING CLAIM STATUS

It is often necessary to send a **"tracer"** to an insurance company to determine the status of a delinquent insurance claim. The accepted practice is to submit the tracer a day or two after the usual turnaround time of the payor, generally 30 to 60 days. A tracer is typically a form letter asking the insurance company about the status of an unpaid insurance claim. An example of a tracer letter is shown in Figure 20-10.

A duplicate copy of all submitted claims should be retained either in paper form or in the computer billing software. A structured routine for following up on claims unpaid within a specific time frame should be created to prevent overlooking a claim that should be filed or that has not been paid. The Insurance Claim Register (Figure 20-11), tickler files, and reports from the insurance database all help to keep track of paid and pending claims. If using software to file claims, an insurance pending report and an insurance aging report (among others) can be generated. The insurance aging report can be sorted by age of the claim, typically 30, 60, 90, and 120 days (or more), and by the payor, such as Medicare, Medicaid, and so on. Any of these methods suggested is useful in the follow-up of claims that have yet to be paid.

If claims are being submitted electronically either directly or through a clearinghouse, the medical assistant might allow 10 business days for claim turnaround time before expecting reimbursement. For paper claims, allow an additional week or two to allow for necessary manual processing and mailing time. Time between when a claim is submitted and when it is paid varies from payor to payor; however, an experienced medical assistant will soon become familiar with individual payment patterns of third-party payors and their claim turnaround times. Most states have laws that require payment within 45 days for clean claims.

Audit Trails

Electronic transactions leave behind a path or trail as they are processed, and this trail can be tracked or audited to provide a

INSURANCE CLAIM TRACER

INSURANCE COMPANY NAME _____ DATE _____

ADDRESS: _____

PATIENT NAME _____ INSURED: _____

POLICY/CERTIFICATE NUMBER _____ GROUP NAME/NUMBER _____

EMPLOYER NAME AND ADDRESS: _____

DATE OF INITIAL CLAIM SUBMISSION _____ AMOUNT: _____

An inordinate amount of time has passed since submission of our original claim as described above. We have not received a request for additional information and still await payment of this assigned claim. Please review the attached duplicate and process for payment within seven (7) days.

If there is any difficulty with this claim, please check one of these below and return this letter to our office.

Claim pending because: _____
Payment of claim in process: _____
Payment made on claim: Date: _____ To whom: _____
Claim denied: (Reason) _____
Patient notified: Yes _____ No _____
Remarks: _____

Thank you for your assistance in this important matter. Please contact _____ in our office if you have any questions regarding this claim.

Office of: _____ M.D.

Address: _____
_____ TELEPHONE NUMBER: _____

Figure 20-10 Example of an insurance claim tracer. (From Fordney MT: *Insurance handbook for the medical office,* ed 9, St Louis, 2006, Saunders.)

INSURANCE CLAIMS REGISTER   Page No. _____

Patient's Name Group/Policy No.	Name of Insurance Company	Claim Submitted Date	Claim Submitted Amount	Follow-Up Date	Follow-Up Date	Claim Paid Date	Claim Paid Amt	Difference
Jones, Bob	BC/BS	1-7-03	319.37			2/28/03	294.82	24.55
Carson, David	BC	1-8-03	268.08	2-10-03	3-10-03			
Linden, Jan	Medicaid	1-9-03	146.15	2-10-03				
Paul, Emma	Medicare	1-10-03	96.28	2-10-03				
Cortez, Jose	Unicare	1-10-03	647.09	2-10-03				
Dimico, Joe	Tricare	2-1-03	134.78	3-10-03				
Coldman, Billy	Aetna	2-4-03	607.67	3-10-03				
Fritz, Renee	Travelers	2-10-03	564.55	3-10-03				
Wong, Chang	Prudential	2-15-03	1515.79					
Billings, Harry	Allstate	2-21-03	121.21					
Green, James	BC	2-24-03	124.99					

Figure 20-11 Insurance claims register.

record. This record, called an **audit trail** (Figure 20-12), can be used to verify that information was processed correctly or to locate the source of an error. If an office uses a computerized accounting program and submits claims electronically, the task of keeping track of claims is simple, because the software is capable of printing out an "insurance aging report" by date, by patient name, or by carrier name. If paper claims are used, however, the medical assistant should establish a follow-up procedure for tracking insurance claims. This can be accomplished by using an insurance claims register or log. This document can be developed and updated with little effort using a spreadsheet computer program, such as Microsoft Excel if the provider's office is computerized. If a physician financial management and billing software is used by the provider, an audit trail report can be generated automatically from the software program.

Blackburn Primary Care Associates
Patient Aging

NAME	CURRENT 0 - 30	PAST 31 - 60	PAST 61 - 90	PAST 91 - 120	PAST over 120	Total Balance
Mary Smith Last Payment on 08/08/XX	$120.00					$120.00
John Payne Last Payment on 07/06/XX		$250.00				$250.00
Jack Desmonde Last Payment on 05/25/XX			$500.00			$500.00
Jill Jayne Last Payment on 04/02/XX		$80.00		$100.00		$180.00
Report Aging Totals Percent of Total Aging	$120.00 11.4%	$330.00 31.4%	$330.00 47.6%	$100.00 9.5%		$1,050.00 100.0%

Figure 20-12 Sample accounts aging record. (From Hunt SA: *Saunders fundamentals of medical assisting,* Philadelphia, 2002, Saunders.)

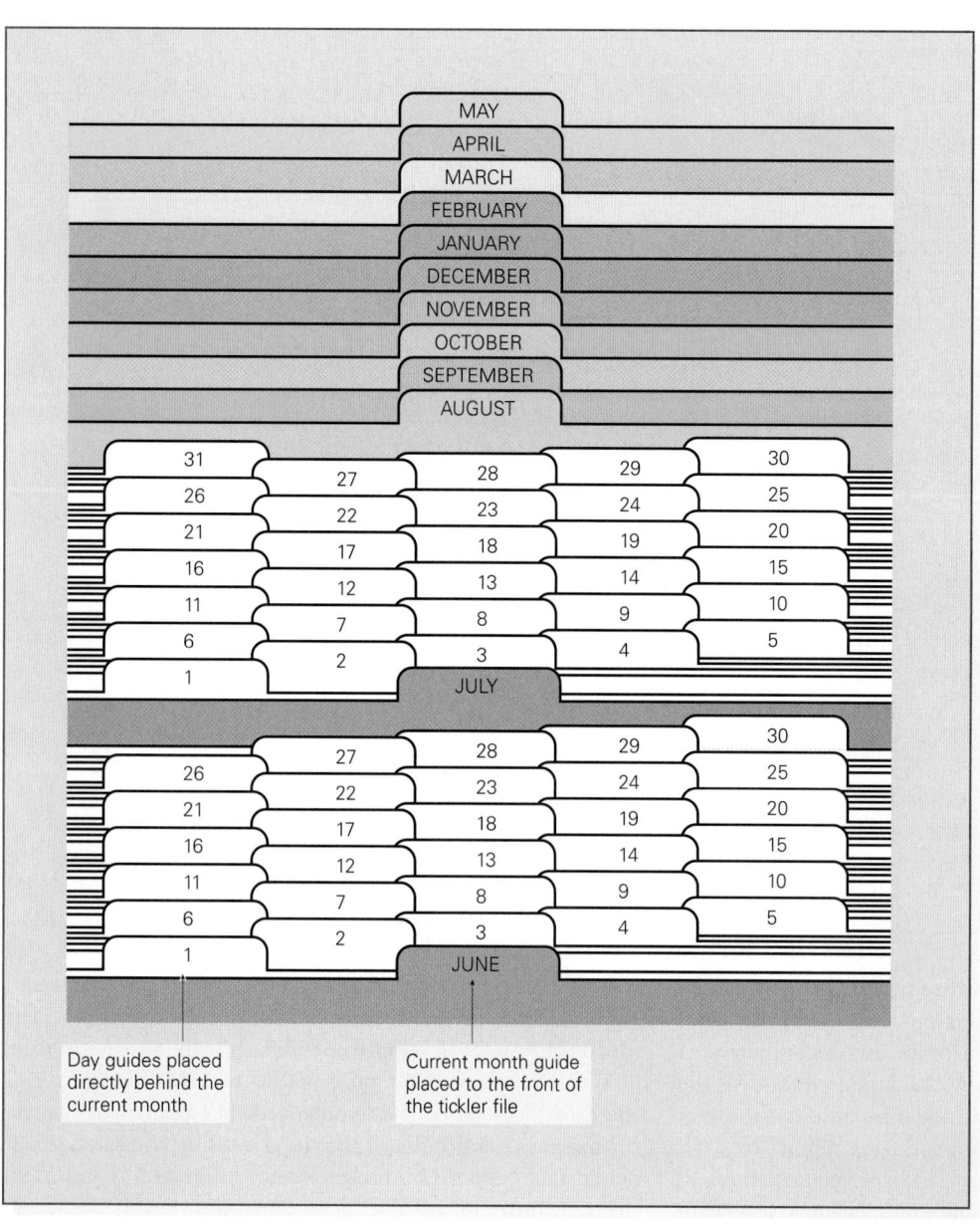

Figure 20-13 Example of an insurance claims tickler file. (From Fordney MT: *Insurance handbook for the medical office,* ed 9, St Louis, 2006, Saunders.)

Day guides placed directly behind the current month

Current month guide placed to the front of the tickler file

Another method of tracking claims is a tickler file (Figure 20-13), also called a *suspense* or *follow-up file*. With this method, a copy of each insurance claim is filed chronologically, and the file is checked periodically for unprocessed (delinquent) claims. When the claim is paid, the copy is removed, and the information is posted on the patient's ledger card.

Delinquent claims remaining in the file after the normal contract time limits are pulled, then traced. If the claim has been denied, a letter may be sent to the insurance carrier's appeals department with a copy to the patient.

Claim Status

Obtaining timely and correct payment from third-party payors is a concern for many medical practices. Lost claims, delayed claims, and dirty claims result in healthcare providers waiting months for payment of professional services rendered. Most providers would agree that claim-processing payment issues are at the heart of most provider-payor conflicts.

Rejected Claims

A rejected claim is one that has missing or incorrect information. Rejected claims subsequently require investigation, need further clarification, and/or possibly require answers to or documentation regarding specific questions.

Denied Claims

Claims can be denied as the result of a technical error but are usually not paid because the medical service submitted is not covered under the policy, is an ineligible service, or must be applied to the deductible in accordance with the policy.

CLOSING COMMENTS

Patient Education

The medical assistant should be able to explain confusing technical issues to patients in simple, understandable terms. Patients, especially elderly ones, quickly become confused and frustrated over insurance issues—especially Medicare rules and regulations, which change nearly every year. The medical assistant should attempt to keep patients fully informed of changes in insurance guidelines and patiently explain why some procedures and services are paid for and others are not.

Legal and Ethical Issues

The practice of medicine and the responsibilities of the medical assistant are greatly affected by the legislative process. It is extremely important to stay current on the laws that affect medicine, federal and state insurance programs, such as Medicare, Medicaid, workers' compensation, and TRICARE, and the completion of the CMS-1500 claim form.

The Health Insurance Portability and Accountability Act of 1996 (HIPAA), developed by CMS, is responsible for the implementation of various acts that protect individuals' health insurance and privacy standards. Medical assistants should familiarize themselves with this important insurance act.

Because of the emphasis on compliance in medical practices today, every medical office must create and implement a plan to identify potential compliance problems and correct them before a liability risk is incurred. It is mandated that all providers avoid fraud and abuse charges by following the regulations and guidelines provided by governmental entities and third-party payors.

SUMMARY OF SCENARIO

Machelle feels that she now has a better understanding of the insurance claims process. Before becoming a medical assisting student, she did not give much thought to what went on behind the scenes when she visited a medical office for her own personal healthcare. She now understands why all of the information is collected at the time of her visits to the doctor, including the patient registration form listing her demographic and insurance information – Machelle has learned that the gathering of accurate data and verification of eligibility and benefits are some of the most important tasks performed, before she even begins to complete an insurance claim form. This information and the procedure to verify eligibility and benefits greatly reduce the chance of insurance claim denials or requests for additional information. No matter where she works and whether or not the office is computerized, organization, communication, dedication, and attention to detail head the list of requirements for becoming successful.

Machelle has asked for her instructor's help in developing a reference manual for the various third-party payors common to her area which will help her understand the requirements of the insurance carriers when submitting an insurance claim form. This too will greatly reduce the number of claims that are returned for more information which will delay reimbursement for services rendered. She is looking forward to more hands-on experience in the medical office where she is doing her externship so she can gain as much knowledge as possible in every facet of medical assisting. She is also establishing positive relationships with the staff at her externship site. She feels the knowledge and expertise they share with her will do much to round out her education in the medical field in preparation for her career.

SUMMARY of LEARNING OBJECTIVES

1. Define, spell, and pronounce the terms listed in the vocabulary.
   - Spelling and pronouncing medical terms correctly adds credibility to the medical assistant. Knowing the definition of these terms promotes confidence in communication with patients and co-workers.

2. Discuss the differences between paper claims and electronic claims.
   - Insurance claims can be submitted in two forms: paper and electronic. Both have advantages and disadvantages; however, electronic claims normally have fewer errors and historically are paid faster.

3. Understand the guidelines for completing the CMS-1500 claim form.
   - The insurance claim cycle begins when the patient first makes an appointment. The medical assistant should follow an established list of guidelines for CMS-1500 form completion, including obtaining a signed authorization to release information and assign benefits, if applicable.

4. Explain how to complete each of the 33 blocks of the CMS-1500 claim form.
   - There are 33 blocks in the CMS-1500 claim form, and, except for a few blocks that ask for standard information, completion requirements vary from payor to payor. The medical assistant should familiarize himself or herself with each major payor's unique requirements in order to maximize reimbursement.

5. Differentiate between "clean" and "dirty" claims.
   - Clean claims are those that can be processed and paid quickly; dirty claims contain errors and/or omissions that often result in rejection, thus greatly slowing the reimbursement process.

6. Discuss methods of preventing claim rejections.
   - Claim rejection and delay cost the medical facility time and money. Proven methods of preventing claim rejections should be established and adhered to.

7. Describe ways of checking the status of claims.
   - It is important to track claims once they are submitted. An insurance claim register, or log, can be created and used as one method of tracking claims. A routine should be established for claims follow-up.

8. Gather information for use on insurance claim forms.
   - The medical assistant who completes claim forms must have accurate, complete information to work with.

9. Complete a CMS-1500 insurance claim form appropriately for various federal, state, and commercial third-party payors.
   - Accuracy in completing insurance claim forms is mandatory. The process for completing claim forms appropriately is outlined in Procedure 20-1.

CONNECTIONS

 Study Guide Connection: Go to Chapter 20 Study Guide. Read the Case Study and Workplace Applications and complete the assignments. Do online research for answers to the questions in the Internet Activities associated with the health insurance claim form.

 CD Connection: Go to the Medical Assisting Competency Challenge CD and do the training activities under Health Insurance Activities.

 Evolve Connection: For more information related to the health insurance claim form, go to evolve.elsevier.com/kinn and visit related weblinks for Chapter 20. Click on the Medical Assisting Exam Review and do the practice questions to sharpen your test-taking skills. To learn more about office software, do the exercises for the Altapoint demo that is on the CD.

Professional Fees, Billing, and Collecting

21

SCENARIO

Myra Morrison has worked for Dr. Jerry Wallace, an endocrinologist, for 3 years. She began as a receptionist, but she always had a knack for mathematics. Dr. Wallace was confident enough in her abilities to place her in charge of the accounting functions for the practice. When patients are ready to leave, Myra totals their bill and enters the charges and payments into the computerized ledger system. She also schedules their return appointments. Myra has learned quite a bit about medical insurance as well, so she can answer the patients' questions about their coverage and the benefits or exclusions of their insurance policies. In many instances, she was able to decipher a confusing insurance claim and explain the reimbursement to the patient. Myra has a great attitude about assisting patients with insurance questions and does not hesitate to call the insurance company to ask questions on behalf of the patient. She provides the patients with exceptional customer service.

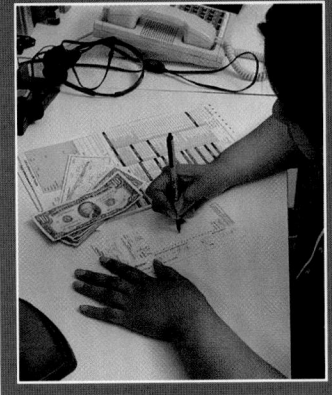

Myra knows that care must be taken when dealing with numeric transactions. Her handwriting is clear and legible, and she writes numbers the same way each time to avoid confusion and errors. She is able to use a manual pegboard but prefers the computer programs that do most of the work for her. Myra has some basic accounting background, so she can find errors easily and correct them. She even enjoys balancing the accounts on a daily basis to be sure all transactions were entered correctly.

Myra provides a valuable service to the patients who visit Dr. Wallace. She can always be counted on to follow up on any detail that needs attention. When patients call her for assistance, she takes no more than 24 hours to respond with the answers to their questions. She is a great patient advocate in the office. Some patients even tease her by asking her to balance their checkbooks! Myra is also willing to help any staff member with other duties whenever necessary. She is an enthusiastic team player who puts the patients first.

While studying this chapter, think about the following questions:

- Why do the provider's usual fees influence the amount of reimbursement received from third-party payors?
- Why is professional courtesy used less frequently than in the past?
- How does the medical assistant effectively explain fees to patients?
- Why might some providers still use a manual pegboard accounting system?

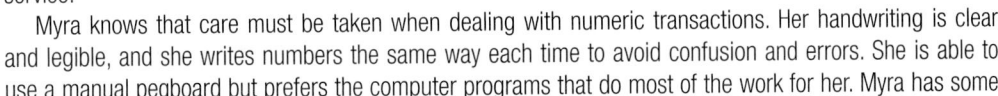

LEARNING OBJECTIVES

1. Define, spell, and pronounce the terms listed in the vocabulary.
2. List three values that are considered in determining professional fees.
3. Distinguish among the terms *usual*, *customary*, and *reasonable*.
4. Discuss the value of estimates for patient treatment.
5. Explain the concept of professional courtesy.
6. Name the ways by which payment for medical services is accomplished.
7. Explain why itemizing statements is important.
8. Discuss why patients fail to pay accounts.
9. Explain how to handle a "skip."
10. Briefly explain some of the guidelines of telephone collecting.
11. Explain professional fees to patients.
12. Effectively use a pegboard system.
13. Establish credit arrangements for patient payment.
14. Prepare accurate monthly statements.
15. Evaluate patient accounts for necessary collection procedures.
16. Perform accounts receivables procedures.
17. Post adjustments to patient accounts.
18. Process a credit balance on a patient account.
19. Process refunds and send overpayments to patients, when appropriate.
20. Post non-sufficient fund checks to patient accounts.
21. Post payments to accounts that have been turned over to a collection agency.
22. Age accounts receivable.

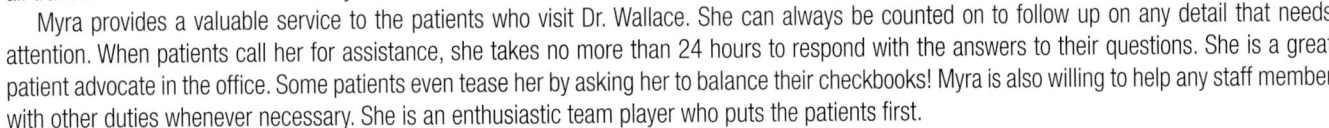
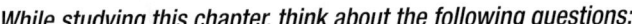

National Accreditation Competencies and Content

CAAHEP COMPETENCIES

Administrative

3.a.(2)(b). Post entries on a day sheet
3.a.(2)(c). Perform accounts receivable procedures
3.a.(2)(d). Perform billing and collection procedures
3.a.(2)(e). Post adjustments
3.a.(2)(f). Process a credit balance
3.a.(2)(g). Process refunds
3.a.(2)(h). Post non-sufficient fund (NSF) checks
3.a.(2)(i). Post collection agency payments

General

3.c.(3)(a). Explain general office policies

ABHES COMPETENCIES

Administrative Duties

3.k. Post entries on a day sheet
3.l. Perform billing and collection procedures
3.o. Post adjustments
3.p. Process credit balance
3.q. Process refunds
3.r. Post NSF checks
3.s. Post collection agency payments
3.x. Use physician fee schedule

Instruction

7.d. Orient patients to office policies and procedures

Financial Management

8.a. Use manual and computerized bookkeeping systems
8.e. Maintain records for accounting and banking purposes

VOCABULARY

account A statement of transactions during a fiscal period and the resulting balance.

account balance The amount owed on an account.

accounts receivable ledger A record of the charges and payments posted on an account.

credit An entry on an account constituting an addition to a revenue, net worth, or liability account; the balance in a person's favor in an account.

debit An entry on an account constituting an addition to an expense or asset account or a deduction from a revenue, a net worth, or a liability account.

debit cards Cards that looks like credit cards and by which money may be withdrawn or the cost of purchases paid directly from the holder's bank account without the payment of interest.

disbursements (dis-buhr'-smunts) Funds paid out.

fee profile A compilation or average of physician fees over a given period of time.

fee schedule A compilation of preestablished fee allowances for given services or procedures.

fiscal agent An organization under contract to the government as well as some private plans to act as financial representatives in handling insurance claims from providers of health care; also referred to as *fiscal intermediary.*

guarantor (gar-uhn-tor') A person who makes or gives a guarantee of payment for a bill.

instigate (in'-stuh-gat) To goad or urge forward; to provoke.

medically indigent Able to take care of ordinary living expenses but not able to afford medical care.

payables Balances due to a creditor on an account.

pegboard system Also called the *write-it-once system;* a method of tracking patient accounts that allows the figures to be proved accurate through mathematic formulas.

posting Transferring or carrying from a book of original entry to a ledger; entering figures in an accounting system.

premium The consideration paid for a contract of insurance.

preponderance (pri-pahn'-duh-rents) A superiority or excess in number or quantity; a majority.

professional courtesy Reduction or absence of fees to professional associates.

receipts (ri-sets') Amounts paid on patient accounts.

receivables Total monies received on accounts.

third-party payor Someone other than the patient, spouse, or parent who is responsible for paying all or part of the patient's medical costs.

transaction (tran-zak'-shun) An exchange or transfer of goods, services, or funds.

The practice of medicine is a business as well as a profession, and the details of conducting the business aspects are often the responsibility of the medical assistant. Although service to the patient is the primary concern of the medical profession, a physician must charge and collect a fee for such services to continue providing medical care. The physician is one of many contributors in determining the amount of the fees. The medical assistant usually has the responsibility of informing the patient about financial matters, collecting the payment, and in some cases making arrangements for deferred payment.

WHY PATIENTS DO NOT PAY

Most patients truly want to pay the bills that they owe. However, there may be times that the patient experiences difficulties in meeting his or her obligations. The patient may have lost a job or insurance coverage. An emergency could arise that depletes finances. When patients are in a position in which they must choose between paying their medical bills or having electricity, the physician is often forced to wait for reimbursement for the services rendered. Although a few patients will absolutely refuse to pay for medical care they have received, most are honest and willing to pay but may need help with a payment plan. Terms can be arranged for collecting payment in full when both the office and the patient cooperate with each other. The medical assistant should attempt to work out a plan that the patient can abide by, and the patient should be expected to make promised payments.

HOW FEES ARE DETERMINED

Setting fees is no simple matter. The physician has three commodities to sell—time, judgment, and services. Yet the value of these commodities is never exactly the same to any two individuals. Medical care has little value except to the patient, and the value may not be consistent with his or her ability to pay. In every case the physician must place an estimate on the value of the services. Such an arrangement is known as *fee for service*. This value may then be modified by other considerations.

Impact of Managed Care

An important consideration in today's atmosphere of managed care is the **preponderance** of patients who are enrolled in health maintenance organization (HMO) insurance contracts. Under managed care the physician agrees to accept predetermined fees for specific procedures and services instead of the fee-for-service arrangement described in the preceding paragraph. The patient may be subject to a copayment that is determined by the insurance contract and is collected at the time of service. A base capitation plan pays the provider a set amount for each patient enrolled that is meant to cover all of the person's healthcare expenses. Usually, capitation plans cover a group of individuals.

Prevailing Rate in the Community

One of the bases for determining charges on the fee-for-service basis is the economic level of the community. Different communities have different living scales, and this situation is reflected in medical fees as well. Consequently, the prevailing rate in the community—the average composite fee—must be taken into consideration by each physician. Strangely enough, fees that are too low drive patients away just as quickly as fees that are too high, because the average person tends to judge worth of a product on its cost—low cost translates as low value.

Usual, Customary, and Reasonable Fees

Most insurance plans base their payments on what has become known as a *usual, customary, and reasonable* (UCR) fee for a given procedure.

- Usual—The physician's usual fee for a given service is the fee that an individual physician most frequently charges for the service.
- Customary—The customary fee is a range of the usual fees charged for the same service by physicians with similar training and experience practicing in the same geographic and socioeconomic area. There is now a growing tendency for fees to be determined by national trends rather than by local custom.
- Reasonable—The term *reasonable* usually applies to a service or procedure that is exceptionally difficult or complicated, requiring extraordinary time or effort on the part of the physician.

To illustrate, let us suppose that Dr. Wallace usually charges patients $100 for a first office visit. The usual fees charged for a first visit by other physicians in the same community with similar training and experience range from $75 to $125. Dr. Wallace's fee of $100 is within the customary range and would therefore be paid by an insurance plan that pays on a usual and customary basis. If, on the other hand, the range of usual fees in the community is from $60 to $85, the insurance plan would allow only the maximum within the range, or $85, to Dr. Wallace.

UCR rates were developed many years ago when indemnity plans were the most common type of health insurance coverage. However, because the majority of insurance plans today are some type of managed care, the UCR rates now are based on the prevailing managed care rate of payment in a region.

CRITICAL THINKING APPLICATION

Myra realizes that many of Dr. Wallace's patients are confused about insurance policies and are easily frustrated when payments are not as high as the patient thinks they should be. How can Myra help patients understand their policies better?

Fee Setting by Third-Party Payors

The physician does not act alone in determining fees. A **third-party payor** may provide the physician with a schedule of predetermined fees that it will approve for payment. Some require preapproval of the fee before service is rendered. A third-party payor may require precertification before it will pay for a specific service. Government programs such as Medicare and Medicaid have strict guidelines regarding reimbursement for fees and the raising of fees.

Physician's Fee Profile

The **fiscal agent,** or fiscal intermediary, for government-sponsored insurance programs as well as some private plans keeps a continuous record of the usual charges submitted for specific services by each physician. When these fees have been compiled and averaged over a given period, usually a year, the physician's **fee profile** is established. This fee profile is then used in determining the amount of third-party liability for services under the program. One of the objections voiced by physicians is the lag between the time of a private fee increase and the time it is reflected in payments by an insurance carrier. It may be as long as 2 to 3 years.

Insurance Allowance

In some individual cases the physician may not wish to charge the patient more than what will be allowed by the patient's insurance. This is often a **professional courtesy** extended to other healthcare professionals. The full fee should be quoted to the patient and charged to the **account,** with the understanding that after the insurance allowance has been received, the balance may be discounted. If a smaller fee is quoted and charged, the following problems may arise:

- The lower fee will alter the physician's fee profile.
- If it becomes necessary to bring suit for payment of the fee, only the reduced fee can be recovered.
- If the insurance allowance is paid on the basis of a certain percentage of the physician's fee and a lower fee is charged, the insurance allowance will be correspondingly lower.
- If the physician does this with many patients, the insurance company may take the position that the reduced fee is the physician's usual fee and base its payments accordingly. It may even be considered fraudulent in some instances.

EXPLAINING COSTS TO PATIENTS

It is natural for the patient, particularly one new to the practice, to wonder, "How much is this going to cost?" However, some patients may be reluctant to voice this concern. Do not wait for the patient to ask about the fees. It is the responsibility of the physician or the medical assistant to approach the subject if the patient does not do so (Procedure 21-1). Be prepared to discuss costs with any patient who is interested, and ask all patients if they have questions about the fees. A good way to open the discussion would be to ask the following:

"Mr. Willardson, do you have any questions about the costs of your operation? If you do, I'll be glad to review them."

In this preliminary discussion of fees the physician or medical assistant must not sidestep the issue by saying, "Don't worry

---

PROCEDURE 21-1

Explain General Office Policies: Explain Professional Fees

CAAHEP COMPETENCY: 3.c.(3)(a)
ABHES COMPETENCY: 7.d

GOAL: *To explain the physician's fees so that the patient understands his or her obligations and rights for privacy.*

EQUIPMENT and SUPPLIES

- Patient's statement
- Copy of physician's fee schedule
- Quiet, private area where the patient feels free to ask questions

PROCEDURAL STEPS

1. Determine that the patient has the correct bill.
   PURPOSE: To make certain that the bill belongs to this patient and that the insurance numbers, the address, and the telephone number are correct.
2. Examine the bill for possible errors.
   PURPOSE: To demonstrate that the patient's concerns are important and that you are willing to make any necessary adjustments.
3. Refer to the fee schedule for services rendered.
   PURPOSE: To explain how physicians determine their fees. If an error has occurred, correct it immediately with a sincere apology.

4. Explain itemized billing:
   - Date of each service
   - Type of service rendered
   - Fee.
   PURPOSE: To make certain that the patient realizes the number and extent of the services rendered.
5. Display a professional attitude toward the patient.
   PURPOSE: To reassure the patient that you have a thorough understanding of the fee schedule and show willingness to answer questions politely and completely.
6. Determine whether the patient has specific concerns that may hinder payment.
   PURPOSE: To provide an opportunity for making special arrangements if needed.
7. Make appropriate arrangements for a discussion between the physician and patient if further explanation is necessary for resolution of the problem.

about the bill; let's just get you well first." The patient may later complain about the bill because he or she misunderstood the complexity of the service.

Even in cases in which the physician quotes a fee, the medical assistant often has the responsibility of explaining the physician's fees to the patient. The medical assistant must know how fees are determined and why charges vary, as well as have a thorough knowledge of the physician's practice and policies, to handle perplexing situations involving fees.

As the medical assistant's understanding of the practice increases, he or she can build respect for the physician's services by educating patients that money spent for medical care is an excellent investment in the future. It is a rare patient who understands the intricate procedures involved in diagnosis and treatment, especially when third-party payors are involved. Be patient and understanding when questions arise in this area.

CRITICAL THINKING APPLICATION

Mr. Reynolds, one of Dr. Wallace's long-standing patients, continually complains about his insurance policies and the small payments made on his medical claims. He frequents the office at least twice a month for checkups and goes into a long speech about the problems with his insurance each time he stops to pay his bill at Myra's desk. He will continue complaining even when other patients come to pay their bills. How can Myra tactfully handle Mr. Reynolds and stop his complaints?

Advance Discussion of Fees

Advance fee discussions help the patient plan ahead for medical expenditures (Figure 21-1). Most patients want to meet their financial obligations but rightly insist on an accurate estimate of those obligations before they contract for purchase of goods

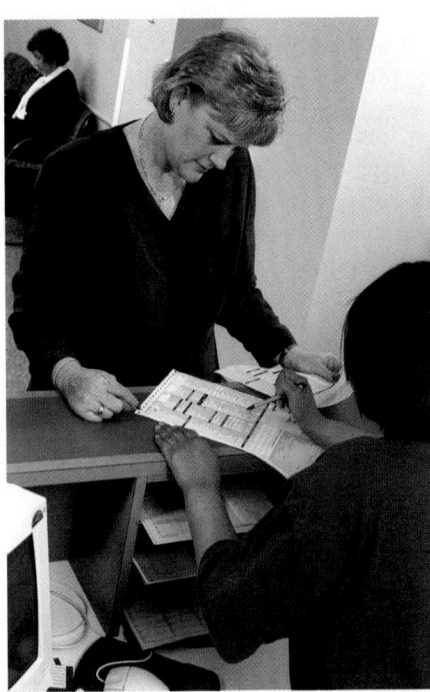

FIGURE 21-1 Taking a short amount of time to explain fees will often result in prompt payment for services.

or services. When a physician frankly discusses fees in advance with patients, even to the point of describing how a fee is established, misconceptions and complaints about overcharging and fee discrepancies are usually eliminated.

Explanation of Additional Costs

Explanations of medical costs should extend beyond the physician's own charges. For example, if a patient is to undergo surgery, the physician should also explain the costs of the operation, the anesthesiologist's and radiologist's charges, the laboratory fees, and the approximate hospital bill. The importance of calling in another physician for consultation should be explained to patients when consultation becomes necessary. It should be made clear, in advance, that there will be a separate bill submitted by the consulting physician. Patients do not always understand that the consultation is for the benefit of the patient, not the physician.

Estimates of Costs

Some physicians give patients an estimate of medical expenses before hospitalization. A few medical societies cooperatively develop estimate sheets or forms with local hospitals. Individual physicians occasionally work up their own estimate forms when a patient is embarking on long-term treatment. The physician should, however, emphasize that it is an estimate only and that the actual cost may vary somewhat.

Estimate slips should be prepared in duplicate so that the patient may have a copy while the original is retained in the patient's file. Using duplicate estimate slips may help in the following ways:

- It may help to avoid forgetting that a fee was quoted.
- It may help eliminate the possibility of later misquoting the fee.
- It may help simplify collection by preventing misunderstanding and confusion over charges.

Guarantor's Ultimate Responsibility: The Bill

Patients must understand that the **guarantor** is the person ultimately responsible for the entire bill. The insurance policy is a contract between the policy holder and the insurance company or between a group of people (such as an employer) and a managed care organization. The actual physician is not a party to that contract. Therefore it is not the responsibility of the physician or staff to pursue insurance payment for the benefit of the patient. However, it is in the best interest of the staff to actively assist the patient if problems occur in securing payment for several reasons.

First, the staff is almost always more knowledgeable about the insurance business than the patient. Many patients have never even read their insurance policies and have no idea what is or is not covered. Some patients expect the insurance to pay all costs simply because they are paying a high **premium.** The medical assistant may need to educate these patients about their policies and offer advice regarding how the patients can effectively work with the insurance company to get answers to questions and make certain that they are receiving all of the benefits to which they are entitled.

Second, it is in the best interest of the staff to assist the patient in collecting from the insurance company so that the physician will be compensated for services rendered. Helping the patient in this area will usually result in the bill for care being paid. Another reason to actively assist the patient is that the medical assistant will gain knowledge about the insurance industry. The more experience the medical assistant has in working with third-party payors, the more helpful he or she can be to the patients of the clinic. It is a good idea to keep a notebook with specific information about each type of policy that the office handles. This reference notebook will provide excellent guidance and suggestions for the medical assistant when working with a particular payor.

Always be sure to secure guarantors in writing. Most patient information sheets have a section that refers to the guarantor. There may be a statement that the guarantor signs indicating an agreement to pay the costs of medical care. States have varying statutes that deal with guarantors, so be sure that the office policies reflect compliance with those laws. It is especially important to secure a written agreement to pay for services when the care will be long term or when a costly treatment or surgical procedure must be done.

CRITICAL THINKING APPLICATION

■ Madeline Amos has a 12-year-old diabetic son, Eric, who is Dr. Wallace's patient. Ms. Amos is divorced from her son's father, but the father is required to keep a medical insurance policy on the son. Myra knows that Ms. Amos has had numerous problems with the father. On a visit to the office, it is discovered that the insurance policy on the son has been cancelled. How does Myra explain this to Ms. Amos?

■ What steps, if any, can be taken to assist Ms. Amos in paying her son's account?

ENCOUNTER FORMS

Encounter forms are the slips that are attached to charts while the patient is in the office; they are used for billing purposes. The encounter form provides information about the patient, such as the name, account number, and previous balance. Current charges and payments for the visit are added after the physician sees the patient. The physician can indicate on the encounter form when the patient should return to the clinic (Figure 21-2). The medical assistant then schedules an appointment and can even use the patient's copy of the encounter form to note the next appointment date and time.

The encounter form normally consists of three parts, with a white top sheet, a yellow sheet, and a pink sheet. The colors can vary, but usually the white copy is kept as a permanent record by the office, and the yellow and pink copies are given to the patient. The yellow copy is used by the patient for insurance billing (if not done by the office), and the pink copy is a receipt for the patient.

Encounter forms are sometimes designed to work with a **pegboard system** or may be available in continuous forms

that can be placed in the printer for computer use. Encounter forms have been known by many aliases throughout the years; these include *superbills, charge slips,* and *multipurpose billing forms.*

PATIENT ACCOUNT TRANSACTIONS

A business **transaction** is the occurrence of an event or of a condition that must be recorded. For example, when a service is performed for which a charge is made, when a debtor makes a payment on account, when a piece of equipment is purchased, or when the monthly rent is paid, a business transaction has been completed.

Each of these examples is a transaction that must be recorded within the accounting system. The medical assistant will very likely encounter various other business transactions as he or she becomes more familiar with the individual needs of the employer's practice.

A patient's financial record is called an *account.* All of the patients' accounts together constitute the **accounts receivable ledger.** Account cards vary in design, but all will have at least three columns for entering figures. In the manual system these columns are as follows:

- **Debit** column—It is on the left, is used for entering charges, and is sometimes called the *charge column.*
- **Credit** column—It is to the right, is sometimes headed *Paid,* and is used for entering payments received.
- Balance column—It is on the far right and is used for recording the difference between the debit and the credit columns.

An adjustment column is available in some systems and is used for entering professional discounts, write-offs, disallowances by insurance companies, and any other adjustments. In a computer system, when a patient is called up by name or identification number, the patient's balance will appear. This is the individual patient's ledger.

Posting means the transfer of information from one record to another. Transactions are posted from the journal to the ledger; this is accomplished in one writing on the pegboard system. The **account balance** is normally a debit balance, which means that the charges exceed the payments on the account. A debit balance is entered by simply writing the correct figure in the balance column. A credit balance exists when payments exceed charges (e.g., when a patient pays in advance). This is common in obstetric practices.

Discounts are also credit entries and are entered in the adjustment column; if there is no adjustment column, the discount is entered in the debit column and enclosed in parentheses. When the entry is made this way, it is recognized as a subtraction from the charges. When columns are totaled, any figure in red or in parentheses is always subtracted. **Receipts** are cash and checks taken in payment for professional services. **Receivables** are charges for which payment has not been received—amounts that are owing. **Disbursements** are cash amounts paid out. **Payables** are amounts owed to others but not yet paid.

LIC. # 999999
S.S. # 111-22-3333
UPIN # A12365

JANE A. SMITH, M.D.
Reproductive Endocrinology
123 FIRST AVENUE
ANYTOWN, N.Y. 22222

TELEPHONE: (212) 555-4444
FAX: (212) 555-4545

PATIENT INFORMATION

PATIENT'S LAST NAME	FIRST	INITIAL	BIRTHDATE / /	SEX ☑ FEMALE	TODAY'S DATE / /	
ADDRESS	CITY	STATE	ZIP	RELATION TO SUBSCRIBER	REFERRING PHYSICIAN	
SUBSCRIBER OR POLICYHOLDER				INSURANCE CARRIER		
ADDRESS	CITY	STATE	ZIP	INS. ID	COVERAGE CODE	GROUP
OTHER HEALTH COVERAGE? ☐ NO ☐ YES IDENTIFY			DISABILITY RELATED TO: ☐ IND. ☐ ACCIDENT ☐ PREGNANCY ☐ OTHER		DATE SYMPTOMS APPEARED, INCEPTION OF PREGNANCY, OR ACCIDENT OCCURRED: / /	

ASSIGNMENT & RELEASE: I hereby assign my insurance benefits to be paid directly to the undersigned physician. I am financially responsible for non-covered services. I also authorize the physician to release any information required to process this claim.
SIGNED: (Patient, or Parent, if Minor) DATE: / /

✓	DESCRIPTION	CODE	FEE	✓	DESCRIPTION	CODE	FEE	✓	DESCRIPTION	CODE	FEE
	OFFICE VISIT				**OFFICE PROCEDURES**				**LABORATORY - IN OFFICE**		
	New Patient				Sperm Wash	58323			Pregnancy Test	85160	
	Consultation	99204			Cauterization of Cervix	57510			Urinalysis	81002	
	Comprehensive	99205			Cervical Biopsy	57500			Stool Occult Blood	82270	
	OFFICE VISIT				Endocervical Curettage	57505			Lyme Titer	86317	
	Established Patient				Endometrial Biopsy	58100			Estradiol	82670	
	Limited	99211			Office Endometrial Curettage	58102			Chemistry	80019	
	Intermediate	99212			Post Coital Test	89300			CBC, pit., Diff.	85024	
	Extended	99213			Artificial Insemination	58310			T3 Uptake	84479	
	Comprehensive	99214			Pelvic Sonogram	76856			T4	84435	
	Comprehensive	99215			Vulvar Biopsy	56600			TSH	84443	
	SURGERY				Bilateral Mammogram	76091			ESR	85650	
	D & C	58120			Unilateral Mammogram	76090			Pregnancy Test	84702	
	Pregnancy Termination	59840			Breast Ultrasound	76645			FSH	83000	
	Laparoscopy	56305			Abdominal Ultrasound	76700			Prolactin	84146	
	Hysteroscopy	56351			Polypectomy	57500					
	Laporotomy	49000									
	Myomectomy	58140									
	Hysterectomy	58150									

DIAGNOSIS: **ICD-9**

☐ Abortion, Incomplete 634.71
☐ Abortion, Spontaneous 634.90
☐ Alopecia 704.09
☐ Amenorrhea 626.0
☐ Anemia 285.9
☐ Anovulation 628.0
☐ Atrophic Vaginitis 627.3
☐ Breast Cyst 610.1
☐ Breast Mass 611.72
☐ Breast Pain 611.71
☐ Cervical Polyp 622.7
☐ Cervicitis 616.0
☐ Condyloma 091.3
☐ Cyclic Adrenal Hyperplasia .255.2
☐ Cystocele 618.0
☐ Cystitis 595.9
☐ Diabetes Mellitus 250.0
☐ Dysmenorrhea 625.3
☐ Dyspareunia 625.0
☐ Dysuria 788.1
☐ Ectopic Pregnancy 633.9
☐ Edema 782.3
☐ Endometrial Hyperplasia ..621.3
☐ Endometriosis 617.0
☐ Fatigue 780.7
☐ Fibrocystic Breast Disease .610.1
☐ Galactorrhea 676.6
☐ Headache 784.0
☐ Hemorrhoids 455.6
☐ Herpes 054.1
☐ Hypercholesterolemia 272.0
☐ Hyperprolactinemia 253.1
☐ Hypertension 401.9
☐ Hyperthyroidism 242.9
☐ Hypothyroidism 244.9
☐ Infertility 628.9
☐ Luteal Phase Insufficiency .628.8
☐ Menometrorrhagia 626.2
☐ Menopausal Syndrome 627.2
☐ Menorrhagia 626.2
☐ Monilial Vaginitis 112.1
☐ Obesity 278.0
☐ Osteoarthritis 715.9
☐ Osteopenia 733.9
☐ Osteoporosis 733.0
☐ Ovarian Cyst 620.2
☐ Ovarian Insufficiency 256.3
☐ Pelvic Pain 625.9
☐ Polycystic Ovary Syndrome 256.4
☐ Postmenopausal Bleeding .627.1
☐ Pregnancy V22.2
☐ Pregnancy Termination ...V72.4
☐ Premature Ovarian Failure .256.3
☐ Premenopausal Menorrhagia .627.0
☐ Prolactinoma 253
☐ Prolapsed Uterus 618.1
☐ Rectocele 569.1
☐ Thyroiditis 245.2
☐ Trichomonas 131.0
☐ Urinary Tract Infection 599.0
☐ Uterine Fibroids 218.9
☐ Vasomotor Instability 780.2
☐ Vaginitis 616.1
☐ Vulvitis 616.1

DIAGNOSIS: (IF NOT CHECKED ABOVE)	ADDITIONAL INFORMATION:	DOCTOR'S SIGNATURE

SERVICES PERFORMED AT: ☐ OFFICE ☐ University Hospital 345 Second Avenue Anytown, N.Y. 23333 ☐ Day Surgery / University Hosp. 678 Third Avenue Anytown, N.Y. 23444

REFERRING PHYSICIAN:

ACCEPT ASSIGNMENT? ☐ YES ☐ NO

TOTAL TODAY'S FEE	
PREVIOUS BALANCE	
AMT. REC'D. TODAY	
NEW BALANCE	

INSTRUCTIONS TO PATIENT FOR FILING INSURANCE CLAIMS:

1. COMPLETE UPPER PORTION OF THIS FORM; SIGN AND DATE.
2. MAIL THIS FORM DIRECTLY TO YOUR INSURANCE COMPANY. YOU MAY ATTACH YOUR OWN INSURANCE COMPANY'S FORM IF YOU WISH, ALTHOUGH IT IS NOT NECESSARY.

PLEASE REMEMBER THAT PAYMENT IS YOUR OBLIGATION, REGARDLESS OF INSURANCE OR OTHER THIRD PARTY INVOLVEMENT.

INSUR-A-BILL ® BIBBERO SYSTEMS, INC. • PETALUMA, CA • © 5/95 (SB M-N) (REV. 9/96)

FIGURE 21-2 An encounter form. The encounter form is used by the physician and staff to document what was done to the patient during an office visit and to indicate when the physician wishes the patient to return. The copies of the form may be used to bill third-party payors. (Courtesy Bibbero Systems, Inc., Petaluma, Calif. 94954, (800) 242-2376, www.bibbero.com.)

Manual Posting

All charges and payments for professional services are posted to the ledger daily. The ledger then becomes a reliable source of information for answering all inquiries from patients about their accounts.

A separate account card or page is prepared for each patient at the time of the first visit or service. The heading of the account should include all information pertinent to collecting the account, such as the following:

- Name and address of person responsible for payment (the guarantor)

- Insurance identification
- Social Security number
- Home and business telephone numbers
- Name of employer
- Any special instructions for billing

Billing statements to the patient and the patient's insurance carrier are prepared from the ledger.

Computer Posting

The patient's name, date, diagnosis, and procedures are posted when the patient leaves the office. The database will retrieve the correct charges and post the charges on the computerized patient record and the accounts receivable ledger.

WRITE-IT-ONCE, OR PEGBOARD, SYSTEM

The initial cost of materials for the pegboard system is slightly more than that for other accounting systems but is still moderate. The system is simple to operate, and training is included in most medical assisting programs.

The system gets its name from the lightweight aluminum or Masonite board with a row of pegs along the side or top that holds the forms in place. The accounting forms are perforated for alignment on the pegs. All of the forms used in any system must be compatible so that they may be aligned perfectly on the board. The pegboard system generates all the necessary financial records for each transaction with one writing, as follows:

- Encounter form
- Receipt
- Ledger card
- Journal entry

It may also include a statement and bank deposit slip.

The system provides current accounts receivable totals and a daily record of bank deposits and cash on hand, in addition to the record of income and expenses. The need for separate posting to patient accounts is eliminated, and the chance for error is decreased.

Using the Pegboard System

The pegboard system provides positive control over cash, collections, and receivables and ensures that every cent is accounted for and properly entered. It provides a record of every patient, every charge, and every payment, plus a daily recap of earnings—a running record of receivables and an audited summary of cash. The system requires a minimum of time. One writing allows a medical assistant to do the following:

- Enter a transaction on the day sheet
- Give the patient a receipt for payment
- Bring the patient's account up to date
- Provide a current statement of account for the patient
- Give the patient a notation of the next appointment

All of these features communicate the money message to patients effectively and courteously and generate good financial records.

Gathering Required Materials

The pegboard may be of inexpensive Masonite construction with pegs down the left side, or it may be a more sophisticated aluminum sliding board that allows flexible positioning of materials. The basic pegboard forms follow:

- Day sheet (Figure 21-3)
- Patient ledger
- Encounter form

All of the forms must be compatible and are available from medical office supply companies. They may be customized to the practice, incorporating the usual services and procedure codes of the practice.

Preparing the Board

At the beginning of each day, place a new day sheet on the accounting board. Some systems have a sheet of clean carbon attached to the day sheet, others use special carbon with holes for the pegs, and some use NCR (no carbon required) paper. The carbon goes on top of the day sheet. Over the carbon, place the encounter form. The receipt has a carbonized writing line that should align with the first open writing line on the day sheet. If the slips are shingled, lay the entire bank of receipts over the pegs, with the top one aligned as mentioned. The remainder will be automatically in place. Receipts should be used in numeric order.

Pulling the Ledger Cards

If a great many patients are to be seen in a day, pull the ledger cards for all scheduled patients in the morning to save time (Figure 21-4). Keep the cards in the order in which the patients are scheduled to be seen.

Entering and Posting Transactions

As each patient arrives, insert the patient's ledger card under the first receipt, aligning the first available writing line of the card with the carbonized strip on the receipt. Enter the receipt number and date, the account balance in the space labeled *previous balance,* and the patient's name. The information recorded on the receipt is automatically posted to the ledger and the day sheet (Figure 21-5). The charge slip is then detached and clipped to the patient chart to be routed to the physician, who now has an opportunity to see how much the patient owes and can discuss the account in privacy, if desired.

After the service has been performed, the physician enters the service on the encounter form and asks the patient or the nurse to return it to the medical assistant. The assistant then has an opportunity to ask the patient whether this is to be a charge or cash transaction before completing the posting. Again, insert the ledger card under the proper receipt, checking the number that was previously entered to make sure the correct card is being used. Record the service by procedure code, post the charge from the **fee schedule,** enter any payment made, and write in the current balance (Procedure 21-2, p. 409). If there is no balance, place a zero or a straight line in the balance column. If another appointment is required, enter the date and time at the bottom of the receipt.

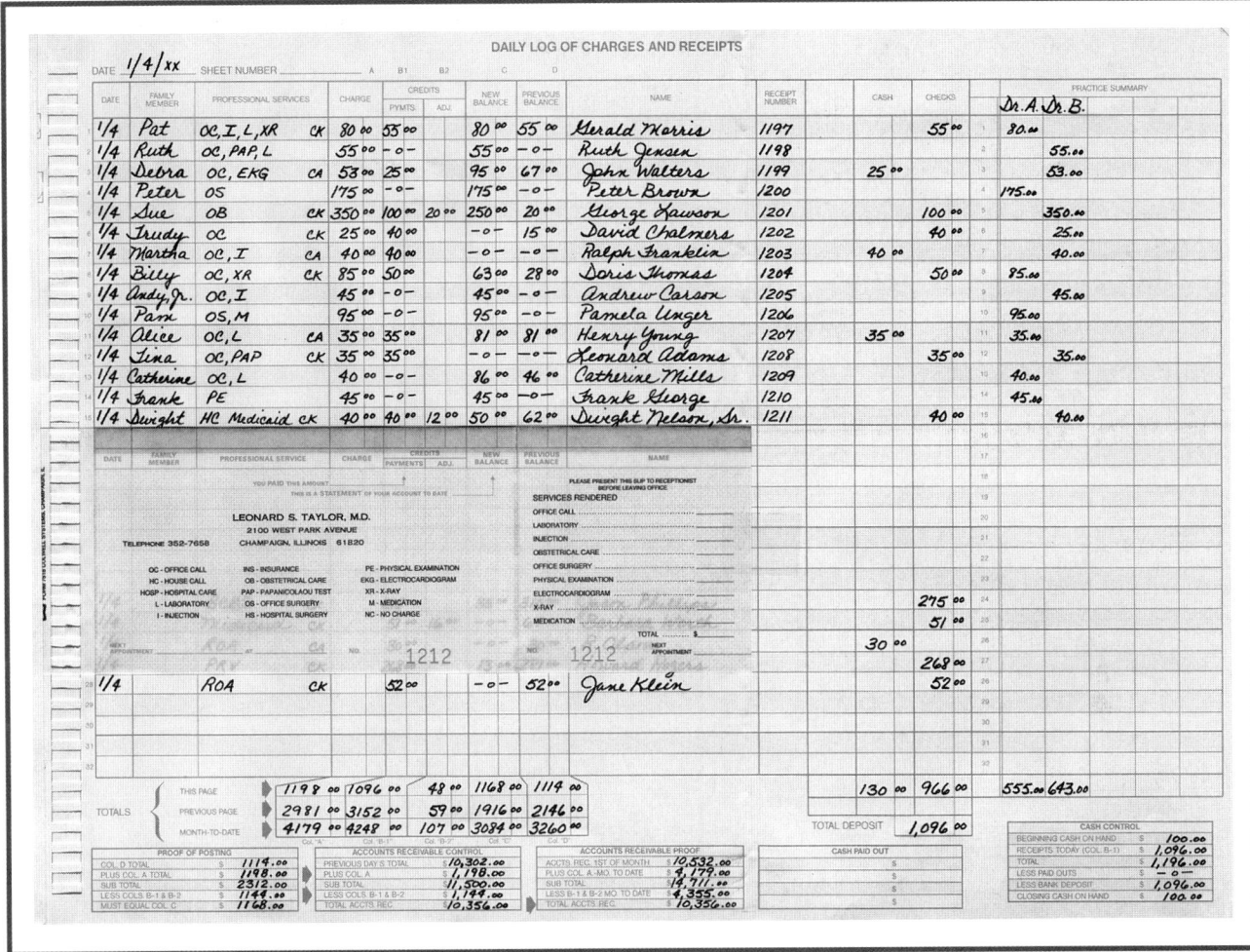

FIGURE 21-3 Sample day sheet for use with a pegboard bookkeeping system. The pegboard system allows the user to write bookkeeping entries once, prepare deposit slips, and perform business analysis functions. (Courtesy Colwell Systems, Inc., Champaign, Ill.)

The transaction has now been posted to the journal and the ledger, and if payment was made by the patient, a receipt has been generated. The service receipt is given to the patient; no other receipt is necessary. The ledger card is ready for refiling.

File the encounter forms in numeric order for any internal audit. At the end of the month, the total of the encounter forms should equal the total of the charges recorded on the day sheets for the month (Figure 21-6, p. 410).

Recording Other Payments and Charges

Payments will be received in the mail and may be brought in by patients some time after a service was performed. These payments are entered on the day sheet and the ledger card in the same manner as previously explained. Payments by mail do not require a receipt.

The physician may have daily charges for visits to patients in a hospital or convalescent facility. Enter these charges on the day sheet and ledger card only. Surgery fees are usually recorded as one entry that includes the surgery and aftercare.

CRITICAL THINKING APPLICATION

- Dr. Wallace sometimes forgets to write down information for billing when he goes to the hospital to check on his patients. Myra has a difficult time entering the charges for hospital visits because Dr. Wallace's records are not reliable in this area. How might Myra rectify this situation?
- How can Myra help Dr. Wallace be more accurate in this area?

Summarizing Accounting Transactions

At the end of the day, all columns must be totaled and proved. Although all bookkeeping is done in ink, it is a good idea to write the totals in pencil until they have been proved. If an error is discovered, correct the entry in which it occurred. Do not attempt to erase or write over the incorrect entry. Simply draw one line through it and make a new entry on the first open writing line. Remember to reinsert the ledger card for these corrections. Also, if the entry included a receipt for the patient, make a new receipt and notify the patient of the correction.

STATEMENT

LEONARD S. TAYLOR, M.D.
2100 WEST PARK AVENUE
CHAMPAIGN, ILLINOIS 61820

TELEPHONE 351-5400

DATE	FAMILY MEMBER	PROFESSIONAL SERVICE	CHARGE	CREDITS		BALANCE
				PAYMENTS	ADJ.	
				BALANCE FORWARD ▷		
5/13/00		Office consult 99203	60 –	60 –		0

Form 1625   PAY LAST AMOUNT IN THIS COLUMN

OC - OFFICE CALL	INS - INSURANCE	PE - PHYSICAL EXAMINATION
HC - HOUSE CALL	OB - OBSTETRICAL CARE	EKG - ELECTROCARDIOGRAM
HOSP - HOSPITAL CARE	PAP - PAPANICOLAOU TEST	XR - X-RAY
L - LABORATORY	OS - OFFICE SURGERY	M - MEDICATION
I - INJECTION	HS - HOSPITAL SURGERY	NC - NO CHARGE

FIGURE 21-4 Patient ledger card. A ledger card showing the charge and payment for an office consultation. (Courtesy Colwell Systems, Inc., Champaign, Ill.)

SPECIAL BOOKKEEPING ENTRIES

The following special entries are necessary occasionally and may be used with a pegboard or any other accounting system:

- Adjustments
- Credit balances
- Refunds
- Insufficient funds checks

Adjustments

At times, it is necessary to enter a credit adjustment. These could be for professional discounts, insurance disallowances, account write-offs, or payments that come to the office after the account has been placed for collection (Procedure 21-3, p. 411). If a patient or guarantor files for bankruptcy, the charge will usually have to be adjusted off the books.

If the system has an adjustment column, enter adjustments there. Otherwise, because the adjustment is actually a subtraction from the charge, enter it in the charge column with the figure enclosed in parentheses or circled and with an explanation of the entry in the description column. When the column of figures is totaled, the circled figure is subtracted rather than added. The learner has a tendency to ignore the circled figures. This is incorrect—they must be subtracted.

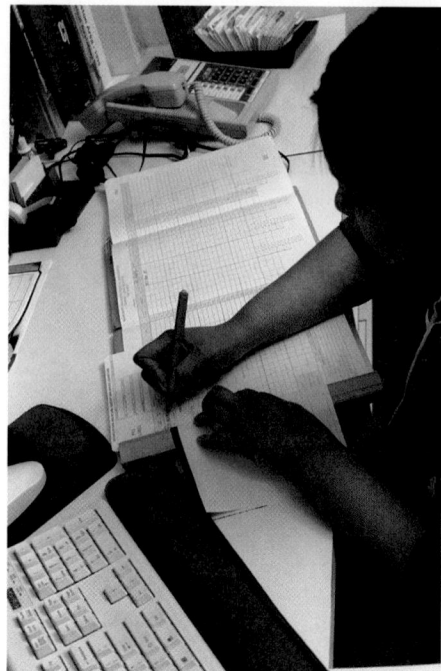

FIGURE 21-5 The pegboard system saves time by allowing several entries to be made at one time.

Credit Balances

A credit balance occurs when a patient has paid in advance or there has been an overpayment or duplicate payment (Procedure 21-4, p. 411). For example, an overpayment occurs if the patient made a partial payment and later the insurance allowance was more than the remaining balance. The difference between the total amount of money received and the amount owed must be entered in the balance column and enclosed within parentheses or circled. This indicates a credit balance. Some credit balances are created when an error has been made in posting.

The credit balance is money owed to the patient. If the patient has paid in advance or wishes to leave the overpayment in the account in anticipation of future charges, care must be taken in figuring the balance on future transactions. Whereas normally a charge increases the balance, it will decrease a credit balance.

Refunds

If a patient wishes to have an overpayment refunded, write a check for the amount due and enter the transaction on the day sheet. In most cases, the refund will result in a patient balance of zero (Procedure 21-5, p. 412).

CRITICAL THINKING APPLICATION

■ Myra receives a phone call from a patient who says that she is due a refund because her insurance company sent her an explanation of benefits for $654.00, and her balance was only $436. She demands an immediate refund, but Myra has not yet received the check. What should she do?

■ Myra suspects that the check sent to pay on the account was an error. What should she do in this situation?

PROCEDURE 21-2

Post Entries on a Daysheet

CAAHEP COMPETENCY: 3.a.(2)(b)
ABHES COMPETENCY: 3.k

GOAL: *To post 1 day's charges and payments and compute the daily bookkeeping cycle using a pegboard.*

EQUIPMENT and SUPPLIES

- Pegboard
- Calculator
- Pen
- Day sheet
- Receipts
- Ledger cards
- Balances from previous day

PROCEDURAL STEPS

1. Prepare the board.
   - Place a new day sheet on the board.
   - Place a bank of receipts over the pegs, aligning the top receipt with the first open writing line on the day sheet.
2. Carry forward balances from the previous day.
   PURPOSE: To keep all totals current.
3. Pull ledger cards for patient being seen that day.
4. Insert the ledger card under the first receipt, aligning the first available writing line of the card with the carbonized strip on the receipt.
   PURPOSE: To ensure that one writing will correctly post the entry to receipt, ledger, and day sheet.
5. Enter the patient's name, the date, the receipt number, and any existing balance from the ledger card.
6. Detach the charge slip from the receipt and clip it to the patient's chart.

PURPOSE: The physician will indicate the service performed on the charge slip and return it to you.
7. Accept the returned charge slip at the end of the visit.
8. Enter the appropriate fee from the fee schedule.
9. Locate the receipt on the board with a number matching the charge slip.
   PURPOSE: To make certain it is the correct receipt.
10. Reinsert the patient's ledger card under the receipt.
11. Write the service code number and fee on the receipt.
12. Accept the patient's payment, and record the amount of payment and the new balance.
    PURPOSE: To bring the patient's account up to date and provide a current statement for the patient.
13. Give the completed receipt to the patient.
14. Follow your agency's procedure for refilling the ledger card.
15. Repeat Steps 4 to 14 for each service of the day.
16. Total all columns of the day sheet at the end of the day.
    PURPOSE: To determine total amount of the charges, receipts, and resulting balances for the day.
17. Write preliminary totals in pencil.
    PURPOSE: To facilitate any necessary changes.
18. Complete proof of totals and enter totals in ink.
19. Enter figures for accounts receivable control.
    PURPOSE: To complete daily accounting cycle.

Insufficient Funds Checks

Sometimes, a patient sends in a check without having sufficient funds to cover it; this check is later deposited to the physician's account. The bank will return the check to you marked NSF ("nonsufficient funds"). Two accounting functions must be performed. First, deduct the amount from the practice's checking account balance. Then add the amount back into the patient's account balance by entering the amount in the paid column in parentheses and increasing the balance by the same amount. Write a brief explanation of the transaction in the description column (Procedure 21-6, p. 412).

Balancing the Accounts Receivable and Accounts Receivable Control

The accounts receivable control is a daily summary of what remains unpaid on the accounts. Most offices also complete an end-of-day summary. These are integral parts of the office accounting system and are discussed in Chapter 23.

PAYING FOR MEDICAL SERVICES AND TREATMENT

The payment for medical services is accomplished in the following four ways:
- Payment at the time of service
- Internal billing when extension of credit is necessary
- Internal insurance or other third-party billing
- Outside billing and collection assistance

Payment at the Time of Service

A large percentage of patients will have some type of health insurance for at least major items. Every practice in which there are patient visits should encourage time-of-service collection. It is especially important to collect co-payments and payment for office visits not covered by insurance. If patients get into the habit of paying their current charges before they leave the office, there are no further billing and bookkeeping expenses. If patients are informed when making an appointment that payment is expected at the time of service, they are not surprised

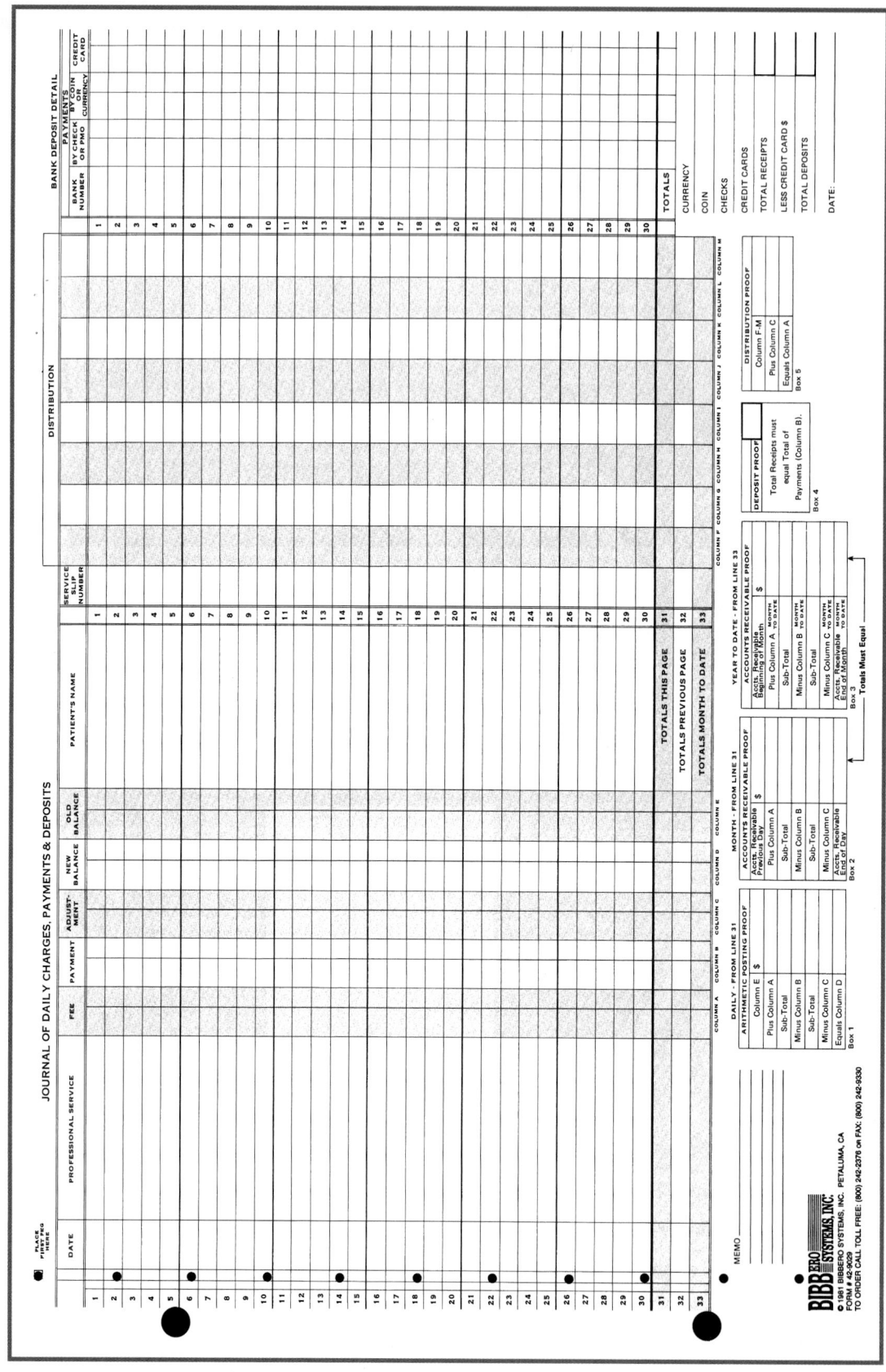

FIGURE 21-6 Sample day sheet used to log patient charges and receipts. (Courtesy Bibbero Systems, Inc., Petaluma, CA 94954, (800) 242-2376, www.bibbero.com.)

PROCEDURE 21-3

Post Adjustments

CAAHEP COMPETENCY: 3.a(2)(e)
ABHES COMPETENCY: 3.o

GOAL: *To process adjustments to patient accounts accurately.*

EQUIPMENT and SUPPLIES

- Patient ledgers
- Office policy manual
- Explanation of benefits and remittance advice
- Bookkeeping system
- Clerical supplies
- Payments
- Calculator

PROCEDURAL STEPS

1. Open checks that arrive in the mail as payment on patient accounts.
2. Paper-clip the check to the explanation of benefits or remittance advice.
   PURPOSE: To keep the check with the EOB as payments are posted.

3. Post the payment to the patient's account.
4. Determine if an adjustment is necessary on the patient account.
   PURPOSE: Adjustments may be necessary in cases of disallowed charges, noncovered services, and so on.
5. Review the office policy manual to ascertain the correct procedure to follow regarding adjustments to patient accounts.
   PURPOSE: To make certain that office policies are followed and are consistent with regard to patient accounts and adjustments.
6. Make sure that the ledger card is aligned with the day sheet correctly.
7. Write the adjustment amount in the adjustment column of the ledger card.
8. Check the math to make certain the adjustment was posted correctly.

PROCEDURE 21-4

Process a Credit Balance

CAAHEP COMPETENCY: 3.a(2)(f)
ABHES COMPETENCY: 3.p

GOAL: *To return overpayments to patients in a timely manner.*

EQUIPMENT and SUPPLIES

- Patient ledgers
- Office policy manual
- Explanation of benefits and remittance advice
- Bookkeeping system
- Clerical supplies
- Payments
- Calculator

PROCEDURAL STEPS

1. Review the office policy manual to determine the guidelines for credit balances.
   PURPOSE: To make certain that office policy is followed.

2. Review the payment received and the explanation of benefits or remittance advice.
3. Post the payment to the patient's account.
4. Determine if an overpayment has been made.
5. Review the account to determine if more insurance is expected on the account.
   PURPOSE: Some credit balances need not be made if more activity exists on the account; only refund amounts that remain after the complete bill has been paid.
6. Adjust the credit balance off of the patient's account.
   PURPOSE: To refund the credit balance if it is due to the patient.

when asked for payment at the end of the visit. Use a phrase, such as the following:

"Your charge for today is $25.00. Will that be cash, check, or credit card?"

Many patients are hesitant to ask about charges and are unsure whether to offer to pay or to wait until asked. Make it easier for the patients by offering to accept their payments, because most people are prepared to pay small bills on a cash basis. If a patient requests to be billed, the medical assistant may say:

"Our normal procedure is to pay at the time of service unless other arrangements are made in advance."

PROCEDURE 21-5

Process Refunds

CAAHEP COMPETENCY: 3.a(2)(g)
ABHES COMPETENCY: 3.q

GOAL: *To process patient refunds in a timely manner.*

EQUIPMENT and SUPPLIES

- Patient ledgers
- Office policy manual
- Explanation of benefits and remittance advice
- Bookkeeping system
- Clerical supplies
- Payments
- Calculator

PROCEDURAL STEPS

1. Determine the amount of the refund to be processed.
   PURPOSE: To make certain that the patient receives a refund in the correct amount.
2. Write a check for the amount of the refund.

PURPOSE: Always use a check to pay refunds so that the patient's name is on the back of the check as endorsement, proving that the patient received the refund.

3. Give the check to the physician for a signature.
   PURPOSE: Most physicians prefer to sign their own checks.
4. Determine the correct mailing address for the patient.
   PURPOSE: To make certain that the patient has not reported a change of address.
5. Make a copy of the check, and place it in the patient medical record.
   PURPOSE: The copy will show that a check was mailed to the patient.
6. Mail the refund check to the patient.

PROCEDURE 21-6

Post Nonsufficient Fund Checks

CAAHEP COMPETENCY: 3.a(2)(h)
ABHES COMPETENCY: 3.r

GOAL: *To correctly note that a patient's check was returned because of insufficient funds.*

EQUIPMENT and SUPPLIES

- Patient ledgers
- Office policy manual
- Bookkeeping system
- Clerical supplies
- Calculator

PROCEDURAL STEPS

1. Pull the ledger card that corresponds with the patient who wrote the check.
   PURPOSE: To post charges to the correct patient account.
2. Determine the amount to be added back to the account as a result of the returned check.

PURPOSE: The physician's bank usually charges a fee for all checks that are returned by the bank because of insufficient funds.

3. Post the total amount onto the patient's ledger card.
   PURPOSE: To account for the original check amount plus the fee for the returned check.
4. Send a certified letter to the patient notifying him or her of the returned check and demanding fast payment.
   PURPOSE: Many states require that certified mail be used when notifying patients about insufficient funds checks.
5. Note this collection activity in the patient medical record.

Many offices accept credit cards for the convenience of their patients. **Debit cards** are now widely accepted for payment as well. Computers have made the electronic transfer of funds easy and convenient.

The medical assistant must believe that the physician and the facility have a right to charge for the services provided. Do not

be embarrassed to ask for payment for the value of the service. When tact and good judgment are used in billing and collecting, patients appreciate the service they receive and the help the medical assistant provides. Give individual attention and personal consideration to each patient, and be courteous, showing a sincere desire to help the patient who has financial problems.

CRITICAL THINKING APPLICATION

■ Mr. Page comes to Myra's desk to pay his account. His credit card is rejected, and a message comes back through the machine, saying that the card should be collected from the patient. How does Myra handle this situation?

■ Mr. Page argues that he recently paid the balance of his account in full. What steps should Myra take in this case?

Billing after Extension of Credit

In some types of practice, particularly those involving large fees for surgery or long-term care, it becomes necessary to extend credit and establish a regular system of billing. This requires informing the patient of what the charges will be, what professional services these charges cover, and what the credit policy of the office is (Procedure 21-7).

Many practices do not have a true credit policy; thus each account continues to be evaluated individually. It is almost impossible to judge accounts objectively and equitably under such circumstances.

The physician and the staff should think through their situation, decide what they expect of patients with respect to payments, and how they will inform the patient. Although there will always be exceptions to any rule, there must be a rule, which should be in writing and conveyed to the patient at the outset of the relationship.

Some medical practices prepare an information booklet that includes the payment policy. New patients are given a copy of the booklet. Any patient who needs special consideration can be counseled by the medical assistant. The medical assistant who has the guidance and support of an established credit policy can perform with confidence when handling patient accounts. The credit policy must be fair and must address the following issues:

- Time when payment is due from patients
- Payment at the time of service
- Times when or if assignment of insurance benefits is accepted
- Completion of insurance forms by the office staff (or not)
- Billing procedures
- Collection protocol
- Length of time an account will be carried without payment
- Telephone collection protocol
- Use of a collection agency

Installment Buying of Medical Services

Because installment buying is so much a part of our economic system today, the physician's office must be prepared to help patients budget for their medical care. Patients expect to use their credit resources and appreciate business-like assistance in establishing a payment plan. The medical profession has too long suffered a poor collection record because of its fear

---

PROCEDURE 21-7

Explain General Office Policies: Make Credit Arrangements with a Patient

CAAHEP COMPETENCY: 3.c.(3)(a)
ABHES COMPETENCY: 7.d

GOAL: *To assist the patient in paying for services by making mutually beneficial credit arrangements according to established office policy.*

EQUIPMENT and SUPPLIES

- Patient's ledger
- Calendar
- Truth in Lending form
- Assignment of benefits form
- Patient's insurance form
- Private area for interview

PROCEDURAL STEPS

1. Answer all questions about credit thoroughly and kindly.
2. Inform the patient of the office policy regarding credit:
   - Payment at the time of first visit
   - Payment by bank card
   - Credit application
   PURPOSE: To ensure complete understanding of mutual responsibilities.
3. Have the patient complete the credit application.
   PURPOSE: To comply with office practices on the extension of credit.

4. Check the completed credit application.
   PURPOSE: To confirm that all the necessary information is included.
5. Discuss with the patient the possible arrangements and ask the patient to decide which of those arrangements is most suitable.
   PURPOSE: To ensure better compliance, which can be expected when the patient makes the choice.
6. Prepare the Truth in Lending form and have the patient sign it if the agreement requires more than four installments.
   PURPOSE: To comply with Regulation Z.
7. Have the patient execute an assignment of insurance benefits.
   PURPOSE: To comply with credit policy.
8. Make a copy of the patient's insurance card, and have the patient sign a consent for release of the information to the insurance company.
   PURPOSE: To ensure that a claim can be processed because consent for the release of information is necessary on most insurance forms.
9. Keep credit information confidential.

of appearing too commercial. The physician should be ready to arrange credit when medical bills will be high or when a patient for some reason is unable to pay at the time of service. In general, fees for routine office calls and small medical bills should be kept on a pay-as-you-go basis.

In recent years companies have begun to offer credit or loans specifically for medical procedures. This is very popular for cosmetic surgeries. Offices that offer these types of procedures may wish to investigate these alternative financing services.

Truth in Lending Act

Regulation Z of the Truth in Lending Act, which is enforced by the Federal Trade Commission, requires that when a bilateral agreement exists between physician and patient for the physician to accept payment in more than four installments, the physician is required to provide disclosure of information regarding finance charges (Figure 21-7). Even if there are no finance charges involved, the form must be completed stating this fact. The physician retains a copy of the form, and the original is given to the patient. Specific wording is required in the disclosure. Have the patient sign the agreement in your presence, because you must have proof of signing. The disclosure statement must be kept on file for 2 years. Although the disclosure statement is designed as protection for the debtor, it can be a good collection tool for the creditor.

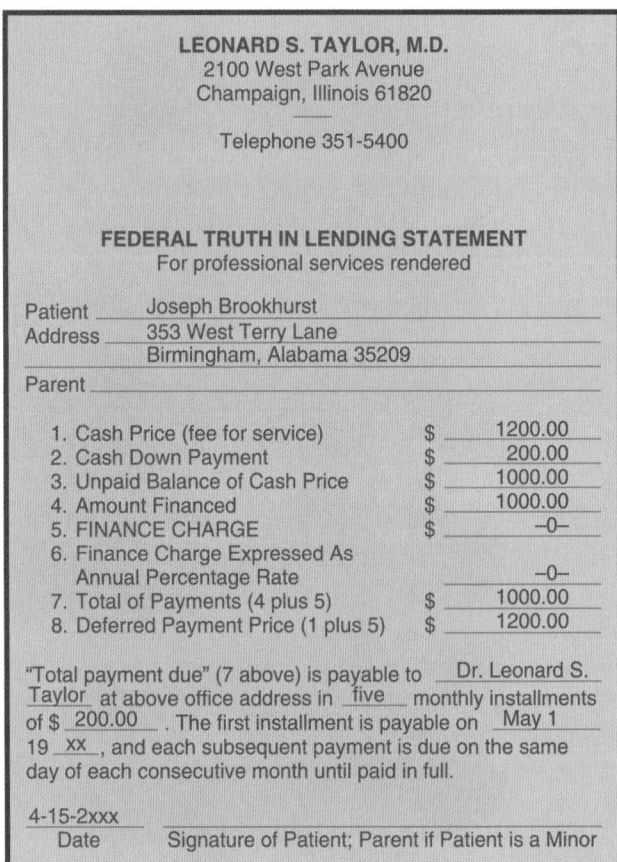

FIGURE 21-7 Disclosure statement. An example of a document for compliance with the Federal Truth in Lending Act. (Courtesy Colwell Systems, Inc., Champaign, Ill.)

It is recognized that physicians generally permit their patients to pay in installments, and as long as no specific agreement has been made for payment to the physician to be made in more than four installments and no finance charge is assessed, the account is not subject to the regulation. If the patient chooses to pay in installments instead of the full amount, this is considered a unilateral action. The physician, in accepting such payments, probably would not be subject to the provisions of the regulation. The physician's office, however, must be certain to bill for the full balance each time. If the statement is for only a partial payment, it then becomes a bilateral agreement and as such is subject to Regulation Z.

Helping patients budget their medical expenses is a rather new aspect of the business side of medical practice. However, it is a real service to patients and demonstrates that the physician and the office staff are sincerely anxious to help patients pay their own way. It may also prevent many collection problems.

Confidentiality

Obtaining Credit Information

Credit information is confidential. It should be guarded as carefully as a confidential medical history and should be disclosed to no one. When asking for credit information from patients in the office, do so in a private area where others cannot overhear the conversation. A desk or table away from the reception area where a patient can sit in total privacy and complete a credit application is a great asset. Credit information is personal—it should be kept that way.

Credit Bureaus

Some physicians join a credit bureau, particularly in large cities where it is more difficult to gauge informally the patients' ability to pay. Credit bureaus gather credit information from many sources, pool it, and make it available to dues-paying bureau members. If the office receives a request for credit information about a patient, it is permissible to furnish it because the debtor, by giving the physician's name as a reference, has given implied consent; otherwise, the credit bureau would not have contacted the office. According to the Fair Credit Practices Act Amendments of 1975, only the following information can be given:

- When the account was opened
- How much the patient now owes
- What the highest amount of the account is at any time
  You should avoid any reference to the following:
- Character
- Paying habits
- Credit rating

Billing Insurance or Other Third Parties

Insurance billing in the medical office is a courtesy to patients. Often, patients do not understand the policies and appreciate the assistance given by the medical office. Information on completing insurance forms and diagnostic and procedure coding is found in Chapters 17 through 20.

Independent Billing and Collection Services

Many healthcare facilities find it advantageous to refer their billing and collections to an independent billing service. The information related to services and fees is sent to the billing service on a daily or weekly basis. The servicing agent then handles all billing and collections, as well as any telephone inquiries. This system frees the regular office staff for more patient-oriented duties. An added advantage is that a person who is not connected with the patient care on a personal basis handles any dispute that may arise.

INTERNAL BILLING BY THE ACCOUNT MANAGER

Billing Methods

In a practice with only a moderate number of accounts, the medical assistant handles the preparation and mailing of statements. This may be accomplished by using the following:

- A computer-generated statement
- An encounter form
- A typewritten statement
- A photocopied statement

The appearance of the statement carries a visual impact just as a letter does, so the statement heads should be carefully chosen and the typing clean and accurate. Statement heads are usually imprinted with the same information as the physician's letterhead. They should be of good quality and large enough to allow itemization of charges. Envelopes should be imprinted with Address Correction Requested under the return address to maintain up-to-date mailing lists. A self-addressed return envelope included with the statement encourages prompt payment. This is mainly for the convenience of patients who do not always have stationery available for sending a return payment or who are less likely to return a payment immediately if they must address an envelope.

Computer-Generated Statement

Patient accounts are generated and stored in the computer, and a statement can be produced whenever needed. The statement can show the service rendered on each date, the charge for each service, the date on which a claim was submitted to the insurance company, the date of payment, and the balance due from the patient. The computer may also be programmed to print messages on the statement, such as "Balance now 30 days past due" or various other messages.

Encounter Form as a Bill

There are variations in style, but encounter forms are usually personalized for the practice. The form has space for all the elements required in submitting medical insurance claims, such as the following:

- Name and address of the patient
- Name of the insurance carrier
- Insurance identification number
- Brief description of each service by code number
- Fee for each service
- Place and date of service
- Diagnosis
- Physician's name and address
- Physician's signature

The encounter form can be used as a charge slip for office treatments if the physician checks the services performed at the completion of the visit and asks the patient to hand it to the medical assistant when leaving. Either the physician or the medical assistant may write in the amount of the fee. If a payment is made, it can be so indicated. Instructions to the patient for filing insurance claims are on the bottom left.

Statements

Statements must be correct and must include the patient's name and address as well as the balance owed. If statements are photocopied or microfilmed, special care must be taken that the ledger card is correct because it will be duplicated in the billing process.

Typewritten Statements

The use of continuous-form billing statements is a timesaver. The statements are printed in a roll with perforated edges for separation. The roll is fed into the typewriter for the first statement and remains until the last statement is typed, eliminating the time and energy necessary for inserting and removing each statement form from the typewriter. These statements are rarely used in this age of computers.

Photocopied Statements

Coordinated ledger cards and copy paper are used in preparing photocopied statements. A perfect statement is ready for mailing in minimal time. Extra care must be used in posting the ledgers. A black pen should be used in making entries on the ledger card, because other ink colors do not reproduce well. Writing must be clear and legible. No personal notes should be made on the ledger cards unless there is something you wish conveyed to the patient. (It is possible to buy pencils with nonreproducible lead if you believe this is necessary for making collection entries.) Usually, a window envelope is used for mailing, which means that the name and address on the ledger must be neat, correct, and positioned correctly for the envelope window.

Internal Billing Procedures

Itemizing the First Statement

If the medical fee has been explained in advance, the monthly statement is merely a confirmation of what is owed, and there should be no misunderstanding. However, it is good business practice and a courtesy to the patient to itemize the charges. This is essential if the statement is to be used for billing the patient's insurance. Patients are entitled to an understanding of the physician's statement for medical services.

Itemizing statements is not difficult, and computerized statements usually automatically itemize the first statement. The simplest method is merely to allow space on the original statement, below the "For Professional Services" line, in which to list the separate charges for office visits, hospital calls, or treatments or tests performed in the medical facility (Procedure 21-8).

PROCEDURE 21-8

Perform Accounts Receivable Procedures

<u>CAAHEP COMPETENCY:</u> 3.a(2)(c)
<u>ABHES COMPETENCY:</u> 8.e

GOAL: *To collect amounts due to the physician or medical facility.*

EQUIPMENT and SUPPLIES

- Patient ledgers
- Office policy manual
- Telephone
- Letterhead and envelopes
- Clerical supplies

PROCEDURAL STEPS

1. Determine the billing cycle for the medical facility according to the office policy manual.
   <u>PURPOSE:</u> The billing cycle specifies which groups of accounts are billed at different times of the month.

2. Determine amounts due to the physician and who owes these amounts.
   <u>PURPOSE:</u> To specify which accounts need to be billed.

3. Group accounts together when necessary.
   <u>PURPOSE:</u> Some physicians prefer to separate regular billings from past-due billings.

4. Print bills using the computer system, or make copies of ledger cards.

5. Mail bills to patients.

6. Post payments to patient accounts as they arrive at the office.
   <u>PURPOSE:</u> To credit the patients' accounts with payments that they submit to the medical facility.

Many physicians have devised their own itemized encounter forms, which are given to the patient when payment is made at the time of service or later mailed in a combination statement-reply envelope. The use of such charge slips simplifies the itemization procedure, because filling out the slips is usually just a matter of checking the procedures listed. Although the itemization of bills may seem tedious, the medical assistant will spend less time in explaining services provided, clearing up misunderstandings with patients, and following up on delinquent accounts by itemizing.

CRITICAL THINKING APPLICATION

Mrs. Deaton is frustrated because she claims she was never sent an itemized statement and now refuses to pay her account. Myra believes that this is a delay tactic, because she specifically recalls sending an itemized statement to the patient. How can this situation be remedied?

Time and Frequency of Billing

A regular system of mailing statements should be put into operation. Most people expect to receive statements from their creditors, and they plan their budgets around first-of-the-month bills received. Punctuality in billing encourages prompt payment.

Statements should be sent at least once each month. Some offices send bills immediately after treatment; others bill all patients on the same day each month. Mailing statements twice a month (e.g., half of the accounts on the tenth and the remaining half on the twenty-fifth) is also a common practice.

Once-a-Month Billing

If a monthly pattern is followed, bills should leave the office in time to reach the patient no later than the last day of each month and preferably before the twenty-fifth of the month. Planning ahead for the preparation of statements can lighten the burden of once-a-month billing (Procedure 21-9). The statement can be prepared at the time of service, postdated, and mailed at the end of the month.

Cycle Billing

Many physicians prefer to use the cycle billing system, which calls for the billing of certain portions of the accounts receivable at given times during the month instead of the preparation of all statements at the end of each month. Cycle billing is used in large businesses such as department stores, banks, and utility companies. Its many advantages include avoiding once-a-month peak workloads and stabilizing the cash flow. In a small office in which billing is done only once a month, the unexpected illness or absence of the medical assistant for any emergency can leave the physician in a financial bind if the statements do not go out.

The accounts are separated into fairly equal divisions, with the number of divisions depending on how many times billing will be done during a month. For example, if the office expects to bill twice per month, divide the accounts into two equal groups; for weekly billing, divide into four groups; and for daily billing, divide into 20 groups.

Small alphabetic groups can be combined to keep the divisions nearly equal in the number of statements to prepare on each billing day. If the files are color-coded, the medical assistant may wish to use the same alphabetic breakdown in billing. Regardless of constant changes in the individual accounts, the mailing dates for accounts in each section remain the same. A schedule for processing and mailing is therefore established, and the workload is apportioned throughout the entire month.

Cycle billing allows the medical assistant to continue all routine duties each day, handling the statements on a day-to-day

PROCEDURE 21-9

Perform Billing Procedures

CAAHEP COMPETENCY: 3.a(2)(d)
ABHES COMPETENCY: 3.I

GOAL: *To bill insurance companies for patient procedures and services and obtain the maximum legal reimbursement.*

EQUIPMENT and SUPPLIES

- Patient ledgers
- Accounting system
- Calculator
- Claim forms
- Encounter forms
- Clerical supplies

PROCEDURAL STEPS

1. Read the medical record or encounter form to determine the procedures and services that are to be billed.
   PURPOSE: To make certain that all procedures and services performed by the provider are billed so that he or she can receive the correct reimbursement.
2. Determine the diagnosis code for each diagnosis noted by the provider.
   PURPOSE: To use the proper code to note each diagnosis.
3. Determine the procedure codes for all procedures noted by the provider.
   PURPOSE: To use the proper code to note each procedure.
4. Complete the insurance claim form, following the directions provided for each block.
5. Determine the amount of money that the provider is billing for on this claim.
   PURPOSE: To bill for the correct amount in reimbursement.
6. Complete the claim form according to the directions for each block.
7. Determine the address where the claim forms should be mailed.
   PURPOSE: To eliminate unnecessary delays in the carrier's receipt of the claim form.
8. Mail the claim form.
9. Note the date that the claim should receive follow-up to make certain it is paid.

---

or weekly schedule rather than in one intensive period at the end of the month. This means that whole days need not be sacrificed from other duties to get statements in the mail. When the billing is spaced throughout the month, more time and consideration can be given to each statement, the itemization of bills is less burdensome, and the likelihood of error is decreased.

Patients generally accept the cycle billing system quickly, often with enthusiasm. However, if your office decides to change from a once-a-month billing system to a cycle billing system, patients should be notified in advance, and the new plan should be explained to them. To explain the new system to established patients, enclose a notice in each statement for 2 months before the transfer, describing the plan and indicating the future dates on which each patient will receive the bill.

Before a physician adopts the cycle billing system, particularly in a small community, several factors should be taken into consideration, such as the following:

- What is the general income level of the community, and how and when does the average patient get paid?
- Do local companies pay employees at various times during the month, or are most paychecks handed out at the beginning of the month?
- Would cycle billing benefit patients as well as the overall operation of the office?

Billing Third-Party Payors

Collection problems may arise if the medical assistant fails to get the necessary insurance information, particularly Medicare and Medicaid information. In some instances, if the insurance forms are not completed correctly the claim may be denied because of minor infractions such as failing to name the responsible party or omitting Social Security information, the policy number, or the group number.

Time limits must also be observed in billing third-party payors. In cases of Medicare patients with a terminal illness, it may be best to accept assignment of benefits. If the physician does not take assignment, he or she may receive nothing because the family is not obligated to pay, and Medicare will not pay after a certain time or if the claim has not been correctly filed.

Billing Minors

Minors cannot be held responsible for payment of a bill unless they are emancipated. Bills for minors must be addressed to a parent or legal guardian. If a bill is addressed to a minor, the parent or parents could take the attitude that they are not responsible because they never received the bill.

If the parents are separated or divorced, the parent who brings the child in for treatment is responsible for payment. Whatever financial agreement exists between the parents is strictly their personal business and should not concern the medical office. The responsible parent should be so informed from the beginning.

If a minor appears in the office and requests treatment and you can ascertain that the person is legally emancipated, the minor is responsible for the bill. It may be wise to make a determination either with the business manager or with the physician as to whether your office wishes to treat this emancipated minor.

CARE FOR THOSE WHO CANNOT PAY

The medical profession has traditionally accepted the responsibility of providing medical care for individuals unable to pay for these services. In spite of the increased scope of government-sponsored care for the **medically indigent,** physicians still donate thousands of dollars' worth of such medical services each year.

In many instances medical care of the indigent is available through social service agencies. The medical assistant should learn about any local organizations and agencies that can aid the patient in obtaining the necessary assistance. The physician can provide only medical services. Other agencies must provide hospitalization, for example, or arrange for paying the costs of special therapy, rehabilitation, or medications. Unfortunately, there is still another segment of the population that consists of uninsured employees who are not eligible for public assistance, are not covered under a group policy, and cannot afford the high premiums for private medical insurance. Special attention must be given to helping these people arrange to pay their medical bills.

If a physician accepts a case for which a fee will not be paid, complete records must still be kept on the patient. The only deviation in procedure is that the financial record indicates no charge (n/c) in the debit column.

Fees in Hardship Cases

Sometimes a physician is faced with the problem of deciding whether to reduce or cancel a fee in a hardship case. Before adjusting or canceling a fee, the physician or the medical assistant should engage in a frank discussion of the patient's financial situation. Find out whether the patient is entitled to an insurance settlement of some kind. For instance, if the patient's injuries are the result of a car accident, there may be insurance through the automobile policy. Circumstances may qualify the patient for local or state public assistance, such as crime victim assistance. If so, the assistant may direct the patient to the appropriate agency.

If the circumstances of hardship are known before the services are rendered, a thorough discussion of what the fee will be and how it will be paid should take place at that time. The physician may suggest that a medically indigent patient seek care at a county hospital with public assistance. A physician should be free to choose his or her form of charity and should not feel obligated to substantially reduce or cancel a fee when the circumstances are known in advance.

After the physician and patient have agreed on a fee, special circumstances may arise that create a hardship. If the physician then agrees to reduce the fee, the patient should be told that the reduction will be effective only after the adjusted amount is paid in full. For instance, if a fee of $500 is reduced to $350, the full amount of the $500 charge should appear on the ledger, and when $350 has been received the remainder can be written off as an adjustment.

PITFALLS OF FEE ADJUSTMENTS

When a physician begins to reduce his or her fees, problems can arise. Patients may begin to expect that fees will be reduced in all circumstances. Patients may even doubt the competency of a physician who habitually reduces fees.

Great care should be taken in reducing the fee for care of a patient who dies. The physician's sympathy is with the family in such instances, but the physician's generosity in reducing a fee could be misinterpreted and result in a suit for malpractice. The family may suspect that the fee was reduced because the physician knows he or she made an error.

If the physician agrees to settle for a reduced fee in a situation in which the patient is disputing the fee, care should be taken to make certain the negotiations are without prejudice. By taking this precaution, the physician protects the right to collect the original sum should the patient refuse to pay the lowered fee. The offer of a discount therefore should be made in writing, with the insertion of the words "without prejudice" and a definite time limit for making payment stated. Prepare two copies of the agreement and have the signatures witnessed. Keep the original for the physician and give a copy to the patient.

A fee should never be reduced on the basis of a poor result or as a means of obtaining payment to avoid the use of a collection agency. A reduction for these reasons degrades the physician and the practice of medicine.

PROFESSIONAL COURTESY

Traditionally, physicians do not charge professional colleagues or their immediate dependents for medical care. Although the concept of professional courtesy is often attributed to Hippocrates, the foundations of professional courtesy today are derived from Thomas Percival's Code of 1803.

In some cases, giving professional courtesy represents the loss of a large amount of potential income. If there is a substantial outlay in the cost of materials, the professional colleague will probably wish to reimburse the physician for the materials used. Most physicians today subscribe to a health insurance plan. If the care they receive is covered by insurance, it is entirely ethical for the attending physician to accept the insurance benefits in payment for services.

If the services are frequent enough to involve a significant portion of the physician's professional time or if they extend over a long time, the physician may wish to charge on an adjusted basis. When professional courtesy has been offered and the recipient still insists on paying, the physician need not hesitate on ethical grounds to accept a fee for service.

Professional courtesy is often extended beyond fellow physicians and their dependents. Most physicians treat their own medical assistants, and often their families, without charge and grant discounts to nurses and medical assistants not in their direct employ. Student externs should never expect to be treated while serving in an externship capacity. Professional courtesy is sometimes extended to others in the healthcare field (e.g., pharmacists and dentists).

CRITICAL THINKING APPLICATION

Dr. Franklin has just finished seeing Dr. Wallace as a patient and insists to Myra that Dr. Wallace always extends him professional courtesy. This is not indicated on the ledger card, because several payments are shown on the record. Dr. Wallace has just left the office and is in an important meeting at the hospital. What should Myra do?

COLLECTION TECHNIQUES

Sometimes, it becomes necessary to aggressively attempt to collect the balances that patients owe the physician (Procedures 21-10 and 21-11). Persuasive collection procedures include telephone calls, collection reminders and letters, and personal interviews.

Telephone Collection Calls

A telephone call at the right time, in the right manner, will be more successful than notes, a statement, or a collection letter. The personal contact of a telephone call will bring in more money than if a call is not made. In the absence of time to make calls, the collection letter is the next best avenue. If collections are a serious problem, it may pay to hire an extra person to do the telephoning. Written notification is a must before making a final demand for payment indicating that legal or collection proceedings will be started. There are no hard and fast rules for pursuing collections by telephone. Each case should be handled individually on the basis of the experience with the person involved.

Collection Letters or Reminders

Some consultants believe that a printed collection letter or reminder enclosed with a statement is more effective than a personal letter. Their attitude is that a patient may be embarrassed by a personal letter and feel that he or she has been singled out for attention. An impersonal printed message will probably encourage the debtor to send a payment. The printed form is a time saver and is recommended if a lack of time is contributing to poor collection follow-up. Standard printed forms are readily available, and the medical assistant can also design original forms.

Letters that are friendly requests for an explanation of why payment has not been made are still effective in many cases. These letters should indicate that the physician is sincerely interested in the patient and wishes to help straighten out the financial obligations. The patient should be invited to visit the office to explain the reasons for nonpayment so that, if possible, special arrangements can be worked out. To give the patient an opportunity to save face, these letters can suggest that the patient may have overlooked previous statements.

PROCEDURE 21-10

Perform Collection Procedures

<u>CAAHEP COMPETENCY:</u> 3.a(2)(d)
<u>ABHES COMPETENCY:</u> 3.l

GOAL: *To collect the maximum amount of funds on each account.*

EQUIPMENT and SUPPLIES

- Patient ledger
- Office policy manual
- Clerical supplies
- Scripts for telephone collections
- Letters for collection efforts
- Telephone
- Letterhead and envelopes
- Copies of claim forms previously filed

PROCEDURAL STEPS

1. Be familiar with office policy regarding turning accounts over to collections.
   <u>PURPOSE:</u> To make certain that policy is followed when accounts are turned over to collection agencies.
2. Review the patient ledger to determine if it needs collection activity.
   <u>PURPOSE:</u> Some accounts may be past due, but patients have made arrangements to pay them; in this case, collection activities should not commence.
3. Determine the type of collection activity the account needs.
   <u>PURPOSE:</u> The account that is only slightly past due does not need a harsh collection letter; determine the best approach for each particular account.
4. Begin collection efforts with telephone calls or postcards.
   <u>PURPOSE:</u> Many patients only need a small reminder that their account is past due.
5. Progress to more stringent collection efforts if the patient does not pay the account as promised.
6. Once all collection efforts have been exhausted, report the account to the physician for further disposition.
   <u>PURPOSE:</u> The physician should decide which accounts are given to collection agencies and which are simply written off as bad debts.
7. Document the final collection activity on the ledger and/or in the patient medical record.

PROCEDURE 21-11

Perform Accounts Receivable Procedures: Age Accounts Receivables

<u>CAAHEP COMPETENCY</u>: 3.a.(2)(c)
<u>ABHES COMPETENCY</u>: 3.l

GOAL: *To determine the age of accounts and decide what collection activity is needed.*

EQUIPMENT and SUPPLIES

- Patient ledger cards with a balance due
- Pen
- Computer
- Calculator

PROCEDURAL STEPS

1. Prompt the computer to compile a report on the age of accounts receivable. Many programs will have this as an easily accessed report option.
   <u>PURPOSE:</u> To determine which accounts have a balance due.

2. Divide the accounts into categories as listed below:
   - 0-30 days old
   - 30-60 days old
   - 60-90 days old
   - 90-120 days old
   - Over 120 days old
   <u>PURPOSE:</u> To determine how old the various accounts are and place the accounts into categories as to when the last payment was made.

3. If the computer program does not perform this function, manually pull all ledger cards that have a balance due and divide them into the categories listed above.

4. Examine the accounts to see which are awaiting an insurance payment. Action need not be taken if an insurance payment is expected and is not long overdue. Return those ledgers to the ledger tray.
   <u>PURPOSE:</u> To avoid collection activity on accounts for which a payment is expected.

5. Follow the office procedure for collections on the accounts left. Collection reminder stickers may be placed on the statements sent to the patient, or a collection letter may be sent. Be sure that the stickers are inside the envelope, not on the outside.
   <u>PURPOSE:</u> To prompt the patient to make a payment by pointing out the age of the account.

6. Call patients whose accounts are over 90 days old. Attempt to make payment arrangements with the patient.
   <u>PURPOSE:</u> To attempt to collect from the patient or determine why the patient has not yet paid the account.

7. Send a collection letter to patients whose accounts are over 120 days old, if indicated, to encourage the patient to pay the bill. If it is the office policy, mention that the account is in danger of being sent to a collection agency.
   <u>PURPOSE:</u> To reach patients who are not available by telephone.

8. Add the total accounts receivable for each category and arrive at a figure outstanding for each. The physician may wish to have a report weekly or monthly on these figures.
   <u>PURPOSE:</u> To have a current accounting of the amounts owed to the physician, and to double-check the amount outstanding according to the pegboard system or software system.

9. Note in the chart and/or on the ledger any arrangements made with patients regarding payment of the accounts. Send a follow-up letter to remind the patients of their payment agreements.
   <u>PURPOSE:</u> To document arrangements made and remind the patients of their obligation and promise to pay.

On receipt of such a letter, most patients make some effort to explain their failure to make payment. If a patient really is having financial difficulties, the physician may be able to get public assistance for him or her. If it is a temporary financial embarrassment, the physician and the patient may together be able to work out a satisfactory installment plan for payment.

The medical assistant often is given a free hand in designing collection patterns and composing collection letters. Many medical assistants compose a series of collection letters, using model letters that they have found to be effective (Figure 21-8). Such a series usually includes at least five letters in varying degrees of forcefulness.

Sometimes even the person with poor paying habits will pay the bill if treated with respect and consideration. The medical assistant should never go beyond the authority granted by the physician in pursuing collections. If there are questions about special collection problems, always check with the physician before proceeding. This is particularly important with patients whom you do not know personally (e.g., patients whom the physician has seen in the hospital or at home and patients with no credit history). It is difficult to say whether the effects of pressing collections too hard (which can result in loss of patient good will) are more detrimental than the effects of not pursuing collections diligently enough (which can result in loss of revenue). The physician and the medical assistant together should agree on general collection policies as outlined earlier in this chapter, then the policies should be followed. In all cases in which an account is to be assigned to a collection agency, be certain that the physician is aware of it.

Signing Collection Letters

In most medical offices, the medical assistant signs collection letters with the identification "Assistant to Dr. Brown" or "Financial Secretary" below the typewritten signature. Some

1. Your account has always been paid promptly in the past, so this must be an oversight. Please accept this note as a friendly reminder of your account due in the amount of $ _____ .

2. Since your care in this office in March, we have had no word from you in regard to how you are feeling or your account due. If it is impossible for you to pay the full amount of $ _____ at this time, please call this office before June 15 so that satisfactory arrangements can be worked out.

3. Medical bills are payable at the time of service unless special credit arrangements are made. Please send your check in full or call this office before June 30.

4. If you have some question about your statement, we will be happy to answer it for you. If not, may we have a payment before the end of this month?

5. Unless some definite arrangement is made to reduce your balance of $ _____ , we can no longer carry your account on our books. Delinquent accounts are turned over to our collection agency on the 25th of the month.

6. **When a payment plan has been established, it can be reinforced by recognizing the first remittance with a letter of acknowledgment:**

   Thank you for the recent payment of $ _____ on your account. We are glad to cooperate with you in this arrangement for clearing your account. We will look for your next check at about the same time next month, and your final payment the following month.

7. **When a payment schedule has been arranged by a telephone call, it can be confirmed by letter.**

   As agreed upon in our telephone conversation today, we will expect you to mail a payment of $50 on February 10; $50 on March 10; and the balance on April 10. If some emergency should prevent your making one of these payments on time, please notify us immediately by telephone.

DO'S AND DON'TS

DO:

1. Individualize letters to suit the situation.

2. Design your early letters as mere reminders of debt.

3. Always imply that the patient has good intentions to pay, until lack of response over a period of time proves otherwise.

4. Send letters with a firmer tone only after you have sent one or two friendly reminders.

DON'T

1. Use the same collection letter for a patient with good paying habits as for one who is known to neglect financial obligations.

2. Place an overdue notice of any kind on a postcard or on the outside of an envelope. This is an **invasion of privacy.**

FIGURE 21-8 Suggestions for composing collection letters. Brief collection letters that ask patients to explain the lack of payment are often effective.

physicians may wish to personally sign these communications, but generally the medical assistant who handles the accounts also signs the collection letters.

Personal Interviews

Personal interviews with patients can sometimes be more effective than a whole series of collection letters. By talking to a patient face to face, the medical assistant can come to an understanding of the problem more quickly, and an agreement about future payment plans can be reached.

Occasionally a patient may undergo a long course of treatment and yet make no attempt to pay anything on account. Perhaps such a patient is only waiting for the physician or the medical assistant to suggest that a payment be made. When there is advance knowledge that the patient will require extensive treatment, the matter of payment should be discussed early in the course of treatment, the credit policy explained, and some agreement reached as to a payment plan.

Because medical services are far more intangible than any commercial service, collection efforts must not be delayed too long. Any responsible, sincere patient will call or write the physician's office after receiving a second statement and explain the delay in payment or ask for a payment plan.

If it becomes necessary to refer the account to a collector, a good agency should have a 35% to 40% recovery rate with an account that is assigned within 4 or 5 months. This may drop to 25% if the account is held only a few more months. If recovery by the agency is greater than 40%, it may indicate that the collection effort by the medical assistant needs to be intensified.

The value of medical accounts diminishes in direct proportion to the length of time that has elapsed since service was rendered.

General Rules to Follow in Telephone Collections

What to Do

- Call the patient when it can be done with privacy.
- Call between 8 am and 9 pm.
- Determine the identity of the person with whom you are speaking. If you ask, "Is this Mrs. Noble?" and she answers, "Yes," it could be the patient's mother-in-law or daughter-in-law, who is also "Mrs. Noble." Use the person's full name.
- Be dignified and respectful. One can be friendly and formal at the same time.
- Ask the patient if it is a convenient time to talk. Unless you have the attention of the called party, there is little to be gained by continuing. If told that it is an inopportune time, ask for a specific time to call back, or get a promise that the patient will call the office at a specified time.
- After a brief greeting, state the purpose of the call. Make no apology for calling, but state the reason in a friendly, businesslike way. The physician expects payment and the medical assistant is interested in helping the patient meet the financial obligation. Open the call with a phrase such as, "This is Alice, Dr. Wallace's financial secretary. I'm calling about your account." A well-placed pause at this point in the call sometimes gets an immediate response from the debtor in regard to the nonpayment.
- Assume a positive attitude. For example, convey the impression that the patient intended to pay and it is only a matter of working out some suitable arrangements.
- Keep the conversation brief and to the point, and avoid threats of any kind.
- Try to get a definite commitment—payment of a certain amount by a certain date.
- Follow up on promises. This is best accomplished by a tickler file or a note on the calendar. If the payment does not arrive by the promised date, remind the patient with another call. If the medical assistant fails to do this, the whole effort has been wasted.

What Not to Do

- Do not call between 9 PM and 8 AM. To do so may be considered harassment.
- Do not make repeated telephone calls.
- Do not call the debtor's place of work if the employer prohibits personal calls.
- If a call is placed to the debtor at work and the person cannot take the call, leave a message asking the debtor to "call Mrs. Black at 727-9238" without revealing the nature of the call; that is, do not state that the call is from "Dr. Wallace's office" or "Dr. Jones's medical assistant."
- Do not show hostility. An angry patient is a poor-paying patient. Insulted patients often do not pay at all.

Do not fight the law of diminishing returns. All collection activity is costly. Know when to stop and call on the services of a professional agency.

Special Collection Situations

Tracing "Skips"

When a statement is returned marked "Moved–no forwarding address," you may consider this account as a "skip." This generally is accepted as an indication that the patient is attempting to avoid liability for debts. Some so-called skips are innocent errors. The person may have been careless in not leaving a forwarding address, or the mistake may have occurred in the physician's office; the wrong name or address may have been placed on the statement. However, immediate action should be taken in regard to returned statements. Do not wait until the next billing time to attempt to trace the debtor.

The tracing of skips is a challenge to any medical assistant. A certified letter can be sent; by paying additional fees, you can ask the Postal Service to obtain a receipt including the address where the letter was delivered. The certified letter may be sent in a plain envelope so that the patient will not refuse to accept the letter because of the return address.

If all attempts fail, turn the account over to a collection agency without delay. Do not keep a skip account too long, because the trail may become so cold as time elapses that even collection experts will be unable to follow it.

Claims Against Estates

A bill owed by a deceased patient may be handled a little differently than regular bills. Courtesy dictates that a bill not be sent during the initial period of bereavement, but do not delay more than 30 days. The person responsible for settling the affairs of the estate will be assembling outstanding accounts and will expect to receive the medical bills along with all others. Address the statement using the following format:

Estate of (name of patient)
c/o (spouse or next of kin, if known)
Patient's last known address

Do not address the statement to a relative unless you have a signed agreement that that person will be responsible. If for some reason the statement cannot be addressed as just suggested (e.g., if the patient was in a convalescent home and there is no name of a relative), seek information from the county seat in the county in which the estate is being settled.

A will is generally filed within 30 days of a death. A request to the Probate Department of the Superior Court, County Recorder's Office, will usually provide the name of the executor or administrator. The time limits for filing an estate claim are determined by the state in which the decedent resided.

After the name of the administrator or executor of the estate has been obtained, a duplicate itemized statement of the account should be sent to that person by certified mail, return receipt requested. If no response is received in 10 days, contact the executor or the county clerk where the estate is being settled and obtain forms for filing a claim against the estate. (Some states do not have special claim forms but will accept simple itemized statements.) This claim against the estate must be made within a certain length of time, varying from 2 to 36 months, depending on the state in which it is filed.

The executor of the estate will either accept or reject the claim and if it is accepted, will send an acknowledgment of the debt. Payment is often delayed because of the legal complications in settling an estate, but if the claim has been accepted, you will receive your money in due time. If the claim is rejected and there is full justification for claiming the bill, file a claim against the executor within a limited time, according to state laws. The time limit in such cases starts with the date on the letter of rejection that was sent in response to the original claim.

Because states have different time limits and statutes in regard to such matters, it is advisable for the medical assistant to contact the physician's attorney or the local court for the exact procedure to follow.

Bankruptcy

Bankruptcy laws were passed to secure equal distribution of the assets of an individual among the individual's creditors. Bankruptcy laws are federal and are applicable in all states. When notified that a patient has declared bankruptcy, do not send statements or make any attempt to collect on the account from the patient.

Chapter VII bankruptcy is usually a "no asset" situation. Because the physician's fee is an unsecured debt, there is little purpose in pursuing collection. Chapter XIII is known as *wage-earner bankruptcy*. Under Chapter XIII, the patient-debtor pays a fixed amount (agreed on by the court) to the trustee in bankruptcy. This is then passed on to the creditors. During this period, none of the creditors can attach the debtor's wages or otherwise attempt to collect the debt. It is sometimes beneficial to file a claim under Chapter XIII because small payments will be made by the debtor under the supervision of the court over a period of 3 years.

USING OUTSIDE COLLECTION ASSISTANCE

When everything possible has been done internally to follow up on an outstanding account and the office has not received payment, the question arises as to what step to take next, as follows:

- Should the facility sue for the payment?
- Should the account be sent to a collection agency?
- Should the account be written off as a bad debt?

Before forcing an account, first consider the time element: Has the patient been given a fair chance to pay this bill? Have statements been sent regularly, and has a systematic method of following the account been used? Ask if there might be a misunderstanding about the fee charged. Was the first statement fully itemized? A large unexplained bill may frighten a patient into making no payments at all because the whole balance looks too large.

If the correct registration forms to secure advance credit information were used, the medical assistant should know the financial abilities of the patient to pay. However, illness may have caused a loss of salary and resulted in temporary inability to pay. Try to thoroughly analyze the situation.

Could the patient have been dissatisfied with the care received? For some unknown reason, a patient may feel that he or she was not treated correctly. Perhaps the patient expected a complete cure too soon. Only an explanation of the condition, prognosis, and care can enlighten such patients, and this is best handled by the physician. If payment of a bill is pressed too hard and the patient is dissatisfied for some reason, a malpractice suit may be filed by the patient to seek retribution against the physician. The court can approve a period longer than 3 years in special cases, but cannot approve a period longer than 5 years.

Collecting Through the Court System

Making the Decision to Sue

Will a physician lose more good will by suing for a bill than by writing it off as a loss? One management official has related that, strangely enough, when a physician-client sued two patients for large amounts, the patients lost the cases, paid up, and were back in the office for treatment very shortly! However, most physicians believe it is unwise to resort to the court to collect medical bills unless there are extraordinary circumstances.

An account must be considered a 100% loss to the physician before legal proceedings are started. Remember to never threaten to **instigate** legal proceedings unless prepared to carry out the

---

Suggestions for Tracing Skips

- Examine the patient's original office registration card.
- Call the telephone number listed on the card. Occasionally a patient may move without leaving a forwarding address but will transfer the old telephone number. The new telephone number may be given when you call the old number.
- If you are unable to contact the individual by telephone, make a few discreet calls to the references listed on the registration card to get leads.
- Check the Internet to secure the names and telephone numbers of neighbors or the landlord, and contact these people to secure information about the debtor's whereabouts.
- Do not inform a third party that the person owes you money. Simply state that you are trying to locate or verify the location of the individual.
- Check the debtor's place of employment for information. If the person is a specialist in his or her field of work, the local union or similar organizations may be contacted. Although they may not give you the person's current address, they will relay the message that you are seeking to contact him or her. Often people will be stirred into paying a bill if they think that their employer may learn of their payment failure.
- Do not communicate with a third party more than once. This is specifically forbidden by law (Public Law 95-109, Sec. 804) unless the third party requests the collector to do so.

threat, and have the physician's consent to such a warning being issued. If the physician decides in favor of a lawsuit, investigate thoroughly before taking action. Litigation to collect a bill is generally in order when the following occur:

- The patient can afford to pay without hardship.
- The physician can produce office records that support the bill.
- The physician can justify the amount of the bill by comparing it with fee practices in the community.
- The patient's general condition after treatment is satisfactory.
- The persuasive powers of an ethical collection agency have been exhausted, and the agency advises suing.
- The patient can be given ample warning of the physician's intention to sue.
- The defendant (whether a patient or a parent or legal guardian) is legally liable for the services rendered to the patient.
- The statute of limitations has ruled out any possible malpractice action.
- The physician is not indignant or in a negative frame of mind.

Small Claims Court

Many medical practices find the small claims court a satisfactory and inexpensive way to collect delinquent accounts. The law places a limit on the amount of debt for which relief may be sought in the small claims court. Because this varies from state to state (from $300 to $5000) and in some instances even within a state, this limit should be checked locally before seeking recovery in this manner.

Parties to small claims actions cannot be represented by an attorney at the trial but may send another person to court in their behalf to produce records supporting the claim. Physicians often send their bookkeeper or medical assistant with records of unpaid accounts to show the judge.

If the court awards a judgment for the amount owed, the plaintiff in small claims court may also recover the costs of the suit. For a very small investment in time and money, the physician who uses this method has done the following:

- Saved the time of a regular court action
- Had no attorney's fee to pay
- Not sacrificed the commission charged by a collection agency

After being awarded a judgment, the medical assistant must still collect the money. The only person in a small claims action who has the right of appeal is the defendant. An appeal by the defendant may have the judgment set aside. The plaintiff cannot file an appeal in a small claims action; the decision of the court is final.

The necessary papers for filing action and full instructions on the course to follow may be obtained from the clerk of the small claims court. The medical assistant who has never appeared in the court would probably be wise to attend once as a spectator to preview the procedure and feel more at ease when appearing for the physician.

A collection agency to which an account may have been assigned may not file or handle a small claims action. It must either sue in the regular municipal or justice court or attempt to collect the debt in some other manner.

Using a Collection Agency

The medical assistant should try every means possible to collect accounts before they become delinquent. As soon as the account is determined uncollectible through the office (i.e., the patient has failed to respond to the final letter or has failed to fulfill a second promise on payment), send the account to the collector without delay. Skips should be assigned immediately.

Even though collection by an agency will mean sacrificing from 40% to 60% of the amount owed, further delay will only reduce the chances of recovery by the professional collector. If the agency finds that the case deserves special consideration, it will seek the physician's advice before proceeding further.

CRITICAL THINKING APPLICATION

- Myra has had several complaints about the collection agency used by the office. Patients have called to report that the collectors are threatening and unprofessional. How should Myra approach the collection agency about these complaints?
- The office manager refuses to take these patients seriously, saying that because they owe the money, the collection agency's job is to collect the account in whatever way necessary. Myra does not agree with her philosophy. What should she do?

Selecting a Collection Agency

A number of agencies are either owned and operated as an integral part of the county medical society or are operated separately from the medical society but supervised by the medical profession. These bureaus provide specialized medical collection services.

Another type of collection agency is a division of the local credit association, recognized by the National Retail Credit Association. If the local credit association does not maintain a collection department, it will be able to recommend a reputable one. A nationally recognized credit association has considerable responsibility and a high standard to maintain. These factors serve as monitors to its reliability.

The most common type of collection agency throughout the United States is the privately owned and operated agency. Many of these work with the local professional societies and strive to adhere to a high ethical standard. Because a few bureaus are unethical and unscrupulous in their tactics, care should be taken to be sure that the one chosen is reliable and ethical. For the sake of comparison, many healthcare facilities use two or three agencies.

Responsibilities to the Collection Agency

When a reputable agency is selected, the medical assistant must be prepared to provide the agency with all the necessary data to enable it to begin prompt collection procedures on overdue accounts. The agency should receive the following:

PROCEDURE 21-12

Post Collection Agency Payments

CAAHEP COMPETENCY: 3.a(2)(i)
ABHES COMPETENCY: 3.s

GOAL: *To post payments received on an account after it has been turned over to a collection agency.*

EQUIPMENT and SUPPLIES

- Patient ledgers
- Office policy manual
- Bookkeeping system
- Clerical supplies
- Calculator

PROCEDURAL STEPS

1. Determine that a payment has been received on an account that is now being serviced by a collection agency.

2. Notify the collection agency that the payment has been made.
   PURPOSE: The collection agency is entitled to a portion of money collected when a payment is sent to the medical office.

3. Send a notice to the patient, if necessary, to explain that the payment has been forwarded to the collection agency for credit.

4. Instruct patients to forward additional payments straight to the collection agency.

- Full name of the debtor
- Name of the spouse
- Last known address
- Full amount of the debt
- Date of the last entry on account (debit or credit)
- Occupation of the debtor
- Business address
- Any other pertinent data

After an account has been released to a collection agency, the office makes no further collection attempts. Once the agency has begun its work, the following guidelines and procedures should be adhered to:

- Send no more statements.
- Mark the patient's ledger or stamp it so that everyone will know it is now in the hands of the collector.
- Refer the patient to the collection agency if he or she contacts the office in regard to the account.
- Promptly report any payments made directly to your office (a percentage of this payment is due the agency).
- Call the agency if any information is obtained that will be of value in tracing or collecting the account.
- Do not push the agency with frequent calls. The representatives of the agency will report regularly and will keep the office posted on collection progress.

Collection Agency Payments

If a patient sends a payment after the account has been turned over to a collection agency, the amount will need to be adjusted on the patient ledger. The collection agency will be due a percentage of the payment (Procedure 21-12).

CLOSING COMMENTS

Billing and collecting are critical duties in the medical office, and a responsible medical assistant is a great asset in this important area. Always maintain a positive attitude with the patients and guarantors. Remember that those who are ill or facing challenges are not always at their best and may not respond in a positive way to calls regarding their accounts. Make every attempt to work with each patient to develop a workable plan to clear his or her account.

Most patients are unaware of the actual coverage they have through their insurance policies. The medical assistant should encourage patients to read the entire policy so that they become familiar with its limitations and exclusions. Tell patients that when calling the company with questions, they should always write down the date, time, and name of the person with whom they spoke. Using email is helpful, because a record of the correspondence can be easily saved or printed. It is well worth the effort to make sure that patients have a general understanding of their health insurance coverage.

Often, patients do not dispute or question the company when a claim is rejected or not paid in the expected amount. Encourage them to call the company and question rejections if they do not understand why the claim was denied. Patients are paying for coverage and they should receive all of the benefits to which they are entitled.

Patients appreciate receiving an office policy brochure or booklet that informs them about payment and credit options. The patient can use the printed booklet as a reference whenever questions arise, and its regular use by most patients will reduce the number of calls made to the office. Encourage patients to use the booklet. Helpful phone numbers or extensions, as well as instructions as to whom the patient should call for answers to questions at the medical facility, should be included.

A patient who has filed for bankruptcy cannot be contacted or billed further. A threat to take collection action must be fulfilled or the creditor is in violation of the federal Fair Debt Collection Practices Act. Never say that the physician intends to take action if he or she does not plan to follow through.

The Federal Equal Credit Opportunity Act of 1977 bars discrimination in all areas of credit. If the physician agrees to extend credit to one credit-worthy patient, then the same arrangement must be offered to any other patient who requests it, as long as the patient is also credit worthy.

Because laws vary greatly from state to state, the medical assistant should review the statutes pertaining to billing and collecting in the area in which he or she lives. Develop a good understanding of what is required of the small business, such as a physician's office, in collecting fees and billing for amounts due. Remember that laws change often, and constantly update policies to reflect current statutes.

SUMMARY OF SCENARIO

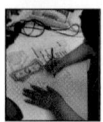

Myra is a well-respected member of Dr. Wallace's office team. Her friendly attitude and flexibility attract patients, and she enjoys the interaction with them. She knows that there are only a few patients for whom she cannot work out some type of payment arrangements. She is professional in her dealings with those whom she contacts about outstanding accounts.

Dr. Wallace has noticed that more and more patients pay their accounts, and he attributes this to the care that Myra shows when working with them. She is never hesitant to ask for payment from patients but is sensitive to their needs and struggles at the same time. She urges her patients to cooperate and make a good attempt to pay their accounts, and in return, Myra arranges a payment schedule that the patient can meet.

Although she was initially nervous about explaining fees to patients and asking for payments, she has become more comfortable in doing this aspect of her job, since she understands the business aspect of the practice. The physician is operating the practice to make a profit and support his family, and the practice is a source of support for the employees' families as well. Patients understand that physicians must charge for their services, and have become used to copayments and coinsurance amounts. Many times, these fees are collected in advance before the patient sees Dr. Wallace. This practice saves time on checkout and most patients feel that the copay is a small cost compared to the entire fee that physicians charge to manage their care in one office visit.

Myra has noticed that the usual, customary, and reasonable fees that Dr. Wallace charges his patients directly affect the reimbursements that are paid by various insurance and managed care companies. She has handled several claims in which the payor questioned the fee when it fell outside of the UCR ranges. Dr. Wallace commented that he uses professional courtesy much less frequently than in the past because of the many rules and regulations placed on providers by managed care companies. He still offers the occasional patient a professional discount when it does not violate the managed care contract that he holds with the insurer or managed care company.

Myra's flexibility as an employee has paid off for Dr. Wallace several times. During a week-long period when the computer bookkeeping system was malfunctioning, Myra was able to retrieve information from her backup disks and use a pegboard system until the system was repaired. Her preparation allowed the office to continue operations without skipping a beat. Most patients did not even notice that the computer was not in use for the week.

Many physicians still use the manual pegboard system out of habit and because it is a reliable method of keeping up with patient accounts. Some simply trust manual, written records more than computerized systems. Since this is a matter of personal choice, either system will work in the physician's office.

Myra has been able to fill in for other employees because of the versatility she gained from her medical assistant training. She has scheduled appointments and even assisted Dr. Wallace with minor office surgery. Myra feels that performing other duties is a nice change periodically, and she keeps her skills sharp. She has proved herself to be a valuable and efficient employee.

SUMMARY of LEARNING OBJECTIVES

1. Define, spell, and pronounce the terms listed in the vocabulary.
   - Spelling and pronouncing medical terms correctly adds credibility to the medical assistant. Knowing the definition of these terms promotes confidence in communication with patients and co-workers.
2. List three values that are considered in determining professional fees.
   - Medical services are valuable to the patient who receives them. The physician sets fees based on three commodities. The physician offers the patient his time and makes the most

accurate judgments possible about the patient's medical condition. The services provided to the patient also figure into the fees that are set for various procedures.
3. Distinguish among the terms usual, customary, and reasonable.
   - Many third-party payors use the UCR method of determining fees for procedures. The usual fee is what the physician normally charges for a given service. The customary fee is the range of fees charged by physicians who have similar experience in the same geographic area. Services or procedures that are exceptionally complicated and that require

Continued

SUMMARY of LEARNING OBJECTIVES

Continued

extra time deserve a reasonable fee and may be higher than the usual fee.

4. Discuss the value of estimates for patient treatment.
   - Providing estimates for medical care helps patients plan their finances when an illness or injury occurs. When estimates are provided, the possibility of later misquoting the fee is avoided. The office staff should keep a copy of the estimate in the patient's chart, which will help to avoid misunderstandings and confusion over charges.

5. Explain the concept of professional courtesy.
   - Some physicians choose to extend professional courtesy to other physicians, medical professionals, and medical staff employees. This means that the physician either discounts or eliminates the charges for all or part of the services provided. The decision to offer professional courtesy should remain with the physician.

6. Name the ways by which payment for medical services is accomplished.
   - Payment for medical services is accomplished in several ways. Most physicians prefer that payment be received at the time of service. When the extension of credit is offered, internal billing is necessary. Some offices contract with external billing services. Often, patients have some type of insurance or managed care policy that pays at least a portion of the bill. When patients fail to meet their obligations, outside collection services may be used.

7. Explain why itemizing statements is important.
   - The first statement should always be itemized. This provides the patient and the guarantor with a record of each procedure and each charge. Insurance companies require itemized bills to reimburse the charges.

8. Discuss why patients fail to pay accounts.
   - Rarely do patients not wish to meet their bill-paying obligations. Some do not have the money to pay for medical services, and if they do not have health insurance, it could be even more difficult to obtain medical care. The financial problem that the patient faces may be temporary, or it may be a long-standing situation. Only a few patients are actually unwilling to pay, so the medical assistant should work with the patient to develop a payment plan that the patient can meet.

9. Explain how to handle a "skip."
   - Immediate action should be taken when the office classifies a patient as a "skip." Search the patient chart for all possible telephone numbers, and call those that the patient has given. Do not reveal that the patient owes money. If it is necessary to leave a message, do not indicate that the call is from a physician's office. The employer may be called if the patient has not given specific permission not to call the place of business. Never communicate with a third party more than once unless invited to call back. A certified letter may be sent, and when address corrections are requested, the new address

is often obtainable. Unless the skip is found quickly, the account is generally turned over to a collection agency.

10. Briefly explain some of the guidelines of telephone collecting.
    - When making collection calls to patients or guarantors, be sure to call within accepted calling hours, which are 8 am to 9 pm. Be sure to correctly identify the person speaking, and always be respectful and courteous. State the purpose of the call, and keep the conversation businesslike and professional. Keep a positive attitude, and convey to the patient that the call is to help devise a way that his or her obligations to the physician can be met. Never threaten the patient, and make every effort to get a commitment as to when payment can be expected. Most important, follow up on collection calls to ensure that patients send in the payment as promised.

11. Explain professional fees to patients.
    - The medical assistant will periodically be required to explain the physician's professional fees to patients. The process for explaining fees to patients is outlined in Procedure 21-1.

12. Effectively use a pegboard system.
    - The pegboard system is effective in allowing the physician to know his or her accounts receivable on a daily basis. The process for posting entries on a daysheet is outlined in Procedure 21-2.

13. Establish credit arrangements for patient payment.
    - From time to time, the medical assistant will be required to make credit arrangements with patients who are unable to pay their accounts in full at the time of service. The process for making credit arrangements with patients is outlined in Procedure 21-7.

14. Prepare accurate monthly statements.
    - Billing statements sent in cycles through the month allow the physician to receive a constant flow of income. The process for preparing billing statements is outlined in Procedure 21-9.

15. Evaluate patient accounts for necessary collection procedures.
    - Some accounts will require collection activities. The process for performing collection procedures is outlined in Procedure 21-10.

16. Perform accounts receivables procedures.
    - The medical assistant may be required to work with receivables in the business office of the practice. The process for performing accounts receivable procedures is outlined in Procedure 21-8.

17. Post adjustments to patient accounts.
    - Various adjustments will be made to patient accounts in situations such as adjusting the allowable charge or writing off bad debt accounts. The process for posting adjustments is outlined in Procedure 21-3.

18. Process a credit balance on a patient account.
    - When an overpayment is made on a patient's account, the patient will receive funds back from the practice. The process for a credit balance is outlined in Procedure 21-4.

SUMMARY of LEARNING OBJECTIVES

Continued

19. Process refunds and send overpayments to patients, when appropriate.
    - Once a credit balance has been discovered, the patient will be due a refund. The process for refunds is outlined in Procedure 21-5.
20. Post non-sufficient fund checks to patient accounts.
    - When a patient writes a check that is returned to the practice for non-sufficient funds, the check must be added back to the patient's ledger account. The process for posting non-sufficient fund checks is outlined in Procedure 21-6.
21. Post payments to accounts that have been turned over to a collection agency.

- Once an account has been turned over to a collection agency, the physician should no notify the collection agency that a payment has been made. The process for posting collection agency payments is outlined in Procedure 21-12.
22. Age accounts receivable.
    - The medical assistant must periodically evaluate patient accounts to determine their age and decide what action needs to be taken on the account. The process for aging accounts receivables is outlined in Procedure 21-11.

CONNECTIONS

 Study Guide Connection: Go to Chapter 21 Study Guide. Read the Case Study and Workplace Applications and complete the assignments. Do online research for answers to the questions in the Internet Activities associated with professional fees, billing, and collecting.

 CD Connection: Go to the Medical Assisting Competency Challenge CD and do the training activities under Financial Management.

 Evolve Connection: For more information related to professional fees, billing, and collecting, go to evolve.elsevier.com/kinn and visit related weblinks for Chapter 21. Click on the Medical Assisting Exam Review and do the practice questions to sharpen your test-taking skills. To learn more about office software, do the exercises for the Altapoint demo that is on the CD.

Banking Services and Procedures 22

SCENARIO

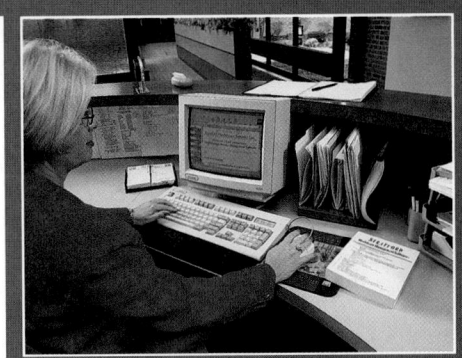

Laura Anderson likes working with figures and has always been interested in bookkeeping. In high school she took all the bookkeeping and accounting courses that were offered, and during the summer months she helped out in the accounting department of the family business. In addition to her schooling and on-the-job experience, Laura wants to learn all she can about the financial transactions common to a medical practice. She is especially interested in electronic banking and all of the possibilities that it has to offer. Once her career in medical assisting is launched, Laura hopes to specialize in helping medical offices set up and run electronic banking systems.

Although Laura has had considerable bookkeeping experience, she realizes that she still has a lot to learn about the daily financial duties in a medical office, including accounts payable, working with the business checkbook, making deposits, reconciling bank statements, and many other banking responsibilities.

Taking on the bookkeeping functions of a medical office involves not only responsibilities to the physician and employer, but also to patients and the vendors from whom the medical office purchases supplies. Laura realizes that to perform well in her upcoming career as a medical assistant, she must learn all she can about the topics pertinent to her special interest areas and stay current with the rapidly changing world of finance.

While studying this chapter, think about the following questions:

- How has banking changed over the years?
- How safe is Internet banking?
- How can an office manager know that an employee can be trusted with banking procedures?
- Why is it a good idea to make daily deposits?

LEARNING OBJECTIVES

1. Define, spell, and pronounce the terms listed in the vocabulary.
2. Explain how the Internet has changed traditional banking practices.
3. State the four requirements of a negotiable instrument.
4. Discuss the advantages of using checks.
5. Identify the three most common types of bank accounts.
6. Explain how you would handle mistakes made in preparing a check.
7. List and discuss eight precautions to observe in accepting checks.
8. Name and compare the four kinds of endorsements.
9. Discuss the actions necessary when a deposited check is returned.
10. Correctly write checks for bill payment.
11. Prepare a bank deposit and appropriate office documents.
12. Accurately reconcile a bank statement with the office checking account.

National Accreditation Competencies and Content

CAAHEP COMPETENCIES	ABHES COMPETENCIES
Administrative 3.a.(2)(a). Prepare a bank deposit	**Administrative Duties** 3.i. Prepare a bank statement and deposit record 3.j. Reconcile a bank statement 3.m. Prepare a check
General 3.c.(4)(c). Utilize computer software to maintain office systems	
	Financial Management 8.e. Maintain records for accounting and banking purposes

clearinghouses Networks of banks that exchange checks with one another.

disbursements Money (funds) paid out.

drawee Bank or facility on which a check is drawn or written.

drawer Person who writes a check.

e-banking Electronic banking via computer modem or over the Internet.

endorser Person who signs his or her name on the back of a check for the purpose of transferring title to another person.

holder Person presenting a check for payment.

m-banking Banking through the use of wireless devices, such as cellular phones and wireless Internet services.

maker In reference to a check, any individual, corporation, or legal party who signs a check or any type of negotiable instrument.

negotiable Legally transferable to another party.

payee Person named on a draft or check as the recipient of the amount shown.

payor Person who writes a check in favor of the payee.

power of attorney A legal statement in which a person authorizes another person to act as his or her attorney or agent. The authority may be limited to the handling of specific procedures. The person authorized to act as the agent is known as the *attorney in fact.*

principal A capital sum of money due as a debt or used as a fund for which interest is either charged or paid.

reconciliation The process of proving that a bank statement and checkbook balance are in agreement.

Uniform Commercial Code (UCC) A unified set of rules covering many business transactions; it has been adopted in all 50 states, the District of Columbia, and most U.S. territories. It regulates the fields of sales of goods; commercial paper, such as checks; secured transactions in personal property; and particular aspects of banking, letters of credit, warehouse receipts, bills of lading, and investment securities.

Financial transactions in the professional office nearly always involve banking services and the use of checks. Therefore a medical assistant must understand the responsibilities involved in accepting payments, endorsing and depositing checks, writing checks, and regularly reconciling bank statements. Payments received in the medical office should be deposited as soon as possible–ideally, on the same day. The medical assistant may very well be in charge of these financial responsibilities; therefore he or she must understand each transaction and what its function is.

BANKING IN TODAY'S BUSINESS WORLD

With the advent of the Internet, banking as we once knew it has changed. People once had to fight traffic and wait in line at crowded banks; today they can sit in the comfort of their own homes and do their banking on the computer at any time of day. It is now possible to conduct such electronic banking transactions as buying and selling shares, paying bills, and transferring funds between accounts. In addition, customers have access to information about stock market prices and news and historical analyses of shares, which makes buying or selling decisions easier.

In fact, it is no longer necessary to sit in front of a computer terminal to conduct banking transactions. Instead, customers can sit on a bus or a train or be waiting for a flight and still make their investments or carry out other bank transactions. All of this is possible by just turning on a mobile telephone.

Online Banking

Online banking is a means to perform banking services via the Internet. It is also called *personal computer (PC) banking, home banking, electronic banking,* **e-banking,** or *Internet banking.* There are many facilities to choose from; most of them offer both basic and advanced services. Basic services usually include these:

• Checking account balances
• Transferring funds between accounts
• Paying bills electronically

Some of the advanced services that banks offer include the following:

• Applying for loans
• Downloading account information
• Trading stocks or mutual funds
• Viewing images of transactions (checks and deposits)

Online banking has advantages and disadvantages. One of the most obvious advantages is the ability to bank at one's own convenience in one's own home or office at any time. This can save considerable time and expense, especially if banking must be done daily. Many people find online banking a convenient and comprehensive method for money management. Other advantages include ease of use, portability, and availability.

Disadvantages of e-banking include having to learn the software—it is less versatile than physical banking—and the fact that service options are often more limited. In addition, some experts believe that there may be a slight increase in risk as compared with conventional banking, although this has been debated by e-banking proponents. Forecasts show, however, that in spite of the disadvantages, banking via the Internet is becoming more popular, with an estimated 20% to 25% of homes and businesses using it.

The cost of online banking varies from bank to bank. Some charge a flat rate (from $5 to $10 per month), with varying fees for additional transactions.

Online Loans

Online lending is becoming more common as well. Loans are available for nearly anything consumers want to purchase—from homes and cars to small business loans and student loans for college tuition. Although online lending still has many loopholes, consumers can save time and money by comparison shopping the dozens of lenders available to find a good rate. Application forms can be downloaded for processing to initiate the process quickly, but the complicated loan process—especially for home mortgages—still requires coordination among many parties, and the sensitive financial and personal information needed for loan approval can raise online security concerns. Despite these issues, many people are "surfing the Web" for loans.

Online Convenience

Convenience is probably the number one reason people and businesses use the Internet for their financial services. There is no frenzied drive to the bank during rush hour, waiting in line, or working around the confines of banking hours. Online banking is available 24 hours a day, 7 days a week. In addition to Internet banking services, consumers can also pay bills online, without the delay of mailing. Credit card holders can check their balances and transaction status. Costly fees can be avoided for financial transactions left until the last minute, because online transactions can be accomplished in a matter of seconds. The need to wait and worry if the mail will get it there in time is eliminated.

Customer-Oriented Banking

Americans are becoming more and more mobile. They want to conduct business and take care of personal concerns over cell phones on their way to and from work. In addition, the rapid pace of life requires rapid or "instant" solutions: people are buying take-out food at a record rate; some churches even offer drive-up services. It is no wonder that today's mobile consumers want the ability to conduct their financial transactions on the go, every day, at any time.

Banks no longer consider customers to be merely account numbers; to stay competitive, banks are being forced to look at the total customer picture. Some banks even offer a type of interactive voice response system that operates through speech recognition, allowing customers to conduct business through a combination of talking into the telephone and using the telephone keypad. The call centers of some banks employ live customer service personnel to answer questions and fulfill requests for all types of bank transactions.

Another customer-oriented innovation is mobile banking, or **m-banking,** which is emerging through the wireless technology market. Through the use of wireless devices such as cellular phones and wireless Internet services, customers can conduct a variety of financial transactions, set up alerts and notifications when bills are due, and make electronic transfers to pay these bills.

CRITICAL THINKING APPLICATION

Laura is excited about all of the possibilities available with e-banking and m-banking. Where can Laura learn more about electronic banking and its advantages and disadvantages compared with conventional banking?

CHECKS

A check is a bank draft or order to pay a certain sum of money payable on demand to a specified person or entity. The concept of writing and depositing checks as a method of conducting financial transactions dates back as far as the Roman Empire. Widespread check-writing didn't become popular, however, until the 1500s, when people in Holland began depositing excess cash with Dutch "cashiers," as a safer alternative than keeping money in their homes. These cashiers then paid the debts of the "depositors" on receipt of a written order. The word "check" was coined in England nearly 200 years later, when serial numbers were marked on these written orders of payment as a way to "check" on them. About 90% of all financial transactions in the United States are said to be accomplished by check.

A check is considered to be a **negotiable** instrument. For a check to be negotiable, it must:

- Be written and signed by a **maker**
- Contain a promise or order to pay a sum of money
- Be payable on demand or at a fixed future date
- Be payable to order or bearer

Types of Checks

A medical assistant is probably familiar with the standard personal check, but there are many additional types of checks used in business transactions. He or she should also be familiar with other types of checks, which are discussed next.

Bank Draft

A bank draft is a check drawn by a bank against funds deposited to its account in another bank.

Advantages of Using Checks

Using checks for the transfer of funds has many advantages:

- Checks are both safe and convenient, particularly for making payments by mail.
- Expenditures are quickly calculated.
- Specific payments can be easily located from the check record.
- A stop-payment order can protect the payor from loss resulting from stolen, lost, or incorrectly drawn checks.
- Checks provide a permanent reliable record of disbursements for tax purposes.
- The deposit record provides a summary of receipts.
- Checking accounts protect the money while on deposit.

Cashier's Check

A cashier's check is a bank's own check drawn on itself and signed by the bank cashier or other authorized official. It is also known as an *officer's* or *treasurer's check*. A cashier's check is obtained by paying the bank cashier the amount of the check, in cash or by personal check. Many banks charge a fee for this service. Cashier's checks are often issued to accommodate the savings account customer who does not maintain a checking account.

Certified Check

A certified check is the depositor's own check, on the face of which the bank has placed the word *certified* or *accepted* with the date and a bank official's signature. Because the bank deducts the amount of the check from the depositor's account at the time it certifies the check, the bank can guarantee that the amount is available. A certified check, like a cashier's check, can be used when an ordinary personal check might not be acceptable. If not used, a certified check should be redeposited promptly, so that the funds previously set aside are credited back to the depositor's account.

Limited Check

A check may be limited as to the amount written on it and as to the time during which it may be presented for payment—30, 60, or 90 days. The limited check is often used for payroll or insurance checks.

Money Order

Domestic money orders are sold by banks, some stores, and the United States Postal Service. Money orders are often used for paying bills by mail when an individual does not have a checking account. The maximum face value varies according to the source. International money orders may be purchased for limited amounts, indicated in U.S. dollars, for use in sending money abroad.

Traveler's Check

Traveler's checks are designed for persons traveling where personal checks may not be accepted or for use in situations in which it is inadvisable to carry large amounts of cash. Traveler's checks are usually printed in denominations of $10, $20, $50, and $100, and sometimes $500 and $1000. They require two signatures of the purchaser, one at the time of purchase and the other at the time of use. They are available at banks and some travel agencies. The use of traveler's checks is becoming less common, because major credit cards are widely accepted throughout the world.

Voucher Check

A voucher check has a detachable voucher form. The voucher portion is used to itemize or specify the purpose for which the check is drawn. It is used for the convenience of the **payor** and shows discounts and various other itemizations. This portion of the check is removed before the check is presented for payment and provides a record for the **payee** (Figure 22-1).

THE BANKING SYSTEM

The Federal Reserve

Wanting to provide the nation with a safer, more flexible, and stable monetary and financial system, Congress created the Federal Reserve in 1913 as the central bank of the United States. It consists of a seven-member Board of Governors with headquarters in Washington, DC and 12 Reserve Banks located in major cities throughout the country.

Figure 22-2 shows how the country is divided into the 12 regional Federal Reserve districts. For additional information on the Federal Reserve System and its regional banks, visit its website; the Web address is found at the end of this chapter.

American Bankers Association Number

The American Bankers Association (ABA) number is part of a coding system originated by the ABA. It appears in the upper right area of a printed check. The number is used as a simple way to identify the area where the bank on which the check is written is located and the particular bank within the area. The code number is expressed as a fraction (Figure 22-3), for example:

$$\frac{90\text{-}1822}{1222}$$

In the top part of the fraction, before the hyphen, the numbers 1 to 49 designate cities in which Federal Reserve banks are located or other key cities; the numbers from 50 to 99 refer to states or territories. The part of the number following the hyphen is a number issued to each bank for its own identification purposes. The ABA number is used in preparing deposit slips, to identify each check. The bottom part of the fraction includes the number of the Federal Reserve district in which the bank is located and other identifying information.

HOW CHECKS ARE PROCESSED

When a check is presented for payment, the **drawee** (bank or facility on which the check is drawn or written) pays the specified sum of money written on the face of the check to the **holder** (person presenting the check for payment). Checks received

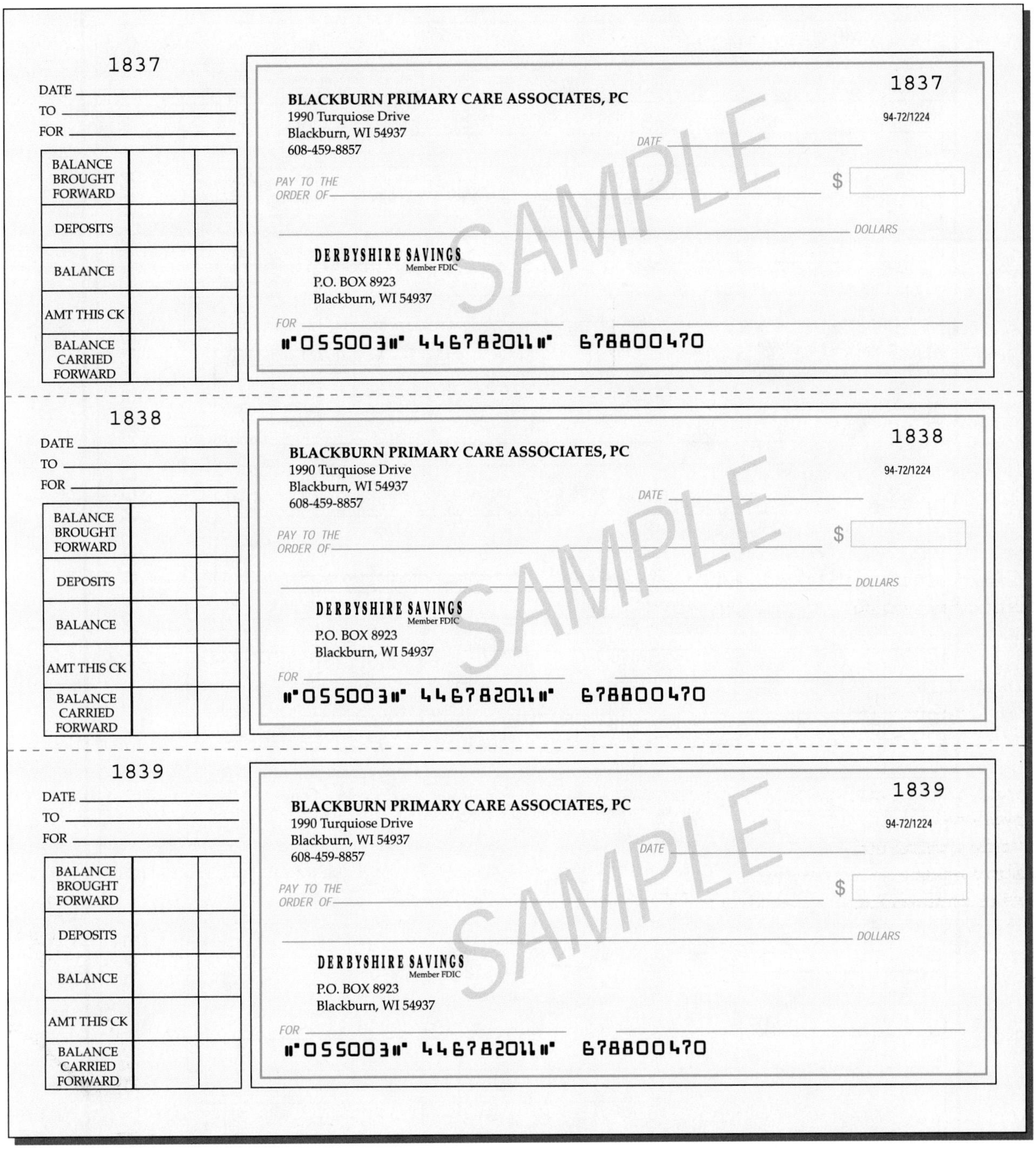

FIGURE 22-5 Example of business checks with stubs. (From Hunt SA: *Fundamentals of medical assisting*, Philadelphia, 2002, Saunders.)

of the check and the date it was paid. Then if any question arises about whether or when the bill was paid, you can readily locate the check stub. The handling and writing of checks must be done with extreme care (Procedure 22-1).

Designated Times

Rather than haphazardly paying bills as they are received in the office, the medical assistant should establish a routine for paying bills at designated times, such as on the fifteenth and thirtieth days of each month. Most vendors allow a 30-day cycle to elapse before adding on interest or late fees.

One method of handling accounts payable is to create a chronologic "tickler file" with dividers for each pay cycle (e.g., the tenth of the month, the twentieth, and the thirtieth). Behind each of the dividers, the invoices can be arranged alphabetically, if desired. When the date arrives, the medical assistant can pull all of the bills from that section and prepare the checks.

Paying Bills to Maximize Money

In establishing the procedure for accounts payable, a medical assistant should keep in mind that most vendors allow 30 days to pay. When each invoice is received, check the "terms," which

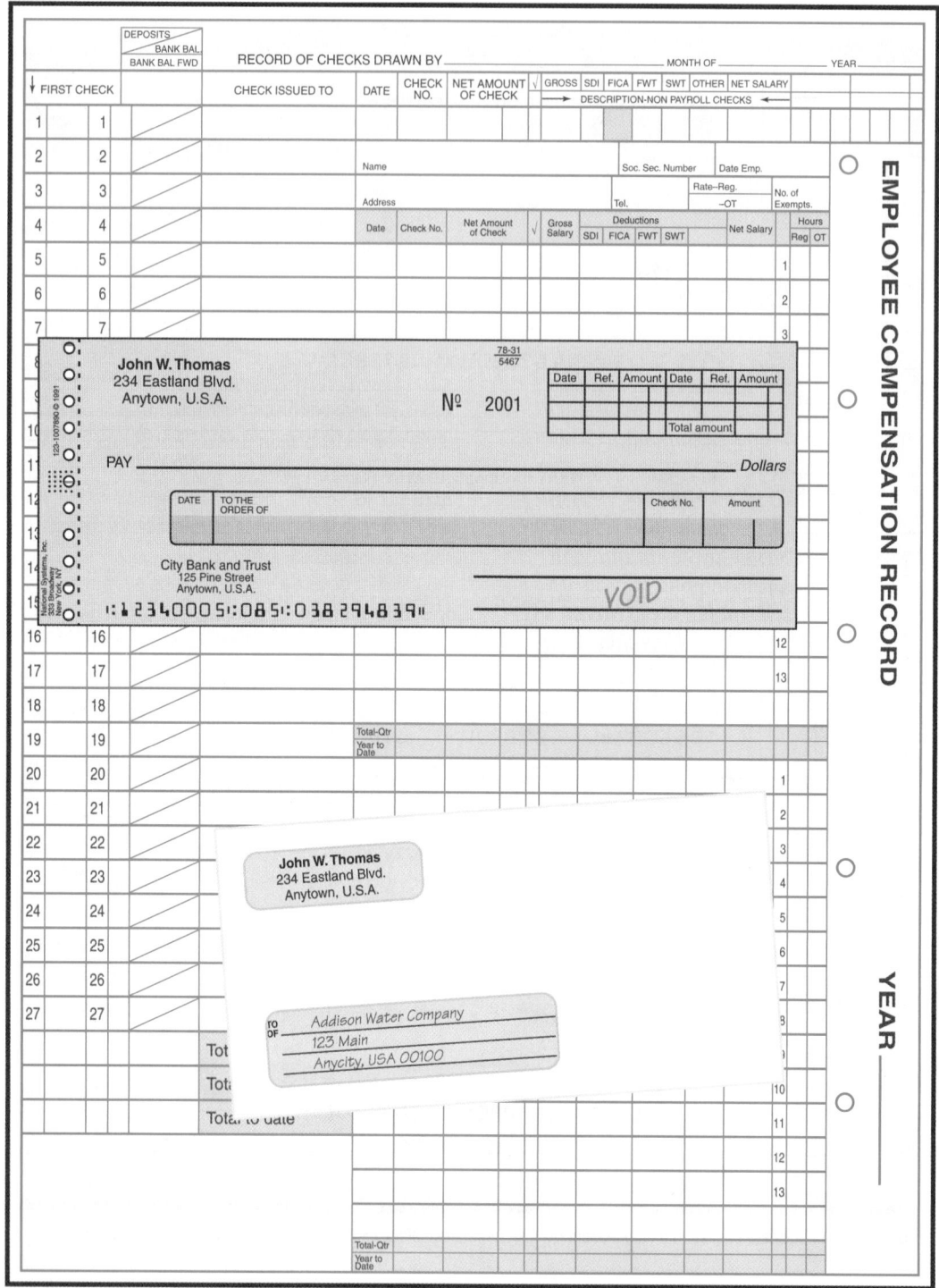

FIGURE 22-6 Pegboard system for check writing. (Courtesy Bibbero Systems, Inc., Petaluma, Calif. 94954, (800) 242-2376, www. bibbero.com.)

are usually located at the top of the document. A few vendors offer a discount (normally 1% to 2%) if bills are paid within a shorter period of time. If the terms say "Net 30," this means the total amount of the bill is due within 30 days. Remember to allow a certain number of days (2 to 5, depending on where payment is to be sent) for mailing. If the business checking account is an interest-bearing one, do not pay bills before their due date. In this way the funds in the account will continue to draw interest until it is time to write the check.

Also, if the practice has a weekly service, such as a laundry or cleaning service that bills several times a month, accumulate the invoices and issue only one check per month. Checks are costly, and some banks charge businesses a fee for each transaction.

PROCEDURE 22-1

Write Checks in Payment of Bills

ABHES COMPETENCY: 3.m

GOAL: *To correctly write checks for payment of bills.*

EQUIPMENT and SUPPLIES

- Checkbook
- Bills to be paid

PROCEDURAL STEPS

1. Locate the first bill to be paid. Before writing the check, fill out the stub or the place designated for recording expenditures. Include the date, name of payee, amount of check, the new balance to be carried forward, and usually, the purpose of the check.
   <u>PURPOSE:</u> To prevent the possibility of delivering or mailing a check without entering the information in the checkbook.
2. Complete both the check and the stub with pen or typewriter.
   <u>PURPOSE:</u> To avoid danger of alteration for any reason.
3. Date the check the day it is written (do not postdate).
4. Write the name of the payee after the printed words, "Pay to the Order of _____ ," with the necessary information following. Do not use abbreviations unless so instructed.
5. Leave no space before the name, and follow it with three dashes if space remains.
6. Omit personal titles from the names of payees.
7. If a payee is receiving a check as an officer of an organization, the name of the office should follow the name. Example: "John F. Jones, Treasurer."
8. Start writing at the extreme left of each space. Leave no blank spaces. Keep the cents notation close to the dollars figure to prevent alteration.
9. Verify that the amount of the check is recorded correctly on the stub, in the box for the dollar ($) amount, and on the line where the amount is written in words.
10. If a check is written for an amount less than 1 dollar, the figures by the $ sign may be circled or enclosed in parentheses ($0.65) to emphasize the amount.

Automatic Withdrawals and Deductions

Some routine bills that occur monthly or on a regular billing cycle, such as insurance premiums, rent payments, and utility bills, can be set up to be paid automatically through prior arrangements with the bank.

Online Bill-Paying

An online bill-paying account can be established with a bank or other business entity. The bank then pays bills by automatically debiting the customer's account and crediting the merchant's account. More banks are offering this service; however, not all vendors accept electronic transfers in payment of bills. If a business decides to take advantage of online bill-paying, the options should be researched carefully, with consideration of the advantages and disadvantages involved.

Writing Checks

Instructions

Writing checks is a routine and basically simple function; however, certain guidelines should be followed to prevent potential problems. Figure 22-7 illustrates several correct methods to use when writing checks.

Figure 22-8 shows the correct method for writing a check for an amount less than a dollar *(top)*. The check on the bottom illustrates an incorrect method of check writing. Note the incomplete name and space for altering (e.g., $6.00 could easily be changed to $26.00 or more, and 00 could be made into 88). When writing in the numeric amount of a check, begin as far to the left in the block as possible. When inserting the written amount of the check, again start as far to the left as possible, allowing no space for added or altered words. Writing checks for less than a dollar is not recommended.

Checkbook Stubs

The check stub (the part that remains in the book after the check has been written and removed) is the depositor's own record of checks written—date, amount, payee, and purpose (Figure 22-9). It is important that the stub be completed before the check is written.

This prevents the possibility of writing a check and neglecting to complete the stub. If the stub is not completed and the check is sent out, you will have no record of the payee and the amount taken from the account until the cancelled check is returned at a later date. Consequently, the account cannot balance nor can one determine the amount on hand until the bank returns those cancelled checks. It is possible to get this information from the bank after the check has been cashed. There may be a charge for this service.

Signing Checks

After all checks have been written, place them along with the invoices or other verifying information on the physician's desk for signature. In some practices, the medical assistant who is in charge of the financial matters is also allowed to sign the checks. This is accomplished by filing a **power of attorney** at the depositor's bank. The power of attorney may limit the check-signing authorization to a certain amount or to a limited time period.

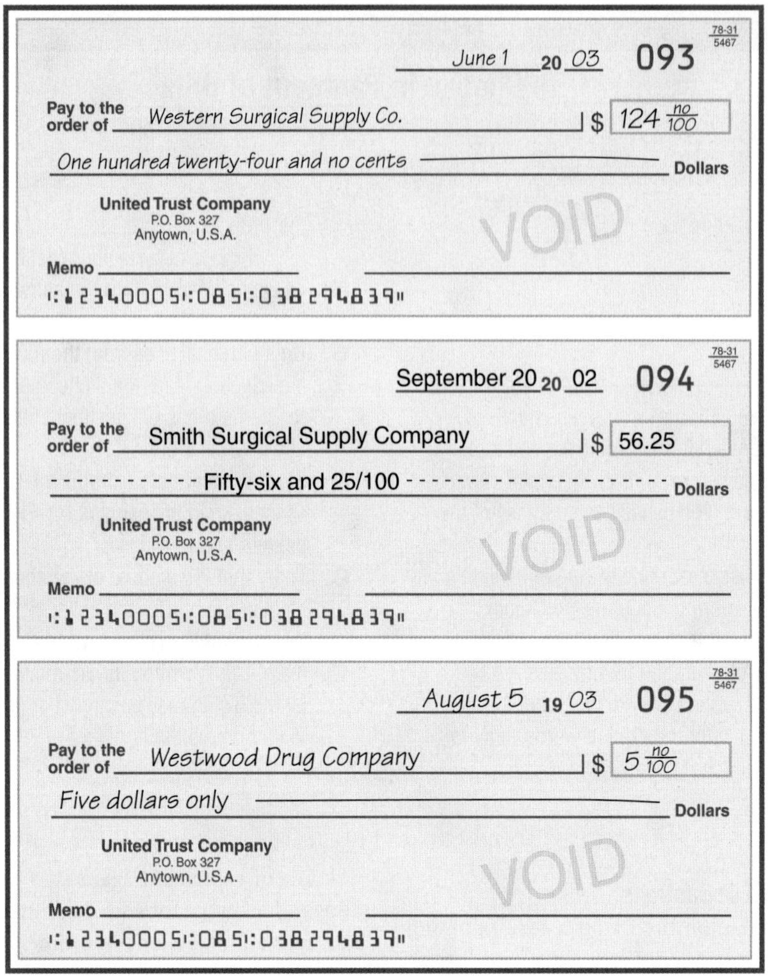

FIGURE 22-7 Correct methods of writing checks.

Handling Corrections

Do not cross out, erase, or change any part of a check. Checks are printed on sensitized paper so that erasures are easily noticeable, and the bank has the right to refuse to pay on any check that has been altered. (See Figures 22-7 and 22-8 for examples of correct and incorrect check writing.) If a mistake is made, write the word "VOID" on the stub and the check, but do not throw out or destroy the check. It should be filed with the canceled checks so that it is available for auditing purposes.

Writing Cash Checks

A cash check is made payable to Cash or Bearer. Such checks are completely negotiable. Because these checks are easily cashed without positive identification, it is poor policy to write cash checks unless they are to be cashed at the time they are written. Some bank personnel may require that the person receiving the cash endorse the check. Many experts in the banking business advise their customers not to endorse a check written for cash or petty cash; often if there is a problem the person who endorses the check is liable. A medical assistant should never endorse a check written for cash or petty cash, as he or she is not a party in the transaction.

Mailing Checks

When checks are sent through the mail, the check should not be visible through the envelope. Either place the check within a letter or fold it into a plain sheet of paper. Checks may be folded at the right end to conceal the amount of money written. Make certain the envelopes are sealed before mailing, and the medical assistant should personally mail all checks as soon as possible after writing.

Special Problems with Checks

Special problems may arise when a check is written on non-existent funds or when a payor wishes, for a legitimate reason, to prevent the payee from cashing a check.

Overdraws or Overdrafts

When a depositor draws a check for more than the amount on deposit in the account, the account becomes overdrawn. In most states it is illegal to issue a check for more than the amount on deposit in the bank. Should this happen through error or oversight, the bank may refuse to honor the check and will return it to the bank that presented it for payment. Such a check is said to "bounce."

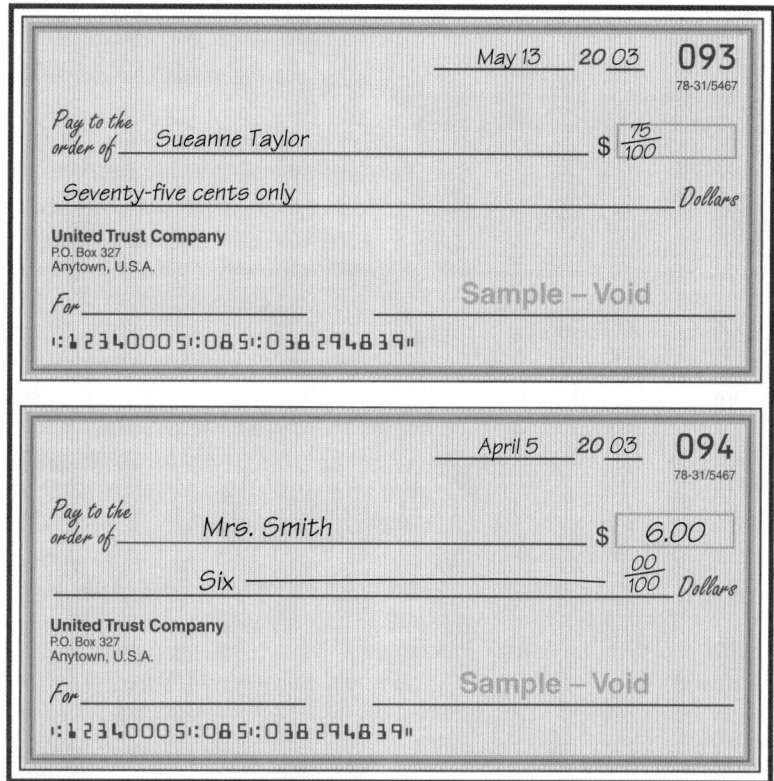

FIGURE 22-8 *Top,* Correct method of writing a check. *Bottom,* Incorrect method of writing a check, with incomplete name and space for altering (e.g., 6.00 could be made into 26.00 or more, and 00 could be made into 88).

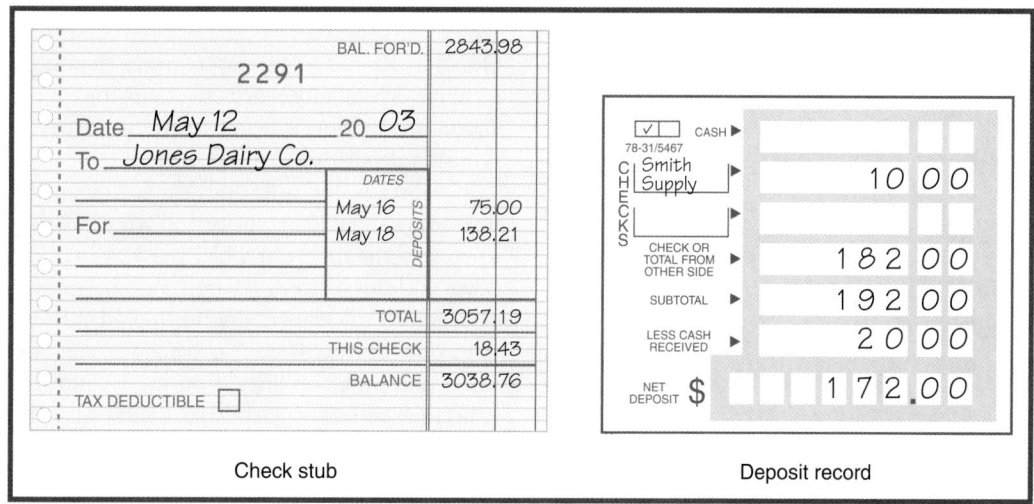

FIGURE 22-9 Methods of filling out a check stub.

If a check is written by an established depositor, the bank may honor the check and notify the depositor that the account is overdrawn. If the bank thus pays or covers the check, it issues an overdraft on the depositor's account. Considerable fees (from $10 to $30) are normally charged when an overdraft occurs. Some accounts allow automatic withdrawals from savings accounts to cover overdrafts without additional charges.

Stop-Payments

A depositor or check writer who wishes to rescind the check has the right to request that the bank stop payment on it. Stop-payment orders should be used only in emergencies. Reasons for stop-payment requests include the following:

- Loss of a check
- Disagreement about a purchase
- Disagreement about a payment

As with overdrafts, most banks charge a fee for stop-payment orders.

CRITICAL THINKING APPLICATION

When Laura arrives at the office on Monday morning, she discovers that a check is missing from the business checkbook, and the stub is blank. What actions should Laura take to solve the problem?

Check Washing

Check washing is the fraudulent process of erasing or "washing out" the ink on a check with common household chemicals, such as bleach, benzene, or correction fluid. The person then rewrites the check to himself or herself, increasing the amount payable by hundreds or even thousands of dollars. It is estimated that check-washing fraud amounts to over $800 million a year in this country, and it is increasing at an alarming rate.

The National Check Fraud Center suggests the following to minimize the chance of check fraud:

- Ask your bank to advise your office when new books of checks are ready, then either pick them up or use a parcel delivery service to deliver them.
- Make sure cancelled checks are in a secured area, such as a bank lock box or a wall safe. Don't throw them in the trash.
- Check bank statements immediately after receiving them. If check fraud is not reported within 30 days of receipt of a monthly statement, the bank does not have to reimburse the loss (**Uniform Commercial Code [UCC]** Code 4-406).
- Print a return address on an envelope. A signature can be traced, duplicated, or forged.
- Don't discard credit card records or bills with trash.

For more information on how to avoid check fraud or what to do when fraud occurs, log onto the National Check Fraud Center's website, listed at the end of this chapter.

ACCEPTING CHECKS

Precautions in Accepting Checks

A medical assistant is presented with checks for payment of physician's services on a daily basis. In most cases these are personal checks.

Acknowledging Payment in Full

If payment in full is to be recognized with regard to a given check, the statement "Payment in Full to Date" must appear on the back of the check, above the endorsement, not on the face of the check. Canceled checks are a receipt for the maker of the check, not for the payee.

CRITICAL THINKING APPLICATION

A new patient wishes to pay for his services at the end of the office visit. The charge is $75. The patient writes the check out for $100 and asks Laura for $25 in currency in return. How should Laura handle the situation?

Guidelines for Accepting Checks

- Scan the check carefully for the correct date, amount, and signature.
- Do not accept a check with corrections on it.
- If you do not know the person presenting a personal check, ask for identification and compare signatures.
- Accept an out-of-town check, government check, or payroll check only if you are well acquainted with the person presenting it and it does not exceed the amount of the payment.
- Acceptance of a third-party check is generally unwise. A third-party check is one made out to your patient by a party unknown to you. A check from the patient's health insurance carrier is an exception.
- When accepting a postal money order for payment, make certain it has only one endorsement. Postal money orders with more than two endorsements will not be honored.
- Do not accept a check marked "Payment in Full" unless it does pay the account in full up to and including the date on which it is received. If a check so marked is less than the amount due, you will be unable to collect the balance on the account once you have accepted and deposited such a check. It is illegal for you to scratch out the words "Payment in Full."
- Accepting checks written for more than the amount due and returning cash for the difference between the amount of the check and the amount owed is poor policy. If the check is not honored by the bank, your office will suffer the loss not only of the amount of the check but also of the amount returned in cash.

Returned Checks

Occasionally the bank may return a deposited check because of some irregularity, such as a missing signature or missing endorsement. More often, it is because the payor has insufficient funds on deposit to cover the check.

If a check is stamped "NSF," indicating insufficient funds, do not delay in contacting the person who gave the check. If unable to contact the maker of a bad check, waste no time in tracking down all leads, such as referrals, numbers obtained from credit cards, driver's license, and so forth. Bad checks may be reported to several places. Credit associations are often a great help when such problems arise. Turn the account over to a qualified collection agency if you do not succeed in collecting on the account yourself within a short time.

If a check is returned to your office marked "No Account" and it is a check that had been deposited promptly, the office has obviously been swindled. This check should be given to the police, the local Better Business Bureau, or a collection agency.

Charging Fees

To cover their overhead costs, most banks currently charge both the payor and payee a fee of $15 to $30 dollars for a check that has been returned because of "insufficient funds." It is customary for the medical assistant to notify the person responsible for writing the check that it has been returned. Often the individual will have a plausible excuse and simply requests that the check be "run through again." If this is the case, it is a wise practice to first call the bank and ask if there are sufficient funds to do this, thereby avoiding additional time delay and fees. Some offices add these charges to the patient's account in an attempt to recoup the expense.

Collecting Returned Checks

There are several options available for collecting returned checks. As mentioned previously, the medical assistant might want to make an initial collection attempt by either telephoning or writing a letter to the patient. Many NSF problems can be cleared up quickly and easily using courtesy and tact, assuming that the situation was simply a mistake or oversight. If this method proves unsuccessful, the office might consider registering with a company that specializes in collecting bad checks. This can be done online or physically, using a local collection agency.

Legal Options

After all reasonable options for collecting NSF checks have been exhausted, a medical assistant may employ a collection method using the court system. Small claims court is a special court in which disputes are resolved inexpensively and quickly; it is a commonly used method that avoids costly attorney fees. Filing fees are in the $20 to $30 range, and there is usually a charge for having the papers served. There are restrictions, however. The amount for which the plaintiff (individual or company initiating the suit) can sue in a small claims lawsuit is limited to $5000. Other limitations vary from state to state. Contact the local Clerk of the District Court for the necessary forms and instructions in completing a small claims suit. For more information on filing small claims, refer to the government legal department's website.

CRITICAL THINKING APPLICATION

When opening the mail, Laura notices a form from the bank with a check attached. It is a check from Elliott Benson, a new patient seen in the office the previous week, being returned for insufficient funds. How should Laura handle this problem?

It is important that the medical assistant learn how to become "proactive" rather than "reactive" when it comes to problem patients. He or she should discuss fees with the patient on the first visit and gather all the financial and insurance information necessary to make a judgment as to whether the patient is able and willing to pay. An experienced medical assistant can often sense a "red flag" during this initial information-gathering process. If this happens, requesting payment in advance might be wise. This practice should not be abused, however, and the medical assistant should follow the established office policy or discuss the matter with the office manager or physician when necessary.

ENDORSEMENTS

An endorsement is a signature plus any other writing on the back of a check by which the **endorser** transfers all rights in the check to another party. Endorsements are made in ink, with either pen or rubber stamp, on the back of the check across the left (or perforated) end.

Why an Endorsement Is Necessary

The Uniform Negotiable Instrument Act, applicable in all states, explains the need for an endorsement as follows:

An instrument is negotiated when it is transferred from one person to another in such a manner as to pass title to another party. If payable to bearer, it is negotiated by delivery. If payable to order, it is negotiated by the endorsement of the holder completed by delivery.

The name of the last endorser of the check shows who last received the money. If a check is cashed for someone who did not endorse it and is returned for some reason, the bank will charge the check to the last endorser, not to the last person receiving the money. For this reason, it is not wise to cash a check made payable to another party without having the endorsement of the person who delivered the check to you for cashing.

Types of Endorsements

There are four principal kinds of endorsements. Blank and restrictive endorsements are the ones most commonly used.

Blank Endorsement

The payee signs only his or her name. This makes the check payable to the bearer. It is the simplest and most common type of endorsement on personal checks but should be used only when the check is to be cashed or deposited immediately.

Restrictive Endorsement

This specifies the purpose of the endorsement. A restrictive endorsement is used in preparing checks for deposit to the physician's checking account. An example is shown in Figure 22-10.

Special Endorsement

This endorsement includes words specifying the person to whom the endorser makes the check payable. For instance, a check naming Helen Barker as the payee may be endorsed to the physician by writing on the back of the check as follows:

Pay to the order of
Theodore F. Wilson, M.D.
Helen Barker

The check is still negotiable but requires Dr. Wilson's signature or endorsement.

> Pay to the Order of
> Midwest National Bank
> Main Branch
> For Deposit Only
> CARLOS MACAULEY
> 301-012697

FIGURE 22-10 Example of a restrictive endorsement.

Qualified Endorsement

The effect of the endorsement is qualified by disclaiming or destroying any future liability of the endorser. Usually the words "without recourse" are written above by an attorney who accepts a check on behalf of a client but who has no personal claim in the transaction.

Methods of Endorsement

Stamp

As checks from patients and other sources arrive, they should be recorded on the ledger and immediately stamped with the restrictive endorsement "For Deposit Only." This is a safeguard against lost or stolen checks.

Any endorsement should agree exactly with the name on the face of the check. If the name of the payee is misspelled, it is usually necessary for the payee to endorse the check the way the name is spelled on the face, followed by the correctly spelled signature. UCC, Section 3-203, states:

Where an instrument is made payable to a person under a misspelled name or one other than his own, he may endorse in that name or his own or both; but signature in both names may be required by a person paying or giving value for the instrument.

Most banks accept routine stamp endorsement that is restricted to deposit only, if the customer is well known and maintains an established account.

Signature

Some insurance checks or drafts require a personal signature endorsement; a stamped endorsement is not acceptable. This will be stated on the back of the check. In such cases, ask the payee to endorse the check, then stamp immediately below the signature the restrictive endorsement "For Deposit Only."

MAKING DEPOSITS

The financial duties of a medical assistant include depositing checks and reconciling the bank statements with the checkbook. Checks should be deposited promptly, for these reasons:

- A stop-payment order may be placed.
- The check may be lost, misplaced, or stolen.
- Delay may cause the check to be returned because of insufficient funds.
- The check may have a restricted time for cashing.
- It is a courtesy to the payor.

Preparing the Deposit

Deposit slips are itemized memoranda of cash or other funds that a depositor presents to the bank with the money to be credited to the account. All deposits must be accompanied by a deposit slip. A carbon or photocopy of the deposit slip should be kept on file (Procedure 22-2).

There are several types of deposit slips, sometimes called *deposit tickets*. The commercial slip is used for the office checking account. The deposit slips are printed with the number of the account in magnetic ink characters to correspond with the checks. Preprinted deposit slips are ordered along with the checks.

Some write-it-once accounting systems include a deposit slip that the bank will accept as the itemization if it is attached to the customer's numbered deposit slip. The deposit slip should be prepared before you go to the bank, with the money organized and ready to present to the bank teller.

PROCEDURE 22-2

Prepare a Bank Deposit

CAAHEP COMPETENCY: 3.a.(2)(a)
ABHES COMPETENCY: 3.i

GOAL: *To prepare a bank deposit for the day's receipts and complete appropriate office records related to the deposit.*

EQUIPMENT and SUPPLIES

- Currency
- Checks for deposit
- Deposit slip
- Endorsement stamp (optional)
- Typewriter
- Envelope

PROCEDURAL STEPS

1. Organize currency.
   PURPOSE: To arrange currency in the best order for speedy and accurate presentation to the teller.
2. Total the currency, and record the amount on the deposit slip.
3. Place restrictive endorsements on the checks, using an endorsement stamp or the typewriter.

PURPOSE: To transfer the title and protect checks from loss or theft.

4. List each check separately on the deposit slip, with the ABA number and the amount.
5. Total the amount of currency and checks, and enter on the deposit slip.
6. Enter the amount of the deposit in the checkbook.
   PURPOSE: To record the current balance in the account.
7. Prepare a copy of the deposit slip for the office record, including the names of the payors.
   PURPOSE: For verification of checks deposited, if necessary.
8. Place the currency, checks, and deposit slip in an envelope for transporting to the bank.

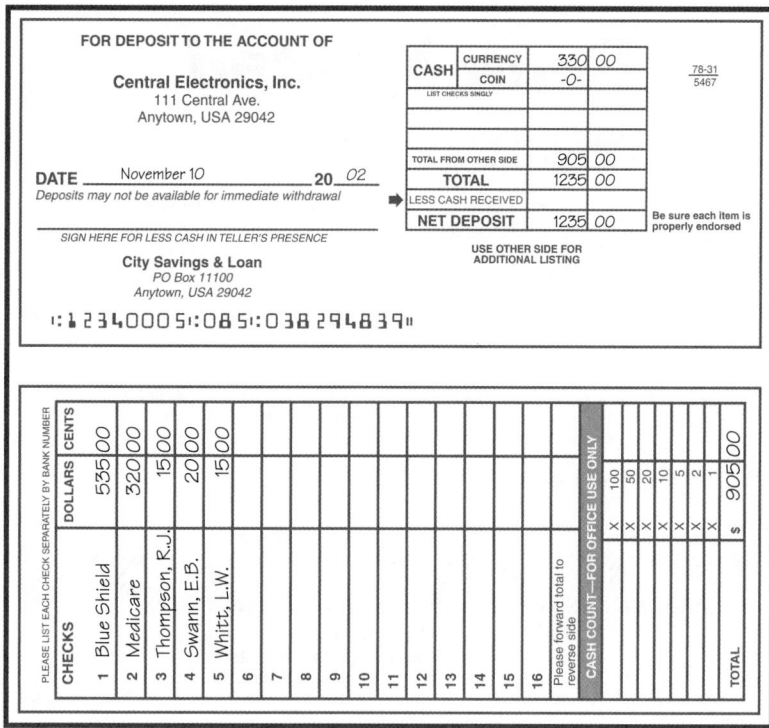

FIGURE 22-11 Front and back of a deposit slip.

Payment on patient accounts is generally made by check, but some payments are made in currency (paper money). Each type of fund is recorded separately on the deposit slip. The currency is usually listed first. Organize the currency so that all of the bills are facing in the same direction—for example, with the black-ink (portrait) side up. Place the largest-denomination bills on top.

Some banks prefer that checks be recorded individually by the ABA number; others use just the maker's name. If the checks are arranged alphabetically by the names of the patient accounts, with these names included on your office copy of the deposit slip, you will have a ready reference of checks deposited should a question arise regarding a patient's payment. Follow the following procedure for preparing a deposit slip (Figure 22-11):

1. List all checks on the back of the deposit slip.
2. Transfer the total to the front of the slip.
3. Enter the amount of the total deposit on the deposit slip stub.

Money orders, either postal, express, or others, are identified by "PO Money Order" or "Express MO." Remember that money orders cannot have more than two endorsements.

The deposit slip should be carefully totaled, and the total entered in the checkbook. Any torn bills should be mended with transparent tape. Clip the currency together, and clip the checks in a separate packet. Then place the entire amount in a heavy envelope for taking to the bank. Deposit the currency and checks daily if possible.

Deposits by Mail

Depositing by mail saves time and is easily accomplished if the deposit consists of checks only. Banks usually supply their customers with special mailing deposit slips and envelopes on request (Figure 22-12). Although the majority of banking that is not done in person is performed on the internet, some offices do still use mail services for banking procedures, especially if the physician has accounts at banks in other cities or states.

Some mailing deposit slips have an attached portion that the bank will stamp and return to the customer as a receipt. Others may provide the customer with a receipt card that is sent along with the deposit each time for the bank's notation. The mailer shown in Figure 22-12 has a peel-off receipt for the depositor's records. Mailed deposits are prepared in the same manner as are regular deposits, but certain precautions should be observed.

Direct Deposits

Direct deposit is a plan in which payments are transferred, usually electronically, by a paying agency directly into the account of a recipient. Direct deposits are commonly used for paying salaries; paychecks are credited to employees' accounts—checking, savings, or any other type of account—at any financial institution.

Precautions for Deposits Made by Mail

- Do not send cash or currency by mail. If this is absolutely necessary, then send it by registered mail.
- Use only a restrictive endorsement; use a deposit stamp or write the notation "For Deposit Only to the account of _____ ."
- If you have not obtained mailing deposit slips or your bank does not provide them, make duplicate slips and mail them with your deposit. Ask the bank to stamp one copy and return it to you as a receipt.

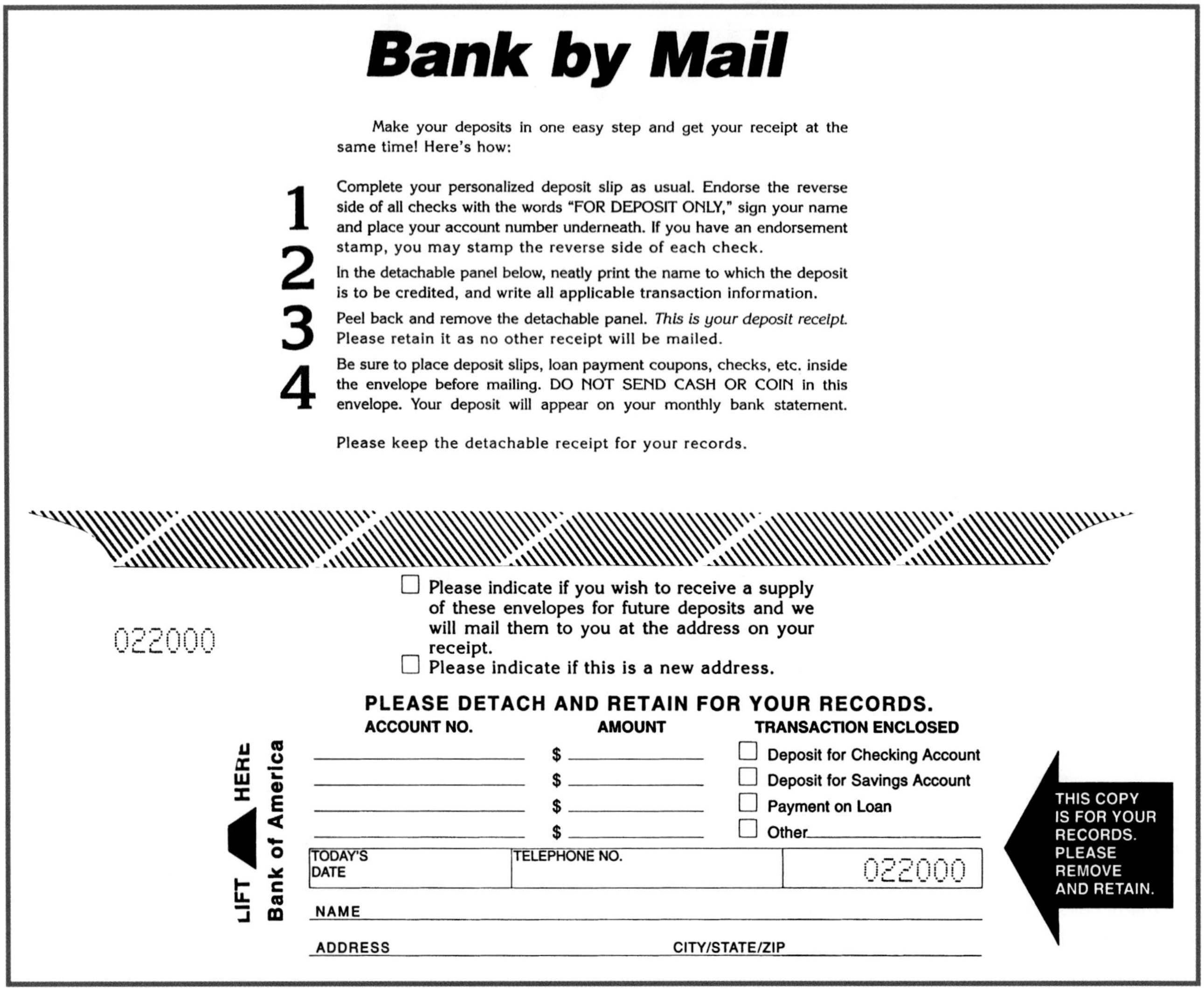

Bank by Mail

Make your deposits in one easy step and get your receipt at the same time! Here's how:

1 Complete your personalized deposit slip as usual. Endorse the reverse side of all checks with the words "FOR DEPOSIT ONLY," sign your name and place your account number underneath. If you have an endorsement stamp, you may stamp the reverse side of each check.

2 In the detachable panel below, neatly print the name to which the deposit is to be credited, and write all applicable transaction information.

3 Peel back and remove the detachable panel. *This is your deposit receipt.* Please retain it as no other receipt will be mailed.

4 Be sure to place deposit slips, loan payment coupons, checks, etc. inside the envelope before mailing. DO NOT SEND CASH OR COIN in this envelope. Your deposit will appear on your monthly bank statement.

Please keep the detachable receipt for your records.

022000

☐ Please indicate if you wish to receive a supply of these envelopes for future deposits and we will mail them to you at the address on your receipt.
☐ Please indicate if this is a new address.

PLEASE DETACH AND RETAIN FOR YOUR RECORDS.

ACCOUNT NO.	AMOUNT	TRANSACTION ENCLOSED
	$	☐ Deposit for Checking Account
	$	☐ Deposit for Savings Account
	$	☐ Payment on Loan
	$	☐ Other

LIFT ▲ HERE Bank of America

TODAY'S DATE

TELEPHONE NO.

022000

THIS COPY IS FOR YOUR RECORDS. PLEASE REMOVE AND RETAIN.

NAME

ADDRESS   CITY/STATE/ZIP

FIGURE 22-12 Example of a bank-by-mail deposit envelope. (Courtesy Valley Bank of Nevada, Las Vegas, Nev.)

Other Methods of Deposit

Advances in computer technology have allowed financial institutions to offer other methods of deposit to consumers and business customers. Some automated teller machines (ATMs) will accept deposits, and there are checking accounts available that allow the customer to conduct the majority of banking services using the computer and ATMs. These types of accounts may limit the amount of times the customer can use teller services without a fee.

Online banking allows customers to view their accounts, make transfers, order checks, pay bills, and perform numerous other transactions simply by logging onto the bank website and accessing the account with a password. Online banking is also an excellent way to research the checks that have cleared the bank and compute accurate bank balances.

BANK STATEMENTS AND RECONCILIATION

A statement is periodically sent by the bank to the customer; it shows the status of the customer's account on a given date. This statement indicates the following:

- Beginning balance
- Deposits received
- Checks paid
- Bank charges
- Ending balance

Mailed Statements

Bank statements, similar to the one illustrated in Figure 22-13, are prepared at regular intervals (usually once a month) and are usually mailed to the bank's customers. These statements may or may not include the accompanying cancelled checks, depending on bank policy and account type. The back of each page of the statement usually includes a reconciliation page so that the customer can determine what checks have still not cleared the bank, what deposits are not yet shown on the statement, and the accurate account balance.

Online Statements

Online statements, or e-statements, are an electronic version of a paper bank statement. Financial establishments that offer online banking services in an attempt to make banking easier

0821-402054

#821

Ilhundhllululululululullhuullhunhlululull

N
2

CALL (888) 555-2932
24 HOURS/DAY, 7 DAYS/WEEK
FOR ASSISTANCE WITH
YOUR ACCOUNT.

PAGE 1 OF 2   THIS STATEMENT COVERS: 6/22/02 THROUGH 7/22/02

**INTEREST
CHECKING**
0821-402054

SUMMARY

PREVIOUS BALANCE	252.10		MINIMUM BALANCE	142.55
DEPOSITS	68.74 +		AVERAGE BALANCE	220.00
INTEREST EARNED	.18 +		ANNUAL PERCENTAGE	
WITHDRAWALS	109.55 −		YIELD EARNED	.96 %
CUSTOMER SERVICE CALLS	.00 −			
INTERLINK/PURCHASE FEE	.00 −		INTEREST EARNED 1994	2.23
MONTHLY CHECKING FEE				
AND OTHER CHARGES	.00 −			

▶ **NEW BALANCE**   **211.47**

USE YOUR EXPRESS CARD TO MAKE UNLIMITED PURCHASES AT RETAILERS DISPLAYING
THE INTERLINK SYMBOL. (A $1 MONTHLY FEE MAY APPLY.)

TRY IT TODAY AT ARCO . . . MOBIL . . . LUCKY . . . RALPHS . . . SAFEWAY & MORE!

**CHECKS AND
WITHDRAWALS**

CHECK	DATE PAID	AMOUNT	CHECK	DATE PAID	AMOUNT
202	7/05	15.05	203	7/15	94.50

DEPOSITS

		DATE POSTED	AMOUNT
CUSTOMER DEPOSIT		7/22	68.74
INTEREST PAYMENT THIS PERIOD		7/22	.18

**BALANCE
INFORMATION**

DATE	BALANCE	DATE	BALANCE	DATE	BALANCE
6/22	252.10	7/05	237.05	7/15	142.55
				7/22	211.47

**24 HOUR
CUSTOMER
SERVICE**

EACH ACCOUNT COMES WITH 3 COMPLIMENTARY CALLS PER STATEMENT PERIOD.

CALLS TO 24 HOUR CUSTOMER SERVICE THIS STATEMENT PERIOD: 0

**INTEREST
INFORMATION**

FROM	THROUGH	INTEREST RATE	ANNUAL PERCENTAGE YIELD (APY)
6/22	7/22	1.00%	1.01%

INTEREST RATE/APY AS OF 7/22/02 IF YOUR BALANCE IS

$ 0 - 4,999 . . . . .1.00%	1.01%
$ 5,000 - 9,999 . . . . .1.00%	1.01%
$ 10,000 AND OVER. 1.00%	1.01%

CALL 1-800-555-2932 IN CALIFORNIA ANYTIME FOR CURRENT RATES.

MEMBER FDIC

STATEMENT

FIGURE 22-13 Example of a regular checking account statement.

for their customers claim that e-statements are a user-friendly way of viewing account balances and checking financial images online.

With e-statements, there is no need to continue receiving paper statements. The benefits include the following:
- Receiving statements quickly and easily
- Being able to save statements in an electronic file for examination and printing at the customer's convenience
- Keeping fees low by minimizing unnecessary paper and mailing costs

Various banks offer different options, and fees vary. If the medical assistant has been authorized to set up an online banking account with the financial institution used by the medical facility, he or she should visit the bank to discuss the details of what is involved.

Reconciling the Bank Statement

The bank statement balance and the customer's checkbook balance usually differ, except in a relatively inactive account. The two balances must be reconciled. The reconciliation discloses any errors that may exist in the checkbook or, on rare occasions, in the bank statement (Figure 22-14).

The bank statement may include an entry for service charges that must be deducted from the checkbook balance. In all types of accounts, the bank may charge a fee for services. Usually in the case of an individual account, it is a flat fee; in a business account, the fee is based on services rendered. If the average or minimum balance is maintained at an established level, the bank may forego a service charge.

Most banks ask to be notified within a reasonable amount of time (e.g., 10 days) of any error found in the statement. The bank statement should be reconciled as soon as it is received. You will usually find a form to follow in carrying out this procedure on the back of the bank statement.

The **reconciliation** procedure may be put in a formula, as shown below.

If the two corrected balances agree, you may stop there. If they do not agree, subtract the lesser figure from the greater figure; the difference will usually give you a clue to the error (Procedure 22-3).

Bank Statement Reconciliation Formula

Bank statement balance	$ _____
Less outstanding checks	$ _____
Plus deposits not shown	$ _____
Corrected bank statement balance	$ _____
Checkbook balance	$ _____
Less any bank charges	$ _____
Corrected checkbook balance	$ _____

SIGNATURE CARDS

When an account is first opened at a banking facility, the depositor will be required to affix his or her handwritten signature to a card, which is then kept on file at the bank. If

Questions to Ask in Searching for a Possible Error

- Is your arithmetic correct?
- Did you forget to include one of the outstanding checks?
- Did you fail to record a deposit or did you record one twice?

a check comes through, and some suspicion arises that the depositor's signature has been forged, the bank personnel compare the signature on the check with the original one on the signature card.

In a business situation, as in a medical office, the physician often delegates the responsibility of paying bills to the medical assistant or other office staff members. In this case, any staff member who has been authorized to sign the medical facility's checks must go to the bank and add his or her handwritten signature to the signature card. Only the people whose names appear on the signature card are authorized to sign checks, and it is the bank's responsibility to verify any questionable signatures.

BONDING

To protect their business establishments from embezzlement or other financial loss caused by employees who handle large sums of money, physicians often purchase fidelity bonds. Fidelity bonds reimburse the physician for any monetary loss caused by employees. The three types of bonding methods are as follows:
- Position-schedule bonding, which covers a specific position rather than an individual, such as bookkeeper or receptionist
- Blanket-position bonding, which covers all employees
- Personal bonding, which covers specific individuals

For individuals to be bonded, a personal background investigation is normally necessary.

CLOSING COMMENTS

Patient Education

Medical assistants might want to encourage patients to pay for professional services rendered with a personal check because of the numerous benefits checks offer. If a patient attempts to pay for services with a third-party check (other than an insurance reimbursement), the medical assistant should tactfully explain why this is not a wise practice. In addition, if a patient makes a mistake when writing a check, it is the responsibility of the medical assistant to point it out and request a new one, as corrections on the face of a check often render the check useless.

When a patient's check is returned from the bank marked "insufficient funds," the medical assistant should immediately call the patient and explain the problem, requesting that he or she correct the matter as soon as possible. It is important to remember, however, that most overdrafts are simply the result of mathematic errors or a delay in deposited funds being available

THIS WORKSHEET IS PROVIDED TO HELP YOU BALANCE YOUR ACCOUNT

1. Go through your register and mark each check, withdrawal, Express ATM transaction, payment, deposit or other credit listed on this statement. Be sure that your register shows any interest paid into your account, and any service charges, automatic payments, or Express Transfers withdrawn from your account during this statement period.

2. Using the chart below, list any outstanding checks, Express ATM withdrawals, payments or any other withdrawals (including any from previous months) that are listed in your register but are not shown on this statement.

3. Balance your account by filling in the spaces below.

ITEMS OUTSTANDING	
NUMBER	AMOUNT
TOTAL	$

ENTER

The NEW BALANCE shown on this statement _ _ _ _ _ _ _ _ _ _ _ _ _ _ _ _ _ _ $_____

ADD

Any deposits listed in your register $_____
or transfers into your account $_____
which are not shown on this $_____
statement.   +$_____

                          TOTAL _ _ _ _ _ _ _ _ +$_____

CALCULATE THE SUBTOTAL _ _ _ _ _ _ _ _ _ $_____

SUBTRACT

The total outstanding checks and withdrawals from the chart at left _ _ _ _ _ _ _ _ _ –$_____

CALCULATE THE ENDING BALANCE

This amount should be the same as the current balance shown in your check register _ _ _ _ _ _ _ _ _ _ _ _ _ _ _ _ _ $_____

IF YOU SUSPECT ERRORS OR HAVE QUESTIONS ABOUT ELECTRONIC TRANSFERS

If you believe there is an error on your statement or Express ATM receipt, or if you need more information about a transaction listed on this statement or an Express ATM receipt, please contact us immediately. We are available 24 hours a day, seven days a week to assist you. Please call the telephone number printed on the front of this statement. Or, you may write to us at United Trust Company, P.O. Box 327, Anytown, USA.

1) Tell us your name and account number or Express card number.

2) As clearly as you can, describe the error or the transfer you are unsure about, and explain why you believe there is an error or why you need more information.

3) Tell us the dollar amount of the suspected error.

You must report the suspected error to us no later than 60 days after we sent you the first statement on which the problem appeared. We will investigate your question and will correct any error promptly. If our investigation takes longer than 10 business days (or 20 days in the case of electronic purchases), we will temporarily credit your account for the amount you believe is in error, so that you may have use of the money until the investigation is completed.

FIGURE 22-14 Reverse side of a bank statement to be used for reconciling a checking account.

PROCEDURE 22-3

Reconcile a Bank Statement

ABHES COMPETENCY: 3.j

GOAL: *To reconcile a bank statement for a checking account.*

EQUIPMENT and SUPPLIES

- Ending balance of previous statement
- Current bank statement
- Canceled checks for current month
- Checkbook stubs
- Calculator
- Pen

PROCEDURAL STEPS

1. Compare the opening balance of the new statement with the closing balance of the previous statement.
   PURPOSE: To determine that the balances are in agreement.
2. Compare the canceled checks with the items on the statement.
   PURPOSE: To verify that they are your checks and that they are listed in the right amount.
3. Arrange the canceled checks in numeric order, and compare with the checkbook stubs.
4. Place a checkmark on each stub for which a canceled check has been returned.
   PURPOSE: To locate any outstanding checks.

5. List and total the outstanding checks.
6. Verify that all previous outstanding checks have cleared.
7. Subtract the total of the outstanding checks from the bank statement balance.
   NOTE: Do not include any certified checks as outstanding because their amount has already been deducted from the account.
8. Add to the total in step 7 any deposits made but not included in the bank statement.
   PURPOSE: To correct the credits in the bank statement balance.
9. Total any bank charges that appear on the bank statement, and subtract them from the checkbook balance. Such charges may include service charges, automatic withdrawals or payments, and NSF checks.
   PURPOSE: To correct the checkbook balance.
10. If the checkbook balance and the statement balance do not agree, match the bank statement entries with the checkbook entries.

---

for withdrawal. So the medical assistant should be patient and courteous when discussing NSF issues with patients. Patients need to know, however, that overdrafts are costly not only to them, but also to the medical facility.

Legal and Ethical Issues

If a mistake is made in preparing a check, do not destroy this check. Rather, write "VOID" across the face of the check, make a note on the check stub, and file the check with the cancelled checks for auditing purposes.

A stop-payment order may be placed with the bank in an emergency, such as when a check is lost or a disagreement occurs with regard to a purchase or payment.

Do not accept a check made payable to another party without having the endorsement of the person who gives the check to you. If the check is returned by the bank for any reason, the check will be charged to the last endorser, not the last person to receive the money.

SUMMARY OF SCENARIO

Laura has gained considerable knowledge through her experiences and work with the various aspects of the banking world. The goals she set for completing the assignments and competencies were accomplished in the time frame allowed by the instructor. She is comfortable now that she can readily apply this knowledge to whatever medical facility she works in.

Laura spent extra time outside of class exploring online banking and bill paying on the Internet and found a wealth of information available. Laura now plans to visit several banks in her area to see what kind of e-banking services they offer.

The versatility of the medical assistant's role and the variety of the opportunities available reinforce to Laura that she has made the right career choice.

SUMMARY of LEARNING OBJECTIVES

1. Define, spell, and pronounce the terms listed in the vocabulary.
   - *Spelling and pronouncing medical terms correctly adds credibility to the medical assistant. Knowing the definition of these terms promotes confidence in communication with patients and co-workers.*

2. Explain how the Internet has changed traditional banking practices.
   - *The Internet has changed conventional banking as we know it, and it offers expansive opportunities without leaving home. As with everything, however, e-banking has both advantages and disadvantages, and these should be thoroughly researched before an online account is opened.*

3. State the four requirements of a negotiable instrument.
   - *For an instrument (e.g., a check) to be "negotiable," it must meet certain criteria: (1) be written and signed by a maker, (2) contain a promise or order to pay a sum of money, (3) be payable on demand or at a fixed future date, and (4) be payable to order or bearer.*

4. Discuss the advantages of using checks.
   - *There are many advantages to using checks. These advantages include safety and convenience, quick calculation of expenditures, and a permanent record for tax purposes.*

5. Identify the three most common types of bank accounts.
   - *The three most common types of bank accounts are checking accounts, savings accounts, and money market savings accounts. Each one is slightly different, and each has its special uses.*

6. Explain how you would handle mistakes made in preparing a check.
   - *Normally, when a mistake is made on a check, it should be marked "VOID" and a new check should be written. Some banks will accept minor errors if the maker initials the error. Erasures are not allowed, nor is the use of correction fluid.*

7. List and discuss eight precautions to observe in accepting checks.
   - *Scan the check carefully for the correct date, amount, and signature.*
   - *Do not accept a check with corrections on it.*
   - *If you do not know the person presenting a personal check, ask for identification and compare signatures.*
   - *Accept an out-of-town check, government check, or payroll check only if you are well acquainted with the person presenting it and it does not exceed the amount of the payment.*
   - *Acceptance of a third-party check is generally unwise. A third-party check is one made out to your patient by a party unknown to you. A check from the patient's health insurance carrier is an exception.*
   - *When accepting a postal money order for payment, make certain it has only one endorsement. Postal money orders with more than two endorsements will not be honored.*
   - *Do not accept a check marked "Payment in Full" unless it does pay the account in full up to and including the date on which it is received. If a check so marked is less than the amount due, you will be unable to collect the balance on the account once you have accepted and deposited such a check. It is illegal for you to scratch out the words "Payment in Full."*
   - *Accepting checks written for more than the amount due and returning cash for the difference between the amount of the check and the amount owed is poor policy. If the check is not honored by the bank, your office will suffer the loss not only of the amount of the check but also of the amount returned in cash.*

8. Name and compare the four kinds of endorsements.
   - *The four kinds of endorsements are (1) blank endorsement, in which the payee simply signs his or her name on the back of the check; (2) restrictive endorsement, which specifies which bank and what specific account the funds are to be deposited in; (3) special endorsement, which names a specific person on the back of the check as payee; and (4) qualified endorsement, which disclaims future liability. This type of endorsement is used when the person who accepts the check has no personal claim in the transaction.*

9. Discuss the actions necessary when a deposited check is returned.
   - *When a deposited check is returned, the maker should be contacted immediately, informed of the situation, and asked to remedy the situation either by immediately depositing funds in his or her account to cover the check or by paying the bill by alternative means—cash or money order.*

10. Correctly write checks for bill payment.
    - *The medical assistant may be required to write checks on the practice account to pay bills. The process for writing a check is outlined in Procedure 22-1.*

11. Prepare a bank deposit and appropriate office documents.
    - *Bank deposits should be made on a daily basis. The process for preparing a bank deposit is outlined in Procedure 22-2.*

12. Accurately reconcile a bank statement with the office checking account.
    - *Bank statements should be reconciled as soon as they arrive at the physician's office or should be printed from the bank's website for reconciliation. The process for reconciling a bank statement is outlined in Procedure 22-3.*

CONNECTIONS

 Study Guide Connection: Go to Chapter 22 Study Guide. Read the Case Study and Workplace Applications and complete the assignments. Do online research for answers to the questions in the Internet Activities associated with banking services and procedures.

 CD Connection: Go to the Medical Assisting Competency Challenge CD and do the training activities under Financial Management.

Evolve Connection: For more information related to banking services and procedures, go to evolve.elsevier.com/kinn and visit related weblinks for Chapter 22. Click on the Medical Assisting Exam Review and do the practice questions to sharpen your test-taking skills. To learn more about office software, do the exercises for the Altapoint demo that is on the CD.

Management of Practice Finances

23

SCENARIO

Brenda Newman is the office manager for Dr. Susan Wilkins, a neurologist who is beginning her second year of practice. Dr. Wilkins is financially savvy and takes care with the money she has invested in her business. She encourages her employees to plan for the future and offers them a retirement plan as well as opportunities for investing in mutual funds through payroll deduction. Her accountant, Grant Schmidt, assists Dr. Wilkins with the financial aspects of her practice and is always willing to counsel the employees of the clinic about finances.

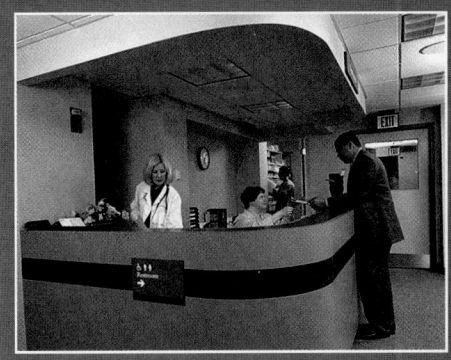

Mr. Schmidt has taught Brenda several methods of keeping track of the practice finances. Brenda is interested in learning more about general accounting rules and bookkeeping. She is able to perform computerized accounting duties and is also able to use a pegboard system. She is able to work with patients when they need to make payment arrangements and has an excellent collection ratio.

Dr. Wilkins is cost conscious and does not order random supplies and equipment. Instead, she and Brenda plan the inventory for a 6-month period and have needed to order supplies only every 6 months. By ordering in precise amounts, Dr. Wilkins saves money and uses the extra funds for staff development events and seminars. Each month, the budget is reviewed to ensure that the office is on track with expenses.

The team effort among Dr. Wilkins, Brenda, and Mr. Schmidt results in a balanced budget for the clinic, and subsequently the staff is able to enjoy more benefits and perks.

While studying this chapter, think about the following questions:

- Why is a constant flow of income preferable to a once-a-month influx for a physician's office?
- Why should the person entering numbers on a manual system make all numerals exactly alike all the time?
- From a legal standpoint, why is positive identification required before hiring individuals to work in the physician's office?
- How do practice finances affect the income of the medical assistant?

LEARNING OBJECTIVES

1. Define, spell, and pronounce the terms listed in the vocabulary.
2. List the four items that all financial records should show at any given time.
3. Distinguish between accounts payable and accounts receivable.
4. List and explain the three most common bookkeeping systems found in physicians' offices today.
5. Explain the importance of a trial balance.
6. State the types of employment records required by the IRS.
7. Discuss the basis for the withholding amounts that are taken from employees' earnings.
8. Name the five common periodic accounting reports.
9. Explain the purpose of the W-4 form.
10. Explain the requirements of the Federal Insurance Contributions Act.
11. Discuss the importance of setting a budget each fiscal year.
12. Maintain a petty cash fund.
13. Accurately process an employee payroll.

National Accreditation Competencies and Content

CAAHEP COMPETENCIES

Administrative
3.a.(2)(c). Perform accounts receivable procedures

General
3.c.(4)(a). Perform an inventory of supplies and equipment
3.c.(4)(c). Utilize computer software to maintain office systems

ABHES COMPETENCIES

Administrative Duties
3.j.   Reconcile a bank statement
3.l.   Perform billing and collection procedures
3.m. Prepare a check
3.n. Establish and maintain a petty cash fund

Office Management
6.c. Inventory equipment and supplies
6.d. Evaluate and recommend equipment and supplies for practice

Financial Management
8.a. Use manual and computerized bookkeeping systems
8.d. Manage accounts payable and receivable
8.e. Maintain records for accounting and banking purposes
8.f.   Process employee payroll

VOCABULARY

accounts payable Debts incurred and not yet paid.

accounts receivable Amounts owed to the physician.

accounts receivable trial balance A method of determining that the journal and the ledger are in balance.

accrual basis of accounting Method of accounting in which income is recorded when earned and expenses are recorded when incurred.

assets The entire property of a person, association, corporation, or estate applicable or subject to the payment of debts.

balance sheet A financial statement for a specific date that shows the total assets, liabilities, and capital of the business.

bookkeeping The recording of business and accounting transactions.

cash basis of accounting Method of accounting in which income is recorded when received and expenses are recorded when paid.

cash flow statement A financial summary for a specific period that shows the beginning balance on hand, the receipts and disbursements during the period, and the balance on hand at the end of the period.

disbursements journal A summary of accounts paid out.

equities The money value of a property or of an interest in a property in excess of claims or liens against it.

fiscal year An accounting period of 12 months.

in balance State in which the total ending balances of patient ledgers equals total of accounts receivable.

invoice A paper describing a purchase and the amount due.

liabilities Things that are owed; debts.

packing slip An itemized list of objects in a package.

petty cash fund A fund maintained to pay small unpredictable cash expenditures.

statement A request for payment.

statement of income and expense A summary of all income and expenses for a given period.

trial balance A method of checking the accuracy of accounts.

A physician's business records are the key to good management practice. The medical assistant who can keep accurate financial records and who will conduct the administrative side of the practice in a businesslike fashion is genuinely needed and appreciated.

Financial records that are complete, correct, and current are essential for the following:

- Prompt billing and collection procedures
- Professional financial planning
- Accurate reporting of income to federal and state agencies

WHAT IS ACCOUNTING?

Accounting is a system of recording, classifying, and summarizing financial transactions. **Bookkeeping** is mainly the recording part of the accounting process. The bookkeeping must be done daily and is the responsibility of the administrative medical assistant in a small practice and of the office manager or financial manager in a larger practice.

Accounting Bases

There are two general bases, or methods, for accounting: the cash basis and the accrual basis. Most physicians use the **cash**

basis of accounting, which means that charges for services are entered as income when payment is received, and expenses are recorded when they are paid. Merchants, on the other hand, generally use an **accrual basis of accounting.** Income is considered earned when services have been performed or goods have been sold, even though payment may not have been received. Expenses are recognized and recorded when incurred, even though they have not been paid.

Financial Summaries

The financial records of any business should at all times show the following:

- How much was earned in a given period
- How much was collected
- How much is owed
- The distribution of expenses incurred

From the daily entries, the accountant can prepare monthly and annual summaries that provide a basis for comparing any given period with another similar period. Periodic analyses of the financial records can result in improved business practices, better management of time, curtailment or elimination of unprofitable services, and better budgeting of expenses. With the appropriate software these analyses can be accomplished using the computer. The medical assistant may notice notations of AP/AR, which stand for **accounts payable** and **accounts receivable.**

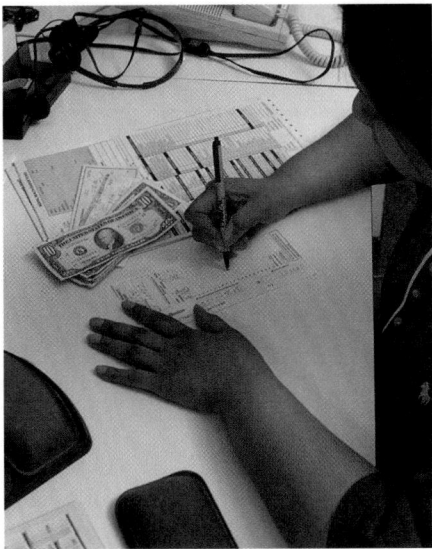

FIGURE 23-1 Accurate records reflect competency in the medical office. The medical assistant should use a calculator when adding figures and should be careful not to transpose numbers.

CRITICAL THINKING APPLICATION

- Brenda has noticed several errors on encounter forms lately. These errors seem to be a result of not using a calculator when adding the charges once the patient checks out. Brenda has approached the person who assists the patients in this area but has not seen any improvement in the errors. How might she convince the employee to follow precautions in adding charges?
- How might Mr. Schmidt educate the staff about the importance of accurate financial records?

The Cardinal Rules of Bookkeeping

There are many rules that apply to bookkeeping that the medical assistant must learn. First, use good penmanship so that the records are clearly legible, even years later. Use the same pen style and type of ink consistently. Keep columns of figures straight, and write well-formed figures (a careless 9 may look like a 7; an open 0 may resemble a 6). Carry decimal points correctly.

Enter all charges and receipts immediately in the daily record or journal. Write a receipt in duplicate for any currency received (Figure 23-1). Writing receipts for checks is optional, but a consistent pattern should be followed. Post all charges and receipts to the patient ledger daily. Checks should be endorsed for deposit as soon as received. Verify that the total of the deposit plus the amount on hand equals the total to be accounted for in the daily journal. The **petty cash fund** should be used to pay for small unpredictable expenses. Pay all other expenses by check. A cancelled check is the best proof of payment. Bills should be

paid before their due dates, after checking them for accuracy. Place date of payment and number of check on paid bills.

Do not erase, write over, or blot out figures. If an error is made, a straight line should be drawn through the incorrect figure, and the correct figure written above it. Bookkeeping procedures are not complicated, but they do require concentration to avoid errors. There is no such thing as almost correct financial records. The books either balance or they do not balance. The bookkeeping is either right or wrong. This is not the place to be creative or take shortcuts.

The medical assistant should set aside a certain time each day for bookkeeping tasks, if possible. Do not attempt to work on financial records when busy attending patients or when other distractions are present.

Kinds of Financial Records

Daily Journal

The daily journal day sheet is the chronologic record of the practice—the financial diary. All information regarding services rendered, charges, and receipts is first recorded in the daily journal. It is important that every transaction be recorded.

In addition to professional services rendered in and out of the office, there may be income from other sources, such as rentals, royalties, interest, and so forth. Usually a special place is provided in the journal for such income. Any income that is not practice related should be recorded separately from patient receipts.

Checkbook

Receipts are usually deposited in the checking account, and a record of the deposit is entered in the journal and on the check stub. A copy of each deposit slip should be kept with the financial records. Bills are usually paid by check or via online bill-paying services, and a record of the payment is entered on the check stub and in the disbursements section of the general journal.

CRITICAL THINKING APPLICATION

■ Brenda has noticed two checks missing from the business checkbook. Dr. Wilkins is out of town for a week and unable to be contacted. How might Brenda determine where the checks are or to whom they were written?

■ What steps can be taken to resolve the problem of not knowing the amount of a missing check?

Disbursements Journal

Manual Posting. In simplified accounting systems, the **disbursements journal** usually consists of a section at the bottom of each day sheet and a check register page at the end of each month, plus monthly and annual summaries. It must show the following:

- Every amount paid out
- Date and check number
- Purpose of payment

Computer Posting. Use the cash or check payments screen. Enter payment information and the computer can print the check, or enter information after the check has been manually prepared.

Petty Cash Records

A petty cash fund and voucher system should be established to take care of minor unpredictable expenditures such as postage due, parking fees, small contributions, emergency supplies, and miscellaneous small items. In the average facility $25 to $50 is sufficient for the petty cash fund. If a larger sum is available, there is a tendency to pay too many bills out of petty cash instead of writing a check.

When the check for this fund is exchanged at the bank for small bills and coins, the money is placed in a cashbox or drawer that can be locked or kept in the safe at night. One person only should be in charge of the petty cash fund. This person must be able to account for the full amount of the fund at any time.

CRITICAL THINKING APPLICATION

■ Brenda has noticed that on several occasions employees have borrowed money from the petty cash fund. Is this an acceptable practice? Why or why not?

■ How might Brenda keep an accounting of money taken from the petty cash drawer if she is not the person actually in control of it?

Payroll Records

The payroll record is an auxiliary disbursement record. A separate page or card for each employee, as well as a summary record, should be kept. This procedure is discussed in more detail later in this chapter.

COMPARISON OF COMMON BOOKKEEPING SYSTEMS

Success in bookkeeping requires a thorough understanding of the system and what it is expected to accomplish. Many variations in bookkeeping systems exist, from simple to complex, no one of which can meet the needs of every physician. The basic principles are the same for all; only the system of recording varies. The three most common systems found in the professional office are as follows:

- Single-entry
- Double-entry
- Pegboard or write-it-once

An overview of the three systems is presented here. More detailed instruction for the pegboard system, the most widely used manual system in medical practices, is found in Chapter 21.

Single-Entry System

Single-entry bookkeeping is inexpensive, is simple to use, and requires very little training. It is the oldest and simplest of bookkeeping systems and includes at least three basic records:

- A general journal, also called a daily log, daybook, day sheet, daily journal, or charge journal
- A cash payment journal, which in its simplest form is a checkbook
- An accounts receivable ledger, which is a record of the amounts owed by all the patients. The accounts receivable ledger may be a bound book, a loose-leaf binder, a card file, or loose pages in a ledger tray

There may also be auxiliary records for petty cash and payroll records.

The records of charges and receipts are usually entered into a bound journal with a page for each day of the year, monthly summary pages, and an annual summary. Daily pages have columns for entering each transaction that show the patient's name, the service performed and the charge, any payments received, and the totals for charges and receipts. The daily totals are entered on the monthly summary, and the monthly totals are carried forward to the annual summary.

The same bound book may also have space for recording cash payments, or the checkbook may be the only cash payment journal. Monthly and annual summaries would be done from the checkbook.

The accounts receivable ledger usually consists of an account card for each patient, on which are entered the charges and payments from the general journal. The patients' statements are prepared from these cards. In a single-entry system, each entry is made separately.

Although the single-entry system may satisfy the requirements for reporting to government agencies, it does have some drawbacks:

- Errors are not easily detected.
- There are no built-in controls.
- Periodic analyses are inadequate for financial planning.

The single-entry system was at one time widely used in healthcare facilities but has been largely replaced by more complete accounting systems.

Double-Entry System

Double-entry bookkeeping is also inexpensive but requires a trained and experienced bookkeeper or the regular services of an accountant. The transactions may be recorded manually or by computer. In addition to the basic journals used in a single-entry system, there may be numerous subsidiary journals. The system is based on the following accounting equation:

Assets = Liabilities + Proprietorship (Capital)

Every transaction requires an entry on each side of the accounting equation, and the two sides must always be **in balance.** For this reason the system is called *double-entry bookkeeping.* It is the most complete of the three systems. An understanding of the basics of double-entry bookkeeping will help to clarify the principles of all systems.

Assets are the properties owned by a business, such as bank accounts, accounts receivable, buildings, equipment, and furniture. The rights to these assets are called **equities.** The equity of the owner is called *capital, proprietorship,* or *owner's equity.* The equities of the creditors to whom money is owed are called **liabilities.** The owner's equity or capital is what remains of the value of the assets after the creditor's equities or liabilities have been subtracted.

For example, if the physician purchased equipment for $1000, paid $250 down, and gave a promissory note for $750, the accounting equation would be as follows:

Assets	$1000 =	Liabilities	$750
		+	
	_____	Capital	250
	$1000		$1000

The total value of the asset is $1000. The owner's equity is $250, and the creditor's equity is $750. The accounting terms *capital, proprietorship, owner's equity,* and *net worth* are used interchangeably.

Few medical assistants are trained in accounting. If a double-entry system is used, a practice management consultant or the accountant who does most of the actual bookwork and reports usually sets it up. The medical assistant in this instance generally maintains only the daily journal, from which the accountant takes the figures once a month.

The double-entry system provides a more comprehensive picture of the practice and its effect on the physician's net worth. Errors show up readily, and there are many built-in accuracy controls; however, because of the time and skill required, it is not frequently used in the small practice.

Pegboard or Write-It-Once System

The pegboard is the most commonly used manual method of accounting in the physician's office. It is discussed at length in Chapter 21.

CRITICAL THINKING APPLICATION

Mr. Schmidt has taught Brenda all three types of accounting systems. Which seems to be the easiest system to use in the medical office? What is the basis for this choice?

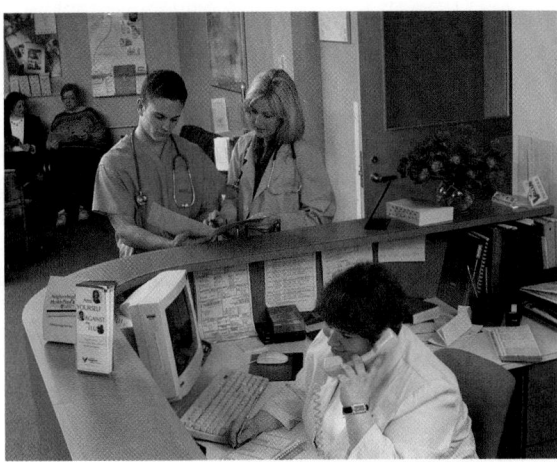

FIGURE 23-2 Ask the physician when unsure about financial information. When an unfamiliar statement arrives, check with the physician to be sure it should be paid.

END-OF-DAY SUMMARIZING

Most computer accounting systems will perform end-of-the-day summarizing automatically. If the office uses the pegboard system, the bottom of the day sheet has three sections to be completed that will show that the accounts have balanced for the day.

The first section is the proof of posting section, which deals with the transactions that occurred that day on the day sheet. The second section is month-to-date accounts receivable proof, and the day's totals being added to the month-to-date totals should balance to the penny. The last section is the year-to-date accounts receivable proof, which adds the accounts, including the day's totals, to the year-to-date total.

Most systems also have a deposit ticket, which can be double-checked when adding the cash receipts and the checks. This is handy when preparing the day's deposit.

The totals at the bottom of the second and third sections must be identical. When the end-of-the-day summarizing does not balance, the medical assistant should first check the addition of each column, both horizontally and vertically. This will result in finding most errors (Figure 23-2). Be sure that the instructions are followed to the letter. To avoid frustrating mistakes, it is best to use a calculator, even when adding small numbers.

TRIAL BALANCE OF ACCOUNTS RECEIVABLE

A **trial balance** should be done once per month after all posting has been completed and before preparing the monthly statements. The purpose of a trial balance is to disclose any discrepancies between the journal and the ledger. It does not prove the accuracy of the accounts. For example, if a charge or payment was posted to the wrong account, or if the wrong amount was entered in the journal then posted to the ledger, the totals would still "balance," but the accounts would not be accurate.

To begin, pull all the account cards that have a balance, enter each balance on the calculator, and total the figures. This should equal the accounts receivable balance figure on the control.

If there is no daily control, total all of the charges, all of the payments, and all of the adjustments for the month, then do the computation illustrated as follows. The end-of-the-month accounts receivable figure must agree with the figure arrived at by adding all the account card balances. The accounts are then said to be *in balance*. If the two totals do not agree, the error must be located.

Example of Balancing End-of-Month Accounts Receivable

Accounts receivable at first of month	$ _____
Plus total charges for month	$ _____
Subtotal	$ _____
Less total payments for month	$ _____
Subtotal	$ _____
Less total adjustments for month	$ _____
Accounts receivable at end of month	$ _____

Locating and Preventing Errors

After checking the tape and verifying that no error in calculation has been made, the first step in locating an error in the trial balance is to find the difference between the two totals. Then search the daily journal pages and the account cards for an entry for the identical amount. Check each one found, and verify that it was posted correctly. Of course, more than one error may add up to this amount.

If only one error has been made and the amount of the error is divisible by 9, a figure may have been transposed. For example, if the difference is $81 (a number divisible by 9), the person who posted to the account may have written $209 instead of $290. If the amount of the error is divisible by 2, the amount may have been posted to the wrong column, reversing a debit and a credit.

A common error is made by entering the wrong amount in the previous balance column or in figuring the new balance. This kind of error will show up on the pegboard daily proof but could easily go undetected in the single-entry system. Carrying forward the wrong amount results in another common error total from one day to the next (e.g., carrying forward the beginning accounts receivable total rather than the ending accounts receivable total). There is always a chance of sliding a number, which means writing the first digit in the wrong column, such as writing 400 for 40 or 60 instead of 600.

Many bookkeepers avoid errors in the cents column by using a line (–) instead of writing two zeros when only even dollars are involved. For example, instead of writing $12.00, the bookkeeper will write $12.–. This eliminates the possibility of misreading zeros as other numbers. It also speeds the adding process when columns must be totaled.

If the medical assistant is unable to locate any numeric error, then an account card may have been lost or overlooked or transferred as paid in full.

CRITICAL THINKING APPLICATION

- What should Brenda do if she has repeatedly reviewed records in search of an error and is still unable to find it?
- To whom should this be reported?

ACCOUNTS PAYABLE PROCEDURES

Invoices and Statements

When an item is not paid for at the time of purchase, the vendor usually includes a **packing slip** with delivery of the merchandise. A packing slip describes the items enclosed. The vendor may also enclose an **invoice.** An invoice describes the items and shows the amount due. Always check to verify that the items listed on the packing slip and invoice are included in the delivery.

Invoices should be placed in a special folder until paid. The facility may be making more than one purchase from the same vendor during the month. Some vendors request that payment be made from the invoice; others expect to send a **statement** later. A statement is a request for payment.

Paying for Purchases

At the time of payment, compare the statement with the invoice to verify accuracy, fasten the statement and invoice together, write the date and check number on the statement, and place it in the paid file.

CRITICAL THINKING APPLICATION

- Brenda does not recall ordering a certain item from the office supply company. However, it was included in her last shipment and listed on the packing list. How can she recount whether the item was ordered?
- How would Brenda correct this problem if the item was in fact not ordered?

Recording Disbursements

Both the pegboard and the single-entry bookkeeping systems provide pages for recording disbursements. This is sometimes called a *check register.* On these pages disbursements are distributed to specific expense accounts such as the following:

- Auto expense
- Dues and meetings
- Equipment
- Insurance
- Medical supplies
- Office expenses
- Printing, postage, and stationery
- Rent and maintenance
- Salaries
- Taxes and licenses
- Travel and entertainment
- Utilities
- Miscellaneous
- Personal withdrawals

Each check should be entered on the disbursement page, showing the date, the name of the company to which the check was written, the number and amount of the check, and the payment allocated to one or more of the expense accounts. It is important to separate personal expenditures from business expenses. Business expenses are tax deductible and are

---

PROCEDURE 23-1

Account for Petty Cash

ABHES COMPETENCIES: 3.m, 3.n

GOAL: *To establish a petty cash fund, maintain an accurate record of expenditures for 1 month, and replenish the fund as necessary.*

EQUIPMENT and SUPPLIES

- Form for petty cash fund
- Pad of vouchers
- Disbursement journal
- Two checks
- List of petty cash expenditures

PROCEDURAL STEPS

1. Determine the amount needed in the petty cash fund.
2. Write a check in the determined amount.
   PURPOSE: To establish a fund.
3. Record the beginning balance in the petty cash fund.
4. Post the amount to Miscellaneous on the disbursement record.
   PURPOSE: To account for the original amount in the fund.
5. Prepare a petty cash voucher for each amount withdrawn from the fund.
   PURPOSE: The vouchers will be used for internal audit.
6. Record each voucher in the petty cash record, and enter the new balance.
   PURPOSE: To record current balance and determine the need for replenishing the fund.
7. Write a check to replenish the fund as necessary.
   NOTE: The total of the vouchers plus the fund balance must equal the beginning amount.
8. Total the expense columns, and post to the appropriate accounts in the disbursement record.
   PURPOSE: To record expenditures in the correct expense category.
9. Record the amount added to the fund.
10. Record the new balance in the petty cash fund.

---

considered in determining net income from the practice, but personal expenditures are not. Although personal expenses are not deductible in determining net income from the practice, some qualify as personal deductions in computing personal income tax, so a careful accounting should be kept. Deductible expenses would include property taxes, interest paid out, contributions, and so on.

Accounting for Petty Cash

The petty cash fund is a revolving fund (Procedure 23-1). It does not change in amount except to increase or decrease the established fund. To establish the petty cash fund, a check is written payable to Cash or Petty Cash and entered in the disbursements journal under Miscellaneous. This is the only time that the petty cash check is charged to Miscellaneous.

Each time the fund is replenished, the amount of the check is spread among the various accounts for which the money was used. This is determined from a record of expenditures. The headings of the columns should correspond to headings in the disbursements journal to which they will be posted.

A pad of petty cash vouchers is kept in or near the cash box. For every disbursement from the fund, the petty cashier should either have a receipt or prepare a voucher. The total of the petty cash vouchers and receipts plus the amount of cash in the box must always equal the original amount of the fund.

At the end of the month, or sooner if the fund is depleted, a check is written to Cash for replenishing the fund, but instead of being charged to Miscellaneous as previously, the amount of the check is divided among the various accounts affected.

Avoid the habit of borrowing from the petty cash fund. This admonition applies to the physician as well as to the medical assistant. If the physician requests cash from the fund, request a personal check or an office check in exchange for cash from the fund. It is also poor policy to use the petty cash fund for making change. In facilities where patients frequently pay with currency, a separate change fund should be kept.

PERIODIC SUMMARIES

Financial summaries are compiled on monthly and annual bases. They may be prepared either by the medical assistant manually or on the computer or by the accountant. Common summary reports include the following:

- **Statement of income and expense**
- **Cash flow statement**
- Trial balance
- **Accounts receivable trial balance** and aging analysis
- **Balance sheet**

The statement of income and expense is also known as the *profit and loss statement* and covers a specific period. It lists all the income received and all expenses paid during the period. The total income is called *gross income* or *earnings*. The income after deduction of all expenses is the *net income*.

A cash flow statement starts with the amount of cash on hand at the beginning of the month (or for any specified period). It then lists the cash income and the cash disbursement made throughout the period and concludes with a statement of the amount of cash remaining on hand at the end of the period.

A trial balance is necessary to determine that the books are in balance. All of the columns on the disbursements journal must be totaled at the end of the month. The combined totals of all the expense columns must be equal to the total of the checks written. If the figures do not balance, it is necessary to recheck every entry until an error is found.

The accounts receivable trial balance is done before the monthly statements are sent out. First, record the total of the accounts receivable ledger at the end of the previous month; then add the charges for the current month and subtract the adjustments and the payments received. The remainder should equal the total of the accounts receivable ledger at the end of the current month.

The balance sheet, also known as a *statement of financial condition*, shows the financial picture of the practice on a specific date. Often, it is done only on an annual basis. The balance sheet is set up using the following accounting equation:

$$\text{Assets} = \text{Liabilities} + \text{Proprietorship}$$

The title of the statement had its origin in the equality of the elements—the balance between the sum of the assets and the sum of the liabilities and proprietorship.

At the end of the accounting year, it is very simple to combine the monthly reports to compile the annual summaries. The annual summaries simplify the reporting of income for tax returns.

PAYROLL RECORDS

Handling payroll records, whether for one employee or dozens of employees, involves frequent reporting activities (Procedure 23-2). Government regulations require the withholding of taxes from employees and payment of certain taxes due from both employees and employers. To comply with government regulations, complete records must be kept for every employee. All records of employment taxes must be kept for at least 4 years. These should be available for review by the Internal Revenue Service (IRS). Such records include the following:

- Social Security number of the employee
- Number of withholding allowances claimed
- Amount of gross salary
- All deductions for Social Security and Medicare taxes; federal, state, and city or other subdivision withholding taxes; state disability insurance; and state unemployment tax, where applicable

CRITICAL THINKING APPLICATION

- On Friday Brenda hired a new employee, who reported to work on Monday. The new employee states that she cannot produce her Social Security card. Can Brenda allow the individual to work?
- Investigate the procedures for verifying a Social Security number.

PROCEDURE 23-2

Process an Employee Payroll

ABHES COMPETENCY: 8.f

GOAL: *To process payroll and compensate employees, making deductions accurately.*

EQUIPMENT and SUPPLIES

- Checkbook
- Computer and payroll software, if applicable
- Pen
- Tax withholding tables
- Federal Employers Tax Guide

PROCEDURAL STEPS

1. Be sure that all information and paperwork have been collected from the employees, including a copy of the Social Security card, a W-4 form, and an I-9 form.
   PURPOSE: To make certain that the employee is eligible to work in the United States and to determine what withholding amounts should be deducted from paychecks.
2. Review the time cards for all employees. Determine if any employees need counseling because of late arrivals or habitual absences.
   PURPOSE: To address problem issues immediately and help to correct habits that can lead to employee termination.

3. Figure the salary or hourly wages that are due the employee for the period worked.
   PURPOSE: To ascertain the amount owed to the employee.
4. Figure the deductions that must be taken from the paycheck. These usually include but are not limited to the following:
   - Federal, state, and local taxes
   - Social Security withholdings
   - Medicare withholdings
   - Other deductions, such as insurance, savings, and so on
   - Donations to organizations, such as the United Way.
   PURPOSE: To comply with federal, state, and local laws and deduct amounts for insurance, savings plans, and so on.
5. Write the check for the balance due the employee. Most software can print the checks and explanations of deductions.
6. Have employees sign for their paychecks, if that is the policy of the office.

Payroll Reporting Forms

Each employee and each employer must have a tax identification number. The Social Security number is the employee's tax identification number. Any person who does not have a Social Security number should apply for one, using Form SS-5, available from any Social Security Administration office.

The employer applies for a number for federal tax accounting purposes using Form SS-4, available at Social Security Administration offices. In states that require employer reports, a state employer number must also be obtained.

Before the end of the first pay period, the employee should complete an Employee's Withholding Allowance Certificate (Form W-4) showing the number of withholding allowances claimed (Figure 23-3). Otherwise, the employer must indicate withholding on the basis of a single person with no exemptions.

The employee should complete a new form when changes occur in marital status or in the number of allowances claimed. Each employee is entitled to one personal allowance and one for each qualified dependent. The employee may elect to take fewer or no allowances, in which case the tax withheld will be greater and a refund may be due when the employee's annual tax report is filed (Figure 23-4). If an employee claims more than 10 withholding allowances or an exemption from withholding and his or her wages would normally be more than $200 per week, the employer is required to send copies of these W-4 forms to the IRS.

A supply of all the necessary forms for filing federal returns, preprinted with the employer's name, will be furnished to an employer who has applied for an employer identification number. Extra forms may be obtained from the IRS office.

CRITICAL THINKING APPLICATION

- Mr. Schmidt has explained to Brenda that the more withholding deductions an employee claims, the less tax is taken from the paycheck. If Brenda's new employee wishes to claim seven deductions and she has only three children and is single, could she do so legally?
- Why or why not?
- Why might it be risky to claim all of the deductions to which a person is legally entitled?

Income Tax Withholding

Employers are required by law to withhold certain amounts from employees' earnings. These amounts must be reported and forwarded to the IRS to be applied toward payment of income tax. The amount to be withheld is based on the following:

- Total earnings of the employee
- Number of withholding allowances claimed
- Marital status of the employee
- Length of the pay period involved

The Federal Employer's Tax Guide includes tables to be used in determining the amount to be withheld. There is one table for single persons and unmarried heads of households and one for married persons. The tables cover monthly, semimonthly, biweekly, weekly, and daily or miscellaneous periods.

Employers Income Tax

The physician who is practicing as an individual is not subject to withholding tax but is expected to make an estimated tax payment four times a year. The accountant prepares four copies of Form 1040-S, Declaration of Estimated Tax for Individuals, for the ensuing year when the annual income tax return is prepared. The first form and the quarterly estimated tax for the next year are filed at the same time as the tax return. The remaining three forms, with the estimated tax due, must be filed on June 15, September 15, and January 15. It may be the business manager's responsibility to see that these returns are filed when due. The employer also contributes to Social Security and Medicare in the form of a self-employment tax.

Social Security, Medicare, and Income Tax Withholding

The Federal Insurance Contributions Act (FICA) provides for a federal system of old age, survivors, disability, and hospital insurance. The tax rate is reviewed frequently and is subject to change by Congress. As of 2001, the wage base for Social Security tax is $84,900 and the tax rate is 6.2% each for employers and employees. All wages are subject to the Medicare tax at a rate of 1.45% each for both employees and employers.

Quarterly Returns

Each quarter of the year, all employers who are subject to income tax withholding (including withholding on sick pay and supplemental unemployment benefits) of Social Security and Medicare taxes must file an Employer's Quarterly Federal Tax Return on or before the last day of the first month after the end of the quarter (Figure 23-5). Due dates for this return and full payment of the tax are April 30, July 31, October 31, and January 31. If deposits equaling full payment of taxes due have been made, the due date for the return is extended 10 days.

Annual Returns

The employer is required to furnish two copies of Form W-2, the Wage and Tax Statement, to each employee from whom income tax or Social Security tax has been withheld or from whom income tax would have been withheld if the employee had claimed no more than one withholding allowance. The forms should be given to employees by January 31. If employment ends before December 31, the employer may give the W-2 form to the terminated employee any time after employment ends. If the employee asks for Form W-2, the employer should give the employee the completed copies within 30 days of the request or the final wage payment, whichever is later.

Employers must file Form W-3, the Transmittal of Income and Tax Statement, annually to transmit wage and income tax withheld statements (Form W-2) to the Social Security Administration. These forms are processed by the Social Security Administration, which then furnishes the IRS with the income tax data that it needs from those forms. Form W-3 and its attachments must be filed separately from Form 941 on or before the last day of February after the calendar year for which the W-2 forms are prepared.

Form W-4 (2002)

Purpose. Complete Form W-4 so your employer can withhold the correct Federal income tax from your pay. Because your tax situation may change, you may want to refigure your withholding each year.

Exemption from withholding. If you are exempt, complete only lines 1, 2, 3, 4, and 7 and sign the form to validate it. Your exemption for 2002 expires February 16, 2003. See **Pub. 505**, Tax Withholding and Estimated Tax.

Note: *You cannot claim exemption from withholding if* **(a)** *your income exceeds $750 and includes more than $250 of unearned income (e.g., interest and dividends) and* **(b)** *another person can claim you as a dependent on their tax return.*

Basic instructions. If you are not exempt, complete the **Personal Allowances Worksheet** below. The worksheets on page 2 adjust your withholding allowances based on itemized deductions, certain credits, adjustments to

income, or two-earner/two-job situations. Complete all worksheets that apply. **However, you may claim fewer (or zero) allowances.**

Head of household. Generally, you may claim head of household filing status on your tax return only if you are unmarried and pay more than 50% of the costs of keeping up a home for yourself and your dependent(s) or other qualifying individuals. See line **E** below.

Tax credits. You can take projected tax credits into account in figuring your allowable number of withholding allowances. Credits for child or dependent care expenses and the child tax credit may be claimed using the **Personal Allowances Worksheet** below. See **Pub. 919**, How Do I Adjust My Tax Withholding? for information on converting your other credits into withholding allowances.

Nonwage income. If you have a large amount of nonwage income, such as interest or dividends, consider making estimated tax payments using **Form 1040-ES**, Estimated Tax for Individuals. Otherwise, you may owe additional tax.

Two earners/two jobs. If you have a working spouse or more than one job, figure the total number of allowances you are entitled to claim on all jobs using worksheets from only one Form W-4. Your withholding usually will be most accurate when all allowances are claimed on the Form W-4 for the highest paying job and zero allowances are claimed on the others.

Nonresident alien. If you are a nonresident alien, see the **Instructions for Form 8233** before completing this Form W-4.

Check your withholding. After your Form W-4 takes effect, use Pub. 919 to see how the dollar amount you are having withheld compares to your projected total tax for 2002. See Pub. 919, especially if you used the **Two-Earner/Two-Job Worksheet** on page 2 and your earnings exceed $125,000 (Single) or $175,000 (Married).

Recent name change? If your name on line 1 differs from that shown on your social security card, call 1-800-772-1213 for a new social security card.

Personal Allowances Worksheet (Keep for your records.)

A Enter "1" for **yourself** if no one else can claim you as a dependent . . . . **A** _____

B Enter "1" if: {
- You are single and have only one job; or
- You are married, have only one job, and your spouse does not work; or
- Your wages from a second job or your spouse's wages (or the total of both) are $1,000 or less.
} . . **B** _____

C Enter "1" for your **spouse.** But, you may choose to enter "-0-" if you are married and have either a working spouse or more than one job. (Entering "-0-" may help you avoid having too little tax withheld.) . . . . **C** _____

D Enter number of **dependents** (other than your spouse or yourself) you will claim on your tax return . . . . **D** _____

E Enter "1" if you will file as **head of household** on your tax return (see conditions under **Head of household** above) . **E** _____

F Enter "1" if you have at least $1,500 of **child or dependent care expenses** for which you plan to claim a credit . . **F** _____

(**Note:** Do **not** include child support payments. See **Pub. 503,** Child and Dependent Care Expenses, for details.)

G **Child Tax Credit** (including additional child tax credit):
- If your total income will be between $15,000 and $42,000 ($20,000 and $65,000 if married), enter "1" for each eligible child plus **1 additional** if you have three to five eligible children or **2 additional** if you have six or more eligible children.
- If your total income will be between $42,000 and $80,000 ($65,000 and $115,000 if married), enter "1" if you have one or two eligible children, "2" if you have three eligible children, "3" if you have four eligible children, or "4" if you have five or more eligible children. . **G** _____

H Add lines A through G and enter total here. **Note:** *This may be different from the number of exemptions you claim on your tax return.* ▶ **H** _____

For accuracy, complete all worksheets that apply.
- If you plan to **itemize or claim adjustments to income** and want to reduce your withholding, see the **Deductions and Adjustments Worksheet** on page 2.
- If you have **more than one job** or are **married and you and your spouse both work** and the combined earnings from all jobs exceed $35,000, see the **Two-Earner/Two-Job Worksheet** on page 2 to avoid having too little tax withheld.
- If **neither** of the above situations applies, **stop here** and enter the number from line H on line 5 of Form W-4 below.

- - - - - - - - - - - - - - - **Cut here and give Form W-4 to your employer. Keep the top part for your records.** - - - - - - - - - - - - - - -

Form **W-4**
Department of the Treasury
Internal Revenue Service

Employee's Withholding Allowance Certificate

▶ **For Privacy Act and Paperwork Reduction Act Notice, see page 2.**

OMB No. 1545-0010

2002

1 Type or print your first name and middle initial	Last name		2 Your social security number

Home address (number and street or rural route)	3 ☐ Single ☐ Married ☐ Married, but withhold at higher Single rate.
City or town, state, and ZIP code	**Note:** *If married, but legally separated, or spouse is a nonresident alien, check the "Single" box.*
	4 If your last name differs from that on your social security card, check here. You must call 1-800-772-1213 for a new card. ▶ ☐

5 Total number of allowances you are claiming (from line **H** above **or** from the applicable worksheet on page 2) | **5** _____

6 Additional amount, if any, you want withheld from each paycheck . . . . | **6** $ _____

7 I claim exemption from withholding for 2002, and I certify that I meet **both** of the following conditions for exemption:
- Last year I had a right to a refund of **all** Federal income tax withheld because I had **no** tax liability **and**
- This year I expect a refund of **all** Federal income tax withheld because I expect to have **no** tax liability.

If you meet both conditions, write "Exempt" here . . . . ▶ | **7** _____

Under penalties of perjury, I certify that I am entitled to the number of withholding allowances claimed on this certificate, or I am entitled to claim exempt status.

Employee's signature
(Form is not valid unless you sign it.) ▶ _____ Date ▶ _____

8 Employer's name and address (Employer: Complete lines 8 and 10 only if sending to the IRS.)	9 Office code (optional)	10 Employer identification number

Cat. No. 10220Q

FIGURE 23-3 IRS Form W-4: Employee's Withholding Allowance Certificate.

Form W-4 (2002)   Page **2**

Deductions and Adjustments Worksheet

Note: *Use this worksheet only if you plan to itemize deductions, claim certain credits, or claim adjustments to income on your 2002 tax return.*

1   Enter an estimate of your 2002 itemized deductions. These include qualifying home mortgage interest, charitable contributions, state and local taxes, medical expenses in excess of 7.5% of your income, and miscellaneous deductions. (For 2002, you may have to reduce your itemized deductions if your income is over $137,300 ($68,650 if married filing separately). See **Worksheet 3** in Pub. 919 for details.) . . .   **1** $ _____

2   Enter: { $7,850 if married filing jointly or qualifying widow(er)
$6,900 if head of household
$4,700 if single
$3,925 if married filing separately } . . . .   **2** $ _____

3   **Subtract** line 2 from line 1. If line 2 is greater than line 1, enter "-0-" . . . .   **3** $ _____

4   Enter an estimate of your 2002 adjustments to income, including alimony, deductible IRA contributions, and student loan interest   **4** $ _____

5   **Add** lines 3 and 4 and enter the total. Include any amount for credits from **Worksheet 7** in Pub. 919.   **5** $ _____

6   Enter an estimate of your 2002 nonwage income (such as dividends or interest) . . . .   **6** $ _____

7   **Subtract** line 6 from line 5. Enter the result, but not less than "-0-" . . . . . .   **7** $ _____

8   **Divide** the amount on line 7 by $3,000 and enter the result here. Drop any fraction . . . .   **8**   _____

9   Enter the number from the **Personal Allowances Worksheet,** line H, page 1 . . . .   **9**   _____

10   **Add** lines 8 and 9 and enter the total here. If you plan to use the **Two-Earner/Two-Job Worksheet,** also enter this total on line 1 below. Otherwise, **stop here** and enter this total on Form W-4, line 5, page 1 .   **10**   _____

Two-Earner/Two-Job Worksheet

Note: *Use this worksheet only if the instructions under line H on page 1 direct you here.*

1   Enter the number from line H, page 1 (or from line 10 above if you used the **Deductions and Adjustments Worksheet**)   **1**   _____

2   Find the number in **Table 1** below that applies to the **lowest** paying job and enter it here . . . . .   **2**   _____

3   If line 1 is **more than or equal to** line 2, subtract line 2 from line 1. Enter the result here (if zero, enter "-0-") and on Form W-4, line 5, page 1. **Do not** use the rest of this worksheet . . . .   **3**   _____

Note: *If line 1 is **less than** line 2, enter "-0-" on Form W-4, line 5, page 1. Complete lines 4-9 below to calculate the additional withholding amount necessary to avoid a year end tax bill.*

4   Enter the number from line 2 of this worksheet . . . .   **4**   _____

5   Enter the number from line 1 of this worksheet . . . .   **5**   _____

6   **Subtract** line 5 from line 4 . . . .   **6**   _____

7   Find the amount in **Table 2** below that applies to the **highest** paying job and enter it here . . . . .   **7** $ _____

8   **Multiply** line 7 by line 6 and enter the result here. This is the additional annual withholding needed . .   **8** $ _____

9   Divide line 8 by the number of pay periods remaining in 2002. For example, divide by 26 if you are paid every two weeks and you complete this form in December 2001. Enter the result here and on Form W-4, line 6, page 1. This is the additional amount to be withheld from each paycheck . . . .   **9** $ _____

Table 1: Two-Earner/Two-Job Worksheet

Married Filing Jointly				All Others			
If wages from **LOWEST** paying job are—	Enter on line 2 above	If wages from **LOWEST** paying job are—	Enter on line 2 above	If wages from **LOWEST** paying job are—	Enter on line 2 above	If wages from **LOWEST** paying job are—	Enter on line 2 above
$0 - $4,000	0	44,001 - 50,000	8	$0 - $6,000	0	75,001 - 95,000	8
4,001 - 9,000	1	50,001 - 55,000	9	6,001 - 11,000	1	95,001 - 110,000	9
9,001 - 15,000	2	55,001 - 65,000	10	11,001 - 17,000	2	110,001 and over	10
15,001 - 20,000	3	65,001 - 80,000	11	17,001 - 23,000	3		
20,001 - 25,000	4	80,001 - 95,000	12	23,001 - 28,000	4		
25,001 - 32,000	5	95,001 - 110,000	13	28,001 - 38,000	5		
32,001 - 38,000	6	110,001 - 125,000	14	38,001 - 55,000	6		
38,001 - 44,000	7	125,001 and over	15	55,001 - 75,000	7		

Table 2: Two-Earner/Two-Job Worksheet

Married Filing Jointly		All Others	
If wages from **HIGHEST** paying job are—	Enter on line 7 above	If wages from **HIGHEST** paying job are—	Enter on line 7 above
$0 - $50,000	$450	$0 - $30,000	$450
50,001 - 100,000	800	30,001 - 70,000	800
100,001 - 150,000	900	70,001 - 140,000	900
150,001 - 270,000	1,050	140,001 - 300,000	1,050
270,001 and over	1,150	300,001 and over	1,150

Privacy Act and Paperwork Reduction Act Notice. We ask for the information on this form to carry out the Internal Revenue laws of the United States. The Internal Revenue Code requires this information under sections 3402(f)(2)(A) and 6109 and their regulations. **Failure to provide a properly completed form will result in your being treated as a single person who claims no withholding allowances; providing fraudulent information may also subject you to penalties.** Routine uses of this information include giving it to the Department of Justice for civil and criminal litigation, to cities, states, and the District of Columbia for use in administering their tax laws, and using it in the National Directory of New Hires.

You are not required to provide the information requested on a form that is subject to the Paperwork Reduction Act unless the form displays a valid OMB control number. Books or records relating to a form or its instructions must be retained as long as their contents may become material in the administration of any Internal Revenue law. Generally, tax returns and return information are confidential, as required by Code section 6103.

The time needed to complete this form will vary depending on individual circumstances. The estimated average time is: **Recordkeeping,** 46 min.; **Learning about the law or the form,** 13 min.; **Preparing the form,** 59 min. If you have comments concerning the accuracy of these time estimates or suggestions for making this form simpler, we would be happy to hear from you. You can write to the Tax Forms Committee, Western Area Distribution Center, Rancho Cordova, CA 95743-0001. **Do not** send the tax form to this address. Instead, give it to your employer.

FIGURE 23-3, cont'd For legend see previous page.

SINGLE Persons—WEEKLY Payroll Period

(For Wages Paid in 2002)

If the wages are—		And the number of withholding allowances claimed is—										
At least	But less than	0	1	2	3	4	5	6	7	8	9	10
		The amount of income tax to be withheld is—										
$0	$55	$0	$0	$0	$0	$0	$0	$0	$0	$0	$0	$0
55	60	1	0	0	0	0	0	0	0	0	0	0
60	65	1	0	0	0	0	0	0	0	0	0	0
65	70	2	0	0	0	0	0	0	0	0	0	0
70	75	2	0	0	0	0	0	0	0	0	0	0
75	80	3	0	0	0	0	0	0	0	0	0	0
80	85	3	0	0	0	0	0	0	0	0	0	0
85	90	4	0	0	0	0	0	0	0	0	0	0
90	95	4	0	0	0	0	0	0	0	0	0	0
95	100	5	0	0	0	0	0	0	0	0	0	0
100	105	5	0	0	0	0	0	0	0	0	0	0
105	110	6	0	0	0	0	0	0	0	0	0	0
110	115	6	0	0	0	0	0	0	0	0	0	0
115	120	7	1	0	0	0	0	0	0	0	0	0
120	125	7	1	0	0	0	0	0	0	0	0	0
125	130	8	2	0	0	0	0	0	0	0	0	0
130	135	8	2	0	0	0	0	0	0	0	0	0
135	140	9	3	0	0	0	0	0	0	0	0	0
140	145	9	3	0	0	0	0	0	0	0	0	0
145	150	10	4	0	0	0	0	0	0	0	0	0
150	155	10	4	0	0	0	0	0	0	0	0	0
155	160	11	5	0	0	0	0	0	0	0	0	0
160	165	11	5	0	0	0	0	0	0	0	0	0
165	170	12	6	0	0	0	0	0	0	0	0	0
170	175	13	6	1	0	0	0	0	0	0	0	0
175	180	13	7	1	0	0	0	0	0	0	0	0
180	185	14	7	2	0	0	0	0	0	0	0	0
185	190	15	8	2	0	0	0	0	0	0	0	0
190	195	16	8	3	0	0	0	0	0	0	0	0
195	200	16	9	3	0	0	0	0	0	0	0	0
200	210	17	10	4	0	0	0	0	0	0	0	0
210	220	19	11	5	0	0	0	0	0	0	0	0
220	230	20	12	6	0	0	0	0	0	0	0	0
230	240	22	13	7	1	0	0	0	0	0	0	0
240	250	23	15	8	2	0	0	0	0	0	0	0
250	260	25	16	9	3	0	0	0	0	0	0	0
260	270	26	18	10	4	0	0	0	0	0	0	0
270	280	28	19	11	5	0	0	0	0	0	0	0
280	290	29	21	12	6	0	0	0	0	0	0	0
290	300	31	22	14	7	1	0	0	0	0	0	0
300	310	32	24	15	8	2	0	0	0	0	0	0
310	320	34	25	17	9	3	0	0	0	0	0	0
320	330	35	27	18	10	4	0	0	0	0	0	0
330	340	37	28	20	11	5	0	0	0	0	0	0
340	350	38	30	21	12	6	1	0	0	0	0	0
350	360	40	31	23	14	7	2	0	0	0	0	0
360	370	41	33	24	15	8	3	0	0	0	0	0
370	380	43	34	26	17	9	4	0	0	0	0	0
380	390	44	36	27	18	10	5	0	0	0	0	0
390	400	46	37	29	20	11	6	0	0	0	0	0
400	410	47	39	30	21	13	7	1	0	0	0	0
410	420	49	40	32	23	14	8	2	0	0	0	0
420	430	50	42	33	24	16	9	3	0	0	0	0
430	440	52	43	35	26	17	10	4	0	0	0	0
440	450	53	45	36	27	19	11	5	0	0	0	0
450	460	55	46	38	29	20	12	6	0	0	0	0
460	470	56	48	39	30	22	13	7	1	0	0	0
470	480	58	49	41	32	23	15	8	2	0	0	0
480	490	59	51	42	33	25	16	9	3	0	0	0
490	500	61	52	44	35	26	18	10	4	0	0	0
500	510	62	54	45	36	28	19	11	5	0	0	0
510	520	64	55	47	38	29	21	12	6	0	0	0
520	530	65	57	48	39	31	22	14	7	1	0	0
530	540	67	58	50	41	32	24	15	8	2	0	0
540	550	68	60	51	42	34	25	17	9	3	0	0
550	560	70	61	53	44	35	27	18	10	4	0	0
560	570	71	63	54	45	37	28	20	11	5	0	0
570	580	74	64	56	47	38	30	21	12	6	0	0
580	590	76	66	57	48	40	31	23	14	7	1	0
590	600	79	67	59	50	41	33	24	15	8	2	0

FIGURE 23-4 Pages from the 2002 Withholding Tax Table.

MARRIED Persons—MONTHLY Payroll Period
(For Wages Paid in 2002)

At least	But less than	0	1	2	3	4	5	6	7	8	9	10
$0	$540	$0	$0	$0	$0	$0	$0	$0	$0	$0	$0	$0
540	560	1	0	0	0	0	0	0	0	0	0	0
560	580	3	0	0	0	0	0	0	0	0	0	0
580	600	5	0	0	0	0	0	0	0	0	0	0
600	640	8	0	0	0	0	0	0	0	0	0	0
640	680	12	0	0	0	0	0	0	0	0	0	0
680	720	16	0	0	0	0	0	0	0	0	0	0
720	760	20	0	0	0	0	0	0	0	0	0	0
760	800	24	0	0	0	0	0	0	0	0	0	0
800	840	28	3	0	0	0	0	0	0	0	0	0
840	880	32	7	0	0	0	0	0	0	0	0	0
880	920	36	11	0	0	0	0	0	0	0	0	0
920	960	40	15	0	0	0	0	0	0	0	0	0
960	1,000	44	19	0	0	0	0	0	0	0	0	0
1,000	1,040	48	23	0	0	0	0	0	0	0	0	0
1,040	1,080	52	27	2	0	0	0	0	0	0	0	0
1,080	1,120	56	31	6	0	0	0	0	0	0	0	0
1,120	1,160	60	35	10	0	0	0	0	0	0	0	0
1,160	1,200	64	39	14	0	0	0	0	0	0	0	0
1,200	1,240	68	43	18	0	0	0	0	0	0	0	0
1,240	1,280	72	47	22	0	0	0	0	0	0	0	0
1,280	1,320	76	51	26	1	0	0	0	0	0	0	0
1,320	1,360	80	55	30	5	0	0	0	0	0	0	0
1,360	1,400	84	59	34	9	0	0	0	0	0	0	0
1,400	1,440	88	63	38	13	0	0	0	0	0	0	0
1,440	1,480	92	67	42	17	0	0	0	0	0	0	0
1,480	1,520	96	71	46	21	0	0	0	0	0	0	0
1,520	1,560	100	75	50	25	0	0	0	0	0	0	0
1,560	1,600	106	79	54	29	4	0	0	0	0	0	0
1,600	1,640	112	83	58	33	8	0	0	0	0	0	0
1,640	1,680	118	87	62	37	12	0	0	0	0	0	0
1,680	1,720	124	91	66	41	16	0	0	0	0	0	0
1,720	1,760	130	95	70	45	20	0	0	0	0	0	0
1,760	1,800	136	99	74	49	24	0	0	0	0	0	0
1,800	1,840	142	105	78	53	28	3	0	0	0	0	0
1,840	1,880	148	111	82	57	32	7	0	0	0	0	0
1,880	1,920	154	117	86	61	36	11	0	0	0	0	0
1,920	1,960	160	123	90	65	40	15	0	0	0	0	0
1,960	2,000	166	129	94	69	44	19	0	0	0	0	0
2,000	2,040	172	135	98	73	48	23	0	0	0	0	0
2,040	2,080	178	141	103	77	52	27	2	0	0	0	0
2,080	2,120	184	147	109	81	56	31	6	0	0	0	0
2,120	2,160	190	153	115	85	60	35	10	0	0	0	0
2,160	2,200	196	159	121	89	64	39	14	0	0	0	0
2,200	2,240	202	165	127	93	68	43	18	0	0	0	0
2,240	2,280	208	171	133	97	72	47	22	0	0	0	0
2,280	2,320	214	177	139	102	76	51	26	1	0	0	0
2,320	2,360	220	183	145	108	80	55	30	5	0	0	0
2,360	2,400	226	189	151	114	84	59	34	9	0	0	0
2,400	2,440	232	195	157	120	88	63	38	13	0	0	0
2,440	2,480	238	201	163	126	92	67	42	17	0	0	0
2,480	2,520	244	207	169	132	96	71	46	21	0	0	0
2,520	2,560	250	213	175	138	100	75	50	25	0	0	0
2,560	2,600	256	219	181	144	106	79	54	29	4	0	0
2,600	2,640	262	225	187	150	112	83	58	33	8	0	0
2,640	2,680	268	231	193	156	118	87	62	37	12	0	0
2,680	2,720	274	237	199	162	124	91	66	41	16	0	0
2,720	2,760	280	243	205	168	130	95	70	45	20	0	0
2,760	2,800	286	249	211	174	136	99	74	49	24	0	0
2,800	2,840	292	255	217	180	142	105	78	53	28	3	0
2,840	2,880	298	261	223	186	148	111	82	57	32	7	0
2,880	2,920	304	267	229	192	154	117	86	61	36	11	0
2,920	2,960	310	273	235	198	160	123	90	65	40	15	0
2,960	3,000	316	279	241	204	166	129	94	69	44	19	0
3,000	3,040	322	285	247	210	172	135	98	73	48	23	0
3,040	3,080	328	291	253	216	178	141	103	77	52	27	2
3,080	3,120	334	297	259	222	184	147	109	81	56	31	6
3,120	3,160	340	303	265	228	190	153	115	85	60	35	10
3,160	3,200	346	309	271	234	196	159	121	89	64	39	14
3,200	3,240	352	315	277	240	202	165	127	93	68	43	18

Header note: If the wages are— / And the number of withholding allowances claimed is— / The amount of income tax to be withheld is—

FIGURE 23-4, cont'd For legend see previous page.

Form 941
(Rev. January 2002)
Department of the Treasury
Internal Revenue Service (99)

Employer's Quarterly Federal Tax Return

▶ **See separate instructions revised January 2002 for information on completing this return.**

Please type or print.

Enter state code for state in which deposits were made **only** if different from state in address to the right ▶ (see page 2 of instructions).

Name (as distinguished from trade name)

Trade name, if any

Address (number and street)

Date quarter ended

Employer identification number

City, state, and ZIP code

OMB No. 1545-0029

| T |
| FF |
| FD |
| FP |
| I |
| T |

If address is different from prior return, check here ▶

IRS Use

1 1 1 1 1 1 1 1 1 1   2   3 3 3 3 3 3 3   4 4 4   5 5 5

6   7   8 8 8 8 8 8 8 8   9 9 9 9 9   10 10 10 10 10 10 10 10 10 10

If you do not have to file returns in the future, check here ▶ ☐ and enter date final wages paid ▶

If you are a seasonal employer, see **Seasonal employers** on page 1 of the instructions and check here ▶ ☐

| 1 | Number of employees in the pay period that includes March 12th . ▶ | 1 | | |

2	Total wages and tips, plus other compensation	2	
3	Total income tax withheld from wages, tips, and sick pay . . .	3	
4	Adjustment of withheld income tax for preceding quarters of calendar year	4	
5	Adjusted total of income tax withheld (line 3 as adjusted by line 4—see instructions) . . .	5	

6	Taxable social security wages	6a		× 12.4% (.124) =	6b	
	Taxable social security tips	6c		× 12.4% (.124) =	6d	
7	Taxable Medicare wages and tips . . .	7a		× 2.9% (.029) =	7b	

| 8 | Total social security and Medicare taxes (add lines 6b, 6d, and 7b). Check here if wages are not subject to social security and/or Medicare tax . . . . ▶ ☐ | 8 | |

| 9 | Adjustment of social security and Medicare taxes (see instructions for required explanation) Sick Pay $ _____ ± Fractions of Cents $ _____ ± Other $ _____ = | 9 | |

10	Adjusted total of social security and Medicare taxes (line 8 as adjusted by line 9—see instructions)	10	
11	**Total taxes** (add lines 5 and 10)	11	
12	Advance earned income credit (EIC) payments made to employees	12	
13	Net taxes (subtract line 12 from line 11). **If $2,500 or more, this must equal line 17, column (d) below (or line D of Schedule B (Form 941))**	13	
14	Total deposits for quarter, including overpayment applied from a prior quarter	14	
15	**Balance due** (subtract line 14 from line 13). See instructions	15	

16 **Overpayment.** If line 14 is more than line 13, enter excess here ▶ $ _____
and check if to be: ☐ Applied to next return   **or**   ☐ Refunded.

- **All filers:** If line 13 is less than $2,500, you need not complete line 17 or Schedule B (Form 941).
- **Semiweekly schedule depositors:** Complete Schedule B (Form 941) and check here . . . . ▶ ☐
- **Monthly schedule depositors:** Complete line 17, columns (a) through (d), and check here . . . . ▶ ☐

17	**Monthly Summary of Federal Tax Liability.** Do not complete if you were a semiweekly schedule depositor.		
(a) First month liability	**(b)** Second month liability	**(c)** Third month liability	**(d)** Total liability for quarter

Third Party Designee

Do you want to allow another person to discuss this return with the IRS (see separate instructions)?   ☐ **Yes.** Complete the following.   ☐ **No**

Designee's name ▶   Phone no. ▶ ( )   Personal identification number (PIN) ▶

Sign Here

Under penalties of perjury, I declare that I have examined this return, including accompanying schedules and statements, and to the best of my knowledge and belief, it is true, correct, and complete.

Signature ▶   Print Your Name and Title ▶   Date ▶

For Privacy Act and Paperwork Reduction Act Notice, see back of Payment Voucher.   Cat. No. 17001Z   Form **941** (Rev. 1-2002)

FIGURE 23-5 IRS Form 941: Employer's Quarterly Federal Tax Return.

Form 941
Payment Voucher

Purpose of Form

Complete Form 941-V if you are making a payment with **Form 941,** Employer's Quarterly Federal Tax Return. We will use the completed voucher to credit your payment more promptly and accurately, and to improve our service to you.

If you have your return prepared by a third party and make a payment with that return, please provide this payment voucher to the return preparer.

Making Payments With Form 941

Make payments with Form 941 only if:

1. Your net taxes for the quarter (line 13 on Form 941) are less than $2,500 and you are paying in full with a timely filed return or

2. You are a monthly schedule depositor making a payment in accordance with the **accuracy of deposits** rule. (See section 11 of **Circular E,** Employer's Tax Guide, for details.) This amount may be $2,500 or more.

Otherwise, you must deposit the amount at an authorized financial institution or by electronic funds transfer. (See section 11 of Circular E for deposit instructions.) Do not use the Form 941-V payment voucher to make Federal tax deposits.

Caution: *If you pay amounts with Form 941 that should have been deposited, you may be subject to a penalty. See Circular E.*

Specific Instructions

Box 1—Employer identification number (EIN). If you do not have an EIN, apply for one on **Form SS-4,** Application for Employer Identification Number, and write "Applied for" and the date you applied in this entry space.

Box 2—Amount paid. Enter the amount paid with Form 941.

Box 3—Tax period. Darken the capsule identifying the quarter for which the payment is made. Darken only one capsule.

Box 4—Name and address. Enter your name and address as shown on Form 941.

● Make your check or money order payable to the United States Treasury. Be sure to enter your EIN, "Form 941," and the tax period on your check or money order. Do not send cash. Please do not staple this voucher or your payment to the return or to each other.

● Detach the completed voucher and send it with your payment and Form 941 to the address provided on the back of Form 941.

▼   Detach Here and Mail With Your Payment   ▼   Form **941-V** (2002)

Form **941-V** Department of the Treasury Internal Revenue Service (99)	**Payment Voucher** ▶ **Do not staple or attach this voucher to your payment.**	OMB No. 1545-0029 20**02**

1 Enter your employer identification number	**2** **Enter the amount of the payment**	Dollars	Cents

3 Tax period	**4** Enter your business name (individual name if sole proprietor)
⦰ 1st Quarter ⦰ 3rd Quarter	Enter your address
⦰ 2nd Quarter ⦰ 4th Quarter	Enter your city, state, and ZIP code

FIGURE 23-5, cont'd For legend see previous page.

Form **940**

Department of the Treasury
Internal Revenue Service (99)

**Employer's Annual Federal
Unemployment (FUTA) Tax Return**

▶ **See separate Instructions for Form 940 for information on completing this form.**

OMB No. 1545-0028

20**01**

**You must
complete
this section.** ▶

Name (as distinguished from trade name)

Trade name, if any

Address and ZIP code

Calendar year

Employer identification number

T	
FF	
FD	
FP	
I	
T	

A Are you required to pay unemployment contributions to only one state? (If "No," skip questions B and C.) . ☐ **Yes** ☐ **No**

B Did you pay all state unemployment contributions by January 31, 2002? ((1) If you deposited your total FUTA tax when due, check "Yes" if you paid all state unemployment contributions by February 11, 2002. (2) If a 0% experience rate is granted, check "Yes." (3) If "No," skip question C.) . . . . ☐ **Yes** ☐ **No**

C Were all wages that were taxable for FUTA tax also taxable for your state's unemployment tax? . . . . . ☐ **Yes** ☐ **No**

If you answered "No" to any of these questions, you must file Form 940. If you answered "Yes" to all the questions, you may file Form 940-EZ, which is a simplified version of Form 940. (Successor employers see **Special credit for successor employers** on page 3 of the instructions.) You can get Form 940-EZ by calling 1-800-TAX-FORM (1-800-829-3676) or from the IRS Web Site at **www.irs.gov**.

If you will not have to file returns in the future, check here (see **Who Must File** in separate instructions), **and complete and sign the return** . . . . ▶ ☐

If this is an Amended Return, check here. . . . . ▶ ☐

Part I   Computation of Taxable Wages

1 Total payments (including payments shown on lines 2 and 3) during the calendar year for services of employees **1**

2 Exempt payments. (Explain all exempt payments, attaching additional sheets if necessary.) ▶ --

-- **2**

3 Payments of more than $7,000 for services. Enter only amounts over the first $7,000 paid to each employee. (See separate instructions.) Do not include any exempt payments from line 2. The $7,000 amount is the Federal wage base. Your state wage base may be different. **Do not use your state wage limitation**. **3**

4 Add lines 2 and 3 . . . . **4**

5 **Total taxable wages** (subtract line 4 from line 1) . . . . ▶ **5**

Be sure to complete both sides of this form, and sign in the space provided on the back.

For Privacy Act and Paperwork Reduction Act Notice, see separate instructions.   ▼ **DETACH HERE** ▼   Cat. No. 11234O   Form **940** (2001)

Form **940-V**

Department of the Treasury
Internal Revenue Service

Form 940 Payment Voucher

Use this voucher only when making a payment with your return.

OMB No. 1545-0028

20**01**

Complete boxes 1, 2, and 3. Do not send cash, and do not staple your payment to this voucher. Make your check or money order payable to the **"United States Treasury."** Be sure to enter your employer identification number, "Form 940," and "2001" on your payment.

1 Enter your employer identification number.

2 **Enter the amount of your payment.** ▶

Dollars	Cents

3 Enter your business name (individual name for sole proprietors).

Enter your address.

Enter your city, state, and ZIP code.

FIGURE 23-6 Employer's Annual Federal Unemployment Tax (FUTA) Return.

Form 940 (2001)   Page **2**

Part II   **Tax Due or Refund**

1	Gross FUTA tax. Multiply the wages from Part I, line 5, by .062	**1**
2	Maximum credit. Multiply the wages from Part I, line 5, by .054 . . **2**	
3	Computation of tentative credit (**Note:** *All taxpayers must complete the applicable columns.*)	

(a) Name of state	(b) State reporting number(s) as shown on employer's state contribution returns	(c) Taxable payroll (as defined in state act)	(d) State experience rate period		(e) State experience rate	(f) Contributions if rate had been 5.4% (col. (c) x .054)	(g) Contributions payable at experience rate (col. (c) x col. (e))	(h) Additional credit (col. (f) minus col.(g)) If 0 or less, enter -0-.	(i) Contributions paid to state by 940 due date
			From	To					

3a Totals . . . ▶

3b   **Total tentative credit** (add line 3a, columns (h) and (i) only—for late payments, also see the instructions for Part II, line 6) . . . . ▶   **3b**

4

5

6   **Credit:** Enter the smaller of the amount from Part II, line 2 or line 3b; or the amount from the worksheet in the Part II, line 6 instructions **6**

7   **Total FUTA tax** (subtract line 6 from line 1). If the result is over $100, also complete Part III . .   **7**

8   Total FUTA tax deposited for the year, including any overpayment applied from a prior year . .   **8**

9   **Balance due** (subtract line 8 from line 7). Pay to the **"United States Treasury."** If you owe more than $100, see **Depositing FUTA Tax** on page 3 of the separate instructions . . . . . . ▶   **9**

10   **Overpayment** (subtract line 7 from line 8). Check if it is to be: ☐ **Applied to next return** or ☐ **Refunded** . . . . ▶   **10**

Part III   **Record of Quarterly Federal Unemployment Tax Liability** (Do not include state liability.) **Complete only if line 7 is over $100.** See page 6 of the separate instructions.

Quarter	First (Jan. 1–Mar. 31)	Second (Apr. 1–June 30)	Third (July 1–Sept. 30)	Fourth (Oct. 1–Dec. 31)	Total for year
Liability for quarter					

Third Party Designee   Do you want to allow another person to discuss this return with the IRS (see instructions page 4)? ☐ **Yes.** Complete the following. ☐ **No**

Designee's name ▶   Phone no. ▶ ( )   Personal identification number (PIN) ▶

Under penalties of perjury, I declare that I have examined this return, including accompanying schedules and statements, and, to the best of my knowledge and belief, it is true, correct, and complete, and that no part of any payment made to a state unemployment fund claimed as a credit was, or is to be, deducted from the payments to employees.

Signature ▶   Title (Owner, etc.) ▶   Date ▶

Form **940** (2001)

FIGURE 23-6, cont'd For legend see previous page.

Federal Unemployment Tax

Employers also contribute under the Federal Unemployment Tax Act (FUTA). Generally, credit can be taken against the FUTA tax for amounts paid into a state unemployment fund up to a certain percentage. Employers are responsible for paying the FUTA tax; it must not be deducted from employees' wages. For 1998 the FUTA tax was 6.2% of the first $7000 in wages paid to each employee during the calendar year.

For deposit purposes, the FUTA tax is figured quarterly, and any amount due must be paid by the last day of the first month after the quarter ends. The formula for determining the amount due is set forth in the Federal Employer's Tax Guide.

An annual FUTA return must be filed on Form 940 on or before January 31 following the close of the calendar year for which the tax is due (Figure 23-6). Any tax still due is payable with the return. Form 940 may be filed on or before February 10 following the close of the year, if all required deposits were made on time and if full payment of the tax due is deposited on or before January 31.

State Unemployment Taxes

All of the states and the District of Columbia have unemployment compensation laws. In most states, the tax is imposed only on the employer, but a few states require employers to withhold a percentage of wages for unemployment compensation benefits. An employer may be subject to federal unemployment tax and not subject to state unemployment tax. In some states, for instance, the employer with fewer than four employees is not subject to the state unemployment tax. The regulations for a specific state should be checked.

State Disability Insurance

Some states require that employees be covered by disability or sick-pay insurance. The employer may be required to withhold

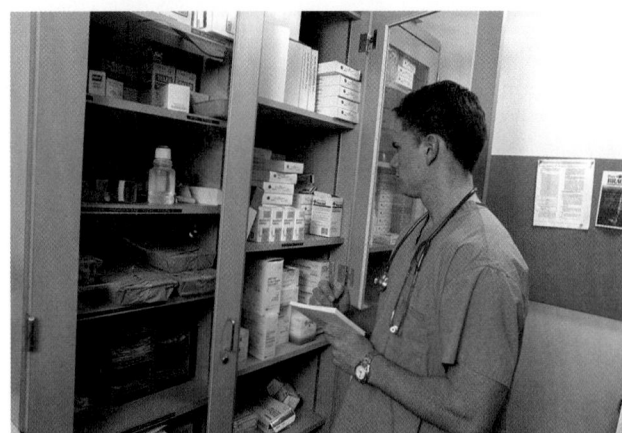

FIGURE 23-7 Inventory supplies and equipment before developing the annual budget. Once a good inventory has been completed, more accurate projections can be made for the expenses for the coming year.

a certain amount from the employee's salary to pay for this insurance.

BUDGETS

Growing businesses must develop budgets that help to plan finances over a certain period. Medical offices should compile a new budget before the beginning of each **fiscal year.** The best way to begin a budget is to look at the expenses from the previous year (Figure 23-7). These expenses should be divided into categories, then a total should be derived for each category. Each month should represent approximately $1/12$ of the total budget, not including large capital expenses.

Within the individual categories, examine expenses for those that could be eliminated or those that were underbudgeted. For example, if $3345 was spent on office supplies and the budget was $3000, either more money needs to be allotted for this category or cuts in spending are necessary. If $3345 was spent and the budget was $4000, the excess may be placed in another category for the next year.

CRITICAL THINKING APPLICATION

- Brenda has developed a preliminary budget. She realizes that several pieces of equipment need to be replaced in the coming year. However, Dr. Wilkins has expressed that she does not wish to make any capital purchases. How might Brenda approach Dr. Wilkins about the needed equipment?
- How might leasing equipment benefit the office? How can Brenda determine if this would be more or less expensive than purchasing the equipment?

By monitoring expenses on a monthly basis, the physician can see if the facility is over budget, under budget, or right on target. Categories in which overspending has occurred can be reconciled by taking funds from another category (for instance, category B) and adding them to the overspent category (category A). However, the amount taken must be subtracted from category B and added to category A. Those subtracted

funds are no longer available in category B. Specific notes should be kept when categories are overspent, so that an adjustment may be made for the next fiscal year.

The following categories should be considered for the physician's operating budget:

- Insurance
- Rent
- Depreciation
- Loan payments
- Advertising and promotions
- Legal and accounting
- Miscellaneous expenses
- Supplies
- Salaries and wages
- Utilities
- Dues, subscriptions, and fees
- Taxes
- Repairs and maintenance
- Medical equipment
- Administrative equipment
- Medication and pharmacy expenses

The physician should investigate whether leasing equipment might be a better option for the facility. Some leasing programs are very progressive and provide service contracts at no additional cost. Because depreciation costs are high, leasing might be the best answer to a new equipment need.

Insurance

Insurance coverage is one of the physician's major expenses. Almost every physician carries some type of malpractice insurance for protection against the cost of legal liabilities. Property and fire insurance are mandatory, and most physicians carry workers' compensation insurance to cover employee injuries and accidents. The medical assistant may be asked to shop for the best insurance rates at the time of renewals.

CLOSING COMMENTS

The physician will come to rely heavily on the person who manages the finances of the office. It is important that this individual keep information confidential. The entire staff must be conscious of the costs involved in operating a medical office and should adhere to their respective budgets as closely as possible. By being conservative, the physician may be willing to spend more money on pay increases and benefits to reward his or her employees.

There may be times when patients do not fully understand the costs involved in providing high-quality medical care. The medical assistant may need to educate the patient about the basic costs involved with the procedures that are performed in the office. Patients do not need a lengthy explanation but may be set more at ease in knowing that the physician does not set his or her fees arbitrarily. The physician's office is a small business, like thousands of other small businesses, and should be able to pay its overhead and expenses.

The keeping of the financial records is a position of great trust and responsibility. Some physicians require the person placed in charge of the office finances to be bonded. This means that the facility has done a security check on an individual and the person was found worthy to be placed in a position of responsibility. A bond is issued by an entity on behalf of a second party, guaranteeing that the second party will fulfill an obligation or series of obligations to a third party. In the event that the obligations are not met, the third party will recover its losses via the bond.

Records must be accurate and completed on a daily basis. Daily journals should be kept indefinitely in support of tax returns.

SUMMARY OF SCENARIO

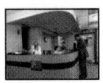

Brenda has learned much about the financial management of a physician's office. She is never hesitant to call the practice accountant, Mr. Schmidt, whenever a question arises. As she gains more experience, she comes to understand the budgeting process, cost management, and the various methods of accounting practice.

There are many things that can affect the finances of a medical practice. However, the physician who is fairly conservative about spending and careful with investments should remain a stable part of the community's healthcare professionals. Dr. Wilkins lives by this philosophy and encourages her employees to manage money wisely, too. This attitude among all the staff members promotes a sense of teamwork and cooperation for the benefit of all.

SUMMARY of LEARNING OBJECTIVES

1. Define, spell, and pronounce the terms listed in the vocabulary.
   - Spelling and pronouncing medical terms correctly adds credibility to the medical assistant. Knowing the definition of these terms promotes confidence in communication with patients and co-workers.
2. List the four items that all financial records should show at any given time.
   - The financial records of any business should at all times show how much was earned in a given period, how much was collected, how much is owed, and the distribution of expenses incurred.
3. Distinguish between accounts payable and accounts receivable.
   - *Accounts payable* refers to the amounts of money owed by a business and not yet paid, whereas *accounts receivable* refers to amounts owed to the business that are not yet paid.
4. List and explain the three most common bookkeeping systems found in physicians' offices today.
   - The three most common bookkeeping systems in use today are the single-entry system, double-entry system, and pegboard system. The single-entry method is the oldest accounting method and uses a general journal, a cash payment journal, and an accounts receivable ledger. Payroll records and petty cash records may also be included. The double-entry system, which is more difficult to use than the single-entry system, requires an entry on each side of the accounting equation, and each side must always balance. The pegboard system requires a moderate initial investment to implement but allows the user to perform several accounting functions at one time. It is often called the *write-it-once system.*

5. Explain the importance of a trial balance.
   - A trial balance will reflect discrepancies between the journal and the ledger. It does not reveal errors in the individual accounts but will show errors in the overall balances of accounts.
6. State the types of employment records required by the IRS.
   - The IRS requires that several employment records be kept for at least 4 years. These records include the Social Security number of the employee; the number of withholding allowances claimed; the amount of gross salary; all deductions for Social Security and Medicare taxes; federal, state, and city or other subdivision withholding taxes; state disability insurance; and state unemployment tax.
7. Discuss the basis for the withholding amounts that are taken from employees' earnings.
   - Several deductions are taken from the employee's wages as required by law. These deductions are based on the total earnings of the employee, the number of withholding allowances claimed, the marital status of the employee, and the length of the pay period involved.
8. Name the five common periodic accounting reports.
   - Five common reports are used for accounting in the small business office: the statement of income and expense, the cash flow statement, the trial balance, the accounts receivable trial balance, and the balance sheet.
9. Explain the purpose of the W-4 form.
   - The Employee's Withholding Allowance Certificate, or Form W-4, specifies the number of withholding allowances that the employee is claiming. The more allowances that are

Continued

SUMMARY of LEARNING OBJECTIVES

Continued

claimed, the less money that is taken from the employee's paycheck.

10. Explain the requirements of the Federal Insurance Contributions Act.
    - FICA requires that a certain amount of money be deducted from an employee's wages and designated for Medicare and Social Security programs. The current percentages are 1.45% for the Medicare contribution and 6.2% for Social Security. Both the employer and the employee contribute these amounts.

11. Discuss the importance of setting a budget each fiscal year.
    - The physician's office must set a budget each fiscal year to prepare for all of the expenses that will be involved in running the office. Without a well-planned budget, the physician cannot control expenses. The expenditures from the past year should be evaluated when the new budget is planned, with particular attention paid to the expense categories that exceeded expected amounts.

12. Maintain a petty cash fund.
    - Most offices pay for small, incidental expenses with petty cash. The process for maintaining a petty cash fund is outlined in Procedure 23-1.

13. Accurately process an employee payroll.
    - Employee payroll is an essential function related to practice finances. The process for employee payrolls is outlined in Procedure 23-2.

CONNECTIONS

 Study Guide Connection: Go to Chapter 23 Study Guide. Read the Case Study and Workplace Applications and complete the assignments. Do online research for answers to the questions in the Internet Activities associated with management of practice finances.

 CD Connection: Go to the Medical Assisting Competency Challenge CD and do the training activities under Financial Management.

 Evolve Connection: For more information related to management of practice finances, go to evolve.elsevier.com/kinn and visit related weblinks for Chapter 23. Click on the Medical Assisting Exam Review and do the practice questions to sharpen your test-taking skills. To learn more about office software, do the exercises for the Altapoint demo that is on the CD.

Medical Practice Management and Human Resources

24

SCENARIO

Katherine Martinson is the office manager for Dr. Michael Collins, a family practitioner in a group practice located in a metropolitan area. The office usually carries a full schedule of patients each day. Katherine has been instrumental in the seamless operation of the facility. Before joining Dr. Collins, Katherine worked for a physician in the same group of doctors, Dr. Grant Bradley, who retired last year. She worked as an administrative medical assistant for 6 years before that. Her strength and ability to motivate employees led Dr. Collins to approach her about becoming his office manager once Dr. Bradley retired.

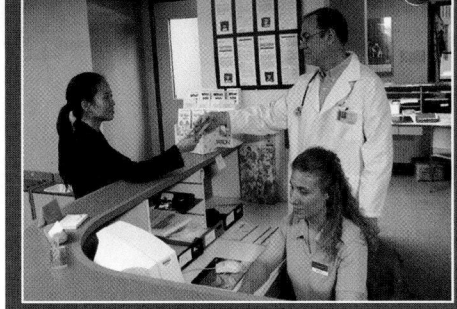

Katherine is a consummate professional but knows the importance of treating each employee as an individual. At weekly staff meetings the employees offer input on the various procedures followed in the office. Katherine regularly consults with the staff members and always asks for input as to how the office can function more effectively. She then implements many of the staff members' suggestions in the day-to-day activities of the office. She knows that employees need to feel a part of the team, and by trying the procedures others suggest she validates them as an asset to the facility.

When a position is open, Katherine is careful about whom she hires, always checking at least three references per applicant and verifying each previous place of employment. She trains each employee on every aspect of the job and keeps checklists that reflect the employee has been given instruction on certain skills.

Katherine makes sure that each person has the tools needed to do his or her job. She also explains overhead costs to employees and helps them to understand what is involved with the daily operation of the practice. With this information the employees are more conservative about use of supplies and care of equipment. Major changes are presented to the entire staff, and although Dr. Collins makes the final decision, he and Katherine seek the input of the employees, too. The cooperative attitude between management and the employees of the office provides a good atmosphere for teamwork, and Katherine and the physician are pleased with the results.

While studying this chapter, think about the following questions:

- How friendly should office managers become with the staff members?
- Why is it important to check references when hiring a new staff member?
- How should negative employee evaluations be handled?
- Why could the patient information folder be considered a management tool?

LEARNING OBJECTIVES

1. Define, spell, and pronounce the terms listed in the vocabulary.
2. Explain the importance of management in the medical office.
3. Discuss the desirable qualities of a medical office manager.
4. List and discuss the three types of leaders.
5. Discuss several types of power and whether power is a positive or negative entity.
6. Identify several ways in which employees are motivated.
7. Explain the difference between intrinsic and extrinsic motivation.
8. List several ways to prevent burnout.
9. Discuss what to look for when reviewing resumes and applications.
10. Explain why the telephone voice of an applicant is important.
11. Identify the follow-up activities the office manager should perform after an interview.
12. Explain the importance of mentors for new employees in the medical office.
13. List the various types of staff meetings.
14. Successfully arrange a group meeting.
15. Interview a job candidate for a position at the facility.
16. Conduct a performance review for an employee.

National Accreditation Competencies and Content

CAAHEP COMPETENCIES

General

3.c.(1)(b). Recognize and respond to verbal communications
3.c.(1)(c). Recognize and respond to nonverbal communications
3.c.(2)(b). Perform within legal and ethical boundaries
3.c.(2)(d). Document appropriately
3.c.(4)(c). Utilize computer software to maintain office systems

ABHES COMPETENCIES

Professionalism

1.d. Be cognizant of ethical boundaries

Communication

2.f. Interview effectively
2.k. [Use] principles of verbal and nonverbal communication

Administrative Duties

3.a. Perform basic secretarial skills
3.d. Apply computer concepts for office procedures

Legal Concepts

5.a. Determine needs for documentation and reporting
5.b. Document accurately

Office Management

6.e. Maintain liability coverage
6.f. Exercise efficient time management

Instruction

7.d. Orient and train personnel

VOCABULARY

affable Being pleasant and at ease in talking to others; characterized by ease and friendliness.

agenda (ah-jen'-duh) A list or outline of things to be considered or done.

ancillary (an'-suh-ler-e) Subordinate; auxiliary.

appraisal An expert judgment of the value or merit of; judgment as to quality.

blatant Completely obvious, conspicuous, or obtrusive, especially in a crass or offensive manner; brazen.

burnout Exhaustion of physical or emotional strength or motivation, usually as a result of prolonged stress or frustration.

chain of command A series of executive positions in order of authority.

circumvention To manage to get around, especially by ingenuity or stratagem.

cohesive Sticking together tightly; exhibiting or producing cohesion.

disparaging (dis-pahr'-uh-jing) Slighting; having a negative or degrading tone.

embezzlement Stealing from an employer; to appropriate goods, services, or funds for personal use without permission.

extrinsic (eks-trin'-zik) External to a thing, its essential nature, or its original character.

impenetrable Incapable of being penetrated or pierced; not capable of being damaged or harmed.

incentives Things that incite or spur to action; rewards or reasons for performing a task.

insubordination Disobedience to authority.

intrinsic Originating with or resulting from causes within a body, organ, or part.

mentors Trusted counselors or guides.

meticulous (meh-tiku'-luhs) Marked by extreme or excessive care in the consideration or treatment of details.

micromanage To manage with great or excessive control or attention to details.

morale The mental and emotional condition, such as enthusiasm, confidence, or loyalty, of an individual or group with regard to the function or tasks at hand.

motivation The process of inciting a person to some action or behavior.

reprimands Criticisms for a fault; severe or formal reproofs.

retention The act of keeping in possession or use; keeping in one's pay or service.

subordinate Submissive to or controlled by authority; placed in or occupying a lower class, rank, or position.

targeted Directed or used toward a target; directed toward a specific desire or position.

The management of a professional medical office can greatly influence the success of the operation. Good management will allow the physician to see and treat his or her patients in a functional environment with the confidence that the business side of the facility is operating as it should be. A well-managed office is not something that just happens. Great effort and teamwork are necessary to ensure that the day-to-day activities are carried out efficiently and that the many details needing attention are handled expeditiously.

WHO'S IN CHARGE?

If the office has only one medical assistant, that person must be able to assume many management responsibilities with cooperation from the physician. When there are two medical assistants, one administrative and one clinical, it is often the administrative medical assistant who is expected to assume management duties. In an office with a larger staff, a line of authority must be established.

A facility with three or more employees should designate one person as supervisor or office manager. This individual should have management skills and the ability to deal with personnel matters (Table 24-1). Other employees answer to the office manager, and the office manager answers to the physician or physicians. A **chain of command** allows the office staff to consult with the physician regarding administrative or clinical problems, complaints, or grievances; however, it prompts employees to allow those individuals whom the physician has placed in charge to have the first opportunity to solve problems. It also allows the physician to check on the operation of the office, disseminate information on policy changes, and correct errors or grievances by dealing with one person instead of all employees.

A medical assisting career is challenging and offers great opportunities for advancement. The recently graduated medical assistant, whose first position may have been as a receptionist, can be given more responsibilities and may eventually become the office manager of a large staff. Executive-level personnel work in one of the most critical areas in healthcare.

Management problems can often be avoided by carefully defining the areas of authority and responsibility of each employee. Many physicians say that friction among workers is their most common personnel problem. The importance of the chain of command cannot be overemphasized, and the physician must not undermine the office manager's authority by **circumvention.** When employees know what is expected of them, they can plan both their daily and long-term work more effectively.

Duties of the Medical Office Manager

The duties carried out by medical office managers vary from place to place and practice to practice. Some physicians take on a much more active role in office management than others. The best management plan for the physician is to hire an office manager who is trustworthy and reliable, then allow him or her to run the business aspects of the office. This frees the physician to concentrate on taking care of patients (Figure 24-1).

Some of the tasks performed by the medical office manager include the following:

- Preparing and updating policy and procedure manuals
- Developing job descriptions
- Recruiting new employees
- Performing orientation and training
- Conducting performance and salary reviews
- Dismissing employees
- Planning staff meetings
- Maintaining staff harmony
- Establishing work-flow guidelines
- Ensuring compliance with all federal and state regulations
- Improving office efficiency
- Supervising the purchase and care of equipment
- Educating patients
- Eliminating time-wasting tasks for the physician
- Marketing the practice
- Performing customer service

TABLE 24-1 Qualities of an Effective Manager
• Uses good judgment
• Has good health
• Has the ability to organize
• Is willing to learn
• Possesses original ideas
• Has leadership ability
• Is fair with all employees
• Is flexible
• Has a sense of fairness
• Cares about employees
• Remains calm during crises
• Is open to constructive criticism
• Has good communication skills
• Uses good listening skills
• Is approachable

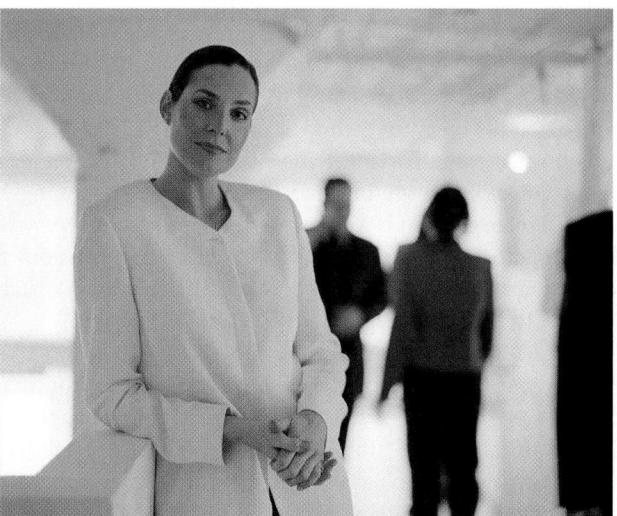

FIGURE 24-1 The office manager ensures that the medical facility runs smoothly so that the physician can concentrate on patient care.

Office management can best be accomplished by developing a thorough office policy and procedure manual. This is discussed later in the chapter.

The Power of Influence

Managers have a great deal of influence over the people they supervise. A successful manager must be interested in people and enjoy working with them on a daily basis. It is said that if one helps others get what they want in life, the individual usually gets what he or she wants as well. An effective manager discovers the **motivation** behind employees' drives to be a part of the profession in which they are employed, then helps them achieve their individual goals. In turn, most employees are enthusiastic about working toward the facility's goals as productive team members.

Successful managers know that their employees should be encouraged to perform at optimal levels, and they are confident enough in their own skills to give credit to those employees who develop ideas and concepts for the team. These managers know how to let their employees help them "look good." A manager with a group of outstanding employees usually is looked on as an effective leader.

CRITICAL THINKING APPLICATION

- When Katherine first began as Dr. Collins's office manager, she found several supportive employees, but a few were concerned about their new boss. How can a new manager help employees be at ease during the first few weeks?
- Katherine scheduled a time with each employee and asked the three things he or she liked best about the office and three things he or she liked the least. How does this help her to manage the office effectively?

The Manager as a Leader

Leaders nurture other people. They take the time to discover what makes people tick, then give them opportunities that will help them rise to new levels of responsibility. Leaders have a strong belief in people, and they express confidence in their abilities, seeing them as successes rather than failures. Often this belief exists before people prove themselves, and that provides motivation for them to reach their potential.

Perhaps most important, leaders listen to their people. Few things are more frustrating than an employee attempting to talk to a manager who is working on some project or typing on the computer. Listening involves eye contact and questions to ensure that the employee is understood. Being willing to take the time to listen is a step toward success as a manager.

Instead of sitting across from employees at a desk, try sitting beside them in the chairs that are usually placed in front of a desk. When discussing issues with employees, this simple change in position places the office manager on an equal plane with the employee and implies more of a team effort. At times this positioning would be inappropriate, such as during discussions about disciplinary matters. Still, when attempting to get an employee to cooperate or come over to the office manager's

way of thinking, position can play a large role in placing people "on the same page."

Types of Leaders

There are three basic types of leaders today, including the charismatic leader, the transactional leader, and the transformational leader. Each has positive qualities, and all can be successful in business.

Charismatic leaders have a special way of inspiring an unswerving allegiance and devotion from their followers. They encourage people to overcome great obstacles and buy into their vision for the organization or business. They also tend to trust people in **subordinate** positions and earn trust in return.

Transactional leaders are structured and organized. They ensure that their subordinates understand their duties and roles. These leaders are fair and provide rewards when they have been earned. The transactional leader is hardworking, a planner, and strict about budgets and time frames.

Transformational leaders are innovative and able to bring about change in an organization. These leaders are relationship builders. They stress shared values and strive to create a common ground among team members. Transformational leaders are the most effective when an organization is experiencing change and reorganization.

Styles of Management

Some managers are democratic and willing to listen to employees. These managers are fair-minded and ask the opinions of the staff when making decisions. In contrast, the autocratic manager is more of a dictator, making demands and insisting tasks be done in a certain way—his or her way. The laissez-faire manager is easygoing and does not make a lot of demands on employees. This is a "go with the flow" manager who lets employees work on their own and does not **micromanage.**

Leading During Transitions and Change

Change is a part of the life of every person and every business. Most people are initially hesitant to face change, and many people try to avoid it completely. However, a business cannot experience growth without change. The manager who is able to lead subordinates through periods of change will be a valuable asset to the organization. Employees will need guidance on maintaining focus on the tasks at hand. The manager should remain visible to the employees during times of change and communicate frequently with status reports and updates on policies and procedures.

The book *Who Moved My Cheese?* by Spencer Johnson, MD, is one of the most innovative stories in recent years. Any manager or employee experiencing a time of change should study this simple, short book. The opening quotes A. J. Cronin, saying:

"Life is no straight and easy corridor along which we travel free and unhampered, but a maze of passages, through which we must seek our way, lost and confused, now and again checked in a blind alley. But always, if we have faith, a door will open for us, not perhaps

one that we ourselves would ever have thought of, but one that will ultimately prove good for us."

Who Moved My Cheese? stresses several points about change that the good manager should remember, including the following:

- Change happens
- Anticipate change
- Monitor change
- Adapt to change quickly
- Move with the change
- Enjoy change
- Be ready to change again quickly, and enjoy it again

The simplicity of this advice does not diminish its truth. Change will happen in any person's job and personal life. Those who learn to adapt quickly and move forward will be the ones who do not become casualties of change.

The Role of Power

Power is the ability to influence employees so that they carry out their directives. Leaders use many types of power.

Coercive power is manipulative, and the leader often makes threats or uses fear to accomplish goals. The fear of losing a job is one manipulation of power.

Granting rewards is a more positive use of power. When the leader is able to give employees some type of reward for a job well done, most strive to reach their goals.

Expert power is a factor when the leader is knowledgeable about a subject. Employees respect leaders who know their job and how things should be done. Most people look up to a person who has a high degree of knowledge about a given subject. When working for someone who knows nothing about procedures or the services offered, employees frequently are frustrated.

Legitimate power is that of position or status. It does not really matter who the President of the United States is—the office itself carries the weight of power. Therefore the individual who serves as President holds legitimate power.

Referent power is granted from subordinates to those who lead by example. It is a power based on the admiration of the leader. **Mentors,** parents, and teachers are often the objects of referent power.

> ### CRITICAL THINKING APPLICATION
>
> ■ Katherine is a respected office manager in the facility where she works, but several other managers are not as well liked. What makes a good office manager?
> ■ Everyone has worked for at least one supervisor whom they did not like. What traits make a poor office manager?

Abuse of Power and Authority

Unfortunately, many managers have the capacity to abuse the power they have. A manager who puts up barriers and erects emotional walls with the employees will have difficulty forming a **cohesive** team. Some managers use other people as tools to get what they want, whereas others stick to their own level or stature, relating only to the inner circle of decision makers in the facility.

When there are no checks and balances in an organization, it is easy to abuse power. It is difficult to work with a manager who cannot look inside himself or herself and see mistakes. Some managers stress rules and conformity, leaving no gray areas where subordinates are concerned. Some show a false humility and pretend to care, but most employees can see right through this half-effort at a relationship. Others only hire "yes" people, who agree with everything that the manager says. All of these are abuses of power and indications of a poor manager.

The Power of Motivation

What motivates a person to reach a goal?

- A challenge
- Money
- Praise
- Satisfaction
- Freedom
- Fear
- Family
- Insecurity
- Competition
- Fulfillment
- Integrity
- Honor
- Reputation
- Responsibility
- Prestige
- Needs
- Love

All of the motivators listed above could prompt an employee to action. There are two general types of motivation. **Intrinsic** motivation is internal or originates within someone. Intrinsic motivation is long term and can be focused toward a lifelong goal. **Extrinsic** motivation is external and more material in nature. Generally, extrinsic motivation is more short-lived and less satisfying than intrinsic motivation.

> ### CRITICAL THINKING APPLICATION
>
> ■ Katherine knows that employees have different reasons and motivations for working. Some must work to help support their families, and others work simply because of a love for their field. How can Katherine discover her employees' motivations for working?
> ■ How does this knowledge benefit the office manager?
> ■ Can this knowledge help Katherine achieve her goals?

CREATING A TEAM ATMOSPHERE

Teamwork is critical in the medical profession. In the physician's office the manager must promote an atmosphere in which the employees are willing to work together toward common goals. Low **morale** may exist in the office because of recent changes in policies or procedures, changes in staff or management,

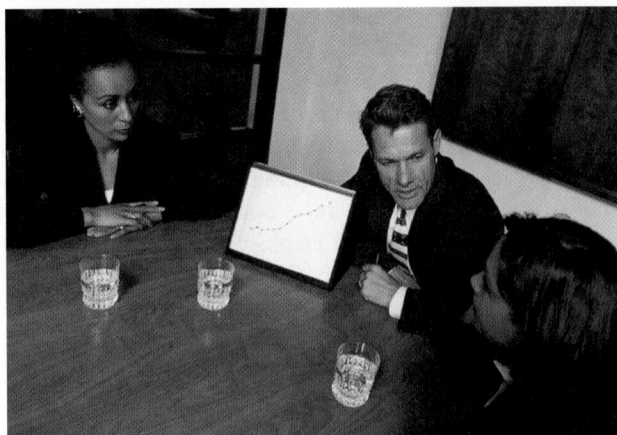

FIGURE 24-2 Communication is vital when building a team. Employees appreciate good communication with management. Sharing good and bad news openly with employees leads to fewer rumors and nervous workers.

Five Essential Elements for Teamwork

- Mutual accountability: Each person on the team holds the others accountable for the success of the organization.
- Common purpose and performance goals: Short-term and intermediate goals must relate to the long-term goals of the group.
- Small size: Most successful teams have a small number of members, and fewer than 10 is optimum.
- Common approach: All of the team members must learn to work together toward the goal.
- Complementary skills: A variety of talents, skills, and abilities is needed for a successful team.

From Katzenbach JR, Smith DK: *Wisdom of teams: creating the high-performance organization*, Boston, 1992, Harvard Business School Publishing.

terminations of recent employees, lack of business, or any number of other reasons. The wise manager will take steps to constantly improve employee morale, including scheduling frequent meetings and keeping the employees abreast of changes and developments that affect them (Figure 24-2). Employees like to be kept "in the loop." Some managers attempt to shield employees from negative information, but this practice can cause rumors to circulate and make morale even worse.

Managers can improve morale by scheduling activities that involve the families of employees and making an obvious effort to include employees in various events. One of the most effective ways to improve employee morale is to communicate. Regular staff meetings are critical for good communication and smooth operation of the medical facility.

Use of Incentives and Employee Recognition

The staff of the physician's office should feel satisfaction with the working conditions and atmosphere in the facility. The office manager plays a part in ensuring that this happens.

Incentives give the employees reason to perform over and above the level expected of them. For instance, if the staff meets or exceeds a goal that has been set, the physician may elect to provide tickets to a sports or entertainment event for the entire staff. A paid day off is always a great incentive for accomplishing a goal. Some physicians have an incentive program that is related to collections for a given period. These ideas provide a goal for the employees to work toward and an opportunity to expand their efforts as a team.

Recognition is a strong method for improving employee morale and encouraging outstanding performance. Certificates for peak performance are a great way to motivate employees. For instance, the office manager may decide to award a certificate each month to the employee who provides the best customer service. Patients could even be involved by allowing them to nominate employees for this honor. When an award is at stake, most employees will enjoy participating and striving to accomplish the goals that have been set.

CRITICAL THINKING APPLICATION

- One of Katherine's employees, Jewel, is very sensitive about performing perfectly on the job. She is an excellent employee, but she does have a few weaknesses. However, she has received a lot of recognition for the good things she has done at work. Katherine still feels that she needs to discuss the areas where Jewel is performing weakly with her but knows that it will upset her. How might Katherine deal with this sticky situation?
- How can Katherine reassure Jewel that she is pleased with her overall performance?

Problem Employees

Occasionally, problem employees disrupt the efficiency of the physician's office. Counseling these employees to find the source of their difficulties is the first step toward resolution. Many employees can be redirected to become productive staff members with a little patience and understanding on the part of the manager. However, some employees have negative attitudes that seem **impenetrable.**

The manager must never hesitate to counsel the employee who is not performing at the expected level, and this includes employees with attitude problems. Establish a set regimen of counseling. Many offices allow one verbal warning before written **reprimands** go into the employee files. If the manager does not make a habit of writing formal reprimands, there may be insufficient documentation of problems with the employee once the manager is ready to terminate him or her. Even small offenses, such as being tardy, should at least be noted in the employee's file. The manager should never be in a position that the termination of an employee cannot be justified by written documents.

Preventing Burnout

Burnout is defined as exhaustion of physical or emotional strength or motivation, usually as a result of prolonged stress or frustration. Medical professionals are particularly susceptible to burnout because of the intensity of their jobs. Even small decisions could affect the life of a patient. Therefore the office

TABLE 24-2 Tips for Preventing Burnout

- Ask for help
- Devote specific times to self-introspection or meditation
- Understand what can be changed and what cannot be changed
- Get some exercise
- Organize and prioritize tasks
- List tasks that are displeasing, and delegate them to others, if possible
- Understand personal limitations
- Take short vacations at least twice a year
- Identify goals, and try to perform only tasks that lead to reaching them
- Consider options, including changing jobs
- Personalize work space with pictures and comforting items
- Get a good understanding of a position and the stress involved before accepting it

manager should take measures to help employees avoid burnout (Table 24-2).

Some of the causes of burnout include a stressful, disorganized home or work environment; poor human relations skills; a feeling of being out of control of one's life; excessive expectations from supervisors or family members; long work hours or time away from family and friends; and not being able to relax either at home or in the work environment.

Keeping the Management Relationship Professional

When people work together for an extended period, they often become **affable,** and sometimes relationships develop into close friendships. This is a normal occurrence, but the office manager must be careful about becoming too close to his or her employees. When the relationship is friendly, it is sometimes difficult to reprimand an employee when needed. Some employees will take advantage of a good relationship with the office manager and may begin to arrive late or call in sick more than usual. A healthy respect for each other must be maintained. The manager can have a good rapport with employees without becoming overly friendly, and this is the best policy. Some facilities have strict rules about fraternization with subordinates outside of the work facility. It is advisable to keep the relationship on a professional level at all times.

CRITICAL THINKING APPLICATION

- The clinical medical assistants usually celebrate payday by going to eat after work every other Friday. After about 6 months on the job, they invited Katherine to join them. Should she go with the employees? Why or why not?
- Most offices plan parties for Christmas or at other times during the year. Are these good for employee morale, or should they be avoided?

SELECTING THE RIGHT STAFF MEMBERS

The most important asset to any medical facility is the staff that cares for the patients. From the doctor to the receptionist,

all play a vital role in the well-being of those who visit the office. Selecting staff members who can be molded into a cohesive team is not an easy task. Care should be taken to choose employees who have the necessary skills and the right personality for the office. Never try to select employees who are all alike. A variety of personality types works better than several similar personalities.

Understanding the Needs of the Office

The office manager should discuss with the physician the type of employee needed when an opening arises. Ask what qualities he or she desires in the person who occupies that particular position and what tasks the person will be responsible for. Once the need has been established and the duties confirmed, the office manager can begin the recruiting process.

One of the most effective methods of finding new employees is through word of mouth. Ask other office managers, physicians, or medical professionals if they are aware of a person looking for employment who has the skills needed in the office. It is a good idea to keep a file of resumes that can be accessed when an opening exists in the office. Often the physician or office manager may know of a person working in another area of the clinic or perhaps in a nearby hospital who may be interested in a job change. Be careful in approaching a person who is already employed. There is no harm in asking if a person is interested, but if the reply is negative, do not pursue the issue further.

Employment agencies can be used to find staff members, but they may charge a fee for their services. The office manager may wish to contact a local medical assistant school to secure an extern. If the extern proves to be an asset to the office, then he or she may be offered the permanent position. Newspaper ads are another option for finding employees, but many resumes may be submitted from people who are not qualified, especially when the economy is not at its best. When creating an ad for the newspaper, list the basic requirements for the position. Briefly describe the office and location and the personality type being sought. Some offices list a few of the benefits offered to attract applicants and may disclose a salary range as well.

Reviewing Resumes and Applications

Once several resumes or applications have been submitted, the office manager should set aside quiet time to review the documents. Place them into one of three stacks—stack one should contain resumes of individuals who will be called for an interview, stack two those of possible candidates but not the strongest, and stack three those of applicants who will not be called.

During this preliminary review process, look for several items. First, be sure the documents are neatly prepared and completely legible (Figure 24-3). The person hired will probably write in the patient charts, so this is a good opportunity to ensure that his or her handwriting can be read clearly. Second, look for gaps between positions. Be sure that any lengthy time of unemployment is explained. The application should be filled out completely, and no notations of "see resume" should be included. The application provides important information,

APPLICATION FOR POSITION / Medical or Dental Office
AN EQUAL OPPORTUNITY EMPLOYER

(In answering questions, use extra blank sheet if necessary)

No employee, applicant, or candidate for promotion, training or other advantage shall be discriminated against (or given preference) because of race, color, religion, sex, age, physical handicap, veteran status, or national origin.

PLEASE READ CAREFULLY AND WRITE OR PRINT ANSWERS TO ALL QUESTIONS. DO NOT TYPE.

Date of Application

A. PERSONAL INFORMATION

Name - Last | First | Middle | Social Security No. | Area Code/Phone No. ( )

Present Address: - Street | (Apt #) | City | State | Zip | How Long At This Address?

Previous Address: - Street | City | State | Zip | Person to notify in case of Emergency or Accident - Name:

From: | To: | Address: | Telephone:

B. EMPLOYMENT INFORMATION

For What Position Are You Applying?: | ☐ Full-Time ☐ Part-Time ☐ Either | Date Available For Employment?: | Wage/Salary Expectations:

List Hrs./Days You Prefer To Work | List Any Hrs./Days You Are Not Available: (Except for times required for religious practices or observances) | Can You Work Overtime, If Necessary? ☐ Yes ☐ No

Are You Employed Now?: ☐ Yes ☐ No | If So, May We Inquire Of Your Present Employer?: ☐ No ☐ Yes, If Yes:
Name Of Employer: | Phone Number: ( )

Have You Ever Been Bonded? ☐ Yes ☐ No | If Required For Position, Are You Bondable? ☐ Yes ☐ No ☐ Uncertain | Have You Applied For A Position With This Office Before? ☐ No ☐ Yes If Yes, When?:

Referred By / Or Where Did You Learn Of This Job?:

Can You, Upon Employment, Submit Verification Of Your Legal Right To Work In The United States?: ☐ Yes ☐ No
Submit Proof That You Meet Legal Age Requirement For Employment? ☐ Yes ☐ No | Language(s) Applicant Speaks or Writes (If Use Of A Language Other Than English is Relevant To The Job For Which The Applicant Is Applying:

C. EDUCATIONAL HISTORY

Name & Address Of Schools Attended (Include Current)	Dates From	Thru	Highest Grade/Level Completed	Diploma/Degree(s) Obtained/Areas of Study
High School				
College				Degree/Major
Post Graduate				Degree/Major
Other				Course/Diploma/License/Certificate

Specific Training, Education, Or Experiences Which Will Assist You In The Job For Which You Have Applied.

Future Educational Plans

D. SPECIAL SKILLS

CHECK BELOW THE KINDS OF WORK YOU HAVE DONE:

		☐ MEDICAL INSURANCE FORMS	☐ RECEPTIONIST
☐ BLOOD COUNTS	☐ DENTAL ASSISTANT	☐ MEDICAL TERMINOLOGY	☐ TELEPHONES
☐ BOOKKEEPING	☐ DENTAL HYGIENIST	☐ MEDICAL TRANSCRIPTION	☐ TYPING
☐ COLLECTIONS	☐ FILING	☐ NURSING	☐ STENOGRAPHY
☐ COMPOSING LETTERS	☐ INJECTIONS	☐ PHLEBOTOMY (Draw Blood)	☐ URINALYSIS
☐ COMPUTER INPUT	☐ INSTRUMENT STERILIZATION	☐ POSTING	☐ X-RAY
OFFICE EQUIPMENT USED: ☐ COMPUTER	☐ DICTATING EQUIPMENT	☐ WORD PROCESSOR	☐ OTHER:

Other Kinds Of Tasks Performed Or Skills That May Be Applicable To Position: | Typing Speed | Shorthand Speed

ORDER # 72-110 • © 1976 BIBBERO SYSTEMS, INC. • PETALUMA, CA. • (REV. 1/95)
TO REORDER CALL TOLL FREE: (800) BIBBERO (800-242-2376) OR FAX (800) 242-9330   MFG IN U.S.A.

(PLEASE COMPLETE OTHER SIDE)

FIGURE 24-3 Application for employment. Candidates for jobs in the medical office should complete applications accurately, leaving no blanks or unanswered questions. (Courtesy Bibbero Systems, Inc., Petaluma, Calif. 94954, (800) 242-2376, www.bibbero.com.)

E. EMPLOYMENT RECORD

LIST MOST RECENT EMPLOYMENT FIRST   May We Contact Your Previous Employer(s) For A Reference?   ☐ Yes ☐ No

1) Employer   Work Performed. Be Specific:

Address   Street   City   State   Zip Code

Phone Number
( )

Type of Business   Dates   Mo. Yr.   Mo. Yr.
                            From   To
Your Position   Hourly Rate/Salary
                            Starting   Final
Supervisor's Name

Reason For Leaving

2) Employer   Worked Performed. Be Specific:

Address   Street   City   State   Zip Code

Phone Number
( )

Type of Business   Dates   Mo. Yr.   Mo. Yr.
                            From   To
Your Position   Hourly Rate/Salary
                            Starting   Final
Supervisor's Name

Reason For Leaving

3) Employer   Worked Performed. Be Specific:

Address   Street   City   State   Zip Code

Phone Number
( )

Type of Business   Dates   Mo. Yr.   Mo. Yr.
                            From   To
Your Position   Hourly Rate/Salary
                            Starting   Final
Supervisor's Name

Reason For Leaving

F. REFERENCES — FRIENDS / ACQUAINTANCES NON-RELATED

(1) _____
    Name   Address   Telephone Number   (☐ Work ☐ Home)   Occupation   Years Acquainted
(1) _____
    Name   Address   Telephone Number   (☐ Work ☐ Home)   Occupation   Years Acquainted

Please Feel Free To Add Any Information Which You Feel Will Help Us Consider You For Employment

READ THE FOLLOWING CAREFULLY, THEN SIGN AND DATE THE APPLICATION

"I certify that all answers given by me on this application are true, correct and complete to the best of my knowledge. I acknowledge notice that the information contained in this application is subject to check. I agree that, if hired, my continued employment may be contingent upon the accuracy of that information. If employed, I further agree to comply with Company/Office rules and regulations."

Signature: _____   Date: _____

FIGURE 24-3, *cont'd*

and an applicant who does not fill it out in its entirety might be classified as lazy and prone to taking shortcuts. Watch for inconsistencies or oversights, including information that seems incomplete. Also look for resumes that are **targeted** toward the job opening available in the clinic. Targeted resumes are written specifically for a certain position. With today's computer capabilities, job seekers can target their resumes for each job applied for, and this strategy tells the manager that the applicant has enough interest in the job to demonstrate that he or she meets the requirements.

Once the entire stack of documents has been reviewed and separated, return to the stack of potential interviews. Careful judgment and objectivity must be used in the search for an employee who is suitable for the practice. Before interviewing any applicant, the manager needs to know several details:

- What personal qualities and abilities must the applicant have?
- What responsibilities are involved with the position?
- What is the salary range that the physician is willing to offer?
- How soon will the position be open?

Once these facts are clear, the manager should review the final resumes and applications with the following questions in mind:

- Do the applicant's appearance and personal grooming meet the standards set forth in the policy manual?
- Has the applicant been employed previously? What duties were performed?
- If previously employed, how long was the applicant in the last position? Why did the applicant leave?
- What are the applicant's skills? Do these meet the requirements for the position as set forth in the office procedure manual?
- Does the applicant seem to accept and enjoy responsibility?
- What is the applicant's formal education? Is he or she registered or certified? If not, is the applicant interested in taking the examination?
- Is the applicant a member of a professional organization? Does he or she attend meetings?

Arranging the Personal Interview

If the applicant sent a letter asking for an interview, note whether the letter was correctly typed and included essential contact information, and whether he or she also provided an attractive resume. Amazingly, many resumes do not include a contact telephone number! Many managers schedule interviews by email, but there are advantages to speaking to applicants directly. By telephoning the applicant, the manager will have an opportunity to judge his or her telephone voice. The manager may wish to prescreen applicants with the telephone call, asking several questions about the person's education and experience. Because the employee probably will speak with patients on the telephone, clarity of speech will be important. Those who perform well during the prescreening should be scheduled for an interview.

CRITICAL THINKING APPLICATION

- Katherine was impressed with Carol Limpken's resume and application, but when scheduling an interview on the telephone she noticed that Carol's grammar was not as professional as Katherine would like. Should this influence Katherine's decision to hire Carol?
- Why is speech such an important issue in the medical office?

Set a time for the personal interview when the applicant can be given undivided attention. An applicant who is being considered for employment should have an opportunity to see the office when there is a fairly normal amount of activity. The prospective employee who is interviewed in a peaceful, quiet office on the physician's day out may not be prepared for the activity on a normal working day.

Before interviewing any applicant, be thoroughly familiar with the federal, state, and local fair employment practice laws affecting hiring practices. Both men and women receive protection from on-the-job discrimination, sexual harassment, mandatory lie detector tests, and unfair discharge. Title VII of the Civil Rights Act of 1964, as amended by the Equal Employment Opportunity Act of 1972, prohibits inquiries into an applicant's race, color, sex, religion, and national origin. Inquiries regarding medical history, arrest records, or previous drug use are also illegal. Most states have laws designed to protect the rights of job applicants, and these laws may impose additional restrictions.

If an application has not been submitted, have the applicant complete it at the time of the interview. The application form can serve as a check of the applicant's penmanship and thoroughness as well as become a permanent record if the individual is hired. Tell the candidate if the form should be completed in the applicant's own handwriting, and be sure to state this on the instructions. Check to see if the applicant was **meticulous** about following instructions and filling in all the blanks. This provides the manager with an indication of the individual's capacity for following directions.

The Interview

The manager's first priority is to make certain that the applicant feels at ease (Figure 24-4). Shake his or her hand and ask a few social questions before starting the interview (Procedure 24-1). In general, use good manners and see that the person to be interviewed is comfortable. Most people feel some butterflies in the stomach when interviewing, but the manager will get a better idea of the person's capabilities if he or she is relaxed and able to discuss strengths and background openly with the manager.

Begin with a few open-ended questions that cannot be answered with a simple "yes" or "no," such as "What were your duties during your last position?" When interviewing a recent graduate who does not have experience, ask questions such as, "What subject did you perform well in at school?" When speaking with the candidate, make a mental note of whether he or she displays essential personal qualities, such as the ability to converse easily, the capacity to listen, and a bright smile. The applicant should be interested enough in the position to ask

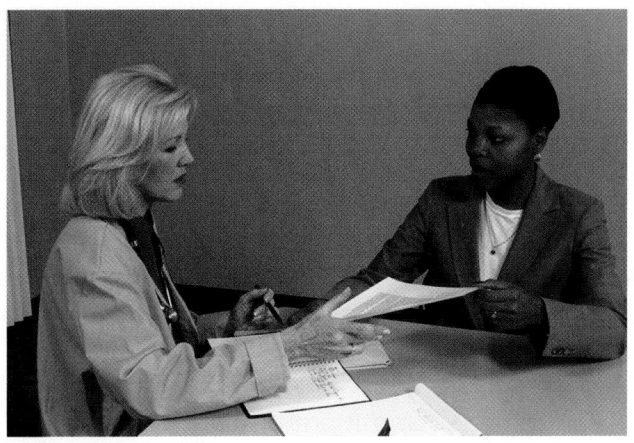

FIGURE 24-4 Put the applicant at ease. Job applicants perform at their peak when relaxed and calm.

Intelligent Questions for Late in the Interview

Interviewers expect candidates to ask intelligent questions concerning the organization and the nature of the work. Always indicate an interest in the position by asking questions. The medical assistant should ask a minimum of two intelligent questions at the end of the interview. Unless a few questions are asked by an interviewee, the interviewer may assume that he or she is not interested in the position. One cautionary note: never allow the first question asked to be about money or benefits. Ask other questions first, and end with a question about money or benefits if that information was not covered in the interview. This way, the interview can progress naturally into a negotiation stage, if the interviewer is ready to move in that direction.

Consider asking some of these questions if they have not been answered earlier in the interview:

- What are the duties and responsibilities of the job?
- How does this position relate to the other positions within the organization?
- How long has this position been a part of the organization, and how long has it been vacant?
- Could you describe the ideal person that you would like to place in this position?
- How have others succeeded or failed in this position in the past?
- With whom would I work?
- What would I be expected to accomplish in the first year?
- How will I be evaluated?
- Are promotions and raises tied to performance evaluations?
- Based on your experience, what type of problems would someone new in this position likely encounter?
- I'm interested in your career with this organization. When did you start? What do you enjoy about your job?
- How can I advance if I am hired at this company?
- What is particularly unique about this organization?
- What does the future look like for this organization?
- What is the salary range for this position? What benefits would I be eligible for, if I am hired?

intelligent questions and appear interested in the office and the physician's specialty.

Avoid inquiries that involve the applicant's privacy. The questions should be related to the available position and the applicant's ability to do the job. An interview is a two-way exchange of information between the applicant and the interviewer. If the applicant appears to be one who will receive serious consideration, explain what will be expected as an employee. Office policies regarding appearance, working hours, overtime, time off, and vacations may be discussed at this stage. Salary and other fringe benefits should be discussed once the manager is ready to offer the job. If the manager fails to mention these items, the applicant may be hesitant to inquire.

Some employers request a credit check before offering employment, especially if the individual will be handling practice finances. It can safely be assumed that one who is unable to handle personal financial affairs will be a poor risk in handling office finances.

Review the job description for the position being filled. The person being interviewed must understand the required duties and responsibilities of the job. Ask if the applicant has any questions, and close the interview on a positive note. Let the candidate know when a decision will be made and what further contact the office will initiate.

During the hiring proceedings, the manager may wish to invite the prospective employee to lunch with the staff or for coffee in the more relaxed atmosphere of the employee lounge. This presents an opportunity to discover whether the applicant's personality will mesh with the atmosphere of the office. Employees appreciate being asked their opinion on those who are potential team members.

An extensive list of interview questions can be found in Chapter 57.

Follow-Up Activities

When the interview is over, immediately take a few moments to rate the applicant while the interview is fresh in the memory. Jot down some notes so that the applicant will be remembered easily when the final decisions are being made as to who will be hired. Do not trust the impressions to memory, especially if several applicants have been interviewed. Never write harmful personal statements; instead, be objective and fair. Should the potential employee ever have cause to bring the physician to court for discrimination in hiring practices, there should be no **disparaging** information written down that would reflect in a negative way on the physician or office manager.

Always carefully check all references and follow through on any leads for information. Use the telephone in checking references, because people are sometimes less than candid in a letter; furthermore, letter writing is time consuming and a reply may never be sent. If the email address for a reference is provided, this is an excellent way to check a reference, and the printed version may be added to the applicant's file.

Prepare a checklist before placing the call. When speaking with the person called, be sure to "listen between the lines." Note the tone of the replies to the questions. Do not ask

PROCEDURE 24-1

Interview a Job Candidate

<u>ABHES COMPETENCY:</u> 2.f

GOAL: *To evaluate job candidates fairly and choose the best person to fill an available position in the medical facility.*

EQUIPMENT and SUPPLIES

- Candidate's completed job application
- Candidate's resume
- Private area in the medical office
- Clerical supplies

PROCEDURAL STEPS

1. Review the job requirements that the candidate will be required to perform.
   <u>PURPOSE:</u> To properly evaluate candidates, one must determine the tasks that the new employee will be expected to perform.
2. Match each job application with the corresponding resume.
3. Separate strong candidates from moderate candidates and poor candidates.
   <u>PURPOSE:</u> To screen the best candidates and invite them to interview for the position.
4. Review each resume and job application again, and determine which candidates should be brought to the office for an interview.
5. Call each candidate and schedule an appointment for an interview.
6. Evaluate the applicant's speaking voice while making the appointment or the interview.
   <u>PURPOSE:</u> To determine the candidate's professionalism and ability to speak clearly and with clarity on the telephone.
7. Select several interview questions in advance to ask all of the applicants.
   <u>PURPOSE:</u> To avoid having to think of questions during the actual interview.
8. Note whether the applicant arrives on time for the interview.
   <u>PURPOSE:</u> If the candidate does not arrive on time for the interview, he or she may be a habitually late employee.
9. Introduce yourself to the applicant, and proceed to a private area to conduct the interview.

10. Make the applicant feel as much at ease as possible.
    <u>PURPOSE:</u> Most individuals are a little nervous during job interviews, and if helped to relax they will be able to present their qualifications and skills confidently.
11. Ask the applicant the chosen questions.
12. Evaluate the answers and make notations about the candidate that are not demeaning or unprofessional.
    <u>PURPOSE:</u> Demeaning comments in an employee file may eventually be seen if there is a subsequent lawsuit, and this can reflect poorly on the person who made the comments.
13. Ask the candidate if he or she has any questions.
    <u>PURPOSE:</u> Evaluate the types of questions that the employee asks; determine whether they are intelligent questions and if they indicate a true interest in the position.
14. Offer strong candidates a brief tour of the facility.
15. Provide a date that a hiring decision will be made, and suggest that the candidate call the facility that day, if desired.
16. Evaluate all applicants fairly according to their experience and training.
17. Select the best three candidates, and call them for a second interview, if desired.
18. Discuss the final hiring decisions with the physician or others with influence.
    <u>PURPOSE:</u> Some physicians want to make the final hiring decisions.
19. Make the final hiring decision.
20. Call the candidate to come to the office to discuss the position.
21. Negotiate salary and benefits.
22. Offer the position.
23. If the offer is declined, call the next candidate to the office to discuss the position until a satisfactory candidate accepts and agrees to a start date.

questions that might incriminate the person answering them. The following questions are effective as an introduction:

- When did (the applicant) work for you?
- For how long?
- What were the duties and responsibilities?
- Did the employee assume responsibility well?

Some employers will provide information only on the date of hire, job title, and date of termination of the employment. Respect the company's policy and do not press for further information.

CRITICAL THINKING APPLICATION

- While checking Carol's references, Katherine speaks to her last employer, who makes the statement, "she is not eligible for rehire." The former employer placed strong emphasis on the word "not." All of Carol's other references were glowing. Should Katherine decide not to hire Carol on the basis of this employer's comment?
- How might Katherine find out more about the situation with the last employer?

Any person who is granted an interview should send a thank-you letter to the person who interviewed him or her. Watch the mail to see if any of the applicants perform this important follow-up task.

A second interview may be granted when the field is narrowed to two or three candidates. The physician may wish to participate in these interviews. Some offices conduct a group interview with several staff members present. Remember that these interviews become more and more stressful for the candidate, and the manager should expect some nervousness. Do not "count off" in the interview for mild nervousness.

Making the Selection

When a decision has been reached to hire someone, it is best to bring the successful candidate back into the office to offer the position and negotiate the final details. The office manager may wish to wait until the first-choice candidate has actually accepted the offer before notifying anyone else that the job has been filled. Don't expect the potential employee to answer the offer on the spot. Twenty-four hours is a reasonable time to consider the offer.

Remember to notify all others who have interviewed for the position that it has been filled so that they can continue their job search. They may have hesitated to accept other interviews, and it is unfair to keep individuals who are seeking employment hoping for a telephone call from the physician's office. Good etiquette requires dropping them a note or calling to say that the position is filled. Although this is a rare practice in today's busy clinics, all of the applicants who interviewed were surely the manager's best candidates and professional individuals. Therefore, they deserve a brief call and a wish for success in their job search. Thank the individual for applying, and offer to keep his or her application on file, if the candidate was especially impressive.

ORIENTATION AND TRAINING—CRITICAL FACTORS FOR SUCCESSFUL EMPLOYEES

Recruitment does not end with the hiring. Orientation and training will help new employees to understand what is expected and to develop to their full potential (Figure 24-5). One of the most critical errors in bringing new staff members aboard is not providing them with a fair orientation and training period. The office manager should develop a checklist of the paperwork needed for newly hired staff and all of the information that should be covered with the new employee at the onset of the job.

Some managers assign a mentor to assist the new employee during the initial probationary period. This is a guide whom the new staff member can approach with questions and concerns (Figure 24-6). Using this type of "buddy" system is a good practice, because the new person does not feel isolated and alone during the first few weeks on the job.

Acquaint the new employee with such aspects of the office as the following:
- Staff members and their names
- Physical environment and layout of the office

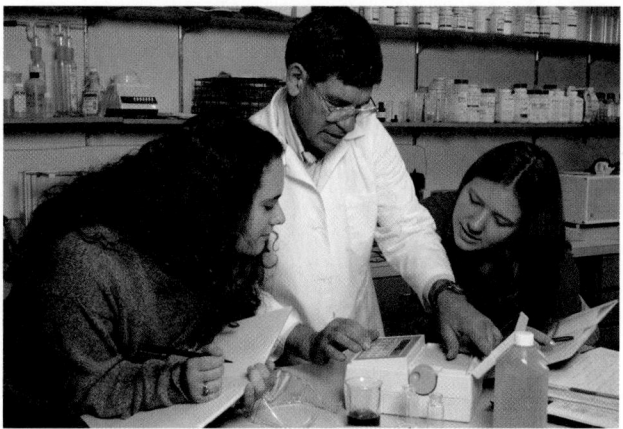
FIGURE 24-5 Training the employee well contributes greatly toward his or her success.

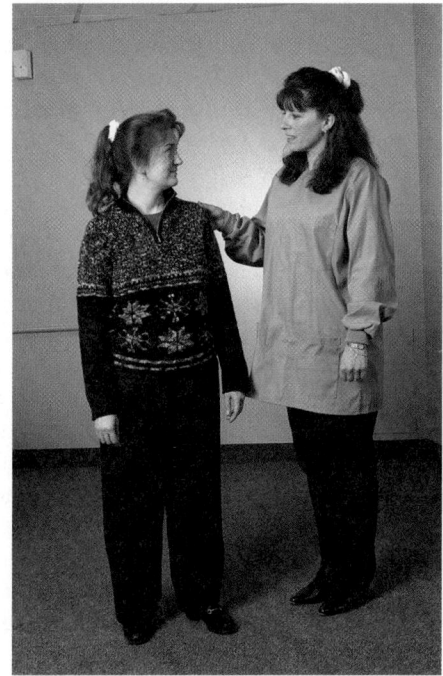
FIGURE 24-6 Mentors are valuable to the new employee. A mentor provides assistance to new employees who are learning their duties and growing accustomed to the medical office.

- Nature of the practice and specialty
- Types of patients seen in the office
- Office policies
- Long-range expectations

All new employees should be required to read the office policy and procedure manual. It is advisable for the manager to require the employee to sign a statement verifying that the manuals were read.

Be sure that all federal and state regulations are met where new employees are concerned. Occupational Safety and Health Administration (OSHA) training must be provided to employees at risk for exposures before they begin any duties. Health Insurance Portability and Accountability Act (HIPAA) training is also required. Certain documents that verify the employee's right to work in the United States must be examined also. It is wise to insist on a fully completed personnel file before allowing the employee to work even 1 hour. Documents that prove worker eligibility are especially important to obtain.

CRITICAL THINKING APPLICATION

Katherine is bringing in a new employee who must begin work on the following Monday, because the staff has been short one person for approximately 2 weeks. However, Katherine will be going on vacation the same day. How can she ensure that the new employee is trained properly?

Job Descriptions

The job description is a tool designed to inform employees about the duties they are expected to perform. Well-written job descriptions list the essential functions of the job and reveal the chain of command that the employee should follow when questions or concerns arise. These documents provide a good guideline for employees so that they will understand exactly what is expected of them and what they are responsible for at work.

The job description should include a statement that says the employee must perform any additional duties as assigned by the supervisor. With this statement in place, the employee cannot say "that is not my job." All employees should be willing to pull together and assist with any tasks, but this statement gives added weight to assignments that are not specified in the written job description.

An effective manager understands the phrase "inspect what you expect." When duties are assigned, the manager should ensure that the tasks were completed correctly and in a timely manner. New employees should be monitored to make certain that their delegated tasks are getting done and getting done right. Without inspection, the manager cannot know that the new employee is meeting expectations. Once employees have earned a degree of trust, inspecting their work is not as necessary as in the beginning. Many managers practice a skill called "management by walking around." By strolling through the areas where subordinates work, managers can observe and hear about issues that might be brewing, while at the same time improve morale by offering encouragement and praise.

Staff Development Training

Continuous training and staff development are vital aspects of any medical office. Constant advancements and technologic changes take place, and employees must be kept up to date on those changes. Meetings should be held at least quarterly to ensure that the staff is using the latest techniques and current regulations when dealing with issues that confront the medical facility.

Delegation of Duties

Delegating duties to subordinates allows managers to concentrate on the most critical aspects of their own jobs. Delegation also provides an opportunity for the employees to grow and learn new skills. Some managers are hesitant to assign duties to employees because they feel the tasks are too important not to be completed by the manager. This hesitation suggests either a refusal to release control or mistrust of the employees. However, this type of manager will soon be overrun with tasks and unable to complete them. Managers should place trust in employees who have earned it and allow them to prove their abilities.

Discover the strengths of individual employees, then assign them tasks that will allow them to use those strengths. If a medical assistant was hired to do administrative duties but is good with phlebotomy, encourage and allow the employee to assist with venipunctures whenever needed.

USING PERFORMANCE EVALUATIONS EFFECTIVELY

A new employee should be granted a probationary period. A period of 60 to 90 days has been traditional, but many employers believe that 2 weeks is sufficient to determine whether the employee will be able to learn and adapt to the position.

Set a definite date for a performance review covering the probationary period at the time of employment. This review should not be squeezed in between patient visits or be given a token few minutes at the end of a day. There should be ample time to relax and talk. At this time, tell the new employee how well expectations have been met and whether there are any deficiencies. Then give the employee an opportunity to ask questions. Sometimes an employee fails to perform because he or she was never told what was expected. Although the probationary period does not always allow time to fully train an individual for a specific position, it is fair to assume that the potential for being a satisfactory employee can be judged at this time. Now is the time to talk out any problems and make suggestions for improvement. Sometimes the employee is released after an unsuccessful probationary period.

The performance **appraisal** includes a judgment of both the quality and quantity of work, personal appearance, attitudes and team spirit, dependability, self-discipline, motivation, attendance, punctuality, and any other qualities essential to satisfactory performance of the job in question (Figure 24-7). The supervisor is responsible for ongoing performance appraisals of all employees, complimenting whenever possible and appropriate and offering helpful criticism when necessary. A formal performance appraisal at the end of the probationary period and at regular 6-month intervals thereafter, with a report to the physician employer, is helpful in the employee's salary review (Procedure 24-2, p. 489).

When negative information is to be relayed to the employee during a performance appraisal, sandwich the negative comment between two positive ones whenever possible. For instance, tell the employee:

"Jewel, you are a pro at greeting patients and making them feel at home. I would like to see you improve your time management skills, however, because I feel you are spending too much time with each individual patient. I must confess that they feel a part of the clinic family. Just watch the time and keep making them feel so welcome!"

PERFORMANCE EVALUATION AND DEVELOPMENT PLAN
(OFFICE AND CLERICAL)

NAME: _____   DATE OF EVALUATION:_____

DATE OF HIRE: _____   DEPARTMENT: _____

JOB TITLE: _____   SUPERVISOR: _____

DATE APPOINTED THIS JOB: _____   MANAGER:_____

LAST REVIEW DATE: _____   LAST REVIEW RATING: _____

NEXT REVIEW DATE: _____   CURRENT REVIEW RATING: _____

PURPOSE

The purpose of this evaluation is to:

1. SET GOALS WITHIN SCOPE OF PRESENT JOB.
2. COMMUNICATE OPENLY ABOUT PERFORMANCE.
3. EVALUATE PAST PERFORMANCE.
4. DISCUSS FUTURE DEVELOPMENT PLANS FOR GROWTH.

INSTRUCTIONS

1. Supervisor to review form prior to completion. If specific items are not applicable they should be left blank.

2. Supervisor and employee to review job description prior to review.

3. In "COMMENTS" section supervisor may indicate which factors should be more heavily weighted in this particular evaluation.

4. Comments should be specific and job-related. All appropriate evaluation factors should be commented on to some degree.

I.   POSITION OBJECTIVES AND MAJOR RESPONSIBILITIES. Summarize specific responsibilities of the job.

_____

_____

_____

II. ACCOMPLISHMENTS AND/OR IMPROVEMENTS. What specific accomplishments and/or improvements has employee made since last review with respect to set goals?

_____

_____

_____

PLEASE CONSIDER THE EMPLOYEE'S DEMONSTRATED PERFORMANCE AND MARK THE CIRCLE WHICH MOST CLOSELY DESCRIBES THAT PERFORMANCE.

4 - Performance consistently far exceeds expectations and requirements.
3 - Performance consistently exceeds normal expectations and job requirements.
2 - Performance consistently meets expectations and job requirements
1 - Performance usually meets expectations and minimum job requirements.
0 - Performance does not meet job requirements.

– CONTINUED, NEXT PAGE –

FORM # 72-119 © 1987 BIBBERO SYSTEMS, INC. PETALUMA, CA

TO REORDER CALL TOLL FREE:
800-BIBBERO /(800 242-2376) OR
FAX: (800) 242-9330 MFG IN U.S.A.

FIGURE 24-7 Performance evaluation and development plan. Performance evaluations should be considered tools that will help employees reach their personal goals and the goals of the organization. (Courtesy Bibbero Systems, Inc., Petaluma, Calif. 94954, (800) 242-2376, www.bibbero.com.)

7. DEPENDABILITY: CONSIDER ATTENDANCE, PUNCTUALITY, IDLE TIME AND RELIANCE WHICH CAN BE PLACED ON EMPLOYEE TO PERSEVERE AND CARRY THROUGH TO COMPLETION ALL ASSIGNED TASKS

○ 0   ○ 1   ○ 2   ○ 3   ○ 4

_____

_____

_____

8. COMPLIANCE WITH COMPANY POLICIES: DOES THE EMPLOYEE COMPLY WITH RULES AND REGULATIONS WHICH APPLY TO SAFETY, FAIR EMPLOYMENT PRACTICES AND GENERAL ADMINISTRATIVE PROCEDURE.

○ 0   ○ 1   ○ 2   ○ 3   ○ 4

_____

_____

_____

9. SPECIFIC PERFORMANCE	1	2	3	4	COMMENTS
A. Ability to handle scheduling:					
B. Willingness to work OT when necessary:					
C. Handling of calls and follow-up:					
D. Maintenance of equipment:					
E. Ability to handle patient complaints:					
F. Tact in dealing with patients:					
G. Speed (in specific technical procedures):					
H. Secretarial accuracy:					
I. Professional terminology:					
J. Assisting procedures:					
K. Laboratory techniques:					
L. X-ray techniques:					
M. Physical therapy:					
N. Collections:					
O. Medical Insurance:					
P. Bookkeeping:					

10. PERSONAL	1	2	3	4	COMMENTS
A. Grooming:					
B. Professional conduct:					
C. Energy, enthusiasm:					
D. Ability to handle stress:					

ADDITIONAL COMMENTS: _____

_____

_____

_____

_____

_____

FORM # 72-119 © 1987 BIBBERO SYSTEMS, INC. PETALUMA, CA

FIGURE 24-7, *cont'd*

PROCEDURE 24-2

Conduct a Performance Review

<u>ABHES COMPETENCY:</u> 7.d.

GOAL: *To evaluate job performance fairly and determine the strengths and weaknesses of employees.*

EQUIPMENT and SUPPLIES

- Employee's file
- Past evaluations of employee
- Notes and/or reports regarding employee behavior
- Private area in the medical office
- Clerical supplies

PROCEDURAL STEPS

1. Set an appointment with the employee to conduct the review.
2. Allow the employee to complete a self-evaluation of his or her own work.
   <u>PURPOSE:</u> To gain insight into how the employee sees his or her own work performance and allow input as to how the employee feels that he or she has performed during the evaluation period.
3. Review the self-evaluation, then document additional information about the employee and his or her performance.
4. Share the information with any other supervisor or the physician, if dictated by office policy or if additional input is necessary.
   <u>PURPOSE:</u> The physician may have additional input that needs to be documented and discussed during the review.
5. Complete the final written review, and proofread it for accuracy and completeness.
6. Discuss the review with the employee during the evaluation appointment.
   <u>PURPOSE:</u> Discussion should promote an understanding of what is expected by the employer.
7. Progress through the interview, and explain the results of the evaluation to the employee.
8. Allow the employee to respond to any of the points raised during the evaluation, but do not allow an argumentative attitude.
   <u>PURPOSE:</u> o gain insight into the employee's reasons for any poor performance without becoming belligerent.
9. Allow the employee to respond in writing to the evaluation for a limited time, such as 5 days.
   <u>PURPOSE:</u> To give the employee a chance to insert his or her input into the performance report.
10. Ask the employee to sign the evaluation to document that it was reviewed with him or her. (The employee does not have to agree with the evaluation to sign it.).
11. Give a copy of the evaluation to the employee.
12. File the evaluation in the employee's file.

Managers also may use the "feel, felt, found" approach when talking with employees about their performance. Consider the following example:

"Jewel, I feel the same way you do about the patients taking up a lot of our time. I know there are some that want to talk with us for hours, and I have felt the pressure of wanting to make them feel comfortable but having so much to do, too. I have found that if I explain that I have a meeting or another patient to assist, they are very understanding and not offended. Perhaps you can try that approach, too."

Peer Evaluations

Some innovative companies use peer evaluations of employees to get a different view of the work performed by a worker. Asking co-workers to assist in the evaluation process can promote teamwork and cooperation. The rare employee will offer a poor evaluation because of a personal problem with another staff member, but for the most part employees will provide fair, unbiased evaluations, knowing that they will also be evaluated when it is their turn.

Evaluations called *360-degree evaluations* are excellent tools for evaluating any employees, including managers. Such evaluations usually consist of a questionnaire that is given to those who work closely with the employee, and they provide input regarding the performance of the person being evaluated.

Poor Evaluations Made Easier

No supervisor enjoys giving an evaluation that is not a positive one. It is difficult to know where to begin when the employee has not performed as expected or hoped. Perhaps the best way to open the conversation is to say,

"Rebecca, your review today is not going to be a positive one. It seems that we do not have a meeting of the minds about your duties and our expectations of you. Let's talk about your performance and discuss whether this position is a good match for you."

The manager should have good documentation of the problems that led to the poor evaluation. If so, these can be reviewed with the employee with specific times, dates, and descriptions of incidents. If the manager does not document these issues, the conversation can become an argument and grow quite heated. Firm dates and times leave little room for argument and place the manager on the offensive.

The employee may be apprehensive or even defensive at this point, but the phrasing will certainly get his or her attention, and the discussion should produce either the motivation to improve or the clarity that termination is in order.

CRITICAL THINKING APPLICATION

- While Katherine gives an evaluation to a particularly poor employee whom Katherine plans to terminate, the employee begins screaming and accusing Katherine of discrimination and harassment. How should Katherine handle this situation?
- What are Katherine's options if the employee does not stop the inappropriate behavior?

Terminating Employees

The necessity for dismissing an employee is unpleasant at best, but if the ground rules are decided on in advance, written into the policy manual, and explained to all employees, the problem is partially solved. The policies must be applied equally and impartially to all. The final decision for dismissal probably will be made by the physician but may be based on the recommendation of the office manager or supervisor. The person who does the hiring should do the firing.

The probationary employee who does not prove satisfactory should be dismissed at the end of the probationary period, with tact and a full explanation of the reasons for dismissal. In all fairness, an individual should be told why the employment is being ended and not be given weak excuses or untruths that do not help to correct deficiencies. If the manager is not straightforward in giving the reason for dismissal, the employee will not have the opportunity to grow and improve his or her performance.

An employee who has been in service for some time and is offering unsatisfactory performance should be warned and given an explanation of the specific improvements expected (Figure 24-8). If a second chance does not produce improvement in performance or attitude, then dismissal must follow. It should be done privately, with tact and consideration.

Most practice consultants believe that firing should come close to the end of the day, after all other employees have left, and that the break should be clean and immediate. If the office policy provides for 2 weeks' notice, the physician may wish to offer 2 weeks' pay unless the circumstances that led to the dismissal were extremely **blatant.** A dismissed employee should never be allowed to train or influence a replacement.

The exit meeting should be planned just as carefully as the employment interview. Be honest with the employee. Discuss the employee's assets as well as liabilities, and give the reasons for the termination. There is no need to dwell on the employee's deficiencies. These should have been thoroughly discussed at the warning interview, and the employee need only be told that the necessary improvements have not been made. Do listen to the employee's feedback, unless it becomes abusive. This may reveal some important administrative problems that need correction.

After dismissing an employee, do not leave that person in the office unattended. Request and get the office keys and any other equipment in the employee's possession before the dismissed employee leaves the building. Most states have strict payday laws that will not allow holding the final paycheck for

any reason. Do not offer to give the employee a good reference unless it can be done sincerely.

Certain breaches of conduct, such as **embezzlement, insubordination,** and violation of patient confidentiality, are grounds for immediate dismissal without warning.

Occasionally an employee voluntarily terminates a job without giving a valid reason. The physician or office manager may wish to follow up with a letter to the former employee to determine whether a problem prompted the resignation.

CRITICAL THINKING APPLICATION

- Katherine has two employees who have never seemed to get along. One of the employees has a history of being vindictive and manipulative, but never in an obvious enough way for Katherine to have sufficient proof to reprimand her in writing. One day, this employee comes to Katherine's office to report that she saw the other employee, who has an exemplary record, taking drugs from the supply cabinet. How does Katherine react to this situation?
- What steps should Katherine take from here?

Fair Salaries and Raises

Medical office managers should recruit employees who will remain with the office for a long period of time. There are always situations when a part-time worker returns to college, or someone working during the summer months goes back to school. However, good employee **retention** is a goal to work toward.

For good employees to be kept, they must be paid a fair salary and will expect regular raises if they are performing as expected. The office manager can find information about salary comparisons on the Internet. Check the job duties and descriptions found on the web, and see if the salary that the medical facility is offering is comparable to other salaries for similar jobs in the area.

Merit raises are increases based on an employee's commendable performance. Cost-of-living increases are given when earned, usually after specific periods or annually, and are based on national statistics and trends. An employee who is being promoted may be awarded a salary increase, also. When the office pays a fair salary for the work being done, the physician will retain happy employees.

STAFF MEETINGS

There must be some formal mechanism for keeping the office manager and other key employees current on the daily business affairs of the practice. One of the most common complaints from office personnel is that of being unable to discuss problems with the physician. The solution to this problem may be to hold regular staff meetings, which may be scheduled as frequently as weekly but should be held no less often than quarterly (Figure 24-9). Some of the best ideas on improvement come from the office staff, and expressing ideas should be encouraged.

The simplest technique is to set aside a specific time for regular meetings at an hour when the most people can attend

TERMINATION / REHIRE EVALUATION FORM

Employee Name_____ Social Security No._____

Department _____ Title _____

Termination Date _____

Reason for Termination: _____Resigned _____Laid Off_____Retired

Evaluation of Job Performance	Excellent	Very Good	Average	Poor	Unacceptable
Quality (accuracy, etc.)	☐	☐	☐	☐	☐
Quantity (productivity, consistency, etc.)	☐	☐	☐	☐	☐
Knowledge of Duties	☐	☐	☐	☐	☐
Reliability (absenteeism)	☐	☐	☐	☐	☐
Punctuality	☐	☐	☐	☐	☐
Ability to Cooperate with Co-workers	☐	☐	☐	☐	☐
Relationship with Patients	☐	☐	☐	☐	☐
Overall Attitude (willingness and commitment)	☐	☐	☐	☐	☐
Initiative	☐	☐	☐	☐	☐
Judgment	☐	☐	☐	☐	☐

Recommendation for Rehiring: _____

_____

_____

Comments:_____

_____

_____

_____

_____

_____

_____

_____

_____ Date _____

Supervisor's Signature

FORM # 72-123 PERSONNEL RECORDS ORGANIZING SYSTEMS • © 1987 BIBBERO SYSTEMS, INC. • PETALUMA, CA.
TO REORDER CALL TOLL FREE: (800) BIBBERO (800-242-2376) OR FAX (800) 242-9330   MFG IN U.S.A.

FIGURE 24-8 Termination form. Document the reasons for terminating employees, and be sure that there is supporting documentation showing warnings and previous counseling efforts. (Courtesy Bibbero Systems, Inc., Petaluma, Calif. 94954, (800) 242-2376, www.bibbero.com.)

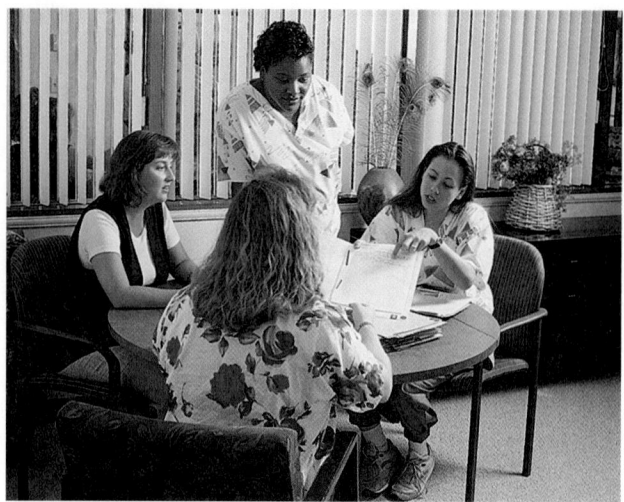

FIGURE 24-9 Periodic staff meetings are important tools for improving communication and resolving problems.

with the least disruption (Procedure 24-3). The meetings need not be long or overly formal, but to be effective they must be planned and organized. There must be a leader, and a secretary should be appointed to take notes. The effectiveness of the leader, a person who can balance firmness with fairness, is an important aspect of the meeting. This is usually either the physician or the office manager or supervisor. All members of the staff should be encouraged to submit ideas for discussion.

Draw up a simple **agenda** listing the issues to be discussed, and prepare any supporting data needed for the meeting. There are many kinds of staff meetings. They may be purely informational, problem-solving, or brainstorming meetings. They may be work sessions for updating manuals, training seminars, or whatever is necessary to that individual practice. Or, meetings may be scheduled to discuss new ideas and any changes in office procedures. Some meetings are held simply to resolve specific problems. The staff meeting must not be allowed to deteriorate into a gripe session. Individual complaints should be handled privately.

The meeting must have a set agenda, with time for topics that need discussion on a regular basis as well as time to handle any current problems. The agenda might be similar to that of any business meeting:

1. Reading of the last meeting's minutes
2. Discussion of any unfinished business
3. Discussion of any problems in the clinical area
4. Discussion of any problems in the administrative area
5. Discussion of any problems in common areas
6. Adjournment

Some physicians like to combine the staff meeting with a breakfast or lunch. The time or place is not important as long as it is neutral and meets the needs of the practice. Meetings should be conducted regularly, democratically, and without interruption. There must be follow-up to the items discussed; otherwise, the only result will be frustration and a reluctance to discuss problems at future meetings.

SEEING THE WHOLE PICTURE

The office manager must keep a bird's-eye view on the office operations. He or she must look at the whole picture when difficulties arise. Remember, there are always two sides to every story, and there is usually truth intermingled with falsity. Do not form the habit of taking every word that an employee says as being 100% accurate. This is not meant to suggest that all employees are not truthful, but to encourage the office manager to look at all sides before making critical decisions.

See issues from the employees' point of view. Try to understand their perspective when dealing with everyday situations in the medical facility. Do not become closed-minded as a manager, unable to grasp what the employees see as important.

OTHER OFFICE MANAGER RESPONSIBILITIES

Patient Information Folder

Only a very small percentage of practices have a booklet that explains the information basic to the operational and service aspects of the practice. Yet, the physician and staff can easily compile a patient information folder cooperatively during a staff meeting. Experience has shown that if such a folder is given to every new patient, the number of incoming telephone calls can be reduced by an average of 20% to 30%. It also can reduce misunderstandings and forgotten instructions. The folder must of necessity be tailored to the specific practice.

The patient information folder should be an introduction to the practice and, if possible, mailed to a new patient before the first visit. A supply also may be left with referring physicians' offices to be given to patients coming to your office. It should be designed to fit easily into a No. 10 business envelope.

The cover should show the name of the practice, its location, and the practice logo, if there is one. Consider using a photo of the medical building for easy identification by the new patient, and a map to the office.

A statement of philosophy frequently is included in the introduction, followed by a description of the practice, such as in the example below:

"The doctors and staff would like to welcome you to our office. We work as a team with the goal of providing prompt and thorough care for your problems. We are always working to improve our care and service in any way possible. Our practice is limited exclusively to the musculoskeletal system and its disorders. Therefore it is important for each patient to have a primary care physician such as a pediatrician, family physician, or internist to oversee the primary medical care for the entire patient. Our role is most effective as a consultant to your primary care physician."

Describe the office policy regarding appointments and cancellations, telephone calls, and the function of the answering service. If a separate business telephone line is available, be sure to include this information, as in the following example:

"This office has two receptionists available to answer telephone calls during regular office hours. The office is very busy, and occasionally you will be asked to hold for a brief period. Please be patient with this. If you wish to speak to a doctor, your call usually will be returned during the next available break period or

PROCEDURE 24-3

Arrange a Group Meeting

ABHES COMPETENCY: 3.a

GOAL: *To plan and execute a productive meeting that will result in achieved goals.*

EQUIPMENT and SUPPLIES

- Meeting room
- Agenda
- Visual aids and equipment
- Handouts
- Stopwatch or clock
- Computer or word processor
- Paper
- List of items for the agenda

PROCEDURAL STEPS

1. Determine the purpose of the meeting, and draft a list of the items to be discussed. Include the desired results of the meeting.
   PURPOSE: To keep the focus on the issues at hand and make the meeting a productive one.

2. Determine where the meeting will be held, the time and date of the meeting, and the individuals who should attend.
   PURPOSE: To have the demographic information about the meeting on hand before posting a notice. Only necessary staff members should attend, so that those not directly involved in the issues to be discussed can continue their regular duties.

3. Send a memo, email, or letter at least 10 days in advance, if possible, to the individuals who should attend the meeting. Send a copy to any supervisors who should be kept informed about the issues to be raised in the meeting.
   PURPOSE: To allow for rescheduling if the key personnel cannot attend on the originally planned time and date. To keep managers informed of important details in areas for which they are ultimately responsible.

4. Be sure that the notice includes the following information:
   - Date
   - Time
   - Place
   - Directions, if not in a common meeting room or if away from the office
   - Speakers and/or meeting topics
   - Cost and registration information, if applicable
   - List of items individuals should bring to the meeting
   PURPOSE: To fully inform those who should attend the meeting of the demographic information and their responsibilities.

5. Finalize the list of items to discuss, and place them in priority order.
   PURPOSE: To keep the focus of the meeting on the issues at hand and to avoid discussion of nonrelated items. To make certain that the time spent in the meeting is productive for all involved.

6. Delegate any tasks that others can accomplish, and follow up to be sure that they fulfill their duties before the meeting.
   PURPOSE: To ensure that all needed information and items are available for the meeting.

7. Assign a staff member the task of taking notes and keeping time during the meeting.
   PURPOSE: To have notes as to what happened so that a permanent record of what was discussed and the decisions that were made can be written after the meeting.

8. Make a list of all items that need to be taken to the meeting, including equipment such as microphones, projectors, screens, computers, disks containing presentations, and so on.
   PURPOSE: To be fully prepared and have all needed items in place during the meeting.

9. Compile the final agenda for the meeting.

10. On the meeting day, transport all items needed to the meeting room. Begin and end the meeting on time. Stay on track, and follow the agenda.
    PURPOSE: Following the plan and being considerate of the time that staff members devote to meetings will promote a positive attitude for meetings and will encourage group participation.

11. Follow up whenever necessary on items discussed in the meetings. Distribute a synopsis of the meeting to all of the individuals who attended, and keep a copy in a binder or folder.
    PURPOSE: To have a permanent record of the meeting and the items discussed and decided.

---

at the end of the office day. We receive many calls during the day, and it is unfair to the patients who have scheduled appointments to continually interrupt the doctor for telephone calls. Therefore the receptionist usually will take a message, and your call will be returned as soon as possible. Please inform the receptionist if your problem is urgent and she will let the doctor know this."

Describe any **ancillary** or laboratory services provided, how test results are reported, and your policy on prescription renewals. Patients need to know the provisions for emergency procedures: What hospitals does the practice use regularly?

What is the night and weekend coverage? Hospitalization procedures and postoperative care and follow-up may also be included:

"One of the doctors in the group is always on call for emergency situations. You may reach him by calling our office telephone number (714) 555-2323, and the answering service will put you in touch with the doctor on call at that time. Our doctors are on staff at St. Joseph Hospital (714) 555-3333 and, for children, Children's Hospital of Orange County (714) 555-4444. In case of emergency, call 911."

List all physicians in the practice; state their educational backgrounds, training, and board certifications; and define their specialties. List the names of key clinical and administrative staff members, such as registered nurses and nurse practitioners, medical assistants, the office manager, and the business manager. Provide the practice address, a map of how to get there, and information about the parking facilities.

Do not just stack these folders in the reception room for patients to pick up. Have the receptionist write the patient's name on the folder, hand it to the patient when he or she registers for the first appointment, and suggest that the patient keep it for future reference.

Financial Policy Folder

A separate small folder covering the financial policies of the office can eliminate many questions and possible misunderstandings. Tailor the financial policy folder to the specific practice. Keep it small enough to fit into the billing envelope, and send it out with the first monthly statement. If the practice sends out a welcome package before the patient's first visit, include the financial policy folder. Otherwise, present one at the first visit.

Spell out policies regarding billing and collection procedures, and make it clear that patients are responsible for the uninsured portion of the fees. If payment is expected at the time of service, put this in the folder. Keep the language simple and straightforward so that the message is clear:

"We ask that our services be paid for at the time they are rendered. You will be provided with an encounter form so that you may bill your insurance company and be reimbursed for services paid at the time of your visit. Simply attach the encounter form to your insurance form and mail it to the insurance company. The appropriate diagnoses and charges will be on the encounter form. There is usually a greater charge for the initial visit, because this involves more time than follow-up visits. If you are sent to an outside office for laboratory testing or special x-ray procedures, you will be billed separately by that office. We will be available to help if special circumstances arise involving difficulty with forms or receiving reimbursement. We will bill your insurance if you have a special situation such as surgery, prepaid health plans, Medicaid, CCS, or Senior Savers. We will complete disability papers as promptly as possible. However, you must obtain the necessary forms from your employer or the disability office."

The financial policy folder should also clearly state that the ultimate responsibility for payment lies with the patient.

Patient Instruction Sheets

In most medical offices there are patient procedures that occur over and over again. Instead of attempting to instruct a patient orally each time, why not develop clearly stated instruction sheets that can be reviewed with the patient, then give the patient the written instructions to take home? The following are suggestions for patient instruction sheets:

- Preparation for x-ray procedure or laboratory tests
- Preoperative and postoperative instructions
- Diet sheets
- Performing an enema
- Dressing a wound
- Taking medications
- Using a cane, crutches, walker, or wheelchair
- Care of casts
- Exercise therapy

Moving a Practice

The thought of moving into a shiny new spacious office can be exciting. However, unless the move is planned in advance, moving day and the weeks that follow can be a nightmare.

Planning the New Quarters

Do some careful measuring to see how the furniture and equipment that will be moved will fit into the new quarters. If possible, draw the rooms to scale and show where each item is to be placed by the mover. Include the location of available electrical outlets in the floor plan. If new furniture, carpets, or equipment is needed, try to have them in place before moving day. Do not expect to have the new carpet installed the day of the move.

Establishing a Moving Date

Decide what day the move will take place and whether the office will close for 1 day or several. Select a mover, and confirm the date. Patients must be notified of the move. As soon as the moving date is established, post a notice in the office and draw the patients' attention to it. Send announcement cards to the active patients. Many physicians place a notice in the local newspapers.

Notifying Utilities and Mailers

At least 60 days in advance of the move, start a change-of-address notification campaign. Notify publishers of journals and suppliers of catalogs. Cards for changes of address are available from the post office. Six weeks' notice generally is required on subscriptions, and postage due on forwarded journals can be very expensive. Notify the telephone company and utility companies well in advance so that there will be no break in service. File a change of address card with the local post office. Order stationery and business cards with the new address.

Packing

The moving company will supply packing cartons. Have each employee be responsible for packing and labeling the items from his or her own work area. Tag each carton with a number, and keep a master list of what is in each numbered carton. This will help in finding items that are needed. Also, if a carton should be lost or mislaid, a record of what was in it will be available. If time allows, just before moving is a good time to cull material from the files and discard old journals, supply catalogs, and any obsolete supplies or equipment.

Moving Day Strategy

Prepare a written outline of the moving day strategy, indicating each person's responsibility, and give each member of the office staff a copy. It may be wise to work in shifts to avoid confusion, but have one person stationed at the new address to direct the movers when they arrive.

Follow-up

After the move, be sure to mention the new address when patients call for appointments. This often is neglected, especially after a few months have passed, and is very upsetting to the patient who tries to check in at the former address.

Closing a Practice

A medical practice may be closed because of retirement, death, a change in geographic location, or a change in profession. If the closing is unexpected, as in the case of sudden death of the physician, much of the burden falls on the staff. If the closing is voluntary and planned for, the physician may wish to consult an attorney or the local medical society for guidelines. The following information is useful in either event.

Advance Notice to Patients

The physician who anticipates retirement can begin cutting back the practice months in advance. Patients can be notified as they come in that the practice will be closing on a specified date and asked to begin arrangements for care from another physician. The physician also can ask that patients pay at the time of service, to minimize accounts receivable at the time of retirement.

Avoiding Abandonment Charge

To avoid a charge of abandonment the physician should notify active patients by letter that the practice is being discontinued. The letter should be sent out at least 3 months in advance, if possible. If a patient has been discharged or has not been given care by the physician for at least 6 years, there is no obligation to send the notice.

Public Announcement

About 1 month after the physician begins telling patients of the closing, an announcement should be placed in a local newspaper, giving the closing date of the office, explaining any arrangements made for continuing care, and thanking patients for their support over the years.

Other Notices

Hospital affiliations should be informed early, particularly if the physician will be leaving the community. If the office space is being rented, be sure to notify the landlord in observance of the rental contract if there is one. Insurance carriers must be advised of the change. The state medical licensure board should be contacted. If the practice is incorporated, an attorney should be consulted about dissolving the corporation.

Patient Transfer and Patient Records

If another physician is taking over the practice, tell the patients about the new physician. However, be sure to explain that a patient's records will be transferred to the physician of his or her choice and that the request for transfer of records must be in writing. For convenience, the physician can have a form available that needs only the patient's signature.

Although the records belong to the physician, they can be transferred legally to another physician only with the consent of the patient. Any records not transferred should be stored, either in bulk or on microfilm or disk, until the statutes of limitations for malpractice and abandonment have run out.

Financial Concerns When a Practice Closes

Income tax returns and supporting documents should be kept for at least 3 years after the tax return was filed. Appoint someone to take care of any remaining outstanding accounts receivable.

Disposition of Controlled Substances

Check with the Drug Enforcement Administration (DEA) for current regulations on disposal of controlled substances and the physician's certificate of registration. Do not simply toss them out. The certificate will have to be sent to the DEA for cancellation, then it will be returned. It may be necessary to produce an inventory of all controlled substances on hand when the practice is terminated, along with duplicate copies of the official order forms that were used to obtain them. Return any unused forms to the DEA. Do not use leftover prescription blanks for note pads. Burn or shred them to prevent misuse.

Professional Liability Insurance

The physician who is discontinuing active medical practice can safely drop the professional liability insurance. However, do not destroy any of the previous policies. Most professional liability claims are covered by the policy that was in effect at the time the alleged act of negligence took place. The suit may be filed many years later, and it is important that the old policy be available.

Furnishings and Equipment

Unfortunately, used office furniture and equipment do not bring much in the marketplace. If another physician is taking over the practice, the value of the furnishings and equipment can be negotiated. Many physicians donate their libraries to the local hospital and declare the gift as an income tax deduction. This is an item to check with the accountant.

A physician may reward loyal employees with severance pay. On average, this equals at least 1 month's salary plus prorated compensation for any unused vacation time. A letter of reference usually is offered.

Many details must be taken care of in closing a medical practice. Contact the local medical society for further guidance.

CLOSING COMMENTS

Successful office managers care about their employees and the vision for the office. They must be strong promoters of the office mission statement. The areas of authority and responsibility must be clearly defined to avoid management problems. A solid office policy and procedure manual will assist the office manager in running an efficient office.

Leadership is an important quality for any manager, and the medical office manager is no exception. The manager should develop good leadership skills, be fair and open-minded, and treat employees and patients as he or she would want to be treated. These actions will help to ensure a pleasant, productive working environment.

Educate patients about the policies and procedures in the office by providing patient information folders or brochures. When these documents are prepared and given to the patients formally, the patient is better informed and fewer calls will come to the office.

Office managers must stay abreast of current employment laws and regulations for all of the different agencies that govern the medical office. Joining an office manager's association will help the manager keep the office up to date and in compliance. Periodic checks on the websites of various organizations, such as OSHA, will help the manager to stay aware of the most recent changes in policies and rules.

Documentation is a critical aspect of the office manager's duties. The manager should keep detailed notes on the performance of employees and always discuss poor performance with employees. Never allow bad habits to go unmentioned. To the extent that it is possible, treat employees in a similar fashion and extend fairness to all.

SUMMARY OF SCENARIO

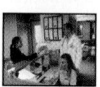 Katherine has made an impact on all of the staff members at Dr. Collins's office. She treats her employees well and is fair regarding office policies and procedures. Her subordinates appreciate her flexibility and professionalism as she deals with the many issues surrounding the operation of a medical office. Katherine treats the employees as team members, never speaking to them as if she were superior to them. She shares vital information with the staff so that they feel a part of the whole team and believes that even some negative information should be related to the staff so that everyone is aware of the challenges the office faces. She makes good hiring decisions and firmly believes in a good orientation and training program. Dr. Collins has placed a great deal of trust in Katherine, and she has performed well, proving to be reliable in her position as office manager.

Katherine knows that she should display a friendly attitude toward her staff members when appropriate to do so. She is kind and considerate and treats the staff as individuals. She does not fraternize with them, but is open to having lunch with the staff at various times and participates in all casual office activities. She maintains a healthy distance so that she can be an effective manager, but she listens to those who are experiencing difficulty and is compassionate about helping whenever possible.

Katherine knows that she must be diligent in checking references so that she brings reliable, qualified individuals on board as staff members. Unless she receives acceptable references, she will not hire a medical assistant to become a part of her team. Once she hires someone, she conducts a thorough training program and takes special care to share the experience and skills of the new staff member with the rest of the team.

When Katherine must give a negative employee evaluation, she states that fact at the beginning of their meeting. Although she is compassionate, she is able to point out a staff member's shortcomings in a detailed, fair way. She is usually willing to give an employee time to improve, but if he or she fails to perform, Katherine does not hesitate to end the employment.

Katherine uses patient information folders as management tools. She has instructed her staff to fully explain the folders to patients and tell them about the information contained within them. Because the staff takes the time to review the folders with patients, calls to the office have been reduced and the staff feels that patients are much more informed. They understand office policies much better, and the staff finds that they repeat basic information much less frequently. Katherine heads a cooperative team that functions well together every day, making the office efficient and the work environment a pleasant one of which to be a part.

SUMMARY of LEARNING OBJECTIVES

1. Define, spell, and pronounce the terms listed in the vocabulary.
   - Spelling and pronouncing medical terms correctly adds credibility to the medical assistant. Knowing the definition of these terms promotes confidence in communication with patients and co-workers.
2. Explain the importance of management in the medical office.
   - Management is an important aspect of running a professional medical office. The physician counts on the office manager to run the business aspects of the office so that he or she can focus efforts on good patient care. A high degree of trust is placed with the office manager.

3. Discuss the desirable qualities of a medical office manager.
   - A good office manager is fair and flexible. Good communications skills are necessary, as well as attention to details. The manager should care about the employees and have a sense of fairness. The ability to remain calm in a crisis is important, as is the use of good judgment and ability to organize tasks.
4. List and discuss the three types of leaders.
   - Charismatic leaders inspire allegiance and dedication and encourage individuals to overcome great obstacles. The transactional leader is structured and organized, hardworking,

Continued

SUMMARY of LEARNING OBJECTIVES
Continued

and a planner. The transformational leader is excellent during times of transition and is effective at building relationships.

5. Discuss several types of power and whether power is a positive or negative entity.
   - Power can be both a positive and a negative entity. Power should not be used in a manipulative or coercive manner. Expert power is based on a high degree of knowledge about a certain subject. Using rewards is one form of invoking power, and legitimate power is that of position or status. Referent power is granted from subordinates to those who lead by example.

6. Identify several ways in which employees are motivated.
   - Employees are motivated by various factors, including money, praise, insecurity, honor, prestige, needs, love, fear, satisfaction, and many others. The effective manager attempts to discover what motivates employees to do a good job.

7. Explain the difference between intrinsic and extrinsic motivation.
   - Intrinsic motivation comes from within the employee. Extrinsic motivation has an outside source.

8. List several ways to prevent burnout.
   - Asking for help, first and foremost, can prevent burnout. Managers often take on too many duties and do not delegate as much as they should. Exercise and rest help prevent burnout, as well as understanding one's personal limitations. Focused goals are important and help keep the manager working toward the most critical tasks.

9. Discuss what to look for when reviewing resumes and applications.
   - Resumes and applications should be reviewed for accuracy and completeness. Gaps in employment dates should be explained fully, and the office manager should verify any references given. Documents should be legible, and the information contained should be consistent and without oversights.

10. Explain why the telephone voice of an applicant is important.
    - The telephone voice of an applicant is important because most employees have occasion to answer the telephone while at work. The employee's voice should be clear and easily

understandable. Good grammar skills must be used to reflect a professional image.

11. Identify the follow-up activities the office manager should perform after an interview.
    - After interviewing a prospective candidate, the office manager should verify the facts on the resume and application and check several references. A comparison should be made between the candidates and the top two or three chosen for a possible second interview. It is wise to involve other staff members when choosing new employees for the office.

12. Explain the importance of mentors for new employees in the medical office.
    - Mentors assist new employees by offering information regarding policies and procedures. The mentor can be a helpful advocate that the new employee can approach when questions arise about any aspect of the medical office.

13. List the various types of staff meetings.
    - Staff meetings may be held to relay information, solve a problem, or brainstorm ideas. Some meetings are designed as work sessions, whereas others may be scheduled to discuss new policies or changes in procedures.

14. Successfully arrange a group meeting.
    - Meetings will be held on at least a monthly basis in most physician offices. The process for arranging a group meeting is outlined in Procedure 24-3.

15. Interview a job candidate for a position at the facility.
    - By making job candidates comfortable during job interviews, the manager will be able to evaluate the candidate as he or she is expressing the skills that will be pertinent to the position. The process for interviewing a job candidate is outlined in Procedure 24-1.

16. Conduct a performance review for an employee.
    - Performance reviews can be productive, positive experiences, or can lead to termination of employment. The process for conducting a performance review is outlined in Procedure 24-2.

CONNECTIONS

Study Guide Connection: Go to Chapter 24 Study Guide. Read the Case Study and Workplace Applications and complete the assignments. Do online research for answers to the questions in the Internet Activities associated with medical practice management and human resources.

CD Connection: Go to the Medical Assisting Competency Challenge CD and do the training activities under General Office Duties.

Evolve Connection: For more information related to medical practice management and human resources, go to evolve.elsevier.com/kinn and visit related weblinks for Chapter 24. Click on the Medical Assisting Exam Review and do the practice questions to sharpen your test-taking skills. To learn more about office software, do the exercises for the Altapoint demo that is on the CD.

Medical Practice Marketing and Customer Service

25

SCENARIO

Monica Ray is a medical assistant who is also pursuing a bachelor's degree in marketing. She has worked for Drs. Julie and Robert Todd for 2 years, and based on her interest in marketing the physicians have agreed to allow her to develop some new strategies for their obstetrics and gynecology office.

Monica is highly computer literate and can design Web pages. She plans to incorporate several ideas that she saw on other physicians' websites, including a method of online scheduling. She is quite creative and is excited about the challenge of providing such a service to the patients of the clinic.

Monica knows that planning is involved in any project, such as the facility's Internet presence. She plans to speak to every employee of the office to get input regarding the design and content of the site. Patients will be able to provide her with additional suggestions as to what features they would like to see.

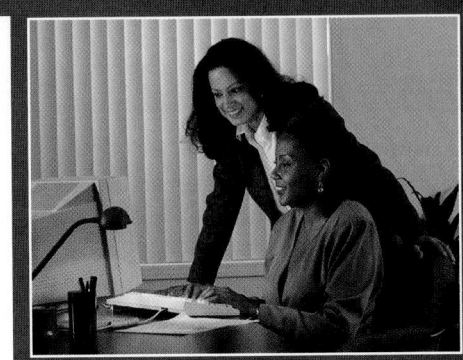

This new development for the office is just one way that Monica hopes to incorporate more formal customer service techniques. She plans to share the information she is learning in the classroom with the physicians and staff at the clinic. Monica and the doctors are fortunate that the staff is enthusiastic and eager to try new methods of customer service. The physicians will set specific goals with the help of the employees and devise a reward system for reaching them. An exciting few months are ahead for this innovative group of medical professionals!

While studying this chapter, think about the following questions:

- How important is an Internet presence to today's medical office?
- Why has *customer service* become a buzzword in the medical industry?
- How do presentation skills enhance the medical assistant's career?
- Which is more important—the internal or the external customer?

LEARNING OBJECTIVES

1. Define, spell, and pronounce the terms listed in the vocabulary.
2. List the three steps to be followed when preparing to implement a medical marketing strategy.
3. Explain the term *target market*.
4. Discuss how suggestion boxes might help the medical facility to make improvements.
5. List and discuss the "four P's" of marketing.
6. Explain the five steps for developing a plan in marketing.
7. Discuss how community involvement can make a difference in marketing efforts.
8. State the difference between advertising and public relations.
9. Determine ways to promote a new practice.
10. Discuss responses that help the medical assistant identify with the patient.
11. Explain the concept of the internal customer.
12. Design a presentation for a marketing event.
13. Prepare a presentation using PowerPoint.

National Accreditation Competencies and Content

CAAHEP COMPETENCIES

General

3.c.(1)(a).   Respond to and initiate written communication
3.c.(1)(b).   Recognize and respond to verbal communications
3.c.(1)(c).   Recognize and respond to nonverbal communications
3.c.(2)(b).   Perform within legal and ethical boundaries
3.c.(2)(d).   Document appropriately

ABHES COMPETENCIES

Communication

2.i. Recognize and respond to verbal and nonverbal communication
2.j. Use correct grammar, spelling, and formatting techniques in written works
2.k. Principles of verbal and nonverbal communication

Legal Concepts

5.b. Document accurately

VOCABULARY

marketing The process or technique of promoting, selling, and distributing a product or service.

objectives Something toward which effort is directed; aims, goals, or ends of action.

outreach The process of using marketing and education strategies to reach and involve diverse audiences through the use of key messages and effective programs.

prosthetic (prohs-thet′-ik) The surgical or dental specialty con-cerned with the design, construction, and fitting of prostheses, which are artificial devices that replace missing parts of the body.

tangible (tan′-juh-buhl) Capable of being appraised at an actual or approximate value; capable of being precisely identified or realized by the mind.

target market A specific group of individuals toward whom the marketing plan is focused.

Each medical office needs a mission statement that defines the reason for the existence of the office. The physician's philosophy of medicine and reasons for pursing medicine as a career greatly influence the mission statement. With this statement in place, the staff develops goals that will assist them in meeting the mission. The goals can be met through a **marketing** and **outreach** plan for the practice and by providing excellent customer service to patients and visitors of the facility.

DEVELOPING MARKETING STRATEGIES

If a business is to grow, marketing strategies are critical. A marketing strategy is designed to promote the services offered by the organization and encourage new business. Three steps are generally followed when preparing to implement or change medical marketing strategies:

- Evaluate what is being done now to increase patient flow.
- Decide what **objectives** are important and how meeting these objectives will be measured.
- Develop a plan with various means of marketing the practice and a specific methodology for implementing each phase.

CRITICAL THINKING APPLICATION

- Monica knows that the office has never attempted any formal marketing in the past. Because no one at her office is familiar with this task, who might she contact for advice and assistance?
- Even though her fellow staff members are not familiar with marketing, could they provide workable ideas?
- What are some ideas for marketing a medical practice?

Knowing the Target Market

During the strategic phase of developing a marketing plan, the physician and office manager must identify the **target market** for the services provided by the clinic. The target market is the group or groups of individuals that the office wishes to reach. Reaching the target market means that the specific groups are made aware of the clinic and what it has to offer. With managed care restrictions and regulations, competition for patients has become keen among physicians, and a facility that does not pursue growth runs a great risk of not surviving.

Several questions must be answered when discussing the target market. Consider the following:

- What specific outcomes do we hope to accomplish?
- What are the needs and desires of our target market?
- What are the characteristics of a typical member of the target market?
- How can the target market be reached in the most cost-effective ways?

Staff meetings are excellent times to brainstorm about reaching target markets. The staff can relate the needs of the patients who are active at the medical office. If patients have made suggestions, they should be discussed and weighed with regard to which most would benefit the patient population of the facility (Figure 25-1).

CRITICAL THINKING APPLICATION

- What community resources could Monica seek as she is determining the target market of the practice?
- What information does she need to begin her search?

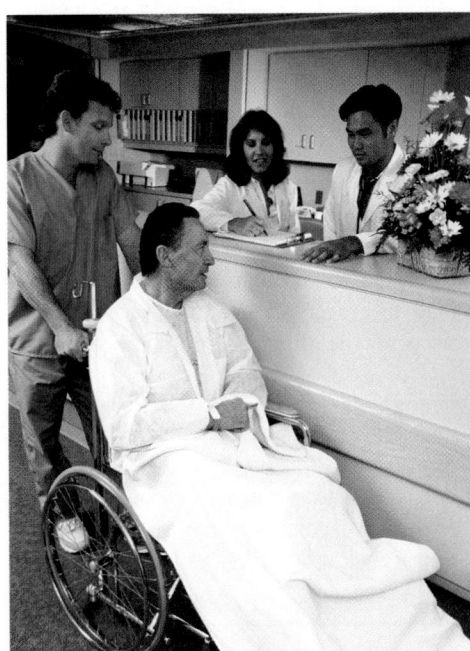

FIGURE 25-1 Friendly staff members are the best marketing tools. A smile is an excellent way to make patients feel welcome in the medical facility.

Suggestion boxes are a great way to solicit patient input. Ask patients for ideas about how the clinic could operate in a smoother fashion and what additional services they would like to see introduced at the facility. Provide and frequently check the suggestion box. If the patient leaves his or her name on the suggestion form, it is a good customer service tactic to reward the patient for the suggestion. Mail the patient a coupon for a free lunch at a local restaurant or a free car wash at a local detailing shop. Involving other businesses in marketing efforts helps both attract new customers.

The "Four P's"

The "four P's" of marketing include product, placement, price, and promotion. A physician's office offers medical services as a product. Some offices have **tangible** retail products that they also offer, such as vitamins, skin-sensitive cosmetics, or **prosthetic** devices. Placement involves the actual location of the medical office. The office may be located in an urban area close to large neighborhoods of young professionals or in a rural area with a few people living several miles apart. Placement can greatly influence the traffic to the facility. Placement can refer also to the setup of the office, the specific suite in a shopping strip where the office is located, or even the placement of retail objects on a shelf.

Price is simply the amount of money charged for goods and services provided. Promotion refers to the methods used to get the product or services to the consumers, or patients in the case of the medical office.

CRITICAL THINKING APPLICATION

- How can Monica investigate the charges for similar procedures at other clinics in her area?
- Why is this information important to Monica?

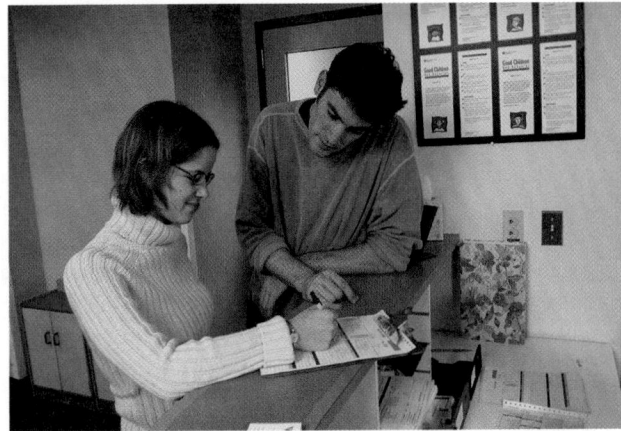

FIGURE 25-2 Offer services that are important in the geographic area of the office. College students may need to see a physician for minor illnesses, and they will appreciate offices that provide short office visits for a reasonable fee.

Deciding What Services to Offer

Once the physician and office manager have identified the target market, decisions can be made regarding what services should be offered to the patients. For instance, suppose the office is situated in a neighborhood of young families. There is a strong possibility that both parents work outside the home, so evening hours would be beneficial to these patients. The physician may decide to extend office hours to 8:00 PM twice a week and to open from 9:00 AM to noon on Saturdays. If there are several schools in the area, particularly junior high and high schools, the physician may wish to offer a special price on sports physicals during the fall. Schools often require physicals, and if the physician offers them at a reasonable price, the entire family may decide to seek medical care from the physician.

If the office is located in a college town, the physician may wish to offer a special student rate for short office visits (Figure 25-2). If a number of senior citizens live in the area, a senior citizen discount might be appropriate. Input from patients and staff members will be valuable in deciding what services to offer in the medical facility.

Developing a Plan

The facility may use several specific planning steps for events, marketing strategies, and any number of other ideas that the physician would like to implement. They are as follows:

- Assessment
- Research
- Planning
- Execution
- Evaluation

Assessment is the phase of planning in which the problem or goals are reviewed. This is another excellent time for brainstorming. Research allows the physician or office manager to investigate the needs of the target market, then decide what the medical office can do to meet those needs. Planning the concept follows, and once a firm plan is in place it is executed or carried out. Afterward, the participants evaluate what went well and what problems occurred so that future efforts will be even more successful.

PROMOTING THE PRACTICE

The physician and office manager should constantly watch for ways to promote the medical practice and keep its name in the public eye. Some of these methods are free of charge, and others will need detailed budgeting and planning. By becoming a member of various civic organizations, such as the Chamber of Commerce, the practice will receive notice of upcoming events and should plan to participate in them on a regular basis. The more that the public sees the physician in the community, the more likely this will affect the growth of the practice.

Tapping into Free Resources

Many good promotional activities are relatively free to the physician. One of the most popular and beneficial to the physician is a professional website. If the physician or an office staff member has sufficient knowledge for website construction, then there is little or no cost to the doctor if one of the free website services is used. Businesses that host websites on the Internet offer very reasonable costs, starting at around $25 per month.

Some newspapers offer an advice column wherein different types of professionals give general medical advice to those who write in with questions. Physicians volunteer to answer these questions in print, and in return the office address, the office telephone number, and often the physicians' pictures are featured. This is an excellent way to generate patient calls and inform the public about the specialties and types of cases the physician handles.

CRITICAL THINKING APPLICATION

- Monica knows there are many opportunities and free resources in her area. Where should she begin to look?
- How might Monica's clinic partner with other businesses and services to provide excellent care to patients and to help one another at the same time?

Community Involvement

Getting involved in the local community is another way to promote a medical practice. Some physicians sponsor Little League football teams, baseball teams, or bowling leagues. Some entire staffs participate in charity events and marathons, wearing T-shirts with the clinic name printed on the back.

The physician or staff may have specific charities that they support on an annual basis, or they may participate in United Way activities, which distribute funds to many different types of worthy organizations through payroll deductions and other gifts. Some medical facilities have volunteer programs in which employees receive recognition for participation in various activities. A good example includes blood donations. Many blood centers offer pins and recognition certificates for the number of pints of blood that volunteers donate. The office staff may set a goal to reach a certain number of donated pints in a year, and as recognition certificates are collected the staff may wish to display them in a prominent place in the office. This is

an indication to patients that the staff is concerned about the community and is volunteer-minded. From a public relations standpoint this is valuable to the medical office, because patients tend to expect medical professionals to be volunteer oriented.

Health fairs are a great avenue for promoting the services offered by the clinic, resulting in name recognition and increasing public visibility. Some health fairs are huge, highly publicized events, whereas others are small, often held at a local shopping mall or grocery store. All of these events could be worthy projects for the physician and the medical office.

CRITICAL THINKING APPLICATION

- What community organizations might help Monica in her efforts to make the office an integral part of the community?
- What resources and community organizations are available in your area that would be good avenues for practice marketing and community service?

Advertising Plans and Agencies

Most physician offices do not use advertising agencies to promote their practices, but on occasion an agency might be useful (Figure 25-3). If a very special event is scheduled that needs extensive planning, then a public relations firm or advertising agency might be consulted. Unfortunately, the cost of these groups is usually high and beyond the reach of sole practitioners or small group practices. However, the investment may be well spent when an event is critical and attendance is important to its success.

There is a difference between advertising and public relations. Advertising could be defined as "creating or changing attitudes, beliefs, and perceptions by influencing people with purchased broadcast time, print space, or other forms of written and visual media." Broadcast time could take the form of television commercials, radio broadcasts, or audiovisual aids. Print could be in a newspaper, magazine, or trade journal, and written and visual media may be a flier, brochure, or billboard. Public relations offerings are influential as well, using news broadcasts, radio reports, and magazine or newspaper articles to reach people. Most public relations efforts are free, but it is often difficult to get others interested enough in the activities the medical office is planning to warrant coverage.

Communication as a Marketing Tool

Many medical offices use communications tools to market the practice and improve customer service. Sending a monthly newsletter through mail or electronically provides health information and news about upcoming events. The newsletter can be very personalized for the office and might even include news about patients and the medical staff, as long as permission is obtained.

Sending birthday cards is an excellent public relations tool. Some offices sign the greetings at staff meetings, and they are placed in a tickler file for the proper mailing date. Sending holiday greetings is another method of wishing patients well.

FINDING A GOOD ADVERTISING AGENCY

1. *Define your objective in hiring an ad agency.* What do you want to achieve? What should be different after the agency goes to work for you? What kind of working relationship do you prefer?

2. *Check out sources.* Consider work you have seen or heard that has impressed you. Call friends and colleagues you trust and get their recommendations. Attend professional or trade association meetings, and talk to members who have used agencies before. Seek out their opinions, and note whose names come up often (both pro and con). Watch for articles about ad agencies in area papers, trade magazines, and related publications, such as chamber of commerce newsletters.

3. *Once you have a list of candidates, screen them by telephone.* Ask about their backgrounds, projects they have worked on, the results they have had, their fees, and anything else important to you. Then set up interviews with the three or four firms that impressed you the most.

4. *Interview the finalists.* Find out the following:
   - *Do they have experience working with your industry?* What is their track record when working with companies like yours? Do they understand your business and the nuances of what you do? If not, are they willing to research the information they need?
   - *Is there chemistry?* You can tell if there is a good "fit" with an ad agency. A good agency will express interest in getting to know you as an individual and learning more about your company. They will be good listeners and quick learners. They will make good suggestions and react quickly to your questions and opinions. They should demonstrate the ability to anticipate what is best for your business and be prepared to disagree with you if they feel you are on the wrong track.
   - *Do they show originality and creativity?* Based on the agency's previous work, do you feel these people understand how best to "sell" your product or service? If you operate a home healthcare agency, for example, you probably do not want an ad campaign that features technology over tenderness. Sensing your clientele, the agency should know enough about you to put together the appropriate message.
   - *Are they reliable and budget conscious?* No amount of chemistry and creativity can make up for a missed deadline or an estimate that is way off. Be sure the agency has not only the creative skills needed but also the time and commitment to devote to your needs. Whether you are the biggest or smallest client in their stable, you should be able to count on consistent attention to detail. Their staff should be available to answer your questions and be accountable for delays and expenses.

FIGURE 25-3 Selecting an advertising or public relations agency. (From Anderson L: *Star makers.* Entrepreneur Magazine, April 1997.)

Automated call distribution is becoming a popular means of communicating with large numbers of people. A computer dials multiple numbers at the same time and plays a recorded message, which can be the actual physician reading a message. Although many people block such calls to their homes and an equal number hang up, the success rate for automatic call distribution is actually quite good.

Many individuals listen and respond to the calls, especially if they come from someone they know and the information is important. For instance, if a medical clinic were planning to move to another part of the city, a program could be initiated to notify all patients with telephone numbers that the office will be moving after a certain date. The message could include the address of the new location, and even prompt patients to "press 1" if they need to schedule an appointment. The same principle could be applied to news about an upcoming health fair, a special seminar about a certain illness, or even an article that will be in the Sunday paper about the clinic.

Promoting a New Practice

Most physicians who open a new practice place an ad in local newspapers to announce the event. Usually a picture of the physician is included, and a map to the exact location may be available on the ad. Some physicians purchase clinics from others who are moving or retiring, but many will open a freestanding clinic in a new building, and the word about the new facility must be spread for the business to be a success.

Providing business cards for all employees is a good way to increase public knowledge about the facility. Some offices offer incentives for patient referrals from the staff or other patients, but the physician must ensure that there are no state statutes or ethical standards that prohibit this. The incentive could be a simple coffee cup with the clinic's logo on it or a book about a healthcare issue. Recognition is the important factor where referrals are concerned. A thank-you card is the minimal acceptable "thanks" for patient referrals.

Some physicians hold an open house when the new facility opens. Often, those individuals who assisted with the business from its inception will attend the open house to lend support to the owners. Bankers, attorneys, accountants, and other physicians will often show their support by attending the open house. Pictures from this event should be placed on the facility's website or in the monthly newsletter.

Developing and Giving Presentations

Today's medical assistant should be comfortable when speaking in front of individuals and groups. By developing additional skills the medical assistant increases his or her value to the physician. Developing and giving presentations is not difficult, although one of the most prevalent fears in the United States is the fear of speaking in public (Procedures 25-1 and 25-2).

There are many different types of speeches, but remember that all public speaking is persuasive. The speaker is attempting to get the audience to do something—whether to buy a new product or convince people to vote. The speaker always has a purpose and must be credible to convince listeners to act. Credibility underlies all persuasion. When the speaker is proficient at persuasion, the audience's questions are answered, their concerns addressed, and their needs fulfilled, while at the same time the speaker's goals are met. If the speaker does a good job, the audience will feel satisfied after hearing a persuasive speech. Persuasion should be nonadversarial and gentle so that the audience feels comfortable in making a decision.

Jerry Weissman, in his book *Presenting to Win: The Art of Telling Your Story*, calls persuasion "audience advocacy"—by that, he means the ability to view the self, a company, a story, or a presentation through the eyes of the audience. Answer the question, "What's in it for me?" which the audience is constantly thinking. To motivate the audience, the speaker must do the following:

- Know the audience
- Research the audience to know their needs, what they care about, and what they want to know
- Link all presentation information to the audience's needs
- Know the purpose of the presentation
- Rehearse the presentation repeatedly

When designing the content of the presentation, keep the audience in mind, and nail down the most important points that must be conveyed to them.

Overcoming Anxiety

Because the fear of public speaking is so common, the speaker must develop ways to overcome the fear and make a successful presentation. Find the actions that promote relaxation, and practice them before giving a speech. Look for a sympathetic face in the audience, and speak directly to that person. Never begin a presentation with an apology of any type such as, "I didn't have much time to prepare" or "I'm not very good at presentations." This undermines the authority of the speaker. Greeting as many of the guests as possible before the presentation helps to develop a rapport and may reduce anxiety. In addition, the guests feel welcome and special because the speaker took the time to make introductions.

During the Presentation

Make certain that the audience can hear everything that is being said. The presentation cannot be effective if it cannot be heard. Make all movements purposeful; if a hand gesture is used, make it then relax the arms. Do not wander around the room. If moving from place to place, go to a spot then stop. Constant movement distracts from the message of the presentation.

Most individuals speak faster when making a presentation, so slow down the pace just a little. Speak so that all the people in the back of the room can hear, but not so loudly that the people in the front rows have to cover their ears. Possibly most important, remember to relax. The physical reactions felt before speaking, such as an increase in pulse rate and a rush of adrenaline, are natural. Do not allow negative thoughts to enter the mind. Instead, deal with fear by knowing the topic and being confident about the message.

Building a Practice Website

Four basic steps are involved in building a website for the medical practice. These steps include the following:

- Define the objectives of the website.
- Design the pages.
- Locate a Web server to which the pages can be uploaded.
- Upload the pages to the server.

Defining Objectives

When defining objectives, important decisions about specific goals must be considered. The physician and staff should discuss who the audience for the website will be and what will be included on the site. Most websites designed for physician offices and clinics are informational, developed mostly for patient and public use. Once the objectives are clearly defined, specific content can be written to place on the website.

Preparing a Presentation

Answer these important questions when preparing a presentation:

- Who is the audience?
- What are the key points?
- When is the presentation?
- How long is the presentation?
- What will the physical surroundings be?
- Why should the audience listen?
- How will the presentation be done?

PROCEDURE 25-1

Design a Presentation

<u>ABHES COMPETENCY:</u> 2.j

GOAL: *To gain skill in designing presentations that can be used for a variety of projects in the medical facility.*

EQUIPMENT and SUPPLIES

- Information about presentation subject
- Software, such as PowerPoint, if needed
- Computer access
- Peripheral computer equipment, if needed

PROCEDURAL STEPS

1. Determine the goals of the presentation.
   <u>PURPOSE:</u> The goals and purpose of the presentation must be determined before beginning so that the presenter is sure to reach those goals.
2. Write an outline of the entire presentation.
   <u>PURPOSE:</u> The outline helps the presenter prepare so that no important points are left out of the presentation.
3. Build the presentation using software, such as PowerPoint, highlighting the major points of the presentation.
4. Evaluate the audience, and adjust the presentation to appeal to that audience.
   <u>PURPOSE:</u> The presenter must know the audience to ensure a successful presentation.
5. Rehearse the presentation several times in front of a mirror.
   <u>PURPOSE:</u> Rehearsing in front of a mirror builds confidence.
6. Make a list of all equipment and materials to take to the presentation.
   <u>PURPOSE:</u> A list will help the presenter to remember all items that need to be taken to the presentation.
7. Arrive for the presentation between 15 to 30 minutes early, depending on the preparation and setup required.
   <u>PURPOSE:</u> Arriving early gives the presenter the opportunity to set up the presentation before the audience arrives.
8. Deliver the presentation within the prescribed time period.
9. Ask the audience if they have any questions about the information in the presentation.
   <u>PURPOSE:</u> A question-and-answer period allows the presenter to interact with the audience.
10. Thank the audience, and remove all equipment and supplies when appropriate.
11. Send a thank-you note to the organization for allowing the presentation, if appropriate.

Designing Presentation Content

Remember these points when designing a presentation:
- Use bulleted points consistently
- Use white space between bullets
- Align text systematically in one area of a slide, and place graphics on the other side
- Make certain that visuals deal with the subject of the presentation and are necessary
- Time the transition between slides
- Make bulleted points appear in a systematic way so that readers see text as the speaker is talking and not before or after the points are mentioned
- If a physical process is demonstrated, use visuals to enhance the demonstration
- Choose the most readable font
- Use hyperlinks effectively
- Use midrange colors for backgrounds
- Rehearse the narration
- Use titles for charts and illustrations
- Organize content well

Designing Pages

Once the objectives are clear, begin developing ideas about what the site will look like on the computer screen. Color choices, animation, and fonts will enhance the look that is being created and make a strong statement about the medical facility. The menus should be designed so that viewers can navigate easily through the site. Most users appreciate a means to go back to the page previously viewed and grow frustrated with sites that have an excessive number of pop-up boxes. Consistency is important, so it is a good idea to keep the same design theme on each page of the website.

The most important part of the website is the text. It has been said that every word in a book must add to the story, and this is a good way to look at the text in a website. Avoid repetition, and remain clear about what is being communicated on the site. Headings and titles help to clarify the theme of each page. Use a spellchecker before uploading the message and making it available for public viewing.

Photographs, graphics, music, and video can add fun to the website, but be careful not to overdo them. Graphics are often large files that take time to download. Most people will not wait more than about 10 seconds for a Web page to load

PROCEDURE 25-2

Prepare a Presentation Using PowerPoint

ABHES COMPETENCY: 2.j

GOAL: *To enhance presentations using PowerPoint as a visual aid.*

EQUIPMENT and SUPPLIES

- Information about presentation subject
- Software, such as PowerPoint, if needed
- Computer access
- Peripheral computer equipment, if needed

PROCEDURAL STEPS

1. Open the PowerPoint program.
2. Have the outline of the presentation available.
3. Click on the "new slide" icon in the program.
4. Create the title slide using the slide layout section on the right side of the screen.
5. Create additional slides using the slide layout section, or design the slides manually.
6. Limit the number of words on the slides so that a concise message results.
   PURPOSE: Too many words on one slide makes the message difficult to understand.
7. Make certain that the font is as large as possible on the slide, beginning with a size 18 font and increasing from there.
   PURPOSE: The font on a presentation must be easy to read from the back of the room.
8. Do not use more than three font types per slide.
   PURPOSE: More than three font types makes the presentation difficult to read.
9. Avoid using more than three text-only slides in a row.
   PURPOSE: Use clip art, photographs, graphs, and other items to enhance the presentation.
10. Insert photos or clip art into the presentation by clicking on "insert," then clicking on "picture," then choosing "clip art" or "from file."
11. Format the background of each slide, or of all slides, by clicking on "format," then "background," then choose a color or fill effects.

PURPOSE: A consistent background makes the presentation look more professional.

12. Click on "slide show," and adjust the slide transitions so that the slides appear and disappear as desired and are timed correctly.
13. Click on "custom animation" to change the entrance and exit of the slides to the effect that is desired.
14. Save the presentation frequently while working on it.
    PURPOSE: Saving the presentation frequently ensures the user that the work will not be lost.
15. Click on "view" in the task bar, then on "slide sorter," which will allow moving the slides around in the presentation.
16. To run the show continuously, click on "slide show," then on "set up show," then click the box labeled "loop continuously until escape" in the "show options" box.
    PURPOSE: Running the show continuously is helpful for situations in which the presentation can be watched while people are passing through an exhibit hall, and so on.
17. Make certain the presentation has been saved.
18. Practice giving the presentation several times to smooth all transitions and to be familiar with the content.
    PURPOSE: The more the presentation is practiced, the more comfortable the presenter will be.
19. Anticipate questions that the audience may ask, and have answers prepared.
    PURPOSE: Anticipating questions will help the presenter to better prepare for the presentation and ensure that the presenter knows the material.
20. Offer other visual aids, such as handouts, if appropriate, when giving the presentation.
    PURPOSE: Visual aids will help the audience to remember the presentation and may prompt them to take any action that the presenter wishes them to take.

---

before clicking elsewhere. When designing Web page graphics, remember that smaller is better. Graphics can be found by searching for "index of GIF files" or "GIF library." Once an appropriate file is found, it should be copied onto the hard drive by "right-clicking" the graphic and selecting "save picture as." Music can be found by searching for "mid" or "midi." The search can even specify a certain singer, song, or composer. Always respect any copyrights that are designated on any file used. Many websites offer these files for free.

For a more professional-looking website, consider purchasing Web development software, such as Macromedia's Dreamweaver or Microsoft's FrontPage. These feature-rich products are fairly

inexpensive and can help the medical assistant create very attractive, easy-to-maintain websites. Most products integrate tutorial and "help" features that explain how to use them.

Hyperlinks are words or graphics on a Web page that, when clicked, take the viewer to another page or another website. To add a hyperlink, simply highlight the text field or graphic, select the hyperlink icon, and specify the destination address (uniform resource locator [URL]). Always specify the full URL.

The main page should always be assigned the file name "index.htm" or "default.htm." Other pages on the website can be assigned any name; however, keep the names short, and avoid using special characters.

Locating a Web Server

At this point the design of the website is complete, but the files reside on the computer hard drive, not on the Internet. Now the pages are ready to be uploaded, or published, to a Web server that will allow them to be viewed on the Internet. The Internet service provider (ISP) that the office uses for email and online services may offer free Web space to its customers. If not, a number of companies will provide Web space at no charge, but the user usually will be required to use banners on the site that advertise the ISP or other services. If no banner ads are desired, the medical facility may wish to use a paid provider. Some Web hosting companies provide other services free of charge, like simple Web page editors and email addresses.

Uploading Pages

When using a free Web server, instructions and passwords will be sent to the users that describe how to upload files to the server. The password is necessary so that other people cannot alter the files. Copying the files from the local hard disk to the Web server is a simple process. The hosting site will prompt the user for the name of the directory on the hard drive where the files are stored and for the names of the specific files to be uploaded. To avoid confusion, make certain that the files saved on the server have the same file names that were used on the hard drive.

Once all of the files have been uploaded, test the page on the Web server and make certain that it functions properly and that all files have been uploaded correctly. It is also a good idea to test the page using a different computer to ensure that graphic files are being read from the server and not from the local hard drive.

Evaluating the Website

Include an email address where viewers of the website can interact with the creator with comments. When viewers have this option, problems with the site can be readily identified and corrected. It is also advisable to check the site every few days to make certain that it is functioning properly.

Counters often can be added to the website that will indicate how many people viewed it. This helpful tool will allow the medical facility to track how many people are viewing which pages.

HIGH-QUALITY CUSTOMER SERVICE IN THE MEDICAL PRACTICE

Treating the Patient as a Customer

The best way to increase the number of patients in a medical office is through word of mouth. When patients are satisfied with the treatment they receive, they will refer other patients to the physician. However, if they are dissatisfied, they will tell everyone they know!

Because patients often have a choice about who provides their healthcare services, it is important that the physician's office become the patient's first choice. Some patients have such loyalty to a certain physician that even if their healthcare coverage would no longer pay for visits, they would continue to see that doctor. This happens because of the attitude of the physician and his or her office staff.

CRITICAL THINKING APPLICATION

- Monica is considering a "Frequently Asked Questions" section of the website. How might this help patients?
- What kinds of questions might be asked in this section?
- How might the inclusion of this section benefit employees?

Helpful Attitudes

The physician and staff probably project a helpful attitude in every contact with the patient. They sincerely ask, "How may I help you?" then take steps to assist the patient in whatever way possible. Instead of pointing in the general direction of the radiology department, they take the patient there and introduce him or her to the receptionist. Instead of telling a patient on the telephone, "Ann handles the insurance billing—I'll transfer you to her," say, "One moment, Mrs. Brown, let me see if Ann is at her desk." Then place Mrs. Brown on hold, call Ann, and let her know that she has a call. Then return to Mrs. Brown and tell her that Ann is at her desk, and transfer the call at that time. Be courteous and kind to every patient and visitor to the office. Good customer relations must be one of the primary goals of the medical facility. Patients count on the staff members to be reliable and available to help them to the best of their abilities.

Phrases That Undermine Successful Customer Service

Several phrases could be considered the "deadly sins" of customer service. These phrases should never be used when relating to patients and visitors:

- "I don't know."
- "I don't care."
- "I can't be bothered."
- "Ask someone else."
- "It's not my job."
- "It's not my fault."
- "I didn't do it."
- "I know that."
- "I'm right, you're wrong."

All of these phrases will give the patient or visitor a negative view of both the office and those who work in the facility.

Identifying with Patients

Patients appreciate staff members who can identify with the problems they are facing. This is especially effective when a patient is upset or angry. For example, if a patient comes to the

---

Customer Service at Nordstrom

- Use your good judgment in all situations
- There will be no additional rules

From the *Nordstrom, Inc., Employee Handbook.* Courtesy Nordstrom, Inc.

office complaining that charges were placed on his account for procedures that were not performed, the medical assistant may respond with a phrase similar to the following:

"Mr. Roberts, I understand that you are upset about these additional charges. I know I would be upset if I were billed for something I didn't receive. Let me help you by doing this...."

Identifying with the patient shows an understanding on the part of the staff member, no matter how upset the patient may be. Always acknowledge and restate the patient's concern. It proves that the medical assistant was listening and is interested in resolving the problem.

Remember, it costs much more to find new customers than to keep existing customers happy. Providing helpful, personal service impresses even the most difficult patient. To patients and visitors to the clinic, whomever they speak to represents the whole company. Perceptions and opinions will likely be formed based on experiences with only one person. Each individual employee must be aware that to the patient, each employee is the healthcare facility.

What Do Patients Expect?

First, patients expect to be treated using the golden rule. They expect their concerns to be met with responsiveness, which means that the medical assistant should have a caring attitude. They also expect that the professionals in the medical office are knowledgeable about their field or specialty. An insurance biller should know more than just the basics of insurance filing. The office manager should have a certain degree of authority to handle problems and complaints. Patients also expect confidentiality and trust from the staff of the medical office. They expect an organized office that runs on schedule, and that if a staff member promises to do something, it is as good as done (Figure 25-4).

Remembering the Internal Customer

Most of us do not have problems figuring out who the external customers are in a medical practice. Patients, their families and friends, and visitors to the office are external customers. But who is the internal customer?

Internal customers are employees and staff members of the facility. Although they work for the business, they also are served by the business. If they are not pleased with the atmosphere of the medical facility, they are sure to look elsewhere for employment. Keeping the internal customer is just as important as keeping the external customer.

CLOSING COMMENTS

Providing good customer service is a commitment that must be made by every employee of the medical facility, every single day. There will be times that the customer is not right, but he or she should be treated with dignity and respect at all times. In addition, the expert customer service provider will have the knack for making the customer think he or she was right all along! The medical office is no exception to the requirements for providing good service to its patients, and doing so will result in an excellent reputation for the clinic, built by those who matter most–the patients.

Endless opportunities for patient education exist through the practice's marketing and public relations efforts. Most physicians agree that a part of the obligation to the medical profession is to educate patients about healthcare issues. The public relations and practice's marketing staffs can work together to provide information to patients of the facility and to the general public.

Many physicians attend health fairs, where brochures and pamphlets can be distributed about conditions such as diabetes, heart disease, hypertension, and other disorders. Screenings for cholesterol and blood pressure checks are good ways to market a practice and gain new patients.

The medical assistant who knows how to build and maintain a simple website can be of great value to the physician. The practice website could provide opportunities for educating patients, as well as special sections for upcoming events, an online newsletter, and appointment setting. The website address should be included on stationery, business cards, and other documents used to promote the facility.

The physician must take care that patients do not use the information in brochures or on the practice website as medical advice or a substitute for the physician's counsel. When attaching links to other websites, be sure they are reputable. The patient may consider information on the practice's website to be an extension of the advice of the physician, so make sure that everything on the website is accurate.

The physician should review carefully all printed information that is used to promote the medical facility. Be sure that no misleading statements are included. A disclaimer should be used to remind patients that the information given in brochures and on websites is only general information. Patients should discuss specific medical issues with the physician.

Todd Family Medical Clinic

Julie Todd, M.D.   Robert Todd, M.D.
3343 Smithson Place
Dallas, Texas 75229

We are interested in the customer service you received today as a patient of our clinic. Please return this form by mail and help us evaluate our service to you!

Date of contact or visit: _____   Day of week: _____

Name of employees with which you made contact (if known):

How was this contact made?   ☐ by phone   ☐ by mail   ☐ in person

This is a (please check appropriate box)   ☐ complaint   ☐ comment

Description of situation:

Has the problem been resolved to your satisfaction, if any?   ☐ yes   ☐ no

If not, how can we resolve the problem?

Please rate the following based on your experience with our staff:

	Excellent	Good	Fair	Poor
Greeting to you by name	☐	☐	☐	☐
Familiarity with your account	☐	☐	☐	☐
Courtesy and willingness to help	☐	☐	☐	☐
Quickness in answering the phone	☐	☐	☐	☐
Time placed on hold	☐	☐	☐	☐
Quickness in locating your chart	☐	☐	☐	☐
All of your questions answered	☐	☐	☐	☐
Phone transfers kept to a minimum	☐	☐	☐	☐

Other suggestions and comments:

Name (optional): _____   Phone Number (optional): _____

FIGURE 25-4 Customer service evaluation form for the medical office. By using this form for patient feedback, the medical office manager can better assess patient expectations.

SUMMARY OF SCENARIO

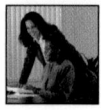

Monica knows that without growth, many businesses eventually fail. She is confident that with a simple marketing plan, the clinic will experience steady, continuous expansion. She has spoken to all of the office staff members and gained input from both employees and the patients of the clinic. Many offered excellent suggestions that Monica can incorporate into her marketing plan.

One of her first activities was to develop an annual calendar of special events and outreach efforts. A monthly newsletter and the practice website will be the main thrusts of her marketing plan. The newsletter will be available both in print and online. The patients in the office database who have email addresses will receive automatically a computer-generated email message containing a link that will take them directly to the online newsletter. Inside, patients will find health information and details about upcoming events.

Monica also planned one special activity for each month of the year. She scheduled a blood drive, a Christmas toy drive, and mini-health fair. Because both Dr. Julie and Dr. Robert Todd are dedicated to students who wish to pursue medicine, Monica even planned a career day for high school students interested in becoming physicians, inviting representatives from the medical school that the Todds attended. Because this is considered a public service, Monica was able to get press coverage on the local radio station and in the newspaper at no cost.

Monica visited a new restaurant located close to the office that serves heart-healthy dishes, met with the manager, and discussed ways that the two businesses could help each other. They decided to provide a "buy one entrée, get one free" coupon to patients who referred other patients to the clinic. In turn, Dr. Robert Todd agreed to hold his free nutrition seminars at the restaurant. This arrangement has proven to work well for both businesses. Monica obtained this new agreement by making an effective presentation to the restaurant manager. Her skills in putting an interesting, informative presentation together helped her secure the agreement.

An Internet presence is important to businesses that wish to grow in today's society. Consumers often look on the Internet first when planning purchases, shopping, or looking for community resources. Monica plans to track responses to each event promoted on the practice website to determine what efforts were the most effective in promoting the clinic. The website will allow her to count the number of times it is accessed, as well as which pages were the most popular within the website. She will keep the physicians informed and be open to their suggestions throughout the year. Monica is anxious to see results of her marketing efforts and feels confident of success.

The staff members understand that no matter what efforts are used to promote the facility and obtain new patients, it is their responsibility to provide exceptional customer service so that the patients will be happy with their experience. In the medical industry today, customer service has become as important as in the retail world. Patients have choices as to who provides their healthcare, so they must be treated cordially and fairly by medical professionals who truly wish to serve their needs. The success and growth of the facility depends on customer service. Monica knows that there is more than one type of customer in the medical office—the internal customers (employees) are critical to clinic success. She includes other employees in marketing decisions and often asks for their input. The more involved employees feel in company decisions, the more they feel as if they are a part of the community that is created in the individual facility. Monica has helped to create a fun, exciting workplace, and she looks forward to going to work every single day.

SUMMARY of LEARNING OBJECTIVES

1. Define, spell, and pronounce the terms listed in the vocabulary.
   - Spelling and pronouncing medical terms correctly adds credibility to the medical assistant. Knowing the definition of these terms promotes confidence in communication with patients and co-workers.
2. List the three steps to be followed when preparing to implement a medical marketing strategy.
   - When preparing to implement marketing strategies, first evaluate what currently is being done toward the marketing effort. Then decide what the objectives of the marketing plan are and how they will be measured. Finally, develop a specific plan and timeline for implementing each phase.
3. Explain the term *target market*.
   - A target market is a very specific group of people or individuals whom the medical facility wishes to serve. Geography, lifestyle, and personality all are ways to classify individuals into specific target markets. When identifying a target market ask, "Who is our patient?" "What does our patient want?" and "Why is it wanted?" These questions will help the medical facility to design a marketing plan to meet the needs of these individuals.
4. Discuss how suggestion boxes might help the medical facility to make improvements.
   - Suggestions from patients and employees should always be welcomed in the medical office. Often these people see the

Continued

SUMMARY of LEARNING OBJECTIVES
Continued

facility from a different point of view, and their suggestions can enhance the atmosphere and services that are offered.

5. List and discuss the "four P's" of marketing.
   - A marketing plan must always address the "four P's," which are product, placement, price, and promotion. The product in a medical office would include the services and any actual retail items that might be sold. Placement relates to the location of the office and its convenience to the patients, and the placement of retail items in the facility. Price represents the charges for goods and services, and promotion entails the ways in which the services are promoted to the general public and the target market.

6. Explain the five steps for developing a plan in marketing.
   - When developing a marketing plan, the facility should first assess the efforts that have been made in the past, then research the results of those efforts. Next the plan is developed, which should include very specific steps for each aspect of the endeavor. After the plan is executed, the staff must evaluate its effectiveness and determine whether the goals were met. The evaluation is important in planning future marketing strategies.

7. Discuss how community involvement can make a difference in marketing efforts.
   - Involvement in the community is an excellent way to give to the medical profession and to remain in the public eye. These efforts can result in new patients for the facility. The public sees medical professionals as caring and compassionate, so volunteer activities reinforce this attitude and help to meet patient expectations.

8. State the difference between advertising and public relations.
   - Advertising is defined as a medium that attempts to create or change attitudes, beliefs, and perceptions through purchased broadcast time, printed material, or other forms of communication. Public relations is a similar field but relies more on news broadcasts or reports, magazine or newspaper articles, and radio reports to reach the audience.

9. Determine ways to promote a new practice.
   - The new medical practice can be promoted by placing an announcement in the newspaper about its opening. Some physicians hold an open house, inviting the public to visit the office. A website is an excellent promotional tool and should be listed on business cards and stationery. Community service and volunteer activities that mention the practice will also help to spread the word about the services that are available.

10. Discuss responses that help the medical assistant identify with the patient.
    - Identifying with the patient is an effective customer service tool. The medical assistant should express his or her understanding about the patient's concerns. Then, tell the patient that the situation can be resolved and how it will be resolved. Four magic words in customer service are, "Let me help you."

11. Explain the concept of the internal customer.
    - External customers are those who visit the facility, such as patients. However, staff members and employees are internal customers who wish to derive a sense of satisfaction from working for the medical office. The internal customers are just as important as the external customers.

12. Design a presentation for a marketing event.
    - A sharp, effective presentation will help the medical assistant to or secure permission to hold or promote a marketing event. The process for designing a presentation is outlined in Procedure 25-1.

13. Prepare a presentation using PowerPoint.
    - PowerPoint is a user-friendly program that will produce effective presentations. The process for preparing a presentation using PowerPoint is outlined in Procedure 25-2.

CONNECTIONS

 Study Guide Connection: Go to Chapter 25 Study Guide. Read the Case Study and Workplace Applications and complete the assignments. Do online research for answers to the questions in the Internet Activities associated with medical practice marketing and customer service.

 CD Connection: Go to the Medical Assisting Competency Challenge CD and do the training activities under Communication.

Evolve Connection: For more information related to medical practice marketing and customer service, go to evolve.elsevier.com/kinn and visit related weblinks for Chapter 25. Click on the Medical Assisting Exam Review and do the practice questions to sharpen your test-taking skills. To learn more about office software, do the exercises for the Altapoint demo that is on the CD.

Infection Control

26

Rosa Lucia is a certified medical assistant working in a multiphysician pediatric practice. She is quite concerned about contracting an infectious disease while caring for her patients. Rosa learned about standard precautions while enrolled in her medical assistant program and now must implement that knowledge in the workplace. An important part of preventing the spread of infection is to understand how to break the chain of infection and to recognize the importance of correct and frequent hand washing.

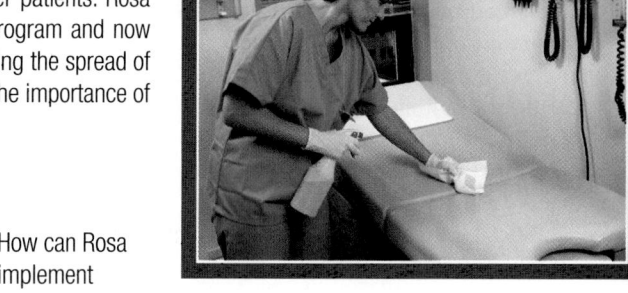

While studying this chapter, think about the following questions:

- How can Rosa achieve these goals?
- What is the significance of an Exposure Control Plan in Rosa's pediatric office?
- What are the important details regarding the office's compliance with OSHA guidelines?

- How can Rosa implement required infection control procedures in the pediatric office where she works?

1. Define, spell, and pronounce the terms listed in the vocabulary.
2. Recognize diseases caused by pathogenic microorganisms.
3. Apply the chain-of-infection process to healthcare practice.
4. Summarize the impact of the inflammatory response on the body's ability to defend itself against infection.
5. Differentiate between humoral and cell-mediated immunity.
6. Analyze the differences among acute, chronic, and latent disease processes.
7. Compare viral and bacterial cell invasion.
8. Specify potentially infectious bodily fluids.
9. Integrate OSHA's requirement for a site-based Exposure Control Plan into office management procedures.
10. Summarize the management of postexposure evaluation and follow-up.

11. Explain the major areas included in the OSHA Compliance Guidelines.
12. Apply the concepts of medical and surgical asepsis to the healthcare setting.
13. Differentiate among sanitization, disinfection, and sterilization procedures.
14. Demonstrate the proper hand-washing technique for medical asepsis.
15. Demonstrate the correct procedure for sanitization of contaminated instruments.
16. Apply patient education concepts to infection control.
17. Discuss the legal and ethical concerns regarding medical asepsis and infection control.

National Accreditation Competencies and Content

CAAHEP COMPETENCIES	ABHES COMPETENCIES
Clinical	**Clinical Duties**
3.b.(1)(a). Perform hand washing	4.c. Apply principles of aseptic techniques and infection control
3.b.(1)(d). Dispose of biohazardous materials	4.q. Dispose of biohazardous materials
3.b.(1)(e). Practice Standard Precautions	4.r. Practice Standard Precautions
General	**Instruction**
3.c.(3)(c). Provide instruction for health maintenance and disease prevention	7.c. Teach patients methods of health promotion and disease prevention

VOCABULARY

anaphylaxis (an-uh-fuh-lak′-sis) Exaggerated hypersensitivity reaction that in severe cases leads to vascular collapse, bronchospasm, and shock.

antibody (an′-ti-bah-de) Immunoglobulins produced by the immune system in response to bacteria, viruses, or other antigenic substances.

antigen (an′-ti-juhn) Foreign substance that causes the production of a specific antibody.

antiseptics (an-ti-sep-tik) Substance, such as alcohol and povidone-iodine solution (Betadine), that inhibits the growth of microorganisms on living tissue.

autoimmune (o-to-im′-yuhn) Pertaining to a disturbance in the immune system in which the body reacts against its own tissue. Examples of autoimmune disorders include multiple sclerosis, rheumatoid arthritis, and systemic lupus erythematosus.

candidiasis (kan-duh-de-uh′-sis) Infection caused by a yeast that typically affects the vaginal mucosa and skin.

coagulate (ko-ag′-yuh-lat) To form into clots.

contaminated Soiled with pathogens or infectious material; nonsterile.

disinfectant Substance such as alcohol or povidone-iodine solution (Betadine) that inhibits the growth of microorganisms on inanimate surfaces or objects.

germicides (jur′-muh-sids) Agents that destroy pathogenic organisms.

hereditary (huh-re′-duh-ter-e) Pertaining to a characteristic, condition, or disease transmitted from parent to offspring on the DNA chain.

interferon (in′-tuhr-fir-on) A protein that forms when a cell is exposed to a virus, blocking viral action on the cell and providing protection against viral invasion.

nosocomial infections Infections acquired during hospitalization or in a healthcare setting; often caused by *Escherichia coli*, hepatitis viruses, *Pseudomonas*, and *Staphylococcus* microorganisms.

palliative Relieving or alleviating symptoms without curing the disease.

parenteral (puh-ren′-tuh-ruhl) Relating to injection or introduction of substances into the body through any route other than the digestive tract such as subcutaneous, intravenous, or intramuscular administration.

pathogen (path′-o-jen) A disease-causing microorganism.

pathophysiology Study of the biologic and physical manifestations of disease as they are related to system abnormalities and physiologic disturbances.

permeable (pur′-me-uh-buhl) Able to be passed or soaked through.

pyemia (pi-em′-e-uh) The presence of pus-forming organisms in the blood.

relapse The recurrence of the symptoms of a disease after apparent recovery.

remission The partial or complete disappearance of the clinical and subjective characteristics of a chronic or malignant disease.

rhinitis (rin-i′-tis) Inflammation of the mucous membranes of the nose.

spores Thick-walled structures formed within certain bacteria, enabling the organism to withstand unfavorable environmental conditions.

sterile (ster′-il) Free of all microorganisms, pathogenic and nonpathogenic.

tinea (tin′-e-uh) Any fungal skin disease that results in scaling, itching, and inflammation.

urticaria (uhr-tuh-kar′-e-uh) A skin eruption creating inflamed wheals; hives.

vectors Animals or insects (e.g., ticks) that transmit the causative organisms of disease.

The concepts of disease transmission and the body's response to infection form the basis for understanding the importance of the first line of defense in preventing disease. Before we can assist in the prevention of disease, we have to look at methods we can use to minimize the chances of being a carrier of disease. One of the simplest ways of preventing the spread of disease is to wash your hands or use alcohol-based handrubs. As you continue through the remainder of this textbook, you should refer to the fundamental concepts of this chapter when faced with an infection control issue. Because of the need for infection control and the impact of Occupational Safety and Health Administration (OSHA) guidelines on medical practice, every procedure must begin and end with hand hygiene practices. The concepts in this chapter are basic to all clinical skills, and following them can lessen the transmission of disease, can reduce the severity of disease, and might save the life of a patient or co-worker, or even your own.

DISEASE

Disease is defined as any sustained, harmful alteration of the normal structure, function, or metabolism of an organism or cell. This pathologic condition of the body presents a group of clinical signs, symptoms, and laboratory findings that set it apart as an abnormal entity, differing from other normal and pathologic conditions. We recognize and categorize many different types of diseases: **hereditary** (genetic), drug-induced, **autoimmune,** degenerative, communicable, and infectious, to name only a few. Sometimes a specific disease may fit two or more categories.

Any disease caused by the growth of pathogenic microorganisms in the body falls into the category labeled *infectious diseases.* The entrance of a living microbe into the body is not disease, because until the infected cell or individual shows a harmful alteration in structure, physiology, or biochemistry,

Conditions Required for Microbial Growth

Certain conditions must exist for microbes to grow and flourish. To maintain a healthcare environment that is as free as possible of pathogenic organisms, the medical assistant must prevent or eliminate as many of these growth requirements as possible.

- Nutrients: Pathogens thrive on contaminated surfaces and equipment. Most microbes need the same nutrients we do—carbohydrates, proteins, and fats.
- Moisture: Microbes require moisture for cellular activities.
- Temperature: Most pathogenic microbes flourish at body temperature (98.6° F or 37° C).
- Oxygen: Some microbes, called *aerobes*, require oxygen to grow and multiply, whereas others, *anaerobes*, thrive in environments without oxygen.
- Neutral pH: pH refers to the acid-base level of a solution on a scale of 1 to 14, with 7 being neutral. The majority of pathogens prefer a neutral pH for optimal growth.

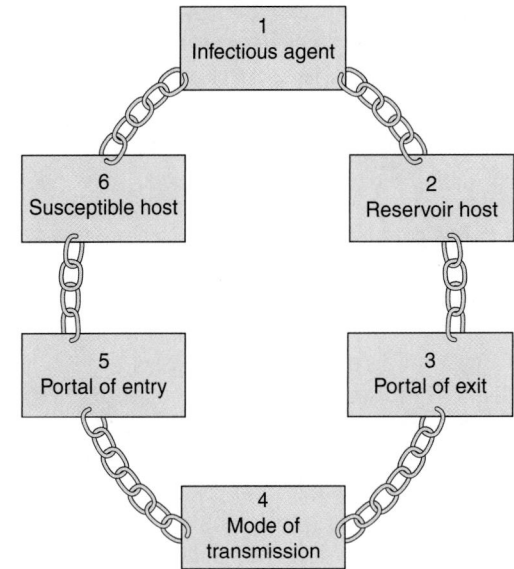

FIGURE 26-1   Chain of infection.

disease is either not detected or not considered present. In fact, a living microbe may be ingested, injected, or inhaled and never cause disease. An unaffected person, however, could still transmit the infection to another person. In this case we call the unaffected person a *carrier*.

Microorganisms are almost everywhere. We carry them on our skin, in our bodies, and on our clothing. They can be in ice, boiling water, the soil, and the air. The only places that are free of microorganisms are certain internal body organs and tissues and the inside of sterilized containers. Organs and tissues that do not connect with the outside by means of mucus-lined membranes are, in the normal state, free from all living microorganisms.

THE CHAIN OF INFECTION

Infectious diseases can spread only if certain factors occur. These factors, or links, make up the chain of infection. Break the chain, and you break the infectious process (Figure 26-1).

The chain of infection starts with the infectious agent. There are five groups of potentially pathogenic agents or microorganisms: viruses, bacteria, protozoa, fungi, and rickettsia. Additional information about typical diseases caused by these pathogens is included in Chapter 54. Infection cannot occur without the presence of an infectious microorganism, so the best way for healthcare workers to prevent the spread of disease is to use adequate infection control procedures such as consistent hand washing and the proper use of **antiseptics** as well as effective disinfection and sterilization methods.

The smallest of all pathogens, viruses, lead the list of important disease-causing agents. Viral microorganisms are intracellular parasites that take over the DNA or RNA of the invaded cell. Viral invasion may not cause significant immediate symptoms, because host cells infected with viruses can produce a substance called **interferon,** which protects nearby cells. Symptoms are delayed because the virus must use the host cell's metabolic and synthetic mechanisms to make more viruses to compound the illness. The interferon leaves the infected cell and acts somewhat like a Paul Revere to warn neighboring cells that "a virus is coming!" With this warning neighboring cells produce antiviral proteins that destroy viruses once they enter. Antibiotics are unable to destroy viral invaders that enter a normal cell and multiply within the cell. Therefore the treatment for viral infections typically focuses on the relief of symptoms or **palliative** treatment. To counteract and slow down the rate of viral replication, interferon and the antiviral agents acyclovir (Zovirax), valacyclovir hydrochloride (Valtrex), penciclovir (Denavir), and famciclovir (Famvir) may be prescribed.

Bacteria are tiny, simple cells that produce diseases in a variety of ways. Pathogenic bacteria can secrete toxic substances that damage human tissues, act as parasites inside human cells, or colonize body surfaces, disrupting normal human functions. Bacteria are classified according to their shape or morphology and include spherical (cocci), rod-shaped (bacilli), and spiral-shaped (spirilla) structures (see Chapter 54). Some bacteria can produce resistant internal structures called **spores** that make treatment difficult. When bacteria invade the body, there are several ways to treat the patient. The most common approach is the use of antibiotics to destroy or inhibit the growth of the invader. We all have normal microbiota, or nonpathogenic bacteria that reside in various body systems, especially the digestive tract, and provide protection from disease by competing for nutrients that pathogenic bacteria require to grow and multiply.

CRITICAL THINKING APPLICATION

Susie Chen, a 3-year-old patient, is being seen today because of complaints of a cough and nasal congestion. Susie's father does not understand why the pediatrician did not order his daughter an antibiotic for her viral infection. Rosa needs to reinforce the doctor's decision. How can she help the father understand the proper use of antibiotics?

The Body's Natural Protective Devices

The body possesses multiple levels of protection against the invasion of pathogenic microorganisms. These include the following:

- Intact skin serves as a natural barrier to disease.
- Mucous membranes lining the openings of the body help protect underlying tissues and trap foreign substances.
- Tiny hairlike projections, called *cilia*, line the respiratory tract and move in a coordinated upward motion to expel the trapped foreign substances.
- These trapped substances can be expelled with sneezing and coughing before the organisms invade underlying tissue.
- Additional bodily secretions, such as tears, have antimicrobial properties that help destroy invading pathogens.
- The natural pH of many of the body's organs discourages the growth of microbes. The acidic pH of urine, the vaginal mucosa, and the stomach helps prevent pathogenic invasion. The body's resident microbes create and maintain this environment.

Protozoa are unicellular parasites that have the ability to replicate and multiply rapidly once inside the host. Examples of protozoa-related diseases include *Giardia,* which is confined to the gastrointestinal tract, and malaria, which invades the blood system. Protozoal infections are frequently seen in tropical climates where a large insect population exists because many of these diseases are transmitted by **vectors.** For example, the mosquito transmits malaria.

Fungi may be unicellular or multicellular and include such organisms as mushrooms, molds, and yeasts. Many forms are pathogenic and can cause such diseases as **candidiasis** and **tinea** infections. Fungi grow best in warm, moist environments. Treatment with antifungal agents includes the application of topical preparations for tinea infections, such as Lotrimin; vaginal suppositories for candidiasis, such as Monistat; or oral medications, such as fluconazole (Diflucan), ketoconazole (Nizoral) and terbinafine (Lamisil). Fungal infections are also called *mycotic* infections.

Rickettsiae are microorganisms that have characteristics of both bacteria and viruses. Like viruses they are obligate parasites that must live within a host cell for growth but are larger than viruses so they can be viewed with a regular microscope. Vectors such as fleas, ticks, and mites usually transmit pathogenic forms of rickettsia. Diseases caused by rickettsia can be treated with antibiotics and include Rocky Mountain spotted fever, which is transmitted by a tick.

The second link in the chain of infection is the reservoir. Reservoirs may be people, insects, animals, water, food, or **contaminated** instruments. Most pathogens must gain entrance into a host or else they will die. The reservoir host supplies nutrition for the organism, allowing it to multiply. The pathogen either causes infection in the host or, in the case of vector-borne diseases, exits from the host in great enough numbers to cause disease in another host. The chain of infection continues with the means or portal of exit—which is how the pathogen escapes the reservoir host. Exits include the mouth, nose, eyes, ears, intestines, urinary tract, reproductive tract, and open wounds.

Again, the use of standard precautions such as latex gloves, masks, proper wound care, correct disposal of contaminated products, and hand washing all help control the ability of the infectious material to spread from one host to another.

After exiting the reservoir host, organisms spread by transmission. Transmission is either direct or indirect. Direct transmission occurs from contact with either an infected person or with discharges from an infected person, such as feces or urine. Indirect transmission occurs from droplets in the air expelled by coughing, speaking, or sneezing; vectors that harbor pathogens; contaminated food or drink; and/or contact with contaminated objects (called *fomites).* Proper sanitation of water and food; use of sanitization, disinfection, and sterilization procedures; and use of **germicides,** such as Wavecide and Cidex, help control the transmission of pathogens.

The next step in the chain of infection is the means or portal of entry. This is how the transmitted pathogen gains entry into a new host. The means of entry, like the means of exit, may be the mouth, nose, eyes, intestines, urinary tract, or reproductive system or an open wound. The first line of defense against pathogenic invasion is the intact *integumentary* system, or skin, which serves as a mechanical barrier to infection. Anatomic defense mechanisms also include tears, cilia, mucous membranes, and the pH of body fluids. The body's second line of defense includes the inflammatory process and immune system response. The immune system responds by producing **antibodies** specifically designed to combat the presence of a foreign substance or **antigen.** This process is called *humoral immunity.* The immune system also reacts at the cellular level with *cell-mediated immunity* by causing destruction of pathogenic cells at the site of invasion. An example of cell-mediated immunity is *phagocytosis,* in which specialized immune system cells called *macrophages* actually ingest and destroy pathogenic microbes (see Chapter 53 for further discussion). If the host is a susceptible host, that is, one that is capable of supporting the growth of the infecting organism, the organism will multiply. Factors affecting host susceptibility include the location of entry, the dose of organisms, and the individual's state of health. If the conditions are right, the organism reaches infectious levels and the susceptible host can start the chain of infection all over again.

Individuals who are effectively immunized against a disease, such as hepatitis B, are not susceptible to the disease even if exposed to the pathogen because their immune systems have created antibodies to protect them. In addition to immunization, other ways to decrease susceptibility to disease are proper nutrition and healthy lifestyles.

CRITICAL THINKING APPLICATION

Tommy Anderson, a 5-year-old patient, is seen in the office because of an outbreak of impetigo. Rosa must apply the concepts of the chain of infection and infection control methods to teach Tommy and his mother how to prevent the spread of the infection to other members of the family. What procedures should she follow after Tommy's visit to prevent the spread of the infection to other patients, other staff members, and herself?

Antibiotic Resistance

Antibiotic resistance is one of the world's most significant public health problems. Infectious microorganisms that were once easily treated with antibiotics are growing increasingly resistant to the actions of the drugs. Resistance occurs when an antibiotic is used inappropriately to treat an infection, resulting in a change or mutation of the pathologic organism that in some way reduces or eliminates the effectiveness of the drug. Because antibiotic medication is prescribed inappropriately (such as for a viral infection) or inaccurately (lower dosage, fewer days than recommended) or perhaps not taken by the patient as prescribed, some of the bacteria that survive the initial antibiotic treatment may mutate, which allows the microorganism to survive even in the presence of the antibiotic. Although mutations are rare, overuse of antibiotics provides more opportunity for them to occur. Antibiotics should be used to treat bacterial infections; however, they are not effective against viral infections such as the common cold, most sore throats, and the flu. Cautious use of antibiotics is the key to preventing the spread of resistance. The CDC recommends that physicians do the following:

- Prescribe antibiotic therapy only when it will benefit the patient.
- Treat the patient with an antibiotic that is specific to the infecting **pathogen.**
- Prescribe the recommended dose and time interval of the medication.

THE INFLAMMATORY RESPONSE

When trauma occurs to the body, it alerts protective mechanisms, and the body responds in a predictable manner, called the *inflammatory response.* To defend itself the body initiates specific responses that destroy and remove pathogenic organisms and their byproducts or, if this is not possible, limit the extent of damage caused by the invading pathogen. This process results in the four classic symptoms of inflammation: *erythema* (redness), *edema* (swelling), pain, and heat.

Figure 26-2 details the inflammatory response. When the body is exposed to an infectious agent or a foreign substance, cellular damage occurs at the site. Inflammation mediators—histamine, prostaglandins, and kinins—are released and cause three different responses at the cellular level. All three actions are designed to increase the number of white blood cells (WBCs) at the injury site.

First, blood vessels at the site dilate, causing an increase in local blood flow, resulting in redness or inflammation and heat. Blood vessel walls become more **permeable,** which assists in the release of WBCs to the site. The WBCs begin to form a fibrous capsule around the site to protect surrounding cells from damage or infection. Blood plasma also filters out of the more permeable vessel walls, resulting in edema, which puts pressure on the nerves and causes pain. Finally, chemotaxis, the release of chemical agents, occurs, attracting even more WBCs to the site. The increased number of WBCs at the site results in phagocytosis, or the engulfing and destruction of microorganisms and damaged cells. Destroyed pathogens, cells, and WBCs collect in the area and form a thick, white substance called *pus.* If the pathogenic invasion is too great for localized control, the infection may collect in the body's lymph nodes, where more WBCs are present to help fight the battle. This causes swollen glands or *lymphadenopathy.* If the body is too weak or the number of pathogens is too great, the infection may spread to the bloodstream. A systemic infection, called *septicemia* or *blood poisoning,* may occur that could ultimately affect the entire body. Another term for septicemia is **pyemia.** Without appropriate medical intervention, death can occur.

CRITICAL THINKING APPLICATION

Rosa's next patient appears to have a localized inflammatory response to a splinter. What signs and symptoms should she expect the patient to exhibit?

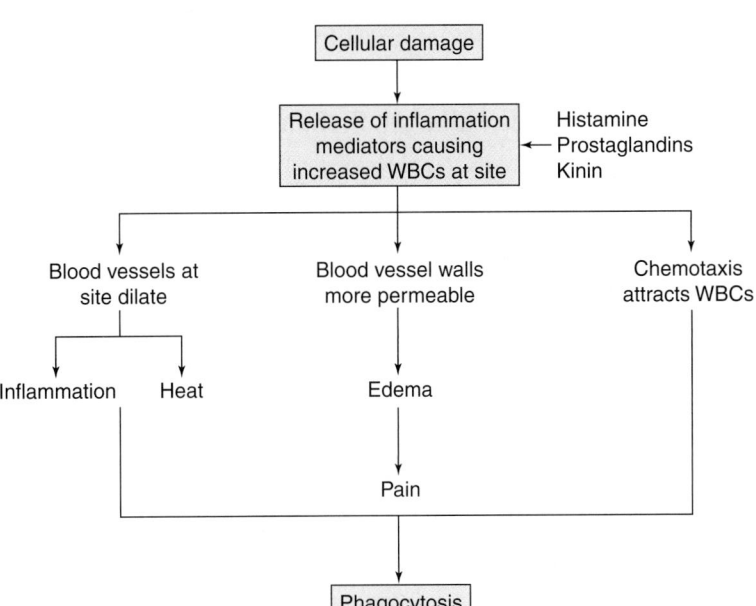

FIGURE 26-2 The inflammatory response.

TYPES OF INFECTIONS

Acute Infection

Acute infections have a rapid onset of symptoms but last a relatively short time. The *prodromal* period is that time when the patient first exhibits vague, nonspecific symptoms of the disease. In an acute viral infection the host cell typically dies within a period of hours or days. Symptoms appear after the tissue damage begins to occur. In most acute infections, such as the common cold, the body's defense mechanisms eliminate the virus within 2 to 3 weeks.

Chronic Infection

Infections that persist for a long period of time, sometimes for life, are called *chronic* infections. In the case of chronic viral hepatitis B, patients are *asymptomatic* or without symptoms, but the virus is detectable with blood tests and remains transmissible throughout their lives. Hepatitis B, or serum hepatitis, is transmitted by blood or blood products as well as all body fluids. It is a serious health hazard to medical personnel. All individuals employed in a healthcare setting should be immunized against hepatitis B.

Latent Infection

A latent infection is a persistent infection in which the symptoms cycle through periods of **relapse** and **remission.** Cold sores and genital herpes are latent viral infections caused by the herpes simplex virus (HSV) types I and II. The virus first enters the body and causes the original lesion. It then lies dormant, in nerve cells away from the surface, until a certain provocation (illness with fever, sunburn, or stress) causes the virus to leave the nerve cell and seek the surface again. Once the virus reaches the superficial tissues, it becomes detectable for a short time and causes a new outbreak at the site. Another herpes virus, varicella- zoster virus, causes chickenpox (varicella). This virus may lie dormant along a nerve pathway for years and later erupt as the painful disease shingles (zoster).

Slow Infections

Slow infections progress over very long periods and typically refer to viral infections of the brain. These conditions include the degenerative neurologic diseases, such as dementia caused by human immunodeficiency virus (HIV) or mad cow disease.

OSHA STANDARDS FOR THE HEALTHCARE SETTING

Chapter 7 introduced the role of OSHA in protecting patients and healthcare personnel from potentially harmful substances in the medical facility. Because of concern about the increasing prevalence of HIV and hepatitis B virus (HBV), in 1987 the Centers for Disease Control (today called the *Centers for Disease Control and Prevention* [CDC]) recommended a new approach to potentially infectious materials called *universal precautions.* The underlying concept of universal precautions was that because it is impossible for healthcare workers to know whether patients have an infectious **disorder,** all blood and certain body fluids must be treated as if they are known to be infectious for blood-borne pathogens. Therefore, precautions should be implemented for all patients, regardless of knowledge of their individual health history. At the same time, use of universal precautions procedures protects patients from any blood-borne infection the healthcare worker may be carrying.

Exposure Control Plan

OSHA recognizes that healthcare employees face significant health risks as the result of occupational exposure to blood or other potentially infectious materials that may contain HBV, hepatitis C virus (HCV), or HIV. In July 1992 OSHA began enforcing work practice controls to reduce or eliminate occupational exposure to blood-borne pathogens. Employers with workers who are at risk for occupational exposure to blood or other infectious materials must implement an Exposure Control Plan that details employee protection procedures. The Exposure Control Plan must identify job classifications and/or specific work-related tasks in which an employee has the potential for being exposed to blood and/or body fluids. The plan must describe how an employer will use a combination of controls, including personal protective equipment (PPE), training, medical surveillance, hepatitis B immunizations, record keeping of occupational injuries, postexposure follow-up, and labeling of hazardous materials. Engineering controls such as safer medical equipment, puncture-proof sharps containers, and shielded needle devices as well as PPE such as gloves, gowns, and face shields are recommended as the primary ways to decrease or eliminate employee exposure.

The plan must be reviewed and updated at least annually to incorporate the use of safer medical devices designed to eliminate or minimize occupational exposure to contaminated waste. In addition, the Exposure Control Plan must be readily available to all employees for review and training. It does not have to be a separate document and may be included as part of the facility's procedure manual or in the health and safety manual developed by the site. Employer failure to comply with the OSHA Bloodborne Pathogens Standard could result in a maximum penalty of $7000 for the first violation and up to $70,000 for repeated violations.

Bloodborne Pathogen Standard

The CDC estimates that medical personnel annually sustain almost 600,000 exposure incidents from contaminated sharps. In response to the CDC's concern about employee risk, the U.S. Congress passed the Needlestick Safety and Prevention Act, which became effective in April 2001. Employers are required to keep a confidential sharps injury log that describes the device involved in the incident and the details of how and where the incident occurred. Employers must also make available to employees effective sharps management devices, such as syringes with self-sheathing needles, needles that retract after use, and needleless intravenous (IV) systems that do not require sharps for **parenteral** administration. Parenteral exposure includes accidental needlesticks, occupation-related human bites, and exposure of potentially infectious material to nonintact skin, as in the presence of cuts and abrasions on employee hands.

The standard also clarifies the use of washing or flushing any exposed body area or mucous membrane immediately or as soon as possible after exposure to potentially infectious materials. This includes hand washing after the removal of gloves or other PPE. The CDC recently made new recommendations regarding hand hygiene in healthcare facilities. Although hands should be washed with antimicrobial soap and warm running water when available, studies have shown that the correct use of alcohol-based handrubs significantly reduces the number of microorganisms on the skin, takes less time than traditional hand washing, and causes less irritation to the skin, especially if the solution is mixed with emollients. The CDC has the following recommendations for adequate hand hygiene:

- Visibly soiled hands should be washed for a minimum of 15 seconds with antimicrobial soap and warm running water.
- Gloves reduce hand contamination by 70% to 80%. Alcohol handrubs should be used before and after attending to each patient as well as after gloves are removed, to prevent cross-contamination among patients and healthcare workers.
- To properly use an alcohol handrub, apply the label-recommended amount to the palm of one hand and rub hands together, covering all surfaces until the hands are dry.
- Studies have shown that even after careful hand hygiene, healthcare workers with artificial nails have more pathogenic microbes under their nails and on their fingertips than workers with natural nails. Artificial nails also cause nail changes that contribute to the transmission of microbes.
- Natural nail tips should be no longer than $1/4$ inch to prevent microbial growth in the nail bed.
- Allergic contact dermatitis from alcohol handrubs is uncommon (Figure 26-3).

The best way to reduce occupational risk of infection is to follow the Pathogen Standards. Healthcare workers must take adequate and consistent precautions to protect themselves and their patients. Figure 26-4 summarizes OSHA standard precautions.

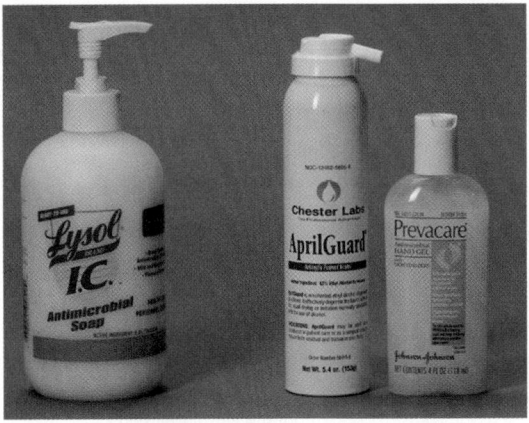

FIGURE 26-3 Antimicrobial soap and alcohol-based handrubs. (From Klieger DM: *Saunders textbook of medical assisting*, St Louis, 2005, Saunders.)

Compliance Guidelines

Because the Pathogen Standards are written to cover employees working in all health fields, it is obvious that only some of the regulations apply to the ambulatory care setting. Safety and infection control fundamentals go beyond hand washing and knowledge of the disease cycle. The information presented here is as it applies to the medical assistant profession.

Barrier Protection

Medical assistants should routinely use appropriate barrier precautions when contact with blood or other body fluids is anticipated. Barrier protection, or PPE, includes specialized clothing or equipment that prevents blood or other potentially infectious material from passing through to reach the healthcare worker. Barrier devices include latex gloves, face masks, face shields, protective glasses, laboratory coats, barrier gowns, mouthpieces, and resuscitation bags (Figure 26-5) that protect you from potentially infectious substances. The purpose of PPE is to prevent or minimize the entry of infectious material into your body.

Since implementation of universal precautions, the use of latex gloves is commonplace in healthcare facilities. As a result there has also been an increase in allergic reactions associated with latex products. Hypersensitive reactions to latex gloves or the powder that lines them may be localized, with **urticaria,** dermatitis, conjunctivitis, and **rhinitis;** or systemic, with asthmatic reactions or an **anaphylaxis** response. If you or a patient shows signs of sensitivity to latex, the healthcare provider is required to provide gloves made of nonallergenic materials as barrier devices.

Gloves must be used if there is any chance that you will be involved in any of the following activities (Procedure 26-1):

- Touching a patient's blood and body fluids, mucous membranes, or skin that is not intact.
- Handling items and surfaces contaminated with blood and body fluids.
- Performing venipuncture, finger sticks, injections, and other vascular procedures.

Potentially Infectious Fluids

- Cerebrospinal fluid (CSF); synovial, pleural, pericardial, peritoneal, mucous, and amniotic fluids
- Liquid or semiliquid blood
- Vaginal and seminal secretions
- Saliva in dental procedures
- Body fluid visibly contaminated with blood
- Unknown body fluid
- Wound drainage
- Human tissue, including tissue culture, cells, or exudates
- HIV has been isolated from CSF and synovial and amniotic fluids; hepatitis antigens have been detected in synovial, amniotic, and peritoneal fluids.
- Items that are contaminated with any of the potentially infectious materials listed above require special handling.

Requirements of Employers: OSHA Bloodborne Pathogens Standard

---

EXPOSURE CONTROL PLAN

Each medical office must develop a written exposure control plan (ECP). The purpose of an ECP is to identify tasks where there is the potential for exposure to blood and other potentially infectious materials.

- A timetable must be published indicating when and how communication of potential hazards will occur.
- The employer must offer employees the hepatitis B vaccine within 10 working days of employment (at no cost to the employee). If employees sign a form to refuse the vaccine, they can change their mind at no cost to the employee.
- The employer must document the steps that should be taken in case of an exposure incident, including a postexposure evaluation and follow-up, strict record keeping, implementation of engineering controls, provision for personal protective equipment, and general housekeeping standards. This plan must be posted in the medical office.
- There must also be written procedures for evaluating the circumstances of an exposure incident.
- Training records must be kept for 3 years.

ENGINEERING CONTROLS AND WORK PRACTICES

The employer must provide engineering controls, or equipment and facilities that minimize the possibility of exposure. Examples of engineering controls include the following:

- Providing puncture-resistant containers for used sharps.
- Providing handwashing facilities that are readily accessible.
- Equipment for sanitizing, decontaminating, and sterilizing.

The employer must also enforce work practice controls. Work practice controls also minimize the possibility of exposure by making sure employees are using the proper techniques while working. Examples include the following:

- Enforcing proper handwashing or sanitizing procedures.
- Enforcing proper technique for using and handling needles to prevent needle sticks.
- Enforcing proper techniques to minimize the splashing of blood.

PERSONAL PROTECTIVE EQUIPMENT

Employers must provide, and employees must use, personal protective equipment (PPE) when the possibility exists of exposure to blood or contaminated body fluids. This equipment must not allow blood or potentially infectious material to pass through to the employee's clothes, skin, eyes, or mouth. Examples of PPE include the following:

- Gowns
- Face shields
- Goggles
- Gloves

If an employee has an allergy to powder or latex, the employer must provide hypoallergenic or powderless gloves. The employee cannot be charged for PPEs.

EXPOSURE INCIDENT MANAGEMENT

An exposure incident is contact with blood or biohazard infectious material that occurs when doing one's job. When an exposure incident is reported, the employer must arrange for an immediate and confidential medical evaluation. The information and actions required are as follows:

- Documenting how the exposure occurred.
- Identifying and testing the "source" individual, if possible.
- Testing the employee's blood, if consent is granted.
- Providing counseling.
- Evaluating, treating, and following up on any reported illness.

Medical records must be kept for each employee with occupational exposure for the duration of employment plus 30 years.

COMMUNICATION OF POTENTIAL HAZARDS TO EMPLOYEESS

A medical assistant will be exposed to hazardous chemicals on the job. Most chemicals handled by assistants are not any more dangerous than those used in the home. In the workplace, however, exposure is likely to be greater, concentrations higher, and exposure time longer.

The **"right to-know" law,** OSHA's hazard communication standard, states that each employee has a right to know what chemicals he or she is working with in the workplace. The right-to-know law is intended to make the workplace safer by making certain that all information regarding chemical hazards is known to the employee. This information is supplied in the **material safety data sheet (MSDS),** a fact sheet about a chemical that includes the following information:

- Identification of the chemical
- Listing of the physical and health hazards
- Precautions for handling
- Identification of the chemical as a carcinogen
- First-aid procedures
- Name, address, and telephone number of manufacturer

Many MSD information sheets can be obtained in repositories on the Internet. An MSDS should be updated at least every 3 years. Employers must ensure that all products have an up-to-date MSDS when they enter the workplace.

Potential hazards are also communicated with labels and color. Any containers with biohazard waste must be orange (or reddish orange) and must display the biohazard symbol. These labels and colors alert employees to the risk of possible exposure.

FIGURE 26-4 Requirements of employers: OSHA bloodborne pathogens standard. (From revision to OSHA's Bloodborne Pathogens Standard, April 2006.)

- Assisting with any surgical procedure. If a glove is torn or an injury occurs during the procedure, the glove should be removed and replaced with a new glove as soon as safety permits.
- Handling, processing, and disposing of all specimens of blood and body fluids.
- Cleaning and decontaminating spills of blood or other body fluids.

SAFETY ALERT PROTECTIVE EQUIPMENT CONTAMINATED WITH BODY FLUIDS OF ANY KIND MUST BE REMOVED AND PLACED IN A DESIGNATED AREA OR BIOHAZARD CONTAINER, AND HANDS OR ANY OTHER EXPOSED AREAS MUST BE WASHED OR FLUSHED AS SOON AS POSSIBLE. PROTECTIVE EYEWEAR AND/OR FACE SHIELDS MUST BE WORN WHENEVER SPLASHES, SPRAYS, OR DROPLETS MAY OCCUR. STANDARD PRESCRIPTION EYEGLASSES ARE NOT

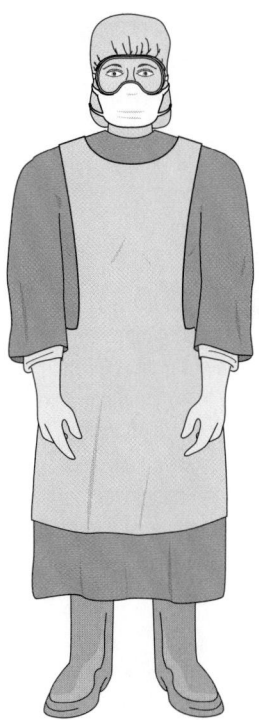

FIGURE 26-5 Personal protective equipment. (From Fuller JK: *Surgical technology: principles and practice*, ed 4, St Louis, 2005, Saunders.)

CONSIDERED EFFECTIVE. UTILITY GLOVES MAY BE REUSED IF THEY ARE INTACT WITHOUT CRACKS, TEARS, OR PUNCTURES. ALL PPE MUST BE REMOVED BEFORE ONE LEAVES THE MEDICAL FACILITY (Figure 26-6).

CRITICAL THINKING APPLICATION

Rosa is caring for an injured 3-year-old child with an open wound on his right knee. She puts on latex gloves to clean the wound, and the mother demands to know why. How can she explain her actions?

Environment Protection

The environment protection section of the compliance guidelines covers controls to minimize the risk of occupational injury by isolating or removing any physical or mechanical health hazard in the medical workplace. Every medical assistant must adhere to these safety rules.

- Observe warning labels on biohazard containers and equipment.
- Minimize splashing, spraying, and spattering of drops of potentially infectious materials. Splattering of blood onto skin or mucous membranes is a proven mode of transmission of HBV.
- Bandage any breaks or lesions on your hands before gloving.
- If exposed body surfaces, such as the eyes, come in contact with body fluids, flush with water and/or scrub with soap and water as soon as possible (Figure 26-7).
- Contaminated needles and other sharps should not be recapped, bent, broken, or resheathed. Needle units are now required to have sliding shields or some other protective device for use after injection.
- Use hemostats to attach and remove scalpel blades from handles.
- Contaminated reusable sharps should not be stored or processed in a way that requires employees to reach into the containers.

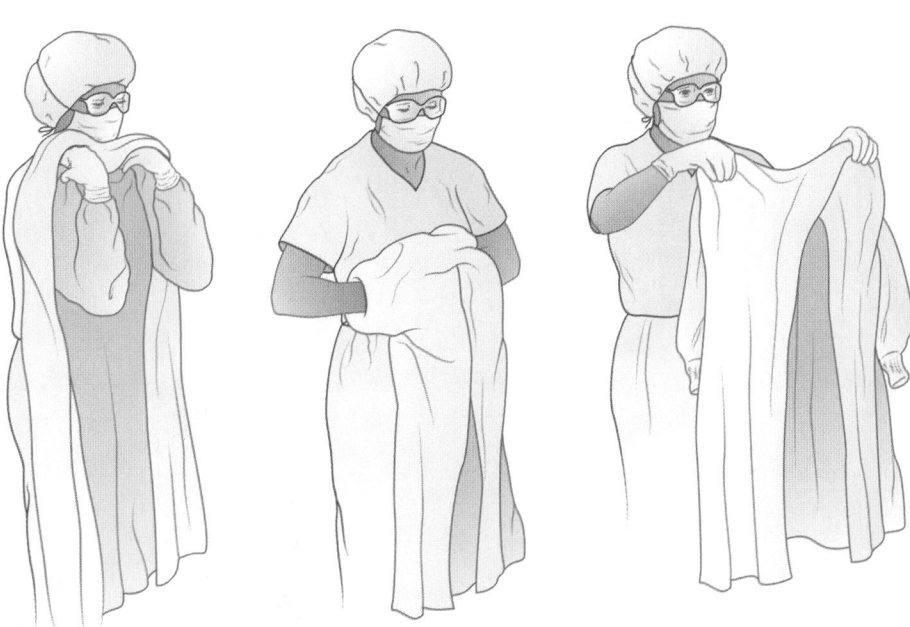

FIGURE 26-6 Removing a contaminated gown. (From Fuller JK: *Surgical technology: principles and practice*, ed 4, St Louis, 2005, Saunders.)

PROCEDURE 26-1

Use Standard Precautions for Removing Contaminated Gloves and Disposal of Biohazardous Material

<u>CAAHEP COMPETENCIES:</u> 3.b.(1)(d), 3.b.(1)(e)
<u>ABHES COMPETENCIES:</u> 4.q, 4.r

GOAL: *To minimize pathogen exposure by aseptically removing and discarding contaminated gloves.*

EQUIPMENT and SUPPLIES

- Latex or alternative disposable examination gloves
- Biohazard waste container with labeled red biohazard bag

PROCEDURAL STEPS

1. With the dominant hand, grasp the glove of the opposite hand near the palm and begin removing the first glove (Figure 1). Arms should be extended from the body, with hands pointed down.

PURPOSE: Having the hands held down and away from the body helps avoid possible contamination.

2. Pull the glove inside out until you reach the fingers, holding the contaminated glove in the dominant gloved hand (Figure 2).
   PURPOSE: Taking the glove off inside out prevents transmission of pathogens to a nongloved surface.

3. Insert the thumb of the nongloved hand inside the cuff of the remaining contaminated glove (Figure 3).

4. Pull the glove down the hand inside out over the contaminated glove being held, leaving the contaminated side of both gloves on the inside.

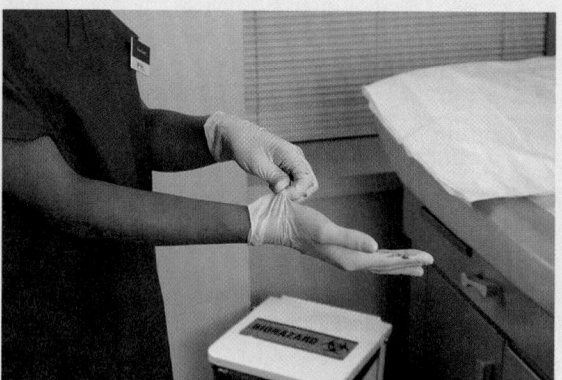

FIGURE 1

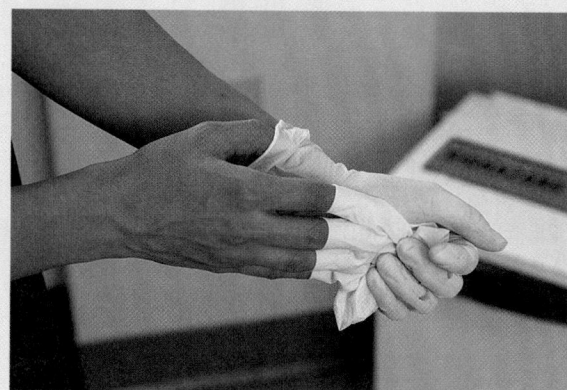

FIGURE 3

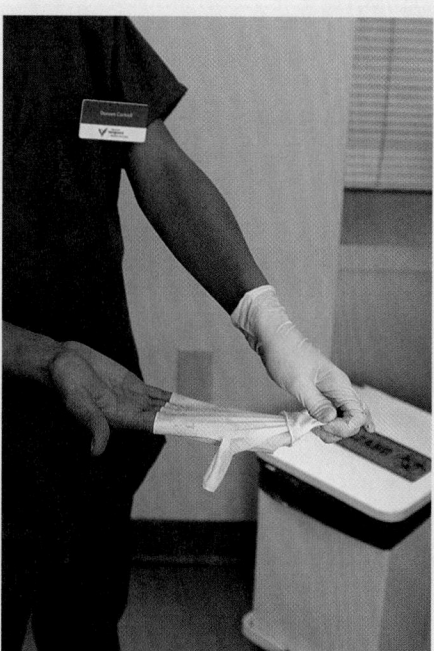

FIGURE 2

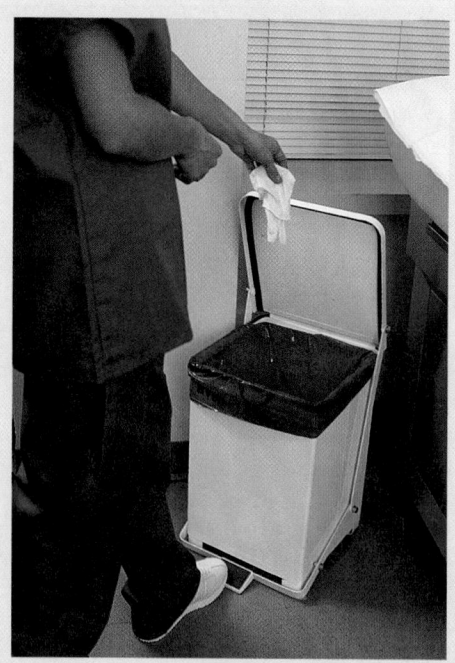

FIGURE 4

Continued

PURPOSE: The medical assistant is now protected from the contaminated surface of both gloves.

5. Properly dispose of the inside-out contaminated gloves in a biohazard waste container (Figure 4).

PURPOSE: To prevent the spread of infection.

6. Perform a medical aseptic hand wash as described in Procedure 26-2.

PURPOSE: To minimize the number of pathogens on your hands, thereby reducing the number of transient bacteria and the risk of pathogenic transmission.

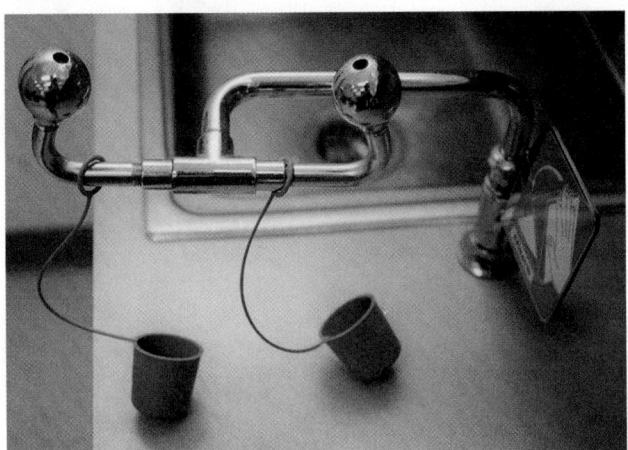

FIGURE 26-7 Eye washing unit.

- Immediately after use, dispose of syringes and needles, scalpel blades, and other sharp items in a labeled, leakproof, puncture-resistant biohazard container. The container must be located as close as possible to the area where the instruments are used.

- All specimens must be placed in a container that prevents leakage during collection, handling, processing, storage, transport, and shipping. Avoid contaminating the outside of the container or the label with the specimen substance. If the outside is contaminated, the container should be disinfected. One method is to use a 1:10 dilution of sodium hypochlorite (household chlorine bleach and water) and place the container in an impervious bag for transport. The container must have a biohazard label that alerts others it holds potentially infectious material. Gloves should be worn throughout this procedure.

- Mouth pipetting or the sucking of blood through tubing is prohibited.

- Contaminated test materials should be decontaminated before reprocessing or should be placed in impervious bags and disposed of according to policy.

- Equipment that has been contaminated with blood or body fluids should be decontaminated before being repaired in the office or transported to the manufacturer. There is no documented evidence of HIV transmission from contaminated environmental surfaces, but surface contamination is a proven mode of transmission for HBV.

- Smoking, eating, drinking, applying cosmetics or lip balm, and handling contact lenses are prohibited in work areas where there is reasonable likelihood of contamination from blood-borne pathogens.

- Food and drink cannot be kept in refrigerators, freezers, shelves, or cabinets or on countertops where blood or other potentially infectious materials could be present.

Housekeeping Controls

The OSHA Standard specifies certain housekeeping measures be followed to promote a work area that is clean and sanitary. One requirement is a posted schedule for cleaning and decontaminating each work area where exposure could occur. This documentation must be specific and include information about the surface cleaned, type of waste encountered, and procedures performed in the designated area.

- Work surfaces must be immediately decontaminated with a **disinfectant** (such as a 1:10 solution of sodium hypochlorite) after accidental spills of blood or body fluids and at the end of each procedure.

- Disinfection and decontamination of all reusable containers must be done on a routine basis.

- Sharps containers are to be maintained in an upright position to keep waste inside and as close as possible to the work area. Never attempt to reach inside a sharps container, and do not overfill them. Replace containers on a routine basis, and be certain that the lid is closed securely before preparing them for biohazard waste disposal.

- Never pick up spilled material or broken glassware with hands. Brooms, brushes, dustpans, and pickup tongs or forceps should be used and the material placed immediately into an impervious biohazard bag or container at the spill site (Figure 26-8). Use an absorbent professional biohazard spill preparation as directed to decontaminate the site.

- Handle soiled linen as little as possible, and always while wearing gloves or other protective equipment. Linens soiled with blood or body fluids should be double-bagged and transported in labeled, leakproof biohazard bags.

- Contaminated materials and/or infective wastes are to be handled with extreme caution to prevent exposure. Biohazard waste must be collected in impermeable red polyethylene or polypropylene biohazard-labeled bags or containers and sealed (Figure 26-9). This waste must

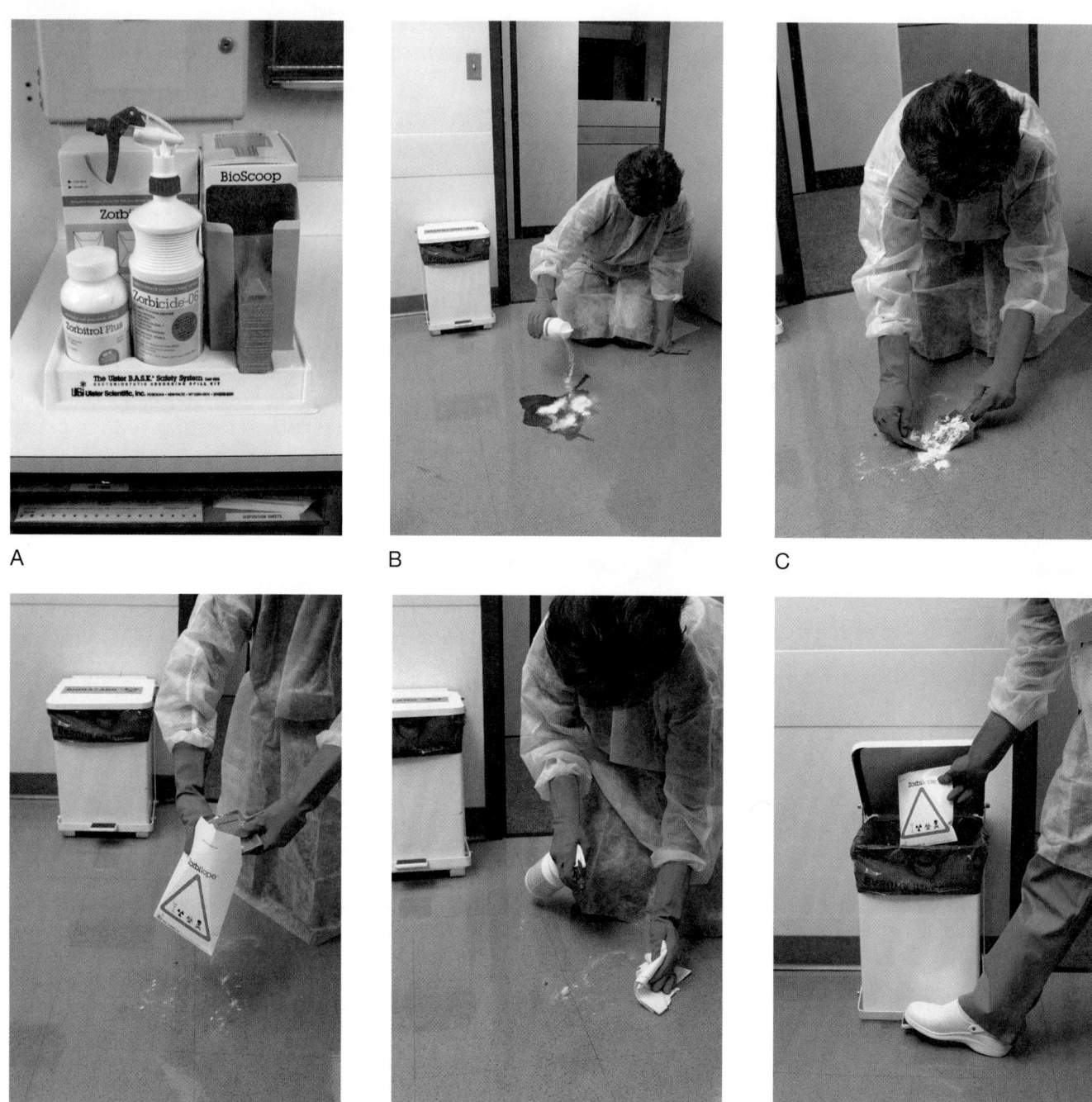

FIGURE 26-8 Cleaning spilled material. **A,** Clean-up kit with printed instructions. **B,** Sprinkle congealing powder over the spill. **C,** Scoop up spill. **D,** Place contents in bag. **E,** Wipe area thoroughly with germicide. **F,** Place all contaminated material in biohazard bag or container.

be disposed of in accordance with all applicable federal, state, and local regulations. Disposal methods include treatment by heat, incineration, steam sterilization, chemical treatment, or other equivalent methods that render the waste inactive before it can be placed in a landfill.

CRITICAL THINKING APPLICATION

Using the techniques learned in Chapter 1, create a mind map that identifies the details of OSHA's Bloodborne Pathogens Standard.

Hepatitis B Vaccination

Hepatitis B vaccine must be available free of charge to all employees who are at risk for occupational exposure to bloodborne pathogens, whether they are full-time or part-time workers, within 10 days of starting employment. The vaccine is administered by intramuscular injection in three doses. The second injection is administered 4 weeks after the first, and the third injection 6 months after the first. The U.S. Public Health Service does not currently recommend routine boosters for hepatitis B immunization. However, if they are recommended

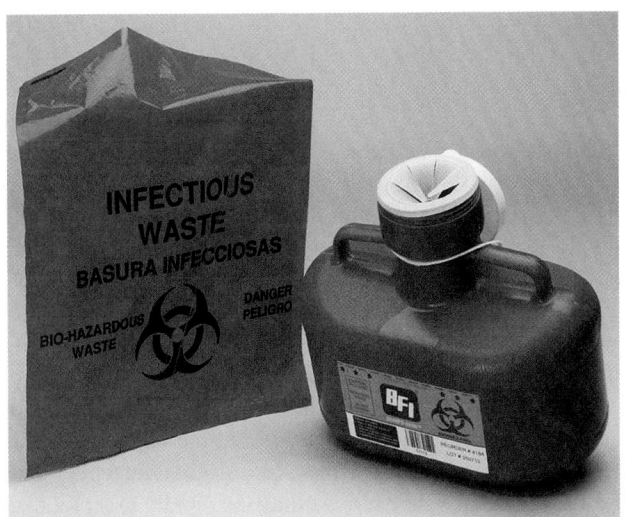

FIGURE 26-9 Biohazard bag and biohazard sharps container.

Hepatitis B Vaccine Declination

I understand that due to my occupational exposure to blood or other potentially infectious materials I may be at risk of acquiring hepatitis B virus (HBV) infection. I have been given the opportunity to be vaccinated with hepatitis B vaccine, at no charge to myself. However, I decline hepatitis B vaccination at this time. I understand that by declining this vaccine, I continue to be at risk of acquiring hepatitis B, a serious disease. If in the future I continue to have occupational exposure to blood or other potentially infectious materials and I want to be vaccinated with hepatitis B vaccine, I can receive the vaccination series at no charge to me.

Name: _____   Date: _____

FIGURE 26-10 Sample hepatitis B declination form. (From OSHA website: www. osha.gov. Accessed May 2006.)

---

in the future, boosters must be made available to eligible employees without cost.

Although the effectiveness rate of vaccination is almost 96%, employees should have a blood titer drawn after completion of the injection cycle to determine whether they have created antibodies against the disease. If the employee did not respond to the first series or if the series was not completed, revaccination with a second three-dose series is recommended. If antibodies still do not develop, no further vaccination is given.

Employees have the right to decline the hepatitis B immunization but are required to sign a declination form that is kept on file as a record of worker refusal. A sample declination form developed by OSHA is shown in Figure 26-10. However, if the employee changes his or her mind, he or she can receive the vaccine at a future date free of charge.

Postexposure Follow-Up

If a worker is exposed through an accidental needlestick, a human bite, exposure to broken skin, or from a splash or splatter onto mucous membranes, such as the eyes, certain procedures must be followed.

- Immediately, or as soon as possible after exposure, the worker should wash or flush the exposed area.
- The exposure incident must be immediately reported to the supervisor.
- The employee must immediately receive a confidential medical evaluation. The physician caring for the exposed employee must receive written details regarding the exposure incident including the route and circumstances surrounding the incident. All documentation related to the exposure must remain confidential, not disclosed to any individual without the employee's express written permission, and kept for at least the duration of the worker's employment plus 30 years.
- An incident report must be filed that documents the details surrounding the exposure incident, the route or

type of exposure, and the identity, if known, of the source individual. The source individual is the person, living or dead, whose blood or potentially infectious material was the source of the occupational exposure.

- The source individual, if known, is immediately screened for HBV and HIV. Depending on state regulations, consent may or may not be required from the source individual to perform the screening. If consent is required but not given, the employer must document that consent was not received from the source individual. State law also determines if the employee may be told the results of the source individual's tests.
- The exposed worker is tested for HBV and HIV if consent is given. If the employee refuses the tests but blood is drawn, the sample must be stored 90 days for the worker to decide whether screening is wanted.
- If not vaccinated against HBV, the employee is offered vaccination.
- The injured employee must receive a copy of the healthcare provider's written opinion within 15 days of the completion of the evaluation.
- The exposed worker must receive health counseling regarding the risk of illness or other adverse outcomes of exposure and the potential for as well as the consequences of transmission of the disease to family, patients, and others.

Because students are not considered employees and are attending an educational institution, OSHA standards do not apply. However, all healthcare students are at risk for blood-borne pathogen exposure and should follow all OSHA guidelines designed to protect individuals from exposure.

A complete unabridged copy of OSHA's Bloodborne Pathogens Standard may be obtained at the OSHA website, www.osha.gov.

CRITICAL THINKING APPLICATION

Rosa's office has been especially busy today. While administering an injection to a frightened 6-year-old child, a co-worker has an accidental needlestick. She tells Rosa about the incident but does not know what to do. What steps should be taken to manage the situation?

ASEPTIC TECHNIQUES: PREVENTION OF DISEASE TRANSMISSION

Asepsis means freedom from infection or infectious material. *Medical asepsis* is defined as the destruction of disease-causing organisms after they leave the body. When we practice the principles of medical asepsis, we are directing our efforts at preventing reinfection of the patient or the cross-infection of other patients or ourselves. The goal is to eliminate or minimize pathogens by following OSHA's Bloodborne Pathogens Standard and disinfecting objects as soon as possible after contamination. This creates a healthcare environment that is as free of pathogens as possible.

Surgical asepsis is the destruction of organisms before they enter the body. This technique is used for any procedure that invades the body's skin or tissues, such as surgery or injections. Any time the skin or mucous membrane is punctured, pierced, or incised (or will be during a procedure), surgical aseptic techniques are practiced. Everything that comes into contact with the patient, such as gowns, drapes, instruments, and the gloved hands of the surgical team, should be **sterile.** Minor surgery, urinary catheterizations, injections, and some specimen collections, such as blood collection and biopsies, are performed using surgical aseptic technique. This technique is presented in Chapter 56.

Because it is not possible to sterilize your hands, the goal of hand washing is to reduce skin bacteria by the use of mechanical friction, antimicrobial soaps, and warm running water. Normally, two types of bacteria are on your skin: transient bacteria, which are surface bacteria that are introduced by fomites and remain with you a short time, and resident bacteria, found under fingernails, in hair follicles, in the openings of the sebaceous glands, and in the deeper layers of the skin. The goal of thorough hand washing is to remove or decrease the numbers of transient bacteria on the surface of the skin, thus preventing transient bacteria from becoming resident bacteria.

The most effective barrier against infection is the unbroken skin. If the skin and mucous membranes are intact, medical asepsis can be practiced for most noninvasive (not penetrating through human tissues) procedures, such as pelvic and proctologic examinations. Instruments and objects used in medical aseptic procedures must be decontaminated or sterilized before being used on another patient. Medical aseptic procedures may also include the use of gowns and masks, but these are not sterile and are worn to protect you more than the patient.

Hand Washing

Hands must be washed, using the correct technique, before and after each patient is examined or treated and also when stipulated in the Bloodborne Pathogens Guidelines. It is not necessary to do an extended scrub each time, but the first scrub in the morning should be extensive, lasting 2 to 4 minutes. Subsequent hand washing may be brief unless hands are excessively contaminated. A good antimicrobial soap with chlorhexidine, such as Hibiclens, which has antiseptic residual action that will last several hours, should be used. Each office sink should be equipped with a liquid soap dispenser. A water-soluble lotion may be rubbed into the hands after they are washed and dried. Dry, cracked, chapped skin interrupts the skin's integrity and can result in transmission of disease.

Proper hand washing depends on two factors: running water and friction. Water should be warm, because water that is too hot or too cold will cause the skin to become chapped. Friction means the firm rubbing of all surfaces of the hands and wrists. Remember that your fingers have four sides and fingernails have two sides. For medical hand washing, all jewelry except a plain wedding band is removed. A wristwatch may be left on if it can be moved up on the forearm away from the wrist area. Hands are washed under running water, with the fingertips pointing downward. Soap and friction are applied to the hands and wrists. Allow the water to wash away debris from the wrists down toward the fingertips (Procedure 26-2).

Remember, the goal of aseptic hand washing is to protect you from infection and prevent cross-contamination of microorganisms from one patient to another. Use this procedure after you finish with one patient and before you attend to another patient; after you finish handling one specimen and before you handle another specimen; before and after you use toilet facilities; whenever you touch something that causes your hands to become contaminated; when you arrive at work and before you leave the office; before and after eating; and at the end of the day.

As stated earlier, alcohol handrubs may substitute for hand washing except if the hands are visibly contaminated. Evidence suggests that hand antisepsis is more effective in reducing **nosocomial infections** than plain hand washing. Using anti-microbial-impregnated wipes (e.g., towelettes) is not a substitute for using an alcohol-based handrub or antimicrobial soap.

Sanitization

Instruments and other items used in office surgery, examination, or treatment must be carefully cleaned before proceeding with the steps of disinfection or sterilization. *Sanitization* is the cleansing process that decreases the number of microorganisms to a safe level as dictated in public health guidelines. This cleansing process removes debris such as blood and other body fluids from instruments or equipment. Blood and debris must be removed so that later disinfection with chemicals or sterilization with steam, heat, or gases can penetrate to all the instrument's surfaces (Procedure 26-3).

The medical assistant should always wear gloves (thick utility gloves if the instruments have sharp or pointed edges) while performing sanitization, to prevent possible personal contamination with potentially infectious body fluids that may be present on the articles being cleaned. The procedure should be completed immediately after use of the instruments in a separate workroom or area to avoid cross-contamination with

PROCEDURE 26-2

Perform Medical Aseptic Hand Washing

<u>CAAHEP COMPETENCY:</u> 3.b.(1)(a)
<u>ABHES COMPETENCY:</u> 4.c

GOAL: *To minimize the number of pathogens on the hands, thus reducing the risk of pathogenic transmission.*

EQUIPMENT and SUPPLIES

- Sink with running water
- Antimicrobial liquid soap in a dispenser (bar soap is not acceptable)
- Nail brush or orange stick
- Paper towels in a dispenser
- Water-based antimicrobial lotion
- Biohazard waste container with labeled red biohazard bag

PROCEDURAL STEPS

1. Remove all jewelry except your wristwatch if it can be pulled up above your wrist and a plain gold wedding ring.
   <u>PURPOSE:</u> Jewelry is capable of concealing microorganisms.

2. Turn on the faucet with a paper towel, and regulate the water temperature to lukewarm.
   <u>PURPOSE:</u> Use a paper towel to prevent touching contaminated surfaces; water that is too hot can cause skin to become dry and chapped.

3. Allow your hands to become wet, apply soap, and lather using a circular motion with friction while holding your fingertips downward (Figure 1). Rub well between your fingers.
   <u>PURPOSE:</u> Friction removes soil and contaminants from your hands and wrists.

4. If this is the first hand washing of the day, use a nail brush or an orange stick and thoroughly inspect and clean under every fingernail during step 3.

5. Rinse well, holding your hands so that the water flows from your wrists downward to your fingertips (Figure 2).
   <u>PURPOSE:</u> Soil and contaminants will wash off your skin and down the drain.

6. Wet your hands again and repeat the scrubbing procedure using a vigorous, circular motion over wrists and hands for at least 1 to 2 minutes.
   <u>PURPOSE:</u> Time is required for friction and motion to eliminate all possible soil and contaminants.

7. Rinse your hands a second time, keeping fingers lower than your wrists.
   <u>PURPOSE:</u> To ensure that the hands are really clean.

8. Dry your hands with paper towels. Do not touch the paper towel dispenser as you are obtaining towels (Figure 3).
   <u>PURPOSE:</u> Touching the dispenser contaminates your hands, and you will need to start over.

9. If faucets are not foot operated, turn off the water faucet with the paper towel (Figure 4).

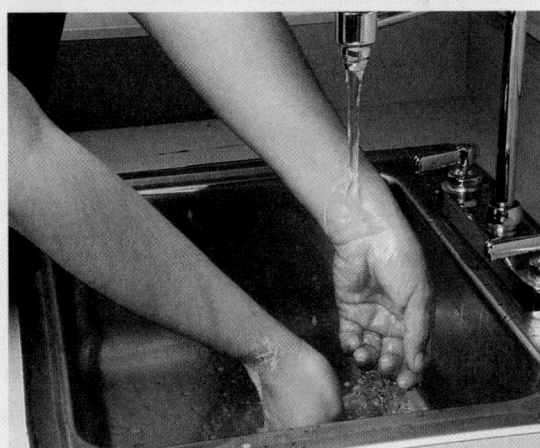

FIGURE 2

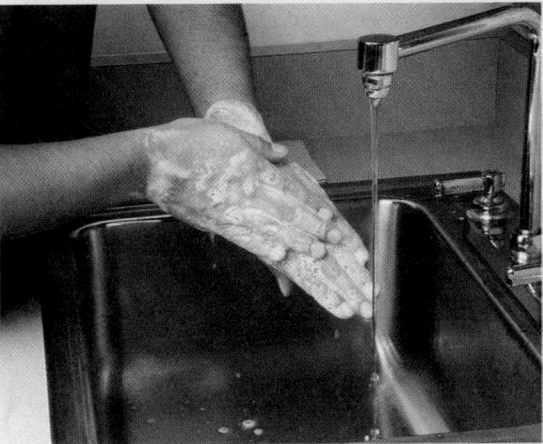

FIGURE 1

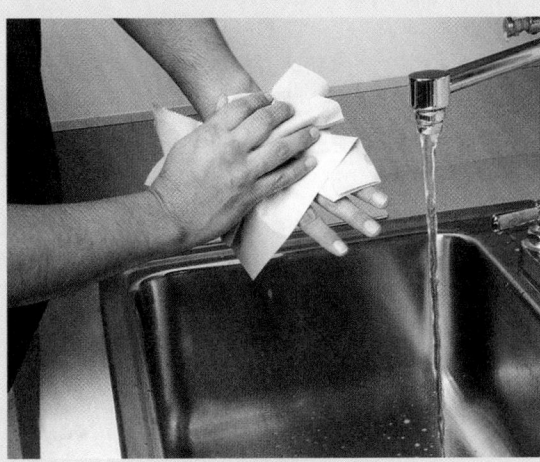

FIGURE 3

Continued

PROCEDURE 26-2—cont'd

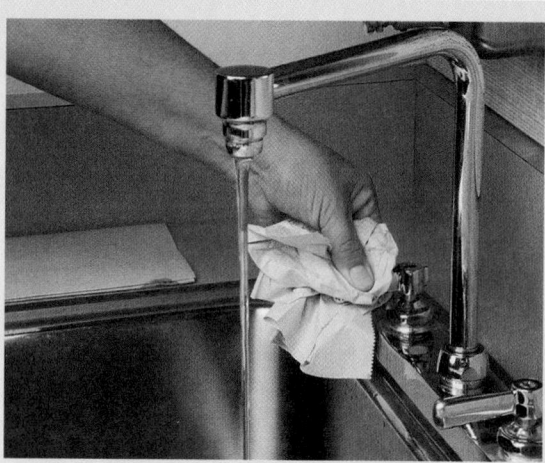

FIGURE 4

PURPOSE: The faucet is dirty and will contaminate your clean hands.

10. After completion of drying your hands and turning off faucets, place used towels into a biohazard waste container.

   PURPOSE: Always discard contaminated waste in a biohazard waste container immediately to eliminate the source of infection.

11. Apply a water-based antibacterial hand lotion to prevent chapped or dry skin.

   PURPOSE: Chapped skin eliminates the first line of defense against infectious organisms.

PROCEDURE 26-3

Use Standard Precautions for Sanitizing Instruments and Disposal of Biohazardous Material

CAAHEP COMPETENCIES: 3.b.(1)(d), 3.b.(1)(e)
ABHES COMPETENCIES: 4.q, 4.r

GOAL: *Following standard precautions, remove all contaminated matter from instruments in preparation for disinfection or sterilization.*

EQUIPMENT and SUPPLIES

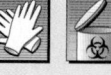

- Sink with hot running water
- Sanitizing agent or low-sudsing soap with enzymatic action
- Utility gloves that are decontaminated and show no signs of deterioration
- Chin-length face shield or goggles and face mask if contamination with droplets of blood-borne pathogens is possible
- Disposable brush
- Disposable paper towels
- Disposable gloves
- Disinfectant cleaner
- Biohazard waste container with labeled red biohazard bag

PROCEDURAL STEPS

1. Put on utility gloves.
   PURPOSE: To provide personal protection against potentially infectious matter and sharp instruments.

2. Put on face shield or goggles and mask if potential for splashing of infectious material exists (Figure 1).
   PURPOSE: To provide personal protection against potentially infectious matter.

3. Separate sharp instruments from other instruments to be sanitized.
   PURPOSE: To prevent possible self-injury and exposure to infectious matter.

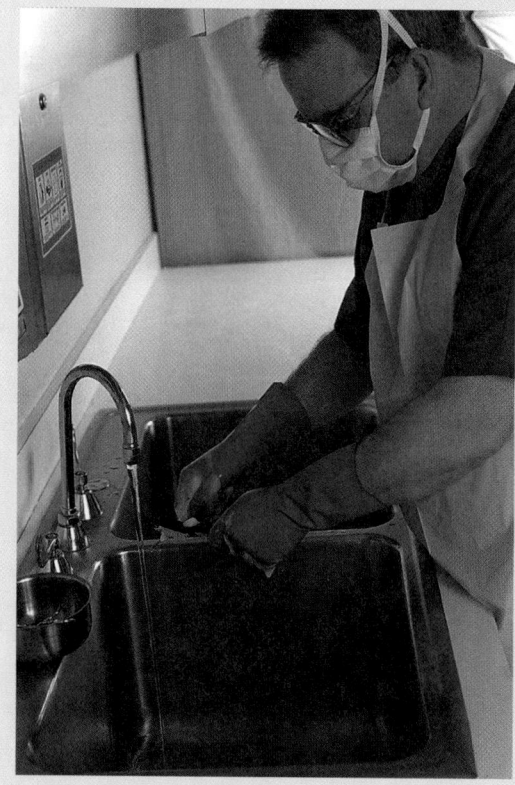

FIGURE 1

Continued

PROCEDURE 26-3—cont'd

4. Rinse the instruments under cold running water.
   PURPOSE: To help remove debris and prevent coagulation of body fluids.

5. Open hinged instruments, and scrub all grooves, crevices, and serrations with a disposable brush (Figure 2).
   PURPOSE: Microorganisms can hide under contaminants and not be destroyed by the disinfection process.

6. Rinse well with hot water.
   PURPOSE: Hot water removes all soap and contaminant residue.

7. Towel dry all instruments thoroughly, and dispose of contaminated towels and disposable brush in a biohazard waste container. Do not touch the paper towel dispenser as you are obtaining towels.

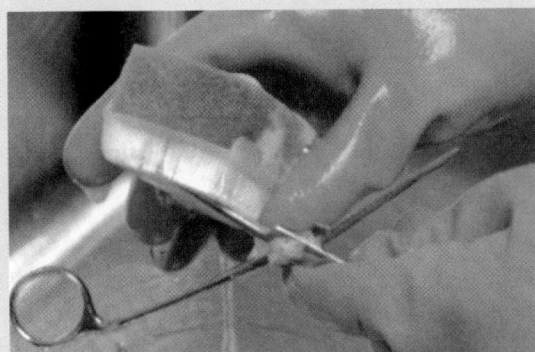

FIGURE 2

PURPOSE: All contaminated material must be disposed of in a labeled biohazard container and/or a labeled red biohazard bag. Touching the dispenser contaminates your hands. Wet instruments can rust or become dull and also dilute disinfectant or sterilizing chemicals.

8. Remove utility gloves and wash hands according to Procedure 26-2.
   PURPOSE: To remove any possible contaminants.

9. Towel dry your hands, and apply disposable gloves. Decontaminate utility gloves and work surfaces using disinfectant cleaner.
   PURPOSE: To prevent personal exposure to contaminants. All equipment and working surfaces should be cleaned and decontaminated with a disinfectant to prevent transmission of infectious material.

10. Dispose of contaminated towels in a biohazard waste container.
    PURPOSE: All contaminated material must be disposed of in a labeled biohazard container and/or a labeled red biohazard bag.

11. Remove disposable gloves according to Procedure 26-1. Dispose of gloves in a biohazard waste container. Wash hands according to Procedure 26-2.
    PURPOSE: To prevent spread of infection and to remove any possible contaminants.

12. Towel dry your hands and place sanitized instruments in a designated area for disinfection or sterilization.
    PURPOSE: Sanitized instruments must be removed from the cleaning area to prevent possible cross-contamination.

clean instruments and equipment. If this is not possible, rinse the used items under cold water, then place them in a low-sudsing, rust-inhibiting, enzyme-containing, detergent solution. Never allow blood or other substances that can **coagulate** to dry on an instrument. When you are ready to sanitize instruments, drain off the soak solution and rinse each instrument in cold, running water. Separate the sharp instruments from the others because metal instruments may damage the cutting edges and sharp instruments may injure the other instruments or you. Clean all the sharp instruments at one time, when you can concentrate on avoiding the dangers of injury to yourself. Open all hinges and scrub serrations and ratchets with a small scrub brush or toothbrush. Rinse the instruments in hot water, then check carefully for proper working order before they are disinfected or sterilized. The items should be hand dried with a towel to prevent spotting. Sanitization is a very important step, and it cannot be overlooked or done carelessly. The use of disposable instruments when working with human blood or giving injections minimizes the need for sanitization, disinfection, and sterilization.

Ultrasonic Sanitization

Sound waves can be used for sanitization of instruments by placing the instruments in an ultrasonic bath of cleaner and water. Sound waves cause the solution to vibrate, thereby loosening the materials attached to the instruments. Ultrasonic cleaners are beneficial because they do not damage even the most delicate instruments, and workers do not run the risk of an accidental sharps injury.

Disinfection

Disinfection is the process of killing pathogenic organisms or of rendering them inactive. It is not always effective against spores, the tubercle bacilli, and certain viruses. Disinfectant chemicals may kill microbes within a short time but are usually very hard on the instruments. Some chemicals, such as Cidex, are effective enough to kill all organisms, but the usual immersion time for these sterilants is 10 or more hours. For equipment and countertop surfaces, the cheapest and most reliable method for disinfection is the use of a 1:10 bleach solution. It is an effective and noncaustic disinfectant that can be used to wipe laboratory countertops where human blood and other body-fluid samples are handled. It can also be used for soaking reusable rubber goods before sanitizing. In addition, bleach solution is an effective disinfectant for surfaces that have come into contact with viruses, including HIV.

Many types of disinfecting agents are available and have varying degrees of effectiveness. It is important to follow manufacturer's guidelines on how to properly use each product, as well as understand its advantages, disadvantages, and the possible sources of error (Figure 26-11).

Disinfection is very difficult to verify, because no convenient indicators ensure destruction of organisms. Even when the manufacturer's directions for chemical strength and immersion times are followed, common errors can cause chemicals to lose their effectiveness:

- Instruments are not thoroughly sanitized, and attached organic matter inhibits or prevents the action of the disinfectant. No chemical can kill unless it reaches all instrument surfaces; therefore complete sanitization is absolutely necessary.
- Sanitized instruments are not dried, and the moisture on the instruments dilutes the disinfectant solution beyond the effective concentration.
- A solution is left in an open container, and evaporation changes its concentration.
- Solutions are not changed after the recommended period for use has expired.
- Solutions are not prepared properly or not mixed properly before using.
- The recommended manufacturer's temperature for use and storage is not maintained.

Alcohol is the most widely used antiseptic, but recent studies indicate that it is not as effective as other products in inhibiting the growth and reproduction of microorganisms on the skin surface. Other antiseptic chemicals, such as povidone-iodine solution (Betadine), are effective antimicrobial agents that are safe to use on patient skin. Disinfection by boiling is both impractical and ineffective in killing many pathogens, including bacterial spores and viruses. In addition, an article must be boiled at a rolling boil for at least 15 minutes to be adequately disinfected.

CRITICAL THINKING APPLICATION

Rosa is responsible for orienting the new medical assistant in the office on sanitization and disinfection procedures. Outline the important concepts and methods of each.

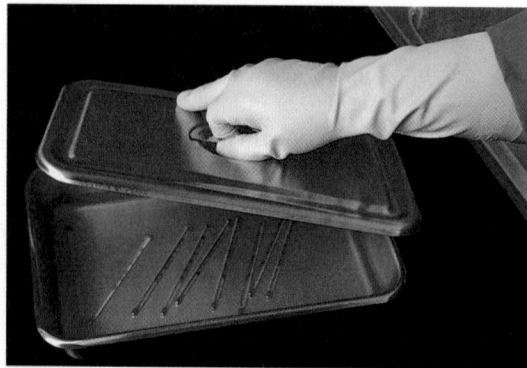

FIGURE 26-11 Instruments soaking in solution for disinfection. (From Klieger DM: *Saunders textbook of medical assisting*, St Louis, 2005, Saunders.)

Sterilization

Sterilization, or the destruction of all microorganisms, is essential when conducting surgical asepsis. To ensure proper sterilization for aseptic procedures, an area should be set aside in each office for just this purpose. The area should be divided into two sections. One section is used for receiving contaminated materials. This area should have a sink as well as receiving basins, proper cleaning agents, brushes, autoclave wrapping paper, sterilizer envelopes and tape, sterilizer indicators, disposable gloves, and designated biohazard waste containers. The other section should be reserved for receiving the sterile items after they are removed from the autoclave. Clear, clean plastic bags in which to store sterile packs may be kept in the sterile area. Both areas should be spotlessly clean and well organized. Sterile technique is addressed in Chapter 56.

ROLE OF THE MEDICAL ASSISTANT IN ASEPSIS

Medical asepsis is one of the few procedures that directly affect the health of the patient, physician, and staff. The spread of pathogens in the ambulatory care setting can be controlled only through effective and consistent application of the Bloodborne Pathogens Standard and proper sanitization, disinfection, and sterilization of supplies, equipment, and work surfaces.

The medical assistant must develop an inner sense for properly performing aseptic procedures. It is important that these techniques be done on such a routine basis that they become an unbreakable habit. The use of disposable items is highly recommended for infection control purposes. However, when disposable equipment is used, the assistant must follow recommended disposal guidelines.

CLOSING COMMENTS

Patient Education

The medical assistant should take every opportunity to educate patients on the infection process and ways of preventing disease transmission. The best time to instruct a patient about aseptic techniques that can be used at home is while performing the aseptic procedure. For example:

- While hand washing, explain to the patient that this routine is part of daily hygiene and is particularly important for patients who are very young or old or who seem to get sick frequently. Discuss with the patient that hands should be washed before and after meals; after sneezing, coughing, or nose blowing; after using the bathroom; before and after changing a dressing; and after changing an infant's diaper.
- Explain to the patient how using disposable tissues to cover the nose and mouth when coughing or sneezing decreases the possibility of transmitting illness among household members.
- Discuss proper ways for disposing of used tissues, especially when one member of the household is suspected of having a communicable disease.

- Instruct the patient regarding the differences between sterile and clean dressings and bandages. Show him or her step by step how to change a dressing properly and how to dispose of contaminated items.

There are many ways that a medical assistant can help the patient. Here are a few more suggestions of ways to educate the patient about asepsis and infection control:

- Set up an information table in the waiting room with take-home pamphlets and literature.
- Mail a periodic newsletter to patients regarding infection control, especially during flu season.
- Demonstrate and explain aseptic procedures to patients and/or family members, inviting them to participate.

Legal and Ethical Issues

Numerous legal and ethical concerns are related to medical asepsis and infection control in the ambulatory care setting. Personal discipline is the primary concern in medical asepsis. Typically you are alone when performing a medical aseptic procedure, so if contamination occurs you are the only one who knows. If contamination should occur, it is your responsibility to start over again with clean supplies. One of the medical assistant's main responsibilities is to carry out disinfection and sterilization procedures with precision and total effectiveness. There is no room for compromise. Patients should have absolute assurance that they are being taken care of in an aseptic atmosphere and under aseptic conditions. This assurance is just as important for the protection of the physician and staff as it is for the patient. Allowing the physician to assume that the correct aseptic techniques have been employed in the preparation of equipment and allowing him or her to use contaminated equipment on a patient can result in possible malpractice. Honesty on the part of the medical assistant builds self-respect and contributes to professional achievement.

One of the primary reasons for performing aseptic procedures completely and effectively is to prevent the development of nosocomial infections in susceptible patients. These infections that are acquired in the healthcare environment can be especially devastating to elderly or debilitated patients. Ignorance of the various aseptic techniques or carelessness can be dangerous and is inexcusable before the law.

More than 36 states have adopted Good Samaritan legislation, which protects bystanders and first responders from liability when they perform lifesaving procedures at the scene of an accident. If the individual acts in good faith, is not compensated, and performs techniques to the best of his or her knowledge, he or she is not liable for civil damages. However, because OSHA regulates employer responsibility for management of blood-borne pathogens, exposure at the scene of an accident will not be covered by employer postexposure incident policies. Therefore healthcare workers who volunteer their assistance in an emergency must enact blood-borne precautions as much as possible without expectation of medical follow-up at the workplace.

SUMMARY OF SCENARIO

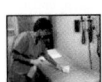

Implementing standard precautions throughout daily practice is crucial to the welfare and protection of both the patient and the healthcare worker. Rosa must be sure to routinely wash hands and/or use an alcohol handrub; familiarize herself with the office's Exposure Control Plan; follow OSHA's Bloodborne Pathogen Standards; use PPE when needed; follow environmental protection guidelines; use appropriate procedures for cleaning up contaminated spills and other housekeeping controls; and understand postexposure follow-up if an accidental exposure occurs. In addition, Rosa must follow guidelines for sanitization, disinfection, and sterilization of appropriate instruments and equipment.

SUMMARY of LEARNING OBJECTIVES

1. Define, spell, and pronounce the terms listed in the vocabulary.
   - Spelling and pronouncing medical terms correctly adds credibility to the medical assistant. Knowing the definition of these terms promotes confidence in communication with patients and co-workers.
2. Recognize diseases caused by pathogenic microorganisms.
   - Pathogenic microorganisms include viruses, bacteria, protozoa, fungi, and rickettsiae.
3. Apply the chain-of-infection process to healthcare practice.
   - The chain of infection represents how infectious disease is spread. It begins with the infectious agent and moves to the host, the means or portal of exit from the host, the mode of

transmission, and the means or portal of entry into a new host and ends with the presence of the infection in a susceptible host. For the spread of infection to be stopped, at least one of these links must be broken.

4. Summarize the impact of the inflammatory response on the body's ability to defend itself against infection.
   - The inflammatory response is one aspect of the body's ability to defend itself against infection. It involves the body's reaction to the introduction of a foreign substance or antigen, with release of inflammation mediators that cause an increase in WBCs at the site. The WBC's isolate and destroy the source of inflammation.

Continued

SUMMARY of LEARNING OBJECTIVES
Continued

5. Differentiate between humoral and cell-mediated immunity.
   - Humoral immunity creates specific antibodies to combat antigens. Cell-mediated immunity attacks the source of the infection at the cellular level.

6. Analyze the differences among acute, chronic, and latent disease processes.
   - Acute diseases have a rapid onset and short duration. Chronic diseases are present over a long period, perhaps a lifetime. Latent diseases cycle through relapse and remission phases.

7. Compare viral and bacterial cell invasion.
   - Bacterial infections can be treated with antibiotics, but viral infections, which involve viral takeover of cellular DNA or RNA material, cannot be treated with antibiotics because viruses are not cells but are parasites within a cell.

8. Specify potentially infectious bodily fluids.
   - Potentially infectious bodily fluids include CSF; synovial, pleural, pericardial, peritoneal, mucous, and amniotic fluids; blood; vaginal and seminal secretions; saliva; and human tissue.

9. Integrate OSHA's requirement for a site-based Exposure Control Plan into office management procedures.
   - OSHA requires incorporation of a site-based Exposure Control Plan into office management procedures. The plan must be revised annually and be available for employee review. It must reflect current safety technology, identify employees at risk for exposure, and contain specifics about protection from blood-borne pathogens including PPE, training, hepatitis B immunization, exposure, follow-up, record keeping, and the labeling and disposal of all biohazard waste.

10. Summarize the management of postexposure evaluation and follow-up.
   - Postexposure evaluation and follow-up are as follows: The site is cleaned and the exposed individual reports to the supervisor immediately. Medical assessment is performed immediately. Examination of the source individual's and worker's blood is conducted if possible and if consent is given. Health counseling is provided. Strict confidentiality of all medical records is maintained.

11. Explain the major areas included in the OSHA Compliance Guidelines.
   - The OSHA Compliance Guidelines include barrier protection devices, environment protection, housekeeping controls, hepatitis B immunization, and postexposure follow-up.

12. Apply the concepts of medical and surgical asepsis to the healthcare setting.
   - Medical asepsis is removal or destruction of pathogens. Medical aseptic techniques are used to create an environment that is as free of pathogens as possible. Surgical asepsis is destruction of all microorganisms. Surgical asepsis is used when the patient's skin or mucous membranes are disrupted.

13. Differentiate among sanitization, disinfection, and sterilization procedures.
   - Sanitization is cleaning of contaminated articles or surfaces to reduce numbers of microorganisms. Disinfection involves the use of physical or chemical means to destroy pathogens or their components on inanimate surfaces or objects. Sterilization removes all living microorganisms.

14. Demonstrate the proper hand-washing technique for medical asepsis.
   - Refer to Procedure 26-2.

15. Demonstrate the correct procedure for sanitization of contaminated instruments.
   - Refer to Procedure 26-3.

16. Apply patient education concepts to infection control.
   - Take every opportunity to demonstrate aseptic techniques, to educate patients about proper management of infectious materials at home, and to emphasize the importance of frequent and consistent hand washing.

17. Discuss the legal and ethical concerns regarding medical asepsis and infection control.
   - The medical assistant is responsible for applying infection control procedures in all situations at all times in order to prevent cross-contamination and the development of nosocomial infections in patients.

CONNECTIONS

Study Guide Connection: Go to Chapter 26 Study Guide. Read the Case Study and Workplace Applications and complete the assignments. Do online research for answers to the questions in the Internet Activities associated with OSHA Bloodborne Pathogens Standards and infection control.

CD Connection: Go to the Medical Assisting Competency Challenge CD and do the training activities under Infection Control. For a better understanding of the inflammatory response and controlling infection, view the animations for antibiotics and phagocytosis.

Evolve Connection: For more information related to infection control, go to evolve.elsevier.com/kinn and visit related weblinks for Chapter 26. Click on the Medical Assisting Exam Review and do the practice questions to sharpen your test-taking skills.

Patient Assessment

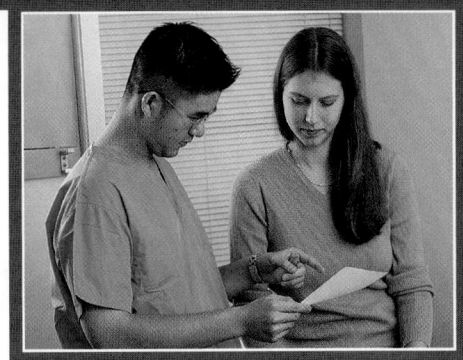

27

SCENARIO

Chris Isaccson, CMA, works in an ambulatory care setting located at the community hospital. He is responsible for initial patient interviews, taking medical histories, and documentation. Chris is having difficulty gathering the information needed from some of the clients. Patients do not always respond openly and honestly to him, and therefore the attending physician is not satisfied with his work. His supervisor is responsible for helping him improve his interview skills.

While studying this chapter, think about the following questions:

- How can Chris learn to develop helping relationships so the patient's medical history is as comprehensive as possible?
- Does Chris need to display greater sensitivity to diverse populations?
- Would using active listening techniques and attending to the patient's nonverbal behaviors better enable Chris to develop therapeutic communication skills?
- How can Chris's supervisor enable him to be a better communicator and demonstrate comprehensive and accurate documentation in the patient chart?

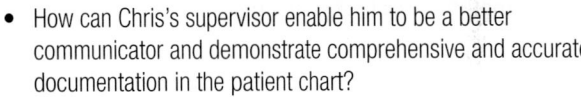

LEARNING OBJECTIVES

1. Define, spell, and pronounce the terms listed in the vocabulary.
2. Employ the components of holistic care in the patient assessment process.
3. Describe the components of the patient's medical history.
4. Define and apply the qualities of a helping relationship.
5. Display sensitivity to diverse patient populations.
6. Demonstrate therapeutic communications including the use of the linear communication model and active listening techniques.
7. Recognize the importance of nonverbal communication when interacting with patients.
8. Identify barriers to communication and their impact on patient assessment.
9. Detect patients' use of defense mechanisms and resultant barriers to therapeutic communication.
10. Apply therapeutic communication techniques with patients across the lifespan.
11. Demonstrate professional patient interview techniques.
12. Integrate detailed information about the chief complaint into concise, accurate documentation methods.
13. Differentiate among various medical record systems employed in the physician's office.
14. Describe the connection between the interview process and implementation of patient education practices.
15. Determine risk management strategies for the ambulatory care setting.
16. Obtain a written medical history from a patient.

National Accreditation Competencies and Content

CAAHEP COMPETENCIES

Clinical

3.b.(4)(c). Obtain and record patient history

General

3.c.(1)(b). Recognize and respond to verbal communications
3.c.(1)(c). Recognize and respond to nonverbal communications
3.c.(2)(a). Identify and respond to issues of confidentiality
3.c.(2)(b). Perform within legal and ethical boundaries
3.c.(2)(c). Establish and maintain the medical record
3.c.(2)(d). Document appropriately

ABHES COMPETENCIES

Communication

2.a. Be attentive, listen, and learn
2.b. Be impartial and show empathy when dealing with patients
2.f. Interview effectively
2.i. Recognize and respond to verbal and nonverbal communication

Clinical Duties

4.a. Interview and record patient history

Legal Concepts

5.a. Determine needs for documentation and reporting
5.b. Document accurately

VOCABULARY

biophysical (bi-o-fi′-zi-kuhl) Pertaining to the science dealing with the application of physical methods and theories to biologic problems.

chief complaint The reason for the patient's seeking medical care.

cognitive (kog′-nuh-tiv) Pertaining to the operation of the mind; referring to the process by which we become aware of perceiving, thinking, and remembering.

congruence (kon-groo′-ents) Agreement; the state occurring when the verbal expression of the message matches the sender's nonverbal body language.

diagnosis Concise technical description of the cause, nature, or manifestations of a condition or problem. *Initial:* Physician's temporary impression, sometimes called a *working diagnosis.*

Differentiated diagnosis: Comparison of two or more diseases with similar signs and symptoms. *Final:* Conclusion physician reaches after evaluating all findings, including laboratory and other test results.

familial Occurring in or affecting members of a family more than would be expected by chance.

present illness The chief complaint, written in chronologic sequence, with dates of onset.

psychosocial Pertaining to a combination of psychologic and social factors.

rapport (ra-por′) Relationship of harmony and accord between the patient and the healthcare professional.

As medical professionals directly involved in gathering information from patients about their health status, medical assistants must remember that a healthy state is more than the absence of disease. The assessment process should be a reflection of the entire patient, not just a report about signs and symptoms. Lifestyles and environmental factors can create disease and therefore should be considered when we gather information about the **chief complaint.** Not just physical data but **cognitive, psychosocial,** and behavioral data are significant for the analysis of a patient's health status. This method of analyzing the development of disease is based on a holistic perspective. Holistic patient care recognizes that illness is the result of many factors, not just physical ones.

Assessment factors are a list of **biophysical** signs and symptoms. The first step in treating a disease process is for the physician to determine the patient's medical **diagnosis.** The identification of disease begins with the physician's

working diagnosis, which he or she has determined through the patient's history, report of the chief complaint, and physical examination. Next the physician orders laboratory tests, diagnostic examinations, and/or a referral visit to another physician to substantiate or refute the working diagnosis. Once the test results are received, the clinical diagnosis is established. The patient is then treated, and after a period of time is reevaluated to see whether the clinical diagnosis has changed. If it has, the new diagnosis is called the differentiated diagnosis. The physician continues to evaluate the progress of the patient and order tests and/or alters treatment as needed.

However, patient care does not start with the physical examination; it begins when the patient makes first contact with the office. Even before the examination, the medical assistant has the opportunity to interact with the patient to ensure that he or she feels comfortable during the process and that all the necessary information is obtained.

Interviewing patients, assisting with examinations, and documentation are important responsibilities for a medical assistant. You must know the components and techniques for securing a medical history that will help the physician in the diagnosis and treatment of the patient. The more complete the medical history, the more efficient the physician's care and treatment will be.

MEDICAL HISTORY

Collecting the History Information

When a new patient calls or comes in for an appointment, the patient is asked to complete a health history form. Besides being useful for diagnosing and treating the patient, the self-history allows the patient more participation in the process. The form may be mailed to the patient's home before the appointment or may be completed in the office during the first visit.

If you are responsible for taking a portion of the medical history, conduct the interview in a private area free from outside interference and beyond the hearing range of other patients (Figure 27-1). Patients will not talk freely where they may be overheard or interrupted. The interview room should be physically comfortable and conducive to confidential communications. Legally and ethically the patient has the right to privacy, and access to the patient's medical record is permitted only to healthcare workers directly involved in the patient's care or to those individuals the patient has specified on his or her Health Insurance Portability and Accountability Act (HIPAA) release form.

Listen to the patient. Do not express surprise or displeasure at any of the patient's statements. Remember, you are there not to pass judgment but to gather medical data. Documentation of information gathered while taking the medical history is included in the Progress Notes section of the medical chart. The medical assistant records the information in an organized manner, exactly as given by the patient, without opinion or interpretation. The note should include the purpose of the patient's visit written as the chief complaint (CC), vital signs (VS) including height and weight if preferred by the physician,

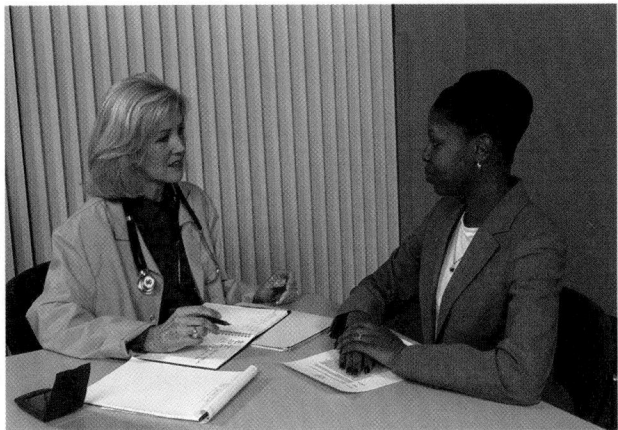

FIGURE 27-1 Private patient interview area.

and if the patient reports pain it should be documented using a scale of 1 to 10, with one being the least and ten being the most amount of pain.

In some facilities the physician takes the medical history during the patient's initial visit. The physician will correlate the physical findings in the examination with the information in the history. The complete medical history and the physical examination form the foundation and starting point for all patient-physician contracts.

Components of the Medical History

Medical history forms vary depending on the physician's preference and the practice specialty (Figure 27-2). The most common medical history method includes these components:

- *Database:* Record of the patient's name, address, date of birth, insurance information, personal data, history, physical examination, and initial laboratory findings. As new information is added, it becomes a part of this database.
- *Chief Complaint (CC):* The purpose for the patient's visit. The medical assistant should gather as much information about the health problem as possible and record it concisely using the patient's own words as much as possible.
- *Past history (PH) or past medical history (PMH):* Summary of the patient's previous health. It includes dates and details regarding the patient's usual childhood diseases (UCD or UCHD), major illnesses, surgeries, allergies, accidents, and immunization record. Each medical practice has a policy on how to document patient allergies, but these are typically written in red ink or with a colored sticker so that all healthcare workers can easily take note of potential allergic reactions. Included in the patient's medication history should be a record of frequently used over-the-counter (OTC) medications, including supplements, as well as currently prescribed drugs.
- *Family history (FH):* Details regarding the patient's mother and father, their health, and, if deceased, the cause and age of death. Hereditary and/or familial diseases and disorders are recorded here and may include information about siblings and offspring. This information is important because certain diseases and disorders have familial and/ or hereditary tendencies.
- *Social history (SH):* Information regarding the patient's lifestyle, hobbies, entertainment preferences, education, occupation, use of tobacco and alcohol, sleeping habits, methods of exercise, diet, last menstrual period (LMP) for female patients, and method of birth control if the patient is sexually active is noted in this section. It may be important to note the patient's cultural and religious background since these could influence certain lifestyle and dietary choices. This information assists the physician in planning treatment for the patient or in determining causative factors for disease. It also provides a holistic picture of the patient's health.
- *Systems review (SR) or review of systems (ROS):* These questions provide a guide to the patient's general health

MEDICAL RECORD

NAME				AGE	SEX	S M D W
ADDRESS			PHONE		DATE	
E-MAIL			CELL PHONE			
SPONSOR		ADDRESS				
OCCUPATION		REF BY			ACKN	

CHIEF COMPLAINT

PRESENT ILLNESS

FAMILY HISTORY		URINARY TRACT	
MOTHER	FATHER	NOCTURIA	FREQUENCY
BROTHERS		PAIN	BURNING
SISTERS		BLEEDING	INFECTION
TB DIAB MALIG		INCONTINENCE	
HT DIS NEPH EPILIP		GENITAL TRACT	
PSYCH		AGE AT MENST	TYPE PERIOD
PAST HISTORY - GENL HEALTH		INTERMEN BLEEDING	
		AMENORRHEA	DYSMENORRHEA
CHILDHOOD DISEASES		VAG DISCH	IRRITATION
SC FEV RHEUM FEV ALLERGY		PAINFUL PERIOD	
OTHER USUAL WEIGHT		L M P	
HAVE YOU EVER TAKEN FEN-PHEN/REDUX? YES NO		CHILDREN-L D S B	
ACCIDENTS		MARRIED YRS. YOUNGEST CHILD	
HABITS COFFEE TOBACCO ALCOHOL		NEURO-MUSCULAR	
REVIEWS OF SYSTEMS		STRENGTH	NERVOUSNESS
E E N T—EYES		SLEEP	WORRY
EARS		MUSCULAR PAIN	
NOSE		JOINT PAIN	
THROAT		ABNORMAL SENSATIONS	
NECK		DEFORMITIES	
BREASTS			
HEART-LUNGS		OPERATIONS	
PAIN			
DO YOU HAVE A PERSISTENT COUGH OR THROAT CLEARING NOT ASSOCIATED WITH A KNOWN ILLNESS (LASTING MORE THAN 3 WEEKS)? YES NO			
BLEEDING DYSPNEA			
IRREG EDEMA		TREATMENTS	
GASTRO-INTESTINAL			
APPETITE DIET			
INDIGESTION PAIN			
NAUSEA VOMITING		COMMENTS	
JAUNDICE BLEEDING			
BOWEL HABITS			
HEMORRHOIDS			
PAIN WITH STOOL ITCHING			
OTHER			

FIGURE 27-2 General medical history form. (From Klieger DM: *Saunders textbook of medical assisting,* St Louis, 2005, Saunders. Courtesy Patterson Office Supplies, Champaign, Ill.)

and help the healthcare worker detect conditions other than those covered under the **present illness.** Often a patient may think certain health problems irrelevant and may fail to mention them. These problems may help the physician in determining the cause of the disorder presently being explored. A systems review is obtained by a logical sequence of questions regarding the state of health of body systems, beginning with the head and proceeding downward. The physician frequently completes this section of the medical history while conducting the physical examination.

UNDERSTANDING AND COMMUNICATING WITH PATIENTS

To provide high-quality patient care, we must communicate effectively with the patient and provide a warm, caring environment. Positive reactions and interactions with the patient are essential. As the patient progresses through the various levels of healthcare, all members of the medical team must exercise a variety of special skills to enhance the process. These skills are not all technical and medical. Many involve the art of caring for the patient as a human being; that is, consistently implementing respectful patient care. Because medical care is of an extremely personal nature, a medical assistant must always remember that each patient is an individual with certain anxieties. These anxieties often cause people to act and react in different ways, making effective verbal and nonverbal communication with each patient absolutely essential.

Healthcare professionals accept the responsibility for developing helping relationships with their clients. The interpersonal nature of the patient–medical assistant relationship carries with it a certain amount of responsibility to detach one's self-interest and focus on the needs of the patients. A medical assistant, simply by the way he or she treats and interacts with patients, can create either a positive or a negative patient response to care. You are usually the first person the patient communicates with and therefore you play a vital role in initiating therapeutic patient interactions (Procedure 27-1).

Sensitivity to Diversity

Demonstrating respectful patient care is extremely important when working with a diverse patient population. Empathy is the key to creating a caring, therapeutic environment. Empathy goes beyond sympathy—if the medical assistant is empathetic he or she respects the individuality of the patient and attempts to see the patient's health problem through the patient's eyes, recognizing the effect of all holistic factors on the patient's well-being. Empathetic sensitivity to diversity first requires those interested in healthcare to examine their own values, beliefs, and actions. It is impossible to treat all patients with caring and respect until you first recognize and evaluate personal biases. There are many reasons why we think and act a certain way. The first step in understanding the process is to evaluate your individual value system. Why do you have certain attitudes or beliefs about the worth of individuals or things?

CRITICAL THINKING APPLICATION

What do you value most in life? What is important to you? What influences you to act in a certain way? Make a list of five "things" you value the most and share them with the class. Try to determine why you feel so strongly about those particular items.

Many different factors shape value system development. Value systems begin as learned beliefs and behaviors. Families, as well as cultural influences, shape the way we respond to a diverse society. To develop therapeutic relationships, you must recognize your own value system to determine whether it could affect your method of interaction. Other factors that influence reactions include socioeconomic and educational backgrounds. Whatever the history of value system development, preconceived ideas about people because of their race, religion, income level, ethnic origin, sexual orientation, or gender can cause serious trouble for the therapeutic relationship. It is impossible to treat your patients empathetically unless you can connect with them in some way. Personal biases, or prejudices, act as overwhelming barriers to the development of therapeutic relationships (Figure 27-3).

CRITICAL THINKING APPLICATION

Honestly evaluate your personal biases. What do you find unacceptable in people? Do you prejudge an individual based on his or her affiliation with a particular group or because of a certain lifestyle decision? Do these biases create barriers to the development of therapeutic relationships? If so, how can you get beyond these barriers?

Therapeutic Techniques

Chapter 5 introduced the communication process. The linear communication model describes communication as an interactive process involving the sender of the message, the receiver, and the crucial component of feedback to confirm the reception of the message. All medical assistants must be effective communicators. You will play a vital role in collecting and documenting patient information. If your methods of collection or recording are faulty, it could seriously affect the quality of patient care.

Active Listening Techniques

Active listeners go beyond hearing the patient's message to concentrating, understanding, and listening to the main points in the discussion. Active listening techniques encourage patients to expand on and clarify the content and meaning of their messages. They are very useful communication tools to implement when a patient is agitated or upset, because these methods help patients clearly hear what the medical assistant is saying.

Three processes are involved in active listening: restatement, reflection, and clarification. Restatement is simply paraphrasing, or repeating, the patient's statements with phrases such as "You are saying…" or "You are telling me the problem is…."

PROCEDURE 27-1

Obtain and Record a Patient History

<u>CAAHEP COMPETENCY:</u> 3.b.(4)c
<u>ABHES COMPETENCY:</u> 4.a

Complete this procedure with another student role playing the patient. To make the experience more realistic, choose a student about whom you know very little. To maintain the privacy of your student partner, he or she does not have to share any confidential information while participating in the role-play.

GOAL: *To obtain an acceptable written background from the patient to help the physician determine the cause and effects of the present illness. This includes the chief complaint (CC), present illness (PI), past history (PH), family history (FH), and social history (SH).*

EQUIPMENT and SUPPLIES

- History form
- Two pens—a red pen for recording patient allergies and a black pen to meet legal documentation guidelines
- A quiet, private area

PROCEDURAL STEPS

1. Greet and identify the patient in a pleasant manner. Introduce yourself and explain your role.
   PURPOSE: To make the patient feel comfortable and at ease.
2. Take the patient to a quiet, private area for the interview, and explain to the patient why the information is needed.
   PURPOSE: A quiet, private area is necessary to protect confidentiality and prevent interruptions. An informed patient is more cooperative and therefore more likely to contribute useful information.
3. Complete the history form by using therapeutic communication techniques. Make sure that all medical terminology is adequately explained. A self-history may have been mailed to the patient before the visit. If so, review the self-history for completeness.
   PURPOSE: Therapeutic communication techniques will assist the medical assistant in gathering complete information; the self-history is designed to save time and to involve the patient in the process.
4. Speak in a pleasant, distinct manner, remembering to maintain eye contact with your patient.
   PURPOSE: Positive nonverbal behaviors create a friendly, caring atmosphere.
5. Record the following statistical information on the patient information form:
   - Patient's full name, including middle initial
   - Address, including apartment number and ZIP code
   - Marital status
   - Sex (gender)
   - Age and date of birth
   - Telephone number for home and work
   - Insurance information if not already available
   - Employer's name, address, telephone number

6. Record the following medical history on the patient history (PH) form:
   - Chief complaint (CC)
   - Past history
   - Social history
   - Present illness
   - Family history
   PURPOSE: This is information that the physician needs to know to make an accurate assessment and diagnosis. The physician usually completes the review of systems (ROS) during the preexamination interview.
7. Ask about allergies to drugs and any other substances, and record any allergies in red ink on every page of the history form, on the front of the chart, and on each progress note page. Some practices apply allergy alert labels to the front of each chart.
   PURPOSE: The presence of an allergy may alter medication and treatment procedures.
8. Record all information legibly and neatly, and spell words correctly. Print rather than writing in longhand. Do not erase, scribble, or use whiteout. If you make an error, draw a single line through the error, write "error" above it, add the correction, and initial and date the entry.
   PURPOSE: To maintain a medical record that is understandable and defensible in a court of law.
9. Thank the patient for cooperating, and direct him or her back to the reception area.
10. Review the record for errors before you pass it to the physician.
11. Use the information on the record to complete the patient's chart. Keep the information confidential.
    PURPOSE: All information concerning the patient must remain in the office. This information may be legally and ethically discussed with only the physician.
    DOCUMENTATION PRACTICE: Mr. Bonski is a new patient being seen today for the first time. His CC is dizziness for 2 weeks. He denies having headaches and has no previous Hx of ear infections or hypertension. He doesn't take any prescribed medications but uses Tylenol as needed for a headache. T 97.6, P 88, R 22, BP 172/94. Document pertinent patient findings using the SOAPE method.
    S: _____
    O: _____
    _____

Reflection involves repeating the main idea of the conversation while also identifying the *feelings* of the sender. For example, if the mother of a young patient is expressing frustration about her child's behavior, a reflective statement identifies that feeling with the response, "You sound frustrated about...." Or, if a new insulin-dependent diabetic patient exhibits anxiety about administering injections, an appropriate reflective statement recognizes the patient's feelings: "You are anxious about...." Reflective statements clearly demonstrate to patients that you are not only listening to their words, but you are also attending to their feelings. Therefore reflection is an excellent method of

communicating concern to your patients. Finally, clarification seeks to summarize or simplify the sender's thoughts and feelings as well as resolve any confusion in the message. Questions or statements that begin with "Give me an example of..." or "Explain to me about..." or "So what you are saying is..." help patients focus on the chief complaint as well as giving you the opportunity to clear up any misconceptions before documenting patient information.

Listening is not a passive role in the communication process; it is active and demanding. You cannot be preoccupied with your own needs or you will miss something important. For the time of the patient interview, no one is more important than this particular patient. Listen to the way things are said, the tone of the patient's voice, and even to what the patient may not be saying out loud but saying very clearly with body language. Listening is probably the most effective communication technique available. It requires the medical assistant's complete attention and a great deal of energy (Figure 27-4).

Nonverbal Communication

Much of what we communicate to our patients is through the use of conscious or unconscious body language. Our nonverbal actions, such as gestures, facial expressions, and mannerisms, are learned behaviors that are greatly influenced by our family and cultural backgrounds. The body naturally expresses our true feelings; in fact, experts say that more than 90% of communication is nonverbal. Most of the negative messages communicated through body language are unintentional; therefore while conducting patient interviews it is important to remember that nonverbal communication behaviors can seriously affect the therapeutic process.

The verbal messages you send are only part of the communication process. You have a specific context in mind when you send your words, but the receiver puts his or her own interpretations on them. The receiver attaches meaning determined by his or her past experiences, culture, and self-concept, as well as the current physical and emotional state. Sometimes these messages and interpretations do not coincide. Feedback from the patient is crucial in determining if the patient understood the message. It takes mutual understanding by both the

---

Sensitivity to Diversity

Regardless of what type of healthcare facility you work in, you will care for a wide variety of patients. Some things to consider about diverse groups include the following:

- Patients with Asian backgrounds may have been raised in a culture that considers it extremely rude to establish eye contact. Americans view an unwillingness to establish eye contact as a sign of distrust or embarrassment, but for those from Japan or China a lack of eye contact may be a way of demonstrating respect.
- Personal space may be an issue for patients from diverse backgrounds. If a patient appears very uncomfortable with touch or lack of personal space, attempt to accommodate him or her as much as possible during the office visit.
- Research has shown that aging persons face unique communication problems in the healthcare environment. When caring for an aging person it is important to focus patient teaching and information toward the patient rather than the family member who may be present. Chapter 47 outlines specific communication techniques that should be implemented with aging persons to assure proper communication if vision and/or hearing deficits are present.
- Patients may use their religious beliefs and values to understand and cope with their health problems. However, using religion to guide healthcare decisions may result in a conflict with physician recommendations. Healthcare workers may need to find a balance between respect for patient beliefs and delivery of high-quality healthcare.

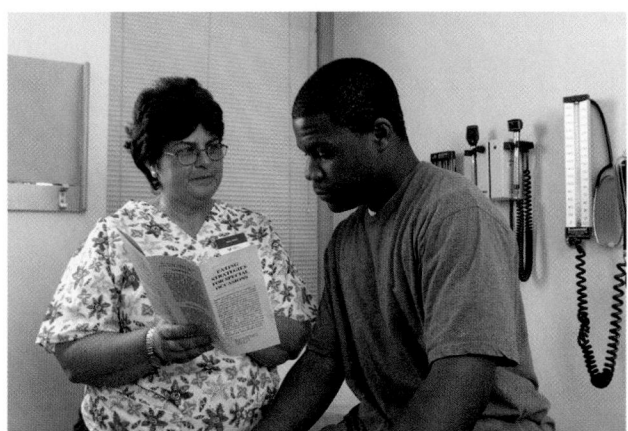

FIGURE 27-3 Respectful patient care.

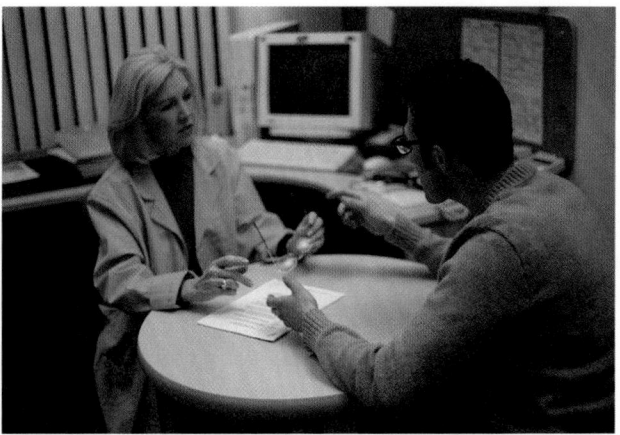

FIGURE 27-4 Active listening.

interviewer and the person being interviewed to have successful communication.

Observing your patient during the interview will foster mutual understanding. The purpose of observing nonverbal communication is to become sensitive to or aware of the feelings of others as conveyed by small bits of behavior, rather than words. This sensitivity enables you to adapt your behavior to these feelings, to consciously select your response, either verbal or nonverbal, and thereby have a favorable effect on others. The favorable effect may consist of providing emotional support, conveying that you care, defusing the other's fear or anger, or providing an invitation to release pent-up feelings by talking about the situation that aroused the feelings. Table 27-1 lists some patient nonverbal behaviors that may indicate anxiety, frustration, or fear.

You can do much to put a patient at ease through the tone of your voice. Facial expression and the ease and confidence of your movements demonstrate to the patient a sincere interest.

Therapeutic use of space and touch are also important ways of sending nonverbal messages to your patients. You should establish eye contact, sit in a relaxed but attentive position, and avoid the use of furniture as a barrier between you and the patient. Give the patient your undivided attention, and let your body language inform each patient that you are interested in his or her medical problems (Figure 27-5). The key to successful patient interaction is **congruence** between verbal and nonverbal messages. Although choosing the correct words is very important, only 7% of the message received is verbal, so to be seen as honest and sensitive to the needs of your patients you must be aware of your nonverbal behavior patterns. The nonverbal message the patient receives by the medical assistant's listening behavior should be, "You are a person of worth, and I am interested in you as a unique individual."

Environmental Factors

Before you meet with the patient, prepare the physical setting. The setting may be an examination room or an office. In any location, optimal conditions are important to have a smooth, productive interview.

Open-Ended Questions or Statements

An open-ended question or statement asks for general information or states the topic to be discussed, but only in general terms. Use this communication tool to begin the interview and to introduce a new section of questions or whenever the person introduces a new topic. It is a very effective method for gathering more details from the patient about the chief complaint or health history.

Helpful Listening Guidelines

- Listen to the main points in the discussion
- Attend to both verbal and nonverbal messages
- Be patient and nonjudgmental
- Do not interrupt
- Never intimidate your patient
- Use active listening techniques: restatement, reflection, and clarification

---

TABLE 27-1 Patient Nonverbal Communication Observations

AREA OBSERVED	OBSERVATION	INDICATION
Breathing patterns	Rapid respirations, sighing, shallow thoracic breathing	Anxiety, boredom, pain
Eye patterns	No eye contact, side-to-side movement, looking down at hands	Anxiety, distrust, embarrassment
Hands	Tapping fingers, cracking knuckles, continuous movement, sweaty palms	Anxiety, worry, fear
Arm placement	Folded across chest, wrapped around abdomen	Anxiety, worry, fear, pain
Leg placement	Tension, crossed and/or tucked under, tapping foot, continuous movement	Frustration, anger

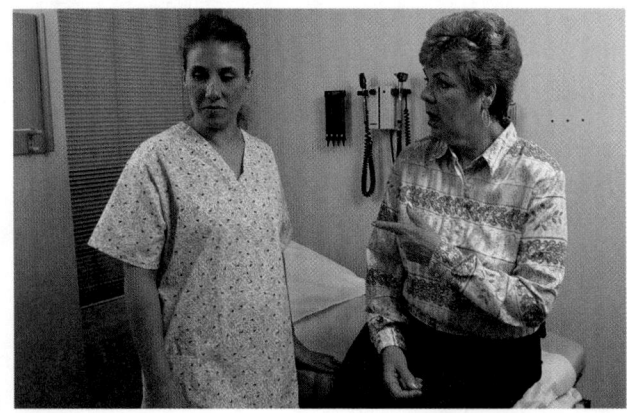
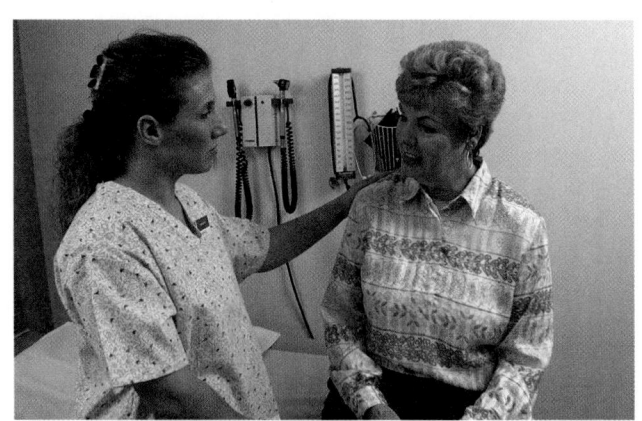

FIGURE 27-5 A, Ineffective nonverbal language. **B,** Therapeutic nonverbal language.

What brings you to the doctor?

How have you been getting along?

You mentioned having dizzy spells. Tell me more about that.

This type of question or statement encourages the patient to respond in a manner that is comfortable for him or her. It allows the patient to express himself or herself fully and provide comprehensive information about the chief complaint.

Closed Questions

Direct or closed questions ask for specific information. This form of questioning limits the answer to one or two words, a yes or no in many cases. Use this form of question when you need confirmation of specific facts, such as when asking about past health problems.

Do you have a headache?

What is your birth date?

Have you ever broken a bone?

INTERVIEWING THE PATIENT

The interview, or gathering the patient's medical history, is the first and most important part of data collection. The medical history identifies patient health strengths and problems and is a bridge to the next step in data collection, the physical examination performed by the physician. At this point the individual knows everything about his or her own health state and you know nothing. Your skill in interviewing will glean the necessary information as well as build **rapport** for a successful working relationship.

Consider the interview as a form of contract between you and your patient. The contract consists of spoken and unspoken language and addresses what the patient needs and expects from the healthcare visit. The patient interview consists of three stages: the initiation or introduction, the body, and the closing.

The initiation of the interview is the time to introduce yourself and identify the patient as well as the purpose of the interview (Figure 27-6). If you are nervous about how to begin, remember to keep it short. The patient is probably nervous, too, and is anxious to get started. Address the patient, using his or her last name, and give the reason for the interview:

> "Mr. Coleman, my name is Stacey and I am a certified medical assistant who works with Dr. Yang. I have some questions to ask you regarding your health history. Would you mind sharing this information with me?"

After the brief introduction, move on to the body of the interview. This is when you use various therapeutic communication techniques to determine why the patient is seeking healthcare, the patient's perception of the problem, the characteristics of the problem, and the patient's expectations of care. During this time use active listening skills, meaningful silence, congruent verbal and nonverbal communication, and a combination of open and closed statements and questions to gather the details of the patient's history and current health problem (Table 27-2).

Conclude the interview by summarizing the results of your interaction. The closing of the interview should clarify the patient's chief complaint, the purpose of the health visit,

---

Preparing the Appropriate Environment

Ensure Privacy

Make sure the room you are using is unoccupied for the entire time allowed for the interview. The patient needs to feel sure that no one can overhear the conversation or interrupt.

Prevent Interruptions

Inform your co-workers of the interview and ask them not to interrupt you during this time. You need to concentrate on the patient and establish rapport. An interruption can destroy in seconds what you have spent many minutes building up.

Prepare Comfortable Surroundings

Conducting the interview in comfortable surroundings reduces patient anxiety. Keep the distance between you and the patient to 4 to 5 feet. Arrange chairs so you and the patient are comfortably seated at eye level and the desk or table does not act as a barrier between you.

Take Judicious Notes

Note taking should be kept to a minimum while you try to focus your attention on the person. Note taking during the interview has disadvantages, such as breaking eye contact and shifting your attention away from the patient, which diminishes the patient's sense of importance. However, it is important to write down pertinent details as you are interviewing, because you may forget important facts if you do not note them at the time of the discussion. With experience you will develop a personal type of shorthand that you can use during the interview process.

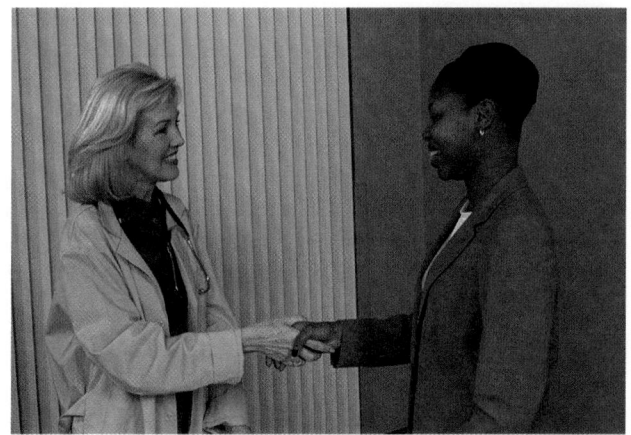

FIGURE 27-6 Greeting the patient.

and the patient's expectations of care. This is the patient's opportunity to add any additional details or to explain further the characteristics of the health problem.

Interview Barriers

In Chapter 5 we discussed barriers to communication. In this chapter we are going to look at the effect of communication barriers on the patient interview. Certain communication behaviors create nonproductive messages that may be misleading or restrict the patient's response.

TABLE 27-2 Therapeutic Communication Techniques

TECHNIQUE	VALUE
Open-ended questions and statements	Encourages the patient to respond in more detail
Direct questions	Asks for specific information; usual reply is a yes or no answer
Listening	Nonverbally communicates your interest in the patient
Silence	Nonverbally communicates your acceptance of the patient and willingness to wait until the patient is ready to answer
Establishing guidelines	Helps the patient know what to expect during the interview
Acknowledgment	Shows the importance of the patient's role and respect for autonomy
Restating	Checks your interpretation of the patient's message for validation
Reflecting	Shows the patient the importance of his or her feelings
Summarizing	Helps patient separate relevant from irrelevant material; provides clarity to the interview

Providing Unwarranted Assurance

Mrs. Miller says to you, "I know this lump is going to turn out to be cancer." The typical reply is almost automatic: "Don't worry, I'm sure everything will be fine." This type of answer indicates her anxiety is insignificant and denies her the opportunity to further discuss her fears. A reflective response, such as, "You sound really worried about…" acknowledges her feelings and demonstrates empathy and a willingness to listen to her concerns.

Giving Advice

Mrs. Thompson has just finished talking to the doctor. She looks at you and says, "Dr. Rowe says I need surgery to get rid of these gallstones. I just don't know. What would you do?" If you tell her how you would handle the situation, you may have shifted the accountability for decision making from her to you, and she has not worked out her own solution. Does this woman really want to know what you would do? Probably not. You could respond to her question with, "Based on what the doctor told you, what do you think you should do?" or "Do you need further information to make your decision?" If the patient continues to question the physician's recommendations, the medical assistant should encourage further discussion with the physician.

Using Medical Terminology

You must adjust your vocabulary to fit the patient. The more the patient understands about what is happening and what the management of the problem will be, the better the outcome. Misinterpreted communication is the most frequent error encountered in patient care. One of the biggest problems for the patient is in understanding medical terminology. Closely observe the patient's body language while he or she receives instructions or patient education. If the patient shows signs of not understanding the procedure, ask the patient to repeat back to you the information or instructions. This demonstration–return-demonstration form of providing feedback ensures that the patient completely understands what is happening. It also gives the medical assistant the opportunity to clarify any misconceptions.

Leading Questions

During the interview, you ask the patient, "You don't smoke, do you?" By asking the patient questions in this manner, you indicate the preferred answer. To tell you that he or she does smoke would surely meet with your disapproval.

Keep your questions positive. A better way of asking would be to say, "Have you ever smoked?" or "Do you use tobacco?"

Talking Too Much

Some medical assistants associate helpfulness with verbal overload. The patient may let the interviewer talk at the expense of his or her own need to explain what is wrong. Always remember that when interviewing a patient you should listen more than you talk. Pay close attention to the patient's body language to make sure you are giving the patient ample opportunity to discuss the health problem.

Defense Mechanisms

In Chapter 5 we discussed the impact of defense mechanisms on professional communications. Many individuals respond to anxiety-provoking situations by automatically relying on defense mechanisms. Because defense mechanisms are used consciously or unconsciously to block an emotionally painful experience, it is understandable why patients facing a traumatic diagnosis or a difficult treatment would need to protect themselves from the reality of the situation. The problem is, how can we ensure compliance with treatment if the patient is in denial, projecting feelings onto the healthcare worker, or repressing the need for treatment or diagnostic follow-up? The medical assistant needs to be sensitive to the use of defense mechanisms by patients and must consistently apply therapeutic communication techniques to patient interactions.

CRITICAL THINKING APPLICATION

Mr. Gonzales, a 48-year-old patient recently diagnosed with hypertension, did not show up today for his follow-up appointment. Chris calls to find out why he failed to keep the appointment, and the

Continued

patient tells Chris he forgot to come, even though an appointment reminder call was made yesterday. He also tells Chris he has not been taking his medicine and does not understand why it is so important for him and his wife to meet with the dietitian. Is this patient exhibiting defense mechanisms? How should Chris respond to the patient? What communication skills might be helpful to promote a therapeutic relationship?

Communication Across the Lifespan

The key to effectively communicating with patients is using an age-specific approach. Given the age and developmental level of your patient, how can you best interact with him or her as well as with significant family members?

For example, Tasha is a 2-year-old patient scheduled for a physical examination. How can you best interact with the child and her father to ensure that the history phase of the visit is complete and accurate? Therapeutic use of nonverbal language is essential when interacting with children of all ages. Getting down on the child's level, establishing eye contact, and using a gentle but firm voice are ways of gaining the child's confidence and cooperation. Children fear the unknown, so it is important to explain all procedures with language the child understands. At the same time the medical assistant needs to continue to communicate to the child's caregiver so he or she can contribute to the intake process (Figure 27-7). Some important guidelines to follow when conducting the health history of a child include the following:

- The environment should be safe and attractive.
- Do not keep children and their caregivers waiting any longer than necessary, because children become anxious and/or distracted quickly.
- Do not offer a choice unless the child can truly make one. If part of the treatment requires that the child receive an injection, asking her if she'd like her shot now will get an automatic "No!" However, giving her a choice of stickers after the injection is appropriate.
- Praising the child during the examination helps decrease anxiety and increase self-esteem. When possible, direct questions to the child so that he or she feels part of the process.

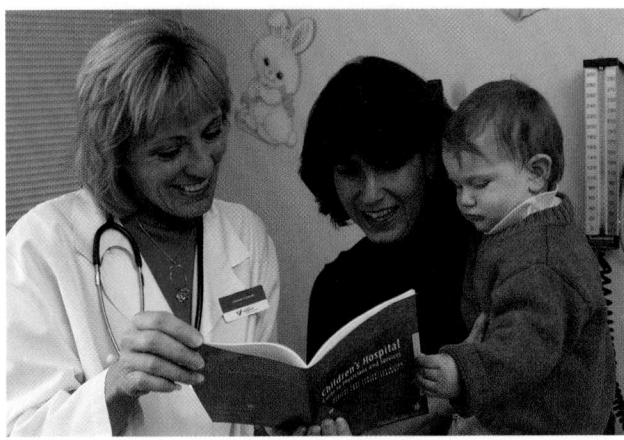

FIGURE 27-7 Interacting with a parent and child.

Defense Mechanisms

Patients may use defense mechanisms to protect themselves from a situation or medical information that they cannot manage psychologically. Defense mechanisms may hide any of a variety of thoughts or feelings: anger, fear, sadness, despair, or helplessness. A patient exhibiting defense mechanisms can be very difficult to deal with; however, if the medical assistant is aware of the patient's need for psychologic protection, he or she may be able to find a way to provide care for the patient while maintaining a therapeutic relationship. For example, Mrs. Alicia Simone, a 48-year-old patient, has just been told she has cancer of the breast. Following are defense mechanisms that she might display to protect herself from the psychologic reality of her disease.

Denial: The patient completely rejects the information.
"I couldn't possibly have breast cancer. You must be mistaken."
Suppression: The patient is consciously aware of the information or feeling but refuses to admit it.
"I don't think the test is accurate. My mammograms are always normal."
Reaction Formation: The patient expresses her feelings as the opposite of what she really feels. For example, if she is angry at the medical assistant for insisting a biopsy be scheduled, the patient may express the opposite emotion.
"I appreciate your trying to help me, but I just can't come to the hospital that day."
Projection: The patient accuses someone else of having feelings she possesses. For example, if the patient is angry about the diagnosis, she may say to the medical assistant, "You don't have to lose your temper about this," even though the medical assistant is acting completely professionally.
Rationalization: The patient comes up with various explanations to justify her response.
"I think the results are wrong. I didn't follow the directions for the tests like I should have, and besides, there's no history of breast cancer in my family."
Undoing: The patient tries to reverse a negative feeling by doing something that indicates the opposite feeling. If the patient feels angry and violated about the diagnosis but she finds those feelings unacceptable, she may say, "Don't worry dear, I'm not upset with you for telling me about this."
Regression: The patient reverts to an old, usually immature behavior to ventilate her feelings. Perhaps instead of discussing the diagnosis and need for treatment, she just storms out of the office. Or she may say, "I can't possibly schedule a procedure without discussing this with my mother."
Sublimation: The patient redirects her negative feelings into a socially productive activity. For example, Mrs. Simone eventually becomes an active member of a local support group for women recovering from breast cancer.

- Involving the child in the examination by permitting him or her to manipulate the equipment may help relieve anxiety. If possible, use your imagination and make a game of the assessment or the procedure.
- A typical defense mechanism seen in sick or anxious children is regression. The child may refuse to leave the

mother's lap or may want to hold a favorite toy during the procedure as a comfort measure. Look for signs of anxiety such as thumb-sucking or rocking during the assessment, and encourage caregivers to be involved in the process to help make the child feel as safe as possible.

- Listen to parents' concerns, and respond truthfully to questions (Figure 27-8).

Older children may also display difficulty during the health visit (Figure 27-9). To help school-age children gain a sense of control, they should be given the opportunity to make certain decisions about treatment. For example, Heather, a 13-year-old diabetic patient, could be given the choice of having her father present during the visit. Or, if she requires an insulin injection, the adolescent could choose the site of the injection or perhaps administer the medication herself. This would give the medical assistant an opportunity to observe her technique as well as permit Heather to exert her independence.

Privacy is also an important issue to consider with older children, especially adolescents. During the physical examination, respect privacy by keeping body exposure to a minimum and adequately preparing the child for procedures and positions. In addition, older children want to know what is going on during the examination, what to expect, and what the findings mean, so it is important to keep them informed in a language they can understand. The teen should always be encouraged to ask questions, which should be answered as completely and clearly as possible. Take every opportunity to teach your patients, regardless of their age, about their disease as well as sharing information about significant wellness factors (Figure 27-10).

Patient education is extremely important when interacting with adult clients. Therefore using language the adult patient understands and involving them in treatment decisions as much as possible are essential criteria for developing a helping relationship with your older patients. Adults are bombarded by multiple responsibilities, which means that stress-related health problems are not unusual in this patient population. Get to know your adult clients and emphasize preventive healthcare when possible (Figure 27-11). Specific communication techniques for therapeutic interactions with aging adults will be addressed in Chapter 47.

Recognizing and Responding to Verbal and Nonverbal Communications

The medical assistant not only must implement therapeutic communication skills but also must observe the patient to determine the patient's message and level of understanding. Based on the following case study, Chris conducts a patient

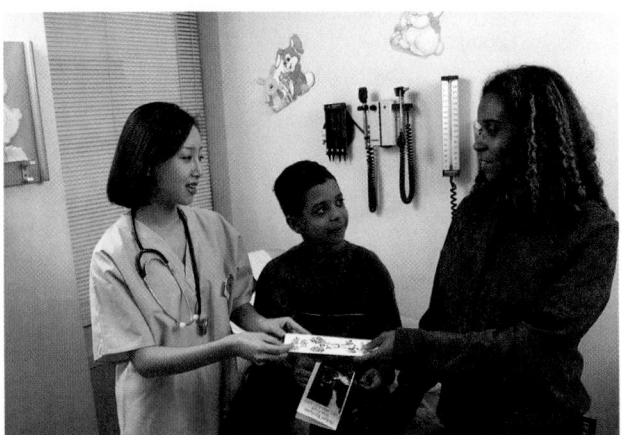

FIGURE 27-8 Responding to parental concerns.

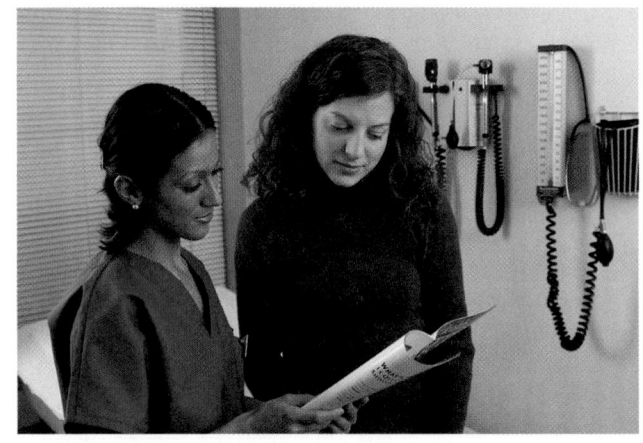

FIGURE 27-10 Interacting with an adolescent.

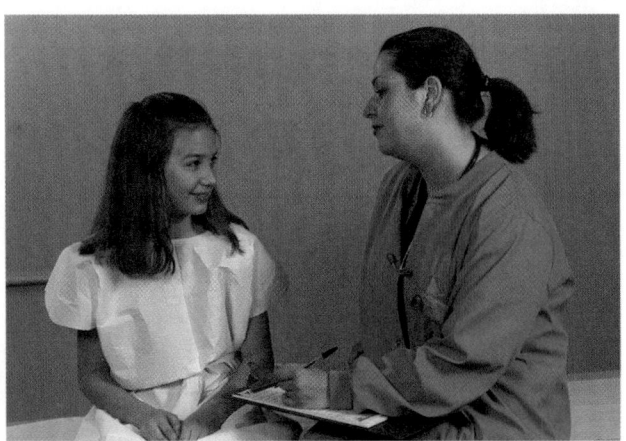

FIGURE 27-9 Interacting with a school-aged child.

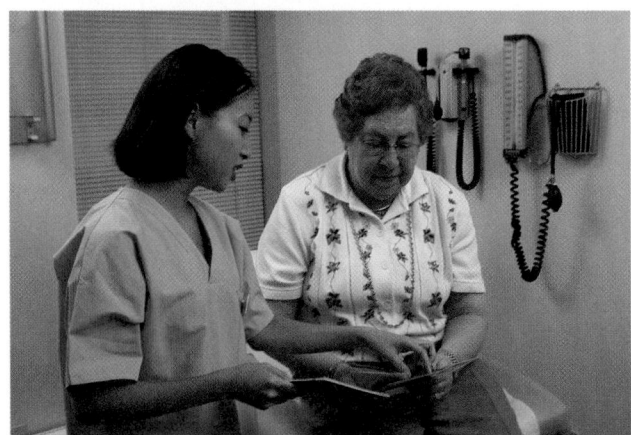

FIGURE 27-11 Adult patient education.

interview implementing the therapeutic communication skills discussed in this chapter including active listening techniques, open and closed questions and statements, use of positive nonverbal interview skills, and effective observation of patient body language.

CRITICAL THINKING APPLICATION

Toby Anderson, a 48-year-old patient, was recently diagnosed with hypertension and prescribed Lotensin bid for treatment. He is being seen today for a follow-up measurement of his blood pressure. Mr. Anderson is 45 pounds overweight and was given information about a reduced-calorie, low-sodium diet 1 month ago but has not lost any weight. He tells you he has been having side effects from the medication. He is sitting with his arms across his chest, tapping his foot and occasionally cracking his knuckles.

Communication approaches Chris should consider include the following:

- What nonverbal language is being used by Mr. Anderson and how should Chris interpret it?
- Mr. Anderson tells Chris he is not following that crazy diet and never will. What therapeutic communication skills can Chris use to get more information out of Mr. Anderson and to reinforce the physician's recommendations?
- During the discussion Mr. Anderson tells Chris he stopped taking the Lotensin because of the side effects. What communication techniques and therapeutic body language can Chris use to emphasize the need for Mr. Anderson to take his medicine as prescribed?

Document the patient interview using the CC method.

CC: _____

_____

_____

ASSESSING THE PATIENT

After completion of the interview the patient is escorted to an examination room and prepared for the physical examination, which is performed by the physician or healthcare professional such as a physician's assistant or nurse practitioner. The medical assistant's role in assisting with the physical examination will be discussed in detail in Chapter 31. During the examination the healthcare provider will methodically check all of the body systems. As this examination is done, the physician is mentally comparing the patient's system with established norms. When something deviates from the accepted normal range, it is documented in the patient's chart. The physician typically starts the examination with the head and progresses through the systems down to the feet. However, depending on the specialty of the physician, the order may vary.

Signs and Symptoms

When the physician completes the examination he or she will document all of the signs and symptoms gathered during the physical assessment process. To better understand the examination procedure, it is important that you know the difference between a sign and a symptom.

Subjective findings, or symptoms, are perceptible only to the patient; they are what the patient feels and can be interpreted only by that patient. For example, only the patient experiences and can define the quality of his or her discomfort, pain, nausea, or dizziness. The typical method of recording a complaint of pain is to quantify the pain by asking the patient, "On a scale of 1 to 10, with 1 being the least amount of pain and 10 being the greatest, how would you describe the pain?" Symptoms of the greatest significance in identifying a disease are called *cardinal symptoms*. For example, crushing chest pain and difficulty breathing are cardinal symptoms for a potential heart attack.

Objective findings, or signs, can be observed and/or measured by the physician or medical assistant. They are the indicators of health or disease that a physician detects when examining a patient. The physician feels, sees, hears, or measures the signs that are often associated with a certain disease or abnormal condition. For example, a mass that a physician palpates, or feels, in the patient's abdomen is an objective finding and a sign of an abnormal condition. In addition, objective data can be measured and recorded, and repeat measurements can be taken to confirm the presence of or changes in the sign. Objective signs that the medical assistant measures and records on a regular basis include the patient's temperature, pulse, respirations, and blood pressure.

You also need to know the difference between a functional versus an organic (physical) disorder. When a condition or disease is functional, it is without organic cause; that is, when inspected the organ appears normal without any evidence of disease even though patient symptoms indicate a problem. An example of a functional problem would be a patient who has repeated bouts of elevated urinary albumin, but all tests on the kidneys show normal, healthy organs. Or a patient is diagnosed with irritable bowel disease even though diagnostic studies have failed to show any evidence of intestinal disease. A functional disorder can be difficult for the patient to deal with, because even though the patient is suffering with certain health problems, all diagnostic tests fail to show that anything is wrong with the system affected. Meanwhile, an organic disease or condition is one in which the abnormality can be seen or felt or clinically proven via laboratory or other diagnostic tests. For example, an electrocardiogram (ECG) confirms that a patient with chest pain is having a heart attack. Or a colonoscopy performed on a patient complaining of bloody stools shows evidence of ulcers in the colon.

DOCUMENTATION

The method used for charting may vary depending on the healthcare provider's preference. However, regardless of the type of documentation used, certain charting procedures have been standardized to meet the necessary legalities of maintaining medical records accurately and concisely. Accurate and complete documentation is one of the primary responsibilities of a medical assistant (Figure 27-12).

Physician's Assessment of Body Systems

Appearance
Body build, posture, and gait
Height and weight fluctuation
Hygiene and grooming
Emotional state and mood

Head and Neck
Size, shape, and contour of head
Hair and scalp
Palpation of neck, thyroid, trachea
Difficulty in swallowing
Change in voice, hoarseness

Eyes
Visual acuity and field
Inspection of eyelids and eyeballs
Pupillary reaction and eye movement
Inspection of internal eye structures
Measurement of ocular pressure

Nose
Size, shape, and symmetry
Deviated septum, nasal congestion
Sense of smell

Ears
Hearing deficits
Inspection of size, symmetry, placement
Discharge, ringing in the ears, infection

Mouth and Throat
Inspection of gums, teeth, tongue, pharynx
Bad breath, changes in salivation
Sense of taste

Respiratory
Size and shape of chest
Phlegm, cough, sneezing, wheezing
Coughing of blood, asthma, emphysema
Upper respiratory tract infections

Cardiovascular
Shortness of breath, chest pain
Heart murmur, palpitations, night sweats
Cold hands, leg cramps, varicose veins
Hypertension, valvular disease

Gastrointestinal
Symmetry, tenderness, pain
Changes in appetite, nausea, vomiting
Jaundice, ulcers, gallstones
Change in bowel habits: diarrhea, constipation, hemorrhoids, stool color

Urinary
Changes in urinary habits: hesitancy, urgency, frequency, night voiding, pain when voiding, loss of stream force
Kidney stones, urinary tract infections
Dribbling, incontinence

Genitalia (Male)
Infertility, sterility, impotency
Testicular pain, penile discharge
Penile enlargement or discomfort
Erections, emissions, hernias
Prostate or testicular enlargement

Genitalia (Female)
Menses regularity, flow, pain, duration
Premenstrual symptoms, menopause
Obstetric history, birth control method
Estrogen therapy, reproductive surgeries
Pain during intercourse, sterility

Lymph Glands
Enlargement, tenderness
Female breasts: symmetry, lumps

Neurologic
Level of consciousness, headaches
Reflex reactions, general weakness
Speech changes, memory loss, seizures
Changes in balance, incoordination

Endocrine
Weight change, fatigue, bulging eyes
Increased thirst or hunger, neck swelling
Excessive sweating, heat or cold intolerance

Skin
Color, turgor, and tone
Lesions or scars
Temperature, rashes, itching
Moles, sores, acne

Arms and Legs
General appearance and symmetry
Palpation of arm muscles
Range of motion, limitation of movement
Inspection of fingernails
Deformities, joint stiffness

Legs and Feet
Symmetry, scars, bruises, swelling
Broken bones, deformity, sprains, strains
Gout, arthritis, osteoporosis
Inspection of toenails

Correct Method of Charting

- Check the name on the record and be certain that the information being charted is recorded on the correct form on the correct patient's chart.
- All charting is done in black ink. Never use pencil.
- Write in a clear, legible manner.
- The month, day, and year must precede the entry; many facilities also require the time of the documentation.
- All unusual complaints, symptoms, or reactions must be noted in detail. Include complete information regarding the *onset* (when problem started), *duration* (how long episodes last), and *frequency* (how often episodes occur) of each reported sign and symptom. Example: Pt reports night cough which started 2 days ago, lasting approximately 10 minutes, occurs 3-4 times per night.
- Describe objective data, such as the presence of a wound, using correct anatomic medical terminology. Example: Observed wound on left distal anterior tibia approximately 2 cm long and 1 cm wide.
- If the patient reports pain, the quality and intensity of the pain should be recorded using a pain scale of 1 to 10. Example: Pt c/o dull pain at wound site, a 4 on a scale of 1-10.
- If patient comments are entered in the patient's own words, enclose them in quotation marks. Example: Pt states, "I fell against a stone foundation while cutting the grass and slashed my leg."
- Document the complete medication history, including both prescription and over-the-counter (OTC) medications taken on a regular basis, the last dose taken of the medication, the effectiveness of the medication, and any other pertinent details. Example: Pt reports taking 2 ibuprofen tablets for pain with moderate relief; last dose taken 45 minutes ago.
- Record details regarding previous history of the current chief complaint (CC). Example: Pt reports having a similar cough 3 weeks ago.
- When entering information on a patient's chart, sign the entry, including the appropriate initials after your name (e.g., CMA).
- Learn to be observant and to note anything that seems pertinent.
- Spelling, abbreviations, symbols, and terminology used must be accurate. Refer to Table 27-3 for typical medical abbreviations.
- Review your documentation immediately after completion so errors can be detected while the information is fresh in your mind.
- Never scribble, erase, or use whiteout on an error. For legal purposes it is crucial that the corrected error can be read.
- Correct the error by drawing one line through it. Write "error" above the corrected word or words and date and initial the correction. Then write in the correction.
- If details are omitted, add information by documenting after the last entry. Record "late entry," include date and time of note, and document the omitted information (see Figure 27-12).

Professional Medical Offices
1722 E. North Avenue Suite 109
Aloha, HI 99751

Patient Name Gastrin, Eleanor C.   DOB 8/15/40   Chart # ___3361___
               Last   First   MI   Allergies ___Iodine___

Date	Time	Progress Note
7/4/07	10 AM	C/O fever x 3 days. Productive cough.
		T-101, P-72, ~~R-6t~~ Error SW 7/4/02
		R-16 S. Watkins, CMA
7/4/07	10:20AM	Late entry ————————
		Denies wheezing, SOB S. Watkins, CMA

FIGURE 27-12 Documentation correction.

Terminology

Medical terminology is a language system that is based on Latin and addresses processes occurring in specific body systems, procedures, diagnostics, and diseases. The system depends on the use of a suffix, which is defined first, a root word, and many times a prefix. The parts of the word are connected using a combining form "o" except in terms that have a suffix beginning with a vowel. For example, osteitis is defined as inflammation (the suffix "itis") of the bone (root word "oste"). The combining form "o" is not needed to connect the suffix and root word because the suffix begins with an "i." However, with the term *osteopathic*, "ic" means pertaining to, the suffix "path" means disease condition of, and the root word "oste" (bone) is connected with the combining form "o."

If a word is unfamiliar to you, it is important to learn the meaning, correct spelling, pronunciation, and proper use of the term. Learning medical terminology is an ongoing process of vocabulary building. Consistent use of a good medical dictionary is essential. To aid your learning, a sample of frequently used medical word parts with their definitions

TABLE 27-3 Medical Abbreviations

ABBREVIATION	DEFINITION	ABBREVIATION	DEFINITION
ABD	abdomen	FBS	fasting blood sugar
ABG	arterial blood gases	f/u	follow up
ac	before eating	FUO	fever of unknown origin
ACLS	advanced cardiac life support	fx	fracture
ad lib	as desired	GC	gonorrhea
AFP	alpha-fetoprotein	GI	gastrointestinal
AKA	above the knee amputation	GTT	glucose tolerance test
ASAP	as soon as possible	GU	genitourinary
ASHD	atherosclerotic heart disease	HCT	hematocrit
BE	barium enema	Hgb	hemoglobin
bid	twice a day	HIV	human immunodeficiency virus
BM	bowel movement	HPI	history of present illness
BMR	basal metabolic rate	hs	at bedtime or hour of sleep
BOM	bilateral otitis media	HTN	hypertension
BP	blood pressure	Hx	history
BUN	blood urea nitrogen	I&D	incision and drainage
bx	biopsy	I&O	intake and output
$\bar{c}$	with	IG	immunoglobulin
C&S	culture and sensitivity	lytes	electrolytes
CA	cancer	MI	myocardial infarction
CABG	coronary artery bypass graft	NG	nasogastric
CAD	coronary artery disease	NKA	no known allergies
CBC	complete blood count	NPO	nothing by mouth
cc	chief complaint	N/V	nausea and vomiting
CHF	congestive heart failure	$\bar{p}$	after
CHO	carbohydrate	PE	pulmonary embolism
CNS	central nervous system	prn	as needed
c/o	complains of	pt	patient
COPD	chronic obstructive pulmonary disease	PE	physical examination
CPK	creatinine phosphokinase	PT	physical therapy
CPR	cardiopulmonary resuscitation	q	every
CSF	cerebrospinal fluid	RBC	red blood cells
CT	computed tomography	R/O	rule out
CVA	cerebrovascular accident	ROM	range of motion
CXR	chest x-ray	Rx	treatment
DAT	diet as tolerated	$\bar{s}$	without
dc	discontinue	SOB	shortness of breath
D&C	dilation and curettage	STD	sexually transmitted disease
DDx	differential diagnosis	stat	immediately
DM	diabetes mellitus	Sx	symptoms
DNR	do not resuscitate	Tx	treatment
DVT	deep vein thrombosis	UA	urinalysis
Dx	diagnosis	URI	upper respiratory infection
ECG	electrocardiogram	UTI	urinary tact infection
ENT	ears, nose, throat	VS	vital signs

is listed in Table 27-4. In addition, a terminology glossary is located in the back of this textbook, a vocabulary section appears at the beginning of each chapter, and Appendix C is an overview of understanding medical terms. Because the physician communicates using medical terminology and the medical assistant should use medical terms when documenting in the patient chart, it is essential that you become comfortable and familiar with the medical language system and its correct use.

Charting Methods

Problem-Oriented Medical Record

The problem-oriented medical record (POMR) is a documentation form that introduces a logical sequence to recording the information obtained from the patient. It is based on the scientific method and was designed to efficiently present the patient's health problem and record systematically how it

TABLE 27-4 Medical Word Parts

WORD PART	MEANING	WORD PART	MEANING	WORD PART	MEANING
a-	without	eu-	good; normal	para	near; beside
-ac	pertaining to	gastr/o	stomach	path/o	disease
aden/o	gland	-genesis	forming	-penia	deficiency
adip/o	fat	gest/o	pregnancy	-pepsia	digestion
-al	pertaining to	-globin	protein	per-	through
-algesia	sensitivity to pain	gloss/o	tongue	peri-	surrounding
-algia	pain	gluc/o	glucose, sugar	-pexy	fixation
angi/o	blood vessel	-gram	recording	-phagia	eating
ankyl/o	stiff	hem/o	blood	-phasia	speech
ante-	before	hemi-	half	phleb/o	vein
anter/o	front	hepat/o	liver	-plasty	repair
anti-	against	hist/o	tissue	-plegia	paralysis
arter/o	artery	hydr/o	water	-pnea	breathing
arthro	joint	hyper-	above; excessive	-poiesis	formation
artucul/o	joint	hyp/o	deficient	poly	many
-ase	enzyme	hyster/o	uterus	post-	after
ather/o	fatty plaque	-iasis	abnormal condition	-prandial	meal
aur/o	ear	infra-	below	pre-	before
auto-	self	inter-	between	proxim/o	near
axill/o	armpit	intra-	within	prurit/o	itching
bi-	two	jaund/o	yellow	pseudo/o	false
bi/o	life	kines/o	movement	-ptosis	drooping; sagging
-blast	immature	lact/o	milk	py/o	pus
blephar/o	eyelid	-lapse	to sag	pyel/o	renal pelvis
brady-	slow	later/o	side	pyr/o	fever
bucc/o	cheek	leuk/o	white	quadric-	four
carcin/o	cancerous	lip/o	fat	ren/o	kidney
cardi/o	heart	lith/o	stone	-rrhage	bursting forth
-cele	hernia	-lithiasis	condition of stones	-rrhea	flow
cephal/o	head	-logy	study of	-sclerosis	hardening
-cide	killing	-lysis	to break down	-scope	instrument to visualize
-clast	to break	macro-	large	semi-	half
colp/o	vagina	mal-	bad	somat/o	body
contra-	against	-malacia	softening	spl/o	spleen

Continued

TABLE 27-4 Medical Word Parts—cont'd

WORD PART	MEANING	WORD PART	MEANING	WORD PART	MEANING
crani/o	skull	mast/o	breast	-stasis	to stop
-crit	to separate	medi/o	middle	-stenosis	tightening
cyan/o	blue	mega-	large	stomat/o	mouth
cyst/o	urinary bladder	-megaly	enlargement	-stomy	new opening
cyt/o	cell	morph/o	shape	sub-	under
-derma	skin	my/o	muscle	supra-	above
dipl/o	double	necr/o	death	tachy-	fast
dors/o	back	neo-	new	thorac/o	chest
-dynia	pain	nephr/o	kidney	thromb/o	clot
dys-	painful, abnormal	neur/o	nerve	-tomy	cutting
-ectasia	dilation, stretching	odyn/o	pain	tox/o	poison
-ectomy	excision	olig/o	scanty	trans-	across; through
-emesis	vomiting	-oma	tumor; mass	-tresia	opening
-emia	blood condition	onych/o	nail	tri-	three
encephal/o	brain	oophor/o	ovary	-tripsy	to crush
endo-	within	ophthalm/o	eye	ur/o	urine
enter/o	small intestine	orch/o	testis	varic/o	varicose veins
eosin/o	red	orth/o	straight	vascul/o	vascular
epi-	above	oste/o	bone	ventr/o	front
erythem/o	flushed; red	ot/o	ear	viscer/o	internal organs
-esis	condition	pan-	all	vit/o	life

was managed. The medical history and physical examination fit into a special format that clarifies the patient's health problems. Each patient problem, or diagnosis, is defined and documented on a problem list sheet at the beginning of the chart. Each time the patient is diagnosed with a new health problem, that diagnosis is added to the problem list in numeric order. If the patient is successfully treated for the health problem and cured, then the physician will document next to that diagnosis on the problem list "Problem resolved" and date it accordingly. By identifying and numbering the patient's diagnoses at the beginning of the chart, the POMR assists with the process of auditing the medical record. In addition, the system is designed for and easily adapted to electronic medical record (EMR) systems. The POMR system includes four basic parts:

1. *Database:* Includes the patient's health history, physical examination, and the results of baseline laboratory and diagnostic procedures. This information allows the physician to compile a health problem list for the patient.
2. *Problem list:* A list of the identified patient problems kept in the front of the patient's chart. It is the table of contents or the index of the chart that defines patient health concerns, including diagnoses, treatment, and educational needs. The problem list takes a holistic approach by including psychosocial as well as physical needs. Each problem entered is numerically listed and dated and is supported by the database. The problems are then identified and referred to throughout progress note documentation by their assigned number. If over time an additional problem is identified, the information is added to the problem list. If the problem is resolved, the date of problem resolution is entered next to the problem. For example, if Mrs. Xu is diagnosed with hypertension and that particular health problem is listed as diagnosis number three, then every time Mrs. Xu comes to the office for follow-up of her blood pressure the documentation piece begins by identifying the diagnosis with the number three (#3). This system makes it very easy for the physician or medical assistant to scan the Progress Notes, review all documentation on diagnosis #3 (hypertension), and obtain a relatively quick and comprehensive history of how her blood pressure is being managed and controlled.

3. *Plan:* A written plan for each problem identified on the problem list, outlining further studies, treatments, and patient education (Figure 27-13).
4. *Progress notes:* Using the first letter of each part of the progress note spells the acronym SOAPE; therefore this portion of the POMR system is called the *SOAP notes* (or

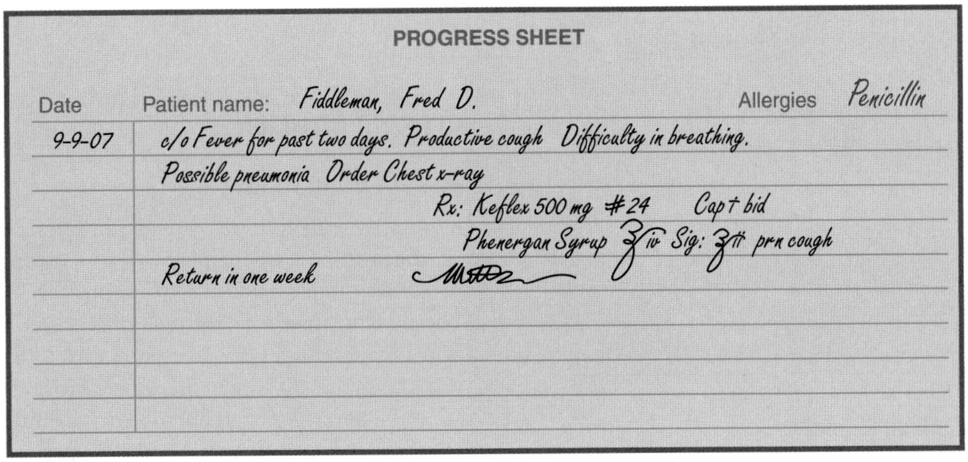

PROGRESS SHEET

Date	Patient name: Fiddleman, Fred D. Allergies Penicillin
9-9-07	c/o Fever for past two days. Productive cough Difficulty in breathing.
	Possible pneumonia Order Chest x-ray
	Rx: Keflex 500 mg #24 Cap ↑ bid
	Phenergan Syrup ℥iv Sig: ℨii prn cough
	Return in one week

FIGURE 27-13 Initial plan for POMR progress notes.

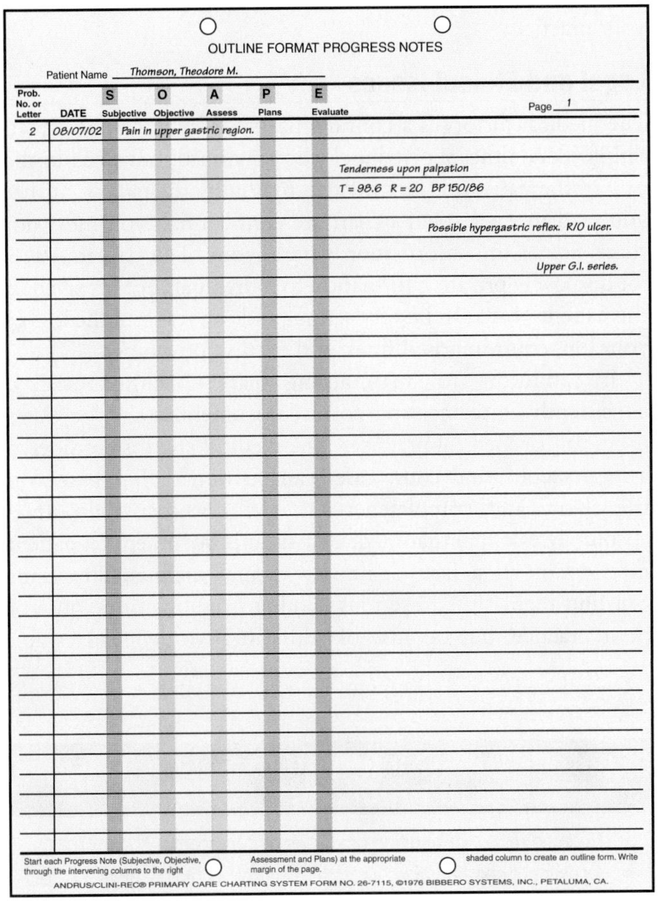

OUTLINE FORMAT PROGRESS NOTES

Patient Name Thomson, Theodore M.

Page 1

Prob. No. or Letter	DATE	S Subjective	O Objective	A Assess	P Plans	E Evaluate
2	08/07/02	Pain in upper gastric region.				
			Tenderness upon palpation			
			T = 98.6 R = 20 BP 150/86			
				Possible hypergastric reflex. R/O ulcer.		
					Upper G.I. series.	

Start each Progress Note (Subjective, Objective, Assessment and Plans) at the appropriate shaded column to create an outline form. Write through the intervening columns to the right margin of the page.

ANDRUS/CLINI-REC® PRIMARY CARE CHARTING SYSTEM FORM NO. 26-7115, ©1976 BIBBERO SYSTEMS, INC., PETALUMA, CA.

FIGURE 27-14 Structured notes for the POMR system. (Courtesy Bibbero Systems, Petaluma, Calif.)

SOAPE notes when evaluation is included) (Figure 27-14). Each progress note uses the following format:

- **S** for *subjective* data–the purpose of the visit, with the patient's words in quotation marks, or a summary of the patient's statement regarding the chief complaint. For example, the subjective note may record exactly what the patient says, such as, "I feel horrible, exhausted, coughing all night long." If the patient's exact words are not documented in quotation marks, the subjective entry typically starts with "Patient states…," "Patient c/o…," or "Caregiver reports…." The medical assistant documents this information based on details gained from the patient interview.
- **O** for *objective* data–anything that is observed or measurable, including vital signs (VS), the exact anatomic location of an injury, difficulty with gait, and so on. Objective data can be repeatedly measured, which means that regardless of how many different healthcare workers observe the patient or document the sign, the same or very similar numbers or explanations would be given. The medical assistant is responsible for documenting complete and accurate objective data about all patient signs. This information should be in such specific detail that even an individual who has not seen the patient can visualize the patient's state of health. Typically the medical assistant charts only the subjective and objective data, leaving the remainder of the documentation to the physician.
- **A** for *assessment* of the problem–usually the physician's preliminary diagnosis or the cause of the patient's chief complaint. The physician or healthcare provider makes a judgment about what is wrong with the patient and documents it in this section; therefore the medical assistant is not involved in this piece.
- **P** for the *plan of care*–the physician's documentation regarding how the health problem will be managed, including diagnostic studies, treatments, and patient education.
- **E** for *evaluation*–assessment of the patient's understanding of the treatment or the ability to comply with the treatment plan. It may also be used to document a follow-up on medication or treatments administered in the physician's office. For example, if an asthmatic patient receives a breathing treatment during the office visit, a note would be made regarding the effectiveness of the treatment.

CRITICAL THINKING APPLICATION

Document the following scenario using the POMR method:
The patient c/o a sore throat with pain of 5 on a 1-10 scale and fever for 2 days. He has been taking OTCs for relief of symptoms. His VS are T 100.4, P 88, R 20. He also has an erythemic papular rash across his chest.

S: _____

O: _____

_____

_____

Source-Oriented Medical Record

The source-oriented medical record (SOMR) is the most common form of record keeping in physicians' office practices. The data in the chart are organized in divided sections including an area for the History and Physical (H&P), Progress Notes, Laboratory Results, Consultations, and so on. All information is filed in reverse chronologic order, with the most recent report or progress note placed on top. Progress notes are made each time the patient is seen or contacted by telephone. Documentation in the Progress Notes section is based on details surrounding the patient's chief complaint (CC) or treatment protocol. For example, if a patient is being seen today for the flu, the note may read, "CC flu-like symptoms, fever Xs 3 days, general discomfort, yellow nasal drainage, productive cough." The primary disadvantage of the SOMR system is that it can be very time consuming to find a back entry regarding a particular problem or treatment.

Electronic Medical Record

Many ambulatory care settings, especially multipractice facilities and health maintenance organizations (HMOs), are using new technology to collect and file patient information as well as link offices together. These EMR systems are usually designed for the particular needs of the practice and are set up so that information is directly entered and downloaded into the patient's computerized file, while the patient is being interviewed or assessed, via personal digital assistants, laptop computers, or computer stations located throughout the facility. Proponents of EMR state that this type of record keeping will reduce practice overhead and improve staff efficiency, will cut the cost of running the practice, and will improve patient care. EMR can cut costs by limiting the physical resources, such as paper, chart material, copiers, and so on, needed to operate the practice and drastically reduces the amount of space needed to store medical records. With an EMR, patient charts are on computerized files and therefore are easily accessible, saving time for the staff, and all documentation pieces are easily legible. In addition, it is possible to link the physician's office system to the hospital or laboratory so that patient diagnostic tests can be downloaded into the file and be readily available for the physician to review and share with the patient. The biggest problem with EMR systems is if the electricity or computer system goes down patient information cannot be accessed. Backup files must be maintained and special attention must be paid to patient confidentiality to prevent the accidental sharing of private information.

CLOSING COMMENTS

Patient Education

Finding time to conduct patient education in a busy healthcare practice can be challenging. Every opportunity to interact with patients should be considered a potential "teaching moment." The perfect time to begin the education process is during the initial patient interview, because this is when you will first become aware of patient lifestyle factors that may negatively affect wellness. Or perhaps during the interview process the patient mentions a financial, social, or psychologic problem that could be helped with referral to a community or hospital-based service. Your interactions with patients and implementation of therapeutic communication skills as well as interview techniques are crucial to the quality of care patients receive in your practice.

Legal and Ethical Issues

The medical history is a confidential record that can be shared only with healthcare personnel who are directly involved in the care of the patient. Data provided to you by the patient or that you read in the patient's chart are confidential; you must not share any of this information with anyone. The consequences for disclosing private information to individuals not involved in the patient's care can be very serious and can result in the loss of your job, court-imposed fines, and even imprisonment.

In addition to maintaining patient confidentiality, consistently implementing correct documentation procedures is crucial for medical practices. The medical chart is considered a legal record, and court cases can be won or lost based on the clarity and completeness of staff documentation. It is absolutely essential that medical assistants document all patient information in a factual, nonjudgmental manner. Physicians can find themselves in serious liability trouble, not because of poor practice, but because of administrative deficiencies and

Factors That Contribute to Sound Risk Management Practices

- Periodic review or auditing of patient office records
- Consistent charting of accurate and complete clinical facts and test results
- Adequate office procedures for informing patients of test results as well as documenting this communication
- Appropriate use of abbreviations and legible recording on the patient chart as well as corrections made in the legally required manner
- Documentation that shows diagnostic tests have been received, reviewed by the attending physician, and filed in a timely manner
- Documented evidence of appropriate discharge and continuing care instructions

poor communications. Risk management practices focus on these problems as a way of reducing the chances of professional liability claims.

Health Insurance Portability and Accountability Act Applications

- The patient has the right to request that the physician practice limit the disclosure of protected health information (PHI) for treatment, payment, and healthcare operations (TPO). For example, if the patient had an abortion 5 years ago, she may request this information not be shared unless absolutely necessary.
- The facility is not required to comply with this request, but if agreement is reached, the restriction on sharing the information must be documented and all employees must comply with the agreement. Therefore if a physician referral includes sending the patient's chart to a consulted physician, the medical assistant must make sure that the restricted information is not included in the material that is sent.
- The patient has the right to request that confidential information be sent in a manner that the patient decides is best. For example, the patient may request that all phone calls from the office be made to a work number rather than home, whereas some patients may give approval for messages to be left on the home answering machine. Whatever the patient's preference, this information must be documented and complied with each time the office attempts to contact the patient.

SUMMARY OF SCENARIO

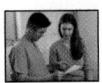

The office supervisor met with Chris and reviewed the essential techniques for gathering patient information. Therapeutic communication includes demonstrating respectful patient care, using active listening skills, observing nonverbal behaviors, and using a combination of both open and closed questions to gather the best possible detail about the patient's chief complaint. The supervisor gave Chris a variety of information on meeting the needs of a diverse patient population and gave him suggestions on how to develop empathetic helping relationships. One of the suggestions she made was that Chris develop a community resource file that he can refer to if a patient needs additional assistance outside of the healthcare setting. Chris learned to identify the parts of the patient interview and became familiar with typical barriers to patient communication so that interviews would run more smoothly and he could gather more specific information from patients. Chris's workplace uses POMR documentation methods, so he reviewed the specifics of this type of record keeping with his supervisor. In conclusion, the significance of patient confidentiality was emphasized, and Chris agreed to work at implementing the techniques for therapeutic communications.

SUMMARY of LEARNING OBJECTIVES

1. Define, spell, and pronounce the terms listed in the vocabulary.
   - Spelling and pronouncing medical terms correctly adds credibility to the medical assistant. Knowing the definition of these terms promotes confidence in communication with patients and co-workers.
2. Employ the components of holistic care in the patient assessment process.
   - Holistic care includes assessing the patient's health status through the collection of physical, cognitive, psychosocial, and behavioral data. The medical assistant should consider all of these factors when collecting data about the patient's health problems.
3. Describe the components of the patient's medical history.
   - The medical history consists of the patient's database, past medical history, family and social histories, and the review of systems.
4. Define and apply the qualities of a helping relationship.
   - Developing a professional helping relationship with patients is the responsibility of all healthcare workers. The helping relationship involves consistent application of respectful patient care that recognizes the impact of patient anxieties on interactions and responses to treatment.
5. Display sensitivity to diverse patient populations.
   - Sensitivity to diverse populations includes the application of empathetic communications and an awareness of the impact of individual value systems and personal prejudices on patient interactions.
6. Demonstrate therapeutic communications including the use of the linear communication model and active listening techniques.
   - The linear communication model illustrates communication as an interactive process between the sender and receiver of the message, with feedback a crucial part of the process. Active listening techniques, which include restatement, reflection, and clarification, help the medical assistant go beyond hearing the message to actually listening to and appropriately responding to the patient's main point.
7. Recognize the importance of nonverbal communication when interacting with patients.

Continued

SUMMARY of LEARNING OBJECTIVES

Continued

- Approximately 90% of patient interactions occur through nonverbal language. The key to successful patient interaction is congruence between verbal and nonverbal messages.

8. Identify barriers to communication and their impact on patient assessment.
   - Certain communication styles can be misleading or restrict the patient's response. A medical assistant must be alert to using such faulty techniques as inappropriately providing reassurance, giving advice, using medical terminology without clarification, asking leading questions, and talking too much. These behaviors interfere with gathering complete data during the interview and are obstacles to developing rapport with your patient.

9. Detect patients' use of defense mechanisms and resultant barriers to therapeutic communication.
   - Patients use defense mechanisms to protect themselves in emotionally challenging situations. A medical assistant must consistently apply nonjudgmental therapeutic communication skills to maintain professional relationships.

10. Apply therapeutic communication techniques with patients across the lifespan.
    - Therapeutic communication techniques vary according to the age and developmental level of the patient. A medical assistant should be aware of how to interact most effectively with various age groups, including young children, adolescents, adults, elderly patients, and family members. Age-specific application of interview styles enables clear communication between the health professional and the patient.

11. Demonstrate professional patient interview techniques.
    - The patient interview is divided into the introduction, the body, and the summary or closing. Throughout the interview the medical assistant should use professional interview techniques, such as empathetic patient care, sensitivity to patient diversity, active listening skills, appropriate nonverbal communication, attention to the interview environment, avoidance of communication barriers, and the framing of questions and statements in an open or closed manner depending on the

information that is needed and the patient's communication behaviors.

12. Integrate detailed information about the chief complaint into concise, accurate documentation methods.
    - The ability to document accurately and completely is an essential skill for all medical assistants. Documentation should describe the patient's chief complaint, identify all pertinent signs and symptoms, and demonstrate the correct use of medical terminology, with appropriate abbreviations. Any error in the medical record must be corrected according to legally approved methods.

13. Differentiate among various medical record systems employed in the physician's office.
    - There are three main forms of medical record systems. These include the POMR method, which uses SOAPE charting to define the patient's health problems; the most frequently used form of medical record keeping, the SOMR, which organizes patient data into specific sections; and the EMR system, which compiles computer records for patient data.

14. Describe the connection between the interview process and implementation of patient education practices.
    - The perfect time to initiate patient education is during the initial patient interview. A medical assistant should take advantage of every "teaching moment" to get to know his or her patients and promote patient wellness.

15. Determine risk management strategies for the ambulatory care setting.
    - Risk management practices focus on reducing the chances of professional liability claims and maintaining compliance with HIPAA standards. Accurate and complete documentation on the patient's chart is crucial for successful risk management. In addition, maintaining strict confidentiality of patient information and factual, nonjudgmental, legible recording of patient data are essential to professional patient care.

16. Obtain a written medical history from a patient.
    - Refer to Procedure 27-1.

CONNECTIONS

 Study Guide Connection: Go to Chapter 27 Study Guide. Read the Case Study and Workplace Applications and complete the assignments. Do online research for answers to the questions in the Internet Activities associated with patient assessment.

 CD Connection: Go to the Medical Assisting Competency Challenge CD and do the training activities under Patient Care and Legal Concepts.

evolve **Evolve Connection:** For more information related to patient assessment, go to evolve.elsevier.com/kinn and visit related weblinks for Chapter 27. Click on the Medical Assisting Exam Review and do the practice questions to sharpen your test-taking skills.

Patient Education

28

SCENARIO

In a busy family-practice office, medical assistant Taylor DiSalvo is working with a patient, Mr. Sam Ignatio, 68 years old, who has just been diagnosed with type 2 diabetes mellitus. Mr. Ignatio knows nothing about his disease or how to manage it; has never seen a glucometer and never handled needles; consumes a high-fat, high-carbohydrate diet; does not exercise on a regular basis; is 50 pounds overweight; has functional deafness in his left ear and decreased sound quality in his right ear; and shows early signs of diabetic-related vision loss. Taylor is responsible for assisting with Mr. Ignatio's patient-teaching plan.

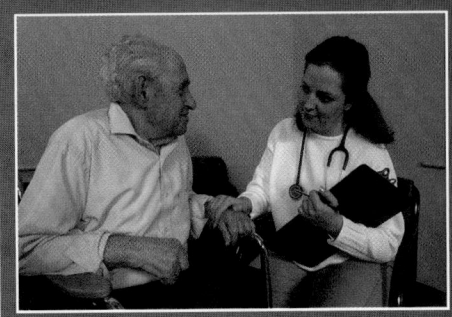

Mr. Ignatio is faced with a serious illness, and his future health depends on compliance with a wide range of lifestyle changes. The methods Taylor chooses to teach this patient about his disease can have a significant impact on his eventual health outcome.

While studying this chapter, think about the following questions:

- How should Taylor begin Mr. Ignatio's patient education?
- What individual characteristics does Mr. Ignatio possess that may affect his ability to learn all of the information required to manage his disease?
- How can Taylor make certain that Mr. Ignatio understands the importance of following treatment and disease-monitoring guidelines?

- What teaching approaches and materials would best meet the needs of this patient?
- Are there any community resources available that could help Mr. Ignatio learn how to manage his disease?

LEARNING OBJECTIVES

1. Recognize the implications of models relating to health and illness on patient education.
2. Illustrate at least five guidelines for patient education that can affect overall patient wellness.
3. Define six patient factors that have an impact on learning.
4. Summarize education approaches for patients with language barriers.
5. Determine potential barriers to patient learning.

6. Implement a variety of teaching methods and strategies that are responsive to individual patient needs.
7. Demonstrate the ability to develop an appropriate and effective patient-teaching plan.
8. Describe the role of the medical assistant in patient education.
9. Integrate the legal and ethical implications of patient teaching into the ambulatory care setting.

National Accreditation Competencies and Content

CAAHEP COMPETENCIES

General

3.c.(1)(b). Recognize and respond to verbal communications
3.c.(1)(c). Recognize and respond to nonverbal communications
3.c.(3)(b). Instruct individuals according to their needs
3.c.(3)(c). Provide instruction for health maintenance and disease prevention
3.c.(3)(d). Identify community resources

ABHES COMPETENCIES

Communication

2.a. Be attentive, listen, and learn
2.b. Be impartial and show empathy when dealing with patients
2.i. Recognize and respond to verbal and nonverbal communication
2.m. Adaptation for individual needs

Instruction

7.b. Instruct patients with special needs
7.c. Teach patients methods of health promotion and disease prevention

This chapter will help students recognize the individual learning needs of patients and provides guidelines for developing effective teaching approaches. The key to patient compliance with prescribed treatments is empowerment—providing the patient with the information and support that enables the patient to take charge of his or her health problem. The concepts in this chapter are basic to all patient education interventions, and following them can positively affect a patient's understanding of the disease process as well as his or her willingness to comply with physician-recommended disease management.

PATIENT EDUCATION AND MODELS OF HEALTH AND ILLNESS

Patient education should begin with the first contact between the patient and the healthcare team (Figure 28-1). A well-informed patient is more likely to comply with treatment and adopt a healthy lifestyle. However, informing a patient about his or her disease is only a portion of the health-teaching process. The key to successful health teaching is that the patient is empowered and therefore willing to implement teaching guidelines.

Decreases in hospital admissions and shorter hospital stays have resulted in the need for patients and families to assume responsibility for care that was once given by hospital staff. This means that those of us who work in ambulatory care settings have an even greater responsibility to meet the educational needs of our patients. To develop an effective teaching approach, we must implement a holistic model that considers not only the patient's physical state but also his or her psychological, social, and spiritual needs (Figure 28-2). The holistic model suggests we look at patients and determine their needs based on a complete view of their lives rather than just as an analysis of their specific diseases. It is our responsibility not only to teach patients about disease processes but also to help them implement related skills and changes in lifestyle to promote recovery and improve function. In the case of Mr. Ignatio, diabetes mellitus is a complicated disease that requires an in-depth understanding of the disease process as well as significant changes in lifestyle. When considering the impact of this diagnosis on the patient, the medical assistant

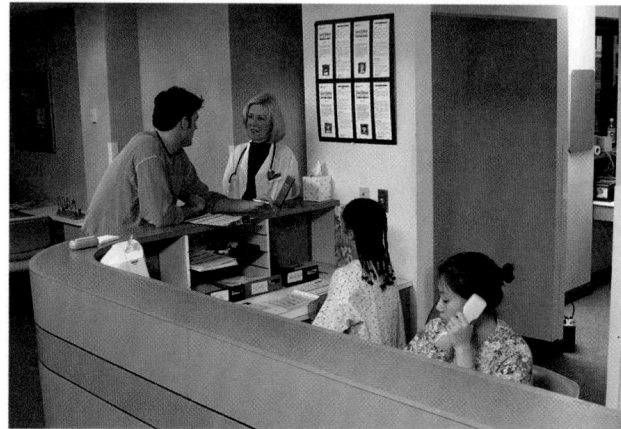

FIGURE 28-1 First contact with a patient.

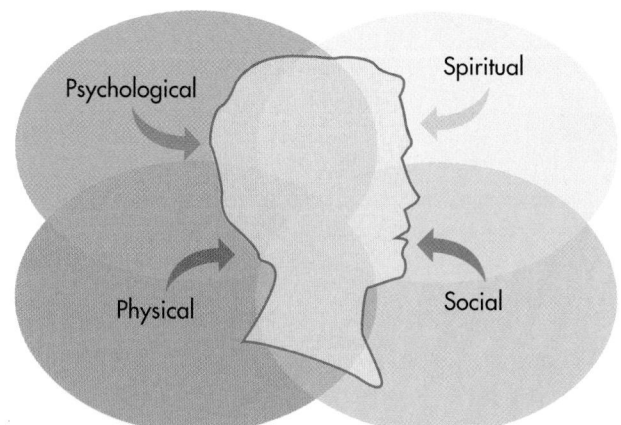

FIGURE 28-2 Holistic approach. (From Sorrentio SA, Gorek B: *Mosby's essentials for nursing assistants*, ed 3, St Louis, 2006, Mosby.)

should keep in mind the following factors because they will affect the patient's response.

- Emotional effect of the disease: Is Mr. Ignatio in shock and denial? Is he angry or depressed?
- Social impact: How will his family and employer respond to the diagnosis? Does he have a support system that will assist him in making healthy lifestyle choices?

- Intellectual impact: Is Mr. Ignatio able to understand the complexities of the disease and treatment recommendations?
- Economic impact: Can he afford the treatment for diabetes? Does he have health insurance to cover the cost, or will he need assistance in paying for ongoing diagnostic and treatment recommendations?
- Spiritual impact: What is Mr. Ignatio's spiritual response to his diagnosis?

The Health Belief Model may be helpful in understanding why individuals do not follow recommended guidelines to maintain health and prevent the development of disease. This model analyzes what people believe to be true about themselves and their health. The model suggests we first consider how the patient perceives his or her risk of developing a disease. For example, even though Mr. Ignatio's mother and sister developed type 2 diabetes in their sixties, he may believe he is not going to have the same problem. Therefore, even though wellness information encouraged him to lose weight, exercise, and eat a healthy diet, he didn't believe he was in danger of developing diabetes so he didn't believe he needed to follow these disease-prevention recommendations. Another factor considered with the Health Belief Model is the patient's perceived benefits of action—whether the patient believes altering health behaviors will prevent him from developing the disease. In this case, because Mr. Ignatio has a strong family history of the disease, he may have decided he was going to get diabetes anyway, so why should he bother exercising and watching his diet? He may have believed he was going to develop diabetes no matter what he did, so why bother trying to prevent it? Until the patient believes that teaching and health promotion guidelines affect him and are worth pursuing, he will not follow suggested health promotion tips or comply with treatment protocols.

Another model that may be helpful in understanding why patients respond the way they do to health threats is Elizabeth Kübler-Ross's stages of grief. When a patient faces a serious health threat, adjusting to the disease and starting to take control of his or her health may be delayed by the grief process. For example, Mr. Ignatio may be responding to the news of his diagnosis with the first stage of the grief process—denial. Perhaps both his mother and sister suffered serious complications from diabetes including blindness and leg amputation, and he may be using denial to psychologically deal with the burden of the diagnosis. Each individual goes through the stages of grief in his or her own way and at his or her own pace. It is a process that can take weeks to months to complete, but until the patient reaches the point at which he or she accepts the diagnosis and possible ramifications of the disease, compliance with patient education is going to be very difficult to achieve. The stages of grief include the following:

Denial and isolation. The patient denies the existence of the disease, may be unwilling to accept the reality of the situation, and refuses to discuss the health problem or remember health teaching interventions. For example, Mr. Ignatio refuses to meet with the dietitian because he says his diet is fine and there is no need to change it.

Suggestions for Therapeutic Interactions for Patients in Grief

Following are suggestions for therapeutic interactions:

Denial and isolation. Reinforce each education intervention with handouts that explain the disease and treatment. Encourage the patient's family to attend physician office visits and be involved in the patient's care.

Anger. Use therapeutic communication techniques, especially reflection, to acknowledge the patient's feelings about the diagnosis. Recognize the patient's need to use defense mechanisms to protect himself or herself from the reality of the disease. Remember, the patient is not angry at you or the physician—he or she is angry about the diagnosis and its accompanying challenges.

Bargaining. Rely on the physician's recommendations regarding postponing certain treatment methods. Discuss the patient's bargaining requests with the physician and other staff members to work out a solution that will promote patient compliance with healthcare recommendations.

Depression. Use available community resources to provide support for the patient and family. The physician may recommend the patient attend a support group, meet with a dietitian, or use professional counseling services to deal with depression.

Acceptance. Take advantage of this time to renew education efforts by providing multiple methods for learning about the disease such as videos, DVDs, professional websites, and community support services.

Anger. The patient may be very angry and hostile when forced to discuss the condition. Mr. Ignatio may say, "Why did this happen to me? I am a good person, why did I get diabetes?"

Bargaining. The patient tries to bargain for privileges or time. Mr. Ignatio may say, "Look, I know I am supposed to start this new diet, but Christmas is coming and I'll meet with the dietitian after the holidays."

Depression. The patient grieves the loss of health. Mr. Ignatio may be very sad about the diagnosis. He doesn't want to have to deal with the complexities of the disease, he just wants it to go away so he can live his life without the fear of diabetic complications.

Acceptance. The patient finally gets to the point where he or she accepts the diagnosis and is ready to make the best of it. At this point, Mr. Ignatio would be willing to use community resources for education and support.

Patient Factors That Affect Learning

Many factors or patient characteristics may affect the patient's ability to learn. Medical assistants must be aware of these factors to develop a patient education approach that best meets the needs of each patient. A summary of these factors follows.

Perception of Disease Versus Actual State of Disease

Patients respond to a particular diagnosis in many different ways. One of the predictors of how a patient will respond, and

Guidelines for Patient Education

- Provide knowledge and skills to promote recovery and health
- Encourage patient ownership and participation in the teaching process
- Include family and significant others in education interventions, with patient approval
- Promote safe and appropriate use of medications and treatments
- Encourage patient adaptation to healthy behaviors
- Provide information about accessing community resources

therefore how he or she will react to health education, is the patient's perception of the disease. Previous life experiences may greatly influence your patient's knowledge base and/or desire to learn about his or her disease. Does the patient recognize and accept the seriousness of the diagnosis? Or, perhaps, does your patient overreact to potential disease risks? Both of these responses will determine the patient's willingness to learn about the disease as well as his or her compliance with treatment recommendations.

How do you think it will affect Taylor's patient education efforts if Mr. Ignatio does not consider diabetes a serious disease?

Patient Need for Information

The patient's perception of the impact of the disease on his or her general health will also determine the need for information about the disease. Does the patient express a desire to learn all he or she can about the disease, or does the patient resist or act indifferent to teaching efforts? A vital part of patient education is encouraging patient ownership of the learning process. To do this you may first have to persuade the patient that he or she does actually need to understand the disease before he or she can improve overall wellness.

What is the appropriate response if Mr. Ignatio tells Taylor his father was a diabetic and had to have both legs amputated because of the disease, so he doesn't think it matters if he controls his blood sugar—he will still have major health complications?

Patient Age and Developmental Level

Depending on the age of patients and/or their ability to understand information about their disease, you may need to adapt the teaching plan to meet their specific learning needs. For example, educating a 9-year-old type 1 diabetic patient about disease management requires an approach that is different from the one used for 68-year-old Mr. Ignatio. The medical assistant should be flexible and creative in providing learning opportunities that support the physician's attempt to educate the patient about disease prevention and health maintenance. Many times the key to patient understanding and compliance is the involvement of family members.

While conducting an assessment of Mr. Ignatio's diet, Taylor learns that his wife cooks all his meals and packs his lunch daily. What should Taylor do to make certain Mr. Ignatio's diet complies with diabetic recommendations?

Patient Mental and Emotional State

Even a well-planned teaching intervention can be ineffective if the patient is unable to pay attention because of anxiety, stress, anger, or denial (Figure 28-3). Frequently patients will use defense mechanisms to protect themselves from the reality of a serious illness. It is important that the medical assistant be sensitive to the mental state of the patient and adapt teaching interventions as needed.

Mr. Ignatio has just been told about his disease. He already shared that his father died of diabetes. Do you think he is able to pay attention to patient teaching about how to give his insulin injections? What should Taylor do to manage this problem?

Influence of Multicultural and Diversity Factors on Patient Education

Culture, family background, and religious beliefs influence patient actions. Working with patients from diverse backgrounds is an exciting challenge; however, for patient education to be successful it is essential that the medical assistant be aware of and sensitive to the impact of these factors on patient learning (Figure 28-4). Some questions you should consider when teaching a patient from a diverse background include the following:

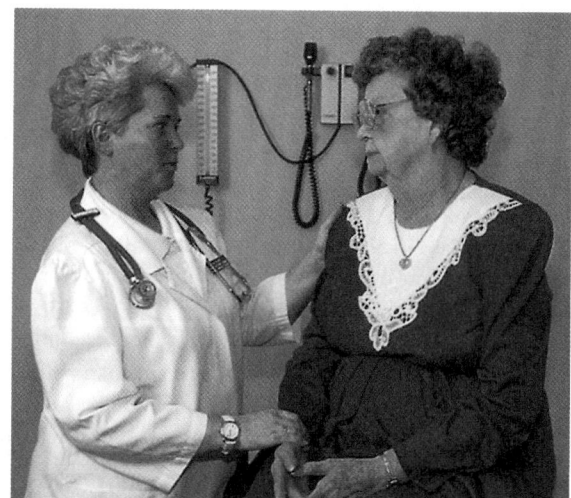

FIGURE 28-3 Demonstrating sensitivity to patient needs.

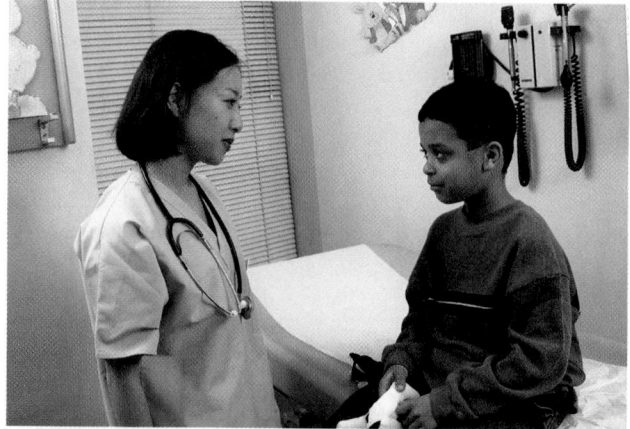

FIGURE 28-4 Considering diversity.

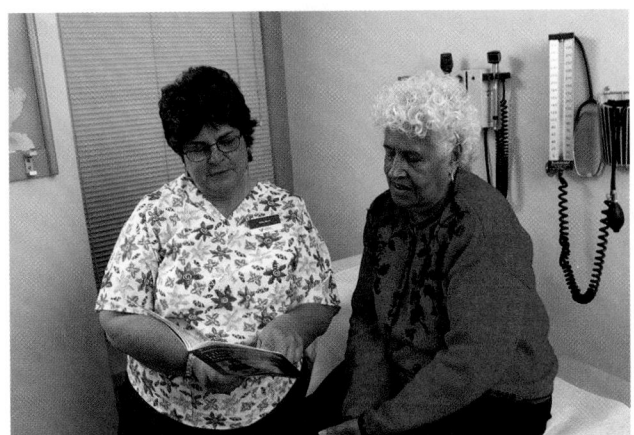

FIGURE 28-5 Managing language barriers.

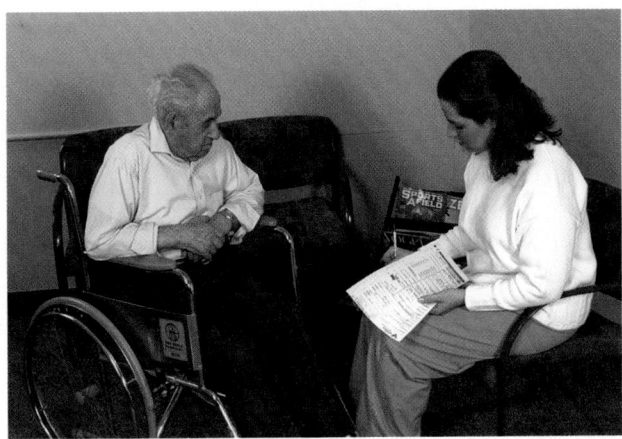

FIGURE 28-6 Assessing learning challenges.

- Is language an issue with your patient (Figure 28-5)? If the patient is unable to understand English verbally or read it correctly, do you have an alternative method for getting the information across?
- Do the patient's culture, ethnic background, or religious beliefs influence the way he or she perceives disease, as well as the role of healthcare workers?
- What strategies or techniques might minimize patient education problems?
- Are there community resources that could facilitate patient learning?

Approaches for Language Barriers

- Address the patient by his or her last name
- Be courteous, and use a formal approach to communication
- Use gestures, tone of voice, facial expressions, and eye contact to emphasize appropriate parts of the discussion
- Integrate pictures, handouts, models, and other aids that visually depict the material
- Monitor the patient's body language, especially facial expression, for understanding or confusion
- Use simple, everyday words as much as possible
- Demonstrate all procedures, and have the patient return the demonstration to check for understanding
- Implement the teaching plan in small manageable steps
- Give the patient written instructions for all procedures and treatments
- Use an interpreter when appropriate, if available

Patient Learning Style

Chapter 1 presented information on individual learning styles that affect you as a student. These same factors will have an impact on your patient's learning preference. Some patients learn best from discussion or lecture, whereas others must think or reflect about the material before understanding it. Some patients can learn from observing; others must act or do something with the material to learn it. Start your teaching

intervention by asking your patient how he or she prefers to learn new material, and pattern your teaching interventions along those lines.

Mr. Ignatio tells Taylor that he could never learn things by listening to someone tell him what to do. What approach to learning would best meet his needs?

Impact of Physical Disabilities

The patient must first be assessed to determine whether he or she can adequately hear instructions, see written material, and manipulate any required treatment equipment. All teaching efforts are lost if disabilities interfere with a patient's capacity to understand information or to properly handle equipment (Figure 28-6). A hearing or speech impairment may require the use of sign language with supplemental written instructions. If the patient is unable to manipulate equipment because of a physical disability or vision problem, family or community resources may be necessary for the patient to manage his or her care.

Mr. Ignatio's physical assessment revealed hearing and vision problems. Is he able to understand verbal instructions clearly? Will he be able to draw up the correct amount of insulin? What can be done to adapt the teaching intervention to meet his needs?

CRITICAL THINKING APPLICATION

Implement the holistic education model and Health Belief Model to determine and respond to Mr. Ignatio's individual learning needs.

THE TEACHING PLAN

What is it that patients need to know to effectively manage a disease? What is it about an individual patient that needs to be addressed for a teaching intervention to work? What are the immediate and long-term goals of patient education? What teaching materials or strategies should be used to meet the learning needs of the patient and also effectively relay the information? How can the teaching plan be implemented successfully? How does the medical assistant manage the limited

Therapeutic Communication with Special Needs Patients

Patients with Vision Loss

- Alert the patient that you are in the room, and identify yourself; do not touch the patient without warning.
- The patient is unable to pick up your body language; use clear and concise verbal language and a normal tone of voice.
- All written material should be in large font or print; often, large-print educational materials can be ordered.

Patients with Hearing Loss

- Stand in front of the patient or within the field of vision before you begin speaking; the patient may be able to lip-read.
- It may be necessary to lightly touch the patient to get her or his attention.
- Use expanded speech; lower the tone of your voice and pronounce each syllable.
- Carefully observe patient body language for understanding or confusion.
- Use gestures or demonstration as needed to get the message across.
- Clearly print information to clarify the patient education information.
- If a patient is wearing a hearing aid, ask the patient if it is on and working before starting the conversation; the patient may turn a hearing aid off to avoid annoying background noise.
- Provide written material that reviews the material being taught.
- Request family assistance in verifying that the patient received and understood the material.

Patients with Language Barriers

- Determine if the patient can read and/or understand English.
- If possible, have an interpreter present; a family member may be able to interpret the material for the patient.
- If available, use a dictionary that translates as many words as possible for the patient.
- Use gestures or demonstration to get the message across.
- Carefully observe the patient's body language to determine level of understanding.
- If available, order educational materials in the patient's native language or send materials home in English if there is a family member who can interpret the material for the patient.

time available for patient teaching? How do you know the patient is learning and actually implementing this knowledge into disease management? One of the most important aspects of patient teaching is to be flexible and to provide information about what patients want to know when patients want to know it. These and other guidelines for developing an appropriate and effective teaching plan follow.

Assess Patient Learning Needs

Developing a teaching plan that works for each individual first requires an assessment of the patient as a learner and consideration of any characteristics that might affect the learning

process. Many of these factors have already been addressed, such as the patient's learning preference, perception of the illness, age, background, multicultural influences, language barriers, and disabilities. The medical assistant must also consider what the patient already knows about the diagnosis and whether that knowledge includes misconceptions about the disease. The goal of the assessment process is to create a teaching plan that meets the needs of the patient to understand and manage his or her illness. The learning assessment therefore should consider what the patient needs to know, what the patient wants to know, and what can be done in the time available for learning.

Before developing a specific approach to patient education, the medical assistant must also consider potential barriers to learning besides those already presented, such as the presence of pain. If a patient is in acute distress, he or she will be unable to concentrate on the information. In this case the amount of material must be adjusted to meet the patient's immediate needs, and time should be planned in the future for a more in-depth transfer of information.

Does Mr. Ignatio exhibit any potential barriers to learning about his disease?

Potential Barriers to Patient Learning

- Individual learning style
- Age and developmental level
- Use of defense mechanisms
- Language
- Motivation to learn
- Physical limitations or disabilities
- Emotional or mental state
- Cultural or ethnic background
- Pain
- Time limitations

Determine Teaching Priorities

Once you have conducted an adequate assessment of your patient as a learner and you understand your patient's learning needs, the next question is, "Where do I start?" A patient such as Mr. Ignatio has a significant amount of information to learn before he can completely manage his disease. The volume of information might seem overwhelming unless priorities are established. How do you figure out what material should be first? The first question to ask is, "What are the patient's immediate versus long-term needs?" What must this patient learn today to be able to take care of himself, and what does he need to know overall about his illness to promote healthy behaviors?

Because the patient learning assessment told you what your patient knows about his or her disease, that is a good place to start. Confirm what the patient knows about the problem, and attempt to correct any potential misconceptions. If you start with something the patient knows and understands, he or she will feel more competent and capable of managing new material. You should then go on to the new material the patient is most anxious about. If the patient is nervous or afraid about a particular item, he or she will be unable to pay attention to any other new material until the anxieties are addressed.

For example, if Mr. Ignatio is most concerned about giving himself injections, that is the first skill he should learn. Once he is confident about that particular part of treatment, he will be able to pay attention to diet and exercise recommendations. You should always begin with the basic details about the disease and add more information during each patient visit.

Every interaction with the patient is an opportunity to conduct health education. One of the major problems with delivering high-quality patient education in an ambulatory healthcare setting is the lack of time. Therefore a medical assistant must take advantage of every "teaching moment." That is, every time you interact with the patient, use it as an opportunity to assess the patient's current education needs and provide as much information or guidance about that specific learning need as possible during the time available (Figure 28-7).

Use the waiting room as a place for learning by providing up-to-date educational materials on a wide variety of health issues. Many offices have video equipment in the waiting room for patient education while the patient is waiting to be seen. These can be specific to the type of physician practice or can provide general health information.

Decide on Appropriate Teaching Materials

What teaching device would best meet the needs of your patient? A wide variety of patient education materials is available, and deciding which materials best meet your patient's needs depends on the patient's learning preference, individual characteristics, and lifestyle factors. Individualized instruction is the key to understanding and patient compliance; however, additional materials will help reinforce the information.

When possible, all patient instruction should include a handout or some type of printed material that reinforces information and can be used by the patient as a resource. Patient factors such as the use of defense mechanisms, emotional state, and language barriers can limit the patient's ability to comprehend and remember information. Printed information is needed to help the patient and the patient's family understand

Identifying Community Resources

One of the roles of the medical assistant in the ambulatory care setting is to assist patients and their families in finding and using community education and support services when needed. The healthcare facility should maintain a current file of area resources that identifies the name of the group and the services provided; the contact person; a telephone number and address; meeting times and location if applicable; and a related website if available. This information may be found in a number of different locations including the blue pages of the local phone book, through the community outreach or speakers bureau of area hospitals, or online by searching for area educational institutions at .edu sites or local chapters of national organizations at .org sites. For example, the American Cancer Society operates local branches throughout the United States and information on local services can be found on the national homepage at *http://www.cancer.org*. An excellent comprehensive Internet site operated by the U.S. National Library of Medicine and the National Institutes of Health is MedlinePlus. Both health professionals and consumers can depend on it for information that is accurate and updated frequently. The site provides a variety of information about health issues, an extensive list of diseases and conditions, a medical encyclopedia and dictionary, health information in Spanish, extensive information on prescription and nonprescription drugs, health information from the media, and links to thousands of clinical trials. It can be bookmarked at the URL: medlineplus.gov.

what is happening and what needs to be done to improve the patient's health (Figure 28-8). Informational flyers can be ordered from medical office suppliers, pharmaceutical company representatives, and health education companies. Many hospitals also offer free educational materials about diagnostic procedures, immunizations, and other disease-related topics. The ambulatory care setting where you are employed may develop its own educational materials. Some guidelines to follow if you are responsible for developing or ordering educational supplies include the following:

* Material should be written using lay language at a sixth- to eighth-grade level to promote general patient understanding.

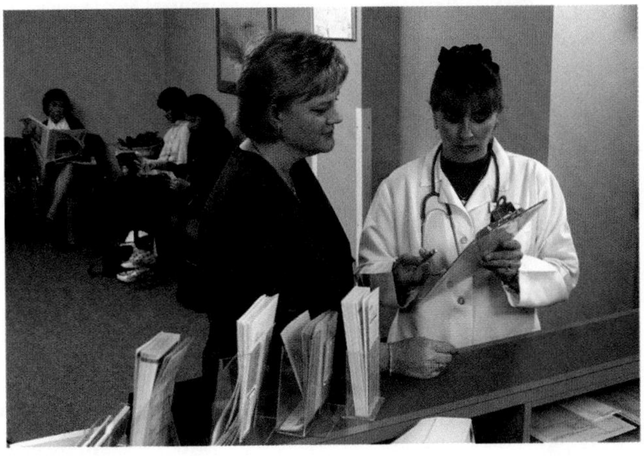

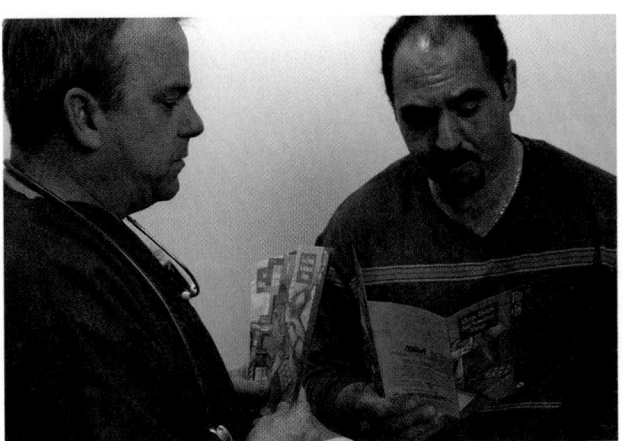

FIGURE 28-7 A teaching moment.

FIGURE 28-8 Reviewing printed information.

- Information should be well organized and clearly described.
- All material should be checked for accuracy.
- Information should be in an appealing and professional format.
- Copies should be available in other languages when possible and in large print for visually impaired clients.

Other teaching materials include videos, DVDs, and Internet sites to reinforce or expand knowledge. These learning aids promote self-directed and self-paced learning. They also permit the patient to access material in a nonstressful environment, which improves patient learning potential. Depending on the patient's age or access to the appropriate technology, using media resources or referring the patient to physician-approved healthcare sites on the Internet will help develop patient ownership of the learning process as well as provide excellent resources for patient referral. However, using the Internet as a resource for patient education information has its drawbacks. It is important that the patient understand there is no oversight or control over information posted on the Web; therefore some sites may offer information that is erroneous, out of date, or misleading. Provide patients with accurate, well-researched sites and/or be informed about what sites patients are accessing to make certain that online recommendations support the physician's treatment protocol.

Decide on Appropriate Teaching Methods

A variety of methods may be used to get the message across to your patients. One of the best ways of managing a large amount of information in a short period of time is to use community resources to reinforce the message. Your local area provides a wide range of education services for your patients to help them better understand and manage their health problems, to promote wellness, and to provide support for treatment compliance. Hospitals and many community agencies and organizations provide patient education opportunities, support groups for specific problems or diseases, and learning materials. These same groups may help the patient by providing professional consultation for many topics including diet, exercise, and emotional support. It is important that a medical assistant be aware of the various resources available in the community for patient education and referral.

Based on your evaluation of Mr. Ignatio's learning needs, what community resources would help him and his family better understand and manage his disease?

Teaching patients specific skills is also an important component of health education. The best way to teach a patient how to accurately manipulate and operate medical equipment is to use demonstration and return demonstration of the skill (Figure 28-9). Using the exact piece of equipment the patient will be using at home, the medical assistant should first demonstrate to the patient how to perform the skill, ask for questions and explain further as needed, then have the patient return the demonstration before leaving the office. This allows the medical assistant to observe the patient performing the task and correct any mistakes or clarify any misconceptions before the patient has to use the equipment at home alone.

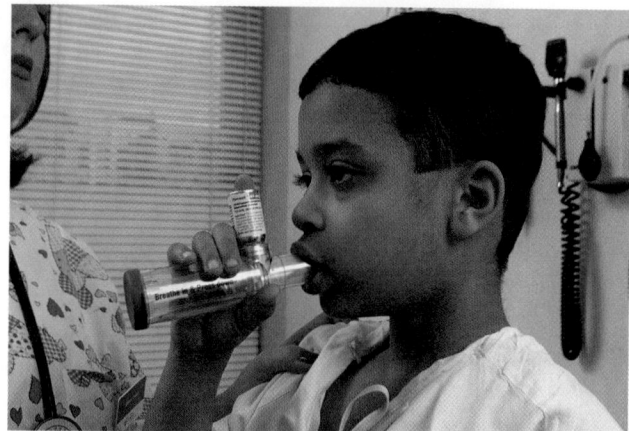

FIGURE 28-9 Demonstration and return demonstration.

For some patients an effective method for monitoring health education is to have the patient keep a journal of his or her activities and response to treatment. For example, a patient who is trying to adapt to a new diet could record daily intake to get a better idea of whether he or she is following through with dietary recommendations. In the case of Mr. Ignatio, recording blood-glucose levels from routine glucometer readings will reinforce the results of compliance with medication and diet therapies.

Another vital link to the success of patient education is family involvement. If the patient is being treated holistically, the family plays an integral role in patient wellness. Involving family members in patient education efforts provides support and understanding for the patient while managing family concerns about the patient's welfare. An educated family member can be an excellent resource for patient concerns as well as a vigilant reinforcer of healthy behaviors (Figure 28-10).

CRITICAL THINKING APPLICATION

The physician recommends that Mr. Ignatio start a 1200-calorie diabetic diet for weight reduction and blood glucose control, monitor glucometer readings three times per day, and start with three injections of insulin daily. After you consider various teaching methods, which strategies do you think would be most useful in helping Mr. Ignatio to learn about his disease and to implement the doctor's recommendations?

Implement the Teaching Plan

After you have completed the patient assessment, decided on teaching materials and methods that match your patient's characteristics and learning needs, and adapted the material and your approach for any potential barriers to learning, it is time to actually implement the plan. Conduct the lesson in a quiet area away from distractions. You must assemble any equipment the patient will need. The patient should learn to handle and practice on the same type of equipment that will be used at home so that no problem occurs in transferring the skill. Time is always an issue in the ambulatory care setting, so it is

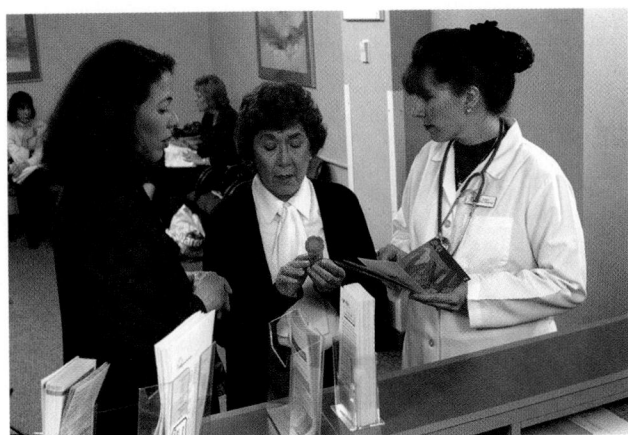

FIGURE 28-10 Family involvement in patient education.

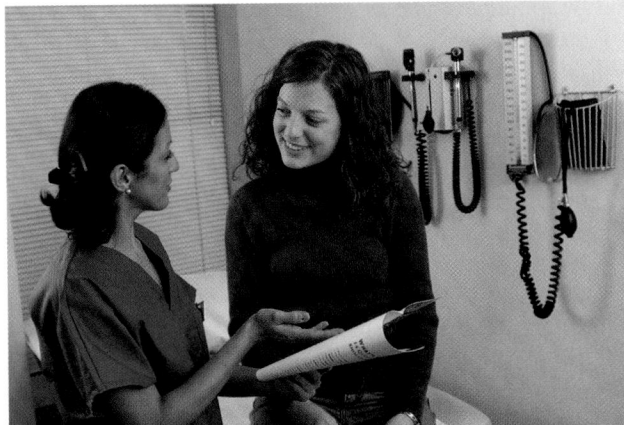

FIGURE 28-11 Patient feedback.

in the progress note about the lesson. In addition, the medical assistant must document details regarding the material covered, the patient's competency or level of skill in learning treatment techniques, and any referral to community or hospital experts or education groups.

Summary of the Teaching Plan

Conduct patient assessment
- Consider pertinent patient factors
- Identify barriers to learning
- Prioritize patient information

Determine the patient's immediate and long-term needs
- Decide on appropriate teaching materials and methods

Prepare the teaching area, and assemble necessary equipment and materials
- Use supplies and equipment the patient will use at home
- Provide positive feedback for correct display of skills

Maintain adequate pace (not too fast)

Repeatedly ask for patient feedback to confirm understanding
- Eliminate barriers to learning
- Address immediate learning needs
- Use repetition and rephrasing to promote understanding

Summarize the material learned or skill mastered at the end of each teaching interaction

Outline a plan for the next meeting

Evaluate the teaching plan
- Was there enough time to complete the lesson?
- Was the patient physically and psychologically ready for the information?
- Were the goals for the session reached?

Document the teaching intervention
- Material covered
- Patient response or level of skill performance
- Plans for next session
- Community referrals

important to present only the material or skill that is possible for the patient to master before the end of the appointment. Throughout the lesson, remember to maintain an adequate pace for learning—not too fast and not too slow—to optimize the patient's understanding.

One of the most important aspects of successful patient teaching is to consistently ask for feedback about the process (Figure 28-11). It also helps to restate, repeat, or rephrase the material to make certain patients understand the process. As patients provide correct feedback about what they are learning or demonstrate skills correctly, it is important to be positive about their progress. It also helps to summarize the material learned or the skills mastered at the end of each teaching intervention as a way of reviewing the material and clarifying important concepts.

The medical assistant should continue to evaluate the teaching plan throughout the process to make certain that the time was adequate for the patient to learn what was needed, that the patient was able to pay attention and understand the process, and that the patient understood the information needed to care for himself or herself at home. In addition, plans should be made for the material that will be covered during the patient's next visit. All of this information needs to be included

Role of the Medical Assistant as Patient Educator

- Reinforce physician instructions and information
- Encourage patients to take an active role in their health
- Use each patient interaction as an opportunity to conduct health teaching
- Keep information relevant to patient needs
- Establish and maintain patient rapport
- Communicate clearly
- Be sensitive to patient learner factors
- Modify the teaching plan as needed to best meet the needs of patients

CRITICAL THINKING APPLICATION

Taylor DiSalvo has just completed the initial patient education session with Mr. Ignatio and his wife. Taylor used demonstration–return demonstration to teach him how to properly check his blood glucose levels with the glucometer he will be using at home. He also demonstrated how to draw up and administer an insulin injection. Taylor answered Mrs. Ignatio's questions about his diet but referred the couple to the dietitian at the hospital for further diet information. Taylor plans to review the skills practiced today at Mr. Ignatio's next appointment and continue the teaching intervention with the importance of checking feet daily for any signs of infection or open areas. Accurately and completely document Taylor's initial education intervention.

CLOSING COMMENTS

Legal and Ethical Issues

Providing adequate, correct, understandable information to patients is integral to the informed consent mandate within the Patient's Bill of Rights. All patients have the right to information before they agree to receive care. An extension of this concept is the right of patients to understand their disease process and manage their health. Another consideration from the Patient's Bill of Rights is the issue of patient confidentiality as it relates to patient education. When developing and implementing the teaching plan, designing teaching interventions and strategies, and referring patients for community assistance, a medical assistant must protect the patient's confidentiality.

Essential factors in risk management for the ambulatory care setting are conducting adequate patient education and follow-up. Integral to risk management is also the importance of completely and accurately documenting each patient education intervention. The patient's chart should clearly describe the education intervention, methods and materials used, the patient's response to the intervention, the date of each session, and the individual who conducted each intervention. Each documentation entry should completely describe the material covered and the patient's feedback regarding the information so there is no doubt the patient understood the information and was able to perform any related skills properly and adequately.

Teaching interventions should demonstrate sensitivity to multicultural factors and diverse populations. Meeting the needs of all patients without evidence of prejudice is a key risk-management step.

Health Insurance Portability and Accountability Act Applications

- The patient has the right to restrict who can receive personal health information (PHI). At the first office visit the patient should complete a release-of-information form that identifies, if the patient agrees, a particular family member, close friend, or any other individual that the patient states can receive disclosures of health information.

- If someone calls the office seeking information about the patient, only the individual(s) identified on the Health Insurance Portability and Accountability Act (HIPAA) release form can be given information about the patient. Therefore, the medical assistant must first check the patient's release form to identify the individual(s) whom the patient has approved before discussing the patient's condition.

- If the physician believes it is in the best interest of the patient that family members be involved in patient health education, the medical assistant can contact the family only if the patient has given approval. This permission should be included in the patient's HIPAA information and should be documented on the medical record so that all employees can read evidence of the patient's approval.

SUMMARY OF SCENARIO

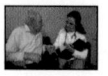

After interacting with Mr. Ignatio, Taylor realizes the significance as well as the complexity of educating patients in the ambulatory care setting. Despite the time constraints that are typical in this particular healthcare setting, patients must still learn how to manage their diseases and follow treatment guidelines. Approaching each patient as an individual learner with particular needs and characteristics is crucial to ultimate success with a teaching plan. Through the use of a holistic model and recognizing the patient's attitude toward his diagnosis from the Health Belief Model, Taylor has considered the ramifications of diabetes mellitus on Mr. Ignatio's life and has made efforts to include family and community resources in the management of the disease.

SUMMARY of LEARNING OBJECTIVES

1. Recognize the implications of models relating to health and illness on patient education.
   - The holistic model suggests patient education should consider all aspects of patient life, including physical, emotional, social, intellectual, economic, and spiritual needs. The Health Belief Model analyzes what people believe to be true about themselves and their health. The model suggests we consider how the patient perceives the risk of developing the disease and whether he or she believes that altering health behaviors will prevent the disease from occurring. Kübler-Ross' stages of grief may also help explain the patient's reaction to a particular diagnosis, especially if the disease requires a drastic change in lifestyle. Grief is an ongoing process, with patients moving through denial, anger, bargaining, depression, and finally resolution at their own pace and in their own way.

2. Illustrate at least five guidelines for patient education that can affect overall patient wellness.
   - The guidelines for patient education include providing knowledge and skills that promote recovery and health; including family in education interventions; encouraging patient ownership of the education process; promoting safe use of medications and treatments; encouraging healthy behaviors; and providing information on how to access community resources.

3. Define six patient factors that have an impact on learning.
   - Patient factors that have an impact on learning include the patient's perception of disease versus the actual state of disease; the need for information; age and developmental level; mental and emotional state; the influence of multicultural and diversity factors; individual learning style; and the impact of physical disabilities on the education process.

4. Summarize education approaches for patients with language barriers.
   - Education approaches for patients with language barriers include addressing the patient formally and courteously; using nonverbal language to promote understanding; integrating pictures or models that illustrate the material; observing the patient for understanding or confusion; using simple lay language; demonstrating procedures; implementing teaching in small, manageable steps; providing written instructions; and using an interpreter when available.

5. Determine potential barriers to patient learning.

   - Potential barriers to patient education include patient learning style; physical limitations; age and developmental level; emotional or mental state that interferes with learning; use of defense mechanisms; cultural or ethnic factors; language; the presence of pain; patient motivation to learn; and limited time for teaching.

6. Implement a variety of teaching methods and strategies that are responsive to individual patient needs.
   - Teaching materials and methods that are effective include the use of printed materials, videos, and approved Internet sites to gather information; referral to community resources and experts; demonstration and return demonstration of medical skills; patient journals of events; and involvement of family members in the education process.

7. Demonstrate the ability to develop an appropriate and effective patient-teaching plan.
   - The parts of the teaching plan include assessing learning needs; eliminating learning barriers; determining teaching priorities; using appropriate teaching materials and methods; gathering feedback repeatedly to ensure patient understanding; summarizing the material at the end of each education session; planning for the next meeting; evaluating the effectiveness of the session; and completely and accurately documenting the details of the teaching intervention.

8. Describe the role of the medical assistant in patient education.
   - The role of the medical assistant in patient education is to reinforce physician instructions and information by encouraging patients to take an active part in their health; using teaching moments effectively; keeping information relevant to the patient; establishing and maintaining patient rapport; communicating clearly; remaining aware of learning factors; being flexible with the teaching plan; and using community resources for learning and support.

9. Integrate the legal and ethical implications of patient teaching into the ambulatory care setting.
   - Appropriate patient education reflects the Patient's Bill of Rights emphasis on patient confidentiality as well as informed consent. Risk management practices related to patient education include accurate and complete documentation of patient education sessions, sensitivity to the diverse needs of the patient, and application of HIPAA practices.

CONNECTIONS

 Study Guide Connection: Go to Chapter 28 Study Guide. Read the Case Study and Workplace Applications and complete the assignments. Do online research for answers to the questions in the Internet Activities associated with patient education.

 CD Connection: Go to the Medical Assisting Competency Challenge CD and do the training activities under Patient Instruction.

Evolve Connection: For more information related to patient education, go to evolve.elsevier.com/kinn and visit related weblinks for Chapter 28. Click on the Medical Assisting Exam Review and do the practice questions to sharpen your test-taking skills.

Nutrition and Health Promotion

29

SCENARIO

Marcia Schwartz, CMA, is employed by an internal medicine practice in her hometown. She recognizes that many of the patients seen in the practice have diseases that are influenced by diet and lifestyle factors. She learned about the importance of good nutrition and wellness in her medical assisting program. In addition, Marcia has continued to attend workshops and read about current trends in nutrition, so she is prepared to provide assistance to her patients as directed by the physician.

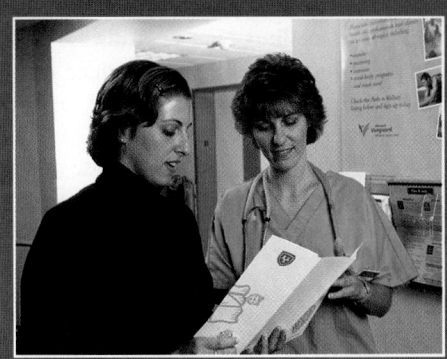

While studying this chapter, think about the following questions:

- How can Marcia help her patients understand the importance of and suggested requirements for the primary nutrients?
- What should Marcia know about dietary guidelines for fat consumption?
- What is the importance of vitamins and nutrients, and in what foods can they be found?
- How can Marcia educate patients about the Food Guide Pyramid?
- Is Marcia able to teach patients the significance of the body mass index (BMI) and how it can be calculated?
- What are the general guidelines for therapeutic nutrition?
- Is it important that Marcia be able to teach patients how to read food labels?
- What factors contribute to a healthy lifestyle?

LEARNING OBJECTIVES

1. Define, spell, and pronounce the terms listed in the vocabulary.
2. Recognize the impact of cultural influences on diet choices.
3. Analyze the relationship between poor diet and lifestyle choices and the risk of developing diet-related diseases.
4. Classify the types and functions of dietary nutrients.
5. Describe the role of carbohydrates, fats, and protein in the daily diet.
6. Explain the function of appropriate amounts of vitamins, minerals, and water in the diet.
7. Apply Food Guide Pyramid guidelines to patient dietary recommendations.
8. Implement nutritional assessment techniques.
9. Compare patient BMI calculations with the risk of diet-related disease development.
10. Demonstrate the concepts of therapeutic nutrition.
11. Interpret food labels and their application to healthy diets.
12. Summarize the causes of eating disorders and obesity and their impact on patient health.
13. Define the concepts of health promotion.
14. Understand the role of the medical assistant in nutrition and health promotion.
15. Demonstrate the nutritional labeling of food products to a patient.

National Accreditation Competencies and Content

CAAHEP COMPETENCIES

General

3.c.(3)(b). Instruct individuals according to their needs
3.c.(3)(c). Provide instruction for health maintenance and disease prevention

ABHES COMPETENCIES

Instruction

7.c. Teach patients methods of health promotion and disease prevention

VOCABULARY

amino acids Organic compounds that form the chief constituents of protein and are used by the body to build and repair tissues.

cholesterol (kuh-les'-tuh-rol) Substance produced by the liver and found in plant and animal fats that can produce fatty deposits or atherosclerotic plaques in the blood vessels.

deficiencies (di-fi'-shun-ses) Conditions caused by a below-normal intake of a particular substance.

diabetes mellitus type 1 A disease in which the beta cells in the pancreas no longer produce insulin. Patients must rely on daily insulin administration to use glucose for energy and prevent complications.

diabetes mellitus type 2 A disease in which the body is unable to use glucose for energy as a result of either a lack of insulin production in the pancreas or resistance to insulin on the cellular level.

digestion Process of converting food into chemical substances that can be used by the body.

diverticulosis (di-vuhr-ti-kyuh-lo'-suhs) Presence of pouchlike herniations through the muscular layer of the colon.

free radicals Compounds with at least one unpaired electron that makes the compound unstable and highly reactive.

hydrogenated (hi-drah'-juh-na-ted) Combined with, treated with, or exposed to hydrogen.

macular degeneration A progressive deterioration of the macula of the eye; causes loss of central vision.

obesity An excessive accumulation of body fat; defined as a body mass index (BMI) of 30 or higher.

osteoporosis (ah-ste-o-puh-ro'-ses) Loss of bone density; lack of calcium intake is a major factor in its development.

psyllium (si'-le-um) Grain that is found in some cereal products, in certain dietary supplements, and in certain bulk fiber laxatives; a water-soluble fiber.

registered dietitian (RD) Person with a minimum of a bachelor's degree in foods and nutrition who is concerned with the maintenance and promotion of health and the treatment of diseases through diet.

triglyceride (tri-gli'-suh-rid) Fatty acid and glycerol compound that combines with a protein molecule to form high- or low-density lipoprotein.

turgor Resistance of the skin to being grasped between the fingers and released; refers to normal skin tension; is decreased in dehydration and increased with edema.

vertigo Dizziness; a sensation of faintness or an inability to maintain normal balance.

Good health is a state of emotional and physical well-being that is determined, to a large extent, by diet and lifestyle factors. Health promotion and disease prevention practices focus on sound nutrition, regular exercise, avoidance of smoking and tobacco, limited alcohol intake, management of stress, and avoidance of environmental contaminants. We are what we eat, because the food we consume is used to build and repair every part of our bodies. A well-nourished person is also better able than a poorly nourished individual to ward off infections. Consequently, a poor diet and risky lifestyle behaviors are directly related to multiple health problems.

The physician, the medical assistant, and the **registered dietitian (RD)** are all closely involved in the nutritive care of a patient. The physician prescribes the diet, and ideally the dietitian instructs the patient in how to follow it. If professional aid is not available, the medical assistant may be asked to discuss the diet with the patient, answer questions, and explain certain aspects of the modifications involved. The patient may hesitate to ask the physician details about a recommended diet, or he or she may call with questions about how to implement the diet after leaving the office. Therefore, the medical assistant is frequently the one the patient turns to for answers. You should be able to answer basic questions on healthy nutrition and should have a fundamental knowledge of the diets that physicians prescribe most often.

Health Problems Related to Poor Nutrition and Lifestyle Factors

- Anemia: Low iron or folate intake
- Cancers: High-fat, low-fiber, low–complex-carbohydrate diet; high alcohol and sodium intake; sedentary lifestyle; tobacco use
- Constipation: Low fiber, inadequate fluids; high-fat diet; sedentary lifestyle
- Type 2 diabetes: High-calorie, high-fat, low–complex-carbohydrate diet; obesity; sedentary lifestyle
- Hypercholesterolemia and atherosclerosis: High-fat, low-fiber diet; high sugar and alcohol intake; tobacco use; sedentary lifestyle
- Hypertension: High-calorie, high-fat diet; high alcohol and sodium intake; tobacco use; sedentary lifestyle; obesity; stress
- Osteoporosis: Low calcium intake; inadequate vitamin D or lack of sun exposure; high alcohol intake; sedentary lifestyle; tobacco use
- Stroke: High-fat, low-fiber, low–complex-carbohydrate diet; high alcohol intake; tobacco use; stress

There are many reasons why people eat the way they do. Encouraging patients to make significant lifestyle changes regarding their diets requires sensitivity to these reasons. The choices people make about what they eat are greatly influenced by their background and relationships. Every culture, religion,

Reasons for Food Choices

- *Convenience.* What is easiest and quickest including eating out and take home meals.
- *Cost.* What you can afford.
- *Emotional comfort.* "Feel good" foods are chosen based on psychological influences.
- *Routine.* You eat what you always eat out of habit, personal preference, and availability.
- *Positive experiences.* A food is associated with a fond memory, eaten by someone you admire, or chosen because of the influence of marketing and advertising.
- *Ethnic or regional influences.* The food is what you grew up with, is associated with your cultural background, or is part of the regional diet in which you live.
- *Health and weight.* You think a particular food is good for you or will help you maintain or lose weight.

Cultural Eating Patterns

- *Asian diets* emphasize whole grains in the form of millet, rice, and noodles as well as fruits, vegetables, legumes, and nuts and seeds; fats are derived largely from vegetable oils, such as peanut or sesame oils. Dairy products are not traditionally eaten. Protein sources are typically broiled or stir-fried fish and seafood, egg whites, tofu, and nuts.
- *Latin American diets* emphasize food from plant sources, especially maize (corn) and potatoes, as well as fruits, vegetables, whole grains, beans, and nuts, at each meal. Poultry, fish, and dairy are typically consumed daily, and meats and eggs weekly.
- *Mediterranean diets* emphasize whole grains, fresh fruits and vegetables, and all types of legumes such as beans, lentils and peas daily; olive oil replaces other fats and oils; fish, poultry and eggs consumed weekly; meat monthly.
- *Mexican diets* emphasize corn or flour tortillas, cabbage, legumes, squash, tomatoes, corn, and potatoes daily. Dairy is used in the form of cheeses, but milk is not regularly consumed. Protein sources are typically fish, beef, poultry, lamb, and many types of beans.

and ethnic group has its own beliefs and practices about food. For example, according to the Hindu religion, eating beef is forbidden. Certain Jewish practices govern the types of foods that are eaten and how they are prepared. Food is also more than sustenance; it represents family and celebrations and has an entire psychologic component that we must be aware of if we are to care for each individual patient most effectively.

NUTRITION AND DIETETICS

Nutrition refers to all the processes involved in the intake and use of nutrients. *Nutrients* are the organic and inorganic chemicals in food that supply the energy and raw materials for cellular activities. Nutrients include carbohydrate, fat, protein, vitamins, minerals, and water. *Metabolism* is the process in which nutrients are used at the cellular level for growth and energy production as well as excretion of waste. Metabolism occurs in two ways. *Anabolism* is the building phase in which smaller molecules, such as **amino acids,** are combined to form larger molecules, such as proteins. An example of anabolism is the creation of *glycogen,* a stored form of glucose, created when many units of glucose combine. *Catabolism* is the breaking-down phase in which larger molecules are broken down and converted into smaller units, such as when stored glycogen is broken down into glucose molecules for energy. **Digestion** is a combination of mechanical and chemical processes occurring in the mouth, stomach, and small intestine that result in reducing nutrients into absorbable forms including amino acids, fatty acids, glycerol, and glucose. Most nutrients are absorbed in the small intestine, then carried by the bloodstream to all parts of the body.

The term *nutrition* is also used to indicate nutritional status, or the condition of the body resulting from the use of nutrients. Public interest in nutrition continues to increase owing to concerns about wellness and health promotion as well as media coverage of the topic. *Dietetics* is the practical application of nutritional science to individuals. It is the combined science and art of feeding individuals or groups, given a wide range of economic factors and/or health conditions, according to the principles of nutrition and dietary management. An RD's role is the promotion of good health through proper diet and the therapeutic use of diet in the treatment of disease.

Nutrients

To nurture life, the nutrients in food must perform one or more of three basic functions in the body: (1) provide a source of fuel or energy, (2) supply material to build and repair tissues, and (3) regulate metabolic processes. No one food supplies all the nutrients required; therefore a combination of different foods is necessary to promote health. With a little planning it is possible to supply all the body's needs from a well-balanced diet. Dietary **deficiencies** result in undernourishment or malnourishment and may lead to a variety of diseases. Good nutrition is an important part of health promotion for all individuals but especially for pregnant women, young children, and the elderly.

The role of diet in supplying energy is crucial to body functions. Every action of the body, whether voluntary or involuntary, requires energy. Even when asleep, the body still needs a source of energy to keep vital organs functioning. *Basal metabolism* is the amount of energy needed to maintain essential body functions. The *basal metabolic rate* (BMR) is the amount of energy used by a fasting, resting individual to maintain vital functions. The rate is determined by the amount of oxygen used and is defined in units of heat energy called *calories* (cal). Because this unit represents a relatively small amount of energy and because metabolism involves much larger quantities of energy, the large calorie (Cal), or kilocalorie (kcal), is commonly used. A kilocalorie is defined as the amount of heat required to raise the temperature of 1 kg of water 1° C. Of the seven food constituents (carbohydrates, proteins, fats, water, minerals, vitamins, and fiber), only carbohydrates, proteins, and fats are capable of furnishing the body with energy. The amount of energy, or kilocalories, needed by a given individual varies according to activity level, basal metabolic requirements, and the presence of disease. Most adults between 20 and 40 years of age require 1800 to 2200 kcal/day. A patient is generally said to be overweight or underweight when his or her present weight is compared with nutritional assessment standards. **Obesity** may be caused by excessive caloric intake in relation to the expenditure of calories or because of certain endocrine imbalances.

One of the ways nutrients are categorized is by whether they are a required part of the diet or whether they can be anabolized in the body. An *essential* nutrient cannot be manufactured by the body and therefore must be part of the diet or a deficiency disease will occur. Examples of essential nutrients are certain amino acids. A *nonessential* nutrient can be created within the body and so does not need to be included in the diet—for example, **cholesterol** is manufactured in the liver and vitamin D is synthesized from sun exposure.

Nutrient Components

Carbohydrates

Carbohydrates (CHO) are chemical organic compounds composed of carbon, hydrogen, and oxygen and are primarily plant products in origin. They are divided into three groups based on the complexity of their molecules: simple sugars such as table sugar, molasses, syrup, honey, candy, baked goods, and milk; complex carbohydrates (starch) including whole-grain products, cereal, pasta, rice, potatoes, legumes, fruits, vegetables, and seeds; and dietary fiber found in bran, oatmeal, whole-grain

---

How Many Terms Can Apply to Bread?

Recent government dietary guidelines recommend consumers eat more whole-grain products rather than refined white bread and wheat products. However, labels can be confusing. How do you know which is a healthy choice? Understanding the following definitions associated with grain foods will help. Review the definitions and see what you think about the healthiest grain choices.

- *Bran*—the tough fibrous covering of a grain that is the primary source of fiber in grain products
- *Enriched or fortified bread*—starting in 1942 and with legislation amended in 1996 to include folate, the U.S. government requires thiamin, riboflavin, niacin, folate, and iron be added to refined grain products because the process of creating white flour destroys these nutrients
- *Refined or white flour or bread*—a process removes the coarse parts of the grain (the fiber and nutrients); the flour is bleached to create the white color
- *Stone ground flour*—the process of grinding the grain; may include white flour
- *Unbleached flour*—similar to white flour in nutritional value and nutrient content
- *Wheat flour or brown bread*—bread made from wheat (white bread is also made of wheat) or any other type of flour that contains molasses to color the bread brown
- *Whole grain or whole wheat flour*—the entire grain kernel is ground; not refined

---

breads, beans, fruits, vegetables, seeds, and dried fruits. Each has a function in health and consists of many variations. With the exception of fiber, carbohydrates are easily digested and absorbed into the body. Simple sugars are quickly absorbed, whereas complex carbohydrates must be processed before they can be absorbed in the intestinal tract. Dietary fiber is indigestible and passes through the gastrointestinal tract unchanged.

The main function of carbohydrates is to supply fuel for energy as well as all basic cellular activities. To meet energy needs, carbohydrate is metabolized at a rate of 4 kcal/g. When digested, carbohydrate is converted into glucose, which is carried by the bloodstream to cells that need energy. A small amount of concentrated glucose is stored in the liver and muscles as glycogen. This stored glucose is available to supplement dietary supplies of carbohydrate. As with all nutrients, excess amounts of carbohydrate are converted into fat and stored in the body as *adipose* tissue. In addition to serving as the body's primary energy source, carbohydrate is also needed to regulate protein and fat metabolism. As long as there are sufficient amounts of dietary carbohydrate available to meet the energy needs of the body, protein and fat are not needed to supply energy. This *protein-sparing* effect allows protein to be used for its intended purpose—the repair and growth of tissues. Carbohydrate is used for energy with limited production of waste materials, whereas protein and fat metabolism creates by-products that are challenging for the body to process and excrete. For example, metabolizing fat for energy results in the production of ketone bodies, which can cause both an increase in the acidic content of the blood as well as potential kidney damage from the excretion of ketones. In addition, the central nervous system (CNS) requires a constant minute-to-minute supply of glucose to function properly. Neurons find it difficult to use fat or protein for energy.

Dietary fiber is commonly called *roughage*. It is defined as the portion of the plant that cannot be digested or absorbed. However, fiber's inability to be digested makes it an important dietary asset. Fiber adds bulk to the intestinal tract that stimulates peristalsis and promotes regular bowel movements. In addition, *water-soluble fiber* found in oat bran, peas, beans, certain fruits, and **psyllium** has been proven to lower blood cholesterol levels and thereby reduce the risk of heart disease. Soluble fiber combines with cholesterol in the intestine and is excreted through the bowel, thereby preventing absorption of cholesterol into the bloodstream. *Insoluble fiber,* which is found in whole grains and beans, promotes regular bowel movements, which prevents constipation and hemorrhoids; prevents **diverticulosis** by stimulating and toning the muscles lining the large intestine; and is thought to help prevent colon cancer. The dietary recommendation for daily fiber intake is 20 to 35 g/day, and 5 to 10 g of this should be soluble fiber. Table 29-1 identifies food sources of both soluble and insoluble fiber. Just keeping the skin on fruit and eating raw vegetables greatly increases the fiber content of the food.

Recommendations for Carbohydrate Consumption

- Carbohydrate intake should range from 55% to 57% of the total calories consumed each day, or 271 to 288 g/day for a 2000-calorie diet.

TABLE 29-1 Food Sources of Fiber

FOOD	SERVING SIZE	TOTAL FIBER (g)	SOLUBLE FIBER (g)	INSOLUBLE FIBER (g)
Spaghetti, cooked	1 cup	2	0.5	1.5
Whole-wheat bread	1 slice	2.5	0.5	2
White rice, cooked	$1/_2$ cup	0.5	0	0.5
Bran flake cereal	$3/_4$ cup	5.5	0.5	5
Corn flake cereal	1 cup	1	0	1
Oatmeal, cooked	$3/_4$ cup	3	1	2
Banana	1 medium	2	0.5	1.5
Apple, with skin	1 medium	3	0.5	2.5
Orange	1 medium	2	0.5	1.5
Pear, with skin	1 medium	4.5	0.5	4
Strawberries	$1/_2$ cup	1	0	1
Broccoli	$1/_2$ cup	2	0	2
Corn	$1/_2$ cup	1.5	0	1.5
Potato, baked with skin	1 medium	4	1	3
Spinach	$1/_2$ cup	2	0.5	1.5
Kidney beans	$1/_2$ cup	4.5	1	3.5
Popcorn	1 cup	1	0	1

From the American Dietetic Association: http://www.eatright.org/cps/rde/xchg/SID-5303FFEA-A120B9BE/ada/hs.xsl/nutrition_5440_ENU_HTML.htm.

- Choose fiber-rich fruits, vegetables, and whole grains as often as possible.
- Should consume 15 g of fiber for every 1000 calories eaten.
- Sugar—reduce the intake of simple sugars, especially sugar-sweetened drinks; limit snacking on sugars and starches.
- Fruits and vegetables—based on the typical 2000-calorie diet, 2 cups of fruit and $2^1/_2$ cups of vegetables daily; consume a variety of dark green, orange, and starchy vegetables and legumes.
- Whole grains—eat at least three servings (3 oz) per day by substituting whole for refined grains; at least half of the daily grain consumption should be from whole grains. One ounce is equal to one slice of bread, 1 cup of dry cereal, or $1/_2$ cup of cooked rice, pasta, or cereal.
- Milk—3 cups of fat-free or low-fat milk or milk products each day; children 2 to 8 should have 2 cups/day, and those 9 and older should have 3 cups. One cup is equal to 1 cup of yogurt, $1^1/_2$ oz of natural cheese, or 2 oz of processed cheese.

CRITICAL THINKING APPLICATION

A patient, George Hawthorne, was recently diagnosed with hypertension and hypercholesterolemia and has a family history of colon cancer. The physician recommends a high-fiber diet. Describe how Marcia could reinforce the physician's information by explaining the purpose of dietary fiber, the difference between soluble and insoluble fibers, and the types of foods he should include in his diet.

Fats

Fats are the storage form of fuel used to back up carbohydrates as an available energy source. Fat is a much more concentrated form of fuel, producing 9 kcal of energy per gram when metabolized. Dietary fats, or *lipids,* provide essential fatty acids and are needed for the absorption of the fat-soluble vitamins, A, D, E, and K. Fat gives food flavor and creates a feeling of *satiety* or satisfaction after eating. *Adipose* tissue, the stored form of fat in the body, supports and protects vital organs, insulates the body to help in the regulation of body temperature, and plays an important role in protecting nerve fibers as well as relaying nerve impulses. Lipids are also crucial to cell membrane development.

Saturated and Unsaturated Fatty Acids. When digested, fats are broken down into fatty acids and glycerol. The main building blocks of fat are *fatty acids,* which can be either saturated or unsaturated. *Unsaturated* fatty acids can take on more hydrogen under the proper conditions and therefore are less heavy and less dense. If fatty acids have one unfilled hydrogen bond, the fat is called *monounsaturated.* Olives and olive oil, peanuts and peanut oil, canola oil, pecans, and avocados contain mono-unsaturated fats. *Polyunsaturated* fats, such as safflower, corn, cottonseed, and soy oils, have two or more unfilled hydrogen bonds. Unsaturated fats are found in plants and are usually liquid at room temperature. Monounsaturated fat should be used as frequently as possible to replace saturated fat in the diet. Research on olive oil indicates it may offer some protection against heart disease and breast cancer, and canola oil is another rich source of monounsaturated fatty acids.

What Is a Trans Fat?

Trans-fatty acids are byproducts that are created when polyunsaturated oils are solidified by the addition of hydrogen. Manufacturers use this process to preserve food products because they are much more resistant to rancidity after hydrogenation. The shelf life of the processed food is increased. In addition, the product tastes better. Trans fats are found naturally in meat and dairy products, but Americans consume most of their trans fats in processed foods such as margarine, crackers, cookies, doughnuts, biscuits, chips, frozen meals, french fries, and other items containing or fried in partially hydrogenated oils. Trans fats raise bad-cholesterol levels (LDL) while lowering good-cholesterol levels in the blood. Scientific evidence indicates that saturated fat, trans fat, and dietary cholesterol combine to raise LDL levels, resulting in an increased risk of coronary heart disease (CHD). According to the National Institutes of Health (NIH), more than 12.5 million Americans have CHD, and more than 500,000 die from its complications each year. Since 1993 nutritional food labels have been required to list the amounts of saturated fat and dietary cholesterol in products. Effective January 1, 2006, manufacturers must also include trans fats on the label if the amount exceeds 0.5 g per serving. Label readers should be cautious however, because eating more than the designated serving size can drastically increase the amount of trans fats consumed.

Foods Containing Antioxidants

Vitamin C	Beta Carotene
Broccoli	Apricots
Cabbage	Broccoli
Cauliflower	Cantaloupe
Grapefruit	Carrots
Lemons	Kale and spinach
Oranges	Mustard greens
Peppers	Pumpkin
Strawberries	Sweet potatoes
Tangerines	Winter squash

Vitamin E	Mixed Antioxidants
Almonds	Cloves
Chick peas	Green tea
Oatmeal	Oregano
Soy beans	Rice
Sunflower seeds	Rosemary
Wheat germ	Sesame
	Thyme
	Wheat bran
	Wine

Benefits of Omega-3 Fatty Acids

Omega-3 fatty acids: Consume two servings of fish weekly.
- Found in large amounts in the cerebral cortex of the brain and help form the retina
- Have antiinflammatory effects including improving the immune response, protecting blood vessels such as the coronary arteries, and inhibiting the formation of blood clots
- Sources: Cold water fish including mackerel, salmon, tuna, and trout; certain oils including canola, flaxseed, soybean, wheat germ; walnuts; soybean kernels; and soy beans

The chemical structure of a *saturated* fatty acid contains all the hydrogen possible and therefore is denser, heavier, and solid at room temperature. Examples of saturated fats are those contained in dairy products, eggs, lard, meat, and **hydrogenated** fats such as margarine. Some saturated fats, such as those in soft margarines, are partially hydrogenated. These fats are usually soft at room temperature. Most saturated fats come from animal sources. The main exceptions are coconut and palm oils, which are of plant origin but are exceptionally high in saturated fat. The primary dietary factor that is associated with high blood cholesterol levels is a high intake of saturated-fat foods.

Foods High in Saturated Fat. Even a fat-free food can become one high in saturated fat depending on how it is prepared—such as a fat-free potato cooked as French fries. Therefore, we not only need to lower our intake of saturated-fat foods, but we also need to be cautious about how foods are prepared. Grill, roast, broil, bake, or microwave foods rather than frying them. Use only lean meats, and cut the visible fat off before eating.

Substitute low-fat or fat-free products when possible. Some foods high in saturated fat include:

Whole-milk dairy products	Cream
Butter	Whole-milk cheeses
Egg yolks	Salad dressing, mayonnaise
Oil-packed fish	Meat, especially red meat
Ice cream	Coconut and palm oils

A **triglyceride** molecule is created when three fatty acids attach to a molecule of glycerol. This structure is the main storage form of lipids. Triglyceride molecules are transported throughout the body via the bloodstream as lipoproteins. Dietary fats determine the saturation level of triglyceride chains. The total amount of triglycerides in the blood is used as a diagnostic tool for determining patient risk for hypertension and heart disease. It is recommended that levels do not exceed 40 to 160 mg/dL in men and 35 to 135 mg/dL in women.

Cholesterol. Cholesterol is a nonessential nutrient that plays a vital role in metabolic activities. It is synthesized only in animal tissue, so it is not found in plant foods. The primary food sources of cholesterol are egg yolks and organ meats, although all animal sources of food contain cholesterol. As a nonessential nutrient, it is also manufactured within the body, particularly in the liver.

The confusion between good and bad fat stems from the distinction between the fat in food and the fat in our bodies. The good fats in our diet are monounsaturated and polyunsaturated fats. The bad dietary fats are cholesterol, trans fats, and saturated fats. The fat in our bodies is divided into two lipoprotein categories. The good fats, or high-density lipoproteins (HDL), carry cholesterol from body tissues or the bloodstream to the liver for metabolism and excretion. The

TABLE 29-2 Recommendations for Total and Low-Density Lipoprotein Cholesterol Levels

	TOTAL CHOLESTEROL (MG/DL)			LOW-DENSITY LIPOPROTEIN (LDL) CHOLESTEROL (MG/DL)		
AGE IN YEARS	ACCEPTABLE	BORDERLINE	HIGH	ACCEPTABLE	BORDERLINE	HIGH
2 to 20	<170	170-199	>200	<110	110-129	>130
>20	<200	200-239	>240	<130	130-159	>160

bad fats, or low-density lipoprotein (LDL) and very–low-density lipoprotein (VLDL), carry cholesterol to the cells. LDL and VLDL form atherosclerotic plaques on arterial walls that frequently result in heart disease, hypertension, and strokes. However, serum LDL levels can often be successfully changed through diet. Using polyunsaturated- and monounsaturated-fat products reduces total serum cholesterol levels. In addition, using monounsaturated fats (olive, peanut, and canola oils) reduces LDL levels. Aerobic exercise is an important tool for lowering total serum cholesterol levels, increasing HDL levels, and decreasing triglycerides. The higher the serum level of HDL, the greater the protection against cardiovascular disease. The normal HDL range is 30 to 80 mg/dL. A level below 40 is considered a major risk for heart disease, whereas a value of 60 or greater is thought to protect against heart disease. Heart experts recommend an LDL level below 100 mg/dL and an HDL level of 60 mg/dL or greater (Table 29-2).

Another potential health risk from a high-fat diet is obesity. Too much fat in the diet is deposited in the body as stored adipose tissue. Currently fats make up 35% to 40% of the total calories in the American diet. Nutritionists and epidemiologists believe that decreasing dietary fat to 30%, with saturated fat and trans fat making up no more than 10% of calories, would decrease the risk of developing cancer, atherosclerosis, hypertension, and heart disease.

Recommendations for Fat Consumption
- Keep total fat intake between 20% and 35%, or at approximately 17 g of fat per day for a 2000-calorie diet.
- No more than 10% of daily calories should come from saturated and trans fats.
- Limit cholesterol to less than 300 mg/day.
- Use only lean cuts and smaller portions of meat; trim visible fat.
- Substitute poultry and fish for red meat; remove poultry skin before eating.
- Avoid adding fat to the cooking process.
- Limit intake of organ meats and egg yolks.
- With elevated serum cholesterol, limit eggs to two or three per week, or use egg substitutes or egg whites only.
- Use low-fat or fat-free milk and milk products.
- Use low-fat or fat-free products.
- Choose liquid monounsaturated oils such as canola or olive oils.

Antioxidants. Cholesterol has been high on the list of dietary villains for years and has been thought to be a serious contributor to the development of heart disease. Recent studies indicate that the problem may lie not with the cholesterol itself but with the way in which it reacts with oxygen, or the process of oxidation, in the bloodstream. The normal body process of using oxygen for energy combined with environmental factors such as pollution and tobacco smoke creates **free radicals** in the body that can lead to cellular damage. Our bodies have developed mechanisms to protect us against oxidizing free radicals through use of antioxidant vitamins C and E and beta carotene, but their amounts are not always sufficient. When enough antioxidants are circulating in the blood, cholesterol is prevented from oxidizing. Without enough, the opposite is true, and damage to arteries begins. Therefore, in addition to lowering cholesterol, saturated fat, and trans fat intake, increasing dietary intake of antioxidants may prove to be of great help in preventing cardiovascular disease. Research indicates a diet rich in antioxidant vitamins may also be linked to protection against some cancers and **macular degeneration.** Naturally occurring antioxidants are found in many fruits and vegetables and certain seasonings.

CRITICAL THINKING APPLICATION

Mr. Hawthorne is attempting to control his hypercholesterolemia with diet and exercise. What recommendations regarding fat intake can Marcia make that will help him lower his total cholesterol and LDL levels as well as raise his HDL level?

Proteins

Proteins are very large, complex molecules. They are composed of units known as *amino acids,* which are the materials that our bodies use to build and repair tissues. Twenty amino acids are

Functions of Protein

- Builds and repairs body tissue including new tissue, blood, enzymes and hormones
- Aids in the body's defense mechanisms against disease by creating antibodies
- Regulates fluid and electrolyte balance
- Provides energy when carbohydrate and fat stores are depleted

Protein Food Sources

- *Complete proteins:* Meat, fish, poultry, eggs, and dairy products
- *Incomplete proteins:* Whole grains such as barley, bulgur, cornmeal, oats, rice, whole-grain breads; cashews, sesame seeds, sunflower seeds, walnuts; soy products, dried legumes, peanuts; broccoli, dark leafy greens

Examples of Nutritionally Balanced Incomplete Protein Combinations

Combine foods from two or more incomplete amino acid sources to obtain complete protein.

- Black beans and rice
- Peanut butter sandwich on whole-grain bread
- Split-pea soup with whole-grain bread
- Lentil soup and cornbread
- Walnuts, peanuts, and rice
- Whole-wheat pasta, broccoli, and spinach
- Sunflower seeds and navy bean soup

necessary for normal growth and maintenance of tissues. Of these, eight are essential amino acids that must be included in the diet because humans do not have the enzymes necessary for their formation.

Proteins are classified according to whether they contain all essential amino acids in good proportion to one another. *Complete* proteins come from animal sources and contain a mixture of all eight essential amino acids. *Incomplete* proteins do not supply the body with all the essential amino acids. These are the vegetable proteins that must be used in specific combinations because each is missing or extremely low in one or more of the essential amino acids.

To prevent the wasting of protein for energy and to permit the creation of needed amino acid compounds dietary protein must be adequate, the diet must supply essential amino acids, and there must be enough carbohydrate and fat to prevent the burning of protein for energy. Fortunately, most foods have a mixture of proteins that supplement one another. Because little, if any, storage of amino acids occurs in the body, it is important that a source of protein be included at each meal. Adult women need approximately 45 g of protein a day, and men need approximately 55 to 60 g. The average North American diet contains twice that amount. Excess protein is metabolized and either converted to glucose, burned as fuel, or stored as fat in adipose tissue.

Recommendations for Protein Consumption

- Consume no more than 18% of daily calories from protein or approximately 91 g of protein per day for a 2000-calorie diet.
- U.S. Department of Agriculture (USDA) Food Guide recommends $5\frac{1}{2}$ to 6 oz of cooked lean meat, poultry, or fish each day.
- One ounce of meat equals one egg, $\frac{1}{4}$ cup of dry beans, 1 tablespoon of peanut butter, $\frac{1}{2}$ cup of cooked beans, or $\frac{1}{2}$ cup of tofu.

If incomplete proteins are the only source of protein in the diet, a food that is protein deficient in one amino acid should be eaten with one that is high in the same amino acid to get the needed mix of essential amino acids. Vegetarianism has become increasingly popular, and many different forms exist. Some vegetarians consume no red meats but will eat fish and poultry. Lactoovovegetarians eat primarily vegetable foods but also include eggs and/or dairy products in their diets. Lactovegetarians will consume milk and milk products in addition to vegetables but no other animal sources of food. Vegans, or strict vegetarians, consume no animal proteins at all, relying solely on vegetable foods for protein.

Those who eat some animal protein in the form of fish, eggs, and milk are generally not at risk nutritionally. However, vegans must include a variety of vegetable foods to ensure the nutritional adequacy of their diets. To supply sufficient protein, vegetables that complement each other must be eaten together to get the correct proportion of amino acids. This is customarily done in the diets of different cultures. For example, in Mexico beans are combined with rice, and in Middle Eastern countries wheat bread is combined with cheese.

Tips for vegetarians from www.mypyramid.gov include the following:

- Build meals around protein sources that are naturally low in fat, such as beans, lentils, and rice, rather than high-fat cheeses.
- Try calcium-fortified soy-based beverages in place of milk.
- Try the following vegetarian products:
  - Soy-based sausage patties or links.
  - Veggie burgers made from soybeans, vegetables, and/or rice.
- Add meat substitutes, such as tempeh (cultured soybeans with a chewy texture), tofu, or wheat gluten (seitan), to soups and stews to boost protein without adding saturated fat or cholesterol.
- Many Asian and Indian restaurants offer a varied selection of vegetarian dishes.

Vitamins (Micronutrients)

Vitamins are organic substances that occur in minute quantities in plant and animal tissues and are essential for specific metabolic processes to proceed normally. Vitamins function as catalysts and help or allow metabolic reactions to proceed. Originally they were lettered or numbered as they were discovered. However, as they have been identified chemically, they have been given more specific names. In many cases their chemical names are as well known as their letter designations.

Vitamins are divided into two groups: *fat-soluble* (A, D, E, and K) and *water-soluble* (B complex and C). Some vitamins can be manufactured in the body. Vitamin A is produced from beta-carotene food sources such as carrots, pumpkin, and sweet potatoes. Ultraviolet light from the sun initiates the production of vitamin D in the skin. Vitamin K is created from intestinal bacteria.

Functions of Vitamins

- Regulate the synthesis of bones, skin, glands, nerves, brain, and blood
- Aid in the metabolism of protein, carbohydrates, and fats
- Prevent nutritional deficiency diseases
- Provide for good health at all ages

Vitamins will not cure a disease or illness, other than one caused by the lack of that nutrient. For example, adding vitamin C to a patient's diet will not cure bleeding gums, unless the condition is specifically caused by a lack of ascorbic acid, the chemical name for vitamin C. It should also be noted that toxic symptoms from excessive ingestion of fat-soluble vitamins can occur, because they are capable of being stored in adipose tissue, compared with water-soluble vitamins, which are typically excreted in the urine. However, large intakes of some water-soluble vitamins may cause adverse effects. Table 29-3 contains complete information on vitamins. Nutrition experts agree that the greatest benefit from vitamins comes from their natural ingestion as part of the diet rather than in supplement form.

Supplements may be needed in the following cases:
- Patients exhibiting signs and symptoms of a vitamin or mineral deficiency
- Folate for women planning on becoming pregnant or in their childbearing years
- Iron and folate for pregnant and lactating women
- Calcium for lactose-intolerant individuals
- Daily vitamins for the elderly, who may have difficulty chewing or malabsorption problems or who may live alone or make poor food choices
- Postsurgical or burn patients, who require more protein and nutrients to grow and repair tissue
- Strict vegetarians, who may need B_{12}, vitamin D, iron, and zinc
- Post–gastric bypass patients, who may require multiple nutrients including B_{12}, protein, and iron

Extensive research is underway regarding the role vitamins play in disease prevention and treatment. Research indicates that antioxidant vitamins (C, E, and A) may prevent cell membrane damage that leads to cancer and heart disease. Vitamins C and E also appear to protect against the development of cataracts. Vitamin E is recommended to help prevent blood clot formation and coronary heart disease (CHD). In addition, B vitamins may help lower LDL levels, and for women planning a pregnancy, folic acid is recommended to prevent neural tube defects.

Because vitamins and dietary supplements are regulated as food and not drugs, there are no standards or regulatory mechanisms for their production. Therefore various brands differ in the amount of substance available, its quality, and its level of absorption. The U.S. Pharmacopoeia (USP), an independent organization that sets standards for drugs, recently developed standards for vitamins. It is recommended that consumers look for the USP label on products that adhere to these standards.

Minerals (Electrolytes)

Minerals are required by the human body in relatively small amounts, but even so, they are absolutely essential for life (Table 29-4). Of the 19 or more that form the mineral composition of the body, at least 13 are needed to maintain a healthy state. Minerals must be supplied by the diet or from supplements. Recommended daily intakes have been established for 12 minerals. Minerals contribute to the body's water-electrolyte balance and acid-base balance and are essential components

---

Sodium, Blood Pressure, and the DASH Diet

Research has proven that individuals with a sodium intake of over 2400 mg/day have a high risk of developing hypertension. It is estimated that adults in the United States consume on average 3300 mg of sodium per day. A healthy body excretes excess sodium through the kidneys, but sodium's attraction for fluid can cause hypertension to develop. How can you cut down on salt intake? You should avoid pickles, olives, and sauerkraut; all processed meats (lunch meat) and processed fish, but especially those that are smoked; salty snacks; fast and processed foods; canned soups; and cheese, especially processed. A recommended diet for lowering blood pressure is the Dietary Approaches to Stop Hypertension (DASH) diet. Daily guidelines for DASH include:

- Four to five servings of both fruits and vegetables
- Seven to eight servings of whole grains
- 6 oz or less of meat, fish, and poultry
- Four to five servings per week of nuts, seeds, and dry beans
- 2 to 3 cups of milk
- 2 to 3 teaspoons of oils
- 5 tablespoons of added sugar per week
- 1500 to 2000 mg of sodium per day
- Total fat should not exceed 22% of calories

---

of enzymes. Minerals also help regulate muscular and nervous activities, blood clotting, and normal heart rhythm.

2005 Food Guide recommendations for daily intake of minerals based on a 2000-calorie diet are approximately as follows:

- Potassium—4000 mg
- Sodium—1800 mg
- Calcium—1300 mg
- Magnesium—400 mg
- Copper—2 mg
- Iron—18 mg
- Phosphorous—1800 mg
- Zinc—14 mg

Minerals present in the largest amounts include sodium, potassium, calcium, chlorine, phosphorus, and magnesium. Those present in very small amounts, the trace elements, include iron, zinc, copper, selenium, chromium, manganese, iodine, and fluorine. The minerals that are needed only in trace amounts seem either to behave as part of hormone or enzyme systems or to work with vitamins in various metabolic reactions throughout the body. For example, iodine is part of the thyroid hormone thyroxine, and another hormone, insulin, has zinc as part of its structure. Cobalt, on the other hand, is an essential part of vitamin B_{12}.

Calcium, iodine, and iron are the minerals most frequently missing in the American diet. Some of the leading causes of disease-related mineral deficiencies include **osteoporosis** from lack of vitamin D and/or calcium as well as iron-deficiency anemia. Meanwhile, high sodium levels are associated with hypertension.

TABLE 29-3 Vitamin Facts

VITAMIN	U.S. RDA*	BEST SOURCES	FUNCTIONS	DEFICIENCY SYMPTOMS†	TOXIC?	PROCESSING TIPS	DID YOU KNOW?
A (carotene)	5000 IU/day	Yellow or orange fruits and vegetables, green leafy vegetables, fortified oatmeal, liver, dairy products	Formation and maintenance of skin, hair, and mucous membranes; helps us see in dim light; bone and tooth growth.	Night blindness, dry and scaly skin, frequent fatigue	Yes, in high doses, but beta-carotene is nontoxic	Serve fruits and vegetables raw and keep covered and refrigerated; steam vegetables; broil, bake, or braise meats.	Low-fat and skim milks are often fortified with vitamin A, which is removed with the fat.
B₁ (thiamine)	1.5 mg/day	Fortified cereals and oatmeals, meats, rice and pasta, whole grains, liver	Helps body release energy from carbohydrates during metabolism; growth and muscle tone.	Heart irregularity, fatigue, nerve disorders, mental confusion	No, high doses are excreted by the kidneys	Do not rinse rice or pasta before and after cooking. Cook in minimal water.	Pasta and breads made of refined flours have B₁ added because it is lost in the milling process.
B₂ (riboflavin)	1.7 mg/day	Whole grains, green leafy vegetables, organ meats, milk and eggs	Helps body release energy from protein, fat, and carbohydrates during metabolism.	Cracks in corners of mouth, rash, anemia	No toxic effects reported	Store food in containers that light cannot enter; cook vegetables in minimal water; roast or broil meats.	Most ready-to-eat cereals are fortified with 25% of the U.S. RDA for B₂.
B₆ (pyridoxine)	2 mg/day	Fish, poultry, lean meats, bananas, prunes, dried beans, whole grains, avocados	Helps build body tissue and aids in metabolism of protein.	Convulsions, dermatitis, muscular weakness, skin cracks, anemia	Long-term megadoses may cause nerve damage in hands and feet.	Serve fruits raw or cook for shortest time in little water; roast or broil meats.	Because B₆ aids in use of protein in the body, the need for B₆ increases with protein intake.
B₁₂ (cobalamin)	6 µg/day	Meats, milk products, seafood	Aids cell development, functioning of the nervous system, and the metabolism of protein and fat.	Anemia, nervousness, fatigue, and, in some cases, neuritis and brain degeneration	No toxic effects reported	Roast or broil meat and fish.	Vegetarians who do not eat any animal products may need a supplement.
Biotin	0.3 mg/day	Cereal/grain products, yeast, legumes, liver	Involved in metabolism of protein, fats, and carbohydrates.	Nausea, vomiting, depression, hair loss, dry, scaly skin	No toxic effects reported	Storage, processing, and cooking do not appear to affect this vitamin.	Biotin deficiency is extremely rare in the United States.
Folate (folacin, folic acid)	0.4 mg/day	Green leafy vegetables, organ meats, dried peas, beans, and lentils	Aids in genetic material development and involved in red blood cell production.	Gastrointestinal disorders, anemia, cracks on lips	Some evidence of toxicity in large doses	Store vegetables in refrigerator and steam, boil, or simmer in minimal water.	Deficiencies can occur in premature infants and pregnant women.
Niacin	20 mg/day	Meat, poultry, fish, enriched cereals, peanuts, potatoes, dairy products, eggs	Involved in carbohydrate, protein, and fat metabolism.	Skin disorders, diarrhea, indigestion, general fatigue	Nicotinic acid form should be taken only under physician's care	Roast or broil beef, veal, lamb, and poultry. Cook potatoes in minimal water.	Niacin is formed in the body by converting an amino acid found in proteins.

Vitamin	RDA	Sources	Functions	Deficiency Symptoms	Toxicity	Tips	Notes
Pantothenic acid	10 mg/day	Lean meats, whole grains, legumes, vegetables, fruits	Helps in the release of energy from fats and carbohydrates.	Fatigue, vomiting, stomach stress, infections, muscle cramps	No toxic effects reported	Eat fruits and vegetables raw.	It is believed some pantothenic acid is produced in the gastrointestinal tract.
C (ascorbic acid)	60 mg/day	Citrus fruits, berries, and vegetables—especially peppers	Essential for structure of bones, cartilage, muscle, and blood vessels; also helps maintain capillaries and gums and aids in absorption of iron.	Swollen or bleeding gums, slow wound healing, fatigue/depression, poor digestion	Intakes of 1 g or more can cause nausea, cramps, and diarrhea.	Do not store or soak fruits and vegetables in water; refrigerate juices and store only 2 to 3 days.	Smokers may benefit from an increased intake of vitamin C.
D	400 IU/day	Fortified milk, sunlight, fish, eggs, butter, fortified margarine	Aids in bone and tooth formation; helps maintain heart action and nervous system.	In children: rickets and other bone deformities. In adults: calcium loss from bones.	High intakes may cause diarrhea and weight loss.	Storage, processing, and cooking do not appear to affect this vitamin.	Sunlight starts vitamin D production in the skin.
E	30 IU/day	Fortified and multigrain cereals, nuts, wheat germ, vegetable oils, green leafy vegetables	Protects blood cells, body tissue, and essential fatty acids from harmful destruction in the body.	Muscular wasting, nerve damage, anemia, reproductive failure	Relatively nontoxic.	Store in air-tight containers away from light.	Most fortified cereals have 40% of the RDA.
K	‡	Green leafy vegetables, fruit, dairy and grain products	Essential for blood clotting functions.	Bleeding disorders in newborns and those on blood-thinning medications	Not toxic as found in food.	Store in containers away from light.	Vitamin K is also formed by bacteria in the colon.

IU, International units; *mg*, milligrams; *µg*, micrograms.

*For adults and children older than 4.

†There is no U.S. RDA for vitamin K; however, the Recommended Dietary Allowance is 1 µg/kg of body weight.

‡Many of the symptoms outlined under this heading can also be attributed to problems other than vitamin deficiency. If you have these symptoms and they persist, consult your physician.

Information for this chart was obtained from the Food and Drug Administration, the American Institute for Cancer Research, and the United States Department of Agriculture/Human Nutrition Information Service. Vitamins A, D, E, and K are fat soluble; the other vitamins in this table are water soluble.

TABLE 29-4 Minerals

FUNCTIONS	SOURCES	DEFICIENCY SYMPTOMS	TOXICITY SYMPTOMS
Mineral and Elemental Symbol: Calcium (Ca^{2+})			
Helps muscles to contract and relax, thereby helping to regulate heartbeat Plays a role in the normal functioning of the nervous system Aids in blood coagulation and the functioning of some enzymes Helps build strong bones and teeth May help prevent hypertension	Primarily found in milk and milk products; also found in dark green, leafy vegetables, tofu and other soy products, sardines, salmon with bones, and hard water	Poor bone growth and tooth development, leading to stunted growth and increased risk of dental caries, rickets (bowing of legs) in children, osteomalacia (soft bones) and osteoporosis (brittle bones) in adults, poor blood clotting, and possible hypertension	Kidney stones
Mineral and Elemental Symbol: Chloride (Cl^-)			
Involved in the maintenance of fluid and acid-base balance Provides an acid medium, in the form of hydrochloric acid, for activation of gastric enzymes	Major source is table salt (sodium chloride); also found in fish and vegetables	Disturbances in acid-base balance, with possible growth retardation, psychomotor defects, and memory loss	Disturbances in acid-base balance
Mineral and Elemental Symbol: Magnesium (Mg^{2+})			
Helps build strong bones and teeth Activates many enzymes Participates in protein synthesis and lipid metabolism Helps regulate heartbeat	Raw, dark green vegetables, nuts and soybeans, whole grains and wheat bran, bananas and apricots, seafood and coffee, tea, cocoa, and hard water	Rare but in disease states may lead to central nervous system problems (confusion, apathy, hallucinations, poor memory) and neuromuscular problems (muscle weakness, cramps, tremor, cardiac arrhythmia)	Drowsiness, weakness, and lethargy and in severe toxicity skeletal paralysis, central nervous system depression, respiratory depression, and ultimately coma and death
Mineral and Elemental Symbol: Phosphorus (PO_4)			
Helps build strong bones and teeth Present in the nuclei of all cells Helps in the oxidation of fats and carbohydrates (energy metabolism) Aids in maintaining the body's acid-base balance	Milk and milk products, eggs, meats, legumes, whole grains, soft drinks (used to make the "fizz")	Rare but with malabsorption can cause anorexia, weakness, stiff joints, and fragile bones	Hypocalcemic tetany (muscle spasms)
Mineral and Elemental Symbol: Potassium (K^+)			
Plays a key role in fluid and acid-base balance Transmits nerve impulses, helps control muscle contractions, and promotes regular hearbeat Needed for enzyme reactions	Apricots, bananas, oranges, grapefruit, raisins, green beans, broccoli, carrots, greens, potatoes, meats, milk and milk products, peanut butter and legumes, molasses, coffee, tea, cocoa	May cause impaired growth, hypertension, bone fragility, central nervous system changes, renal hypertrophy, diminished heart rate, and death	Hyperkalemia (excess potassium in the blood) with cardiac function disturbances
Mineral and Elemental Symbol: Sodium (Na^+)			
Plays a key role in the maintenance of acid-base balance Transmits nerve impulses and helps control muscle contractions Regulates cell membrane permeability	Salt (sodium chloride) is the major dietary source; minor sources occur naturally in foods such as milk and milk products and several vegetables	Hyponatremia (too little sodium in the blood)	May cause hypertension, which can lead to cardiovascular diseases and renal (kidney) disease; in the form of salt tablets, can cause gastric irritation
Mineral and Elemental Symbol: Chromium (Cr^{3+})			
Activates several enzymes Enhances the removal of glucose from the blood	Liver and other meats, whole grains, cheese, legumes, and brewer's yeast	Weight loss, abnormalities of the central nervous system, and possible aggravation of diabetes mellitus	Inhibited insulin activity

TABLE 29-4 Minerals—*cont'd*

FUNCTIONS	SOURCES	DEFICIENCY SYMPTOMS	TOXICITY SYMPTOMS
Mineral and Elemental Symbol: Copper (Cu²⁺)			
Aids in the production and survival of red blood cells Parts of many enzymes involved in respiration Plays a role in normal lipid metabolism	Shellfish—especially oysters—liver, nuts and seeds, raisins, whole grains, and chocolate	Anemia, central nervous system problems, abnormal electrocardiograms, bone fragility, impaired immune response; may be a factor in failure to thrive in premature infants	In Wilson's disease and Huntington's chorea (both hereditary diseases), copper accumulation causes neuron and liver cell damage
Mineral and Elemental Symbol: Fluorine (F⁻)			
Helps the formation of solid bones and teeth, thereby reducing incidence of dental caries, and may help prevent osteoporosis	Fluoridated water (and foods cooked in fluoridated water), fish, tea, gelatin	Increased susceptibility to dental caries	Fluorosis and mottling of teeth
Mineral and Elemental Symbol: Iodine (I⁻)			
Helps regulate energy metabolism through being part of thyroid hormones Essential for normal cell functioning, helps to keep skin, hair, and nails healthy	Primarily from iodized salt, also found in saltwater fish, seaweed products, vegetables grown in iodine-rich soils	Goiter, cretinism in infants born to iodine-deficient mothers, with accompanying mental retardation and diffuse central nervous system abnormalities	Little toxic effect in individuals with normal thyroid gland functioning
Mineral and Elemental Symbol: Iron (Fe³⁺)			
Essential to the formation of hemoglobin, which is important for tissue respiration and ultimately growth and development Part of several enzymes and proteins in the body	Heme sources: organ meats—especially liver, red meats, and other meats Nonheme sources: iron-fortified cereals, dark green leafy vegetables, legumes, whole grains, blackstrap molasses, dried fruit, and foods cooked in iron pans	Iron-deficiency anemia and possible alterations that impair behavior	Idiopathic hemochromatosis, which can lead to cirrhosis, diabetes mellitus, skin pigmentation, arthralgias (joint pain), and cardiomyopathy
Mineral and Elemental Symbol: Manganese (Mn²⁺)			
Needed for normal bone structure, reproduction, normal functioning of cells and the central nervous system A component of some enzymes	Nuts, whole grains, vegetables and fruits, coffee, tea, cocoa, and egg yolks	None observed in humans	Iron-deficiency anemia through inhibiting effect on iron absorption; pulmonary changes, anorexia, apathy, impotence, headaches, leg cramps, and speech impairment; in advanced stages of toxicity resembles Parkinson's disease
Mineral and Elemental Symbol: Selenium (Se)			
Part of an enzyme system Acts as an antioxidant with vitamin E to protect the cell from oxygen	Protein-rich foods (meat, eggs; milk), whole grains, seafood, liver and other meats, egg yolks, and garlic	Keshan disease (a human cardiomyopathy) and Kashin-Bek disease (an endemic human osteoarthropathy)	Physical defects of the fingernails and toenails and hair loss
Mineral and Elemental Symbol: Zinc (Zn²⁺)			
Plays a role in protein synthesis Essential for normal growth and sexual development, wound healing, immune function, cell division and differentiation, and smell acuity	Whole grains, wheat germ, crabmeat, oyster, liver and other meats, brewer's yeast	Depressed immune function, poor growth, dwarfism, impaired skeletal growth and delayed sexual maturation, acrodermatitis	Severe anemia, nausea, vomiting, abdominal cramps, diarrhea, fever, hypocupremia (low blood serum copper), malaise, fatigue

From Poleman CM, Peckenpaugh NJ: *Nutrition essentials and diet therapy*, ed 6, Philadelphia, WB Saunders, 1991, pp 128-129. Data from Garrison RH, Somer E: *The nutrition desk reference*, New Canaan, Conn, Keats Publishing, 1985; and Griffeth HW: *Complete guide to vitamins, minerals and supplements*, Tucson, Fisher Books, 1988.

Functions of Water

- Plays a key role in the maintenance of body temperature
- Acts as a solvent and the medium for most biochemical reactions
- Acts as the vehicle for transport of substances such as nutrients, hormones, antibodies, and metabolic waste
- Acts as a lubricant for joints and mucous membranes

Water

Water is all too often overlooked when nutritional status is evaluated. The body is approximately 80% water and can survive longer without food than it can without water. Water is part of almost every vital body process.

Water is lost daily from the body in urine, feces, sweat, and expiration. Extensive water losses from diarrhea, vomiting, burns, or perspiration can lead to electrolyte losses that result in life-threatening imbalances. Water is contained in almost all foods; however, a healthy diet should include about eight glasses of water a day.

THE FOOD GUIDE PYRAMID

In 1992, to reflect the new dietary guidelines that called for more consumption of grains and less consumption of meat, sweets, and fats, the Food Guide Pyramid was introduced by the USDA. In 2005 the Pyramid was revised by flipping it on its side and depicting an individual climbing stairs next to the pyramid. For the first time, dietary recommendations recognize the importance of exercise in maintaining a healthy weight; the narrowing of each food group up the pyramid represents the importance of choosing more foods with limited added sugars and fats; the potential exists for multiple guidelines based on age and activity level, which provides an individualized approach to choosing foods that best fit individual characteristics and lifestyles; the widths of the food groups represent how much should be consumed from each food group daily; and the emphasis is on the importance of choosing a variety of nutritious foods each day. Students should refer to the USDA website www.mypyramid.gov to investigate the many learning opportunities available to enhance understanding of the new guidelines. Figure 29-1 represents the 2005 Food Guide Pyramid.

Explaining this food pyramid to patients will encourage healthful eating habits. Many patients have never been educated in nutrition and do not know how to plan a healthy diet for themselves or their families. Good nutrition is a balance between carbohydrates, protein, vitamins, minerals, fiber, and water, with limited amounts of fat, sodium, sugar, and alcohol. Calorie intake must be balanced with energy output in order to maintain a healthy body weight.

NUTRITIONAL STATUS ASSESSMENT

During the physician's examination of the patient, he or she will assess the patient's nutritional status. The physician considers the patient's age; height and weight; body mass index (BMI) level; overall health status; any recent changes in weight; diet and exercise habits; and lifestyle, culture, and educational background. In addition to this information, the physician may check the patient's skin **turgor** to determine the level of hydration and perform various techniques to assess the percentage of body fat.

Body Fat Measurement

The location of body fat may be related to increased risk of developing diabetes, stroke, hypertension, and coronary artery disease. Studies indicate that the body has two different places to store fat: at the hips and in the abdomen. Fat at the hips is more common in women and is used to store energy for special purposes, such as during pregnancy and breastfeeding. Abdominal fat, or central obesity, seems to be more dangerous to overall health. Health risks related to weight vary in an increasing amount from no increased risk with normal weight to severe risk from central obesity, with the risk from other types of obesity falling somewhere in between. To determine the patient's status, the waist and hips of the patient are measured and correlated with the waist-to-hip ratio (the bigger the belly, the higher the ratio). Normal ratios are less than 0.75 in women and are 0.9 to 0.95 in men. Waist measurements can also predict the risk of developing a weight-related disease. Using a nonelastic measuring tape, measure your waist at the level of the umbilicus. Men at increased risk for disease have waist measurements greater than 40 inches (102 cm) and women greater than 35 inches (88 cm).

At the physician's request the medical assistant may perform body fat measurements on a patient. The percentage of body fat may be an indicator of overall health as well as risk for cardiovascular disease. Body fat can be measured by several methods. A reliable method of measuring body fat uses a specially designed caliper to measure the thickness of a fold of tissue in three areas: the triceps, the subscapular, and the suprailiac regions (Figure 29-2, p. 583). However, an increasing number of patients have fat folds that are too large for calipers to measure. The physician may also order a dual energy x-ray absorptiometry (DEXA) scan that uses two x-ray beams to give accurate feedback on body fat percentage, where the fat is distributed, and bone density.

Body Mass Index

To determine how healthy the patient's weight level is, the physician may want you to calculate the patient's BMI. The BMI is the relationship of weight to height, and it mathematically correlates the patient's measurements with health risks. It is a more accurate predictor of weight-related diseases than traditional height/weight charts because it provides a good estimate of the degree of body fat. There are two methods for determining a patient's BMI. The nomogram in Figure 29-3 (p. 585) can be implemented using the patient's weight in kilograms or pounds and the height in centimeters or inches. To practice using the nomogram, angle the edge of a piece of paper or a ruler from your weight (on the left) to your height (on the right). Then read the BMI where the edge crosses the centerline. The BMI can also be calculated mathematically by dividing the

Anatomy of MyPyramid

One size doesn't fit all

USDA's new MyPyramid symbolizes a personalized approach to healthy eating and physical activity. The symbol has been designed to be simple. It has been developed to remind consumers to make healthy food choices and to be active every day. The different parts of the symbol are described below.

Activity

Activity is represented by the steps and the person climbing them, as a reminder of the importance of daily physical activity.

Moderation

Moderation is represented by the narrowing of each food group from bottom to top. The wider base stands for foods with little or no solid fats or added sugars. These should be selected more often. The narrower top area stands for foods containing more added sugars and solid fats. The more active you are, the more of these foods can fit into your diet.

Personalization

Personalization is shown by the person on the steps, the slogan, and the URL. Find the kinds and amounts of food to eat each day at MyPyramid.gov.

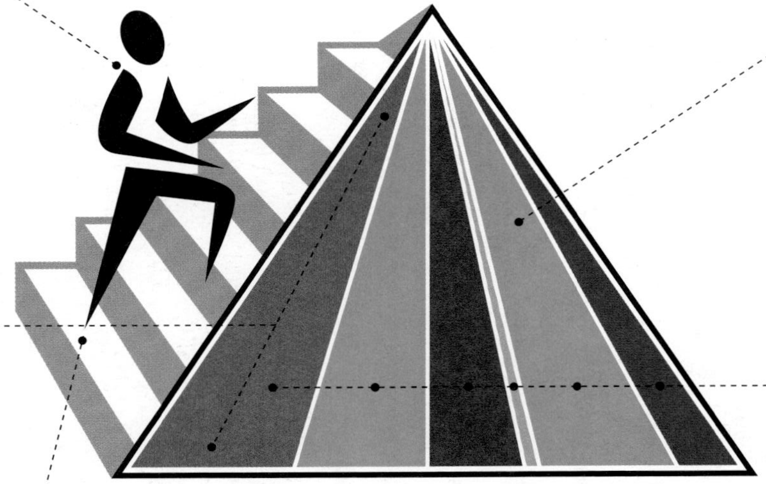

Proportionality

Proportionality is shown by the different widths of the food group bands. The widths suggest how much food a person should choose from each group. The widths are just a general guide, not exact proportions. Check the Web site for how much is right for you.

Variety

Variety is symbolized by the 6 color bands representing the 5 food groups of the Pyramid and oils. This illustrates that foods from all groups are needed each day for good health.

Gradual Improvement

Gradual improvement is encouraged by the slogan. It suggests that individuals can benefit from taking small steps to improve their diet and lifestyle each day.

MyPyramid.gov
STEPS TO A HEALTHIER YOU

GRAINS   VEGETABLES   FRUITS   OILS   MILK   MEAT & BEANS

USDA U.S. Department of Agriculture
Center for Nutrition Policy
and Promotion
April 2005 CNPP-16

USDA is an equal opportunity provider and employer.

FIGURE 29-1 Food Guide Pyramid. (From U.S. Department of Agriculture, www.mypyramid.gov.)

Highlights of the 2005 USDA Dietary Recommendations

Adequate Nutrients within Caloric Needs

Consume a variety of nutrient-dense foods while limiting saturated and trans fats, cholesterol, added sugars and salts, and alcohol.

Meet dietary recommendations by adopting a balanced eating pattern.

Most Americans need to increase consumption of vitamin E, calcium, potassium, and fiber.

Childbearing women should increase the intake of iron-rich and folic acid foods or take supplements.

Those over 50 should consume B_{12}-fortified foods.

Aging individuals, those with dark skin, and people not exposed to sunlight should eat fortified vitamin D foods or take a supplement.

Weight Management

Balance the intake of calories with those expended.

With aging, calories should be decreased and physical activity increased to prevent gradual weight gain over time.

Those who need to lose weight should do so slowly.

Reducing intake by 50 to 100 calories per day will prevent weight gain, reduction by 500 calories per day will promote weight loss. Control portion sizes; reduce the intake of saturated fats, added sugars, and alcohol.

Carbohydrates

Choose fiber-rich fruits, vegetables, and whole grains.

Limit the use of added sugar and sweeteners.

Practice good dental hygiene, and limit sugary snacks to reduce dental caries.

Sodium and Potassium.

Consume less than 2300 mg of sodium per day (approximately 1 teaspoon of salt).

Consume potassium-rich foods.

Alcoholic Beverages

Moderate consumption—one drink per day for women, and two for men.

Avoid alcohol if you are or may become pregnant or if lactating.

Food Safety

Clean all fruits, vegetables, and cooking surfaces.

Keep raw, cooked, and ready-to-eat foods separate.

Cook foods to the recommended temperature to kill microbes.

Chill perishable foods, and defrost foods properly.

Avoid unpasteurized milk products, raw eggs, and raw or undercooked meats.

Physical Activity

Engage in 30 to 60 minutes of moderate physical activity per day to prevent weight gain and 60 to 90 minutes for weight loss.

Children and adolescents should be physically active 60 minutes per day.

Aging people should participate in regular exercise to maintain function.

Include aerobic activity, stretching, and weight training.

Food Groups to Encourage

Consume 2 C fruit and $2\frac{1}{2}$ C vegetables per day for a 2000-calorie diet.

Eat dark green and orange vegetables, legumes, and starches several times per week.

At least half of the grains consumed should be whole grains.

Consume 3 C fat-free or low-fat milk or milk products; children 2 to 8 years should consume 2 C/day.

Fats

Less than 10% of calories should come from saturated fats, and less than 300 mg of cholesterol should be consumed each day; keep trans fats as low as possible.

Consume less than 35% of calories from fat.

Choose low-fat or fat-free milk products and lean meats.

---

weight in kilograms by the square of the height in meters (BMI = weight [kg] ÷ height [m²]). However, most physician's offices will either have a wheel device that the medical assistant can use to determine the patient's BMI or have a BMI chart available (Table 29-5, p. 585) for reference. The majority of physicians require the medical assistant to record the patient's BMI after the height and weight are measured because decisions related to patient health status will be based on the patient's BMI level. Table 29-6 (p. 585) correlates BMI rates with risks for disease.

Individuals with BMIs between 19 and 22 are thought to live the longest. Death rates are significantly higher for people with indexes of 25 and above. If the risk is anything other than acceptable, it may indicate a need for dietary modifications. This will have to be decided by the physician when all of the information on the patient is evaluated.

CRITICAL THINKING APPLICATION

The physician encourages Mr. Hawthorne to lose weight to lower his at-risk BMI index of 29. Explain how Marcia should teach Mr. Hawthorne about the importance of his BMI, how it is measured, and how he can calculate his index at home.

THERAPEUTIC NUTRITION

Although a majority of patients are treated medically without the use of a therapeutic diet, some illnesses and diseases can be cured and some patients' recovery can be facilitated by the use of special diets. For example, patients with hypertension, hypercholesterolemia, certain gastrointestinal diseases, and

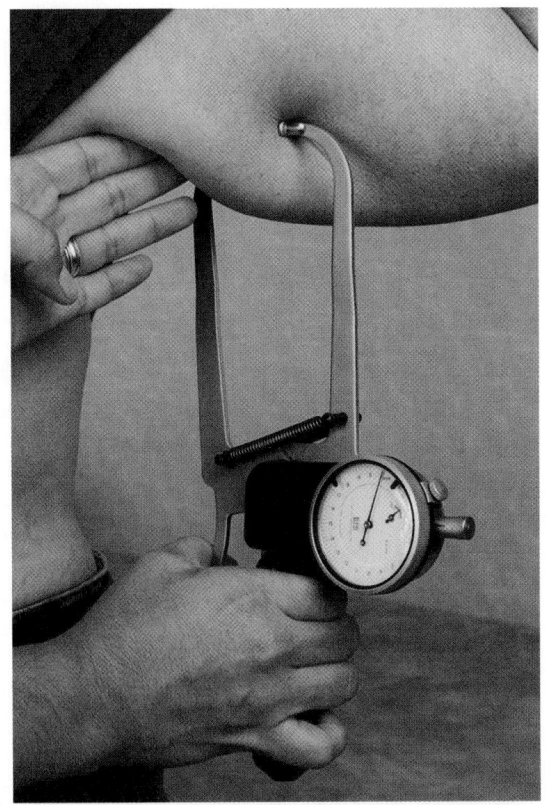

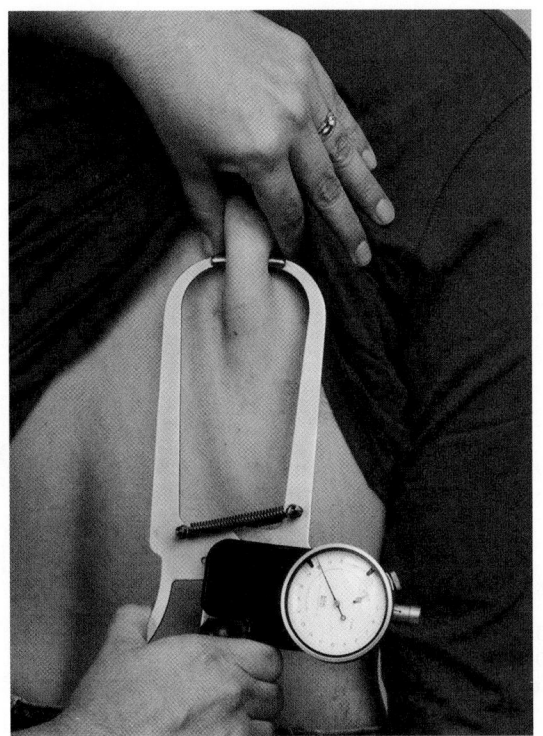

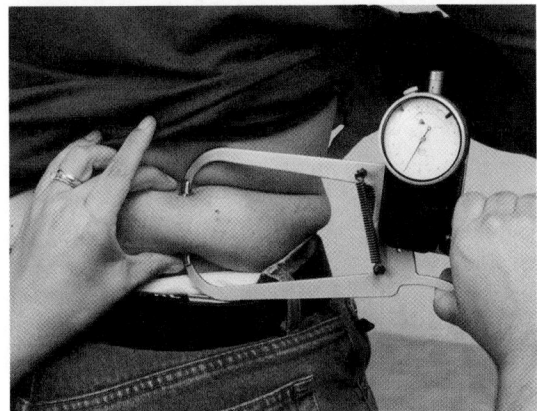

FIGURE 29-2 Determining fat-fold measurements. **A,** Triceps. **B,** Subscapular. **C,** Suprailiac.

diabetes mellitus types 1 and 2 all benefit from a therapeutically planned diet. It is important to take into consideration the patient's lifestyle, cultural influences, and background to ensure cooperation.

Modifying a Diet

The normal diet can be modified with regard to the following features (or combination thereof) to create a therapeutic diet:

- Consistency
- Calorie level
- Amounts of one or more nutrients
- Degree of bulk or fiber
- Spiciness
- Levels of specific foods

In general the normal diet is modified by either restricting or increasing the foods that are sources of the nutrient involved in the disease process. Except for the nutrient in question, the recommended daily allowances can usually be met. However, if several restrictions are ordered for the same patient, a nutrient supplement may be necessary.

Liquid Diet

Two types of liquid diets are used. A clear liquid diet includes only broth soups, tea, and gelatin. In some cases, apple juice and cranberry juice may be allowed. A full liquid diet includes all foods allowed on a clear liquid diet plus milk, custards, strained cream soups, refined cereals, eggnog, milkshakes, and all juices. This diet may be indicated as part of preparation for certain

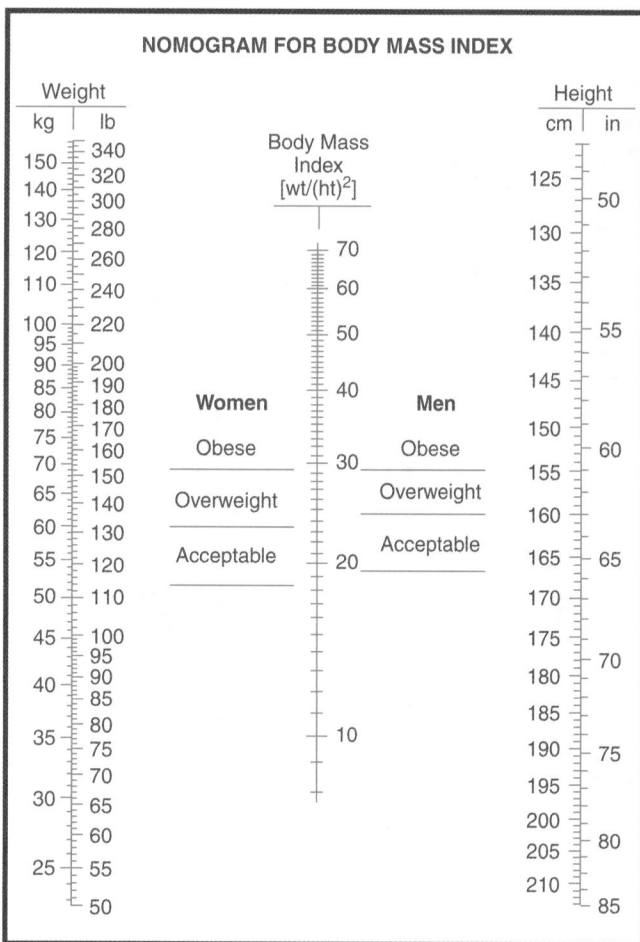

FIGURE 29-3 Nomogram for body mass index.

diagnostic tests (such as a colonoscopy) or for the first several days after major surgery.

Soft or Light Diet

When a soft or light diet is prescribed, foods with roughage are eliminated (no raw fruits or vegetables). No strongly flavored or gas-forming vegetables are allowed (onions, beans, broccoli, and cauliflower), and spices may also be limited. Often this diet is used after surgery to place less strain on the gastrointestinal system or for patients with certain gastrointestinal disorders.

Mechanical Soft Diet

A mechanical soft diet is a regular diet in which the food is chopped, ground, or pureed, depending on the degree of texture change required. No foods or spices are restricted. This diet may be used after dental or oral surgery or for patients who have difficulty chewing or swallowing.

Bland Diet

A bland diet restricts the dietary components that are classified as gastrointestinal irritants. Such a diet limits any foods that are chemically irritating (e.g., caffeine, pepper, chili, nutmeg, and alcohol) or mechanically irritating (e.g., high-fiber foods).

No fried foods or highly concentrated sweets are allowed. Gas-forming vegetables belonging to the onion and cabbage family are also eliminated. A bland diet is commonly used for problems occurring in the gastrointestinal tract. Such a diet should supply sufficient nutrients for the individual to meet the recommended daily allowances, unless fruits and vegetables are eliminated.

Elimination Diet

Diets that modify the levels of specific foods are most frequently used to treat allergies of various kinds. There are two basic elimination regimens. A simple elimination diet removes only one or two foods that are suspected of causing the allergy. The Rowe elimination diet involves a more extensive program. With this method the basic diet consists of a few hypoallergenic foods such as rice cereal, apples, pears, carrots, sweet potatoes, lamb, and milk substitutes. If no allergic reaction is observed, single food-family groups are added slowly in periods of about 10 days while the child is observed for the onset of allergic symptoms. In children the most common allergies are to chocolate, wheat, eggs, and milk. In some cases it may be difficult to meet the recommended daily allowances for all nutrients. When this situation occurs, supplements should be ordered.

High- or Low-Fiber Diet

The amount of bulk or fiber in the diet is either increased or decreased, depending on the specific disorder of the colon or large bowel. In either case foods high in cellulose are considered to be high in fiber, because the body does not digest this carbohydrate well and a residue is left in the colon. In some instances a low-residue diet is distinguished from a low-fiber diet. In this case a low-fiber diet eliminates those foods with a high cellulose content, and a low-residue diet restricts milk, in addition to fiber content. Either diet should supply all the nutrients needed; however, if milk is restricted drastically, the calcium level must be watched carefully. Low-fiber diets are prescribed for patients with certain gastrointestinal disorders such as diverticulitis. High-fiber diets are recommended for patients with hypercholesterolemia or diabetes mellitus and to prevent certain forms of cancer.

Diabetic Diet

The specific diet for a diabetic patient is determined by the individual's health needs. The basic goal of managing the disease is to maintain consistent control of blood-glucose levels. When developing a diabetic diet plan, the physician or RD must consider additional factors such as weight control methods, individual patient preferences, exercise patterns, and lifestyle factors. General guidelines for a healthy diabetic diet include the following:

- Five servings of dark-colored fruits and vegetables and six of whole grains each day
- Two weekly servings of fatty fish (salmon, cod, mackerel)
- Complex carbohydrates that are high in fiber, such as whole grains
- Monounsaturated fats (olive and canola oil)
- Daily serving of nuts, seeds, or legumes
- Fish or soy over poultry or other meat

TABLE 29-5 Body Mass Index Chart*

HEIGHT (IN)	19	20	21	22	23	24	25	26	27	28	29	30	31	32	33	34	35
	BODY WEIGHT (LB)																
58	91	96	100	105	110	115	119	124	129	134	138	143	148	153	158	162	167
59	94	99	104	109	114	119	124	128	133	138	143	148	153	158	163	168	173
60	97	102	107	112	118	123	128	133	138	143	148	153	158	163	168	174	179
61	100	106	111	116	122	127	132	137	143	148	153	158	164	169	174	180	185
62	104	109	115	120	126	131	136	142	147	153	158	164	169	175	180	186	191
63	107	113	118	124	130	135	141	146	152	158	163	169	175	180	186	191	197
64	110	116	122	128	134	140	145	151	157	163	169	174	180	186	192	197	204
65	114	120	126	132	138	144	150	156	162	168	174	180	186	192	198	204	210
66	118	124	130	136	142	148	155	161	167	173	179	186	192	198	204	210	216
67	121	127	134	140	146	153	159	166	172	178	185	191	198	204	211	217	223
68	125	131	138	144	151	158	164	171	177	184	190	197	203	210	216	223	230
69	128	135	142	149	155	162	169	176	182	189	196	203	209	216	223	230	236
70	132	139	146	153	160	167	174	181	188	195	202	209	216	222	229	236	243
71	136	143	150	157	165	172	179	186	193	200	208	215	222	229	236	243	250
72	140	147	154	162	169	177	184	191	199	206	213	221	228	235	242	250	258
73	144	151	159	166	174	182	189	197	204	212	219	227	235	242	250	257	265
74	148	155	163	171	179	186	194	202	210	218	225	233	241	249	256	264	272
75	152	160	168	176	184	192	200	208	216	224	232	240	248	256	264	272	279
76	156	164	172	180	189	197	205	213	221	230	238	246	254	263	271	279	287

From National Institutes of Health/National Heart, Lung, and Blood Institute: *Clinical guidelines on the identification, evaluation, and treatment of overweight and obesity in adults: the evidence report,* June 1998.

*To use the table, find the appropriate height in the left-hand column. Move across to a given weight. The number at the top of the column is the BMI at that height and weight. Pounds have been rounded off.

TABLE 29-6 Body Mass Index and Disease Risk

BODY MASS INDEX	CLASSIFICATION	DISEASE RISK
18.5 or less	Underweight	Low
18.5-24.9	Normal weight	Low
25-29.9	Overweight	Increased
30-34.9	Obese	High
35-39.9	Obese	Very high
40 or greater	Extremely obese	Extremely high

- Avoid fad diets, especially those with high-protein, low-carbohydrate foods
- Reduce salt intake
- Avoid of saturated fats (animal fat) and trans fats

Traditionally, the diabetic diet has been based on exchange lists, which include foods grouped according to similar calorie, carbohydrate, protein, and fat content. The objective of the exchange lists is to achieve the proper balance of carbohydrates, proteins, and fats while maintaining healthy weight and blood-glucose levels. Menus are developed based on the food groupings and the optimal number of daily calories needed to meet the patient's needs. Foods can be substituted for one another within an exchange list but not among lists. You can get a copy of the exchange list by contacting the American Diabetes Association. Table 29-7 lists the number of exchanges per day allowed within certain calorie-restricted diabetic diets.

However, diabetic educators agree that the simplest way to teach patients about the relationship between diet and blood-glucose levels is to focus on the total number of carbohydrates they can consume daily while maintaining recommended blood-glucose levels. Patients can then decide how they want to distribute carbohydrate intake throughout the day. The number of grams of carbohydrate that a diabetic can eat each day is determined by a combination of the following: the patient's weight and whether or not weight loss or maintenance is part of the treatment plan; the level of exercise, because physical activity lowers blood-glucose levels; prescribed diabetic medications including insulin; and other factors such as age and blood-lipid levels. Therefore people with diabetes can eat sugary foods as long as they restrict themselves to the total number of carbohydrates allowed for that snack or meal and the decision to eat that food adheres to the rules of healthy nutrition. In other words, a diabetic can have a whole-wheat raisin bagel for

TABLE 29-7 Diabetic Diet Exchanges per Day

EXCHANGE GROUPS AND SERVING SIZES	NO. OF EXCHANGES OR SERVINGS IN EACH GROUP				
	1200*	1500*	1800*	2000*	2200*
Starch or breads: One exchange equals 1 oz bread and 1/2 C cooked cereal, grain, or pasta	5	8	10	11	13
Meat and cheese: One exchange equals 1 oz; high fat exchanges should be used no more than three times per week	4	5	7	8	8
Vegetables: One exchange equals 1/2 C cooked, 1 C raw, and 1/2 C juice	2	3	3	4	4
Fruits and sugar: No more than 10% of total daily carbohydrates; each exchange equals 15 g carbohydrate	3	3	3	3	3
Milk products: One exchange equals 1 C or 8 oz; skim and very–low-fat milk products are recommended	2	2	2	2	2
Fats: One exchange equals 1 tsp fat	3	3	3	4	5

*Number of calories in the prescribed diabetic diet.

TABLE 29-8 Carbohydrate Grams in Breakfast Foods

FOOD TYPE	SERVING SIZE	CARBOHYDRATE GRAMS
1% reduced fat milk	1 C	12
Bran Chex	2/3 C	23
Frosted Flakes	3/4 C	26
Apples and cinnamon instant oatmeal	1 packet	27
Low-fat granola	1/2 C	30
Toast	1 slice	15
White table sugar	1 tsp	4
Pancakes	2	15
Pancake syrup	2 Tbsp	30
Light pancake syrup	2 Tbsp	4
Fruit yogurt	1 C	40
Fruit yogurt with NutraSweet	1 C	19
Fruit juice	1/2 C	15
Banana	1/2	15

The glycemic index places carbohydrate foods on a scale from slowest to fastest effects on blood-glucose levels. One of the scales is based on 100 glycemic units, which is equivalent to the number of units in a glucose tablet. The glycemic index of foods helps diabetics understand the impact of different carbohydrates on blood-glucose levels, but it can be a complicated tool to understand and it must be used in conjunction with a dietary plan that considers the nutritional guidelines for all foods.

Glycemic Index of Some Foods Based on 100

Honey	91	Oatmeal cookies	57
Puffed rice	90	Potato chips	56
White potato	87	Oatmeal	53
Corn chips	72	Sweet potato	50
White rice	72	Spaghetti	38
Whole-wheat bread	72	Yogurt	38
Shredded wheat	70	Milk	34
Brown rice	66	Kidney beans	33
Refined sugar	64	Fructose	22
Rye bread	64	Soy beans	14

breakfast as long as the total carbohydrate grams for that food do not exceed the number of carbohydrates that should be eaten for that particular meal. Refer to Table 29-8 to choose a breakfast for a diabetic person that is restricted to a total of 50 g of carbohydrates.

All carbohydrates will raise blood-glucose levels to a similar degree. In general, 1 g of carbohydrate raises the blood sugar of someone who weighs 200 pounds by 3 points and for someone who weighs 150 pounds, by 4 points. However, not all carbohydrates raise the blood-glucose level at the same rate. Choosing a carbohydrate that takes longer to affect blood-glucose levels helps control the hyperglycemic peaks associated with the complications of diabetes mellitus. Another rating system, the glycemic index of foods, may help solve this problem.

CRITICAL THINKING APPLICATION

Samantha Rashad was recently diagnosed with diabetes mellitus type 2. She has met with the dietitian, but she has some questions about her 1200-calorie diabetic diet. The goal of her treatment is to maintain blood-glucose levels within normal range, but also to help her lose weight. Based on Marcia's knowledge of the components of a healthy diet, what recommendations can she make to Ms. Rashad?

Heart-Healthy Diet

The goals of a heart-healthy diet are to eat foods that reduce overall cholesterol levels, decrease LDL, increase HDL, and keep blood pressure within normal limits. Other factors that must be

The American Heart Association Eating Plan for Healthy Americans

Five or more servings per day of a variety of fruits and vegetables.

Six or more servings per day of a variety of grain products, including whole grains.

Eat fish at least twice a week, particularly fatty fish such as salmon.

Include fat-free and low-fat milk products, legumes, skinless poultry, and lean meats.

Choose fats and oils with 2 g saturated fat or less per tablespoon, such as canola and olive oils.

Limit the intake of foods high in calories or low in nutrition.

Limit foods high in saturated fat, trans fat, and/or cholesterol

Eat less than 6 g of sodium per day.

Women should limit alcoholic intake to one drink per day, and men not more than two.

Balance calorie intake with the number used each day. If overweight or obese, multiply your ideal body weight by 15 (active) or 13 (nonactive) to find the number of calories you should eat to gradually achieve your ideal body weight.

Get enough physical activity to keep fit. Exercise at least 30 minutes every day.

From the AHA website: www.americanheart.org.

considered for patients at risk for heart disease are the presence of obesity and the level of exercise. Obesity is associated with elevated lipid levels, so weight management, when a factor, must be part of the patient's dietary plan. In addition, researchers report that an aerobic exercise program must be included for cholesterol levels to be maintained at healthy levels.

CRITICAL THINKING APPLICATION

Ms. Rashad's blood pressure at this visit was 182/94. She is concerned about lowering her blood pressure and the potential risks for heart disease. What facts should Marcia share with her about heart-healthy diets that will help her understand the importance of nutrition in overall wellness?

READING FOOD LABELS

The USDA requires that all food products carry a nutritional fact label (Figure 29-4). These labels are on the back or side of the package and are a source of nutrition information and facts about the nutrients within the package. When planning or implementing a designated diet, the food label can be used as a valuable source of nutritional information (Procedure 29-1).

Under the label's "Nutrition Facts" panel, manufacturers are required to provide information about certain nutrients. The mandatory (underlined) and voluntary components and the order in which they must appear are as follows:

- Serving size
- Calories per serving

Nutrition Facts

Serving Size 1/12 package
(44g, about 1/4 cup dry mix)
Servings Per Container 12

Amount Per Serving	Mix	Baked
Calories	190	280
Calories from Fat	45	140

	% Daily Value**	
Total Fat 5g*	**8%**	**24%**
Saturated Fat 2g	**10%**	**13%**
Trans Fat 1g		
Cholesterol 0mg	**0%**	**23%**
Sodium 300mg	**13%**	**13%**
Total Carbohydrate 34g	**11%**	**11%**
Dietary Fiber 0g	**0%**	**0%**
Sugars 18g		
Protein 2g		
Vitamin A	0%	0%
Vitamin C	0%	0%
Calcium	6%	8%
Iron	2%	4%

*Amount in Mix
**Percent Daily Values are based on a 2,000 calorie diet. Your Daily Values may be higher or lower depending on your caloric needs:

	Calories:	2,000	2,500
Total Fat	Less than	65g	80g
Sat Fat	Less than	20g	25g
Cholesterol	Less than	300mg	300mg
Sodium	Less than	2,400mg	2,400mg
Total Carbohydrate		300g	375g
Dietary Fiber		25g	30g

FIGURE 29-4 Nutritional facts label. (From FDA website, www.cfsan.fda.gov/)

- Calories from fat in each serving
- Grams of total fat
- Grams of saturated fat
- Grams of trans fat
- Polyunsaturated fat
- Monounsaturated fat
- Milligrams of cholesterol
- Milligrams of sodium
- Milligrams of potassium
- Grams of total carbohydrate
- Grams of dietary fiber
- Soluble fiber
- Insoluble fiber
- Grams of sugars
- Sugar alcohol (e.g., the sugar substitutes xylitol, mannitol, and sorbitol)
- Other carbohydrate (the difference between total carbohydrate and the sum of dietary fiber, sugars, and sugar alcohol if declared)
- Grams of protein
- Percent of Daily Value of vitamin A

Provide Instruction for Health Maintenance and Disease Prevention: Teach the Patient to Read Food Labels

<u>CAAHEP COMPETENCIES:</u> 3.c.(3)(b), 3.c.(3)(c)
<u>ABHES COMPETENCY:</u> 7.c

GOAL: *To accurately explain the nutritional labeling of food products to the patient.*

EQUIPMENT and SUPPLIES

- One each of three bars: Snickers candy bar, granola bar, fat-free fruit bar
- Pencil and paper

PROCEDURAL STEPS

1. Explain to the patient that you are going to teach him or her how to read a food label. Be sure to include reasons why food labels are a valuable source of nutritional information in diet planning.

2. Using the labels on each bar, point out the nutritional information according to the guidelines in the text.
   <u>PURPOSE:</u> Using actual labels assists in learning and reinforces practical application.

3. Give the patient the pencil and paper to write down the serving size of each type of bar.
   <u>PURPOSE:</u> Writing information down aids in memory retention.

4. Compare the similarities and differences among the bars.
   <u>PURPOSE:</u> Comparing the results reinforces learning.

5. Have the patient write down the total caloric amount for each product serving.
   <u>PURPOSE:</u> To reinforce the significance of high-calorie snacks on overall nutritional health.

6. Compare the similarities and differences among the bars.

7. Write down the percentage of total, saturated, trans, and unsaturated fats.
   <u>PURPOSE:</u> To review the importance of a low-fat diet and the role of saturated and trans fats in disease.

8. Compare the similarities and differences among the bars.

9. Together, analyze the nutritional level of each.

10. Discuss any new information that was learned.
    <u>PURPOSE:</u> To gather feedback regarding the learning experience so that the patient's learning needs are clarified.

11. Ask the patient if he or she will use this information when shopping and how it will be implemented in nutritional planning.
    <u>PURPOSE:</u> Role-play implementation of information to determine the level of learning.

- Percent of vitamin A present as beta carotene
- <u>Percent of Daily Value of vitamin C</u>
- <u>Percent of Daily Value of calcium</u>
- <u>Percent of Daily Value of iron</u>
- Other essential vitamins and minerals

If a claim is made about any of the optional components, or if a food is fortified or enriched with any of them, nutrition information for these components becomes mandatory. These mandatory and voluntary components are the only ones allowed on the Nutrition Facts panel. The required nutrients were selected because they address today's health concerns. The order in which they must appear reflects the priority of current dietary recommendations.

How to Use Label Information

Start with serving size information, which is listed in both household and metric units. The amount of each nutrient in the food is expressed in two ways: in terms of weight per serving and as a percentage of the daily value. By using the percentage of daily value, you can determine whether a food contributes a lot or a little of a particular nutrient. However, if you eat more or less than the serving size on the label, you will need to adjust the amounts of nutrients accordingly. Keep in mind that the percentage of daily value is based on the amount of food usually eaten in 1 day. The goal is to choose foods that total 100% of your daily nutrition needs.

The ingredient list also can help you learn more about the foods you eat. Ingredients are listed in descending order of weight. That helps you get an idea of the proportion of an ingredient in a food (Figure 29-5). Artificial colors have to be named in the ingredient list; they no longer can be stated as "color added." This is an important item for individuals with food allergies or certain specialized diets. In addition, the total percentage of juice in juice drinks must be declared so that you can see exactly how much juice is in the product.

The front label is where manufacturers often place statements describing the nutritional qualities of their product. The

---

INGREDIENT LABEL

INGREDIENTS: COOKED WHITE RICE, WATER, COOKED CHICKEN TENDERLOINS, GREEN BEANS, CARROTS, RED PEPPERS, BROWN SUGAR. CONTAINS LESS THAN 2% OF MODIFIED FOOD STARCH, MUSTARD (VINEGAR, MUSTARD SEED, SALT, SPICES, TURMERIC), DIJON MUSTARD (WATER, MUSTARD SEED, DISTILLED VINEGAR, SALT, WHITE WINE, CITRIC ACID, TARTARIC ACID, SPICES), HONEY, MALTODEXTRIN (FROM CORN), SALT, EGG YOLK SOLIDS, SODIUM PHOSPHATE, VINEGAR POWDER (MALTODEXTRIN, MODIFIED FOOD STARCH, VINEGAR SOLIDS), XANTHAN GUM FLAVORS, SPICES, LEMON JUICE CONCENTRATE

FIGURE 29-5 Ingredient label. (Courtesy Weight Watchers International, Inc.)

Regulated Nutritional Claims for Food Labels

- Light: One third fewer calories than in the regular product
- Fresh: Raw; never frozen, processed, or preserved
- Calorie-free: Less than 5 calories per serving
- Sugar-free: Less than 0.5 g of sugar per serving
- Sodium-free: Less than 5 mg of sodium per serving
- Fat-free: Less than 0.5 g of fat per serving
- Saturated fat–free: Less than 2 g of saturated fat per serving
- High: Provides more than 20% of the recommended daily consumption of the nutrient, as in "high-fiber"
- Lean: Cooked meat or poultry with less than 10.5 g of fat, of which less than 3.5 g is saturated fat
- Extra lean: Cooked meat or poultry with less than 4.9 g of fat, of which less than 1.8 g is saturated fat
- Low-sodium: Less than 140 mg of sodium
- Low-calorie: Less than 40 calories
- Low-fat: 3 g or less of fat
- Low saturated fat: 1 g or less of saturated fat, and not more than 15% of calories from saturated fat
- Low cholesterol: 20 mg or less of cholesterol and 2 g or less of saturated fat

From U.S. Food and Drug Administration.

government has set strict conditions under which statements such as "low fat," "cholesterol free," and "good source of fiber" can be used as part of the front label. The Food and Drug Administration (FDA) permits claims linking a nutrient or food to the risk of a disease or health-related condition, but only those health claims that are supported by scientific evidence are allowed.

Organic Foods Production Act

In 1990 the USDA initiated regulations regarding food that was organically grown, and in 2002 the agency revised regulations governing the production and labeling of organic foods. Until then, organizations from state governments to trade and consumer groups contributed to the regulation of organic products, resulting in often conflicting standards about which products could be labeled organic. Under the new guidelines, foods labeled as organic must have been produced without exposure to pesticides, chemical fertilizers, or sewage sludge. To be identified as an organic product, the food cannot have been irradiated to extend shelf life, nor can it contain any ingredients that are genetically modified. In addition, animals raised for organic meat, eggs, and milk cannot be given antibiotics or growth hormones, must receive organic feed, and must have had access to the outdoors.

The 2002 regulations extend the rules to cover labeling for organic foods. Products with a "100 percent organic" label are limited to strictly organic ingredients. Products simply labeled "organic" identify the food as being made up of 95% organic materials. Products that fall into these two categories can display a "USDA Organic" seal. Foods containing at least 70% organic ingredients may be labeled "made with organic ingredients" and may list up to three of them on the package. Under the new regulations, any product containing less than 70% organic ingredients may not be marketed as an organic food.

FOODBORNE DISEASES

Eating or drinking contaminated food can result in a foodborne disease. Many different types of bacteria, viruses, and parasites can contaminate food, but the most common are *Escherichia coli*, *Salmonella*, and *Campylobacter*. Patients may experience a variety of symptoms, but the first are typically gastrointestinal—nausea, vomiting, stomach pain, and/or diarrhea. Usually a delay of several hours to days occurs after ingestion of the contaminated substance before symptoms begin. This is the *incubation period*, when the microbes are attaching to the intestinal walls and beginning to multiply. Diagnosis is confirmed with laboratory tests, the most frequent being a stool sample. However, more-sophisticated tests may be needed to diagnose viral pathogens. Treatment depends on patient symptoms; if diarrhea and vomiting are severe, one of the biggest concerns is dehydration, especially in young children and older adults. In such cases replacing fluid and electrolytes is the most important part of care. Other treatments include the use of antidiarrheal medications (e.g., Imodium) and drugs that coat the gastrointestinal tract (e.g., Pepto-Bismol). When doing phone triage with patients experiencing gastrointestinal symptoms, these are some of the items to consider:

- Presence of a fever of 38.6° C (101.5° F) or higher
- Diarrhea for more than 3 days
- Prolonged vomiting
- Blood in the stools
- Signs of dehydration: decrease in urination, dry mouth, **vertigo**

EATING DISORDERS

Eating disorders are defined as any eating behavior pattern that can lead to a health problem. The two problems that cause the most serious health risks are anorexia nervosa and bulimia. These disorders can damage all of the body systems and can cause death. Although 90% of reported cases occur in adolescent and young adult women, the incidence in males and middle-aged women is increasing.

Anorexia nervosa is characterized by self-induced starvation. Anorexic individuals are typically adolescents when first diagnosed and tend to be perfectionists who are extremely sensitive to failure and any criticism. They use avoidance of food as a way of controlling their feelings and fear becoming grossly overweight if they allow themselves to eat. As a result, they lose an excessive amount of weight, usually 15% to 60% of their normal body weight, resulting in extreme malnourishment. They can die without medical intervention. If necessary, patients are fed intravenously or by nasogastric tube feedings to establish an immediate level of nourishment to the body systems. Patients with anorexia nervosa have a significantly distorted body image and require psychotherapy to alleviate depression, to deal with their emotional issues, and for assistance in forming a positive self-image.

Bulimia is more common than anorexia and is characterized by cycles of binging and purging. This behavior pattern usually begins in adolescence when an individual who is slightly overweight diets but fails to achieve the expected results. Psychologically the person believes that self-worth is related to being thin. Usually the pattern begins with some form of stress that upsets the individual, who then turns to food for consolation. Intake during a binge period can reach as high as 20,000 calories. The eating binge is followed by self-induced punishment in the form of vomiting, using laxatives and enemas, excessive exercise, and food abstinence. Most individuals with bulimia have normal or above-normal body weight, but their weight can vary as much as 10 pounds during binging and purging cycles. Treatment programs are a combination of medication, psychotherapy, and nutritional counseling. The goal is to establish healthy eating patterns and to develop an improved self-image.

CRITICAL THINKING APPLICATION

A close friend of Marcia's sister is visiting at their home, and she hears the friend tell her sister that she is using Ex-Lax after every meal and secretly exercising for 3 hours at night after the rest of the family is asleep. She is 5 feet 6 inches tall and determined not to weigh over 100 pounds at graduation. What should Marcia do?

OBESITY

Overweight and obesity affect over 60% of the American population. Obese individuals are at risk for a wide range of health problems, including hypertension, diabetes mellitus type 2, coronary artery disease, stroke, gallbladder disease, osteoarthritis, sleep apnea, and certain types of cancer. The physician's assessment of patients with weight problems includes an evaluation of the BMI and/or the patient's waist-to-hip ratio as well as the presence or risks of conditions associated with obesity. Research evidence indicates the risk for cardiovascular disease rises significantly if the BMI is over 25, and risk of death increases if the BMI is 30 or above. In addition, as BMI levels increase, so do the risks for hypertension and hypercholesterolemia.

Gastrointestinal surgery, or *bariatric* surgery, may be an option for people who are severely obese, have attempted unsuccessfully to lose weight by traditional means, and who have been diagnosed with obesity-related health problems. The operation promotes weight loss by reducing the size of the stomach to the point that food intake is restricted and/or interrupting the digestive process by surgically circumventing part of the small intestine. Three different types of surgical procedures can be performed: restrictive, which decreases the size of the stomach and slows the movement of food through it; malabsorptive, which bypasses most of the small intestine, thereby affecting nutrient digestion and absorption; and combined restrictive-malabsorptive surgery, which uses both techniques to decrease the amount of food ingested as well as decrease the digestion and absorption of nutrients. Patients seeking bariatric surgery must meet certain criteria including a BMI of 40 or greater or a BMI of 35 to 39.9 along with a diagnosed obesity-related health problem such as type 2 diabetes mellitus or severe sleep apnea. The patient must also undergo counseling and psychiatric evaluation because bariatric surgery requires a lifelong commitment to dietary change. The procedure will be successful for long-term weight loss only if the individual is willing to commit to making drastic behavioral changes and undergoing regular medical checkups for the rest of his or her life. In addition, the cost of the procedure—$20,000 to $35,000—may be prohibitive, and insurance coverage varies by state and insurance provider.

According to the Harvard School of Public Health, 100,000 cases of cancer a year can be directly linked to obesity including the following distributions:

- Breast—11%
- Colon—14%
- Esophageal—39%
- Kidney—31%
- Non-Hodgkin's lymphoma—20%
- Pancreatic—14%

Medications for Obesity

Weight-loss medications fall into two categories: appetite suppressants or lipase inhibitors. Appetite-suppressant medications, such as phentermine (Adipex-P, Fastin, Ionamin, Oby-Trim, Pro-Fast, Zantryl) and sibutramine (Meridia), promote weight loss by decreasing appetite or increasing the feeling of being full. Orlistat (Xenical), a lipase inhibitor, blocks the release of the enzyme lipase, which metabolizes fat for absorption. If fat is not broken down, it cannot be absorbed, which results in a decrease in dietary fat absorption by about one third. Most weight-loss medications have been approved by the FDA for short-term use only, typically restricted to a few weeks. Meridia and Xenical are the only weight-loss medications that have been approved for use longer than 2 years. The response to medications for weight loss varies among patients, but the average weight loss is 5 to 22 pounds more than might have been lost without medication. The majority of the weight is lost in the first 6 months of treatment, after which the patient's weight is stabilized or may even increase. The use of weight-loss medications must be combined with improvement in overall nutrition and exercise to have long-lasting effects and reduce weight-related health risks.

HEALTH PROMOTION

The concept of health promotion includes such aspects as adequate nutrition, a healthy environment, ongoing health education, and an overall attempt to prevent disease and maintain optimum wellness. Wellness goes beyond the absence of disease to a state of moving toward fitness, managing stress, and maximizing individual potential. Health promotion employs immunizations, appropriate personal hygiene, environmental sanitation standards, protection against occupational hazards, nutritious diets, and periodic health screenings and examinations to safeguard patients and promote wellness.

The medical assistant plays a key role in assisting the physician in many of these areas. The medical assistant can work as a patient advocate by interacting with local social service agencies or insurance companies on behalf of the patient. The medical assistant also plays an important role in scheduling and assisting the physician with health screenings and physical examinations as well as assisting with health teaching.

The remainder of this chapter discusses components of wellness that all medical assistants should promote.

Exercise

Exercise is defined as physical exertion for the maintenance or improvement of health or for the correction of a physical handicap. Exercise improves cardiorespiratory endurance; maintains musculoskeletal health by improving or maintaining strength, flexibility, and bone integrity; and relieves stress. Although most Americans say they know about the benefits of exercise, only 20% to 25% of adults exercise enough to gain significant health benefits. Twenty-five percent are not active at all, and more than half of all American youths 12 to 21 years of age are not vigorously active on a regular basis.

A well-balanced diet is only half of the fitness equation; to ensure good health, adequate exercise and sufficient rest form the other half of the equation. As with special diets, exercise programs must be approved for each individual by the physician. It is the physician who determines the patient's exercise needs and tolerance levels to safeguard the patient from overexertion and potential injury.

Many forms of exercise are available. Some patients may find that it is best to go to a gym and develop a formal program of physical fitness. Others may purchase home exercise equipment so they can exercise in privacy. Many feel just getting out in the fresh air and walking is the best form of exercise. All of these are acceptable, because all have one thing in common: physical activity. Each individual should find the outlet that brings enjoyment and enrichment to his or her life. It is not the form of exercise that is important, but the participation in physical activity that promotes wellness.

If you are working with a patient who cannot engage in a full physical exercise program, you can suggest range-of-motion exercises. These exercise patterns are designed to improve circulation and promote muscle tone by putting each joint through its full range of motion. Patients with disabilities such as partial paralysis, arthritis, bursitis, and musculoskeletal deformities may be helped with these exercises. Range-of-motion exercises are presented in Chapter 42.

CRITICAL THINKING APPLICATION

The physician tells Mr. Hawthorne he must exercise to maintain a healthy lifestyle. What can Marcia tell him about the benefits of exercise and possible methods that might help him follow through with the physician's recommendation?

Stress Management

Stress stimulates the fight-or-flight response that physically prepares us to either fight off a stressor or run away from it. Unfortunately, most of the stress we experience on a daily basis is not something we can either physically battle or effectively run away from. Therefore the stress response can lead to multiple health problems if it is not therapeutically managed. The stress response results in the release of epinephrine (adrenaline), which increases the heart and respiratory rates, slows down peristalsis, increases blood supply to the skeletal muscles while decreasing blood to the periphery, causes overall muscular tension, and raises the blood pressure. If stress is permitted to build without release, multiple health problems can occur, some of which can lead to chronic disorders.

Health Screening

Routine physical examinations and health screenings are important components of health promotion. The patient scheduled for a physical examination should have a health

Benefits of Exercise

- Increases self-esteem
- Improves mood
- Boosts energy
- Strengthens heart
- Strengthens muscles
- Burns calories
- Improves cholesterol levels
- Relieves stress
- Prevents bone loss
- Decreases risk of some cancers

Stress Management Strategies

- Engage in regular aerobic exercise
- Apply time-management strategies
- Use assertive communication as needed
- Practice relaxation and visualization exercises
- Avoid caffeine and cigarettes
- Eat a balanced nutritious diet and get adequate sleep
- Make time for yourself

Stress-Related Health Problems

Muscular tension	Anxiety
Headaches	Hypertension
Gastric discomfort	Back pain
Diarrhea	Heart disease
Fatigue	Gastrointestinal disorders
Insomnia	Autoimmune disorders
Depression	

history completed or updated and should be weighed; blood pressure, temperature, pulse, and respirations recorded; and any complaints documented on the chart. Assisting with the physical examination will be covered in Chapter 31. The physician may order the following studies as part of the health screening process:

- Tuberculin skin test
- Papanicolaou (Pap) smear
- Prostate-specific antigen (PSA) levels
- Hemoccult test after age 50
- Colonoscopy or sigmoidoscopy every 3 to 5 years after age 50
- Mammogram yearly after age 50
- Urinalysis
- Serum cholesterol
- Chest x-ray films
- Electrocardiogram (ECG)

CLOSING COMMENTS

Patient Education

The medical assistant may be called on to discuss a diet plan with a patient, so it is extremely important to have a thorough knowledge of diet therapy. The patient must understand the diet and the rationale behind its use. If the patient feels uneasy or questions are unanswered, he or she may be less motivated to follow a diet plan. You can be a valuable asset to the physician, the dietitian, and the patient when implementing a specific diet.

When talking to patients about a diet, the medical assistant may find the following helpful:

- Use charts and diagrams to illustrate diets.
- Consider the patient's dietary likes and dislikes.
- Remember that ethnic and cultural foods are important.
- Encourage the patient to play an active role in the learning process.
- Suggest local support groups that can help in diet maintenance.

You can also play a vital role in health promotion by making sure that patients are scheduled for annual examinations and that they follow up with the physician's recommendations for dietary changes, exercise programs, stress management approaches, and health screening procedures. The medical assistant is the link between the patient and the physician as well as between the patient and available community resources.

Legal and Ethical Issues

Always remember that you are not a physician, nor are you a dietitian. Follow the physician's instructions, and if the patient has a question for which you are not sure of the answer, always ask the physician for his or her advice in handling the question. If your workplace employs an RD, refer questions involving meal patterns and food selection changes to him or her. When seeking advice in the field of nutrition and exercise programs, direct patients to someone who is a qualified expert. Use community resources as needed.

SUMMARY OF SCENARIO

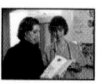
This chapter has emphasized the influences of nutrition and health promotion practices on patient wellness. As a certified medical assistant working in an internal medicine practice, Marcia must be familiar with the types and functions of dietary nutrients, the Food Guide Pyramid, how nutritional assessments are conducted, the concepts of therapeutic nutrition, how to apply interpretation of food labels to patient practice, and the concepts of health promotion. Recommendations for nutrition are constantly changing as research is done on the dietary needs of healthy people. Marcia can refer her patients to the USDA site, www.mypyramid.gov, for updated information on the revised Food Guide Pyramid as well as educational material on nutrition. For the first time, dietary recommendations are linked to the importance of regular exercise and the individual's BMI. Physicians are now relying on BMI levels to determine the patient's risk for diet-related diseases. In addition, medical assistants working in a physician office practice must be familiar with the various diets included in therapeutic nutrition so patient questions can be answered about foods that should be included or avoided. As a certified medical assistant it is important that Marcia make a commitment to lifelong learning so she is able to provide her patients with up-to-date information on these topics and to use community resources to support patient care.

SUMMARY of LEARNING OBJECTIVES

1. Define, spell, and pronounce the terms listed in the vocabulary.
   - Spelling and pronouncing medical terms correctly adds credibility to the medical assistant. Knowing the definition of these terms promotes confidence in communication with patients and co-workers.

2. Recognize the impact of cultural influences on diet choices.
   - People eat the way they do for many reasons. Encouraging patients to make significant lifestyle changes regarding their diets requires sensitivity to these reasons. The choices people make about what they eat are greatly influenced by their background and relationships. Every culture, religion, and ethnic group has its own beliefs and practices about food.

3. Summarize the relationship between poor diet and lifestyle choices and the risk of developing diet-related diseases.
   - Research has made direct correlations between the development of certain diseases and disorders with individual lifestyle and dietary habits. These include certain types of anemia, constipation, type 2 diabetes mellitus, hypercholesterolemia, atherosclerosis, hypertension, osteoporosis, and cerebrovascular accidents.

4. Classify the types and functions of dietary nutrients.
   - Nutrients consist of carbohydrates, fats, proteins, vitamins, minerals, and water. Their primary functions are to provide the body with energy, protection, and insulation; build and repair tissues; and regulate metabolic processes.

5. Describe the role of carbohydrates, fats, and protein in the daily diet.
   - The primary function of carbohydrates is to provide the body with a ready source of energy. Dietary fiber plays an important role in maintaining regularity and helping to prevent cancer and heart disease. Dietary fat provides essential fatty acids and is needed for the absorption of fat-soluble vitamins. Adipose tissue helps protect the organs of the body, insulates, and serves as a concentrated form of stored energy. Protein builds and repairs tissue and assists with metabolic functions.

6. Explain the function of appropriate amounts of vitamins, minerals, and water in the diet.
   - Vitamins are essential for metabolic functions and are classified as either fat- or water-soluble. They regulate the synthesis of body tissues and aid in the metabolism of nutrients. Vitamins also play a vital role in disease prevention. Minerals help maintain electrolytes and acid-base balance as well as regulate muscular action and nervous activities throughout the body. Water is part of almost every vital body process.

7. Apply Food Guide Pyramid guidelines to patient dietary recommendations.
   - In 2005 the Pyramid was revised, and for the first time dietary recommendations are linked to the importance of exercise in maintaining a healthy weight. The narrowing of each food group up the pyramid represents the importance of choosing more foods with limited added sugars and fats. Individually designed guidelines are available based on age and activity level. The widths of the food groups represent how much should be consumed from each group daily. Emphasis is on the importance of choosing a variety of nutritious foods each day. Refer to the USDA website, www.mypyramid.gov, to investigate the many learning opportunities available to enhance understanding of the new guidelines.

8. Implement nutritional assessment techniques.
   - The physician's assessment of the patient's nutritional status includes an evaluation of the patient's current health and lifestyle habits as well as body fat measurements. Body fat can be measured by using the waist-to-hip ratio, by using calipers to measure fat folds, or by calculating the BMI.

9. Compare patient BMI calculations to the risk of diet-related disease development.
   - BMI is the relationship of weight to height; the patient's measurements are correlated with health risks. BMI is a more accurate predictor of weight-related diseases than traditional height/weight charts because it provides a good estimate of the degree of body fat. Individuals with BMIs between 19 and 22 are thought to live the longest. Diet-related disorders as well as mortality rates are significantly higher for people with indexes of 25 and above.

10. Demonstrate the concepts of therapeutic nutrition.
    - Therapeutic nutrition uses various diets to help treat or prevent disease. There are many ways diets can be modified, including changes in consistency and taste, monitoring caloric levels, altering amounts and types of specific nutrients, and managing the fiber content of foods. Two examples of diet therapies are the diabetic diet and the heart-healthy diet, both of which can have a significant impact on patient wellness.

11. Interpret food labels and their application to healthy diets.
    - The federal government requires all food manufacturers to follow certain guidelines when labeling packages. Labels provide facts on the nutritional value of foods. The food label can be a valuable tool in patient compliance with specialized diets.

12. Summarize the etiology and impact of eating disorders and obesity on patient health.
    - *Eating disorders* are defined as any eating behavior pattern that can lead to a health problem. The chapter discusses both anorexia nervosa, in which profound malnutrition occurs because of an individual's attempt to control life by not eating, and bulimia, which is characterized by bingeing and purging episodes. Obesity has become a national health emergency, with obese individuals at increased risk for a wide range of health problems including hypertension, diabetes mellitus type 2, coronary artery disease, stroke, gallbladder disease, osteoarthritis, sleep apnea, and certain types of cancer.

13. Define the concepts of health promotion.
    - Health promotion considers all aspects of patient care, including the concepts of general wellness, adequate nutrition, environmental health and safety, health education needs, and disease prevention. The components of health promotion

Continued

SUMMARY of LEARNING OBJECTIVES

Continued

include exercise, stress management, regular physical examinations, and health screening.

14. Understand the role of the medical assistant in nutrition and health promotion.
    • A medical assistant plays a key role in nutrition and health promotion, serving as a patient advocate and liaison between the patient and community resources. It is important for

the medical assistant to understand various implications of nutrition and specific diets so he or she is capable of answering patient questions and thereby promoting compliance with treatment.

15. Demonstrate the nutritional labeling of food products to a patient.
    • Refer to Procedure 29-1.

CONNECTIONS

Study Guide Connection: Go to Chapter 29 Study Guide. Read the Case Study and Workplace Applications and complete the assignments. Do online research for answers to the questions in the Internet Activities associated with nutrition and health promotion.

CD Connection: Go to the Medical Assisting Competency Challenge CD and do the training activities under Patient Care. For a better understanding of the digestive process, view the animation for the digestive tract.

Evolve Connection: For more information related to nutrition and health promotion, go to evolve.elsevier.com/kinn and visit related weblinks for Chapter 29. Click on the Medical Assisting Exam Review and do the practice questions to sharpen your test-taking skills.

Vital Signs

30

SCENARIO

Dr. Susan Xu is part of a multiphysician primary care practice. Each physician in the practice has a medical assistant who works directly with him or her. Carlos Ricci, CMA, is Dr. Xu's assistant. Carlos graduated from a medical assistant program 3 years ago and enjoys the variety of patients seen in Dr. Xu's practice. One of Carlos' primary responsibilities is to accurately monitor and record each patient's vital signs before the patient is seen by Dr. Xu.

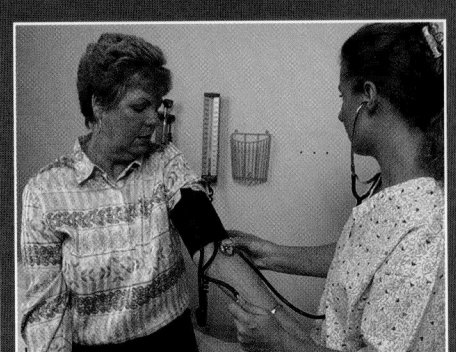

While studying this chapter, think about the following questions:

- What factors might alter a patient's vital signs?
- What methods can Carlos use to gather and record patient temperature, pulse, respirations, blood pressure, height, weight, and BMI?
- What are the most recent guidelines for diagnosing and treating hypertension?

LEARNING OBJECTIVES

1. Define, spell, and pronounce the terms listed in the vocabulary.
2. Cite the average body temperatures, pulse rates, respiratory rates, and blood pressures for various age groups.
3. Describe emotional and physical factors that cause body temperature to increase or decrease.
4. Obtain and record an accurate patient temperature using three different sites.
5. Describe pulse rate, volume, and rhythm.
6. Locate and record the pulse at multiple sites.
7. Demonstrate the best way to obtain an accurate respiration count.
8. Specify physiologic factors that affect blood pressure.
9. Differentiate between essential and secondary hypertension.
10. Interpret revised hypertension guidelines and treatment.
11. Identify the different Korotkoff phases.
12. Accurately measure and document blood pressure.
13. Accurately measure and document height and weight.
14. Convert kilograms to pounds and pounds to kilograms.
15. Identify patient education opportunities when measuring vital signs.
16. Determine legal and ethical responsibilities in obtaining vital signs.

National Accreditation Competencies and Content

CAAHEP COMPETENCIES	ABHES COMPETENCIES
Patient Care 3.b.(4)(b). Obtain vital signs	**Clinical** 4.d. Take vital signs

VOCABULARY

apnea Absence or cessation of breathing.

arrhythmia (ar-rith'-me-uh) Irregular heart rhythm.

bounding Describes a pulse that feels full because of increased power of cardiac contractions or as a result of increased blood volume.

bradycardia A slow heartbeat; a pulse below 60 beats per minute.

bradypnea Respirations that are regular in rhythm but slower than normal in rate.

cerumen (see-room'-men) A waxy secretion in the ear canal; commonly called *ear wax.*

chronic obstructive pulmonary disease (COPD) A progressive and irreversible lung condition that results in diminished lung capacity.

diurnal rhythm Patterns of activity or behavior that follow day-night cycles.

dyspnea Difficult or painful breathing.

essential hypertension Elevated blood pressure of unknown cause that develops for no apparent reason; sometimes called *primary hypertension.*

febrile (feb'-ril) Pertaining to an elevated body temperature.

homeostasis Internal adaptation and change in response to environmental factors.

hyperpnea Increase in the depth of breathing.

hypertension High blood pressure (systolic pressure consistently above 140 mm Hg and diastolic pressure above 90 mm Hg).

hyperventilation Abnormally prolonged and deep breathing usually associated with acute anxiety or emotional tension.

hypotension Blood pressure that is below normal (systolic pressure below 90 mm Hg and diastolic pressure below 50 mm Hg).

intermittent pulse Pulse in which beats are occasionally skipped.

orthopnea Condition in which an individual must sit or stand to breathe comfortably.

orthostatic (postural) hypotension Temporary fall in blood pressure when a person rapidly changes from a recumbent position to a standing position.

otitis externa Inflammation or infection of the external auditory canal.

peripheral Pertaining to an area that is outside or away from an organ or structure.

pulse deficit Condition in which the radial pulse is less than the apical pulse; may indicate peripheral vascular abnormality.

pulse pressure Difference between the systolic and the diastolic blood pressures (30 to 50 mm Hg is considered normal).

rales Abnormal or crackling breath sounds during inspiration.

rhonchi (ron'-ki) Abnormal rumbling sounds on expiration that indicate airway obstruction by thick secretions or spasms.

secondary hypertension Elevated blood pressure resulting from another condition.

sinus arrhythmia Irregular heartbeat originating in the sinoatrial node (pacemaker).

spirometer Instrument that measures the volume of inhaled and exhaled air.

stertorous (stuh-tuh'-rus) Describes a strenuous respiratory effort that has a snoring sound.

syncope Fainting; a brief lapse in consciousness.

tachycardia Rapid but regular heart rate exceeding 100 beats per minute.

tachypnea Respirations that are rapid and shallow; hyperventilation.

thready Describes a pulse that is scarcely perceptible.

vertigo Dizziness.

Measurement of vital signs is an important aspect of almost every patient visit to the medical office. These signs are the human body's indicators of internal **homeostasis** and represent the general state of health of the patient. Because the medical assistant is chiefly responsible for obtaining these measurements, it is imperative to have confidence in the theoretic and practical applications of vital sign measurement. A medical assistant who understands the principles of and the reasons for these measurements will become a valuable asset to any medical office.

Accuracy is essential. A change in one or more of the patient's vital signs may indicate a change in general health. Variations may suggest the presence or disappearance of a disease process and therefore may lead to alteration of the treatment plan. Although the medical assistant obtains vital signs routinely, it is a task that requires consistent attention to accuracy and detail. These findings are crucial to a correct diagnosis, and vital signs should never be measured with indifference or casualness. In addition to accurate measurement, care must be taken when charting the findings on the patient's medical record.

Vital signs are the patient's temperature, pulse, respiration, and blood pressure. These four signs are abbreviated *TPR* and *BP* and may be referred to as *cardinal signs.* It is a medical assistant's duty to understand the significance of the vital signs and to accurately measure and record them. *Anthropometric* measurements are not considered vital signs but are usually obtained at the same time as the vital signs. These measurements include height, weight, body mass index (BMI), and other body measurements, such as fat composition and head and chest circumference.

FACTORS THAT MAY INFLUENCE VITAL SIGNS

Vital signs are influenced by many factors, both physical and emotional. A patient may have consumed a hot or cold beverage just before the examination or may be angry or afraid of what the physician may find. For example, a patient has been asked to return to have a repeat Papanicolaou (Pap) smear because the first one showed the presence of suspicious cells. The medical assistant measures the patient's blood pressure and finds it to be significantly elevated when compared with previous readings. It is possible that this individual is anxious and apprehensive about the test results and that the elevated blood pressure readings reflect her anxiety. What temperature reading might be expected in a patient who could not find a parking place and had to walk four blocks to the office knowing he would be late for his appointment? If you said it would be elevated, you are right. Certainly, this patient would have an increase in his metabolism because of the physical exercise, and as a result, his temperature would be elevated, along with his pulse, respirations, and blood pressure.

Most patients, for one reason or another, are apprehensive during an office visit. These emotions may alter the vital signs, and the medical assistant must help the patient relax before taking any readings. It sometimes is necessary to obtain measurements a second time, after the patient is calmer or more comfortable. For a better picture of the patient's vital signs, the medical assistant may be asked to record the vital signs twice: at the beginning of the visit and just before the patient leaves the office.

TEMPERATURE

Physiology

Body temperature is defined as the balance between the heat lost and the heat produced by the body. It is measured in either degrees Fahrenheit (F) or degrees Celsius (C). The process of chemical and physical change within our bodies that produces heat is called *metabolism*. Body temperature is a result of this process. The core body temperature is maintained within a normal range by the thermoregulatory center in the hypothalamus. The average body temperature varies from person to person and is at different levels at different times in each person. This **diurnal rhythm** in a healthy adult varies from 97.6° F to 99° F (36.4° C to 37.3° C); the average daily temperature is 98.6° F (36.8° C). The body temperature is lowest in the morning and highest in the late afternoon. Factors that may affect body temperature include the following:

- *Age.* The body temperature of infants and young children fluctuates more rapidly in response to external environmental temperatures. Teething may cause a slight elevation in temperature but should not be the cause of a fever. Aging adults lose their ability to therapeutically respond to environmental temperature extremes, making them more susceptible to hypothermic or hyperthermic reactions.
- *Stress and physical activity.* Both exercise and emotional stress can increase the metabolic rate, causing an elevation in temperature.
- *Gender.* Hormone secretions result in fluctuations of core body temperature in women throughout the menstrual cycle.
- *External factors.* Smoking, drinking hot fluids, and gum chewing can temporarily elevate an oral temperature.

In illness an individual's metabolic activity is increased; this causes internal heat production to increase, which in turn increases body temperature. The increase in body temperature is thought to be the body's defensive reaction, because heat inhibits the growth of some bacteria and viruses.

When a fever is present, superficial blood vessels (near the surface of the skin) constrict. The small papillary muscles at the base of hair follicles also constrict and create goose bumps. Chills and shivering may follow, causing internal heat to be produced. As this process repeats itself, more heat is produced, and the body temperature becomes elevated or increases above normal levels. When more heat is lost than is produced, the opposite effect occurs, and body temperature drops below normal levels.

Fever

Infection, either bacterial or viral, is the most common cause of fever in both children and adults. It is unusual for infants to develop **febrile** illnesses during the first 3 months of life, but if one is present it is usually very serious. However, fever in young children is very common and accounts for an estimated 26% of office visits. Fevers are classified according to the 24-hour pattern they follow. The three most commonly seen patterns include the following:

- *Continuous fever* rises and falls only slightly during a 24-hour period. Temperature consistently remains above the patient's average normal temperature range and fluctuates less than 3 degrees.
- *Intermittent fever* comes and goes, alternating between elevated and normal levels.
- *Remittent fever* has great fluctuation—more than 3 degrees—and never returns to the normal range.

Variation from the patient's average body temperature range may be the first warning of an illness or change in the patient's present condition. Patients with a fever usually have loss of appetite or *anorexia*, headache, thirst, flushed face, hot skin, and general malaise. A serious complication for young children with high fevers is the potential of developing a febrile seizure. Medication to reduce the fever—*antipyretic* drugs such as Tylenol—should be taken as instructed to prevent dangerous spikes in temperature. Age-related normal values for temperature readings are in Table 30-1.

TABLE 30-1 Age-Related Temperature Norms

AGE	FAHRENHEIT SCALE (DEGREES)	CELSIUS SCALE (DEGREES)
Newborn	98.2	36.8 (axillary)
1 year	99.7	37.6
6 years to adult	98.6	37 (oral)
Elderly over age 70 years	96.8	36 (oral)

Temperatures That Are Considered Febrile

- Rectal or aural (ear) temperatures over 100.4° F (38° C)
- Oral temperatures over 99.5° F (37.5° C)
- Axillary temperatures over 98.6° F (37° C)
- *Fever of unknown origin* (FUO) is a fever over 100.9° F (38.3° C) that lasts for 3 weeks in adults and 1 week in children without a known related diagnosis

Temperature Readings

A clinical thermometer is used to measure body temperature and is calibrated in either the Fahrenheit or the Celsius scale. The Fahrenheit (F) scale is used most frequently in the United States to measure body temperature, but hospitals and many ambulatory care settings use the Celsius (c) scale. The formulas for conversion from one system to the other are as follows:

$$°C = (°F - 32) \times {}^5/_9$$
$$°F = (°C \times {}^9/_5) + 32$$

CRITICAL THINKING APPLICATION

Using the formulas given, convert the following temperatures from one system to the other.

99° F = _____ ° C   102° F = _____ ° C
40° C = _____ ° F   45° C = _____ ° F

The thermometer is placed under the tongue, in the ear, or in the axilla, because large blood vessels are near the surface at these points. The average temperature values for adults at these three sites are shown in Table 30-2.

Axillary temperatures are approximately 1° F or 0.6° C lower than accurate oral readings because axillary readings are not taken in an enclosed body cavity. The tympanic (ear) temperature is considered the most accurate because it records the temperature of the blood that is closest to the hypothalamus and therefore reflects a true measure of the core body temperature. It is also the fastest, least invasive, and easiest method to perform.

When obtaining temperatures using the oral method of measurement, you do not have to indicate the site when documenting the reading in the patient's chart. However, you should record a (T) for tympanic or an (A) for axillary readings after the temperature is recorded to clarify an alternative site. It is impossible to accurately measure oral temperatures in young

TABLE 30-2 Average Adult Temperature Values		
SITE	FAHRENHEIT SCALE (DEGREES)	CELSIUS SCALE (DEGREES)
Oral	98.6	37
Axillary	97.6	36.4
Tympanic	98.6	37

children because the technique requires patients to hold the thermometer under the tongue and keep the mouth closed. The American Academy of Pediatricians no longer recommends the taking of rectal temperatures because of the danger of rectal perforation. Therefore, for children under the age of 3 years or in any patient who is unable to properly hold the thermometer in the mouth during the procedure, a tympanic thermometer should be used if possible; if not, an axillary temperature can be obtained.

CRITICAL THINKING APPLICATION

The mother of a 3-year-old calls the office to report that the child had an axillary temperature of 101° F at 9 o'clock this morning. The schedule is very full today, so Carlos has to decide whether the child should be seen today or first thing tomorrow. When should Carlos schedule the appointment?

Types of Thermometers and Their Uses

Digital

Digital thermometers are battery operated and are available in both Fahrenheit and Celsius scales. Disposable covers fit snugly over the probes and are easily and quickly removed by pushing in the colored end of the probe. The instrument sounds an audible "beep" when the process is completed (between 10 and 60 seconds), and the reading appears on an LED screen on the face of the instrument (Procedure 30-1). Because the only part of the instrument that comes in contact with the patient is the probe, and that is sheathed, the risk of cross-infection is greatly reduced. Another type resembles the old mercury thermometers that the U.S. Occupational Safety and Health Administration (OSHA) no longer permits in healthcare facilities. These thermometers also have a digital screen on which the temperature is read and should always be covered by a disposable sheath (Figure 30-1).

An oral temperature should not be taken if the patient has recently had something hot or cold to eat or drink or has just smoked, because these factors may artificially alter the patient's temperature.

Tympanic

The tympanic membrane of the ear can also be used for quick, accurate, and safe assessments of patient temperatures. It shares the blood supply that reaches the hypothalamus, which is the brain's temperature regulator. The ear canal is a protected cavity, so the aural temperature is not affected by factors such as an open mouth, hot or cold drinks, or even a stuffy nose that would prevent a patient from keeping the mouth closed during the procedure. In addition, the covered probe is designed to bounce an infrared signal off the eardrum without touching it, so the risk of spreading communicable diseases during temperature measurement is greatly reduced.

The tympanic measurement system consists of a hand-held processor unit equipped with a tympanic probe that is covered with a disposable speculum when being used (Figure 30-2).

PROCEDURE 30-1

Obtain Vital Signs: Obtain an Oral Temperature Using a Digital Thermometer

CAAHEP COMPETENCY: 3.b.(4)(b)
ABHES COMPETENCY: 4.d

GOAL: *To accurately determine and record a patient's temperature using a digital thermometer.*

EQUIPMENT and SUPPLIES

- Digital thermometer
- Probe covers
- Biohazard waste container
- Disposable gloves as appropriate
- Patient record

PROCEDURAL STEPS

1. Wash your hands and assemble equipment and supplies.
   PURPOSE: Infection control.
2. Identify your patient and explain the procedure. Be sure that the patient has not eaten, consumed any hot or cold fluids, smoked, or exercised during the 30 minutes before the temperature is measured.
   PURPOSE: Identification of the patient prevents errors, and explanations are a means of gaining implied consent and patient cooperation. The temperature will be inaccurate if food or fluids have been ingested or the patient has exercised within 30 minutes.
3. Prepare the probe for use as described in package directions (Figure 1). Make certain probe covers are always used.
   PURPOSE: Infection control.

4. Place the probe under the patient's tongue (Figure 2), and instruct the patient to close the mouth tightly. Assist the patient by holding the probe end.
   PURPOSE: Air seeping into the mouth interferes with an accurate body temperature reading.
5. When the "beep" is heard, remove the probe from the patient's mouth and immediately eject the probe cover into the appropriate biohazard waste container.
   PURPOSE: The probe cover is contaminated and must be placed in a biohazard waste container.
6. Note the reading in the LED window of the processing unit you are holding.
7. Record the reading on the patient's medical record (e.g., T = 97.7°).
   PURPOSE: Procedures that are not recorded are considered not done.
8. Wash your hands, and disinfect the equipment as indicated.
   PURPOSE: Infection control and standard precautions.

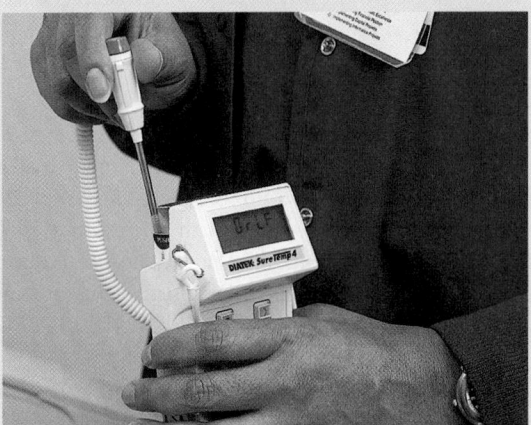

FIGURE 1

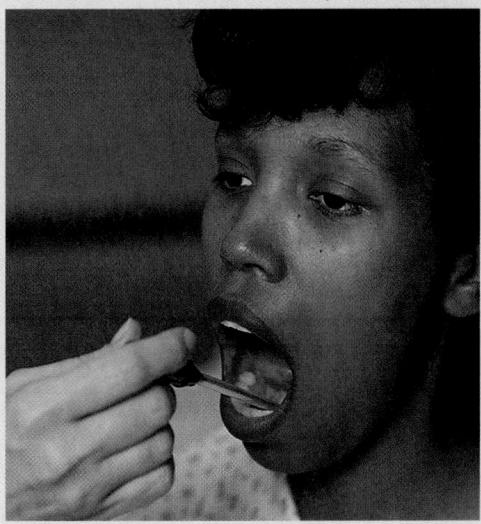

FIGURE 2

When the probe is placed into the ear canal, it gently seals the external opening of the canal, and the infrared energy emitted by the tympanic membrane is gathered. This signal is then digitized by the processor unit and shown on the display screen. Accurate readings are obtained in less than 2 seconds (Procedure 30-2). The speed and patient comfort of the tympanic thermometer have greatly influenced its popularity. This unit should not be used (1) if the patient has bilateral **otitis externa,** because the procedure would be uncomfortable for the patient, or (2) if impacted **cerumen** is present in both ears, because the reading may be inaccurate.

Disposable

Disposable thermometers (those that are used only once) are also available for obtaining body temperatures. They are frequently used in the home on small children. The reading is obtained

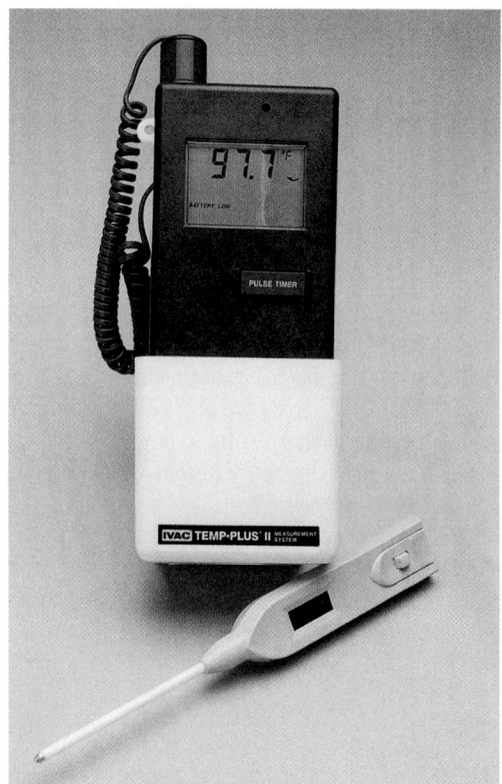

FIGURE 30-1 Digital thermometers.

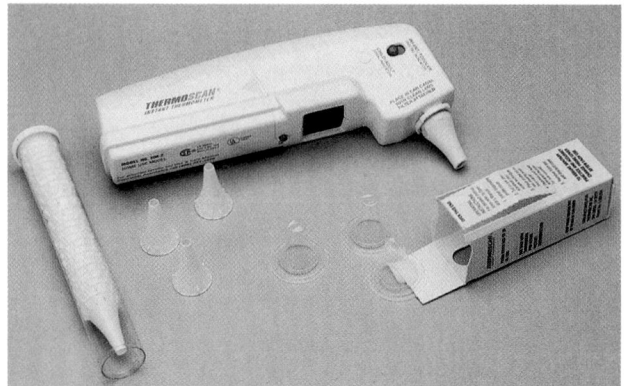

FIGURE 30-2 Tympanic thermometer.

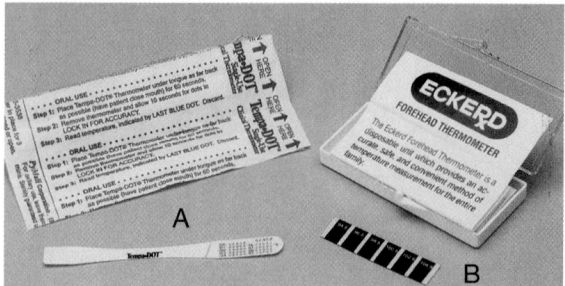

FIGURE 30-3 A, Tempa-Dot disposable oral strip thermometer. **B,** Eckerd forehead disposable thermometer. (*A,* Courtesy Tempa-Dot, Sommerville, NJ; *B,* Courtesy Eckerd, San Jose, Calif.)

time to register the correct body temperature, but the method is safe, simple, and easily accessible (Procedure 30-3). Axillary temperatures are taken using a digital thermometer that is placed into the axillary fold. If the digital thermometer has more than one probe, the oral (blue) probe with a disposable probe cover should be used. Because tympanic thermometers are relatively expensive, the axillary method may be a viable way for parents of young children to get accurate temperature readings.

Cleaning Thermometers

Digital

The digital unit or individual digital thermometers should be routinely cleaned with disinfectant. When ejecting the probe shield or removing the sheath, be careful not to contaminate the probe or the processing unit. If there is a chance that a patient's body fluids touched the unit, wipe it with disinfectant before returning it to the storage area.

Tympanic

Clean a tympanic thermometer by following the same guidelines as for the digital unit. When using the device on a small child, be conscious of what the child touches. If the processing unit is touched, be sure to wipe it with disinfectant after use. However, be careful not to get the tip of the probe surface wet, and always use probe covers, because disinfectant can ruin the probe surface.

by a heat-sensitive material that changes color according to the elevation of body temperature. Two types of disposable thermometers are frequently used by parents of young children. One type is placed under the child's tongue (Figure 30-3, *A); the* other is placed on the forehead (Figure 30-3, *B). Although both* types are fairly reliable, the temperature-sensing materials have expiration dates that are often overlooked and may have specific storage requirements. Disposable thermometers are considered good screening devices but not as accurate as oral or tympanic thermometers.

Axillary

Studies indicate that axillary temperatures are very accurate when performed correctly. Axillary temperatures take more

---

CRITICAL THINKING APPLICATION

How should the medical assistant adapt temperature-taking techniques in the following scenarios?

- A patient who is continuously talking with the thermometer in his or her mouth.
- A 7-year-old child with bilateral otitis externa
- A 3-month-old infant when a tympanic thermometer is not available
- A 46-year-old patient with a severe asthma attack
- A 72-year-old patient with bilateral impacted cerumen
- A 28-year-old patient who has just smoked a cigarette

PROCEDURE 30-2

Obtain Vital Signs: Obtain an Aural Temperature Using the Tympanic Thermometer

CAAHEP COMPETENCY: 3.b.(4)(b)
ABHES COMPETENCY: 4.d

GOAL: *To accurately determine and record a patient's temperature using a tympanic thermometer.*

EQUIPMENT and SUPPLIES

- Tympanic thermometer
- Disposable probe covers
- Biohazard waste container
- Disposable gloves as appropriate
- Patient record

PROCEDURAL STEPS

1. Wash your hands.
   PURPOSE: Infection control.
2. Gather the necessary equipment and supplies.
3. Identify your patient and explain the procedure.
   PURPOSE: Identification of the patient prevents errors, and explanations are a means of gaining implied consent and patient cooperation.
4. Place a disposable cover on the probe (Figure 1).
   PURPOSE: To ensure a clean surface and prevent cross-contamination.
5. Follow the package directions to start the thermometer.
6. Insert the probe into the ear canal far enough to seal the opening. Do not apply pressure (Figure 2). For children under the age of 3, gently pull the ear lobe down and back; for patients over the age of 3, gently pull the top of the ear up and back.
   PURPOSE: The external ear must be pulled gently to open the external auditory canal for an accurate reading.
7. Press the button on the probe as directed. The temperature will be on the display screen in 1 to 2 seconds.
8. Remove the probe, note the reading (Figure 3), and discard the probe cover into a biohazard container without touching it.
   PURPOSE: The probe cover will be contaminated and must be disposed of in a biohazard waste container.

9. Wash your hands and disinfect the equipment if indicated.
   PURPOSE: Infection control.
10. Record the temperature results (e.g., T = 98.6° [T]) on the patient's medical record.
    PURPOSE: Procedures that are not recorded are considered not done.

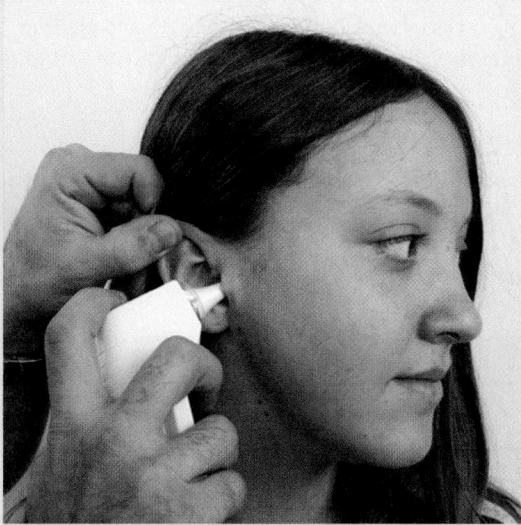

FIGURE 2

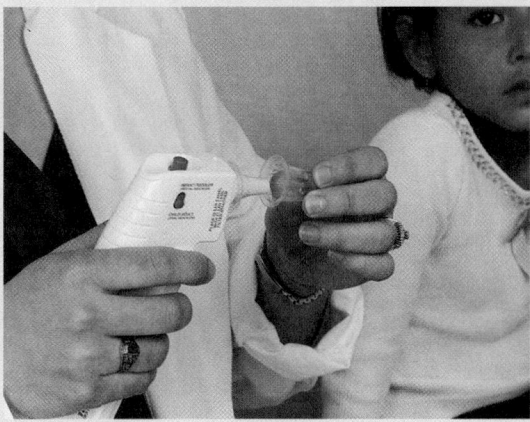

FIGURE 1

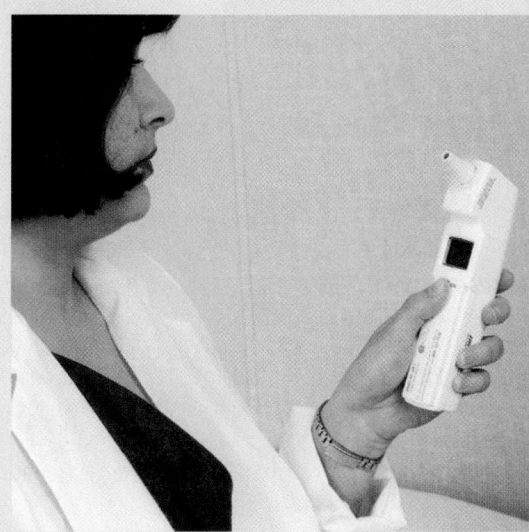

FIGURE 3

Disposable

Always discard a disposable thermometer in the appropriate waste container immediately after use to avoid contamination and the spread of pathogens to other patients. If you are instructing a parent in the use of a disposable thermometer at home, be sure to emphasize that it should be discarded immediately in a childproof container.

PULSE

A patient's pulse rate reflects the palpable beat of the arteries throughout the body as they expand in response to the contraction of the heart. With every beat, the heart pumps an amount of blood, known as the *stroke volume*, into the aorta. Arteries branch off of the aorta as it travels down through the center of the abdomen, transferring the pulse beat throughout the body. When the pulse is measured, an artery that is close to the body surface that can be pushed against a bone is used. Palpating a **peripheral** pulse gives the rate and rhythm of the heartbeat, as well as local information about the condition of the artery being used.

Pulse Sites

A pulse rate may be counted any place where an artery is near the surface of the body and the vessel can be pressed against a bone. The most common sites that are used to feel this rhythmic throbbing are at the following arteries: temporal, carotid, apical, brachial, radial, femoral, popliteal, and dorsalis pedis (Figure 30-4).

The *temporal* pulse is located at the temple area of the skull, parallel and lateral to the eyes (Figure 30-5). It is seldom used as a pulse site but may be used as a pressure point to assist in controlling bleeding from a head injury.

The *carotid* artery is located between the larynx and the sternocleidomastoid muscle in the front and to the side of the neck (Figure 30-6). It is most frequently used in emergencies and to check the pulse during cardiopulmonary resuscitation (CPR). It can be felt by pushing the muscle to the side and pressing against the larynx.

The *apical* heart rate, or the heartbeat at the apex of the heart, is heard with a stethoscope. It is often used for infants and young children or in adults if the radial pulse is difficult to feel or is irregular. An apical count may be requested if the patient is taking cardiac drugs or has either **bradycardia** or **tachycardia.** To determine the presence of a **pulse deficit,** the physician may listen to the apical beat while the medical assistant counts the pulse at another site. The apex of the heart is located in the left fifth intercostal space on the midclavicular line, that is, between the fifth and sixth ribs on a line with the midpoint of the left clavicle. The stethoscope is placed just below the left nipple between the fifth and sixth ribs. The pulse should be counted for 1 full minute and documented with an (AP) beside the recorded count (Procedure 30-4).

PROCEDURE 30-3

Obtain Vital Signs: Obtain an Axillary Temperature

CAAHEP COMPETENCY: 3.b.(4)(b)
ABHES COMPETENCY: 4.d

GOAL: *To accurately determine and record a patient's temperature using the axillary method.*

EQUIPMENT and SUPPLIES

- Digital unit
- Thermometer sheath or probe cover
- Supply of tissues
- Biohazard waste container
- Disposable gloves as appropriate
- Patient gown as needed
- Patient record

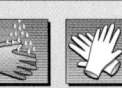

PROCEDURAL STEPS

1. Wash your hands.
   PURPOSE: Infection control.
2. Gather equipment and supplies.
3. Introduce yourself, identify your patient, and explain the procedure.
   PURPOSE: Identification of the patient prevents errors, and explanations are a means of gaining implied consent and patient cooperation.
4. Prepare the thermometer or digital unit in same manner as for oral use.
5. Remove the patient's clothing and gown the patient as needed to access the axillary region.

6. Pat the patient's axillary area dry if needed.
   PURPOSE: To ensure an accurate reading. Do not rub the area, because this may cause an elevated reading.
7. Cover the thermometer or probe and place the tip into the center of the armpit, pointing the stem toward the upper chest, making sure the thermometer is touching only skin, not clothing.
   PURPOSE: To obtain the most accurate axillary reading; contact with clothing will alter the reading.
8. Instruct the patient to hold the arm snugly across the chest or abdomen until the thermometer beeps.
   PURPOSE: Prevents air from leaking in and interfering with the temperature reading.
9. Remove the thermometer, note the digital reading, and dispose of the cover in the biohazard waste container
10. Disinfect the thermometer if indicated.
11. Wash your hands.
12. Record the axillary temperature on the patient's medical record (e.g., T = 97.6° [A]).
    PURPOSE: Procedures that are not recorded are considered not done.

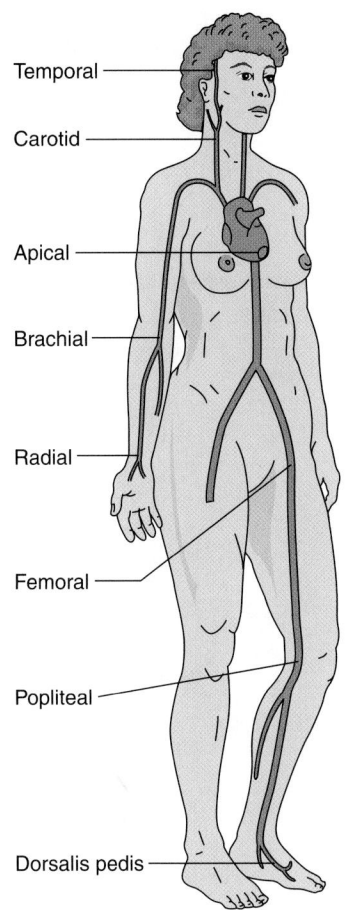

FIGURE 30-4 Pulse sites.

Temporal
Carotid
Apical
Brachial
Radial
Femoral
Popliteal
Dorsalis pedis

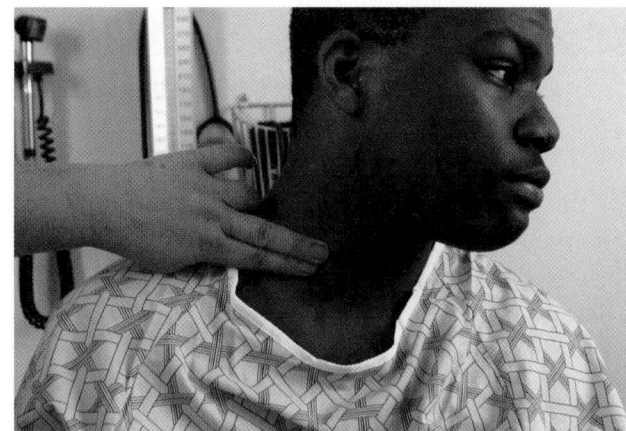

FIGURE 30-6 Carotid pulse.

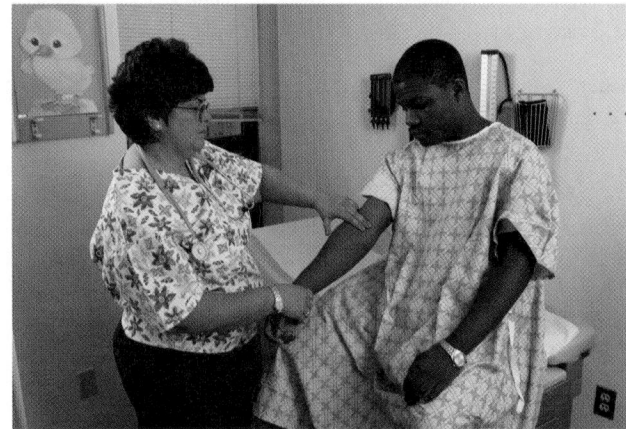

FIGURE 30-7 Brachial pulse.

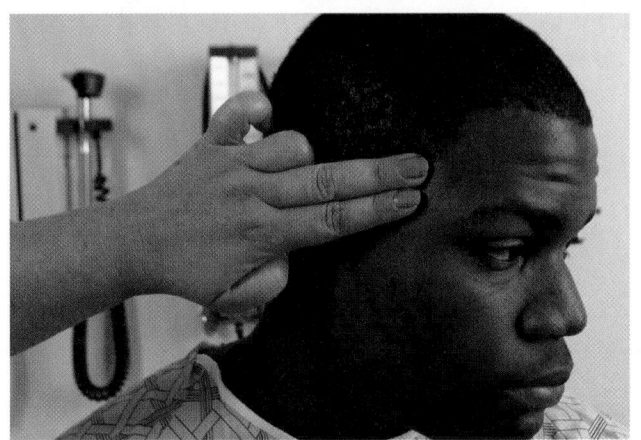

FIGURE 30-5 Temporal pulse.

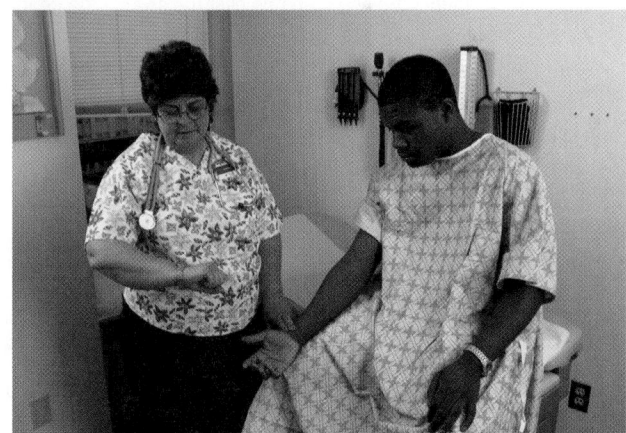

FIGURE 30-8 Radial pulse.

The *brachial* pulse is felt at the inner *(antecubital)* aspect of the elbow. It is the artery felt and heard when determining blood pressure (Figure 30-7). It can also be felt in the groove between the biceps and triceps muscles on the inner surface of the mid-upper arm. This is the pulse that is checked on infants and young children when performing CPR.

The *radial* artery is the most frequently used site for counting the pulse rate. It is best found on the thumb side of the wrist, 1 inch below the base of the thumb (Figure 30-8).

The *femoral* pulse is located at the site where the femoral artery passes through the groin. One must press deeply below the inguinal ligament to palpate this pulse.

The *popliteal* pulse is found at the back of the leg behind the knee. The patient must be in a recumbent position, with the knee slightly flexed, for this pulse to be palpated. The popliteal artery is deep and difficult to feel. This artery is palpated and listened to with the stethoscope when a leg blood pressure reading is necessary. The physician will check the blood flow

PROCEDURE 30-4

Obtain Vital Signs: Obtain an Apical Pulse

<u>CAAHEP COMPETENCY:</u> 3.b.(4)(b)
<u>ABHES COMPETENCY:</u> 4.d

GOAL: *To accurately determine and record the patient's apical heart rate.*

EQUIPMENT and SUPPLIES

- Watch with a second hand
- Stethoscope
- Alcohol wipes
- Patient gown as needed
- Patient record

PROCEDURAL STEPS

1. Wash your hands, and clean the stethoscope earpieces and diaphragm with alcohol swabs.
   <u>PURPOSE:</u> Infection control and standard precautions.
2. Introduce yourself, identify your patient, and explain the procedure.
   <u>PURPOSE:</u> Identification of the patient prevents errors, and explanations are a means of gaining implied consent and patient cooperation.
3. If necessary, assist the patient in disrobing from the waist up and provide the patient with a gown, open in the front.
   <u>PURPOSE:</u> To expose the chest and provide for patient privacy and warmth.
4. Assist the patient to the sitting or supine position.
   <u>PURPOSE:</u> Easier access to apical site at the apex of the heart.
5. Hold the stethoscope diaphragm against the palm of your hand for a few seconds.
   <u>PURPOSE:</u> Warms the diaphragm, promoting patient comfort.
6. Place the stethoscope just below the left nipple in the intercostal space between the fifth and sixth ribs over the apex of the heart (Figures 1 and 2).
   <u>PURPOSE:</u> This is the point of maximum contractile strength, where the heartbeat can be heard best.
7. Listen carefully for the heartbeat.
8. Count the pulse for 1 full minute. Note any irregularities in rhythm and volume.
   <u>PURPOSE:</u> The apical pulse is always measured for 1 full minute to determine the most accurate reading.
9. Assist the patient to sit up and dress.

10. Wash your hands.
11. Record the pulse in the patient chart as AP (e.g., AP = 96), and record any arrhythmias.

See Appendix D for a charting example.

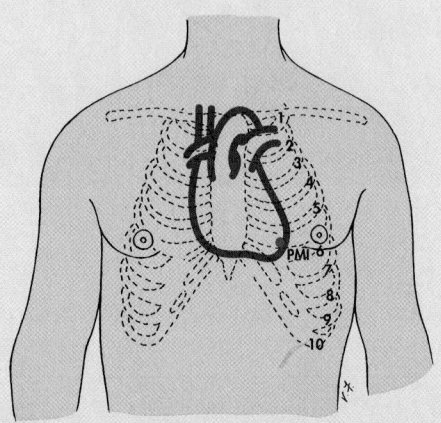

FIGURE 1

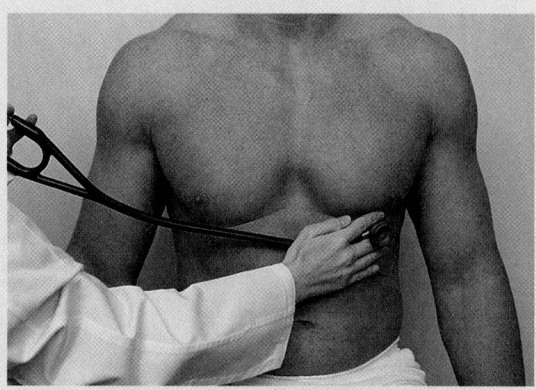

FIGURE 2

---

through the popliteal artery if a circulatory system problem, such as a blood clot, is suspected in the lower leg.

The *dorsalis pedis* (pedal) artery is felt across the arch of the foot, just slightly lateral to the midline, beside the extensor tendon of the great toe. This pulse may be congenitally absent in some patients. A good pulse rate at this site is an indicator of normal lower limb circulation and arterial sufficiency so pedal pulses are checked by the physician in patients with peripheral vascular problems such as those with diabetes mellitus.

Characteristics of Pulse

When you are measuring a pulse, there are three important characteristics to note: the rate, rhythm, and volume of the

pulse. These characteristics depend on the size and elasticity of the artery as well as the strength and regularity of the heart's contractions. A patient's pulse may reveal valuable information about the cardiovascular system.

Rate

The pulse rate is a measure of the number of heartbeats felt from the movement of blood through an artery. When the heart contracts, pressure throughout the arteries increases and the arteries expand. When the heart relaxes, arterial pressure decreases and the arteries relax. Each contraction and relaxation of the heart muscle is a heartbeat, and each resulting expansion and relaxation of the arteries is the pulse rate. Normally the heartbeat (rate) and pulse rate are the same. The rate of the pulse is the number of heartbeats (pulsations) that occur in 1 minute. Because the body must balance heat loss by increasing circulation (a faster heart rate), the pulse rate is proportionate to the size of heart the body. The smaller the body, the greater the heat loss and the faster the heart must pump to compensate. Therefore, infants and children normally have a faster pulse than do adults; as the aging process progresses, the pulse rate decreases.

Pulse rates normally vary as a result of a person's age, body size, gender, and health status. The rate is affected by an individual's activities, psychologic state, and certain medications and is usually faster in women (70 to 80 beats per minute) than in men (60 to 70 beats per minute). Children tend to have more rapid pulse rates than adults do. When a person is sitting, the rate is more rapid than when lying down, and it increases when an individual stands, walks, or runs. During sleep or rest, the pulse rate may drop as low as 45 to 50 beats per minute. Well-conditioned athletes tend to have pulse rates of 50 to 60 beats per minute because consistent aerobic exercise strengthens the heart muscle (the myocardium) so that each heart contraction is capable of ejecting an increased volume of blood into the arterial system. Table 30-3 lists the normal pulse ranges for various age groups of patients.

Rhythm

The pulse rhythm is the time between each pulse beat. A normal rhythm pattern has an even tempo, indicating that the time intervals between the beats are of equal duration. An abnormal rhythm, or **arrhythmia**, is described according to the rhythm pattern that is detected. An **intermittent pulse** may occur in healthy individuals during exercise or after drinking a beverage containing caffeine. A common irregularity found in children and young adults is **sinus arrhythmia**, in which the heart rate varies with the respiratory cycle, speeding up at the peak of inspiration and slowing to normal with expiration. If beats are frequently skipped or if the beats are markedly irregular, the physician should be advised, because this may indicate heart disease. If an irregular rhythm is detected, the apical pulse should be measured for a full minute to ensure accuracy, and the rate should be recorded for the physician's review. A note should also be made that the patient's pulse was irregular.

Volume

The volume (pulse amplitude) reflects the strength of the heart when it contracts. It can be assessed by feeling the strength

TABLE 30-3 Age-Related Pulse Ranges

AGE	APPROXIMATE RANGE	APPROXIMATE AVERAGE
Newborn	120-160	140
1-2 years	80-140	120
3-6 years	75-120	100
7-11 years	75-110	95
Adolescence to adulthood	60-100	80

Three-Point Scale for Measuring Pulse Volume

3+ = Full, bounding	Pulsation is very strong and does not disappear with moderate pressure.
2+ = Normal pulse	Pulsation is easily felt but disappears with moderate pressure.
1+ = Weak, thready	Pulsation is not easily felt, and slight pressure causes it to disappear.

of the pulse as the blood flows through the vessel. The force of each pulse beat is described as **bounding** or full; strong or normal; or **thready** or weak. The force of the heartbeat and the condition of the arterial wall, whether it is hard or soft, influence the volume. It is possible for the pulse to vary only in intensity and otherwise be perfectly regular. This condition can also indicate heart disease. The pulse force is recorded using a three-point scale.

Determining Pulse Rate

Radial, Brachial, and Apical

The patient should be in a comfortable position, with the artery to be used at the same level as or lower than the heart (Procedure 30-5). The limb should be well supported and relaxed. The patient may be lying down or sitting. As with all pulse readings, the pads of the first three fingers are placed over the artery. The thumb should never be used to determine the pulse rate, because the thumb has its own pulse and the medical assistant's pulse rate may be confused with the patient's. Push until the strongest pulsation is felt. The pulse should be counted for 1 full minute. The 15- or 30-second interval may be used once the medical assistant becomes proficient at performing the skill.

Variations from the normal quality, such as an arrhythmia or a pulse that is thready or bounding, should be noted. Some pulses are more difficult to feel than others, and the correct pressure to be used for each patient and site requires repeated practice and experience.

Both the medical assistant and the patient should be in relaxed positions. The sensitivity in your counting fingers is greatly reduced if you are in an awkward position. Too much pressure obliterates the patient's pulse, and too little pressure prevents detection of irregularities or of all of the beats. Record the number of beats in 1 minute. Assess the pulse, including rate, rhythm, and volume. If the pulse rate is counted at any site other than the radial, the rate should be recorded along with a notation of the site used.

CRITICAL THINKING APPLICATION

Mrs. Arnez has a documented thready pulse. What site should Carlos use to measure the pulse?

Femoral, Popliteal, and Pedal

Pulses in the lower extremities may be difficult to find and equally difficult to hear. A Doppler unit, which is an ultrasound unit that magnifies the pulsation, may be used to locate and

PROCEDURE 30-5

Obtain Vital Signs: Assess the Patient's Radial Pulse

CAAHEP COMPETENCY: 3.b.(4)(b)
ABHES COMPETENCY: 4.d

GOAL: *To accurately determine and record a patient's radial pulse rate, rhythm, and volume.*

EQUIPMENT and SUPPLIES

- Watch with a second hand
- Patient record

PROCEDURAL STEPS

1. Wash your hands.
   PURPOSE: Infection control.
2. Introduce yourself, identify your patient, and explain the procedure.
   PURPOSE: Identification of the patient prevents errors, and explanations are a means of gaining implied consent and patient cooperation.
3. Place the patient's arm in a relaxed position, palm downward, at or below the level of the heart.
   PURPOSE: The patient's radial artery is more easily palpated when the patient is relaxed and in this position.
4. Gently grasp the palm side of the patient's wrist with your first three fingertips approximately 1 inch below the base of the thumb (Figure 1).
   PURPOSE: This position puts your fingertips directly over the artery. Press firmly, but if you press too hard, you will occlude the artery and feel nothing.
5. Count the beats for 1 full minute, using a watch with a second hand.
   PURPOSE: Counting for 1 full minute allows you to obtain an

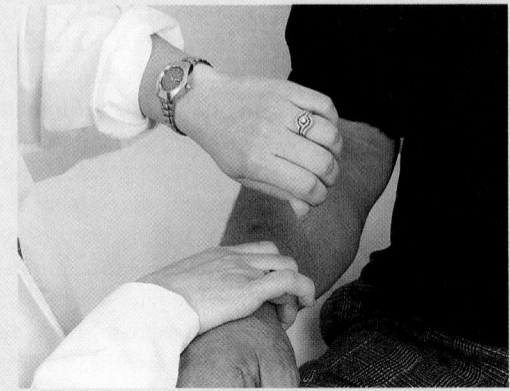

FIGURE 1

accurate count, including any irregularities in rhythm and volume.

6. Wash your hands.
   PURPOSE: Infection control.
7. Record the count and any irregularities on the patient's medical record (e.g., P = 72). Pulse is usually recorded immediately after temperature.
   PURPOSE: Procedures that are not recorded are considered not done.

*See Appendix D for a charting example.

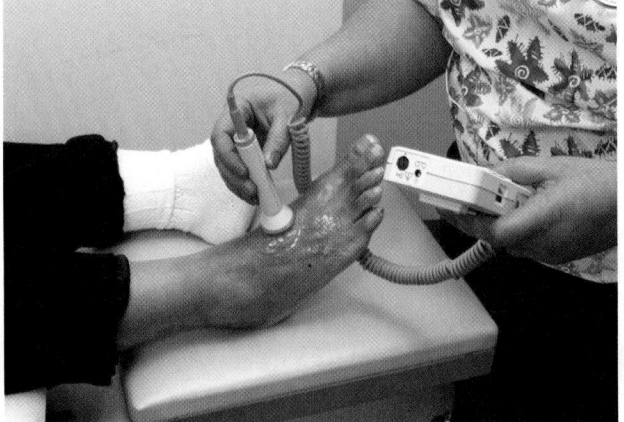

FIGURE 30-9 Doppler ultrasound unit measuring pedal pulse.

count these pulses accurately (Figure 30-9). This unit is battery operated and can be attached to a stethoscope so only you hear the beat, or it can be set so that both you and your patient can hear the pulsations.

RESPIRATION

Physiology

The purpose of respiration is to provide for the exchange of oxygen and carbon dioxide among the atmosphere, the blood, and the body cells. Oxygen is taken into the body to be used for life-sustaining body processes, and carbon dioxide is released as a waste product.

One complete inspiration and expiration is called a *respiration*. During the inspiration phase the diaphragm contracts, causing the lungs to expand and fill with air. During the expiration phase the diaphragm returns to its normal, elevated position, causing the lungs to expel the waste air back into the atmosphere.

Respiration is both internal and external. *External respiration* is the exchange of oxygen and carbon dioxide in the lungs. *Internal respiration* occurs at the cellular level, when oxygen in the bloodstream is transferred into the cells for energy and carbon dioxide is released as a waste product, then transported back to the lungs for exhalation.

When there is a buildup of carbon dioxide in the blood, a message is sent to the medulla oblongata, which is located in the brain between the top of the spine and the brainstem. This respiratory control center sends a message that triggers respiration. Therefore, respiration is controlled by the involuntary nervous system; this means we breathe automatically. Because a person can control respiration to a certain extent, it is also a voluntary body function. However, breathing is ultimately under the control of the medulla oblongata, which is why we can hold our breath only for a given length of time. Once the blood carbon dioxide level increases to the point at which cells become oxygen starved, a stimulus is sent and breathing begins involuntarily.

Characteristics of Respirations

Normally a person's breathing is relaxed, automatic, and silent. When determining the respiratory rate of a patient, you must note three important characteristics: rate, rhythm, and depth.

- *Rate.* The rate of respiration is the number of respirations per minute and is described as normal, rapid, or slow. Figure 30-10 shows sample rate patterns as recorded using a **spirometer. Dyspnea** occurs in patients with pneumonia, asthma, or **chronic obstructive pulmonary disease (COPD).** It also occurs after physical exertion or at very high altitudes. Other alterations in breathing are **bradypnea, apnea, tachypnea,** and **hyperpnea.** Hyperpnea is usually accompanied by **hyperventilation** and is often found when the patient is extremely anxious or in pain. **Orthopnea** frequently occurs in patients with congestive heart failure (CHF) and COPD. There is typically a ratio of four pulse beats to one respiration. As a rule, both pulse and respiration rates respond to exercise or emotional upsets. Table 30-4 lists normal respiratory ranges for various age groups of patients.

TABLE 30-4 Age-Related Respiration Ranges

AGE	APPROXIMATE RANGE	APPROXIMATE AVERAGE
Newborn	30-50	40
1-3 years	20-30	25
4-6 years	18-26	22
7-11 years	16-22	19
Adolescence to adulthood	12-20	16

- *Rhythm. Rhythm* refers to the breathing pattern. A regular breathing pattern is normal in adults; however, the breathing pattern for infants varies. Automatic interruptions, such as sighing, are also considered normal.
- *Depth.* The *depth of respiration* refers to the amount of air being inhaled and exhaled. When a patient is at rest, normal respirations have a consistent depth, which can be noted as you watch the rise and fall of the chest. Rapid, shallow breathing at rest occurs with some disease states, such as asthma and emphysema.

Normally no noticeable breath sounds occur during the breathing process; the exception is snoring. Noticeable breath sounds are a sign of certain diseases, such as pneumonia, asthma, and pulmonary edema. Descriptive characteristics for breath sounds are indicated with specific terminology (e.g., **rales, rhonchi,** and **stertorous** breathing) by the physician.

When an individual cannot inspire enough oxygen to supply all of the body's cells with oxygenated blood, the normal skin coloring, particularly around the mouth and the nail beds, turns a bluish, dusky color. This coloration, which represents the increased level of carbon dioxide present in the blood, is called *cyanosis.* The patient may display other signs and symptoms including **vertigo,** chest pain *(angina),* and numbness in the fingers and toes.

Counting Respirations

Because most people are unaware of their breathing, do not mention that you will be counting the respirations (Procedure 30-6). The respiratory rate is easily controlled, and patients self-consciously alter their breathing rates when they are being watched. Therefore, count the respirations while appearing to count the pulse. Keep your eyes alternately on the patient's chest and your watch while you are counting the pulse rate, and then, without removing your fingers from the pulse site, determine the respiration rate. It may be easier to count the respirations first, because that number is not as hard to remember (Figure 30-11). If the patient is lying supine, the arm may be crossed over the chest so the respirations can be felt with the rise and fall of the chest. Another way of observing respirations is to watch the movement of the patient's shoulders with each inspiration. Count the respirations for 30 seconds and multiply the number by 2. Avoid using the 15-second interval, because this count can vary by a factor of +4 or −4, which is significant when dealing with such a small number. Note any variation or irregularity in the rate. Record the respiration count on the medical record.

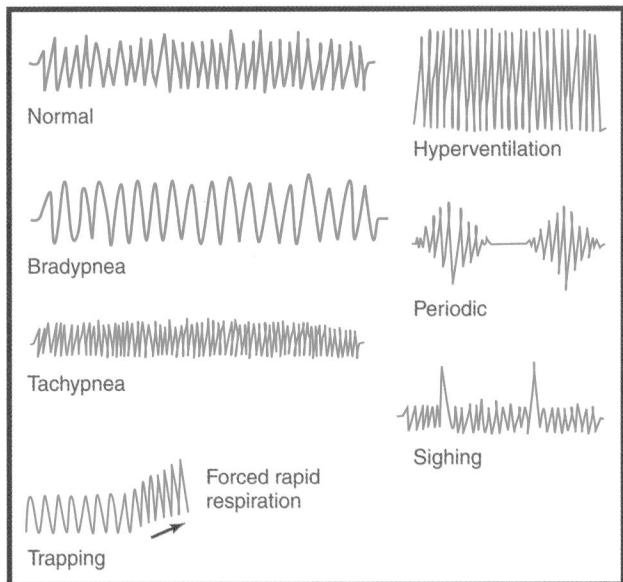

FIGURE 30-10 Respiration rate patterns, called *spirograms*, which are recorded using a spirometer.

PROCEDURE 30-6

Obtain Vital Signs: Determine Respirations

CAAHEP COMPETENCY: 3.b.(4)(b)
ABHES COMPETENCY: 4.d

GOAL: *To accurately determine and record a patient's respirations. Remember that the respiration count may be altered if the patient is aware that you are counting his or her breaths. Respirations are typically counted immediately after taking the pulse while fingers are still at the radial site.*

EQUIPMENT and SUPPLIES

- Watch with a second hand
- Patient record

PROCEDURAL STEPS

1. Wash your hands.
   PURPOSE: Infection control.
2. Identify your patient.
   PURPOSE: Identification of the patient prevents errors.
3. The patient's arm will be in the same position as when counting the pulse. If having difficulty noticing breathing, place the arm across the chest to pick up movement.
   PURPOSE: This position allows you to feel or see the rise and fall of the chest wall.
4. Note the rise and fall of the patient's chest.

   PURPOSE: Inspiration and expiration make up one complete breathing cycle or respiration.
5. Count the respirations for 30 seconds, using a watch with a second hand, and multiply by 2.
   PURPOSE: Counting for 30 seconds allows you to obtain an accurate count and determine any irregularities in rhythm or depth or unusual breathing patterns. If respirations are abnormal in any way, count for 1 full minute.
6. Release the patient's wrist.
7. Wash your hands.
   PURPOSE: Infection control.
8. Record the respirations on the patient's medical record after the pulse recording (e.g., R = 18).
   PURPOSE: Procedures that are not recorded are considered not done.

*See Appendix D for a charting example.

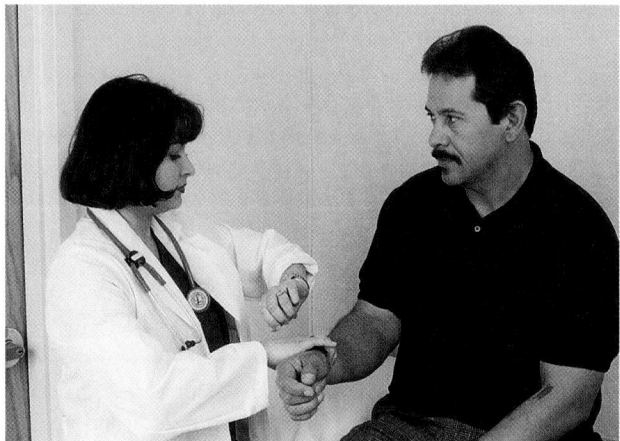

FIGURE 30-11 Hand position when counting respirations. The hands should be left in place as if still counting the patient's pulse.

CRITICAL THINKING APPLICATION

Tina Anderson, a 36-year-old obese patient, is wearing a heavy knit sweater and Carlos needs to obtain a respiration count. What could he do to accurately record Tina's respiration count?

BLOOD PRESSURE

Blood pressure is a reflection of the pressure of the blood against the walls of the arteries. Each time the ventricles contract, blood is pushed out of the heart and into the aorta, exerting pressure on the walls of the arteries. There are actually two blood pressure

TABLE 30-5 Age-Related Blood Pressure Ranges	
AGE	**APPROXIMATE RANGE**
Newborn	60-96/30-62
1-3 years	78-112/48-78
4-6 years	78-112/50-79
7-11 years	85-114/52-79
Adolescent	94-119/58-79
Adult	100-119/60-79

readings: the *systolic* pressure is the highest pressure level that occurs when the heart is contracting and the pulse beat is first heard, and the *diastolic* pressure is the lowest pressure level when the heart is relaxed and the last sound is heard. Systole (heart contraction) and diastole (heart relaxation) together make up the cardiac cycle. The difference between the systolic and diastolic pressures is the **pulse pressure.**

Blood pressure is read in millimeters of mercury, abbreviated *mm Hg*. However, the abbreviations do not have to be included when you document the reading on the patient's medical record. Blood pressure is recorded as a fraction, with the systolic reading the numerator (top) and the diastolic reading the denominator (bottom) (e.g., 130/80). Table 30-5 lists the normal blood pressure ranges for various age groups of patients.

Factors Affecting Blood Pressure

The physiologic factors that determine blood pressure include blood volume, peripheral resistance created by blood viscosity (the thickness of the blood), vessel elasticity, and the condition of the heart muscle and the arterial walls.

Volume is the amount of blood in the arteries. An increased blood volume raises the blood pressure, and a decreased blood volume lowers the blood pressure. Therefore if extensive bleeding or hemorrhage occurs, the blood volume drops and so does the blood pressure.

Peripheral resistance of blood vessels refers to the relationship of the lumen or diameter of the vessel and the amount of blood flowing through it. The smaller the lumen, the greater the resistance to blood flow. Blood pressure is higher with a small or reduced-size lumen and lower with a large lumen. Vessels affected by fatty cholesterol deposits called *atherosclerotic plaques* become narrower over time, resulting in smaller vessel lumens and higher blood pressure levels.

Vessel elasticity is an artery's ability to expand and contract to supply the body with a steady flow of blood. With age, lifestyle factors, or the presence of arteriosclerosis, vessel elasticity may decrease, causing the arterial walls to become firm and resistant; as a result, blood pressure will increase.

The condition of the myocardium is of primary importance to the volume of blood flowing through the body. A strong, forceful contraction empties the heart and tends to keep the blood pressure within normal limits. If the myocardium becomes weak, pressure in the vessels begins to increase in an attempt to maintain an adequate level of circulating blood to meet the oxygen and nutrient needs of the body.

Evaluating Blood Pressure

When a patient's blood pressure is being tracked, frequent readings should be taken at about the same time of day and by the same person. **Secondary hypertension** is caused by another underlying pathologic condition, such as renal disease, complications of pregnancy, endocrine imbalances, obesity, arteriosclerosis, atherosclerosis, and brain injuries. Temporary hypertension may occur with stress, pain, exercise, and exhaustion. Many patients experience white-coat **hypertension**: their blood pressure becomes elevated in the medical environment, although it is normal away from the healthcare facility. An adult is diagnosed with **essential hypertension** (primary hypertension) with a systolic pressure of 140 mm Hg or higher and/or a diastolic pressure of 90 mm Hg or higher. Essential hypertension is the most common type of hypertension. It has no single identified cause but is associated with obesity, a high blood level of sodium, elevated cholesterol levels, and family history.

In 2003 the American Heart Association (AHA) published new guidelines for the diagnosis and management of hypertension. For the first time a new category of blood pressure,

prehypertension, was identified, and normal blood pressure levels were lowered to less than 120/80. Table 30-6 identifies the categories of normal, prehypertensive, and hypertensive blood pressures.

The goal of the new recommendations is to decrease the number of people who die each year from hypertension-related illnesses such as coronary artery disease, which leads to heart attacks, heart failure, kidney disease, and strokes. Hypertension can occur in children or adults, but those of African American descent, middle-aged and elderly people, those with diabetes, and those with kidney disease are at greatest risk. Hypertension has been called the "silent killer," because it frequently has no symptoms and individuals may go for long periods without knowing that they have a problem. Often hypertension is discovered during the medical treatment of another problem. Signs and symptoms may include blurred vision, angina, vertigo, dyspnea, fatigue, headaches, flushing, nosebleeds or *epistaxis,* and palpitations. The revised treatment guidelines have four basic aspects:

1. Diagnose individuals with prehypertension, and encourage lifestyle changes before they require medical treatment and/ or move into the hypertensive category. The AHA recommends limiting the intake of salt and eating a diet rich in potassium, calcium, magnesium, and protein while decreasing total fat intake, especially saturated fat and cholesterol. Prehypertensive individuals should also restrict their alcohol intake, engage in regular physical activity, and lose weight if necessary to maintain a healthy BMI range. Many times just losing weight lowers blood pressure readings.

2. Systolic pressures are more important than diastolic readings in people over the age of 50. Individuals over 50 should be treated if they have a systolic pressure of 140 mm Hg or greater regardless of their diastolic blood pressure level. Medical treatment at this age can result in less cardiac and kidney disease later in life.

3. Most hypertensive patients will require two or more antihypertensive medications to achieve desired blood pressure levels. The goal of treatment is to maintain blood pressures below 140/90 mm Hg, or less than 130/80 mm Hg in patients with diabetes or kidney disease. Most patients will require a combination of diuretics to help the body excrete excess amounts of fluid and sodium as well as a form of antihypertensive medication.

4. Implement a patient-centered treatment approach to motivate patients and gain compliance with hypertension management. The medical assistant can play an active role in establishing a therapeutic relationship with the patient by providing ongoing education and support to maintain compliance with physician-recommended treatment.

TABLE 30-6 Hypertension Categories			
BLOOD PRESSURE	**NORMAL**	**PREHYPERTENSION**	**HYPERTENSION**
Systolic (mm Hg)	Less than 120	120-139	140 or higher
Diastolic (mm Hg)	Less than 80	80-89	90 or higher

CRITICAL THINKING APPLICATION

Mr. Samuel Long is a 43-year-old patient who was recently diagnosed with essential hypertension. What should Carlos discuss with Mr. Long to emphasize the dangers of his disease and to educate him about possible lifestyle modifications he needs to initiate to improve his health? Are there any community resources that might help Mr. Long and his family effectively manage his disease?

Hypotension is abnormally low blood pressure and may be caused by emotional or traumatic shock; hemorrhage; central nervous system disorders; and chronic wasting diseases. Persistent readings of 90/60 mm Hg or below are usually considered hypotensive. **Orthostatic (postural) hypotension** can cause patients to experience vertigo or **syncope.** Some medications can cause orthostatic hypotension.

Measuring Blood Pressure

The instrument used to measure blood pressure is called the *sphygmomanometer.* The term *manometer* refers to an instrument used to measure the pressure of a liquid or a gas. *Sphygmo-* means pulse. Therefore *sphygmomanometer* means an instrument used for measuring blood pressure in the arteries. The instrument consists of an inflatable cuff, an inflation bulb with a control valve, and a pressure gauge. The blood pressure mechanism consists of an aneroid dial attached to an inflatable cuff (Figure 30-12, *A)* or a floor model with a large angled face (Figure 30-12, *B).*

Sphygmomanometers are delicately calibrated instruments and must be handled carefully. They should be recalibrated regularly and checked for accuracy, either by you or by a medical supply dealer. The needle on the aneroid dial sphygmomanometer should rest within the small square or circle at the bottom of the dial. The dial can be calibrated by connecting it to a calibrated manometer. Pump both manometers to 250 mm Hg and record readings on both machines at least four different times as the pressure is released. A correctly calibrated mechanism shows no more than a 3–mm Hg difference between the two readings at any time during the deflation period. If the sphygmomanometer is not correctly calibrated, the patient's blood pressure reading will be inaccurate.

The sphygmomanometer must be used with a stethoscope. The objective of the procedure is to use the inflatable cuff to obliterate (cause to disappear) circulation through an artery. The stethoscope is placed over the artery just below the cuff, then the cuff is slowly deflated to allow the blood to flow again. As blood flow resumes, cardiac cycle sounds are heard through the stethoscope, and gauge readings are taken when the first (systolic) and the last (diastolic) sounds are heard (Procedure 30-7).

Blood pressure cuffs and stethoscopes are available in drug stores and retail stores for patients to use to measure their own blood pressure at home. These units can be aneroid, electronic, or computerized sphygmomanometers (Figure 30-13). If you have patients who are monitoring their pressures at home, be sure that they understand the mechanics of accurately obtaining a reading. It is best to have the patient bring his or her equipment

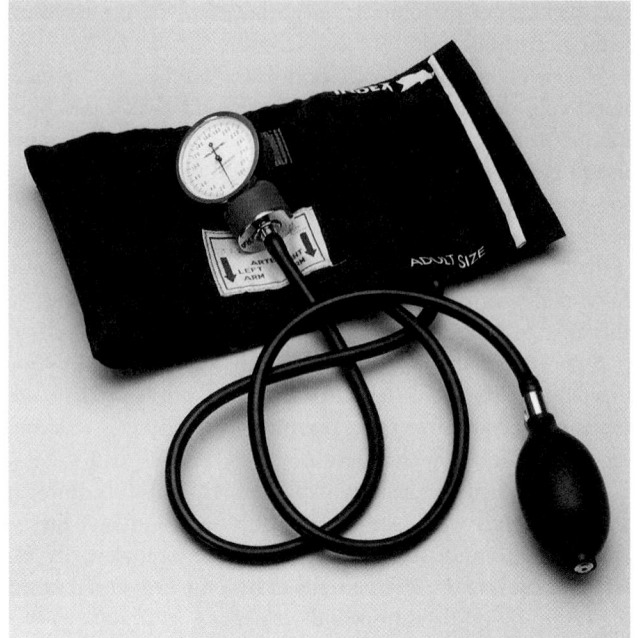

A

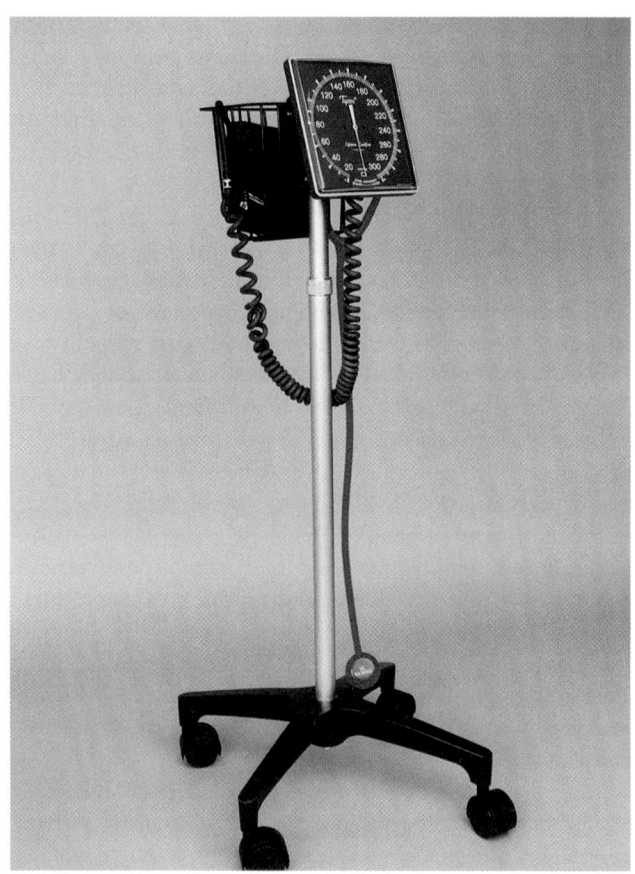

B

FIGURE 30-12 A, Aneroid dial system, with inflatable cuff. **B,** Aneroid floor model, with a large slanted face.

to the office and demonstrate its use. While the patient is showing you the home equipment, you will have an ideal time to check technique and calibration and answer any questions the patient might have regarding the use of the equipment. This is

PROCEDURE 30-7

Obtain Vital Signs: Determine a Patient's Blood Pressure

<u>CAAHEP COMPETENCY:</u> 3.b.(4)(b)
<u>ABHES COMPETENCY:</u> 4.d

GOAL: *To perform a blood pressure measurement that is correct in technique, accurate, and comfortable for the patient.*

EQUIPMENT and SUPPLIES

- Sphygmomanometer
- Stethoscope
- Antiseptic wipes
- Patient record

PROCEDURAL STEPS

1. Wash your hands.
   <u>PURPOSE:</u> Infection control.
2. Assemble the equipment and supplies needed. Clean the earpieces and diaphragm of the stethoscope with alcohol swabs.
   <u>PURPOSE:</u> Standard Precautions.
3. Introduce yourself, identify the patient, and explain the procedure.
   <u>PURPOSE:</u> Identification of the patient prevents errors, and explanations are a means of gaining implied consent and patient cooperation.
4. Select the appropriate arm for application of the cuff (no mastectomy on that side, without injury or disease).
   <u>PURPOSE:</u> The pressure of the cuff will temporarily interfere with circulation to the limb.
5. Seat the patient in a comfortable position with legs uncrossed and the arm resting at heart level on the lap or a table with the palm upward.
   <u>PURPOSE:</u> To promote patient relaxation and ensure obtaining a true reading. Crossed legs may increase the blood pressure, and the arm above the heart level may cause an inaccurate reading. This position exposes the brachial artery.
6. Roll up the sleeve to about 5 inches above the elbow, or have the patient remove his or her arm from the sleeve.
   <u>PURPOSE:</u> Tight clothing interferes with an accurate reading.
7. Determine the correct cuff size (Figure 1).

<u>PURPOSE:</u> An incorrect cuff size prevents accurate measurement of blood pressure. The cuff should fit comfortably around the patient's arm, and the bladder should be located over the brachial artery between the lines designated on the cuff.

8. Palpate the brachial artery at the antecubital space in both arms. If one arm has a stronger pulse, use that arm. If the pulses are equal, select the right arm (Figure 2).
   <u>PURPOSE:</u> A stronger pulse is easier to measure; the right arm is the universal arm of choice.
9. Center the cuff bladder over the brachial artery, with the connecting tube away from the patient's body and the tube to the bulb close to the body (Figure 3).
   <u>PURPOSE:</u> Pressure must be applied directly over the artery for an accurate reading. The cuff and its tubing should not touch the stethoscope. Noise from the tubing can interfere with a correct reading.

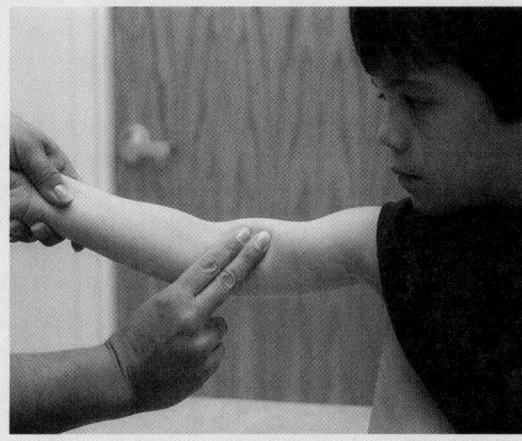

FIGURE 2

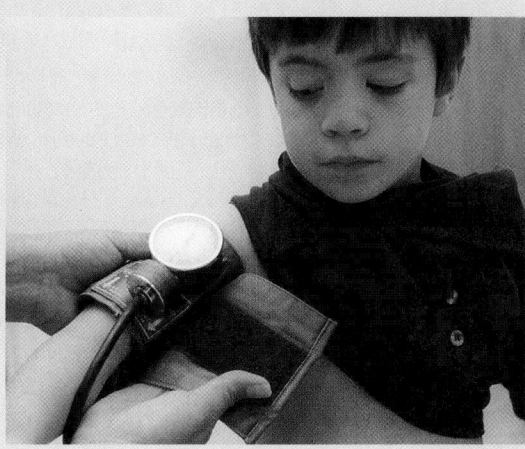

FIGURE 1

FIGURE 3

Continued

PROCEDURE 30-7—cont'd

10. Place the lower edge of the cuff about 1 inch above the palpable brachial pulse, normally located in the natural crease of the inner elbow, and wrap it snugly and smoothly.
    PURPOSE: This helps ensure an accurate reading. The cuff should be high enough on the arm that the stethoscope does not touch it, so that cuff sounds do not interfere with listening to the blood pressure sounds. A loose cuff results in an inaccurate reading.

11. Position the gauge of the sphygmomanometer so that it is easily seen.
    PURPOSE: An aneroid gauge should show the needle within the zero mark.

12. Palpate the brachial pulse, tighten the screw valve on the air pump, and inflate the cuff until the pulse can no longer be felt. Make a note at the point on the gauge where the pulse could no longer be felt. Mentally add 30 mm Hg to the reading. Deflate the cuff, and wait for 15 seconds.
    PURPOSE: The point where the brachial pulse is no longer felt provides an estimate of the systolic pressure. Pumping the cuff above that level assures that phase I of the Korotkoff sounds will be heard.

13. Insert the earpieces of the stethoscope turned forward into the ear canals.
    PURPOSE: With the earpieces in this position, the openings follow the anatomic line of the ear canal and the blood pressure will be accurately heard.

14. Place the stethoscope bell or diaphragm over the palpated brachial artery firmly enough to obtain a seal, but not so tightly that you constrict the artery.
    PURPOSE: The bell magnifies the low-pitched sounds better than the diaphragm and also forms a better seal.

15. Close the valve, and squeeze the bulb to inflate the cuff at a rapid but smooth rate to 30 mm above the palpated pulse level, which was previously determined (Figure 4).

16. Open the valve slightly, and deflate the cuff at the constant rate of 2 to 3 mm Hg per heartbeat.
    PURPOSE: Careful, slow release allows you to listen to all of the sounds.

17. Listen throughout the entire deflation; note the point on the gauge at which you hear the first sound (systolic) and the last sound (diastolic) until the sounds have stopped for at least 10 mm Hg. Read the pressure to the closest even number.

18. Do not reinflate the cuff once the air has been released. Wait 30 to 60 seconds to repeat the procedure if needed.

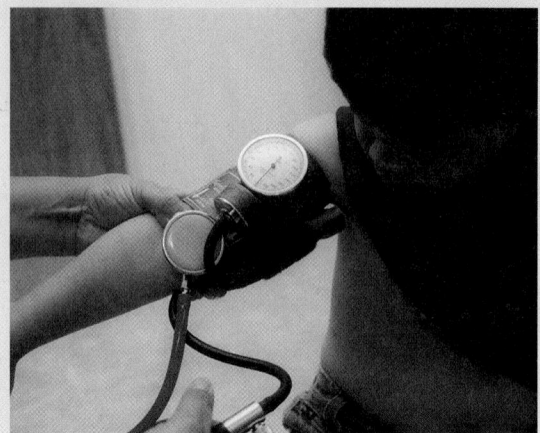

FIGURE 4

PURPOSE: Not permitting the blood to refill in the brachial artery will result in inaccurate readings.

19. Remove the stethoscope from your ears, and record the systolic and diastolic readings as BP systolic/diastolic (e.g., BP 120/80).
    NOTE: It is recommended that the blood pressure be checked and recorded in each arm during the initial assessment of the patient and then periodically after that for patients with hypertension.

20. Remove the cuff from the patient's arm and return it to its proper storage area. Clean the earpieces of the stethoscope with alcohol and return it to storage.

21. Wash your hands.
    PURPOSE: Infection control.
    ADDENDUM: The physician may direct the medical assistant to record patient blood pressure in two different positions to determine the presence of orthostatic hypotension. To perform this skill:
    • Measure and record the patient's blood pressure (as detailed earlier) while the patient is either supine or sitting.
    • Leave the cuff in place.
    • Have the patient stand, and immediately measure the blood pressure again.
    • Record the second blood pressure as well as any patient symptoms, such as complaints of (c/o) vertigo or light-headedness.

See Appendix D for a charting example.

---

also a good opportunity to reinforce treatment plans, such as medication, diet, and exercise. It is helpful for a patient who is monitoring blood pressure readings at home to keep a log and review it with the physician during visits to help detect blood pressure variations during normal daily activities.

Heart Sounds

There are two basic heart sounds produced by the functioning of the heart during the cardiac cycle. The first sound, produced at systole (contraction), is dull, firm, and prolonged and is heard as a *lubb* sound. The second sound, produced at diastole (relaxation), is shorter and sharper and is heard as a *dupp* sound. Therefore *lubb-dupp* is the sound of one heartbeat.

Korotkoff sounds are the sounds heard during the measurement of the blood pressure. These sounds are produced by the vibrations of the arterial wall when the blood surges back into the vessel after it has been compressed by the blood pressure cuff. The sounds were first discovered and classified

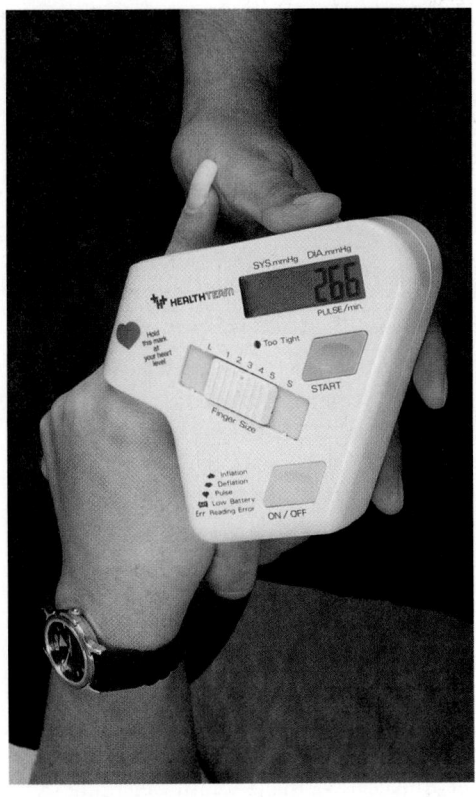

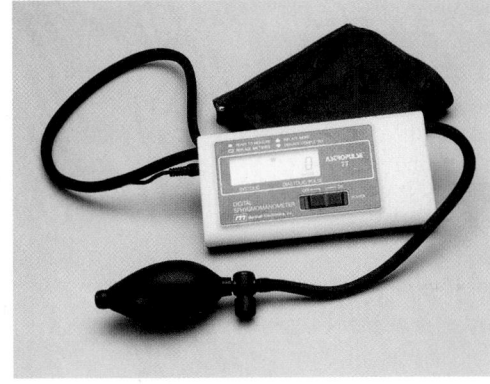

A

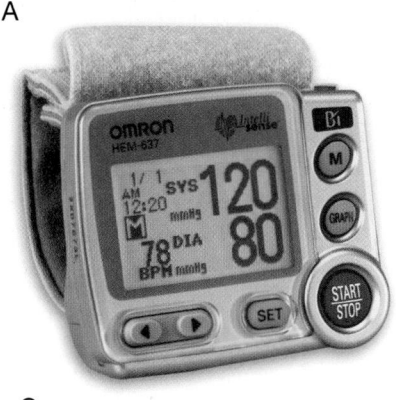

B   C

FIGURE 30-13 Personal blood pressure systems. **A,** Home system finger cuff. **B,** Digital blood pressure home system arm cuff. **C,** Wrist cuff. (**C,** Courtesy Omron Healthcare, Inc.)

into five distinct phases by Nikolai Sergeyevich Korotkoff, a Russian neurologist.

Phase I

Phase I is the first sound heard as the cuff deflates. The blood is resurging into the patient's artery and can be heard quite clearly as a sharp, tapping sound. Note the gauge reading when this first sound is heard. Record this as the systolic pressure.

Phase II

As the cuff deflates, even more blood flows through the artery. The movement of the blood makes a swishing sound. If you do not follow proper procedure in inflating the cuff, you may not hear these sounds because of their soft quality. Occasionally blood pressure sounds completely disappear during this phase. The loss of the sounds and their reappearance later is called the *auscultatory gap.* The silence may continue as the needle falls another 30 mm Hg. Auscultatory gaps occur particularly in hypertension and certain heart diseases, so if you notice such a gap, be certain to report it to the physician.

Phase III

A great deal of blood is now pushing down into the artery. The distinct, sharp tapping sounds return and continue rhythmically. If you do not inflate the cuff enough, you will miss the first two phases completely and you will incorrectly interpret the beginning of phase III as the systolic blood pressure (phase I).

Phase IV

At this point the blood is flowing easily. The sound changes to a soft tapping, which becomes muffled and begins to grow fainter. Occasionally these sounds continue to zero. This may occur in children, in patients of any age after exercise or with a fever, or in pregnant patients if anemia is present. The AHA recommends that the beginning of phase IV be recorded as the diastolic reading for a child. Some physicians call the change at phase IV the *fading sound* and want it recorded between the systolic and the diastolic recordings (e.g., 120/84/70, with the 84 representing the gauge reading when the sounds of phase III have ended and those of phase IV are beginning). Other physicians consider phase IV the true diastolic pressure.

Phase V

All sounds disappear in this phase. Note the gauge reading when the last sound is heard. Record this as the diastolic pressure.

Palpatory Method

The systolic pressure may be checked by feeling the radial pulse rather than hearing it with the stethoscope. Place the cuff in the usual position and palpate the radial pulse, noting the rate and rhythm. Inflate the cuff until the pulse disappears, and then add 30 mm Hg more of inflation to get above the systolic pressure. Do not remove your fingers from the pulse or change the pressure of your fingers. Then slowly release the pressure in the cuff and wait for the pulse to be felt again. Note

Common Causes of Errors in Blood Pressure Readings

- The limb being used is not at the same level as the heart.
- The rubber bladder in the cuff has not been completely deflated before a reading is started or retaken.
- The pressure in the cuff is released too rapidly, resulting in an inaccurate reading.
- The patient is nervous, uncomfortable, or anxious, which may cause a reading higher than the patient's actual blood pressure.
- The patient drank coffee or smoked cigarettes within 30 minutes of the elevation.
- The cuff is improperly applied.
- The cuff is too large, too small, too loose, or too tight.
- The cuff is not placed around the arm smoothly.
- The bladder is not centered over the artery, or it bulges out from the cover.
- The practitioner has failed to wait 1 to 2 minutes between measurements.
- Instruments are defective:
  - Air leaks in the valve
  - Air leaks in the bladder
  - Aneroid needle that is not calibrated to zero

Occupational Safety and Health Administration Guidelines for Measuring Vital Signs

- Wash hands before and after each procedure.
- Always use protective disposable sheaths on all forms of thermometers.
- Immediately disinfect any equipment that has become contaminated during the procedure.
- Wear gloves if the potential exists for contacting any open areas or body fluids.
- When caring for a patient with a known respiratory infectious disorder, such as tuberculosis, use protective clothing, including a face shield or mask as indicated.
- Dispose of all contaminated material, including thermometer covers, gloves, and disinfectant swabs, in the proper biohazard waste containers.

the reading on the gauge, and record the first pulse felt as the systolic pressure. For example, if you first felt the radial pulse at 52 mm Hg, the palpated blood pressure is recorded as 52/P, with P indicating that the systolic reading was palpated. The diastolic and the Korotkoff phases cannot be determined by this method. This method can be very useful in times of a medical emergency, such as shock, when the patient's blood pressure cannot be auscultated.

CRITICAL THINKING APPLICATION

Vital signs are documented with temperature (T) first, pulse (P) second, and respirations (R) last, with the blood pressure recorded after the TPR. Correctly document the following vital signs:

1. Oral temperature of 101.2°, apical pulse of 90, respirations 22, and orthostatic blood pressure of 138/88 supine and 110/70 standing
2. Tympanic temperature of 36.8°, radial pulse of 66, respirations 18, and bilateral blood pressure of 128/76 in the left arm and 132/80 in the right arm
3. Axillary temperature of 97.7°, carotid pulse of 58, respirations 24, and palpated blood pressure of 62

ANTHROPOMETRIC MEASUREMENT

Anthropometry is the science that deals with the measurement of the size, weight, and proportions of the human body. These measurements are often included in the initial recording of vital signs and before the physician conducts a physical examination or does a well-baby check. Because they are indicators of the state of health and well-being of a patient, the measurements of height and weight and associated BMI are discussed as part

of the vital signs. Other measurements are discussed when pertinent in the specialty chapters.

Measuring Weight and Height

A patient's weight and height can be helpful in diagnosis, and the medical assistant must determine these readings with accuracy and empathy (Procedure 30-8). Weight and height are often routinely measured in many medical settings as the patient is being escorted to the examination room. If this is the patient's first visit, the anthropometric measurements will be written in the history database and used as reference information during future visits as needed. Many physicians are now using BMI levels to determine risk for certain diseases, so the medical assistant may have to use measured height and weight to determine the patient's BMI level as discussed in Chapter 29.

Certain medical specialties and specific medical problems may require continuous monitoring of weight. Hormone disorders (e.g., diabetes), growth patterns (seen in children), and eating disorders (e.g., obesity and bulimia) necessitate accurate weight checks as part of every medical visit. In addition, maternity patients and heart patients with fluid retention also need weight monitoring. Some scales are calibrated in kilograms, whereas others are in pounds. When it is necessary to convert a weight, use the formulas shown later in the chapter.

Weight

Some patients are sensitive or secretive about their body weight, so the scale should be located in an area that provides privacy from staff and other patients. Your manner and approach are very important in keeping patients from feeling embarrassed or shy. As explained in Chapter 29, healthcare specialists are depending more on BMI ratios than on traditional height and weight tables, but there still must be an accurate measurement of height and weight to accurately determine a patient's BMI. If patients are unstable, assist them onto the scale and help them to balance themselves. A walker can be placed over the scale for the patient to use as hand support when getting on or off or to balance on the scale (Figure 30-14).

PROCEDURE 30-8

Obtain Vital Signs: Measure a Patient's Weight and Height

<u>CAAHEP COMPETENCY:</u> 3.b.(4)(b)
<u>ABHES COMPETENCY:</u> 4.d

GOAL: *To accurately weigh and measure a patient as part of the physical assessment procedure.*
<u>NOTE:</u> Be sure the scale is located in an area away from traffic to maintain patient privacy.

EQUIPMENT and SUPPLIES

- Balance scale with a measuring bar
- Patient record

PROCEDURAL STEPS

1. Wash your hands.
   <u>PURPOSE:</u> Infection control.
2. Identify your patient, and explain the procedure.
   <u>PURPOSE:</u> Identification of the patient prevents errors, and explanations are a means of gaining implied consent and patient cooperation.
3. If the patient is to remove his or her shoes for weighing, place a paper towel on the scale platform. The patient may be given disposable slippers to wear.
4. Check to see that the balance bar pointer floats in the middle of the balance frame when all weights are at zero.
   <u>PURPOSE:</u> A floating pointer indicates that the scale is properly adjusted and in balance.
5. Help the patient onto the scale. Make certain that the female patient is not holding a purse and that the male or female patient has removed any heavy objects from pockets.
6. Move the large weight into the groove closest to the estimated weight of the patient. The grooves are calibrated in 50-lb

increments. If you choose a groove that is more than the patient's weight, the pointer will immediately tilt to the bottom of the balance frame. You then must move it back one groove (Figure 1).

7. While the patient is standing still, slide the small upper weight to the right along the pound markers until the pointer balances in the middle of the balance frame.
   <u>PURPOSE:</u> The pointer will float between the bottom and the top of the frame when both lower and upper weights together balance the scale with the patient's weight.
8. Leave the weights in place.
9. Ask the patient to stand up straight and to look straight ahead. On some scales the patient may need to turn with the back to the scale.
10. Adjust the height bar so that it just touches the top of the patient's head (Figure 2).
11. Leave the elevation bar set, but fold down the horizontal bar.
    <u>PURPOSE:</u> Maintain the height recording while protecting the patient from possible injury.
12. Assist the patient off the scale. Make certain that all items removed for weighing are given back to the patient.

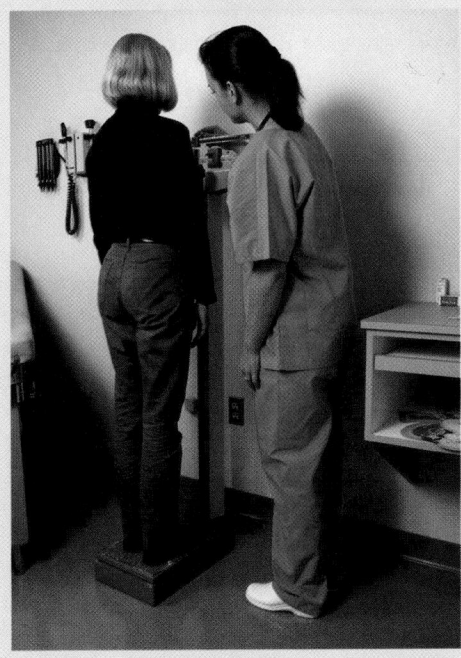

FIGURE 1

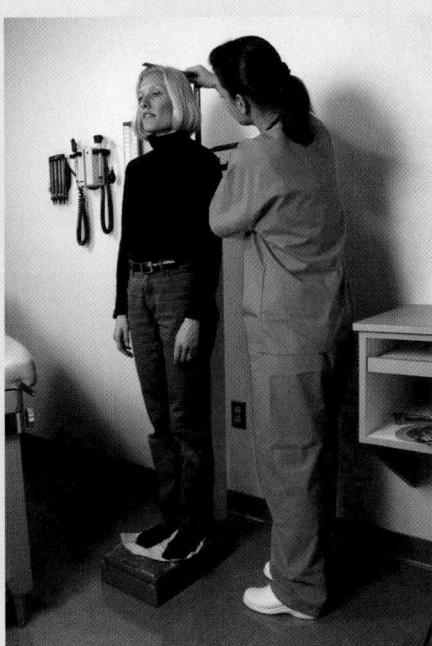

FIGURE 2

Continued

PROCEDURE 30-8—cont'd

13. Read the weight scale. Add the numbers at the markers of the large and the small weights, and record the total to the nearest ¼ lb on the patient's medical record (e.g., Wt: 136½).

14. Record the height. Read the marker at the movable point of the ruler, and record the measurement to the nearest quarter inch on the patient's medical record (e.g., Ht: 64 ¼).

15. Use the patient's weight and height to record the BMI level if part of office procedure.

16. Return the weights and the measuring bar to zero.

17. Wash your hands.

18. Record the results on the patient's medical record.

*See Appendix D for a charting example.

Conversion Formulas

To Convert Kilograms to Pounds
1 kg = 2.2 lb
Multiply the number of kilograms by 2.2.

Example
If a patient weighs 68 kg, multiply 68 by 2.2 = 149.6 lb.

To Convert Pounds to Kilograms
1 lb = 0.45 kg
Multiply the number of pounds by 0.45, or divide the number of pounds by 2.2 kg.

Example
If a patient weighs 120 lb, multiply 120 by 0.45 = 54 kg, or divide 120 by 2.2 = 54.5 kg.

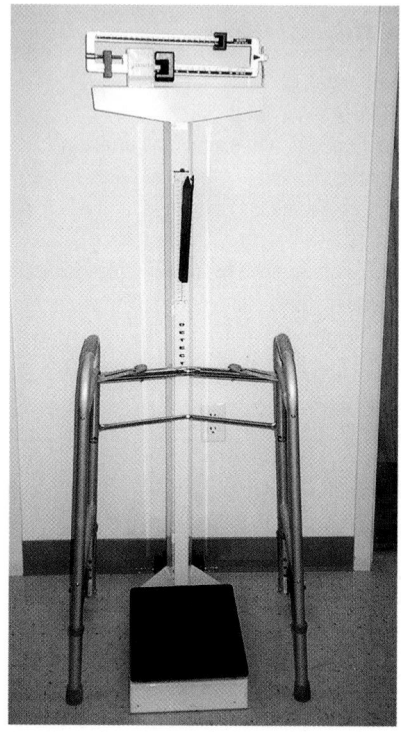

FIGURE 30-14 Walker over a scale to aid the patient in balancing.

If the physician prescribes weight measurement at home, make certain that the patient understands the importance of weighing himself or herself each day at the same time in clothing of similar weight. Body weight may vary considerably from early morning to late afternoon. Teach the patient how to record the weight on a graphic record and how to make any other important notations.

CRITICAL THINKING APPLICATION

- A patient weighs 87 kg; how many pounds does he weigh?
- A patient weighs 148 lb; how many kilograms does she weigh?

Height

Height can be measured in inches or in centimeters. Measurement is easily accomplished by moving the parallel bar attached to a wall ruler or on the scale. Length measurements used in pediatrics are discussed in Chapter 41.

CRITICAL THINKING APPLICATION

Mrs. Johnson is being seen for the first time by Dr. Xu. In what order should Carlos take her vital signs and her anthropometric measurements? Should the blood pressure be measured in both arms, with the patient both sitting and standing? What is the rationale?

CLOSING COMMENTS

Patient Education

All patients should know how to use a thermometer safely and accurately and the preferred site based on age and other patient factors. Because many types of temperature-reading equipment are sold, ask the patient what type of equipment he or she uses at home to obtain temperature readings. Inexpensive digital models have greatly simplified home temperature taking.

To teach a patient how to assess the pulse rate, familiarize the patient with counting the beats and how to determine the rate, rhythm, and regularity of the beat. Use diagrams to teach pulse points, and have the patient measure your pulse to assess the patient's accuracy and to provide any needed assistance.

If a patient is to keep track of respirations, a family member or helper will need to do this for the patient. The patient and all caregivers should also be taught self-assessment of impending complications as well as preventive breathing exercises.

The Role of the Medical Assistant in Obtaining Vital Signs

- Monitoring vital signs is a key responsibility of the medical assistant.
- It is crucial to correctly measure and describe all facets of each vital sign.
- The medical assistant must accurately and clearly document this information.
- The medical assistant should take advantage of all opportunities to answer questions and help the patient understand the significance of healthy vital signs.
- Patient privacy must be maintained throughout all procedures.
- Family members or caregivers should be included in patient care and education as indicated.
- Community resources should be used to promote holistic patient care.
- The medical assistant should be sensitive to cultural and socioeconomic factors that may affect patient compliance with physician recommendations, such as diet, exercise, weight control, and the use of medication.

Monitoring blood pressure at home has become very common. Suggest that the patient bring his or her equipment to the office and practice with it. In this way, you can be certain that the patient is using the equipment correctly and is recording the results accurately in a record book.

Weight management can be a trying and emotional experience for a patient. Understanding how weight is affected by the time of day, by a particular activity, or by the type of scale used can help the patient to maintain a positive attitude. Have an assortment of weight-management literature available for the patient to take home, and use community resources when indicated to help the patient with weight-related issues (see Chapter 29 for further details).

Legal and Ethical Issues

A medical assistant must remember that as the physician's agent he or she plays an important role in preventing legal claims against the physician and the medical office. The medical assistant must always function within the legal boundaries of the profession. When obtaining vital signs, carefully select your response to a patient who asks about the results. Remember, medical assistants are not qualified to diagnose a patient problem; that is, never evaluate or give an opinion of what the results may mean. For example, if a patient asks, "Is my blood pressure better?" you might reply, "The reading is 160/90 today." You have not said that it is worse, the same, or better but have informed the patient of the current blood pressure reading.

Always be accurate in transcribing results onto the patient's medical record. If the results are incorrectly recorded, there is a chance that the patient will be incorrectly diagnosed or treated. This can result in legal action that may implicate you. A careless attitude toward the assessment of vital signs and toward documentation can lead to possible legal entanglement. In every procedure in this chapter there is a reminder to record the test results. If no entry has been made, the assumption is that the procedure was not done. Cultivate sensitivity toward proper conduct and performance so that you can protect yourself and your physician-employer.

SUMMARY OF SCENARIO

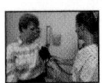

Carlos recognizes the significance of measuring and recording patient vital signs and anthropometric measurements. Dr. Xu relies on Carlos to accurately provide this information. Carlos has never let these procedures become routine or done them without focusing on the task, because the patient's vital signs are an important reflection of his or her health status. He recognizes that a number of factors can alter patient vital signs including the external environment, smoking, drinking hot beverages, exercise, and patient anxiety and pain. Carlos evaluates patient factors such as age, gender, level of compliance, and the presence of disease to determine the best method for accurately measuring vital signs. In addition, Carlos is sensitive to the need for safeguarding patient privacy. He was concerned about privacy and confidentiality when first hired by Dr. Xu when he discovered the patient scale in the hall next to the waiting room. After discussing this with the office manager, the scale was moved to an examination room so patients could be weighed in privacy. Carlos attended a workshop last year on the revised AHA guidelines for diagnosis and treatment of hypertension and is prepared to explain those recommendations to patients if asked. He recognizes his role in motivating patients diagnosed with prehypertension to stick with recommended lifestyle changes and follow the physician's treatment protocol. Carlos continues to care for patients while providing valuable assistance to Dr. Xu in her busy primary care practice.

SUMMARY of LEARNING OBJECTIVES

1. Define, spell, and pronounce the terms listed in the vocabulary.
   - Spelling and pronouncing medical terms correctly adds credibility to the medical assistant. Knowing the definition of these terms promotes confidence in communication with patients and co-workers.

2. Cite the average body temperatures, pulse rates, respiratory rates, and blood pressures for various age groups.
   - The normal ranges for vital signs are summarized in Tables 30-1 through 30-5. The normal pulse, respiratory rate, and blood pressure averages vary according to age, whereas temperature values vary according to age and the site used.

3. Describe emotional and physical factors that cause body temperature to increase or decrease.
   - Multiple factors affect the body temperature, including the external environment, age, stress, physical exercise, gender, and illness.

4. Obtain and record an accurate patient temperature using three different sites.
   - The patient's temperature can be measured orally with a digital thermometer, in the ear using an aural thermometer, and in the axillary region. Axillary temperatures are approximately 1° F or 0.6° C lower than accurate oral readings because the reading is not taken in an enclosed body cavity. The tympanic temperature is considered the most accurate because it records the temperature of the blood that is closest to the hypothalamus. Record a (T) for tympanic or an (A) for axillary readings after the temperature is recorded to clarify an alternative site.

5. Describe pulse rate, volume, and rhythm.
   - The pulse rate reflects the number of times the heart contracts over a period of 1 minute. The pulse volume is the amount of force placed on the arterial walls when the heart beats; the rhythm of the pulse is the length of time between each beat. Monitor and record the pulse rate, noting whether the rhythm is regular or arrhythmic, and if the volume is bounding, normal, or thready.

6. Locate and record the pulse at multiple sites.
   - The most common sites that are used to feel the pulse are at the temporal, carotid, apical, brachial, radial, femoral, popliteal, and dorsalis pedis arteries. Refer to Procedures 30-4 and 30-5 for specifics on recording the apical and radial pulses.

7. Demonstrate the best way to obtain an accurate respiration count.
   - Count the number of respirations in a 30-second period and multiply by 2. Should be done immediately after taking the patient's pulse, while still holding the pulse point, and without warning the patient, because the patient may inadvertently alter the respiratory rate if he or she is aware you are counting breaths.

8. Specify physiologic factors that affect blood pressure.
   - Physiologic factors that affect blood pressure include the amount or volume of blood in circulation; the condition of the blood vessels, including the presence of atherosclerosis and arteriosclerosis; the degree of blood viscosity; and the strength of the myocardium.

9. Differentiate between essential and secondary hypertension.
   - The cause of essential hypertension is unknown; it is diagnosed when a patient has a systolic reading greater than 140 mm Hg and/or a diastolic reading greater than 90 mm Hg. Secondary hypertension is caused by another underlying condition, such as renal disease, pregnancy, or congenital heart defects.

10. Interpret revised hypertension guidelines and treatment.
    - AHA guidelines for the diagnosis and management of hypertension include a new category, prehypertension, and normal blood pressure is identified with readings less than 120/80. Table 30-6 identifies the categories of normal, prehypertensive, and hypertensive blood pressures. The goal of the new recommendations is to decrease the number of people who die each year from hypertension-related illnesses. Treatment includes a combination of weight management, sodium reduction, lifestyle changes, and the use of two or more antihypertensive medications.

11. Identify the different Korotkoff phases.
    - Korotkoff sounds are the sounds heard during the measurement of the blood pressure. These sounds are produced by the vibrations of the arterial wall when the blood surges back into the vessel after it has been compressed by the blood pressure cuff. Phase I is the first sound heard as the cuff deflates and is the systolic reading; phase II is the swishing sound made by the movement of the blood through the artery, but you may have an auscultatory gap in which sounds completely disappear; phase III involves distinct, sharp tapping sounds made as the blood rushes through the artery; in phase IV the sound changes to a soft tapping, which becomes muffled and begins to grow fainter; and in phase V sound completely disappears. The last sound heard is the diastolic reading.

12. Accurately measure and document blood pressure.
    - The sphygmomanometer is used with a stethoscope to hear the systolic over diastolic sounds. (Procedure 30-7 outlines the method for performing this skill.)

13. Accurately measure and document height and weight.
    - Patient height and weight are anthropometric measurements that are recorded during the initial patient visit and periodically after that, depending on patient needs and physician preference. The scale should be in a private location. Variations in weight may indicate physical or emotional disorders, including diabetes, CHF, hormone abnormalities, depression, and eating disorders. Procedure 30-8 describes the techniques involved. Determine the patient's BMI level as indicated. Chapter 29 discusses BMI in more detail.

14. Convert kilograms to pounds and pounds to kilograms.
    - To convert kilograms (kg) to pounds (lb) multiply the number of kilograms by 2.2. To convert pounds to kilograms divide the

Continued

SUMMARY of LEARNING OBJECTIVES

Continued

number of pounds by 2.2 kg or multiply the number of pounds by 0.45 kg.

15. Identify patient education opportunities when measuring vital signs.
   - Patient education regarding vital signs includes confirming the ability of the patient to monitor vital signs at home as needed, providing assistance in working home equipment systems, and confirming understanding of the need to comply with physician recommendations.

16. Determine legal and ethical responsibilities in obtaining vital signs.
   - Legal and ethical implications for the medical assistant include following physician guidelines with patient disclosure, monitoring and recording vital signs accurately, and being consistently alert to inaccurate readings or potential carelessness.

CONNECTIONS

 Study Guide Connection: Go to Chapter 30 Study Guide. Read the Case Study and Workplace Applications and complete the assignments. Do online research for answers to the questions in the Internet Activities associated with vital signs.

 CD Connection: Go to the Medical Assisting Competency Challenge CD and do the training activities under Patient Care.

Evolve Connection: For more information related to vital signs, go to evolve.elsevier.com/kinn and visit related weblinks for Chapter 30. Click on the Medical Assisting Exam Review and do the practice questions to sharpen your test-taking skills.

Assisting with the Primary Physical Examination

31

SCENARIO

Felicia Grand, a newly hired certified medical assistant (CMA), works for Dr. Anna Kosto, who is a member of a busy multiphysician primary care practice. One of Felicia's chief responsibilities is to assist Dr. Kosto with physical examinations. Her duties include preparing and maintaining the examination room and equipment; getting the patient ready for specific physical examinations; and gowning, draping, and positioning the patient as needed. Felicia must be familiar with the physical examination procedure and the order in which the physician will need various pieces of medical equipment. It is also important that Felicia protect herself from possible injury by using appropriate body mechanics throughout her day in the office.

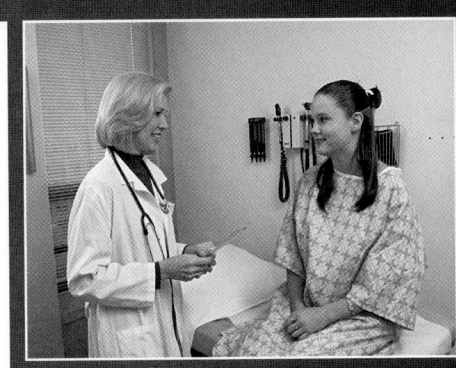

While studying this chapter, think about the following questions:

- What measures can Felicia take to prevent injury from lifting heavy items or assisting with the transfer of patients?
- What examination and treatment positions should Felicia be familiar with, and when should the various positions be used?
- What equipment does Felicia need to gather before the physician enters the examination room to make sure the examination goes smoothly and without interruption?

LEARNING OBJECTIVES

1. Define, spell, and pronounce the terms listed in the vocabulary.
2. Describe the structural development of the human body.
3. Differentiate among the 11 body systems and the major organs and structures in each.
4. Outline the medical assistant's role in preparing for the physical examination.
5. Summarize the instruments and equipment typically used by the physician during a physical examination.
6. Describe the six methods of examination, and give an example for each.
7. Outline the basic principles of properly gowning and draping a patient for examination.
8. Compare and contrast the various positions that may be used during an examination, and identify the purpose of each.
9. Position and drape a patient in six different examining positions while remaining mindful of patient privacy and comfort.
10. Demonstrate proper body mechanics in transferring a patient from a chair to the examination table and back.
11. Outline the sequence of a routine physical examination.
12. Prepare for and assist in the physical examination of a patient, correctly completing each step of the procedure in the proper sequence.
13. Summarize the role of the medical assistant in the physical examination process.
14. Determine the role of patient education during the physical examination.
15. Discuss the legal and ethical implications of the physical examination.

National Accreditation Competencies and Content

CAAHEP COMPETENCIES

Clinical

3.b.(4)(d). Prepare and maintain examination and treatment areas
3.b.(4)(e). Prepare patient for and assist with routine and specialty examinations

General

3.c.(4)(b). Perform routine maintenance of administrative and clinical equipment.

ABHES COMPETENCIES

Clinical Duties

4.b. Prepare patients for procedures
4.g. Prepare and maintain examination and treatment areas
4.h. Prepare patient for and assist physician with routine and specialty examinations

Office Management

6.b. Operate and maintain facilities and perform routine maintenance of administrative and clinical equipment safely

VOCABULARY

bruit (bruh-e′) Abnormal sound or murmur heard on auscultation of an organ, vessel, or gland.

clubbing An abnormal enlargement of the fingertips; usually seen with advanced heart and lung disease.

colonoscopy Examination of the large intestine with a fiberoptic scope.

electrocardiogram (i-lek-tro-kar′-de-uh-gram) A graphic record of electrical conduction through the heart.

emphysema (em-fuh-ze′-muh) Pathologic accumulation of air in the tissues or organs; in the lungs the bronchioles become plugged with mucus and lose elasticity.

gait The manner or style of walking.

hematopoiesis (hi-ma-tuh-poi-e′-suhs) Formation and development of blood cells in the bone marrow.

intercellular Between cells.

manipulation Moving or exercising a body part via an externally applied force.

mastication (mas-tuh-ka′-shun) Chewing.

murmur Abnormal sound heard when auscultating the heart that may or may not have a pathologic origin.

nodules (nah′-juhls) Small lumps, lesions, or swellings felt when palpating the skin.

peristalsis (per-uh-stahl′-suhs) Rhythmic contraction of involuntary muscles lining the gastrointestinal tract.

sclera White part of the eye that forms the orbit.

transillumination Inspection of a cavity or organ by passing light through its walls.

trauma Physical injury or wound caused by an external force or violence.

vasoconstriction (va-zo-kuhn-strik′-shun) Contraction of the muscles lining blood vessels that results in decreased lumen size.

The human body is so complex that it is hard to imagine that science will ever entirely unravel its mysteries. Imagine billions of microscopic parts, each with its own functioning identity, yet all working together in a systematic, organized manner for the perfect harmony of the entire organism. To promote health maintenance, healthcare professionals must understand the anatomy and physiology of the body, what role each part plays, how each component functions, and what happens to the body when disease occurs in the body systems.

ANATOMY AND PHYSIOLOGY

Anatomy is the study of how the body is shaped and structured. It encompasses a wide range of subjects, including structural development, levels of organization, relationships among microscopic parts, and the interrelationship of structure and function.

Physiology is the study of body functions. This field is also subdivided into areas of study; some physiologists spend their entire lives studying only one function, such as how cells work or how a single organ such as the small intestine is interrelated in function with the stomach and the large intestine.

It is almost impossible to separate these two sciences, because one continuously influences the other. Function affects structure, and structure affects function; for example, an infant has the ability to suck effortlessly because of the lack of teeth in its mouth. Once teeth appear, sucking becomes more tiresome, and the child now begins to chew and bite. Phenomena in structure and function affect the interrelationship of all body systems.

Structural Development

Cells

The basic unit of life is the cell. Cells determine the functional and structural characteristics of the entire body. Cells are microscopic in size, come in a variety of shapes, and perform a vast array of functions. It is estimated that the human body is composed of approximately 100 trillion living, functioning cells. A cell is made up of three primary parts: the plasma membrane that surrounds the cell, creating an outer covering; the cytoplasm inside the cell, which contains the living material that carries on the cell's function; and the nucleus of the cell, which contains the genetic code of the cell that determines the cell's function.

Tissues

When cells with similar structure and function are placed together, they form tissues. The study of tissues is known as *histology.* All of the body tissues are grouped into four types. The types of tissues distributed throughout the body and where they are located are as follows:

- *Epithelial:* Skin, glands, lining of body cavities and organs; packed closely together with little or no **intercellular** material; classified according to shape as either *squamous* (flat), *cuboidal* (square), *columnar* (long and narrow), or *transitional* (varying shapes that can stretch). Epithelial cells may be arranged in a single layer of cells that are the same shape, called *simple epithelium,* or *stratified epithelium,* which consists of many layers of cells named according to the shape of the cells in the outer layer.
- *Connective:* Supports and binds other body tissues. Types include collagen, bone, cartilage, adipose, ligaments, tendons, blood, and lymph. It is the most frequently occurring tissue in the body, with the widest distribution.
- *Muscle:* Produces movement. Classified as either skeletal (striated, voluntary) muscle, which is attached to bones and produce voluntary body movements when contracted; cardiac (striated and involuntary) muscle, which forms the heart muscle wall; or smooth muscle (nonstriated and involuntary), which forms the walls of blood vessels and hollow organs and causes such actions as **peristalsis** and **vasoconstriction.**
- *Nervous:* Conducts nerve impulses between the periphery and the central nervous system; creates rapid communication between body structures and controls body functions to maintain homeostasis; made up of neurons as well as supportive structures called *neuroglial* cells.

Organs

An *organ* is composed of two or more types of tissue bound together to form a more complex structure for a common purpose or function. An organ may have one or many functions—for example, the pancreas has an endocrine function because it produces the hormone insulin and a digestive function because it produces digestive enzymes. Organs may also be part of one or several systems. For example, in the male system the urethra is part of both the urinary and the reproductive systems.

Systems

A *body system* is composed of several organs and their associated structures. These structures work together to perform a specific function within the body. The human body has 11 systems. Each system has specific units within it, and each performs specific functions. Table 31-1 summarizes the body systems; their primary cells, organs, and structures; and the major functions of each.

PRIMARY CARE PHYSICIAN

Primary care physicians (PCPs) treat patients of all ages for a broad range of diseases and complaints. A PCP is qualified to provide continuing healthcare for the entire family, from birth to old age. Within the healthcare system of today, many health insurance programs have converted to the primary care referral system. This means that most patients are required to have a PCP as their gatekeeper in personal healthcare. In this role the PCP must first be contacted before the patient can be referred to specialty physicians for care.

The PCP evaluates a patient's total healthcare needs, provides personal medical care within one or more fields of medicine, and refers the patient to a specialist when an advanced or serious condition warrants additional expertise. The medical assistant's clinical responsibilities in the primary care office encompass assisting with patients who may have problems in any of the body systems and with procedures in all age groups. With such a diversified scope of practice, the physician and medical assistant must work as a team to use their time efficiently and still provide patient-centered healthcare.

PHYSICAL EXAMINATION

The purpose of a physical examination is to determine the overall state of well-being of the patient. All major organs and body systems are checked during a physical examination. As the physician examines the entire body, findings are interpreted, and by the time the examination is completed the physician will have formed an initial diagnosis regarding the patient's condition. Frequently, laboratory and other diagnostic tests are ordered to supplement the physician's initial diagnosis. The results of these tests are used to refine the patient's diagnosis, to aid the physician in planning or revising treatment for the patient, to evaluate and maintain current drug therapy, and/or to determine the patient's progress.

Preparing for the Physical Examination

The Medical Assistant's Role in the Physical Examination

Assessment of the patient begins with the first contact to the office. Before the examination the medical assistant has the opportunity to interact with the patient to ensure that he or she feels comfortable during the examination process and that all the necessary medical information is obtained. As part of patient preparation the medical assistant should verify the patient's current medications and allergies. The medical assistant's duties include preparing and maintaining the examination room and equipment, preparing the patient, and assisting the physician during the physical examination.

TABLE 31-1 Organization of Body Systems

BODY SYSTEM	CELLS, ORGANS, AND STRUCTURES	FUNCTIONS
Blood	Arteries, arterioles, veins, venules, lymphocytes, white blood cells, red blood cells, platelets, plasma	Transports materials and collects wastes throughout the body; white blood cells fight infection; red blood cells carry oxygen; platelets help form clots; plasma carries dissolved nutrients and other materials
Cardiovascular	Heart, valves, arteries, arterioles, veins, venules	Circulatory system transports materials in blood throughout the body; veins return deoxygenated blood to the heart, which pumps it into lungs; oxygenated blood is pumped into aorta and branching arteries to cells throughout the body
Endocrine	Pituitary, pineal, hypothalamus, thyroid, pancreas, adrenal cortex and medulla, parathyroid, thymus, ovaries, testes	Produce hormones that circulate in the blood to target tissue to stimulate a particular action
Integumentary	Skin, subcutaneous tissue, sweat and sebaceous glands, hair, nails, sense receptors	Protection, temperature regulation, senses organ activity
Gastrointestinal	Mouth, teeth, pharynx, esophagus, stomach, small intestine, large intestine, liver, gallbladder, pancreas, appendix	**Mastication**, swallowing, digestion, absorption of nutrients, excretion of waste materials
Lymphatic and immune	Lymph, lymph vessels, lymph nodes, thymus, tonsils, spleen, phagocytes, lymphocytes, antibodies	Maintains fluid balance; protects internal environment; defends against foreign cells and disease; provides immunity to some diseases
Musculoskeletal	Bones, joints, muscles, tendons, ligaments, cartilage	Movement, posture, heat production, support, protection, mineral storage, **hematopoiesis**
Nervous	Brain, spinal cord, neurons, neuroglial cells, peripheral nerves, autonomic nerves	Controls body structures to maintain homeostasis; higher-order thinking and reflex centers that control autonomic processes; carries sensory stimulus to the brain and motor impulses to the periphery
Reproductive	Female: estrogen and progesterone, ovum, ovaries, fallopian tubes, uterus, vagina, vulva, mammary glands Male: testosterone, sperm, epididymis, vas deferens, prostate gland, testes, scrotum, penis, urethra	Produces hormones, reproduction
Respiratory	Nose, sinuses, pharynx, larynx, trachea, bronchi, lungs, bronchioles, alveoli	Responsible for inhalation of oxygen and exhalation of carbon dioxide externally and exchange of oxygen and carbon dioxide internally at cellular level; acid-base regulation
Sensory	Eyes, ears, taste buds, olfactory receptors, sensory receptors	Helps sense changes in external and internal environments via vision, hearing, balance, taste, smell
Urinary	Nephron unit, bilateral kidneys, ureters, urinary bladder, urethra	Filters waste material from blood; reabsorbs fluid and electrolytes as needed; excretes waste in urine; maintains electrolyte, water, acid-base balances; regulates blood pressure; activates red blood cells

Room Preparation. It is the medical assistant's responsibility to make sure that the examination room is ready for any procedure that might be performed during the physical examination. The area should also be as comfortable as possible for the patient and free from any potential dangers (Procedure 31-1). Preparation of the examination room includes the following:

- The area should be checked at the beginning of each day and between patients to make sure that it is completely stocked with equipment and supplies and that equipment is functioning properly. The medical assistant must understand how to take care of and operate all equipment and instruments, referring as needed to operation manuals supplied by manufacturers.

- Expiration dates must be checked on all packages and supplies on a regular basis. Dispose of expired materials when indicated.

- The room should be private, well lit, and at a comfortable temperature for the patient during the physical examination.

- Clean and disinfect the area daily, and between patients as needed, to prevent the spread of infection and to ensure patient comfort. Restock supplies and clean all potentially contaminated surfaces, including the examination table, between patients with an appropriate disinfectant (Figure 31-1). After cleaning the table, change the examination paper by unrolling a new piece.

- Arrange drapes, gowns, and any other patient supplies before the patient enters the room so they are ready for use.

PROCEDURE 31-1

Prepare and Maintain Examination and Treatment Areas

CAAHEP COMPETENCY: 3.b(4)(d)
ABHES COMPETENCY: 4.g

GOAL: *Prepare an examination room for a patient procedure, maintain equipment and supplies needed for the physical examination, and demonstrate maintenance of the room after a patient visit.*

EQUIPMENT and SUPPLIES

- Examination table
- Patient gown
- Drape
- Stethoscope
- Ophthalmoscope
- Scale with height measurement bar
- Tongue depressor
- Cotton balls
- Examination light
- Percussion hammer
- Lubricating gel
- Examination gloves
- Sphygmomanometer
- Otoscope with disposable speculum
- Tape measure
- Gauze sponges
- Pen light
- Nasal speculum
- Tuning fork
- Biohazard container
- Laboratory request forms
- Specimen bottles/lab requisitions
- Thermometer
- Cotton-tipped applicators
- Hemoccult supplies
- Table paper
- Spray disinfectant

PROCEDURAL STEPS

1. Check the examination room at the beginning of each day and between patients to make sure that it is completely stocked with equipment and supplies and that equipment is functioning properly.
   PURPOSE: Room must be ready for patient services.
2. Check all equipment and instruments to make sure they are operational, referring to manuals supplied by manufacturers as needed.
3. Check expiration dates on all packages and supplies on a regular basis, disposing of expired materials as needed.
   PURPOSE: To maintain patient safety.
4. The room should be private, well lit, and at a comfortable temperature for the patient during the physical examination.
   PURPOSE: To maintain patient confidentiality, safety, and comfort.
5. Prepare the examination room before and between patients according to acceptable medical aseptic rules.
   PURPOSE: Room must be aseptically clean to prevent spread of infection.
6. After each patient use, apply disposable examination gloves, spray the table and any other contaminated surface with a disinfectant, clean the area with disposable towels, dispose of waste in an appropriate biohazard container, and apply clean paper to the table.
7. Wash your hands.
   PURPOSE: Infection control. Prevent transmission of pathogens from one patient to another.
8. Inventory the supplies needed after each patient visit and restock as needed.
   PURPOSE: Room must be maintained and ready for each examination.

- Prepare instruments and equipment needed for the examination, and arrange these items for easy access before the physician enters the room to save the time spent on the actual examination.
- The examination room should contain all required materials for standard precautions, including disposable gloves, sink with antibacterial hand-washing agent, paper towels, biohazard waste containers, sharps containers, and impervious gowns and face guards. Replace biohazard containers when they are two-thirds full, following standard precautions as explained in Chapter 26.

Patient Preparation. Getting the patient ready for the examination includes taking care of paperwork before the patient enters the examination room as well as performing related clinical skills.

- Make sure the medical record is complete and that any needed consent forms are signed. It is not the medical assistant's responsibility to obtain informed consent, but he or she should review the paperwork to make sure that informed consent forms were reviewed by the physician and that the patient signed the forms.
- Introduce yourself and address the patient by his or her preferred name, making sure to maintain respect at all times. Use the communication skills presented in Chapter 27, and pay close attention to the patient's nonverbal language to make sure the patient understands what to expect.

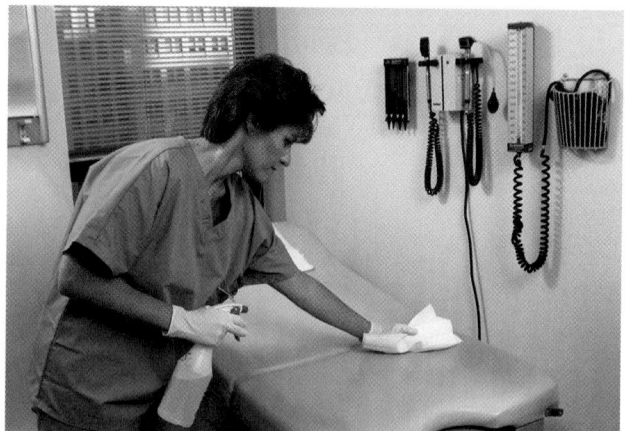

FIGURE 31-1 Disinfecting the examination table.

- Gather insurance information according to office policy. In most facilities the policy is to make a copy of the patient's insurance card when the patient first enters the office or to ask if there have been any changes in insurance information if the patient has been to the office regularly.
- Obtain specimens such as urine and blood if they have been preordered by the physician.
- Measure and record height, weight, body mass index (BMI), and vital signs.
- Conduct the initial investigation into the reason for the visit, and explain to the patient the examination procedure. Be prepared to answer patient questions about the procedure and allay any fears.
- Ask the patient if he or she needs to empty the bladder before the examination, because a full bladder may interfere with the examination as well as be uncomfortable for the patient.
- Help the patient physically prepare for the examination. Explain to the patient what clothing should be removed, in what direction to put on the gown (open either to the front or to the back depending on the type of examination), and provide a drape to ensure patient privacy. Offer assistance as needed.
- Throughout this entire sequence of events, explain what is happening and consistently maintain patient privacy and confidentiality.
- Document patient data in the chart, completing all forms required.
- Place the patient's chart in the designated area for the physician, usually in a chart holder on the examination room door, making sure that no identifiable patient information is visible. According to the Health Insurance Portability and Accountability Act (HIPAA), patient information must be protected at all times.

Assisting the Physician. The medical assistant should be prepared to help the physician complete the physical examination as comprehensively and efficiently as possible. You have already prepared the room so all equipment and supplies are available and in good working order and prepared the patient by gathering the needed information and measuring

and recording vital signs. During the examination, the physician may expect the medical assistant to do the following:

- Hand instruments and equipment as requested and provide supplies as needed.
- Alter the position of a gooseneck lamp to better illuminate the area being examined, and turn lights off and on during specific phases of the examination.
- Position and drape the patient during the different phases of the examination.
- Assist in collecting and properly labeling specimens such as urine, Pap smear samplings, and throat cultures.
- Conduct follow-up diagnostic procedures as ordered including an **electrocardiogram** (ECG), eye or ear screening, urinalysis, and phlebotomy.
- Schedule postexamination diagnostic procedures such as a mammogram, x-ray examination, or **colonoscopy.**

CRITICAL THINKING APPLICATION

Felicia's first patient for the day is Harry Garcia, a 51-year-old truck driver who is scheduled for a complete physical examination. Mr. Garcia's insurance has changed since his last visit. The physician ordered an ECG to be performed and a complete blood panel to be drawn before the physical. What does Felicia need to complete before Dr. Kosto sees the patient?

Supplies and Instruments Needed for the Physical Examination

The instruments typically used during the physical examination are displayed in Figure 31-2. They enable the physician to see, feel, inspect, and listen to parts of the body. All equipment must be in good working order, properly disinfected, and readily available for the physician's use during the examination. The instruments most frequently used for the physical examination are described in the following paragraphs. Physical examinations are typically conducted from the head to the feet; the instruments are listed in the order in which the physician would typically request them.

Ophthalmoscope. An ophthalmoscope is used to inspect the inner structures of the eye. It has a stainless-steel handle containing batteries, onto which a head is attached. The head is equipped with a light and magnifying lenses and an opening through which the eye is viewed. Examination rooms are usually equipped with wall-mounted electrical units for the ophthalmoscope and otoscope, a dispenser for disposable speculums, and a wall-mounted sphygmomanometer (Figure 31-3).

Tongue Depressor. A tongue depressor is a flat, wooden blade used to hold down the tongue when examining the throat (Figure 31-4).

Otoscope. An otoscope is used to examine the external auditory canal and tympanic membrane. It has a stainless-steel handle containing batteries or is part of a wall-mounted electrical unit (see Figure 31-3). The head of the otoscope contains a light that is focused through a magnifying lens and should be covered with disposable ear speculum. The light may also be used to illuminate the nasal passages and throat.

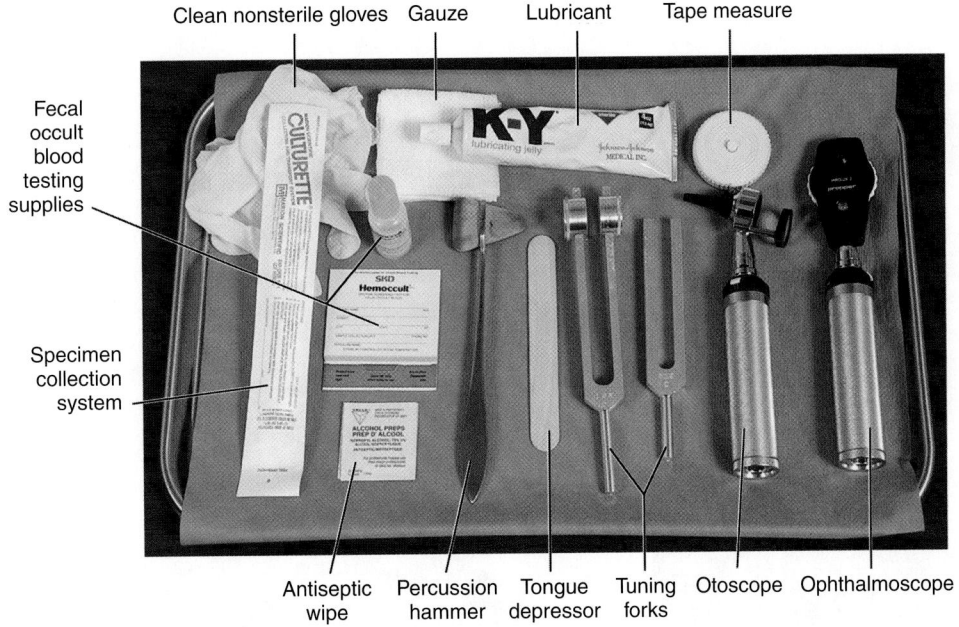

Clean nonsterile gloves Gauze Lubricant Tape measure

Fecal occult blood testing supplies

Specimen collection system

Antiseptic wipe Percussion hammer Tongue depressor Tuning forks Otoscope Ophthalmoscope

FIGURE 31-2 Instruments for the physical examination. (From Bonewit-West K: *Clinical procedures for medical assistants*, ed 6, Philadelphia, 2004, Saunders.)

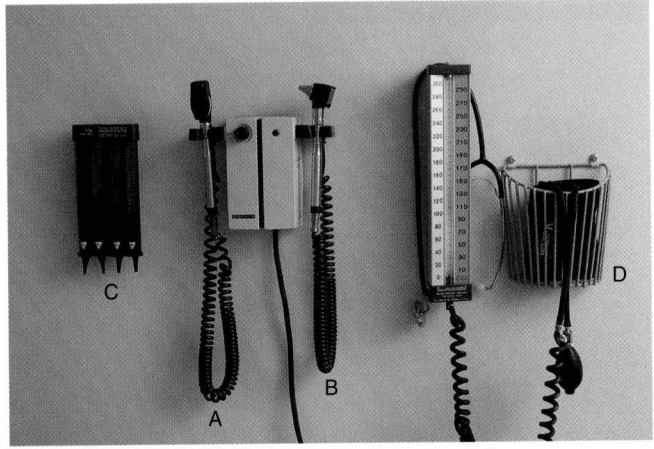

FIGURE 31-3 Examination room wall unit. **A,** Ophthalmoscope. **B,** Otoscope. **C,** Disposable speculums. **D,** Sphygmomanometer.

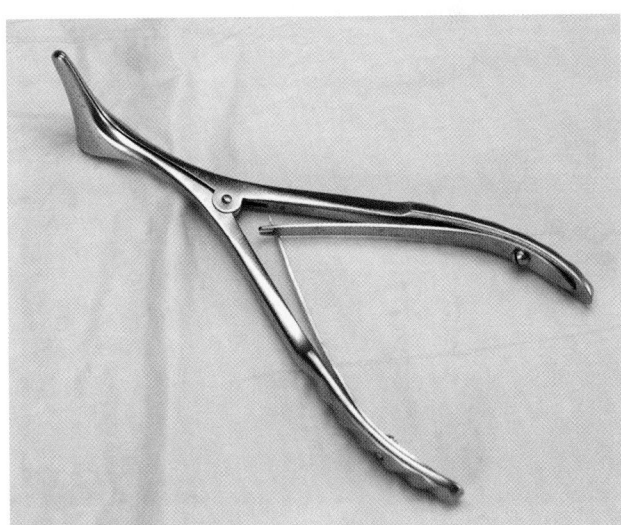

FIGURE 31-5 Nasal speculum.

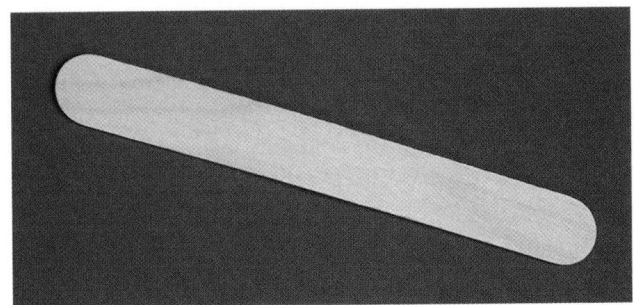

FIGURE 31-4 Disposable tongue depressor.

Nasal Speculum. A nasal speculum is a stainless-steel instrument used to inspect the lining of the nose, nasal membranes, and internal septum (Figure 31-5). When the handles of the nasal speculum are squeezed, the tips spread apart to dilate the nostrils, allowing the physician to visualize the internal aspects. An otoscope with a special attachment may also be used for nasal visualization.

Tuning Fork. Tuning forks come in different sizes, and each size produces a different pitch level (Figure 31-6, *A*). A tuning fork is used to check a patient's auditory acuity (Figure 31-6, *B*) and to test bone vibration (Figure 31-6, *C*). This aluminum instrument consists of a handle and two prongs that produce a humming sound when the physician strikes the prongs against his or her hand.

Tape Measure. A tape measure is a flexible ribbon ruler usually printed in inches and feet on one side and in centimeters and meters on the opposite side (Figure 31-7). Measurement is used to assess length and head circumference in infants, wound size, and so on.

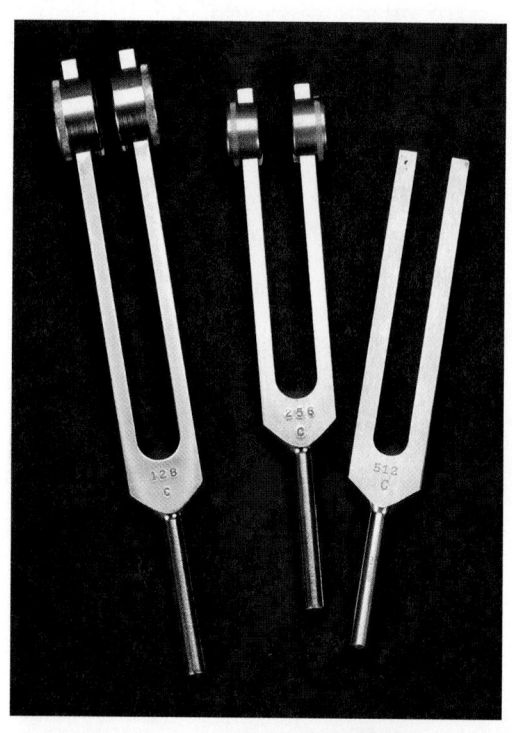

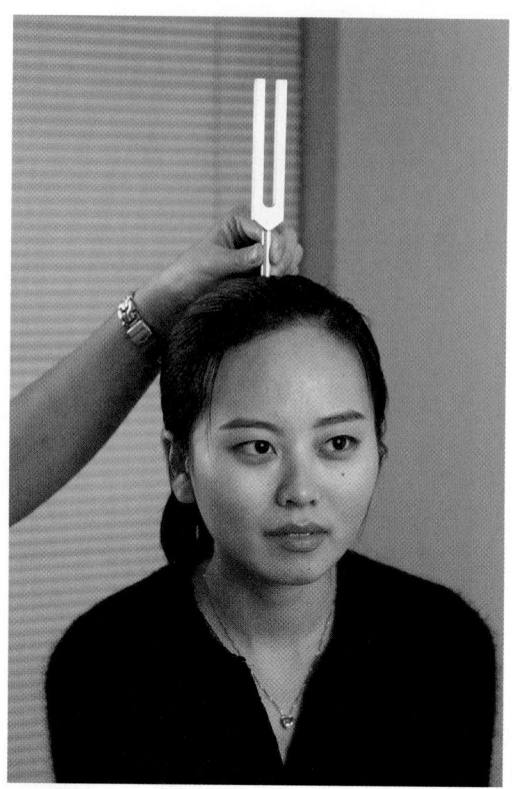

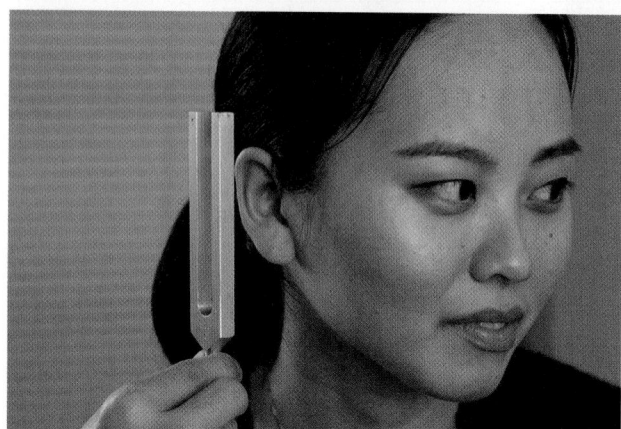

FIGURE 31-6 A, Tuning forks. **B,** Sound vibration test. **C,** Bone vibration test.

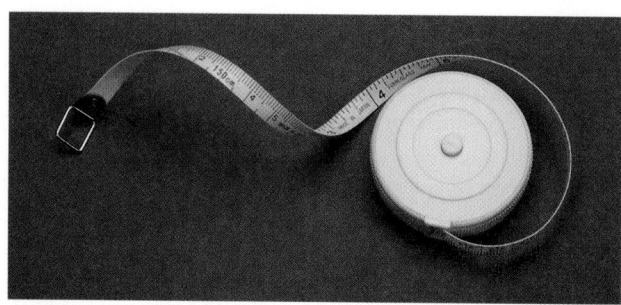

FIGURE 31-7 Tape measure.

Stethoscope. A stethoscope is a listening device used when auscultating certain areas of the body, particularly the heart and lungs. This instrument comes in many shapes and sizes. All have two earpieces that are connected to flexible rubber or vinyl tubing (Figure 31-8). At the distal end of the tubing is a diaphragm or bell (many have both) that when placed securely on the patient's skin enables the physician to hear internal body sounds.

Reflex Hammer. A reflex hammer is sometimes called a *percussion hammer.* This stainless-steel instrument has a hard rubber head used to test neurologic reflexes of the knee and elbow when the tendons are struck (Figure 31-9).

Gloves. Disposable latex gloves protect the healthcare worker and the patient from microorganisms. Under standard

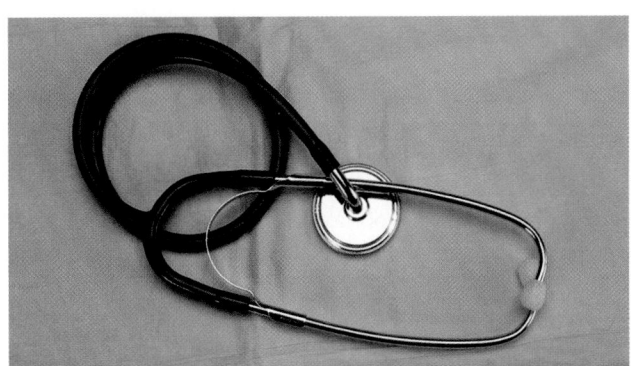

FIGURE 31-8 Stethoscope.

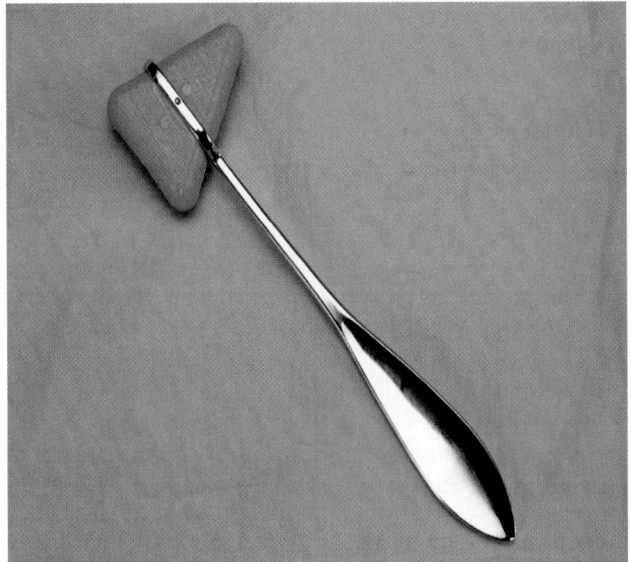

FIGURE 31-9 Reflex hammer.

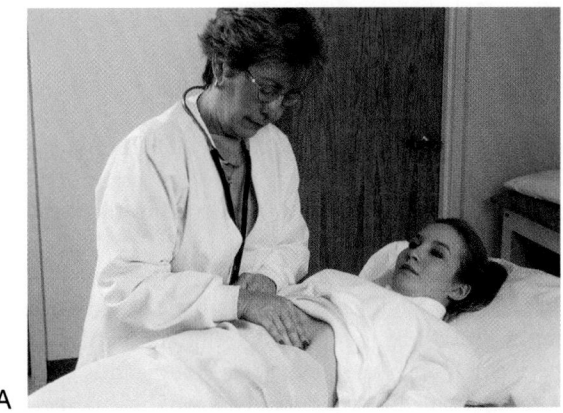

A

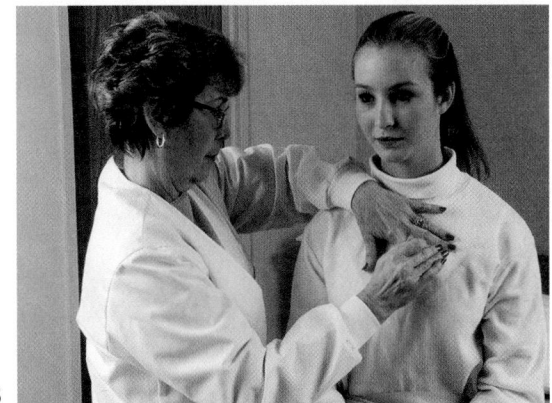

B

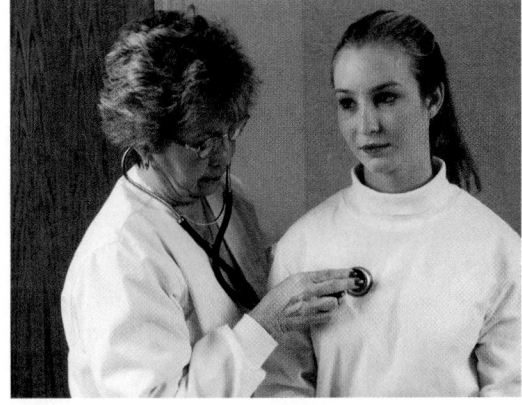

C

FIGURE 31-10 A, Demonstration of palpation. **B,** Demonstration of percussion. **C,** Demonstration of auscultation. (From Zakus SM: *Mosby's clinical skills for medical assistants*, ed 4, St Louis, 2001, Mosby.)

precautions, gloves are to be worn whenever there may be contact with any body fluids, broken skin or wounds, or contaminated items.

Additional Supplies. Gauze squares, cotton balls, cotton-tipped applicators, specimen containers, hemoccult packets, Pap smear supplies for female patients, K-Y jelly for vaginal and rectal examinations, and laboratory request forms should be easily accessible for use during the examination.

Assisting with the Physical Examination

Methods of Examination

Examinations are performed as both a routine confirmation of the absence of illness and a means of diagnosing disease. Six methods of examining the human body are used by healthcare providers. All six methods are part of a complete physical examination.

Inspection. During inspection the examiner uses observation to detect significant physical features or objective data. This method of examination ranges from focusing on the patient's general appearance (the general state of health, including posture, mannerisms, and grooming) to more-detailed observations

including body contour, **gait,** symmetry, visible injuries and deformities, tremors, rashes, and color changes.

Palpation. In palpation the examiner uses the sense of touch (Figure 31-10). A part of the body is felt with the hand to determine its condition or the condition of an underlying organ. Palpation may include touching the skin or a firmer exploration of the abdomen for underlying masses. This technique involves a wide range of perceptions: temperature, vibrations, consistency, form, size, rigidity, elasticity, moisture, texture, position, and contour. Palpation is performed with one hand, both hands (bimanual), one finger (digital), the fingertips, or the palmar aspect of the hand. A pelvic examination is done bimanually, whereas an anal examination is performed digitally.

Do not confuse palpation with *palpitation,* which is a throbbing pulsation felt in the chest.

Percussion. Percussion involves tapping or striking the body, usually with the fingers or a small hammer, to elicit sounds or vibratory sensations. Percussion aids in the determination of the position, size, and density of an underlying organ or cavity. The effect of percussion is both heard and felt by the examiner. It is helpful in determining the amount of air or solid matter in an underlying organ or cavity. The two basic methods of percussion are *direct* and *indirect.* Direct (immediate) percussion is performed by striking the body with a finger. Indirect (mediate) percussion is used more frequently and is done by the physician placing his or her own hand on the area and then striking the placed hand with a finger of the other hand (Figure 31-10, *B).* Both a sound and a sense of vibration are evident. The examiner quantifies the sound in terms of pitch, quality, duration, and resonance.

Auscultation. In auscultation the physician uses a stethoscope to listen to sounds arising from the body (not the sound produced by the physician, as in percussion, but sounds that originate within the patient's body). Auscultation is a difficult method of examination, because the physician must distinguish between a normal and an abnormal sound (Figure 31-10, *C).* It is particularly useful in evaluating sounds originating in the lungs, heart, and abdomen, such as a **murmur**, a **bruit,** and bowel sounds.

Mensuration. Mensuration is the process of measuring. Measurements are recorded of the patient's height and weight, the length and diameter of an extremity, the extent of flexion or extension of an extremity, the size of the uterus during pregnancy, the size and depth of a wound, or the pressure of a grip. Measurements are taken using a flexible tape measure or a circular wound measurement device and are usually recorded in centimeters.

Manipulation. **Manipulation** is the forceful, passive movement of a joint to determine the range of extension or flexion of a part of the body. Manipulation may or may not be grouped with palpation. It is usually considered separate from the four standard methods of examination (inspection, palpation, percussion, and auscultation) and is grouped with mensuration, especially by an orthopedist or a neurologist. Insurance and industrial reports often request this information in detail. For example, a patient involved in a work-related accident that caused joint damage may have to perform assisted range-of-motion (ROM) exercises to the joint, with subsequent measurements of joint flexion and extension.

Positioning and Draping for Physical Examinations

Various patient positions are used to facilitate a physical examination. The medical assistant instructs the patient about, and assists the patient into, these positions with as much ease and modesty as possible and helps the patient to maintain the position during the examination with as little discomfort as possible. Do not place a patient into a position that is uncomfortable or compromises the patient's privacy until it is necessary to complete that part of the examination. Never leave the patient's side if he or she is in a position that could result in a fall.

Draping the patient with an examination sheet protects the patient from embarrassment and keeps the patient warm. However, the sheet must be positioned so that it allows complete visibility for the examiner and does not interfere with the examination. During the general examination, each part of the body is exposed one portion at a time. For gynecologic and rectal examinations, the sheet is positioned on the diagonal across the patient, or in a diamond shape, to provide maximum comfort for the patient while allowing the physician to conduct the examination. The following positions are used for medical examinations.

Fowler's. In Fowler's position the patient sits on the examination table with the head of the table elevated 90 degrees or simply sits at the edge of the table. This position is useful for examinations and treatments of the head, neck, and chest or for patients who find it difficult to breathe lying down. The drape will vary according to the exposure of the patient (Procedure 31-2).

Semi-Fowler's. The semi-Fowler's position is a modification of Fowler's position. Instead of the head of the table being at a full 90-degree angle, it is lowered to a 45-degree angle. This position is useful for postsurgical examinations, for patients with breathing disorders, and for patients who have an elevated temperature or are suffering from head **trauma** or pain (see Procedure 31-2). The drape and/or gown should cover the entire patient from the nipple line down.

Supine (Horizontal Recumbent). In the supine position the patient lies flat, with the face upward and the lower legs supported by the table extension (Procedure 31-3). This position is used for the examination of the frontal portion of the body, including the heart, breasts, and abdominal organs. The patient's gown should be open down the front, and the drape placed over any exposed area that is not being examined.

Dorsal Recumbent. In the dorsal recumbent position the patient lies face upward, with the weight distributed primarily to the surface of the back. This is accomplished by flexing the knees so that the feet are flat on the table. This position relieves muscle tension in the abdomen and may be used for examination and/or inspection of the rectal, vaginal, and perineal areas. This position can be used for digital examinations of the vagina and rectum but is not used if an instrument such as a speculum is needed. To ensure the patient's privacy, it is important to keep the patient completely draped, with the drape in a diamond shape until the physician is present (see Procedure 31-3).

Lithotomy. The patient should not be placed into this position until the physician is in the examination room and is ready for this portion of the examination. Place the patient on the back, with the knees sharply flexed, the arms placed at the sides or folded over the chest, and the buttocks at the bottom edge of the table. Support the feet in stirrups placed wide apart and somewhat away from the table. If the heels are too close to the buttocks, the possibility of leg cramps increases and it is more difficult for the patient to relax the abdominal muscles. Make certain that the stirrups are locked in place. Place a drape diagonally over the patient's abdomen and knees. The drape should be large enough to cover the breasts if the patient

PROCEDURE 31-2

Prepare Patient for and Assist with Routine and Specialty Examinations: Fowler's and Semi-Fowler's Positions

<u>CAAHEP COMPETENCY:</u> 3.b.(4)(e)
<u>ABHES COMPETENCY:</u> 4.h

GOAL: *To position and drape the patient for examinations of the head, neck, and chest or for patients who have difficulty breathing when lying flat.*

EQUIPMENT and SUPPLIES

- Examination table
- Table paper
- Patient gown
- Drape

PROCEDURAL STEPS

1. Prepare the examination room according to acceptable medical aseptic rules.
   <u>PURPOSE:</u> Room must be aseptically clean to prevent spread of infection.
2. Wash your hands.
   <u>PURPOSE:</u> Infection control.
3. Greet and identify the patient, and determine whether the patient understands the procedure. If the patient does not understand, explain what to expect.
   <u>PURPOSE:</u> To promote patient understanding and cooperation during the examination.

4. Give the patient a gown, and explain the clothing that must be removed for the particular examination being done and whether the gown should be open in the front or the back. Provide assistance as needed. Give the patient privacy while changing. Knock on the examination room door before reentering to make sure the patient has completed undressing and gowning.
5. Either elevate the head of the bed 90 degrees or instruct the patient to sit at the end of the table (Figure 1). Extend the footrest for patient comfort. The patient may be more comfortable in a semi-Fowler's position. This modification of Fowler's position has the head of the table elevated 45 degrees and may be used for postsurgical follow-up or for patients with fevers, head injuries, or pain. It is also a comfortable, supported position for patients with breathing disorders (Figure 2).
6. Drape the patient according to the type of examination and the needed patient exposure.
   <u>PURPOSE:</u> Draping the patient provides warmth and privacy while giving the physician access to the examination site.
7. After the examination is completed, assist the patient as needed to get off of the table and get dressed.
8. Clean and disinfect the examination room according to standard precautions. Roll clean paper over the table.
   <u>PURPOSE:</u> Infection control. Prevent transmission of pathogens from one patient to another.
9. Wash hands.
10. Follow up with physician orders regarding scheduling of diagnostic studies, collection of specimens, and/or scheduling of future appointments.

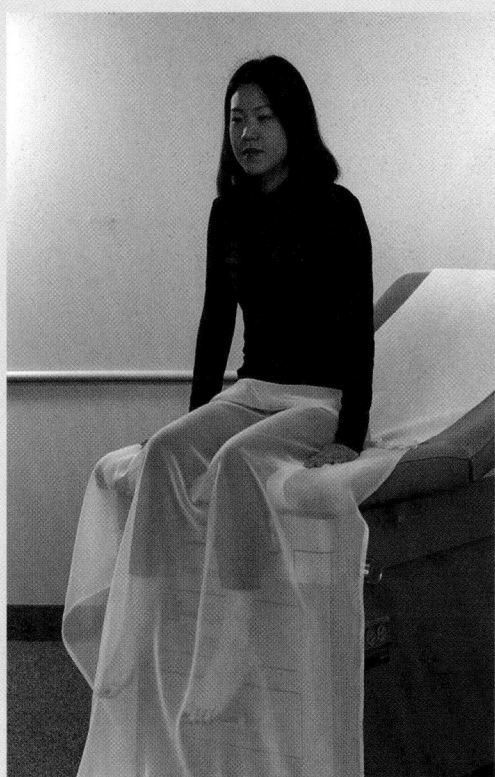

FIGURE 1

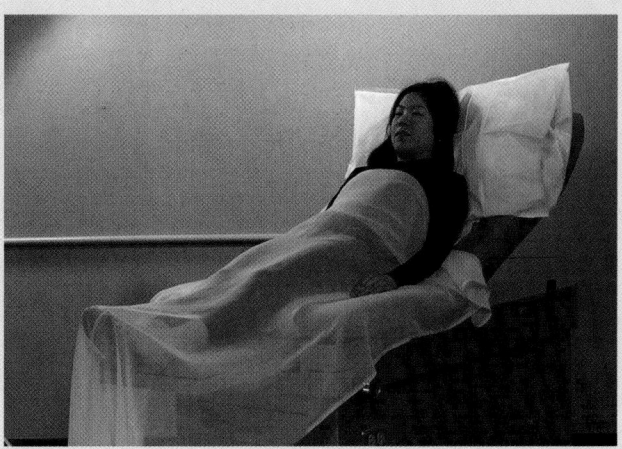

FIGURE 2

PROCEDURE 31-3

Prepare Patient for and Assist with Routine and Specialty Examinations: Horizontal Recumbent and Dorsal Recumbent Positions

<u>CAAHEP COMPETENCY:</u> 3.b.(4)(e)
<u>ABHES COMPETENCY:</u> 4.h

GOAL: *To position and drape the patient for examinations of the abdomen, heart, and breasts in the horizontal recumbent (supine) position and the rectal, vaginal, and perineal areas in the dorsal recumbent position.*

EQUIPMENT and SUPPLIES

- Examination table
- Table paper
- Patient gown
- Drape

PROCEDURAL STEPS

1. Prepare the examination room according to acceptable medical aseptic rules.
   <u>PURPOSE:</u> Room must be aseptically clean to prevent spread of infection.
2. Wash your hands.
   <u>PURPOSE:</u> Infection control.
3. Greet and identify the patient, and determine whether the patient understands the procedure. If the patient does not understand, explain what to expect.
   <u>PURPOSE:</u> To promote patient understanding and cooperation during the examination.
4. Give the patient a gown, and explain the clothing that must be removed for the particular examination being done and whether the gown should be open in the front or the back. Provide assistance as needed. For the horizontal recumbent position, the gown should be open in the front. Give the patient privacy while changing. Knock on the examination room door before reentering to make sure the patient has completed undressing and gowning.

5. Do not place the patient in these positions until the physician is ready for that part of the examination.
   <u>PURPOSE:</u> To promote patient privacy, comfort, and modesty.
6. Pull out the table extension that supports the patient's legs. For the horizontal recumbent (supine) position, help the patient lie flat on the table with the face upward (Figure 1). For the dorsal recumbent position, have the patient lie flat on the back and flex the knees so the feet are flat on the table (Figure 2). If needed, help the patient move down toward the foot of the table for the examination.
7. Drape the patient from nipple line to feet in the supine position, and diagonally with the point of the drape between the feet for the dorsal recumbent position.
   <u>PURPOSE:</u> Draping the patient provides warmth and privacy while giving the physician access to the examination site.
8. After the examination is completed, assist the patient as needed to get off of the table and get dressed.
9. Clean and disinfect the examination room according to standard precautions. Roll clean paper over the table.
   <u>PURPOSE:</u> Infection control. Prevents transmission of pathogens from one patient to another.
10. Wash hands.
11. Follow up with physician orders regarding scheduling of diagnostic studies, collection of specimens, and/or scheduling of future appointments.

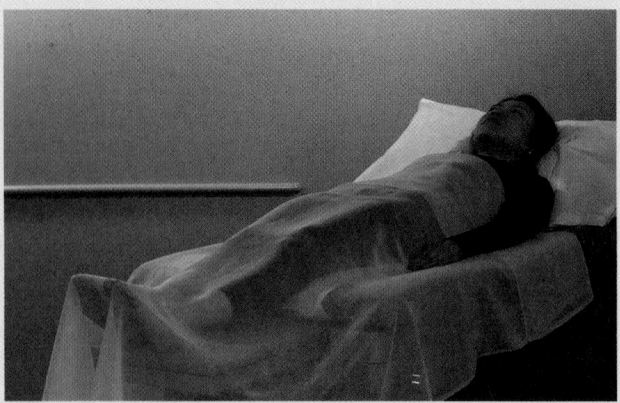

FIGURE 1

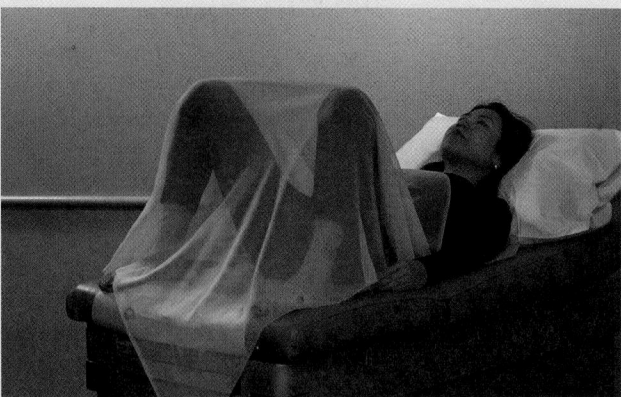

FIGURE 2

is not wearing a gown. The drape must be long enough to cover the knees and touch the ankles and wide enough to prevent the sides of the thighs from being exposed. The physician will lift the drape away from the pubic area when the examination begins (Procedure 31-4). The lithotomy position is primarily used for vaginal examinations that require the use of a speculum and for Pap smears.

Sims'. Sims' position is sometimes called the *lateral position*. The patient is placed on the left side; the left arm and shoulder are drawn back behind the body so that the body's weight is predominantly on the chest. The right arm is flexed upward for support. The left leg is slightly flexed, and the buttocks are pulled to the edge of the table. The right leg is sharply flexed upward. The drape extends diagonally from under the arms to below the knees. The physician can raise a small portion of the sheet from the back of the patient to sufficiently expose the rectum. The remaining portion of the sheet covers the patient's chest area and thighs. This position is used for rectal

---

PROCEDURE 31-4

Prepare Patient for and Assist with Routine and Specialty Examinations: Lithotomy Position

<u>CAAHEP COMPETENCY:</u> 3.b.(4)(e)
<u>ABHES COMPETENCY:</u> 4.h

GOAL: *To position and drape the patient primarily for vaginal and pelvic examinations and Pap smears.*

EQUIPMENT and SUPPLIES

- Examination table
- Table paper
- Patient gown
- Drape

PROCEDURAL STEPS

1. Prepare the examination room according to acceptable medical aseptic rules.
   <u>PURPOSE:</u> Room must be aseptically clean to prevent spread of infection.
2. Wash your hands.
   <u>PURPOSE:</u> Infection control.
3. Greet and identify the patient, and determine whether the patient understands the procedure. If the patient does not understand, explain what to expect.
   <u>PURPOSE:</u> To promote patient understanding and cooperation during the examination.

4. Give the patient a gown, and instruct the patient to undress from the waist down with the gown open in the back. If the physician will also be doing a breast examination, the gown should be open in the front. Provide assistance as needed. Give the patient privacy while changing. Knock on the examination room door before reentering to make sure the patient has completed undressing and gowning.
5. Do not place the patient in this position until the physician is ready for that part of the examination.
   <u>PURPOSE:</u> To promote patient privacy, comfort, and safety.
6. Pull out the table extension that supports the patient's legs, and help the patient lay face upward on the table. Pull out the stirrups, adjusting their extension length for patient comfort, and lock them in place.
7. Reinsert the table extension and have the patient move toward the foot of the table with her buttocks on the bottom table edge. Gently place the patient's legs in the stirrups, checking for comfort. Some offices may stock cloth or paper stirrup covers to protect the patient and make the position more comfortable. The patient's arms can be placed alongside the body or across the chest (Figure 1).
8. Drape the patient diagonally with the point of the drape between the feet. The drape should be large enough to cover the patient from the nipple line to the ankles and wide enough so the patient's thighs are not exposed.
   <u>PURPOSE:</u> Draping the patient provides warmth and privacy while giving the physician access to the examination site.
9. After the examination is completed, assist the patient as needed to get off of the table and get dressed.
10. Clean and disinfect the examination room according to standard precautions. Roll clean paper over the table.
    <u>PURPOSE:</u> Infection control. Prevents transmission of pathogens from one patient to another.
11. Wash hands.
12. Follow up with physician orders regarding scheduling of diagnostic studies, collection of specimens, and/or scheduling of future appointments.

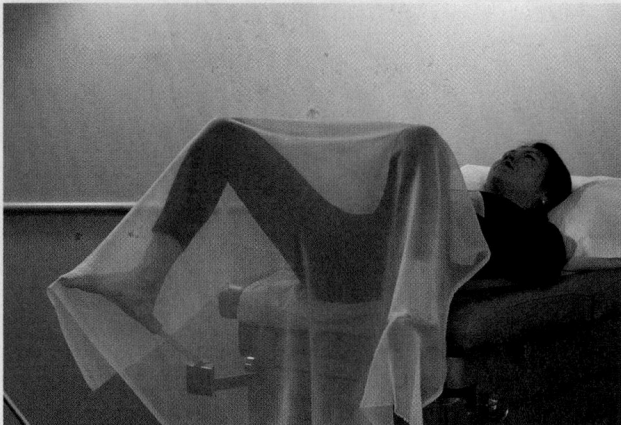

FIGURE 1

examinations, instillation of rectal medications, and perineal and some pelvic examinations (Procedure 31-5).

Prone. The patient lies face down on the table, on the ventral surface of the body. This is the opposite of the supine position and is another one of the recumbent positions. The drape should cover from the middle of the back to below the knees, with the gown open to the back. The drape on a female patient should extend high enough to cover her breasts if she is to be turned over to the dorsal recumbent position during the examination (Procedure 31-6). This position is used for examinations of the back and for certain surgical procedures.

Knee-Chest. The patient rests on the knees and the chest with the head turned to one side. The arms can be placed under the head for support and comfort or bent and at the sides of the table near the head. The thighs are perpendicular to the table and are slightly separated. The buttocks extend up into the air, and the back should be straight. The patient will need assistance to do the knee-chest position correctly. It is difficult for most patients to maintain this position, so they should not be placed into it until the point in the examination that it is required. The medical assistant must remain next to the patient for assistance and support the entire time that the knee-chest position is needed. If the correct knee-chest position cannot be obtained, the patient may have to be placed in a knee-elbow position. This position puts less strain on the patient and is easier to maintain. These positions are used for proctologic examinations

PROCEDURE 31-5

Prepare Patient for and Assist with Routine and Specialty Examinations: Sims' Position

<u>CAAHEP COMPETENCY</u>: 3.b.(4)(e)
<u>ABHES COMPETENCY</u>: 4.h

GOAL: *To position and drape the patient for examinations of the rectum, rectal thermometer readings, instillation of rectal medications, perineal examinations, and some pelvic examinations.*

EQUIPMENT and SUPPLIES

- Examination table
- Table paper
- Patient gown
- Drape

PROCEDURAL STEPS

1. Prepare the examination room according to acceptable medical aseptic rules.
   <u>PURPOSE:</u> Room must be aseptically clean to prevent spread of infection.

2. Wash your hands.
   <u>PURPOSE:</u> Infection control.

3. Greet and identify the patient, and determine whether the patient understands the procedure. If the patient does not understand, explain what to expect.
   <u>PURPOSE:</u> To promote patient understanding and cooperation during the examination.

4. Give the patient a gown and explain the clothing that must be removed for the particular examination being done. Tell the patient to open the gown in the back. Provide assistance as needed. Give the patient privacy while changing. Knock on the examination room door before reentering to make sure the patient has completed undressing and gowning.

5. Do not place the patient in this position until the physician is ready for that part of the examination.
   <u>PURPOSE:</u> To promote patient privacy, comfort, and safety.

6. Help the patient turn onto the left side; the left arm and shoulder should be drawn back behind the body so that the patient is tilted onto the chest. Flex the right arm upward for support, slightly flex the left leg, and sharply flex the right leg upward. Help the patient move the buttocks to the side edge of the table (Figure 1).

7. Drape the patient diagonally in a diamond shape, with the point of the diamond dropping below the buttocks. Make sure that the drape is large enough that the patient is not exposed.
   <u>PURPOSE:</u> Draping the patient provides warmth and privacy while giving the physician access to the examination site.

8. After the examination is completed, assist the patient as needed to get off of the table and get dressed.

9. Clean and disinfect the examination room according to standard precautions. Roll clean paper over the table.
   <u>PURPOSE:</u> Infection control. Prevent transmission of pathogens from one patient to another.

10. Wash hands.

11. Follow up with physician orders regarding scheduling of diagnostic studies, collection of specimens, and/or scheduling of future appointments.

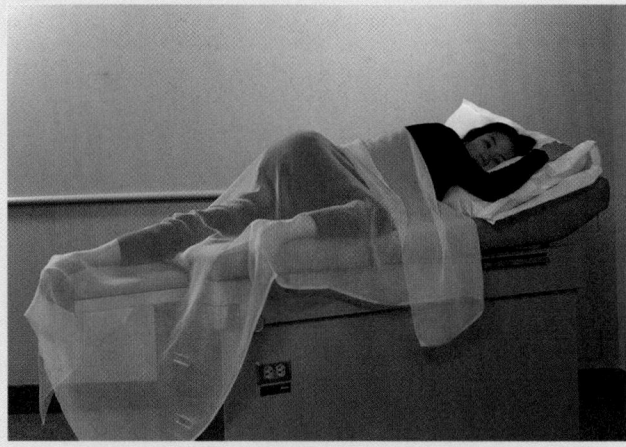

FIGURE 1

PROCEDURE 31-6

Prepare Patient for and Assist with Routine and Specialty Examinations: Prone Position

<u>CAAHEP COMPETENCY:</u> 3.b.(4)(e)
<u>ABHES COMPETENCY:</u> 4.h

GOAL: *To position and drape the patient for examinations of the back and certain surgical procedures.*

EQUIPMENT and SUPPLIES

- Examination table
- Table paper
- Patient gown
- Drape

PROCEDURAL STEPS

1. Prepare the examination room according to acceptable medical aseptic rules.
   <u>PURPOSE:</u> Room must be aseptically clean to prevent spread of infection.
2. Wash your hands.
   <u>PURPOSE:</u> Infection control.
3. Greet and identify the patient, and determine whether the patient understands the procedure. If the patient does not understand, explain what to expect.
   <u>PURPOSE:</u> To promote patient understanding and cooperation during the examination.
4. Give the patient a gown, and explain the clothing that must be removed for the particular examination being done. Tell the patient to open the gown in the back. Provide assistance as needed. Give the patient privacy while changing. Knock on the examination room door before reentering to make sure the patient has completed undressing and gowning.
5. Do not place the patient in this position until the physician is ready for that part of the examination.
   <u>PURPOSE:</u> To promote patient privacy, comfort, and safety.
6. Pull out the table extension if necessary, and help the patient lie down on his or her stomach (Figure 1).
7. Drape the patient over any exposed area that is not included in the examination. For female patients the drape should be large

enough to cover from the breasts to the feet so if the patient is asked to roll over she is not exposed accidentally.
   <u>PURPOSE:</u> Draping the patient provides warmth and privacy while giving the physician access to the examination site.
8. After the examination is completed, assist the patient as needed to get off of the table and get dressed.
9. Clean and disinfect the examination room according to standard precautions. Roll clean paper over the table.
   <u>PURPOSE:</u> Infection control. Prevent transmission of pathogens from one patient to another.
10. Wash hands.
11. Follow up with physician orders regarding scheduling of diagnostic studies, collection of specimens, and/or scheduling of future appointments.

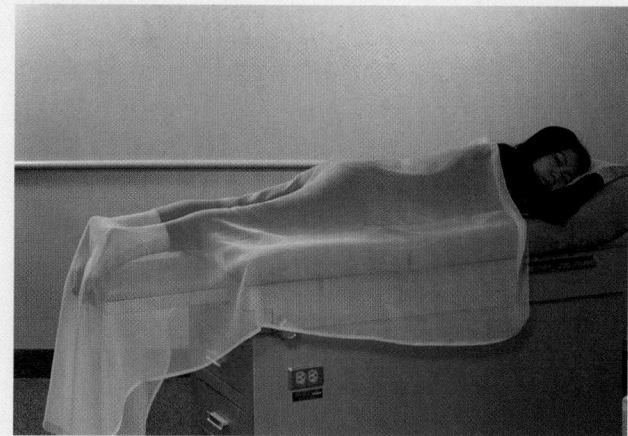

FIGURE 1

---

and sigmoid, rectal, and occasionally vaginal examinations. The patient's gown should open in the back, with a fenestrated (opening) drape or a single sheet draped diagonally over the patient's back at the sacral area (Procedure 31-7).

CRITICAL THINKING APPLICATION

Determine the correct patient position and method of gowning and draping for the following examinations:
- Instillation of a rectal suppository
- An annual Papanicolaou (Pap) smear
- Examination of the back
- Patient with dyspnea
- Breast examination

PRINCIPLES OF BODY MECHANICS

Proper body mechanics should be used consistently throughout the work environment when sitting or standing, lifting or carrying objects, pushing or pulling, or transferring patients. Without consistent application of correct anatomic alignment, it is very easy for injuries, especially lower back injuries, to occur.

Proper body alignment begins with good posture. Maintaining posture requires a combination of muscle efforts. Good posture keeps the spine balanced and aligned while sitting and standing. A person in good body alignment can maintain balance without undue strain on the musculoskeletal system.

When reaching for an object, avoid twisting or turning; instead, move the feet to face the object needed. This will avert

PROCEDURE 31-7

Prepare Patient for and Assist with Routine and Specialty Examinations:
Knee-Chest Position

<u>CAAHEP COMPETENCY:</u> 3.b.(4)(e)
<u>ABHES COMPETENCY:</u> 4.h

GOAL: *To position and drape the patient for examinations of the back and certain surgical procedures.*

EQUIPMENT and SUPPLIES

- Examination table
- Table paper
- Patient gown
- Drape

PROCEDURAL STEPS

1. Prepare the examination room according to acceptable medical aseptic rules.
   <u>PURPOSE:</u> Room must be aseptically clean to prevent spread of infection.
2. Wash your hands.
   <u>PURPOSE:</u> Infection control.
3. Greet and identify the patient, and determine whether the patient understands the procedure. If the patient does not understand, explain what to expect.
   <u>PURPOSE:</u> To promote patient understanding and cooperation during the examination.
4. Give the patient a gown and explain the clothing that must be removed for the particular examination being done. Tell the patient to open the gown in the back. Provide assistance as needed. Give the patient privacy while changing. Knock on the examination room door before reentering to make sure the patient has completed undressing and gowning.
5. Do not place the patient in this position until the physician is ready for that part of the examination.
   <u>PURPOSE:</u> To promote patient privacy, comfort, and safety.
6. Pull out the table extension if necessary, and help the patient lie down on his or her back then turn over to the prone position. Ask the patient to move up onto the knees, spread the knees apart, and lean forward onto the head so that the buttocks are raised. Tell the patient to keep the back straight and turn the face to either side. The patient should rest his or her weight on the chest and shoulders (Figure 1).

7. If the patient has difficulty maintaining this position, an alternative is to place weight on bent elbows with head off of the table.
8. Drape the patient diagonally so that the point of the drape is on the table between the legs.
   <u>PURPOSE:</u> Draping the patient provides warmth and privacy while giving the physician access to the examination site.
9. After the examination is completed, assist the patient as needed to get off of the table and get dressed.
10. Clean and disinfect the examination room according to standard precautions. Roll clean paper over the table.
    <u>PURPOSE:</u> Infection control. Prevent transmission of pathogens from one patient to another.
11. Wash hands.
12. Follow up with physician orders regarding scheduling of diagnostic studies, collection of specimens, and/or scheduling of future appointments.

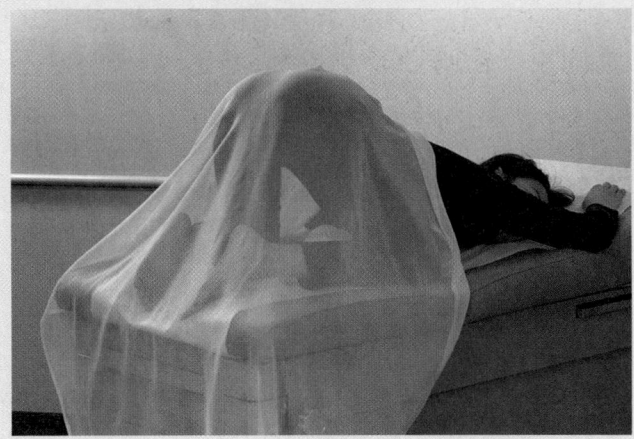

FIGURE 1

undue strain on the lumbar region. Do not cross the legs while sitting, because it interferes with circulation to the legs and feet. When sitting, keep the popliteal area (behind the knees) free from the edge of the chair. Pressure in this area interferes with circulation and may cause damage to nerves located behind the knees. Do a mental check of posture on a regular basis. Hold the head erect, with the face forward and chin slightly up, the abdominal muscles contracted up and in, shoulders relaxed and back, feet pointing forward and slightly apart, and weight evenly distributed to both legs, with the knees slightly bent. Always

be on alert for poor body mechanics that may cause injuries (Figures 31-11, 31-12).

Transferring a Patient

Frequently patients need assistance to move from a chair to the examination table or back again. There are multiple ways to transfer patients, but all should focus on correct body mechanics. If the patient is in a wheelchair, move the chair close to the examination table, lock the wheels, and lift the foot rests of the wheelchair out of the way (Figure 31-13). Explain the

Safe Lifting Techniques

- Always get help if the load is too heavy.
- Maintain correct body alignment with legs spread apart for a broad base of support.
- Do not reach for items. Clear barriers out of the way and get as close as possible to what needs to be lifted.
- Bend at the knees with the feet shoulder-width apart, and *keep the back straight.* Use the major muscle groups of the arms and legs to help lift a heavy item rather than the weaker ones of the back (see Figure 31-11).
- Keep the weight as close as possible to the body when carrying a heavy item (see Figure 31-12).
- Move feet in the direction of the lift. *Do not twist or turn on fixed feet.*
- Bend knees while keeping the back straight when lowering an item at the completion of the lift.
- If there is a choice, slide, roll, or push a heavy item rather than pulling it.

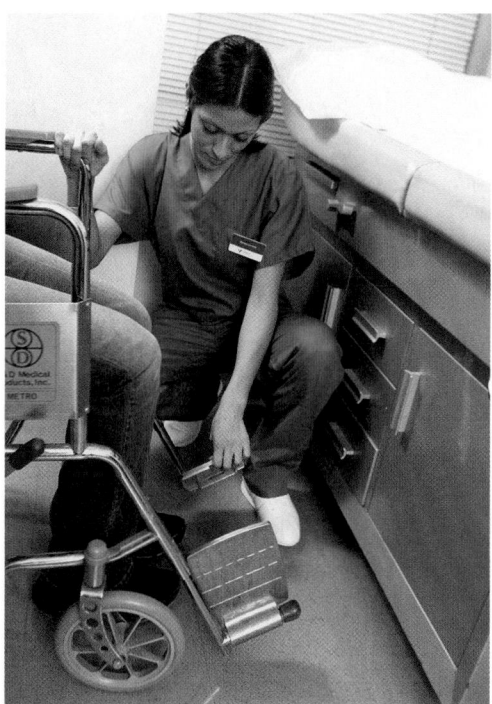

FIGURE 31-13 Wheels locked and foot rests elevated.

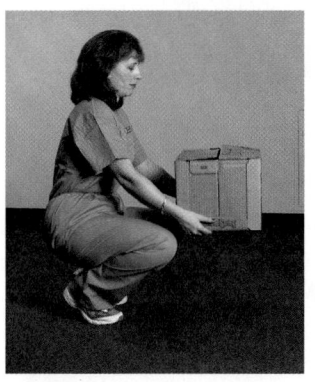 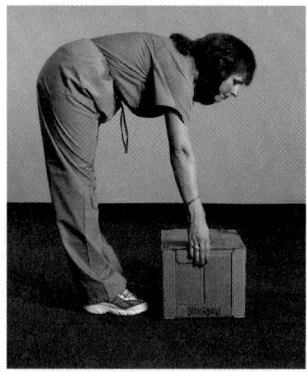

A   B

FIGURE 31-11 A, Proper lifting technique. **B,** Improper lifting technique.

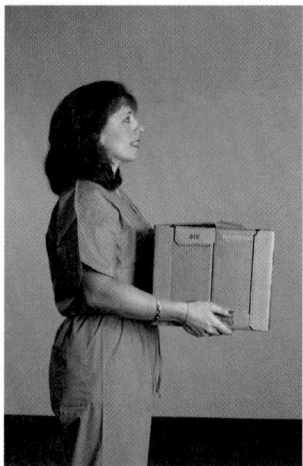 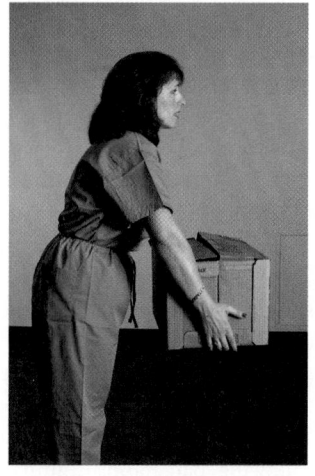

A   B

FIGURE 31-12 A, Carrying item close to body. **B,** Improper carrying technique.

procedure to the patient, and ask for his or her assistance.

If one side of the patient is stronger than the other, always provide support on the strong side. Place a step stool in front of the wheelchair next to the side of the examination table.

Support the patient close to your body on the strong side, with one hand under the axillary region and the other either grasping the patient's hand or holding the forearm. When bending, always bend at the knees and maintain the back's three natural curves, allowing the leg muscles to help in lifting. Give the patient a signal and lift as the patient assists. Anchor the step stool with one foot, and help the patient step up onto the stool with the strong leg, then pivot (Figure 31-14). Ease the patient down onto the table, bending your knees while keeping your back aligned. Make sure the patient is comfortable and safely positioned on the table (Figure 31-15). It may be necessary to remain with the patient until the examination is completed to ensure patient safety. If the physician prefers that the patient be in a supine position, place one arm across the patient's shoulders and the other under the knees and smoothly lower the patient's upper body to the table while raising the legs. Use the same pivoting techniques with proper body mechanics to help transfer the patient from the examination table back to the locked wheelchair. If the patient must hold onto you, have him or her hold your waist or shoulders, not your neck.

EXAMINATION SEQUENCE

The physical examination sequence is fairly standard; however, variations may occur, depending on the physician's specialty, the medical necessity for the examination, and the physician's preference. The medical assistant can do much to facilitate high-quality patient care and maintain the physician's schedule. A successful medical assistant develops a routine that is organized yet flexible enough to adjust to individual needs.

Give the patient a brief explanation of the examination process. Patients are more cooperative and less anxious if

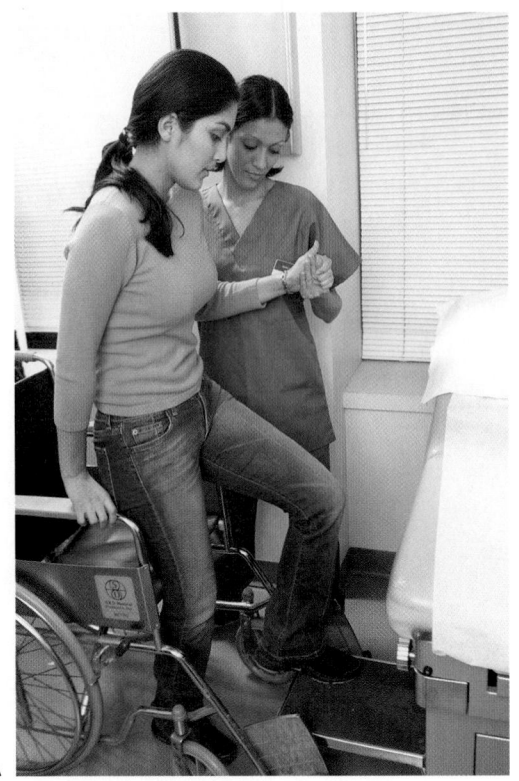

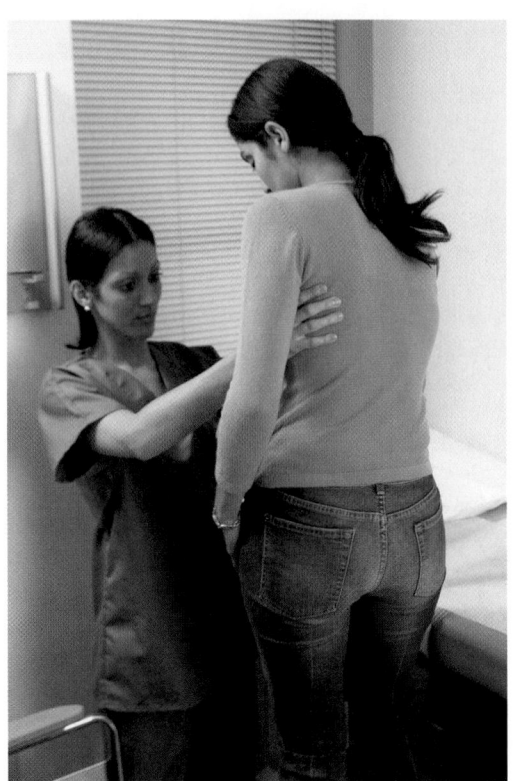

FIGURE 31-14 A, Strong side support. **B,** Pivot with support.

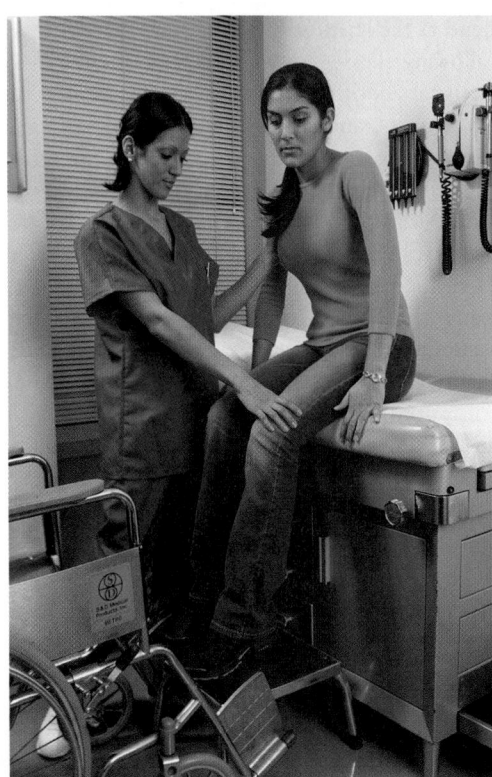

FIGURE 31-15 Sitting on table with support.

they understand what is expected of them. Assemble all the supplies and instruments needed for the examination before the physician enters the room. As the physician proceeds with the examination, make sure the patient remains unexposed by adjusting the drape and gown as needed. In every examination, the medical assistant assists the physician by handing him or her the correct instruments and supplies needed.

A female assistant in the room during the examination of a female patient can avert potential lawsuits. If the physician is male, a female medical assistant must remain with a female patient throughout the examination unless the physician excuses the medical assistant from the room.

When the physician begins the examination, the medical assistant should keep conversation to a minimum and remain inconspicuous. The examination usually starts with the patient seated on the examining table. If the physician uses reflected light, the light source should be behind the patient's right shoulder. If illuminated instruments are used, then the standard overhead lights are sufficient. Be careful not to shine a light directly into the patient's eyes. Turning on lights while they are directed away from the patient and carefully moving the light toward the area to be examined can accomplish this. The following paragraphs summarize areas that are observed and evaluated.

Presenting Appearance (General Appearance)

The physician starts the physical examination by observing the patient's appearance. Either *presenting appearance* or *general appearance* may be used on the medical record. These terms note whether the patient appears well and in good health (e.g., the patient appears disoriented or in distress; well or undernourished; may answer questions with ease or confusion).

The patient's gait often provides important information. The patient may limp, walk with the feet wide apart, exhibit a shuffle step, or have difficulty in maintaining his or her balance. In addition to gait, the patient's entire body movements are observed for possible muscle actions that the physician deems unusual. Posture is also checked for indications of pain, stiffness, or difficulty with limb movement. If the medical assistant notes any of these observations or the patient reports any complaints, these should be recorded in the patient's chart with the vital signs before the physician begins the examination.

Nutrition and Stature

The patient's height and weight are measured by the medical assistant before the examination begins and are recorded in the patient chart along with the BMI level. During the examination the physician notes the body build and proportions. Any *gross* (immediately obvious) deformities are recorded. Sometimes abnormalities in height or body proportion may be caused by hormonal imbalances.

Speech

Speech may reveal a pathologic condition. Some basic speech defects include *aphonia*, the inability to speak because of a loss of the voice, commonly seen with severe laryngitis or overuse of the voice; *aphasia*, the loss of expression by speech or writing because of an injury or disease of the brain centers; and *dysphasia*, a lack of coordination and failure to arrange words in proper order, usually caused by a brain lesion. *Motor aphasia* occurs when the patient knows what she or he wants to say but cannot use muscles properly to speak, such as slurred or incoherent speech that might occur after a cerebrovascular accident (CVA). *Sensory aphasia* is when the patient pronounces words easily but uses them inaccurately, such as in jumbled speech.

Breath Odors

Breath odors may or may not be diagnostic, although they are often associated with poor oral hygiene or dental care. Acidosis will give the strong odor of acetone, which is sweet and fruity, and may result from diabetes mellitus, starvation, or renal disease. A musty odor is usually associated with liver disease, and the odor of ammonia may be found in cases of uremia.

Skin

The condition of the skin can be a good reflection of the patient's nutritional status and hydration level. If dehydration is suspected, skin *turgor* is checked by pinching the skin on the posterior surface of the hands. The tissue is then observed to see how quickly it returns to the normal location. A delay indicates a decrease in tissue fluid, confirming the diagnosis of dehydration. Extreme dryness, scaling, extended time for wound healing, or frequent breaks in the skin may indicate systemic disease.

Fingernails and toenails often give some indication of a person's health. Brittle, grooved, or lined nails may indicate either local infection or systemic disease. **Clubbing** of the fingertips is associated with some congenital heart or lung diseases. *Spooning* of the nail is seen in some patients with severe iron-deficiency anemia. *Beau's lines* appear after an acute illness but will grow out and disappear. The PCP may refer the patient with skin disorders to a dermatologist for diagnosis and treatment.

Head

Once the physician makes overall observations of the patient's general condition, the physical examination typically begins with the head and face and moves downward toward the feet. The face reflects the patient's state and tells the physician a great deal about how the patient handles stress and illness. The skull, scalp, and face are palpated for size, shape, and symmetry. The distribution or the lack of hair and the hair texture may indicate hormonal changes. Excessive hair, especially facial hair in females, indicates a hormonal imbalance. As the head is examined the physician assesses possible **nodules,** masses, or signs of trauma.

Eyes

The pupils are checked for reaction by shining a light into the eye. If the pupils constrict equally and smoothly to the light stimulus the physician will document "PEARL" (which means the pupils are equal and respond to light). The **sclera** is checked for color, which ranges from white to pale yellow. The movements of the eyes are tested by having the patient follow the physician's finger. If the movement is within average range, the note "extraocular movement (EOM) intact" is written. The physician uses the ophthalmoscope to examine the interior of the eye, including the retina and the intraocular vessels. Some diseases, such as diabetes mellitus, cause damage to the blood vessels of the retina.

Ears

The ears are examined with the use of the otoscope. The external ear is first checked for inflammation of the external auditory canal or the presence of ear wax *(cerumen).* The tympanic membrane (eardrum) is examined and should appear pearly gray. Scars appearing on the eardrum are frequently the result of earlier, chronic ear infections or perforations. The color of the eardrum is important to the diagnosis, because it may indicate fluids such as blood or pus behind the eardrum in the middle ear. The patient may be asked to swallow several times to allow observation of movement of the tympanic membrane, which occurs because of pressure changes in the eustachian tube. The eustachian tube equalizes air pressure between the middle ear and the throat. The ability of the tympanic membrane to move is crucial to the hearing process.

Nose and Sinuses

The mucosa of the nasal cavity is examined for color and texture. The sinuses cannot be seen, but the frontal and maxillary sinuses may be examined by firm palpation over the area and by **transillumination.** When disorders in the eyes, ears, nose, and throat are observed, and the physician believes that the condition warrants the attention of a specialist, the patient is referred to an ophthalmologist or an otorhinolaryngologist (ear, nose, and throat specialist).

Mouth and Throat

The mouth, or oral cavity, is usually thought of in terms of oral hygiene and dental care. Dental hygiene includes the condition of the teeth, how the patient cares for the teeth and gums, and whether the teeth of the upper and lower jaws meet properly (occlude) for chewing. Healthy gums are pale pink, glossy, and smooth and do not bleed when pressure from a tongue depressor is applied. The palatine tonsils are usually visible. The physician may use a tongue depressor and a piece of gauze to grasp the tongue for careful examination of it. The floor of the mouth is examined by both inspection and palpation for enlarged lymph nodes, salivary gland function, and ulcerations. The insides of the cheeks are also examined for any abnormal marks or color.

Neck

The neck is examined for ROM by having the patient move the head in various directions. The thyroid gland is given special attention for symmetry, size, and texture. The physician manually palpates the thyroid area, and the patient is asked to swallow several times. The carotid artery is palpated and auscultated for possible bruit. The lymph nodes are palpated. *Lymphadenopathy* (condition in which lymph nodes are enlarged) is usually present if there is an infection of the face, head, or neck.

Reflexes

The patient's reflexes are checked with the patient in the high Fowler's and supine positions. While the patient is sitting, the biceps are checked with the patient's arm flexed and supported by the examiner. The knee jerk (patellar reflex) and the ankle jerk (Achilles reflex) are checked using *tapotement* (a tapping or percussing movement) with either the fingers or the reflex hammer. The plantar reflexes (Babinski and Chaddock reflexes) are tested with the patient in either an upright or supine position.

Chest

While the patient is still in the sitting position, the chest, heart, and lungs are examined. The chest is examined for symmetric expansion. A tape measure may be used, especially if variation exists between the upper and lower chest expansion. A patient with a history of **emphysema** may have a barrel-shaped chest. The physician may use percussion to determine the density of lung tissues.

With the stethoscope to the patient's back, the examiner auscultates lung sounds. The patient is asked to take deep and regular breaths. This may produce slight dizziness, but the patient should be assured that it is only the result of the deep respirations and will rapidly pass. The physician notes the types of respirations and the presence of lung sounds in all lobes.

Because it takes considerable concentration to interpret heart sounds, the physician must have complete silence when listening to the patient's heart. The heart is examined using a stethoscope from both the anterior and posterior approaches to the patient. Further examination may include auscultation on the left lateral side. In patients with heart disease the physician may spend an extended period of time listening to heart sounds. If chest or heart abnormalities are found, the physician typically orders further diagnostic tests, including blood analysis, x-ray evaluation, and an ECG. Once the results of these studies are analyzed, the physician may refer the patient to a cardiologist for treatment of a heart condition or a pulmonologist or respiratory care specialist for treatment of a breathing disorder.

Abdomen

The patient is lowered to the dorsal recumbent position, and the drape is lowered to the pubic hair line. The gown is raised to just under the breasts. The physician stands to the patient's right side if at all possible. The patient's arms may be placed at the side, or the hands may be crossed over the chest or under the head. Relaxation of the abdominal muscles is absolutely essential for the abdominal examination. An alternative position is to place the patient supine with a small pillow under the head and knees. The physician auscultates the abdomen in all quadrants to confirm the presence of complete bowel sounds and palpates the abdomen for any abnormalities. The physician may also use percussion to determine the density, position, and size of underlying abdominal organs.

Breast and Testicular Examinations

A careful breast examination is part of the physical examination for every female, whether or not she is symptomatic. The breasts are examined both visually and by palpation in a high Fowler's position and then again in the supine position. Breast cancer is the most common malignancy occurring in women, and early detection is the key to successful treatment. This is a good opportunity to discuss and reinforce the consistent use of monthly self-breast examination (SBE). This technique is presented in Chapter 40. For male patients who have reached puberty or are 15 years of age or older the physician will perform a testicular examination. This is an important self-examination for all males to perform on a monthly basis because testicular carcinoma is a major health risk. The technique is presented in Chapter 39.

Rectum

The rectal examination usually follows the abdominal examination or may be part of the examination of the male or female genitalia. The patient's comfort and dignity are vital. For this part of the examination the physician needs examination gloves and lubricating jelly. The examination light must be directed at the perineal area during the examination.

Hemoccult test specimens are often collected at the time of the digital rectal examination. If this is a procedure that the physician performs, be sure to include the necessary collection folder with the examination equipment. Patients diagnosed with gastrointestinal (GI) disorders may be referred to a gastroenterologist. GI disorders are discussed in Chapter 38. See Procedure 31-8 for the steps involved in assisting with the physical examination.

PROCEDURE 31-8

Prepare Patient for and Assist with Routine and Specialty Examinations: Prepare Patient for and Assist with the Physical Examination

<u>CAAHEP COMPETENCY:</u> 3.b.(4)(e)
<u>ABHES COMPETENCY:</u> 4.h

GOAL: *To help the physician examine patients by preparing the patient and the necessary equipment and ensuring patient safety and comfort during the examination.*

EQUIPMENT and SUPPLIES

- Stethoscope
- Ophthalmoscope
- Scale with height measurement bar
- Tongue depressor
- Cotton balls
- Examination light
- Percussion hammer
- Lubricating gel
- Examination gloves
- Sphygmomanometer
- Otoscope with disposable speculum
- Tape measure

- Gauze sponges
- Pen light
- Nasal speculum
- Tuning fork
- Biohazard container
- Laboratory request forms
- Specimen bottles and laboratory requisitions
- Patient gown
- Drapes
- Thermometer
- Cotton-tipped applicators
- Hemoccult supplies

PROCEDURAL STEPS

1. Prepare the examining room according to acceptable medical aseptic rules.
   <u>PURPOSE:</u> Room must be aseptically clean to prevent spread of infection.
2. Wash your hands.
   <u>PURPOSE:</u> Infection control.
3. Locate the instruments for the procedure. Set them out in order of use within reach of the physician and cover them until the physician enters the examination room.
   <u>PURPOSE:</u> Promotes time management and ensures that all needed equipment and supplies are ready.
4. Identify the patient, and determine whether the patient understands the procedure. If the patient does not understand, explain what to expect.
   <u>PURPOSE:</u> To promote patient cooperation during the examination.
5. Review the medical history with the patient, and investigate the purpose of the visit. Record interview results.
   <u>PURPOSE:</u> To verify that all information is current and complete.
6. Measure and record the patient's vital signs, height, weight, and BMI.
   <u>PURPOSE:</u> To gather data needed before the examination begins.
7. Instruct the patient on how to collect a urine specimen if ordered, and hand the patient the properly labeled specimen container (see Chapter 51). Obtain blood samples for any tests that are ordered (see Chapter 52). Obtain resting ECG if ordered (see Chapter 48).

<u>PURPOSE:</u> To obtain all specimens and perform all tests as ordered by the physician.

8. Hand the patient a gown and drape. Instruct the patient regarding what clothes should be removed for the examination and whether the gown should be open in the front or back. Help the patient with undressing as needed; however, most patients prefer to undress in privacy. Knock on the door before reentry to protect patient privacy.
   <u>PURPOSE:</u> To assist the patient in preparing for the examination and safeguard patient privacy, comfort, and safety.
9. Assist the patient in sitting at the foot examination table; place the drape over the patient's lap and legs. If the patient is elderly, confused, or feeling faint or dizzy, do not leave him or her alone.
   <u>PURPOSE:</u> To provide for the patient's warmth and privacy and to prevent a fall or injury.
10. Place the patient chart in the chart holder on the door, or inform the physician that the patient is ready. Be careful to place patient identity information out of sight to protect patient privacy.
11. Assist during the examination by handing the physician each instrument as it is needed and by positioning and draping the patient.
12. When the physician has completed the examination, allow the patient to rest for a moment, then help the patient from the table. Assist with dressing, if necessary. Use proper body mechanics if assistance in transfer is needed.
    <u>PURPOSE:</u> To ensure patient's stability and safety.
13. Return to the patient and ask if he or she has any questions. Give the patient any final instructions, and schedule tests as ordered by the physician and/or the next appointment.
    <u>PURPOSE:</u> To clarify directions, eliminate any misunderstandings, and allow the patient to discuss any concerns. If there are misunderstandings or concerns beyond your scope of experience or skill, arrange for the physician to speak with the patient again.
14. Put on gloves and dispose of used supplies and linens in designated biohazard waste containers. Clean surfaces with disinfectant. Disinfect all equipment.
    <u>PURPOSE:</u> To prevent cross-contamination with any potential infectious materials.
15. Remove gloves, discard them in the biohazard waste container, and wash hands.
    <u>PURPOSE:</u> Infection control.
16. Replace used supplies and prepare room for next patient.

THE ROLE OF THE MEDICAL ASSISTANT

The physical examination establishes a baseline from which a patient's healthcare needs are determined. The examination should never be considered routine. Each patient's needs are special, and the medical assistant must be prepared to assist when needed. Throughout the procedure the medical assistant must treat the patient with respect and guard individual privacy as much as possible.

The primary role of the medical assistant regarding the physical examination is to have the room, equipment, and supplies stocked and ready; the patient prepared, with vital signs, height, weight, and BMI measured and recorded; documentation completed regarding the patient's chief complaint or reported data; and the patient properly gowned and in position for the examination. During the examination the medical assistant should be prepared to hand the physician needed equipment or assist in any other way necessary. After the examination is completed, the medical assistant should provide assistance to the patient as needed; complete any diagnostic procedures ordered by the physician; assist in the patient's discharge; answer patient questions or complete patient education; and disinfect and restock the room for the next patient.

CRITICAL THINKING APPLICATION

Alice Greenbaum is a 68-year-old patient of Dr. Kosto's who is scheduled for an annual physical examination, including a breast check and Pap smear. Mrs. Greenbaum appears anxious about the examination and asks Felicia if the gynecologic examination is necessary. How should Felicia answer this patient? What might be helpful in easing the patient's fears and preparing her for the examination?

CLOSING COMMENTS

Patient Education

To improve the overall health status of individuals and to enlist the patient as an ally in the examination process, the medical assistant can educate the patient in many different ways. Patient education contributes to the patient's holistic care. The physical examination process is an excellent time for the medical assistant to assess the need for patient education. This assessment should be performed to identify the best way to meet the needs of the patient. When identifying these needs, consider the following:

- The information that the patient needs to know
- How to convey the information so that the patient will understand
- How the patient will use the information once he or she has it

Develop a plan to teach the patient. Think about the different modalities available, such as pamphlets, pictures, DVDs, demonstrations, and community resources. The more interesting the information, the more fun it is to teach the patient, and the more enjoyment the patient will get out of learning. Many facilities maintain patient education files containing handouts on a wide range of health issues. The medical assistant should always review teaching plans with the physician and follow the physician's direction in patient education. Chapter 28 offers details on how to create an effective patient education intervention.

CRITICAL THINKING APPLICATION

Dr. Kosto serves as the PCP in the area for residents of group homes for the developmentally delayed. Jimmy Cosgrove, a 38-year-old patient who is severely retarded, is being seen today for an abdominal postsurgical visit. Felicia is responsible for preparing the patient for the examination as well as educating Jimmy's caregiver on how to assist in his recovery. Describe how Felicia should prepare the patient and the room and develop a teaching plan that meets the needs of the patient and his caregiver.

Legal and Ethical Issues

The medical assistant must recognize that a legal and ethical contract exists between the patient and the physician. As the physician's employee the medical assistant is part of that contract. Information gained during the physical examination is confidential and must remain that way. The medical assistant must uphold ethical responsibilities as written in the Code of Ethics of the American Association of Medical Assistants (AAMA): to render service, respect confidential information, and uphold the honor and high principles of the profession.

Health Insurance Portability and Accountability Act Applications

- Remember that conversations occurring in the office may be overheard. Guard patient confidentiality when gathering information about the chief complaint, scheduling diagnostic tests, or processing samples. If there is a privacy glass at the front desk, make sure it remains closed; turn your back away from the waiting room when talking on the phone; and avoid any conversation about the patient that has the potential of being overheard.
- Place patient charts on the examination room door with identifying information facing the door to prevent those passing by from recognizing the patient's name.
- Place the physician's schedule away from patient areas and maintain patient confidentiality during the admissions procedure in the facility. Many offices no longer use sign-in sheets, but if they are used, the staff must completely block the previous patient names from sight to maintain confidentiality.

SUMMARY OF SCENARIO

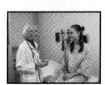

As a new medical assistant, Felicia Grand has a great deal of responsibility when it comes to assisting with physical examinations. She must prepare the room for the particular examination ordered and also prepare and care for the patient during the procedure. Preparing the room includes making sure appropriate supplies and equipment are readily available, as well as planning for the privacy of the patient during the examination. Each examination is different, just as each patient has his or her own set of needs. Felicia helps patients into a variety of positions depending on the examination being conducted by the physician, remembering to properly gown and drape the patient to safeguard privacy. It is Felicia's responsibility to make sure the examination runs smoothly for the physician and to support the patient throughout the process. To protect herself against potential injury, Felicia needs to use proper posture and body alignment, remembering to bend at the knees and use her arm and leg muscles to lift heavy items rather than her back. She should always ask for help if the load is too heavy and should push a heavy item rather than lifting it.

SUMMARY of LEARNING OBJECTIVES

1. Define, spell, and pronounce the terms listed in the vocabulary.
   - Spelling and pronouncing medical terms correctly adds credibility to the medical assistant. Knowing the definition of these terms promotes confidence in communication with patients and co-workers.
2. Describe the structural development of the human body.
   - The human body is made up of trillions of microscopic cells that determine the functional and structural characteristics of the entire body. A cell is made up of three primary parts: the plasma membrane, the cytoplasm, and the nucleus. When cells with similar structures and functions combine, tissues are formed. There are four types of tissues in the body: epithelial, connective, muscular, and nervous. A combination of two or more types of tissues creates an organ, and a number of organs joined together form a body system.
3. Differentiate among the 11 body systems and the major organs and structures in each.
   - A body system is composed of several organs and their associated structures. These structures work together to perform a specific function within the body. The human body has 11 systems. Each system has specific units within it, and each performs specific functions. Table 31-1 summarizes the body systems; their primary cells, organs, and structures; and the major functions of each.
4. Outline the medical assistant's role in preparing for the physical examination.
   - Before the examination the medical assistant has the opportunity to interact with the patient to ensure that he or she feels comfortable during the examination process and that all the necessary medical information is obtained. The medical assistant's duties include preparing and maintaining the examination room and equipment; preparing the patient by conducting the initial interview and measuring vital signs; and assisting the physician with positioning and draping and by providing instruments and supplies as needed during the physical examination.
5. Summarize the instruments and equipment typically used by the physician during a physical examination.

- Instruments and supplies that are typically used in the physical examination include the nasal speculum, ophthalmoscope, otoscope, tongue depressor, reflex hammer, various tuning forks, stethoscope, sphygmomanometer, thermometer, examination gloves, tape measure, scale, examination light, disposable gloves, biohazard container, specimen bottles, lab requisitions, hemoccult test supplies, patient gown, drapes, and lubricating gel.

6. Describe the six methods of examination, and give an example for each.
   - The examiner uses inspection to detect significant physical features such as the patient's general appearance. Palpation uses the sense of touch to feel the brachial pulse before taking a blood pressure reading. Percussion involves tapping or striking the body to elicit sounds or vibratory sensations such as in the percussion of the chest to detect fluid in the lungs. The physician uses a stethoscope auscultate or listen to the lungs and heart. Mensuration is the process of measuring the patient's height and weight. Manipulation is the forceful, passive movement of a joint to determine the range of extension or flexion of a joint.
7. Outline the basic principles of properly gowning and draping a patient for examination.
   - The patient should be instructed on whether to wear the gown open in the front or open in the back depending on the type of examination that will be done. Draping requires constant attention to maintaining the privacy of the patient throughout the examination while assisting the physician with exposure of the area being examined. The general rule is to cover all exposed body parts until the point in time during the examination when the physician must evaluate that particular area.
8. Compare and contrast the various positions that may be used during an examination, and identify the purpose of each.
   - The position assumed by the patient during the examination depends on the part of the body that is being examined or the procedure being done. Possible patient positions include the sitting positions of Fowler's, with the patient sitting straight

Continued

SUMMARY of LEARNING OBJECTIVES
Continued

up, and semi-Fowler's, with the patient elevated 45 degrees; dorsal recumbent, in which the patient is on the back with the legs bent; supine, in which the patient is lying flat on the back; lithotomy, in which the patient has the buttocks at the bottom of the table and legs positioned in stirrups; prone, in which the patient is lying on the stomach; Sims', in which the patient is on the left side with the limbs flexed so the weight of the body is tilted toward the chest; and knee-chest, in which the patient is on the knees with the buttocks elevated and the weight of the body tilted downward toward the chest and turned head.

9. Position and drape a patient in six different examining positions while remaining mindful of patient privacy and comfort.
   - Procedures 31-2 through 31-7 outline the steps for positioning and draping patients.

10. Demonstrate proper body mechanics in transferring a patient from a chair to the examination table and back.
   - Good body mechanics principles include maintaining balanced posture, bending the knees while maintaining the back's three natural curves, and using leg muscles to help lift. Move the wheelchair close to the examination table, lock the wheels, and lift the foot rests of the wheelchair out of the way. Provide patient support close to your body on the patient's strong side. Place a step stool in front of the wheelchair next to the side of the examination table and with one hand under the axillary region and the other grasping the patient, anchor the step stool with one foot. Help the patient step up onto the stool with the strong leg, then help the patient pivot into a sitting position on the table.

11. Outline the sequence of a routine physical examination.
   - The examination sequence is dependent on the type of examination and physician preference. The physician typically begins the examination by noting the patient's general health appearance, nutrition status, speech, breath odor, skin condition, and reflexes. The physician then begins the physical examination, starting at the head and working the way down through the body to the rectum. Any abnormalities are noted and may be further investigated with diagnostic tools after the examination is completed.

12. Prepare for and assist in the physical examination of a patient,

correctly completing each step of the procedure in the proper sequence.
   - Prepare the examination room and the patient; complete initial patient interview, and measure and record vital signs; gather needed equipment, and place in order of use; gown and drape the patient as needed; provide patient instruction, and check for understanding throughout the process; assist during the examination by handing the physician instruments, managing changes in light, collecting samples as ordered, and conducting diagnostic procedures as ordered; assist the patient when the examination is done, including scheduling further diagnostic tests as ordered, helping the patient dress, and answering patient questions. Complete the documentation, disinfect the examination room and equipment, and restock supplies to make the room ready for the next patient.

13. Summarize the role of the medical assistant in the physical examination process.
   - The medical assistant must pay attention to the individual needs of the patient as well as assist the physician with the procedure. This includes preparing the room and supplies, preparing the patient, documenting pertinent patient information, and assisting the physician throughout the process. After the examination is completed, the medical assistant should provide assistance to the patient as needed, complete diagnostic procedures as ordered, and disinfect and restock the examination room for the next patient.

14. Determine the role of patient education during the physical examination.
   - Before, during, and after the physical examination are excellent times to provide appropriate patient education. The medical assistant should clarify or reinforce any information provided by the physician as well as take advantage of "teaching moments" to promote patient well being.

15. Discuss the legal and ethical implications of the physical examination.
   - The medical assistant is part of the legal contract established between the patient and physician that begins at the time of the first visit to the ambulatory care facility. Maintaining confidentiality and providing respectful service are crucial to the integrity of that patient contract.

CONNECTIONS

Study Guide Connection: Go to Chapter 31 Study Guide. Read the Case Study and Workplace Applications and complete the assignments. Do online research for answers to the questions in the Internet Activities associated with assisting with the primary physical examination.

CD Connection: Go to the Medical Assisting Competency Challenge CD and do the training activities under Patient Care.

Evolve Connection: For more information related to assisting with the primary physical examination, go to evolve.elsevier.com/kinn and visit related weblinks for Chapter 31. Click on the Medical Assisting Exam Review and do the practice questions to sharpen your test-taking skills.

Principles of Pharmacology

32

SCENARIO

Kathy Augustino, CMA, was hired recently to work for a primary care physician in her hometown. Her responsibilities include administering medications to a wide range of patients. To correctly and safely give patients medications in the ambulatory setting, she must understand the basic principles of pharmacology.

While studying this chapter, think about the following questions:

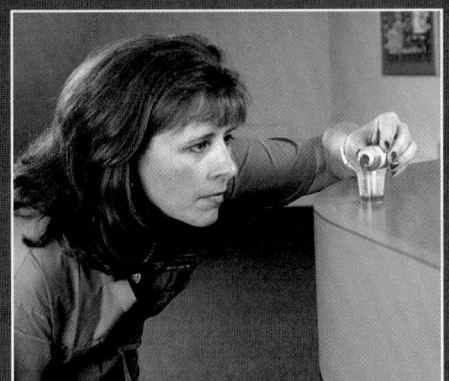

- What should Kathy know about the management of controlled substances in the ambulatory care setting?
- If Kathy is not familiar with a medication how can she learn about the properties of the drug?
- Is it important that Kathy understand the clinical uses of prescribed drugs as well as OTCs?
- One of Kathy's responsibilities will be phoning in drug orders to the pharmacy.
- What parts of the prescription should she recognize?
- Clients in the physician practice will be of all ages. What are factors that might affect the action of medications on her patients?

LEARNING OBJECTIVES

1. Define, spell, and pronounce the terms listed in the vocabulary.
2. Distinguish among the government agencies that regulate drugs in the United States.
3. Cite the Drug Enforcement Administration (DEA) regulations for the management of controlled or regulated substances.
4. List the DEA regulations for prescription drugs under each of the five schedules of the Controlled Substance Act.
5. Explain the medical assistant's role in the prevention of drug abuse.
6. Differentiate among a drug's chemical, generic, and trade names.
7. Describe the use of drug reference materials.
8. Summarize the clinical uses of drugs.

9. Cite safety measures for the use of over-the-counter drugs.
10. Diagram the parts of a prescription.
11. Demonstrate the ability to accurately transcribe a prescription.
12. Relate the principles of pharmacokinetics to drug usage.
13. Describe factors affecting drug action.
14. Differentiate among the therapeutic classifications of medications.
15. Examine the role of the medical assistant in drug therapy education.
16. Identify the legal ramifications of medication management for the medical assistant in an ambulatory care setting.

National Accreditation Competencies and Content

CAAHEP COMPETENCIES	ABHES COMPETENCIES
Clinical	**Clinical Duties**
3.b.(4)(g). Apply pharmacology principles to prepare and administer oral and parenteral medications	4.m. Prepare and administer oral and parenteral medications as directed by physician
3.b(4)(h). Maintain medication and immunization records	4.n. Maintain medication and immunization records
General	**Legal Concepts**
3.c.(2)(e). Demonstrate knowledge of federal and state health care legislation and regulations	5.e. Dispose of controlled substances in compliance with government regulations

VOCABULARY

angina pectoris (an-ji'-nuh/pek'-tuh-ruhs) Spasm-like pain in the chest caused by myocardial anoxia.

bronchodilator (brahn-ko-di'-la-tuhr) A drug that relaxes contractions of the smooth muscle of the bronchioles to improve lung ventilation.

cirrhosis (suh-ro'-suhs) A chronic degenerative disease of the liver that interferes with normal liver function.

colloidal (kah-loid'-uhl) Pertaining to a gluelike substance.

enteric-coated Drug formulation in which tablets are coated with a special compound that does not dissolve until the tablet is exposed to the fluids of the small intestine.

generic Not protected by trademark.

hypercholesterolemia (hi-per-kuh-les-tuh-ruh-le'-me-uh) Elevated blood levels of cholesterol.

lumen Space within a vessel or tube.

metabolic alkalosis Condition characterized by the significant loss of acid in the body or an increased amount of bicarbonate; severe levels can lead to coma and death.

over-the-counter (OTC) drugs Medications sold without a prescription.

parenteral Denoting any medication route other than the gastrointestinal (oral).

spermicide (spuhr'-muh-sid) A chemical substance that kills sperms cells.

therapeutic range Blood concentration of a drug that produces the desired effect without toxicity.

vertigo Dizziness.

Pharmacology is the broad science of the origin, nature, chemistry, effects, and uses of drugs. *Clinical pharmacology* is the study of the biologic effects of a drug on a patient when used as a medical treatment and the actions of a drug in the body over time, including the rate at which body tissues absorb a drug; where a drug is distributed or localized in the tissues; the route by which a drug is excreted; and the drug's toxicity or poisonous effect.

Medical assistants need to have a general understanding of the types of drugs that are available as well as their uses. For every medication administered, a medical assistant must understand the drug's action, typical side effects, route of administration and recommended dose, and individual patient factors that can alter the drug's effect and elimination. Drugs are constantly being developed and released for patient treatment; therefore, medical assistants must continually update their knowledge of specific drugs used in the ambulatory care setting. Correct management of drug administration and patient education are crucial factors in providing safe drug therapy for all patients.

GOVERNMENT REGULATION

Several federal agencies combine forces to regulate, safeguard, and manage the development and use of medications in the United States. The Food and Drug Administration (FDA), a division of the Department of Health and Human Services, regulates the development and sale of all prescription and **over-the-counter (OTC) drugs.** Pharmaceutical companies developing new medications must first gain FDA approval before the drugs can be sold to consumers. The approval process begins with chemical testing in the laboratory and progresses to toxicity testing in laboratory animals and finally to human clinical trials, which involve volunteers participating in controlled drug studies. Only one of 10 new drugs ever reaches the clinical testing phase. If the drug is found to have

an acceptable *benefit-to-risk ratio*, meaning it is effective without causing an unacceptable level of harm to the user, then the FDA approves the medication for release.

The original manufacturer of the drug is awarded copyright protection on that particular chemical compound for 17 years. Therefore, other pharmaceutical companies are unable to produce **generic** copies of the drug until the 17-year period is over. Besides approving new drugs for the marketplace, the FDA is also responsible for establishing standards for their purity and strength while being manufactured and ensuring that generic brands are effective and safe.

Standards for Both Brand and Generic Drug Manufacturers

- The generic version must have the same active ingredients, labeled strength, route of administration, and dosage form (tablet, patches, etc.).
- Generics do not have to replicate the human clinical trials of the brand-name drugs but applicants must prove that the product performs exactly as the brand-name version.
- Generic versions must act in the same period of time as the brand-name version, delivering the same amount of active ingredient into the bloodstream in the same amount of time.
- The FDA has found no difference in the rates of reported side effects between brand name and generic drugs.
- The generic drug's label must contain the same information for patient education.
- The generic manufacturing process must have comparable quality and production standards. Brand-name firms produce approximately 50% of the generic drugs on the market, making generic versions of their own products or other brand-name products.

Other Federal Agencies Involved in the Regulation of Drugs

- Drug Enforcement Administration (DEA)—Federal law enforcement agency responsible for the control of narcotics and drug abuse, investigation of the illegal sale of dangerous substances, and drug abuse prevention through public education.
- Federal Trade Commission (FTC)—Regulates advertising of over-the-counter drug preparations

Controlled Substances

The Drug Enforcement Administration (DEA) was established in 1973 as part of the Department of Justice to enforce federal laws regarding the use of illegal drugs. According to the federal Controlled Substances Act (CSA), a drug or other substance that has potential for illegal use and abuse must be placed on the controlled substance list. Any new medication that has a similar action to a drug already on the controlled substance list is also considered one that has potential for abuse.

Most controlled drugs provide significant assistance to patients in need of their particular actions such as pain relief or anesthesia for surgery. However, certain guidelines must be followed to comply with the storage of, record keeping surrounding, and security for controlled substances. In addition, federal law requires that all medical personnel, including medical assistants, share the responsibility for managing controlled substances on site. Precautions must be taken to monitor the drug use of patients, protect prescription pads, maintain the records required by law, and report any known or suspected drug diversion or theft.

Based on guidelines set forth in the CSA, controlled substances are divided into five sections or *schedules* according to their addictive abilities and degree of abuse. The classifications range from Schedule I drugs, which are illegal and cannot be prescribed, to Schedule V medications, which have the least potential for addiction and abuse.

Every medical practice that stores and administers medications that fall into any of the schedule categories should have a copy of the controlled substances regulations. A medical assistant may secure this list from a regional office of the DEA. It is also important to be on the DEA's mailing list to receive updates as drugs are added, deleted, or moved from one schedule to another. Table 32-1 summarizes the classification of controlled substances.

Regulation of Controlled Substances

There are specific CSA regulations governing the record keeping, physician registration, and inventory of controlled substances. Complete and accurate records must be maintained on the purchase and management of scheduled drugs in the

TABLE 32-1 Classification of Controlled Substances

SCHEDULE	GUIDELINES	DRUG EXAMPLES
I	No accepted medical use High potential for abuse Possession of these drugs is illegal	Heroin, lysergic acid diethylamide (LSD), marijuana, methaqualone (Quaalude), mescaline (peyote), amphetamine variations, phencyclidine (PCP), fentanyl, acetylcodone, Dipipan
II	Accepted for medical use but with severe restrictions High potential for abuse May cause severe psychologic or physical dependence	Opium extracts, morphine, methadone, cocaine precursors, amphetamine, cannabis, barbiturates, methylphenidate (Ritalin), oxycodone (Percocet or OxyContin), hydromorphone HCl (Dilaudid), meperidine HCl (Demerol), codeine, alfentanil (Alfenta), alphaprodine (Nisentil), Burgodin, secobarbital (Seconal)
III	Accepted for medical use Potential for abuse less than with schedule I or II drugs May cause moderate to low physical dependence or high psychologic dependence Includes combination drugs that contain limited amounts of narcotics or stimulants	Paregoric, acetaminophen and codeine (Tylenol with codeine), benzphetamine, suppositories with barbiturates, anabolic steroids, testosterone, butabarbital (Butisol), Fiorinal, Voranil, Empirin, hydrocodone (Vicodin),
IV	Accepted for medical use Low potential for abuse May cause limited physical or psychologic dependence in comparison with schedule III drugs Includes minor tranquilizers and hypnotics	Meprobamate (Equanil), chlordiazepoxide (Librium), diazepam (Valium), flurazepam (Dalmane), chloral hydrate, propoxyphene napsylate (Darvon), pentazocine lactate (Talwin), alprazolam (Xanax), triazolam (Halcion), temazepam (Restoril), chlorazepate dipotassium (Tranxene), lorazepam (Ativan), zolpidem tartrate (Ambien), barbital, Lexatin, Urbanyl, clonazepam (Klonopin), diethylpropion (Tenuate), Motofen, Capla, midazolam (Versed), Donnatal, Meridia, zolpidem tartrate (Ambien), eszopiclone (Lunesta)
V	Accepted for medical use Low potential for abuse May cause limited physical or psychologic dependence in comparison with schedule IV drugs Includes drug mixtures containing limited amounts of narcotics	Cough medicines containing codeine (Robitussin A-C), alkaloids, kaolin and pectin belladonna (Donnagel), diphenoxylate with atropine (Lomotil), buprenorphine

ambulatory care setting. These records must be kept separate from the patient chart for 2 years and be readily available for inspection by the DEA at all times. Every time a controlled substance is dispensed and administered in the office, documentation of that process includes the number of doses of the drug on site both before and after the medication is dispensed. Medical practices that dispense and administer controlled substances on site have forms developed for this purpose. Any discrepancy in the count of the amount of medication available must be documented and cosigned by two employees.

Each physician who prescribes or who has controlled substances on site must register with the DEA for a Controlled Substance Registration Certificate and will receive a specific DEA registration number that must be included on all controlled substance prescriptions. The certificate is renewable every 3 years and is specific to a particular site of practice. Therefore, if the physician dispenses or prescribes scheduled drugs at more than one site, a DEA registration number must be obtained for each site.

All controlled substances must be stored in a security safe or immovable locked cabinet. Prescription forms should be kept out of areas that are used by patients and preferably secured in an area that prohibits unauthorized or illegal use. DEA Prescription Form 222 and the state triplicate forms also need to be kept in a locked area.

Many ambulatory practices no longer keep controlled substances on site. However, if drugs are lost, it must be reported to the regional DEA office and local law enforcement authorities immediately. If a controlled substance is damaged or must be disposed of (e.g., a pill falls to the floor during dispensing), two employees must be present to witness the medication being flushed down the sink or toilet, and both must document the procedure on the controlled substance inventory form used by that office. If a large quantity of scheduled drugs must be disposed of, the local DEA office should be contacted for guidance.

CRITICAL THINKING APPLICATION

Kathy is responsible for maintaining the inventory of the controlled substances in the office. While checking the supply of meperidine she notices the expiration date of the medication is today. She must dispose of the remaining two pills. According to DEA regulations, how should she dispose of the medication?

Individual states may also regulate controlled substances; therefore it is essential that a medical assistant know his or her state's legal requirements.

There are specific guidelines for prescription orders of controlled substances. These include the following:

- Must be written in ink or typed.
- Must include the date prescribed; the name and address of the patient; and the name, address, and DEA number of the physician.
- Amount prescribed must be written out ("ten" rather than "10"), and usually the prescription is for small quantities of the drug.

- The physician must manually sign all prescriptions for controlled substances, although the medical assistant can prepare the prescription for the physician signature.
- Drugs in Schedules II, III, and IV must bear this label when dispensed by the pharmacy: *Federal law prohibits the transfer of this drug to any person other than the patient for whom it is prescribed.*

There are also specific rules depending on the designated schedule of the prescribed controlled substance. Symbols C-II, C-III, C-IV, and C-V are used to indicate the specific schedule:

- Schedule II (C-II) prescriptions:
  1. Must be written unless an absolute emergency exists that requires a telephone prescription order. The amount in the phone order is limited to that needed during the emergency, and the physician must deliver a written prescription to the pharmacy within 72 hours.
  2. Cannot be refilled.
  3. Certain states require the use of multiple-copy prescriptions.
- Schedule III (C-III) and IV (C-IV) prescriptions:
  1. May be oral or written.
  2. May be refilled up to five times within 6 months of the original order.
- Schedule V (C-V) prescriptions:
  1. May be oral or written.
  2. May be refilled up to five times within 6 months of the original order.
  3. Depending on the state, may be dispensed by the pharmacist without a prescription.

CRITICAL THINKING APPLICATION

Kathy is responsible for orienting a new medical assistant to the practice. Summarize the important points about government regulation of controlled substances that she should include in the orientation.

DRUG ABUSE

Any drug, from aspirin to alcohol, may be misused or abused. There has been a tremendous increase in the use of illegal and legal drugs. Treatment programs are available throughout the United States for people from all walks of life. Programs include detoxification, rehabilitation, and long-term rehabilitation maintenance.

Medical assistants may encounter patients who are misusing or abusing drugs. It is important to be alert to the symptoms of drug dependence and to notify the physician when you suspect a patient, or a co-worker, of having a problem with drug or alcohol dependency.

Drug *misuse* is the improper use of common drugs that can lead to dependence or toxicity. Examples of persons with chronic dependencies include people who cannot have a bowel movement unless they take a laxative; those who have used nasal decongestants for so long that they cannot breathe without the use of nasal sprays; and those who take so many antacids that they suffer systemic **metabolic alkalosis.**

Drug *abuse* is the continuous or periodic self-administration of a drug that could result in addiction (physical dependence). Drug *dependency* is the inability to function unless under the influence of a substance, and it may be either psychologic or physical. *Psychologic dependency* is the compulsive craving for the effects of a substance. *Habituation* is a mild form of psychologic dependency, such as the need for caffeine. *Physical dependency*, or addiction, is a person's need to use a substance continuously so the body can function and also to prevent physical discomfort. This type of dependency occurs when abused substances produce biochemical changes in cells and tissues, most commonly in the nervous system. Discontinuing a substance that causes physical dependency results in withdrawal symptoms. Withdrawal symptoms may be mild or potentially serious, leading to convulsions and possibly death.

Regardless of the type of drug abused, it will have two effects on the person: acute and chronic. The acute effect is what the person feels when intoxicated, or directly under the influence of a particular substance. Chronic effects include the temporary or permanent physical and mental changes that result from long-term abuse.

The medical assistant is often called on to answer patient questions concerning drug abuse. The medical assistant should read and keep up to date on drug-related issues. Pamphlets and agency referral names should be available for patients. Patient concerns and questions regarding drug abuse should also be conveyed to the physician.

DRUG NAMES

A single drug may have up to three names: chemical, generic, and trade. The chemical name represents the drug's exact formula. For example, the chemical name of the analgesic acetaminophen is N-(4-hydroxyphenyl). Acetaminophen is the generic name, and one of its trade names is Tylenol. All drugs have a generic or nonproprietary (official) name assigned to them. This name is much simpler than the chemical name, and it is not protected by copyright. The trade or brand name is assigned by the manufacturer and is protected by copyright. The use of generic names is encouraged over trade names to avoid confusion. Drugs are also classified by their use. For example, Advil is a brand name of the generic drug ibuprofen, which is classified as an analgesic and an antiinflammatory agent.

APPROACHES TO STUDYING PHARMACOLOGY

A pharmaceutical glossary could be a book in itself. Many terms are combinations of the condition to be treated, with the prefix *anti* (e.g., antianginal, antianxiety, antiarrhythmic, anticoagulant, anticonvulsant, antidiarrheal). Notice how these names emphasize the drug's effect (use) rather than its action in the body. More recent classifications, such as parasympathomimetic and cholinesterase inhibitors, describe the pharmacologic action rather than the therapeutic use. However, both viewpoints are necessary for a more complete understanding of drugs and what they do in the human body. No one can remember all there is to know about clinical pharmacology. The number of new drugs being introduced into use far exceeds the number of older drugs being replaced or discontinued. The number of drugs available for clinical use grows beyond the ability to learn all there is to know about each medication. Therefore, it is essential that a medical assistant understand how to use pharmacology resource books as references.

Reference Materials

Reference books that are updated annually or periodically should be available for easy reference at all medical facilities. Most references list drug information in the following sequence:

1. *Action:* How the drug provides the therapeutic results in the body or the use of the drug.
2. *Indication:* The conditions for which the drug is used.
3. *Contraindications:* Conditions that make the administration of a drug improper or undesirable.
4. *Precautions:* Actions necessary because of special conditions of the patient, drug, or environment that need to be considered for the drug to be successful or not harmful. The pregnancy risk category is included in this section as well as precautions for nursing mothers (Table 32-2).
5. *Adverse reactions:* Commonly observed side effects on a tissue or organ system other than the one being sought by the administration of a medication. Adverse reactions include *hypersensitivity*, which causes an allergic reaction to the drug; *idiosyncrasy*, or an unexplained, unusual response to the drug; psychologic dependence or habituation to the drug; or physical dependence to the compound, causing signs and symptoms of withdrawal in the patient if the medication is removed.
6. *Dosage and administration:* The usual route, dosage, and timing for administering the drug.
7. *How supplied:* Description of how the medication is packaged and specifics on how it should be administered.

The Medical Assistant's Role in Prevention of Drug Abuse

- Carefully monitor patients who repeatedly call for prescription refills of controlled substances.
- Request medical records for patients who report previous prescriptions for scheduled drugs.
- Keep prescription blanks in a safe place away from patient treatment areas, and minimize the number of prescription pads in use at any given time.
- Never use prescription pads for notepads, and never use preprinted or presigned forms.
- Keep only a limited supply of controlled substances on hand.
- Maintain complete and accurate records of controlled substances that are dispensed on site as well as those prescribed. Include specific documentation in the patient chart for all prescribed controlled substances.

TABLE 32-2 Pregnancy Risk Categories

CATEGORY OF RISK	CATEGORY DESCRIPTION
A	Remote risk Controlled studies in women have failed to demonstrate risk to fetus
B	Slightly more risk than A Animal studies show no risk but controlled human studies have not been done or animal studies show risk, but controlled studies in women have shown no risk
C	Greater risk than B Animal studies have shown risk, but no controlled human studies have been done or no studies have been done in animals or women
D	Proven risk of fetal harm Human studies show proof of fetal damage, but the potential benefits of use during pregnancy may make its use acceptable
X	Proven risk of fetal harm Studies in women or animals show definite risk of fetal abnormality Risks outweigh any possible benefit

Package Inserts

Every drug package contains an insert describing all the significant aspects of using the drug, including information on the chemical formulation of the drug and clinical studies. The information in the insert is controlled by the FDA and is an excellent quick reference on new medications in the ambulatory setting.

Physicians' Desk Reference

The *Physicians' Desk Reference* (PDR) is published annually by Thomson Medical Economics Company (Oradell, NJ). For physicians who subscribe to *Medical Economics* magazine, a PDR is provided free. Copies can be purchased through the publisher or in local bookstores. Supplements are published quarterly throughout the year. This reference contains information on approximately 2500 drugs, and the product descriptions are identical to the package inserts. The drug manufacturers pay for this space, so the PDR could be called the yellow pages of the drug industry. The PDR is the most commonly used drug reference book and should be available in all healthcare settings.

The book's sections are color-coded and cross-referenced for easy use. The various sections allow you to begin searching for information concerning a drug from any starting point. You can start with the usage, classification, generic name, manufacturer's name, or trade name of a drug or what the drug looks like. There is a special photographic section for visual product identification. Once you know which drug you want to study, the product information section lists the actual package insert information alphabetically, first by the manufacturer, then by the brand name. Also, a separate PDR volume, the *Physicians' Desk Reference for Nonprescription Drugs*, is published annually for OTC drugs and dietary supplements. The six sections of the PDR are color-coded into the following areas:

- Manufacturer's index—white
- Brand and generic section—pink (this is the one you will typically use to research unknown drugs alphabetically)
- Product category index—blue (alphabetic listing according to drug classification)
- Product identification section—gray
- General and diagnostic product information area—white

U.S. Pharmacopeia/National Formulary

The *U.S. Pharmacopeia/National Formulary* (USP/NF) is the official source of drug standards for the United States. The Pharmacopeia was combined with the *National Formulary,* which lists the chemical formulas for all accepted drugs. This combined reference lists and describes all the approved medications in the United States that are considered useful and therapeutic in the practice of medicine. Single drugs rather than combined products (compound mixtures) are listed. If a drug name is the same as the official name in this volume, the drug will have the initials USP after it (e.g., digitoxin, USP).

Learning about Drugs

The study of pharmacology is difficult at best. However, there are a few ways you can make it easier.

First, take opportunities to observe the use of drugs in patient care. Studying about atorvastatin calcium (Lipitor) becomes more meaningful when you see how its lipid-lowering action actually affects a patient's blood cholesterol level.

Second, concentrate on the most important drugs in each classification. As you expand your knowledge to other drugs in each classification, you will easily understand new drugs by noting the similarities and differences between them and the basic, important drugs you studied first.

Third, learn about a drug's primary action and use, then expand your knowledge to its other actions and uses. Soon you will be able to name the drug that is usually indicated for a particular condition. Then, by knowing a drug's secondary effects, you will be able to understand what side effects are likely to occur during the use of the drug. More important, you will be aware of the contraindications for the drug (conditions that make the use of the drug improper or undesirable). Knowledge of the drug's actions will also enable you to predict what toxic reactions could occur from an overdose.

Dispensing Drugs

There are two methods of dispensing drugs: OTC and by prescription. OTC drugs are available to the public for self-medication without a prescription. These drugs have been approved by the FDA for general consumer use, but patients on prescription drugs should keep their healthcare providers informed about their OTC drug use.

A medical assistant who is directly involved in patient care should have an understanding of some basic facts regarding OTC drugs. Today patients are better informed about their personal healthcare, and many want to be active participants in healthcare decisions. They need facts to make informed choices when using OTC preparations. Most OTC preparations are safe if used as directed on the package; however, patient education contributes greatly to the safe and correct use of OTCs. Patients should be encouraged to do the following when choosing or using an OTC:

- Carefully read the package label and insert for use guidelines.
- Take only the recommended dose.
- Monitor the expiration date, and discard the medication when appropriate.
- Never combine an OTC with a prescription drug without the knowledge of the physician.
- Recognize that many OTC drugs are contraindicated in pregnancy, nursing mothers, and young children and in the presence of certain diseases.
- Check with the pharmacist if questions or concerns arise.

The number of prescription drugs that have been granted OTC status is constantly increasing, and as the list of OTC drugs increases, so does the need for consumer education. Many OTC medications influence the safety and effectiveness of prescription drugs, so gathering a complete and accurate pattern of the use of OTCs should be part of every visit the patient makes to the physician.

Terminology Describing Drug Uses

diagnostic Helps determine the cause of a particular health problem (e.g., injecting antigen serum for allergy testing).

palliative Indicates that the drug does not cure but provides relief from pain or symptoms related to the disorder (e.g., the use of an antihistamine for allergic symptoms or narcotics for pain relief).

prophylaxis Prevents the occurrence of a condition (e.g., vaccines prevent the occurrence of specific infectious diseases).

replacement Provides patients with substances needed to maintain health (e.g., insulin for patients with diabetes or levothyroxine sodium [Synthroid] for patients with hypothyroidism).

therapeutic Drugs used to treat the disorder and cure it (e.g., antibiotics cure bacterial infections).

Prescription Drugs

Federal law makes drugs that are dangerous, powerful, or habit-forming illegal to use except under a physician's order. A *prescription* is an order written by the physician for the dispensing of a particular medication by the pharmacist and its administration to the patient. Sometimes an order may be written by the physician on the patient's medical record; however, most often it is a written order on a prescription blank for the pharmacist to fill. A prescription must be signed by the physician or the order cannot be carried out (Procedure 32-1). If the medical assistant is requested to phone in a prescription to the pharmacy for the physician, all of the pertinent information must be written down and reviewed by the physician for accuracy before the call is made. A note is also made in the patient's chart that a medication order was phoned into the pharmacy, with all of the pertinent information about the order included (see Procedure 9-3).

Table 32-3 lists the top 50 prescribed drugs in the United States in 2004. Appropriate medical terminology and abbreviations must be used to complete the prescription. The more common terms and abbreviations are listed in Table 32-4.

CRITICAL THINKING APPLICATION

Dr. Simon requests that Kathy prepare the following prescription for his signature. "Take one 20-mg tablet of Lipitor daily at bedtime. Dispense 4 weeks' worth, and the prescription may be refilled 2 times." How would Kathy write the prescription using the correct format, medical terminology, and abbreviations?

DRUG INTERACTIONS WITH THE BODY

Pharmacology is the study of drugs, their desired effect, and what happens to a drug while it is in the body. Different patients may react to the same dose of a drug in very different ways, and the same patient may react to the same dose of a drug differently at various times. Therefore the management of medication therapy is primarily concerned with the effectiveness of a drug's action as well as the medication's potential side effects. *Pharmacokinetics* is the study of the movement of drugs throughout the body. Four basic actions occur when a drug is taken: absorption, distribution, metabolism, and excretion. By knowing what happens to the drug in the body, we can know the *onset* of a drug's activity (when the drug action starts), when the effects of the drug are likely to peak, the minimum amount of the drug needed to bring about the desired effect (therapeutic dose), and the *duration* of a particular drug's activity. All of these factors help the physician determine the appropriate form, amount, route, and frequency of administration of a medication for a given patient.

Drug Absorption

The rate at which drugs are absorbed from the site of administration into the bloodstream depends on many factors including the drug's ability to be dissolved, the characteristics of the medication, the concentration of the dose, and the route of administration. Liquid oral medications are dissolved more

PROCEDURE 32-1

Maintain Medication and Immunization Records: Prepare a Prescription for the Physician's Signature

<u>CAAHEP COMPETENCY:</u> 3.b.(4)(h)
<u>ABHES COMPETENCY:</u> 4.n

GOAL: *To accurately prepare a prescription for the physician's signature using appropriate abbreviations and prescription format.*

EQUIPMENT and SUPPLIES

- Prescription pad
- Drug reference materials if needed
- Black pen
- Patient chart

PROCEDURAL STEPS

1. Refer to the physician's written order for the prescription. If the physician gives a verbal order to write a prescription, write down the order and review it with the physician for accuracy.
   <u>PURPOSE:</u> To ensure accuracy in writing the ordered medication.

2. If unfamiliar with the medication, look up the drug in a drug reference book (such as the PDR).
   <u>PURPOSE:</u> The medical assistant should be familiar with the details about the drug, including correct spelling, how it is dispensed, strength, recommended dose, storage guidelines, drug-to-drug interactions, and possible side effects to make sure the transcription is correct and to be prepared to answer the patient's questions about the medication.

3. Ask the patient about drug allergies.
   <u>PURPOSE:</u> The patient should be asked about drug allergies each time a medication is prescribed or dispensed, because these can change over time.

4. Using a prescription pad that has the physician's name, address, telephone number, and DEA registration number preprinted on the slip, begin to transcribe the physician order.

5. Record the patient's name and address and the date on which the prescription is being written.

6. Next to the Rx, write in legible handwriting the name of the drug (correctly spelled), the dosage form (such as tablet, capsule, and so forth, using correct abbreviations), and the strength ordered. For example, if the physician orders Lipitor, 40-mg tablets, by mouth, one tablet at bedtime, then the first line of the prescription should read: Lipitor 40 mg tabs. This is the inscription.

7. On the next line write Disp. This is the subscription, which includes directions to the pharmacist on the amount to be dispensed and the form of the drug. For the Lipitor order, the subscription would read: Disp: #30.

8. Next comes the signature. This includes directions for the patient, such as how and when to take the medicine, and is usually preceded by the symbol Sig. For the Lipitor order the signature would read: Sig: Ī tab po hs.

9. The physician tells you the patient can get three refills of the prescription, so this information should be added at the bottom of the prescription on the designated line.

10. The physician must review and sign the prescription before it is given to the patient.

11. Document on the patient's chart the medication order and any pertinent details, including patient education and refill information.
    <u>PURPOSE:</u> All patient education should be documented for future reference, and the details about the prescription as well as refill information must be included for future prescriptions and/or refill orders.

---

rapidly than solid forms because they do not have to be dissolved by gastrointestinal (GI) fluids. In addition, drugs that are soluble in fat pass more readily through the cell membrane because cell membranes have a fatty acid layer. More acidic drugs are absorbed well in the stomach, whereas others can't be absorbed until they reach the small intestine. For some medications, such as antibiotics, the physician may order an initial *loading dose* of the drug, usually twice the typical amount, so that the patient's blood levels reach the **therapeutic range** more quickly.

An important point to remember is that regardless of the route of administration, a drug can have one of two actions on the body: *local* (restricted to one spot or part; not general) or *systemic* (affecting the body as a whole). Most drugs are used for their systemic effects. Even when drugs are used for local purposes, we know that no drug remains completely localized in the body. Any chemical that comes into contact with even

the most superficial surface, such as the skin, has the potential to be absorbed into the bloodstream and to circulate to other tissues and organs.

Oral Route

Oral medications are convenient, safe, and relatively inexpensive. However, drugs that can be destroyed in any way by the digestive tract must be given by injection. Insulin and heparin are examples of drugs that are destroyed by the digestive process. Injection of medications leads to rapid absorption into the bloodstream, but this increases the danger of overdose or possible infection. Most oral medications are absorbed by the small intestine, but a few are absorbed more rapidly in the stomach. After absorption into the bloodstream from the small intestine, drugs are carried to the liver. In this organ much of the drug's potency is inactivated before the drug circulates to the

TABLE 32-3 Top 50 Prescribed Drugs in the United States in 2004

BRAND NAME	GENERIC NAME	CLASSIFICATION BY USE
Hydrocodone w/APAP	Hydrocodone w/APAP	Analgesic and antitussive
Lipitor	Atorvastatin calcium	Lipid-lowering agent
Prinivil	Lisinopril	Long-acting angiotensin-converting enzyme inhibitor
Tenormin	Atenolol	Beta-blocker: antihypertensive and treatment of myocardial infarction
Synthroid	Levothyroxine	Thyroid replacement hormone
Amoxicillin	Amoxicillin	Antibiotic
Hydrochlorothiazide	Hydrochlorothiazide	Diuretic and antihypertensive
Zithromax	Azithromycin	Antibiotic
Furosemide	Furosemide	Diuretic
Norvasc	Amlodipine	Calcium channel blocker; antihypertensive; used for treatment of myocardial infarction
Toprol-XL	Metoprolol	Beta-blocker, extended release
Xanax	Alprazolam	Antianxiety and hypnotic
Albuterol Aerosol	Albuterol	Bronchodilator
Prilosec	Omeprazole	Inhibits gastric acid secretion
Zoloft	Sertraline	Antidepressant
Zocor	Simvastatin	Lipid-lowering agent
Glucophage	Metformin HCl	Oral hypoglycemic
Motrin	Ibuprofen	Nonsteroidal antiinflammatory agent
Dyazide	Triamterene/HCTZ	Diuretic and antihypertensive
Ambien	Zolpidem tartrate	Hypnotic; sleep agent
Keflex	Cephalexin	Antibiotic
Nexium	Esomeprazole	Antacid; inhibits gastric acid secretion
Prevacid	Lansoprazole	Inhibits gastric acid secretion
Lexapro	Escitalopram	Antidepressant
Prednisone	Prednisone	Steroid, antiinflammatory
Zyrtec	Cetirizine	Seasonal allergic rhinitis
Singulair	Montelukast sodium	Antiinflammatory
Celebrex	Celecoxib	Antiarthritic
Prozac	Fluoxetine HCl	Antidepressant
Fosamax	Alendronate	Osteoporosis
Metoprolol	Metoprolol tartrate	Beta-blocker, antihypertensive, antianginal
Premarin	Conjugated estrogens	Estrogen: hormone replacement therapy
Levoxyl	Levothyroxine	Thyroid hormone replacement
Ativan	Lorazepam	Antianxiety
Allegra	Fexofenadine	Antihistamine
Plavix	Clopidogrel bisulfate	Antiplatelet agent
Effexor XR	Venlafaxine hydrochloride	Extended release antidepressant
Micro-K Extencaps	Potassium chloride	Extended release potassium chloride replacement
Protonix	Pantoprazole	Inhibits gastric secretion
Propoxyphene N/APAP	Propoxyphene N/APAP	Analgesic
Advair Diskus	Salmeterol xinafoate	Steroidal inhalant with bronchodilator
Coumadin	Warfarin sodium	Anticoagulant
Tylenol w/Codeine	Acetaminophen w/codeine	Analgesic, antipyretic

TABLE 32-3 Top 50 Prescribed Drugs in the United States in 2004—*cont'd*

BRAND NAME	GENERIC NAME	CLASSIFICATION BY USE
Klonopin	Clonazepam	Anticonvulsant
Neurontin	Gabapentin	Partial seizure disorders
Flonase	Fluticasone propionate	Corticosteroid inhalant; allergic rhinitis, asthma
Elavil	Amitriptyline HCl	Antidepressant
Zantac	Ranitidine HCl	Antiulcer agent
Desyrel	Trazodone HCl	Antidepressant
Naproxen	Naproxen	Nonsteroidal antiinflammatory agent, treatment of arthritis
Augmentin	Amoxicillin and clavulanate	Antibiotic

Six Parts OF A Prescription (Figure 32-1)

Superscription: Patient's name and address, the date, and the symbol ℞ (for the Latin recipe, meaning "take").

Inscription: Main part of the prescription; name of the drug, dosage form, and strength.

Subscription: Directions for the pharmacist; size of each dose, amount to be dispensed, and the form of the drug, such as tablets or capsules.

Signature: Directions for the patient; usually preceded by the symbol *Sig:* (for the Latin *signa*, meaning "mark"). This is where the physician indicates what instructions are to be put on the label to tell the patient how, when, and in what quantities to use the medication.

Refill information: May be regulated by federal law if the drug is a controlled substance; must write number of times refill allowed on the script.

Physician's signature: Must include the manual signature of the physician and the DEA number when indicated.

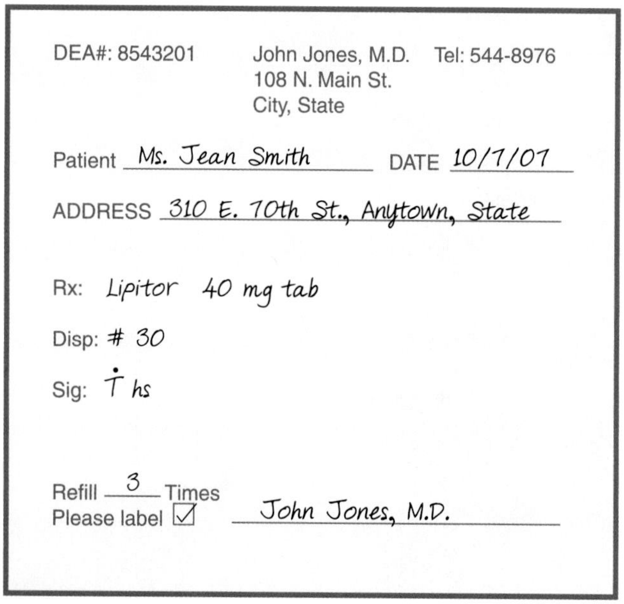

Terms Related to Drug Interactions

antagonism The action of one drug decreases the intensity or shortens the duration of action of another drug.

synergism One drug increases the intensity or prolongs the action of another drug. This can have a positive effect, as in using two different antibiotics to treat an infection, or a negative effect, as when two drugs lower blood pressure to dangerous levels.

potentiation A form of synergism in which the action of one of the drugs is increased by the presence of another drug. In this case the two drugs have different actions, but one increases the effect of the other.

tissues. This inactivation by the liver often makes it necessary to administer higher doses orally than when given by injection.

Food slows the absorption of drugs. Therefore many medications are absorbed best when taken either 1 hour before or 2 hours after the ingestion of food. Food may also bind with medication or in some other way destroy the drug. Tetracycline, for example, is destroyed by milk products and antacids containing calcium salts. Therefore patients receiving tetracycline should be advised not to eat dairy products or ingest liquid or solid forms of antacids. Stomach acid that naturally occurs during digestion may destroy certain drugs. Because some drugs are destroyed by the components of the digestive tract or irritate the empty lining of the stomach, oral drugs may be **enteric-coated** to keep them intact for passage into the small intestine or to prevent gastric irritation or vomiting.

Some drugs are not affected by the digestive processes but cannot be absorbed through the intestinal walls into the bloodstream. For example, neomycin has no therapeutic effect when taken orally (unless it is used to sterilize the bowel before bowel surgery). Other drugs may be unable to cross the bowel mucosa because of their poor solubility in lipids (fats), or because they are inactivated by the pH of the GI tract.

It is important to remember these absorption factors when administering medication by the oral route. If a patient has previously responded to a drug but is no longer responding, it may be important to question the patient's food-medication

---

DEA#: 8543201   John Jones, M.D.   Tel: 544-8976
108 N. Main St.
City, State

Patient _Ms. Jean Smith_   DATE _10/7/01_

ADDRESS _310 E. 70th St., Anytown, State_

Rx: *Lipitor*   *40 mg tab*

Disp: # 30

Sig: T̄ hs

Refill _3_ Times
Please label ☑   _John Jones, M.D._

FIGURE 32-1 A sample prescription.

TABLE 32-4 Common Prescription Abbreviations

ABBREVIATION	MEANING	ABBREVIATION	MEANING	ABBREVIATION	MEANING
aa	of each	noct	at night	tid	three times a day
ac	before meals	N/S	normal saline	tinct	tincture
ad lib	as desired	O₂	oxygen	TO	telephone order
agit	shake, stir	OD	overdose	tus	cough
am	morning	OD	right eye	U	unit
amp	ampule	OS	left eye	vag	vagina
AD	right ear	OU	both eyes	ves	bladder
AS	left ear	OTC	over-the-counter (drugs)	VO	verbal order
AU	both ears	pc	after meals	W/O	water in oil
aq	water	PL	placebo	cm	centimeter
bid	twice a day	pm	afternoon	mcg, µg	microgram
c̄	with	PMI	patient medication instruction	Fe	iron
cap	capsule	mg	milligram	Gm, g	gram
DC	discontinue	po	by mouth	kg	kilogram
EENT	eye, ear, nose, throat	pr	per rectum	cc	cubic centimeter
K	potassium	pulv	powder	mL	milliliter
dil	dilute	q	every	L	liter
disp	dispense	qd	every day	gr	grain
ext	extract	qh	every hour	dr	dram
FDA	Food and Drug Administration	q2h	every 2 hours	oz	ounce
fl	fluid	q3h	every 3 hours	lb	pound
h	hour	q4h	every 4 hours	℥	minim
hs	at bedtime	qid	four times a day	gtt	drops
inj	injection	qm	every morning	t, tsp	teaspoon
IM	intramuscular	qn	every night	T, tbs	tablespoon
ID	intradermal	qod	every other day	C	cup, Celsius
IV	intravenous	qs	quantity sufficient	pt	pint
med	medicine	R	rectal	qt	quart
meq	milliequivalent	Rx	take, treatment	gal	gallon
MLD	minimum lethal dose	S, Sig	give the following directions	F	Fahrenheit
mn	midnight	s̄	without	VO	verbal order
MO	mineral oil	SC, SQ	subcutaneous	ung	ointment
MOM	milk of magnesia	TAB	tablet		
MS	morphine sulfate	sub-q	subcutaneous		
MTD	maximum tolerated dose	s̄s̄	one-half		
NPO	nothing by mouth	stat	immediately		

cycle. It could be that the patient is no longer taking the medication on an empty stomach as directed.

Parenteral Route

Parenteral refers to the administration of drugs by injection. The parenteral route results in the fastest action, because the medication is administered directly into the bloodstream or into tissues with a rich blood supply. However, several factors determine the effectiveness and rate of absorption of injected medications.

The absorption of a drug in an aqueous (water) solution is faster in an area with more blood vessels. Therefore drugs deposited in the muscle will be absorbed faster than drugs given subcutaneously. The *intramuscular* (IM) route is chosen in an emergency for fast action or when larger amounts of the medication must be absorbed. The *subcutaneous* (SC) route is chosen when a slower, prolonged effect is desired.

A second way that parenteral drug absorption may be controlled is physically. A drug's absorption may be quickened by hand massage after injection. Absorption may also be slowed by pharmaceutical preparation of the drug in a physical form that slows absorption. These methods include suspending the drug in a solution that prolongs absorption, such as **colloidal** substances, fatty substances (oil), or insoluble salts or esters. Drugs suspended in these substances slowly dissolve in the tissues over a long time, and the patient can be spared costly, frequent, and sometimes painful injections. Penicillin G is suspended with procaine (hydrochloride) salts for this purpose. In addition, local anesthetics are sometimes mixed with epinephrine to keep the medication and its effects in an area longer, because epinephrine (adrenalin) constricts blood vessels at the site, thus decreasing circulation and the rate of absorption.

The third parenteral route is *intravenous* (IV), which injects the medication directly into the vein. Because of the dangers of IV administration, only those members of the medical team who are licensed to do so may inject medication intravenously.

SAFETY ALERT A medical assistant is not licensed to perform the IV administration of medications to patients. Because IV administration is so dangerous, medications given intravenously are usually administered in small doses through an IV infusion (IV drip) so that the effects in the body can be monitored.

Other forms of parenteral routes include *intradermal* injection, which is below the dermal layer of the skin but superficial to the subcutaneous tissues. This route is used mostly for allergy testing and skin testing, such as testing for tuberculosis. *Intrathecal,* or *intraspinal,* injections are used for spinal anesthesia and for administering certain medications into the spinal column. *Intraarticular* or *intralesional* injections are used for administering corticosteroids into joints and lesions or anticancer drugs into cancerous tumors.

Mucous Membrane Absorption

Drugs may be absorbed by the mucous membranes of the mouth, throat, nose, eyes, rectum, vagina, and respiratory tracts. Some applications, such as nasal sprays, eye drops, and rectal suppositories for constipation, have a local effect. Others, such as a rectal suppository to control vomiting or a nitroglycerin tablet dissolved under the tongue (*sublingual*) to dilate coronary arteries and relieve the pain of **angina pectoris,** have a systemic effect. *Inhalation* is used to concentrate drugs locally in the lower respiratory passages or to produce systemic effects, such as general anesthesia. For example, a **bronchodilator** such as metaproterenol sulfate (Alupent) is inhaled by an asthmatic during an asthma attack to relieve bronchospasms.

Topical Absorption

Topical routes include the application of medications to the skin, eyes, and ears. Drugs in ointments, creams, lotions, and aerosols can be applied for the treatment of skin itching, inflammation, or other discomforts and for the treatment of skin infections with antibiotics. Nitroglycerin (for angina) is a drug that can be absorbed through the skin via a dermal patch, which releases it systemically. Hormones such as testosterone and estrogen can also be absorbed via a dermal patch for systemic purposes.

Drug Distribution

Once a drug is absorbed, it must be transported by the circulatory system to the area where it will have its effect. In the bloodstream, drugs can attach to plasma proteins then be freed to pass from the blood into the site of action. Drugs are then carried through the fluids into the cells of the tissues and organs. The amount of blood supply to a part affects the speed with which drugs reach certain tissues.

The blood-brain barrier is a functional barrier between the brain cells and the capillaries circulating blood through the brain. The barrier is poorly permeable to water-soluble materials, making it difficult for dissolved substances in the blood to pass through. For the substances that do cross through, the barrier regulates the degree and rate of their absorption into the brain tissue. The general anesthetic thiopental (Pentothal) is able to cross the blood-brain barrier immediately and produces sleep within seconds, whereas other sleep-producing drugs, such as the barbiturates, cross slowly and may take as long as 30 minutes to 1 hour to produce the same effect. The presence of the blood-brain barrier is a mixed blessing. It provides a physical barrier that protects the brain from potentially dangerous chemicals but at the same time makes it very difficult to treat central nervous system (CNS) disorders. In contrast, the placenta has no method for blocking substances, so whatever the mother consumes is readily passed through the placenta to the developing fetus. This means that childbearing women must be extremely careful of all chemicals that are consumed or inhaled because they are quickly transferred to the bloodstream of the baby.

Drug Action

Multiple theories explain why drugs act the way they do. Drugs are believed to combine with body chemicals on the cell surface or within the cell itself. Pharmaceutical developers create compounds that have an affinity for a specific target cell. The target cell recipient is called a *receptor,* and the drug that has the affinity for it and produces a functional change in the cell is called the *agonist.* Not all drugs that bind to specific cells cause a functional change in the cell. These drugs act as an *antagonist* to the natural process and work by blocking a sequence of biochemical events.

Some drugs are believed to act by affecting the enzyme functions of the body. Drugs attach to enzyme substances and rob the enzymes from cells. As a result, the enzyme products needed for normal cellular function are not supplied, and the cell fails to function properly.

Certain antiinfective drugs have a selected toxicity for pathogens or parasites that have invaded the body. Penicillin and sulfonamides work because they poison, or interfere with the life processes of, bacteria without affecting the life processes of normal human cells. Research scientists continue to look for differences between cancer cells and normal cells so they can apply the principle of selected toxicity in cancer treatment. Only recently have anticancer drugs been produced that are selective and therefore not toxic to human cells.

Both drugs that have a selective affinity for cells and those that bind with enzymes may be counteracted by administering large amounts of natural substances with which the drugs compete. This process is known as administering an *antidote* to a drug that may be acting as a poison. For example, an antidote such as naloxone hydrochloride (HCl) (Narcan) can be administered if a patient receives too much anesthesia or has taken a drug overdose.

Some drugs alter the function of a cell by affecting the physical properties of the cell membrane rather than altering the biochemical processes within the cell itself. This is especially true of drugs, such as anesthetics and alcohol, which affect nerve cells. A change in the cell membrane alters the permeability of the membrane, which in turn changes the flow of ions in and out of the cells. This change in ion flow alters the *polarity* (opposite effects at two extremities, the two extremities being inside and outside the cell membrane) on which nerve pulses are conducted, resulting in general sleep or stupor.

Drug Metabolism

After the drug is absorbed and distributed it is then metabolized for excretion. During metabolism the drug is converted into harmless byproducts. These byproducts are then more easily eliminated by the kidneys. Most drugs are broken down by the enzyme activity of the liver. For oral medications that are absorbed in the small intestine, this process begins in the liver before distribution.

The ability to break down the chemical components of a drug varies among individuals. Factors that determine this ability include age, the presence of other drugs, and liver disease. Infants and aging individuals have an increased problem with effectively metabolizing medications. Patients taking multiple medications may also be at increased risk for liver-related problems with metabolism because of the sheer number of chemicals the liver is exposed to on a daily basis. Individuals with chronic liver disease, such as **cirrhosis,** may not be able to metabolize even normal doses of medications. Because of these factors drug therapy must be closely monitored in very young and aging patients, those taking multiple medications, and patients with chronic liver disease. In contrast, patients receiving long-term drug therapy may develop overstimulation of the enzyme activity of the liver. This results in rapid destruction of the drug, and the patient has to take larger and larger doses for the drug to be effective. This situation is called tolerance.

Drug Excretion

After the drug is metabolized, its byproducts must be excreted from the body. The kidneys are the most important route for the elimination of drugs. Most drugs are filtered out of the blood circulating through the kidneys and excreted in the urine. Because the kidneys are so important in the elimination of chemicals from the body, drug therapy must be carefully monitored in patients with kidney disease or malfunction. Drugs are also eliminated through the sweat glands, saliva, and feces. Exhalation, another mechanism for drug elimination, is the basis for measuring alcohol concentrations in the blood by the breathalyzer test. Drugs may be eliminated through the milk glands of a lactating mother, which means a breastfeeding woman must be extremely careful about taking medications.

The combination of metabolism and excretion decreases the amount of drug in the body at any given time. The therapeutic dose of a medication is dependent on many factors including the drug's half-life. The half-life is the amount of time it takes for half a dose of the medication to be excreted from the body. Some drugs have extremely short half-lives (only minutes), whereas others can take days to leave the body. The amount of drug that is lost during one half-life depends on how much drug is present. The half-life of a drug is used by the physician to determine the time of medication administration, or the dosage intervals. The shorter the half-life of the drug, the closer together the times in which it should be administered. If the next dose of the drug is not given within the half-life, then blood levels will drop and the patient will not receive adequate therapeutic effects from the treatment.

FACTORS THAT AFFECT DRUG ACTION

As stated earlier, different people react to the same dose of medication in different ways, and the same patient can react to the same dose of the same drug differently on various occasions. The following factors are important in determining the correct medication for a patient.

Body Weight

A person's weight has a direct relationship to the effect of a medication. Basically, the same dose has a lesser effect on a patient who weighs more and a greater effect on a person who weighs less. Manufacturers of adult medications calculate dosages based on a normal adult weight (approximately 150 pounds). Sometimes the physician will adjust the dose to better suit the patient's body size. Pediatric medications are designed for the body weight or body surface area of children. If adult medications are used for children, the correct dose must be calculated and adjusted for the child's body weight (see Chapter 33).

Age

The greatest effect of age on the body's response to a drug occurs in newborns and in elderly individuals. This usually is because of immature or deteriorating body systems. In addition, both groups are particularly sensitive to drugs that affect the CNS and are at risk for developing toxic drug levels. Dosage calculations for these two groups must be carefully decided, and therapy usually begins with very small doses. Table 32-5 summarizes the altered effects of medications on aging persons. Chapter 47 discusses the effects of aging on body systems in more detail.

TABLE 32-5 Effects of Medications on Geriatric Patients

PHYSIOLOGIC CHANGES ASSOCIATED WITH AGING	RESULTS
Stomach takes longer to empty, and level of gastric acidity is decreased	Increases risk of stomach irritation and ulceration
Increased percent of *adipose* (fat) tissue in the body	Increases likelihood of drug storage in fat; may lead to drug toxicity
Fewer protein-binding sites available in bloodstream	Decreases drug passage through cell membranes; increases drug blood level; may lead to toxicity
Decline in liver function	Slows rate of drug metabolism; increases risk of toxicity
Decreased kidney function	Slows rate of elimination of drug byproducts; increases risk of toxicity and complications
Peripheral vascular disease; decreased venous tone	Decreases distribution of drug to periphery; may cause orthostatic hypotension
Fat-soluble medications pass through blood-brain barrier more easily	May affect central nervous system; increases risk of *vertigo* and confusion.

Sex

Drugs may affect men and women differently. As previously mentioned, a pregnant woman has to be extremely cautious when taking medications to avoid damage to the developing fetus. In addition, some drugs have side effects that can stimulate uterine contractions, causing premature labor and delivery. Intramuscular medications are absorbed faster by men because they generally have higher levels of muscle mass that are rich in blood vessels. Because women typically have a higher body fat content and less muscle (therefore fewer blood vessels in peripheral tissues in comparison with men), intramuscular drugs remain in their tissues longer. However, the majority of clinical trials in the past have been conducted only on men, so until newer trial results are released that include women, it is impossible to accurately predict the effect of sex on the action and safety of medications.

Time of Day

Diurnal refers to during the day or time of light. Diurnal body rhythms play an important part in the effects of some drugs. Sedatives given in the morning will not be as effective as when administered before bedtime, because the CNS is more stimulated and more resistant to the effects of the drug. Corticosteroid administration is preferred in the morning, because this best mimics the body's natural pattern of corticosteroid production and elimination.

Pathologic Factors

Patients may adversely respond to drugs in the presence of liver or kidney disease because the body will not be able to detoxify and excrete chemicals properly. Drugs may also produce pathologic conditions of the liver or kidney, and patients may need monitoring to alert the physician to potentially serious drug complications. For example, patients on statin medications such as atorvastatin calcium (Lipitor) for **hypercholesterolemia** should have liver function studies done routinely because these drugs are very hard on liver cells. Patients with liver or kidney disease have an increased risk of drug toxicity, which may result in unconsciousness or death. Reactions in patients with other diseases or disorders may be quite different from the expected

response. Therefore a thorough medical history of the patient must always be taken before medications are prescribed and administered.

Immune Responses

The presence of a drug can stimulate a patient's immune response, causing the patient to develop antibodies to a particular chemical. If the same drug is again administered, the patient will have an allergic reaction to the drug, ranging from a mild reaction to *anaphylaxis,* which is a serious respiratory and circulatory emergency. The group of drugs that most commonly causes allergic responses is antibiotics.

Psychologic Factors

People may respond differently to a drug because of the way they feel about the drug. If a patient believes in the therapy, even a *placebo* (sugar pill or sterile water thought to be a drug) may help or bring about relief. A patient's personality can affect whether he or she will be cooperative in following the directions for a particular drug, and a patient's negative mindset, or mental attitude, can reduce an expected response to a drug.

Tolerance

Tolerance is the phenomenon of reduced responsiveness to a drug. Acquired tolerance occurs after a particular drug has been taken for a period of time. Cross-tolerance occurs when a patient acquires a tolerance to one drug and becomes resistant to other, similar drugs. Physical dependence often accompanies tolerance. The body becomes so adapted to the presence of the drug that it cannot function properly without it. To withdraw the drug is to throw the body out of its equilibrium, causing withdrawal symptoms.

Accumulation

When a drug is taken too frequently to allow for proper elimination, it accumulates in the tissues. The result is a more intense effect and a longer duration. Accumulation can cause overdose and/or toxic effects. Proper dosage and timing of administration are the best methods for preventing drug accumulation.

Idiosyncrasy

Occasionally a person reacts to a drug in a manner that is unexpected and peculiar to that individual only. An idiosyncratic response may manifest in many different ways, such as a hypnotic drug keeping a person awake, acting as a stimulant to this person rather than as a depressant. Usually these reactions cannot be explained.

Drug-Drug Interactions

Special care must be taken with patients who are taking more than one drug on a regular basis. One medication may increase or decrease the effects of another or cause unexpected side effects. To safeguard patients from potentially negative drug interactions, it is important to record a complete list at each visit of all the drugs the patient is taking, including OTC medications. However, because many patients do not know or get confused about the names and dosages of their medications, the best way to maintain an accurate record is to ask that patients bring their medication containers with them to each office visit. This way you can list information about their medications on their charts and at the same time ask if they have any questions about their treatment. It is also a good idea to advise patients to fill prescriptions at the same pharmacy, because the pharmacist can monitor medications for potential drug interactions.

An example of a drug interaction is the effect of some antibiotics on oral contraceptives. Certain antibiotics can interact with birth control pills, making birth control pills less effective and pregnancy more likely. Patients should be told that spotting—or midcycle bleeding—may be the first sign that an antibiotic is interfering with the effectiveness of birth control pills. Examples of antibiotics that interact with birth control pills include penicillin (Veetids), amoxicillin (Amoxil), ampicillin (Omnipen), cotrimoxazole (Septra or Bactrim), tetracycline (Sumycin), minocycline (Minocin), metronidazole (Flagyl), and nitrofurantoin (Macrobid or Macrodantin). For prevention of pregnancy while a patient is taking an antibiotic the physician may recommend women use a condom or **spermicide** as a backup birth control method while taking the medication and for at least 1 week after treatment is completed.

CRITICAL THINKING APPLICATION

Sylvia Kramer is a 72-year-old patient of Dr. Simon's who calls today and asks Kathy about how she should be taking her heart medicine, diltiazem HCl (Cardizem). Mrs. Kramer is a diabetic patient with hypertension and a history of heart disease. She also is overweight, has the potential for kidney disease, and takes a number of other prescriptions. What factors may have an impact on the potential effect of Mrs. Kramer's medication?

CLASSIFICATIONS OF DRUG ACTIONS

Clinical pharmacology is a complex subject. To make the subject easier, drugs are classified into groups according to their actions on the body (e.g., diuretics or emetics), the symptoms they relieve (e.g., antihistamine), or the body system that they affect

(e.g., drugs acting on the cardiovascular system). The following is a glossary of terms describing some basic drug actions. As you read some of the examples, remember that a drug classified as one type of agent may have other uses and actions on other systems of the body. For example, a drug classified as a diuretic may also be an antihypertensive drug, and a vasodilator may also be a respiratory antispasmodic. It takes time to understand not only the basic classification of a particular drug but also the many secondary uses and effects the drug has on the human body.

These are just a few examples of the different classifications of medications. Remember to research and review all medications before they are administered.

Examples of Drug Classifications

Adrenergics

Action: Constricts blood vessels, narrows the **lumen** of a vessel; vasoconstrictor; dilates pupils and bronchioles; relaxes muscles of GI and urinary tracts.

Examples: Epinephrine: Phenylephrine (Neo-Synephrine); pseudoephedrine (Sudafed); isoproterenol (Isuprel); oxymetazoline (Visine).

Primary uses: Stops superficial bleeding; raises and sustains blood pressure; relieves nasal congestion; relieves bronchospasm; treatment of allergic reaction.

Adrenergic Blocking Agents

Action: Vasodilation; decreases blood pressure; increases muscle tone of GI walls.

Examples: Lisinopril (Prinivil); amlodipine (Norvasc); metoprolol (Toprol-XL); methyldopa (Aldomet); propranolol (Inderal); atenolol (Tenormin).

Primary uses: Control of hypertension and peripheral vascular disease.

Analgesics

Action: Lessens the sensory function of the brain; blocks pain receptors.

Examples: Nonnarcotic: aspirin; acetaminophen (Tylenol); ibuprofen (Advil, Motrin). Narcotic: hydrocodone w/ APAP (Tylenol with codeine); Propoxyphene N/APAP

Pharmacokinetic Terms

absorption How a drug is absorbed into the body's blood stream. The rate of absorption depends on many factors, including the route of administration.

distribution How a drug is transported from the administration site to the location in the body where it is meant to act, the *target tissue*.

metabolism How the drug is inactivated, including the time it takes for a drug to be detoxified and broken down into byproducts. The liver typically metabolizes medications.

excretion The route by which a drug is eliminated from the body and the amount of time such a process requires. The kidneys typically excrete drug metabolites.

(Darvocet); meperidine (Demerol); hydrocodone (Vicodin); propoxyphene (Darvon).

Primary use: Pain relief.

Anesthetics

Action: Produces insensibility to pain or the sensation of pain; blocks nerve impulses to the brain, resulting in unconsciousness; dilates pupils; lowers blood pressure; decreases respiration and pulse rates.

Examples: Local: lidocaine (Xylocaine); bupivacaine (Marcaine). General: thiopental (Pentothal).

Primary uses: Local (absence of sensation without loss of consciousness) or general (loss of consciousness) anesthesia.

Antacids

Action: Decrease the acidity in the stomach.

Examples: Omeprazole (Prilosec); esomeprazole (Nexium); lansoprazole (Prevacid); pantoprazole (Protonix); magaldrate (Riopan); calcium carbonate (Maalox).

Primary use: Treatment of gastric hyperacidity.

Antianxiety

Action: Reduces anxiety and tension.

Examples: Chlordiazepoxide (Librium); diazepam (Valium); alprazolam (Xanax).

Primary uses: Produces calmness and releases muscle tension.

Antibiotics

Action: Kills or inhibits the growth of microorganisms.

Examples: Azithromycin (Zithromax); cefaclor (Ceclor); tetracycline (Achromycin); amoxicillin (Augmentin); ciprofloxacin (Cipro); cephalexin (Keflex).

Primary use: Treatment of bacterial invasions and infections.

Anticholinergics

Action: Parasympathetic blocking agent; reduces spasms in smooth muscles.

Examples: Scopolamine; atropine sulfate.

Primary use: Dry secretions before surgery.

Anticoagulants

Action: Delays or blocks the clotting of blood.

Examples: Heparin; warfarin sodium (Coumadin).

Primary uses: Treatment of blood clots, thrombophlebitis; prevention of clot formation.

Anticonvulsants

Action: Prevents seizures; reduces excessive stimulation of the brain.

Examples: Clonazepam (Klonopin); gabapentin (Neurontin); phenytoin (Dilantin); phenobarbital; carbamazepine (Tegretol).

Primary use: Treatment of epilepsy and other neurologic disorders.

Antidepressants

Action: Treats depression.

Examples: Sertraline (Zoloft); escitalopram (Lexapro); trazodone HCl (Desyrel); fluoxetine (Prozac); imipramine pamoate (Tofranil); amitriptyline (Elavil).

Primary use: Mood elevator.

Antiemetics

Action: Acts on hypothalamus center in the brain.

Examples: Prochlorperazine (Compazine); trimethobenzamide (Tigan); metoclopramide (Reglan).

Primary use: Prevents and relieves nausea and vomiting.

Antifungals

Action: Slows or retards the multiplication of fungi.

Examples: Miconazole (Monistat); nystatin (Mycostatin).

Primary use: Treatment of systemic or local fungal infections.

Antihistamines

Action: Counteracts the effects of histamine by blocking action in tissues; may be used to inhibit gastric secretions.

Examples: Cetirizine (Zyrtec); fexofenadine (Allegra); chlorpheniramine (Chlor-Trimeton); diphenhydramine (Benadryl); promethazine (Phenergan); cimetidine (Tagamet); ranitidine (Zantac).

Primary uses: Relief of allergies; prevention of gastric ulcers.

Antihypertensives

Action: Blocks nerve impulses that cause arteries to constrict; slows heart rate, decreasing its contractility; restricts the hormone aldosterone in the blood.

Examples: Amlodipine (Norvasc); atenolol (Tenormin); doxazosin mesylate (Cardura); metoprolol (Lopressor or Toprol); methyldopa (Aldomet).

Primary use: Reduces and controls blood pressure.

Antiinflammatories

Action: Reduces inflammation.

Examples: Nonsteroidal antiinflammatory agents (NSAIDs): ibuprofen (Advil, Motrin); naproxen (Naprosyn); Steroidal: dexamethasone (Decadron); prednisone (Cortisone); montelukast sodium (Singulair); fluticasone propionate (Flonase).

Primary use: Treatment of arthritis and other inflammatory disorders including asthma and allergic rhinitis.

Antineoplastic

Action: Inhibits the development of and destroys cancerous cells.

Examples: Interferon alfa-2a (Roferon-A); hydroxyurea (Hydrea); cyclophosphamide (Cytoxan); fluorouracil (Adrucil); chlorambucil (Leukeran); cytarabine (Cytosar-U).

Primary use: Cancer chemotherapy.

Antipruritics

Action: Relieves itching.

Examples: Calamine lotion; hydrocortisone ointment; Benadryl.

Primary use: Treatment of allergies or topical exposures that cause itching.

Antipyretics

Action: Reduces body temperature.
Examples: Aspirin, acetaminophen; ibuprofen.
Primary use: Reduces fever.

Antispasmodics

Action: Relieves or prevents spasms from musculoskeletal injury or inflammation.
Examples: Methocarbamol (Robaxin); carisoprodol (Soma).
Primary use: Treatment of sports injuries.

Antitussives

Action: Inhibits the cough center.
Examples: Narcotic: codeine sulfate. Nonnarcotic: dextromethorphan (Romilar, Robitussin DM).
Primary use: Temporarily suppresses a nonproductive cough; reduces the thickness of secretions.

Bronchodilators

Action: Relaxes the smooth muscle of the bronchi.
Examples: Salmeterol xinafoate (Advair Diskus); aminophylline (Aminophyllin); theophylline (Theo-Dur); epinephrine (Adrenalin, Sus-Phrine); albuterol (Ventolin, Proventil); isoproterenol (Isuprel).
Primary uses: Treatment of asthma, bronchospasm; promotes bronchodilation.

Cathartics (laxative)

Action: Increases peristaltic activity of the large intestine.
Examples: Magnesium hydroxide (Milk of Magnesia); bisacodyl (Dulcolax); casanthranol (Peri-Colace); psyllium hydrophilic mucilloid (Metamucil).
Primary use: Increases and hastens bowel evacuation (defecation).

Contraceptives

Action: Inhibits conception.
Examples: Medroxyprogesterone acetate (Depo-Provera); norgestrel (Ovrette); ethinyl estradiol and ethynodiol diacetate (Demulen 1/35).
Primary use: Prevents pregnancy.

Decongestants

Action: Relieves local congestion in the tissues.
Examples: Ephedrine or phenylephrine (Neo-Synephrine); pseudoephedrine (Sudafed); oxymetazoline (Afrin).
Primary use: Relief of nasal and sinus congestion caused by common cold, hay fever, or upper respiratory tract disorders.

Diuretics

Action: Inhibits the reabsorption of sodium and chloride in the kidneys; promotes excretion of excess fluid in the body.
Examples: Hydrochlorothiazide (Dyazide, Esidrix, Hydro-DIURIL); furosemide (Lasix); triamterene (Dyrenium).
Primary uses: Increases urinary output, decreases blood pressure.

Expectorants

Action: Liquefies secretions in the bronchial tubes so that the secretions can be coughed out.
Examples: Diphenhydramine (Benylin); guaifenesin guaiacolate (Fenesin, Robitussin).
Primary use: Relieves upper respiratory tract congestion.

Hematopoietic Agents

Action: Promotes red blood cell production.
Examples: Epoetin alfa (Epogen, Procrit).
Primary use: Treatment of anemia in chemotherapy patients.

Hemostatic Agents

Action: Controls bleeding; acts as a blood coagulant.
Examples: Phytonadione, vitamin K (Konakion); absorbable hemostatic agents, such as Gelfoam and Surgicel, are applied directly to a wound.
Primary uses: Control of acute or chronic blood-clotting disorder; formation of absorbable, artificial clot.

Hormone Replacement

Action: Replaces hormones or compensates for hormone deficiency.
Examples: Insulin (Humulin); levothyroxine sodium (Synthroid or Levoxyl); estrogen (Premarin); vasopressin (Pitressin).
Primary use: Maintenance of adequate hormone levels.

Hypnotics (sedatives)

Action: Induces sleep and lessens the activity of the brain.
Examples: Zolpidem tartrate (Ambien); Secobarbital (Seconal); flurazepam (Dalmane); temazepam (Restoril).
Primary uses: Insomnia; lower doses sedate.

Lipid-Lowering Agents

Action: Decreases blood cholesterol levels and/or increases HDL levels.
Examples: Atorvastatin calcium (Lipitor); simvastatin (Zocor).
Primary use: Management of high blood cholesterol.

Miotics

Action: Causes the pupil of the eye to contract.
Examples: Carbachol (Isopto Carbachol); isoflurophate (Floropryl); pilocarpine (Isopto Carpine).
Primary use: Counteracts pupil dilation.

Mydriatics (anticholinergic)

Action: Dilates the pupil of the eye.
Examples: Atropine sulfate (Isopto Atropine).
Primary use: Ophthalmologic examinations.

Narcotics

Action: Depresses the CNS and causes insensibility or stupor.
Examples: Natural narcotics: opium group (codeine phosphate, morphine sulfate). Synthetic narcotics: meperidine (Demerol), methadone (Dolophine), and propoxyphene HCl (Darvon).
Primary use: Pain relief.

Oral Hypoglycemics

Action: Decreases blood glucose levels by increasing insulin production and/or decreasing target cell resistance to insulin or by delaying glucose absorption.

Examples: Metformin HCL (Glucophage); acarbose (Precose); chlorpropamide (Diabinese); glimepiride (Amaryl); glipizide (Glucotrol); glyburide (Micronase).

Primary use: Management of type 2 diabetes mellitus.

Osteoporosis Treatment

Action: Inhibits bone reabsorption and/or promotes use of calcium.

Examples: Alendronate (Fosamax); calcitonin (Miacalcin nasal spray and Calcimar); dihydrotachysterol; etidronate (Didronel).

Primary use: Promotes bone mineral density and reverses the progression of osteoporosis.

CLOSING COMMENTS

Patient Education

It is important for the patient to be aware of the effects a drug may have and should have on his or her system. The medical assistant plays an important role in helping patients understand their medications, promoting compliance with treatment, and preventing complications. The following items should be considered when interviewing a patient and documenting on the patient chart:

- Make a comprehensive list of all medications, including OTC agents, that the patient is taking on a regular basis.
- Ask the patient if she is pregnant.
- Preassess the patient for any adverse effects such as drug allergies and drug-to-drug or drug-to-food interactions.
- Observe the patient for any adverse effects for a minimum of 20 minutes after the administration of a medication in the office, and inform the patient of possible adverse reactions to the medication that may occur at home.
- Discuss with the patient how and when the prescribed drug is to be taken and if there are any special storage precautions.
- Reassess that the patient is taking the medication properly.
- Provide comfort, encouragement, and guidance to patients to ensure their understanding, safety, and cooperation while on drug therapy.
- Answer any questions asked. Remember: If you are not certain of the answer, consult the prescribing physician.

Therapeutic Communications with Patients from Diverse Cultures

Health beliefs can affect compliance with medication therapy. Patients from various cultures may be using home remedies or herbal treatments that could interfere with the effectiveness and safety of medications prescribed by the physician. Guidelines that the medical assistant may find helpful include the following:

- Investigate the healing practices of the primary cultures in your area so you are better equipped to discuss these practices with your patients.
- Encourage cultural sensitivity in your co-workers.
- Provide patients with educational materials in their native language.
- Ask patients if they are using home remedies or are consulting a healer from their culture. If so, get as much detail as possible so you can share this information with the physician.

Legal and Ethical Issues

The medical assistant plays a key role in the management of controlled substances in the ambulatory care setting. It is important that all rules regarding record keeping, inventory, prescribing, dispensing, and documentation of scheduled drugs be followed according to state and federal regulations. The medical assistant may be responsible for filing for the initial DEA registration as well as the certification renewal. He or she should contact the area DEA office for instructions. Each DEA number is specific to a site, so multiple practice locations will require a DEA number for each facility.

Accurate and complete documentation is essential for correct management of patient medications. Each time the patient is prescribed or administered a medication, complete details must be included in the patient chart. Failure to do so may result in a serious error that could potentially harm the patient and result in litigation.

Health Insurance Portability and Accountability Act Applications

Patients have the right to request restrictions on the disclosure of protected health information (PHI) for treatment, payment, and health care operations (TPO). For example, if a patient has a history of substance abuse and this information is not pertinent to current TPO circumstances, then the patient can request that this information not be disclosed. The facility does not have to agree to the patient's request; however, there must be a process established within the practice to review the demand and explain the physician's decision to the patient. If the physician agrees not to release this information then the specific restriction must be documented in the patient's chart, and staff must review and comply with the restrictions each time material is sent out of the facility for TPO purposes.

Pharmacology Math

33

SCENARIO

Heather Izacco, a recent graduate from a medical assistant program in the area, has just been hired by a local cardiologist, Dr. Angio. One of her responsibilities will be to administer medications under the supervision of Dr. Angio. Heather is confident about her ability to administer medication but is unsure of her accuracy in pharmacology math. Heather never did well in math at school and had a difficult time calculating accurate doses and converting between math systems during her medical assisting training. Her supervisor, Mrs. Allison, suggests that Heather review the math section of her textbook at home and be prepared to work out some sample problems next week.

While studying this chapter, think about the following questions:

- How can Heather be sure she has calculated the correct dosages?
- What are the parts of the drug label, and why are they important?
- Should she be able to convert dosages from one system to another?
- What is the standard formula for determining the correct dose of a drug?
- Are there any differences in calculating an adult versus a pediatric dose?

- How would Heather go about reconstituting an injectable powder?
- Heather must be prepared to answer these questions and accurately perform the calculations involved.

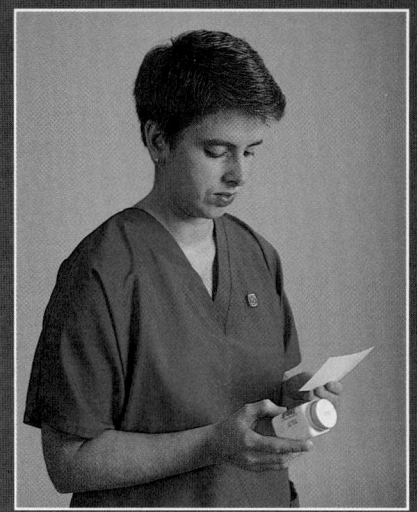

LEARNING OBJECTIVES

1. Define, spell, and pronounce the terms listed in the vocabulary.
2. Demonstrate methods for verifying the accuracy of calculations.
3. Differentiate among the terms used in dosage preparation.
4. Summarize the important parts of a drug label.
5. Describe and perform conversions among the various systems of measurement.
6. Calculate the correct dose of a drug using the standard formula.
7. Determine accurate pediatric doses of medication.
8. Diagram how to reconstitute powdered injectable medications.
9. Specify the legal responsibilities of a medical assistant in calculating drug dosages.

National Accreditation Competencies and Content

CAAHEP COMPETENCIES	ABHES COMPETENCIES
Clinical	**Clinical Duties**
3.b.(4)(g). Apply pharmacology principles to prepare and administer oral and parenteral medications	4.m. Prepare and administer oral and parenteral medications as directed by physician
3.b.(4)(h). Maintain medication and immunization records	4.n. Maintain medication and immunization records

dispense To prepare a drug for administration.
nomogram A graph on which variables are plotted so that a particular value can be read on the appropriate line.
stat Immediately.

surface area The total area of the body exposed to the outside environment.
unit dose Method of preparing individual doses of medications by the pharmacy.

It is a medical assistant's responsibility to be absolutely certain that the medication prepared and administered to a patient is exactly what is ordered by the physician. Although many times drugs are delivered by the pharmacy or supplied by pharmaceutical representatives in **unit dose** packs, the dosage ordered may differ from the dosage on hand. In this case the medical assistant must be prepared to accurately calculate the correct dose before dispensing and administering the medication. There is never a margin of error in drug calculations, because even a minor mistake may result in serious complications for the patient. Therefore the medical assistant must take meticulous care in calculating all drug dosages.

If the dosage ordered by the physician is different from the dosage on hand, there are three basic steps the medical assistant must complete for accurate calculation of the prescribed dose:

1. Based on the type of system printed on the label, determine whether the physician's order is in the same mathematic system of measurement. If the systems vary (the order is in teaspoons but the label states the medication is prepared in milliliters), then accurately convert the order so that it matches the system used on the label.
2. Perform the calculation in equation form, using the appropriate formula.
3. Check your answer for accuracy, and ask someone you trust to confirm your calculations.

All three of these steps must be completed before the medication is dispensed and administered. Confirm your calculations with the physician if you have any doubt of their accuracy.

DRUG LABELS

The first step in safely calculating a drug dosage is to accurately read the label of the drug on hand to determine whether the physician's order and the packaged drug are in the same system of measurement. Starting at the top of the label is the drug's name with the brand name capitalized in bold print and the generic name under this in smaller print in all lowercase letters. If a medication has been on the market for a long time the generic name may be the only one listed (for example, meperidine instead of Demerol or diazepam rather than Valium). If the medication is ordered from the pharmacy and

stocked as a generic drug, then only the generic name will be on the label (Figure 33-1).

Under the name of the drug you will see the dosage strength of the medication. Whether listed in milligrams (mg), milliliters (mL), or another unit of measure, the label identifies how much of the drug is contained in each of the identified units. This is what you must compare with the physician's order to determine if a calculation will be needed to administer the ordered dose of the drug. For example, if the physician has ordered 250 mg of cephalexin and the label states that there are 250 mg per 5 mL, then no calculation is needed—you would administer 5 mL of the medication. However, if the physician orders 500 mg of the medication for a *loading dose* of the antibiotic, then you would have to make sure you administer the correct amount of the medication to match the order. Sometimes the label may help by providing different but equivalent units of measurement for the dosage strength. For example, if the physician orders 250 mg of cephalexin and asks you to make sure the mother understands how much of the medication she should administer to her sick child, the label may state that 5 mL is equivalent to 1 teaspoon (there are 250 mg of the drug in each 5 mL), so you can confirm with the parent that the child should receive 1 teaspoon without having to do any calculation.

The label identifies the *route* or method of administration for the drug. If the medication is packaged as a tablet or capsule you can assume it should be given orally; however, liquid medication will be labeled if it is for oral or parenteral use. If it is a powdered drug *(solute)* and it must be mixed with liquid *(solvent)* before administration, then the label provides instructions on how to prepare the medication. Special storage precautions such as light or heat sensitivity are identified as well. At the bottom of the label is the total amount of the drug that is contained in the package. For example, a multidose vial of liquid cephalexin may contain as much as 200 mL of the drug (e.g., 250 mg in each 5 mL of solution), and a single-dose vial may contain only 5 mL.

The drug manufacturer is identified on the label as well as an expiration date that must be checked each time the medication is dispensed. All drugs whose labeled expiration date has passed must be disposed of. The label also has a lot number stamped on the package so it can be identified as belonging to a batch of drugs that were manufactured at the same time. This number becomes important if problems are noted with a particular

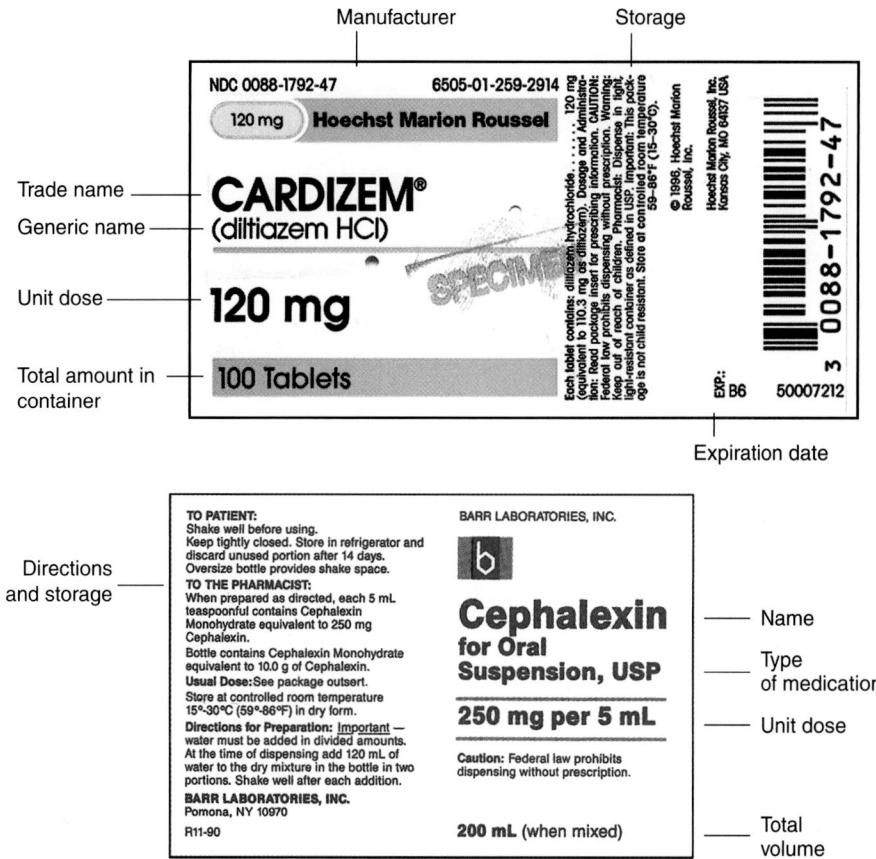

FIGURE 33-1 Drug labels. (From Brown M, Mulholland JM: *Drug calculations: process and problems for clinical practice*, ed 7, St Louis, 2004, Mosby.)

batch and the medication is recalled. Depending on employer preferences, you may need to include the lot number in the documentation of the medication on the patient chart. And finally, federal law requires that all labels contain a national drug code (NDC) that identifies that particular drug.

Some of the basic terms used on drug labels include:

- *Strength:* The potency of the drug stated as a percentage of drug in the solution (2% epinephrine), as a solid weight (grams, milligrams, pounds, grains), or as a milliequivalent or unit.
- *Dose:* The size or amount of the drug available in the drug package. This could be in milliliters, teaspoons, or the number of tablets. For example, the label may read "Imitrex, 6 mg/0.5 mL," which means that there are 6 mg of the drug in each 0.5 mL.
- *Solute:* The pure drug that is dissolved in a liquid to form a solution.
- *Solvent or diluent:* The liquid, usually sterile water or sterile saline, which dissolves the solute.

SYSTEMS OF MEASUREMENT

Sometimes the physician will order a medication in a strength that is totally different from the one on the label. For example, the physician may order 1 gr (grain) of a drug, but the available dosage form is in milligrams. Before the medical assistant can

use the ratio and proportion formulas to arrive at the amount to administer, he or she first must convert to one system or the other. The medical assistant must convert the ordered dose to the measurement system that is on the label (what is available), because that is the system that will have to be used to **dispense** the drug. Three different systems of measurement for medications are used: the metric system, the apothecary system, and the household system.

Metric System

The metric system of weights and measures is used throughout the world as the primary system for weight (mass), capacity (volume), and length (area). In the United States the metric system is used for scientific work, including most tasks involving pharmaceuticals. However, some medication forms still use the older apothecary system, which necessitates learning the two systems and the relationships (conversions) between them.

The metric system of weights and measures is a decimal system based on the number 10, and all calculations are completed by moving decimal points to either the right or the left. Each higher measure is 10 times the measure at hand; each lower measure is 0.1 ($^1/_{10}$) the measure. The basic units are either multiplied or divided by units of 10. The fraction is always written as a decimal, and the number precedes the letters designating the actual measure. Thus $1^1/_2$ liters would be written 1.5 L (Table 33-1). The cubic centimeter (cc) and the

TABLE 33-1 Abbreviations and Symbols for Selected Weights and Measures

APOTHECARY SYSTEM			METRIC SYSTEM	
	ℳ	Min (M) minim	g	gram
	℈	scr scruple	L	liter
	ℨ	dr dram	cc	cubic centimeter
fl	ℨ	f dr fluid dram	mL	milliliter
	℥	oz ounce		
fl	℥	fl oz fluid ounce		
	O	pt pint		
	C	gal gallon		
		gr grain		

the label gave the contents in milliliters. How many milliliters should Heather have given? Review the examples below. Make sure if your answer is *less than* a whole number that you place a zero before the decimal point so the number is not mistaken for a whole number.
Examples:

6 g	= 6.000 g = 6000 mg	3200 mL = 3200.0 mL = 3.2 L
0.6 g	= 0.600 g = 600 mg	320 mL = 320.0 mL = 0.32 L
0.06 g	= 0.060 g = 60 mg	32 mL = 32.0 mL = 0.032 L

Convert the following problems:

2.5 g	= _____ mg	42 g	= _____ mg
0.21 g	= _____ mg	150 µg	= _____ mg
1.7 g	= _____ mg	55 mg	= _____ g
3 mg	= _____ µg	74 L	= _____ mL
0.28 L	= _____ mL	950 mL	= _____ L

milliliter (mL) are interchangeable. In the metric system, 1 cc is a measurement of area, and an area this size holds exactly 1 mL or 0.001 ($^1/_{1000}$) of a liter of fluid. The milliliter measures the *amount* of liquid medication, or the volume, that is to be given orally or by injection. The gram (g) measures the weight, or *strength,* of a solid medication such as a tablet, powder, or topical preparation. The units of measurement in the metric system are based on their prefixes, with *kilo-* meaning 1000 and *milli-* meaning 0.001. The prefixes mean the same whether used to measure volume or weight. For example, a kilogram (kg) is 1000 grams (g) and a kiloliter (kL) is 1000 liters (L), whereas a milligram (mg) is 0.001 ($^1/_{1000}$) of a gram and a milliliter (mL) is 0.001 ($^1/_{1000}$) of a liter.

Conversions within the metric system may be necessary if the physician orders a unit that is different from the one on the label. Units within the metric system are converted by moving the decimal point in multiples of 10. When going from *larger to smaller units of measurement,* as in converting grams to milligrams, the answer will be a larger number, so the *decimal point is moved to the right.* Therefore 0.35 g = 350 mg. When *smaller units of measurement are converted to larger ones,* the answer will be a smaller number, so the *decimal point is moved to the left.* For example, 150 mL = 0.15 L. The following equivalents can be used to make conversions within the metric system.

1 kg = 1000 g	1 kL = 1000 L
1 g = 1000 mg	1 L = 1000 mL
1 mg = 1000 µg (microgram)	1 mL = 1000 µL (microliter)
1 dg = 0.1 g or $^1/_{10}$ of a gram	1 dL = 0.1 L or $^1/_{10}$ of a liter
1 cg = 0.01 g or $^1/_{100}$ of a gram	1 cL = 0.01 L or $^1/_{100}$ of a liter
1 mg = 0.001 g or $^1/_{1000}$ of a gram	1 mL = 0.001 L or $^1/_{1000}$ of a liter

CRITICAL THINKING APPLICATION

The first problems Heather reviewed were conversions within the metric system. Yesterday Dr. Angio ordered 0.45 L of a drug, but

The Apothecary System

In the apothecary system the basic unit of weight for a solid medication is the *grain,* and the basic unit of volume for a liquid medication is the *minim.* As in the metric system, these two units are related: the grain is based on the weight of a single grain of wheat, and the minim is the volume of water that weighs 1 grain (gr). Either Roman or Arabic numerals may be used, but it is not proper to use them together in the same prescription. Either symbols or abbreviations are used; for example, 1½ drams might be written ℨiss or dr 1½. The number follows the symbol or abbreviation. Table 33-2 compares the units of weight and volume in the metric and the apothecary systems. Fluid ounces (oz) are used to differentiate liquids from solid weight.

Household Measurements

The household system is used in most American homes. This system of measurement is important for a patient at home who has no knowledge of the metric or apothecary system; however, household measurements are not precisely accurate, so they should never be used in the medical setting. Nevertheless, a medical assistant must understand the conversions between medical and household measurements so the patient can be instructed on how to most accurately measure the medication at home.

The basic measure of weight in the household system is the pound (lb); the basic measure of volume is the drop (gtt). The household drop is equal to an apothecary minim, so these two systems are sometimes easily interchangeable. Both the household and the apothecary systems use the terms *dram* and *ounce* as units of measurement, so always be sure which system you are using. Medications are not measured in household weights, but many prescriptions contain directions using the household measurements of volume. Liquid oral medications are taken by the drop, teaspoon, or tablespoon and are supplied in bottles labeled in ounces or pints. Pediatric medications are frequently packaged as liquids, and the label gives instructions for the medication to be given in household measurements, for example, a teaspoon or tablespoon. The medical assistant should know that 60 gtt = 1 tsp = 5 cc and that 180 gtt = 3 tsp = 1 Tbsp = 15 cc. Tables 33-3 and 33-4 show the household

TABLE 33-2 Approximate Equivalents for Some Commonly Used Measures

GRAINS	GRAMS	MILLIGRAMS	APOTHECARY		METRIC (mL [cc])	
15	1.0	1000	1	quart	1000	mL (cc)
10	0.6	600	1	pint	500	mL
7½	0.5	500	8	fl oz	250	mL
5	0.3	300	7	fl oz	200	mL
4½	0.25	250	3.5	fl oz	100	mL
3	0.2	200	1	fl oz	30	mL
2	0.12	120	4	fl dr	15	mL
1½	0.1	100	2.5	fl dr	10	mL
1	0.06	60	2	fl dr	8	mL
¾	0.050	50	1	fl dr	4	mL
½	0.030	30	45	M	3	mL
⅜	0.025	25	30	M	2	mL
¼	0.015	15	15	M	1	mL
⅙	0.010	10	12	M	0.75	mL
⅛	0.008	8	10	M	0.6	mL
1/10	0.006	6	8	M	0.5	mL
1/12	0.005	5	5	M	0.3	mL
1/20	0.003	3	4	M	0.25	mL
1/30	0.002	2	3	M	0.2	mL
1/60	0.001	1	1.5	M	0.1	mL
1/100	0.0006	0.6	1	M	0.06	mL
1/120	0.0005	0.5	0.75	M	0.05	mL
1/150	0.0004	0.4	0.5	M	0.03	mL
1/200	0.0003	0.3				
1/250	0.00025	0.25				
1/300	0.0002	0.2				
1/400	0.00015	0.15				
1/500	0.00012	0.12				
1/600	0.0001	0.1				

Weight conversions: 1 lb = 0.45 kg; 1 kg = 2.2 lb; 10 lb = 4.5 kg; 10 kg = 22 lb; 30.0 g = 1 oz; 15.0 g = 4 dr; 7.5 g = 2 dr; 4 g = 1 dr; 4 g = 60 gr.
Domestic equivalents: 1 tsp = 5 mL (cc) = 1 fl dr; 1 Tbsp = 15 mL = 0.5 fl oz; 1 measuring cup = 250 mL = 8 fl oz; 4 measuring cups = 1000 mL = 1 quart.

system of measurement. Based on these equivalents, convert the following orders:

2 tsp = _____ cc   120 gtt = _____ tsp
10 mL = _____ tsp   20 mL = _____ Tbsp
3 mL = _____ tsp   4 Tbsp = _____ cc

Conversions Among Systems of Measurement

Medication orders may need to be converted from one system to another if the order is written in one system and the drug label is in another. Using the conversions in Table 33-2, it is possible to directly convert many measurements or choose an equivalent and mathematically convert the order to the system on the drug label. The conversion is calculated by either multiplication or division. For example, if the physician orders 30 grains of the drug but the label states that each tablet is equivalent to 2 grams, you must convert the order in grains to grams to know how many tablets to give the patient. To convert grains to grams, Table 33-2 tells us that 15 grains equals 1 gram. Therefore, to calculate the amount of the dose in tablets, knowing that 15 grains equals 1 gram and the physician has ordered 30 grains, you must divide the order by the conversion factor.

TABLE 33-3   Common Household Measures

60	drops*	1 teaspoon
1	dash	Less than 1/8 teaspoon
3	teaspoons	1 tablespoon
2	tablespoons	1 ounce
4	ounces	1 juice glass
6	ounces	1 teacup
8	ounces	1 glass or cup
16	tablespoons or 8 ounces	1 measuring cup
2	cups	1 pint
2	pints	1 quart
4	quarts	1 gallon

*Drop (gtt) = Approximate liquid measure, depending on kind of liquid measured and the size of the opening from which it is dropped.

TABLE 33-4   Household Equivalents

60	gtt	=	1 t or tsp		
3	t or tsp	=	1 T		
180	gtt	=	1 T	=	1/2 oz
2	T	=	1 oz	=	6 t or tsp
360	gtt	=	2 T		
1	oz	=	30 cc or 30 mL		
6	oz	=	1 tcp		
8	oz	=	1 C or 1 glass		
2	C	=	1 pt	=	16 oz
2	pt	=	1 qt	=	32 oz
4	C	=	1 qt	=	32 oz
4	qt	=	1 gal	=	128 oz

$$30 \text{ gr} \div 15 \text{ gr} = 2 \text{ g}$$

Each tablet contains 2 grams of the medication, so the patient would be given one tablet.

Conversions between units of measurement can also be done by placing the numbers into an algebraic formula. We know that 15 grains equals 1 gram, and what we are looking for is the number of grams that is equivalent to 30 grains. If the amount ordered is placed on the left side of the equation and the conversion factor on the right side, similar units can be cancelled when cross-multiplied, and we can determine the dose.

$$30 \text{ gr} \times \frac{1 g}{15 \text{ gr}}$$

Cross-multiply, and the grain unit cancels out:

$$30 \times \frac{1 g}{15} = \frac{30 g}{15} = 2 \text{ g}$$

Another example is an order that states the patient should be given 2 tablespoons of a medication, but the label indicates that there are 100 milligrams of the drug in each milliliter. To administer this drug correctly the medical assistant must convert the physician's order of 2 tablespoons to milliliters. As stated previously, 1 tablespoon equals 15 milliliters. Therefore, you can determine the answer in two ways. Either multiply the order by the conversion factor:

$$2 \text{ Tbsp} \times 15 = 30 \text{ mL}$$

or set the problem up as an equation with the ordered amount on the left side of the equation and the conversion factor on the right side:

$$2 \text{ Tbsp} \times \frac{15 \text{ mL}}{1 \text{ Tbsp}}$$

Cross-multiply, and the tablespoon unit cancels out, so you have:

$$2 \times \frac{15 \text{ mL}}{1} = 30 \text{ mL}$$

Complete the following conversion problems:

1. A patient with risk factors for heart disease is told to take a baby aspirin equivalent to gr 5 every morning. How many milligrams is the patient taking?
2. A patient scheduled for urinary tract diagnostic tests needs to drink a minimum of 2 L of water over the next 12 hours. How many ounces should the patient drink?
3. A pediatric patient is ordered 8 cc of amoxicillin qid for 10 days. What is the equivalent dose in household measurements?

CALCULATING DRUG DOSAGES FOR ADMINISTRATION

The correct dosage of a medication may depend on the patient's age, weight, and state of health or on what other drugs the patient may be taking. Frequently the physician orders a medication in a dosage that is different from that of the medications in stock. The difference may be in the system of measurement, the strength, or the form. Formulas and mathematic tables of conversion are available for calculating the correct dosage of medication to be administered. It is helpful to look at how the correct calculation is arrived at, one step at a time.

Mathematic Equivalents

You may need to review some basics of arithmetic before you begin to tackle drug calculations. You must thoroughly understand the addition, subtraction, multiplication, and division of fractions and decimals; the relationship of decimals and fractions; and how they are converted from one to the other. In addition, you need to review how decimals and percentages are converted back and forth. Table 33-5 provides some examples of these relationships.

The table shows that a fraction is, in another sense, a ratio. For example, 1/4 (a fraction) is the same as the ratio 1:4 (one to four). If you have one apple and four oranges, then the number of apples that you have is 1/4 the number of oranges, and the ratio of apples to oranges is 1:4. Now, divide the numerator 1

TABLE 33-5 Mathematic Equivalents			
PERCENTAGE	**DECIMAL**	**FRACTION**	**RATIO**
25	0.25	$^1/_4$	1:4
50	0.5	$^1/_2$	1:2
60	0.6	$^3/_5$ ($^6/_{10}$)	3:5
0.5	0.005	$^1/_{200}$	1:200
0.1	0.001	$^1/_{1000}$	1:1000
85	0.85	$^{17}/_{20}$	17:20
1	0.01	$^1/_{100}$	1:100

by the denominator 4 (a fraction is also an automatic division problem waiting to be solved):

$$4\overline{)1.00} = 0.25$$

The act of dividing a fraction results in a decimal number. Decimal numbers can then be converted to percentages by moving the decimal two spaces to the right:

$$0.25 = 25.0\% \text{ (commonly written 25\%)}$$

Using the example of apples and oranges, you can see that 1 is 0.25, or 25%, of 4. Therefore the number of apples is 0.25, or 25%, of the number of oranges. If you need to review any of these concepts, please stop now and practice these arithmetic steps.

Determine the following equivalents:
1. 0.20 = _____ (percent) = _____ (fraction) = _____ (ratio)
2. 37% = _____ (decimal) = _____ (fraction) = _____ (ratio)
3. 2/3 = _____ (ratio) = _____ (percent) = _____ (decimal)
4. 3:4 = _____ (fraction) = _____ (decimal) = _____ (percent)

Ratio and Proportion

A ratio is one way of expressing a fraction, or division problem, and shows the relationship of the numerator to the denominator. The comparison of two ratios is called a *proportion*. A proportion is written as follows:

$$\frac{4}{16} = \frac{1}{4} \text{ or } 4:16 = 1:4$$

This is read as 4 divided by 16 equals 1 divided by 4, or 4 is to 16 as 1 is to 4. The physician's order for a medication may be a ratio different from that of the medication that is in stock. To determine the correct proportion for administration, we must compare the ordered ratio with the available ratio (what is in stock).

The preceding proportion example has all the answers in it; there is nothing to solve. In calculating dosages, mathematic proportions are used, but with one element unknown. We must solve for that unknown, or x. For example:

$$\frac{4}{16} = \frac{1}{x}$$

Always in a proportion we solve the problem by *cross-multiplication*. Do not confuse this with plain multiplication. If you see an equals sign (=) between two fractions, that indicates this is an equation to be cross-multiplied.

$$4 \times x = 16 \times 1$$

Therefore:

$$4x = 16$$

We know what $4x$ equals, but next we must find what $1x$, or x, equals. To find the value of x, we must find a way to leave x (or $1x$) alone on the left side of the equation. We can change $4x$ to $1x$ by dividing the number 4 by itself:

$$4x \div 4 = 1x$$

But what we do on one side of an equation, we must do on the other side, or the equation will not be equal anymore. Therefore we divide 16 by 4:

$$16 \div 4 = 4$$

Therefore

$$x = 4 \text{ and } \frac{4}{16} = \frac{1}{4}$$

Calculating Dosages

For calculating dosages a standard set of formulas is used (Procedures 33-1 and 33-2). These formulas use the *strength* (potency) and *dose unit* (amount) of the drug. If the drug label reads "5 gr/tab," the strength is 5 grains and the dose unit is one tablet. For liquids the drug strength is an amount of *solute*, which is dissolved in a liquid called the *solvent*. Therefore, if a vial of injectable material reads "500 mg/mL," 500 mg (strength) of the drug is present in every milliliter (amount) of liquid.

We can use these two examples and the proportion formula previously reviewed to work out two problems: (1) filling a syringe and (2) administering oral medications.

Problem 1

Order: Give 250 mg of cefalexin IM
Available: A vial marked 500 mg/mL
Standard formula:

$$\frac{\text{Available strength}}{\text{Ordered strength}} = \frac{\text{Available amount}}{\text{Amount to give}}$$

Problem: Given the strength of the drug needed (the physician's order of 250 mg), the amount of fluid to be withdrawn must be determined.

Set up a proportion with the three known quantities: (1) the strength of the drug in the vial, (2) the unit of fluid in which that strength is contained, and (3) the strength of the drug the physician has ordered for administration.

Apply the problem to the standard formula:

$$\frac{500 \text{ mg}}{250 \text{ mg}} = \frac{1 \text{ mL}}{x \text{ mL}}$$

The mg units in the numerator and denominator on the left side of the equation cross each other out. Cross-multiply the equation.

$$500 \times x = 250 \times 1$$
$$500x = 250 \text{ mL}$$

PROCEDURE 33-1

Apply Pharmacology Principles to Prepare and Administer Oral And Parenteral (Excluding IV) Medications: Calculate the Correct Dosage for Administration

CAAHEP COMPETENCY: 3.b.(4)(g)
ABHES COMPETENCY: 4.m

GOAL: *To calculate the correct dose amount and choose the correct equipment when the physician orders 2.4 million IU of penicillin G benzathine (Bicillin).*

EQUIPMENT and SUPPLIES

- Premixed syringes of Bicillin in the following two strengths are available:
  - 0.6 million IU/syringe
  - 1.2 million IU/syringe

PROCEDURAL STEPS

1. Read the order in quiet surroundings to make sure that you fully understand it.
2. Write out the order.
3. Examine the drug labels to see what strengths and amounts are available.

4. Write down the standard formula.

$$\frac{\text{Available strength}}{\text{Ordered strength}} = \frac{\text{Available amount}}{\text{Amount to give}}$$

   PURPOSE: To eliminate the chances of error, orders should never be carried out unless the calculations are completed in writing.
5. Rewrite the formula, replacing the unknown values with the known quantities. The unknown x will be the amount of the drug to give.
6. Work the proportion problem by cross-multiplying to solve for x.
7. State your answer by filling in the blanks, as follows:
   To administer 2.4 million IU of Bicillin, I would select _____ _____ of the premixed syringes labeled _____ .

PROCEDURE 33-2

Apply Pharmacology Principles to Prepare and Administer Oral And Parenteral (Excluding IV) Medications: Calculate the Correct Dosage for Administration Using Two Systems of Measurement

CAAHEP COMPETENCY: 3.b.(4)(g)
ABHES COMPETENCY: 4.m

GOAL: *To choose the correct system of measurement and calculate the correct dose amount when the physician orders 120 mg of a drug to be administered to a patient. (Tablet label reads 1 gr each.)*

EQUIPMENT and SUPPLIES

- Tablets labeled 1 gr (grain) each
- Standard mathematic formula:

$$\frac{\text{Available strength}}{\text{Ordered strength}} = \frac{\text{Available amount}}{\text{Amount to give}}$$

- Conversion equivalent: 1 gr = 60 mg

PROCEDURAL STEPS

1. Read the order in quiet surroundings to make sure that you fully understand it.
2. Write out the order.
3. Examine the drug labels to see what strengths and amounts are available.
4. Convert the ordered system of measurement to the system of measurement on the label.
5. Place the amount ordered on the left side of the equation and the conversion factor on the right side so that similar units can be cancelled when cross-multiplied.

$$120 \text{ mg} \times \frac{1 \text{ g}}{60 \text{ mg}} = 120 \text{ gr} \div 60 = 2 \text{ gr.}$$

6. Write down the standard formula.

$$\frac{\text{Available strength}}{\text{Ordered strength}} = \frac{\text{Available amount}}{\text{Amount to give}} .$$

   PURPOSE: To eliminate the chances of error, orders should never be carried out unless the calculations are completed in writing.
7. Rewrite the formula, replacing the unknown values with the known quantities and using the system of measurement on the label. The unknown x will be the amount of the drug to give (amount to give).

$$\frac{1 \text{ gr}}{2 \text{ gr}} \times \frac{1 \text{ tab}}{x \text{ tab}}$$

8. Work the proportion problem by cross-multiplying to solve for x.
9. State your answer by filling in the blank, as follows:
   To administer 120 mg of a drug from tablets labeled *1 gr* (grain) *each*, give _____ tablet(s).

To determine what x equals you must divide each side of the equation by 500.

$$\frac{500x}{500} = \frac{250\ \text{mL}}{500}$$

$$x = \tfrac{1}{2}\ \text{mL} = 0.5\ \text{mL}$$

Solution: Administer 0.5 mL of cephalexin.

Problem 2

Order: Give 10 gr (grains) of a drug
Available: A bottle with tablets labeled 5 gr each
Standard formula:

$$\frac{\text{Available strength}}{\text{Ordered strength}} = \frac{\text{Available amount}}{\text{Amount to give}}$$

Problem: Given the strength of the drug needed, the number of tablets to be administered must be determined.

Set up a proportion with the three known quantities: (1) the strength of the drug in each tablet, (2) the unit amount that is in one tablet, and (3) the strength of the drug the physician has ordered for administration.

Apply the problem to the standard formula:

$$\frac{5\ \text{gr}}{10\ \text{gr}} = \frac{1\ \text{tablet}}{x\ (\text{number of tablets})}$$

The grain units in the numerator and denominator on the left side of the equation cross each other out. Cross-multiply the equation.

$$5 \times x = 10 \times 1$$
$$5x = 10$$

To determine what x equals you must divide each side of the equation by 5.

$$\frac{5x}{5} = \frac{10}{5}$$

$$x = 2\ \text{tablets}$$

Solution: Administer two tablets.

Use the standard formula for any type of calculation. You may be using strengths that are measured in international units (IU), as with penicillin, grams, milligrams, grains, or percentages. The forms in which drugs may be prepared include cubic centimeters (cc) or milliliters (mL), minims, drops, drams, ounces, pints, gallons (for making up diluted stock solutions from concentrated solutions, such as with alcohol and hydrogen peroxide), or spoonfuls.

Follow the steps previously shown, and, above all, discipline yourself to write down each step with complete calculations. This is the only way to ensure maximum accuracy and the safety of your patients. If you have difficulty with the calculation, or the answer does not seem quite right, ask the physician to check your calculation. A double check is always preferred.

Calculate the following doses.

1. Administer 0.25 mg Lanoxin. The label reads 0.125 mg/tab. How many tablets should you give?
2. The patient is ordered 15 mEq of KCl, and the label reads 5 mEq/5 mL. How many cc should the patient receive?
3. The phenobarbital label states 15 mg/5 cc. The patient is ordered 40 mg of the drug. How many cc should be administered?

4. The physician orders 25 mg of Compazine IM. The label reads 10 mg/mL. How much medicine should be injected?

Rounding Calculations

What should you do if the dose of the supplied drug does not exactly match your calculation? For example, what if you calculate a tablet dose as 1.75 tabs but you only have whole tablets available? First, check your calculation for accuracy, then check the stocked supply of the drug to make sure no other dosages are available. If the calculation is correct and there are no other dosages of the drug available, then you will have to round your answer to the nearest amount that matches the dose available. *If the calculation is 0.5 or greater, then round up to the next whole number.* Therefore the patient should be given two tabs of the medication. Determine the correct doses for the following examples:

1.2 tabs = _____ tablet(s)	1.55 tabs = _____ tablet(s)
1.37 tabs = _____ tablet(s)	0.56 tab = _____ tablet
1.64 tabs = _____ tablet(s)	0.81 tab = _____ tablet

If a tablet is *scored,* meaning the medication is manufactured with an impression or groove down the center of the tablet, then the tablet can be accurately divided into two equal parts so calculations can be rounded to the closest half tab (Figure 33-2). For example, 0.4 tab would be half of a scored tab, and 1.7 would be two tabs. *Never* give a partial dose of a tablet unless it is scored.

If administering a liquid medication, it is usually acceptable to round the dose to the *nearest tenth.* For example, if the correct calculation for an injection of an antibiotic is 1.46 mL, then administer 1.5 mL of the drug (the calculation is greater than 0.05). The *exception* to this rule is in pediatrics, where accurate doses for children may be much smaller than an adult dose, or if you are using a syringe that is marked in hundredths, in which case the medication is administered in hundredths. What are the correct doses of the following medications, rounded to the nearest tenth?

1.47 cc = _____ cc	1.33 mL = _____ mL
2.62 mL = _____ mL	2.15 cc = _____ cc
0.08 mL = _____ mL	0.15 mL = _____ mL

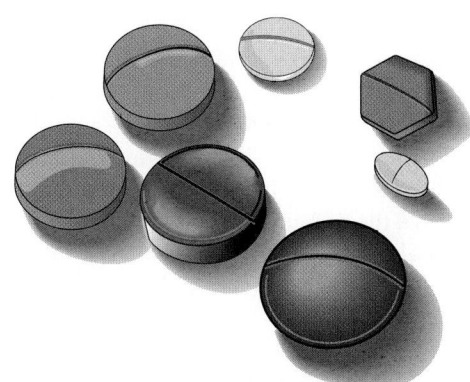

FIGURE 33-2 Examples of scored tablets. (From Fulcher EM, Fulcher RM, Soto CD: *Pharmacology: principles and applications,* St Louis, 2007, Saunders.)

CRITICAL THINKING APPLICATION

At work the next day Dr. Angio orders Heather to administer Acetaminophen Elixir 70 mg stat to a 6-year-old patient with a fever of 102.6° F. Heather checks the label of the Acetaminophen Elixir in the drug cabinet and discovers the bottle contains 120 mg per 5 mL in a 100-mL bottle. Using the standard formula presented earlier, how many milliliters should the child receive? If Heather is concerned about her calculation, what should she do?

PEDIATRIC DOSE

Calculating Dose

Pediatric doses are different from those in other age groups because of multiple factors, including differences in absorption and drug metabolism. Although there have been formulas used in the past that base dose calculation on age, pediatric doses are much more accurate when based on weight, because children of any age can vary greatly in size and body weight. Therefore, the factors used in calculating pediatric doses are either body **surface area** (BSA) or weight. You must be especially careful in calculating dosages for children, because even a minor miscalculation may be dangerous.

Clark's Rule

Clark's rule is based on the weight of the child. It uses 150 pounds (70 kg) as the average adult weight and assumes that the child's dose is proportionately less. The formula is as follows:

$$\text{Pediatric dose} = \frac{\text{Child's weight in pounds}}{150 \text{ pounds}} \times \text{Adult dose}$$

For example: A child weighing 32 pounds is ordered Tylenol. The normal adult dose of the drug is 240 mg. How much Tylenol should the child be given?

$$\text{Dose} = \frac{32 \text{ pounds}}{150 \text{ pounds}} \times 240 \text{ mg} \text{ (First divide 32 by 150 then}$$
$$\text{multiply that figure by}$$
$$240 \text{ mg)}$$
$$= 0.2 \text{ (rounded from 0.213)} \times 240 \text{ mg}$$
$$= 48 \text{ mg}$$

West's Nomogram

West's **nomogram** uses a calculation of the body surface area (BSA) of infants and young children to determine the pediatric dose. Many physicians use the nomogram as a quick reference for pediatric doses (Figure 33-3). The formula is based on the estimated adult BSA of 1.7 m². If the child is of normal height and weight, then the BSA in square meters is the point at which the child's weight in pounds intersects with the surface area in the box on the left. Therefore if the child weighs 15 pounds (and that is normal for his age and height), then his BSA is 0.36 m². If the child is underweight or overweight according to standard growth charts (these will be discussed in Chapter 41) the BSA is determined by intersecting the point on the nomogram between the child's height in either centimeters or inches and the child's

weight in either pounds or kilograms in the right column. For example, if a child is overweight at 45 pounds and 40 inches in height, the BSA is 0.78 m². After the child's BSA is determined from the nomogram, it should be divided by 1.7 m² and that calculation multiplied by the adult dose to determine the amount of medication for the child (Procedure 33-3).

$$\text{Pediatric dose} = \frac{\text{BSA of child in m}^2}{1.7 \text{ m}^2 \text{ (average adult BSA)}} \times \text{Adult dose}$$

Sample problem: A child who weighs 10 pounds and who is 30 inches long (underweight for height) is ordered erythromycin. The normal adult dose of the drug is 400 mg. How much of the antibiotic should the child receive in a single dose?

1. According to the nomogram the child's BSA is 0.31 m²
2. $\frac{0.31 \text{ m}^2}{1.7 \text{ m}^2} = 0.18$ (Because this is a pediatric dose, round to the nearest hundredth for greater accuracy)
3. $0.18 \times 400 \text{ mg} = 72 \text{ mg}$

Dosages Based on Body Weight

Although Clark's rule and West's nomogram provide quick methods for determining pediatric doses, the most frequently used calculation method relies on the child's accurate weight in kilograms. Kilogram measurements are necessary because the majority of pediatric medication dosages are based on a designated number of milligrams to kilogram weight (mg/kg). Several steps are involved in this type of calculation, but if they are followed closely you will determine the most accurate amount of medication to administer to a child (Procedure 33-4).

1. Carefully weigh the child before beginning to calculate the dose to make sure you have an accurate weight. If the scale provides a reading in pounds, convert the child's weight to kilograms by dividing the number of pounds by 2.2 kg (1 kg = 2.2 lb). For example, 36 lb is equal to 16.4 kg (36 ÷ 2.2 = 16.36 = 16.4 kg rounded up). If the child's weight is in pounds and ounces, then you must convert the ounces to pounds as a decimal and add it to the pounds. For example, if an infant weighs 9 lb 7 oz, first convert 7 oz to the nearest tenth of pounds (1 lb = 16 oz; 7 oz ÷ 16 = 0.4 lb) then add it to 9 lb so the baby weighs 9.4 lbs. Then convert pounds to kilograms by dividing 9.4 by 2.2 (9.4 ÷ 2.2 = 4.3 kg).
2. Calculate the total daily dose of the medication.
3. Calculate a single dose of the drug based on how frequently the medication is ordered throughout the day. For example, if the drug is ordered qid, divide the total daily dose by 4; if the medication is ordered every 8 hours, then divide the total daily dose by 3 because there are three 8-hour periods in a 24-hour day.
4. After calculating the amount of a single dose, compare the ordered amount to the drug label. If needed, apply the standard formula to calculate the amount of the medication that should be administered.

Example: An infant that weighs 12 lb, 6 oz is ordered erythromycin q6h. The label states there are 200 mg of the drug in 5 cc of suspension. The recommended range of the medication for

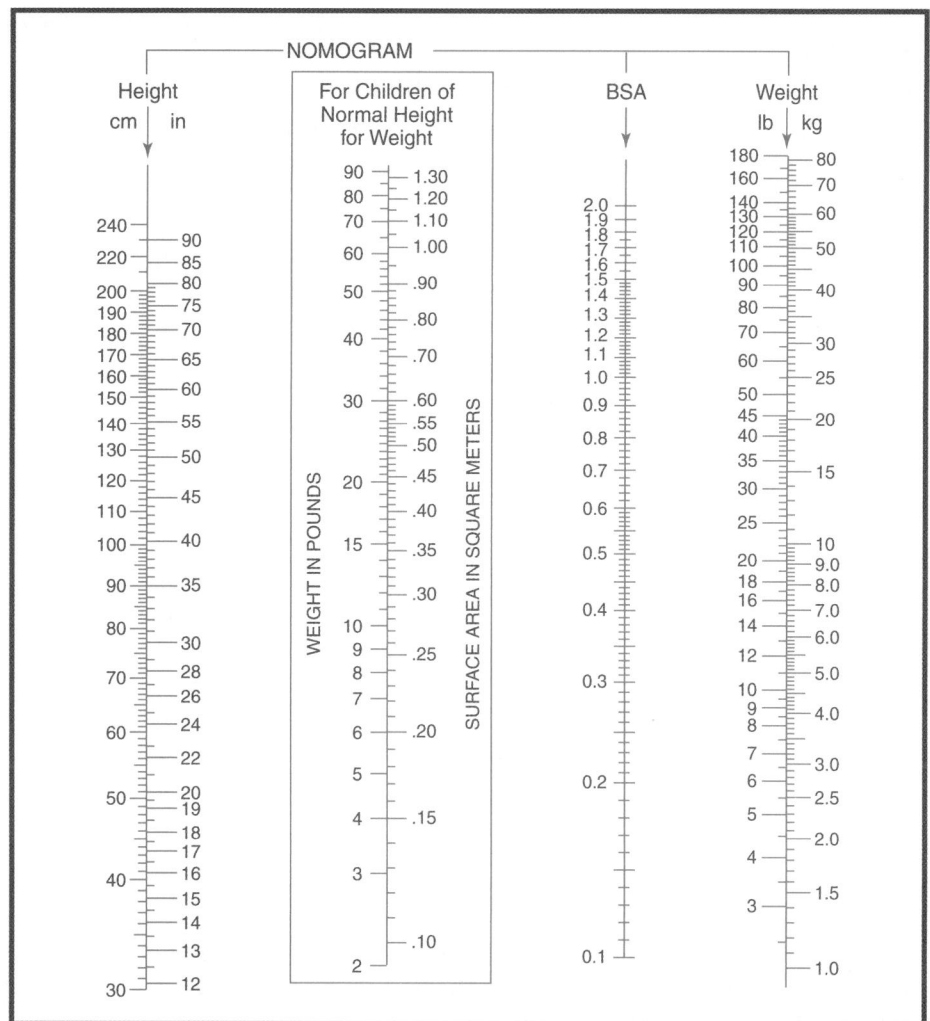

FIGURE 33-3 West's nomogram for estimation of body surface area. (From Behrman RE, Kliegman R, Jenson HB, editors: *Nelson textbook of pediatrics*, ed 16, Philadelphia, 2000, Saunders.)

infants is 30 mg/kg/day. How much should the child receive per dose?

1. Convert 12 lb 6 oz to kg.

$$6 \text{ oz} \div 16 \text{ oz} = 0.375 \text{ converted to the nearest tenth} =$$
$$0.4 \text{ lb} + 12 = 12.4 \text{ lb}$$
$$12.4 \div 2.2 = 5.6 \text{ kg}$$

2. The total daily dose of the medication = 30 mg times the weight in kilograms.

$$30 \times 5.6 = 168 \text{ mg/day}$$

3. A single dose of the drug is the total daily dose divided by 4 (there are four 6-hour time periods in a 24-hour day).

$$168 \text{ mg} \div 4 = 42 \text{ mg/dose}$$

4. The amount of the medication that should be administered in a single dose is determined by the drug label, which states there are 200 mg in every 5 cc of the suspension. Using the standard formula:

$$\frac{\text{Available strength}}{\text{Ordered strength}} = \frac{\text{Available amount}}{\text{Amount to give}}$$
$$\frac{200 \text{ mg}}{42 \text{ mg}} = \frac{5 \text{ cc}}{x \text{ (number of cc)}}$$
$$200x = 210$$
$$x = 210 \div 200$$
$$x = 1.05 \text{ or } 1.1 \text{ cc}$$

RECONSTITUTING POWDERED INJECTABLE MEDICATIONS

Some medications are packaged as crystals or powder (solute) in a vial that must be mixed with sterile isotonic saline or sterile distilled water (solvent) to form a solution before it can be injected. In this case it is essential to carefully read the label directions to determine how much sterile solvent must be added to the solute to create the ordered dosage strength.

PROCEDURE 33-3

Apply Pharmacology Principles to Prepare and Administer Oral and Parenteral (Excluding IV) Medications: Calculate the Correct Pediatric Dosage Using the Body Surface Area Method

CAAHEP COMPETENCY: 3.b.(4)(g)
ABHES COMPETENCY: 4.m

GOAL: *To calculate the correct dose amount using the body surface area (BSA) method for a 90-lb child who is 48 inches tall when the adult dose is 250 mg.*

EQUIPMENT and SUPPLIES

- Accurate scale with length measurement
- West's nomogram
- Adult dose 250 mg/mL

$$\text{Pediatric dose} = \frac{\text{BSA of child in m}^2}{1.7 \text{ m}^2 \text{ (average adult BSA)}} \times \text{Adult dose}$$

PROCEDURAL STEPS

1. Read the order in quiet surroundings to make sure that you fully understand it.
2. Write out the order.
3. Examine the drug labels to see what strengths and amounts are available.
4. Write down the BSA formula.
   <u>PURPOSE:</u> To eliminate the chances of error, orders should never be carried out unless the calculations are completed in writing.
5. Using the BSA method, determine the BSA in m² by intersecting the child's weight and height on the right column (child is overweight).
6. Divide the child's BSA by 1.7 m² (the average adult BSA).
7. Multiply this calculation by the adult dose (250 mg).
8. State your answer by filling in the blank, as follows:
   To administer an adult medication labeled 250 mg/mL to a 90-lb child, give _____ mg.

PROCEDURE 33-4

Apply Pharmacology Principles to Prepare and Administer Oral and Parenteral (Excluding IV) Medications: Calculate the Correct Pediatric Dosage for Administration Using Body Weight

CAAHEP COMPETENCY: 3.b.(4)(g)
ABHES COMPETENCY: 4.m

GOAL: *To calculate correct dosage by using body weight method.*
Ordered: Zithromax suspension, 5 mg/kg bid times 5 days for a patient who has a diagnosis of otitis media. The patient weighs 22 lb. The suspension is labeled 100 mg/5 mL.
Weight conversion: 2.2 lb = 1 kg

EQUIPMENT and SUPPLIES

- Suspension labeled 100 mg/5 mL
- Balance scale
- Formula for conversion of pounds to kilograms
- Standard math formula:

$$\frac{\text{Available strength}}{\text{Ordered strength}} = \frac{\text{Available amount}}{\text{Amount to give}}$$

- Paper and pencil

PROCEDURAL STEPS

1. Read the order in quiet surroundings to make sure that you fully understand it.
2. Write out the order.
3. Examine the drug label to check the strength and amount.
4. Convert the patient's weight from pounds to kilograms.
   22 lb ÷ 2.2 lb/kg = 10 kg.
5. Calculate the total daily amount of medication by multiplying the weight in kilograms by the mg/kg factor.
   10 kg × 5 mg = 50 mg of Zithromax daily for 5 days.
6. Calculate the individual dose of Zithromax; divide the daily dose by 2 (bid is twice a day).
7. Compare the ordered daily dose to the dose information on the medication label (100 mg = 5 mL).
8. Write down the standard formula.
   <u>PURPOSE:</u> To eliminate the chances of error.
9. Rewrite the formula, replacing the unknown values with the known quantities. The unknown *x* will be the amount of the drug to give.
10. Work the problem by cross-multiplying to solve for *x*.
11. State your answer by filling in the blank as follows:
    To administer 5 mg of Zithromax per kilogram of body weight from the suspension labeled 100 mg/5 mL, I would give
    _____ _____ mL.

Example

The physician orders 500 mg of a drug.

The label reads "Add 5.5 mL of sterile water to make 250 mg/mL; total volume of available solution will be 6 mL."

First: Inject 5.5 mL of sterile water into the vial of medication. Rotate the vial between the hands to mix the solutes and solvent. The total volume in the vial is now 6 mL.

Second: According to the label, every milliliter in the vial contains 250 mg of the drug.

Third: Write on the vial the date and time of reconstitution because, according to the particular drug guidelines, once the medication is mixed it must be discarded in a short period of time.

Fourth: Calculate the number of milliliters to withdraw from the vial to fulfill the physician's order for 500 mg of the drug using the standard formula.

$$\frac{\text{Available strength}}{\text{Ordered strength}} = \frac{\text{Available amount}}{\text{Amount to give}}$$

$$\frac{250\ \text{mg}}{500\ \text{mg}} = \frac{1\ \text{mL}}{x}$$

$$250x = 500$$

$$x = 500 \div 250 = 2\ \text{mL}$$

Answer: To administer 500 mg from a vial labeled "250 mg/mL," administer 2 mL of medication.

CLOSING COMMENTS

Legal and Ethical Issues

A medical assistant who is responsible for medication administration must have complete mastery in calculating dosages, whether the prescribed dose is for a child or an adult. If there is ever any doubt about the accuracy of a calculation, the medical assistant should always have a trusted colleague or the physician check the calculations.

The medical assistant who prepares and administers medications is ethically and legally responsible for his or her own actions. Laws vary from state to state; therefore it is essential that the medical assistant become familiar with the laws in the state of employment before giving medications. Legislation in some states gives physicians broad authority to delegate responsibility for giving medications. In this case the medical assistant acts as the "agent" of the physician. However, the assistant is responsible and accountable for the acts performed and may be subject to penalties.

Regardless of the differences in state authorization laws, the courts will not permit the carelessness of healthcare workers to go unpunished, especially when such actions result in harm to or death of the patient.

SUMMARY OF SCENARIO

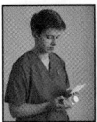

Heather recognizes how important it is to be able to calculate drug dosages correctly. To do so she must understand the terms involved in dosage preparation, be able to read a drug label correctly, and follow the various steps in calculating a correct dose. The drug label contains a great deal of information including the brand and generic names; dosage strength; route of administration; instructions on mixing solvents if appropriate; storage guidelines; total amount of the drug in the container; name of the drug manufacturer; expiration date; and both the lot numbers and the NDC identification number. Heather must also be able to make conversions within and between measuring systems; use the standard formula to determine drug doses; accurately calculate pediatric doses based on the child's weight; and reconstitute powdered drugs for administration by following the label directions regarding the amount of solvent that should be added to the solute. She continues to ask either Mrs. Allison or Dr. Angio to check her calculations for accuracy before dispensing and administering any drug order that differs from the medication label.

SUMMARY of LEARNING OBJECTIVES

1. Define, spell, and pronounce the terms listed in the vocabulary.
   - Spelling and pronouncing medical terms correctly adds credibility to the medical assistant. Knowing the definition of these terms promotes confidence in communication with patients and co-workers.
2. Demonstrate methods for verifying the accuracy of calculations.
   - Verifying the accuracy of calculations is essential before dispensing and administering all medications. First, the medical assistant must check the drug label with the physician's order to verify the systems of measurement. If the physician's order is in a different unit of measurement, the ordered dose must be converted to match the system on the label. Next, the calculation is completed using the appropriate formula. Finally, the calculation is checked for accuracy.
3. Differentiate among the terms used in dosage preparation.
   - Drug label terms must be understood to implement pharmacology math formulas. The strength of the drug is its potency; the dosage is the amount available in the drug package; the solute is the crystal or powdered form of the drug; the solvent is the sterile liquid that is combined in the vial with the solute to create the drug solution.
4. Summarize the important parts of a drug label.

Continued

SUMMARY of LEARNING OBJECTIVES
Continued

- The drug label contains a great deal of information including the brand and generic names; dosage strength; route of administration; instructions on mixing solvents if appropriate; storage guidelines; total amount of the drug in the container; name of the drug manufacturer; expiration date; and both the lot numbers and the NDC identification number.

5. Describe and perform conversions among the various systems of measurement.
   - Three systems of measurement are used for drugs. The metric system is based on units of 10. The liter is a measure of the liquid volume of a drug, and the gram is a measure of the weight or strength. Units within the metric system are converted by moving the decimal point either to the right or the left. The apothecary system measures liquid volume in minims and weight in grains. Household measurements are based on pounds and drops. Table 33-2 can be used to convert from one system of measurement to another, or drug measurements can be converted by using the conversion formula.

6. Calculate the correct dose of a drug using the standard formula.
   - The correct dose of an ordered drug can be calculated by using basic arithmetic involving fractions, ratios, and proportions. The standard formula for calculating drug dosage uses the information about the drug's strength and amount (which is on the label) and the strength of the drug ordered, with the unknown (x) being the answer sought. The only way to gain confidence in using the standard formula is to practice dose calculation frequently until you become comfortable with the math.

7. Determine accurate pediatric doses of medication.
   - The medical assistant must be especially vigilant in calculating pediatric doses, because even a minor error may be dangerous to a child. West's nomogram can be used to determine the pediatric dose if the child's height and weight and the adult dose of the drug are known. However, the most accurate method for determining a pediatric dose is based on the child's weight. Procedure 33-4 describes how to calculate a pediatric dose based on weight.

8. Diagram how to reconstitute powdered injectable medications.
   - In reconstituting powdered injectable medications, the medical assistant must add a particular amount of solvent (as recommended on the drug label) to a vial of powdered or crystalloid medication. Once the solute and solvent are combined and mixed in the vial, a solution of medication is formed; the strength is based on equivalents printed on the drug label. After mixing the medication it is important for the medical assistant to carefully read the label to determine how much of the drug must be withdrawn to equal the physician's order. This process frequently requires the use of the standard conversion formula to determine the accurate dose for administration.

9. Specify the legal responsibilities of a medical assistant in calculating drug dosages.
   - A medical assistant who prepares, dispenses, and administers medications is ethically and legally responsible for his or her own actions. If there is any doubt regarding the accuracy of calculations, it is absolutely essential that the medical assistant have the physician or another trusted employee review the math before the medication is dispensed and administered. It is important for medical assistants to be aware of state laws that monitor medication administration by allied health workers.

CONNECTIONS

 Study Guide Connection: Go to Chapter 33 Study Guide. Read the Case Study and Workplace Applications and complete the assignments. Do online research for answers to the questions in the Internet Activities associated with pharmacology math.

 CD Connection: Go to the Medical Assisting Competency Challenge CD and do the training activities under Diagnostic Testing.

evolve **Evolve Connection:** For more information related to pharmacology math, go to evolve.elsevier.com/kinn and visit related weblinks for Chapter 33. Click on the Medical Assisting Exam Review and do the practice questions to sharpen your test-taking skills.

Administering Medications

34

SCENARIO

Dr. Anna Thau just opened a new primary care office in the community. She is in the process of hiring office staff, and Dorothy Gaston, CMA, is being interviewed for a clinical assisting position. One of Dr. Thau's chief concerns is that the medical assistants working in the clinical area be familiar with medications and competent with their administration. Her primary concern is the safety of her patients, so she requires that employees perform appropriate safety measures when dispensing and administering oral, topical, and parenteral drugs.

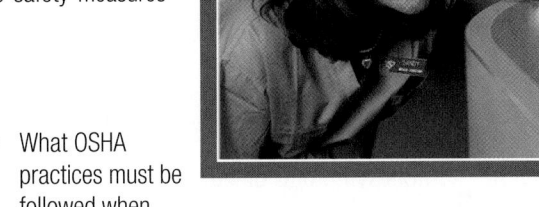

While studying this chapter, think about the following questions:

- What safety guidelines should Dorothy incorporate into her practice each time she receives a drug order from Dr. Thau?
- What information must be included in comprehensive documentation of the administration of medication?
- Are there patient assessment factors that might affect medication administration?
- Why does Dorothy have to understand and be able to apply details regarding various drug forms and their administration guidelines?

- What OSHA practices must be followed when preparing and administering medications?
- Are there IV principles Dorothy should understand?
- Does Dorothy need to be aware of the legal implications of drug administration?

LEARNING OBJECTIVES

1. Define, spell, and pronounce the terms listed in the vocabulary.
2. Analyze safety guidelines for specific patient populations.
3. Perform documentation of medication administration.
4. Apply safety precautions to the management of medication administration in the ambulatory healthcare setting.
5. Summarize patient assessment factors that have an impact on medication administration.
6. Identify various drug forms and their administration guidelines.
7. Specify parenteral administration equipment including details regarding needles and syringes.

8. Employ OSHA guidelines in the management of parenteral administration.
9. Describe and demonstrate parenteral administration types and locations.
10. Outline the principles of IV therapy.
11. Recognize the role of the medical assistant in patient education for drug administration.
12. Assess legal and ethical issues in drug administration in the ambulatory care setting.

National Accreditation Competencies and Content

CAAHEP COMPETENCIES

Clinical
3.b.(4)(g). Apply pharmacology principles to prepare and administer oral and parenteral (excluding IV) medications
3.b.(4)(h). Maintain medication and immunization records

General
3.c.(1)(a). Respond to and initiate written communications
3.c.(2)(b). Perform within legal and ethical boundaries
3.c.(2)(c). Establish and maintain the medical record
3.c.(2)(d). Document appropriately

ABHES COMPETENCIES

Professionalism
1.d. Be cognizant of ethical boundaries

Communication
2.i. Recognize and respond to verbal and nonverbal communication
2.k. [Apply] principles of verbal and nonverbal communication

Clinical Duties
4.m. Prepare and administer oral and parenteral medications as directed by physician
4.n. Maintain medication and immunization records

Legal Concepts
5.b. Document accurately

VOCABULARY

asymptomatic Without symptoms of a disease process.

bevel Angled tip of a needle.

bronchoconstriction Narrowing of the bronchiole tubes.

edema Abnormal accumulation of fluid in the interstitial spaces of tissues.

enteric-coated Referring to an oral medication to which a coating has been added that resists the effects of stomach juices; designed so that medicine is absorbed in the small intestine.

hermetically sealed Sealed so that no air can enter.

hypotension Low blood pressure.

immunosuppressant Pertaining to a substance that suppresses or prevents an immune system response.

immunotherapy Administering repeated injections of diluted extracts of a substance that causes an allergy; also called *desensitization.*

induration An abnormally hard, inflamed area.

loading dose A double dose administered as the first dose of a medication; usually used with antibiotic therapy so that therapeutic blood levels are reached quickly.

meniscus (meh-nis′-kus) The curved surface of liquids in a container.

phlebitis (fluh-bi′-tis) Inflammation of a vein, with the possible complication of clot formation at the site *(thrombophlebitis).*

polyuria (pah-le-yur′-e-uh) Excretion of an unusually large amount of urine.

scored Slashed; for example, describes a tablet that is manufactured with an indentation for division through the center.

sterile Free of all living microorganisms.

vasodilation Increase in the diameter of a blood vessel.

viscosity (vis-kos′-uh-te) The quality of being thick and of lacking the capability of easy movement.

volatile Capable of vaporizing at a low temperature; describes an explosive substance.

wheal Localized area of edema or a raised lesion.

In previous medication chapters you learned about general pharmacologic principles and pharmacology math. In this chapter you will learn about safety factors in drug administration, documentation guidelines, and the forms of medications and how they are administered. It is important to remember that medications have the potential to cause serious harm to the patient. Therefore the process of dispensing and administering medication orders must always be treated with great care. Each member of the healthcare team involved in medication administration must be constantly vigilant to prevent errors and deliver high-quality patient care.

No matter what types of medications are administered, the order must first come from the physician. If the physician delegates drug administration to the medical assistant, it must be allowable under state laws. Every state has a medical practice act that defines whether a medical assistant can administer drugs under the supervision of a physician. Some states allow medical assistants to administer only certain types of medications; some prohibit medical assistants from giving injections. Information concerning the scope of practice for medical assistants in your particular state should be obtained from your local government or medical society. You should know what the law states and how your duties fit into that law.

SAFETY IN DRUG ADMINISTRATION

To ensure patient safety in drug administration, the medical assistant must perform certain procedures every time a medication is ordered. First, it is absolutely essential that the medical assistant understand the physician's order. Safety starts with a written order that can be clearly read and understood. Ask the physician to clarify any questions you have regarding the medication, dose, strength, or route of administration. Once the order is clarified, it is the medical assistant's responsibility to look up the drug in a pharmacology reference, such as the *Physicians' Desk Reference* (PDR) (see Chapter 32). A medication should never be given until its purpose, possible side effects, precautions, and recommended dose are known. After the medical assistant learns about the drug ordered, it is time to dispense and administer the medication. Safeguarding the patient during this process involves using the "seven rights" of proper drug administration:

1. *The right patient.* The easiest way to make sure the medication is being given to the patient ordered is to ask the patient his or her name or call the patient by name before administering the drug.

2. *The right drug.* This begins with clarifying the physician's order if needed. *Every* time a drug is dispensed, the label must be checked *three* times to confirm the right drug, dose, and strength. You must be competent in reading and understanding the information on the drug label. To make sure you are dispensing the exact medication ordered, compare the physician's written order with the label when:
   - Taking the medication from the storage area
   - Dispensing the medication from the container
   - Replacing the container to storage or before discarding the used container

3. *The right dose.* If the dose ordered does not match the dose available according to the drug label, perform appropriate pharmacology math procedures to determine the accurate dose. *Remember to have calculations checked if you have any doubt about the dose accuracy.*

4. *The right route.* Check the physician's order to clarify the route of administration, whether it is oral, via mucous membrane, or parenteral. Patient assessment includes determining whether this is an appropriate route for that particular patient.

5. *The right time.* In the ambulatory care setting, most medications are ordered *stat.* However, it is important to check the physician's order to clarify the time of administration and refer to this information when looking up the drug to clarify any patient questions about home administration of the drug.

6. *The right technique.* A medical assistant must be familiar with the proper techniques for all routes of administration. If you have any doubts about your ability to administer a particular drug, always ask for help.

7. *The right documentation.* Immediately after giving the drug to the patient, document the date and time of administration; the drug's name, strength, dose, and route of administration; any patient reactions to the medication; and details of patient education regarding the drug. For parenteral medications the site of injection should be inspected before administration for scarring, altered pigmentation, or any other indication that there might be

Additional Safety Steps for Medication Administration

- Prepare medications in a quiet, well-lit area.
- Pay close attention to all the steps involved in dispensing drugs.
- Never substitute a drug or drug strength. Consult the physician for any discrepancy between the medication ordered and the medication available.
- Store medications as ordered on the package, and return containers to the proper storage area immediately after dispensing the dose.
- *The person who administers the medication is responsible for any drug errors.* Never administer a medication you have not personally prepared.
- If ordered to prepare a medication for the physician to administer, place the container with the dispensed drug so that the physician can verify the seven rights.
- The physician should write every medication order before the medication is dispensed.
- Routinely check expiration dates when verifying the seven rights. Properly discard expired drugs.
- Discard medications with damaged labels to avoid errors caused by inaccurately reading label information.
- If a medication is not administered after it is dispensed, discard it rather than returning it to the container.
- Before administering any medication, ask the patient about drug allergies. These can change over time.
- Patients should be observed for untoward effects for 20 to 30 minutes after a medication is administered. Any reactions must be reported to the physician and documented on the patient's chart.
- Always provide and document patient education about the medication, time of administration, side effects, and so on when administering a drug.

a problem with medication absorption. The exact site of administration must be charted. If the patient calls in for a prescription refill, document all pertinent information on the patient chart as well. Refer to Procedures 34-1 and 34-2 to apply safety measures in preparing and administering a medication and documenting it properly.

CRITICAL THINKING APPLICATION

Dr. Thau asks Dorothy what safety precautions she would routinely follow when administering a dose of omeprazole (Prilosec). Based on the information you have learned about safe drug administration, what steps should Dorothy follow in dispensing and administering the ordered medication?

Patient Assessment Factors

Although medications are given only under the direct order and supervision of the physician, the medical assistant is part of the assessment and problem-solving processes in the care of the patient. In medicine, assessment never ends, and never is it the responsibility of just one person. A physician gives the order to administer medication to a patient based on a medical

Apply Pharmacology Principles to Prepare and Administer Oral and Parenteral (Excluding IV) Medications: Safety Measures in Preparing, Administering, and Documenting Medication

CAAHEP COMPETENCIES: 3.b.(4)(g), 3.b.(4)(h), 3.c.(1)(a), 3.c.(2)(b), 3.c.(2)(c), 3.c.(2)(d)
ABHES COMPETENCIES: 1.d, 2.i, 2.k, 4.m, 4.n, 5.b

Dr. Thau writes the following order: Administer Recombivax 10 mcg IM to Chris MacCarthy.

GOAL: *To safely prepare, administer, and document completion of a medication order.*

EQUIPMENT and SUPPLIES

- Written physician order, including the drug name, strength, dose, and route of administration
- PDR reference
- Container of ordered medication
- Correct equipment for dispensing the drug
- Patient chart

PROCEDURAL STEPS

1. Read the order and clarify any questions with the physician.
2. If you are unfamiliar with the drug, refer to the PDR or the package insert to determine the purpose of the drug, common side effects, typical dose, and any pertinent precautions or contraindications. Recombivax is a hepatitis B immunization. Use the "seven rights" to prevent errors.
3. Take the written order with you to the medication room, and compare the Recombivax label with the physician's order. Based on the information printed on the medication label, perform calculations needed to match the physician's order. Confirm the answer with the physician if you have any questions.
4. Dispense medication in a well-lit, quiet area.
   PURPOSE: To avoid distractions and possible errors.
5. Wash your hands.
6. Compare the written order with the label on the multidose vial when you remove it from storage. Check the expiration date on the container, and dispose of the medication if it has expired.
   PURPOSE: To check the medication the first of three times.
7. Compare the order with the label on the multidose vial just before drawing it up into the appropriate syringe unit. Make certain that the strength on the label matches the order or that you dispense the correctly calculated dose.
   PURPOSE: To check the medication the second of three times.

8. Compare the label and the physician order before returning the vial to storage.
   PURPOSE: To check the medication the third of three times.
9. Greet and identify Chris by name and inform him you are going to administer a hepatitis B immunization.
   PURPOSE: To be sure that you have the right patient.
10. Mention the name of the drug and why it is being given and ask the patient if he has any allergies to the medication.
    PURPOSE: To educate the patient about drug treatment and verify the patient is not allergic to the prescribed medication.
11. If necessary, help the patient into a sitting position.
12. Administer the medication into the left deltoid muscle using correct administration techniques and Occupational Safety and Health Administration (OSHA) precautions.
13. Conduct patient education on the purpose of the drug, typical side effects, and dosage and storage recommendations. Refer to the physician to clarify information if needed.
    PURPOSE: To ensure compliance with home drug therapy and to monitor for side effects.
14. The patient must remain in the office for 20 to 30 minutes after drug administration as a precaution against untoward effects.
15. If the patient experiences any discomfort after taking a medication, the physician should be notified immediately and the incident documented completely and accurately.
16. Wash your hands.
17. Document the administration of the drug, including the date and time; the drug name, dose, strength, and route of administration; any patient side effects; and patient education conducted about the drug.

See Appendix D for a charting example.

---

assessment, but you also must continue to assess the patient and the patient's environment as you follow through with that order. The physician depends on the medical assistant to be alert to patient changes or new information that could mean that the use of a particular drug should be reconsidered. For example, perhaps the patient denied having any allergies to medications, but right before you administer an injection of penicillin the patient mentions she developed a rash after receiving the last penicillin shot. You should stop right then and go back to the physician with this new information. It is vital to continuing patient safety that you assess the patient, the drug, and the environment before giving any medication.

Drug therapy should be based on a holistic approach to patient treatment. The patient is more than a particular disease. Many factors may have an impact on patient compliance with drug treatment as well as the safety and effectiveness of medication therapy. The first step in holistic medication treatment is collecting a complete and accurate history. This includes gathering details regarding the patient's health history, current and past use of both prescription and over-the-counter (OTC) drugs, and any negative responses to drugs, especially drug allergies. Every time a patient is seen in the office, he or she should be asked about drug allergies. Most medical practices have a specific place on the patient's chart to document drug

PROCEDURE 34-2

Apply Pharmacology Principles to Prepare and Administer Oral and Parenteral (Excluding IV) Medications: Maintain Medication Records

CAAHEP COMPETENCIES: 3.b.(4)(h), 3.c.(1)(a), 3.c.(2)(b), 3.c.(2)(c), 3.c.(2)(d)
ABHES COMPETENCIES: 1.d, 2.i, 2.k, 4.n, 5.b

Dr. Thau writes the following orders for control of Mrs. Lange's hypertension:

Lasix 20 mg PO qd

Potassium Chloride 20 mEq PO qd to Alice Lange.

You reviewed the orders for clarification, completed the three label checks, confirmed the identity of the patient, asked the patient about drug allergies, administered the medications as ordered, and answered patient questions about the continuation of drug therapy at home. You must now document this process in the patient chart.

GOAL: *To document completion of medication orders.*

EQUIPMENT and SUPPLIES

- Written physician order, including the name, strength, dose, and route of administration of the medication ordered
- PDR reference
- Patient chart

PROCEDURAL STEPS

1. Greet and identify Alice by name and inform her you are going to administer a diuretic and potassium supplement.
   UNDERLINE PURPOSE: To be sure that you have the right patient.

2. Mention the names of the drugs and why they are being given, and ask Alice if she has any allergies to the medication.
   PURPOSE: To educate the patient about drug treatment and verify the patient is not allergic to the prescribed medication. Follow office policy to update the patient's chart regarding any newly reported medication allergies.

3. Administer the medications orally as ordered, making sure Alice swallows the pills without difficulty.

4. Conduct patient education about the purpose of the drugs, typical side effects, and dosage and storage recommendations. Refer to the physician to clarify information if needed.
   PURPOSE: To ensure compliance with home drug therapy and to monitor for side effects.

5. The patient must remain in the office for 20 to 30 minutes after drug administration as a precaution against untoward effects.

6. If the patient experiences any discomfort after taking a medication, the physician should be notified immediately and the incident documented completely and accurately.

7. Wash your hands.

8. Document the administration of the medications, including the date and time; the drug names, dose, strength, and route of administration; any patient side effects; and patient education conducted about the drug.
   Practice documenting the following orders:

   1. Tylenol elixir 120 mg PO to Anthony Baker, 8 years old, for a fever

   _____

   2. Gantrisin Pediatric 500 mg PO to Samantha Carpassi, 3 years old, for a urinary tract infection

   _____

   3. Dilaudid cough syrup 2 mg PO to Roberto Alphonse, 43 years old, for bronchitis

   _____

   4. Diflucan 400 mg PO loading dose to Anastasia Smith, 19 years old, for a vaginal yeast infection

   _____

See Appendix D for a charting example.

allergies, such as in red ink in the upper right corner of each documentation sheet, as well as a special label on the front of the patient's chart that alerts the physician and staff to medication allergies. It is crucial that the physician have current and accurate information regarding drug allergies to avoid serious complications and possibly death.

Patient assessment does not end with the administration of the drug. Observe patients carefully for drug reactions after the administration of all medications but especially those that are injected. Patients receiving penicillin (a drug with a high incidence of allergic response) or **immunotherapy** must remain in the office for 20 to 30 minutes in case of acute anaphylactic reaction. An acute anaphylactic reaction can result in respiratory failure and circulatory collapse within minutes if not reversed with epinephrine. Lesser allergic reactions include hives, swelling, and itching. The physician may order an antihistamine, such as diphenhydramine (Benadryl), if these reactions occur.

Because patient factors such as age, weight, and height may be used to determine the correct therapeutic dose, accurate recordings of this information should be documented on the chart. As discussed in Chapter 32, chronic conditions, especially liver and kidney disease, may affect the body's ability to metabolize and excrete medications. Therefore, a complete and accurate medical history is crucial to patient safety.

Besides the patient's physical state, other holistic factors also play a role in successful drug therapy. The patient must understand the drug regimen, may require family support to follow treatment guidelines, and must be able to afford the prescribed medication. Unless these criteria can be met, the patient may be unable to follow through with treatment protocol. It is important that the medical assistant investigate these issues and offer appropriate community support, if available, to help the patient maintain proper drug therapy.

Approaches to Special Patient Populations

Pregnant and breastfeeding women must be especially careful in taking OTC and prescription drugs, because medications are known to cross the placenta and may affect the developing fetus. A pregnant woman should not take any medication without the knowledge and approval of her physician. As discussed in Chapter 32, the Food and Drug Administration (FDA) has determined five pregnancy risk categories of drugs. The medical assistant should be familiar with the specific drug category before administering any medication to a pregnant woman. Besides passing through the placenta, medications are also transferred through breast milk. Therefore similar precautions must be used when the physician prescribes medications to a lactating mother.

As discussed in Chapter 33, special precautions must be followed when determining the correct dose of medication for children. Pediatric doses are primarily determined by the child's weight; therefore it is important to measure and record accurate weights of all children at each office visit. A child's body manages drug absorption, distribution, metabolism, and excretion differently than an adult's body does, and the physician considers these factors when prescribing pediatric doses.

Aging people are also more sensitive to the effects of medications, so certain factors must be considered when prescribing and administering drugs to this population group. The metabolic rate typically slows with the aging process, resulting in an increased susceptibility to a buildup of chemicals in the body that may lead to toxic conditions. Part of the normal aging process is loss of subcutaneous fat, which may affect the route of administration of some medications, especially parenteral sites. In addition, many elderly people have accompanying chronic diseases, such as circulatory, liver, or kidney disease, that may affect the distribution, metabolism, and excretion

of medications. It is not uncommon for geriatric patients to be on multiple medications prescribed by more than one practitioner, which increases the risk of drug contraindications and interactions. A holistic approach to aging patients should include a nutritional evaluation, because a poor diet or restricted fluid intake will have an impact on drug actions. Another very real concern for aging patients is the cost of drug therapy. Many patients on fixed incomes may not be able to afford the ordered drug but hesitate to inform the physician of this problem. It may be up to the medical assistant to ask the patient about his or her ability to pay for the ordered medication, and offer available assistance for prescription drugs. This includes offering stocked drug samples with physician approval and/or investigating drug coverage offered by pharmaceutical companies.

CRITICAL THINKING APPLICATION

Dr. Thau serves both pediatric and geriatric patients. Summarize key items Dorothy should consider when administering medications to these specialty patient population groups.

Assessment of the Patient's Environment

The patient's surroundings affect the success of medication therapy. The patient may become hysterical or uncooperative about receiving the medication, or the patient's family may protest the use of the drug. Administration of certain medications requires the presence of the physician. For example, because of the risk of anaphylactic shock, allergy injections should not be given unless the physician is present. In addition, the environment must be safe for drug administration. Be certain that the patient is comfortable and protected from accidental injury. If a patient is to receive an injection, take care to place

Suggestions for Successful Medication Administration to Children

- Explain why the medication is needed and how it will make the child feel.
- Attempt to gain cooperation by getting down on the child's level and using a soft but firm voice.
- When possible, offer choices of care, such as, "Would you like your medicine in your leg or in your arm?"
- Divert the child to relieve stressful moments.
- If the child refuses to cooperate, get help as needed to restrain the child so the medication can be given safely.
- Encourage parents to participate as much as possible, and make sure both the parent and child (if of an appropriate age) understand the prescribed drug therapy.
- Offer a "treat," such as a sticker, at the end of the visit.

Guidelines for Administration of Medication to Geriatric Patients

- Educate the patient and family about the purpose of the drug; the time, dose, and route of administration; and common side effects. Instructions should be written clearly for home reference.
- If the patient has difficulty swallowing the medication, either crush (if allowed) the medication or mix it into applesauce or pudding.
- Encourage the patient to drink plenty of fluids (at least eight glasses of water per day) while taking the medication.
- Reinforce that the patient should take the medication as prescribed and should not skip or double doses.
- Request that patients bring to every physician visit all of the medications they are currently taking in their labeled containers, including OTCs, so a current medication record can be accurately maintained on the patient's chart.
- If patients are taking multiple medications, suggest the use of daily or weekly medication dispensers. These can be purchased in drugstores and restocked by family members on a weekly basis.
- Encourage patients not to share or "save" medications. All leftover medications should be discarded to avoid use beyond the expiration date.

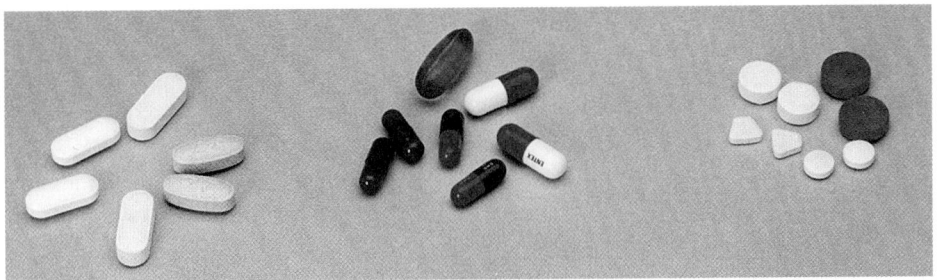

FIGURE 34-1 *Left to right,* Caplets, capsules, and tablets.

the patient in a position that best exposes the site and protects the patient from injury in case he or she faints or has a drug reaction. If the patient is to take an oral medication with water, be certain that he or she is seated in a position that will prevent choking. Because any medication is potentially dangerous to a patient, emergency drugs must be readily available to counteract any adverse effects that might occur immediately after the administration of a medication. Emergency drugs should be in injectable form for rapid effect. Typically emergency carts include adrenergics, such as epinephrine; anticholinergics, such as atropine; bronchodilators; and histamine blockers. The pharmaceutical management of emergencies is discussed in Chapter 35.

Refer to the following list for suggestions of questions that can be asked to get as much information as possible from the patient regarding medication therapy. Any information gathered should be included in your documentation note.

Suggested Questions for Gathering Medication Information

- *What physician-prescribed drugs are you currently taking?* Record the names, doses, strengths, and routes of administration.
- *Do you take any OTC drugs on a regular basis?* Record the purpose, amount, and frequency of use. If appropriate, ask when the last dose was taken. For example, if a mother reports her child has a fever but the temperature is normal at the time of the visit, perhaps she gave the child a dose of Tylenol before the visit.
- *What medications, including OTC drugs, have you taken over the last 6 months to 1 year, and why?* Ask this question to gather a history of medication use and perhaps discover health problems that have not been previously recorded.
- *Do you regularly use any alternative or herbal products? What are they? How much do you use, and how frequently are they used? For what purpose are they used?*
- It is important that patients take their medications as prescribed, so focus a few questions on how currently prescribed drugs are being taken. *What time of day do you take your medicine? How do you remember to take it? Are you having any problems or noticeable side effects from the medication? Can you afford to take the medication as prescribed? Are you having the desired response to the medication (relief of pain, breathing better, lowered blood pressure, and so on)?*
- *Where do you store your medications at home?* Review if there are any special storage precautions for prescribed drugs. The

majority of medications should be stored away from any heat source and sunlight.
- *Have you checked the expiration dates on your containers?* Patients often neglect to dispose of unused medications and may take them after they are expired if not warned about this precaution.
- *Can you tell me why you are taking the prescribed medication?* You should periodically check on the need for patient education about drug therapy. Patients are more likely to be compliant with treatment protocols if they understand the importance of taking the medication as prescribed.
- *Do you use the same pharmacy to fill all of your prescriptions?* Patients may see more than one physician. An excellent method of keeping track of all prescribed drugs, their contraindications, and possible drug-to-drug interactions is to strongly suggest the patient use only one pharmacy. The pharmacist will then be able to monitor overall medication safety.

DRUG FORMS AND ADMINISTRATION

As discussed in Chapter 32, the chosen route of drug administration determines the rate and intensity of the drug's effect. A drug prepared for one route but administered by another route may not have any effect at all and is potentially dangerous. Each route requires different dosage forms.

Solid Oral Dosage Forms

The basic forms for solid oral dosage are tablets, capsules, and lozenges (troches). Figure 34-1 depicts typical caplets, capsules, and tablets. Tablets are compressed powders or granules that, when wet, break apart in the stomach—or in the mouth if they are not swallowed quickly. Tablets may be sugar-coated to taste better, or **enteric-coated,** such as Ecotrin, to protect the stomach mucosa. Buffered tablets are also designed to prevent stomach irritation by combining the drug with a buffering agent that decreases the amount of acidity in the compound. Buffered or enteric-coated tablets should never be crushed or dissolved. Only **scored** tablets can be cut in half. This is accomplished with a pill cutter, as shown in Figure 34-2.

Some tablets are coated with a **volatile** liquid that helps the medication quickly dissolve in the mouth, such as certain antacid tablets or Claritin RediTabs, which are prescribed to dissolve on the tongue rather than to be swallowed. Caplets are tablets that are solid and oblong, similar in shape to capsules but without any coating.

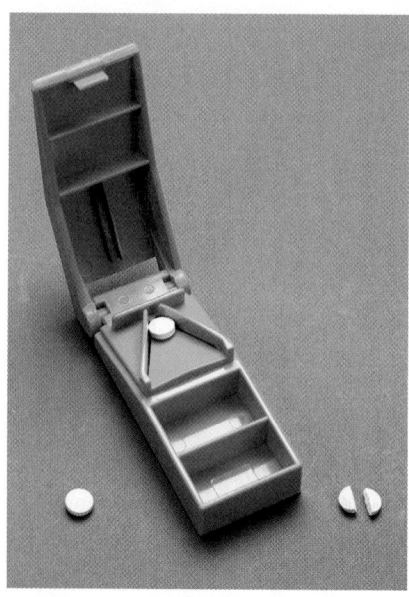

FIGURE 34-2 Pill cutter.

Capsules are gelatin-coated and dissolve in the stomach, or they may be enteric-coated to protect them from the acid action of the stomach. Timed- or sustained-release (SR) capsules or spansules are designed to dissolve at different rates over a period of time, to reduce the number of times a patient has to take a medication. These drugs should never be crushed or dissolved, because this would negate their timed-release action. Another form of oral medication, the lozenge or troche, is a flattened disk that is dissolved in the mouth for coating the throat, such as a lozenge for a sore throat.

Liquid Oral Dosage Forms

Many liquid forms of medication are available. They differ mainly in the type of substance used to dissolve the drug: water, oils, or alcohol.

Solutions are drug substances contained in a homogeneous mixture with a liquid. Liquid forms include the following:

- *Syrups:* A syrup is a solution of sugar and water, usually containing flavoring and medicinal substances. Cough syrups, such as Robitussin, are the most common.

Suspensions are insoluble drug substances contained in a liquid. Examples include the following:

- *Emulsions:* An emulsion is a mixture of oil and water that improves the taste of otherwise distasteful products, such as cod liver oil.
- *Gels and magmas:* Gels and magmas consist of minerals suspended in water. Minerals settle; therefore products containing minerals must be shaken before use. Milk of magnesia is an example.

A drug substance can be mixed with alcohol to enhance the drug's properties. Examples include the following:

- *Fluid extracts:* Fluid extracts are combinations of alcohol and vegetable products that are more potent than tinctures. For example, belladonna fluid extract has a higher percentage of the powdered belladonna leaf than tincture of belladonna.
- *Tinctures:* A tincture is an alcoholic preparation of a soluble drug or chemical substance, usually from plant sources. Examples include tincture of benzoin and tincture of iodine, which are applied externally.
- *Extracts:* Extracts are very concentrated combinations of vegetable products and alcohol or ether that are evaporated until a syrupy liquid, solid mass, or powder is formed. Extracts are many times stronger than the crude drug itself.
- *Elixirs:* An elixir is an aromatic, alcoholic, sweetened preparation. Elixir of phenobarbital is one example; the alcoholic cough medicines terpin hydrate with codeine and plain elixir of codeine are two more. Elixirs differ from tinctures in that they are sweetened. They should be used with caution in patients with diabetes or a history of alcohol abuse. Some pediatric medications retain the name *elixir,* although they no longer contain alcohol.

CRITICAL THINKING APPLICATION

Dorothy is ordered to administer a **loading dose** of cephalexin to a 17-year-old patient with acute bronchitis. The physician's order reads, "Administer cephalexin 500 mg tab PO stat." The patient is sent home with a prescription for Keflex, 250 mg tab q6h times 7 days. Document the details that should be included in Dorothy's note.

_____

_____

_____

_____

_____

Oral Administration

If the drug is not intended to coat the oral cavity or throat, oral medications should be taken with enough water to transport the drug to the stomach. Make certain that the patient is able to swallow the medication. It may be helpful to place the medication on the back part of the tongue. Liquid medications are ideal for children. Solid drugs should not be administered to children until they reach the age at which they can safely swallow a solid drug form without the danger of aspirating the drug. Oral syringes are the best way to give liquid medications to children, because there is less likelihood of spilling the medication (Figure 34-3). Liquid medications, especially those that stain the teeth, can be taken through a straw. If the patient has been vomiting or is nauseated, an alternative route of administration may be necessary. Always remain with the patient until all of the medication has been swallowed. Procedure 34-3 outlines how to dispense and administer oral medications.

Mucous Membrane Forms

Some mucous membranes are selected for their ability to absorb medication for a systemic effect. The most commonly used areas are the gums, the cheeks (buccal), under the tongue (sublingual), the rectum, and the respiratory mucosa (inhalation). Nasal, ophthalmic, rectal, and vaginal preparations may also be applied to these mucous membranes for their localized effects. Inhalation drugs are discussed in Chapter 45.

PROCEDURE 34-3

Apply Pharmacology Principles to Prepare and Administer Oral and Parenteral (Excluding IV) Medications: Dispense, Administer, and Document Oral Medications

CAAHEP COMPETENCIES: 3.b.(4)(g), 3.b.(4)(h), 3.c.(1)(a), 3.c.(2)(b), C.3.c.(2)(c), 3.c.(2)(d)
ABHES COMPETENCIES: 1.d, 2.i, 2.k, 4.m, 4.n, 5.b
ORDER: Administer hydrochlorothiazide (HydroDIURIL) 100 mg PO tab stat for hypertension.

GOAL: To safely dispense, administer to a patient, and document the administration of an oral medication.

EQUIPMENT and SUPPLIES

- Container of ordered medication
- Calibrated medication cup
- Written physician order, including the drug name, strength, dose, and route
- Water if appropriate
- Patient medical record

PROCEDURAL STEPS

1. Read the order and clarify any questions with the physician.
2. If you are unfamiliar with HydroDIURIL, refer to the PDR or the package insert to determine the purpose of the drug, common side effects, typical dose, and any pertinent precautions or contraindications. Be prepared to answer patient questions about the medication. Use the "seven rights" to prevent errors.
3. Perform calculations needed to match the physician's order. Confirm the answer with the physician if you have any questions.
4. Dispense medication in a well-lit, quiet area.
   PURPOSE: To avoid distractions and possible errors.
5. Wash your hands.
6. Compare the order with the label on the container of medicine when you remove it from storage. Check the expiration date on the container, and dispose of the medication if it has expired.
   PURPOSE: To check the medication label and order the first of three times.
7. Compare the order with the label on the container of medicine just before dispensing the ordered dose. Make certain that the strength on the label matches the order or that you dispense the correctly calculated dose.
   PURPOSE: To check the medication label and order the second of three times.

TO DISPENSE SOLID ORAL MEDICATIONS (HydroDIURIL Tablet)

8. Gently tap the prescribed dose into the lid of the medication container. Avoid touching the inside of the lid as well as the medication (Figure 1).
   PURPOSE: Touching the medication or the inside of the container will contaminate the drug.
9. Empty the medication in the container lid into a medicine cup.

TO DISPENSE LIQUID ORAL PREPARATIONS (HydroDIURIL Solution)

10. Shake medication well if required.
11. When liquid medications are poured, the label should be held in the palm of the hand.
    PURPOSE: To protect the label from medication spills. The medication must be discarded if staff members are unable to clearly read the drug label.
12. Place the medicine cup on a flat surface and, at eye level, pour the medication to the prescribed dose mark on the medicine cup (Figure 2).
    PURPOSE: At eye level the base of the meniscus is where the prescribed dose should be measured.

FOR BOTH SOLID AND LIQUID ORAL MEDICATIONS

13. Recap the container and compare the label and the physician order before replacing the container in storage.
    PURPOSE: To check the medication label and order the third of three times.
14. Transport the medication to the patient.

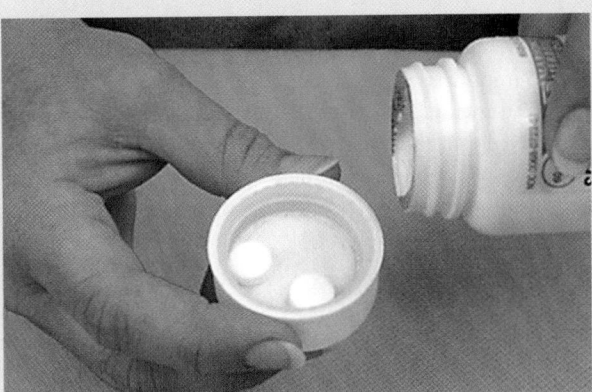

FIGURE 1

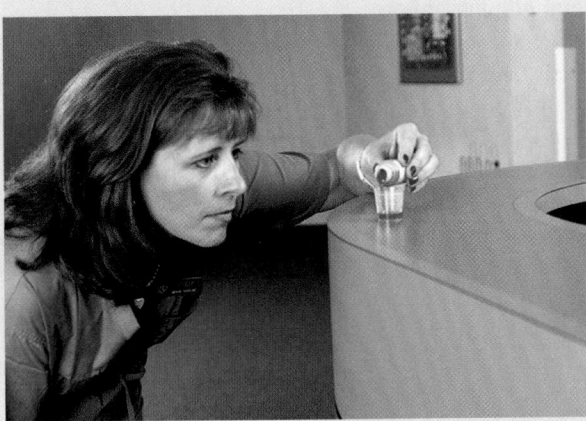

FIGURE 2

Continued

15. Greet and identify the patient by name.
   PURPOSE: To be sure that you have the right patient.
16. Mention the name of the drug and why it is being given, and ask the patient if she or he has any allergies to the medication.
   PURPOSE: To educate the patient about drug treatment and verify the patient is not allergic to the prescribed medication.
17. If necessary, help the patient into a sitting position.
18. Administer tablets, capsules, or caplets with water. If the patient is receiving liquid medication, offer water after the medication is taken if appropriate. Make sure the patient swallows the entire dose.
19. Conduct patient education regarding the purpose of the drug, typical side effects, and dosage and storage recommendations. Refer to the physician to clarify information if needed.

PURPOSE: To ensure compliance with home drug therapy and to monitor for side effects.
20. The patient must remain in the office for 20 to 30 minutes after drug administration as a precaution against untoward effects.
21. If the patient experiences any discomfort after taking a medication, the physician should be notified immediately and the incident documented completely and accurately.
22. Wash your hands.
23. Document the administration of the drug, including the date and time; the drug name, dose, strength, and route of administration; any patient side effects; and patient education conducted about the drug.

See Appendix D for a charting example.

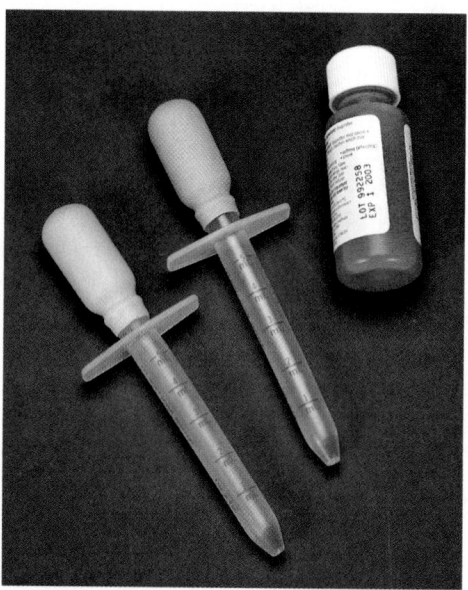

FIGURE 34-3 Sample oral syringes.

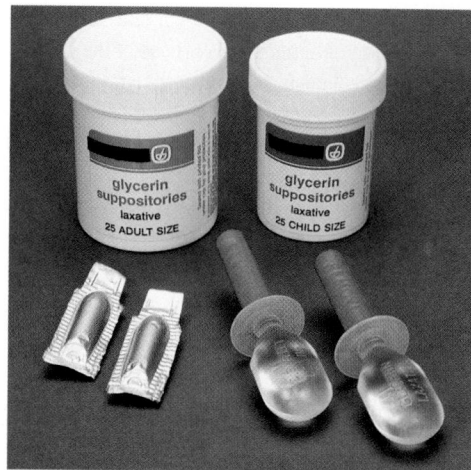

FIGURE 34-4 Sample rectal suppositories.

Rectal Administration

The rectal mucosa provides rapid absorption of a drug, even though the surface of the rectum is small. Drugs are absorbed directly into the bloodstream without being altered as they would be by the digestive processes and without irritating the patient's gastric mucosa. Rectal medications are useful if the patient is nauseated, vomiting, or unconscious. For example, Tylenol or Compazine suppositories may be prescribed for a child who has a fever, nausea, and vomiting. Manufacturers supply rectal medications in the form of gelatin or cocoa butter–based suppositories, which melt in the warmth of the rectum and release the medication (Figure 34-4). Suppositories may be used to soften the stool or stimulate evacuation of the bowel; enemas are used to cleanse and evacuate the bowel.

The best time to administer a rectal drug intended for a systemic effect is after a bowel movement or enema. The patient should be cautioned to remain lying down for 20 to 30 minutes to prevent accidental evacuation of the drug by a bowel movement or elimination of the enema. Of course, suppositories intended to treat constipation are administered to bring about bowel evacuation. The patient should be instructed to insert the suppository approximately 2 inches above the rectal sphincter muscles; a little mineral oil or vegetable oil may be used as a lubricant. If suppositories are individually wrapped in foil, make certain the patient knows that the foil is the wrapper and is not part of the treatment. Suppositories are typically stored in the refrigerator to keep them firm.

Vaginal Administration

Vaginal suppositories, tablets, creams, and fluid solutions are used to treat local infections. Irrigating solutions (douches) may be used as antiinfective treatments. Creams and foams are available as local contraceptives. Vaginal instillation is most effective if the patient remains lying down after administration to prevent leakage; many preparations are therefore intended to be used at bedtime. The patient may need to wear a pad to absorb drainage. Solid suppositories and tablets may be lubricated or moistened with water and inserted by hand or with an applicator. Creams are instilled with applicators. Prepackaged, disposable irrigation kits are available for douching.

When instructing patients, confirm that the patient can differentiate the urinary meatus from the vaginal orifice and the rectum. Mistakes could result in vaginal infections or in damage or infection to the urinary tract. A simple drawing and explanation may be required.

Oral Administration

Mouth and throat agents come in the form of sprays, swabs, sublingual tablets, and buccal tablets. The mouth and throat membranes may be treated locally with antiseptics for oral hygiene and local infections, with anesthetics for relief of pain, and with astringents that form a protective film over the mucous membranes. The patient may have to gargle, or the area may be painted or sprayed. To paint or spray the throat, first look for the area of inflammation to be treated. Otherwise, the part needing treatment may be missed entirely. Avoid touching the posterior pharynx (back of the throat); this causes gagging and possibly vomiting.

Sublingual (SL) tablets are placed under the tongue, where they are rapidly absorbed into the bloodstream by the rich supply of capillaries. Sublingual absorption is systemic and bypasses the acids in the stomach. Nitroglycerin, used for treating the chest pains of angina pectoris, may be administered sublingually. Patients should not chew or swallow sublingual medications. The patient should be instructed not to smoke, eat, or drink immediately before administration of these drugs. Buccal tablets are placed between the cheek and the upper molars and are also quickly absorbed by the oral capillaries.

Nasal Administration

Nose drops and nasal sprays may be used for localized effect, but, like the inhalation drugs, they can spill over into the bloodstream. Some nasal preparations, such as decongestants, can cause an increased heart rate, elevated blood pressure, or central nervous system stimulation. Nasal medications are commonly used for blocked nasal passages (decongestants) and nosebleeds (hemostatics). Instillation of nasal medications is covered in Chapter 36. Nasal decongestant sprays are often misused by patients. Be sure to teach the patient not to exceed the amount or frequency ordered by the physician. If too much is used, these drugs can dry the mucosa and make congestion worse. Nasal inhalants can also be used for their systemic effect, such as the corticosteroid Flonase, which may be prescribed as part of asthmatic treatment.

Topical Forms

Topical drugs are prescribed for both local and systemic effects. Skin medication forms include lotions, liniments, ointments, and transdermal patches. The medical assistant should wear gloves when applying any topical treatment, to prevent self-administration of the drug.

Lotions

Often used to control itching, lotions are applied by dabbing with a soft cloth, cotton ball, or tongue blade. Calamine is an example. Some lotions are used to relieve inflammation and pain in muscles and joints. After the lotion is applied, the area may be covered with a thick cloth to retain heat. However, the therapeutic value of these preparations is controversial. Many believe that the effects of musculoskeletal lotions are limited to the skin surface where the medication is applied.

Liniments

Liniments (emulsions) have a higher portion of oil than do lotions, and volatile active ingredients may be added. Liniments are often used to protect dried, cracked, or fissured skin.

Ointments

Ointments, such as bacitracin, are semisolid medications containing bases such as petrolatum and lanolin. An ointment should be removed from a jar or tube with a tongue blade to prevent contamination of the remaining medication.

Transdermal Patches

Certain medications can be absorbed slowly through the skin to create a constant, time-released systemic effect (Figure 34-5). The nitroglycerin patch is particularly useful for patients

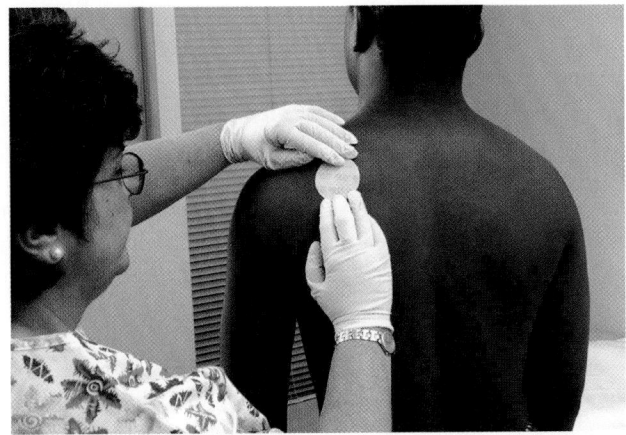

FIGURE 34-5 Transdermal patch.

Patient Teaching Recommendations for Transdermal Patches

- The patient may shower with the patch in place.
- Rotate sites to prevent skin irritation. Follow package insert directions on where to apply the patch, avoiding scars and areas with a great deal of body hair.
- If the patch is to remain on for 24 hours for an extended number of days, apply a new patch at the same time every day and keep the old patch on for 30 minutes after applying the new patch to maintain blood levels of the medication.
- Dispose of used patches appropriately, out of the reach of children or pets, because the old patch may still contain some of the medication.

with frequent attacks of angina. Hormone patches, such as estrogen and testosterone, can also be absorbed slowly through the skin. With dermal patches, drugs can be administered in a time-released manner for up to 3 days. The date and time the patch was applied should be written on the patch as well as documented in the patient's record.

Parenteral Medication Forms

Injectable medications must be **sterile** and in liquid form. The medications may come in an ampule, a single-dose vial, or a multidose vial (Figure 34-6). The drug is usually in a solution that is minimally irritating to human tissues, such as physiologic saline solution or sterile water, and may contain a preservative or a small amount of antibiotic to prevent bacterial growth in the vial. All injectable medications are dated. Before use, check the expiration date and examine the solution for possible deterioration. If the medication is discolored or if any sediment has formed at the bottom of the vial, the vial should be discarded. A parenteral medication is administered with a sterile syringe and needle. Occupational Safety and Health Administration (OSHA) guidelines must be followed when any sharp is used, including all types of needles because every needle used on a patient is contaminated with blood and body fluids. A medical assistant must wear disposable gloves when administering parenteral injections, immediately dispose of the needle and syringe unit into a sharps container after use, and never recap used needles.

Ampule

An ampule is a small **hermetically sealed** glass flask that contains a single dose of medication. Ampules have a neck with a scored weak point that is broken just before use (Figure 34-6, *A*). Procedure 34-4 explains the special technique required for opening an ampule of medication and withdrawing medication for administration.

Single-Dose Vial

A single-dose vial is a small bottle with a rubber stopper through which a sterile needle is inserted to withdraw the single dose of medication inside. Before a sterile syringe and needle unit

can be introduced into the solution, the rubber stopper must be wiped in a circular motion with alcohol or another suitable disinfectant.

Multidose Vial

A multidose vial is a bottle with a rubber stopper that contains enough medication for multiple injections. Because multidose vials are used more than once, extreme caution must be taken every time a needle is inserted into the medication to protect the medication from contamination, which could cause very serious infections in future patients. If at any time you feel that an error has been made or you suspect possible contamination, discard the vial. Never return unused medication to the vial. Learn to withdraw fluids to the correct mark. If you have more medication than you need in the syringe, eject the excess after you remove the unit from the vial. Vials are vacuum sealed. Each time you withdraw medication from a vial, you must first replace the portion of withdrawn medication with the same portion of air. Not enough replaced air will make it difficult to withdraw the medication, and too much replaced air will increase the pressure within the vial and force the medication into the syringe without your having to pull back on the plunger. Procedure 34-5 describes how to safely and accurately withdraw medication from a vial.

Prefilled Syringe

A prefilled syringe is a sterile, disposable syringe and needle unit packaged by the manufacturer with a single dose of medication that is ready to administer. Some prefilled syringe units are designed to fit into a reusable cartridge injection system (Figure 34-7). Tubex and Carpuject are two examples of

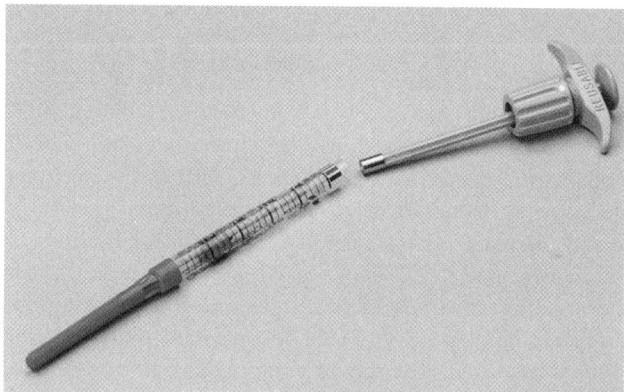

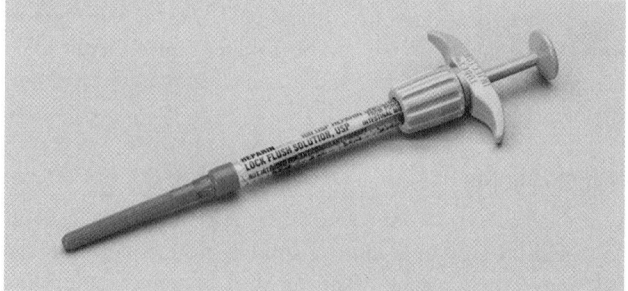

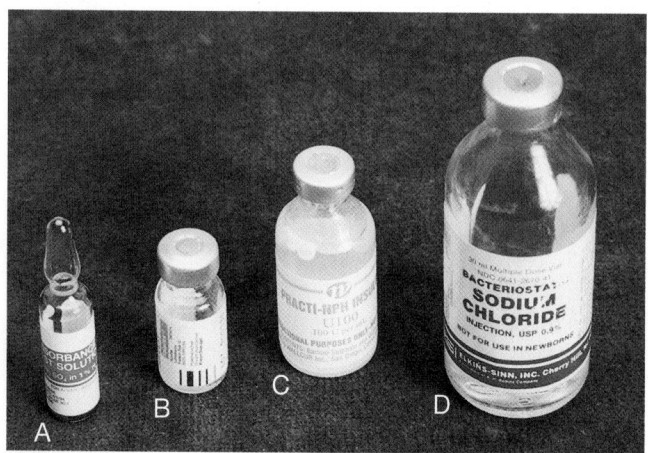

FIGURE 34-6 A, Ampule. **B,** Single-dose vial. **C** and **D,** Multidose vials.

FIGURE 34-7 The Tubex injector system with disposable sterile medication cartridge.

PROCEDURE 34-4

Apply Pharmacology Principles to Prepare and Administer Oral and Parenteral (Excluding IV) Medications: Fill a Syringe Using an Ampule

<u>CAAHEP COMPETENCY:</u> 3.b.(4)(g)
<u>ABHES COMPETENCY:</u> 4.m

GOAL: *To correctly and safely remove medication for administration from a glass ampule.*

EQUIPMENT and SUPPLIES

- Syringe and needle unit
- Filter needle
- Sterile gauze squares
- Sharps container
- Biohazard waste container
- Medication ampule
- Physician order
- Alcohol squares
- Disposable gloves

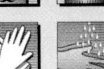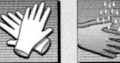

PROCEDURAL STEPS

1. Review physician's medication order for clarity. If unfamiliar with the drug, look it up in a reference book.
   PURPOSE: The medical assistant should never dispense or administer a drug without making sure the physician order is legible and the details of the drug are known.

2. Wash hands and assemble equipment.

3. Perform medication label and physician order check when removing the ampule from storage. Check the expiration date on the ampule.
   PURPOSE: To complete the first check of the order. Dispose of any medication whose expiration date has passed.

4. Gently tap the top of the ampule with your fingers to settle all the medication to the bottom portion of the flask (Figure 1).

5. Thoroughly disinfect the neck of the ampule with alcohol squares. Check the label against the order a second time.
   PURPOSE: Disinfection is done to prevent possible contamination of the medication.

6. Wrap the top of the ampule with a gauze square to protect yourself from the glass. Hold the covered ampule between your thumb and finger, in front of you and above waist level (Figure 2).

PURPOSE: To protect your fingers and maintain eye contact with the medication ampule at all times.

7. Push the top of the ampule away from your body to break the neck. You will hear a pop because the ampule is vacuum sealed. The glass is designed not to shatter, and the medication will not spill out. Dispose of the gauze square and glass top in the sharps container.

8. Open the sterile syringe and needle unit. Touching the needle covers only, unscrew the needle from the syringe, place it on the counter, and attach the sterile filter needle.
   PURPOSE: To maintain the sterility of the unit, only the needle covers are touched. The filter needle is needed to withdraw the medication from the ampule to prevent the accidental aspiration of glass fragments into the injection unit.

9. Without touching the sides of the opened ampule, insert the syringe unit with the filter needle attached into the ampule and withdraw the ordered dose. Then recover the needle.
   PURPOSE: Touching the needle with anything except the sterile interior of the ampule will contaminate the needle. If this happens, start over again with a new filter needle.

10. Before discarding the ampule in the sharps container, check the physician order against the label one more time to complete the three label checks. If you are drawing the medication up for the physician to administer, take the ampule and the syringe unit to the physician for the final safety check.

11. Change the filter needle, safeguarding the sterility of the injection unit, for an appropriate length and gauge needle based on the physician-ordered route of administration and patient characteristics. Discard the used filter needle into the sharps container.

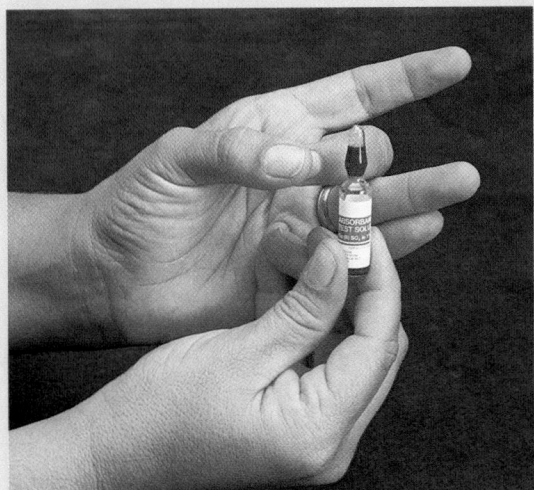

FIGURE 1

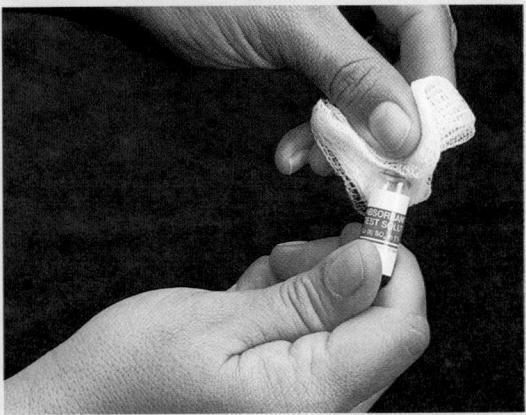

FIGURE 2

Continued

PROCEDURE 34-4—*cont'd*

PURPOSE: A new needle is applied to prevent the possible injection of glass particles on or inside the filter needle.

12. Dispose of used alcohol and gauze squares.
13. Transport ordered medication in the injection unit to the patient. Identify the patient. Apply gloves and administer the medication

as ordered. Discard the used syringe unit into a sharps container in the patient room. Remove gloves and discard in biohazard waste container and wash hands.

14. Answer patient questions and document the procedure on the patient chart.

PROCEDURE 34-5

Apply Pharmacology Principles to Prepare and Administer Oral and Parenteral (Excluding IV) Medications: Fill a Syringe Using a Vial

CAAHEP COMPETENCY: 3.b.(4)(g)
ABHES COMPETENCY: 4.m

GOAL: *To fill a syringe from a multidose vial, using sterile technique.*

EQUIPMENT and SUPPLIES

- Multidose vial containing the medication ordered
- Alcohol wipes
- Sterile needle and syringe unit
- Written order, including the drug name, strength, and route of administration

PROCEDURAL STEPS

1. Wash your hands.
2. Read the order, and choose the correct vial of medication.
   PURPOSE: To check the medication label and order the first of three times.
3. Choose the correct syringe and needle size, depending on the site and the quantity of medication to be injected (Figure 1).
4. Compare the order with both the name of the drug on the vial of medication and the amount to be withdrawn in the syringe.

PURPOSE: To check the medication label and order the second of three times.

5. Gently agitate the medication by rolling the vial between your palms (Figure 2).
   PURPOSE: To mix any medication that may have settled.
6. Check the quality of the medication and the expiration date.
   PURPOSE: Dispose of the medication if it appears contaminated, contains sediment, or is outdated.
7. Cleanse the rubber stopper of the vial with the alcohol wipe, using a circular motion (Figure 3). Place the vial on a secure flat surface, leaving the alcohol swab over the rubber stopper.
8. With the needle cover in place, grasp the syringe plunger and draw up an amount of air equal to the amount of medication ordered.
   PURPOSE: Not enough replaced air will make it difficult to withdraw the medication; too much replaced air will increase the pressure within the vial so that medication is forced into the syringe without pulling on the plunger to withdraw it.

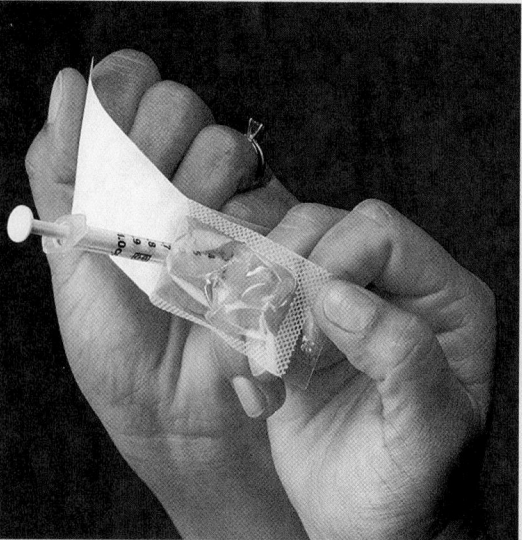

FIGURE 1

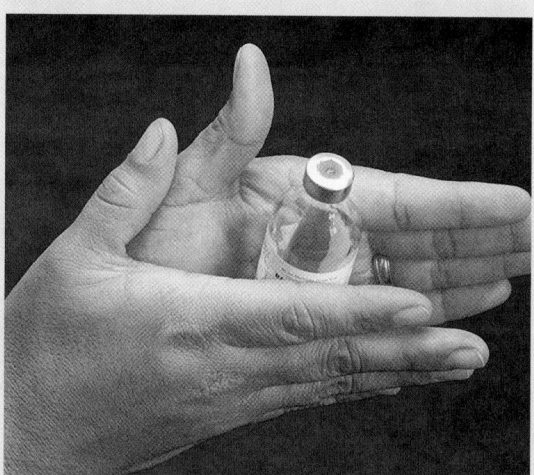

FIGURE 2

Continued

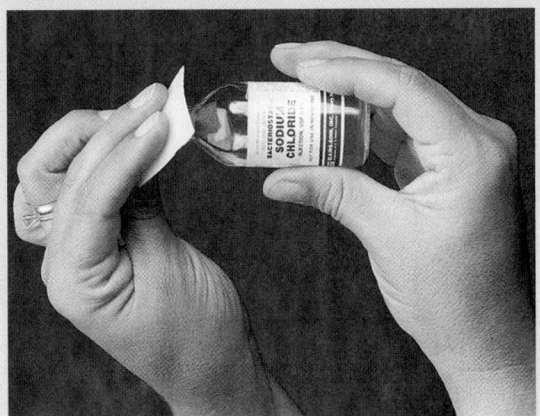

FIGURE 3

9. Remove the needle cover and insert the needle into the center of the rubber stopper. Hold the vial firmly against a flat surface, and watch carefully that the needle touches only the cleaned rubber area.
   PURPOSE: To maintain the sterility of the needle.
10. Inject the aspirated air in the syringe into the vial.
11. Keeping the syringe unit in the vial, pick up and invert them (Figure 4). Slowly pull back on the plunger with the unit at eye level until the proper amount of medication is withdrawn.
    PURPOSE: Withdrawing medication rapidly will cause air bubbles to form in the syringe.
12. While the needle is still in the vial, check that no air bubbles are in the syringe.
    PURPOSE: Air bubbles displace medication, and the patient will not receive the proper amount of medication.
13. If air bubbles are present, slip the fingers holding the vial down to grasp the vial and syringe as a single unit.
    PURPOSE: This frees your dominant hand.
14. With your free hand, tap the syringe until the air bubbles dislodge and float into the tip of the syringe.

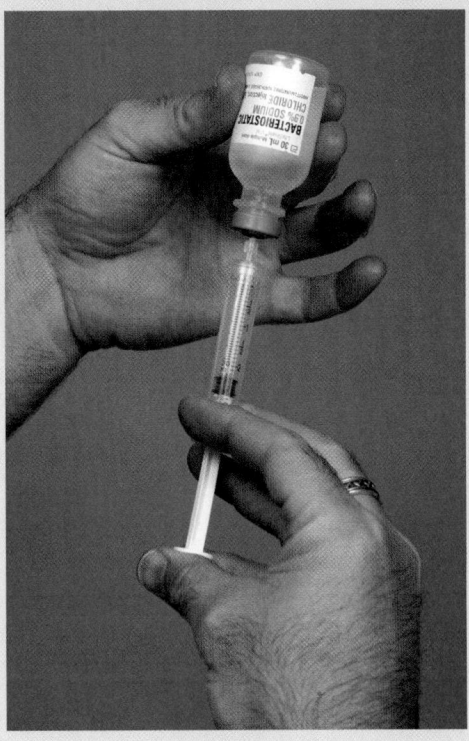

FIGURE 4

15. Gently expel these tiny air bubbles through the needle, then continue withdrawing until the accurate amount of medication has been withdrawn.
16. Withdraw the needle from the vial, and carefully replace the needle cover without letting the needle touch the outside of the cover.
17. Return the medication to the shelf or the refrigerator, checking that you have the correct drug and dosage.
    PURPOSE: This is the third of the three drug label and order checks.

cartridge systems. Most prefilled syringe units are overfilled with medication or may contain more medication than what was ordered by the physician. Before administration carefully check the unit and expel any excess medication or air to be sure that the patient is receiving an accurate dose.

Parenteral Medication Equipment

Syringes and needles are manufactured in countless varieties for specific purposes and sometimes for specific medications. For example, there is a special syringe for insulin. Hypodermic needles are manufactured in many lengths and widths, depending on the depth of the injection, the **viscosity** of the medication to be injected, the ordered route of administration, and patient characteristics. Needles may be purchased separately or as part of a needle-syringe unit. Figure 34-8 shows the parts of a needle

and the three common types of **bevel** points. Needles are measured for length from where the cannula or shaft joins the hub to the tip of the point.

Needle Gauge

The diameter or lumen size of a needle is called its *gauge,* and needle gauges range in size from 14 (the largest) to 28 (the smallest). *The larger the gauge number, the smaller the diameter of the needle.* The smallest gauges (27 to 28) are used for intradermal (ID) injections, such as screening for tuberculosis (TB), when a very small opening is desired. These fine needle widths leave a small amount of medication just below the surface of the skin, with a minimum amount of injury. Gauges 25 and 26 are commonly used for subcutaneous (SC) injections, such as for insulin. Medications in an aqueous solution and with

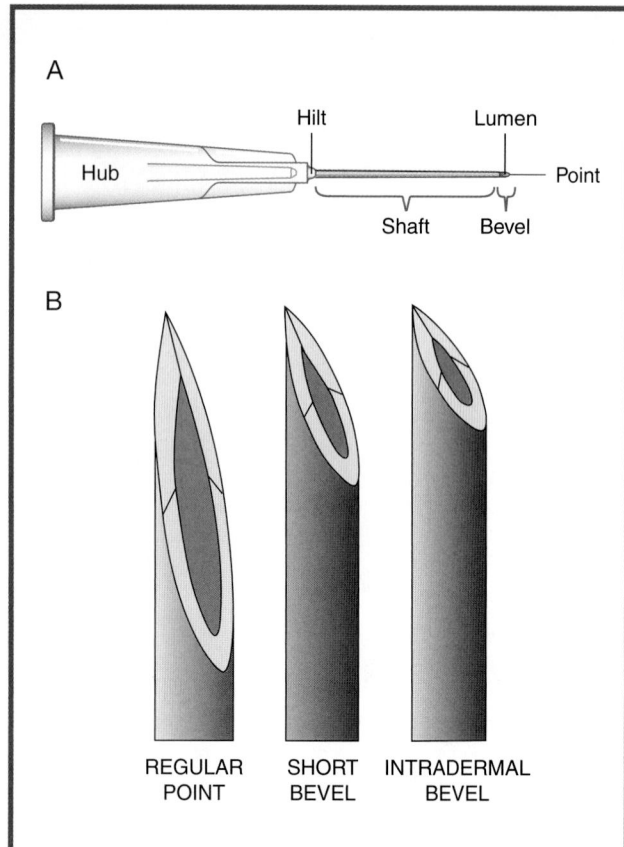

FIGURE 34-8 A, The construction of a hypodermic needle. **B,** Needle points. (A, from Bonewit-West K: *Clinical procedures for medical assistants,* ed 6, Philadelphia, 2004, Saunders.)

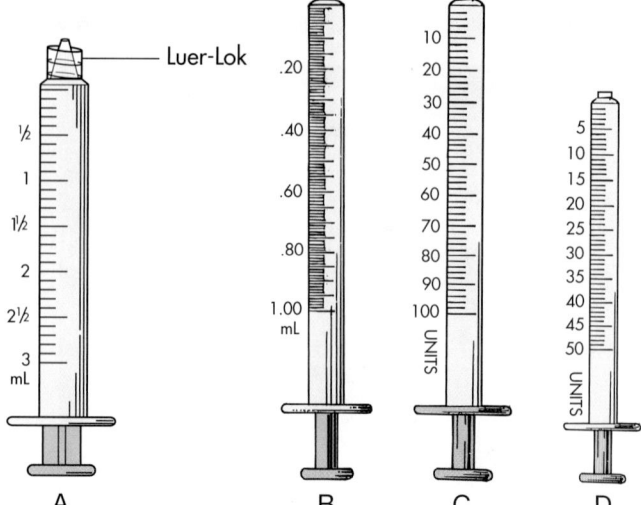

FIGURE 34-9 Parts of a syringe. (From Perry AG, Potter PA: *Clinical nursing skills and techniques,* ed 6, St Louis, 2006, Mosby.)

low viscosity are easily injected through a small opening. In addition, these two gauges cause minimal tissue damage and the patient experiences less pain. Larger needles (gauges 20 to 23) are usually necessary for intramuscular (IM) injections when the medication is thick, such as penicillin, or the length of the needle requires the extra support of a thicker gauge. A patient cannot feel the difference between a 20- and a 22-gauge needle. In fact, the medication is not forced as strongly into the tissues with the larger 20-gauge needle as with the 22-gauge one, and the patient actually experiences less pain. Needles larger than 20-gauge are not used for drug therapy. They are mostly used for venipuncture, blood donations, and blood transfusions.

Needle Length

Needle lengths vary from $3/8$ inch to 4 inches, depending on the area of the body to be injected and the route (depth) used. ID injections require only the short $3/8$-inch needle. Needles that are $1/2$ or $5/8$ inch long are used for SC injections. Longer needles are necessary for depositing drugs intramuscularly. The choice of a 1-inch, $1 1/2$-inch, 2-inch, $2 1/2$-inch or 3-inch length depends on both the muscle being used and the size of the patient.

Syringes

The parts of a syringe are its barrel, a calibrated scale (or scales), plunger, and tip. The typical syringe holds up to 3 mL and is usually calibrated with two scales: milliliters (cubic centimeters),

with each calibrated line marked at 0.1 cc, and minims (Figure 34-9, *A*). Larger syringes are calibrated in milliliters only. The tuberculin syringe is used for small quantities of drug and holds up to 1 mL of injectable material, with each calibrated line marked at 0.01 cc (Figure 34-9, *B*). The insulin syringe is calibrated in units specifically for diabetic use. Insulin syringes are calibrated to hold 30 U, 50 U, or 100 U of insulin (Figures 34-9, *C* and *D*). The type of calibration chosen depends on the total amount of insulin that is to be injected in one dose. When drawing up less than 30 U use the 30-U syringe, for 30 to 50 units use the 50-U syringe, and use the 100-U syringe for amounts greater than 50 units. With the establishment of standard precautions and the danger of needlesticks, syringes with retractable needle covers have been developed and must be made available to employees as an OSHA safeguard against accidental needlesticks. A sample of one type of retractable needle cover and the parts of the syringe are shown in Figure 34-10.

Disposable syringe and needle units are packaged in either sealed, rigid plastic containers or in peel-apart paper wrappers. Both individual needles and syringe-needle units are color coded for easy identification. Table 34-1 summarizes the needle and syringe sizes used for injections.

Specialty Syringe Units

With all of the concerns regarding needlesticks, proper disposal of needles, and cross-contamination of individuals through needle misuse, devices are now available for patients who must give themselves injections that do not require needle disposal. One of the possible answers is the injector pen. Different types are available, depending on the amount of medication to be dispensed per injection and the type of medication being used. Administering insulin away from home has become easier with the development of the insulin pen (Figure 34-11). It contains a predetermined type and amount of insulin that can be injected by the diabetic patient with minimal preparation. The different types of insulin are discussed in Chapter 44.

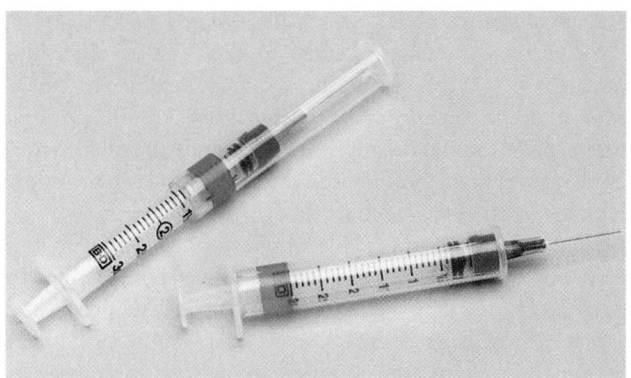

FIGURE 34-10 Disposable syringe with retractable needle cover.

TABLE 34-1 Needle and Syringe Sizes for Injections			
ROUTE	**GAUGE**	**LENGTH (INCHES)**	**SYRINGE**
Intradermal	27-28	$^3/_8$	1 mL; tuberculin
Subcutaneous	25-26	$^1/_2$, $^5/_8$	2 mL; insulin
Intramuscular	20-30	1-3	2-5 mL

FIGURE 34-11 NovoPen.

In addition, EpiPens are automatic injector systems that contain a dose of epinephrine (Figure 34-12). These must be prescribed by the physician and come packaged with the correct dose for either an adult (0.3 mg of epinephrine) or child (0.15 mg of epinephrine). They are carried as a safety precaution by individuals who have anaphylactic reactions to such allergens as bee stings or certain types of foods. Anaphylactic reactions can be fatal if not treated immediately, so patients or their family members should be educated on the signs and symptoms of anaphylaxis and how to manage the EpiPen administration.

The steps for EpiPen injection are quite simple:
1. Pull back the gray end of the auto-injector. This sets the device for use.
2. The injector can go through clothing. Firmly press the black tip on the outer aspect of the thigh and hold in place for 10 seconds. The injector automatically administers the prepackaged dose.
3. Remove the EpiPen and massage the injection area for a few minutes to promote absorption of the epinephrine.
4. The patient should still call a physician or go to the emergency department of a nearby hospital for follow-up care.
5. It is important that patients or family members periodically check the expiration date of the auto-injector device. If the device is near its expiration date, another prescription should be filled and the old unused device discarded. To be of service in an emergency, the EpiPen must be readily available at all times.

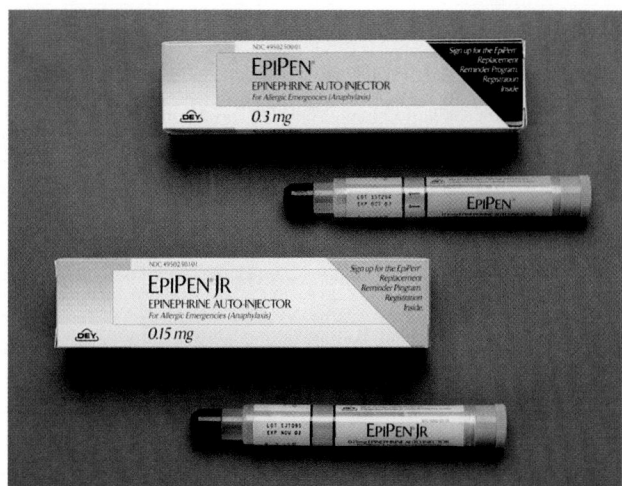

FIGURE 34-12 EpiPen prepackaged auto-injector.

Parenteral Administration

With practice, giving medications by injection will become easy and even automatic. However, the medical assistant must always follow the physician's orders, perform the three order and label checks while dispensing the medication, and strictly adhere to the seven rights throughout the procedure.

Practice developing techniques that provide maximum safety and comfort for the patient. Injections are least painful when the needle is inserted swiftly, the medication is injected slowly, and the needle is removed quickly with counterpressure when needed. Remember that the same aseptic conditions necessary for minor surgery are necessary whenever you penetrate the protective skin barrier with an injection.

Never give an injection near bones or blood vessels. Avoid areas where there is scar tissue; a change in skin pigmentation or texture; or excess tissue growth, such as a mole or a wart. The point of injection should be as far as possible from any major nerve, and the site selected should be capable of holding the amount of medication that is injected. Large doses of medication are given in muscle because muscles have a larger tissue mass than SC tissue and also a more extensive blood supply, allowing for faster absorption and systemic distribution.

Make certain that all materials are ready for use. Many offices have a central room where medications are prepared. The medication is then taken to the waiting patient in another room. Handling medication administration in this way has many advantages, but care must be taken that the syringe and

---

Signs and Symptoms of an Anaphylactic Reaction

- **Hypotension** resulting from systemic **vasodilation**
- Hives or *urticaria*
- Difficulty breathing *(dyspnea)*, resulting from **bronchoconstriction**
- Difficulty swallowing, as a result of **edema**
- Vomiting and diarrhea

Guidelines for Parenteral Administration of Medication

1. Use a professional approach and explain what you are going to do.
2. Small talk can keep the patient's mind off the procedure.
3. Never tell a patient that it will not hurt; you may destroy your credibility.
4. Make the patient as comfortable as possible, and allow for privacy.
5. Never allow the patient to stand during the procedure.
6. Keep the syringe unit out of the patient's sight as much as possible.
7. Always wear disposable gloves.
8. Immediately after the injection, cover the contaminated needle with the syringe unit safety device and dispose of it in a sharps container.
9. *Never* recap a contaminated needle.
10. Wash your hands before and after the procedure.
11. Provide patient education as needed.
12. Document complete details about the procedure in the patient record.

needle unit are transported with sterile technique. After a syringe is filled, the cap is replaced for transport to the patient, taking care to keep the needle sterile. Never transport more than one injection at a time, unless two or more are for the same patient or unless you have a special medication tray that has a named position for each syringe. Never combine two medications in a single syringe unless specifically ordered to do so by the physician and you have checked in the PDR or medication package insert for contraindications on mixing different types of medications. If you are preparing a medication for the physician to give, place the vial or empty ampule beside the filled syringe. This shows what medication is in the syringe and offers a double check for safety (see Procedure 34-5).

Some medications for injection are packaged in vials as sterile powders or crystals that must be mixed with sterile water or saline before they can be administered. This process was discussed in Chapter 33; the amount of solvent to be added to the dry form of the drug (solute) depends on the physician's order and the label directions. After calculating the correct amount of liquid that must be added to the dry form of the drug to create the dose ordered by the physician, follow the guidelines in Procedure 34-6 to prepare the drug and administer it to the patient.

Intradermal Injections

ID injections are given within the skin layers (Figure 34-13 and Procedure 34-7). The ID site is used for allergy testing and tuberculin screening. The tine test is no longer used to screen for TB because it was found to be unreliable in diagnosing exposures to the TB bacillus. The Mantoux (purified protein derivative [PPD]) ID test is now used routinely to screen for tuberculosis (TB) exposure. It is the only widely used test for detecting **asymptomatic** TB infection, currently termed *latent tuberculosis infection* (LTBI). With the Mantoux test, a 0.1-mL solution of PPD is injected into the ID layers. If the person being tested was infected with the TB bacillus in the past, his

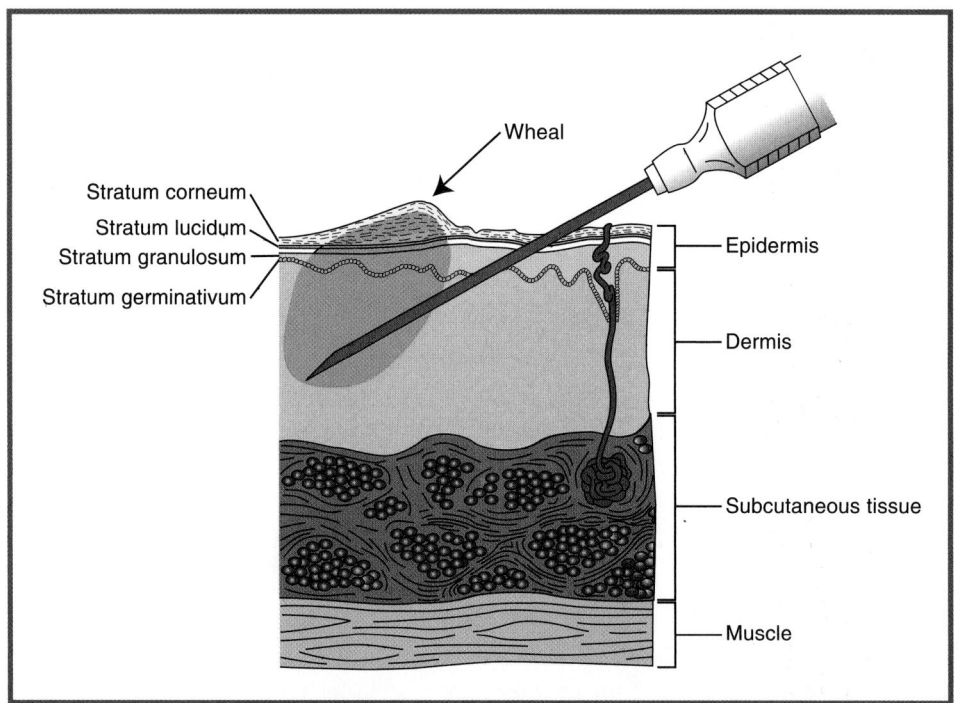

FIGURE 34-13 The intradermal injection is administered just under the epidermis. The drug is dispersed in an area where many nerves are present; therefore it causes momentary burning or stinging. Minute amounts of medication are injected. This method is used to test for allergies, drug sensitivities, and susceptibility to some diseases.

PROCEDURE 34-6

Apply Pharmacology Principles to Prepare and Administer Oral and Parenteral (Excluding IV) Medications: Reconstitute a Powdered Drug for Administration

<u>CAAHEP COMPETENCY:</u> 3.b.(4)(g)
<u>ABHES COMPETENCY:</u> 4.m

GOAL: *To reconstitute a powdered drug for intramuscular injection as ordered by the physician.*

EQUIPMENT and SUPPLIES

- Vial containing the ordered powdered medication
- Diluent: Sterile saline
- Alcohol wipes
- Cotton ball
- Two sterile needle and syringe units
- Disposable gloves
- Sharps container
- Written order, including the patient's name, when to give the drug, the route of administration, and the name and strength of the drug

PROCEDURAL STEPS

1. Wash your hands. Follow standard precautions.
2. Select the correct vial of powdered medication from the shelf and the recommended diluent for reconstitution. Perform the three drug label and physician order checks during preparation, and verify the seven rights throughout the procedure.
3. Read the label to determine the correct amount of diluent to add to create the dose ordered by the physician. (Refer to Chapter 33 for help with calculations.) Calculate the correct dose, if necessary, and continue with the three label checks.
4. Remove the tops from each vial, and clean each with an alcohol wipe. Leave the wipes in place on top of each vial.
5. Using one of the syringe units with the needle cover in place, grasp the syringe plunger and draw up the amount of air equal to the amount of diluent needed to reconstitute the drug.
   <u>PURPOSE:</u> Not enough replaced air will make it difficult to

withdraw the diluent; too much replaced air will force the diluent into the syringe without pulling on the plunger to withdraw it.
6. Remove the needle cover, and insert the needle into the center of the rubber stopper of the diluent. Hold the vial firmly against a flat surface, and watch carefully that the needle touches only the cleaned rubber area.
7. Inject the aspirated air in the syringe into the diluent vial.
8. Invert the diluent vial, and aspirate the calculated or recommended amount of diluent.
9. Remove the needle from the diluent vial, and inject the diluent into the center of the rubber stopper of the drug vial. Remove the needle from the vial, and discard the syringe unit into the sharps container.
   <u>PURPOSE:</u> An unused syringe unit should be used to administer the medication to the patient since the needle on the used unit may not be as sharp as that on a new syringe unit.
10. Roll the vial with the drug and diluent mixture between the palms of your hands to mix it thoroughly. Do not shake the vial unless directed to do so on the drug label. When the medication is completely mixed there is no residue or crystals on the bottom of the vial.
11. Aspirate air into the second syringe unit that is equal to the calculated amount of medication to be administered.
12. Inject the air into the mixed drug vial, invert the vial, and withdraw the ordered amount of medication.
13. Proceed as outlined in steps 6 to 22 in Procedure 34-9 to administer the medication.

PROCEDURE 34-7

Apply Pharmacology Principles to Prepare and Administer Oral and Parenteral (Excluding IV) Medications: Give an Intradermal Injection

<u>CAAHEP COMPETENCIES:</u> 3.b.(4)(g), 3.b.(4)(h), 3.c.(1)(a), 3.c.(2)(b), 3.c.(2)(c), 3.c.(2)(d)
<u>ABHES COMPETENCIES:</u> 1.d, 2.i, 2.k, 4.m, 4.n, 5.b
ORDER: Administer 0.1 mL PPD ID for a Mantoux test for TB screening

GOAL: *To inject 0.1 mL of purified protein derivative (PPD) ID to perform a Mantoux test as ordered by the physician.*

EQUIPMENT and SUPPLIES

- Vial of tuberculin PPD
- Alcohol wipes
- 27-gauge, 3/8-inch sterile needle and syringe unit with safety needle cover device

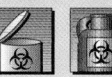

- Physician order, including the patient's name, when to give the drug, the route of administration, and the name and strength of the drug
- Disposable gloves
- Gauze squares
- Sharps container

Continued

PROCEDURE 34-7

- Patient medical record
- Written patient instructions for follow-up

EQUIPMENT and SUPPLIES

- Vial of tuberculin PPD
- Alcohol wipes
- 27-gauge, 3/8-inch sterile needle and syringe unit with safety needle cover device
- Physician order, including the patient's name, when to give the drug, the route of administration, and the name and strength of the drug
- Disposable gloves
- Gauze squares
- Sharps container
- Patient medical record
- Written patient instructions for follow-up
  ORDER: Administer 0.1 mL PPD SC for a Mantoux test for TB screening.

PROCEDURAL STEPS

1. Wash your hands. Follow standard precautions.
2. Select the correct medication from the shelf or the refrigerator.
   PURPOSE: Some medications must be refrigerated.
3. Read the label to be sure that you have the right drug (PPD) and the right strength. Perform the three label and order checks as the medication is dispensed.
   PURPOSE: Confirm that the medication label matches the physician's order. One medication may be manufactured and prepackaged in different strengths; for instance, an allergen may be available in 1:1000, 1:100, and 1:10 dilutions.
4. Warm refrigerated medications by gently rolling the container between your palms.

5. Prepare the syringe as described in Procedure 34-5, withdrawing the correct dose of 0.1 mL.
6. Transport the medication to the patient.
7. Greet and identify the patient by name.
   PURPOSE: To be sure that you have the right patient.
8. Ask the patient if he or she has ever had a positive reaction to a PPD (TB test) injection before. If yes, then report this information to the physician before administering the test. An individual who has a history of a positive PPD test result will always have a positive result because of antibody action.
9. Apply gloves, and position the patient comfortably.
   PURPOSE: To successfully create a wheal, it is easier if the patient is sitting and the medical assistant is lower than the patient (such as on a stool) with the anterior surface of the patient's arm extended straight out and angled downward.
10. Locate the antecubital space, then find a site several fingerwidths down the midanterior aspect of the forearm. Avoid any scarred, discolored, or pigmented areas.
11. Cleanse the patient's skin with an alcohol wipe using a circular motion, moving from the center outward (Figure 1).
12. Allow the antiseptic to dry.
13. Remove the cap from the needle.
14. Wrap the thumb and first two fingers of your nondominant hand around the patient's forearm, pulling downward and apart to stretch the skin of the forearm taut at the location of the injection.
    PURPOSE: Stretching the skin tightens the surface and facilitates the insertion of the needle with minimal discomfort to the patient. You will know if you do not have the skin stretched tight enough if the skin begins to wrinkle as you start to inject the needle.
15. Grasp the syringe between the thumb and first two fingers of your dominant hand, palm down, with the needle bevel upward. Hold the syringe close to the plunger end.
16. At a 15-degree angle, with the syringe unit parallel to the surface of the skin, carefully insert the needle just until the bevel point is under the skin surface (Figure 2).

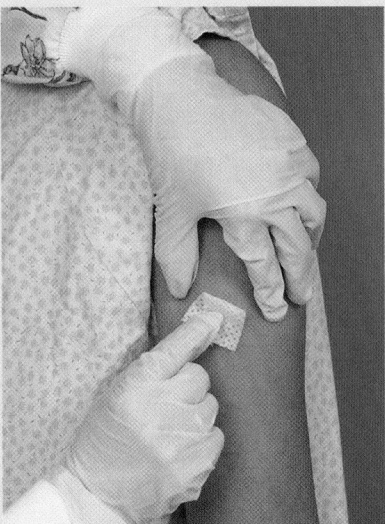

FIGURE 1

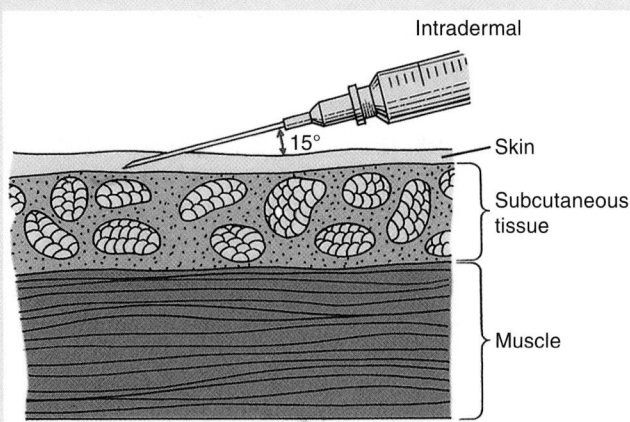

FIGURE 2

Continued

PROCEDURE 34-7—cont'd

17. Slowly and steadily inject the medication by depressing the plunger with your little finger. Do not aspirate. A wheal should appear.
PURPOSE: A rapid injection may force the substance through to the surface.

18. After administering all of the medication (0.1 mL), withdraw the needle.

19. Immediately cover the contaminated needle with the safety device and dispose of the syringe unit in a sharps container.

20. Do not massage, but you may blot the area with a cotton ball or gauze square. Do not cover the site with a bandage.
PURPOSE: Massaging will disturb the wheal and interfere with intended results.

21. Make sure that your patient is comfortable and safe.

22. Observe the patient for any adverse reaction.

23. Dispose of the gloves in the biohazard container, and wash your hands.

24. Record the procedure and any reactions that occurred at the site of the injection on the patient's medical record. Include the exact site of the injection.
PURPOSE: A procedure is not considered done until it is recorded. The exact site must be known to monitor reactions to the PPD in 48 to 72 hours.

25. Tell the patient when to return to the office for any reaction to be read, or give the patient a postcard to be completed and returned.
PURPOSE: Patient education must be done to get intended results.

Reading the Mantoux Test Results

26. Apply latex gloves; using good lighting and with the patient's arm slightly flexed, measure the induration at the site of the injection. Measure only the raised area; do not include any areas of inflammation.
PURPOSE: A positive Mantoux reaction occurs if the induration is inflamed, raised, and 15 mm or larger; in some patients a reaction larger than 5 mm or 10 mm is considered positive (Figure 3). Further diagnostic tests are ordered to either rule out or confirm the diagnosis of tuberculosis. These will be discussed in Chapter 45.

27. Discard the gloves in the biohazard waste container, and wash your hands.

28. Document the results of the Mantoux test in the patient chart, including a complete description of the size of the induration, if any, and the appearance of the test site. Notify the physician.

See Appendix D for a charting example.

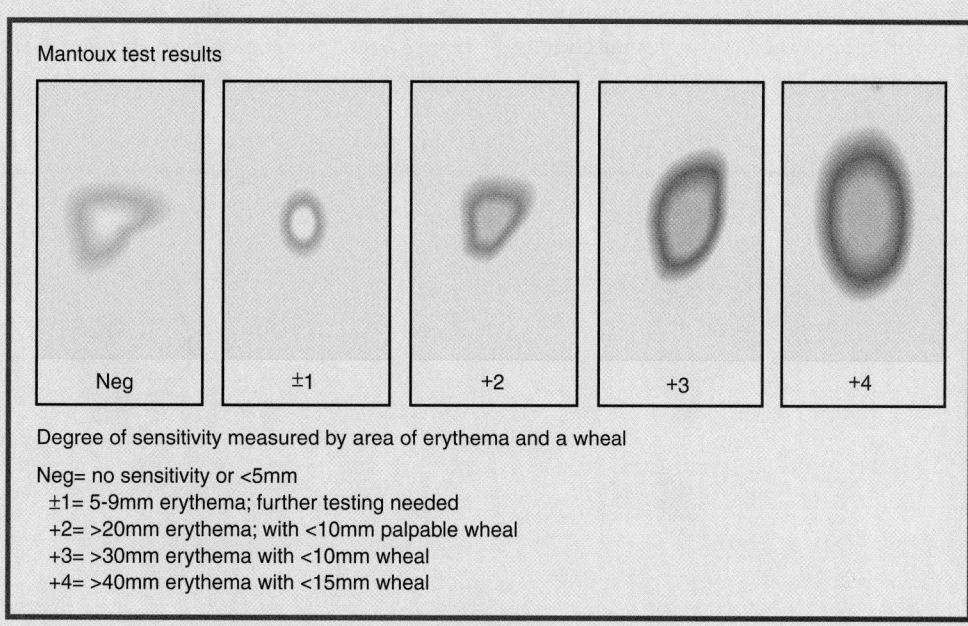

Mantoux test results

| Neg | ±1 | +2 | +3 | +4 |

Degree of sensitivity measured by area of erythema and a wheal

Neg= no sensitivity or <5mm
±1= 5-9mm erythema; further testing needed
+2= >20mm erythema; with <10mm palpable wheal
+3= >30mm erythema with <10mm wheal
+4= >40mm erythema with <15mm wheal

FIGURE 3

or her immune system developed antibodies that recognize and fight the bacteria. When a PPD skin test is performed, these antibodies move to the injection site to try to stop the infection. This immune reaction causes swelling, or **induration,** in the area approximately 48 hours after the skin test is administered. An induration of 5 mm or greater is considered positive in patients who are at increased risk for being infected and in persons who are most likely to develop active disease if they are infected with the TB bacteria. This would include those infected with the human immunodeficiency (HIV) virus; anyone in close contact with a newly diagnosed patient (such as family members); and patients who have undergone recent organ transplants or are taking **immunosuppressant** medications. A 10-mm or greater induration is read as positive if the person has a moderate likelihood of TB exposure and infection, including recent immigrants from countries in which TB is prevalent; intravenous (IV) drug users; residents and employees of correctional institutions, homeless shelters, and healthcare facilities (including medical personnel); and children under 4 years of age. Regardless of risk factors, anyone with an induration of 15 mm or greater in diameter is considered positive. Patients may be given a postcard with pictures having accurate measurements of indurations that can be completed and sent back to the office, or they may be instructed to return to the office after the specified period for the staff to read the results (see Procedure 34-7, Figure 3). TB is discussed further in Chapter 45.

When an ID injection is correctly administered, a small **wheal** is raised on the skin. A $^3/_8$-inch, 27- or 28-gauge needle is used for ID injections. The angle of insertion is 15 degrees, almost parallel to the skin surface. The best site for injection is the center of the anterior forearm, but the upper chest and back

are frequently used for allergy testing (Figure 34-14). Allergy testing is discussed in Chapter 37.

CRITICAL THINKING APPLICATION

Dorothy is ordered to give her first Mantoux test since being hired by Dr. Thau. Document the details that Dorothy should include on the patient's chart. She administered 0.1 mL of PPD by ID injection into the patient's right midforearm and instructed the patient on how to read the results of the test and send the accompanying postcard back into the office.

_____

_____

_____

Subcutaneous Injections

Subcutaneous injections are given between the epidermis and the muscle, into the fatty areolar layer called *adipose tissue* (Figure 34-15 and Procedure 34-8). Smaller doses, no more than 2 mL, of less irritating drugs are given by this method. A $^1/_2$- to $^5/_8$-inch, 25- or 26-gauge needle is used for SC injections. The angle of insertion is 45 degrees; however, heparin and insulin may be administered at a 90-degree angle when using a microneedle or if the patient is obese. The posterior upper arm is the typical injection site, but the abdomen, anterior aspect of the thighs, and upper back may be used as well (Figure 34-16). When multiple or frequent injections are ordered, such as routine insulin injections, the sites must be rotated to prevent tissue damage and problems with absorption of the medication. It is best to keep a rotation record (Figure 34-17, p. 704). It might be helpful for patients to mark the site of the last injection with

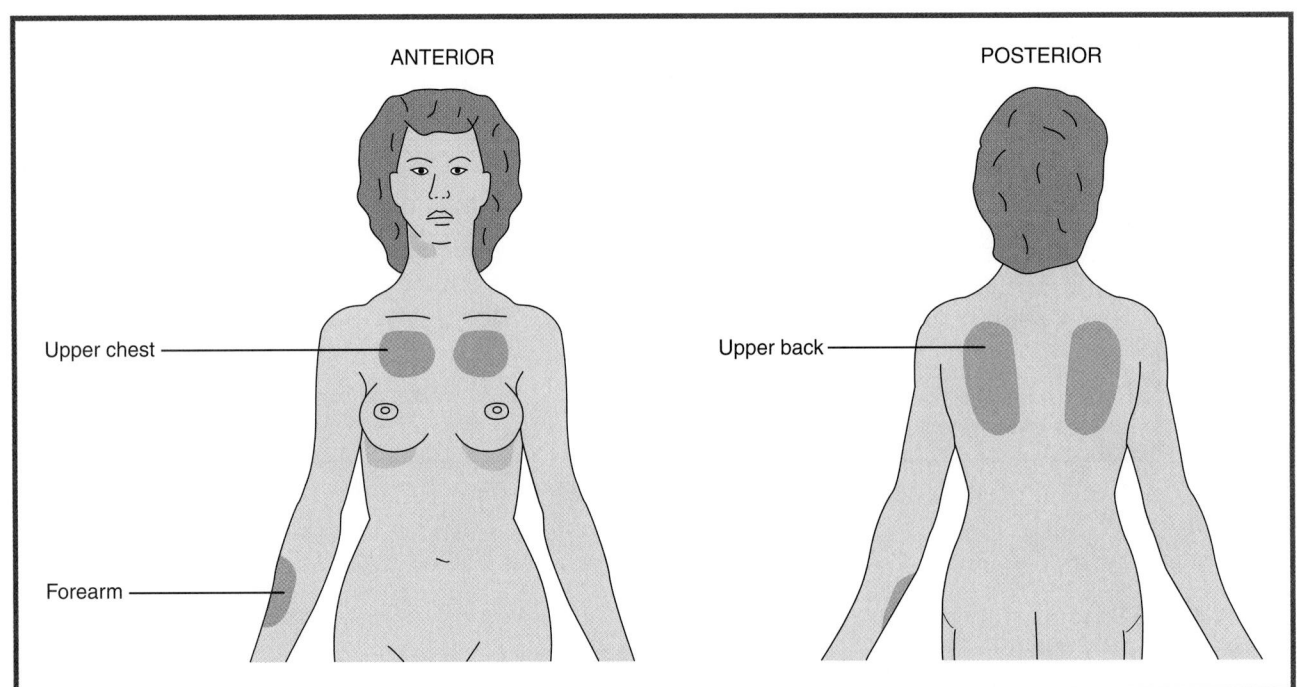

FIGURE 34-14 Sites recommended for intradermal injections.

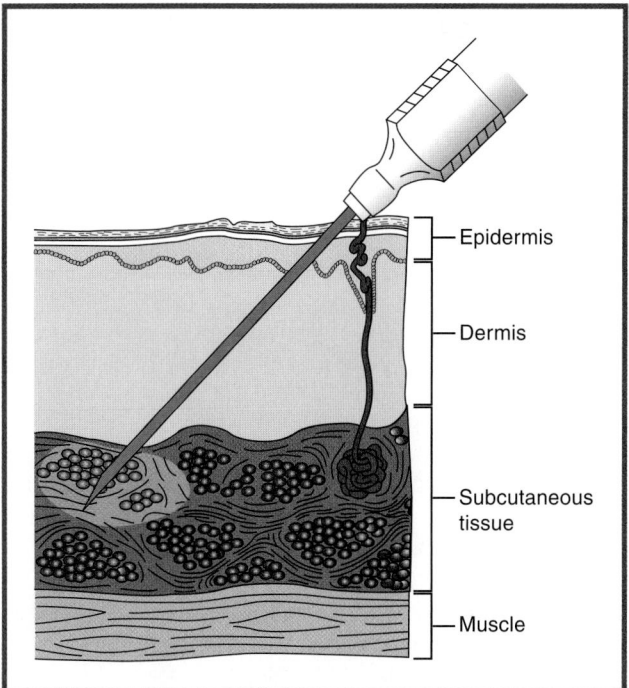

FIGURE 34-15 The subcutaneous injection is administered with a 25- or 26-gauge, $1/2$- or $5/8$-inch needle. The method is used for small amounts of nonirritating medications in aqueous solution. It is injected at a 45-degree angle (at a 90-degree angle for insulin and heparin). The most common site is the posterior upper arm.

Insulin Administration Guidelines

- Typically more than one type of insulin is ordered for immediate administration. Check labels carefully, and follow office policy when mixing insulins in the same syringe.
- Insulin is always ordered in unit amounts. Use the appropriate insulin syringe, either 30 U, 50 U or 100 U, depending on the total amount of insulin ordered.
- Insulin should be stored in the refrigerator and gently rotated between hands to warm before dispensing.
- Do not massage the site after injection.

a spot bandage or a piece of tape. The easiest way to rotate sites is to give subsequent injections in a circular pattern around the site of the first injection in a particular location, such as the right anterior thigh. The goal is that the same location will not be used again for another month.

Intramuscular Injections

IM injections are given into the muscle when drugs will irritate the SC tissues, a more rapid absorption is desired, or the volume of the medication to be injected is large. The angle of insertion is 90 degrees (Figure 34-18, p. 704), and the preferred sites are the vastus lateralis, deltoid, ventrogluteal, and gluteus medius muscles of the adult (Figure 34-19, p. 705) and the vastus lateralis of the infant and child. It is important to select a needle that is long enough, especially for obese patients, that the medication is injected into the muscle and not deposited into the upper adipose tissue. Fatty tissue does not absorb medications well, and the medication may remain at the site of the injection rather than being distributed systemically as intended. The recommended gauge is 20- to 23-gauge, and the length of the needle could be from 1 to 3 inches, depending on the size of the patient.

In adults the deltoid region can hold up to 2 mL of medication, whereas the vastus lateralis and gluteal sites can contain up to 5 mL. Infants and children should be given no more than 2 mL in the vastus lateralis or ventrogluteal sites. The most important criterion in choosing an IM site is to use one that is away from large nerves, bones, and blood vessels. If any of these structures are damaged by the injection it is possible to cause nerve injuries with lingering pain, abscesses, and bone inflammation with infection.

When locating a site for an IM injection, expose the site so that you are able to see and palpate the landmarks correctly. If it is necessary for the patient to receive repeated IM injections, the sites should be rotated to prevent damage to the muscle and surrounding tissues.

Deltoid Site. The deltoid muscle, the muscular cap of the shoulder, is located at the top of the upper arm. The muscle mass is somewhat limited, so it can only hold 1 to 2 mL of medication. This triangular muscle is located between the acromion and deltoid tuberosities, and the injection site is approximately two fingerbreadths below the acromial process (Figure 34-20, p. 706). The major nerves and blood vessels, especially the radial nerve and artery, must be avoided. Aqueous medications, such as vitamin B_{12}, are most appropriate here; hepatitis B and flu vaccinations are also given in the deltoid.

If frequent injections are ordered, rotate the site and alternate the right and left arms. The deltoid site is acceptable for adults and older children, but it should not be used when the muscle is small or underdeveloped. For a small arm, you may need only a 25-gauge $5/8$-inch needle; the 23-gauge 1-inch needle is most often used for an average-sized arm. The patient may be seated or lying down. When injecting, expose the entire shoulder rather than rolling up the sleeve. Rest the palm of your hand across the shoulder, and grasp the muscle before injecting the medication at a 90-degree angle (Procedure 34-9, p. 707).

Vastus Lateralis (Thigh) Site. The vastus lateralis muscle is part of the quadriceps group of the thigh. It is one of the body's largest muscles, and because it is developed at birth, it is considered the safest IM injection site for infants. Many experts believe that as a site for adult IM injections the vastus lateralis is better than either the deltoid or the dorsogluteal sites, because fewer major nerves and blood vessels are in the vastus lateralis. The vastus lateralis muscle fills the midportion of the upper, outer thigh. In an adult, it can be located from one hand's width below the proximal end of the greater trochanter to one hand's width above the top of the patella (knee cap), or the mid third of the upper outer leg.

Injecting infants and small children requires some special considerations. The choice of a site is based on muscular development, as well as the absence of major nerves and blood vessels. As mentioned previously, the most popular site for IM

PROCEDURE 34-8

Apply Pharmacology Principles to Prepare and Administer Oral and Parenteral (Excluding IV) Medications: Give a Subcutaneous Injection

CAAHEP COMPETENCIES: 3.b.(4)(g), 3.b.(4)(h), 3.c.(1)(a), 3.c.(2)(b), 3.c.(2)(c), 3.c.(2)(d)
ABHES COMPETENCIES: 1.d, 2.i, 2.k, 4.m, 4.n, 5.b
ORDER: Administer 0.5 mL varicella vaccine SC stat to Mandy Leno, age 11.

GOAL: To inject 0.5 mL of medication into the subcutaneous tissue using a 25-gauge, $^5/_8$-inch needle and syringe of correct size and type, as directed by the physician.

EQUIPMENT and SUPPLIES

- A vial of ordered medication
- Alcohol wipes
- Gauze squares or cotton balls
- A sterile needle and syringe unit with safety cover device
- Disposable gloves
- Sharps container
- A written order, including the patient's name, when to give the drug, the route of administration, and the name and strength of the drug
- Patient's medical record

PROCEDURAL STEPS

1. Wash your hands. Follow standard precautions.
2. Select the correct medication from the shelf or the refrigerator.
   PURPOSE: Some medications must be refrigerated or stored under special conditions.
3. Read the label to be sure that you have the right drug and the right strength. Perform the three label and order checks while dispensing the medication, and verify the seven rights. Perform any necessary dose calculations.
   PURPOSE: To promote safety and accuracy in drug therapy. One medication may be manufactured and prepackaged in different strengths. For instance, a particular drug may be available in vials of both 250 mg/mL and 500 mg/mL.
4. Warm refrigerated medications by gently rolling the container between your palms.
5. Prepare the syringe, withdrawing the correct dose.
6. Document the vaccine dose on the vaccination log. Each physician office will have a policy regarding vaccination documentation.
   PURPOSE: The immunization record or vaccination log must be completed each time a vaccination is administered. Information includes the manufacturer; batch and lot numbers, which are stamped on the container; expiration date; dose administered; route of administration; and whether there was a patient reaction. More details about immunization records are presented in Chapter 41.
7. Transport the medication to the patient.
8. Greet and identify the patient by name. Explain the purpose of the immunization.
   PURPOSE: To be sure that you have the right patient and to gain cooperation.
9. Ask the patient to sit upright, and help position her comfortably if necessary.
10. Expose the upper posterior arm.
11. Apply gloves, and with the thumb and fingers of your nondominant hand, grasp the tissue of the posterior upper arm. Cleanse the patient's skin with the antiseptic sponge, using a circular motion, moving outward from the center.
12. Remove the cap from the needle.
13. Hold the syringe between the thumb and the first two fingers of your dominant hand, and with one swift movement, insert the entire needle up to the hub at a 45-degree angle.
    PURPOSE: The depth of the injection is determined by the choice of needle length, not by how far you insert the needle. Once the needle is at the tissue layer, do not move the needle while injecting the medication.
14. Aspirate (except when administering heparin or insulin) by withdrawing the plunger slightly to be sure that no blood enters the syringe.
    PURPOSE: Blood in the syringe means that the needle is in a blood vessel and not in the subcutaneous tissue.
15. If blood appears, immediately withdraw the unit without injecting the medication and dispose of it in the sharps container. Compress the injection site with an alcohol swab or gauze bandage.
    PURPOSE: To minimize bleeding and bruising.
16. Begin again with step 1.
17. If no blood appears in the syringe, push in the plunger slowly and steadily until all medication has been administered.
    PURPOSE: A rapid injection may damage the tissues and be uncomfortable for the patient.
18. Place the gauze square next to the needle, and withdraw it at the same angle of insertion. Immediately place the safety device over the contaminated needle.
19. Gently massage the site with the gauze square (do not massage insulin or heparin injections).
    PURPOSE: Massage helps to increase absorption and to decrease pain.
20. Discard the needle and syringe into the sharps container.
21. Make sure that your patient is comfortable and safe.
22. Dispose of the gloves in the biohazard waste, and wash your hands.
23. Observe the patient for any adverse reaction. You may need to keep the patient under observation for 20 to 30 minutes.

Continued

PROCEDURE 34-8—*cont'd*

24. Record the drug administration on the patient's medical record, including the exact injection site, and on the immunization record.

<u>PURPOSE:</u> A procedure is not considered done until it is recorded. It is important to keep an accurate record of vaccination administration. Include in the documentation the name of the vaccination, dose, route of administration and location, lot number, and any observed patient reactions. The caregiver must be given a Vaccine Information Sheet (VIS), and it must be documented that the VIS was received.

See Appendix D for a charting example.

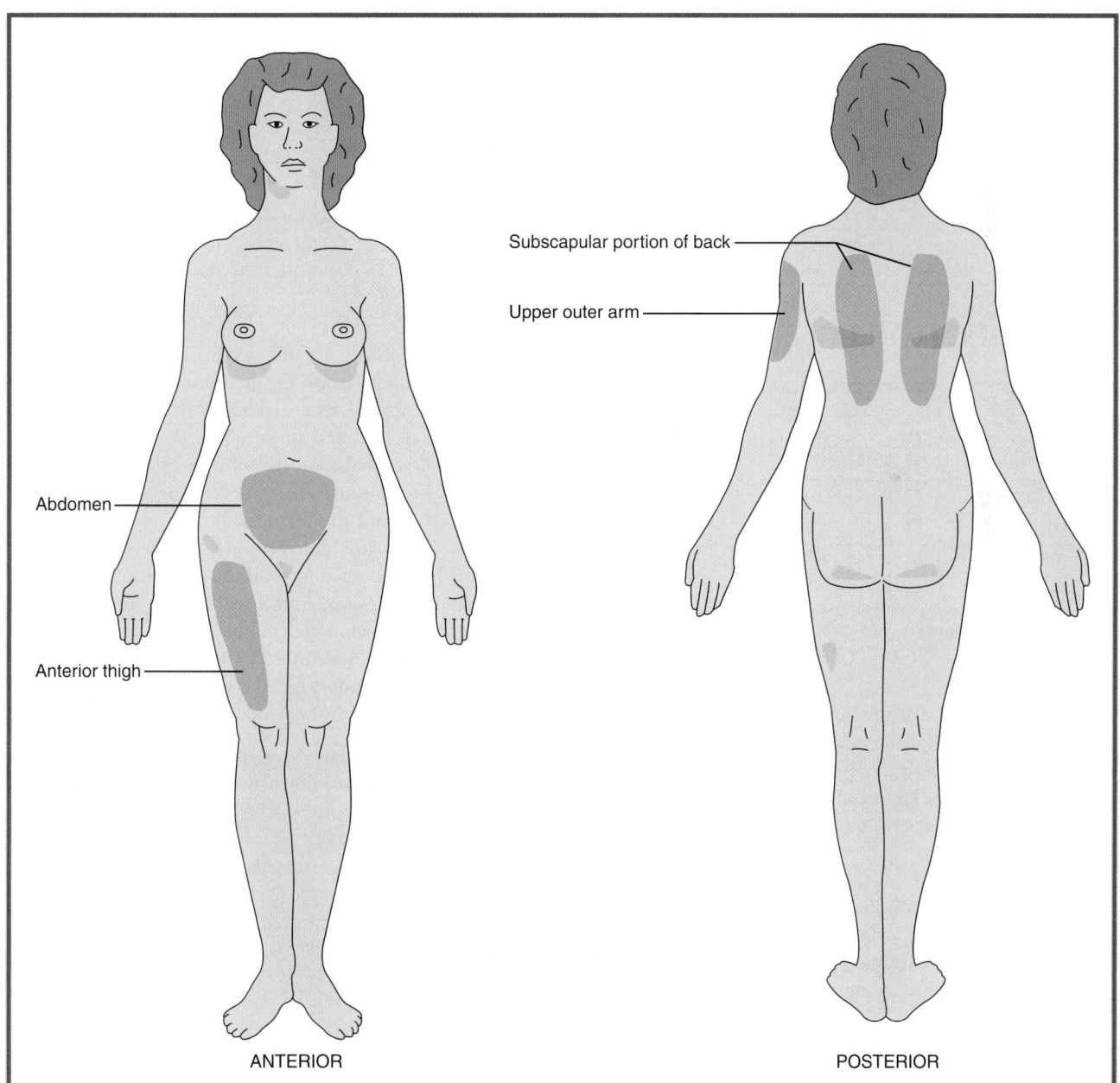

ANTERIOR

POSTERIOR

Subscapular portion of back
Upper outer arm
Abdomen
Anterior thigh

FIGURE 34-16 Areas of the body commonly used for subcutaneous injections.

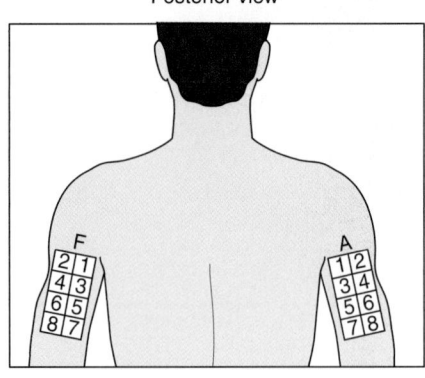

Posterior view

Anterior view

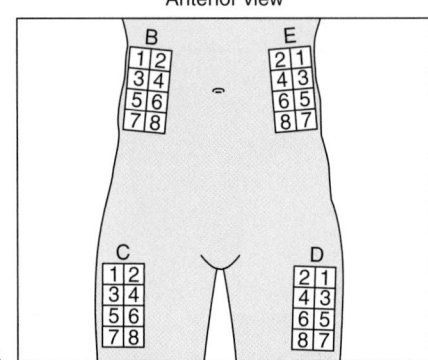

A

INJECTION LOG

SITE		1	2	3	4	5	6	7	8
Right arm	A								
Right abdomen	B								
Right thigh	C								
Left thigh	D								
Left abdomen	E								
Left arm	F								

B

FIGURE 34-17 A, Rotation sites for insulin injections. **B,** Rotation log.

injection in children and infants is the vastus lateralis muscle. Other sites are avoided for the following reasons:

- Infants do not have well-developed deltoid muscles.
- The sciatic nerve, located near the dorsogluteal site, is proportionately larger in the infant.
- The gluteus medius is not well developed until the child is walking.

If you have any doubts, the best policy is to ask the physician to show you exactly where to inject the medication or vaccine. Any site selected for infants and children has a greater margin for error because the muscles are smaller than the muscles of adults.

Infants should be restrained by a co-worker or parent to avoid injury. If the child is old enough to understand, be honest and explain that the injection may sting for a minute, but that it is important to hold very still. Always get help if giving an injection to an uncooperative child.

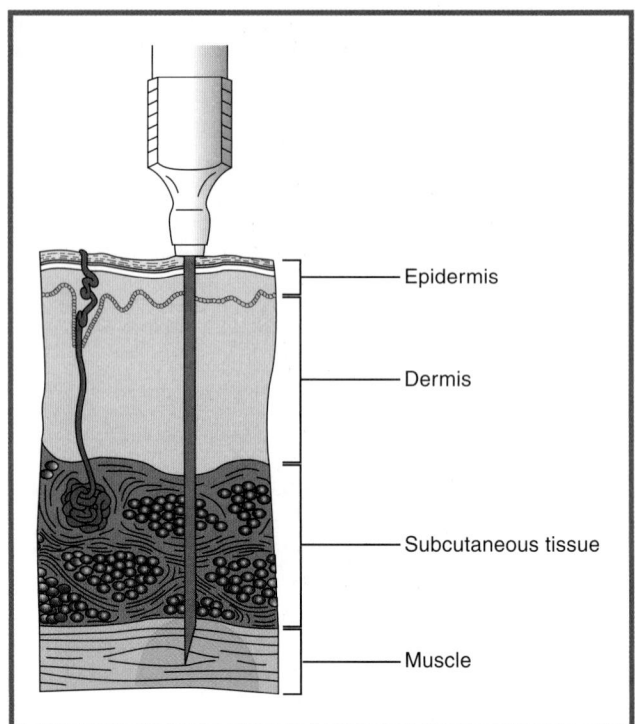

FIGURE 34-18 Anatomic illustration of the intramuscular injection. Note that the needle is inserted at a 90-degree angle, which deposits the medication into the large central part of the muscle.

The recommended site for vastus lateralis injections in infants and children is below the greater trochanter of the femur but within the upper lateral quadrant of the thigh. When the vastus lateralis site is used in an adult, the needle should be injected at a 90-degree angle, but with infants and children the needle should be injected at a 45-degree angle, with the needle point directed toward the feet. Needle gauges for adults range from 20 to 23, lengths range from 1 to $1\frac{1}{2}$ inches, and the muscle can hold as much as 5 mL of medication. In pediatric patients the needle gauge should be 22 to 25, length should be $\frac{5}{8}$ of an inch, and the muscle can hold 0.5 mL in infants and 0.5 to 2 mL in children (Procedure 34-10, p. 708). An adult patient may sit or lie supine, but it is easier to locate the vastus lateralis in pediatric patients with the child lying down.

CRITICAL THINKING APPLICATION

Dr. Thau wants to make certain that Dorothy is comfortable with the procedure for administering IM injections to infants. She orders Dorothy to give the first dose of Diphtheria, Tetanus, Pertussis (DTaP) IM to a 2-month-old infant in the office today for a well-baby check up. Dorothy administers the injection in the right vastus lateralis. Document the information Dorothy should include on the child's record.

_____

_____

_____

Dorsogluteal (Gluteus Medius) Site. The dorsogluteal region is the traditional site for deep IM injections. However,

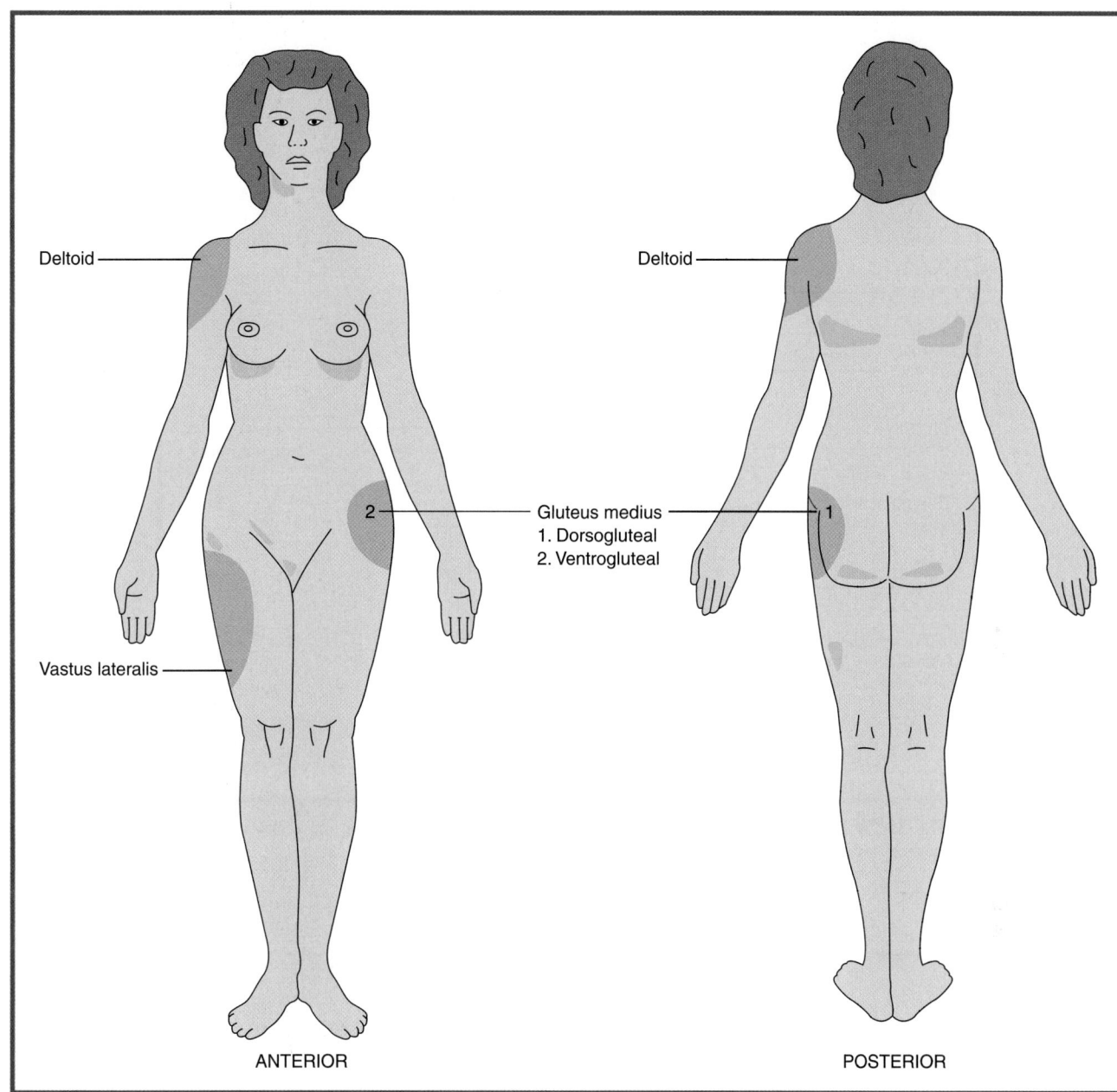

FIGURE 34-19 The muscles commonly used for intramuscular injection.

complications from sciatic nerve injury are frequent enough that experts are suggesting that use of this site be abandoned and replaced with use of the vastus lateralis and ventrogluteal sites. Regardless, the dorsogluteal site continues to be popular, and it is still acceptable for adults if care is taken to locate the exact site. It is recommended that this site not be used for pediatric patients.

The patient should lie in Sims' position with the bottom leg straight and the top leg slightly bent. To locate the site, put the palm of your hand on the greater trochanter of the femur and point your fingers toward the posterior iliac spine. Palpate these bony prominences to make certain that you are at the correct site, and draw an imaginary line between these two anatomic markings. The injection is made into the gluteus medius muscle above the imaginary line (Figure 34-21). Needle gauges 20 to 23 should be used, with length 1 to 3 inches, and the site can hold as much as 5 mL of medication. Refer to Procedure 34-11 to practice finding the dorsogluteal site.

Ventrogluteal (Gluteus Medius) Site. Although considered safe, the ventrogluteal region is not used as frequently as the others previously discussed. This technique uses a larger mass of the gluteus medius muscle than when using the dorsogluteal site. The area is free of major nerves and blood vessels, and it is considered safe for both infants and adults (Figure 34-22, p. 709). All types of IM medications can be injected here, including thick, oily preparations. Needle gauges 20 to 23 should be used, with length 1 to 3 inches, and the site can hold as much as 5 mL of medication.

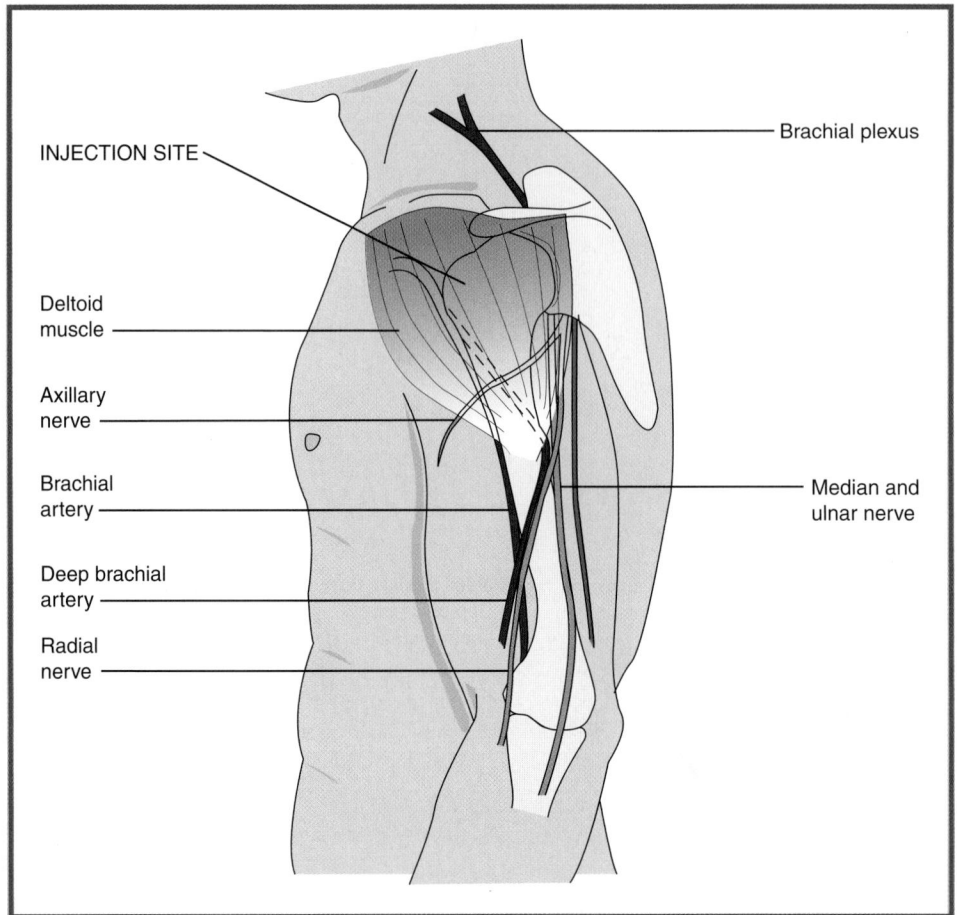

FIGURE 34-20 The deltoid muscle intramuscular site. This site is not recommended for infants, because the muscle is not well developed until later in childhood.

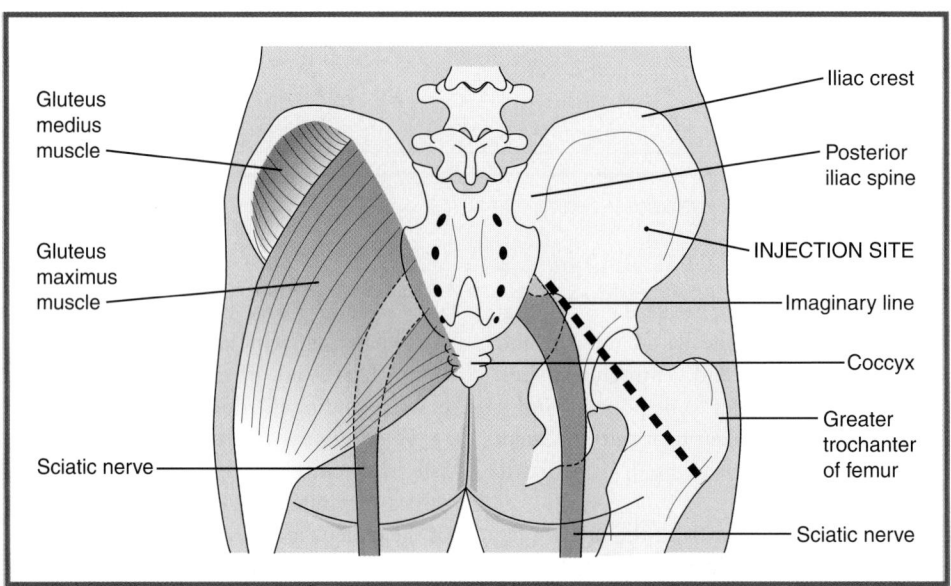

FIGURE 34-21 The dorsogluteal (gluteus medius) site is still preferred by many physicians.

PROCEDURE 34-9

Apply Pharmacology Principles to Prepare and Administer Oral and Parenteral (Excluding IV) Medications: Give an Intramuscular Injection into the Deltoid

CAAHEP COMPETENCIES: 3.b.(4)(g), 3.b.(4)(h), 3.c.(1)(a), 3.c.(2)(b), 3.c.(2)(c), 3.c.(2)(d)
ABHES COMPETENCIES: 1.d, 2.i, 2.k, 4.m, 4.n, 5.b
ORDER: Administer 300,000 U penicillin G IM stat to Ramon Diez, age 23.

GOAL: To inject ordered medication into the muscle, using a 22-gauge, 1½-inch needle and 3-mL syringe, as directed by the physician.

EQUIPMENT and SUPPLIES

- A vial containing ordered medication
- Alcohol wipes
- Cotton ball
- Sterile needle and syringe unit with safety needle cover
- Disposable gloves
- Sharps container
- Written order, including the patient's name, when to give the drug, the route of administration, and the name and strength of the drug
- Patient medical record

PROCEDURAL STEPS

1. Wash your hands. Follow standard precautions.
2. Select the correct medication from storage.
3. Read the label to be sure that you have the right drug and the right strength.
   PURPOSE: To perform the first of three drug label and order checks; one medication may be manufactured and prepackaged in different strengths; for instance, penicillin G is packages in both 300,000-U/mL and 600,000-U/mL vials.
4. Warm refrigerated medications by gently rolling between your palms.
5. Calculate the correct dose if necessary, and continue with the three label checks while drawing the medication into the syringe.
6. Transport the medication to the patient.
7. Greet and identify the patient by name.
   PURPOSE: To be sure that you have the right patient.

8. Ask patient if he is allergic to penicillin or any other antibiotics.
   PURPOSE: Antibiotics, especially the penicillin family, are the most likely groups of drugs to cause allergies. The patient's response can change over time, so it is important to request allergy information before each administration of an antibiotic.
9. Help the patient into an upright sitting position.
10. Apply gloves, and expose the deltoid site. The mid-deltoid site is located approximately two to three fingerwidths below the acromial process.
11. Cleanse the patient's skin with the alcohol wipe using a circular motion, moving outward from the center (Figure 1).
12. Remove the needle cover. Place your nondominant hand on the patient's shoulder, and with the thumb and first two fingers spread the skin tightly. (At the deltoid and vastus lateralis sites pinching of the tissue is also acceptable, as in Figure 2.)
13. Grasp the syringe as you would a dart, and with one swift movement, insert the entire needle up to the hub, at a 90-degree angle, into the muscle (Figure 3).

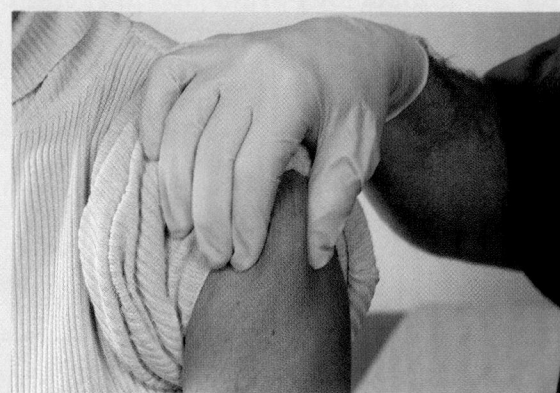

FIGURE 2

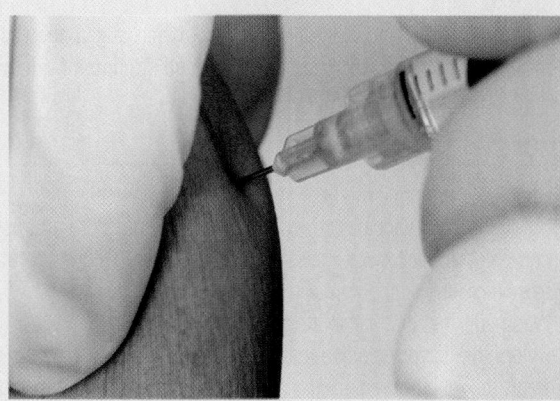

FIGURE 3

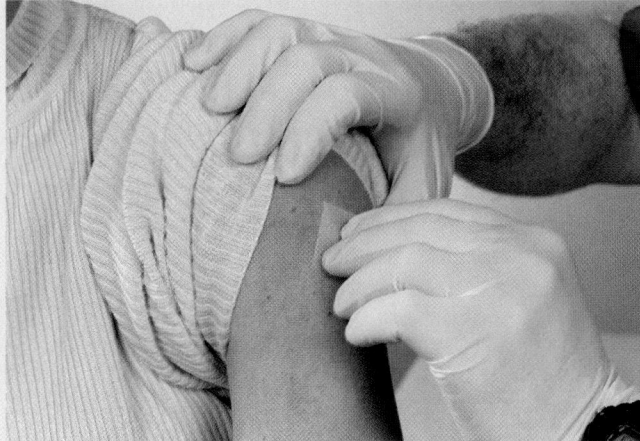

FIGURE 1

Continued

PROCEDURE 34-9—cont'd

PURPOSE: The depth of the injection is determined by the choice of needle length, not by how far you insert the needle. Once the needle is at the tissue layer, do not move the needle while injecting the medication. Being in as far as the hub helps to keep the needle in one place.

14. Aspirate: Withdraw the plunger slightly to be sure that no blood enters the syringe.
    PURPOSE: Blood in the syringe means that the needle is in a blood vessel and is not in the muscle tissue. You may not administer an intramuscular medication by the intravenous route.

15. If blood appears, immediately withdraw the syringe, discard it in the sharps container, and compress the injection site with the cotton ball.

16. Begin again with step 1.

17. If no blood appears in the syringe, push in the plunger slowly and steadily until all medication has been administered.
    PURPOSE: A rapid injection is uncomfortable for the patient.

18. Place the cotton ball next to the needle and apply counter pressure to the area while you withdraw the needle at the same angle of insertion. Immediately place the safety cover over the contaminated needle and discard the syringe unit into the sharps container.

19. Gently massage the site with the cotton ball.
    PURPOSE: Massage helps to increase absorption and to decrease pain.

20. Make sure that your patient is comfortable and safe.

21. Observe the patient for any adverse reaction. You may need to keep the patient under observation for 20 to 30 minutes.

22. Dispose of the gloves in the biohazard waste, and wash your hands.

23. Record the drug administration on the patient's medical record and on the required Drug Enforcement Agency (DEA) record if the medication is a controlled substance.
    PURPOSE: A procedure is not considered done until it is recorded.

See Appendix D for a charting example.

PROCEDURE 34-10

Apply Pharmacology Principles to Prepare and Administer Oral and Parenteral (Excluding IV) Medications: Administer a Pediatric Intramuscular Vastus Lateralis Injection

CAAHEP COMPETENCIES: 3.b.(4)(g), 3.b.(4)(h), 3.c.(1)(a), 3.c.(2)(b), 3.c.(2)(c), 3.c.(2)(d)
ABHES COMPETENCIES: 1.d, 2.i, 2.k, 4.m, 4.n, 5.b
ORDER: Administer 0.5 mL of Haemophilus influenzae (Hib) vaccine IM to Lizzy Dearborne, age 4 months, stat.

GOAL: To inject 0.5 mL of vaccine into the vastus lateralis muscle using a 22-gauge, $^5/_8$-inch needle.

EQUIPMENT and SUPPLIES

- A vial containing Hib vaccine
- Alcohol wipes
- Cotton ball or 2 × 2 gauze square
- Sterile needle and syringe unit with safety device
- Disposable gloves
- Sharps container
- Written order, including the patient's name, when to give the drug, the route of administration, and the name and strength of the drug
- Patient's medical record

PROCEDURAL STEPS

1. Check the patient's medical record for a previous allergic reaction to Hib vaccine; check the baby's temperature and ask caregiver about recent illnesses, because those with moderate to severe illness should not receive the vaccination.

2. Wash your hands. Follow standard precautions.

3. Select the correct medication from storage.

4. Read the label to be sure that you have the right drug and the right strength, and check the expiration date.

   PURPOSE: To perform the first of three drug label and order checks.

5. Warm refrigerated medications by gently rolling between your palms.

6. Calculate the correct dose if needed, and continue with the three label checks while drawing the medication into the syringe. Follow the steps explained in Procedure 34-5 to correctly draw up the vaccination.

7. Complete the vaccination log according to office procedure.
   PURPOSE: The immunization record or vaccination log must be completed each time a vaccination is administered. Information includes the manufacturer; batch and lot numbers, which are stamped on the Hib container; expiration date; dose administered; route of administration; and whether there was a patient reaction. More details about immunization records are presented in Chapter 41.

8. Transport the medication to the patient.

9. Greet and identify the patient's caregiver and child by name.
   PURPOSE: To be sure that you have the right patient.

10. Explain the procedure to the child's caregiver.

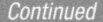
Continued

PROCEDURE 34-10—*cont'd*

<u>PURPOSE:</u> Promotes cooperation and is a form of implied consent to the procedure.

11. Position the infant on her back. Ask the caregiver to remove any clothing necessary to expose the infant's thighs. Choose either the right or the left thigh for the injection.
<u>PURPOSE:</u> It is important to expose the entire vastus lateralis muscle to prevent injury to the child. The pediatric vastus lateralis site is located below the greater trochanter of the femur but within the upper lateral quadrant (fourth) of the thigh.

12. Apply gloves, and cleanse the patient's skin with the alcohol wipe using a circular motion, moving outward from the center.

13. Ask for caregiver assistance in holding the child still if necessary.

14. Remove the needle cover, and with the thumb and first two fingers of your nondominant hand spread the skin at the site tightly.

15. Grasp the syringe as you would a dart, and with one swift movement insert the needle at a 45-degree angle into the muscle, with the needle pointing toward the feet.
<u>PURPOSE:</u> Once the needle is at the tissue layer, do not move the needle while injecting the medication.

16. Aspirate: Withdraw the plunger slightly to be sure that no blood enters the syringe.
<u>PURPOSE:</u> Blood in the syringe means that the needle is in a blood vessel and is not in the muscle tissue. You may not administer an intramuscular medication by the intravenous route.

17. If blood appears, immediately withdraw the syringe, discard it in the sharps container, and compress the injection site with the cotton ball. Begin again with step 2.

18. If no blood appears in the syringe, push in the plunger slowly and steadily until all medication has been administered.
<u>PURPOSE:</u> A rapid injection is uncomfortable for the patient.

19. Place the cotton ball next to the needle, and apply counterpressure to the area while you withdraw the needle at the same angle of insertion. Immediately place the safety cover over the contaminated needle and discard the syringe unit into the sharps container.

20. Gently massage the site with the cotton ball.
<u>PURPOSE:</u> Massage helps to increase absorption and to decrease pain.

21. Make sure that the infant is safely held by the caregiver.

22. Dispose of gloves in the biohazard waste, and wash your hands.

23. Record drug administration in the patient's medical record and on the vaccination log according to office procedure.
<u>PURPOSE:</u> A procedure is not considered done until it is recorded. It is important to keep an accurate record of vaccination administration so that the next dose is timed properly. Include in the documentation the name of the vaccination, dose, route of administration and location, lot number, and any observed patient reactions. The caregiver must be given a Vaccine Information Sheet (VIS), and it must be documented that the VIS was received.

24. Observe the patient for 20 to 30 minutes for any adverse reaction.

See Appendix D for a charting example.

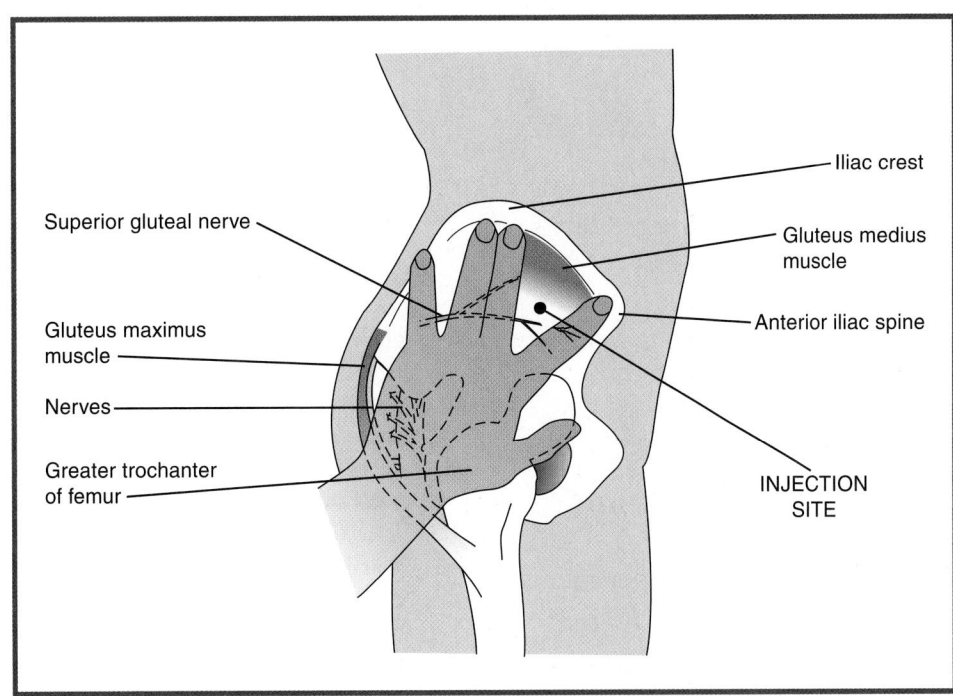

FIGURE 34-22 The ventrogluteal site can be used for most intramuscular injections.

TABLE 34-2 Parenteral Administration of Medication

ROUTE OF ADMINISTRATION	SITE	NEEDLE GAUGE	NEEDLE LENGTH (INCHES)	SYRINGE	DRUG AMOUNT	EXAMPLE DRUGS
Intradermal	Mid anterior forearm	27-28	3/8	1 mL; tuberculin	0.1 mL Allergy tests	Tuberculosis skin test (Mantoux)
Subcutaneous	Posterior upper arm, thigh, abdomen	25-26	1/2, 5/8	2-3 mL; insulin	Adult: 0.1 to 2 mL Child: 0.5 mL	Insulin Heparin Vaccinations
Intramuscular	Adult deltoid	20-23	1-3	2-5 mL	1-2 mL	Epinephrine
	Child deltoid	20-23	5/8-1	1-3 mL	0.5-2 mL	Hepatitis B Vitamin B$_{12}$ Antibiotics
	Adult vastus lateralis, dorsogluteal ventrogluteal	20-23	1-1½ 1-3 1-3	3-5 mL	2-5 mL	Penicillin Meperidine Morphine
	Infant or child vastus lateralis	22-26	5/8	1-3 mL	0.5-2 mL	Immunizations Antibiotics

PROCEDURE 34-11

Apply Pharmacology Principles to Prepare and Administer Oral and Parenteral (Excluding IV) Medications: Give a Z-Track Intramuscular Injection into the Dorsogluteal Site

CAAHEP COMPETENCIES: 3.b.(4)(g), 3.b.(4)(h), 3.c.(1)(a), 3.c.(2)(b), 3.c.(2)(c), 3.c.(2)(d)
ABHES COMPETENCIES: 1.d, 2.i, 2.k, 4.m, 4.n, 5.b

GOAL: *To inject 1 mL of medication into the muscle using a 23-gauge, 2-inch needle and 3-mL syringe and the Z-track method, as directed by the physician.*

EQUIPMENT and SUPPLIES

- Vial containing the ordered medication
- Alcohol wipes
- Cotton ball
- Disposable gloves
- Sharps container
- Sterile needle and syringe unit with safety needle cover
- Additional sterile needle
- Written order, including the patient's name, when to give the drug, the route of administration, and the name and strength of the drug
- Patient medical record

PROCEDURAL STEPS

1. Wash your hands. Follow standard precautions.
2. Select the correct medication from the shelf or the refrigerator.
3. Perform the three order and label checks as well as verifying the seven rights.
4. Warm refrigerated medications by gently rolling the container between your palms.
5. Draw up the ordered amount of medication into the syringe unit.
6. Replace the needle cover, and give a slight turn to loosen the needle. Secure a new needle, still in its sheath, to the tip of the syringe, being careful not to contaminate the needle or hub of the syringe. Discard the contaminated needle.
   PURPOSE: The needle that was used to withdraw the medication is covered with the drug that might be irritating to the skin and subcutaneous tissues.
7. Transport the medication to the patient.
8. Greet and identify the patient by name.
   PURPOSE: To be sure that you have the right patient.
9. Position the patient comfortably in Sims' position.
10. Expose the site, and apply gloves.
11. The dorsogluteal site is found by placing the palm of the nondominant hand on the greater trochanter of the femur, pointing your fingers toward the posterior iliac spine and index finger toward the anterior iliac spine. The injection site is in the upper outer area of the gluteus medius. Visualize the area for the Z-track injection.
12. Cleanse the patient's skin with the alcohol wipe, using a circular motion, moving outward from the center. Make sure to clean the actual area of injection.
13. Remove the needle cover.
14. Push the skin to one side, and hold it firmly in place. If the skin is slippery, use a dry gauze sponge to hold the skin in place.
    PURPOSE: Displacing the skin prevents medication from leaking back to the surface. This method is used for medications that irritate or stain surface tissues.

Continued

PROCEDURE 34-11—cont'd

15. Grasp the syringe as you would a dart, and with one swift movement insert the entire needle up to the hub at a 90-degree angle into the upper outer area of the gluteus medius muscle.
    PURPOSE: The depth of the injection is determined by the choice of needle length, not by how far you insert the needle. Once the needle is at the tissue layer, do not move the needle while injecting the medication. Being in as far as the hub helps to keep the needle in one place.

16. Aspirate: Withdraw the plunger slightly to be sure that no blood enters the syringe.
    PURPOSE: Blood in the syringe means that the needle is in a blood vessel and not in the muscle tissue. You may not administer an intramuscular medication by the intravenous route.

17. If blood appears, immediately withdraw the syringe, dispose of the syringe unit in the sharps container, and compress the injection site with a gauze square or cotton ball.
    PURPOSE: To minimize bleeding and bruising.

18. Begin again with step 1.
    PURPOSE: Blood is now mixed with the medication, and the medication is considered contaminated. Blood may interact with the drug and may be irritating to the intramuscular tissues.

19. If no blood appears in the syringe, push in the plunger slowly and steadily until all medication has been administered.

20. Wait 10 seconds for medication to be dispersed, then withdraw the needle at the same angle of insertion. As the needle is being withdrawn, release the displaced skin to prevent the tracking of medication to the surface.

21. If the manufacturer recommends it, gently massage the site with the gauze square or cotton ball. Many medications requiring Z-track administration should not be massaged.

22. Immediately place the safety needle cover over the contaminated needle and dispose of the needle and syringe unit into a sharps container.

23. Make sure your patient is comfortable and safe.

24. Dispose of gloves in the biohazard waste, and wash your hands.

25. Observe the patient for any adverse reaction. You may need to keep the patient under observation for 20 to 30 minutes.

26. Record the drug administration on the patient's medical record, including the exact site of injection.

See Appendix D for a charting example.

To locate the site, position the patient in Sims' position and place the palm of your hand on the greater trochanter of the femur, pointing your index finger toward the anterior iliac spine. Spread your middle finger back as far as possible from your index finger to form a triangular injection area. For a child, you will need a 1-inch needle, whereas in an obese adult patient, you may need a $2\frac{1}{2}$- to 3-inch needle to reach the depth of the muscle. Table 34-2 summarizes the details of parenteral administration of medication.

Z-Track Intramuscular Injection

Some IM medications are irritating to the skin and SC tissues or leak to the surface, staining surrounding tissues. These medications should be injected in such a way as to prevent any leakage back from the deep muscle into the upper SC layers. The Z-track method displaces the upper tissue laterally before the needle is inserted.

The medication is prepared according to safety guidelines, and gloves are donned. The site is palpated using anatomically correct markings, and the injection site is localized visually. The skin is pushed to one side and cleaned as described for IM injections. Then the needle is injected into the anatomically correct location and the medication is slowly released into the deep muscular tissue (Procedure 34-11). After the needle is withdrawn, the tissue is released so that the needle track is to the side of where the medication was deposited into the muscle. This process prevents a direct pathway to the surface for the medication, thus protecting the SC and surface tissues from the irritating and/or staining properties of the drug.

The medications for which Z-track injection is appropriate require a large muscle mass, so they should be injected only into the dorsogluteal site. Because the medication is so irritating to tissues, the needle should be changed after drawing up the medication from the vial and before drug administration to the patient. Some facilities require personnel to use the Z-track method when administering abdominal heparin injections because leakage of the drug at the site may cause localized bleeding. Although heparin is administered via an SC injection, the technique of pushing the surface tissue to the side before injection is the same.

Many medications that require the Z-track method (such as heparin) should not be massaged after injection because massaging will encourage the spread of the medication. Use alternate sides for multiple or frequent injections to prevent tissue damage.

PRINCIPLES OF INTRAVENOUS THERAPY

Administration of IV fluids or medication bypasses the absorption phase of pharmacokinetics because the fluid and/or medication is placed directly into the bloodstream. IV therapy is often the route of choice because the physician wants to speed up the action of a drug. After installation into a vein, the medication is quickly distributed to the target tissue by the circulatory system and, depending on the medication and its purpose, may start acting within seconds to minutes. This very quality makes IV drug administration the most dangerous route of administration; one minor mistake could be life-

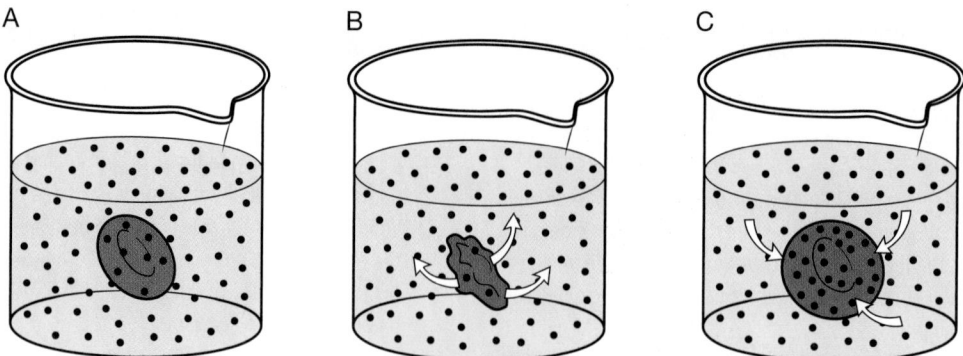

FIGURE 34-23 Basic types of fluids for IV therapy. **A,** Isotonic. **B,** Hypertonic. **C,** Hypotonic. (From Applegate E: *The anatomy and physiology learning system,* ed 3, Philadelphia, 2006, Saunders.)

threatening to a patient. Therefore state medical practice acts and individual healthcare facility policies strictly define the types of individuals who are qualified to perform IV-related procedures and administer IV medication. The medical assistant must be familiar with both legal restrictions and employer policies before having anything to do with IV therapy. However, whether you are responsible for IV therapy or not, you may work in a facility where patients have IV lines operating, so it is important that you understand some basic IV principles.

Intravenous Terminology and Practices

Administration of IV fluid is closely monitored by the physician to assist with maintenance of homeostasis. Three basic types of fluids are used for IV therapy (Figure 34-23):

- *Isotonic* solutions, such as 0.9% sodium chloride (also called *normal saline),* contain the same salt level as normal body fluids. Isotonic fluids are used for patients who need replacement of lost body fluids, such as patients with gastrointestinal disease or burns. If the patient needs glucose for nutrients, dextrose can be added in either water (D5W) or saline (D5NS) to meet the patient's caloric needs. Another type of isotonic IV solution is Ringer's lactate, which contains no dextrose (or calories) but provides electrolytes including sodium, potassium, calcium, and chloride ions.
- *Hypertonic* solutions contain higher concentrations of NaCl than those found in normal body fluids, causing extracellular fluid to shift from the cells into the bloodstream. For example, 3% or 5% NaCl solution may be used in a patient with extensive peripheral edema. The concentrated solution in the blood vessels will attract excess intracellular and interstitial fluid into the bloodstream to dilute the highly concentrated plasma. These solutions are helpful in decreasing edema but also may lead to increased pressure in the blood vessels from the increased volume of fluid and ultimately cause hypertension.
- *Hypotonic* solutions, including 10% dextrose in water (D10W) and 5% dextrose in 0.3% sodium chloride, contain less salt (sodium chloride or NaCl) than body fluids. Hypotonic IV fluids promote cellular hydration by shifting fluid from blood vessels into the interstitial

spaces surrounding cells and are administered to maintain fluid intake when the patient does not require electrolyte replacement.

The physician carefully prescribes the type of IV solution based on the systemic needs of the patient. It is crucial that anyone responsible for hanging, changing, or replacing IV fluids carefully follow the physician's orders to prevent serious complications for the patient.

Dangers of Intravenous Treatment

Infection or inflammation at the IV site and/or systemic infection may occur because of poor aseptic technique. Healthcare workers must be extremely careful when dealing with IV equipment or fluids, because material is being injected directly into the bloodstream.

Localized **phlebitis** may lead to clot formation at the site *(thrombophlebitis).* Local inflammation of the vein typically occurs because of poor aseptic technique when the IV is started or use of a contaminated bandage over the injection site. A vein may also become inflamed because of irritation from the IV solution or patient movement of the site. Signs of phlebitis must be reported to the physician immediately because it could lead to serious complications including *thrombus* formation and/or systemic infection. Indicators of phlebitis include inflammation, edema, warmth, and tenderness at the site; the vein feels hard and ropelike.

Fluid overload may be caused by too rapid infusion of the solution. It may cause serious complications in patients with hypertension, heart disease, or congestive heart failure.

Medication errors may occur. IV fluids and/or medication will circulate throughout the entire body within 1 minute after administration. It is not possible to take back an error in IV therapy.

Intravenous Equipment

The medical assistant may be asked to gather supplies for starting the IV infusion, so it is important that you be familiar with the various pieces of equipment that are needed. Whoever is starting the IV infusion must follow strict sterile technique. All IV infusion equipment is individually packaged and disposable. This equipment includes skin-cleansing solution;

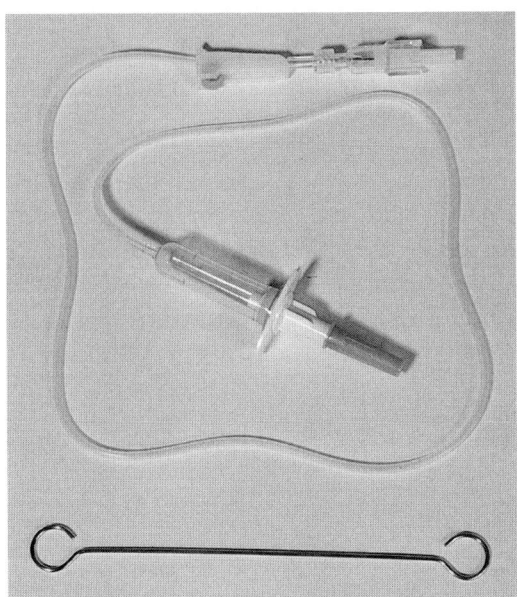

FIGURE 34-24 Intravenous administration set. (From Klieger DM: *Saunders textbook of medical assisting*, St Louis, 2005, Saunders.)

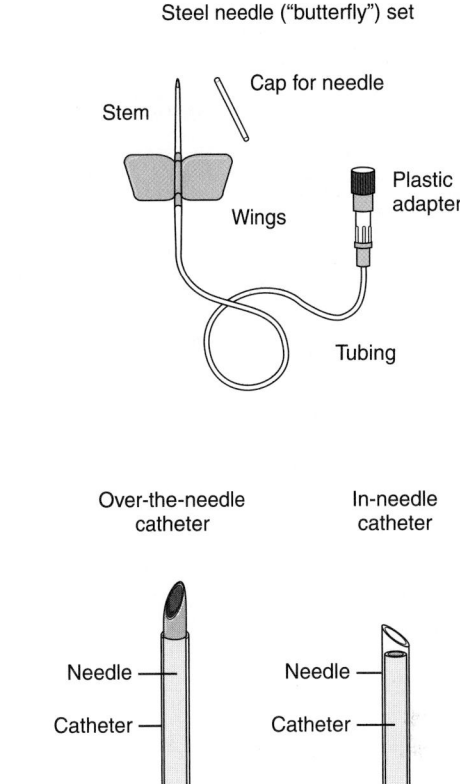

FIGURE 34-25 Intravenous cannulas: steel needle ("butterfly"), over-the-needle catheter, and in-the-needle catheter. (From Klieger DM: *Saunders textbook of medical assisting*, St Louis, 2005, Saunders.)

needle or catheter; tubing with a spike at the end to insert into the IV bag; dressings; and IV fluids. Typically everything you need except for the ordered IV fluid is packaged in a sterile IV infusion kit. Check the package for the desired needle and catheter gauge, infusion rate of administration, expiration date, and package integrity (if the package is moist or torn it is no longer considered sterile and must be discarded) (Figure 34-24). Additional supplies include a tourniquet, disposable gloves, biohazard waste container, and IV pole. Most ambulatory care facilities do not use infusion pumps, but one may be needed depending on your facility's practice.

Most infusion sets in ambulatory care settings contain butterfly infusion needles that have winged extensions for grasping during placement of the needle into the vein (Figure 34-25). They are available in a variety of gauges and lengths (25- to 17-gauge, 0.5- to 1-inch length) and are used for short-term IV administration, such as with a single dose of IV medication. The short, hard needle is relatively easy to dislodge from the vein when the patient moves, causing *infiltration* of IV fluids (IV fluid flows into surrounding tissues). Catheters are used if fluid administration is going to last longer than 24 hours. Over-the-needle catheters have a plastic sheath that covers the point of the needle. The needle serves as a guide into the vein, and after insertion the needle is removed leaving the soft, flexible catheter in place.

The physician prescribes a certain number of drips per minute of the IV solution depending on the patient's condition and reason for fluid administration. The macrodrip size, which delivers 8 to 20 drops/mL is used for adult fluid replacement, whereas the microdrip unit (50 to 60 drops/mL) is used for children and/or the slow administration of medications to patients of any age. The length of the IV tubing that connects the fluid bag to the venous catheter varies according to the patient's need for mobility and freedom. To prepare the solution

for administration, the spike at the end of the IV tubing is inserted into the ordered fluid bag. Just below the spike there is a drip chamber in the tubing that is an enlarged flexible plastic container that is squeezed so it fills partially with fluid. The drop orifice leading into the drip chamber determines the size of the fluid drops. The rate at which the drops fall into the chamber, and from there through the filled tubing into the patient, is regulated by compressing the roller clamp on the tubing until the number of drops per minute prescribed by the physician is dripping into the drip chamber (Figure 34-26). The distal end of the tubing is connected to the needle or catheter after the needle is in place and the tube has been filled with IV fluid so that all air bubbles are expressed. This step prevents the injection of air into the vein. If the patient is receiving medication, the IV tubing will have an injection port, which is a rubber extension to which either another IV bag of medication can be connected or through which the caregiver can inject medication by inserting a needle into the port.

Starting and Disconnecting an Intravenous Line

The procedure for starting an IV line is very similar to that for performing phlebotomy. The most common sites used are the veins in the forearm and the posterior hand. First the infusion fluid should be prepared by inserting the spike end of the tubing into the fluid that was ordered by the physician, being careful not to contaminate the equipment. It is important to completely fill the IV tubing with fluid so that all air has been

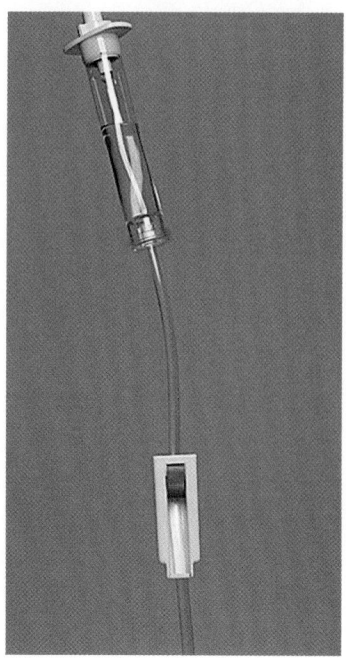

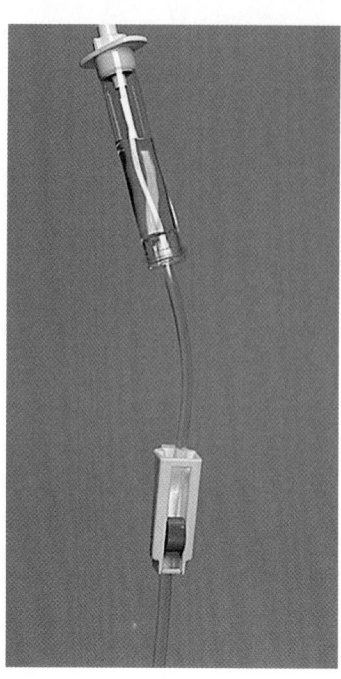

A   B

FIGURE 34-26 A, Roller clamp in the open position. **B,** Roller clamp in the closed position. (From Perry AG, Potter PA: *Clinical nursing skills and techniques,* ed 6, St Louis, 2006, Mosby.)

expressed. To do this, squeeze the drip chamber until it is filled about halfway, then remove the cover on the distal end of the chamber, release the sliding clamp, and run the fluid through the tubing to remove all air pockets.

Once all air bubbles have been removed, recap the tip of the tubing and clamp it tightly. Pick your injection site in either arm; open the appropriate infusion set, maintaining content sterility; apply gloves; and place the tourniquet several inches above the selected site. Prepare the site according to facility policy, anchor the desired vein with either your thumb or pointer finger on your nondominant hand, and insert the needle and catheter. Make sure there is blood return in the needle so you know you are in the vein. Untie the tourniquet, stabilize the needle, and attach the fluid-filled tubing. Secure the needle hub and tubing with tape, and apply a dressing. Open the clamp and adjust the number of drops per minute according to the physician order by rolling the clamp to occlude the tubing as needed.

After cleaning up used equipment and supplies, removing gloves, and washing hands, the final step is to document the details of the procedure. Documentation should include the type of IV fluid, the flow or drop rate, vital signs if assessed, and any adverse reactions. Monitor the patient periodically to assess for equipment problems, drip rate confirmation, and any signs of complications including inflammation, swelling, heat, infiltration, and/or elevated blood pressure.

When the desired fluid or medication infusion is completed, the IV system must be disconnected. To do this, apply gloves before clamping the IV tubing, carefully remove the dressing, and gently slide the needle and catheter out of the vein. Apply pressure to the site with a sterile gauze square to prevent the formation of a hematoma. Discard the contaminated materials in a biohazard waste container (the needle or catheter in a sharps container), and chart the completion of IV therapy.

Role of the Medical Assistant in Assisting with Intravenous Therapy

- Follow state practice acts; whether legal or not, the medical assistant should not perform any task unless he or she understands the principles behind the procedure and has the technical skill to safely perform it.
- Gather a comprehensive health history to determine indications for IV therapy.
- Weigh patient before and monitor vital signs during infusion to alert physician of possible complications; do not take blood pressure in arm with IV.
- Be alert for signs of infiltration and phlebitis.
- Monitor equipment for problems.
- Watch for the too rapid infusion of fluids, which might lead to circulatory overload.
- Document all pertinent information in the patient record.

CLOSING COMMENTS

Patient Education

It is extremely important that the patient receive instruction on how to take a prescribed drug and that he or she understands the medication's purpose. Ideally the patient is informed by the physician, but the medical assistant should be prepared to reinforce the physician's information or explain parts of the information that the patient did not understand. When a patient does not understand the need for the medication or the directions regarding how to take it, there is a greater risk that the medication will be taken incorrectly. As a result, the physician's orders will not be carried out, and the desired therapeutic effect will not be achieved. The patient should fully understand the type of medication, its route of administration, its desired effect, and the side effects that need to be reported if they occur.

If the patient receives medication in the physician's office, he or she should understand the expected results or possible side effects. For example, if a patient is given a diuretic in the office, he or she needs to know what the immediate effect is going to be. This prepares the patient for the urinary urgency and **polyuria** that will occur within a relatively brief period. When a pain medication is given, the patient should have full knowledge so that the possibility of personal injury can be avoided. Any medication given in the ambulatory care setting that affects the patient's ability to walk or drive must be used with caution. The patient must be able to get home safely, and if that is not possible then the medication should not be given.

The medical assistant should instruct the patient to take all of the medication prescribed. Often if a prescription is not completed the treatment objectives may not be achieved. Patients should also be instructed to take their medication in the time sequence prescribed. This keeps the optimal level of the drug circulating in the bloodstream.

When sample medications are dispensed in the office to the patient, the package contains inserts that can be helpful in education efforts. If there are certain parts of the inserts that the patient should review, highlight this information for quick reference. If the physician has specific written instructions for the patient to follow, read over the material with the patient before discharge so that any areas of confusion can be cleared up before the patient leaves the facility. Always remember that the more the patient knows and understands about how to take the medication and why it is prescribed, the greater the chances are that the patient will comply with medication therapy, and the more likely the drug treatment will be successful.

This would also be a good time to suggest that the patient check the status of medications at home. The National Association of Retail Druggists recommends that the medicine cabinet be checked once a month to determine the age and quality of medications. At that time the patient should dispose of any medications falling into the following categories:

- Medicines for past illnesses
- Any expired medicines, unidentified medications, or medications that are more than 2 years old
- Hydrogen peroxide that no longer bubbles or has changed color, ointments or salves that have separated or are crumbly, vinegar-smelling aspirin, antiseptic solutions that are cloudy or have a solid residue on the bottom, and any medicine of uncertain quality

The Association also suggests the following:

- Keep medicines stored away from light, heat, air, and moisture.
- Use medicine from the original container until it is completely used or expired.
- Do not combine medicines from several containers.
- Keep medicine locked away from children.
- Make sure that childproof medicine caps are used properly.

Legal and Ethical Issues

A medical assistant must be extremely knowledgeable when administering medications in the physician's office. Follow all physician orders exactly as written. If you have a question about the order, ask for clarification before you proceed. It is advisable to give a medication only after the order is written in the patient's chart. This helps eliminate errors and possible omissions in medication therapy.

Legal responsibilities in medication practice include prevention of error by carefully following safe practice procedures in pouring and administering drugs. Always implement the seven rights and perform the three drug order and label checks when dispensing and administering medications. Anyone administering a drug must know the possible serious complications related to the drug and be alert for side effects. The medical assistant must demonstrate compliance with individual state laws governing medications and their administration. Precise charting of the administration of medications as well as the management of prescriptions cannot be overemphasized.

The administration of drugs also involves ethical principles. The patient always comes first. With that foremost in mind, never risk giving an incorrect medication. There is no such thing as a small error, because any mistake may result in serious harm or possible death. If an error is made, it must be reported immediately to the physician so that measures can be taken to help the patient. It is difficult to admit that a mistake has been made, but it is absolutely necessary. For that reason, be sure to double-check your calculations with a co-worker or the physician before dispensing the drug. If a mistake is made, it must be completely documented, including the details of the error, to whom the error was reported, any action taken, and subsequent observations of the patient.

SUMMARY OF SCENARIO

Dorothy understands the importance of careful management of medications. Because of her concern for patient safety, she asks Dr. Thau to check all of her calculations and refers to the physician if she has any questions about medication orders or patient education. Because Dr. Thau is a primary care physician, it is important for Dorothy to understand the factors that affect the administration of medication to all age groups of patients. She routinely employs the standard three label checks when dispensing medications and implements the seven rights throughout medication administration procedures. Dorothy also recognizes the importance of complete and accurate documentation of medications, whether they are administered in the physician's office or as a prescription order. In addition, she consistently applies the rules of standard precautions when preparing and administering parenteral medications. Although as a medical assistant Dorothy cannot administer IV medication, she understands the principles of IV therapy just in case there is a patient in the facility who is receiving IV fluids or medications. All those administering a drug must know the possible serious complications related to the drug and be alert for side effects. The medical assistant must demonstrate compliance with individual state laws governing medications and their administration. Precise charting of the administration of medications as well as the management of prescriptions cannot be overemphasized.

SUMMARY of LEARNING OBJECTIVES

1. Define, spell, and pronounce the terms listed in the vocabulary.
   - Spelling and pronouncing medical terms correctly adds credibility to the medical assistant. Knowing the definition of these terms promotes confidence in communication with patients and co-workers.
2. Analyze safety guidelines for specific patient populations.
   - Safety precautions in the management of medication administration should be consistently applied. Safe drug administration includes understanding the physician order, looking up the drug if it is unknown, and using the three label checks and the seven rights every time a drug order is completed.
3. Perform documentation of medication administration.
   - Immediately after administering the drug, document date and time of administration; drug's name, strength, dose, and route of administration; patient reactions; and patient education regarding the drug. For parenteral medications, the exact site of administration must be charted.
4. Apply safety precautions to the management of medication administration in the ambulatory healthcare setting.
   - Perform the three label checks and seven rights routinely. Prepare medications in a quiet, well-lit area. Never substitute a drug or drug strength. Store medications as ordered on the package. Never administer a medication you have not personally prepared. If preparing a medication for the physician to administer, place the container with the dispensed drug. Follow only written physician orders. Check expiration dates, and discard expired drugs. Discard medications with damaged labels. Discard dispensed medication that is not given. Consistently ask patients about drug allergies. Observe patients at least 20 minutes after medication administration. Report and document drug reactions. Provide and document patient education about drug therapy.

5. Summarize patient assessment factors that have an impact on medication administration.
   - Patient assessment factors include the continual evaluation of the patient's physical condition as well as such holistic factors as the impact of the patient's history, an accurate list of drug allergies, the patient's ability to understand the drug regimen and to be able to afford the treatment, and special patient factors based on age, weight, and condition.
6. Identify various drug forms and their administration guidelines.
   - Drugs are packaged in a variety of forms, with a variety of administration guidelines. Oral medications include both solid and liquid preparations; mucous membrane medications are absorbed rectally, vaginally, orally, nasally, or topically through the skin. Each form of medication has specific guidelines for administration, but all require the consistent use of the three label checks and the seven rights.
7. Specify parenteral administration equipment including details regarding needles and syringes.
   - Parenteral medications are manufactured in ampules or single-dose or multidose vials. The ordered route of administration, drug characteristics, and individual patient factors determine the correct gauge and length of needle needed for administration. The appropriate syringe is determined by the type of medication ordered and the amount of drug to be administered. Specialty syringe units, such as the insulin pen and the EpiPen, are designed for the quick administration of certain medications. Tables 34-1 and 34-2 provide further details.
8. Employ OSHA guidelines in the management of parenteral administration.
   - OSHA guidelines include using syringe units with safety needle covers; wearing disposable, nonsterile gloves and other appropriate protective gear when administering any medication

Continued

SUMMARY of LEARNING OBJECTIVES

Continued

that involves coming into contact with blood or body fluids; never recapping a contaminated needle and immediately discarding it into a sharps container; disposing of contaminated nonsharp materials in biohazard containers; disinfecting contaminated work areas; and washing hands before and after procedures.

9. Describe and demonstrate parenteral administration types and locations.
   - Parenteral routes of administration include intradermal (ID), subcutaneous (SC), and a variety of intramuscular (IM) sites. The type of medication, the physician's order, and the unique characteristics of individual patients determine the route and site of administration. Each requires specific administration practices, which are described in Procedures 34-2 through 34-11.

10. Outline the principles of IV therapy.
    - IV therapy bypasses the absorption phase of pharmacokinetics because the fluid and/or medication is placed directly into the bloodstream. After installation into a vein, medication is quickly distributed to target tissue by the circulatory system and, depending on the medication and its purpose, may start acting within seconds to minutes. State medical practice acts and individual healthcare facility policies strictly define the types of individuals who are qualified to perform IV-related procedures. IV fluids are isotonic, hypotonic, or hypertonic. IV equipment

must be handled to maintain sterility. Starting an IV infusion is very similar to performing phlebotomy.

11. Recognize the role of the medical assistant in patient education for drug administration.
    - Patient education is absolutely crucial to the correct administration of medication by patients at home. The patient should understand the purpose of the drug; the time, frequency, and amount of the dose; any special storage requirements; and the typical side effects that occur. The more the patient knows and understands about how to take the medication and why it is prescribed, the greater the chances that the drug treatment will be successful.

12. Assess legal and ethical issues in drug administration in the ambulatory care setting.
    - The medical assistant must be extremely knowledgeable when preparing and administering medications in the physician's office. If there are any questions about the order, ask for clarification before proceeding. Legal responsibilities include the prevention of error by carefully following safe practice procedures in dispensing and administering drugs. The medical assistant must comply with individual state laws governing medications and their administration. Precise charting of the administration of medications as well as the management of prescriptions cannot be overemphasized.

CONNECTIONS

 Study Guide Connection: Go to Chapter 34 Study Guide. Read the Case Study and Workplace Applications and complete the assignments.

 CD Connection: Go to the Medical Assisting Competency Challenge CD and do the training activities under Patient Care and Diagnostic Testing. For a better understanding of the inflammatory response and controlling infection, view the animations for antibiotics and phagocytosis.

 Evolve Connection: For more information related to administering medications, go to evolve.elsevier.com/kinn and visit related weblinks for Chapter 34. Click on the Medical Assisting Exam Review and do the practice questions to sharpen your test-taking skills.

Assisting with Medical Emergencies

35

SCENARIO

Cheryl Skurka, CMA, has been working for Dr. Peter Bendt for approximately 6 months. During that time a number of patient emergencies have occurred in the office, and even more potentially serious problems have been managed by the telephone screening staff. Cheryl is concerned that she is not prepared to assist with emergencies in the ambulatory care setting. She decides to ask Dr. Bendt for assistance, and he suggests she work with the experienced screening staff to learn how to manage phone calls from patients calling for assistance.

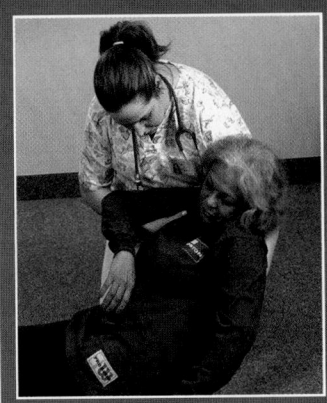

While studying this chapter, think about the following questions:

- What should Cheryl learn about the medical assistant's responsibilities in an emergency situation?
- What are some of the general rules for managing a medical emergency in an ambulatory care setting?
- What types of questions are asked by the phone triage staff if a patient calls with a medical emergency?
- What information from these phone calls should be documented?
- Is it important that Cheryl be able to recognize and be prepared to respond to life-threatening emergencies?

- What are some of the typical patient emergencies that occur in a healthcare facility?
- How should Cheryl instruct a patient to control bleeding from a hemorrhaging wound?
- Are there patient education areas related to common health emergencies that Cheryl should be prepared to share?
- What legal factors should Cheryl be aware of when handling ambulatory care emergencies?

LEARNING OBJECTIVES

1. Define, spell, and pronounce the terms listed in the vocabulary.
2. Describe the medical assistant's responsibilities in an emergency.
3. Identify supplies and equipment for emergency situations.
4. Demonstrate the use of an automated external defibrillator.
5. Summarize the general rules for managing emergencies.
6. Demonstrate screening techniques and documentation guidelines for ambulatory care emergencies.
7. Recognize and respond to life-threatening emergencies in the ambulatory care setting.
8. Perform adult rescue breathing and CPR.

9. Administer oxygen through a nasal cannula to a patient in respiratory distress.
10. Identify and assist a patient with an obstructed airway.
11. Determine appropriate action and documentation procedures for common ambulatory care emergencies.
12. Assist and monitor a patient who has fainted.
13. Control a hemorrhagic wound.
14. Apply patient education concepts to medical emergencies.
15. Discuss legal and ethical concerns regarding medical emergencies.

National Accreditation Competencies and Content

CAAHEP COMPETENCIES

Clinical
3.b.(4)(a). Perform telephone and in-person screening

General
3.c.(1)(d). Demonstrate telephone techniques
3.c.(2)(b). Perform within legal and ethical boundaries
3.c.(2)(d). Document appropriately

ABHES COMPETENCIES

Professionalism
1.d. Be cognizant of ethical boundaries

Communication
2.e. Use proper telephone techniques

Clinical Duties
4.e. Recognize emergencies
4.f. Perform first aid and CPR

Legal Concepts
5.b. Document accurately

VOCABULARY

asystole (ay-sis'-toh-le) The absence of a heartbeat.

bradycardia Slow heart rate; pulse is below 60 beats per minute.

cyanosis (si-an-oh'-sis) Blue color of the mucous membranes and body extremities caused by lack of oxygen.

dyspnea Difficult or painful breathing.

ecchymosis (e-ki-moh'-sis) A hemorrhagic skin discoloration commonly called *bruising*.

emetic (eh-met'-ik) A substance that causes vomiting.

fibrillation Rapid, random, ineffective contractions of the heart.

hematuria (hi-ma-tuhr'-e-uh) Blood in the urine.

idiopathic Pertaining to no known cause of a condition or disease.

mediastinum (meh-de-ast'-uhn-um) Space in the center of the chest under the sternum.

myocardium (my-oh-kar'-de-um) The muscular lining of the heart.

necrosis (neh-kroh'-sis) The death of cells or tissue.

photophobia Visual sensitivity to light.

polydipsia Excessive thirst.

polyuria Excreting large amounts of urine.

thrombolytics Agents that dissolve blood clots.

transient ischemic attack Temporary neurologic symptoms caused by a gradual or partial occlusion of a cerebral blood vessel.

First aid is defined as the immediate care given to a person who has been injured or has suddenly taken ill. Knowledge of first aid and related skills can often mean the difference between life and death, temporary and permanent disability, and rapid recovery and long-term hospitalization. The medical assistant may be responsible for initiating first aid in the office and continuing to administer first aid until the physician or trained medical team arrives. Every medical assistant should successfully complete a course for the professional in cardiopulmonary resuscitation (CPR) and should continue to hold a current CPR card as long as employed (see Procedure 35-2). Basic knowledge of CPR and life-support skills needs to be updated on a regular basis because of changes in procedures as new techniques are developed. For example, both the American Red Cross and the American Heart Association now recommend the inclusion of automated external defibrillator (AED) training for all healthcare workers (see Procedure 35-1). Medical assistants need up-to-date training in current emergency practices and should encourage

their local professional chapters to offer workshops on the management of emergencies in the ambulatory care setting.

Medical assistants are not responsible for diagnosing emergencies but are expected to make decisions regarding emergency situations based on their medical knowledge and training. If any doubt exists about how to manage a particular situation or emergency phone call, do not hesitate to refer to the physician, office manager, or a more experienced member of the healthcare team.

The Medical Assistant's Role in Performing Emergency Procedures

- Perform only the emergency procedures in which you are trained.
- If an emergency occurs in the office, notify the physician.
- If a physician cannot be located, contact the local emergency medical services (EMS) team.

MAKING THE FACILITY ACCIDENT-PROOF

Usually it is the medical assistant's responsibility to make the office as accident-proof as possible by keeping cupboard doors and drawers closed, wiping up spills immediately, and picking up dropped objects. All medications should be kept out of sight and away from busy patient areas; dangerous drugs should be kept in locked cupboards. If children are in the office, all sharp objects and potentially toxic substances must be kept out of reach. A medical assistant should never leave a seriously ill patient or a restless, depressed, or unconscious patient unattended.

PLANNING AHEAD

Every healthcare facility should have a standard policy with specific procedures for the management of emergencies on site. When starting a new job, part of the orientation process will be to review the site's policy and procedures manual. Be sure to clarify any questions you have regarding emergency management in that particular facility.

Staff members should discuss possible emergencies that may occur and have an emergency action plan for rapid, systematic intervention. For instance, local industries may present unique problems that call for very specialized care. Plan for these, and ask the physician's advice on what procedures to follow and what supplies to have on hand. If the facility has several employees, each should be assigned specific duties in the event of an emergency. Organization and planning make the difference between systematic care for the patient and complete chaos.

Using Community Emergency Services

Most communities have an emergency medical services (EMS) system. This system includes an efficient communications network, such as the emergency telephone number 911, well-trained rescue personnel, properly equipped ambulances, an emergency facility that is open 24 hours a day to provide advanced life support, and a hospital intensive care unit for the victims.

More than 100 poison control centers in the United States are ready to provide emergency information for treating victims of poisonings. Every healthcare facility is required to post a list of local emergency numbers. This list should be in plain sight and should be known to all office personnel. A good place to post this vital information is next to all of the phones in the facility. Include on the list the local EMS system, poison control center, ambulance and rescue squad, fire department, and police department numbers.

SUPPLIES AND EQUIPMENT FOR EMERGENCIES

Emergency Supplies

Emergency supplies consist of a properly equipped "crash cart" or kit of items needed for a variety of emergencies (Figure 35-1). The contents will vary to some degree according to the type of emergencies each office might expect to encounter. Emergency supplies should be kept in an easily accessible place that is

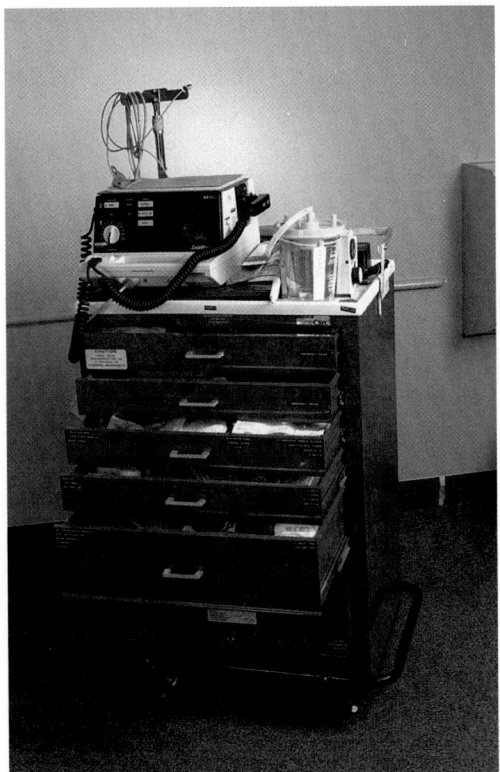

FIGURE 35-1 Office emergency cart with defibrillator. Drawers are marked for easy retrieval of emergency supplies.

known to all personnel in the office, with inventories of supplies completed on a regular basis. Expiration dates of medication and sterile supplies must be checked either weekly or monthly, along with the status of available oxygen tanks and related supplies, and the cart should be replenished with fresh supplies after every use.

Emergency pharmaceutical supplies should include certain basic drugs, such as epinephrine, which has multiple uses in emergency situations. As a vasoconstrictor, it controls hemorrhage, relaxes the bronchioles to relieve acute asthma attacks, and is an emergency heart stimulant used to treat shock. Epinephrine should be in a ready-to-use cartridge syringe and needle unit. These are supplied in 1-ml cartridges.

Additional drugs used are atropine, digoxin (Lanoxin), nitroglycerin (Nitrostat), and lidocaine (Xylocaine). Atropine decreases secretions, increases respiration and heart rate, and is a smooth-muscle relaxant. It is administered in a cardiac emergency for **asystole** or can be used to treat **bradycardia.** Digoxin is a cardiac drug that treats arrhythmias and congestive heart failure (CHF) and is good for emergency use because it has a relatively rapid action. Nitroglycerin is a vasodilator that is given to relieve angina. It acts by dilating the coronary arteries so an increased volume of oxygenated blood can reach the **myocardium.** Lidocaine is used intravenously to treat a cardiac arrhythmia and locally as an anesthetic, and sodium bicarbonate corrects metabolic acidosis that typically occurs after a cardiac arrest.

Emergency medicine supplies should also include an **emetic** such as syrup of ipecac, which causes vomiting soon after swallowing, as well as activated charcoal, an antidote that is swallowed to absorb ingested poisons. Narcan is a narcotic antidote that is administered intravenously for drug overdoses and acts to raise blood pressure and increase respiratory rate. In addition, antihistamines for the treatment of allergic reactions and anaphylaxis need to be available to treat potential allergic responses to medication administered in the facility. These include Benadryl for minor reactions and Solu-Medrol, a corticosteroid, for a severe anaphylactic response.

Other medications that may be found on a crash cart are isoproterenol (e.g., Isuprel, Medihaler-Iso, Norisodrine), an antispasmodic that is used to treat bronchospasms (such as those experienced during an asthma attack) and is also effective as a cardiac stimulant; metaraminol (Aramine) (50%, in a prefilled syringe) for severe shock; phenobarbital, amobarbital sodium (Amytal), and diazepam (Valium) for convulsions and/or sedative effects; furosemide (Lasix) for CHF; and glucagon, primarily used to counteract severe hypoglycemic reactions in diabetic patients taking insulin.

Defibrillators

The medical assistant may be required to assist the healthcare team with defibrillation of emergency patients. Defibrillation is indicated when a patient is in ventricular **fibrillation** (VF). VF is a severe cardiac arrhythmia that is caused by an uncoordinated, rapid firing of the electrical system of the heart, making it impossible for the ventricles to empty. In the absence of ventricular emptying, the patient has no pulse, the blood pressure drops to zero, and the patient could die within 4 minutes unless help is given immediately.

Defibrillators are devices that send an electrical current through the myocardium by means of hand-held paddles or self-adhesive pads applied to the chest. This electrical shock causes momentary asystole, giving the heart's natural pacemaker an opportunity to resume the heart rate at a normal rhythm. The AED has a computerized system that analyzes a cardiac rhythm and delivers voice-prompt instructions on how to operate the device (Figure 35-2 and Procedure 35-1). An AED uses self-

Basic Emergency Supplies

Equipment

- Adhesive tape in 1- and 2-inch widths
- Airways—variety of types and sizes
- Alcohol wipes
- Ambu bag with assorted sizes of facial masks
- Antimicrobial skin ointment
- Bandage scissors
- Cotton balls and cotton swabs
- CPR masks—both adult and pediatric
- Defibrillator
- Elastic bandages in 2- and 3-inch widths
- Filter needles
- Flashlight with batteries
- Gauze pads, 2- × 2- and 4- × 4-inch widths, and roller bandage—both sterile and nonsterile
- Gloves, sterile and nonsterile, in multiple sizes
- Hot and cold packs (instant type)
- Intravenous catheters, tubing, solutions (variety of types including D5W and Ringer's lactate), and tourniquet
- Laryngoscope with blades
- Lubricant
- Personal protective equipment (PPE), including impervious gowns, splash-guards or goggles, and booties
- Portable oxygen tank with regulator, mask, and nasal cannula
- Roller gauze (Ace bandages and gauze dressing) in various sizes
- Sharps container
- Sphygmomanometer—both pediatric and adult regular and large sizes
- Splints—various sizes
- Sterile dressings—miscellaneous sizes, including two abdominal pads

- Steri-Strips or suturing material
- Suction machine and catheters
- Syringes and needles in assorted sizes and gauges
- Tongue blades
- Tubex cartridge system
- Venipuncture supplies and butterfly units

Medications

- Activated charcoal, bottle of 30-50 g
- Amobarbital (Amytal)
- Antihistamine, injectable and oral
- Atropine
- Dextrose
- Diazepam (Valium)
- Digoxin (Lanoxin), injectable
- Diphenhydramine (Benadryl)
- Epinephrine (Adrenalin), injectable
- Furosemide (Lasix)
- Glucagon and/or glucose tablets
- Ipecac syrup
- Isoproterenol (Isuprel), aerosol inhaler and injectable
- Lidocaine (Xylocaine), injectable and spray
- Metaraminol (Aramine)
- Narcan
- Nitroglycerin tablets
- Phenobarbital, injectable
- Sodium bicarbonate, injectable
- Solu-Medrol
- Sterile water and saline for injection

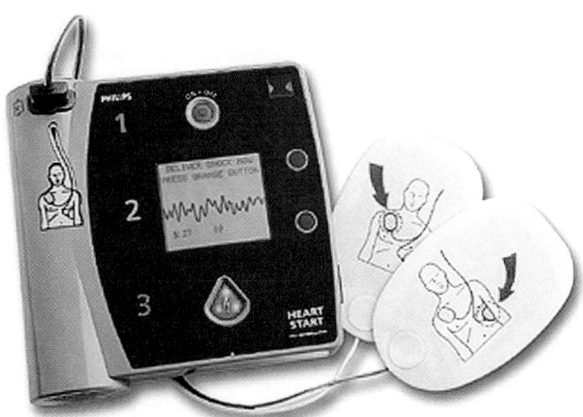

FIGURE 35-2 Fully automated external defibrillator. (From Aehlert B: *Mosby's comprehensive pediatric emergency care*, St Louis, 2005, Mosby.)

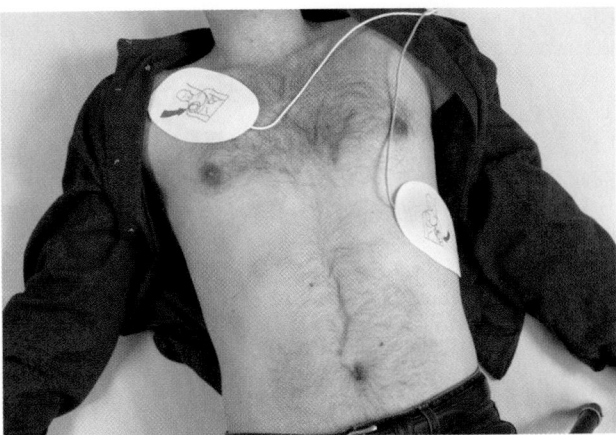

FIGURE 35-3 Connect the adhesive pads to the AED cables, then apply the pads to the patient's chest at the upper-right sternal border and the lower-left ribs over the cardiac apex. (From Chapleau W: *Emergency medical technician: making the difference*, St Louis, 2007, Mosby.)

adhesive pads that record and monitor the cardiac rhythm, and the device instructs the rescuer when to deliver the electrical charge. The apex-anterior position is the most commonly used paddle position, with the anterior (sternum) paddle or pads placed to the right of the upper sternum and the apex one under the patient's left nipple at the left mid-axillary line (Figure 35-3). For defibrillating a female patient, the apex paddle or pad is placed either next to or underneath the left breast.

Automated External Defibrillator Precautions

- Both patient and caregiver should not be in contact with any metal during defibrillation. Do not place the AED pad over jewelry, and remove patient's glasses to avoid injuries.
- A pediatric dose AED system should be used when available for children 1 to 8 years of age. These systems deliver a reduced shock dose for victims up to about 8 years of age or 55 pounds in weight.
- All clothing (including bras) must be removed; pads must be applied directly to the skin. If there is a great deal of hair on the chest, try to push the hair aside before applying the pads, or it may be necessary to shave the areas for complete paddle contact. The machine will prompt you by stating "check electrode" if the connection is poor.
- Make sure the patient is lying on a dry surface and that the chest is dry before applying the paddles, to avoid burns.
- If the patient has an implanted defibrillator or pacemaker it will be obvious from the bulged area under the surface of the skin on the chest. Apply AED pads at least 1 inch away from implants to avoid interference.

GENERAL RULES FOR EMERGENCIES

A medical assistant will face two types of emergencies in the ambulatory care setting: office emergencies and home emergencies. Common office emergencies and their management are discussed later in this chapter. Besides dealing with actual emergency situations on-site, a medical assistant is frequently the first person to interact with patients facing potential emergencies at home. It is estimated that one third of the telephone calls received in a physician's office are for some type

of problem that requires attention. An immediate decision must be made on how to manage that problem—by giving home care advice, scheduling an appointment, or in extreme emergencies notifying EMS personnel. When faced with an emergency, either on the phone or in the facility, the medical assistant should follow some general rules:

- It is most important to stay calm. Reassure the patient, and make him or her as comfortable as possible.
- Assess the situation to determine the nature of the emergency. Decide whether the need is immediate. This decision requires calm judgment and medical knowledge.
- Obtain as much information as possible to determine the appropriate action.
- Immediately refer any concerns to the office supervisor or physician.

Telephone Screening

Each time the phone rings in a healthcare setting there could be a potential life-or-death situation on the other end of the line. One of the most important tasks performed by medical assistants every day is answering the phones and managing patient needs efficiently and appropriately. *Triage* is the process of sorting patients, in this case patient phone calls, according to the patients' need for care. Emergency action principles serve as a guide for managing emergency phone calls in the ambulatory care setting:

- If the patient's situation is life-threatening, activate EMS/911.
  - *Never put the caller with a life-threatening emergency on hold, and always be the last to hang up.*
  - Remain on the line until help arrives and you have talked to EMS personnel.
- Immediately record the name of the caller and that of the patient, location, and phone number in case the connection is lost.
- If you are unsure how to manage the emergency situation, contact the physician.
- If the patient is referred to an emergency department (ED) or emergency room (ER), call the ER to notify them of the

PROCEDURE 35-1

Use an Automated External Defibrillator

<u>ABHES COMPETENCY:</u> 4.f.

GOAL: *To defibrillate adult victims with cardiac arrest. The majority of adult victims in sudden cardiac arrest are in ventricular fibrillation. Survival rates for victims with ventricular fibrillation are as high as 90% when defibrillation occurs within the first minute of collapse. Survival rates for cardiac arrest caused by ventricular fibrillation decrease by 7% to 10% with every minute that defibrillation does not occur.*

EQUIPMENT and SUPPLIES

- Practice automated external defibrillator (AED)
- Approved mannequin

PROCEDURAL STEPS (To be performed on an approved mannequin only)

If the healthcare worker witnesses a cardiac arrest, an AED should be used as soon as it is available. If an arrest is not witnessed, five cycles of CPR should be administered before using an AED. One cycle of CPR consists of 30 compressions and two breaths. When compressions are delivered at a rate of about 100 per minute, five cycles of CPR should take roughly 2 minutes.

1. Place the AED near the victim's left ear. Turn the AED on.
2. Attach electrode pads as pictured on the AED. Place electrodes at the sternum and apex of the heart. Make sure pads have complete contact with the victim's chest and they do not overlap (see Figure 35-3).
3. All rescuers must clear away from the victim. Press the ANALYZE button. The AED will analyze the victim's coronary status, will announce if the victim is going to be shocked, and automatically charges the electrodes (Figure 1*).
4. All rescuers must clear away from the victim. Press the SHOCK button if the machine is not automated. May repeat three analyze-shock cycles.
5. Deliver one shock, leaving the AED attached, and immediately resume CPR, starting with chest compressions.
6. After five cycles (about 2 minutes) of CPR, repeat the AED analysis and deliver another shock if indicated. If a nonshockable

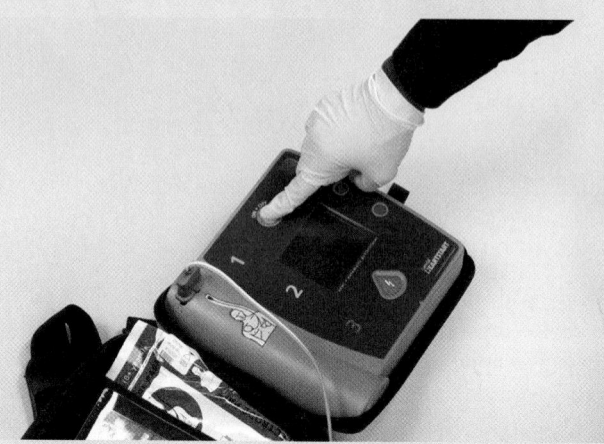

FIGURE 1

rhythm is detected, the AED should instruct the rescuer to resume CPR immediately, beginning with chest compressions.

7. If the machine gives the "no shock indicated" signal, assess the victim. Check the carotid pulse and breathing status and keep the AED attached until emergency medical services arrives.
   <u>PURPOSE:</u> Continue to monitor breathing and circulation because these can stop at any time. Keep AED pads in place to quickly diagnose ventricular fibrillation if it occurs.

*From Chapleau W: *Emergency medical technician: making the difference*, St Louis, 2007, Mosby.

---

patient's arrival and make a follow-up call to determine the patient's condition.

- Gather as much information as possible about what is wrong with the patient and when the problem started. Obtain details regarding the patient's condition, including:
  - Level of consciousness: Alert, responsive, lethargic, or confused? Did the patient lose consciousness at any time? If so, for how long?
  - Character of respirations (and pulse if the caller is able to determine this): normal, rapid, shallow, or difficult?
  - Is there bleeding? If so, how much, and from where?
  - Is there a suspected head or neck injury? If so, has the patient been moved? Is there a suspected fracture? Where?
  - Does the patient have a history of this problem?
  - Any other symptoms, such as fever, vomiting, diarrhea, or pain?

- Details regarding what has been done for the patient:
  - Medication: What, when? Dose, effectiveness? Current allergies?
- Thoroughly document the information gathered and any actions taken, including notification of EMS, whether the patient was sent to the ER or an appointment was scheduled, all home care recommendations, and whether the physician was notified and when.

Based on the outcome of the telephone interaction, a decision is made about when the practitioner will see the patient (Procedure 35-2). Emergency calls require either activation of EMS or immediate attention as soon as the patient arrives. Urgent calls require a same-day appointment if the patient has an acute condition or is in severe discomfort. This would include a young child with a high fever or a patient complaining of moderate to severe abdominal pain. The new patient will

PROCEDURE 35-2

Perform Telephone Screening and Appropriate Documentation

CAAHEP COMPETENCY: 3.b.(4)(a), 3.c.(1)(d), C.3.c.(2)(d)
ABHES COMPETENCY: 2.e., 5.b.

GOAL: *To asses the direction of emergency care and document information appropriately in the patient record.*

EQUIPMENT and SUPPLIES

- Note pad with pen or pencil
- Patient record
- Facility's emergency procedures manual
- Appointment book or program
- Area emergency numbers

PRACTICE SCENARIO

Cheryl is working with the phone triage staff when they receive a call from the mother of a 5-year-old patient; the mother reports that her son fell and cut his arm. What type of information should Cheryl gather about the injury? What action should be taken? How should the incident be documented?

PROCEDURAL STEPS

1. Stay calm and reassure the caller.
   PURPOSE: To enable gathering of accurate details regarding the patient's condition.
2. Verify the identity of the caller and the injured patient.
3. Immediately record the name of the caller and the patient, location, and phone number.
   PURPOSE: To be able to contact them if the connection is lost.
4. Determine if the patient's condition is life-threatening. Quantify the amount of blood loss, if the patient is alert and responsive, if breathing is normal. Notify EMS if necessary.
   PURPOSE: Immediately notify emergency services if the patient is in danger.
5. If EMS is notified, stay on the line with the caller until EMS personnel arrive at the scene.
   PURPOSE: Never break a phone connection in the case of a life-threatening emergency.

6. If emergency services are not needed, gather details about the injury to determine if the patient can be seen in the office or should be referred to an emergency room (ER). Consider the following questions:
   - Is there a suspected head or neck injury? Has the patient been moved?
   - Is there a possible fracture? If so, where?
   - Are there any other symptoms?
   - Is there anything pertinent in the patient's health history that would complicate the situation?
   - Has the caller administered any first aid? What?
7. Based on information gathered, determine when the patient should be seen in the office if he or she has not been referred to an ER.
   PURPOSE: The majority of emergencies would be scheduled for an immediate office visit. This may require altering the current appointment schedule.
8. At any point in this process, do not hesitate to consult the physician or experienced staff or refer to the facility's emergency procedures manual to determine how to manage the patient's problem.
9. Always allow the caller to hang up first, just in case more information or assistance is needed.
10. Document information gathered, actions taken or recommended, any home care recommendations, and whether the physician was notified.
    PURPOSE: To have a legal record of the management of the emergency and a comprehensive description of the patient's condition and recommended management.

See Appendix D for a charting example.

---

have to be worked into the day's schedule, which may cause a delay in currently scheduled appointments. Patients with other, less urgent problems can be scheduled for appointments within the next 3 to 4 days.

Management of On-Site Emergencies

An emergency can occur at any time to anyone. Always implement Occupational Safety and Health Administration (OSHA) standard precautions when at risk for coming into contact with blood and/or body fluids. When an emergency occurs, it is impossible to determine the level of infection. All body fluids must be considered infectious, and the appropriate

Documentation of an On-Site Emergency

1. Patient's name, address, age, and health insurance information
2. Allergies, current medications, and pertinent health history
3. Name and relationship of any person with the patient
4. Vital signs and chief complaint
5. Sequence of events, beginning with how the problem occurred, any changes in the patient's overall condition, and any observations made regarding the patient's condition
6. Details regarding procedures or techniques performed on the patient

precautions must be employed to prevent cross-contamination. If the situation is life-threatening, notify EMS and stay with the patient until you are relieved by the EMS provider or the physician. It is important to document all details regarding the incident in the patient record.

CRITICAL THINKING APPLICATION

Cheryl is working the front desk when a patient comes into the office limping, saying she fell in the parking lot and hurt her ankle. Role-play the situation with a classmate, and make a list of at least 10 questions Cheryl should ask the patient.

Life-Threatening Emergencies

If a patient in the facility exhibits any signs of nonresponsiveness, the clinician must be brought to the patient immediately. If there is no clinician in the facility, EMS should be activated. Even in situations in which a physician is present, the physician may order you to call 911 for immediate emergency care. Before beginning assessment of the patient, put on gloves, because any emergency situation may necessitate exposure to blood or body fluids.

Nonresponsive Patient

If the patient is nonresponsive, the physician must be notified immediately. The physician may instruct the medical assistant to activate EMS.

If a patient is able to talk to you, then you know that he or she has an open airway. If the patient does not respond to a simple question such as "Are you OK?" then gently shake the shoulder to check responsiveness. If the patient does not respond, then you must assume that the patient is unconscious. Immediately call for help and activate EMS if that is office policy.

Caring for a patient who is nonresponsive first requires assessing the patient's respirations to determine the presence of breathing. Perhaps when the patient collapsed, the tongue went limp and occluded the trachea. Just by changing the individual's position and opening the airway you may provide all the assistance the patient needs to breathe independently.

Position the patient on the back, and apply the head tilt–chin lift movement to open the airway. The tongue is attached to the lower jaw, so moving the jaw forward will automatically open the patient's airway. If there is a suspected head or neck injury, the neck should be manipulated as little as possible, so open the airway with the jaw thrust maneuver. Both of these actions relieve possible obstruction of the trachea by the tongue. Check for breathing by looking for a rise in the chest and either listening or feeling for air exchange (Figure 35-4). Breathing may suddenly cease for a variety of reasons, including shock, disease, and trauma. If no breaths are detected, artificial ventilation must be started immediately, because death may occur within 4 to 6 minutes. There should be barrier devices on hand for artificial respirations (Figure 35-5), which should be used if rescue breaths are required (Procedure 35-3).

After giving the patient two slow breaths, check for signs of normal breathing or movement. If there are still no signs of

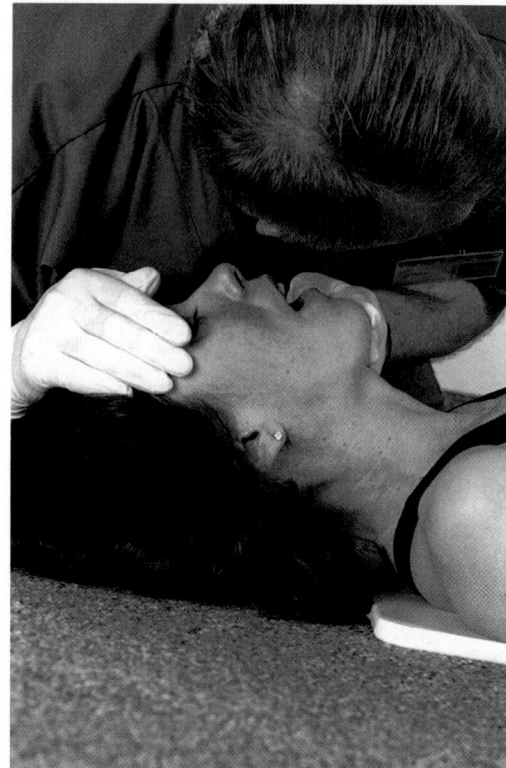

FIGURE 35-4 Checking for breathing in an unconscious patient.

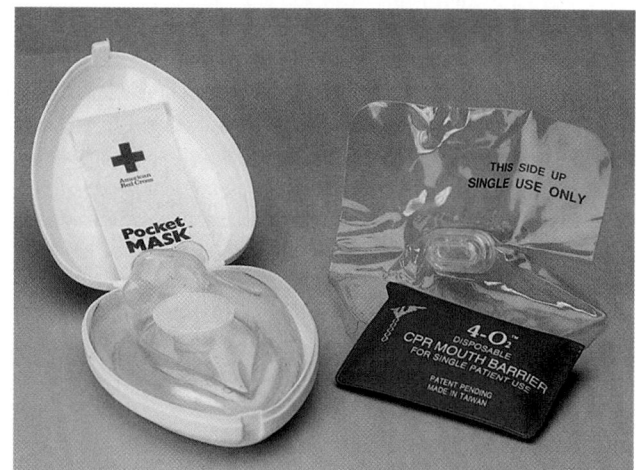

FIGURE 35-5 CPR mouth barriers.

responsiveness, check for cardiac circulation at the carotid pulse in the adult or child or the brachial pulse in the infant (Figure 35-6). Gently feel for the pulse while continuing to assess the patient for possible signs of recovery for 5 to 10 seconds. If the pulse is present, continue ventilating the lungs with slow breaths every 4 to 5 seconds in an adult or every 3 seconds in a child or infant. If the pulse is absent, begin cycles of 30 chest compressions followed by two slow breaths.

When both breathing and pulse stop, the victim has suffered sudden death. There are many causes of sudden death, including heart disease, choking, drowning, poisoning, suffocation, electrocution, and smoke inhalation. CPR must be started immediately in an attempt to revive the patient and

PROCEDURE 35-3

Perform Adult Rescue Breathing and One-Rescuer CPR

<u>ABHES COMPETENCY:</u> 4.f.

GOAL: *To restore a victim's breathing and blood circulation when respiration, pulse, or both stop.*

EQUIPMENT and SUPPLIES

- Disposable gloves
- CPR ventilator mask
- Approved mannequin

PROCEDURAL STEPS (To be performed on an approved mannequin only)

1. Establish unresponsiveness. Tap the victim and ask, "Are you OK?" Wait for victim to respond.
   <u>PURPOSE:</u> To determine whether the victim is conscious.

2. Activate the emergency response system. Put on gloves and get ventilator mask.
   <u>PURPOSE:</u> As soon as it is determined that an adult victim requires emergency care, immediately activate EMS. Most adults with sudden, nontraumatic cardiac arrest are in ventricular fibrillation. The time from collapse to defibrillation is the single most important predictor of survival.

3. Tilt the victim's head by placing one hand on the forehead and applying enough pressure to push the head back and with the fingers of the other hand under the chin, lift up and pull the jaw forward. Look, listen, and feel for signs of breathing. Place your ear over the mouth and listen for breathing. Watch the rising and falling of the chest for evidence of breathing (Figure 1*). If breathing is absent or inadequate, open the open airway and place the ventilator mask over the victim's nose.
   <u>PURPOSE:</u> To open the airway and determine if the victim is breathing.

4. Give two slow breaths (1½ to 2 seconds per breath for an adult and 1 to 2 seconds per breath for an infant or child), holding the ventilator mask tightly against the face while tilting the victim's chin back to keep the airway open (Figure 2*). Remove your mouth from the mouthpiece between breaths to allow time for patient exhalation between breaths.

5. Check the patient's pulse (at the carotid artery for an adult or older child or brachial artery for an infant). If a pulse is present, continue rescue breathing (one breath every 4 to 5 seconds, about 10 to 12 breaths per minute for an adult, or one breath about every 3 seconds, about 12 to 20 breaths per minute, for an infant or child). If no signs of circulation are present, begin cycles of 30 chest compressions (at a rate of about 100 compressions per minute for an adult) followed by two slow breaths.

6. To deliver chest compressions, kneel at the victim's side a couple of inches away from the chest. Move your fingers up the ribs to the point where the sternum and the ribs join in the center of the lower part of the sternum but above the xiphoid process.

7. Place the heel of your hand on the chest over the lower part of the sternum.

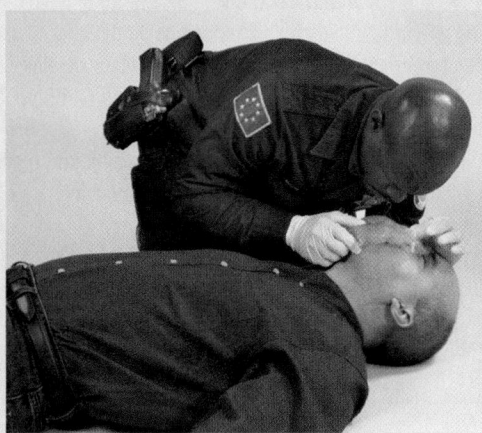

FIGURE 2

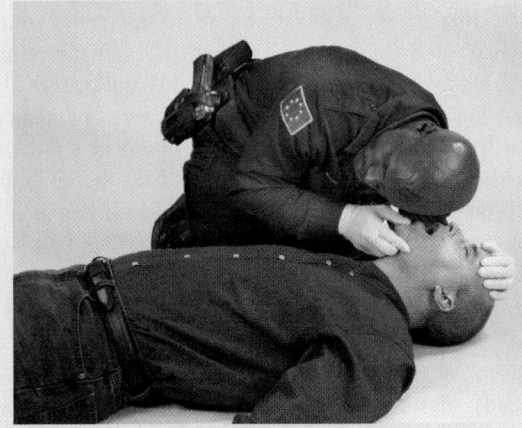

FIGURE 1

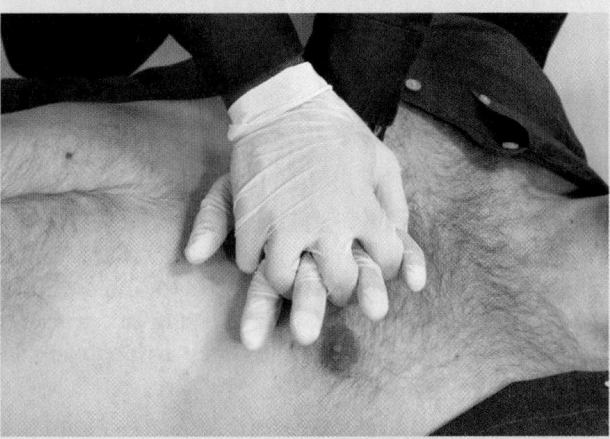

FIGURE 3

Continued

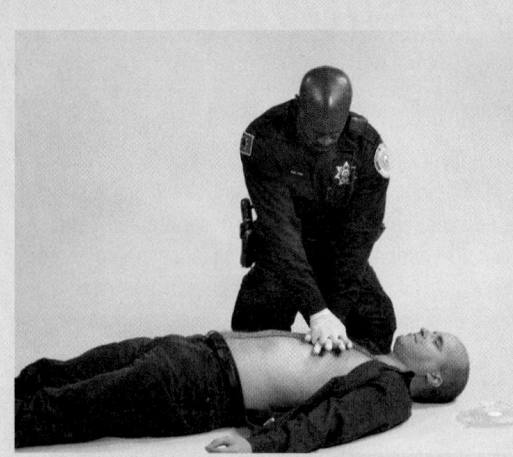

FIGURE 4

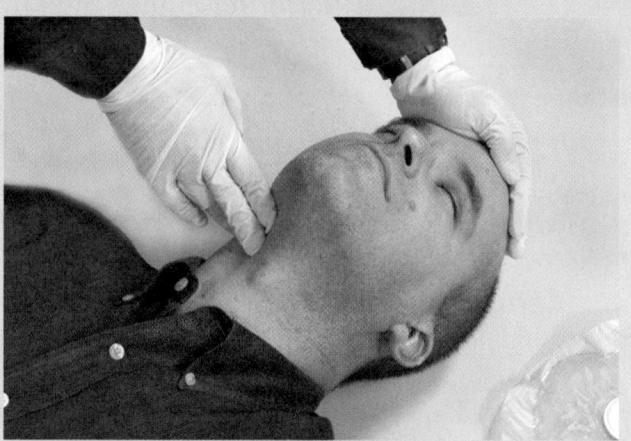

FIGURE 5

8. Place your other hand on top of the first, and either interlace or lift your fingers upward off of the chest (Figure 3*).
   PURPOSE: This position gives you the most control, allowing you to avoid injuring the victim's ribs as you compress the chest.

9. Bring your shoulders directly over the victim's sternum as you compress downward, and keep your elbows locked (Figure 4*).

10. Depress the sternum 1½ to 2 inches in an adult victim. Relax the pressure on the sternum after each compression, but do not remove your hands from the victim's sternum.
    PURPOSE: The depth of compression is needed to circulate blood through the heart. Movement of the hands may cause injury to the victim.

11. After performing 30 compressions (at a rate of about 100 compressions per minute), open the airway and give two slow rescue breaths.

12. After five cycles of compressions and breaths (30:2 ratio, about 2 minutes) recheck breathing and carotid pulse (Figure 5). If there is a pulse but no breathing, continue rescue breathing (one breath every 5 seconds, about 10 to 12 breaths per minute) and reevaluate the victim's breathing and pulse every few minutes. If no signs of circulation are present, continue 30:2 cycles of compressions and ventilations, starting with chest compressions. Continue giving CPR until an AED is available or EMS relieves you.

13. Remove gloves and the ventilator mask valve and dispose in the biohazard container. Disinfect the ventilator mask per manufacturer recommendations. Wash hands.

14. Document the procedure and patient condition.

From Chapleau W: *Emergency medical technician: making the difference,* St Louis, 2007, Mosby.

prevent permanent damage to body organs, especially the brain. After five cycles of compressions and ventilations in the adult patient, recheck the pulse. If no signs of circulation are present, continue CPR until help arrives. If there is a pulse but no breathing, continue rescue breathing and occasionally monitor the pulse until help arrives.

Refer to the American Red Cross *Standard First Aid Manual* or *American Heart Association CPR Manual,* or the organizations' websites for specific procedures and precautions in the management of respiratory and cardiac emergencies. As stated earlier, all healthcare workers must have current CPR Certification for the Professional.

Cardiac Emergencies

Chest pain or angina can be associated with heart and lung disease, as well as a few other conditions. It can be quite serious; a patient with chest pain is treated as a cardiac emergency until a physician has ruled this out. The patient is often sweating and may have a gray, ashen appearance. The lips and fingernails may be blue, which is a sign of **cyanosis** (Figure 35-7). Frequently the patient will clutch the chest in pain. This pain may radiate from the **mediastinum** down the left arm and up the left side of the neck. The pulse may be rapid and weak, and the patient often complains of nausea.

If a patient has any of these signs or symptoms, report this to the clinician immediately. If the physician is not available, activate EMS. Use a wheelchair to move the patient to an examination room. Breathing will be easier if the patient's head is slightly elevated or in Fowler's position. Keep the patient quiet and warm. Loosen all tight clothing. Take vital signs, including both apical and radial pulses. The physician may order oxygen started on the patient to relieve **dyspnea**

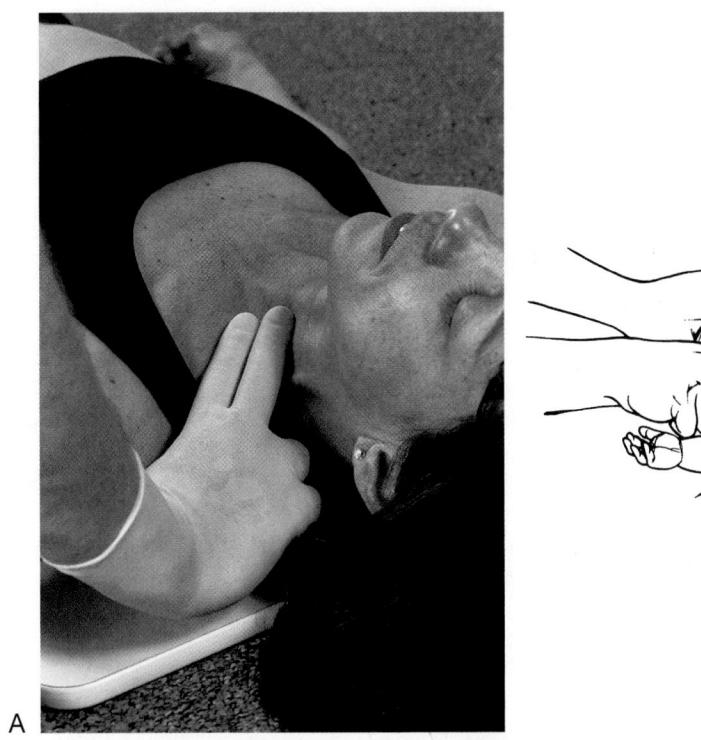

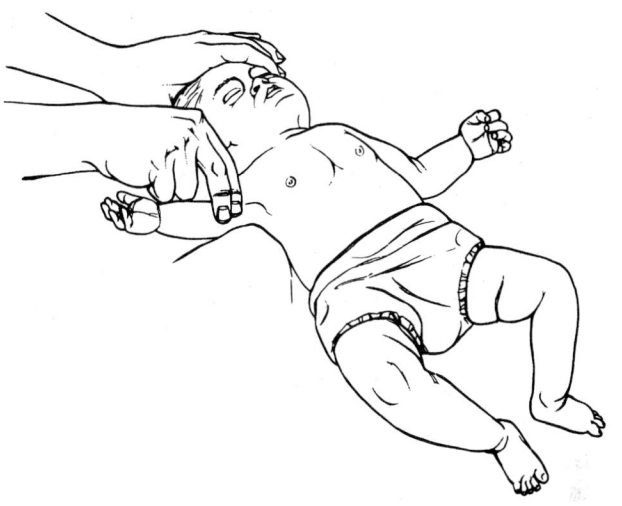

FIGURE 35-6 A, In an adult, check for carotid pulse. **B,** In an infant, check for brachial pulse.

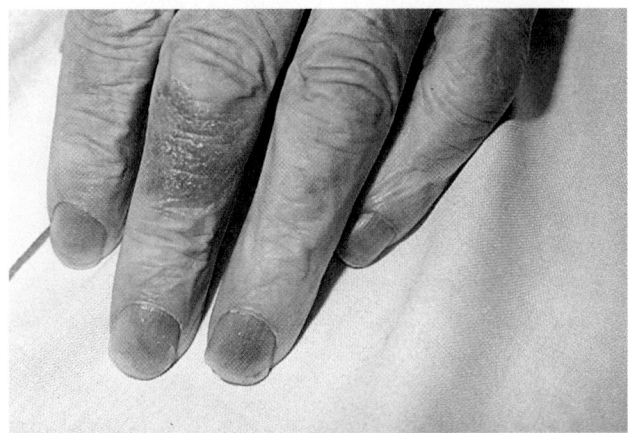

FIGURE 35-7 Cyanosis of nail beds. (From Henry MC, Stapleton ER: *EMT prehospital care*, ed 3, Philadelphia, 2004, Saunders.)

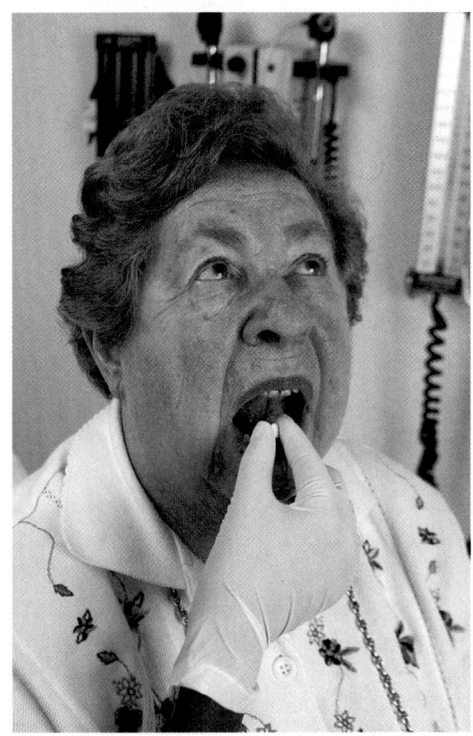

FIGURE 35-8 Nitroglycerin is administered beneath patient's tongue.

(Procedure 35-4). Bring the emergency cart into the room and open the medication drawer so the physician is able to quickly prepare the medications needed. These may include epinephrine (adrenaline), atropine, digitalis, calcium chloride, or morphine.

If the patient is conscious, ask about any medication that he or she has recently taken or is carrying. If the patient has an established heart disorder, the patient may be carrying nitroglycerin tablets. Nitroglycerin tablets are administered sublingually and may be given with the patient's consent (Figure 35-8). If the physician is in the office or is on the way, connect the patient to the electrocardiograph and record a few tracings. If the patient becomes unresponsive before the physician or EMS arrives, it may be necessary to start rescue breathing if there is no evidence of respirations. If chest pain progresses to cardiac arrest and loss of circulation, CPR must be performed until help arrives.

Signs of a Heart Attack

A heart attack, or *myocardial infarction*, is usually caused by a blockage of the coronary arteries that decreases the amount of

PROCEDURE 35-4

Administer Oxygen

ABHES COMPETENCY: 4.f.

GOAL: *To provide oxygen for a patient in respiratory distress.*

EQUIPMENT and SUPPLIES

- Portable oxygen tank
- Pressure regulator
- Flow meter
- Nasal cannula with connecting tubing
- Physician order
- Patient chart

PROCEDURAL STEPS

1. Gather equipment and wash hands.
2. Identify the patient and explain the procedure.
   PURPOSE: A nasal cannula is applied with a nasal prong in each nostril and the tab resting above the upper lip. Patients who will be using oxygen at home need to be taught how to open an oxygen tank or to use an oxygen compressor. It is vital that patients and their families understand the dangers of oxygen use in the home. They must avoid open flames and not smoke when oxygen is in use, because it is combustible. The physician will typically write an order for the number of liters of oxygen to be delivered and for home healthcare services to set up the equipment in the patient's home.
3. Check the pressure gauge on the tank to determine the amount of oxygen in the tank.
4. If necessary, open the cylinder on the tank one full counterclockwise turn, then attach the cannula tubing to the flow meter.

5. Adjust the administration of the oxygen according to the physician's order. Usually the flow meter is set at 12 to 15 liters per minute (LPM). Check to make sure oxygen is flowing through the cannula.
6. Insert cannula tips into the nostrils, and adjust the tubing around the back of the patient's ears (Figure 1).
7. Make sure the patient is comfortable and answer any questions.
8. Wash hands.
9. Document the procedure, including the number of liters of oxygen being administered and the patient's condition. Continue to monitor the patient throughout the procedure, and document any changes in condition.

See Appendix D for a charting example.

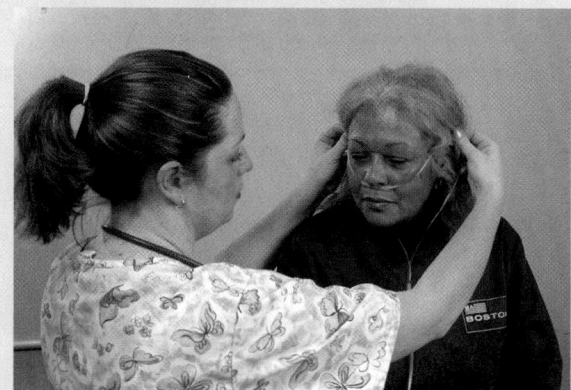

FIGURE 1

Signs and Symptoms of Myocardial Infarction in Women

Women may experience different symptoms than those traditionally associated with a heart attack. These include a combination of the following:
- Back pain or aching and throbbing in the biceps or forearms
- Shortness of breath (SOB)
- Clammy perspiration
- Dizziness (*vertigo*)—unexplained lightheadedness or *syncopal* episodes
- Edema—especially of the ankles and/or lower legs
- Fluttering heartbeat or tachycardia
- Gastric upset
- Feeling of heaviness or fullness in the mediastinum

blood being delivered to the myocardium. The most common signal of a heart attack is an uncomfortable pressure, squeezing, fullness, or pain in the center of the chest. This may spread to the shoulder, neck, jaw, or arms. The pain may not be severe. Other symptoms include sweating *(diaphoresis),* nausea or indigestion, shortness of breath (SOB), cold and clammy skin, and a feeling of weakness *(general malaise).* If these signs persist longer than 5 minutes, the patient should activate EMS. However, the vast majority of people will deny that the problem is serious until they require immediate medical attention.

Choking

Choking is usually caused by a foreign object, often a bolus of food, lodged in the upper airway. The victim may clutch the neck between the thumb and index finger (Figure 35-9). This universal distress signal should be viewed as a sign that the

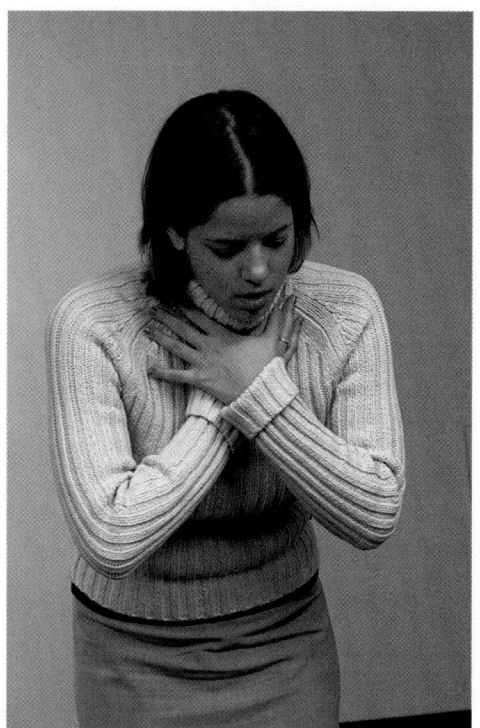

FIGURE 35-9 Universal sign of choking.

need help. If the patient is unable to speak, breathe, or cough, a complete airway obstruction exists and quick action must be taken to clear the airway. With a complete obstruction the patient will eventually lose consciousness from lack of oxygen to the brain. This condition may lead to respiratory and cardiac arrest. If the object is not removed, the victim may die within 4 to 6 minutes. Refer to Procedure 35-5 to learn the steps involved in clearing an obstructed airway on an adult. The procedure for removal of a foreign airway obstruction is exactly the same for a child over the age of 1 year.

To dislodge a foreign object from the airway of an infant up to age 1 year, place the baby face down over your forearm and across your thigh. The head should be lower than the trunk, and you should support the baby's head and neck with one hand. Using the heel of your other hand, deliver five blows to the back, between the infant's shoulder blades (Figure 35-10, A). Holding the baby between your arms, turn the infant face up, keeping the head lower than the trunk. Using two fingers, deliver five thrusts to the midsternal area at the infant's nipple line (Figure 35-10, B). Examine the infant's mouth, and if the object is visible, pluck it out with your fingertips, but never perform a finger sweep on an infant. A baby's oral cavity is too small for a finger sweep; such an action may only lodge the obstruction farther into the airway. If the obstruction is not visible, administer two rescue breaths by covering both the baby's nose and mouth with your mouth or use a pediatric ventilator mask if available. Repeat the sequence until the foreign body is expelled or help arrives.

It is possible to perform the abdominal thrust maneuver on yourself if you are choking and no one is nearby to help you. Press your fist into your upper abdomen with quick upward thrusts, or lean forward and press the abdomen quickly against a firm object, such as the back of a chair. In the case of a woman

victim needs help. If the victim has good air exchange or only partial airway obstruction and can speak, cough, or breathe, do not interfere but encourage the patient to continue coughing until the object is expelled. Monitor the patient for signs of respiratory distress, such as pallor and cyanosis. If the patient has a pronounced wheeze or a very weak cough, he or she has a partial airway obstruction with poor air exchange and may

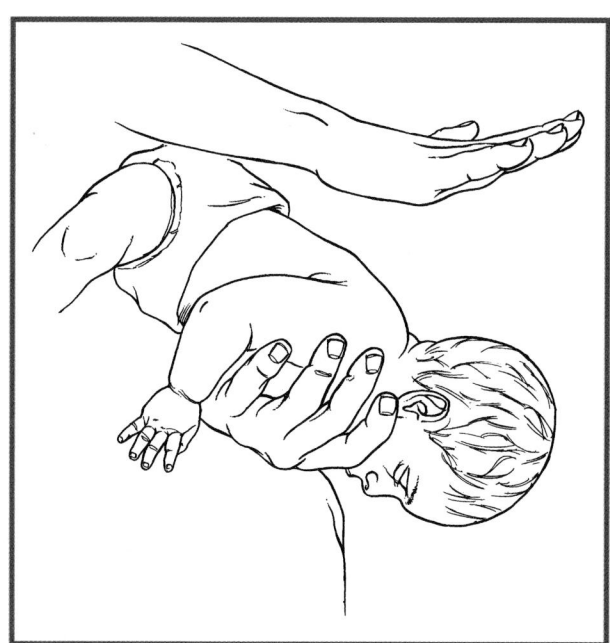

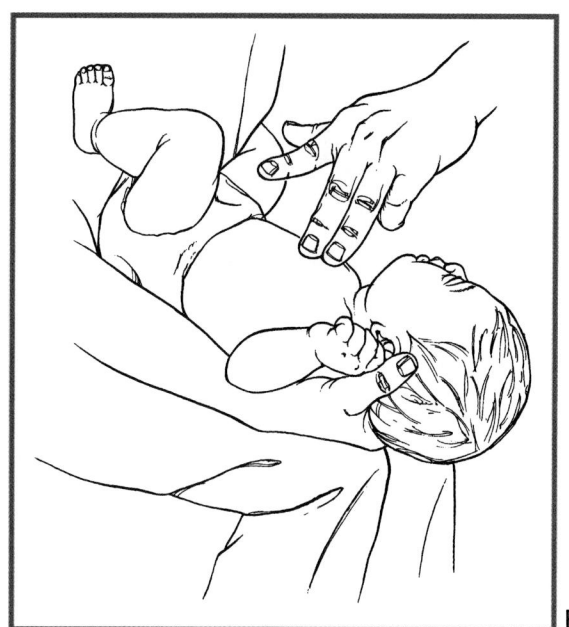

A   B

FIGURE 35-10 A, Back blows are administered to an infant supported on the arm and thigh. **B,** Chest thrusts are administered in the same position as for cardiac compressions. (From Henry MC, Stapleton ER: *EMT prehospital care*, ed 3, Philadelphia, 2004, Saunders.)

PROCEDURE 35-5

Respond to an Adult with an Obstructed Airway

<u>ABHES COMPETENCY:</u> 4.f.

GOAL: *To remove an airway obstruction and restore ventilation.*

EQUIPMENT and SUPPLIES

- Disposable gloves
- Ventilation mask (for unconscious victim)
- Approved mannequin to practice unconscious foreign body airway obstruction (FBAO)

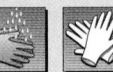

PROCEDURAL STEPS (Unconscious maneuver to be performed on an approved mannequin only)

1. Ask "Are you choking?" If victim indicates yes, ask "Can you speak?" If the victim is unable to speak, tell the victim you are going to help.
   <u>PURPOSE:</u> If the victim is unable to speak, is coughing weakly, and/or is wheezing, there is an obstructed airway with poor air exchange and the obstruction must be removed before respiratory arrest occurs.
2. Stand behind the victim with feet slightly apart.
   <u>PURPOSE:</u> With an obstructed airway, the victim may lose consciousness at any time. The rescuer must be prepared to safely lower the unconscious victim to the floor.
3. Reach around the victim's abdomen and place an index finger into the victim's navel or at the level of the belt buckle. Make a fist of the opposite hand (do not tuck the thumb into the fist) and place the thumb side of the fist against the victim's abdomen above the navel. If the victim is pregnant, place the fist above

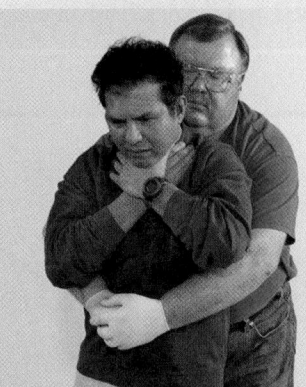

FIGURE 1

the enlarged uterus. If the victim is obese, it may be necessary to place the fist higher in the abdomen. It may be necessary to perform chest thrusts on a victim who is pregnant or obese.
<u>PURPOSE:</u> The fist should be placed in the soft tissue of the abdomen to avoid injury to the sternum or rib cage.

4. Place the opposite hand over the fist, and give abdominal thrusts in a quick inward and upward movement (Figure 1*).
   <u>PURPOSE:</u> Abdominal contents pushing against the diaphragm force trapped air out of the lungs and with it the obstruction.
5. Repeat the abdominal thrusts until the object is expelled or the victim becomes unresponsive.

UNRESPONSIVE ADULT VICTIM

6. Carefully lower the patient to the ground, activate the emergency response system, and apply disposable gloves.
7. Immediately begin CPR with 30 compressions and two breath cycles.
   <u>PURPOSE:</u> Higher airway pressures are maintained with chest compressions rather than abdominal thrusts.
8. Each time the airway is opened to deliver a rescue breath during CPR, look for an object in the victim's mouth and remove it if visible. If no object is found, immediately return to the cycle of 30 chest compressions.
9. A finger sweep should only be used if the rescuer can see the obstruction.
10. Continue cycles of 30 compressions to two rescue breaths until either the obstruction is removed or EMS arrives.
11. If the obstruction is removed, assess the victim for breathing and circulation. If a pulse is present, but the patient is not breathing, begin rescue breathing.
12. Once either the patient is stabilized or EMS has taken over care, remove gloves and the ventilator mask valve and dispose in the biohazard container. Disinfect the ventilator mask per manufacturer recommendations. Wash hands.
13. Document the procedure and patient condition.

*From Chapleau W: *Emergency medical technician: making the difference,* St Louis, 2007, Mosby.
See Appendix D for a charting example.

---

in the late stages of pregnancy, chest compressions should be delivered to prevent possible trauma to the infant.

Cerebrovascular Accident (Stroke)

A cerebrovascular accident (CVA), or stroke, is a disorder of the cerebral blood vessels that results in an impairment of the blood supply to part of the brain. This interruption in normal circulation of blood through the brain leads to some degree of neurologic damage, either temporary or permanent, depending on the severity of the oxygen deprivation to the brain cells.

A minor stroke or **transient ischemic attack** (TIA) usually does not cause unconsciousness, and symptoms depend on the location of the circulatory problem in the brain as well as the amount of brain damage. TIA symptoms are temporary and may include headache, confusion, vertigo, ringing in the ears *(tinnitus)*, temporary paralysis or weakness of one side of the body, transient limb weakness, slurred speech, and vision problems. TIA episodes indicate that the patient is at risk for a major stroke.

Symptoms of a major stroke include unconsciousness, paralysis on one side of the body, difficulty in breathing and swallowing, loss of bladder and bowel control, unequal pupil size, and slurring of speech.

Home recommendations for a patient who has suffered a major stroke should begin with notifying the physician and/or activating EMS. Keep the patient lying down and lightly covered. Maintain an open airway. Position the head so that any secretions will drain from the side of the mouth to prevent choking. If the patient did not fall and no indications of a head or neck injury are present, the patient can be placed in the recovery position, which uses gravity to drain fluids from the mouth and keep the trachea clear. Do not give the patient anything to eat or drink. Vital signs should be measured at regular intervals and recorded for the physician.

The recovery position is used as follows:

1. Place the patient on the left side. If the patient is lying on his or her back, raise the left arm above the head and cross the right leg over the left. Roll the patient toward you while keeping the head and neck in alignment.
2. Place the left arm behind the patient (similar to Sims' position).
3. Bend the right arm, and place the right hand under the side of the face.

Advances made in the early treatment of strokes show great promise in preventing long-term neurologic deficits. However, to prevent permanent brain damage, **thrombolytics** must be administered intravenously within 3 hours of the onset of symptoms. If a patient does not know when symptoms began, for example if he or she woke up with the symptoms, or if the patient cannot accurately tell the physician when the symptoms started, then the time allotted for administration begins from when the patient was last known to be asymptomatic. Intracranial hemorrhage must be ruled out before treatment begins. The earlier the treatment starts, the better the neurologic outcomes. The best possible outcomes are seen in those patients who received thrombolytic therapy within 90 minutes of the onset of symptoms.

CRITICAL THINKING APPLICATION

Thomas Antonio, a 67-year-old patient, calls to report that when he woke up this morning the left side of his face was drooping and he had difficulty seeing out of his left eye. The symptoms went away in about 2 hours, and he is feeling fine now. There are not any openings in the schedule for 2 days. When should Cheryl make Mr. Antonio an appointment? What questions should Cheryl ask Mr. Antonio?

Shock

Shock is a state of collapse resulting from failure of the circulatory system to deliver enough oxygenated blood to the body's vital organs. An injury, hemorrhage, infection, anesthesia, drug overdose, burns, pain, fear, or emotional stress may cause this

Types and Causes of Shock

- Anaphylactic—a severe allergic reaction
- Insulin—overdose of insulin causing severe hypoglycemia
- Psychogenic or mental—excessive fear, joy, anger, or emotional stress
- Hypovolemic or hemorrhagic—excessive loss of blood
- Cardiogenic—myocardial infarction, pulmonary embolism, or severe congestive heart failure
- Neurogenic—dilation of blood vessels resulting from brain or spinal cord injuries
- Septic—systemic infection

physiologic reaction. Shock can be immediate or delayed or mild or severe and is potentially fatal. Many different types of shock may occur, but the signs and symptoms are universal. The most common indicators of shock are a pale, gray, or cyanotic appearance; moist but cool skin; dilated pupils; weak and rapid pulse; marked hypotension; shallow and rapid respirations; lethargy or restlessness; nausea and vomiting; and extreme thirst.

If a patient exhibits signs of shock, maintain an open airway and check for breathing and circulation. Place the patient supine with the legs elevated approximately 1 foot to return the blood from the legs to vital organs. Loosen all tight clothing, and cover the patient with a blanket for warmth. Do not move the patient unnecessarily. Fluids may be given by mouth if the patient is alert. Because shock can develop into a life-threatening situation, it is advisable to administer only basic first aid care and to have the patient transported to the hospital as soon as possible.

COMMON OFFICE EMERGENCIES

The remainder of the chapter highlights typical emergencies seen either in the ambulatory care setting or in telephone triage situations. Table 35-1 summarizes common emergencies, the questions that should be asked, and possible home care advice.

Fainting (Syncope)

Fainting or *syncope* is a common emergency problem. Syncope is usually caused by a transient loss of blood flow to the brain, such as a sudden drop in blood pressure, which results in a temporary loss of consciousness. It can occur without warning, or the patient may appear pale; may feel cold, weak, dizzy, or nauseated; and may have numbness of the extremities before the incident. The greatest danger to the patient is an injury from falling during the attack. Therefore if the patient presents with syncopal symptoms, immediately place the patient in a supine position. Loosen all tight clothing and maintain an open airway. Apply a cold washcloth to the forehead. Measure the patient's pulse, respiration rate, and blood pressure, and report the findings to the physician. Keep the patient in a supine position for at least 10 minutes after consciousness has been regained. A complete patient history helps diagnose the possible

TABLE 35-1 Telephone Triage Approach

EMERGENCY SITUATION	SCREENING QUESTIONS	HOME CARE ADVICE
Syncope	Was the patient injured? Does the patient have a history of heart disease, seizures, or diabetes?	Does not necessarily indicate a serious disease. If injured from a fall, the patient may need to be evaluated and treated. The patient should get up very slowly to prevent a recurrence, take it easy, and drink plenty of fluids. If the patient is to be seen, someone should accompany him or her to the clinician's practice.
Animal bites	What kind of animal (pet or wild)? How severe is the injury? Where are the bites? When did the bite occur?	The health department or police should be notified. Every effort must be made to locate the animal and monitor its health. If the skin is not broken, wash well and observe for signs of infection.
Insect bites and stings	Does the patient have a history of anaphylactic reaction to insect stings? Does the patient have difficulty breathing, have a widespread rash, or have trouble swallowing?	If there is a history of anaphylaxis and the patient has an EpiPen, it should be administered immediately and EMS notified. Activate EMS if the patient is having systemic symptoms. An antihistamine (Benadryl) relieves local pruritus.
Asthma	Does the patient show signs of cyanosis? Has the patient used the prescribed inhalers?	If a patient with asthma is unable to speak in sentences, has poor color, and is struggling to breathe even after inhaler use, he or she should be seen immediately or EMS should be activated.
Burns	Where are the burns located, and what caused them? Are there signs of shock (moist, clammy skin, altered consciousness, rapid breathing and pulse)? Are there signs of infection (foul odor, cloudy drainage) in a burn more than 2 days old?	Activate EMS for burns on the face, hands, feet, or perineum, those caused by electricity or a chemical, or burns associated with inhalation. Activate EMS if there are signs of shock. The patient must receive a tetanus shot if it has been more than 10 years since the last one. Schedule an urgent appointment if signs of infection are reported.
Wounds	Is the bleeding steady or pulsating? How and when did the injury occur? Does the patient have any bleeding disorders or is the patient on anticoagulant drugs? Is the wound open and deep?	Pulsating bleeding usually indicates arterial damage; activate EMS. If the injury was caused by a powerful force, other injuries may exist. For patients taking anticoagulants or with diabetes or anemia, schedule an urgent appointment. A gaping, deep wound requires sutures.
Head injury	Did the patient pass out or have a seizure? Is the patient confused or vomiting? Is there clear drainage from nose or ears?	If the answer is 'yes' to any of these symptoms, EMS should be activated.

causes of the attack, such as history of heart disease or diabetes. Document the details of the episode and how long it took for complete recovery (Procedure 35-6).

If the patient does not recover quickly, the physician may activate EMS for transport to the hospital. Syncope might be a brief episode in the development of a serious underlying illness, such as an abnormal heart rhythm, that may lead to sudden cardiac death.

Poisoning

Poisonings are considered medical emergencies and are the sixth leading cause of accidental pediatric deaths in the United States. Poisoning can occur by oral intake, absorption, inhalation, or injection. Over-the-counter medications such as acetaminophen, detergents and bleach, plants, cough and cold medicines, and vitamins cause the majority of poisoning cases seen in young children. Other typical household poisons include drain cleaners, turpentine, kerosene, furniture polish, and paints (Figure 35-11). Signs and symptoms of poisoning vary greatly and include burns on the hands and mouth, stains on the victim's clothing, open bottles of medicines or chemicals, changes in skin color, nausea or stomach cramps, shallow breathing, convulsions, heavy perspiration, dizziness or drowsiness, and unconsciousness.

What to Ask When a Poisoning Is Reported

- The name, weight, and age of the victim
- The name of the poison taken and any information on the label
- How much was taken
- How long ago the poison was ingested
- Whether vomiting has occurred
- Any pertinent symptoms, such as difficulty breathing or an altered state of consciousness
- Any first aid given

PROCEDURE 35-6

Care for a Patient Who Has Fainted

ABHES COMPETENCY: 4.f.

GOAL: *To provide emergency care for and assessment of a patient who has fainted.*

EQUIPMENT and SUPPLIES

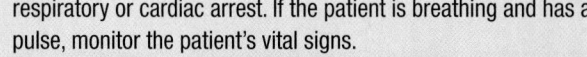

- Patient record
- Sphygmomanometer
- Stethoscope
- Watch with second hand
- Blanket
- Foot stool or box
- Pillows
- Oxygen equipment, if ordered by physician:
    - Portable oxygen tank
    - Pressure regulator
    - Flow meter
    - Nasal cannula with connecting tubing

PROCEDURAL STEPS

1. If warning is given that the patient feels faint, have the patient lower the head to the knees to increase the blood supply to the brain (Figure 1*). If this does not stop the episode, either have the patient lie down on the examination table or lower the patient to the floor. If the patient collapses to the floor when fainting, treat with caution because of possible head or neck injuries.

2. Immediately notify the physician of the patient's condition, and assess the patient for life-threatening emergencies such as respiratory or cardiac arrest. If the patient is breathing and has a pulse, monitor the patient's vital signs.

3. Loosen any tight clothing and keep the patient warm, applying a blanket if needed.

4. If there is no concern about a head or neck injury, elevate the patient's legs above the level of the heart using the footstool with pillow support if available (Figure 2*).
    PURPOSE: Elevating the legs will assist with venous blood return to the heart. This may relieve symptoms of fainting by elevating the blood pressure and increasing blood flow to vital organs.

5. Continue to monitor vital signs, and apply oxygen via nasal cannula if ordered by the physician.

6. If vital signs are unstable or the patient does not respond quickly, activate emergency medical services.
    PURPOSE: Fainting may be a sign of a life-threatening problem.

7. If the patient vomits, roll the patient on his or her side to avoid aspiration of vomitus into the lungs.

8. Once the patient has completely recovered, assist the patient into a sitting position. Do not leave the patient unattended on the examination table.

9. Document the incident, including a description of the episode, patient symptoms, vital signs, length of time, and any complaints. If oxygen was administered, document the number of liters and length of administration.

---

*From Bonewit-West K: *Clinical procedures for medical assistants*, ed 5, Philadelphia, 2000, Saunders.
See Appendix D for a charting example.

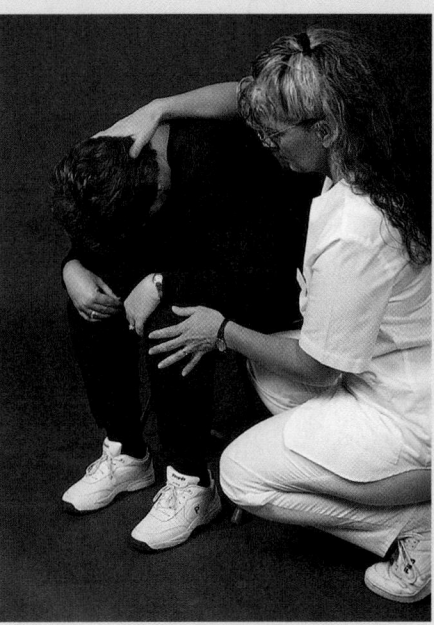

FIGURE 1

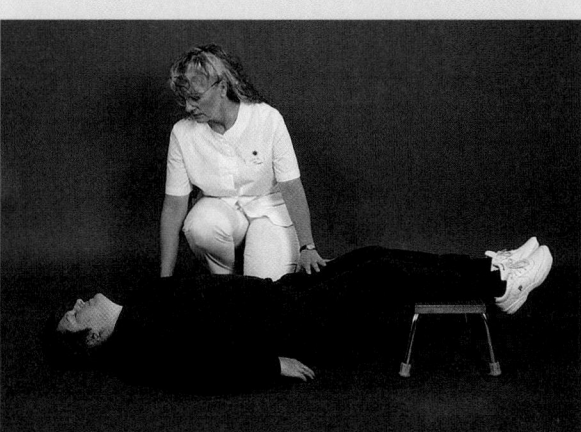

FIGURE 2

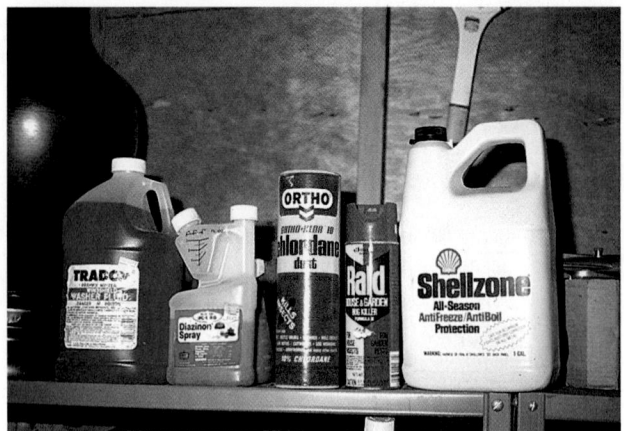

FIGURE 35-11 Hazardous household materials. (From Henry MC, Stapleton ER: *EMT prehospital care*, ed 3, Philadelphia, 2004, Saunders.)

Instruct the caller not to hang up and not to leave the victim unattended. Call the local poison control center, and forward all directions to the caller. Syrup of ipecac, which will cause vomiting within 15 to 20 minutes, should be used only if ordered by the physician or poison control center, because some substances can cause irritation to the tissues when vomited. Do not induce vomiting if the victim is either not alert or having a convulsion because of the risk of aspiration. If syrup of ipecac is recommended, give 2 teaspoons to infants 9 to 12 months old after the child has drunk about 4 oz of warm water. For a child 1 to 4 years old, administer 1 tablespoon after the child has drunk 4 to 8 oz of warm water. If the patient is to be seen by the physician or sent to the hospital, tell the caller to bring the container of poison or sample of vomitus with them so the chemical contents of the substance can be verified.

CRITICAL THINKING APPLICATION

A young mother calls in a panic to report her 18-month-old daughter swallowed at least half a bottle of cough syrup. The child is fussy and very sleepy, and the mother wants to give her ipecac immediately. What should Cheryl do?

Animal Bites

Potential complications from animal bites include rabies, tetanus, and local skin infections. Any animal bite that is extensive or deep should be seen by a physician. Human infection with rabies is rare, but if the bite occurs from a domestic animal, it is recommended that the animal be kept quarantined and under observation for 10 days to monitor for signs of the disease. The animal should not be killed, because a positive rabies identification is almost impossible to make if the animal has been dead for a period of time. If the bite is from a bat, raccoon, or any other wild animal, the animal is assumed to be rabid and the patient must undergo a series of rabies vaccine injections. Local skin infections can be prevented by immediately cleansing the area with antimicrobial soap and water. If the bite (including human) breaks the skin, the patient's tetanus immunization status must be checked and, if needed, a booster or the entire four-dose tetanus series must be administered as indicated.

Insect Bites and Stings

The bite or sting of an insect can be irritating and painful because of the chemical toxin injected from the insect, but it usually is not serious. Typical symptoms—inflammation, itching *(pruritus)*, and edema—are local and confined to the area of the bite. Rarely a severe allergic reaction occurs, which is a potentially dangerous situation that can lead to anaphylaxis. Signs and symptoms of a systemic allergic reaction include a dry cough, feeling of tightening in the throat or chest, swelling or itching around the eyes, widespread hives *(urticaria)*, wheezing, dyspnea, and hypotension. Difficulty in talking is a sign of urticaria or edema in the throat and may indicate the onset of complete airway obstruction. This is a sign of a true emergency. Epinephrine and oxygen should be ready for immediate administration on the physician's orders. Antihistamines may be used, as well as corticosteroids, but the action of these agents is considerably slower than that of epinephrine. If the patient develops acute anaphylactic shock, death may occur within 1 hour unless medical intervention is initiated.

If the stinger is still lodged in the skin, scrape it off with a dull knife, credit card, or fingernail. Be careful not to squeeze the stinger, because that will inject more venom into the skin. Apply an ice bag to the site to relieve pain and slow the absorption of the venom. Calamine lotion or hydrocortisone cream may be applied to relieve itching. If the patient has a history of allergies, especially to insect venom, he or she should have access to an EpiPen injection system and use it immediately after the sting occurs and should be transported to the nearest hospital for immediate care.

Tick Removal

Ticks can cause a number of diseases, including Rocky Mountain spotted fever and Lyme disease. They embed their heads in the skin to obtain blood and should be removed intact by the following method:

1. Do not handle ticks with uncovered fingers; use tweezers to prevent personal contamination.
2. Place the tips of the tweezers as close as possible to the area where the tick has entered the skin.
3. With steady slow motion, pull the tick away from the skin. Try not to squeeze or crush the tick. If the entire tick's body is not removed, make a physician's appointment to evaluate the site.
4. After removal, place the tick directly into a sealable container. Disinfect the area around the bite site using standard procedures.
5. The physician may suggest the tick be brought to the office to be tested for disease.

Asthma Attacks

Asthma is a condition characterized by expiratory wheezing, coughing, a feeling of tightness in the chest, and SOB. During an asthma attack two different physiologic responses occur. The lining of the respiratory tract becomes inflamed and edematous and produces mucus, which results in a narrowing of the air passages. At the same time, bronchospasms occur that also constrict the airways. The quality and severity of attacks vary greatly among patients, and treatment must be individualized to minimize or eliminate chronic symptoms. (Treatment of asthma will be addressed in Chapter 45.) If the patient is prescribed a bronchodilator inhaler, it should be used at the first indication of symptoms. Depending on the severity of the attack, give the patient an appointment for the same day of the call or consult the physician. The physician may recommend the patient go directly to the ER for emergency respiratory care.

Seizures

Seizures may be **idiopathic** or may result from trauma, injury, or metabolic alterations, such as hypoglycemia or hypocalcemia. A *febrile* seizure is transient and occurs with a rapid rise in fever over 101.8° F (38.8° C). Febrile seizures typically occur in children between 6 months and 5 years of age. Many different types of seizures occur, but they all are caused by a disruption in the electrical activity of the brain. The different types of seizures are discussed in Chapter 43.

If a patient suffers a grand mal seizure, which involves uncontrolled muscular contractions, the most important factor is protecting the patient from possible injury. Clear everything away from the patient that could cause accidental injury, and observe the patient until the seizure ends. Do not place anything in the patient's mouth, because it may damage the teeth or tongue. Do not hold the patient down, because that may result in muscle injuries or fractures. If the patient remains unconscious after the seizure has subsided, place the patient in the recovery position to maintain an open airway and allow drainage of excess saliva. After the seizure is over, let the patient rest or sleep, but never leave the patient alone. If the physician is not in the office, check the office procedure manual to determine how to manage the situation.

Call 911 for emergency assistance in any of the following situations:

- The patient has not regained consciousness within 10 to 15 minutes.
- The seizure does not stop within a few minutes.
- The patient begins a second seizure immediately after the initial one.
- The patient is pregnant.
- Signs of head trauma are present.
- The patient is a known diabetic.
- The seizure was triggered by a high fever in a child.

Abdominal Pain

Abdominal pain is a symptom caused by many different problems and may range from acute discomfort to life-threatening complications. The clinician should see every patient who reports abdominal pain; the question is how soon the patient should be seen. A patient with acute onset of severe and persistent abdominal pain, especially when this is accompanied by fever, should receive medical attention as soon as possible. Abdominal pain has a variety of causes, including intestinal infections, appendicitis, ectopic pregnancy, inflammation, hemorrhage, obstruction, and tumors.

Triage Guidelines for Assessing Abdominal Pain

- Investigate the presence of shock-related signs and symptoms—diaphoresis; cold, clammy skin; cyanosis or gray pallor; rapid respirations; altered state of consciousness.
- Is the pain severe and constant, or does it come in waves?
- Has the patient had any bloody or tarry stools?
- Is there a fever greater than 101° F?
- Could the patient be pregnant, or has she missed a menstrual period?
- Has the patient experienced continuous vomiting or severe constipation?
- Are there any urinary symptoms such as frequency, **hematuria,** or flank pain?
- Does the patient have chest pain, SOB, or continuous cough?
- Is there a history of serious illness such as diabetes, heart disease, or cancer?

Treatment in the ambulatory care setting depends on the cause of the pain; however, the medical assistant should observe the following general guidelines:

- Keep the patient warm and quiet
- Have an emesis basin available
- Administer nothing by mouth (NPO)
- Do not apply heat to the abdomen unless so instructed by the physician
- Administer analgesics as ordered
- Check and record the patient's vital signs, and follow the physician's orders

Sprains and Strains

Sprains are tears of the ligaments that support a joint, and *strains* are injuries to a muscle and its tendons. Both types of injury may also cause damage to surrounding soft tissue, blood vessels, and nearby nerves. With a sprain the victim develops edema and **ecchymosis** around the injury, and any movement of the joint, especially a twisting one, results in pain. There usually is no swelling or discoloration with a strain and only mild tenderness unless the injured muscle or tendon is used. Tendon strains and ligament sprains take several weeks to heal, whereas muscle tears usually heal in 1 to 2 weeks, because muscle has such a rich blood supply. Details regarding orthopedic injuries are discussed in Chapter 42. These injuries are treated by elevating the affected area and applying mild compression and ice. Swelling is reduced if ice is applied within 20 to 30 minutes of the injury. After 24 to 36 hours, alternately applying mild heat and ice is usually indicated. The patient may be advised to immobilize the part.

Fractures

A fracture is a break or crack in a bone and can result from trauma or disease. Fractures are very painful and affect the patient's ability to freely move the injured part. When a patient with a fracture is brought into the office, the medical assistant should make the patient as comfortable as possible. Place the patient in a position that does not place strain on the area. Notify the physician immediately, and proceed according to the orders given. Emergency treatment for fractures includes preventing movement of the injured part through splinting, elevation of the affected extremity, application of ice, and control of any bleeding. If a patient with an open fracture is seen in an ambulatory care setting, he or she should be transported to the ER. Fractures are discussed in more detail in Chapter 42.

Burns

Burns are among the most frequent causes of injuries in the United States. Burn injuries can result from flame, heat, scalds, electricity, chemicals, or radiation. The skin surface may be reddened, blistered, or charred. The depth and extent of burns are the major determinants in classifying the severity of the burn. The extent of the pain is directly proportional to the extent of the surface area burned, as well as the depth and nature of the burn.

To triage a burn injury, it is necessary to understand what caused the burn, its location and approximate size, the depth of the burn, and whether any additional injuries also occurred. The percentage of the body surface area burned can be estimated using the Rule of Nines (Figure 35-12). This is an assessment tool that helps caregivers make a quick calculation of the amount of burnt tissue. With the Rule of Nines, the body is divided into areas approximately equal to 9% of the total body surface area. When a burn victim is assessed, the affected regions are combined to estimate the total percentage of burned tissue. Partial-thickness burns over 15% of the total body surface and full-thickness burns of less than 2% can be treated in the

ambulatory care setting if the patient can be seen immediately. Patients with larger body surface area involvement or other complications should be immediately transported to a hospital, preferably one with a burn unit. A complete description of burns and their management is given in Chapter 37.

Lacerations

Lacerations are a common presentation in a primary care physician's office. A lacerated wound displays a jagged or irregular tearing of the tissues. The severity depends on the mechanism, site, and extent of the injury and the presence of foreign bodies or contamination in the wound. The injury that caused the laceration may also have caused damage to blood vessels, nerves, bones, joints, and organs within the body cavities.

When the patient arrives at the facility, apply gloves and notify the physician immediately. Have the patient lie down. Cover the injured area with a sterile dressing; use a dressing that is thick enough to absorb the bleeding (Procedure 35-7). Reassure the patient and explain your actions as much as possible. Ask the patient when he or she last received a tetanus inoculation, and record the date in the patient's record. If it has been more than 10 years, the physician will probably want a booster injection given.

Wounds that are not bleeding severely and that do not involve deep tissue damage should be cleansed with antimicrobial soap and water to remove bacteria and other foreign matter. If the laceration is extremely dirty, the physician may want the area irrigated with a sterile normal saline solution.

A butterfly closure strip may be used over small lacerations to hold the edges together. If the wound is superficial and has straight edges, it may be closed with a microporous tape (such as Steri-Strips), which eliminate the discomfort of suturing and suture removal. Other wound closure devices include Dermabond fluid, which forms a strong, flexible closure that is similar in strength to nylon suture material. It is very useful for the closure of simple lacerations in children and provides an antimicrobial and waterproof coating to the wound site that will last for several days even with repeated washing.

After the clinician has completed the wound closure, the medical assistant typically applies a sterile dressing to the site. The dressing will vary in size and thickness according to the wound. Various wound dressings and techniques for their application are discussed in Chapter 56.

Figure 35-13 shows a patient handout from an ER on potential danger signs as well as instructions for follow-up care. Patient education forms should be printed in different languages for non–English-speaking patients.

Nosebleeds (Epistaxis)

A nosebleed, or *epistaxis*, is a hemorrhage that usually results from the rupture of small vessels within the nose. Nosebleeds can be caused by injury, disease, hypertension, strenuous activity, high altitudes, exposure to cold, overuse of anticoagulant medications such as aspirin, or nasal recreational drug use. Bleeding from the anterior nostril area is usually venous while that in the posterior region is usually arterial and more difficult

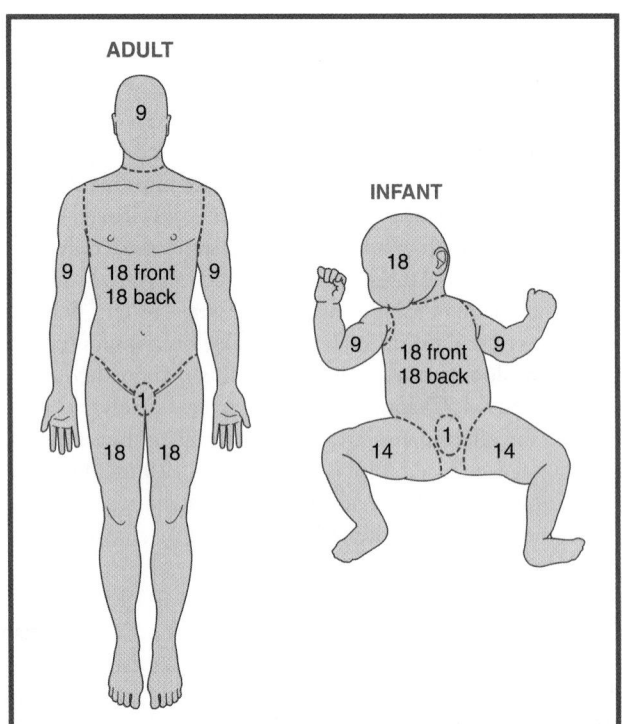

FIGURE 35-12 Rule of Nines classification of burns.

PROCEDURE 35-7

Control Bleeding

<u>ABHES COMPETENCY:</u> 4.f.

GOAL: *To stop hemorrhaging from an open wound.*

EQUIPMENT and SUPPLIES

- Gloves, sterile if available
- Appropriate personal protective equipment (PPE) according to OSHA guidelines including:
  - Impermeable gown
  - Goggles or face shield
  - Impermeable mask
  - Impermeable foot covers if indicated
- Sterile dressings
- Bandaging material
- Biohazard waste container
- Patient record

PROCEDURAL STEPS

1. Wash hands, and apply appropriate personal protective equipment.
   <u>PURPOSE:</u> To meet OSHA standard precautions.
2. Assemble equipment and supplies.
3. Apply several layers of sterile dressing material directly to the wound, and exert pressure.
   <u>PURPOSE:</u> Direct pressure to the wound will slow down or stop bleeding. Sterile supplies are needed to prevent wound infection.
4. Wrap the wound with bandage material. Add more dressing and bandaging material if bleeding continues.
5. If bleeding persists and the wound is located on an extremity, elevate the extremity above the level of the heart. Notify the physician immediately if bleeding cannot be controlled.
6. If bleeding still continues, maintain direct pressure and elevation; also apply pressure to the appropriate artery. If bleeding is in the arm, apply pressure to the brachial artery by squeezing the inner aspect of the mid-upper arm. If bleeding is in the leg, apply pressure to the femoral artery on the affected side by pushing with the heel of the hand into the femoral crease at the groin. If bleeding cannot be controlled, it may be necessary to activate the emergency medical system.
7. Once the bleeding is controlled and the patient is stabilized, dispose of contaminated materials into the biohazard waste container.
8. Disinfect the area, remove gloves, and dispose into biohazard waste.
9. Wash hands.
10. Document the incident, including the details of the wound, when and how it occurred, patient symptoms, vital signs, physician treatment, and the patient's current condition.

---

to stop. Treatment of epistaxis varies according to the amount of bleeding and the presence of other conditions or the use of anticoagulant medications.

If the bleeding is mild to moderate and from one side of the nose, the patient should sit up, lean slightly forward, and apply direct pressure to the affected nostril by pinching the nose. Continue constant pressure for 10 to 15 minutes to allow clotting to take place. Repeat if bleeding cannot be controlled, insert a clean pad of gauze into the nostril, and notify the physician. If the physician is not available, proceed with standard EMS protocols. Bleeding that is bilateral and continuous or in a patient with a bleeding disorder or on anticoagulant therapy should be considered a medical emergency.

Head Injuries

The severity of a head injury can vary greatly. The history of the injury–details about what it is and how it happened–is crucial for determining appropriate management. With a head injury, the patient may appear normal; may experience dizziness, severe headache, mental confusion, or memory loss; or may even be unconscious. The loss of consciousness may be brief or prolonged; it may appear immediately or may be delayed. The victim may experience vomiting; loss of bladder and bowel control; and bleeding from the nose, mouth, or ears. The pupils of the eyes may be unequal and nonreactive to light.

All head injuries must be considered serious. Notify the physician or contact EMS immediately. If there is evidence of neck injury, stabilize the neck and do not attempt to move the victim. Do not administer anything by mouth. Keep the patient warm and quiet. Watch the pupils of the eyes, and record any changes. Measure vital signs and record the extent and duration of any unconsciousness. If the patient is at home or is sent home after physician assessment, he or she should be watched closely for 24 hours after the injury for any change in mental status.

Foreign Bodies in the Eye

The eye is a delicate organ whose unique structure demands special handling. This kind of emergency is most uncomfortable, and it is often extremely difficult to keep the patient from rubbing the eye. Tell the patient not to touch the eye in any way. The physician may order ophthalmic topical anesthetic drops to relieve the patient's pain. The patient should be placed in a darkened room to wait for the physician, because **photophobia** is common with eye irritations. If a contusion and swelling are present, cold, wet compresses will help. Ask the patient to close both eyes and cover them with eye pads until the physician arrives. The physician may order an eye irrigation to remove the object. Unless the foreign object is clearly visible, do not attempt to search for it or to remove it. Eye care is presented in greater detail in Chapter 36.

LACERATIONS

What you need to know . . .

It is important to prevent infection and to allow your cut to heal. Call your doctor or return to him or her immediately if any of the "danger signs" occur.

Return for recheck in _____ days
Return for suture removal in _____ days

Danger signs to watch for . . .

1. Increasing pain, swelling, redness, and warmth in the injured area.
2. Pus in or around the cut.
3. Fever greater than 100°F (38°C).
4. Blood soaking through the dressing.

If any of these signs occur, contact your doctor or return to the Emergency Department.

What to do at home . . .

1. Take all medicines exactly as directed.
2. Raise the injured area above your heart level for 1 to 2 days.
3. Keep the wound and bandage clean and dry. For cuts on the face, a bandage is often not necessary. All finger dressings must be changed within 24 hours.
4. Remove the bandage/dressing in 24 hours.
5. After 24 hours, you may shower or bathe. Begin cleaning the wound with clear water twice each day to remove crusting and scabbing. Then apply ointment (Polysporin).
6. Prevent sunburn. Use a sunscreen for 6 months (e.g., Pre-Sun or Eclipse).
7. If you have a private doctor or are a member of an HMO (e.g., Kaiser), you should call for an appointment for your recheck and suture removal. If you can't get an appointment, you are welcome to return here to complete your care.

Please remember . . .

1. The exam and treatment you have just received are not intended to provide complete medical care. You need to call your doctor to schedule a follow-up visit.

2. The X-rays or ECG taken today will be reviewed by a specialist. If there is any change in your diagnosis, we will contact you.

FIGURE 35-13 Educational materials about lacerations for home care of a wound.

Heat and Cold Injuries

Exposure to extremes in temperature can cause minor to severe injuries. Heat injuries occur most often on hot, humid days and result in cramps, heat exhaustion, or heat stroke. Heat-related muscle cramps may be the first sign of *heat exhaustion*, which is a serious heat-related condition. Patients with heat exhaustion appear flushed and report headaches, nausea, vertigo, and weakness. *Heat stroke,* the most dangerous form of heat-related injury, results in a shutdown of body systems. Patients with heat stroke have red, hot, dry skin; altered levels of consciousness; tachycardia; and rapid, shallow breathing. This is a true medical emergency. If heat-related problems are recognized in the early stages and adequately treated, the patient does not usually develop heat stroke. Management of heat-related illnesses includes getting the person out of the heat; loosening clothing or removing perspiration-soaked clothing; and giving the person cool drinks if he or she is alert. An effective way to lower the victim's temperature is to apply cool, wet cloths and to fan the moist skin so heat is released from the body by evaporation.

There are two types of cold-related injuries: frostbite and hypothermia. *Frostbite,* which is the actual freezing of tissue, occurs when the skin temperature falls to a range of 14° to 25° F. Prolonged exposure of the skin to cold causes damage similar to a burn. The tissue may appear gray or white, be swollen, have clear blisters, or, in full-thickness frostbite, show signs of tissue **necrosis,** including blackened areas and severe deformity. The more advanced the frostbite, the more serious the tissue damage, and the more likely the body part will be lost. There is no feeling in tissue that is frozen, but as thawing occurs, the patient reports itching, tingling, and burning pain. Mild frostbite can be managed by applying constant warmth to the affected areas either by immersing the area in warm water (no warmer than 105° F) or wrapping it in warm, dry clothing. Friction should never be used, because this would increase tissue damage. If blisters have formed or if there is evidence of full-thickness frostbite, the patient should be transported to the nearest ER.

Hypothermia is a medical emergency that may result in death unless the patient receives immediate assistance. Systemic hypothermia occurs when the core body temperature, preferably taken with an Ototemp (tympanic thermometer), is less than 95° F. Signs and symptoms of hypothermia include shivering, numbness, apathy, and loss of consciousness. If hypothermia is suspected, activate EMS and care for any life-threatening conditions until help arrives. Remove the victim's wet clothing and wrap the victim in blankets while moving him or her to a warm place. If the victim is alert, give warm liquids and apply heating pads (using a barrier to avoid burns) to help slowly warm the core body temperature.

Dehydration

A person dehydrates when he or she excretes more water than is taken in. Dehydration can be a very serious health emergency, leading to convulsions, coma, and even death. Infants, young children, and older adult patients are at greatest risk for developing serious complications from dehydration. Severe dehydration may be caused by excessive heat loss, vomiting, diarrhea, or lack of fluid intake. Symptoms include vertigo; dark yellow urine or no urine output for 8 to 10 hours; extreme thirst; lethargy or confusion; and abdominal or muscle cramps. If the patient exhibits any of these symptoms and is not able to retain fluids, schedule an urgent appointment or recommend the patient be taken to the ER. Replacing lost fluids is vital, so the patient should be encouraged to drink water, tea, sports drinks, fruit juice, or Pedialyte.

Diabetic Emergencies

Diabetes mellitus is covered in Chapter 44. The disease is caused by either a malfunction in the production of insulin in the pancreas or an inability of the cells to use insulin. Insulin is required on the cellular level so that glucose can be used for energy. Two different diabetic emergencies are caused by either *hyperglycemia* (high blood glucose levels) or *hypoglycemia* (low blood glucose levels).

Insulin shock is caused by severe hypoglycemia, because the diabetic patient has taken too much insulin, has not eaten enough food, or has exercised an unusual amount. Signs and symptoms have a rapid onset and include tachycardia, profuse sweating (diaphoresis), headache, irritability, vertigo, fatigue, hunger, seizures, and coma. It is important to provide glucose immediately, preferably in the form of glucose tablets, because they have a known concentrated quantity of glucose.

Diabetic coma results from severe hyperglycemia, which develops because the body is not producing enough insulin; the patient ate too much food or is very stressed; or the patient has an infection. Symptoms of impending diabetic coma develop more slowly than those of insulin shock; these include general malaise, dry mouth, **polyuria, polydipsia,** nausea, vomiting, SOB, and acetone- or "fruity"-smelling breath. If the patient or caregiver calling for an appointment reports these symptoms, notify the physician immediately, because the patient would typically be admitted to the hospital.

In an emergency situation, if a patient who has been diagnosed with diabetes mellitus exhibits signs and symptoms of a diabetic emergency, the patient should be given glucose. If the problem is caused by insulin shock (hypoglycemia), the patient will improve quickly after receiving glucose; if it is caused by diabetic coma (hyperglycemia), a small amount of added glucose will not affect the patient's condition, and he or she will need to be transported to the hospital regardless.

CLOSING COMMENTS

Patient Education

Emergencies can occur anywhere. Patients need to learn how to handle emergency situations both by the example of healthcare workers and through instruction. The medical assistant must remain calm, triage the situation, call for help, and be prepared to administer appropriate first aid intervention. Brochures regarding home safety can be used to help educate patients about methods for avoiding accidents in the home.

All patients, even children, should understand how to contact EMS. This is especially important for families with members who have chronic diseases that are potentially life-threatening, such as heart conditions, severe allergic reactions, diabetes, and asthma. Patients should be encouraged to post emergency numbers, such as for the local EMS, poison control center, and their primary care physician, next to the telephone. Families with young children need to "childproof" their homes, being especially careful to keep potentially poisonous substances stored where children cannot get into them. "Mr. Yuk" stickers placed on poisonous containers can be an excellent educational tool for young children.

Remember to keep your American Red Cross and American Heart Association certifications current. Take advantage of community workshops to maintain and extend your skills. Post a list of community safety workshops in an area where it can be seen by patients, and encourage them to attend. Your participation in emergency care workshops and your encouragement to have others participate may help to save lives.

Legal and Ethical Issues

The medical assistant works in the healthcare environment as the physician's agent. Although you are responsible for your own actions, the physician is legally responsible for the care you administer to patients while working in the healthcare facility. You are responsible for knowing the limitations placed on medical assistants in your state and for strictly adhering to your employer's emergency care policies and procedures. Medical assistants are not qualified to diagnose a patient problem but are responsible for acting appropriately in a medical emergency. In addition to legal responsibilities, you have an ethical responsibility to your patients to provide the highest standard of care. Always act in the best interest of the patient, and never hesitate to ask the physician and/or office manager for immediate assistance when faced with a medical emergency.

Most states have enacted Good Samaritan laws to encourage healthcare professionals to provide medical assistance at the scene of an accident without fear of being sued for negligence. These statutes vary greatly, but all have the intent of protecting the caregiver. A physician or other healthcare professional is not legally obligated to give emergency care at the site of an accident, regardless of the ethical and moral considerations. Legal liability is limited to gross neglect of the victim or willfully causing further injury to the victim. As a caregiver, you are required to act as a reasonable person and cannot be held liable for personal injury resulting from an act of omission. Good Samaritan statutes provide for the evaluation of the caregiver's judgment but are only in effect at the site of an emergency, not at your place of employment.

If you have never been trained in CPR, you cannot be expected to perform the procedure at the emergency site. However, in many states a healthcare provider with CPR training and skills who is present at the scene can be declared negligent if cardiac arrest occurs and he or she does not administer CPR to the victim.

If the victim is conscious or if a member of his or her immediate family is present, obtain verbal consent to perform emergency care. Consent is implied if the patient is unconscious and no family member is present.

Many types of emergencies can be handled in the physician's office. In an emergency situation, decisions that must be made quickly can determine whether the patient lives. A medical assistant must be prepared to act calmly and efficiently in all emergency situations.

SUMMARY OF SCENARIO

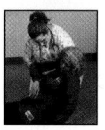

Cheryl has learned through her work with the triage team and involvement with emergencies in the office how important it is to gather complete information about emergency situations as well as to act calmly and knowledgeably when managing patient problems. She knows she must maintain her certification in CPR for the Professional and continue to participate in workshops on emergency care to be prepared for the wide variety of patient problems seen in the ambulatory care setting. Working with the screening staff has also reinforced the need to document all interactions on the telephone as well as information gathered during patient visits. Cheryl recognizes that medical assistants in the office must follow the facility's policy and procedure manual for handling emergencies, plan ahead and complete her designated duties if an emergency occurs, use community emergency services as needed, and keep emergency supplies and equipment well stocked and ready for any potential emergency situation. She recognizes that understanding first aid practices for common patient emergencies allows her to assist patients either through instruction by phone or by performing specific skills when emergencies occur in the facility. Cheryl has investigated her legal standing as a medical assistant in her home state and recognizes her responsibilities when a patient either calls or shows up at the office with a medical emergency. She will continue to refer to the more experienced screening staff or Dr. Bendt when she has questions, but she now feels more confident in managing emergency situations at work.

SUMMARY of LEARNING OBJECTIVES

1. Define, spell, and pronounce the terms listed in the vocabulary.
   - Spelling and pronouncing medical terms correctly adds credibility to the medical assistant. Knowing the definition of these terms promotes confidence in communication with patients and co-workers.
2. Describe the medical assistant's responsibilities in an emergency.
   - A medical assistant should be familiar with the healthcare facility's policy and procedures on the management of emergencies and must maintain certification in CPR. Perform only the procedures in which you are trained, always notify the physician or activate EMS if the physician is unavailable. The medical assistant must make sure the facility is accident-proof to prevent patient injuries on site, participate in planning for emergency situations, and post emergency telephone numbers for reference during an emergency.
3. Identify supplies and equipment for emergency situations.

   - A physician's office must have a centrally located crash cart or emergency bag for all emergency supplies, equipment, and medication. This material must be consistently inventoried and maintained. The chapter provides a detailed list of materials that should be readily available for an on-site emergency, including a defibrillator if indicated by the physician's practice.
4. Demonstrate the use of an automated external defibrillator.
   - Procedure 35-1 describes the use of an AED.
5. Summarize the general rules for managing emergencies.
   - Managing emergencies requires a calm, efficient approach to the situation. Assess the nature of the emergency and determine whether EMS should be activated or whether the patient requires an immediate or urgent appointment. Gather as many details as possible about the situation, and refer to the physician when in doubt.

Continued

SUMMARY of LEARNING OBJECTIVES
Continued

6. Demonstrate screening techniques and documentation guidelines for ambulatory care emergencies.
   - Telephone screening is one of a medical assistant's most important tasks. Emergency action principles should be used to determine the level of a patient's emergency. These include determining whether the situation is life-threatening and obtaining the patient's contact information as well as all pertinent information regarding the injury and patient signs and symptoms. This information must be shared with the physician, and all details must be documented in the patient's chart.

7. Recognize and respond to life-threatening emergencies in the ambulatory care setting.
   - Life-threatening emergencies require immediate assessment, referral to the physician, and, if the physician is not present, activation of EMS. While waiting for assistance, determine the presence of breathing and circulation. Administer rescue breaths or CPR if indicated. Depending on the patient's signs and symptoms, monitor the patient for signs of a heart attack; administer the Heimlich maneuver if there is an obstructed airway; evaluate for signs of a CVA; and assess for shock. Ask for assistance when indicated, and perform appropriate skills based on the patient's presenting condition.

8. Perform adult rescue breathing and CPR.
   - Procedure 35-3 describes how to perform adult rescue breathing and CPR.

9. Administer oxygen through a nasal cannula to a patient in respiratory distress.
   - Procedure 35-4 describes how to administer oxygen with a nasal cannula.

10. Identify and assist a patient with an obstructed airway.
    - Procedure 35-5 demonstrates how to respond to and assist an adult with an obstructed airway. Infants with an obstructed airway should receive alternating back blows and chest thrusts with attempted rescue breaths until the item is dislodged or help arrives.

11. Determine appropriate action and documentation procedures for common ambulatory care emergencies.
    - Always follow standard precautions when caring for a patient with a medical emergency. Documentation of emergency treatment should include information about the patient; vital signs; allergies, current medications, and pertinent health history; the patient's chief complaint; the sequence of events, including any changes in the patient's condition since the incident; and any physician's orders and procedures performed.

12. Assist and monitor a patient who has fainted.
    - Procedure 35-6 demonstrates the steps for caring for a patient who has fainted.

13. Control a hemorrhagic wound.
    - Procedure 35-7 describes how to control wound hemorrhage.

14. Apply patient education concepts to medical emergencies.
    - Patients should know how to contact emergency personnel, and families with young children should have poison control telephone numbers posted. Educating patients about how to care for minor emergencies at home is an important part of telephone triage in the ambulatory care setting. Encouraging patients to participate in community safety workshops and to become CPR certified may help them to avoid emergencies as well as save lives.

15. Discuss legal and ethical concerns regarding medical emergencies.
    - Good Samaritan laws vary from state to state but are designed to protect any individual, whether a healthcare professional or layperson, from liability if he or she provides assistance at the site of an emergency. The law does not require a medically trained person to act, but if emergency care is given in a reasonable and responsible manner, the healthcare worker is protected from being sued for negligence. This protection, however, does not extend to the workplace.

CONNECTIONS

Study Guide Connection: Go to Chapter 35 Study Guide. Read the Case Study and Workplace Applications and complete the assignments. Do online research for answers to the questions in the Internet Activities associated with assisting with medical emergencies.

CD Connection: Go to the Medical Assisting Competency Challenge CD and do the training activities under Patient Care. For a better understanding of cardiopulmonary function when assisting with medical emergencies, view the animation for normal cardiopulmonary physiology.

Evolve Connection: For more information related to assisting with medical emergencies, go to evolve.elsevier.com/kinn and visit related weblinks for Chapter 35. Click on the Medical Assisting Exam Review and do the practice questions to sharpen your test-taking skills.

Assisting in Ophthalmology and Otolaryngology

36

SCENARIO

Kim Tau, CMA, works in an outpatient clinic that specializes in the diagnosis and treatment of eye and ear disorders. Kim has been asked by her supervisor to help orient Amy Ling to the practice. Amy recently graduated from a medical assistant program and is familiar with basic eye and ear procedures but has many questions regarding her responsibilities at the clinic. Amy will be responsible for performing initial Snellen and Ishihara screening examinations on new patients and assisting the ophthalmologist and optician in the practice with eye treatments. She will also have to be comfortable performing audiometry hearing screening on pediatric patients, performing ear irrigations, and administering otic medications. Kim recognizes that it is important that Amy be able to perform these skills with accuracy and confidence, but she must also be sensitive to the communication and patient education needs of patients with eye and ear disorders.

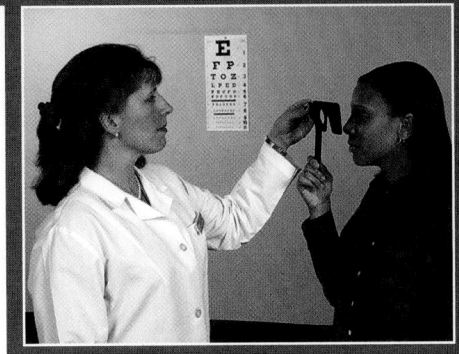

While studying this chapter, think about the following questions:

- What is the basic anatomy and physiology of the eye and ear?
- What are the major types of refractive errors?
- What disorders of the eye and ear does Amy need to be familiar with?
- How is a Snellen test done?
- What are the important steps Amy should follow when performing eye and ear irrigations and medication applications?
- How is an audiometer examination conducted?
- How should Amy perform a throat culture?
- How should Kim prepare Amy to care for patients with sensory loss?

LEARNING OBJECTIVES

1. Define, spell, and pronounce the terms listed in the vocabulary.
2. Explain the differences among an ophthalmologist, optometrist, and optician.
3. Identify the anatomic structures of the eye.
4. Describe how vision occurs.
5. Differentiate among the major types of refractive errors.
6. Summarize typical disorders of the eye.
7. Define the various diagnostic procedures for the eye.
8. Conduct a vision acuity test using the Snellen chart.
9. Assess color acuity.
10. Illustrate the purpose of eye irrigations and the instillation of medication.
11. Properly irrigate a patient's eyes.
12. Accurately instill eye medication.
13. Identify the structures and explain the functions of the external, middle, and internal ear.
14. Describe the conditions that can lead to hearing loss, including conductive, neurogenic, and congenital hearing losses.
15. Define the major disorders of the ear, including otitis, impacted cerumen, and Ménière's disease.
16. Explain the various otic diagnostic procedures.
17. Accurately measure the hearing acuity of a patient by using an audiometer.
18. Identify the purpose of ear irrigations and instillation of ear medication.
19. Demonstrate ear irrigations.
20. Accurately instill otic drops.
21. Summarize the nose and throat examination.
22. Perform a throat culture.
23. Describe the effect of sensory loss on patient education.

National Accreditation Competencies and Content

CAAHEP COMPETENCIES	ABHES COMPETENCIES
Clinical	**Clinical**
3.b.(4)(e). Prepare patient for and assist with routine and specialty examinations	4.b. Prepare patients for procedures
3.b.(4)(f). Prepare patient for and assist with procedures, treatments, and minor office surgeries	4.h. Prepare patient for and assist physician with routine and specialty examinations
3.b.(4)(g). Apply pharmacology principles to prepare and administer oral and parenteral (excluding IV) medications	4.m. Prepare and administer oral and parenteral medications as directed by physician.

VOCABULARY

accommodation Adjustment of the eye for seeing various sizes of objects at different distances.

amblyopia (am-ble-o'-pe-uh) Reduction or dimness of vision with no apparent organic cause; often referred to as *lazy eye syndrome.*

audiologist (au-de-ah'-lah-jist) An allied healthcare professional specializing in evaluation of hearing function, detection of hearing impairment, and determination of the anatomic site of impairment.

cones Structures found in the retina that make the perception of color possible.

fovea centralis (fo'-ve-uhl/sen-trah'-luhs) A small pit in the center of the retina that is considered the center of clearest vision.

hertz A unit of measurement used in hearing examinations; a wave frequency equal to one cycle per second.

miotic (mi-ah'-tik) Any substance or medication that causes constriction of the pupil.

optic disc Region at the back of the eye where the optic nerve meets the retina; considered the blind spot of the eye, because it contains only nerve fibers and no rods or cones and thus is insensitive to light.

optic nerve Second cranial nerve, which carries impulses for the sense of sight.

otosclerosis (o-tuh-skluh-ro'-suhs) Formation of spongy bone in the labyrinth of the ear, often causing the auditory ossicles to become fixed and unable to vibrate when sound enters the ears.

ototoxic (o-tuh-tahk'-sik) A medicine or substance that is capable of producing damage to the eighth cranial nerve or the organs of hearing and balance.

photophobia Abnormal sensitivity to light.

psoriasis (suh-ri'-uh-suhs) Usually chronic, recurrent skin disease marked by bright red patches covered with silvery scales.

rods Structures located in the retina of the eye and forming the light-sensitive elements.

seborrhea (se-buh-re'-uh) Excessive discharge of sebum from the sebaceous glands forming greasy scales or cheesy plugs on the body.

A medical assistant is responsible for performing a wide variety of procedures in an ophthalmologic or otorhinolaryngologic practice. First, the medical assistant must be familiar with the normal anatomy and physiology of the eyes, ears, nose, and throat. With the understanding of how these specialty sensory organs function, it is possible to master the skills needed to be a valuable asset to the physician who specializes in the treatment of eye and ear disorders.

The conditions covered in this chapter are those that are most frequently seen in the ambulatory care setting. Many subspecialty areas within the eye, ear, nose, and throat (ENT) medical practice arena are available for medical assistants to enter. Learning the fundamental procedures now provides a base on which to build the advanced techniques that will be needed if you choose to concentrate your expertise in these areas.

EXAMINATION OF THE EYE

Ophthalmology is the science of the eye and its disorders and diseases. A physician who specializes in the diagnosis and treatment of the disorders and diseases of the eye is an *ophthalmologist.* An ophthalmologist is a licensed medical physician who can diagnose eye disorders, prescribe medication, conduct eye screenings and prescribe glasses or contact lenses, and perform optic surgery. An *optometrist* is not a medical doctor but is licensed and has earned a degree as a Doctor of Optometry (OD). An optometrist can conduct eye examinations, diagnose vision problems and eye diseases, and treat visual defects through corrective lenses and eye exercises. *Opticians* are trained to fill prescriptions written by ophthalmologists and optometrists for corrective lenses by grinding the lenses and dispensing eyewear.

Anatomy and Physiology of the Eye

The eyes are the smallest yet most detailed and complex organs of the body. They are located within a bony orbit or cavity within the skull. This bony *orbit* provides protection and support to the eye. Only approximately one sixth of the eye lies outside this orbit. The eyelid assists in protecting the eye from physical trauma. The eyebrows help to keep irritants out of the eyes. The eyelashes line the margins of the eyelids and help trap foreign particles.

The *conjunctiva* is a thin mucous membrane that lines the eyelid and covers the outside of the eyeball, except for the most central portion of the eyeball, which is covered by the *cornea*. The mucus secreted from the conjunctiva helps to keep the eye moist. The eye blinks every 2 to 3 seconds, causing the *lacrimal gland*, which is located in the superior outer portion of the upper eyelid, to secrete tears. Tears move across the eyes, cleansing and moistening the surface of the eye, and drain into the *lacrimal canals* in the medial corner of the eye. The tears then drain into the nasal cavity through the nasolacrimal duct. Thus, when you cry, the excess tears ultimately empty into your nose, producing a watery nasal discharge.

Eyeball

The eyeball consists of three layers. The outermost layer is made up of the white, opaque *sclera* and the transparent *cornea*. The sclera is a tough, fibrous lining that protects the entire eyeball lying within the orbit, whereas the transparent cornea covers the exposed one sixth of the eyeball. The cornea acts as a clear window that allows light to enter the eye. The cornea also *refracts* or changes the direction of light rays after they enter the eye. The cornea was one of the first tissues to be transplanted, and now corneal transplants are common. Long-term success after corneal implant surgery is excellent.

The *choroid* is the posterior portion of the middle layer of the eye. It is the vascular layer of the eye and contains many blood vessels that supply nutrients to the outer layers of the *retina*. The choroid also contains a brown pigment that absorbs excess light rays that could interfere with vision. In the anterior part of this layer, the choroid creates the *iris* and the *ciliary body*. The iris is the colored portion of the eye. It is doughnut shaped, with the opening of the pupil in the center. The iris contains muscles that regulate the size of the pupil according to the intensity of the light; it becomes smaller in bright light and opens wider in dim light. The ciliary body contains both the *ciliary muscle*, which regulates the shape of the lens, and the *ciliary processes*, which secrete aqueous humor.

The inner layer of the eye includes the retina in the posterior portion and the lens in the anterior portion. It is in the retina where the **rods** and **cones, optic nerve, optic disc,** and **fovea centralis** are located. The delicate tissue of the retina is composed of light-sensitive neurons that convert light into neurologic impulses. These impulses travel by means of the optic nerve to the brain, where they are converted into a visual picture. Any damage to the retina has the potential for causing partial or complete blindness, because this is where the neurologic center of vision is located.

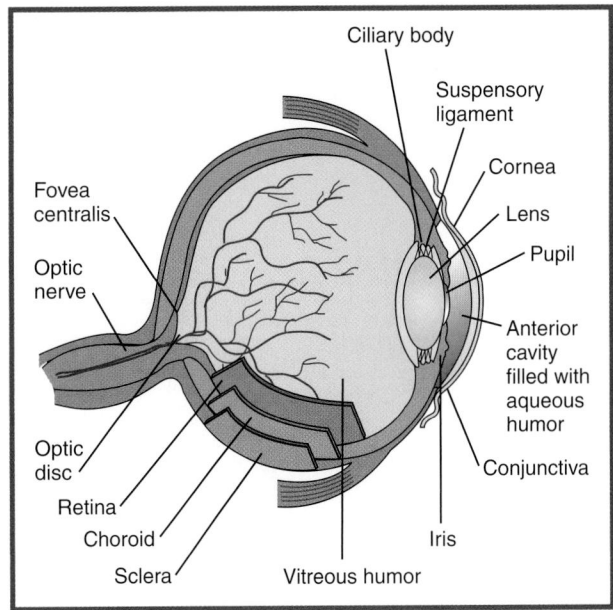

FIGURE 36-1 Anatomy of the eye.

The *lens* is a transparent, biconvex body that helps focus light after it passes through the cornea. The lens and the ciliary body divide the eye into two cavities. The posterior cavity is between the lens and the retina and contains the transparent, gel-like *vitreous humor*. Vitreous humor maintains the shape of the posterior eyeball. The anterior cavity, between the cornea and the lens, is filled with *aqueous humor*, which is continuously produced by the ciliary processes. Aqueous humor helps maintain normal pressure within the eye and provides nutrients to the lens and cornea (Figure 36-1).

Vision

Vision requires light and depends on the proper functioning of all parts of the eye (Table 36-1). A visual impulse begins with the passage of light through the cornea, where it is refracted then passes through the aqueous humor and pupil into the lens. The ciliary muscle adjusts the curvature of the lens to again refract the light rays so they pass into the retina, triggering the photoreceptor cells of the rods and cones. At this point, the light energy is converted into an electrical impulse that is sent through the optic nerve to the visual cortex of the occipital lobe of the brain, where interpretation of the light impulse occurs and a picture is created.

Disorders of the Eye

Refractive Errors

Four major types of refractive errors result when the eye is unable to focus light effectively on the retina. *Refraction* refers to the ability of the lens of the eye to bend parallel light rays coming into the eye so the rays are simultaneously focused on the retina. An error of refraction means that the light rays are not being refracted or bent properly and thus do not focus correctly on the retina. Defects in the shape of the eyeball may cause a refractive error. Most refractive errors can be corrected by wearing corrective lenses (Figure 36-2).

TABLE 36-1 Functions of the Major Parts of the Eye

STRUCTURE	FUNCTION
Sclera	External protection
Cornea	Light refraction
Choroid	Blood supply
Iris	Light absorption and regulation of pupil width
Ciliary body	Secretion of vitreous fluid; changes the shape of the lens
Lens	Light refraction
Retinal layer	Light receptor that transforms optic signals into nerve impulses
Rods	Distinguish light from dark and perceive shape and movement
Cones	Color vision
Central fovea	Area of sharpest vision
Macula lutea	Center of the retina; contains the fovea centralis, the area of most highly acute vision
External ocular muscles	Move the eyeball
Optic nerve	One of a pair of nerves that transmit visual stimuli to (cranial nerve II) the brain
Lacrimal glands	Produce tears
Eyelid	Protects eye

Modified from Damjanov I: *Pathology for the health-related professions*, Philadelphia, 1996, Saunders.

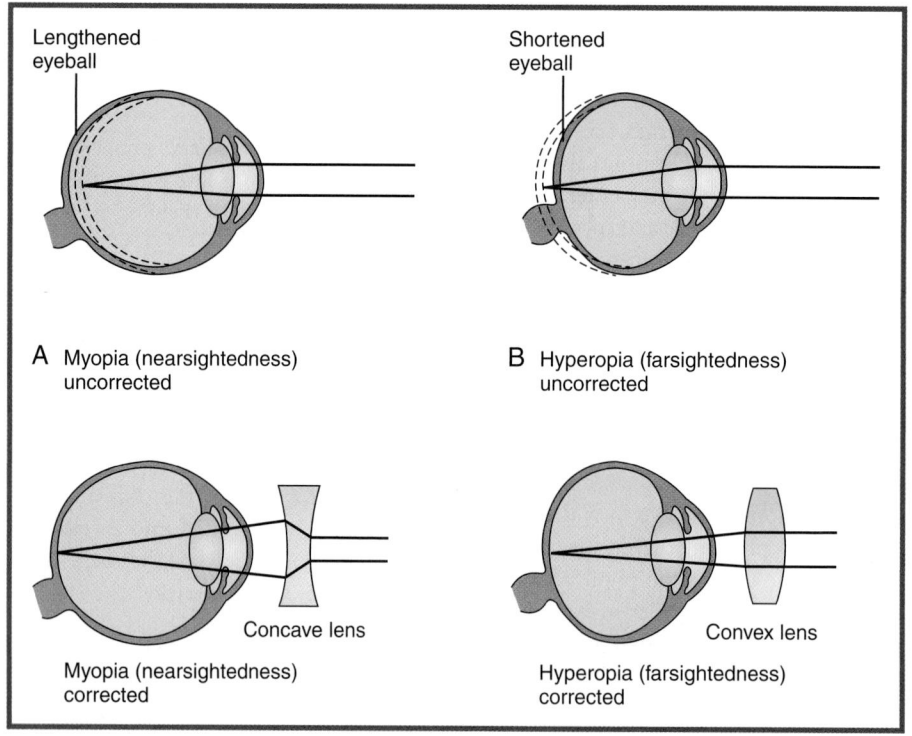

FIGURE 36-2 Errors in refraction. **A,** Myopia. **B,** Hyperopia.

Hyperopia (Farsightedness). When light enters the eye and focuses behind the retina, the person has hyperopia. This disorder is caused by an eyeball that is too short from the anterior to posterior wall. A hyperopic person has difficulty seeing objects that are close, at reading or working level. A convex corrective lens helps the eye's internal lens place objects directly on the retina and create a sharp, detailed image, or refractive surgery may be done to correct the shape of the lens.

Myopia (Nearsightedness). Myopia occurs when light rays entering the eye focus in front of the retina, causing objects at a distance to appear blurry and dull. Objects viewed at reading or working level are seen clearly. In this disorder the eyeball is elongated from the anterior to the posterior walls and the image cannot be sharpened by the internal lens of the eye. A concave corrective lens is used to focus the light rays on the retina, or surgery can be done to change the shape of the lens. However, the surgery is performed only on adults who have had a stable eye prescription for at least 1 year.

Presbyopia. As people age, the lens of the eye becomes less flexible and the ciliary muscles weaken, causing the eye to have difficulty changing the point of focus from distance to near. The condition results in difficulty seeing at reading level. A combination corrective lens, known as a *bifocal lens* or *progressive lens correction,* is used to focus both distal and proximal objects directly on the retina. Presbyopia actually starts at approximately age 10, but most people do not report an alteration in vision until the early forties. Refractive laser surgeries do not correct the effects of presbyopia.

Astigmatism. Astigmatism occurs when the focusing of light rays entering the eye is irregular. This is usually caused by the cornea or the lens not being a smooth sphere but instead having an irregular shape. Ophthalmologists describe the lens as being shaped like a football rather than a spheric shape like a basketball. This causes the light rays to be unevenly or diffusely focused on the retina, resulting in blurred vision. It is like attempting to focus on objects seen through a wavy piece of window glass. Astigmatism can be corrected with glasses or contacts or surgically. Surgical correction attempts to reshape the cornea into a more spherical or uniformly curved surface.

Signs and Symptoms of Refractive Errors

Refractive errors in vision can lead to squinting, frequent rubbing of the eyes, and headaches. The individual notices

---

Surgical Correction of Refractive Errors

- **Photorefractive Keratectomy:** The first surgical procedure developed to treat refraction errors was photorefractive keratectomy (PRK). The procedure uses a laser to reshape the central cornea into a flatter surface for people who are myopic and create a more curved surface for people who have hyperopia.
- **Laser-Assisted In-Situ Keratomileusis:** Laser-Assisted In-Situ Keratomileusis (LASIK) is a more advanced laser procedure that reshapes the central cornea to treat myopia, hyperopia, and astigmatism. A thin, hinged flap of cornea is created, the flap is lifted, and the exposed surface of the cornea is reshaped using a laser. After the corneal curvature is corrected, the flap is replaced and the area heals without stitches.
- **Laser-Assisted Epithelium Keratomileusis:** The most recent laser surgery development is Laser-Assisted Epithelium Keratomileusis (LASEK), which softens the eye's surface epithelial cells with an alcohol solution, allowing the epithelial layer to be rolled back and the cornea to be exposed. Laser energy is then used to reshape the cornea and treat myopia, hyperopia, and astigmatism. The epithelium flap is returned back to its original position, and a contact lens is placed on the cornea as a bandage for several days to aid in healing and decrease pain.

---

blurring of vision and/or fading of words at reading level. Some refractive errors are familial in nature.

Treatment of Refractive Errors

Eyeglasses and contact lenses are the traditional treatments for visual acuity problems caused by refractive errors. However, surgical procedures are available to correct problems with the shape of the lens. The surgery is performed on an outpatient basis and requires only a short stay in the facility. Medical assistants employed in an outpatient eye surgery facility would have to be trained to fulfill this specialized role.

CRITICAL THINKING APPLICATION

Amy is assisting Dr. Hanser with visual acuity examinations when he asks her if she understands the cause of refractive errors. Amy asks Kim over lunch what the different refractive disorders are and why they occur. What information should Kim include in the answer?

Strabismus

Strabismus is failure of the eyes to track together, which means both eyes do not look in the same direction at the same time. Adult development of strabismus is caused by a condition or disease elsewhere in the body, such as diabetes mellitus, muscular dystrophy, hypertension, or a head injury. In children it is caused by weakness in the muscles that control eye movement. If it appears in infancy or childhood, it is most commonly associated with **amblyopia.** Amblyopia is often correctable until approximately 7 years of age or until the retina is fully developed. Treatment involves the child wearing a patch over the unaffected eye so that the muscles of the "lazy" eye are strengthened. The main symptom in all age groups is *diplopia* (double vision).

Nystagmus

A constant, involuntary movement of one or both eyes is called *nystagmus.* The eye movement can be in any direction and is accompanied by blurred vision. A child may be born with the problem (congenital nystagmus), or it may be acquired because of a brain tumor, an inner ear lesion, or multiple sclerosis or because of substance abuse. Nystagmus is caused by an abnormal function in the part of the brain that controls eye movements. Congenital nystagmus is more common than acquired nystagmus, is usually a milder form, does not get worse over time, and is not associated with any other disorder. A patient with the signs and symptoms of nystagmus should first have a neurologic evaluation to determine the cause of the disorder, with treatment based on the underlying reason for the condition. However, congenital nystagmus has no cure. Affected people are typically not aware of the eye movements, but they may have a decrease in visual acuity that can be corrected with surgery or corrective lenses.

Infections of the Eye

Many acute disorders of the eye are seen in the ophthalmology office. These include the following:

- *Hordeolum* (stye): A localized purulent infection of a sebaceous gland of the eyelid; the area is inflamed, swollen, and painful; usually caused by a staphylococcal infection; treated with warm compresses and either topical or systemic antibiotics.
- *Chalazion:* A small cyst resulting from the blockage of a meibomian gland (sebaceous gland) that lubricates the posterior margin of the each eyelid; can become infected, inflamed, swollen, and painful; may disappear spontaneously, or may need to be surgically removed.
- *Keratitis:* Inflammation of the cornea of the eye resulting in superficial ulcerations; caused by the herpes simplex virus, bacteria, or fungi, or may develop as a result of corneal trauma, such as intense light; symptoms include inflammation, tearing, pain, and **photophobia;** it is treated with ophthalmic ointments, eye drops, and the use of an eye patch.
- *Conjunctivitis:* Inflammation of the conjunctiva; caused by irritation, allergy, or bacterial infection; bacterial conjunctivitis (pinkeye) is highly contagious and produces a purulent discharge; symptoms include inflammation, swelling and itching of the sclera, photophobia, and tearing; bacterial infections are treated with antibiotic ophthalmic preparations.
- *Blepharitis:* Inflammation of the glands and lash follicles along the margins of the eyelids; symptoms include itching and inflammation along the eyelash margins; may be caused by a staphylococcal infection, allergies, or irritation; treated with antibiotic ophthalmic ointment.

Disorders of the Eyeball

Corneal Abrasion

The cornea is the transparent outer covering of the eye and is prone to abrasion because of its location. Symptoms include pain, inflammation, tearing, and photophobia. It is usually caused by a foreign body in the eye or by direct trauma such as from contact lenses that fit poorly or are dirty. A corneal ulcer may also form and could become infected.

Diagnosis is based on patient signs and symptoms but can be confirmed with the instillation of a fluorescein stain after which the physician will use a cobalt-blue filtered light to visualize the abrasions. If the abrasions are caused by a foreign body, it must be removed first; then the eye may be treated with antibiotic ophthalmic ointment to prevent infection. Although patching the affected eye has been recommended in the past, studies are now showing that patching does not decrease the patient's pain and may actually prolong the healing time. Corneal abrasions are quite painful, so the patient may be prescribed prescription analgesics. Most corneal abrasions heal in 24 to 72 hours, but the patient should be aware that symptoms can get worse if the affected eye is exposed to bright light, if excessive blinking occurs, or if the patient rubs the injured surface of the cornea against the inside of the eyelid.

Cataract

A cataract is a cloudy or opaque area in the normally clear lens of the eye that blocks the light into the retina, causing impaired vision. This condition may result from injury to the eye, exposure to extreme heat or radiation, or inherited factors. However, the majority of cataracts develop slowly and progressively as a result of the natural aging deterioration of the lens of the eye and typically occur after the age of 60. With advanced cataracts the pupil of the eye appears white or gray.

Blurred and dimmed vision are the first symptoms of a cataract. The patient may need a brighter reading light or must hold objects closer to the eyes for better viewing. The continued clouding of the lens may cause diplopia. The patient also needs frequent changes of eyeglass prescriptions. Patients with cataracts report difficulty with night vision (nyctalopia), seeing halo images around lights, and an increased sensitivity to glare.

When the patient's vision becomes distorted or appears to be deteriorating, the ophthalmologist performs a *slit lamp* procedure, in which he or she examines the structures at the front of the eye through the use of a combination of a low-power microscope and a high-intensity light that shines into the eye as a slit beam. The only known effective treatment for a cataract is the surgical removal of the lens. This is performed as an outpatient procedure in a clinic or hospital. After the eye is anesthetized, the inner portions of the lens—the nucleus and cortex—are removed. The physician may use an extracapsular extraction, which removes the cataract in one piece, or phacoemulsification which employs an ultrasonic probe to break up the cataract and then aspirate the pieces before an artificial intraocular lens (IOL) is implanted. The incision may be closed with fine sutures, or it may be sutureless and self-sealing. The procedure usually takes 15 minutes, and the patient can typically leave the facility after 1 hour. Patients should be aware that they will not be able to drive until cleared by the ophthalmologist and that they may need help at home until their vision is clear. Postoperatively, patients are seen in the office the day after surgery and as frequently as needed in the next month. Their vision will gradually improve until it stabilizes, usually within 2 to 6 weeks, which is when they will be fitted with new corrective lenses to match their improved vision.

Glaucoma

One of the most common and severe ocular disorders is a group of diseases known as *glaucoma.* It is characterized by increased intraocular pressure (IOP), resulting in damage to the optic nerve and blindness if not treated. It rarely occurs in people younger than 40 years of age and usually is seen in people older than 60. The cause is unknown, but there is a hereditary tendency toward the development of the most common forms. Glaucoma is responsible for approximately 12% of all cases of blindness, is the leading cause of blindness among African Americans, and strikes approximately 2% of all persons older than 40 in the United States.

The ciliary body constantly produces aqueous humor, which should circulate freely between the anterior and posterior chambers of the eye and eventually empty into the general circulation. A healthy eye is filled with fluid in an amount carefully regulated to maintain the shape of the eyeball. In chronic open-angle glaucoma, the channels that drain the fluid malfunction, and over time aqueous humor builds up, resulting

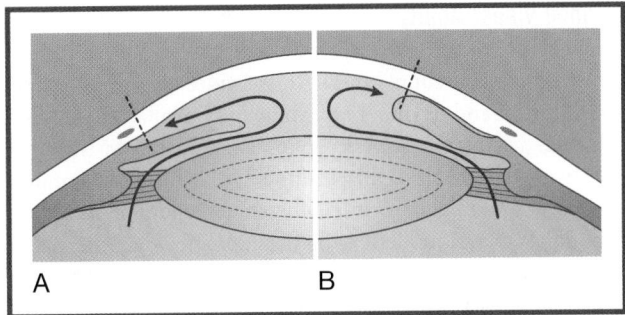

FIGURE 36-3 **A,** Open-angle glaucoma. **B,** Closed-angle glaucoma. (From Damjanov I: *Pathology for the health-related professions,* ed 3, Philadelphia, 2006, Saunders.)

in increased pressure, which affects the blood supply to the retina and the optic nerve. With acute closed-angle glaucoma, the opening of the drainage system narrows or closes completely, causing a sudden increase in IOP (Figure 36-3).

Patients can have chronic open-angle glaucoma for a considerable length of time before symptoms occur. Early detection through regular ophthalmic examinations that include IOP measurements is crucial for prevention of permanent vision loss. The frequent need to change eyeglass prescriptions, a loss of peripheral vision, mild headaches, and impaired dark adaptation are some of the signs and symptoms that may be seen with chronic glaucoma.

Acute closed-angle glaucoma has more obvious symptoms; the patient complains of severe pain, headaches, inflammation, photophobia, and seeing halos around light. If untreated, acute glaucoma can cause permanent blindness in a matter of days.

Screening for glaucoma is conducted during a complete eye examination. The ophthalmologist first uses a *tonometer* with a slit lamp to measure IOP. The air-puff tonometer records the degree of indentation of the cornea from a puff of pressurized air without touching the eye. An applanation tonometer records the pressure needed to indent the cornea when the instrument is applied to the front surface of the eye. Gonioscopy can also be used to examine the aqueous fluid drainage system and determine whether the glaucoma is the open- or closed-angle type. An ophthalmoscopic examination can also identify cupping of the optic disc, which indicates atrophy of the optic nerve.

Open-angle glaucoma can be relieved with **miotic** eyedrops or beta-blocker drugs. The combinations of drugs used to treat glaucoma can vary considerably. It is imperative that prescribed eyedrops and oral medications be taken on an uninterrupted basis. Laser surgery may be performed to create an opening or build a new channel for drainage of the aqueous humor. The goal of treatment in any type of glaucoma is to diagnose the disease early and effectively treat its progression, because any loss of sight that has occurred because of increased IOP cannot be regained. In closed-angle glaucoma, medications to lower IOP are prescribed so that surgery can be performed to create a channel for aqueous fluid to circulate. This is a medical emergency, because the pressure must be relieved within a few hours or permanent vision damage will occur.

Macular Degeneration

The macula lutea is the part of the retina that is near the optic nerve and defines the center of the field of vision. Macular degeneration is a progressive deterioration of the macula lutea that causes loss of central vision so that the patient can see only the edges of the visual field. It affects more than 10 million Americans and is the leading cause of blindness in those over 55. There are two types of macular degeneration. The dry form accounts for 90% of the cases, is painless, and develops slowly, affecting sharp vision over time so that reading or other activities that require fine detailed vision become impossible. Wet macular degeneration causes 90% of all severe vision losses from the disease and has a very acute onset and rapid progression. Dry macular degeneration is caused by the breakdown of light-sensitive cells in the macula region, and the wet form occurs when new blood vessels behind the retina form and leak blood and fluid into the macula. The condition is age related, but additional risk factors include cigarette smoking, family history, cardiovascular disease, elevated blood cholesterol levels, light eye color, and excessive sun exposure. The disease has no known cure, but recent research indicates that antioxidants including carotene, selenium, zinc, and vitamins C and E may prevent the condition or slow its progress.

Diagnostic Procedures

A complete examination of the eye is technical and requires expensive equipment and the expertise of an ophthalmologist. However, a primary care physician performs some basic examinations and treatments of the eye. The ophthalmoscope is used for examining the interior of the eye. It projects a bright, narrow beam of light through the lens that shows the interior parts of the eye and retina. It is helpful in detecting disorders of the eyes as well as certain systemic disorders, such as diabetes mellitus.

The eyelids are examined for edema, which may be the result of nephrosis, heart failure, allergy, or thyroid deficiency. *Blepharoptosis,* also called *ptosis,* is a drooping of the upper eyelid that can be caused by a disorder of the third cranial nerve, muscular weakness as seen in muscular dystrophy, or myasthenia gravis.

The pupils of the eyes are normally round and equal. Normal pupils constrict rapidly in response to light. This is demonstrated by shining a bright pinpoint light into one eye from the side of the patient's head. The pupil of an illuminated eye constricts, and the pupil of the other eye constricts equally. This test is called *light and* **accommodation** (L&A). An older patient's eyes do not accommodate as well as a younger person's do. Each eye is checked this way. Then the patient is asked to look at the physician's finger as it is moved directly toward the patient's nose to check for eye coordination. If the pupils are equal and round, respond normally to light, and adjust and focus on objects at different distances in a reasonable length of time, the physician will chart the acronym PERRLA.

Special techniques employed in the ophthalmologist's office include the use of a slit lamp biomicroscope (Figure 36-4). This device is used to view the fine details in the anterior segments of the eye. It may be used to view a foreign body, because it gives a well-illuminated and highly magnified view of the area. The patient with *exophthalmia* (abnormal protrusion of the eye possibly resulting from an overactive thyroid or from a tumor behind the eyeball) is checked with an exophthalmometer. This instrument measures how far the eye protrudes beyond the edge of the eye socket and helps determine the level of tissue swelling and enlargement behind the eye.

PERRLA	
P	Pupils
E	Equal
R	Round
R	Reactive to
L	Light and
A	Accommodation

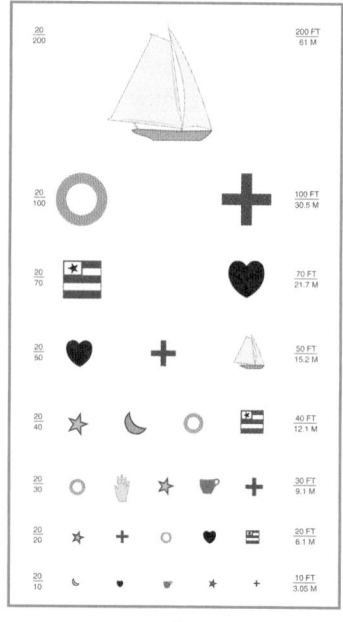

FIGURE 36-4 Slit lamp.

Distance Visual Acuity

Distance visual acuity is frequently part of a complete physical examination (Procedure 36-1). It is widely used in schools and industry and is the best single test available for visual screening. Many cases of myopia, astigmatism, or hyperopia have been detected by this routine test. The most common chart used is the Snellen alphabetic chart (Figure 36-5, *B*). This chart displays various letters of the alphabet that the patient must identify in ever smaller font sizes. However, patients with limited knowledge of the English alphabet can be tested with the E chart (Figure 36-5, *C*). In addition, a chart is available that uses pictures as symbols (Figure 36-5, *A*). This chart is used for young children or individuals who do not know the alphabet. The symbol on the top line of the chart can be read by persons with normal vision at 200 feet. In each of the succeeding rows, from the top down, the size of the symbols is reduced so that a person with normal vision can see them at distances of 100, 70, 50, 40, 30, and 20 feet, consecutively.

The patient must not be allowed to study the chart before the test. The room or hall should be long enough so that the 20-foot distance can be marked off accurately and without interruptions from patient and staff traffic. The chart should be hung at eye level and illuminated with maximum light, without glare on the chart. Most adults do not need the standard Snellen chart explained, but if the E chart is used, an explanation must be given as to how the Es are to be read. The patient may point up or down or right or left towards the part of the letter that is open. If the E chart is going to be used for a child, practice with an index card that has a large E drawn on it before the child is tested. Turn the card in different directions to simulate the position of the "fingers" of the E on the chart, and give the child the opportunity to demonstrate what direction the fingers are pointing by pointing his or her own fingers in the same direction (Figure 36-6).

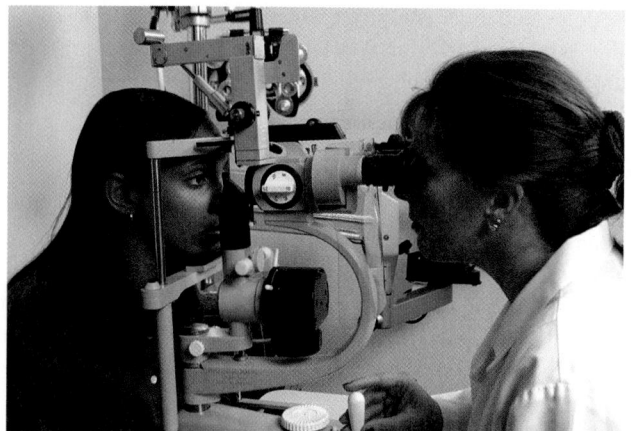

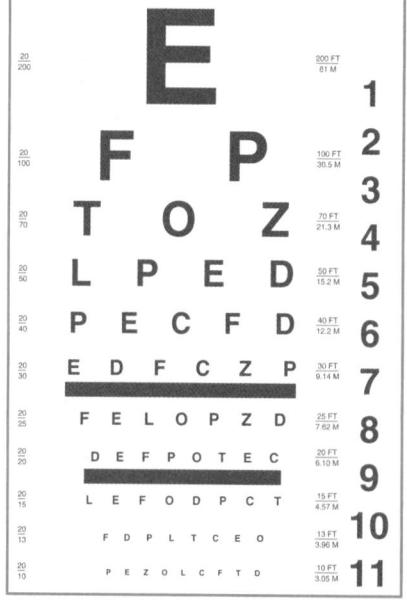

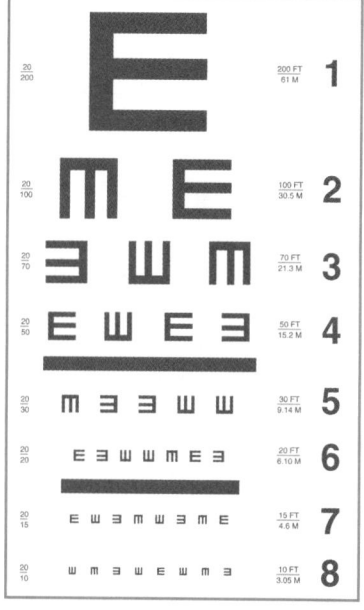

A   B   C

FIGURE 36-5 Different types of Snellen charts.

PROCEDURE 36-1

Prepare Patient for and Assist with Routine and Specialty Examinations:
Measure Distance Visual Acuity Using the Snellen Chart

CAAHEP COMPETENCY: 3.b.(4)(e)
ABHES COMPETENCIES: 4.b, 4.h

GOAL: *To determine the patient's degree of visual clarity at a measured distance of 20 feet using the Snellen chart.*

EQUIPMENT and SUPPLIES

- Snellen eye chart
- Eye occluder
- Pen or pencil and paper
- Patient record

PROCEDURAL STEPS

1. Wash your hands.
   PURPOSE: Infection control.

2. Prepare the examination room. Make sure that the room is well lit, a distance marker is 20 feet from the chart, and the chart is placed at the eye level of the patient.

3. Identify the patient and explain the procedure. Instruct the patient not to squint during the test, because this temporarily improves vision. The patient should not have an opportunity to study the chart before the test is given. If the patient wears corrective lenses, they should be worn during the test.
   PURPOSE: Explanations help gain patient cooperation and alleviate apprehension.

4. Position the patient in a standing or sitting position at the 20-foot marker.
   PURPOSE: Twenty feet is the standard testing distance.

5. Position the Snellen chart at eye level to the patient.

6. Instruct the patient to cover the left eye with the occluder and to keep both eyes open throughout the test to prevent squinting (Figure 1).

PURPOSE: The right eye is traditionally tested first.

7. Stand beside the chart and point to each row as the patient orally reads down the chart, starting with the 20/70 row (Figure 2).
   PURPOSE: Starting with larger letters allows the patient to gain confidence and allows accommodation of vision.

8. Proceed down the rows of the chart until the smallest row the patient can read with a maximum of two errors is reached. If one or two letters are missed, the outcome is recorded with a minus sign and the number of errors (e.g., 20/40 − 2). If more than two errors are made, the previous line should be documented.

9. Record any patient reactions in reading the chart.
   PURPOSE: Reactions such as squinting, leaning, tearing, or blinking may indicate that the patient is experiencing difficulty with the test.

10. Repeat the procedure with the left eye.

11. Document the date and time, the procedure, visual acuity results, and any patient reactions on the patient's record. Also record whether corrective lenses were worn.
    PURPOSE: Procedures that are not recorded are considered not done.
    DOCUMENTATION EXERCISE: The medical assistant conducted a Snellen exam on Truman Anderson, who wears contacts. The results were: right eye 20/60; left eye 20/30, but he missed one letter at the 20/30 line; both eyes 20/40. Truman did not squint or strain during the exam.

_____

_____

_____

See Appendix D for a charting example.

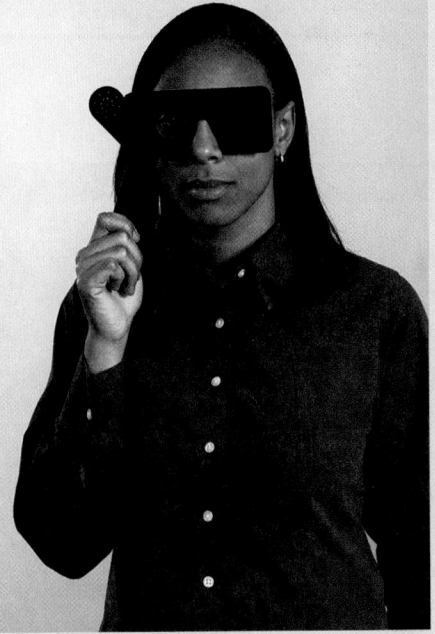

FIGURE 1

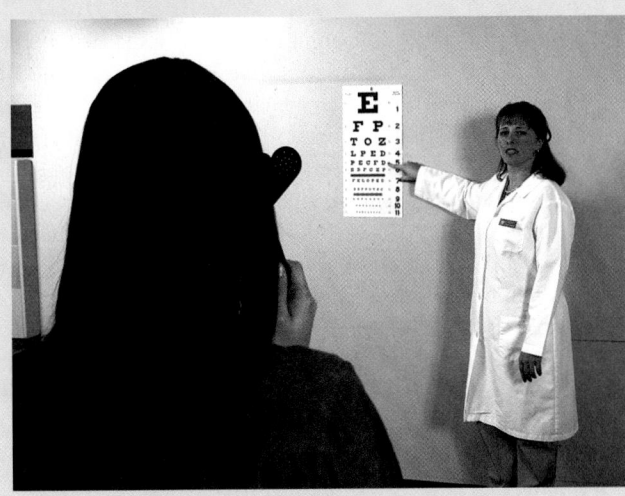

FIGURE 2

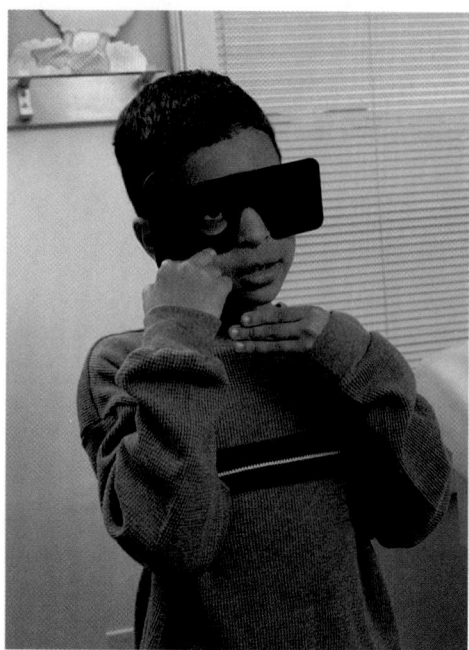

FIGURE 36-6 Visual acuity test with the E chart.

Practice Interpreting Snellen Outcomes

- The patient always stands 20 feet away from the chart.
- Each outcome is a record of how well the patient can see in comparison with normal vision.
- Example: A patient with a 20/40 reading can see that line correctly standing at 20 feet, but an individual with normal vision can see the same line correctly at 40 feet.
- Example: A patient with a 20/15 reading can see that line accurately standing at 20 feet, but a person with normal vision must stand at 15 feet to have the same vision.

60

Nothing can take the place of "the only pair of eyes you will ever have." That is why you are exercising such good judgment in taking care of them as you are now doing.

50

For this reason, you will welcome the suggestion about lenses which are designed and made to give you "greater comfort and better appearance." In man's earliest days he had little use for glasses. He used his eyes chiefly for long distance.

40

He worked by daylight and at tasks with little detail. But now, you use your eyes for much close work—reading, writing, sewing and many other uses which the eyes of primitive man did not know. Now your eyes meet all sorts of lighting conditions, artificial and natural.

30

Many of these conditions produce "overbrightness" or glare. Sometimes it is the direct or reflected glare of sunlight; often it is direct or reflected from artificial light. And very often this glare is uncomfortable—impairs your efficiency. But special lenses, developed by America's leading optical scientists, combat this glare.

25

These lenses give you more comfortable vision and blend harmoniously with your complexion. These lenses are less conspicuous. We are glad to rec- commend them because they will give you greater comfort and better appearance. Thousands of satisfied wearers testify to their real benefits.

20

You are wise in taking good care of "the only pair of eyes you will ever have." You know how valuable they are, that you can never have another pair. For this reason, you will welcome the suggestion about lenses which are designed and made to give you "greater comfort and better appearance." In man's earliest days he had little use for glasses.

The above letters subtend the visual angle of 5' at the designated distance in inches.

FIGURE 36-7 Near-vision acuity chart.

Because this is a gross screening of distance visual acuity, the eyes are typically tested with corrective lenses, so the patient should not remove glasses or contact lenses unless ordered by the physician. Indicate on the patient's record whether the assessment was done with or without corrective lenses. Record the results of each eye separately and as fractions. The numerator (top number) is the distance of the patient from the chart (always 20 feet) and the denominator (bottom number) is the lowest line read satisfactorily by the patient. For example, if the patient reads the 20 line at 20 feet, the fraction 20/20 is recorded for that eye. The last line the patient can read without squinting or straining and with no more than two mistakes is the line recorded in the patient's chart for that eye. The medical assistant should document the outcomes of the test with appropriate abbreviations, using OD (right eye), OS (left eye), and OU (both eyes).

CRITICAL THINKING APPLICATION

Susie Anthony, a 19-year-old patient, is seen today for a general eye examination. The physician orders a routine Snellen test, and Kim administers it. Susie wears contacts and with the right eye reads without errors to the 20/25 line but squints and makes three errors at the 20/20 line. With the left eye Susie makes two mistakes at the 20/30 line. How should Kim document this procedure?

Near Visual Acuity

Near visual acuity can be tested with the near-vision acuity chart (Figure 36-7). This is frequently given to patients to initially screen for presbyopia or hyperopia. If the patient wears corrective lenses, they should be worn during the test. The size of the type on the card varies from newspaper headlines to print similar to that found in telephone books. The test should be given in a well-lit room, with the patient holding the card approximately 14 to 16 inches away. As with the Snellen examination, the near-vision acuity test is given in each eye, starting with the right eye. The eye not being tested should be covered but left open. The patient should be monitored for indications of difficulty, such as squinting or tearing. The patient reads the card, starting at the top, until reaching the smallest print that can be read. The medical assistant should document the number at which the patient stopped reading for each eye, whether corrective lenses were worn, and any signs of eye strain exhibited by the patient.

The Ishihara Color Vision Test

Defects in color vision are classified as either congenital or acquired. Congenital defects are caused by an inherited color vision defect and are found most often in males. Acquired defects in color vision occur because of an eye injury or disease. The Ishihara test is a simple, convenient, and accurate procedure that detects total colorblindness as well as the red-green blindness that is prevalent in congenital blindness (Procedure 36-2). The test assesses the perception of primary colors as well as shades of colors.

The test booklet contains polychromatic plates made up of colored dots in numerical patterns. The numbers are one color, and the background dots are a different color. Patients with average visual acuity will be able to read the numbers within the dot matrix without difficulty. Patients with color vision defects will not be able to read the number or will see a totally different number. There is also a section of plates that contain colored line trails through a background of dots. These plates are designed to be used with children or adults who are not able to read numbers. In this situation, the patient is asked to take his or her finger and follow the dotted trail through the picture.

The test should be administered in a quiet room that is well illuminated by sunlight and not artificial lighting. If this is not possible, create the best situation possible. If there is a quiet outside patio area, use it or try to set the electric lights to create an artificial sunlight effect. The test uses 14 color plates. The basic test consists of plates 1 through 11. Plates 12 through 14 are used if the patient appears to be having difficulty with the red-green differentiations. The medical assistant records the number of plates that were read correctly. If the results are 10 or greater, the patient is within the average range. If the score is 7 or less, the patient is suspected of having a color deficiency, and the ophthalmologist will perform additional assessment tests using more precise color vision testing equipment.

Treatment Procedures

Eye Irrigation

The eye is irrigated to relieve inflammation, remove drainage, dilute chemicals, or wash away foreign bodies. Sterile technique and equipment must be used to avoid contamination (Procedure 36-3). Follow the procedure as prescribed, making sure that the patient is comfortable. Always record the treatment on the patient's chart immediately after completing it. Remember, if it is not recorded, it has not been done.

Foreign bodies in the eye are very irritating and may cause considerable pain. Most foreign bodies are superficial and can be easily removed. Occasionally, foreign particles may be deeply embedded and require eye surgery. When a patient comes into the office and has something in his or her eye, notify the physician immediately.

The first objective of the physician's examination will be inspection. The patient is asked to look to either side and up and down so that the anterior surface can be inspected. For the physician to fully inspect under the upper lid, the patient must cooperate by looking downward while the physician everts the upper lid using a cotton-tipped applicator. While the lid is maintained in an everted position, any foreign materials may be rinsed away with sterile water or saline solution. If the physician gives the order for you to remove the foreign body, do so with irrigation only. If this technique is unsuccessful, cover both of the patient's eyes with a gauze dressing and notify your supervisor immediately.

SAFETY ALERT Never attempt to remove a foreign body from the cornea using an applicator, as scratches to the cornea may result, causing scar formation and impairment of vision.

CRITICAL THINKING APPLICATION

The physician tells Kim to irrigate the left eye of a 22-year-old patient for removal of a foreign body. She is to irrigate it with normal saline solution until clear. How should Kim document this procedure?

Instillation of Medication

Medication may be instilled into the eye for treatment of an infection, to soothe an eye irritation, to anesthetize the eye, or to dilate the pupils before examination or treatment (Procedure 36-4). Ophthalmic medications come in several forms. Liquid drops are usually in small squeeze bottles with tips that allow one drop at a time to be dispensed, or the bottle may contain a dropper with a small rubber attachment used to dispense the medication by drops. Eye ointments are dispensed in small metal or plastic tubes with an ophthalmic tip that allows you to dispense a small stream of ointment directly into the bottom eyelid (Table 36-2, p. 759).

SAFETY ALERT Whatever the medication, the dispenser should never touch the eye while the prescribed amount of medication is administered.

CRITICAL THINKING APPLICATION

Amy is ordered to administer Humorsol 0.25% one drop to the left eye in a 75-year-old patient recently diagnosed with glaucoma. How should Amy document this procedure?

PROCEDURE 36-2

Prepare Patient for and Assist with Routine and Specialty Examinations:
Assess Color Acuity Using the Ishihara Test

CAAHEP COMPETENCY: 3.b.(4)(e)
ABHES COMPETENCIES: 4.b, 4.h

GOAL: *To correctly assess a patient's color acuity and record the results.*

EQUIPMENT and SUPPLIES

- Room area with natural light
- Ishihara color plate book
- Pen, pencil, and paper
- Watch with a second hand
- Patient record

PROCEDURAL STEPS

1. Assemble the necessary equipment and prepare the room for testing. The room should be quiet and illuminated with natural light.
   PURPOSE: For testing colors to be seen correctly, natural light is needed.

2. Identify the patient, and explain the procedure. Use a practice card during the explanation, and be sure that the patient understands that he or she has 3 seconds to identify each plate.
   PURPOSE: An informed patient is a cooperative patient. The first plate is a practice plate and is designed to be read correctly.

3. Hold up the first plate at a right angle to the patient's line of vision and 30 inches from the patient. Be sure both of the patient's eyes are kept open during the test (Figure 1).

4. Ask the patient to tell you what number is on the plate, and record the plate number and the patient's answer (Figure 2).

5. Continue this sequence until all 11 plates have been read. If the patient cannot identify the number on the plate, place an X in the record for that plate number. Your record should look like this: Plate 1 = pass, Plate 2 = pass, Plate 3 = X, Plate 4 = pass, and so on.

6. Include any unusual symptoms in your record, such as eye rubbing, squinting, or excessive blinking.

7. Place the book back into its cardboard sleeve, and return the book to its storage space.
   PURPOSE: The Ishihara color plates need to be stored in a closed position away from external light to protect the colors.

8. Record the procedure, including the date and time, the testing results, and any patient symptoms exhibited during the test in the patient's record.
   PURPOSE: Procedures that are not recorded are considered not done.

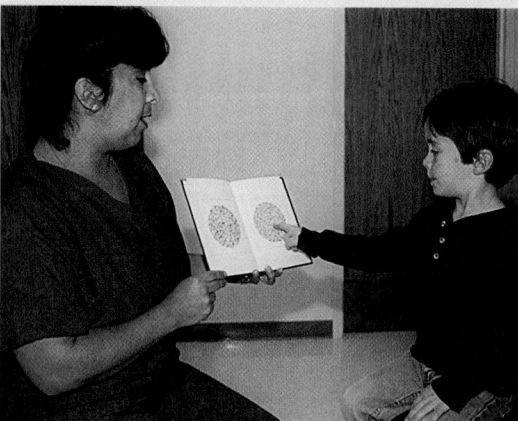

FIGURE 1

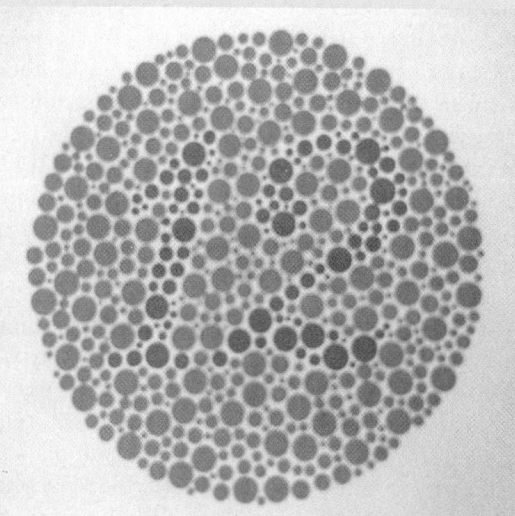

FIGURE 2

Aseptic Procedures in Ophthalmology

A major concern in ophthalmologic procedures is the contamination of eye medication applicators. Because of the concern of cross-contamination, the use of stock ophthalmic medications is discouraged. The sterility of all eye medications is critical for good patient care. Newly opened sterile solutions should be used for each patient and either disposed of after instillation or given to the patient for home use. All instruments used for the removal of a foreign body should be sterile.

EXAMINATION OF THE EAR

Otorhinolaryngology is the medical specialty that deals with the ear, nose, and throat. It is frequently referred to as *otolaryngology*

PROCEDURE 36-3

Prepare Patient for and Assist with Procedures, Treatments, and Minor Office Surgeries: Irrigate a Patient's Eyes

<u>CAAHEP COMPETENCY:</u> 3.b.(4)(f)
<u>ABHES COMPETENCY:</u> 4.b

GOAL: *To cleanse the eye (or eyes), as ordered by the physician.*

EQUIPMENT and SUPPLIES

- Prescribed sterile irrigation solution
- Sterile irrigating bulb syringe and sterile basin or prepackaged solution with dispenser
- Basin for drainage
- Sterile gauze squares
- Disposable drape
- Towel
- Nonsterile disposable gloves
- Biohazard waste container
- Patient record

PROCEDURAL STEPS

1. Wash your hands.
   <u>PURPOSE:</u> Infection control.
2. Check the physician's orders to determine which eye requires irrigation (or whether both eyes require it) and the type of solution to be used.
   <u>PURPOSE:</u> To check the abbreviations: OD (right eye), OS (left eye), OU (both eyes).
3. Assemble the materials needed.
4. Check the expiration date of the solution, and read the label three times.
   <u>PURPOSE:</u> To follow the rules for administering medications.
5. Identify the patient, and explain the procedure.
   <u>PURPOSE:</u> Explanations help gain patient cooperation and alleviate apprehension.
6. Assist the patient into a sitting or supine position, making certain that the head is turned toward the side of the affected eye. Place the disposable drape over the patient's neck and shoulder.

<u>PURPOSE:</u> This position causes the solution to flow away from the unaffected eye so as to reduce the chances for cross-contamination of the healthy eye.

7. Put on gloves, and rinse your gloved hands under warm water to remove all powder from the gloves, or wear powder-free gloves.
   <u>PURPOSE:</u> Gloves assist you in holding the eye open, but powder may irritate the patient's eyes.
8. Place or have the patient hold a drainage basin next to the affected eye to receive the solution from the eye. Place a polylined drape under the basin to avoid getting the solution on the patient.
9. Moisten a gauze square with solution, and cleanse the eyelid and lashes. Start at the inner canthus (near nose) to the outer canthus (farthest from nose) and dispose of the gauze square in the biohazard container after each wipe (Figure 1).
   <u>PURPOSE:</u> Debris on the lids or lashes must be cleansed away before the conjunctiva is exposed.
10. If using a bulb syringe, pour the required volume of body-temperature irrigating solution into the basin and withdraw solution into the bulb syringe. If using an irrigating solution in a prepackaged dispenser, remove the lid.
    <u>PURPOSE:</u> Cold solution will cause the patient pain and discomfort.

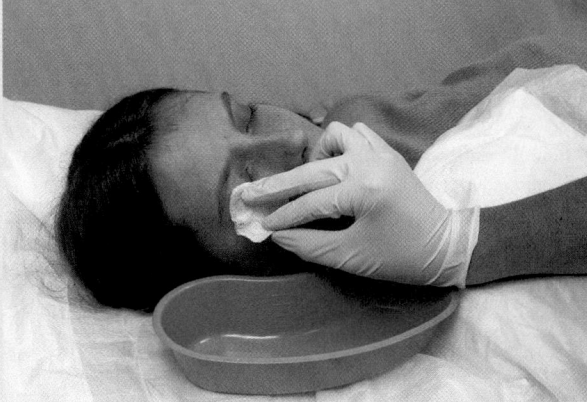

FIGURE 1

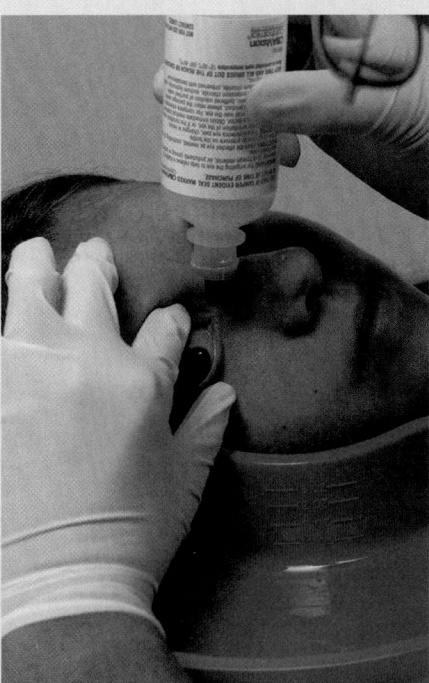

FIGURE 2

Continued

PROCEDURE 36-3—cont'd

11. Separate and hold the eyelids with the index finger and thumb of one hand. With the other hand, place the syringe or dispenser on the bridge of the nose parallel to the eye.
    PURPOSE: To support and steady the dispenser.

12. Squeeze the bulb or dispenser, directing the solution toward the lower conjunctiva of the inner canthus, allowing the solution to flow steadily and slowly from the inner to outer canthus. Do not touch the eye or eyelids with the applicator (Figure 2).
    PURPOSE: Prevents possible injury to the eye.

13. Refill the syringe or continue to gently squeeze the prepackaged bottle, and continue the procedure until the amount of solution ordered by the physician has been administered or until drainage from the eye is clear.

14. Dry the eyelid from the inner to outer canthus with sterile gauze. Do not use cotton balls because fibers might remain in the eye.

15. Dispose of the irrigation results, and clean the work area.

16. Remove gloves and wash your hands.
    PURPOSE: Infection control.

17. Document the procedure using appropriate abbreviations including the date and time, the type and amount of solution used, which eye was irrigated, any significant patient reactions, and the results in the patient's record.
    PURPOSE: Procedures that are not recorded are considered not done.
    DOCUMENTATION EXERCISE: Toby Kramer is ordered eye irrigations until clear because of sand in both eyes. You use 50 mL of irrigation solution in the right eye and 125 cc in the left eye. After the procedure is complete the sclera appears red and Toby complains of irritation in both eyes.

    _____

    _____

    _____

See Appendix D for a charting example.

PROCEDURE 36-4

Prepare Patient for and Assist with Procedures, Treatments, and Minor Office Surgeries: Instill Eye Medication

CAAHEP COMPETENCIES: 3.b.(4)(f), 3.b.(4)(g)
ABHES COMPETENCIES: 4.b, 4.m

GOAL: *To apply medication to the eye(s), as ordered by the physician.*

EQUIPMENT and SUPPLIES

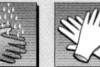

- Sterile medication with sterile eye dropper or ophthalmic ointment
- Disposable drape
- Sterile gauze squares
- Disposable nonsterile gloves
- Patient record

PROCEDURAL STEPS

1. Wash your hands.
   PURPOSE: Infection control.

2. Check the physician's order to determine which eye requires medication (or whether medication is ordered for both eyes) and the name and strength of the medication you will be using.
   PURPOSE: To prevent possible medication error.

3. Assemble equipment and supplies.

4. Read the label of the medication three times.
   PURPOSE: To follow the rules for administering medications.

5. Identify the patient, and explain the procedure.
   PURPOSE: Explanations help gain patient cooperation and alleviate apprehension.

6. Put on nonsterile gloves, and rinse your gloved hands under warm water to remove all powder from the gloves, or wear powder-free gloves.
   PURPOSE: Gloves help you hold the eye open, but powder may irritate the patient's eyes.

7. Assist the patient into a sitting or supine position. Ask the patient to tilt the head backward and look up.
   PURPOSE: Looking up helps to prevent touching the cornea with the tip of the applicator. It also helps keep the patient from blinking as the medication is instilled. For eyedrops, draw the medication into the dropper. For eye ointment, remove the cap.

8. Pull the lower conjunctival sac downward (Figure 1).
   PURPOSE: Creates a pocket for the medication.

9. Insert the prescribed number of drops or amount of ointment into the eye. For eyedrops, place drops in the center of the lower conjunctival sac, with the tip of the dropper held parallel to the eye and $1/2$ inch above the eye sac. For eye ointment (ung), squeeze a thin ribbon along the lower conjunctival sac from inner to outer canthus, making sure not to touch the eye with the applicator.
   PURPOSE: Placing the medication in the conjunctival sac rather than on the eyeball prevents injury to the cornea. Touching the eye with the applicator could injure the eye as well as contaminate the applicator (Figure 2).

Continued

PROCEDURE 36-4—*cont'd*

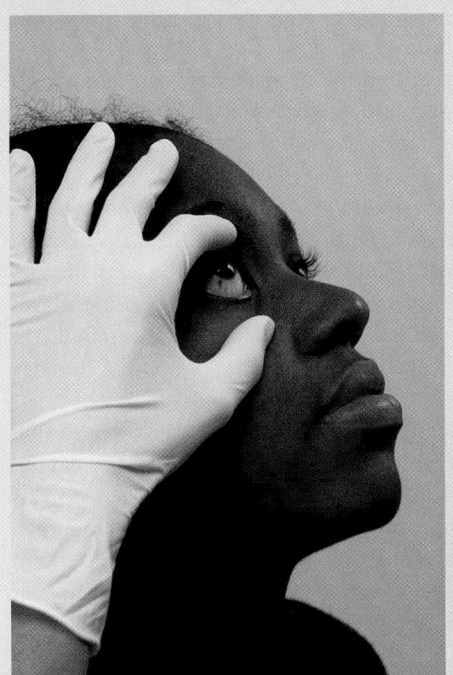

FIGURE 1

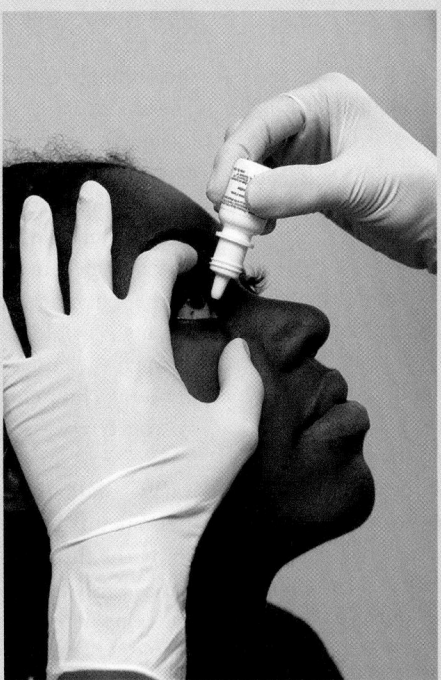

FIGURE 2

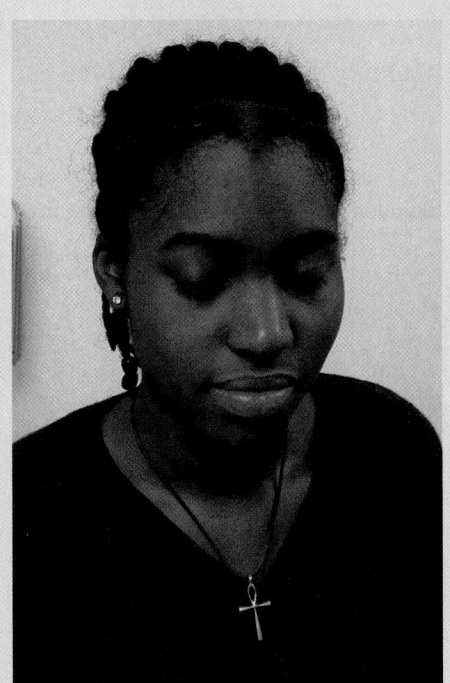

FIGURE 3

10. Instruct the patient to gently close the eye and rotate the eyeball.
<u>PURPOSE:</u> Gently closing the eye prevents the medication from being dispelled, and rotating the eyeball distributes the medication evenly (Figure 3).

11. Dry any excess drainage from inner to outer canthus, and explain that the medication may temporarily blur vision.

12. Discard the unused medication, and clean the procedure area.

13. Remove gloves, and wash hands.
<u>PURPOSE:</u> Infection control.

14. Record the procedure on the patient's chart, including the date and time, the name and strength of the medication, the amount of the dose administered, which eye was treated, teaching instructions given if the treatment is to continue at home, and any observations.
<u>PURPOSE:</u> Procedures that are not recorded are considered not done.

See Appendix D for a charting example.

TABLE 36-2 Ophthalmic Medications

DRUG NAME	CLASS AND USE
Neosporin	Antiinfective and steroid combination
Cetamide	Antibacterial
Viroptic	Antiinfective, antiviral
Pred-G TobraDex	Antiinflammatory agents, corticosteroids
Ocufen Voltaren	Antiinflammatory agents, nonsteroidal antiinflammatory drugs
Isopto atropine	Mydriatic
Iopidine	Glaucoma treatment
Eserine sulfate Isopto carbachol	Mydriatic glaucoma treatments

or even as a single specialty of otology or laryngology. Usually, the specialty otorhinolaryngology is referred to simply as *ear, nose, and throat* (ENT).

Anatomy and Physiology of the Ear

The ears are only a small portion of the actual organ of hearing. Most of this structure lies hidden in the temporal bone. Anatomically the organ of hearing is divided into three sections: the outer ear, the middle ear, and the inner ear (Figure 36-8).

Outer or External Ear

The outer ear consists of the auricle or pinna, the fleshy part of the ear that you see on the side of the head, and the external auditory canal, the tube that extends from the auricle to the tympanic membrane (eardrum). The auricle collects the sound waves and sends them down the auditory canal.

The skin that lines the auditory canal contains numerous hair follicles, many nerve endings, and ceruminous glands that secrete cerumen (commonly called *ear wax),* which lubricates the canal. Both the hair and the waxy cerumen help prevent foreign objects from reaching the eardrum. The canal has a slight S shape to it and is approximately 2.5 cm or 1 inch long.

Middle Ear

The middle ear, which is sometimes called the *tympanic cavity,* is an air-filled chamber that begins with the tympanic membrane and terminates at the oval window. The middle ear contains the auditory ossicles or bones—the malleus, incus, and stapes. These three tiny bones are linked together through minute ligaments to form a bridge across the space of the tympanic cavity. The malleus is next to the tympanic membrane, and the stapes is against the oval window. The eustachian tube opens into the middle ear cavity and connects to the nasopharynx. It is designed to equalize pressure in the middle ear with that in the external auditory canal. This equalized pressure makes hearing possible. Throat infections may spread to the middle ear through the eustachian tube; this is a very common occurrence in young children.

The tympanic membrane is a thin, disk-shaped tissue that totally seals off the outer ear from the middle ear. Sound waves conducted through the external auditory canal hit this membrane and cause it to vibrate. These vibrations are picked up by the three ossicles and changed from air-conducted sound waves to bone-conducted sound waves. The ossicles transmit the bone-conducted sound waves through the middle ear to

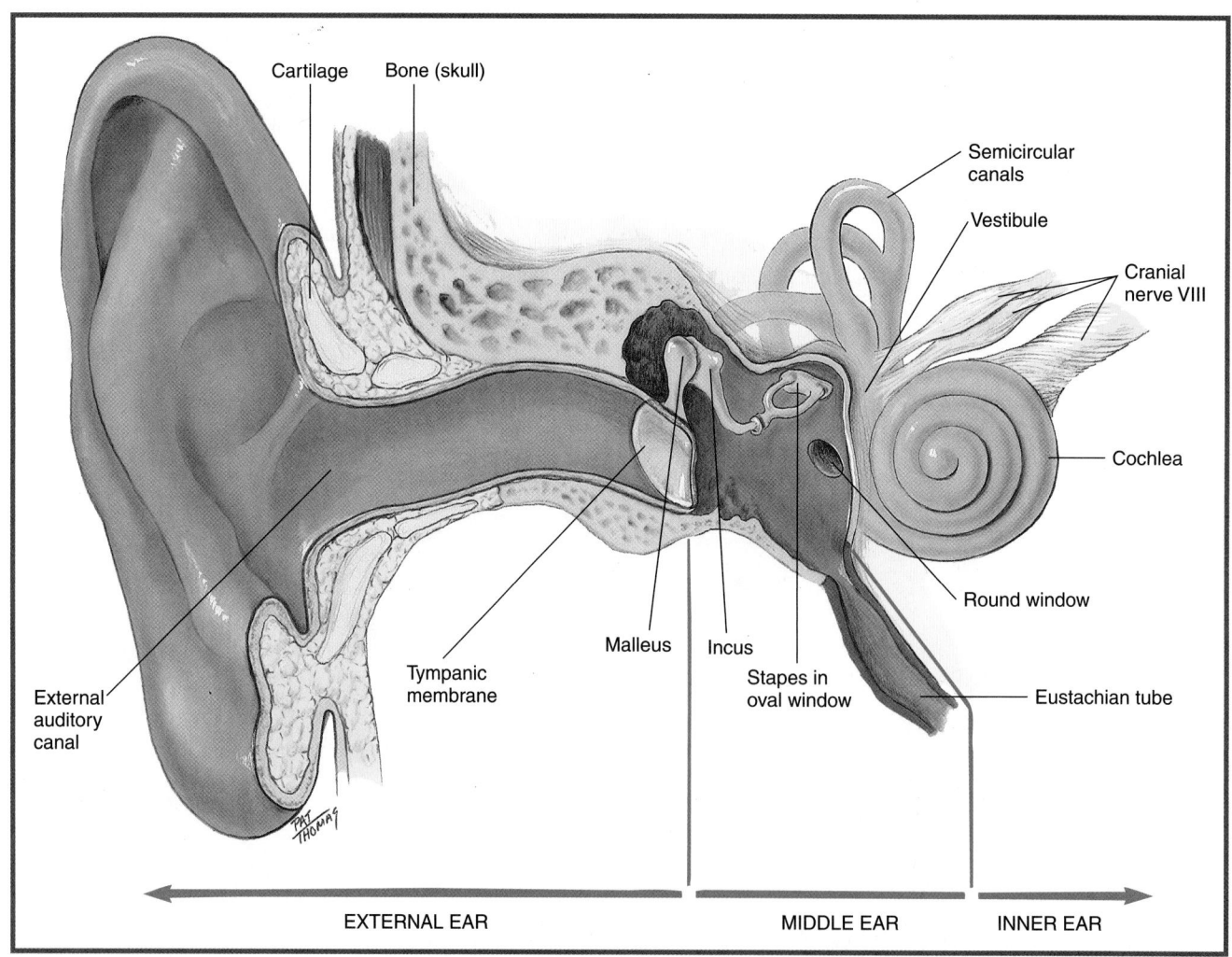

FIGURE 36-8 Anatomy of the ear. (Modified from Jarvis C: *Physical examination and health assessment,* ed 4, Philadelphia, 2004, Saunders.)

the oval window, which is the membrane that connects the middle and inner ear. At the oval window the sound waves move into the fluids of the inner ear. This fluid motion excites the receptors, changing the bone-conducted sound into sensory-neural impulses.

Inner Ear

The inner ear is called the *labyrinth* and is divided into the cochlea and semicircular canals, which are joined by the vestibule. The semicircular canals function to maintain equilibrium, and the cochlea is responsible for the sense of hearing.

The organ of Corti, which contains the receptors for sound, is located within the cochlea. It is made up of hairlike sensory cells surrounded by sensory nerve fibers that form the cochlear branch of the eighth cranial nerve. Sound impulses cause the hairs to bend and rub against the nerve fibers, which initiate stimuli to travel through the cochlear nerve into the brain for sound interpretation.

The eighth cranial nerve transmits auditory impulses to the medulla oblongata. Then impulses travel to the thalamus and on to the auditory cortex of the temporal lobe of the brain, where they are interpreted into audible sound and speech patterns.

The semicircular canals are responsible for evaluating the position of the head in relation to the pull of gravity. The three canals are positioned at right angles to one another, on different planes (Figure 36-9). When the head turns rapidly, these fluid-filled canals must rapidly adjust and send the stimulated change into the central nervous system, which interprets the information and initiates the desired response to maintain balance. With repetitive or excessive stimulation to the equilibrium receptors, some people become nauseated and may vomit. This condition is known as *motion sensitivity* or *motion sickness*.

Disorders of the Ear

Hearing Loss

Hearing loss occurs because of two problems: either a conduction problem or a sensorineural impairment. Some individuals experience both conditions.

A conductive hearing loss is caused by a problem that originates in the external or middle ear that prevents sound

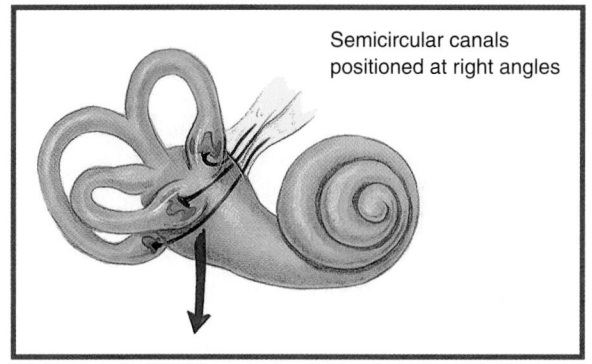

FIGURE 36-9 Semicircular canals. (From Applegate EJ: *The anatomy and physiology learning system*, ed 3, Philadelphia, 2006, Saunders.)

vibrations from passing through the external auditory canal, limits the vibration of the tympanic membrane, or interferes with the passage of bone-conducted sound in the middle ear. Some of the common causative factors for a conduction related hearing loss include impacted cerumen; trauma to the tympanic membrane, especially with scar formation; hemorrhage or fluid in the middle ear; **otosclerosis;** and recurrent chronic ear infections. It is the patient with conductive hearing loss who receives the greatest benefit from a hearing aid. If the hearing loss is caused by a malfunction or congenital abnormality of the ossicles, a surgical procedure can be performed to replace the damaged ossicles with manufactured models.

A sensorineural hearing loss results from an abnormality of either the organ of Corti or the auditory nerve. Viral infections such as rubella, influenza, and herpes can result in hearing loss, as can head trauma or certain **ototoxic** medications. The first sign of ototoxic drug complications is usually *tinnitus*, a ringing in the ears. This sometimes occurs with high doses of aspirin, certain antibiotics (erythromycin and vancomycin), and chemotherapeutic agents. A sensorineural hearing loss can also occur because of prolonged exposure to loud noise, such as repetitive noise in the workplace or loud music, which damages the delicate hairs of the organ of Corti. *Presbycusis,* the hearing loss that affects aging people, is caused by a reduced number of receptor cells in the organ of Corti and is also classified as a sensorineural loss. Children can be born with a congenital hearing deficit or deafness because of intrauterine infection or trauma (Figure 36-10).

If the sensorineural hearing loss cannot be improved by hearing aids, an option is surgically implanting an artificial cochlea. Cochlear implants are complex devices that use electrical impulses to stimulate the auditory nerve, which then carries the current to the brain to be interpreted as sound. The implants do not create normal hearing but provide increased sound for a person with profound or complete hearing loss.

A mixed hearing loss is a combination of conductive and sensory deafness. This type of loss can result from tumors, toxic levels of certain medications, hereditary factors, and stroke.

Otitis

Two common types of otitis are seen in patients in an otology or family practice. The first affects the external ear canal and is called *otitis externa,* or swimmer's ear. Otitis externa may be caused by dermatologic conditions, such as **seborrhea** or **psoriasis,** trauma to the canal, or the continuous use of earplugs or earphones. Swimmers frequently have otitis externa because water collects in the ears and mixes with cerumen to form an ideal culture medium for bacteria and fungus. Patients with otitis externa complain of severe pain with inflammation and swelling of the external auditory canal, hearing loss, and possibly *purulent* (containing pus) or serous drainage. The inflammation is treated with antibiotic or steroid eardrops, and the canal must be kept clean and dry or the condition can become chronic.

Otitis media is an inflammation of the normally air-filled middle ear, resulting in a collection of fluid behind the tympanic membrane. Otitis media can be either serous or suppurative. Serous otitis media occurs because of a buildup of clear fluid in

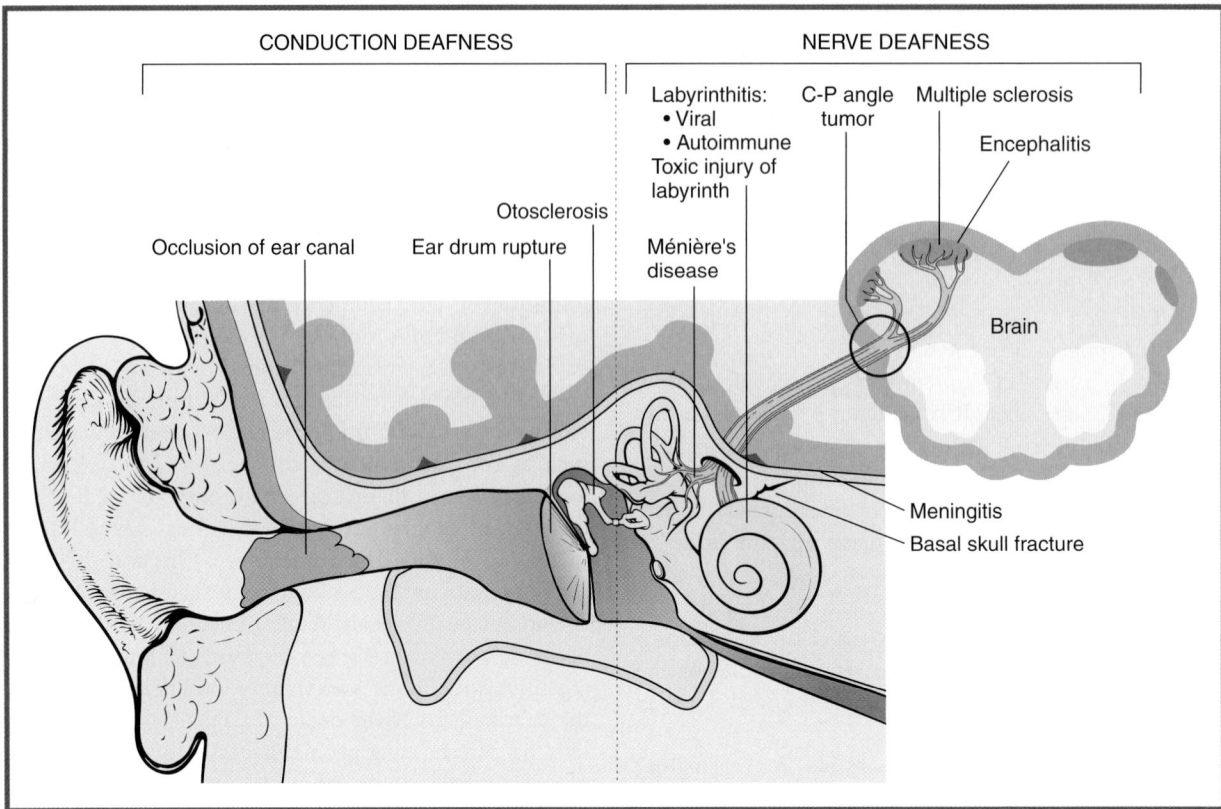

FIGURE 36-10 Causes of deafness. (From Damjanov I: *Pathology for the health-related professions*, ed 3, Philadelphia, 2006, Saunders.)

Recommendations for Treatment of Otitis Media

Because of increased concerns about the development of drug-resistant strains of bacteria as a result of the overprescription of antibiotics, the American Academy of Pediatrics has the following recommendations regarding treatment of otitis media:

- Delay treatment with antibiotics, giving the child's immune system a chance to fight the infection by itself, for 24 hours in children 6 to 24 months old and 72 hours for older children. Approximately 61% of children improve within 24 hours whether or not they are treated. If the child does not improve, then prescribe an appropriate antibiotic.
- The child will typically improve within 48 to 72 hours, but the parent should understand how important it is to complete the antibiotic medication as ordered to prevent the infection from recurring.

- The physician may decide to treat otitis media with a short course of antibiotics—5 days—but with a higher dose. The drugs of choice include amoxicillin (Amoxil), azithromycin (Zithromax), and cefuroxime (Rocephin).
- Antibiotics will not help if otitis is caused by a virus. Pediatricians recommend observing the child for possible complications and administering analgesics for pain control. Viral otitis media typically resolves itself within 7 to 14 days.
- The medical assistant plays a key role in helping parents understand why antibiotic therapy may not be recommended and in educating parents about the importance of administering a prescribed antibiotic at the time ordered using the correct dose and completing the entire prescription.

the middle ear, with patients complaining of a full feeling and some hearing loss. In suppurative otitis media, purulent fluid is present in the middle ear, with fever, pain, and hearing loss. The cause is often associated with an upper respiratory tract infection that has spread through the eustachian tube into the middle ear or with an allergic reaction (Figure 36-11).

An otoscopic examination reveals that the normally pearly gray tympanic membrane is inflamed and bulging. Fluid or pus areas may be visible through the membrane. A *tympanogram* may be done to determine the air pressure of the middle ear and the

mobility of the tympanic membrane. If fluid is present in the canal, it can be cultured to determine the causative pathogen. The individual may be given antibiotics, analgesics, and often a decongestant to promote drainage. If this condition becomes chronic, the physician may recommend a *myringotomy*, which is the creation of a surgical incision in the tympanic membrane to drain the fluid, followed by the insertion of a tympanostomy tube to continually drain the middle ear of fluid. This may be necessary to prevent permanent hearing loss because of damage to the ossicles (Figure 36-12).

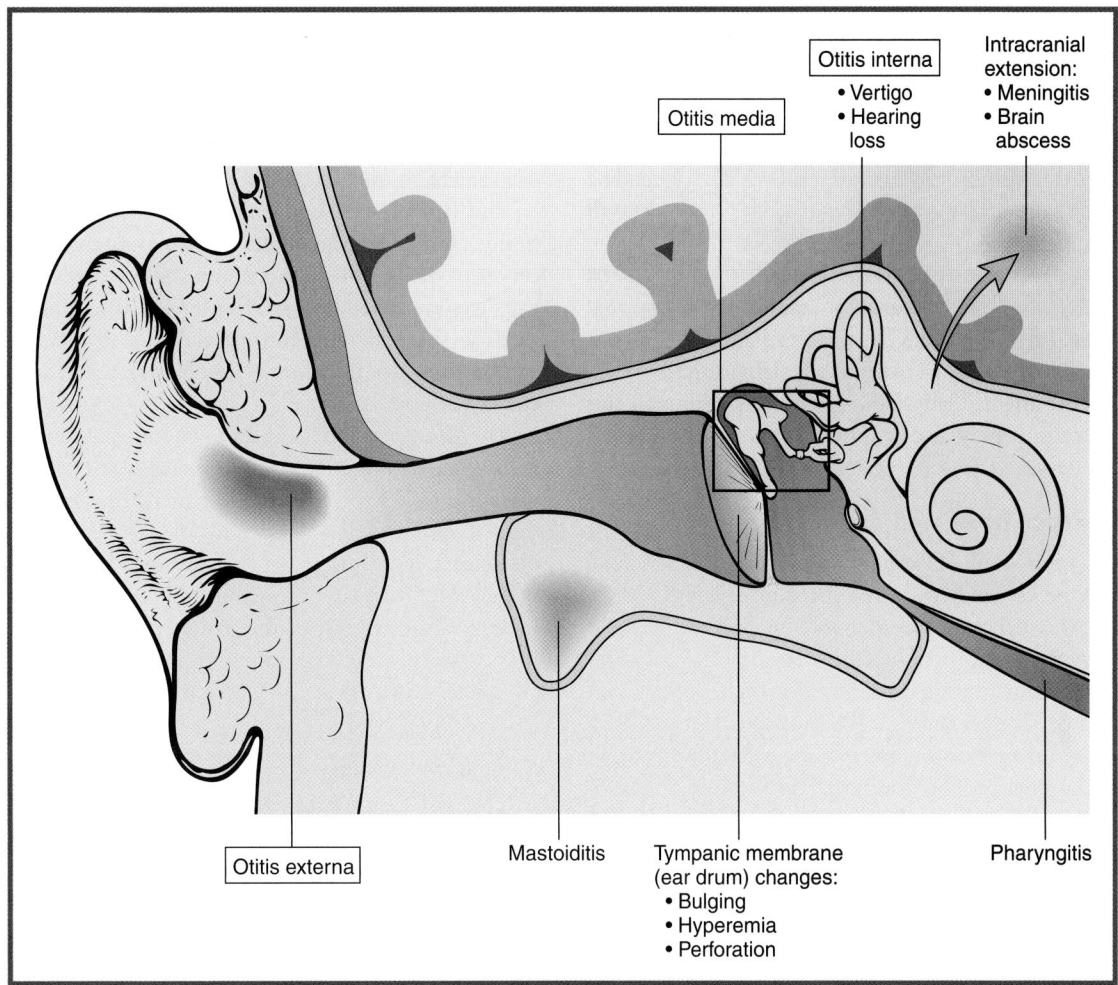

FIGURE 36-11 Inflammations and infections of the ear and surrounding tissues. (From Damjanov I: *Pathology for the health-related professions*, ed 3, Philadelphia, 2006, Saunders.)

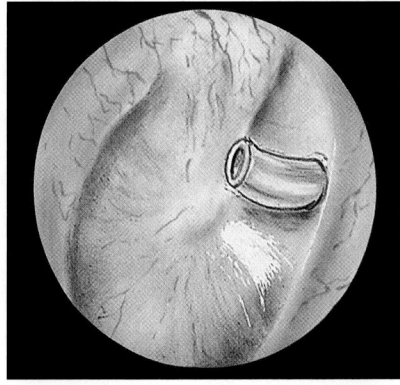

FIGURE 36-12 Insertion of tympanostomy tubes. (From Jarvis C: *Physical examination and health assessment*, ed 4, Philadelphia, 2004, Saunders.)

Impacted Cerumen

Cerumen is normally a soft, yellowish waxy substance created to lubricate the external auditory canal. An excessive secretion of cerumen can gradually cause hearing loss, tinnitus, a feeling of fullness, and *otalgia* (ear pain). Impacted cerumen that has pushed tightly up against the eardrum is a frequent cause of conductive hearing loss because sound vibrations cannot pass through the cerumen to initiate movement of the tympanic membrane. Individuals with psoriasis, abnormally narrow ear canals, or an excessive amount of hair growing within the ear canals are more prone to this condition.

An otoscopic examination quickly reveals this problem. If impacted cerumen is found, it must be removed. This can be done by softening the wax with oily drops, such as carbamide peroxide (Debrox), then irrigating the ear with warm water until the plug is removed. Because this condition can recur, the patient may need to schedule periodic examinations. If the patient is experiencing hearing loss because of the impaction, it is immediately remedied with removal of the cerumen.

Ménière's Disease

The semicircular canals of the inner ear in coordination with the eighth cranial nerve controls balance and gives a sense of how the body is positioned. The canals contain fluid—the endolymph—whose filtration and excretion is controlled by the part of the canal called the *endolymphatic sac.* Ménière's disease causes swelling and edema in this part of the semicircular canals, with an overproduction or collection of excess endolymph.

When this occurs the patient exhibits signs. Although the cause of this problem is unknown, Ménière's disease is a chronic, progressive condition that triggers episodes of recurring attacks of vertigo, tinnitus, a sensation of pressure in the affected ear, and advancing hearing loss. During an acute attack, patients experience nausea, vomiting, and problems with balance. The attacks can last from a few hours to several days, increasing in severity over time.

During the active periods of the disease the patient is treated symptomatically with medications for nausea and vomiting. A salt-restricted diet, diuretics, and antihistamines may be prescribed to control edema within the labyrinth. Surgical destruction of the affected labyrinth is an option. Although this relieves symptoms, it may also result in permanent deafness if the cochlea is damaged.

Diagnostic Procedures

An ear examination involves viewing the external auditory canal with an otoscope covered by an ear speculum (Figure 36-13). Disposable plastic speculum covers should be used each time to prevent disease transmission. A normal otoscopic examination reveals an external auditory canal with a small amount of cerumen and a pearly gray and concave tympanic membrane. In addition to performing the otoscopic examination, the physician will palpate the area around the pinna for abnormalities or sensations. A number of tests are used to assess hearing acuity, ranging from simple tuning fork tests to quantitative and qualitative audiometric testing. If a hearing loss is suspected, the next test is usually performed with a tuning fork.

Tuning Fork Testing

Tuning fork tests, as mentioned in Chapter 31, measure hearing by air conduction and bone conduction. In bone conduction the sound vibrates through the cranial bones to the inner ear. There are different-sized tuning forks, each with a different frequency. The most commonly used fork is the C, which has a frequency of 1024 hertz (Hz), because this frequency reflects the level of normal speech patterns. To activate the fork, the physician holds it by the stem and strikes the tines softly on the palm of the hand. Striking the tines too forcefully will create a tone that is too loud for diagnostic use. The two testing evaluations that are used to evaluate hearing are the Weber and the Rinne tests. Both of these procedures are commonly used to evaluate conductive and sensory losses.

The *Weber* test is used if the patient reports hearing is better in one ear than in the other. The vibrating fork is placed in the center of the top of the head, and the patient is asked in which ear the tone is louder or if the tone is the same in both ears. Because the patient is hearing the tone by bone conduction through the head, a normal result is that the sound is heard equally in both ears.

The *Rinne* test is designed to compare air conduction sound with bone conduction sound. In this test the stem of the vibrating fork is placed on the patient's mastoid process, and the patient is advised to raise his or her hand when the sound disappears. The fork is quickly inverted so that the vibrating tines are approximately 1 inch in front of the external ear canal. If the hearing is normal, the patient should still hear a sound. In normal hearing the sound is heard twice as long by air conduction as by bone conduction.

Audiometric Testing

An audiometric test may be done in an otology or family practice and is performed by medical assistants who have received additional training (Figure 36-14, *A*). Audiometry measures the lowest intensity of sound that an individual can hear. The patient, frequently a child, is assisted in placing headphones over the ears. Each ear is tested by delivering a single frequency at a specific intensity, starting with low frequency tones and going up to very high frequencies (Figure 36-14, *B*). The patient is asked to signal when he or she hears the sound. The results are printed on a graph called an *audiogram,* or the medical assistant charts the results on a graph sheet (Procedure 36-5).

If initial screening indicates a hearing deficit the physician may recommend an appointment with an **audiologist** for audiometric evaluation. The evaluation consists of a battery of tests that assess the level of hearing impairment and provide valuable information as to how the patient may be helped. The first test evaluates speech comprehension and assesses the patient's ability to follow verbal instructions. Once this evaluation is completed, the patient is placed in a soundproof booth with earphones over the ears. From this point on, the audiologist speaks to the patient and conducts all testing through the earphones. The assessment includes testing the frequency, intensity, and audibility of sound. This process takes approximately an hour.

Aseptic Procedures in Otology

Routine examination instruments should be disinfected or sterilized according to office policy after each use and stored in a clean area. Surgical asepsis must be practiced when changing dressings, placing packs, and performing minor surgery. Medications, such as eardrops and nose drops, must be handled carefully to avoid contamination.

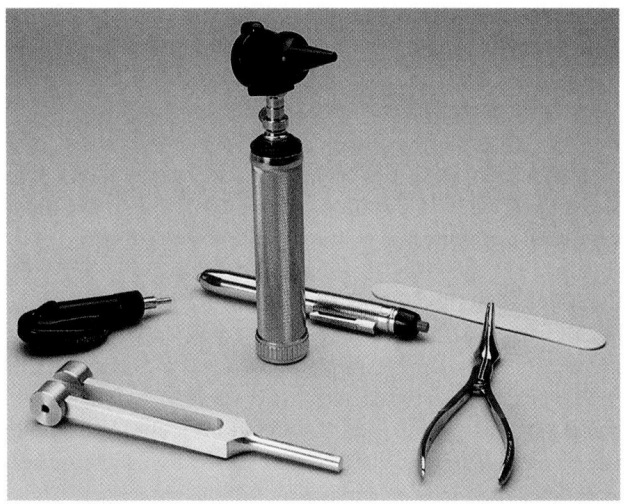

FIGURE 36-13 Otoscopy examination instruments.

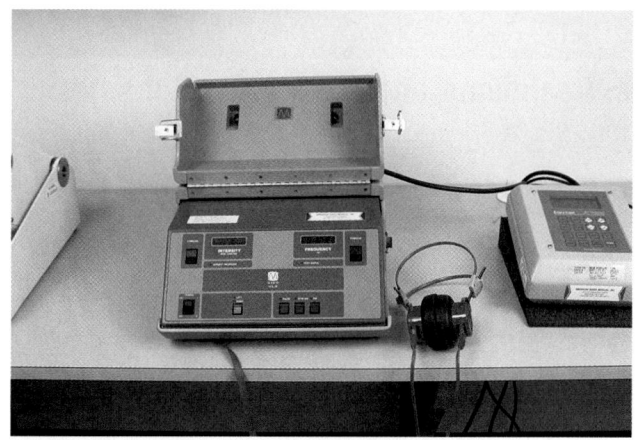
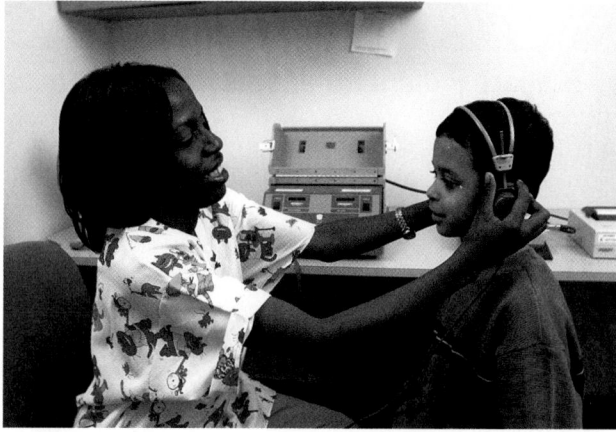

FIGURE 36-14 A, Audiometer. **B,** Placing headphones.

PROCEDURE 36-5

Prepare Patient for and Assist with Routine and Specialty Examinations: Measure Hearing Acuity Using an Audiometer

<u>CAAHEP COMPETENCIES:</u> 3.b.(4)(e), 3.b.(4)(f)
<u>ABHES COMPETENCIES:</u> 4.b, 4.h

GOAL: *To perform audiometric testing of hearing acuity.*

EQUIPMENT and SUPPLIES

- Audiometer with adjustable headphones
- Quiet area
- Patient record

PROCEDURAL STEPS

1. Wash hands, assemble the equipment, and conduct the patient into a quiet area (see Figure 36-14, *A*).
   <u>PURPOSE:</u> The testing room should be free from distractions and noise to allow the patient to completely concentrate on the hearing evaluation.
2. Explain that the audiometer will measure whether the patient can hear various sound wave frequencies through the headphones. Each ear will be tested separately. When the patient hears a frequency, he or she should raise a hand to signal the medical assistant.
   <u>PURPOSE:</u> Patient education is needed for compliance with the examination.

3. Place the headphones over the patient's ears, making sure the headphones are adjusted for comfort (see Figure 36-14, *B*).
4. The audiometer tests each ear separately, starting at a low frequency. If the results are not automatically recorded by the machine, the medical assistant documents the patient response to the frequencies on a graph or audiogram. The medical assistant requires specialized training to conduct this test.
5. Frequencies are gradually increased to test patient ability to hear. The medical assistant continues to document each response by the patient.
6. The other ear is then tested, and the results are documented using the appropriate abbreviations—AU (both ears), AD (right ear), AS (left ear).
7. Patient results are given to the physician for interpretation.
8. Disinfect the equipment according to the manufacturer's guidelines.
9. Wash hands.

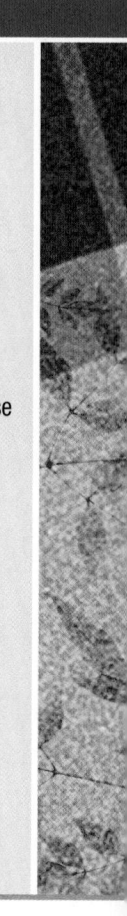

Treatment Procedures

Ear Irrigation

An ear irrigation is performed to remove excessive or impacted cerumen; to remove a foreign body; or to treat the inflamed ear with an antiseptic solution (Procedure 36-6). When an ear irrigation is ordered by the physician, the medical assistant may perform the procedure if proper training has been completed and the assistant is competent in the technique. To prevent patient discomfort it is important to insert the irrigating solution at an angle so the solution is not directed toward the tympanic membrane. Some of the discomforts the patient may experience during an ear irrigation include vertigo, ear discomfort, coughing, or a tickle in the back of the throat. Follow the procedure as prescribed, making sure that the patient is comfortable. Always chart the treatment and its results immediately after completion.

PROCEDURE 36-6

Prepare Patient for and Assist with Procedures, Treatments, and Minor Office Surgeries:
Irrigate a Patient's Ear

<u>CAAHEP COMPETENCIES:</u> 3.b.(4)(e), 3.b.(4)(f)
<u>ABHES COMPETENCIES:</u> 4.b, 4.h

GOAL: *To remove excessive or impacted cerumen from a patient's ear (or ears).*

EQUIPMENT and SUPPLIES

- Irrigating solution
- Basin for irrigating solution
- Bulb syringe or an approved otic irrigation device
- Gauze squares
- Otoscope
- Drainage basin
- Disposable drape with polylined barrier
- Cotton-tipped applicators
- Disposable gloves
- Patient record

PROCEDURAL STEPS

1. Wash your hands.
   <u>PURPOSE:</u> Infection control.

2. Check the physician's order and assemble the materials needed (Figure 1).

3. Check the label of the solution three times: (a) when you remove it from the shelf, (b) when you pour it, and (c) when you return it to the shelf.
   <u>PURPOSE:</u> To prevent possible medication error.

4. Prepare the solution as ordered. The solution temperature should be at body temperature to help loosen the cerumen.
   <u>PURPOSE:</u> Solutions at 100° F are most comfortable to the patient. Ask the patient if the solution temperature is comfortable.

5. Identify the patient, and explain the procedure.

6. View the affected ear with an otoscope to locate cerumen impaction.

7. Place the patient in a sitting position with the head tilted toward the affected ear. A water-absorbent towel is placed over a polylined barrier on the patient's shoulder, and the collecting basin is placed on the towel at the base of the ear. The patient can assist you by holding the collecting basin in place (Figure 2).
   <u>PURPOSE:</u> This technique will minimize the risk of getting the patient's clothing wet and will aid the water flow into the collecting basin.

8. Apply gloves, and wipe any particles from the outside of the ear with gauze squares.
   <u>PURPOSE:</u> This prevents the introduction of foreign materials into the ear canal.

9. Test to be certain that the solution is warm, fill the syringe, and expel air.
   <u>PURPOSE:</u> Trapped air in the syringe will increase the pressure of the irrigation, causing discomfort.

10. Straighten the external ear canal. For adults and children over the age of 3, gently pull the pinna of the ear up and back; for children younger than 3, pull the ear lobe down and back (Figure 3).
    <u>PURPOSE:</u> Straightening the canal allows the irrigating fluid to circulate through the canal.

11. Place the tip of the syringe into the meatus of the ear.

12. Gently direct the flow of the solution toward the roof of the canal.
    <u>PURPOSE:</u> This will help to prevent injury to the tympanic membrane, will aid in the removal of the embedded material, and is most comfortable for the patient.

13. Refill the syringe with warm solution, and continue until the material has been removed. Note the particles in the collecting basin to evaluate when the material has been successfully removed.

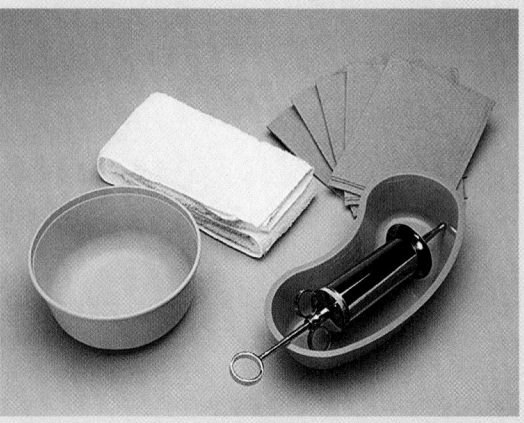

FIGURE 1

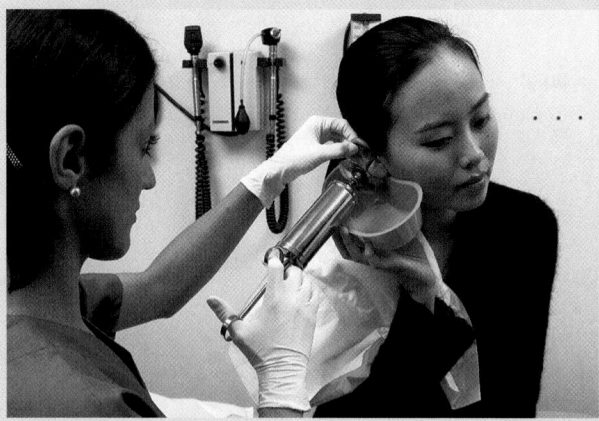

FIGURE 2

Continued

PROCEDURE 36-6

14. Dry the patient's external ear with gauze squares and the visible ear canal gently with cotton-tipped applicators.
    PURPOSE: Inserting the applicator into the canal may cause serious trauma.
15. Inspect the ear with an otoscope to determine the results.
16. Place a clean, absorbent towel on the examination table, and allow the patient to rest quietly with the head turned to the irrigated side while you wait for the physician to return to check the affected ear.
17. Clean the work area, and return all equipment after it has been properly disinfected. Wash your hands.
    PURPOSE: Infection control.
18. Record the procedure, including the date and time; which ear was irrigated, using the appropriate abbreviations—AU (both ears), AD (right ear), AS (left ear); the type and amount of irrigating solution used; the characteristics of the material

returned from the irrigation; the visibility of the tympanic membrane after irrigation; and any patient reactions.
PURPOSE: Procedures that are not recorded are considered not done.
DOCUMENTATION EXERCISE: You are ordered to perform an irrigation of both ears on Mrs. Ophelia Black because of impacted cerumen. Otoscopic examination before the irrigation revealed a large amount of dark brown ear wax in both ears. After irrigation both tympanic membranes were visible and Mrs. Black had no complaints of discomfort.

_____

_____

_____

See Appendix D for a charting example.

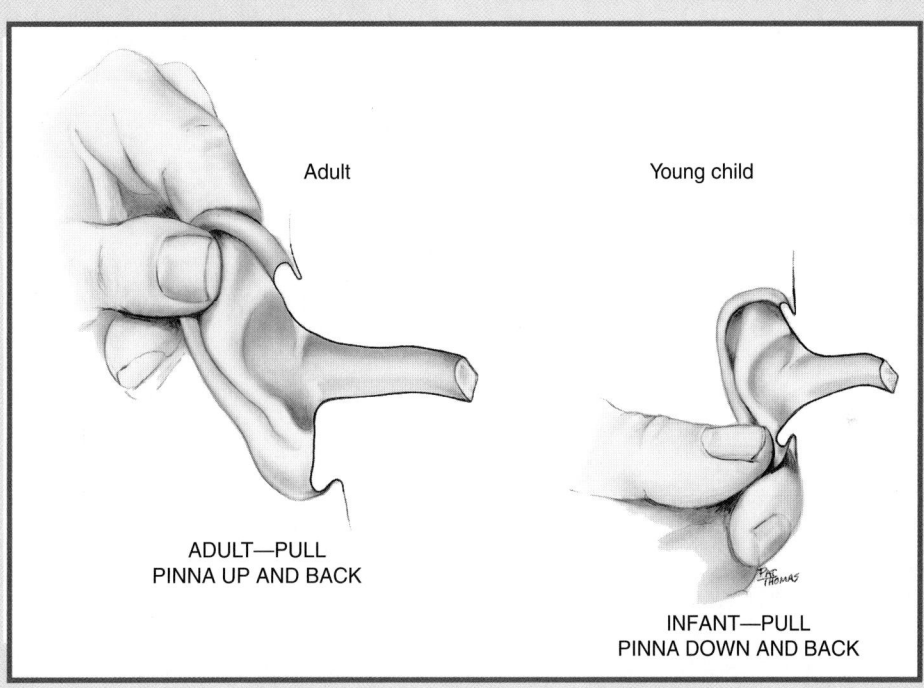

Adult

Young child

ADULT—PULL
PINNA UP AND BACK

INFANT—PULL
PINNA DOWN AND BACK

FIGURE 3

CRITICAL THINKING APPLICATION

Kim is ordered to perform a bilateral ear irrigation on a 68-year-old patient with impacted cerumen. She checks the auditory canals before the procedure with an otoscope and sees a large amount of dark brown cerumen in the right ear completely covering the tympanic membrane. The left ear has a moderate amount of golden brown cerumen covering the bottom half of the tympanic membrane. After the procedure both membranes are visible, and the patient tolerated the procedure without complaints. How should Kim document the procedure?

Instilling Otic Medications

Medication ordered for ear instillation is given to soften impacted cerumen, to relieve pain, or as an antibiotic drop for an infectious pathogen (Procedure 36-7). Patients with ear conditions may be in considerable pain as well as having difficulty hearing, which makes health teaching a challenge. Wait until after the procedure is completed and the patient is more comfortable to reinforce health behaviors.

PROCEDURE 36-7

Prepare Patient for and Assist with Procedures, Treatments, and Minor Office Surgeries: Instill Medicated Ear Drops

CAAHEP COMPETENCIES: 3.b.(4)(f), 3.b.(4)(g)
ABHES COMPETENCIES: 4.b, 4.m

GOAL: *To instill the correct medication in the accurate dose directly into the external auditory canal.*

EQUIPMENT and SUPPLIES

- Prescribed otic drops in dispenser bottle
- Cotton balls
- Disposable gloves
- Patient record

PROCEDURAL STEPS

1. Wash hands, and gather the needed equipment and supplies.
   PURPOSE: To control infection and to reduce procedure time.
2. Check the medication label three times: (a) when you remove it from the shelf, (b) when you prepare it, and (c) when you return it to the shelf.
   PURPOSE: To avoid possible medication error.
3. Identify your patient, and explain the procedure.
4. Have the patient sit up and tilt head away from the affected ear or lie down on the side with the affected ear upward.
   PURPOSE: Exposes the ear for treatment, allows gravity to help the medication flow into the canal, and ensures patient comfort.
5. Check the temperature of the medication bottle. If it feels cold, gently roll the bottle back and forth between your hands to warm the drops.

PURPOSE: Cold medication may increase the pain level or cause symptoms of nausea and vertigo.

6. Hold the dropper firmly in your dominant hand. With the other hand, gently pull the pinna up and back if the patient is an adult or the ear lobe down and back if the patient is younger than 3 years old.
   PURPOSE: To straighten the ear canal and make it easier for the medication to reach its designated position.
7. Place the tip of the dropper in the ear canal meatus, and instill the medication drops along the side of the canal (Figure 1).
8. Instruct the patient to rest on the opposite side of the affected ear and to remain in this position for approximately 3 minutes.
   PURPOSE: Helps the medication reach the base of the canal and prevents it from immediately running out of the ear (Figure 2).
9. If instructed by the physician, place a moistened cotton ball into the ear canal.
   PURPOSE: Protects the ear canal and prevents medication from leaking out of the ear.
10. Clean the work area, and wash your hands.
    PURPOSE: Infection control.
11. Record the procedure using the appropriate abbreviations, including the date and time; name, dose, and strength of the medication; which ear was treated; and patient reactions on the chart.
    PURPOSE: Procedures that are not recorded are considered not done.

See Appendix D for a charting example.

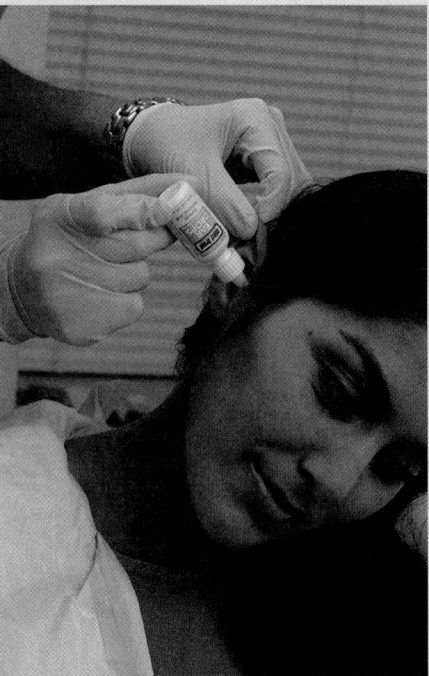

FIGURE 1

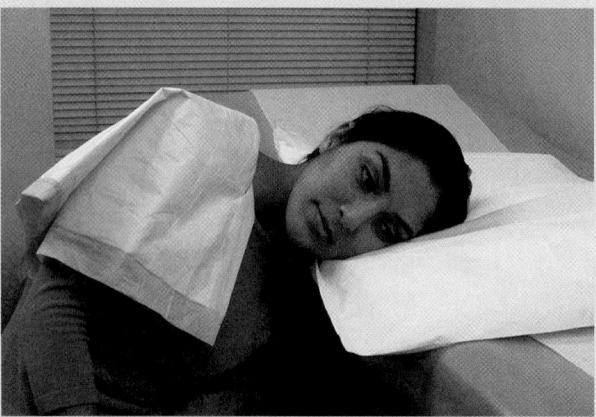

FIGURE 2

EXAMINATION OF THE NOSE AND THROAT

If you are working in an ENT specialty office, you will also be assisting in the examination of the nasal cavity and the throat. The nasal cavity is examined to inspect the mucous membrane of the nostrils. The common cold and allergies are the main causes of changes in the mucosa. The physician may use a nasal speculum to visualize the nostrils and examines the nasal sinuses by palpation and transillumination.

The throat is the area that includes the larynx and pharynx; it can be viewed with the aid of a mirror and either a tongue depressor or a gauze square to grasp the tongue. In the nasopharynx, the physician looks for enlarged adenoids (pharyngeal tonsils) and for the orifices of the eustachian tubes. The physician may spray the patient's throat with a topical anesthetic before the examination to prevent the gag reflex.

Throat specimens are frequently collected in the physician's office to assist in the diagnosis of strep throat infections. Strep throat is caused by the group A *beta-hemolytic Streptococcus* bacteria and if left untreated can cause serious complications. Throat cultures are collected by gently swabbing the back of the throat and the surfaces of the tonsils with a sterile swab. The mouth and tongue should be avoided to prevent contamination of the swab with the normal flora of the mouth (Procedure 36-8).

PROCEDURE 36-8

Prepare Patient for and Assist with Procedures, Treatments, and Minor Office Surgeries: Collect a Specimen for a Throat Culture

CAAHEP COMPETENCY: 3.b.(4)(f)
ABHES COMPETENCIES: 4.b, 4.h

GOAL: *To collect a throat culture, using sterile technique, for either immediate testing or transportation to the laboratory.*

EQUIPMENT and SUPPLIES

- Nonsterile gloves
- Face protection barrier if the patient is coughing or if there is danger of splattering of body fluids
- Sterile swab
- Sterile tongue depressor
- Transport medium
- Biohazard waste container
- Laboratory requisition if sample is being sent out for examination
- Patient record

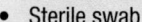

PROCEDURAL STEPS

1. Wash and dry your hands.
   PURPOSE: T Infection control.
2. Gather the materials needed.
3. Don gloves and face protection if needed.
   PURPOSE: Standard precautions.
4. Position the patient so that the light shines into the mouth.
   PURPOSE: Illumination of the area to be swabbed.
5. Remove the sterile swab from the sterile wrap with your dominant hand, and grasp the sterile tongue depressor with your nondominant hand.
   PURPOSE: Better control of the swabbing process.
6. Instruct the patient to open the mouth and say "ah." Depress the tongue with the depressor (Figure 1).
   PURPOSE: Saying "ah" helps elevate the uvula and reduces the tendency to gag. The tongue is depressed so that you can see the back of the throat and avoid contamination of the sterile swab.
7. Swab the back of the throat between the tonsillar pillars and especially any reddened, patchy areas of the throat, white pus pockets, purulent areas, and the tonsils.

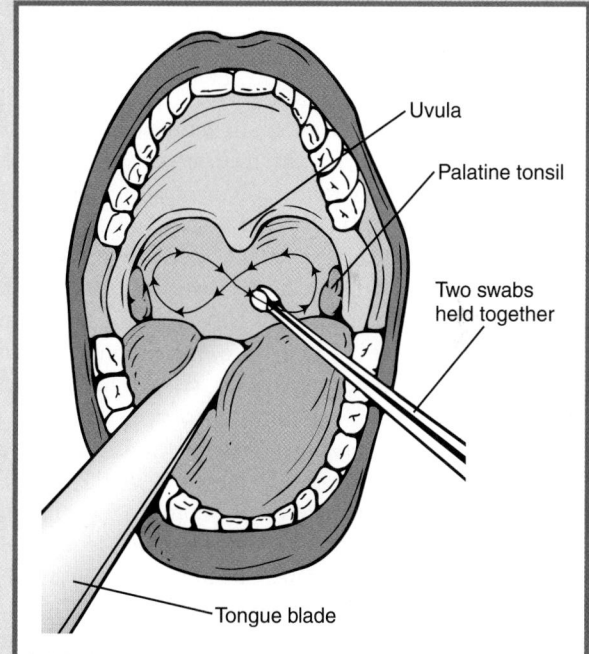

FIGURE 1

PURPOSE: Pathogenic organisms are found in the back of the throat and on the tonsils.
8. Place the swab into the transport medium, label it, and send it to the laboratory. If direct slide testing is requested, return the labeled swab to the laboratory (Figure 2). (Rapid strep test procedure is described in Chapter 54.)
   PURPOSE: Transport medium prevents the swab from drying. Labeling immediately after collection prevents mixing up specimens.

Continued

PROCEDURE 36-8—cont'd

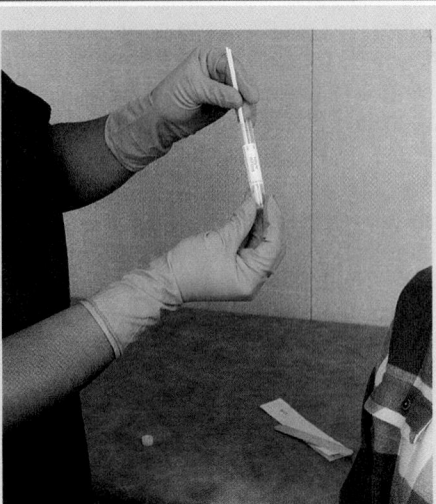

FIGURE 2

9. Dispose of contaminated supplies in biohazard waste container.
   <u>PURPOSE:</u> Prevents the spread of infection.
10. Disinfect the work area.
11. Remove gloves; place in a biohazard waste container.
12. Wash your hands.
   <u>PURPOSE:</u> Infection control.
13. Record procedure in the patient's record.
   <u>PURPOSE:</u> Procedures that are not recorded are considered not done.

See Appendix D for a charting example.

CLOSING COMMENTS

Patient Education

Patients with vision or hearing impairments face serious challenges. For these patients the medical assistant must use good listening skills, appropriate nonverbal methods, and touch to communicate empathy and understanding. Teaching may have to be adapted to meet the special needs of these patients. A person with a vision loss will benefit from large-print forms and handouts, increased levels of lighting, and verbal instructions rather than written ones to reinforce learning. An individual with a hearing deficit should have printed instructions, demonstrations of how to manage treatments, or even sign language interpretation available to assure accurate communications. Including family members in the patient's treatment plan and offering referrals to appropriate community or professional resources may be very beneficial to a patient with sensory loss. Each patient must be individually assessed to determine his or her level of needed adaptation.

An important part of home care for patients receiving eye medications is stressing the need for maintaining the sterility of the medication. Patients and/or family members must be taught how to apply the medication and prevent trauma to the eye as well as contamination of the applicator. Patients receiving ear treatments must also understand how to instill the medication.

Legal and Ethical Issues

Diminished sight or hearing may render the patient seriously impaired. To avoid possible accidents and office injuries, always ask a sight- or hearing-impaired patient if he or she requires assistance. When you escort the patient to an examination room, offer your arm and tell the patient the approximate distance that you will be walking. If the patient is to have an examination that will involve local anesthesia or eye drops that dilate the pupil, be sure the patient has recovered and someone is available to take the patient home before allowing him or her to leave the office. Never assume that the patient is capable of leaving alone. If the patient insists on leaving before the designated recovery time, inform the physician and record the time and circumstances surrounding the event in the patient's chart. This information should be signed and witnessed. The physician may want a refusal of care form signed by the patient and placed in the chart.

Health Insurance Portability and Accountability Act Applications

Regardless of the patient's disability, the ambulatory care center must follow Health Insurance Portability and Accountability Act (HIPAA) guidelines for Notice of Privacy Practices (NPP). The NPP is a form developed by the facility that outlines the patient's rights and the facility's legal responsibilities to safeguard the patient's protected health information. The facility must give the NPP to each new patient at the first office visit. To comply with HIPAA guidelines, the document must be in a language that the patient easily understands. The staff is responsible for obtaining a patient signature on the form that indicates the patient's agreement with the stipulations of the facility's privacy practice. An individual with a vision deficit may require a large print form or a staff member to read the document and answer any questions. The staff must also make sure patients with hearing deficits understand the form before signing.

SUMMARY OF SCENARIO

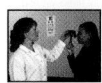

After observing Kim and asking many questions, Amy is beginning to understand her special responsibilities in the ophthalmology and otorhinolaryngology clinic. She recognizes the need to be familiar with the anatomy and physiology of both the eye and the ear as well as to be able to perform specialty-related skills, such as irrigations, medication instillations, and diagnostic procedures. Amy has become quite proficient at performing Snellen and Ishihara screening examinations and accurately documenting each. Kim has taught her to use the audiometer and assisted her with the first few screenings, so she is now ready to do hearing tests on her own. Although she learned about eye and ear medications in her medical assistant program, instilling these medications

in an actual patient is different than working on mannequins and classmates. Kim has reinforced the skills she learned in her program, continually emphasizing infection control procedures and reinforcing patient education information. Amy realizes she needs to understand the pathologic conditions that can occur in the sensory organs so she will be able to assist the physician as needed and answer patient questions. After working with patients who have vision and hearing deficits, Amy understands the importance of adapting communication techniques to meet the needs of each patient. Amy has decided to take advantage of educational opportunities at the hospital and through her professional organization so she can continue to learn about this special area of practice.

SUMMARY of LEARNING OBJECTIVES

1. Define, spell, and pronounce the terms listed in the vocabulary.
   - Spelling and pronouncing medical terms correctly adds credibility to the medical assistant. Knowing the definition of these terms promotes confidence in communication with patients and co-workers.
2. Explain the differences among an ophthalmologist, optometrist, and optician.
   - An ophthalmologist is a medical doctor specializing in the diagnosis and treatment of the eye, an optometrist can examine and treat visual defects, and an optician fills prescriptions for corrective lenses.
3. Identify the anatomic structures of the eye.
   - The anatomy of the eye begins with the outer covering, the conjunctiva, and three layers of tissue: the sclera, choroid, and retina. The retina is where light rays are converted into nervous energy for interpretation by the brain.
4. Describe how vision occurs.
   - Vision begins with the passage of light through the cornea, where it is refracted. It then passes through the aqueous humor and pupil into the lens. The ciliary muscle adjusts the curvature of the lens to again refract the light rays so they pass into the retina, triggering the photoreceptor cells of the rods and cones. Light energy is converted into an electrical impulse that is sent through the optic nerve to the brain, where interpretation occurs.
5. Differentiate among the major types of refractive errors.
   - Refractive errors include hyperopia, myopia, presbyopia, and astigmatism. All are caused by a problem with bending light so it can be accurately focused on the retina. They are usually caused by defects in the shape of the eyeball and can be corrected with glasses, contacts, or surgery.
6. Summarize typical disorders of the eye.
   - Eye disorders can range from problems with eye movement, as in strabismus and nystagmus, to infections of the eye,

including hordeola, chalazions, keratitis, conjunctivitis, and blepharitis. Disorders of the eyeball include corneal abrasions, cataracts, glaucoma, and macular degeneration.

7. Define the various diagnostic procedures for the eye.
   - Diagnostic procedures for the eye begin with a visual examination of the eye using an ophthalmoscope. Next, the eyelids are examined for abnormalities and the pupils are tested for PERRLA. More advanced techniques include the use of a slit lamp to view the fine details of the eye and the exophthalmometer to measure the distance of the eyeball from the orbit. Distance visual acuity is typically assessed with the use of a Snellen chart; near visual acuity is tested with a near-vision acuity chart. A patient can be tested for a color vision defect with the Ishihara test.
8. Conduct a vision acuity test using the Snellen chart.
   - Procedure 36-1 explains the Snellen evaluation.
9. Assess color acuity.
   - Procedure 36-2 outlines the color acuity examination.
10. Illustrate the purpose of eye irrigations and the instillation of medication.
    - Eye irrigations relieve inflammation, remove drainage, dilute chemicals, or wash away foreign bodies. Sterile technique and equipment must be used to avoid contamination. Medication may be instilled into the eye for the treatment of an infection, to soothe an eye irritation, to anesthetize the eye, or to dilate the pupils before examination or treatment.
11. Properly irrigate a patient's eyes.
    - Procedure 36-3 describes the method for performing an eye irrigation.
12. Accurately instill eye medication.
    - Procedure 36-4 explains how to administer eye medications.
13. Identify the structures and explain the functions of the external, middle, and internal ear.
    - The external ear consists of the auricle or pinna and the

Continued

SUMMARY of LEARNING OBJECTIVES

Continued

external auditory canal, which transmits sound waves to the tympanic membrane. The middle ear is an air-filled cavity that contains the ossicles. The sound vibration passes through the tympanic membrane, causing the ossicles to vibrate. This bone-conducted vibration passes through the oval window into the inner ear. The organ of Corti in the cochlea of the inner ear converts the sound waves into nervous energy that is sent to the brain for interpretation. The semicircular canals in the inner ear maintain equilibrium.

14. Describe the conditions that can lead to hearing loss, including conductive, neurogenic, and congenital hearing losses.
    - Conductive hearing loss is caused by a problem that originates in the external or middle ear preventing sound vibrations from passing through the external auditory canal, limiting tympanic membrane vibrations, or interfering with the passage of bone-conducted sound in the middle ear. A sensorineural hearing loss results from damage to the organ of Corti or the auditory nerve and prevents vibrations from being converted into nervous stimuli.

15. Define the major disorders of the ear, including otitis, impacted cerumen, and Ménière's disease.
    - Otitis externa is an inflammation of the auditory canal, and otitis media is an inflammation of the normally air-filled middle ear, resulting in a collection of fluid that is either serous or suppurative behind the tympanic membrane. Impacted cerumen is a frequent cause of conductive hearing loss. Ménière's disease is a chronic, progressive condition that affects the labyrinth and causes recurring attacks of vertigo, tinnitus, a sensation of pressure in the affected ear, and advancing hearing loss.

16. Explain the various otic diagnostic procedures.
    - The ear examination begins with an otoscopic examination and can include various tuning fork tests to determine either conductive or sensorineural hearing deficits and more advanced audiometric testing.

17. Accurately measure the hearing acuity of a patient by using an audiometer.
    - Procedure 36-5 explains the audiometry examination.

18. Identify the purpose of ear irrigations and instillation of ear medication.
    - An ear irrigation is performed to remove excessive or impacted cerumen, remove a foreign body, or treat the inflamed ear with an antiseptic solution. Medication instilled into the ear is given to soften impacted cerumen, relieve pain, or fight an infectious pathogen.

19. Demonstrate ear irrigations.
    - Procedure 36-6 describes how to perform an ear irrigation.

20. Accurately instill otic drops.
    - Procedure 36-7 explains how to administer otic drugs.

21. Summarize the nose and throat examination.
    - Examination of the nose and throat begins with viewing of the nasal cavity followed by visual examination of the throat and the nasopharynx. Throat cultures may be done to determine the presence of a streptococcal infection. The anterior and posterior neck regions are palpated for abnormalities.

22. Perform a throat culture.
    - Procedure 36-8 explains how to perform a throat culture.

23. Describe the effect of sensory loss on patient education.
    - Patients with vision and hearing impairments face serious challenges and require individualized attention to meet their health education needs. Patients with vision losses may need large print forms and handouts, increased levels of lighting, or verbal instructions rather than written ones. Individuals with hearing deficits may benefit from printed instructions, demonstrations on how to manage treatments, or even sign language interpretation. Family members should be included in the patient's treatment plan, and referrals to appropriate community or professional resources may be very beneficial.

CONNECTIONS

Study Guide Connection: Go to Chapter 36 Study Guide. Read the Case Study and Workplace Applications and complete the assignments. Do online research for answers to the questions in the Internet Activities associated with assisting in ophthalmology and otolaryngology.

CD Connection: Go to the Medical Assisting Competency Challenge CD and do the training activities under Diagnostic Testing. For a better understanding of the structure of the eye, view the animation for anatomy of the eye.

Evolve Connection: For more information related to assisting in ophthalmology and otolaryngology, go to evolve.elsevier.com/kinn and visit related weblinks for Chapter 36. Click on the Medical Assisting Exam Review and do the practice questions to sharpen your test-taking skills.

Assisting in Dermatology

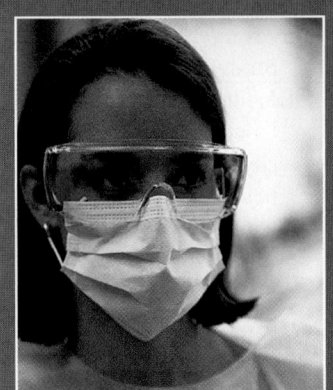

37

SCENARIO

Dr. Sam Lee is a dermatologist who employs several medical assistants in his busy private practice. Melissa Bauman, CMA, has worked for Dr. Lee since graduating from a medical assisting program last year. Melissa works as a clinical specialist whose primary responsibilities are to perform telephone screening, prepare patients for procedures, and assist Dr. Lee as needed. To fulfill her responsibilities in the dermatology practice Melissa must be familiar with common diseases and disorders that affect the skin as well as be prepared to reinforce patient education regarding the treatment and prevention of dermatologic conditions.

While studying this chapter, think about the following questions:

- What is the basic anatomy and physiology of the integumentary system?
- What are the common diseases and disorders that affect the integumentary system?
- How can Melissa determine the difference between the levels of burn injuries?
- Why is it important that Melissa understand the concepts of staging and grading malignant tumors?

- What are the primary malignancies of the skin?
- What dermatologic procedures should Melissa be prepared to perform?

LEARNING OBJECTIVES

1. Define, spell, and pronounce the terms listed in the vocabulary.
2. Explain the major functions of the skin.
3. Diagram the anatomic structures of the skin.
4. Compare various skin lesions, and give examples of each.
5. Describe typical integumentary system infections.
6. Differentiate among various inflammatory and autoimmune integumentary disorders.
7. Recognize thermal injuries to the skin.
8. Compare the characteristics of benign and malignant neoplasms.

9. Define grading and staging of malignant tumors.
10. Conduct patient education on the warning signs of cancer.
11. Describe skin malignancies and their treatment.
12. Define the ABCD rule for identifying a malignant melanoma.
13. Summarize allergy testing procedures.
14. Explain dermatologic procedures conducted in the ambulatory care setting.
15. Accurately obtain an exudate sample from a wound for laboratory analysis.

National Accreditation Competencies and Content

CAAHEP COMPETENCIES

Clinical

3.b.(2)(c). Obtain specimens for microbiological testing

ABHES COMPETENCIES

Clinical Duties

4.h. Prepare patient for and assist physician with routine and specialty examinations

alopecia (al-o-pe′-se-uh) Partial or complete lack of hair.

anaplastic Relating to alteration in cells to a more primitive form; describes cancer-producing cells.

autoimmune Describing the development of an immune response to one's own tissues, in which the body acts against its own cells to cause localized and systemic reactions.

bilirubin (bih-luh-roo′-bin) Orange pigment in bile that when it accumulates leads to jaundice.

cryosurgery Technique of exposing tissue to extreme cold to produce a well-defined area of cell destruction.

debridement Removal of foreign material and dead, damaged tissue from a wound.

ecchymosis Bluish-black skin discoloration produced by hemorrhagic areas.

electrodesiccation Destruction of cells and tissue by means of short high-frequency electrical sparks.

exacerbation An increase in the seriousness of a disease marked by greater intensity in the signs and symptoms.

excoriated Having undergone injury to the skin caused by scratching; abraded.

glomerulonephritis (glo-mer′-yoo-loh-nih-fri′-tuhs) Inflammation of the glomerulus of the kidney.

hyperplasia An increase in the number of normal cells.

idiopathic Having no known cause.

jaundice Yellow discoloration of the skin and mucous membranes resulting from deposits of bile pigments because of excess bilirubin in the blood.

keloid A raised, firm scar formation caused by overgrowth of collagen at the site of a skin injury.

keratin Very hard, tough protein found in hair, nails, and epidermal tissue.

keratinocytes Any one of the skin cells that synthesizes keratin.

leukoderma Lack of skin pigmentation, especially in patches.

opaque Not translucent or transparent; murky.

palliative Relating to a substance that alleviates or eases a painful condition without curing it.

petechiae (peh-te′-ke-uh) Small, purplish hemorrhagic spots on the skin.

Raynaud's phenomenon Intermittent attacks of ischemia of the extremities; results in cyanosis, numbness, tingling, and pain.

remission Partial or complete disappearance of the signs and symptoms of a disease.

teratogen (te-rah′-tuh-jen) Any substance that interferes with normal prenatal development.

The skin, the largest organ in the human body, covers a total area of about 20 square feet in an average-sized adult. Forming the outer boundary of the body, the skin performs several essential functions: it acts as a barrier to protect vital internal organs against infection and injury; it helps dissipate heat and regulate body temperature; and it synthesizes vitamin D when exposed to ultraviolet (UV) light. In addition, the various sensory receptors present throughout the skin enable it to respond to such sensations as heat, cold, pain, and pressure.

The specialty of dermatology deals with the skin and its accessory structures, the hair, nails, and sweat glands, and the subcutaneous tissue that lies beneath the skin. A physician specializing in dermatology is called a *dermatologist.*

ANATOMY AND PHYSIOLOGY

The integumentary system is composed of the skin and its accessory organs. Each square inch of the skin contains millions of cells, numerous specialized nerve endings, hair follicles, muscles, sweat glands to cool the body, and sebaceous glands, which release *sebum,* an oily substance that lubricates the skin. These diverse structures and glands are nourished by a permeating, elaborate network of blood vessels. The thickness of human skin varies markedly on different parts of the body, ranging from fairly thin over protected areas, such as the eyelids, to very thick over areas subject to abrasion, such as the palms of the hands and the soles of the feet.

Skin is composed of three layers: the epidermis, which is the thin, uppermost layer; the dermis, which is the thicker layer beneath, makes up about 90% of the skin mass, and is often referred to as the *true skin;* and the subcutaneous layer, which is composed primarily of fatty or adipose tissue (Figure 37-1).

Epidermis

New skin cells called **keratinocytes** are found in the basal cell layer of the epidermis and migrate upward over a period of about 4 weeks. As the cells move toward the surface, they grow flatter and scalier, eventually losing their nuclei and changing into dead skin cells that contain an inert protein called **keratin.** Keratin, which makes up the outermost layer of the epidermis, forms a protective barrier across the surface of the skin that helps control water loss from the body. Ultimately the outermost keratin layer sloughs off as a result of washing and friction. Hair and nails, which are also composed of keratin, are products of the epidermis.

About 95% of the cells in the epidermis are keratinocytes. The other 5% of epidermal cells are pigmented cells, or melanocytes. Melanin is a protein manufactured in the body that gives coloring to the skin and also protects the body from UV radiation. Skin coloring is determined not by the total number of melanocytes, which is relatively constant for all races, but rather by the rate at which these cells produce melanin. The amount of melanin produced depends on genetics as well as exposure to UV light. Individuals with albinism, an inherited recessive trait, are unable to produce melanin, so they have

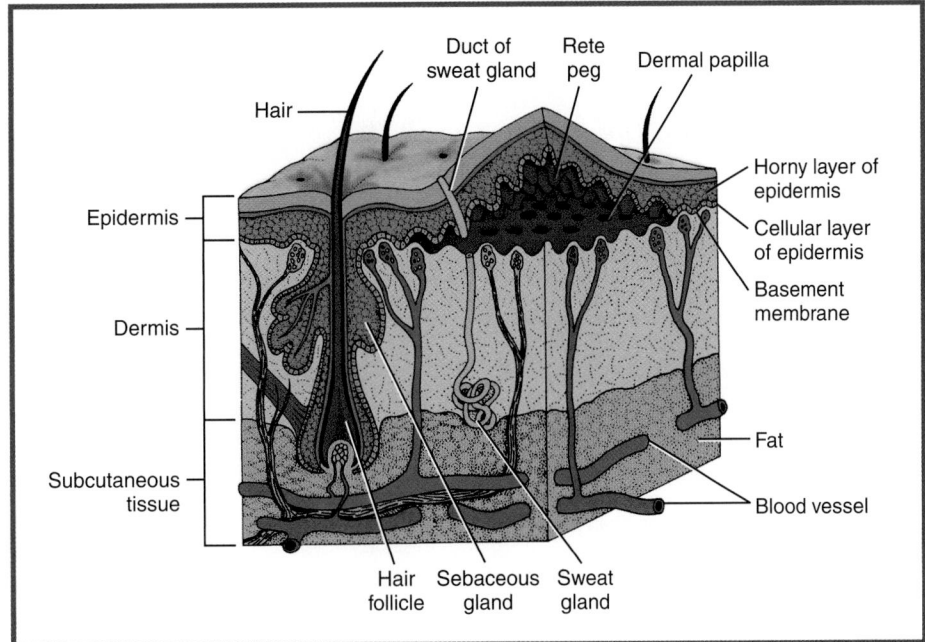

FIGURE 37-1 The three layers of the skin.

white hair and skin and lack pigment in the iris. They have no protection from UV light, so they must stay out of the sun.

Dermis

The underlying dermis is a thick layer of connective tissue that contains collagen and elastin fibers as well as water and jelly-like materials that make the skin compressible. Collagen fibers help to prevent tearing of the skin, and elastin is a flexible fiber that makes the skin resilient. Distributed throughout the dermis are blood vessels, lymph vessels, muscle cells, hair follicles, and sebaceous and sweat glands. Two types of sweat glands exist: *exocrine glands,* which excrete sweat through skin pores to release heat or create sweat in response to stress, and *apocrine glands,* which open into hair follicles and are located in specific areas, including the axilla, scalp, face, and genitalia. Sweat is odorless when excreted, but bacterial action results in odor.

A variety of microorganisms called *normal* or *resident flora* are found on the skin and may increase the risk for integumentary system infections. Healthcare workers are encouraged to perform hand washing before and after each procedure to prevent *transient* microbes picked up throughout the day when interacting with sick patients from becoming resident flora. If transient microorganisms are not destroyed and/or removed by good hand-washing techniques, they will eventually become part of the individual's resident flora. Sensory receptors for the nervous system that detect pain, temperature, pressure, or texture are also located in the dermis.

Subcutaneous Layer

The subcutaneous layer consists of fat cells, which provide insulation and serve as a depository for reserve calories. It also contains blood vessels, nerves, and the base of the appendages of the skin. Subcutaneous tissue is unevenly distributed, and

as the human body ages, it thins considerably, which can make administering injections to or drawing blood from aging patients more difficult. This loss of subcutaneous tissue is one of the reasons why elderly people are unable to compensate for changes in temperature, so they are colder when temperatures drop and hotter when temperature rise. Aging skin is also very fragile—easily traumatized and damaged by such things as tourniquets used for blood draws and bandage adhesives. You need to be very careful to avoid causing injury to the skin of an elderly person.

DISEASES AND DISORDERS

Skin is continuously exposed to the environment and may be affected by a wide range of disorders including infections, inflammatory processes, allergic reactions, and tumors. Many skin problems resolve spontaneously; others can be managed with drug therapy; and still others, such as tumors, large cysts, or moles, may require surgical intervention.

Skin Lesions

Skin lesions can result from a systemic problem, such as an allergic reaction to medication, or may develop from a localized infection. Figure 37-2 describes primary and secondary lesions and gives examples of each. When communicating with the physician, documenting in the patient chart, or conducting telephone screening, always use correct medical terminology to describe skin lesions, such as, "The patient reports a widespread maculopapular rash across anterior trunk" rather than reporting, "The patient has a red raised rash on his stomach."

When the medical assistant is gathering details from the patient regarding the characteristics of lesions, some questions that should be considered include the following:

PRIMARY LESIONS

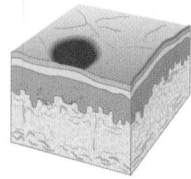

MACULE
Flat area of color change (no elevation or depression)

Example: Freckles

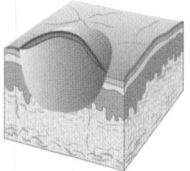

PAPULE
Solid elevation less than 0.5 cm in diameter

Example: Allergic eczema

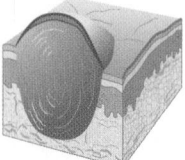

NODULE
Solid elevation 0.5 to 1 cm in diameter. Extends deeper into dermis than papule

Example: Mole

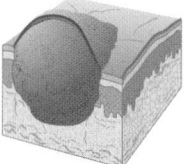

TUMOR
Solid mass—larger than 1 cm

Example: Squamous cell carcinoma

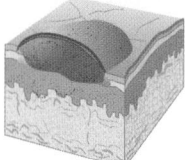

PLAQUE
Flat elevated surface found on skin or mucous membrane

Example: Thrush

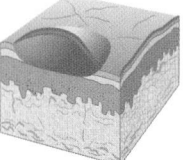

WHEAL
Type of plaque. Result is transient edema in dermis

Example: Intradermal skin test

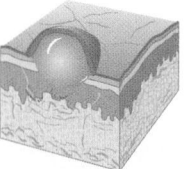

VESICLE
Small blister—fluid within or under epidermis

Example: Herpesvirus infection

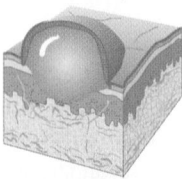

BULLA
Large blister (greater than 0.5 cm)

Example: Burn

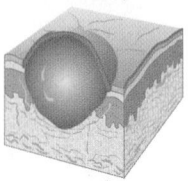

PUSTULE
Vesicle filled with pus

Example: Acne

SECONDARY LESIONS

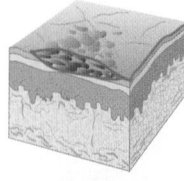

SCALES
Flakes of cornified skin layer

Example: Psoriasis

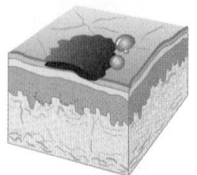

CRUST
Dried exudate on skin

Example: Impetigo

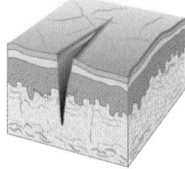

FISSURE
Cracks in skin

Example: Athlete's foot

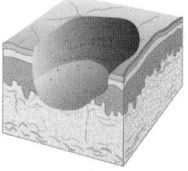

ULCER
Area of destruction of entire epidermis

Example: Decubitus (pressure sore)

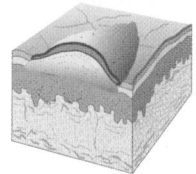

SCAR
Excess collagen production after injury

Example: Surgical healing

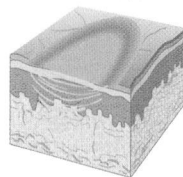

ATROPHY
Loss of some portion of the skin

Example: Paralysis

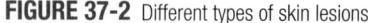

FIGURE 37-2 Different types of skin lesions.

- What are the color, elevation, and texture of the lesion?
- Is there any pain or *pruritus* (itching)? If pruritus is present, is the area **excoriated** or inflamed?
- Is there any drainage? If so, what are its characteristics?
- What is the exact anatomic location of the lesion? Have there been changes over time?

Primary lesions are those that appear immediately. Macules, papules, plaques, nodules, cysts, wheals, and pustules are all primary lesions. *Secondary lesions* are the result of alterations in a primary lesion. Examples of secondary lesions are scales, crusts, fissures, erosions, ulcerations, and scars. For instance, vesicles from a second intention burn are primary lesions, but if the blisters break and ulcerations form, healing ends in a scar. Ulceration and scar formation are secondary lesions.

Infections

Bacterial Infections

Impetigo. Impetigo is a common, contagious, superficial infection caused by streptococci or *Staphylococcus aureus*. It usually affects children and initially looks like small vesicles on the face, especially around the nose and mouth, which quickly enlarge and rupture, excreting a honey-colored exudate. The exudate forms crusty lesions, and beneath the crust the area is inflamed and moist (Figure 37-3). Pruritus accompanies the infection, and scratching helps spread the lesions at the site. Impetigo is contagious and is transmitted by direct contact with the drainage to other sites or to other children by sharing toys and touching. Consistent hand washing is needed to help break the chain of infection. It is also important to keep personal items, such as washcloths, linens, and drinking glasses, that may be contaminated away from other members of the family. If the areas of infection are limited, topical treatment with an antibiotic ointment may be effective. However, impetigo caused by streptococci may result in **glomerulonephritis,** so for more involved infections treatment with oral antibiotics may be indicated.

CRITICAL THINKING APPLICATION

Mrs. Allio calls the office with concerns about her family because of exposure to a child in the neighborhood who was diagnosed with impetigo. She tells Melissa that her 3-year-old woke up this morning with blisters around his mouth. Dr. Lee prescribes polymyxin-bacitracin-neomycin (Neosporin) ointment to be applied three times daily to the affected areas. What should Melissa tell Mrs. Allio about preventing the spread of the infection to her other children?

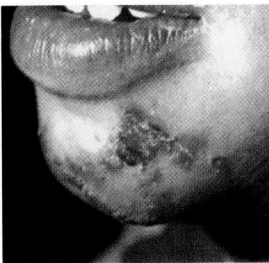

FIGURE 37-3 Impetigo. (From Marks J, Miller J: *Lookingbill's principles of dermatology,* ed 4, Philadelphia, 2006, Saunders.)

Acne. *Acne vulgaris* typically begins at puberty and is caused by a number of factors including inherited predisposition, hormonal fluctuations, exposure to heat and humidity, and the use of oily creams (Figure 37-4). Acne is a disorder of the hair follicle and sebaceous gland unit. It develops when sebum, which reaches the skin surface through the hair follicles, stimulates the follicle walls, causing a more rapid shedding of skin cells. The cells and sebum stick together and form a plug that promotes the growth of staphylococcal organisms in the follicles. The result is the formation of comedones (blackheads), pimples, pustules, or larger abscesses at the site.

Antiacne medications include the use of topical tretinoin (Retin-A) gel or antibacterial creams, such as benzoyl peroxide. Oral antibiotics, such as tetracycline and erythromycin, at a maintenance dose of 250 mg once or twice daily, can be prescribed to control comedones and pustules. Severe cystic acne can be treated with isotretinoin (Accutane), but it is a strong **teratogen** and should never be prescribed for pregnant women or women not using contraceptives. The use of oral contraceptives may reduce acne outbreaks as well. Dermabrasion can be performed to remove the scars that form from extreme cases of acne vulgaris.

Acne conglobata is a severe form of acne that typically occurs later in life and results in lesions across the back, buttocks, thighs, face, and chest. Abscesses or cysts may form between affected sites, and healing frequently results in **keloid** formation. This type of acne requires more aggressive treatment with systemic corticosteroids such as Prednisone, oral antibiotics, oral retinols (Accutane), and dermabrasion or **debridement** to treat excessive scarring.

Rosacea. Rosacea is a chronic disease that is seen most frequently in women between the ages of 30 and 60. It causes inflammation and pustule formation and originates as a frequent flushing across the nose, forehead, cheeks, and chin. As the condition progresses, capillaries of the face dilate and

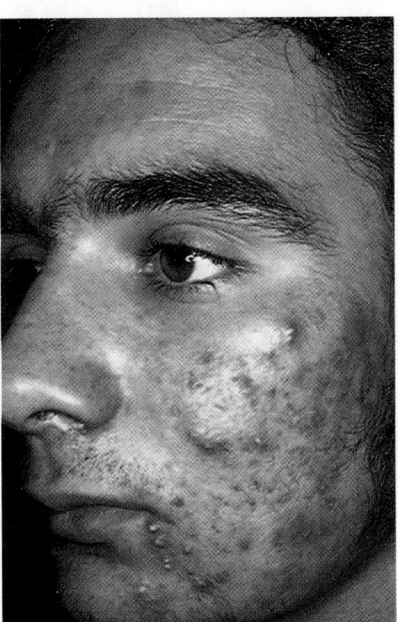

FIGURE 37-4 Acne. (From Paller A, Mancini A: *Hurwitz clinical pediatric dermatology: a textbook of skin disorders in childhood and adolescence,* ed 3, Philadelphia, 2006, Saunders.)

are visible across affected areas as small, red, edematous lines accompanied by eye inflammation and photosensitivity. Over time the face appears red, eye inflammation is more apparent, and painful nodules and pustules form. Men with rosacea may develop *rhinophyma*—a large, inflamed, bulbous nose caused by **hyperplasia** of sebaceous nasal tissue (Figure 37-5). Individuals with rosacea may eventually develop an obvious thickening of the skin across the forehead, nose, cheeks, and chin. Treatment is with topical antibiotics and, as symptoms progress, with oral antibiotics such as tetracycline, erythromycin, or doxycycline. Antibiotics help treat the pustule formation but do not affect the redness and flushing, which may be of most concern to the patient with the condition.

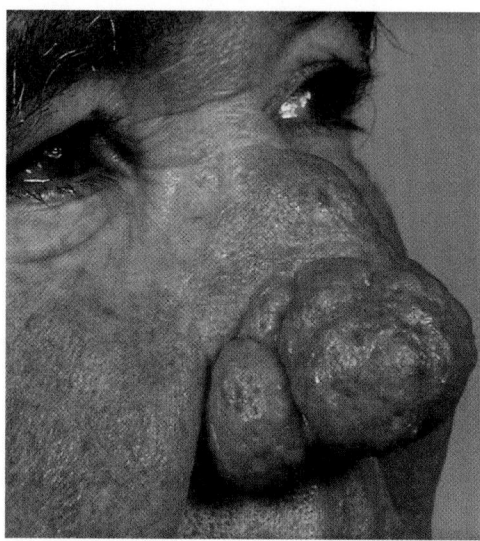

FIGURE 37-5 Rhinophyma. (From du Vivier A: *Atlas of clinical dermatology*, ed 2, London, 1993, Gower Medical Publishing.)

Furuncles and Carbuncles. A *furuncle* or boil is a localized staphylococcal infection that begins as an inflammation of a hair follicle *(folliculitis)* or a skin gland. The affected area is raised, inflamed, and painful and may eventually produce purulent drainage. A *carbuncle* is a collection of furuncles that have joined to form a large infected area that may drain through multiple sites or form an abscess. Both infections are treated by oral antibiotics, frequent cleansing of the area, the application of antibiotic ointment, and in some cases surgical incision and drainage of the purulent material.

Cellulitis. Cellulitis or *erysipelas* is an acute infection of the skin and subcutaneous tissue caused by either staphylococci or streptococci that begins from a small cut, as result of an injury to the skin, or at the site of a furuncle or ulcer. The area surrounding the site becomes inflamed, edematous, and painful with red streaks along the lymph vessels that lead from the infection. Oral antibiotic medications are needed to cure the disease, warm compresses applied locally aid with healing, and analgesics may be needed to relieve discomfort. Cellulitis must be treated with caution because a systemic infection can develop if the lymph glands become involved.

Fungal Infections (Dermatophytoses)

Fungal or mycotic infections, such as *tinea pedis* (athlete's foot) (Figure 37-6, *A)*, *tinea cruris* (jock itch) (Figure 37-6, *B)*, and *tinea corporis* (ringworm) (Figure 37-6, *C)*, are extremely common. These pathogens tend to live off dead tissue located in the keratin layer of the epidermis, the hair, or nails and cause almost no inflammation in the underlying skin. The fungus invades the skin where it has been damaged or is consistently moist. All of these lesions are pruritic and are characterized by a distinct border with scaling areas that have a clear center. Secondary bacterial infections may occur with excoriation.

FIGURE 37-6 Fungal infections. **A,** Tinea pedis. **B,** Tinea cruris. **C,** Tinea corporis. (From Callen J, Greer K, Hood A, et al: *Color atlas of dermatology*, ed 2, Philadelphia, 2000, Saunders.)

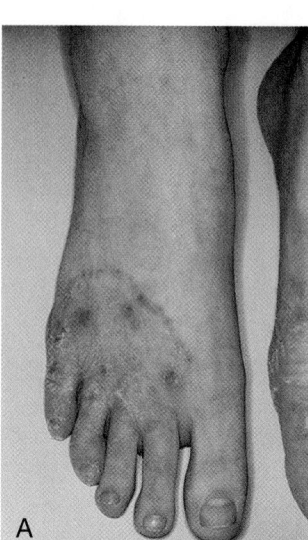

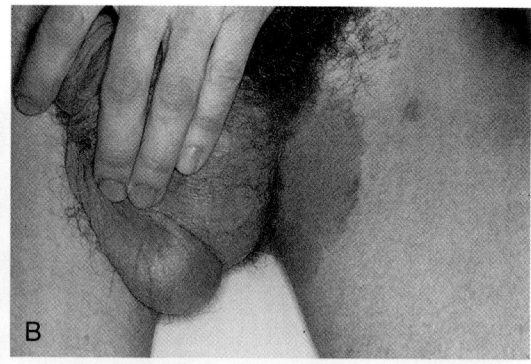

Treatment consists of antifungal topical agents, such as clotrimazole (Lotrimin), ketoconazole (Nizoral), econazole (Spectazole), or nystatin (Mycostatin). Antibiotics may be necessary if a secondary infection occurs. Because mycotic infections thrive in dark, moist areas, the patient should be advised to keep the site clean and dry and to wear loose clothing if possible. All types of dermatophytosis can become chronic infections if not managed carefully.

Tinea unguium, or *onychomycosis,* is a fungal infection of the toenails and fingernails. Unlike athlete's foot, which occurs on the skin's surface, nail fungus lives in the nail bed and the nail plate. The nail provides the fungus with an extremely well-protected place to live, which is why nail fungus may be especially hard to treat. The primary sign of nail fungus is in the appearance of the nail, which turns yellow, white, or **opaque.** The texture of the nail also changes, becoming thick and brittle. If the fungus has been present for a long time, the nail can even become twisted or distorted. The most effective way to treat nail fungus is with oral terbinafine hydrochloride (Lamisil), which inhibits the production of fungal cells. However, it requires administration for 6 weeks to treat fungal infection of a fingernail and 12 weeks for a toenail and carries the risk of liver complications.

Viral Infections

Warts. Warts, or *verrucae,* are caused by the human papillomaviruses (HPV) resulting in hyperplasia of the epidermis and a raised, cauliflower-like appearance. Verrucae can develop anywhere, but the most common sites are the fingers or the soles of the feet (plantar warts). Genital warts are addressed in Chapter 40. Most warts resolve themselves over time but they can be treated with topical chemicals, excised surgically, vaporized with lasers, or removed with **cryosurgery.**

Herpes Simplex (Cold Sores). Cold sores or fever blisters are caused by the herpes simplex virus type I (HSV-1). The initial infection may be asymptomatic or may cause painful ulcers along the gum lines of the mouth or on the lips. After the primary infection, the virus remains dormant in the trigeminal nerve and can be reactivated by exposure to sun, cold, or the presence of another infection such as an upper respiratory infection or when the patient is under stress. The patient reports a feeling of burning, tingling, or numbness before the eruption of vesicles. The blisters heal in 2 to 3 weeks, but the process may be speeded up by the use of topical antiviral drugs, such as acyclovir (Zovirax) or penciclovir cream (Denavir), or with oral antivirals including Zovirax or valacyclovir (Valtrex). These antiviral creams, if applied at the first indications of a cold sore, will limit the duration and severity of the outbreak.

Herpes Zoster (Shingles). *Herpes zoster* is an acute inflammatory disorder that is characterized by highly painful vesicle eruptions on the trunk of the body and occasionally on the face (Figure 37-7). The lesions develop on one side of the body and follow the course of the peripheral nerve, or *dermatome,* that has been infected by the varicella virus, the same virus that causes chicken pox. The virus lies dormant in the affected dorsal root ganglia and becomes reactivated in later years as a result of stress or aging.

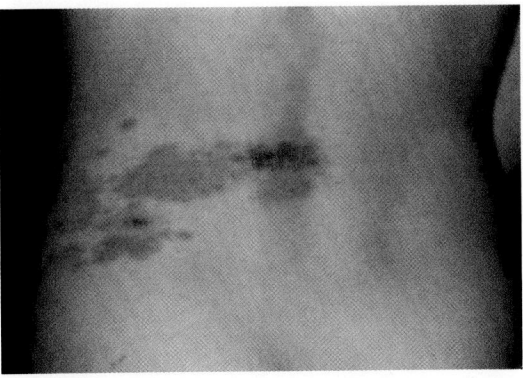

FIGURE 37-7 Herpes zoster (shingles). (From Callen J, Greer K, Hood A, et al: *Color atlas of dermatology,* ed 2, Philadelphia, 2000, Saunders.)

The onset of the disorder is usually marked by pain along the nerve pathway, and in approximately 3 days lesions appear. The duration of the inflammation ranges from 10 days to 5 weeks. The patient is diagnosed with the presence of a characteristic pattern of painful lesions, and the diagnosis may be confirmed by isolating the virus in cell cultures. It can also be detected by the presence of varicella zoster antibodies in the blood. Treatment focuses on promoting patient comfort with analgesic and antipruritic medications. Corticosteroid medications (Prednisone) and antiviral drugs, including topical or oral acyclovir (Zovirax) and oral famciclovir (Famvir) or valacyclovir (Valtrex), can also be prescribed. One of the most serious complications of herpes zoster is *postherpetic neuralgia,* which causes chronic pain after resolution of the initial outbreak and may require treatment with a combination of medications including topical calamine (Caladryl) lotion, capsaicin cream (Zostrix), topical lidocaine (Xylocaine), narcotics, tricyclic antidepressants (such as Elavil or Tofranil), and anticonvulsants (including Dilantin, Tegretol, and Neurotin).

Other Infections

Scabies and Pediculosis. Scabies (itch mite) and pediculosis (lice) are the two most common parasites to infest individuals. Scabies are tiny organisms, barely visible with the eye, that burrow into the epidermis (Figure 37-8). Pediculosis consists of three species of lice: the head louse (Figure 37-9, *A*), the body louse, and the pubic louse (Figure 37-9, *B*). Both types of infestations are highly contagious. Diagnosis of scabies may require scraping the skin at an inflamed area and examining the mites under a low-power microscope. Lice can be seen on the hair shafts. Patients describe symptoms of intense itching, possible body rash, and a sensation of something crawling on the skin.

Treatment consists of ridding the body of the parasite, controlling the pruritus, and disinfecting the home environment to prevent reinfestation. Scabies are treated with a single application of 5% permethrin cream (Elimite). Medicated shampoo, creams, and/or lotions are used to kill head lice. The treatment must be repeated in 7 to 10 days to destroy the nits (eggs). If a secondary infection has begun, antibiotics may also be prescribed. All family members and other individuals who have had direct personal contact with the infested person must also be treated. Lindane lotion (Kwell) should be used only if permethrin treatment has failed, because it carries the risk of neurotoxicity including seizures in children.

The medical assistant can assist the patient through explanations regarding the washing and/or dry cleaning of all clothing and bedding. All items need to be washed and dried in hot cycles. If clothes worn by the infested person have been placed back into a closet, all items in the closet must be washed or dry cleaned. Furniture and carpets should be washed or vacuumed (the bag disposed of) and sprayed with a surface disinfectant.

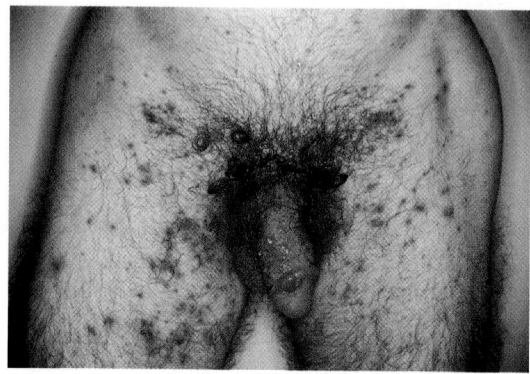

FIGURE 37-8 Scabies rash. (From Callen J, Greer K, Hood A, et al: *Color atlas of dermatology*, ed 2, Philadelphia, 2000, Saunders.)

CRITICAL THINKING APPLICATION

Melissa's young daughter brought home a note today warning of a scabies outbreak in her school. Melissa has a few red marks on her forearms and the areas are quite itchy. Dr. Lee does a skin scraping of one of the areas and views itch mites under the microscope. How should Melissa and her family be treated? Should Melissa remain at work? How should the office and Melissa's home be disinfected to prevent reinfestation?

Inflammatory and Autoimmune Disorders

Seborrheic Dermatitis

Seborrheic dermatitis is one of the most common, chronic, inflammatory conditions of the sebaceous glands. The disorder alters the amount and quality of sebum, resulting in dry or moist greasy-appearing scales and yellowish crusts on the scalp, eyebrows, eyelids, and sides of the nose, behind the ears, and in the middle of the chest. The disease has many different forms, including cradle cap in infants and dandruff in adults. Seborrheic dermatitis of the scalp can be treated with tar- or sulfur-based shampoos; inflammations of the skin are usually treated with topical corticosteroids, such as triamcinolone diacetate (Aristocort), betamethasone valerate (Valisone), or fluocinolone acetonide (Synalar). *Seborrheic keratosis* (age spots)

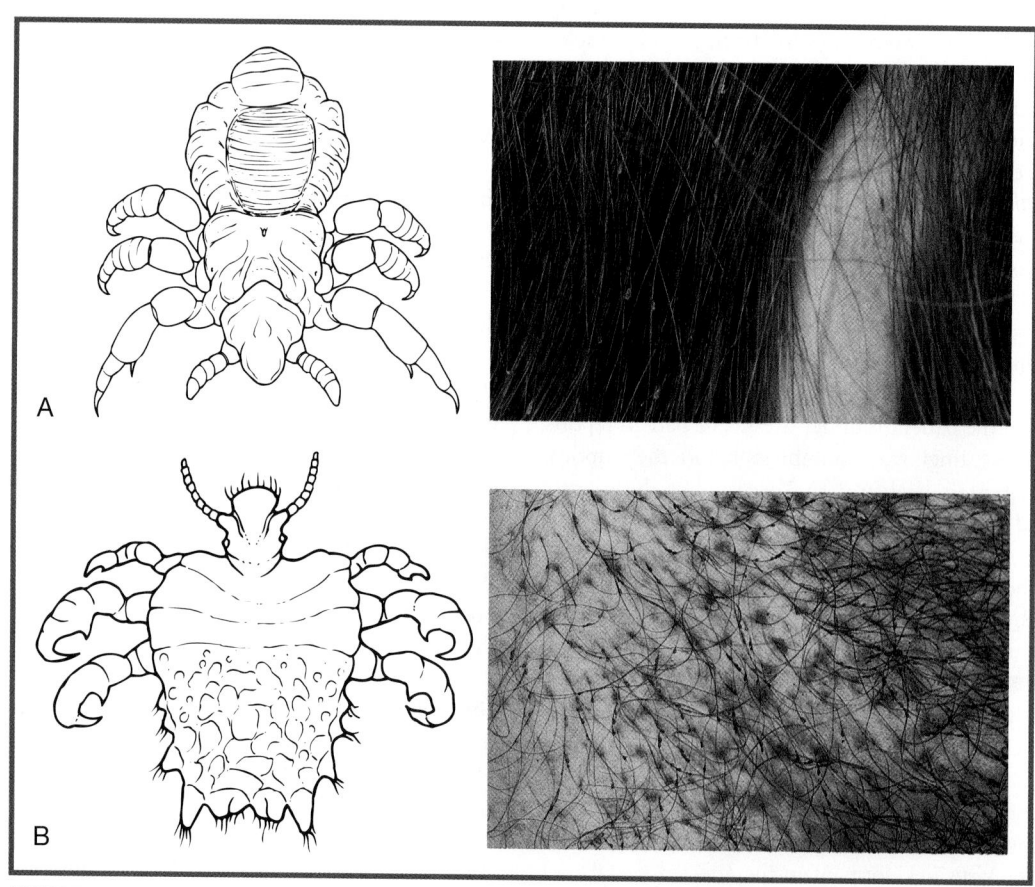

FIGURE 37-9 Pediculosis. **A,** *Pediculus humanus capitis* (head louse) and lice in hair. **B,** *Phthirus pubis* (pubic or crab louse) and pubic lice rash. (From Callen J, Greer K, Hood A, et al: *Color atlas of dermatology*, ed 2, Philadelphia, 2000, Saunders.)

are characterized by benign, slightly raised, tan to black lesions that occur with aging.

Contact Dermatitis

Contact dermatitis is an acute inflammatory response to a skin irritant or exposure to a substance that causes an allergic reaction. An individual who is allergic to latex gloves or who has been exposed to poison ivy will exhibit the signs and symptoms of contact dermatitis. The patient complains of redness *(erythema)*, edema, pruritus, and vesicles. The patient should be encouraged to wash the affected area immediately after exposure to remove the irritant if possible. Medical treatment includes the application of corticosteroid cream or the use of oral corticosteroid medications, such as prednisone or methylprednisolone (Medrol) if the symptoms are severe.

Eczema (Atopic Dermatitis)

Eczema is an **idiopathic** inflammatory skin disease that tends to occur in patients with a family history of allergies. Its appearance in young children may be caused by food allergies, whereas stress or extremes in temperature can trigger flare-ups in older children. The condition usually improves and may disappear as the child ages. Eczema is characterized by a vesicular rash located on the face, neck, and elbows and behind the knees and ears. It causes pronounced pruritus, which results in excoriation of the affected area from constant scratching if not treated.

Eczema is diagnosed with a comprehensive family history and examination of the skin. The patient may be asked to investigate possible allergens by making a list of all of items that might be responsible for the outbreak, or the physician may recommend allergy testing. The goal of treatment is to reduce the frequency and number of eruptions and relieve the pruritus so affected areas do not become excoriated. The primary inflammation is usually treated with topical corticosteroids and oral antihistamines (such as Benadryl, Zyrtec, or Allegra) to control itching. Inflamed plaques indicate a secondary staphylococcal infection and should be treated with an oral antibiotic.

Psoriasis

Psoriasis is a chronic skin disease that produces discrete pink or red lesions covered with silvery scales (Figure 37-10). The disease

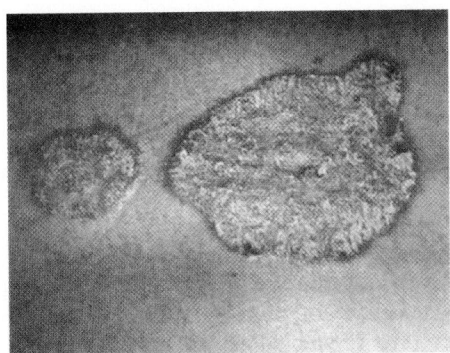

FIGURE 37-10 Psoriasis. (From Callen J, Greer K, Hood A, et al: *Color atlas of dermatology*, ed 2, Philadelphia, 2000, Saunders.)

may begin at any age, although the majority of patients develop the problem before the age of 40. The lesions are noninfectious and the disease is characterized by periodic flare-ups throughout the life of the affected individual. Psoriasis is caused by an **autoimmune** reaction that speeds up the maturation rate of skin cells. Normal skin cells mature, die, and are shed every 28 to 30 days, but in patients with psoriasis cells mature in 3 to 6 days, and instead of sloughing off the surface of the skin they build up and form the classic psoriasis silvery patch. Affected skin is dry, cracked, and encrusted. Psoriasis lesions may appear on the scalp, chest, buttocks, and extremities.

Psoriasis is diagnosed by observations of the skin, a careful patient history (because there is a familial link), and/or a skin biopsy. Treatment is **palliative** because the disease has no cure. Exposure to UV light may slow down cell production, and coal tar preparations help relieve irritation when applied to affected areas. The physician may also order a combination of therapies including methotrexate; a retinoid such as acitretin (Soriatane); the immunosuppressant cyclosporine (Neoral); low-dosage antihistamines; and oatmeal baths to promote patient comfort. More recent approaches include excimer laser treatments that localize high-intensity wavelengths of UV light to targeted plaques, causing a decrease in both cellular production and inflammation.

Systemic Lupus Erythematosus

Systemic lupus erythematosus (SLE) is a chronic autoimmune inflammatory disease of the connective tissue of the body. The cause is unknown, although women are nine times more likely to develop the disease than men. It can affect any connective tissue in the body but typically causes inflammatory changes in the skin, joints, muscles, and kidneys. SLE usually involves more than one organ, with the patient experiencing periods of **exacerbation** and **remission.** One of the diagnostic characteristics of the disease is a "butterfly" rash that is evident from one cheek and across the nose to the other cheek. Other integumentary system symptoms include erythematous patches and plaques, **alopecia,** and photosensitivity.

The prognosis for SLE depends on organ involvement but is poor for those patients experiencing renal, cardiovascular, or neurologic complications. Treatment includes the use of nonsteroidal antiinflammatory drugs (NSAIDs) including Voltaren and Lodine or controlled low doses of corticosteroids (prednisone) when needed. Serious cases are treated with cytotoxic drugs (Cytoxan) and antimalarial drugs such as hydroxychloroquine (Plaquenil) or chloroquine hydrochloride (Aralen) as needed to control inflammatory reactions.

Scleroderma

Scleroderma is a chronic, progressive, autoimmune disease that affects the blood vessels and connective tissues of the skin, lungs, and internal organs. The disease causes generalized inflammation of blood vessels throughout the body, leading to the narrowing and destruction of smaller arteries and ultimately fibrotic circulatory changes. The heart, lungs, and kidneys are most affected by the resultant decrease in circulation. Integumentary system symptoms include fibrous changes in the skin that result in *sclerosis* (hardening) of the skin, edema, pallor, pigmentation, and fixation to subcutaneous tissues. These same sclerotic changes can occur in any organ in the body. **Raynaud's phenomenon** may be the first symptom of the disease. The cause of scleroderma is unknown, but it usually occurs in middle-aged women.

The disease has no cure and no specific treatment. Drugs are used to treat the inflammation and circulatory symptoms of the disease, and analgesics are prescribed for pain. Physical therapy helps maintain muscle strength, but the prognosis is poor. Patients with scleroderma usually die from cardiac, pulmonary, or renal involvement.

Thermal Injuries

Skin can be damaged and injured by exposure to moderately high or low temperatures over an extended period. It also can be injured in a relatively short time when exposed to very high or low temperatures. The most frequent thermal injuries are burns, which are classified as superficial-thickness (first-degree), partial-thickness (second-degree), or full-thickness (third-degree) burns depending on the depth of the wound (Figure 37-11). With severe burns it is common to have all three types of burns in the same location—superficial burns along the edges, partial-thickness burns with vesicles closer to the center, and full-thickness burns at the center of the area.

Superficial (First-Degree) Burn

A superficial-thickness burn affects only the epidermis, is erythemic (red), blanches with pressure, and is painful but without blisters at the site. A mild sunburn and a steam burn without vesicle formation are examples of superficial burns.

Partial-Thickness (Second-Degree) Burn

A partial- thickness burn destroys the entire epidermal layer and varying depths of the dermis, with blister formation and subcutaneous edema and pain. There is also danger of infection in the blistered area. If a burn is deep enough, there may be some destruction of the hair follicles and the sebaceous glands.

Treatment of Minor Burns

Because burns damage the natural protection of the skin, preventing infection at the site is of primary concern. Superficial burns typically heal on their own within a week as long as they are kept clean and infection does not occur. Medical treatment of partial-thickness burns includes gentle cleansing of the site with a bactericidal solution and debridement of broken blisters or dead skin. Blisters that are intact should be left alone. Partial-thickness burns may be treated with a thin layer of silver sulfadiazine cream and a nonadherent multilayered dressing applied for several days to 1 week. The patient's tetanus immunization status should be reviewed and a tetanus injection

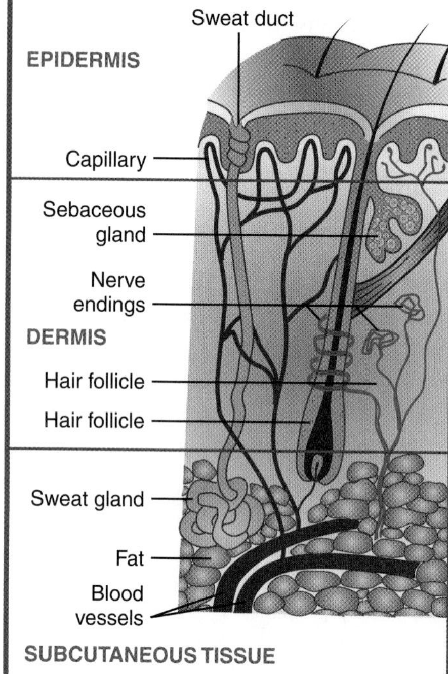

		APPEARANCE	SENSATION	COURSE
EPIDERMIS — Sweat duct, Capillary	**SUPERFICIAL BURN**	Mild to severe erythema; skin blanches with pressure Skin dry Small, thin-walled blisters	Painful Hyperesthetic Tingling Pain eased by cooling	Discomfort lasts about 48 hours Desquamation in 3–7 days
DERMIS — Sebaceous gland, Nerve endings, Hair follicle, Hair follicle	**PARTIAL-THICKNESS BURN**	Large thick-walled blisters covering extensive area (vesiculation) Edema; mottled red base; broken epidermis; wet, shiny, weeping surface	Painful Hyperesthetic Sensitive to cold air	Superficial partial-thickness burn heals in 10–14 days Deep partial-thickness burn requires 21–28 days for healing Healing rate varies with burn depth and presence or absence of infection
SUBCUTANEOUS TISSUE — Sweat gland, Fat, Blood vessels	**FULL-THICKNESS BURN**	Variable, e.g., deep red, black, white, brown Dry surface Edema Tissue disrupted	Little pain Anesthetic	Full-thickness dead skin suppurates and liquefies after 2–3 weeks Spontaneous healing impossible Requires removal of eschar and skin grafting Scarring deformities and function loss Beneath eschar capillary tufts and fibroblasts organize into granulating tissue

FIGURE 37-11 Classification of burns.

Patient Education for Burn Care

- Warning signs of infection include fever, malaise, inflammation, swelling, increased pain, odor, and drainage from the burn area. Any of these should be reported to the physician immediately.
- Review care of the wound, including gentle cleansing with bactericidal solution (such as povidone-iodine solution [Betadine]) and covering of the wound with an antibiotic ointment (silver sulfadiazine) so the dressing does not stick to the burn.
- The patient should consume a high-calorie, high-protein diet to maintain weight and promote healing.
- For partial-thickness burns, new skin development takes 6 weeks, with complete healing in 6 to 12 months, depending on the extent of the burn.

administered if needed, and the physician may also order analgesics for pain relief. Patients with partial-thickness burns (those reporting blisters at the site of the burn) should be seen by the physician for treatment.

CRITICAL THINKING APPLICATION

Thomas Rangoso, a 66-year-old patient, calls the office to report a burn to his right hand and forearm. He fell while passing the stove and burned himself on the hot surface. Mr. Rangoso tells you the area is very red and painful with blisters in the center. He wants to break the blisters and put butter on the burn. Should Mr. Rangoso be seen by Dr. Lee, and what should Melissa tell him about the care of the burn?

Full-Thickness (Third-Degree) Burn

A full-thickness burn destroys all layers of the skin and may involve underlying fat, muscle, nerves, blood supply, and bone. The area appears charred or white, with a firm, leathery texture. The patient feels no pain because nerve endings are destroyed. Full-thickness burns have the potential for causing major complications including dehydration, circulatory collapse, respiratory distress, and septic shock. Treatment of major burns includes maintaining the patient's airway, replacing fluids, preventing infection, and administering oxygen. Debridement of affected tissue and skin grafts are required for wound healing. Depending on the extent of the burns, the patient may be hospitalized in an intensive care unit or a specialty burn unit.

Burns are also classified according to the percentage of body surface involved, based on the Rule of Nines, as discussed in Chapter 35.

Cold Injuries

Cold injuries are usually less severe than burns, but prolonged exposure to cold temperatures can result in infection, gangrene, amputation, and in severe situations, death. Frostbite is caused by exposure to subfreezing temperatures. Damage occurs at the level of the capillaries, which become permanently dilated and unable to regulate local blood flow. The signs and symptoms of superficial frostbite include burning, tingling, numbness, and a white or grayish color of the skin. With deep frostbite blisters form and the area is hard, mottled, edematous, and blue or gray after thawing.

The extent of injury is determined by visual examination and based on the history of the exposure. Treatment consists of warming the area with immersion in water at 38° to 41° C (100° to 106° F). The affected site should never be rubbed because that will increase cellular destruction. Vital signs should be monitored and the physician's orders followed explicitly.

Benign and Malignant Neoplasms

A neoplasm is an abnormal growth or tumor that may be either benign or malignant. Table 37-1 outlines the differences between benign and malignant tumors. Invasion and metastasis are the principal criteria used to distinguish between cancerous and noncancerous tumors. Benign masses are encapsulated, and although they may increase in size they remain within a confined shell, whereas malignant tumors invade and take over surrounding tissues. Local invasion of surrounding tissue occurs when malignant cells break through the basement membrane that separates epithelial cells from connective tissue. Here the cancerous cells can invade blood and lymph vessels, which carry the malignant cells to organs throughout the body. Patients diagnosed with *carcinoma in situ* have a malignant tumor that is confined to the original site of growth without invasion of the basement membrane. Patients with regional spread have evidence of malignant cells in surrounding tissues but no evidence of lymph node involvement. Patients with distant spread, or *metastasis,* show positive lymph node involvement locally with the development of secondary tumors at other organs including the lungs, liver, brain, or bones.

Malignant tumors are classified according to grading and staging. After a biopsy sample of the tumor is obtained, the sample is sent to a pathologist for microscopic examination. The pathologist examines the biopsied cells under a microscope and *grades* the sample according to its histologic, or cellular, classification of differentiation. Differentiation is the process normal cells go through to mature. Immature, or primitive,

TABLE 37-1 Differences Between Benign and Malignant Tumors

CHARACTERISTIC	BENIGN TUMOR	MALIGNANT TUMOR
Cellular structure	Same as surrounding tissue	Anaplastic changes and level of differentiation
Type of growth	Encapsulated mass that expands over time	Infiltrates and metastasizes; can have distant spread through the bloodstream or lymph system to other body tissues and organs
Rate of growth	Usually slow; rarely fatal	May be slow, rapid, or very rapid; almost always fatal if untreated
Destruction of localized tissue	None	Ulceration and necrosis of surrounding tissue common

cells never mature and are classified as **anaplastic** or cancerous in nature. Therefore, the more poorly *differentiated* the cells, meaning the less they look like normal cells, the more likely the biopsy is cancerous. If the physician receives a grading report that indicates anaplastic cancerous cells the next step is to determine if the cancerous cells have spread from the original site. This is called *staging* the tumor. Staging involves using physical examination and diagnostic tests (such as bone or liver scans) to determine the degree of tumor spread to a secondary location. The size and depth of the primary tumor, the degree of lymph node involvement, and the presence of metastatic spread determine whether the patient has a carcinoma in situ, a tumor that is localized to the organ of origin, a direct spread beyond the primary organ, lymph node metastasis, or a confirmed secondary tumor growth in a distant metastatic site. Grading and staging determine the extent of malignant involvement so the physician can plan appropriate treatment.

Three methods are used to obtain a small piece of tissue for examination under a microscope. In an excision biopsy, such as a mole removal, the entire lesion may be removed for analysis. A punch biopsy involves the removal of a small section from a designated location within the lesion; usually the center is the optimal site. This is done with a scalpel-like circular punch instrument if the lesion is on the surface of the skin, as with a mole, or a large-gauge needle and syringe unit that is used to aspirate cells and fluid from a suspicious area such as in a breast biopsy. A shave biopsy is done with a scalpel by cutting or shaving off the growth or lesion just above the skin line. This method is used to biopsy a possible squamous cell carcinoma lesion. The medical assistant may help the physician perform these procedures.

The protocol for treatment of cancer depends on the staging, grading, and type of carcinoma. Possible treatments include surgical removal of the tumor, radiation therapy, chemotherapy, hormone therapy, and immune system boosters. These approaches may be used singly or in combination and are usually determined by a specialist in the study and treatment of cancer, the oncologist.

Assisting with a Tissue Biopsy

1. Assemble the supplies needed for the procedure.
2. Prepare the patient with proper gowning, draping, and positioning, and make sure the patient understands the procedure.
3. Confirm that the physician has obtained the patient's informed consent.
4. Prepare the site of the biopsy according to office protocol.
5. Assist the physician as needed, using appropriate personal protective equipment according to standard precautions.
6. Label the sample container and prepare it for transport to the testing laboratory. Remember to include laboratory request forms.
7. Clean the procedure area, properly dispose of all waste materials, and disinfect and sterilize equipment used in the procedure.
8. Wash hands, and document the procedure including patient education on biopsy site care.

Cancer's Seven Warning Signs The initial letters of the warning signs spell out the word CAUTION. Any of these warning signs should be reported to the physician immediately. Early detection and self-examination are crucial to cancer survival.

- **C**hange in bowel or bladder habits
- **A** sore that does not heal
- **U**nusual bleeding or discharge
- **T**hickening or a lump in the breast or elsewhere
- **I**ndigestion or difficulty in swallowing
- **O**bvious change in a wart or mole
- **N**agging cough or hoarseness

Neoplasms of the Skin

Neoplasms of the skin may be benign or malignant. Examples of benign tumors include birthmarks and moles *(nevi)*. However, a tumor may be benign but have a predisposition to be cancerous, which means it can go from a benign state to a malignant one. Whenever a neoplasm is discovered, the physician usually performs a biopsy of the lesion to establish the type of cells involved.

Three cancerous lesions of the skin may occur: basal cell carcinoma, squamous cell carcinoma, and malignant melanoma. Basal cell carcinoma is very slow growing and is the most frequently seen form of skin cancer. The most common sites are areas of the body that are exposed to the sun, such as the face and forearms. It appears as a painless, smooth, small, waxy, translucent nodule that may become inflamed and ulcerated. It can be white, brown, or black and has ill-defined borders (Figure 37-12).

Squamous cell carcinoma grows rapidly and is more serious because it has a tendency to metastasize. It appears as a firm, red nodule with visible scales and may ulcerate and form a crust (Figure 37-13). Patients typically report both basal and squamous cell skin cancers as sores that persist and never heal.

Malignant melanoma develops from a change in a mole. Sunburns increase the risk of melanoma, and individuals with more moles than average (more than 100) are also at greater risk. Persons with *congenital nevi* (moles present at birth) are more likely to develop a melanoma. Additional risk factors include an

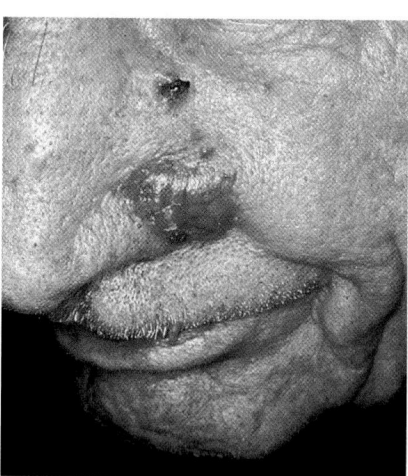

FIGURE 37-12 Basal cell carcinoma. (Modified from Damjanov I: *Pathology for the health-related professions,* ed 3, Philadelphia, 2006, Saunders.)

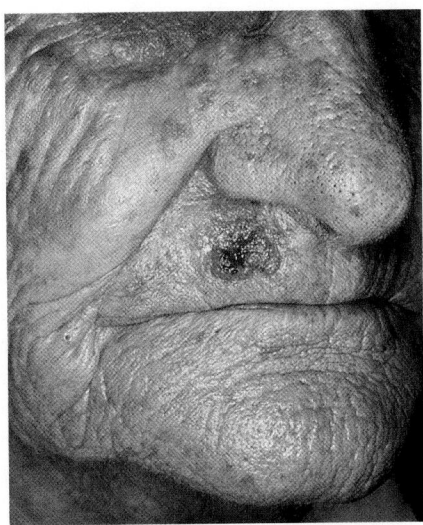

FIGURE 37-13 Squamous cell carcinoma. (Modified from Damjanov I: *Pathology for the health-related professions*, ed 3, Philadelphia, 2006, Saunders.)

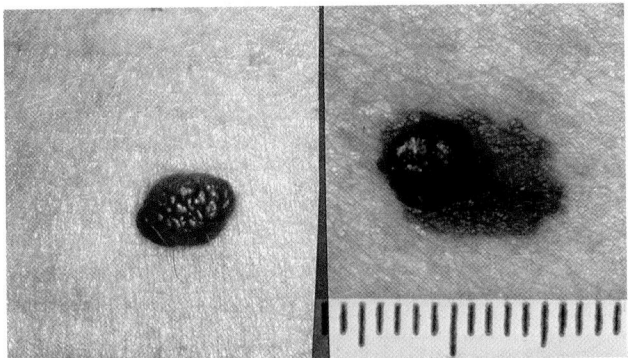

FIGURE 37-14 Pigmented skin lesions. *Left*, Benign pigmented nevus (mole). *Right*, Malignant melanoma. (Courtesy National Cancer Institute, Bethesda, Md.)

inability to tan, light or red hair, fair skin, family history, and the number of childhood sunburns. Many forms of melanoma occur, but all are pigmented lesions (usually brown, tan, blue, red, black, or white) that are asymmetric with irregular borders and are usually larger than 6 mm (Figure 37-14). The staging of the disease is dependent on the depth of the growth of the mass, not on the surface size of the mole. The incidence of malignant melanoma has doubled in the past 10 years and results in more deaths than all other skin diseases. Melanomas often recur or metastasize within 5 years of diagnosis. The patient should be routinely examined for at least 10 years after removal of the melanoma.

All skin cancers are diagnosed by the appearance of the lesions with confirmation through biopsy. Treatment methods depend on the type, level of invasion, and location of the mass. The physician may choose to surgically remove the tumor or eradicate the tumor with cryosurgery, **electrodesiccation,** or the application of chemotherapeutic agents.

The National Cancer Institute recommends the best way to prevent skin cancer is to protect yourself, starting with children at a young age, from the sun. People of all ages should do the following:

Early Warning Signs of Malignant Melanoma: ABCD Rule

If a mole displays any of these characteristics, a dermatologist should examine it immediately.

A	Asymmetry	One half of the mole does not match the other half.
B	Border	Edges of the mole are blurred or irregular.
C	Color	Color of the mole is not the same throughout, with shades of tan, brown, black, red, white, or blue.
D	Diameter	Mole is larger than 6 mm, about the size of a pencil eraser.

- Stay out of the midday sun (from 10 AM to 4 PM).
- Protect yourself from UV rays reflected off of water and snow.
- Even on cloudy days you will be exposed to UV radiation.
- Use protective clothing and a wide-brimmed hat when in the sun, and protect your eyes with sunglasses.
- Use a sunscreen that filters both UVB and UVA rays with a sun protection factor (SPF) of at least 15.
- Do not use artificial lamps and tanning beds.

DERMATOLOGIC PROCEDURES

The integumentary system can reflect both internal and external reactions and disease processes. The skin holds information about the body's circulation, nutritional status, and signs of systemic diseases. It also acts as a mirror, reflecting aging changes that are present in all organs of the body. For many people, self-esteem is linked to a youthful appearance and dermatologic conditions may be very threatening to feelings of self-worth. As patients are prepared for a dermatologic examination, allow them to express their anxieties. The impairments that most frequently bring a patient to the dermatologist's office are cosmetic disfigurements caused by a skin disease, pain and pruritus, and interference with sensations or movements.

Assisting with a Dermatologic Examination

During a dermatologic examination the physician visually inspects the entire body, beginning with the scalp and continuing through to the soles of the feet, including the genital area. Inspection of the skin is followed by detailed examination of suspicious areas through palpation, diascopy, and special tests. The *diascope* is a glass plate held firmly against the skin to permit observation of changes produced in underlying areas when pressure is applied. Inspection may include using a magnifying lens and a bright light to closely examine a suspicious lesion or growth. The dermatologist frequently asks the medical assistant to take photographs of moles and/or chart specific measurements and locations of suspicious lesions. These are placed in the chart for comparison when the patient returns for follow-up visits.

In the physical examination, concerns about the integumentary system include abnormal coloring, such as cyanosis, pallor, erythema, **leukoderma,** or excessive brown patches. **Jaundice** may indicate an increase in the level of **bilirubin** in the blood. Decreased pigmentation is found in *vitiligo,* which is an acquired loss of melanin characterized by blotchy white patches on the skin. Lesions, ulcers, and bruises may be the result of pathologic conditions. Localized red or purple changes may be the result of vascular neoplasms, birthmarks, or subcutaneous hemorrhages (**petechiae** and **ecchymoses).** Palpation helps confirm findings seen with inspection. Therefore inspection and palpation are interrelated in confirming the diagnosis of an integumentary system disorder. Palpated findings may include the skin's texture or elasticity or the presence of edema or a neoplasm.

Draping a patient for a skin examination depends on the area to be examined. Remember to expose the area adequately, but protect the patient's privacy. Try to make the patient as comfortable as possible and offer support when it is needed.

Skin Testing for Allergies

Skin testing to determine allergies requires either percutaneous application or intradermal injection of a small amount of antigen (or groups of antigens) and later examination of the test sites for a visible reaction. The larger the localized skin reaction, the more profound the patient's allergic response to the allergen.

Percutaneous Test. A percutaneous or scratch test may be performed on any smooth surface of the skin; however, the back is favored in young children because of the large area of skin available. It is also easier to immobilize the child in this position. The skin surface is labeled or numbered in rows 1 1/2 to 2 inches apart. A short scratch is made with a needle or lancet and a drop of allergen is placed on each open area. Fifty or more tests may be done at one time. It is essential that a pattern is followed so that the site of each allergen is easily identified. This type of allergy testing is used for allergic rhinitis, asthma, and food allergy detection.

A reaction usually occurs within 10 to 30 minutes after allergen exposure. If the reaction is positive, a *wheal* (hive) will form at the site of the scratch. The interpretation of the test should always be based on a comparison of this reaction with that of the control, which is a scratch with a plain base fluid,

free of any allergy-producing extract.

The interpretation, or reading, of the skin tests is performed by the physician or a trained technician. Reactions are commonly graded from 2 to 4. No precise definition of a reaction can be given, and the intensity of the response may vary among individuals. However, as a general rule, a 2 reaction implies a wheal that is definitely larger than that of the control. A larger wheal is interpreted as a 3, whereas the presence of *pseudopods* (finger-like extensions around the periphery of the wheal) may be read as a 4. If a strong reaction is occurring, the allergen extract should be carefully wiped off to prevent any further exposure. Erythema around the wheal is usually disregarded in the interpretations. Frequently, large or significant reactions are accompanied by local itching. Patients should remain in the office for a minimum of 30 minutes after the completion of the allergy testing procedure in case of a delayed systemic allergic response.

Intradermal (Intracutaneous) Test. The intradermal test is more sensitive than the percutaneous test and is usually used to diagnose allergies to penicillin and insect venom such as bee stings. Extracts are injected into the intradermal layer of the skin in doses of 0.1 to 0.2 ml. This method is also used for the tuberculin (purified protein derivative [PPD]) test and the Valley Fever coccidioidomycosis test. When using intradermal injections for allergy testing, 10 to 15 allergens may be tested at one time on each arm. The reaction time is identical to that of the scratch test; however, the antigen is more dilute.

Radioallergosorbent Test. The radioallergosorbent (RAST) test is a laboratory procedure performed on a blood sample that identifies specific allergens that cause allergic responses such as rashes, hay fever, asthma, and drug reactions. The RAST test is easier to perform than skin testing because it requires a single venipuncture. It is also less painful and less dangerous for the patient and more specific than skin testing. Although skin testing remains the preferred method of diagnosing hypersensitivity, the RAST test may be indicated when the patient cannot stop antihistamine medications, if a skin disorder makes accurate interpretation of skin test results difficult, or if skin test results are negative but the patient's signs and symptoms support further investigation.

Guidelines for Skin Testing

- The patient should stop taking all antihistamines or allergy medication 3 to 10 days before testing to avoid false-negative results.
- Recommended sites for allergen injection or application are the anterior forearm and the back.
- Allergen sites must be specifically labeled and spaced approximately 1 1/2 to 2 inches apart.
- If the patient exhibits signs of anaphylaxis, notify the physician immediately and prepare emergency supplies. Allergy testing should be performed only when the physician is on-site.
- Skin testing may cause a mild systemic allergic response resulting in rhinitis, wheezing, and sneezing. The patient should contact the physician if a more severe reaction occurs.

CRITICAL THINKING APPLICATION

A new employee in the practice asks Melissa's help in understanding the different methods for testing for allergies. What should Melissa tell her about the various skin tests performed in the office and the venipuncture RAST test?

Treatment of Allergies. The classic treatment of allergies is to encourage the patient to avoid known or suspected allergens. Unfortunately, this is not always possible, so the physician may prescribe antihistamine medications such as cetirizine hydrochloride (Zyrtec), fexofenadine hydrochloride (Allegra), or over-the-counter medications for relief of allergy symptoms. Another option is the use of *immunotherapy,* a series of injections in which minute doses of known allergens are administered subcutaneously over time to desensitize the patient's immune system and ultimately develop a resistance to the immune response. This usually requires weekly or bimonthly injections over several years. Some patients are cured, whereas others have only a minor reduction in allergic symptoms. Immunotherapy is controversial because it is an expensive, invasive, and potentially dangerous treatment with unpredictable results. It is recommended only for patients with severe allergic symptoms that are not relieved by antihistamine medications.

If you are responsible for administering allergy injections, you must take great care to dispense the correct dose of each allergen; administer each subcutaneous injection in a separate site; accurately document the procedure and exact location of each injection; record any patient local or systemic reactions; and observe the patient for a minimum of 20 to 30 minutes after the injections to determine possible systemic allergic responses including urticaria, wheezing, or hypotension. If the patient exhibits any localized or systemic reactions, the physician should be notified.

Obtaining a Wound Specimen for Culture

A wound culture specimen is obtained to perform a microscopic analysis of the organisms at the site of a lesion to determine the causative infectious agent. The physician may order a culture if the wound is inflamed or has purulent drainage or the patient has a fever. *Aerobic* cultures are performed to detect organisms that grow in the presence of oxygen and are usually found on the superficial surfaces of the wound. *Anaerobic* cultures check for the presence of organisms that require little or no oxygen and appear in deeper wound sites or areas that have a poor blood supply, such as ulcers or compound fractures (Procedure 37-1). Wound culture results help the physician prescribe the most effective antibiotic for the infection.

Procedures for Appearance Modification

Chemical Peel (Chemexfoliation). Topical agents are used in chemical peels to minimize or remove minor skin features, such as acne scars, hyperpigmentation, and fine wrinkles. Agents used for chemical peels include tretinoin cream 0.05% to 0.1% concentration (Retin-A), alpha hydroxy acid, trichloroacetic acid, or phenol (carbolic acid). During application, care must be taken to prevent the solution from entering the eyes. The use of chemical exfoliating agents may cause the skin to appear inflamed and dry with crusting and edema. The patient may complain of stinging and burning at the beginning of the treatment regimen. The patient should avoid sun exposure for the length of treatment and use a sunscreen with a minimum SPF of 15 because *photophobia* (light sensitivity) is a typical side effect of treatment.

Dermabrasion. A *dermabrader* is a hand-held device that mechanically evens the layers of dermal tissue and is effective in the treatment of scars from acne vulgaris. Either topical anesthetics such as ethyl chloride or locally injected anesthetics are used for the procedure. Besides the dermabrader, the dermatologist may use a variety of wire brushes, abrasive discs, or other devices to smooth scar tissue. Standard precautions must be employed, including the use of face and eye guards to avoid aerosol or splatter contamination from the site.

The patient should be educated about wound care, signs of infection, and the presence of photophobia for 6 to 12 months after the procedure.

Laser Resurfacing (Photothermolysis). Laser therapy may be used for fine lines and wrinkles, pigmented areas, shallow scars, and tattoo removal. Typically, the patient is instructed to prepare the site 3 to 6 weeks before the procedure with tretinoin (Retin-A), alpha hydroxy solutions, or bleaches. Laser procedures are performed with the patient under local, regional, or general anesthesia. During the procedure it is extremely important that both the patient and all personnel wear the type of eye protection recommended by the laser manufacturer. After the procedure, cool packs are applied to help reduce swelling and topical antibiotic ointment is used to prevent infection. The treated area will appear inflamed and edematous and can take up to 2 weeks to heal, and as long as 6 months for the inflammation to fade.

Botox Injections. Botox is a strong neurotoxin (toxic to nerves) produced by *Clostridium botulinum*, a bacterium that causes food poisoning. Two strains of the botulism bacterium are used in dermatologic procedures for appearance modification. Botox treatments involve injection of the substance around the eyes, mouth, and forehead. The toxin interferes with nervous stimulation, which temporarily paralyzes the muscles of the face that cause wrinkles to form. It also smoothes out the skin and makes it look younger and fresher. The effects are short term, so treatments must be repeated every 3 to 4 months, and some patients complain of an inability to show facial expression because of muscle paralysis.

CLOSING COMMENTS

Patient Education

There are many opportunities and topics for patient education in the dermatology field. Skin care products are advertised in the newspaper, on billboards, in magazines, and on television. Consult the dermatologist you work for and get approval of skin care products that the office can recommend to patients. Sometimes companies that manufacture skin care products will give you samples if you write and tell them that your office recommends a certain product's use to patients. Patients enjoy receiving samples and encouragement to try a new skin care technique.

Another area of patient education involves the potentially dangerous effects of sunlight and tanning beds. Obtain literature showing how UV rays cause premature aging and may cause cancerous lesions later in life. You can explain the meaning of the sun protective factor in sun-tanning lotions. Tanning beds should be avoided, especially by persons who have a skin disorder and by individuals taking certain medications that cause photophobia. In addition, providing patients with information about the warning signs of cancer is a vital part of patient education in a dermatology office.

Legal and Ethical Issues

When working in a dermatology office you will hear many patients express concerns regarding skin disorders. Allowing

PROCEDURE 37-1

Obtain Specimens for Microbiological Testing: Collect a Wound Specimen for Testing and/or Culture

CAAHEP COMPETENCY: 3.b.(2)(c)
ABHES COMPETENCY: 4.h

GOAL: *To obtain an adequate sample for culture without contaminating the specimen.*

EQUIPMENT and SUPPLIES

- Sterile culture kit containing tube, swabs, and transport media (for swabbing)
- Sterile culture kit containing syringe and transport media (for aspirating)
- Laboratory requisition
- Sterile gauze squares
- Recommended wound-cleansing solution
- Sterile dressing
- Gloves
- Biohazard container
- Face guard
- Patient record

PROCEDURAL STEPS

1. Wash your hands, gather supplies (Figure 1), and don gloves and face protection.
   PURPOSE: Standard precautions.
2. Remove dressing from the wound, and dispose of it in a biohazard waste container.
   PURPOSE: Infection control.
3. Observe the wound, and make note of the color, odor, and amount of exudate present.
   PURPOSE: Information will be noted for the physician on the patient's record when the procedure is completed.

4. Swabbing. Remove the swab from the culture kit, insert the swab into the wound, and saturate it with the exudate. If necessary, use more than one swab, properly labeling each container, to obtain exudates from the entire wound. If preparing an anaerobic culture, place the specimen in the culture tube as quickly as possible to avoid oxygen exposure and possible destruction of microbes.
5. Aspirating. Remove the syringe from the kit, insert the tip into the wound exudate, and draw back the plunger, drawing the exudate up into the syringe.
6. Place the swab into the culture tube, and crush the transport media ampule, which is in the transport tube, by squeezing the walls of the transport tube slightly, or place the exudate-filled syringe directly into the transport tube (Figure 2).
7. Label the culture tube accurately. Include on the laboratory slip the patient's recent antibiotic therapy, the wound site, and the suspected organism.
8. Clean the wound as ordered by the physician, and apply a sterile dressing to the area. See Chapter 56 for sterile dressing procedure.
9. Clean the area, disposing of all waste materials in a biohazard waste container. Remove gloves and wash your hands.
   PURPOSE: Infection control.
10. Place culture tube in the laboratory collection area. Chart the procedure and all wound data on the patient's record.
    PURPOSE: A procedure is not done until it is recorded.

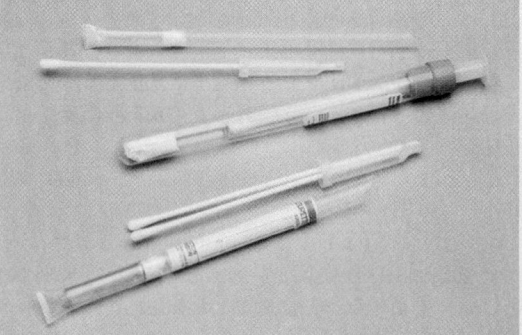

FIGURE 1

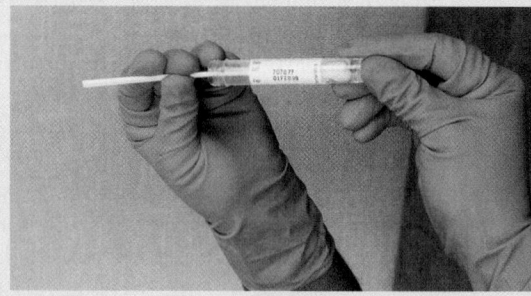

FIGURE 2

patients to express their concerns and using therapeutic listening techniques is always helpful; however, be careful when offering encouragement about the course and outcome of treatment. No treatment can restore youth. The improvement achieved may be slow and gradual. Keep encouragement on a positive level. Compliment the patient on small improvements, but it is the physician's role to explain potential treatment outcomes.

SUMMARY OF SCENARIO

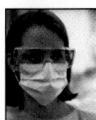

Melissa enjoys her work with Dr. Lee but recognizes the need to keep up with new developments in the field of dermatology. She has learned the importance of giving patients accurate information while conducting telephone screening and always refers questions or concerns to Dr. Lee. Melissa especially enjoys the patient education aspects of working for a dermatologist, including the importance of using sunscreen, controlling sun exposure, and informing patients about the warning signs of cancer. Melissa has also learned how to assist Dr. Lee with dermatologic procedures, including performing allergy skin testing, obtaining wound cultures, and assisting with biopsies, chemical peels, dermabrasions, and laser resurfacing.

SUMMARY of LEARNING OBJECTIVES

1. Define, spell, and pronounce the terms listed in the vocabulary.
   - Spelling and pronouncing medical terms correctly adds credibility to the medical assistant. Knowing the definition of these terms promotes confidence in communication with patients and co-workers.

2. Explain the major functions of the skin.
   - The skin acts as a barrier to protect vital internal organs against infection and injury; helps dissipate heat and regulate body temperature; and synthesizes vitamin D when exposed to UV light. In addition, various sensory receptors throughout the skin enable the body to respond to heat, cold, pain, and pressure.

3. Diagram the anatomic structures of the skin.
   - The skin is made up of three layers: the epidermis, which is the thin uppermost layer; the dermis is the thicker layer beneath making up approximately 90% of the skin mass; and the subcutaneous layer is primarily fatty or adipose tissue.

4. Compare various skin lesions, and give examples of each.
   - Refer to Figure 37-2 for descriptions of skin lesions. The diagnosis of skin lesions is based on the color, level of elevation, and texture of the lesion; the presence of pruritus, excoriation, pain, or drainage; and whether the lesion is a primary or secondary growth.

5. Describe typical integumentary system infections.
   - Integumentary system infections include bacterial infections, such as impetigo, acne vulgaris, furuncles, carbuncles, and cellulitis; fungal infections, including a variety of tinea growths; viral infections, which cause warts, herpes simplex, and herpes zoster outbreaks; and scabies or pediculosis infestations.

6. Differentiate among various inflammatory and autoimmune integumentary disorders.
   - Inflammatory and vascular integumentary system disorders include a variety of seborrheic dermatitis inflammations; contact dermatitis; eczema; and autoimmune disorders.

7. Recognize thermal injuries to the skin.
   - The most frequent thermal injuries are burns, which are classified as superficial, partial-thickness, or full-thickness burns, depending on the depth of the wound. The most important concern in the treatment of burns is the prevention of infection. Cold injuries are usually less severe than burns, but prolonged exposure can result in infection, gangrene, amputation, and death.

8. Compare the characteristics of benign and malignant neoplasms.
   - Benign masses are encapsulated, whereas malignant tumors invade and take over surrounding tissues. Local invasion of surrounding tissue occurs when malignant cells break through the basement membrane that separates epithelial cells from connective tissue. Here the cancerous cells can invade blood and lymph vessels, which can then carry the malignant cells to organs throughout the body.

9. Define grading and staging of malignant tumors.
   - Grading is the histologic, cellular classification of the tumor. The more poorly differentiated the cells from the tumor, the closer the biopsy to an anaplastic cancerous mass. Staging involves using physical examination and diagnostic tests (such as bone or liver scans) to determine the presence of tumor spread.

10. Conduct patient education on the warning signs of cancer.
    - The warning signs of cancer include any change in bowel or bladder habits; a sore that does not heal; unusual bleeding or discharge; a thickening or a lump in the breast or elsewhere; indigestion or difficulty in swallowing; an obvious change in a wart or mole; or a nagging cough or hoarseness. Any of these warning signs should be reported to the physician immediately. Early detection and self-examination are crucial to cancer survival.

11. Describe skin malignancies and their treatment.
    - Three cancerous lesions of the skin occur: basal cell carcinoma is very slow growing and is the most frequently seen form of skin cancer; squamous cell carcinoma grows rapidly and is more serious because it has a tendency to metastasize; melanomas are pigmented lesions that are asymmetric with irregular borders and are usually larger than 6 mm. Treatment depends on the type of lesion, the level of invasion, and the location. The physician may surgically remove the tumor or destroy it with cryosurgery, electrodesiccation, laser treatment, or the application of chemotherapeutic agents.

SUMMARY of LEARNING OBJECTIVES

Continued

12. Define the ABCD rule for identifying a malignant melanoma.
    - The ABCD rule includes examination of the site for any of the following: asymmetry, irregular border, change in color, and an increase in the diameter. If a mole displays any of these characteristics, a dermatologist should check it immediately.

13. Summarize allergy testing procedures.
    - Allergy testing is done by exposing the patient either through a scratch on the skin or an intradermal injection to suspected allergens and observing the exposure site afterwards to see if there is a localized allergic reaction. The patient must be off antihistamine drugs several days before testing, the sites for allergen exposure are the forearms and back, and a physician must be present in the facility while allergy testing is being done since there is the potential for local or systemic allergic reactions in sensitized patients.

14. Explain dermatologic procedures conducted in the ambulatory care setting.
    - Dermatologic procedures include allergy skin testing that can be done with scratch or intradermal tests; drawing blood for a RAST test; treating allergies with immunotherapy; performing a wound culture; and assisting with appearance modification procedures, including chemical peels, dermabrasion, and laser resurfacing.

15. Accurately obtain an exudate sample from a wound for laboratory analysis.
    - Procedure 37-1 summarizes the steps for collecting a wound sample for culture.

CONNECTIONS

Study Guide Connection: Go to Chapter 37 Study Guide. Read the Case Study and Workplace Applications and complete the assignments. Do online research for answers to the questions in the Internet Activities associated with assisting in dermatology.

CD Connection: Go to the Medical Assisting Competency Challenge CD and do the training activities under Patient Care.

Evolve Connection: For more information related to assisting in dermatology, go to evolve.elsevier.com/kinn and visit related weblinks for Chapter 37. Click on the Medical Assisting Exam Review and do the practice questions to sharpen your test-taking skills.

Assisting in Gastroenterology

38

SCENARIO

Joan Rothman, CMA, was recently hired by United Community Hospital to work for a group of internists. Joan works primarily with Dr. Raj Sahani, a physician who specializes in gastroenterology. Although Joan did very well in school, she has had to learn more advanced information about disorders of the gastrointestinal tract so she can manage patient questions and understand the diagnostic procedures ordered by Dr. Sahani. Dr. Sahani has asked Joan to research and develop educational packets for common gastrointestinal studies as well as work with other staff members on understanding procedures related to the gastrointestinal system. Part of the role of the medical assistant working in a gastroenterology practice is to conduct routine patient education so that patients are properly prepared for diagnostic procedures. Joan is also expected to assist with orienting new staff to the practice.

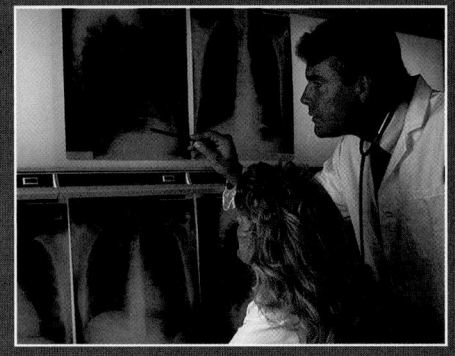

While studying this chapter, think about the following questions:

- What does Joan need to include in the educational packets so that patients are prepared for GI examinations?
- What are some of the GI disorders Joan can expect to see in this specialty practice?
- What information should Joan include in a pamphlet on infectious viral hepatitis?
- What should a new MA know about the GI examination, including instructing patients in the collection of fecal specimens?

LEARNING OBJECTIVES

1. Define, spell, and pronounce the terms listed in the vocabulary.
2. Describe the primary functions of the gastrointestinal system.
3. Identify the anatomic structures that make up the system, and describe the physiology of each.
4. Differentiate among the abdominal quadrants and regions.
5. Summarize the typical symptoms and characteristics of gastrointestinal complaints.
6. Perform telephone screening using a gastrointestinal complaint.
7. Distinguish among cancers of the gastrointestinal tract.
8. Explain common esophageal and gastric disorders, their signs and symptoms, diagnostic tests, and treatments.
9. Define intestinal disorders and their signs and symptoms, diagnostic tests, and treatments.
10. Classify disorders of the liver and gallbladder and their signs and symptoms, diagnostic tests, and treatments.

11. Describe the similarities and differences among the various forms of infectious viral hepatitis.
12. Summarize the medical assistant's role in the gastrointestinal examination.
13. Explain the common diagnostic procedures for the gastrointestinal system.
14. Perform the procedural steps for assisting with the collection of a fecal specimen, including the necessary patient education for preparation for the examination and collection of stool samples at home.
15. Describe the medical assistant's role in the proctologic examination.
16. Demonstrate assisting with an endoscopic colon examination.

National Accreditation Competencies and Content

CAAHEP COMPETENCIES	ABHES COMPETENCIES
Clinical	**Clinical Duties**
3.b.(2)(e). Instruct patients in the collection of a fecal specimen	4.b. Prepare patients for procedures
3.b.(4)(a). Perform telephone and in-person screening	4.h. Prepare patient for and assist physician with routine and specialty examinations
3.b.(4)(e). Prepare patient for and assist with routine and specialty examinations	4.j. Collect and process specimens
	4.x. Instruct patient in collection of fecal specimen
General	4.ff. Perform telephone and in-person screening
3.c.(3)(c). Provide instruction for health maintenance and disease prevention	**Instruction**
	7.c. Teach patients methods of health promotion and disease prevention

VOCABULARY

adhesions (ad-he´-zhuns) Bands of scar tissue that bind together two anatomic surfaces that are normally separate.

anastomosis (uh-nas-tuh-mo´-suhs) The surgical joining together of two normally distinct organs.

anorexia (a-nuh-rek´-se-uh) Lack or loss of appetite for food.

ascites (uh-si´-tez) An abnormal collection of fluid in the peritoneal cavity that contains high levels of protein and electrolytes.

carcinogens (kar-si´-nuh-juhns) Substances or agents that cause the development of or increase the incidence of cancer.

cryosurgery Subfreezing temperature is used to destroy tissue.

diaphoresis (di-uh-fuh-re´-sis) The profuse excretion of sweat.

endemic (en-de´-mik) Disease or microorganism that is specific to a particular geographic area.

esophageal varices (i-sah-fuh-je´-uhl/var´-uh-sez) Varicose veins of the esophagus occurring as a result of portal hypertension; vessels can easily hemorrhage.

fecalith (fe´-kuh-lith) A hard, impacted mass of feces in the colon.

fissures Narrow slits or clefts in the abdominal wall.

fistulas (fis´-chuh-luhz) Abnormal, tubelike passages within the body tissue, usually between two internal organs.

flatus Gas expelled through the anus.

gangrene Death of body tissue as a result of loss of nutritive supply and followed by bacteria invasion and putrefaction.

hematemesis (hi-mat-uh-me´-sis) Vomiting of bright red blood, indicating rapid upper gastrointestinal bleeding; associated with esophageal varices or peptic ulcer.

hematocrit Volume percentage of erythrocytes in whole blood.

hemoglobin (he´-muh-glo-buhn) Protein found in erythrocytes that transports molecular oxygen in the blood.

hepatomegaly (he-puh-to-me´-guh-le) Abnormal enlargement of the liver.

ileostomy Surgical formation of an opening of the ileum onto the surface of the abdomen through which fecal material is emptied.

jaundice Yellowness of the skin and mucous membranes caused by deposition of bile pigment; not a disease but a sign of a number of diseases, especially liver disorders.

lithotripsy (li´-thuh-trip-se) A procedure for eliminating a stone by crushing or dissolving it in situ through the use of high-intensity sound waves.

lymphadenopathy (lim-fa-duh-nah´-puh-the) Any disorder of the lymph nodes or lymph vessels.

peristalsis (per-uh-stahl´-sis) Wavelike movement by which the gastrointestinal tract moves food downward.

polyps (pah´-lips) Tumors on outgrowths found in the mucosal lining of the colon; considered precancerous.

portal circulation Pathway of blood flow through the portal vein from the gastrointestinal system to the liver.

portal hypertension An increased venous pressure in the portal circulation caused by cirrhosis or compression of the hepatic vascular system.

sclerotherapy (skluh-rah-ther´-ah-pe) Injection of sclerosing solutions in the treatment of hemorrhoids, varicose veins, or esophageal varices.

Valsalva's maneuver Occurs when one strains to defecate and urinate, uses the arms and upper trunk muscles to move up in bed, or strains during laughing, coughing, or vomiting; causes a trapping of blood in the great veins, preventing it from entering the chest and right atrium, and may cause heart attack and death.

Internal medicine is a nonsurgical specialty with several subspecialties. Gastroenterology is one of these subspecialties and covers an extremely wide area known as the *gastrointestinal (GI) system* or the *alimentary canal*. Gastroenterologists are concerned with the diseases and disorders of the stomach, small intestine, large intestine (colon), appendix, and the accessory organs of the liver, gallbladder, and pancreas. Proctology, a subspecialty of gastroenterology, is concerned with disorders of the rectum and anus. The major purpose of the GI system is to prepare, digest, and absorb the necessary nutrients to maintain homeostasis and excrete waste products through the feces.

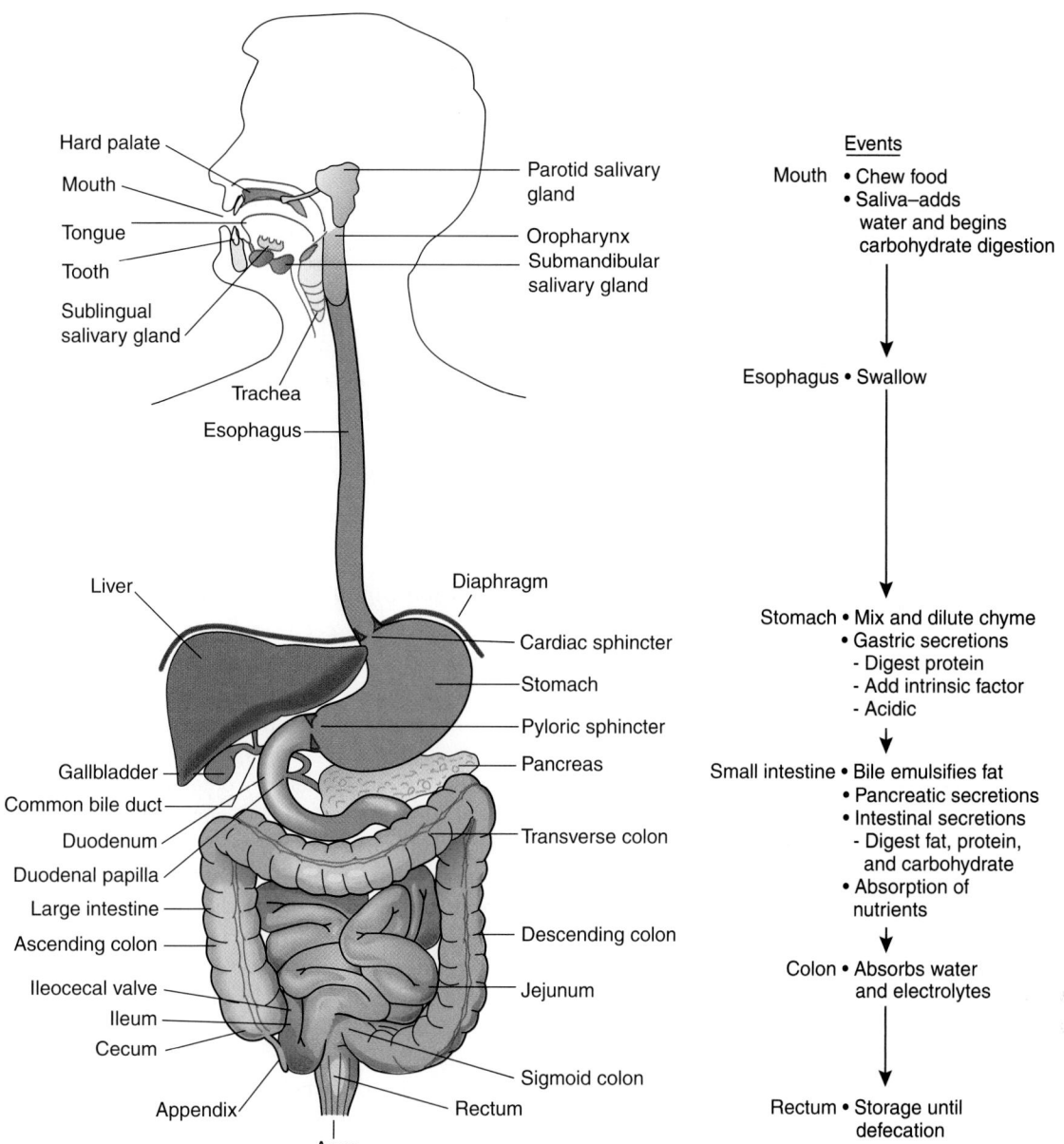

FIGURE 38-1 Anatomy of the digestive system with associated events. (From Gould B: *Pathophysiology for the health professions*, ed 3, Philadelphia, 2006, Saunders.)

ANATOMY AND PHYSIOLOGY

The GI system is basically a long hollow tube that has the same structural organization from its beginning to its termination (Figure 38-1). The muscles lining the GI tract are closely governed by the autonomic nervous system, which gives the entire system its unique ability to move slowly in some locations and to have increased movement in other sections. It is divided into two parts: the upper digestive system includes the mouth, esophagus, and stomach; the lower section consists of the small and large intestines. The GI tract is rich in lymphatic tissue, which is very important for the absorption of nutrients from ingested food. Unfortunately, the lymphatic vessels are also the main route for the spread of cancers.

The primary functions of the GI organs are threefold; digestion, absorption, and elimination. When food is taken in through the mouth, it is chewed or *masticated* and moistened with saliva. An enzyme released by the salivary glands, salivary amylase, mixes with the food and begins carbohydrate digestion. This mass, now called a *bolus,* is swallowed, and the food enters the esophagus. Contractions of the smooth muscles are activated, and the bolus is now moved by **peristalsis** down the esophagus and into the stomach.

At the distal end of the esophagus is the gastroesophageal or cardiac sphincter, which relaxes as the bolus is swallowed so it can pass into the stomach. The muscular walls of the stomach overlap in folds, or *rugae,* which permit the stomach to expand and hold as much as 1 to 1.5 L of food and liquid. The gastric glands located in the stomach mucosa secrete hydrochloric acid, pepsinogen (begins the digestion of protein), and intrinsic factor, which is needed for the absorption of vitamin B_{12}. The gastric contents, now called *chyme*, are slowly emptied through the pyloric sphincter into the small intestine. The small intestine is made up of the duodenum at the proximal end, the jejunum, and the ileum at the distal end.

The common bile duct delivers bile, which is produced in the liver and stored in the gallbladder, to the duodenum. Bile acids *emulsify* fat, or break down large fat molecules into smaller molecules that can be chemically digested by fat enzymes. The pancreatic duct delivers digestive enzymes to the duodenum, including *amylase* for carbohydrate digestion, *trypsin* for protein breakdown, and *lipase* for fats. This mixture of bile and pancreatic enzymes in the duodenum completes digestion of nutrients converting carbohydrates into glucose, protein into amino acids, and fats into fatty acids and glycerol.

Once digestion is completed in the duodenum the second function of the GI tract, absorption of nutrients, begins. The small intestine is lined with transverse folds of tissue called *villi*. There are approximately 25,000 of these overlapping projections, which greatly increase the surface area available in the small intestine for nutrient absorption. Each villus is rich with blood vessels that absorb digested nutrients into the **portal circulation** system and carry them directly to the liver for processing. Lymph vessels along the villi absorb fat and deposit it into the systemic circulation. By the time the chyme reaches the terminal end of the small intestine, every nutrient that your body needs should have been absorbed. This mass enters the colon or large intestine, which is made up of the cecum (extending from it is the vermiform appendix), ascending colon, transverse colon, descending colon, sigmoid colon, rectum, and anus. The colon absorbs large amounts of fluids and electrolytes to prevent dehydration of body tissues. Once fluid has been reabsorbed, the remaining solid waste materials, called *feces*, are moved into the sigmoid colon and rectum, and elimination occurs through the anus. This final function is called *defecation*.

CRITICAL THINKING APPLICATION

Dr. Sahani is concerned that some staff members do not understand the role of the GI system in digestion, absorption, and excretion. He asks Joan to prepare an in-service training on the anatomy and physiology of the GI tract. What should Joan include in the workshop?

DISEASES OF THE GASTROINTESTINAL SYSTEM

GI disorders are probably the most common problems seen in a medical office. Most GI system conditions are managed by a primary care physician. Between 5% and 10% of GI problems are referred to a gastroenterologist for diagnosis and treatment. It is assumed that problems that stem from dental disorders are cared for by the dental professions. This chapter concentrates on the GI problems most frequently seen, diagnosed, and treated in an ambulatory care center.

Characteristics of the Gastrointestinal System

- The abdominal cavity can be divided into four quadrants or nine regions (Figure 38-2).
- The *peritoneum* is a membrane that lines the abdominal wall and covers the organs of the abdominal cavity.
- The *mesentery* is a dorsal peritoneal fold that attaches the jejunum and ileum to the posterior abdominal wall.
- The *omentum* is a fold of fatty peritoneal tissue that contains multiple lymph nodes and hangs from the stomach like an apron covering the anterior transverse colon and the small intestine. Inflammation of the omentum results in the formation of scar tissue and **adhesions.**
- The gastrointestinal system digests and absorbs nutrients for the entire body; if it becomes diseased, all other systems are affected.

Common Signs and Symptoms

A patient with a GI problem may complain of multiple discomforts including nausea, vomiting, **anorexia,** diarrhea, constipation, and abdominal pain. It may be difficult for a medical assistant to identify the exact location and quality of the patient's discomfort. When discussing abdominal pain with the patient, ask the patient to point to or touch the area where the pain is located. This is one way of making sure that the correct quadrant or region is identified and the patient is properly prepared for the physician to examine. If possible, document the location of the patient's complaint using the abdominal regions method, because this is most accurate. For example, if the patient complains of heartburn after eating, this can be charted as, "Pt c/o epigastric discomfort after meals; 6 on a pain scale of 1-10."

Table 38-1 outlines the typical signs, symptoms, and characteristics that would be seen in patients with GI complaints. Using Procedure 38-1, outline how you would respond to the scenarios in the following Critical Thinking Application.

CRITICAL THINKING APPLICATION

Two days a week Joan works in the telephone screening area of the practice, where she is responsible for the initial management of calls from Dr. Sahani's patients. The following problems from patients are typical of a call day. What are some of the questions Joan should ask and subsequently document on each patient's chart?

- The mother of a 7-year-old patient is concerned because her son has been vomiting since yesterday.
- The father of an 18-month-old infant reports that the child has had diarrhea for 2 days.
- A 72-year-old patient is concerned about constipation that is not relieved with laxatives.

Cancers of the Gastrointestinal Tract

Any organ of the digestive tract can develop cancer. The features of malignant tumors and their treatments were described in Chapter 37. These characteristics, including the abilities to

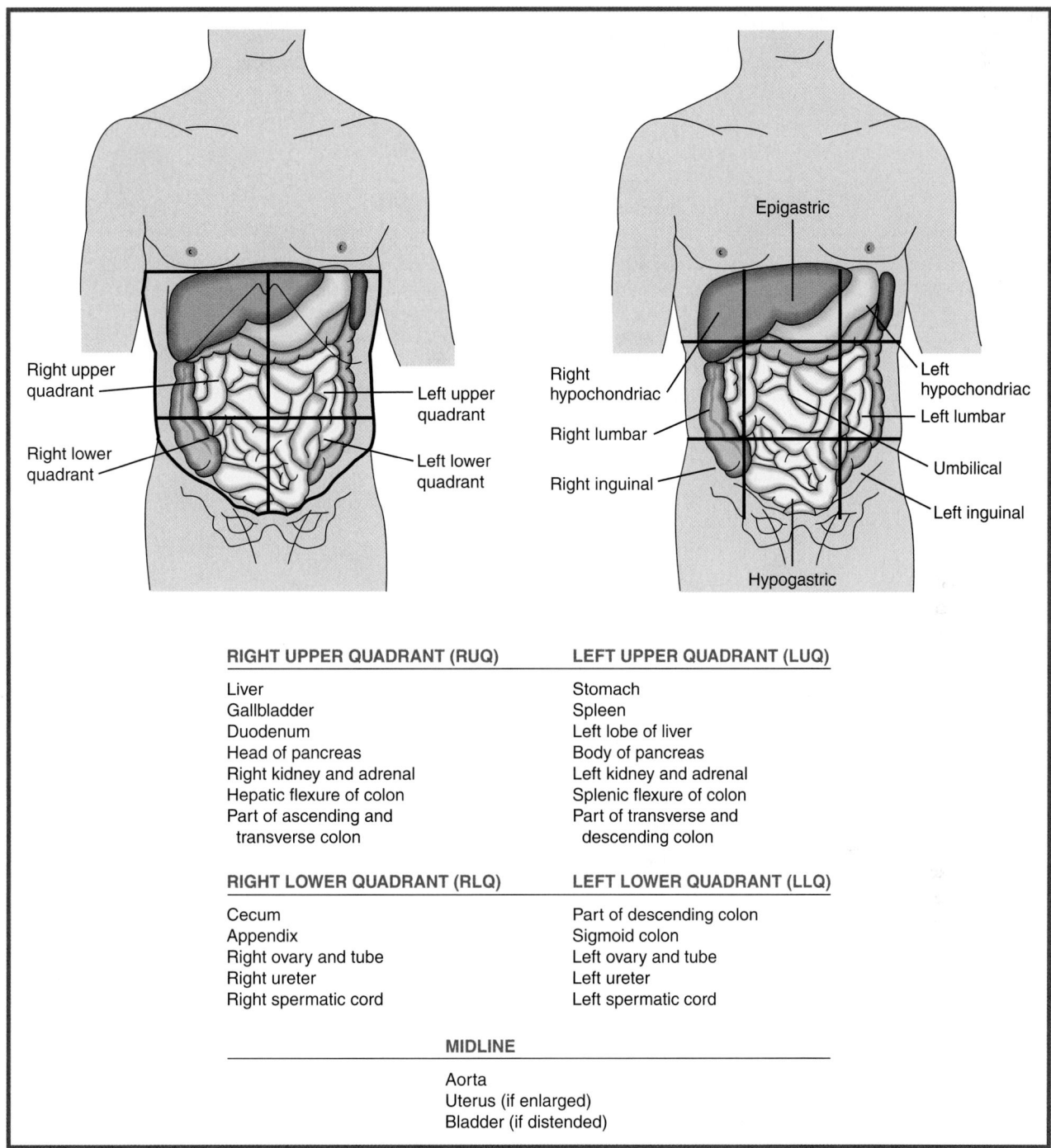

FIGURE 38-2 Abdominal quadrants and regions and the organs located in each.

invade surrounding tissues and metastasize through the blood or lymph systems, are true of all cancerous tumors.

Table 38-2 describes some of the common malignant tumors found in the GI system. The exact cause of a malignancy may not be known, but exposure to **carcinogens** increases the risk of developing a cancerous tumor. Examples of carcinogens include tobacco and alcohol as well as exposure to chemicals and radiation. Family history and lifestyle factors, such as consuming a diet high in fat and low in fiber, can also increase the risk for developing certain types of cancer.

Disorders of the Esophagus and Stomach

Hiatal Hernia

A *hernia* is the abnormal protrusion of part of an organ or tissue through the structures normally containing it. These protrusions can develop in various parts of the body but most frequently are seen in the abdominal region. Causes of herniation include congenital weakness of the structures, trauma, relaxation of ligaments and skeletal muscles, and increased upward pressure from the abdomen. Herniation is most often found in middle-

TABLE 38-1   Characteristics of Common Gastrointestinal Complaints

GASTROINTESTINAL COMPLAINT	CHARACTERISTICS

Nausea
Vomiting (emesis)
	Patient exhibits pallor, **diaphoresis**, tachycardia
	Caused by:
	    Gastrointestinal irritation
	    Pain or stress
	    Inner ear disturbance
	    Increased intracranial pressure
	
	Important characteristics that should be reported and recorded:
	    Onset, frequency, duration of the problem
	    Yellow or greenish color indicates bile from the duodenum
	    Pyloric stenosis causes vomiting of undigested food
	    Projectile vomiting may indicate increased intracranial pressure
	    Hematemesis produces coffee-grounds–appearing vomitus

Diarrhea	Caused by:
	    Infections or inflammation
	    Food allergies
	    Malabsorption syndromes
	
	Important characteristics that should be reported and recorded:
	    Onset, frequency, duration of the problem
	    Dehydration may occur if diarrhea is persistent; occurs more frequently in infants and older adults
	    Presence of blood, mucus, pus
	    Steatorrhea: large, foul-smelling, greasy stools
	    Melena: tarry stools from higher digestive tract bleeding

Constipation	Caused by:
	    Lack of dietary fiber
	    Inadequate intake of fluids
	    Lack of exercise
	    Neurologic disorders including spinal cord injuries and multiple sclerosis
	    Side effect of medications (codeine, iron, antacids)
	    Bowel obstructions or tumors
	
	Important characteristics that should be reported and recorded:
	    Onset, frequency, duration of the problem
	    Treatment and effectiveness of over-the-counter medications
	    Diet and fluid intake
	    Presence of watery diarrhea (may indicate fecal impaction)

Abdominal pain	Caused by:
	    Ulcerative diseases
	    Tumors
	    Appendicitis
	    Bowel obstruction
	    Food poisoning
	    Infections or inflammatory process
	
	Important characteristics that should be reported and recorded:
	    Onset, frequency, duration
	    Exact location (using either quadrants or abdominal regions)
	    Quality of the pain (burning, cramping, sharp, dull, etc.)
	    Degree of pain on a scale of 1 to 10

aged or older individuals. The location of the hernia determines the term by which the protrusion is identified.

In patients with a hiatal hernia, the upper part of the stomach protrudes through the esophageal opening, the hiatal sphincter of the diaphragm (Figure 38-3). With a sliding hiatal hernia, part of the stomach moves above the diaphragm when supine and slides back down into the abdominal cavity when standing.

Part of the fundus of the stomach moves through the weakened hiatus in a paraesophageal hiatal hernia. Food may lodge in the herniated part of the stomach, causing reflux of highly acidic stomach contents into the esophagus, dysphagia, and chronic esophagitis, which may cause fibrosis and stricture. Patients complain of heartburn, frequent belching, and increased discomfort when they cough, bend over, or lie down after

PROCEDURE 38-1

Perform Telephone Screening of a GI Patient Complaint

CAAHEP COMPETENCY: 3.b.(4)(a)
ABHES COMPETENCY: 4.ff

GOAL: *To answer the telephone professionally and manage patient phone calls according to physician guidelines.*
SCENARIO: A 22-year-old woman reports acute abdominal pain.

EQUIPMENT and SUPPLIES

- Telephone
- Message pad
- Pen
- Access to appointment schedule
- Access to patient records
- Physician policy manual for managing patient phone calls

PROCEDURAL STEPS

1. Answer the telephone by the third ring, speaking directly into the mouthpiece.
   PURPOSE: Answering promptly conveys interest in the caller. Proper positioning of the mouthpiece allows for audible tone.
2. Speak distinctly with a pleasant tone and expression, at a moderate rate, and with sufficient volume.
3. Greet the caller, identify the office and/or physician as well as yourself, and offer to help the caller.
   PURPOSE: The patient will know that the correct number has been reached and the identity of the staff member.
4. Verify the identity of the caller, and access the patient's record.
   PURPOSE: To have the patient's chart ready for reference regarding health history and recent care.
5. Determine the needs of the caller.
6. Considering the patient's complaint, formulate questions that are designed to gather the information required to make a decision about when the patient should be seen and the physician notified. Given the patient's sex, age, and complaint of acute abdominal pain, consider the following questions:

- What are the onset, frequency, and duration of the abdominal pain?
- What is the exact anatomic location of the discomfort?
- What is the quality of the pain? Is it sharp, dull, stabbing, etc.?
- On a scale of 1 to 10, what is the patient's level of pain?
- Does the patient have a history of this occurrence? Does she have a history of gynecologic or pelvic disorders?
- Has she taken any medication for the discomfort, and has it been effective?

7. Refer to the physician's policies regarding patient phone calls as needed.
8. Depending on the patient's answers to your questions and the physician's policies regarding the management of abdominal discomfort, refer to the appointment schedule and make her an appointment or take a message for the physician to return her call.
9. Document the details of the interaction and the results in the patient's chart.
   PURPOSE: All communications with a patient, including phone calls, are part of the record of care.
   DOCUMENTATION PRACTICE: _____

   _____

   _____

   _____

   _____

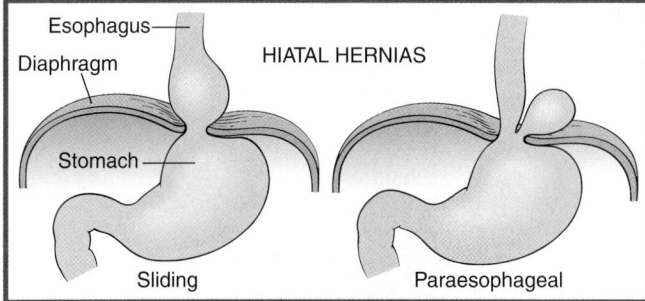

FIGURE 38-3 Hiatal hernias. (From Damjanov I: *Pathology for the health professions*, ed 3, St Louis, 2006, Saunders.)

eating. Patients with hiatal hernias are treated medically with omeprazole (Prilosec), esomeprazole (Nexium), famotidine (Pepcid), cimetidine (Tagamet), or ranitidine (Zantac). The treatment may also include diet modifications such as avoidance of caffeine, cigarettes, and alcohol; eating six small meals a day; weight loss; avoiding lying down after meals; and raising the head of the bed 6 to 8 inches.

Gastroesophageal Reflux Disease

Gastroesophageal reflux disease (GERD) occurs when the gastroesophageal sphincter (cardiac sphincter) at the distal end of the esophagus does not close properly, allowing acidic stomach contents to leak back, or reflux, into the esophagus. The regurgitated acidic contents of the stomach irritate the esophageal lining, causing heartburn symptoms. Occasional heartburn is not a problem but a patient experiencing heartburn more than twice a week is diagnosed with GERD. All age groups can be diagnosed with GERD; however, it is seen most frequently in adults and is associated with alcohol use, pregnancy, and smoking and occurs frequently in overweight patients. Besides persistent heartburn, patients may report chest pain associated

TABLE 38-2 Cancers of the Gastrointestinal Tract

TUMOR	CHARACTERISTICS	CAUSE OR CONTRIBUTING FACTORS
Oral tumors	White mass in or on mouth that bleeds easily Ulcer or fissure that does not heal Mass is usually not painful	Cancer of the lip—pipe smoking Cancer of the tongue or gums—chewing tobacco
Esophageal cancer	Typically found in the distal esophagus Initial sign is dysphagia (difficulty swallowing)	Associated with chronic irritation resulting from chronic esophagitis, alcohol abuse, or smoking
Gastric cancer	Asymptomatic in early stages Usually not diagnosed until well advanced Prognosis is poor Anorexia, indigestion, weight loss, fatigue Positive occult blood in the stool	Food preservatives, chronic use of nitrates, smoked foods Genetic association Chronic gastritis
Liver cancer	Primary malignant tumors rare; usually a metastasized secondary tumor Initial symptoms mild; anorexia, vomiting, weight loss, fatigue, hepatomegaly, splenomegaly, **portal hypertension** Usually advanced when diagnosed	Primary tumor caused by cirrhosis from hepatitis or chemical exposure
Pancreatic cancer	Weight loss, jaundice Usually advanced when diagnosed Metastasis occurs early; no effective treatment	Cigarette smoking
Colorectal cancer	Usually develops from **polyps** in the colon Metastasis to the liver is common Initial signs depend on location of tumor; changes in the character of stool, iron-deficiency anemia, fatigue, weight loss, frank bleeding, or melena	Genetic or familial link Diet high in fat, sugar, red meats, and low in fiber Usually occurs in patients over 55 years of age

with hoarseness in the morning, difficulty swallowing, a feeling of tightness in the throat or a choking sensation, dry cough, and bad breath from the reflux of partially digested food. GERD is frequently seen in patients with hiatal hernias, and treatment protocols are similar in the two conditions.

Laparoscopic repair of the gastroesophageal sphincter may be recommended if lifestyle changes and medication are not effective in curing the problem. The FDA recently approved an Enteryx implant which is laparoscopically placed next to the sphincter and releases a solution that helps strengthen the muscle. The biggest concern with chronic GERD is the potential for developing a condition called *Barrett's esophagus*. Long-term exposure of esophageal cells to gastric contents can result in precancerous changes in the cells lining the esophagus. Patients diagnosed with GERD are followed regularly by a gastroenterologist so that these abnormal cells can be detected early and removed before cancerous changes occur.

Gastric and Duodenal Ulcers

Peptic ulcers occur most frequently in the proximal duodenum (duodenal ulcer) but may also be found in the stomach (gastric ulcer). Both types are characterized by an area of breakdown of mucosal membrane that leads to ulceration of the epithelial lining of the duodenum or stomach (Figure 38-4).

The first sign of a peptic ulcer may be iron-deficiency anemia or a positive stool for occult blood resulting from the erosion of blood vessels in the organ wall. Patients typically complain of gnawing or burning pain in the epigastric area between meals. Gastric ulcers may cause loss of weight, whereas duodenal lesions often produce nausea and vomiting. If the ulcerative

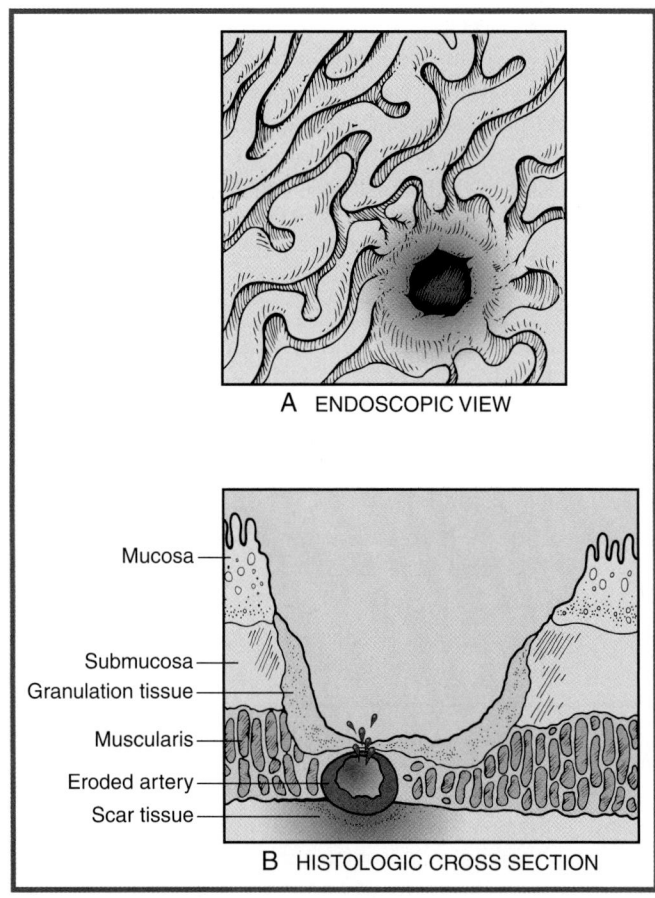

A ENDOSCOPIC VIEW

Mucosa
Submucosa
Granulation tissue
Muscularis
Eroded artery
Scar tissue

B HISTOLOGIC CROSS SECTION

FIGURE 38-4 Peptic ulcer.

area is bleeding internally, the patient may have *hematemesis* (blood in the vomitus) or *melena* (coffee-ground and/or tarry black stools).

The description of the patient's pain gives the physician a suspicion of the disorder. The examination often shows that the patient is guarding the painful area, characterized by clutching of the upper abdominal area and drawing the knees up toward the chest. A definitive diagnosis is based on an upper GI series (x-ray evaluation) or endoscopy (visualization) of the upper GI tract (Figure 38-5). A biopsy of the affected area may be taken during the endoscopy to rule out possible cancer. A stool test may be ordered to check for the presence of occult blood. Blood tests will also be ordered to establish **hemoglobin** and **hematocrit** levels.

Peptic ulcers can appear under a variety of predisposing circumstances, including the use of alcohol, nonsteroidal anti-inflammatory drugs (NSAIDs) and corticosteroids (prednisone), and genetic predisposition. However, research indicates that 80% of gastric ulcers and 90% of duodenal ulcers are caused by the *Helicobacter pylori* bacterium. *H. pylori* can be diagnosed by either a blood test that measures the presence of antibodies to the bacteria or a breath test that is done after the patient swallows a drink containing urea and carbon. Expired air is examined to determine the presence of bacteria. The diagnosis is confirmed with a biopsy of gastric and duodenal mucosa obtained during an endoscopic examination.

H. pylori peptic ulcers are treated with a combination of medications including antibiotics to kill the bacteria and drugs to decrease the production of hydrochloric acid and protect the stomach lining. The most effective treatment is a triple therapy method lasting 2 weeks with two antibiotics (such as amoxicillin, tetracycline, or Biaxin) plus either Tagamet or Zantac, or a proton pump inhibitor (Prilosec or Pepcid). In severe cases, such as those with perforation of the gastric wall, surgery may be indicated. Any nonhealing ulcer is periodically reevaluated through gastroscopy to rule out cancer.

Pyloric Stenosis

Pyloric stenosis, which is the narrowing and hardening of the pyloric sphincter at the distal end of the stomach, can be caused by scar tissue from chronic conditions but is typically seen as a congenital defect in infants. The difficulty becomes apparent in newborns within 2 to 6 weeks of birth with projectile vomiting immediately after feeding because of the inability of the stomach to effectively empty. As a result, the baby displays symptoms of failure to thrive, becomes dehydrated, has small and infrequent stools, and is very irritable. Congenital pyloric stenosis typically occurs in first-born males and can be corrected by surgery.

Intestinal Disorders

Food Poisoning

Food poisoning is a disorder resulting from the ingestion of food that contains bacteria or toxic material. This includes poisoning from eating mushrooms, foods that contain poisonous insecticides, and foods that have been contaminated with bacteria or have partially decomposed. The disease is usually self-limiting and subsides within 48 hours of onset. Occasionally, it can be much more severe and even life threatening. The more severe cases are usually seen in young children and individuals in a weakened state of health. Food poisoning causes generalized gastroenteritis, with sudden and intense symptoms (Table 38-3).

A complete patient history is crucial in determining the diagnosis. Stool and blood cultures may be performed to verify the causative pathogen. If the patient has a remaining portion of the suspected ingested food, it should be sent to the laboratory for analysis. The physician may order an endoscopic examination of the GI system in severe cases to determine the extent of the damage or the condition of the mucosal lining of the system.

The patient is stabilized and symptoms are treated so that dehydration is minimized and electrolyte balance is maintained. Antiemetics, such as prochlorperazine (Compazine) and trimethobenzamide (Tigan) rectal suppositories, may be prescribed to control vomiting. Other medications, such as Furoxone, loperamide (Imodium), or diphenoxylate with atropine (Lomotil) may be used to control diarrhea. If vomiting and diarrhea cannot be corrected within a reasonable time (determined by age, body size, and health condition), the patient may be hospitalized so that intravenous fluid replacement can be administered.

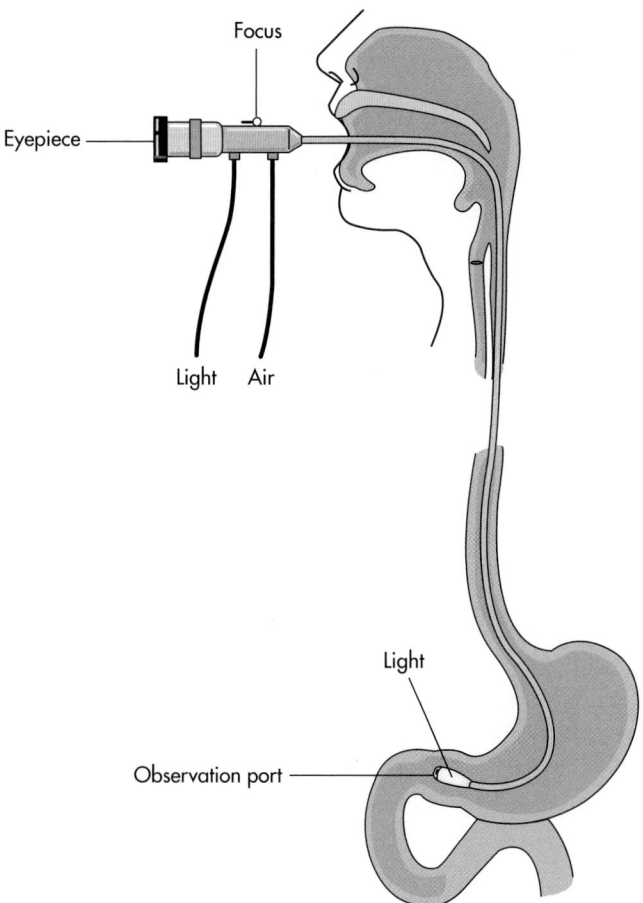

FIGURE 38-5 Fiberoptic endoscopy of the stomach. (From Phipps WJ, Sands JK, Marek JF, editors: *Medical-surgical nursing: health and illness perspectives*, ed 7, Philadelphia, 2003, Saunders.)

TABLE 38-3 Food-Related Gastrointestinal Disorders

MICROORGANISM	CAUSE	INCUBATION PERIOD	SIGNS AND SYMPTOMS
Staphylococcus aureus	Improper hand washing by food handlers; insufficient refrigeration of salads or improper cooking of meats	4-6 hr	Low body temperature; hypotension; acute severe nausea, vomiting, cramps
Escherichia coli	Fecal contamination of food or water; improper cooking of meat or washing of fruits and vegetables	24-72 hr	Vomiting; abdominal cramps; diarrhea, may contain blood or mucus
Salmonella	Fecal contamination of food; contaminated work areas; undercooked or raw poultry, eggs, or shellfish	8-48 hr	Acute diarrhea; sometimes vomiting; abdominal cramping and pain; fever
Campylobacter jejuni	Eating or drinking contaminated food or water; often raw poultry, fresh produce, or unpasteurized milk	2-4 days	Cramping abdominal pain; watery diarrhea; fever
Clostridium botulinum	Bacterial spores in improperly canned or prepared food	12-36 hr	Vomiting or diarrhea possible; neurologic complications of vision problems, paralysis, respiratory failure

Dumping Syndrome

One of the postsurgical complications of procedures for weight loss is rapid gastric emptying or dumping syndrome. This occurs when the jejunum fills too quickly with undigested food, resulting in intestinal distention and increased intestinal motility. Signs and symptoms include nausea, abdominal cramps, diarrhea, vertigo, tachycardia, and **diaphoresis.** Patients undergoing weight loss surgery should be instructed to eat frequent small meals that are high in protein and low in simple sugars as well as drink fluids between meals rather than with meals. These dietary modifications usually prevent the occurrence of dumping syndrome.

Irritable Bowel Syndrome

Irritable bowel syndrome (IBS) is described as a recurrent *functional* bowel disorder—meaning the bowel does not work as it should, but diagnostic studies fail to show an organic cause for the symptoms. The diagnosis of IBS is made if the patient complains of recurrent abdominal discomfort of at least 3 months; abdominal pain that is relieved by defecation; feeling bloated; a change in bowel habits with constipation, diarrhea, and mucous discharge; and increased flatulence. The most frequent site of abdominal pain is the left lower quadrant. Diagnostic studies, such as a complete blood count, stool for hemoccult, urinalysis, barium enema, and colonoscopy, are performed to rule out other GI diseases that have an organic base.

IBS is more common in women. Symptoms usually appear in late adolescence or early adulthood. There appears to be a familial pattern, and IBS may account for up to 50% of referrals to gastroenterologists because of concern about possible organic disease. IBS is quite common, with an estimated 9% to 20% of the adult population affected. The syndrome is associated with food intolerances, menstruation, and stress levels. Treatment is primarily pharmaceutical, with bulk-forming agents (Metamucil); loperamide (Imodium) or diphenoxylate and atropine (Lomotil) for diarrhea episodes; Lactaid if the patient is lactose intolerant; antispasmodic agents (such as dicyclomine [Bentyl]) for cramping; anticholinergic agents (hyoscyamine [Levsin]); and simethicone (Mylicon) for bloating and flatulence. The patient should be encouraged to keep a food diary in an attempt to identify foods that exacerbate the symptoms; to increase fluid and fiber intake; and to avoid spicy and fatty foods as well as caffeine. Routine exercise can also be very helpful in relieving symptoms.

Weight Loss Surgery

Bariatric or weight loss surgeries are surgical weight loss methods that create a smaller stomach pouch and bypass the duodenum, where the majority of digestion is completed. After surgery, patients can eat only small amounts of food at one time, which reduces the number of calories consumed. Because the duodenum is bypassed, fewer nutrients are absorbed. The most common gastric bypass surgery is the Roux-en-Y procedure, in which a small pouch is created at the top of the stomach using surgical staples or a plastic band. The smaller stomach is then anastomosed to the jejunum. This surgery can be done either as an open procedure or with a laparoscope, although the laparoscopic procedure is preferred because it is associated with fewer surgical risks and complications. Bariatric surgery is an option for patients who have a body mass index (BMI) of 40 or higher or those who have a BMI greater than 35 with a serious medical condition such as diabetes, hypertension, and sleep apnea. Individuals investigating the procedure must complete a battery of examinations including a psychologic evaluation and must show that they have been unable to lose weight with other methods. Patients begin to lose weight shortly after the procedure and continue to lose for approximately 12 to 24 months. Most individuals lose 60% to 80% of their excess body weight, and the majority experience resolution of weight-related health issues as the weight comes off, including relief of heartburn, decreased musculoskeletal discomforts, lower blood glucose levels in people with type 2 diabetes, improved breathing, decreased sleep apnea, and lowered blood pressure. Owing to malabsorption problems, patients are prone to develop vitamin B_{12} deficiencies that may necessitate B_{12} injections on a regular basis; iron deficiency anemia; lack of calcium absorption, which may contribute to osteoporosis; and other vitamin and mineral deficiencies. Patients should take daily vitamin and mineral supplements to decrease the effects of these malabsorption problems.

Patients with IBS can become very frustrated and need confirmation that this is a real problem, even though no organic or anatomic changes are apparent. Patients should be encouraged to follow lifestyle recommendations, including actively working to reduce stress. The medical assistant plays an important role in providing understanding and support to the IBS patient.

CRITICAL THINKING APPLICATION

Dr. Sahani frequently sees patients with IBS. He asks Joan to prepare a handout for patients describing the disorder, making sure to include possible treatments. What should Joan include?

Acute Appendicitis

The vermiform appendix is a narrow pouch approximately 3½ inches long that extends off of the cecum of the large intestine. It has no known function but can become inflamed and ultimately infected because of obstruction by a **fecalith** or by foreign material. As bacteria multiply the appendix becomes inflamed and swollen, causing *ischemia* and *necrosis* of the appendix wall. If the infectious material leaks out or bursts from the appendix, a localized infection forms that may become regional if the abdominal peritoneum becomes involved, resulting in peritonitis. Peritonitis is a serious infection that may become life-threatening.

Classic signs of appendicitis include right lower quadrant pain; nausea and vomiting; tenderness at McBurney's point, which is located between the umbilicus and the right anterior superior iliac spine; low-grade fever; and *leukocytosis* (increase in the white blood cell count). The condition is confirmed with either a computed tomography (CT) scan or ultrasound. The infected appendix is surgically removed *(appendectomy)*, and the patient is treated with broad-spectrum antibiotics.

Crohn's Disease

Crohn's disease, also called *regional ileitis* or *regional enteritis,* is an inflammation that may be located anywhere in the alimentary tract but is most commonly found in the ileum. The inflammation begins with a localized area of ulcer development that manifests as healthy tissue interspersed with areas of affected tissue. Inflammation results in the formation of ulcers that eventually invade deeper into the walls of the intestine, creating scar tissue and partial or complete obstruction at the affected site. If in the small intestine, the damaged wall decreases the ability of the intestine to digest and absorb nutrients; if in the colon, increased motility prevents reabsorption of fluids. Scar tissue from the localized ulceration can ultimately lead to a bowel obstruction, or the ulcer may completely invade the intestinal wall, resulting in perforation and leakage of intestinal contents into the abdominal cavity. Adhesions may develop from chronic inflammation, or **fistulas** may form between two loops of the intestine or between the intestine and adjacent organs.

Signs and symptoms of Crohn's disease include loose, semi-formed stool; melena if the ulcers break through blood vessels;

pain or tenderness in the right lower quadrant; anorexia; weight loss; anemia; and fatigue. Most patients cycle through periods of remission and relapse. The cause of the disease is unknown, although some theories associate the disease with either a viral or bacterial immune response or a genetic predisposition. Risk factors include age (most cases are diagnosed between ages 15 and 35), Jewish or European descent, presence of family history, and residence in a developed country or urban area. Diagnosis is made from a barium enema, small bowel series, abdominal CT scan, and colonoscopy and is confirmed with a biopsy. The goals of treatment are to decrease inflammation, manage symptoms, and provide nutritional support. Antiinflammatory drug therapy includes sulfasalazine (Azulfidine), mesalamine (Asacol), and corticosteroids (such as prednisone or Entocort), which are used during acute phases. Immune system suppressors, including Imuran and Remicade, are also recommended to control the immune system's reaction to the inflammatory process. Metronidazole (Flagyl) and Cipro are antibiotics prescribed for fistulas, and antidiarrheal agents (Imodium or Lomotil) may also be used for symptomatic relief. Surgical intervention that involves resection of the diseased bowel and **anastomosis** may be necessary if an intestinal obstruction occurs, a fistula is present, or there is abscess formation. Unfortunately, the disease usually recurs at the site of the anastomosis. The patient may require dietary supplements with a high-protein and high-calorie diet to maintain normal weight.

Ulcerative Colitis

Ulcerative colitis causes inflammation that usually starts in the rectum and moves proximally through the colon, affecting the lining of the colon in a continuous pattern. The disease causes ulcer formation that invades the mucosal and submucosal layers but does not advance through the entire wall of the colon (Figure 38-6). Ulcerative colitis can affect people of any age; although a familial tendency exists, the cause is unknown. The patient complains of abdominal pain, mucoid stools, and intermittent episodes of bloody diarrhea. As the disease progresses, the patient may experience as many as 10 to 20 stools per day, with weight loss, fever, and general malaise.

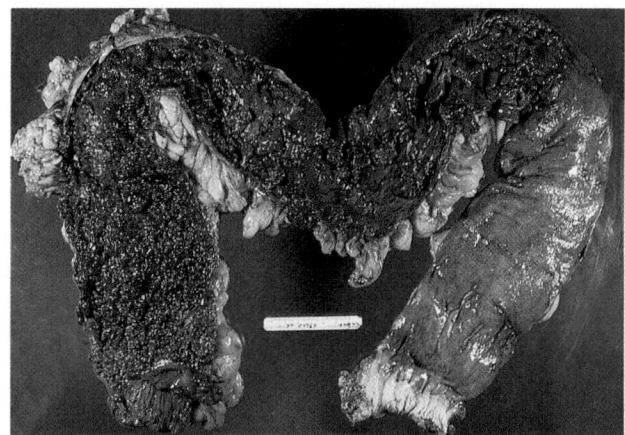

FIGURE 38-6 Ulcerative colitis. (From Damjanov I: *Pathology for the health professions,* ed 3, St Louis, 2006, Saunders.)

Drug therapy is similar to that for Crohn's disease, but surgical removal of the colon with an **ileostomy** is considered curative for ulcerative colitis. A new surgical procedure–the ileoanal anastomosis–has been developed that forms a pouch out of the ileum that is then connected directly to the anus. This results in multiple watery bowel movements a day because the colon is not there to absorb fluid, but the patient has a continuous GI tract without the need to wear a collection bag on the abdomen. Patients with ulcerative colitis must be screened annually with a colonoscopy because they have an increased risk of colon cancer.

Celiac Disease

Celiac disease, also known as *celiac sprue,* is a malabsorption syndrome that is caused by a genetic defect in the intestinal enzyme that metabolizes gluten. Gluten is found in all grains, including any products made from wheat, barley, rye, and possibly oats. If the affected individual eats a product that contains gluten, even a small amount, an antigen-antibody reaction occurs that causes destruction of the villi in the small intestine. The intestine is unable to absorb nutrients; therefore malnutrition occurs. The patient exhibits steatorrhea, abdominal pain, and weight loss. Celiac disease can be treated with strict adherence to a gluten-free diet substituting rice, soy, corn, and potato flours for gluten products. Although oats may not be harmful, oat products are frequently contaminated with wheat, so these should be avoided as well.

Diverticular Disease

Diverticula are outpouchings or herniations of the muscular lining of the colon, usually the sigmoid colon. Diverticula develop because of chronic constipation and muscular hypertrophy in the colon and become more common as people age. *Diverticulosis* is asymptomatic diverticular disease in which multiple diverticula are present in the colon but the patient has no complaints other than mild discomfort, diarrhea, constipation, or flatulence. However, if the herniations become blocked with feces and inflammation develops, *diverticulitis* occurs. Patient signs and symptoms include lower left quadrant cramping, tenderness, or pain; nausea and vomiting; low-grade fever; and leukocytosis. A barium enema or colonoscopy may be done to confirm the presence of diverticula.

Patients with diverticulosis are encouraged to eat a diet that is high in roughage, drink plenty of fluids, and avoid foods with kernels or seeds such as nuts, popcorn, and sunflower, pumpkin, and sesame seeds. Keeping a food diary may help the patient identify problem foods. The goals of dietary management are to prevent collection of waste in the herniations and encourage regular, soft bowel movements. The physician may recommend the patient take a daily fiber product such as Citrucel or Metamucil to increase the amount of fiber regularly consumed. If diverticula become inflamed, antibiotics are prescribed to treat the infection. An acute attack with severe pain and infection may require hospitalization with intravenous antibiotic therapy and pain management. Surgery may be necessary if the colon perforates.

Hernias of the Abdomen

Hernias can develop in various parts of the body but most frequently are seen in the abdomen when an organ or part of an organ protrudes through a weakened area in the abdominal muscle wall. The causes of herniation include congenital weakness of the structures, trauma, relaxation of ligaments and skeletal muscles, and increased upward pressure from the abdomen. They are most often found in middle-aged or older persons. The location of the hernia establishes the term by which the protrusion is identified. The types of hernias include umbilical; incisional at the site of a previous surgery; and inguinal, which is when a loop of the bowel protrudes into the inguinal canal (Figure 38-7).

The usual sign of an abdominal hernia is an abnormal lump or bulge that the patient finds while bathing. This bulge is tender, but the pain is mild. The patient may also discover that the bulge can be pushed back into the abdomen, and it will stay that way until some type of moving activity is performed, then it reappears. If severe pain is present, the hernia may be trapped or strangulated if blood flow has been compromised. If immediate surgical intervention is not performed, the tissue may die and **gangrene** may set in.

The physician uses palpation to assess an abdominal or inguinal hernia for size and inspects the area with the patient standing and lying down. An inguinal hernia can be detected in a male by having him perform **Valsalva's maneuver.** The most frequent treatment is surgical repair in the form of a *herniorrhaphy* or hernioplasty.

Hemorrhoids

Hemorrhoids are varicose veins of the anus and rectum and affect approximately 5% of all adults. There is a familial, hereditary predisposition to the disorder, and it is common in persons with varicose veins of the lower extremities and inguinal hernias. Hemorrhoid formation is related to increased pressure in the rectum often caused by constipation. If the swollen veins are within the rectal wall, they are considered to be internal hemorrhoids; and if they are firm and protruding, and can be felt and/or seen, they are external.

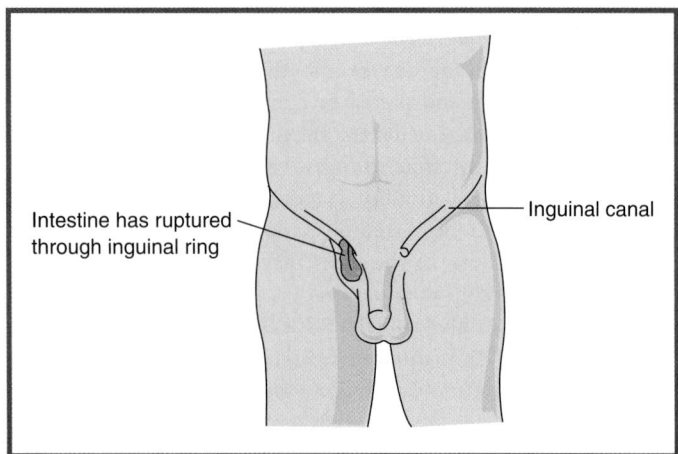

FIGURE 38-7 Herniated inguinal canal.

Some patients experience no pain, whereas other patients experience rectal irritation and discomfort. Frequently, the patient reports that anal itching and burning occur immediately after a bowel movement. If the patient must strain to defecate, bleeding and a protrusion of the swollen mass can occur. Often patients will state that it is necessary to bathe the anal area with warm water or even soak in warm water after every bowel movement to relieve the itching and pain.

A proctologic examination and inspection of the anal area will reveal external hemorrhoids. Proctoscopy is performed to see internal hemorrhoids of the rectum. A hemoglobin level and red blood cell count may be ordered to determine whether there has been any significant blood loss. Hemorrhoids are treated with stool softeners, such as docusate sodium (Colace); fiber supplements such as Metamucil or Citrucel; a high-fiber diet; increased fluid intake; and an analgesic ointment applied locally or by suppository to relieve swelling. If these measures do not correct the problem, the next step may be **sclerotherapy** with a chemical injection, **cryosurgery,** infrared coagulation to burn hemorrhoidal tissue, ligation, or hemorrhoidectomy.

DISEASES OF THE LIVER AND GALLBLADDER

Cirrhosis

The liver is located in the right upper quadrant of the abdomen, and its primary functions are to metabolize nutrients and detoxify drugs or other harmful substances. The liver also excretes proteins that aid in blood clotting and produces bile for fat metabolism. Cirrhosis is a chronic liver disease in which the lobes of the liver become fibrous and hard and liver cells degenerate, causing deterioration in liver function. Cirrhosis is the twelfth leading cause of death by disease and the fourth most common cause of death in men between the ages of 40 and 60. The primary causes of the disease in the United States are chronic alcoholism and hepatitis C. Cirrhosis is also a result of chronic hepatitis B; nonalcoholic steatohepatitis (NASH), which is characterized by a buildup of fat in the liver, eventually causing scar formation and loss of function; blocked bile ducts; and severe reactions to prescription drugs or exposure to environmental toxins.

The patient is asymptomatic in the early stages of cirrhosis, but as scar tissue replaces normal hepatocytes the liver begins to fail and the patient will exhibit fatigue, anorexia, weight loss, and abdominal pain. Complications associated with advanced cases of liver failure include dependent edema (fluid retention in the legs); **ascites** (Figure 38-8); bleeding abnormalities; **jaundice;** pruritus from deposits of bile salts on the skin; sensitivity to medication because the liver is unable to metabolize drugs; portal hypertension; **esophageal varices;** insulin resistance, with the development of type 2 diabetes mellitus; and cancer of the liver. Treatment is based on the cause of the problem, but avoiding alcohol and eating a nutritious diet are key factors. With advanced cases the only cure is a liver transplant.

Hepatitis

Inflammation of the liver, or hepatitis, may be caused by a localized infection (viral hepatitis), a systemic infection, chemical exposure, or a complication of drug metabolism. Mild inflammation temporarily impairs function, but severe inflammation may lead to necrosis and serious complications.

Viral Hepatitis

Acute viral hepatitis is an infection of the liver that causes a sudden onset of hepatocyte inflammation. There are several forms of this virus, known as hepatitis A, B, C, D, E, and G. Hepatic cells are capable of regeneration; therefore, depending on the degree of liver involvement, the patient may recover completely or could develop widespread necrosis, cirrhosis, and liver failure. Chronic inflammation, defined as the presence of the disease for more than 6 months, can occur with hepatitis B, C, and D. This usually results in permanent liver damage and an associated increased risk for liver cancer. Individuals infected with hepatitis B, C, and D may also become lifelong carriers of the disease. Hepatitis carriers are asymptomatic but can transmit the virus to others.

Table 38-4 describes the overall characteristics of the types of hepatitis. Hepatitis A virus (HAV) is transmitted through contaminated water or shellfish. Some parts of the world are **endemic** for the disease, and a vaccine is available. Hepatitis B virus (HBV) has a relatively long incubation period, which makes it more difficult to track the source of the infection. Because the virus is found in all blood and body fluids, it can be transmitted in many ways including needlesticks, human bites from individuals infected with the virus, sexual contact, and fetal transmission. Immunization of persons who are at increased risk is highly recommended. All healthcare personnel are included in this group, because they are at increased risk for infection through exposure to blood or blood products and body fluids. HBV immunizations are also included as part of pediatric immunizations, which is discussed in Chapter 41.

As a healthcare professional a medical assistant cares for sick people on a daily basis who may be carriers of the hepatitis virus. Changing dressings, collecting specimens, holding a patient's hand that was just used to cover the mouth, and discarding a wet baby diaper are all possible ways that exposure can occur. The first line of defense, whether the medical assistant is immunized or not, is employing frequent hand washing and wearing gloves when the possibility of exposure to blood or body fluids exists.

Diagnosis and Treatment

Hepatitis A, B, and C are diagnosed by identifying the virus or the antibodies to the virus in the blood. Another diagnostic test that is very useful is a liver biopsy for tissue examination. Once diagnosed, liver function tests are done periodically throughout the course of the disease to determine the degree of liver damage. Patients with hepatitis B, C, and D must be monitored for possible chronic hepatitis and the formation of a carrier state. Interferon and ribavirin (Rebetol), a broad-spectrum antiviral agent, may be prescribed to control hepatic cell destruction. Otherwise the treatment for all forms of hepatitis generally consists of bed rest and a high-protein diet.

The best form of treatment for hepatitis B is prevention by being vaccinated against the disease. The vaccine is given intramuscularly in three doses. The first two are given 30

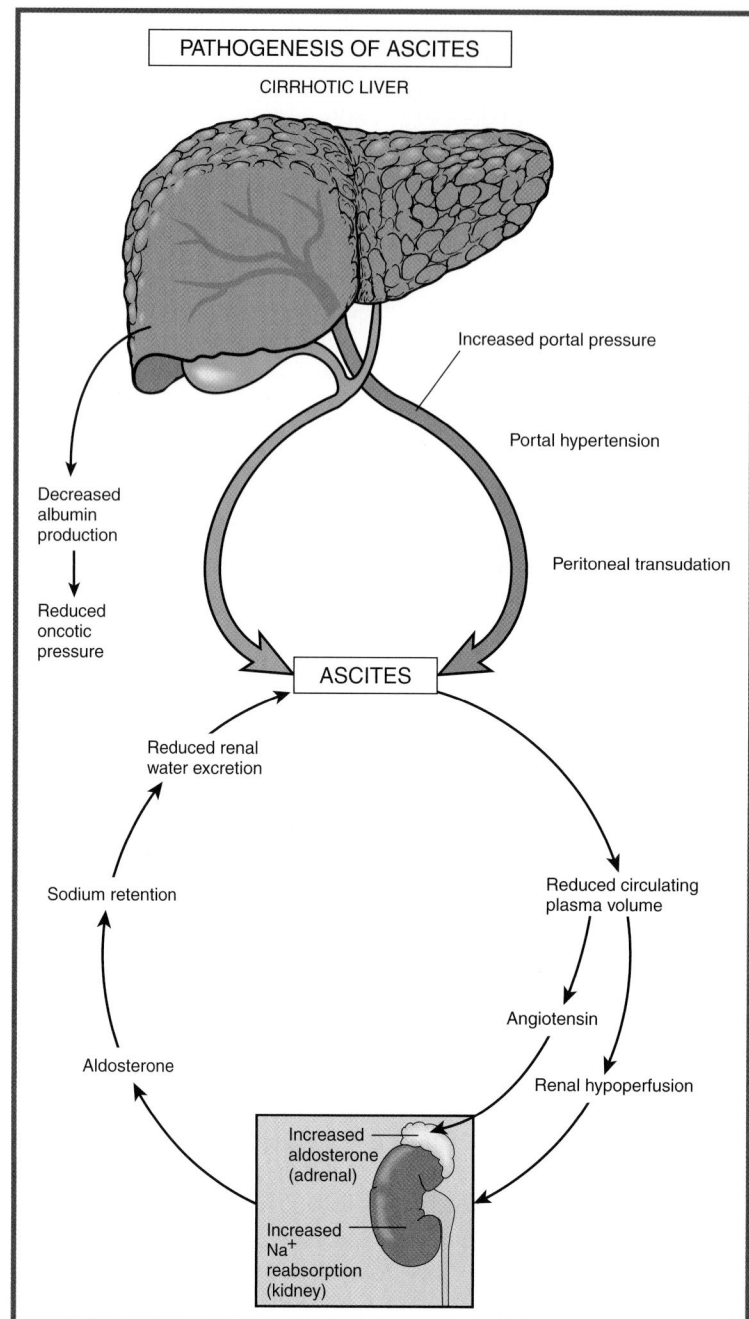

FIGURE 38-8 Pathology of ascites. (From Damjanov I: *Pathology for the health professions,* ed 3, St Louis, 2006, Saunders.)

days apart, and the third is given 6 months after the first. As discussed in Chapter 26, the Occupational Safety and Health Administration (OSHA) requires healthcare employers to make the vaccine available to employees free of charge. Medical assistant programs encourage students to become vaccinated because they are also at risk for contracting the disease.

CRITICAL THINKING APPLICATION

As a healthcare worker who has the potential for being exposed to blood and body fluids, Joan is quite concerned about contracting viral hepatitis. What types of hepatitis is she at risk for in Dr. Sahani's office? What can she do to reduce her risk and safeguard herself from contracting these diseases?

Cholelithiasis (Gallstones)

The gallbladder is an accessory organ of the GI system that stores the bile excreted by the liver. Cholelithiasis, or gallstones, form in the gallbladder from insoluble cholesterol and bile salt and vary in size and number. The reasons for formation are not always clear, although occurrence is more frequent with a high-calorie, high-cholesterol diet and is associated with obesity

TABLE 38-4 Characteristics of Viral Hepatitis Types

HEPATITIS TYPE	MODE OF TRANSMISSION	INCUBATION PERIOD	SYMPTOMS
A	Fecal-oral (food or water contaminated by feces from infected person); contaminated raw shellfish; infected household members or sexual partners	2-7 weeks	Fatigue, weakness, anorexia; some patients have joint pain, hepatomegaly, lymphadenopathy, jaundice
B (serum hepatitis)	Blood and body fluids; placental transfer	1-6 months	General malaise, joint swelling, pruritic rash, hepatomegaly, anorexia, nausea, vomiting, dark yellowish-brown urine, jaundice; may become chronic
C (non-A non-B)	Blood and body fluids; most frequent type of posttransfusion hepatitis	2 weeks-6 months	Acute onset of fever, chills malaise, nausea, vomiting; frequently becomes chronic
D (delta virus)	Blood and body fluids	Seen only in patients with hepatitis B	Similar to HBV; increases the severity of HBV disease
E	Fecal-oral	2-9 weeks	Symptoms similar to hepatitis A; seen in India, Asia, Africa, Central America; mild form but can cause death in pregnant women
G	Blood and blood products	Not known	Similar to HCV; may become chronic but does not appear to be an important cause of clinical liver disease

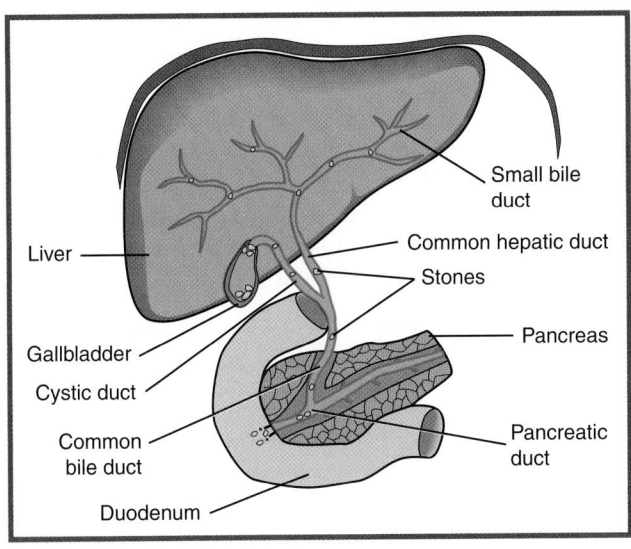

FIGURE 38-9 Gallstones.

Groups at Risk for Hepatitis A, B, and C

- Hepatitis A: Day care workers and clients, institutionalized residents, individuals traveling to infected areas
- Hepatitis B: Intravenous drug users, homosexual men, hemodialysis patients, hemophiliacs, healthcare personnel, those with a history of frequent sexual partners
- Hepatitis C: Patients receiving frequent blood transfusions, homosexual men, intravenous drug users, healthcare personnel

(Figure 38-9). It is estimated that 20% of people older than age 65 years develop cholelithiasis, with women three times more at risk than men.

Signs and Symptoms

Most gallstones are asymptomatic and are incidentally discovered during a routine radiograph. Pain usually occurs when the stones move and obstruct the cystic or common bile ducts. The pain is in the epigastric region and right upper quadrant, often radiating into the right upper back area, and gets worse after the patient eats a high-fat meal. Nausea and vomiting may accompany the pain. The pain hits in a wavelike pattern and is called *colicky pain* or *biliary colic*. If the obstruction is not corrected, jaundice may appear.

Diagnosis and Treatment

The physician will base the preliminary diagnosis on the signs and symptoms noted on palpation of the upper right quadrant. To confirm the diagnosis, blood tests may be taken to determine signs of infection, obstruction, pancreatitis, or jaundice, and an abdominal sonogram is used to visualize the stones. A CT scan may show gallstones, and magnetic resonance (MR) cholangiography may be ordered to diagnose blocked bile ducts. In addition, cholescintigraphy (a hepatobiliary iminodiacetic acid [HIDA] scan) can be ordered to diagnose biliary tract obstruction. The patient is given an intravenous injection of radioactive material (HIDA) that is taken up by the liver and excreted into the biliary tract. A nuclear scanner then takes pictures of the biliary tract over a 2-hour period.

Treatment is surgical removal of the gallbladder (cholecystectomy), which is usually done by laparoscopy. Cholelithiasis may also be fragmented by **lithotripsy** procedures.

THE MEDICAL ASSISTANT'S ROLE IN THE GASTROINTESTINAL EXAMINATION

Emotional factors play an important part in many GI problems, often making the separation of functional disorders and organic disorders difficult. Some forms of GI disease may demand immediate attention, as in acute appendicitis or acute gastritis with possible hemorrhage. Both may require surgical therapy. Careful questioning is needed to guide the patient to a more precise description of the symptoms. The medical assistant's role as the liaison between the patient and the physician can help the physician make the diagnosis and get the patient the treatment needed.

General abdominal discomfort (colic) is common because abdominal pain is frequently referred pain (Figure 38-10)—that is, pain that is felt in the abdomen but is actually being generated from an organ elsewhere. The pain's location may not be directly over the involved organ or over the point of the disorder. In this case, the patient's pain is referred to the site where the organ was located during fetal development. Even though the organ moves during fetal development, its nerves persist in referring sensations to its primitive location.

Assisting with the Examination

When a patient describes and points to the location of the pain being felt, it is important to know the underlying organs that may be involved in the problem. Record the quadrant or region in which the pain is located so the physician can immediately assess this area when the examination begins. The inspection of the abdomen begins with noting any change in skin color, such as jaundice. *Striae* (silver stretch marks), *petechiae* (small purple hemorrhagic spots), scars, and visible masses may be observed.

The contour of the abdomen may be flat, rounded, or bulging in localized areas.

The physician will use palpation and percussion to evaluate the entire abdominal area. As this is done, the medical assistant should remove the drape from the area to be examined and redrape the patient once the physician has completed this segment of the examination. In addition, the physician may want notations made of findings as the examination is being done. If the physician wants to examine the anal area, have the patient turn onto his or her left side and assist the patient into Sims' position. As this is done, be sure the patient remains draped. After the position is achieved, adjust the drape on an angle so that it can be easily lifted for the final part of the examination.

CRITICAL THINKING APPLICATION

Joan is responsible for initially questioning patients about complaints and clearly documenting this information on the patient chart. What information should Joan include that details each patient's problem and would be helpful in determining the patient's diagnosis?

Diagnostic Procedures

Typical diagnostic procedures for the GI system are summarized in Table 38-5. Although the majority of these procedures are not performed in the ambulatory care setting, the medical assistant must still understand the procedure and the recommended patient preparation so adequate patient education can be conducted. If the patient does not adequately prepare for these procedures, the results will be inconclusive and an expensive, time-consuming, uncomfortable test may have to

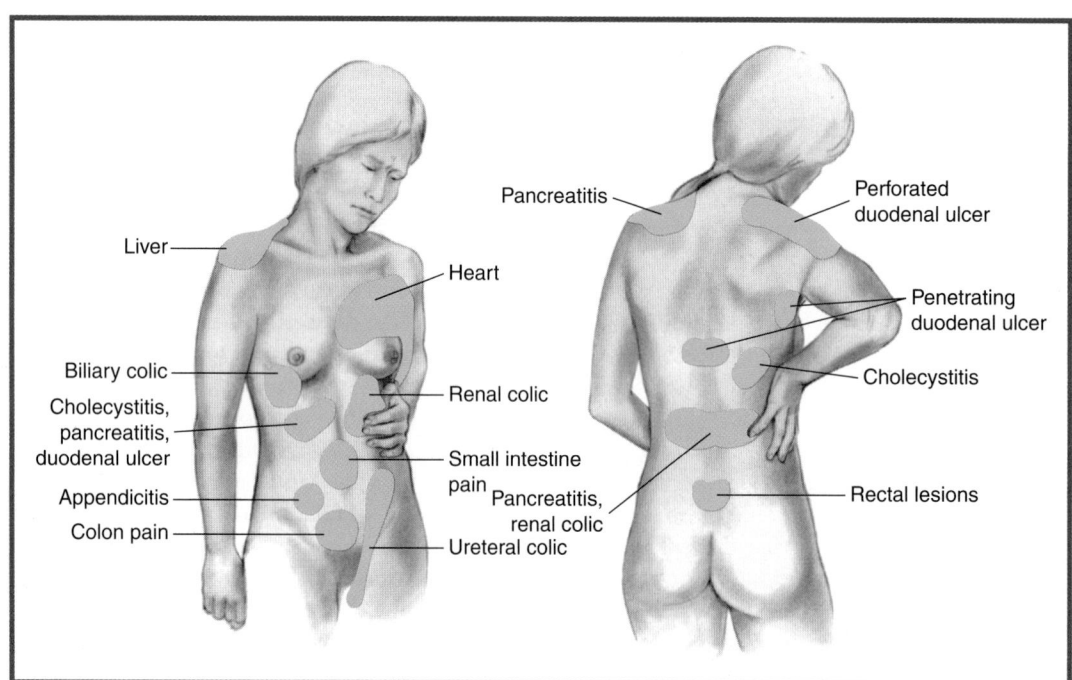

FIGURE 38-10 Common site of referred abdominal pain. (From Jarvis C: *Physical examination and health assessment*, ed 4, Philadelphia, 2004, Saunders.)

TABLE 38-5 Common Diagnostic Procedures for the Gastrointestinal System

TEST	DESCRIPTION AND PURPOSE	PATIENT PREPARATION
Barium swallow	X-ray or fluoroscopic examination of the pharynx and esophagus after patient has swallowed barium sulfate; to diagnose hiatal hernia, esophageal varices, strictures, and tumors. Takes 15-20 minutes.	NPO after midnight; remove all metal objects; do not take medication for GERD. Cathartics given after examination to help with excretion of barium.
Upper gastrointestinal and small bowel series (UGI) Air-contrast UGI	X-ray and fluoroscopic examination of esophagus, stomach, and small intestine after patient has swallowed barium sulfate; to diagnose ulcers, tumors, regional enteritis, and malabsorption syndrome. Takes approximately 30 minutes.	Low-fiber diet 2-3 days before, NPO after midnight, no smoking before test. No medications unless approved by physician after midnight. Remove all metal objects. Stool will be chalky and lightly colored 24-72 hr after the test. Cathartics given after examination to help with excretion of barium. Patient swallows a carbonated powder that creates carbon dioxide in the stomach; helps visualize stomach mucosa.
Barium enema Air contrast barium enema (ACBE)	X-ray evaluation of large intestine after rectal instillation of barium sulfate; to diagnose colorectal cancer, inflammatory disease of the colon; to detect polyps, diverticula, or obstructions. Takes approximately 45 minutes.	No dairy products and liquid diet 24 hr before the test. Take bowel preparation as supplied by radiology department; enemas until clear in the morning. No breakfast; mild laxative or enema after procedure to remove barium. Light colored stool for 24-72 hr after test. Air insufflated into colon after instillation of barium; helps visualize colonic mucosa.
Cholescintigraphy (HIDA scan)	Nuclear scan following IV injection of radioactive material. Pictures of biliary tract taken over a 2-hr period to determine presence of obstruction from cholelithiasis. Best tool to diagnose acute cholecystitis in patients with acute RUQ pain. Gallbladder visualized 60 minutes after injection of radionuclide. Takes 4 hr to get all images. IV morphine during nuclear scanning speeds up bile movement to decrease scanning time to 1 hr.	NPO 2 hr before the test; assure patient there is minute exposure to radioactivity during the procedure. Patient may be given a fatty meal during scanning to determine gallbladder ejection fraction (measures percentage of isotope ejected when gallbladder empties).
Ultrasonography of the liver, gallbladder, biliary system, pancreas	High-frequency sound waves from a transducer penetrate the organ, bounce back to the transducer, and are electronically converted into an image that is recorded on film. Used to diagnose neoplasms of the liver; cholelithiasis in the gallbladder or ducts; pancreatic tumors, abscesses, or inflammation.	Does not use contrast or radiation; useful in patients who are allergic to contrast media or who are pregnant. Must be performed before barium contrast studies because barium and gas distort sound waves and alter test results. Patient must fast before gallbladder and biliary ultrasound.
Sigmoidoscopy	Endoscopic examination of distal sigmoid colon, rectum, and anal canal. Used to diagnose inflammatory, infectious, and ulcerative bowel disease and tumors; to detect hemorrhoids, polyps, fissures, fistulas, abscesses in the rectum and anal canal. Air insufflated to distend and visualize the lower intestinal tract. Biopsy specimens may be collected and polyps removed. Takes 15-20 minutes.	Light breakfast the morning of the examination; oral cathartic and 2 Fleet enemas. Usually done without sedation in the physician's office or outpatient clinic. May experience gas pains after procedure from air instillation. May have slight rectal bleeding if specimen collected.
Colonoscopy	Endoscopic examination of the large intestine. To detect or monitor inflammatory or ulcerative diseases; to locate the site of gastrointestinal bleeding; to diagnose tumors or strictures. Air insufflated for better visualization. Biopsies collected and polyps removed. Recommended for patients with positive Hemoccult test result or at high risk for colon cancer. Takes 30-60 minutes.	Clear liquid diet for 48 hr before the test; laxatives; enemas until clear or 1 gallon of Colyte the day before. Large intestine must be completely cleansed. Monitor vital signs before and during procedure. Done with IV sedation in a hospital or outpatient clinic. May have presedation injection of Demerol and Versed. Must drink large amount of fluids to prevent dehydration from test preparation. Patients with valvular heart disease should have prophylactic antibiotics.

GERD, gastroesophageal reflux disease; *HIDA*, hepatobiliary iminodiacetic acid; *IV*, intravenous; *NPO*, nothing by mouth; *RUQ*, right upper quadrant.

be rescheduled. It is very important that patients completely understand what is required and a handout be given for review at home to confirm verbal instructions given in the office. Physicians may vary in their preferences for patient preparation for GI diagnostic tests. It is important that the medical assistant refer to the office procedure manual or ask the physician his or her preference before conducting patient education.

The most conclusive diagnostic procedure of the GI system is an endoscopic analysis. The upper GI system is examined by passing a soft, flexible tube down the esophagus into the stomach.

The colon is examined through an ascending technique, with entrance through the anus. Fiberoptic technology allows the examiner to view the tissues, take images, and collect laboratory samples, such as tissue biopsies, gastric fluid, pathogens, bile crystals, and cytology samples, during the procedure with only minor discomfort to the patient.

Endoscopic procedures can be used to observe the functioning gallbladder, biliary ducts, and pancreatic ducts by injecting a dye directly into the vessel ducts of the gallbladder and the pancreas. The examination can then render definitive results regarding patency and function of the organs.

Sigmoidoscopy and Colonoscopy Examinations

Sigmoidoscopy is used to diagnose hemorrhoids, polyps, and diverticular disorders. The sigmoidoscope is a flexible fiberoptic instrument that allows the physician to complete this examination with very little discomfort to the patient. The entire examination can be done with the patient in Sims' position, which is less traumatic for the patient to maintain than the proctologic position. This scope is very thin and bendable so that it can be maneuvered around the curves of the sigmoid colon (Figure 38-11). Because the flexible sigmoidoscope is easier to insert and move, the entire sigmoid colon can be examined (see Procedure 38-3). This procedure can be performed in an ambulatory care setting. To examine the entire length of the large intestine, the colonoscope is used. The American Cancer Society recommends that all patients over the age of 50 have a colonoscopy performed for screening of colorectal cancer. This procedure is usually performed in a hospital outpatient area because it requires the use of an IV sedative.

Laboratory Tests

Many of the diagnostic tests for GI disorders are noninvasive. The patient may be asked to have various radiographs taken of the digestive system, which are summarized in Table 38-5. The urine is tested for bilirubin and urinary amylase levels. The stool is tested for occult blood, intestinal ova and parasites, fat excretion, and color.

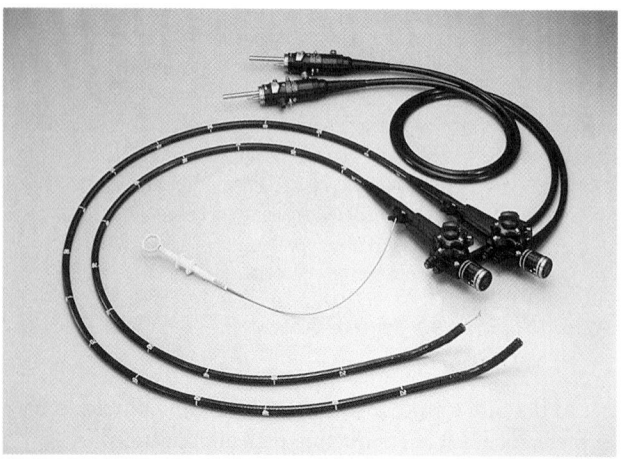

FIGURE 38-11 Flexible colon fiberscopes. (From Phipps WJ, Sands JK, Marek JF, editors: *Medical-surgical nursing: health and illness perspectives*, ed 7, Philadelphia, 2003, Saunders.)

Occult Blood Screening

Fecal examination is one means of evaluating patients with GI bleeding, obstruction, parasites, dysentery, colitis, or increased fat excretion. The test for ova and parasites is described in Chapter 54. The American Cancer Society recommends that all patients older than 50 years of age be screened for occult blood in the stool. This test may be performed on younger patients if a family history indicates a need. Blood is not found in the stool of healthy individuals. If the person is experiencing bleeding of the intestinal wall, the blood is likely to be occult or hidden, which means it cannot be seen with the naked eye. A hemoccult test is done to screen for microscopic bleeding that might occur because of precancerous or cancerous changes in the bowel.

The physician may collect a random stool sample during a routine examination (Procedure 38-2), but if it is suspected that the patient has GI bleeding, the recommendation is to test three different samples for the presence of occult blood. Seven days before the test the patient should stop taking aspirin and NSAIDs such as ibuprofen and Naprosyn. Starting 72 hours before the stool collections the patient should not take any more than 250 mg of vitamin C per day; avoid eating red meats including processed meats or cold cuts; and avoid raw fruits and vegetables, especially melons, radishes, turnips, and horseradish. These restrictions should continue throughout the time it takes the patient to collect the ordered fecal samples. Failure to adhere to dietary guidelines or the use of identified medications can cause false-positive test results.

CRITICAL THINKING APPLICATION

Dr. Sahani wants to update patient handouts on the preparations necessary for common GI tract diagnostic procedures. He asks Joan to do the initial research and gather pertinent information that should be included. What should Joan include regarding patient preparation for these examinations?

Proctologic Examination

Proctology is the branch of internal medicine concerned with the diseases and disorders of the colon, rectum, and anus. The examination of the anal area is done with a proctoscope, which permits the detection of hemorrhoids, polyps, **fissures, fistulas,** and abscesses. The rectum and the sigmoid colon are examined with a flexible sigmoidoscope, and the descending, transverse, and ascending colon sections (or the entire colon) are examined with a colonoscope.

Many persons are apprehensive about colorectal examinations. To alleviate anxiety, the patient needs to be instructed in exactly what to do before the examination, with reinforcement during the procedure. Let the patient know that some discomfort such as cramping can be experienced. Furthermore, the sensations of expelling **flatus** or of an impending bowel movement may be felt. These sensations are caused by the instrument and the procedure.

The patient must prepare the colon for any endoscopic examination. Specific patient preparations for common digestive system diagnostic tests are summarized in Table 38-5. You

PROCEDURE 38-2

Instruct Patients in the Collection of a Fecal Specimen: Assist with Hemoccult Screening

CAAHEP COMPETENCIES: 3.b.(2)(e), 3.c.(3)(c)
ABHES COMPETENCIES: 4.x, 7.c

GOAL: *To assist the physician with collection of a fecal sample and process the sample for hemoccult screening; to instruct the patient on hemoccult screening at home.*

EQUIPMENT and SUPPLIES

- Hemoccult slides
- Hemoccult developer
- Applicator sticks
- Patient record

PROCEDURAL STEPS

1. Wash your hands, and assemble all needed equipment and supplies.
   PURPOSE: Infection control.
2. Identify the patient, and explain the procedure.
3. Give the patient an examination gown, and instruct him or her to remove all clothing below the waist and put on the gown with the opening to the back. Provide a drape for additional privacy.
4. Assist the patient onto the table. When the physician is ready, place the patient in the appropriate position for the type of examination ordered.
5. Drape the patient so that only the anus is exposed. A fenestrated drape (drape with a circular opening placed over the anus) may be used in place of the rectangular drape.
6. Don gloves, and assist the physician as requested during the examination. This includes the following:
   - Handing the needed supplies to the physician
   - Collecting specimens by holding the container to accept the sample
   - Placing a thin smear of fecal material inside Box A
   - Applying a second sample from a different part of the stool inside Box B
   - Closing the cover and disposing of contaminated supplies as you are given them by the physician.
7. On completion of the examination, remove gloves, wash hands, and assist the patient into a sitting position.
8. Wait 3 to 5 minutes before developing the sample.
9. Don gloves, and open the flap in the back of the slides. Apply 2 drops of Hemoccult Developer directly over the smear.
10. Interpret the results in 60 seconds.
11. The hemoccult test is negative if there is no detectable trace of color on or at the edge of the smear, and it is positive if there is any trace of blue on or at the edge of the smear.
12. Apply gloves and clean the work area and all equipment used. Dispose of gloves in biohazard waste container, and wash your hands.
    PURPOSE: Infection control.

13. Record the procedure and any pertinent information on the patient's record.
    PURPOSE: Procedures that are not recorded are considered not done.
    Patient Instructions for Home Collection of Hemoccult Samples.
14. Give the patient a kit for collecting stool samples as ordered by the physician. Typically the physician will order a sample from three different bowel movements. The patient must follow the recommended medication restrictions and dietary guidelines throughout the testing period.
    - No aspirin or nonsteroidal antiinflammatory drugs (NSAIDs) for 7 days before the test
    - No more than 250 mg of vitamin C per day; avoid eating red meats including processed meats or cold cuts; and avoid raw fruits and vegetables, especially melons, radishes, turnips, and horseradish, for 72 hours before the stool collections.
    PURPOSE: False-positive results can occur if recommended medication and dietary restrictions are not followed.
15. Store the kit in the bathroom at home or carry it with you while you are away from home until the 3 different stool samples are collected.
16. Write your name and other required information on the front of the collection slides.
17. Flush the toilet twice before your bowel movement or cover the toilet with plastic wrap to collect the stool specimen.
18. Use one of the applicator sticks to collect a small fecal sample. Place a smear of stool on the designated area in the first slide.
19. Close the slide and store it away from heat, light, and strong chemicals such as bleach. Do not place it in a plastic bag.
    PURPOSE: Strong chemicals will affect the slide. Stool sample must air dry to be processed properly.
20. Repeat this procedure for 2 more days or two more bowel movements as ordered by the physician, using a different card for each sample.
    PURPOSE: To test multiple stool samples for detection of minute amounts of bleeding.
21. After collecting all samples as ordered, seal the test envelope and return the kit to the physician's office. Do not send stool samples in the mail unless you have a special envelope from the physician.
    PURPOSE: To avoid contamination of mail.

should refer to your employer's procedure manual to determine the preferred method of patient preparation for each test, because physician orders may vary.

The flexible sigmoidoscopy can be done in the physician's office because the patient does not receive anesthesia for the procedure. The patient is positioned in a left-lying Sims' position and draped appropriately. The physician inserts a short, flexible, lighted tube into the rectum and slowly guides it into the sigmoid colon. The scope transmits an image of the inside of the rectum and colon, so the physician can carefully examine the lining of these organs. The scope also blows air into the colon to inflate the organ and aid in visualization. The physician may remove polyps or take samples of tissue for biopsy during the procedure. The procedure takes 10 to 20 minutes, during which the patient may complain of pressure and slight cramping in the lower abdomen (Procedure 38-3).

CLOSING COMMENTS

Patient Education

The GI system is responsible for the nourishment of the entire body. When disease interferes with this process, the individual may become ill and develop serious pathologic disorders. Listen for patient concerns that may indicate a possible problem within this system and its accessory organs. Report these concerns to the physician or note them on the patient's medical record for the physician to read. If the office has information that may assist the patient in dealing with a particular problem, lay out the information for the physician to give to the patient; or with the physician's authorization, talk to the patient and offer suggestions that might help in dealing with a particular concern. Learning to perform and assist with diagnostic procedures allows the medical assistant to aid the physician in the diagnostic sequence and assist the patient in maintaining a healthy GI system.

Legal and Ethical Issues

Legally and ethically the medical assistant's responsibility is to assist the physician and act as the patient's advocate. All information that is discussed between the patient and the physician as well as all testing procedures ordered and done must remain confidential. Confidentiality and trust are very closely linked, and these two issues form the basis for a sound patient-physician relationship. The medical assistant is an important part of that relationship and can strengthen it through ethical professional conduct.

PROCEDURE 38-3

Prepare Patient for and Assist with Routine and Specialty Examinations: Assist with a Colon Endoscopic Examination

<u>CAAHEP COMPETENCIES:</u> 3.b.(4)(e)
<u>ABHES COMPETENCIES:</u> 4.b, 4.h, 4.j

GOAL: *To assist the physician with the examination, to prepare collected specimens as requested, and to promote patient comfort and safety.*

EQUIPMENT and SUPPLIES

- Nonsterile gloves (for medical assistant and physician)
- Appropriate instrument: sigmoidoscope or proctoscope
- Water-soluble lubricant
- Drape and patient gown
- Long cotton-tipped swabs
- Suction source
- Sterile biopsy forceps
- Rectal speculum
- Specimen containers with appropriate preservative added
- Laboratory requisition forms
- Tissue wipes
- Biohazard container
- Patient record

PROCEDURAL STEPS

1. Wash your hands, and assemble all needed equipment and supplies.
   <u>PURPOSE:</u> Infection control.

2. Identify the patient and explain the procedure. Be sure the patient has completed the proper preparation procedures.

3. Ask the patient to empty his or her bladder.
   <u>PURPOSE:</u> Aids in patient comfort during the examination.

4. Give the patient an examination gown, and instruct him or her to remove all clothing below the waist and put on the gown with the opening to the back. Provide a drape for additional privacy.

5. Obtain and record the patient's vital signs.
   <u>PURPOSE:</u> Baseline vital signs allow detection of variations that might occur during the examination.

6. Assist the patient onto the table. When the physician is ready, place the patient in the appropriate position for the type of examination ordered.

7. Drape the patient so that only the anus is exposed. A fenestrated drape (drape with a circular opening placed over the anus) may be used in place of the rectangular drape.

8. Don gloves, and assist the physician as requested during the examination. This includes the following:
   - Lubricating the physician's gloved index finger for the digital examination

Continued

PROCEDURE 38-3—cont'd

- Lubricating the obturator tip of the instrument before insertion
- Plugging in the scope's light source when the physician is ready
- Handing the needed supplies to the physician
- Collecting specimens by holding the container to accept the sample
- Labeling specimens immediately, because several specimens may be taken from different areas
- Disposing of contaminated supplies as you are given them by the physician

9. Throughout the examination, observe the patient for any undue reactions. Encourage the patient to breathe slowly through pursed lips to facilitate relaxation.

10. On completion of the examination, provide the patient with tissues to cleanse the anal area. Remove gloves, wash hands, and assist the patient into a resting position; allow the patient time to recover from the procedure. Monitor the patient's blood pressure if indicated.

PURPOSE: A drop in blood pressure often occurs after an invasive procedure, and this may cause fainting.

11. Once the patient's condition is stabilized, assist the patient off the table and instruct him or her to get dressed. Show the patient where the sink, towels, and tissues are, and provide assistance if needed.

12. Complete all laboratory request forms and specimen-container labels, and place specimens in the appropriate location for laboratory pickup.

13. Apply gloves, and clean the work area and all equipment used. The endoscope is first sanitized, then sterilized according to the manufacturer's recommendations. Dispose of gloves in biohazard waste container, and wash your hands.

PURPOSE: Infection control.

14. Record the procedure and any pertinent information on the patient's record.

PURPOSE: Procedures that are not recorded are considered not done.

SUMMARY OF SCENARIO

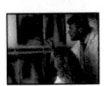

Joan enjoys working with Dr. Sahani and his GI patients but is constantly challenged to maintain and update information about diseases and disorders of the GI system as well as their diagnosis and medical management. Joan must consistently work at applying correct medical terminology when documenting patient complaints and use her knowledge of GI disorders to ask pertinent and detailed questions when gathering patient information.

Joan has also had to update her knowledge of patient preparation for diagnostic procedures so that patients are adequately educated and prepared for scheduled examinations. She participates in workshops offered by her local professional organization to stay up to date on medications and treatments for GI diseases, especially current research on infectious hepatitis. Joan is looking forward to active involvement in patient care as she continues to prepare patient education materials and to assist Dr. Sahani as needed to provide high-quality patient care.

SUMMARY of LEARNING OBJECTIVES

1. Define, spell, and pronounce the terms listed in the vocabulary.
   - Spelling and pronouncing medical terms correctly adds credibility to the medical assistant. Knowing the definition of these terms promotes confidence in communication with patients and co-workers.
2. Describe the primary functions of the gastrointestinal system.
   - The GI system is responsible for the digestion of food, the absorption of nutrients, and the excretion of waste materials.
3. Identify the anatomical structures that make up the system and describe the physiology of each.
   - The GI system begins at the mouth and ends at the anal canal. The digestive process starts in the mouth with mastication and enzyme action; the bolus of food is swallowed and passed from

the esophagus into the stomach, where digestion continues with the addition of hydrochloric acid and further enzyme action. Digestion ends in the duodenum, with pancreatic juices and emulsification of fat by bile, which is excreted by the liver and stored in the gallbladder. Absorption of nutrients takes place in the ileum and jejunum with absorption of fluids in the large intestine. Ultimately waste materials are excreted through the anus.

4. Differentiate between the abdominal quadrants and regions.
   - The abdominal cavity can be divided into four sections or quadrants: the right and left upper quadrants and right and left lower quadrants. Another, more specific method of dividing the abdominal cavity is with nine regions: the right hypochondriac,

Continued

SUMMARY of LEARNING OBJECTIVES

Continued

epigastric, and left hypochondriac; the right lumbar, umbilical, and left lumbar; and the right inguinal, hypogastric, and left inguinal. The purpose of these anatomic markers is to be able to clearly identify the location of a GI problem.

5. Summarize the typical symptoms and characteristics of gastrointestinal complaints.
   - Patients with GI disorders may complain of nausea with pallor, diaphoresis, and tachycardia; vomiting because of pain, stress, GI upset, or an inner ear or intracranial pressure disturbance; diarrhea resulting from an infection, allergy, or malabsorption problem; constipation because of a low-fiber diet or inadequate fluids, as a side effect of medication, or because of a bowel obstruction or tumor; and abdominal pain that varies in intensity and quality. It is important for the medical assistant to identify the location of the patient's discomfort using either abdominal quadrants or regions and to note the onset, duration, and frequency of all symptoms.

6. Perform telephone screening using a gastrointestinal complaint.
   - Telephone screening for GI complaints involves following the physician's policy manual for management of disorders; gathering detailed information about the onset, duration, and frequency of the problem and pertinent patient history; recording the interaction in the patient's chart, including use of medications for relief, pain scale if appropriate, and course of action based on physician recommendations.

7. Distinguish among cancers of the gastrointestinal tract.
   - Cancers of the GI tract can occur in any of the primary or accessory organs of the system. Table 38-2 summarizes the characteristics of GI tumors. These can include oral tumors, which manifest as either a white mass or an ulcer; esophageal tumors, which causes dysphagia; gastric tumors, which cause anorexia and weight loss but are difficult to diagnose in the early stages; liver tumors, which are usually secondary to metastasis from another cancerous site, with hepatomegaly and portal hypertension; pancreatic cancer, which is usually advanced when diagnosed; and colorectal cancer, with changes in bowel function and anemia.

8. Explain common esophageal and gastric disorders, their signs and symptoms, diagnostic tests, and treatments.
   - Esophageal and gastric disorders include hiatal hernias, in which part of the stomach pushes through the hiatal sphincter of the diaphragm, causing GERD; peptic ulcers, associated with *H. pylori* infections, which are treated with a combination of antibiotics and proton pump inhibitors; and pyloric stenosis, which is seen most frequently in firstborn male infants, causes projectile vomiting, and must be corrected by surgery. These disorders are usually diagnosed symptomatically and with the use of a barium swallow or upper GI series of x-ray films. Medical treatment includes the use of omeprazole (Prilosec), esomeprazole (Nexium), famotidine (Pepcid), cimetidine (Tagamet), or ranitidine (Zantac). Surgery may be indicated

for repair of a hiatal hernia or gastric ulcers if perforation occurs.

9. Define intestinal disorders, their signs and symptoms, diagnostic tests, and treatments.
   - Intestinal disorders include a diverse variety of conditions. Food poisoning causes mild to severe gastroenteritis; symptoms are controlled with antiemetics and antidiarrheal medications. Dumping syndrome, which may occur as a postsurgical complication of weight loss surgery, results in widespread GI complaints. IBS is a recurrent functional bowel disorder that causes alternating bouts of diarrhea, flatulence, and constipation; it is treated pharmaceutically with bulk-forming agents, antidiarrheals, antispasmodics, and anticholinergics. Acute appendicitis is diagnosed through a positive McBurney's sign and ultrasonography or CT scan and is treated surgically. Regional enteritis, or Crohn's disease, causes localized areas of ulceration in the intestinal tract and is treated medically to decrease inflammation, manage symptoms, and maintain nutritional status. Ulcerative colitis causes inflammatory ulcers from the anus that move proximally through the colon; it is treated as Crohn's disease is, but surgical removal of the colon is curative. Celiac disease is a malabsorption disorder caused by a genetic defect in the ability to metabolize gluten. Diverticular disease consists of small herniations of the muscular lining of the colon and is managed with dietary changes and surgery if diverticulitis is advanced. Abdominal musculature can become weakened and hernias can develop that require surgical repair. Hemorrhoids, which are varicose veins of the anus, are treated with stool softeners, high-fiber diets, or surgical repair.

10. Classify disorders of the liver and gallbladder, their signs and symptoms, diagnostic tests, and treatments.
    - Disorders of the liver include hepatitis, either from viral infection or a chemical reaction, such as alcohol abuse or a complication of drug metabolism. Mild inflammation temporarily impairs liver function, but severe inflammation may lead to necrosis and serious complications, including jaundice, cirrhosis, and portal hypertension. The gallbladder stores bile that is excreted by the liver to aid in fat metabolism. If cholelithiasis or cholecystitis develops, the gallbladder may have to be surgically removed to relieve symptoms.

11. Describe the similarities and differences among the various forms of infectious viral hepatitis.
    - Viral hepatitis is an infection of the liver that causes acute inflammation of hepatocytes. Several forms of this virus occur: A, B, C, D, E, and G. Hepatic cells are capable of regeneration, so, depending on the degree of liver involvement, the patient may recover or develop widespread necrosis, cirrhosis, and liver failure. Chronic inflammation can occur with hepatitis B, C, and D. This usually results in permanent liver damage and an associated increased risk of liver cancer. Table 38-4 describes

Continued

SUMMARY of LEARNING OBJECTIVES

Continued

the overall characteristics of the types of hepatitis. Vaccinations are available for hepatitis A and B.

12. Summarize the medical assistant's role in the gastrointestinal examination.

- The medical assistant's role in the GI examination includes providing patient support and education, gathering and recording specific details about the patient's complaints, and assisting the physician with the examination and diagnostic procedures performed in the ambulatory care setting.

13. Explain the common diagnostic procedures for the gastrointestinal system.

- Diagnostic procedures for the GI system include laboratory studies, such as liver panels and urinary tests for bilirubin and amylase; and stool tests for occult blood, intestinal parasites, and fat excretion. Radiologic and endoscopic tests, detailed in Table 38-5, include barium swallow, upper GI series, barium enema, cholescintigraphy, sigmoidoscopy, and colonoscopy.

14. Perform the procedural steps for assisting with the collection of a fecal specimen including the necessary patient education for preparation for the examination and collection of stool samples at home.

- The procedural steps for assisting with the collection of a fecal specimen are listed in Procedure 38-2. Patient education includes proper dietary and drug restrictions and collecting three different stool specimens for analysis of hidden blood in the stool.

15. Describe the medical assistant's role in the proctologic examination.

- The role of the medical assistant in the proctologic examination includes supporting and preparing the patient; positioning and draping the patient for the procedure; monitoring vital signs before and during the procedure; and assisting the physician with the procedure.

16. Demonstrate assisting with an endoscopic colon examination.

- The endoscopic colon examination is described in Procedure 38-3. The medical assistant is responsible for preparing the room, equipment, and patient for the procedure; assisting the physician throughout the procedure by positioning the patient, monitoring vital signs as indicated, helping with equipment, and labeling specimens for transport to the lab; assisting the patient after the examination; cleaning the equipment and room; and documenting the procedure on the patient's chart.

CONNECTIONS

Study Guide Connection: Go to Chapter 38 Study Guide. Read the Case Study and Workplace Applications and complete the assignments. Do online research for answers to the questions in the Internet Activities associated with assisting in gastroenterology.

CD Connection: Go to the Medical Assisting Competency Challenge CD and do the training activities under Diagnostic Testing. For a better understanding of the digestive system, view the animation for digestive tract.

Evolve Connection: For more information related to assisting in gastroenterology, go to evolve.elsevier.com/kinn and visit related weblinks for Chapter 38. Click on the Medical Assisting Exam Review and do the practice questions to sharpen your test-taking skills.

Assisting in Urology and Male Reproduction

39

SCENARIO

Sara Ricci, a CMA with 10 years' experience, works for Dr. Samuel Fineman, a urologist who also manages male reproductive disorders. Dr. Fineman relies on Sara to handle telephone calls from patients, have a clear understanding of the anatomy and physiology of the renal system, and assist him in the clinical area of the practice. Although Sara has worked for Dr. Fineman for almost 2 years, occasionally problems still arise that she is not sure how to manage. Sara attends workshops and conferences to earn continuing education units to maintain her CMA credential and tries to choose topics that focus on urologic issues. In addition, she keeps up to date on new diagnostic procedures and treatments for STDs including HIV and AIDS. Sara helps train other medical assistants in the practice and makes sure there are adequate patient education supplies for self-testicular examination.

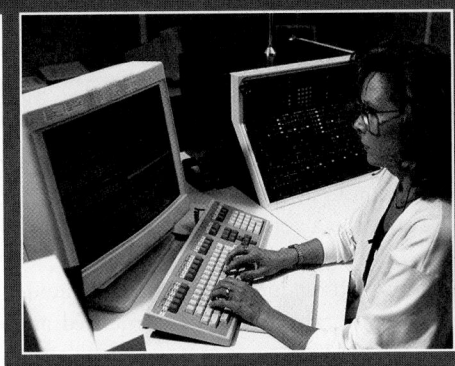

While studying this chapter, think about the following questions:

- What is the basic anatomy and physiology of the renal and male reproductive systems?
- What should Sara know about typical adult and pediatric urologic disorders so that she is able to both assist the physicians in the practice and answer patient questions?
- What are some of the typical genital pathologic conditions seen in men?
- What are the typical signs, symptoms, and treatments for sexually transmitted diseases in men?
- How can Sara provide patient education and support for individuals with renal and male system disorders?

LEARNING OBJECTIVES

1. Define, spell, and pronounce the terms listed in the vocabulary.
2. Describe the organs of the urinary system and their functions.
3. Explain the susceptibility of the urinary system to diseases and disorders.
4. Identify the primary signs and symptoms of urinary problems.
5. Detail common urinary system diagnostic procedures.
6. Compare and contrast infections and inflammations of the urinary system.
7. Describe urinary tract disorders and cancers.
8. Distinguish between the two methods of treating renal failure.
9. Summarize typical pediatric urologic disorders.
10. Illustrate the organs of male reproduction.
11. Determine the causes and effects of prostate disorders.
12. Outline common types of genital pathologic conditions in men.
13. Perform patient education for the testicular self-examination.
14. Analyze the effects of sexually transmitted diseases in the male patient.
15. Summarize the characteristics of HIV infection, diagnostic criteria, and treatment protocols.
16. Describe the medical assistant's role in urologic and male reproductive examinations.

National Accreditation Competencies and Content

CAAHEP COMPETENCIES

Clinical

3.b.(4)(e) Prepare patient for and assist with routine and specialty examinations

3.b.(4)(f) Prepare patient for and assist with procedures, treatments, and minor office surgeries

General

3.c.(3)(c) Provide instruction for health maintenance and disease prevention

ABHES COMPETENCIES

Clinical

4.b. Prepare patients for procedures

4.h. Prepare patient for and assist physician with routine and specialty examinations

Instruction

7.c. Teach patients methods of health promotion and disease prevention

VOCABULARY

albuminuria (al-byu-muh-nur-e′-uh) Abnormal presence of albumin in the urine.

azotemia (a-zo-te′-me-uh) Retention in the blood of excessive amounts of nitrogenous wastes.

casts Fibrous or protein material molded to the shape of the part in which it has accumulated and thrown off into the urine in kidney disease.

copulation Sexual intercourse.

creatinine (kre′-a-tuhn-en) Nitrogenous waste from muscle metabolism excreted in urine.

erythropoietin (i-rith-ruh-poi-e′-tuhn) Substance released from the kidney and liver that promotes red blood cell formation.

Kaposi's sarcoma A malignant tumor that begins as brown or purple papules on the feet and slowly spreads in the skin.

opportunistic infections Infections caused by a normally non-pathogenic organism in a host whose resistance has been decreased.

urgency Sudden, compelling desire to urinate and the inability to control the release of urine.

wasting syndrome Physical deterioration resulting in profound weight loss, fatigue, anorexia, and mental confusion.

Urology is the study of the urinary tract in both male and female patients. The physician who specializes in the diseases and disorders of the urinary system is a urologist. Urologists also specialize in conditions associated with the male reproductive system. A wide variety of medical treatments from radiologic to surgical is available to urologists to treat the diseases and disorders of the urinary system.

ANATOMY AND PHYSIOLOGY OF THE URINARY SYSTEM

The urinary tract consists of bilateral kidneys and ureters, the urinary bladder, and the urethra (Figure 39-1). The main function of the urinary system is to remove waste products from the body. Various wastes are produced as byproducts of the body's metabolic processes and if left to accumulate can become toxic. The urinary system removes salts and nitrogenous wastes (nitrogen is the product of protein metabolism), in the form of soluble urea, from the blood and excretes it through the renal organs. The urinary system also helps to maintain homeostasis by regulating water, electrolytes, and acid-base levels; activates vitamin D, which is needed for calcium ion absorption; secretes the hormone **erythropoietin,** which helps control the rate of red blood cell formation; and helps maintain blood pressure by the secretion of the enzyme renin.

The kidneys are red-brown, bean-shaped glandular organs. They are located posterior to the peritoneum (retroperitoneal) and against the muscles of the back, roughly between the T12 and L3 vertebrae. The left kidney is located approximately 2 cm higher than the right because of the location of the liver.

The kidneys remove unwanted substances from the blood and form urine for excretion. To perform this crucial function a great deal of blood circulates through the kidneys—approximately 15% to 30% of the total cardiac output. The blood is delivered to the two kidneys by the renal artery and is distributed through the kidneys by a highway of smaller arteries. The blood is then returned through a pathway of veins, including the renal vein, which flows into the inferior vena cava in the abdominal cavity.

The outer layer of the kidney, the *cortex,* contains the functional unit of the kidney, the *nephron,* where urine is formed as fluid and dissolved substances move between its vascular and tubular structures. There are three processes involved in urine formation: filtration, reabsorption, and excretion. The nephron consists of the *glomerulus,* which is a cluster of capillaries extending from the distal renal artery that are partially surrounded by the *Bowman's capsule.* Fluid and dissolved substances move from the glomerulus to the Bowman's capsule and then into the proximal convoluted tubules, where most of the fluid is reabsorbed by venules and arterioles surrounding the tubules and sent back into the general circulation. Based on the homeostatic needs of the body, the kidneys determine the type and quantity of substances that are reabsorbed. Finally, the remaining substances are passed through the distal convoluted

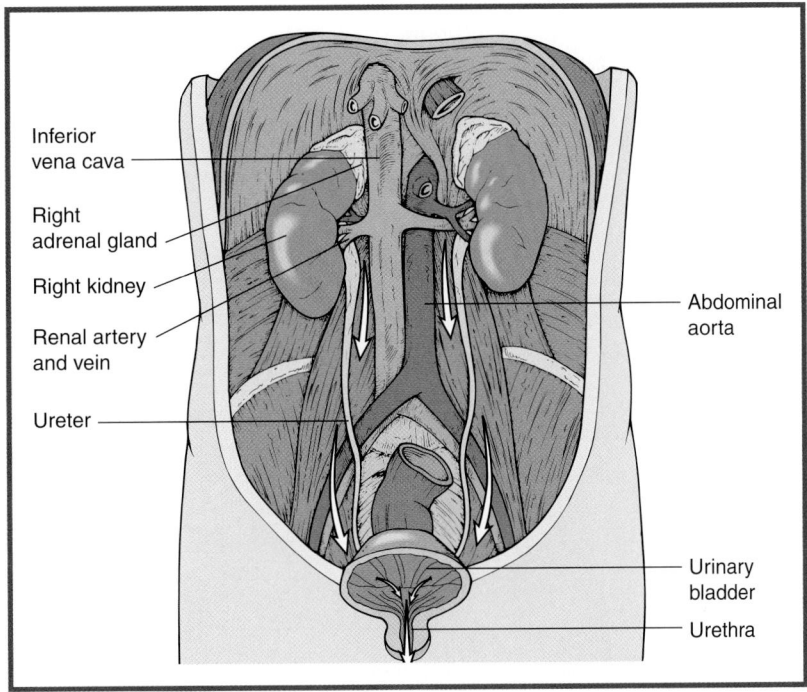

FIGURE 39-1 The urinary system. (From Frazier MS, Drzymkowski JA, Doty SJ: *Essentials of human diseases and conditions*, ed 3, Philadelphia, 2004, Saunders.)

tubules to the collecting tubules, then on to the *medulla* of the kidney, which contains the distal collection area of the *renal pelvis* called the *calyx* (Figure 39-2).

By the time the waste material reaches the calyx it is in the form of urine, which is emptied out of the kidneys through bilateral *ureters*. The ureters are tubular organs approximately 25 cm long; and with the aid of peristaltic waves generated by the ureters' muscle layer, they move the urine from the kidneys to the urinary bladder. The urinary *bladder* is a hollow organ that is lined with smooth muscle that overlaps in rugae formation, which enables the bladder to expand as it fills. When the bladder is full, sphincters open and urine flows into the *urethra*. The urethra is lined with a mucous membrane and in the male functions both as the urinary canal and as a passageway for cells and secretions from various reproductive organs. The male urethra is about 20 cm long and is divided into three sections: the prostatic urethra (passing through the prostate gland at the base of the bladder), the membranous urethra, and the penile urethra. In a female the urethra is 3 to 4 cm long. Its proximity to the vagina and anus exposes the renal system to microorganisms that can cause infection. The urethra conveys the urine from the bladder to the *urinary meatus* and outside the body. The process of urination is known as *voiding* or *micturition*.

CRITICAL THINKING APPLICATION

Dr. Fineman wants Sara to review a number of pamphlets on the anatomy and physiology of the urinary system for patient education purposes. Sara has researched those available and needs to make a decision about which one is best suited for the practice. What material should be included for the pamphlet to be comprehensive? Are diagrams important for patient understanding?

DISORDERS OF THE URINARY SYSTEM

The urinary tract is made up of a continuous mucosal lining that gives organisms entering the urethra a direct pathway through the system. Of the wide range of symptoms that occur in patients with disorders of the renal system, the most common symptoms involve changes in the frequency of urination. Dysuria (difficult or painful urination), **urgency,** retention, and incontinence are all common symptoms. Abnormal functions of any part of the urinary tract can often be determined with urinalysis, blood urea nitrogen (BUN) levels, and analysis of **creatinine** clearance. Urinalysis is discussed in Chapter 51. Radiologic and endoscopic studies are also important in detecting urinary tract diseases. Table 39-1 summarizes common urinary system diagnostic tests.

Urinary Incontinence

Urinary incontinence, which is a temporary or chronic loss of urinary control, can be the result of many conditions. Infections of the urinary tract, brain disorders, and tissue damage can all lead to urinary incontinence. This disorder can also be caused by straining or coughing in postsurgical patients and in patients with weak pelvic musculature; in such situations the condition is called *stress incontinence.*

Treatment methods for incontinence depend on the causative factor. Behavioral approaches include bladder or habit training

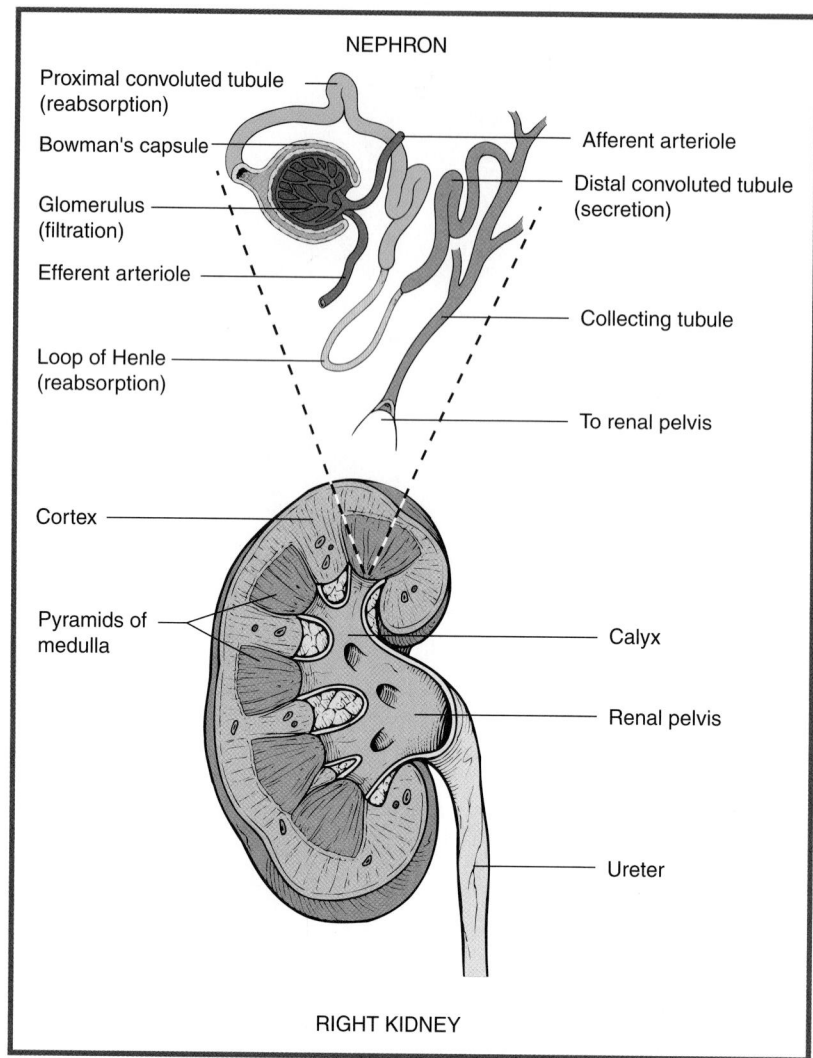

NEPHRON

Proximal convoluted tubule (reabsorption)

Bowman's capsule

Glomerulus (filtration)

Efferent arteriole

Loop of Henle (reabsorption)

Afferent arteriole

Distal convoluted tubule (secretion)

Collecting tubule

To renal pelvis

Cortex

Pyramids of medulla

Calyx

Renal pelvis

Ureter

RIGHT KIDNEY

FIGURE 39-2 The kidney. (From Frazier MS, Drzymkowski JA, Doty SJ: *Essentials of human diseases and conditions*, ed 3, Philadelphia, 2004, Saunders.)

that teaches the patient to urinate according to an established schedule rather than when he or she has the urge to void. This is helpful for patients who are incontinent as a result of strokes, Parkinson's disease, Alzheimer's disease, central nervous system lesions, or cystitis. Pelvic muscle exercises (Kegel exercises), in which the patient simulates stopping the flow of urine and holding that contraction for 10 seconds in sets of 20 three times a day, are helpful for patients with stress incontinence because of weak musculature in the pelvic floor.

Patients with neurologic bladders who have lost control of urination because of central nervous system trauma or disease may have to be catheterized to artificially remove urine from the bladder. Intermittent catheterization to empty the bladder is preferable to indwelling catheters because the use of indwelling catheters often leads to infection. External (condom) catheters can be used for male patients, but they also are associated with an increased incidence of urinary tract infections (UTIs).

Chronic incontinence can be treated pharmacologically with antispasmodic preparations including tolterodine (Detrol) or oxybutynin chloride (Ditropan). When all other treatments have failed, surgical intervention may be the answer. Several

different suburethral sling procedures are successful in treating female incontinence. The surgeon uses either a piece of abdominal tissue or a strip of synthetic material to compress the urethra so urine does not leak during a stressful event such as jumping or coughing. An artificial urinary sphincter is helpful for men with incontinence. A device shaped like a doughnut is implanted around the neck of the bladder, which keeps the urinary sphincter closed until the patient presses a valve implanted under the skin. This deflates the ring and releases urine from the bladder.

CRITICAL THINKING APPLICATION

Sara is responsible for scheduling and providing patient preparation instructions for diagnostic radiologic and endoscopic procedures. With Dr. Fineman's approval, she has prepared patient handouts that summarize the correct procedures to follow when scheduled for specific urologic tests. Today she has a patient who needs to be scheduled for both a cystogram and an intravenous pyelogram (IVP). How should the patient prepare for both of these examinations?

TABLE 39-1 Common Urinary System Diagnostic Tests

TEST	DESCRIPTION	PATIENT PREPARATION
Kidney-ureter-bladder (KUB) x-ray	Flat plate films of the abdomen; shows the size, shape, location, malformations of kidneys and bladder; used to visualize calculi.	No specific patient preparation; contraindicated in pregnancy.
Renal scanning	Nuclear scans to determine size, shape, and function of the kidney or to diagnose obstruction or hypertension. Intravenous administration of a radioisotope, with images taken to see how the isotope is distributed.	Patient should void before the procedure; no sedation or fasting required; drink two to three glasses of water before scanning; contraindicated in pregnancy.
Cystography and voiding	X-ray evaluation with contrast dye to study bladder structure or function.	Clear liquids for breakfast; Foley catheter cystourethrogram inserted; may take x-ray films while patient is voiding (voiding cystourethrogram); after procedure force fluids to eliminate dye and prevent infection.
Intravenous pyelography (IVP); may be called intravenous urography (IUG)	Dye injected intravenously, with x-ray films taken at intervals to show passage through kidneys, ureters, and into bladder. Used to diagnose tumors, calculi, obstructions, and congenital renal problems.	Contraindicated in pregnancy and iodine allergies; laxative evening before; liquid diet 8 hours before; adequate fluids after; may have enema morning of the study.
Arteriography (angiography)	Injection of dye into the renal artery; computerized fluoroscopy permits visualization of the blood flow dynamics of the kidneys, and serial x-ray films are taken. Used to diagnose stenosis of the renal artery and highly vascular renal cancers.	Nothing by mouth (NPO) 2 to 8 hours before procedure; administer preprocedure medications as ordered; void before the study; warm flush may occur when dye is injected; check for allergies to iodine and shellfish.
Renal computed tomography (CT)	Can be done with or without contrast dye. Transverse views of the kidney are taken by CT to detect tumors, abscesses, cysts, and hydronephrosis.	If contrast medium is used, fast 4 hours before procedure; scanner may make loud clicking sounds as it rotates; dye may cause flushing, metallic taste, and headache; check for allergies to iodine and shellfish; remove all metal objects.
Renal ultrasonography	High-frequency sound waves are transmitted through the kidneys to allow detection of abnormalities; used to determine kidney size and diagnose hydronephrosis, polycystic kidneys, and obstructions of ureters and bladder.	No food or fluid restrictions; noninvasive and painless.
Cystoscopy	Endoscopic view of urethra and bladder for biopsy; used to measure bladder capacity; to find or remove calculi; for dilation of urethra and ureters; for placement of ureteral stents.	Enemas to clear bowel; force fluids before procedure if local anesthesia is to be used; for general anesthesia, NPO after midnight; preprocedure sedative to reduce bladder spasms; aftercare: monitor urinary output for 24 hours
Retrograde pyelography	Dye can be injected into the bladder, ureters, and kidneys through a cystoscope to detect stones and other obstructions; also can replace an IVP for patients with renal failure, obstructions, or allergies to IV dye.	Same as cystoscopy; check for iodine and shellfish allergies.

Urinary Tract Infections and Inflammations

UTIs occur frequently because the urinary system has a direct opening to the outside and urine is an excellent medium for bacterial growth. Most UTIs are ascending, starting with pathogen exposure in the perineal area that infects the continuous mucosa of the urinary system, allowing the pathogen to travel up through the urethra, bladder, and ureters to the kidneys. Infection and inflammation of the urethra is called *urethritis* and that of the bladder is *cystitis*. The resident flora of the colon, *Escherichia coli*, is the usual causative agent.

Because of the anatomic structure of women—a short urethra and the close relation of the anus—and irritation from the use of tampons, taking bubble baths, and sexual activity, they are more susceptible to UTIs than men are. Older men with prostatic hypertrophy and resultant urinary retention are also at risk for frequent urinary infections.

CRITICAL THINKING APPLICATION

Tabitha Allison, a 22-year-old patient of Dr. Fineman's, was diagnosed today with her third UTI in as many months. Patient education on the prevention and treatment of UTIs is needed. What should Sara tell her?

General Signs and Symptoms of Urinary Tract Infection

- Overwhelming urge to urinate (urgency)
- Burning on urination (dysuria)
- Urgency with frequent, small amounts of urine
- Blood in the urine (hematuria) or cloudy, dark, foul-smelling urine

Urethritis

Urethritis is an inflammation of the urethra and is more common in men. It typically is caused by chlamydia or gonorrhea bacteria. The symptoms include discharge of pus, an itching sensation at the opening of the urethra, and burning on urination. Infectious urethritis can cause cystitis in women, so sexual partners should be treated, as well. Urinalysis may show hematuria as well as *pyuria* (pus in the urine).

Cystitis

Cystitis, an infection of the urinary bladder, causes inflammation of the bladder wall and urinary urgency. Symptoms vary from very mild to acute discomfort in the lower abdomen, urinary frequency, and painful urination (dysuria). The patient may have systemic infection signs, including fever, general malaise, and leukocytosis. A diagnostic urinalysis shows more than 100,000 bacteria per milliliter of urine, pyuria, and hematuria. An infection of the urinary bladder is especially hard to eliminate because of the overlapping rugae walls. To prevent a recurrence of the infection, it is very important that patients know they must complete the entire antibiotic prescription to destroy all of the bacteria in the folds of tissue.

Pyelonephritis

Pyelonephritis, an inflammation of the renal pelvis and kidney, is the most common type of renal disease. It is caused by bacteria that ascend from the lower urinary tract and is associated with conditions such as urinary retention or obstruction that promote urinary stasis and the growth of bacteria. It frequently is preceded by urethritis and cystitis. With pyelonephritis, pus collects in the renal pelvis, and abscesses form. Symptoms include fever, chills, nausea, vomiting, and flank (lateral lumbar) pain. The patient reports foul-smelling, dark urine with frequency and urgency.

Diagnostic studies include urinalysis of a clean catch urine sample. It reveals hematuria, pyuria, increased white and red blood cells, **albuminuria, casts,** and the presence of bacteria. Urine cultures are usually done to determine the causative agent.

Treatment of Urinary Tract Infections

UTIs are treated with antibiotics, such as amoxicillin (Amoxil, Trimox), ciprofloxacin (Cipro), nitrofurantoin (Macrodantin, Furadantin), and sulfamethoxazole (Bactrim, Septra). Patients are encouraged to force fluids to dilute the urine and flush the urinary tract. A follow-up urinalysis should be run to confirm the effectiveness of antibiotic therapy in curing the infection. UTIs tend to recur unless the cause of the infection is removed.

The medical assistant should instruct the patient to finish the entire antibiotic prescription as ordered, to maintain proper hygiene, to completely empty the bladder when the urge to void arises, and for female patients to wipe the bottom from front to back to discourage the spread of *E. coli* in the urethral region. Cranberry juice may be recommended as a prophylactic measure because it contains substances that discourage *E. coli* growth and helps maintain the acidity of urine.

Glomerulonephritis

Acute glomerulonephritis, the degenerative inflammation of the glomeruli, usually develops in children and adolescents about 2 weeks after a streptococcal infection, such as strep throat or scarlet fever. Its symptoms include low-grade fever, anorexia, general malaise, and flank pain. Hypertension and edema may occur because of reduced renal function. Urinalysis shows hematuria and proteinuria. Diuretics such as triamterene and hydrochlorothiazide (Dyazide) or furosemide (Lasix) may be given to control hypertension and reduce edema. The prognosis is usually good; most patients recover spontaneously, but in some patients the condition progresses to renal failure.

Chronic glomerulonephritis may also be called *nephritis* or *nephrotic syndrome.* It typically develops over many years and may be associated with chronic diseases that affect the blood vessels such as systemic lupus erythematosus and diabetes mellitus. Chronic glomerulonephritis causes progressive, irreversible nephron damage that frequently results in renal failure. At first the patient is asymptomatic, but as the disease progresses and more glomerular damage occurs, the patient will develop anorexia, fatigue, hypertension, hematuria, proteinuria, *oliguria* (scanty urination), and edema. The cause of chronic glomerulonephritis is unknown but it may be associated with an antigen-antibody reaction within the glomerular capsule that ultimately destroys the nephron unit. Treatment is supportive, with an attempt to control symptoms by administering antihypertensives and diuretics as well as prescribing a diet that is low in protein with limited sodium and potassium to slow the progression of the disease. Glomerulonephritis is one of the leading causes of kidney failure; ultimately many patients require kidney dialysis. The only cure for the disease is a kidney transplant.

Urinary Tract Disorders and Cancers

Renal Calculi

Renal calculi, or kidney stones, are created when crystals in the urine—such as calcium, oxalate, and uric acid—collect in the kidney, or when fluid intake is low, creating a highly concentrated filtrate. The tendency to develop kidney stones runs in families, and patients with a history of renal calculi are at increased risk for developing more in the future. Small stones usually do not cause any difficulty until they grow large enough to lodge in the ureters or renal pelvis. If a stone blocks the flow of urine, then infection can develop from the resultant stasis. This blockage can also result in *hydronephrosis,* a backup of urine that causes dilation of the ureters and calyces and increased pressure on the nephron units. Other signs and symptoms include hematuria; cloudy, foul-smelling urine; nausea and vomiting; persistent urge to urinate; and fever and chills if an infection is present.

If stones are located in the kidney or bladder, the patient is often asymptomatic, with frequent infections being the only presenting problem. If the calculi begin to move or are lodged in the ureters, the patient experiences *renal colic,* which is severe pain in the flank region that fluctuates in intensity over periods of 5 to 15 minutes. As the calculi progress down the ureter, the pain radiates to the lower abdomen, groin, and genital areas on the affected side. If the stone stops moving, the pain stops until it starts to move again. This pattern continues until either the stone is passed or it is medically treated. The patient may be able to pass small stones by drinking large amounts of fluid—2 to 3 quarts of water a day—but larger stones or calculi that are causing bleeding, kidney damage, or persistent infection require medical intervention.

The physician may perform a cystoscopy to visualize the urethra and bladder and to remove any stones found (Figure 39-3). The most common procedure for treating calculi is extracorporeal shockwave lithotripsy (ESWL), which uses vibrations of powerful sound waves to break the stones into fragmented pieces that can be easily passed through the urine. Diagnostic studies are performed to identify the exact location of the calculi, and either x-rays or ultrasound is used during the procedure to keep track of the calculi and treatment progress. The patient may be immersed in water during the procedure or may lie on a soft cushion as the shock waves are passed through the body toward the exact location of the calculi (Figure 39-4).

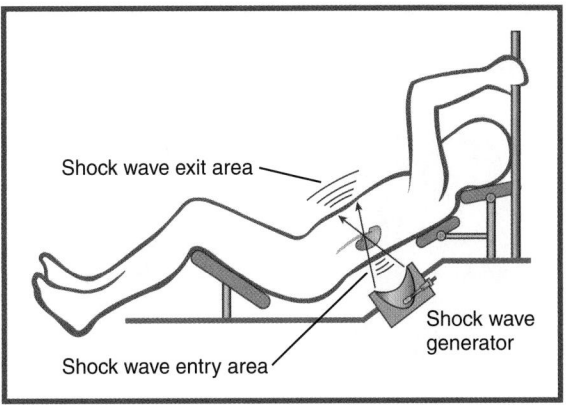

FIGURE 39-4 Extracorporeal shock-wave lithotripsy.

The procedure causes moderate pain, so the patient is usually given either presedation or a light anesthetic and wears earphones during the treatment because of the loud noise created each time a shock wave is generated. Posttreatment side effects include flank tenderness, hematoma formation across the treatment site, and hematuria. Measures for prevention of recurrence include drinking 3 to 4 quarts of fluid daily, preferably water, and following a low-sodium, low–animal protein diet.

Hydronephrosis

Hydronephrosis, the swelling of the kidney caused by the inability of urine to drain out of the renal pelvis, is usually caused by blockage from renal calculi but may also result from an enlarged prostate or a tumor. Hydronephrosis can occur bilaterally or unilaterally. The condition is frequently asymptomatic, or patients may complain of mild flank pain as the renal capsule is distended. Urine testing detects hematuria and, if infection develops from stagnant urine, pyuria. It is important to treat hydronephrosis aggressively, because continued pressure from blocked urine flow can cause tissue necrosis and ultimately lead to irreversible kidney damage. Removing the blockage will correct the condition (Figure 39-5).

Polycystic Kidneys

Polycystic kidney is typically an autosomal dominant genetic disorder, meaning one parent has the disease and each child has a 50% chance of inheriting it. No indications of the disease occur in children, but as time goes on normal renal tissue in both kidneys is replaced with multiple benign cysts filled with fluid (Figure 39-6). The nephrons and collecting tubules become dilated, fused, and infected. As the cysts enlarge they compress the surrounding tissue, causing necrosis, uremia, and renal failure. Symptoms do not usually become apparent until the individual reaches adolescence or adulthood. Patients with polycystic disease have a family history of kidney disease or renal failure, flank pain, hematuria, and hypertension. They are also more likely to develop UTIs and renal calculi. Because cyst formation is progressive, these patients will eventually require either renal dialysis or a kidney transplant.

Bladder Cancer. The most common cancer of the urinary tract affects the bladder (Figure 39-7) and is two to three times more

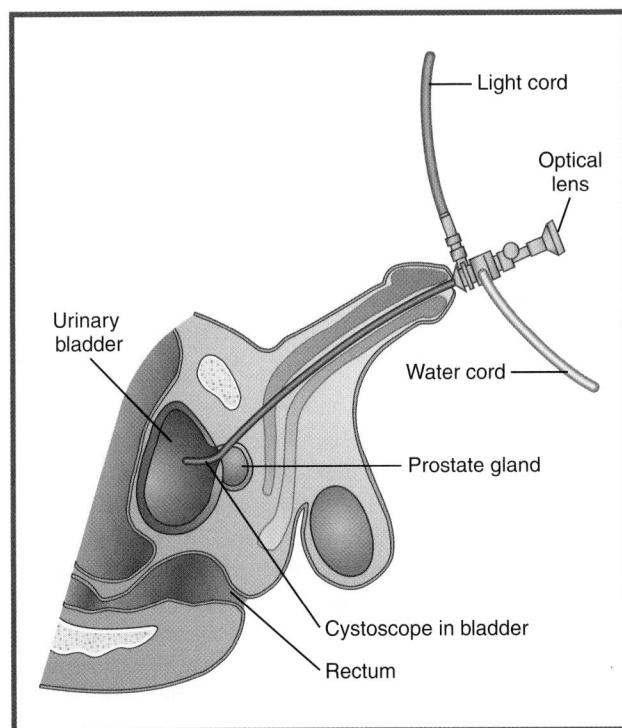

FIGURE 39-3 Cystoscopy.

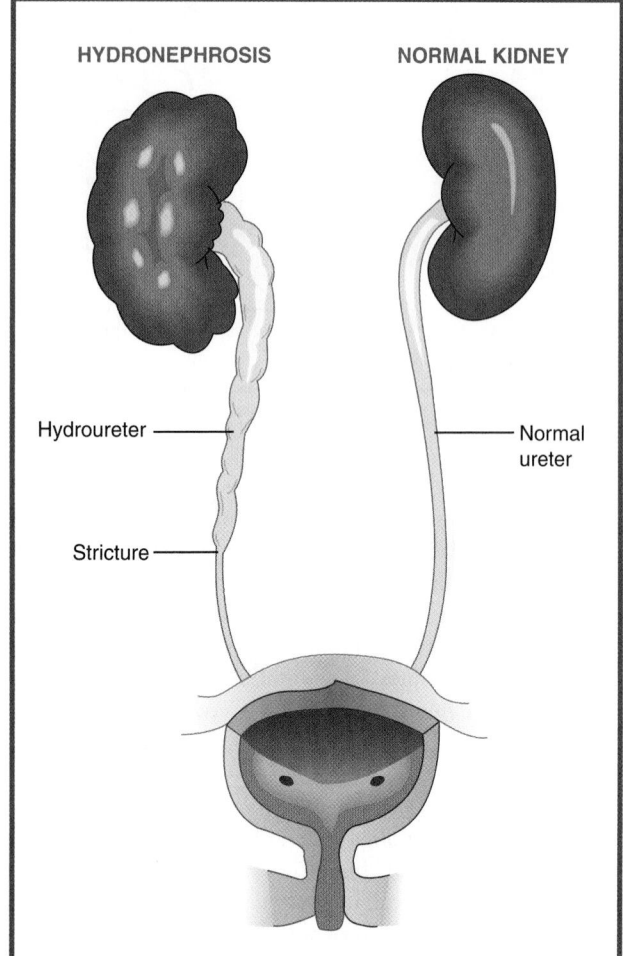

FIGURE 39-5 Hydronephrosis.

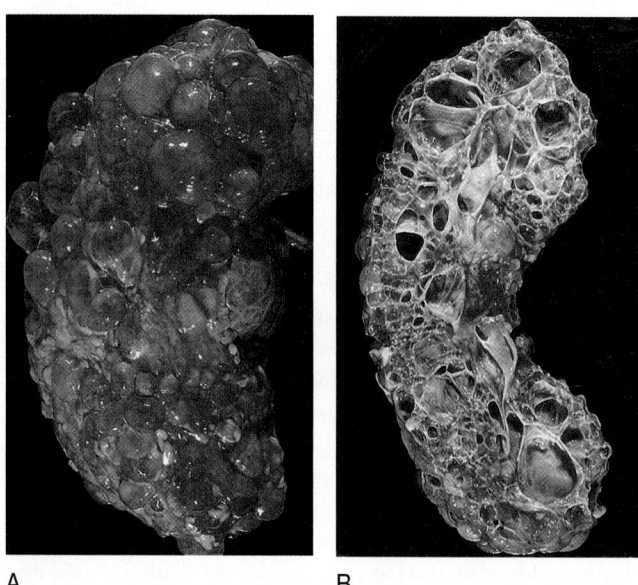

FIGURE 39-6 Polycystic kidney (adult autosomal dominant). **A,** External surface of enlarged kidney, showing cysts. **B,** Bisected, shows large interior cysts. (From Cotran RS, Kumar V, Collins T: *Robbin's pathologic basis of disease*, ed 6, Philadelphia, 1999, Saunders.)

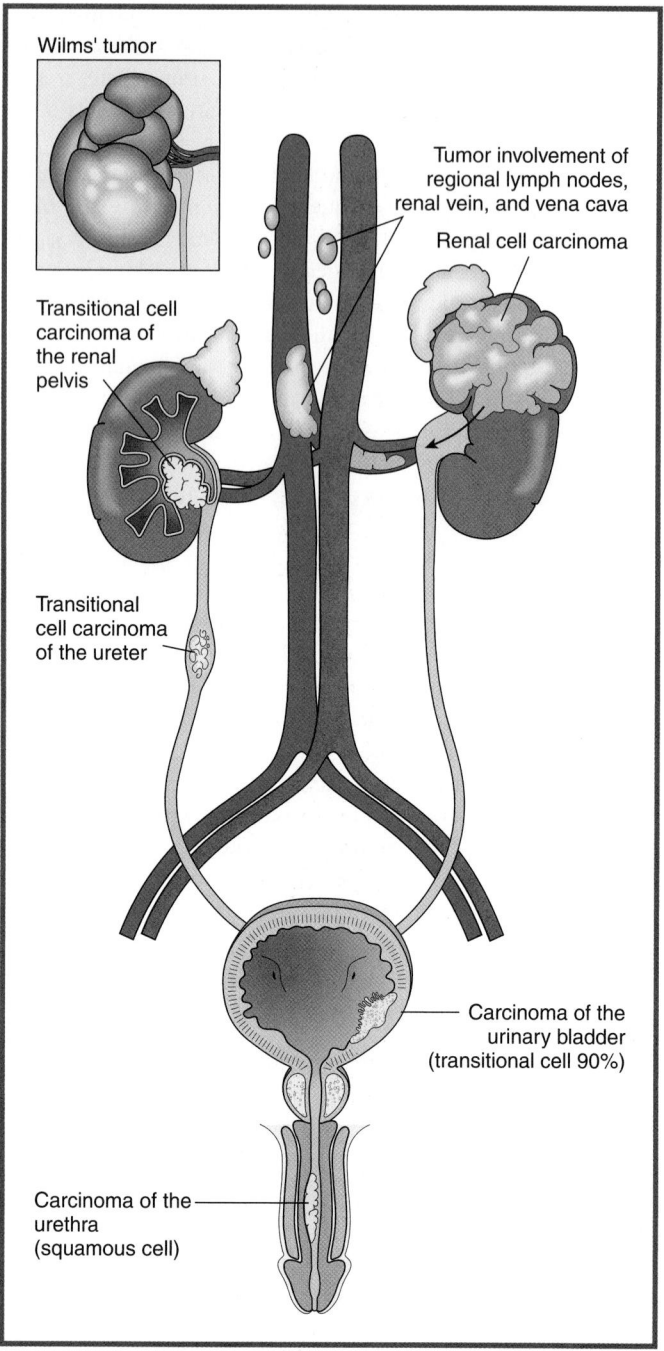

FIGURE 39-7 Neoplasms of the urinary tract. (From Damjanov I: *Pathology for the health-related professions*, ed 3, Philadelphia, 2006, Saunders.)

common in men than in women. Bladder cancer is characterized by one or more tumors that can metastasize through the blood or surrounding pelvic lymph nodes. Because 50% to 90% of patients experience a recurrence of bladder tumors, follow-up testing that can identify recurrence is extremely important. NMP22 is a urine test that identifies recurrence of the disease. This test is twice as sensitive as urine cytology and is painless and inexpensive. It works by identifying the nuclear matrix protein present in the transitional cells of the bladder. Ninety percent of bladder cancers are attributed to these particular cells, called *transitional cells* because of their ability to be cubelike when the bladder is empty and flat when it is full. The test can be performed in the physician's office, with results available in 1 hour. If the NMP22 test results are positive, the patient undergoes a cystoscopy to confirm the presence of abnormal cells.

Smoking is the greatest single risk factor for developing cancer of the bladder because the carcinogens from tobacco become concentrated in the bladder and eventually cause cellular changes in the walls of the organ. Other risk factors include occupational exposure to chemical carcinogens such as oil, rubber, and dyes; drinking pesticide-contaminated water; treatment with certain anticancer drugs; and recurrent parasitic infections of the bladder. Treatment for cancer of the bladder includes surgical removal of the tumor, possibly a complete *cystectomy* (removal of the bladder), radiation, chemotherapy, and the use of interferon to boost the patient's immune system.

Renal Carcinoma. Adenocarcinoma of the kidney, or renal cell cancer, is a primary tumor that can be cured if it is diagnosed and treated in the early stages. However, affected patients are frequently asymptomatic, giving the tumor the opportunity to metastasize to the lungs, liver, male urogenital system, bone, or brain before it is diagnosed. Renal cell carcinoma typically occurs in patients over 50 years of age and is seen more often in men and in smokers. Signs and symptoms of the disease include flank pain, anorexia, anemia, hematuria, and an increased white blood cell count. Surgical nephrectomy is the treatment of choice. Although the prognosis for patients with the tumor has improved, the 5-year survival rate is still only approximately 40%.

Wilms' Tumor. Wilms' tumor, or nephroblastoma, is cancer of the kidney in children. Although the condition appears to be caused by a genetic defect, very few of the children diagnosed with Wilms' tumor have a family history of the disease. It usually occurs unilaterally, is diagnosed most frequently at age 3, and rarely occurs after age 8. The tumor may be noticed by parents as a mass in the child's abdomen or by a physician during a routine physical examination. Preferred treatment is a partial or complete nephrectomy combined with chemotherapy. Children diagnosed and treated for Wilms' tumor have a survival rate of more than 90%.

Renal Failure

Acute renal failure has a sudden, severe onset caused by exposure to toxic chemicals or severe or prolonged circulatory or cardiogenic shock that might occur from serious burns or heart disease, acute bilateral kidney infection or inflammation, or occlusion of the renal arteries or after a complicated surgery. Blood tests will show elevated BUN and creatinine levels, and the patient will experience acute onset of oliguria. The primary problem must be resolved as quickly as possible to avoid necrosis and permanent kidney failure.

Chronic renal failure is a slowly progressive process that is caused by the gradual destruction of the ability of the kidneys to filter waste materials. Diabetes mellitus is the leading cause of chronic renal failure in the United States, but it may also be caused by hypertension; glomerulonephritis; polycystic kidneys; long-term hydronephrosis resulting from urinary obstruction; lead poisoning; or renal artery stenosis. Symptoms of the condition may not be evident until as much as 75% of the kidney is no longer functioning.

Patients with chronic renal failure pass through several stages, starting with an early stage of decreased reserve when there are no apparent clinical signs but serum creatinine levels are consistently higher than average. The middle stage of renal insufficiency is marked by hypertension, an elevation in BUN and creatinine levels, and a low specific gravity of the urine. End-stage renal failure *(uremia)* is marked by oliguria that progresses to *anuria* (no urine output), edema, hypertension, acidosis, and **azotemia.** The end result is that the kidneys can no longer remove waste products from the blood, and toxicity develops. To survive, the patient must be placed on dialysis or receive a kidney transplant.

Treatment

Dialysis, or cleansing of the blood, is used to treat acute renal failure until the problem is reversed or for those patients in end-stage renal disease until a transplant can be performed. There are two forms of dialysis: hemodialysis and peritoneal dialysis (Figure 39-8). Hemodialysis is usually done in an outpatient clinic or a hospital. The process uses a machine known as an *artificial kidney,* or *dialyzer,* to filter out waste products in the blood and return the cleansed blood to the body. The patient has a cannula or shunt surgically placed in an artery, usually in the arm, which creates an internal fistula. During the procedure, approximately 1 cup of blood at a time passes from the shunt through a tube to the semipermeable membrane of the dialysis machine. The membrane filters waste out of the blood, which then is returned to the patient's vein. Patients on hemodialysis require anticoagulant therapy to prevent the formation of clots during the blood transfer process. Hemodialysis is usually needed three times a week; the procedure takes approximately 3 to 4 hours each time.

Peritoneal dialysis uses the capillaries in the peritoneal cavity to filter the blood by infusing the patient's abdomen with a dialyzing fluid that is inserted through a surgically implanted catheter with both entry and exit points. The highly concentrated dialyzing fluid attracts and absorbs waste products from the blood vessels and is then drained from the abdominal cavity by gravity into a container. This procedure can be done at home in two different ways. With continuous ambulatory peritoneal dialysis (CAPD) the patient exchanges the dialysis solution in the abdomen four times a day, 7 days a week. The continuous cycling peritoneal dialysis (CCPD) uses a cycler machine at night to automatically infuse the dialysis solution into and out of the peritoneal cavity. This process takes 10 to 12 hours but can be accomplished while the patient is sleeping.

Although a successful kidney transplant is curative for end-stage renal failure, finding the right donor can be a problem. Donors are matched by blood type, cell surface proteins, and antibodies. Siblings are the best donors, but other blood relatives may also match. If no blood relative donors are available then an adult donor who matches the patient's criteria is the next best fit.

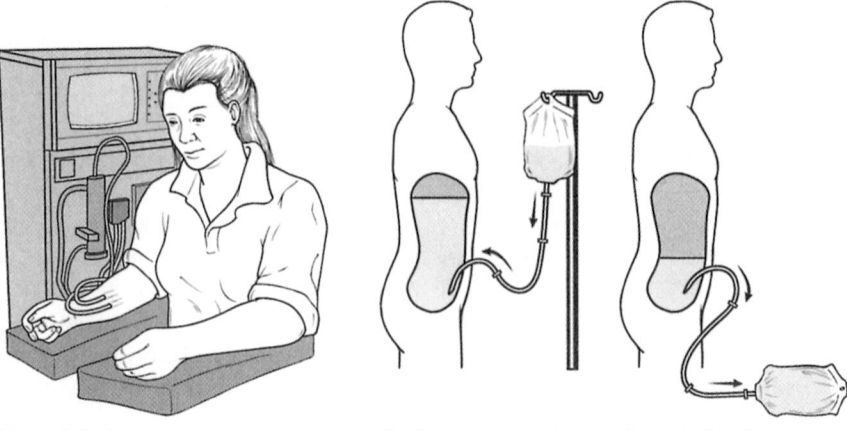

Hemodialysis   Continuous ambulatory peritoneal dialysis

FIGURE 39-8 Dialysis. (From Frazier MS, Drzymkowski JA, Doty SJ: *Essentials of human diseases and conditions*, ed 3, Philadelphia, 2004, Saunders.)

CRITICAL THINKING APPLICATION

Aloysius Gonzales, a 59-year-old patient, is in chronic renal failure. His family is trying to decide whether their father should be brought to the dialysis clinic for hemodialysis or whether they should try to keep him at home and assist with peritoneal dialysis. Sara explains the mechanism of each procedure to the family. What should she include in her description?

PEDIATRIC UROLOGIC DISORDERS

Early detection and treatment of the many urologic disorders that occur in children can drastically reduce permanent physical damage to the urinary system.

Nocturnal Enuresis

One of the most common reasons that parents bring a child to a pediatric urologist is enuresis, or bed-wetting. Enuresis is the lack of voluntary control of urination at night or during the day by a child considered to be beyond the age (usually after 6 years old) when control should be acquired. This problem has a familial tendency and is more common in boys than in girls. The urologist first determines whether the problem is physical or psychologic. With primary enuresis, bladder control was never established in the child. It may be caused by a physiologic problem with bladder control, such as an immature bladder with small capacity, a neurologic deficit, diabetes mellitus or insipidus, a UTI, or sleep apnea, or it may be a result of stressful events. Secondary enuresis, when there is a loss of bladder control in a child who has been consistently dry for at least 6 months, can develop because of stressful events, UTIs, diabetes, or sexual abuse.

A physical and neurologic examination and urinalysis with culture helps determine whether any physical abnormality or disease process is causing the problem. If a psychologic problem is suspected, help from a pediatric mental health professional may be needed. If no known causative factors are present, medications that relax the bladder muscles or that decrease urine production at night may be useful. Unfortunately, these may have side effects, so parents may decline drug therapy. Parents should positively reinforce dryness and should avoid punishing or embarrassing the child. A moisture alarm can be used to help train the child to get up at night to go to the bathroom. This is a small, battery-operated device that connects to a moisture-sensitive pad placed in the pajamas or on the bed that beeps when the pad becomes wet. The goal is to wake the child just as he or she starts to urinate so he or she can stop urinating and get to a toilet. The success rate is high (80%), but the device must be used for at least 2 weeks before any change occurs and up to 12 weeks to stop accidents.

Urinary Reflux Disorder

Another reason for pediatric urology referrals may be a urinary reflux disorder. Reflux nephropathy occurs if the kidneys are damaged by a backward flow of urine into the kidneys. Each ureter has a one-way valve where it enters the bladder that is designed to prevent urine from flowing backward. Reflux may be caused by faulty formation or damage to the valves or may be associated with cystitis, neurogenic bladder, or bladder overfilling because of an obstruction. It may be detected with ultrasonography, computed tomography (CT) scan of the kidneys, or with a voiding cystourethrogram (VCUG) (Figure 39-9). A VCUG is performed by placing a urinary catheter in the bladder and injecting a contrast medium that helps visualize the bladder and the flow of urine. X-ray films are taken in several positions, the catheter is removed, and the child is asked to void. X-ray films are taken while the bladder empties to determine if urinary reflux is present. Although a VCUG is an uncomfortable procedure, the benefit of early detection and decreased damage to the kidneys makes the screening worthwhile. Untreated reflux nephropathy can lead to renal failure.

Treatment of reflux is usually determined by grading severity on a 1 to 5 scale, with 5 being the highest. Prophylactic antibiotics may be given in low doses daily to avoid damaging kidney infections, which can cause low-grade reflux. However, with higher-grade reflux that persists after 4 or 5 years of age

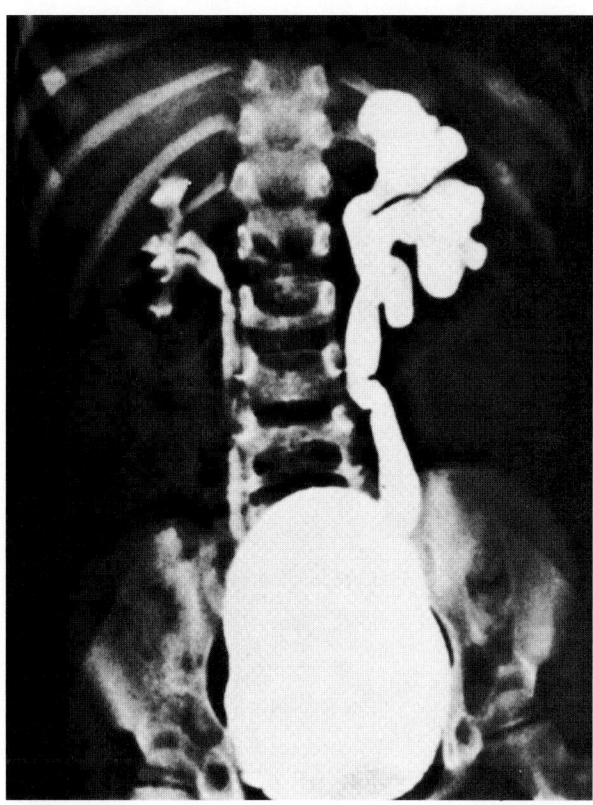

FIGURE 39-9 Voiding cystourethrogram. (From James AE Jr, Squire LF: *Nuclear radiology*, Philadelphia, 1973, Saunders.)

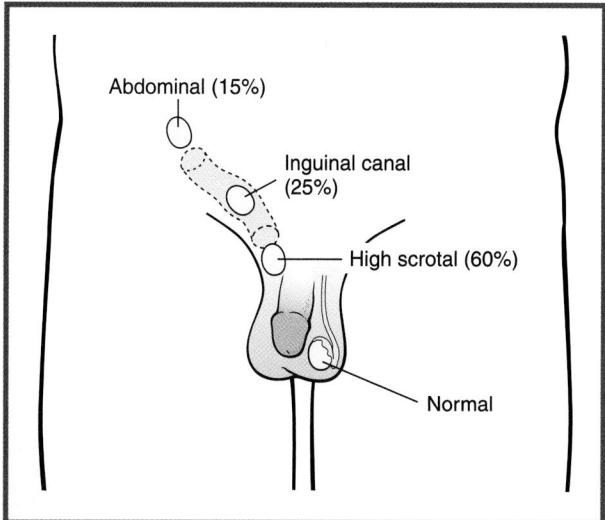

FIGURE 39-10 Cryptorchidism. (From Damjanov I: *Pathology for the health-related professions*, ed 3, Philadelphia, 2006, Saunders.)

or for patients who have breakthrough infections despite the antibiotics, surgical repair of the ureters is necessary. Parents and physicians may also opt for surgery because the procedure has a high success rate of 95% and poses little risk.

Cryptorchidism

Cryptorchidism, or undescended testicles, is fairly common in premature infants and occurs in about 4% of full-term infants (Figure 39-10). The testes develop in the abdominal cavity of the fetus, then descend into the scrotum near the end of the pregnancy. If an infant is born with an undescended testicle, it usually drops without treatment by 9 months of age. However, persistent cryptorchidism should be treated, because infertility may result from the effect on sperm of the slightly warmer temperatures in the abdominal cavity and because the child has an increased risk of developing testicular cancer as an adolescent. It is now recommended that surgical attachment of the testicle should be done by 1 year of age to decrease the chance of permanent testicular damage. Parents need to recognize that this child is considered at increased risk for testicular carcinoma even after treatment and should be taught testicular examination procedures.

The outpatient surgical procedure, known as *orchiopexy*, involves suturing the undescended testicle in the scrotum. If the testicle is impalpable (cannot be felt), laparoscopic surgery is necessary to locate it. This procedure includes inserting the instrument into the abdomen by way of a small incision near the navel. Once found, the testicle is either moved into proper

position or is removed. Success rates decrease with testes that are placed higher.

ANATOMY AND PHYSIOLOGY OF THE MALE REPRODUCTIVE SYSTEM

The male reproductive system plays an important role in the continuation of the human species (Figure 39-11). Although not necessary for individual survival, the production, sustenance, and transport of male sex cells are vital to the creation of life.

The primary reproductive organs in the male are a pair of *testes*. Each testis is an oval structure 4 to 5 cm in length and 2.5 to 3 cm in diameter. Each is surrounded by a white, fibrous capsule, and they are contained together in the retractable saclike *scrotum*. The testes consist of lobules that contain the *seminiferous tubule*, which is where *spermatozoa*, the male sex cells, are produced. These cells contain 23 chromosomes, or half of the DNA chain needed to form a complete cell. The sperm cells are tadpole-like structures less than 0.1 mm long that are carried to the *epididymis* for maturation (Figure 39-12).

The epididymis is a long (approximately 6 meters), coiled tube that rests on the top and lateral side of each testis. Peristaltic waves in the epididymis help the sperm move into the *vas deferens*, where the sperm, which is now capable of movement, is stored until ejaculation. Each vas deferens is a muscular, 45-cm tunnel that connects to the epididymis at the base of the structure and passes along the side of the testes. The vas deferens forms into the spermatic cord that passes through the pelvic cavity and ends behind the urinary bladder. Uniting there with the seminal vesicle just outside the prostate gland, it passes through the prostate and into an ejaculatory duct that empties its contents into the urethra. The male urethra is an organ of two body systems—the urinary and reproductive systems.

The adult *prostate gland* is roughly 4 cm wide and 3 cm thick and surrounds the urethra at the base of the bladder. It is about the size of a pea at birth but grows rapidly at puberty

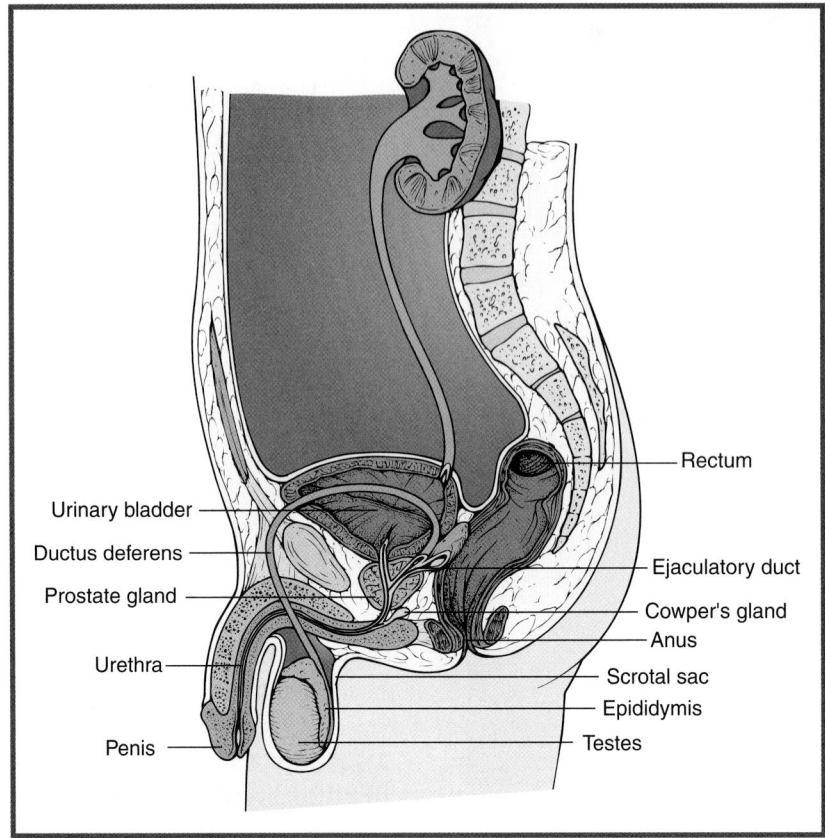

FIGURE 39-11 Male reproductive anatomy. (From Frazier MS, Drzymkowski JA, Doty SJ: *Essentials of human diseases and conditions*, ed 3, Philadelphia, 2004, Saunders.)

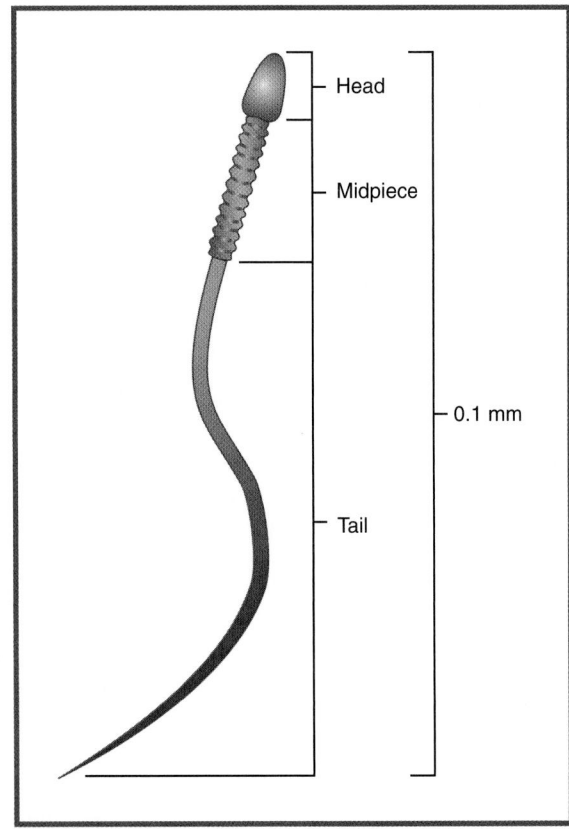

FIGURE 39-12 Sperm.

to its full size by age 20. The central part of the gland may start to grow again after the age of 45. The primary function of the prostate gland is to secrete a thin fluid with an alkaline pH that neutralizes the acidic sperm-containing fluid as well as vaginal secretions to provide an optimal pH for fertilization. Secretions from the prostate gland, vas deferens, seminal vesicles, and bulbourethral glands combine with sperm cells to form *semen*. The volume of semen in one ejaculate varies from 2 to 6 mL and averages roughly 100 to 200 million sperm.

Penis

The organ of male **copulation** is the penis. It is a cylindric organ consisting of an elongated body with a slightly enlarged end, called the *glans penis*. Around the glans penis is a fold of skin that begins just behind the glans and extends forward to cover it like a sheath. This is called the *prepuce,* or foreskin, and is sometimes removed in a surgical procedure known as *circumcision.* The penis conveys urine and semen through the urethra and outside the body. When transmitting semen to the female tract, the penis must enlarge and stiffen for insertion. This is done when three columns of erectile tissue within the penis become stimulated. The arteries within the penis dilate, and the veins compress. This compression of the veins allows a reduction of blood flow away from the penis, causing it to swell. Motor impulses are stimulated by the swelling of the urethra as a result of semen collection, and the contraction of the urethra causes the semen to be ejaculated through the penis.

Hormone Production

Hormone production is also an important aspect of the male reproductive system. As a group the male sex hormones are called *androgens*. Testosterone is the primary male hormone. During pubescence, when the male becomes reproductively functional, the anterior pituitary gland produces gonadotrophic hormones that stimulate the testes to produce testosterone. Testosterone in turn stimulates the testes to enlarge, increases body hair growth, thickens skin and bone, increases muscle growth, and matures sperm cells.

DISORDERS OF THE MALE REPRODUCTIVE TRACT

There are many diseases and disorders of the male reproductive tract. The most common of these involve enlargement or inflammation of certain organs and malignant tumors. The prostate is the most widely affected organ.

Prostatic Diseases

Prostatitis

The cause of inflammation of the prostate is not always known, but it usually develops in the presence of infection. Bacterial causes may be either *E. coli* or gonococci in patients with gonorrhea. Infection or inflammation of the prostate gland puts pressure on the urethra, causing dysuria, tenderness, and secretion of pus from the tip of the penis. Treatment is usually with an antibiotic, such as penicillin. Chronic prostatitis may develop from repeated UTIs, urethral obstruction, or urinary retention.

Benign Prostatic Hyperplasia (BPH)

As men age, the cells of the prostate gland that surround the urethra can start to reproduce more rapidly, causing an increase in the size of the organ *(hypertrophy)*. This nonmalignant process is seen in about half of men in their 60s and over 90% of men in their 70s and 80s. Enlargement of the prostate gland partially blocks the flow of urine, creating a medium for bacterial infection that can lead to cystitis. Signs and symptoms include urinary urgency and frequency; difficulty starting urination; hematuria; and repeated UTIs. The diagnosis is made from patient complaints and a digital rectal examination (DRE) during which the physician can palpate the enlarged gland (Figure 39-13).

Treatment includes the use of alpha-adrenergic blockers, such as doxazosin mesylate (Cardura) or terazosin (Hytrin), which relax the smooth muscles of the bladder, making it easier to urinate. Finasteride (Proscar, Propecia) may also be prescribed to reduce the size of the prostate, increasing urine flow and providing symptomatic relief. Nonsurgical therapies include laser treatment or prostatic stent placement to keep the urethra open, but these do not involve taking a biopsy of the gland for possible cancer. Because one of the signs of prostate cancer is enlargement of the gland, it is important that the patient be screened for this as well as treated for the disorder. If drug therapy and alternative treatments are not successful in relieving the patient's prostate enlargement, surgery is recommended. Transurethral resection of the prostate (TURP), the most common surgical treatment, involves threading a small instrument (resectoscope) through the urethra to the prostate and scraping away the excess tissue.

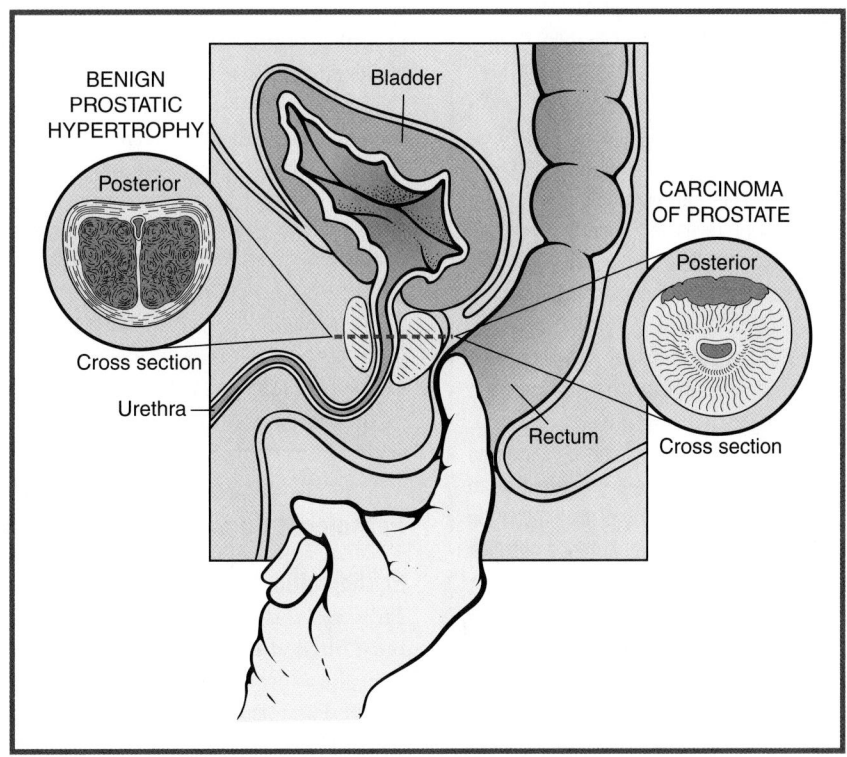

FIGURE 39-13 Benign prostatic hypertrophy and carcinoma of the prostate. (From Damjanov I: *Pathology for the health-related professions*, ed 3, Philadelphia, 2006, Saunders.)

Prostate Cancer

Cancer of the prostate is common in men older than 50 years of age and ranks as the second highest cause of cancer deaths in men, behind lung cancer. The patient is asymptomatic in the early stages and may not become symptomatic until the cancer has spread outside of the prostate gland. Once symptoms do develop, they include urinary obstruction with difficulty urinating; frequent UTIs and *nocturia* (the need to void at night); hematuria; and generalized pain in the pelvic region. Prostate cancer spreads locally to the bladder, rectum, and lymph nodes of the pelvis, causing metastasis to the bones, lungs, and brain. The prognosis is poor unless the tumor is discovered in its early stages of development, when it is still confined to the prostate gland.

The first indication of a problem may come with a routine digital rectal examination (DRE) when the physician notices a firm or irregular area in the prostate. The primary screening tool for cancer of the prostate is the prostate-specific antigen (PSA) blood test. Blood levels of PSA, a protein produced by the prostate, are elevated in the presence of prostatitis, benign prostatic hyperplasia, and cancer of the prostate. The higher the PSA level, the more likely the man has prostate cancer. However, because the level can be elevated in the presence of other disorders, one abnormal screening is not adequate to diagnose cancer. The test should

be repeated over time and if levels continue to rise, further diagnostic studies should be done. If tests indicate cancer, the physician may order a transrectal ultrasound, which involves inserting a small transducer into the rectum to bounce sound waves off of the prostate and create a picture. The ultrasound pictures are used to help pinpoint areas of concern during a tissue biopsy. If the transrectal ultrasound does not indicate any suspicious areas, the physician will take multiple biopsies, usually eight, from different sections of the prostate gland. Tissue samples are sent to the pathologist for analysis and diagnosis.

The American Cancer Society recommends that the PSA test be used in conjunction with a DRE annually for all men older than 50 years of age. In addition, PSA screenings should be performed yearly on men over the age of 40 with a family history of the disease and African American males over 40 because they are at increased risk for developing the disease.

The extent of the prostate cancer will dictate treatment options. Radiation may be delivered directly to the cancer cells through external-beam radiation therapy (EBRT) which uses high-powered x-rays to kill the cancer cells. An alternative procedure is radioactive seed implantation, a variant of radiation therapy. In this procedure, between 40 and 100 rice-sized radioactive seeds are implanted directly into the prostate gland through a precisely placed hollow needle. The radiation is quite strong but has a very short range, so that it destroys the tumor and minimizes damage to surrounding tissue. Testosterone can stimulate the growth of the tumor, so hormone therapy is frequently prescribed to block the action of testosterone or to stop its production. Surgical treatment options include removal of the prostate gland by transurethral resection; orchiectomy, in which the testosterone-producing testicles are removed; or radical prostatectomy, in which the prostate and local lymph nodes are removed. These are debilitating surgical procedures that have serious side effects so are typically used as a last measure. As with all cancers, chemotherapy may be prescribed in advanced cases or in recurrences.

Important Details About Prostate-Specific Antigen Studies

- There are no specific normal or abnormal prostate-specific antigen PSA levels.
- Because there are many possible reasons for PSA elevation, if no other indicators of cancer are present the physician may recommend repeating the DRE and PSA studies to see if the level increases over time.
- Values between 2.6 and 10 ng/mL are slightly to moderately elevated; levels of 10 to 19.9 ng/mL are moderately elevated; and levels of 20 ng/mL or more are significantly elevated.
- If the PSA level increases or the DRE reveals an abnormal prostate, then additional diagnostic studies should be done.
- If cancer is suspected, a biopsy, typically needle aspiration, is done.
- Part of the controversy with PSA testing is that it may diagnose a slow-growing tumor that is not life threatening, which can result in aggressive and life-changing surgery.
- The PSA test has a significant false-positive outcome (patients who do not have cancer are told they do). False-positive results lead to further diagnostic testing that is both expensive and stressful for the patient and his family. Only 25% to 30% of biopsies done because of elevated PSAs actually reveal cancer.
- At this point it is not clear if PSA screening saves lives or if the benefits of screening outweigh the risks of follow-up diagnostic studies and cancer treatment for potentially slow-growing tumors that are not life-threatening.
- The most frequent complications of prostate surgery include erectile dysfunction and urinary incontinence.

CRITICAL THINKING APPLICATION

Dr. Fineman frequently sees patients for prostate-related conditions. Sara decides to review the information on the disorders that affect the prostate gland so she is better able to assist the physician and answer patient questions. What are the important details of prostate disease that Sara should remember?

Pathologic Conditions of the Genital Organs

Epididymitis

Epididymitis is an inflammation of the tubular epididymis. It is most often attributed to a UTI in men over 40, but in younger men the most common cause is a sexually transmitted disease (STD). Patients experience severe low abdominal and testicular pain as well as swelling and tenderness of the scrotum. If abscesses form and produce scar tissue, sterility can occur. Antibiotics are prescribed for treatment, including ceftriaxone

(Ceftin), ciprofloxacin (Cipro), doxycycline (Vibramycin), and azithromycin (Zithromax).

Balanitis

The inflammation of the glans penis and of the mucous membrane beneath it is known as *balanitis*. It occurs most often in uncircumcised patients with narrow foreskins that do not retract easily and in diabetic men. It has many causes, including allergic reaction to certain chemicals, such as contraceptive foam; buildup of skin secretions, called *smegma;* and urinary tract and yeast infections. Treatment follows causative factors. Antibiotics are used for infections, and cleansing for buildup, as well as avoidance of chemicals that cause reactions can help prevent the problem.

Hydrocele

During the descent of the testes, a small canal develops for them to pass through. If the canal does not close after birth, fluid from the peritoneal cavity may pass through and form in the scrotum. This is called a congenital *hydrocele* and must be corrected surgically (Figure 39-14). Acquired hydroceles usually occur after middle age because of a scrotal injury or tumor and can form in men who sit for extended periods of time, such as aging men in long-term care facilities, causing painful scrotal swelling.

Testicular Cancer

Testicular carcinoma is the most common cancer occurring in white males between the ages of 15 and 34. The cause is unknown, but the primary predisposing factor for development of testicular cancer is cryptorchidism. The patient complains of a mass in either testicle; a heavy sensation in the scrotum accompanied by a sudden collection of fluid; pain in a testicle, scrotum, abdomen, or groin; and unexplained fatigue. Testicular cancer can be successfully treated if diagnosed early, with survival rates for stage I at approximately 95%. Unfortunately, because young men may hesitate to go to the physician to report a mass in the testicle, the cancer may have reached an advanced stage before it is diagnosed. Treatment is usually a combination of orchiectomy, radiation therapy, and chemotherapy in advanced stages. Testicular cancer can be detected early with monthly self-examination. Men should be taught to do this

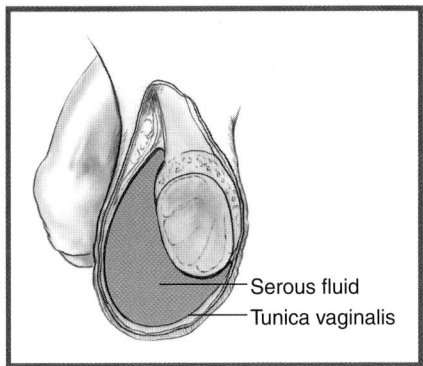

FIGURE 39-14 Hydrocele. (From Jarvis C: *Physical examination and health assessment*, ed 4, Philadelphia, 2004, Saunders.)

3-minute examination beginning in puberty or by 15 years of age (Procedure 39-1).

The physician may provide pamphlets or a shower card on testicular self-examination (Figure 39-15). The medical assistant can approach this teaching intervention in two ways. One way is to take the information to the patient, tell him to follow the pictures, and if he has any questions to call for clarification. Will he call? Would you? The second way is to take the pamphlet in and go over the instructions with the patient. Demonstrate the procedure on a model if one is available, or a male medical assistant could observe the patient doing the examination for the first time and provide feedback to clarify any patient questions.

Erectile Dysfunction

The inability to achieve and maintain an erection sufficient for intercourse is a condition known as *erectile dysfunction* (ED). It has many causes, both psychologic and physiologic. Stress, anxiety, and fear of unsatisfactory performance as well as physical diseases that affect the vascular system, including arteriosclerosis, alcoholism, and diabetes mellitus, can all lead to ED. As men age it is normal for them to have changes in erectile function. Certain medications, such as some hypertensive treatments, have impotency as a side effect. ED can be treated pharmaceutically with sildenafil (Viagra), tadalafil (Cialis), or vardenafil (Levitra). However, these medications are contraindicated in patients with a history of *myocardial infarction* (heart attack), a *cerebrovascular accident* (stroke), or a life-threatening arrhythmia. In addition, they cannot be taken if the patient is prescribed nitrate drugs such as nitroglycerin, because the combination of these medications can cause heart complications.

Infertility

Fertility peaks in men at the age of 25. Infertility may be caused by a problem in the man, a problem in the woman, or a combination of the two. In 10% to 20% of male infertility cases, there is no known cause. For the remaining cases, there can be many causative factors. Cryptorchidism, stricture, and *varicoceles* (dilated spermatic cord veins); low sperm count and motility; obstruction of the vas deferens; and hormonal imbalances are all factors in infertility.

Examination of semen specimens is helpful in making a diagnosis of infertility. These tests determine the presence of sperm, the number of sperm in an ejaculation, and the health and motility of the sperm. The use of ultrasonography is also helpful for detecting blockages of the vas deferens.

Sexually Transmitted Diseases

Diseases of the male reproductive system can also be acquired during sexual intercourse. No one is immune from these diseases, and it is possible to be infected with more than one at a time. There is no cure for viral STDs, such as human immunodeficiency virus (HIV) infection, herpes, and venereal warts; and bacterial infections are becoming increasingly resistant to antibiotic therapy. STDs are frequently asymptomatic in men, although they have the potential for causing serious health

PROCEDURE 39-1

Provide Instruction for Health Maintenance and Disease Prevention:
Teach Testicular Self-Examination

CAAHEP COMPETENCY: 3.c.(3)(c)
ABHES COMPETENCY: 7.c

GOAL: *To instruct the patient in the steps of testicular self-examination.*

EQUIPMENT and SUPPLIES

- Self-examination pamphlet and shower card
- Demonstration model
- Nonsterile gloves
- Patient record

PROCEDURAL STEPS

1. Wash your hands and collect needed supplies.
   PURPOSE: Infection control.
2. Explain to the patient what you are going to do.
   PURPOSE: Understanding helps with cooperation.
3. Begin by explaining to the patient that testicular cancer may produce no symptoms in the early stages, so it is important to examine the testes once a month for abnormal changes and early detection of the disease. This should begin at puberty or approximately 15 years of age. It is best to do the examination in the shower or in a warm bath. The total examination takes about 3 minutes.
   PURPOSE: Heat causes the scrotal skin to relax, making the examination easier.
4. Examination of the testes: Start by holding the scrotum in the palms of the hands. Then feel one testicle. Apply a small amount of pressure. Slowly roll it between the thumb and fingers and feel for any hard, painless lumps (Figure 1).
5. Examination of the epididymis: This comma-shaped cord is found behind the testis. Its job is to store and transport sperm. Tender when touched, it is the location of most noncancerous problems. Check for hard spots and lumps (Figure 2).

6. Examination of the vas deferens: Continue by examining the sperm-carrying tube that runs up the epididymis. Normally the vas feels like a firm, movable, smooth tube (Figure 3).
7. Now repeat the entire examination on the other side, beginning with the opposite testis.
8. After completing the examination on the model, ask the patient to do a return-examination using the model. A male assistant can have the patient do a self-testicular examination.
9. Give the pamphlet to the patient, along with the shower card, with instructions to hang it in the shower as a monthly reminder and guide.
10. Record the instructional interaction in the patient's medical record.
    PURPOSE: If it is not recorded, it was not done.

See Appendix D for a charting example.

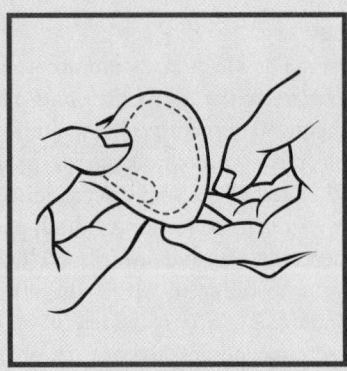

FIGURE 2

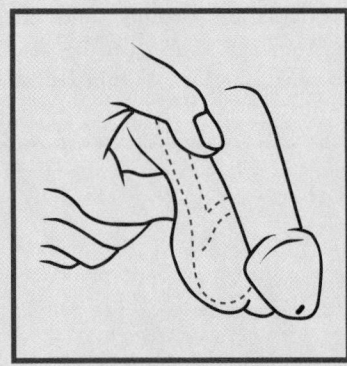

FIGURE 3

FIGURE 1

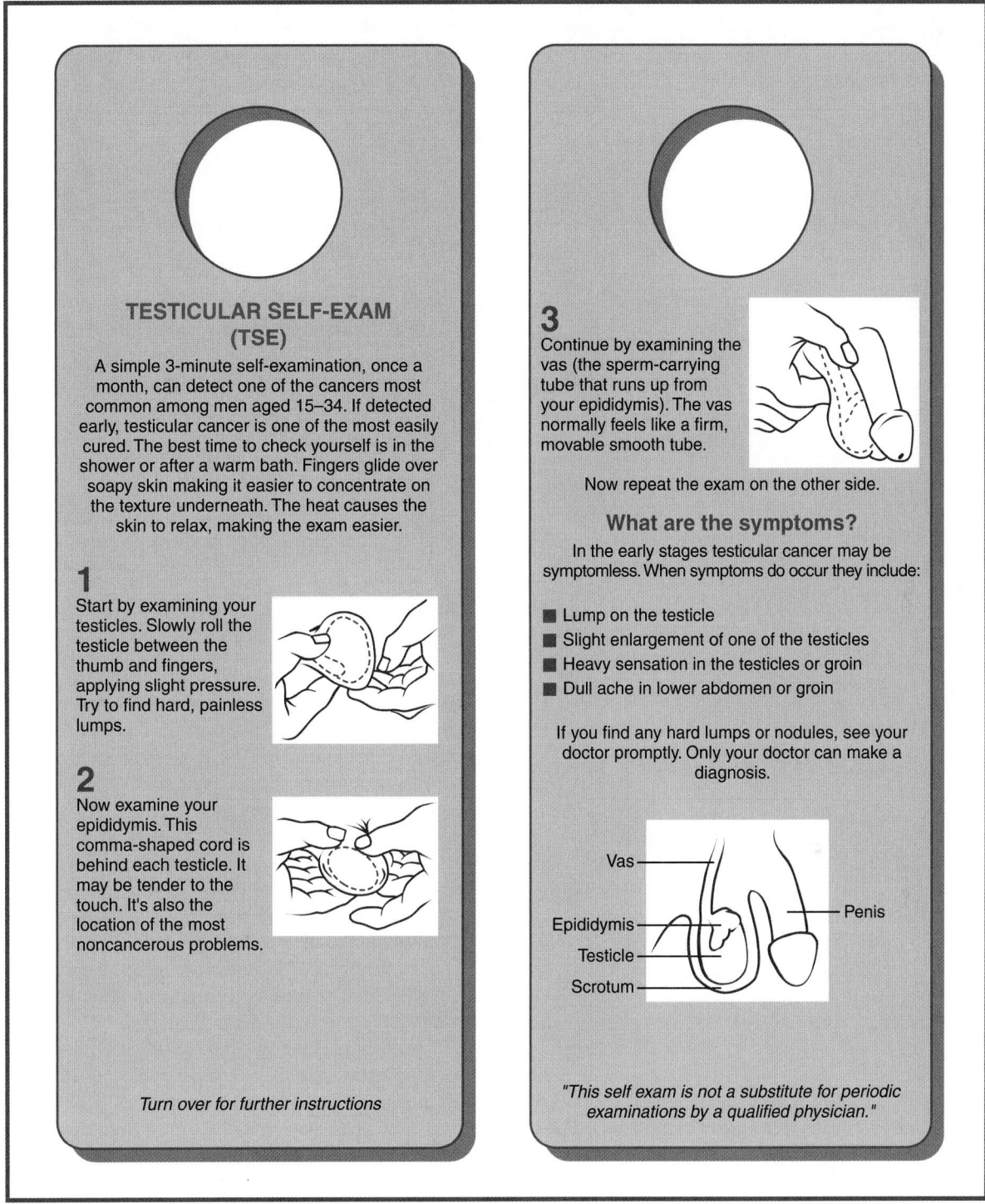

FIGURE 39-15 Self-examination shower card.

problems and are infectious whether symptoms are present or not (see Chapter 40 for gynecologic pathologic conditions). In this chapter we will discuss the signs and symptoms of and treatments for STDs in men (Table 39-2).

Bacterial STDs

Infections with *Gonorrhea* and *Chlamydia* organisms tend to coexist. An affected man develops symptoms associated with acute urethritis and epididymitis. Early detection is done by culturing discharge from the penis for the presence of the pathogen. Chlamydia is resistant to penicillin; therefore a regimen of antibiotics other than penicillin should be used if the patient has been diagnosed with both conditions.

A syphilitic lesion, called a *chancre*, develops on the male genitalia, usually the penis, within a few days to a few weeks after exposure (Figure 39-16). Syphilis is initially diagnosed through either the Venereal Disease Research Laboratory (VDRL) or Rapid Plasma Reagin (RPR) antibody blood test. If results of

TABLE 39-2 Sexually Transmitted Diseases in Men

DISEASE (CAUSATIVE ORGANISM)	SIGNS AND SYMPTOMS	TREATMENT
Chlamydia (*Chlamydia trachomatis*)—bacterial	May be asymptomatic; dysuria; itching and white discharge from penis; testicular pain	Curable with antibiotic therapy: single dose of Zithromax or 1 week of doxycycline (Vibramycin)
Genital herpes simplex virus (herpes simplex virus [HSV]-2)	Painful genital vesicles and ulcers; erythema and pruritus; tingling or shooting pain 1 to 2 days before cycle through episodes. Viral shedding may occur during asymptomatic periods	No cure, but antiviral therapy during episodes shortens duration of lesions: acyclovir (Zovirax), famciclovir (Famvir), or valacyclovir (Valtrex)
Genital warts (human papillomavirus [HPV])	Most prevalent STD; period of communicability is unknown; pinhead lesions may or may not be visible; warts tend to recur	Goal of treatment is to remove symptomatic warts; cryotherapy for lesions; Podoflox (Condylox) solution or Imiquimod (Aldara) cream to lesions
Gonorrhea (*Neisseria gonorrhoeae*)—bacterial	Dysuria; thick, cloudy, or bloody discharge from penis; dysuria and urinary frequency	Curable with antibiotic therapy: cefixime (Suprax), azithromycin, doxycycline
Syphilis (*Treponema pallidum*)—Spirochete bacteria	Six stages that can affect multiple body systems; 10- to 90-day incubation; initial sign is a painless lesion, or *chancre*, at the exposure site (penis); serous discharge from chancre; lymphadenopathy. If not diagnosed and treated, will advance to later stages	Penicillin G (Wycillin); if patient is allergic to penicillin, doxycycline or tetracycline
Trichomoniasis (*Trichomonas vaginalis*)—protozoa	Asymptomatic in men	Single oral dose of metronidazole (Flagyl)

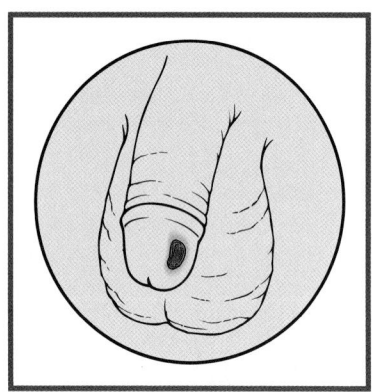

FIGURE 39-16 Syphilitic chancre. (From Frazier MS, Drzymkowski JA, Doty SJ: *Essentials of human diseases and conditions*, ed 3, Philadelphia, 2004, Saunders.)

these are positive, the diagnosis is confirmed with a Fluorescent Treponema Absorption (FTA) test that is specific for antibodies to the *Treponema* microorganism. It can be treated successfully with penicillin but may go unnoticed or unreported. Without treatment, syphilis advances to a secondary phase indicated by a low-grade fever, headache, sore throat, and a rash that does not itch but that can affect any part of the body. The secondary phase is highly contagious but is still treatable with penicillin. The more advanced stages of the disease can remain undetected or dormant for years. Symptoms that appear years after the primary infection show multisystem involvement.

Viral STDs

Genital herpes causes a blistered, inflamed, painful rash on the penis, scrotum, and urethra. After several days the vesicles rupture, resulting in a painful, ulcerated area. The lesions heal in 3 to 4 weeks, but the herpes virus then migrates to a nerve dermatome. Many factors can reactivate the disease at any time (e.g., stress and upper respiratory infections).

Genital warts are often asymptomatic in men and require preliminary treatment with acetic acid to be seen. The incubation period for infections from the human papillomavirus (HPV) may be as long as 6 months. HPV infections in women greatly increase the risk of cervical cancer. This will be discussed in greater detail in Chapter 40.

Acquired Immunodeficiency Syndrome

The most deadly STD is acquired immunodeficiency syndrome (AIDS), which is caused by the human immunodeficiency virus (HIV). The virus invades CD4 T lymphocytes, destroying their ability to fight infection on the cellular level. It is not unusual to be asymptomatic when first exposed to HIV. Those individuals who do have symptoms may complain of a fever, arthralgia (joint pain), myalgia (muscle pain), lymphadenopathy, rash, night sweats, and malaise approximately 2 to 6 weeks after transmission of the virus.

The goal of HIV treatment is to reduce the amount of virus in the body with antiretroviral drugs so the destruction of the immune system is slowed. With advanced drug therapy it is unclear how many years, perhaps as many as 17, that individuals with an early diagnosis and consistent and appropriate medical treatment will remain HIV positive before developing AIDS. AIDS is diagnosed when there is evidence of a wide range of **opportunistic infections** that develop because of depressed T-cell counts. These include *Pneumocystis carinii* pneumonia, candidiasis (yeast infection), **Kaposi's sarcoma,** dementia, and **wasting syndrome.** A patient is considered to be HIV positive when antibodies to the virus have been detected but not to have AIDS until the CD4 T-cell count is below 200 mm^3 and/or opportunistic infections have been diagnosed. Current HIV management includes monitoring CD4 T-cell counts at diagnosis and every 3 to 6 months thereafter.

HIV is transmitted when infected blood or blood products, semen, or vaginal secretions come into contact with the mucous membranes or broken skin of an uninfected person. It can also be passed in utero from an infected mother to her fetus, during delivery, or by breastfeeding. Intravenous drug users who share needles and anyone having unprotected sex of any kind are at increased risk for contracting HIV. Healthcare workers are also at risk for accidental exposure in the workplace and should consistently employ standard precautions to protect themselves and their patients from this deadly disease. The HIV virus is fragile, cannot survive outside the body, and is easily destroyed by chemical disinfectants such as household bleach.

All HIV tests screen for the presence of antibodies to the virus, and any positive result, regardless of the type of test used, is followed up with the more definitive Western Blot test before a positive diagnosis is made. The most widely used screening test for HIV is the enzyme immunoassay (EIA), which is typically performed on a venous blood sample. However, EIA tests can be done with other body fluids, including oral fluid tests and urine tests, although urine screening is not as accurate or sensitive to antibody levels.

Newer developments in rapid HIV screening uses either blood or oral fluid (not the same as saliva) and can produce results within 20 to 60 minutes with accuracy rates similar to those of traditional EIA screening tests. The U.S. Food and Drug Administration (FDA) recently approved the OraQuick Advance HIV1/2 Antibody Test for use on both oral fluid and plasma specimens. To perform the oral test, a single gentle swab is done around both upper and lower outer gums, the swabbing device is inserted into a vial containing a developer solution, and the test is considered positive if there are two reddish-purple lines in a small window in the test device after 20 minutes. This test is not designed for home screening because it is restricted for use by trained individuals, such as medical assistants. However, an FDA-approved home test called the *Home Access HIV-1 Test System* is available at most drug stores. It is actually a kit that provides the materials for collection of a specimen at home rather than in a healthcare facility. To perform the test, the individual pricks a finger, places a blood drop onto a specially treated card, then mails the card to a licensed laboratory for testing. The individual uses an identification number provided with the kit to call the laboratory for results. As with all other HIV screening tools, a positive result must be followed by a Western Blot test to confirm the diagnosis.

HIV can be treated with medications but cannot be cured. Once patients begin antiretroviral treatment they must continue to take these drugs for the rest of their lives. The medications must be taken at the time and frequency prescribed to be effective in controlling the spread of the virus and to prevent drug-resistant strains from developing. The FDA currently has approved 21 medications for the treatment of HIV in adults and adolescents. Guidelines recommend a combination of three or more antiretroviral drugs in a regimen called *highly active antiretroviral therapy* (HAART). Four classes of FDA-approved antiretroviral medications are designed to either prevent HIV replication or block the entry of the virus into the body's T cells. Examples of these drugs include delavirdine (Rescriptor, DLV), zidovudine (Retrovir, AZT, ZDV), amprenavir (Agenerase, APV), and enfuvirtide (Fuzeon, T-20).

Unfortunately, HIV medications can cause multiple side effects including fever, nausea, fatigue, liver abnormalities, diabetes mellitus, hypercholesterolemia, decreased bone density, skin rash, pancreatitis, and neurologic disorders. Patients must be educated on the importance of strictly following their prescribed treatment regimen as well as immediately reporting any side effects to the physician.

The psychosocial needs of a patient diagnosed with HIV are far reaching. Treatment is designed to control the duplication of the virus in the body, but the patient will always be infectious. Prevention of disease transmission includes sexual abstinence or the consistent use of condoms and precautions with blood spills; these options must be discussed and consistently reinforced with the patient. Community organizations can serve as a source of counseling and support for HIV-positive patients and their families. All information regarding the HIV status of a patient must be kept in strict confidence, and there can be no documentation on the chart indicating the patient's HIV or AIDS status.

CRITICAL THINKING APPLICATION

The number of patients seen weekly in Dr. Fineman's practice who have STDs continues to rise. Sara is responsible for telephone screening as well as clinical medical assisting practices. She is constantly being asked questions about the signs and symptoms of STDs and their treatment. What should Sara know about bacterial and viral STDs and their treatment?

THE MEDICAL ASSISTANT'S ROLE IN UROLOGIC AND MALE REPRODUCTIVE EXAMINATIONS

Much of the diagnosis of urinary dysfunction depends on the patient's history, which may include frequency or urgency of urination, dysuria, or incontinence. A major part of the urologic examination is urinalysis. The medical assistant must be able to instruct the patient in how to obtain a clean-catch urine specimen (see Chapter 51). It is best to have the patient collect the specimen during an office visit so it can be examined immediately. The urologist may need to examine a catheterized specimen, which is collected using sterile technique. This procedure requires advanced training.

Assisting with a Urologic Examination

No special instrument setup is required for a routine urologic examination unless a special procedure, such as obtaining a catheterized urine specimen or obtaining a specimen for culture, is to be performed. Most offices use prepackaged disposable units for catheterization and for bladder irrigation.

Trends in Reportable Sexually Transmitted Diseases

- Chlamydia is the most frequently reported infectious disease in the United States, with almost 2.5 million cases reported in 2004; the Centers for Disease Control and Prevention (CDC) estimates that there are approximately 2.8 million new cases each year; improved testing and treatment among men could help reduce transmission to women; can be diagnosed with a urine test; complications among men are rare.
- Gonorrhea is the second most commonly reported infectious disease in the United States, with over 330,000 cases reported in 2004, the lowest level since reporting began; CDC estimates twice as many new infections occur each year; blacks have 19 times more reported cases than whites; antibiotic resistance (especially to such drugs as ciprofloxacin [Cipro] and Levaquin) is a serious concern; untreated infections can cause epididymitis and possibly infertility.
- Syphilis is highly infectious in the early stages but easily curable; untreated it can lead to serious long-term complications, including nerve, cardiovascular, and organ damage, and even death; incidence is increasing in homosexuals.
- Most individuals are asymptomatic or have minimal signs or symptoms of herpes infections; with symptoms the initial outbreak consists of one or more blisters on or around the genitals that break, leaving tender ulcers that last 2 to 4 weeks; may have less-severe outbreaks over time; the virus is present in the body indefinitely, but the frequency of outbreaks decreases over time; transmission can occur from an infected partner who does not have a visible sore and may not know that he or she is infected.
- Herpes simplex virus (HSV)–1 can cause genital herpes, but it more commonly causes oral herpes or cold sores; HSV-1 infection of the genitals can be caused by oral-to-genital contact with a person who has an HSV-1 infection; condoms do not completely prevent transmission of genital herpes.
- Most HPV infections are asymptomatic; may be unaware of the infection but can transmit it to a sex partner; genital warts may disappear without treatment; there are no HPV diagnostic tests available for men, so diagnosis is based on the visible presence of wart development; condoms do not completely prevent transmission.
- HIV is unable to reproduce outside a living host, and there is no record of infection from environmental contact; there is no evidence it can be transmitted by insects; latex or polyurethane condoms used consistently and correctly provide a highly effective mechanical barrier to HIV. Currently the greatest incidence of new HIV cases is seen in 35- to 39-year-olds; 50% of the new cases in 2004 were in African Americans; 73% of individuals with HIV are male.

Both male and female patients disrobe and are given a gown. A woman is placed in the dorsal recumbent position, and a man is seated on the examining table. The physician instructs the patient about what is required. If the patient is a woman and the physician is a man, a female medical assistant must remain in the room with the patient while the patient's genital area is exposed and examined. The primary responsibility during the examination process is to assist the physician with any supplies and equipment needed and to maintain proper draping of the patient.

Assisting with a Male Reproductive Examination

The medical assistant needs to understand the male reproductive system and provide patient support throughout the examination. The patient should empty his bladder and disrobe before the physician begins the examination. A drape sheet is placed around the patient's waist, covering the lower extremities. A female medical assistant assists only if requested by the physician. The physician inspects the foreskin (if the patient is not circumcised) and the glans penis. The penis and scrotum are palpated for possible masses and tenderness. If the physician uses a transilluminator, the assistant may be asked to darken the room. The patient is also examined for possible inguinal hernias, and a rectal examination of the prostate gland completes the physical assessment.

If the assistant is a man, he may be needed to assist the physician with the examination and aid the patient with draping and positioning. The assistant should watch the patient for signs of discomfort and anxiety; if these signs are noted, he should notify the physician immediately. Answering the patient's questions and reinforcing understanding of the physician's orders are among the assistant's responsibilities.

Vasectomy

A vasectomy is a surgical procedure for sterilizing a male patient (Figure 39-17). It is performed by surgically removing a section of each vas deferens to stop sperm from reaching the prostate and mixing with semen. The sexual characteristics of the patient remain the same, and the ability to have an erection is entirely unchanged.

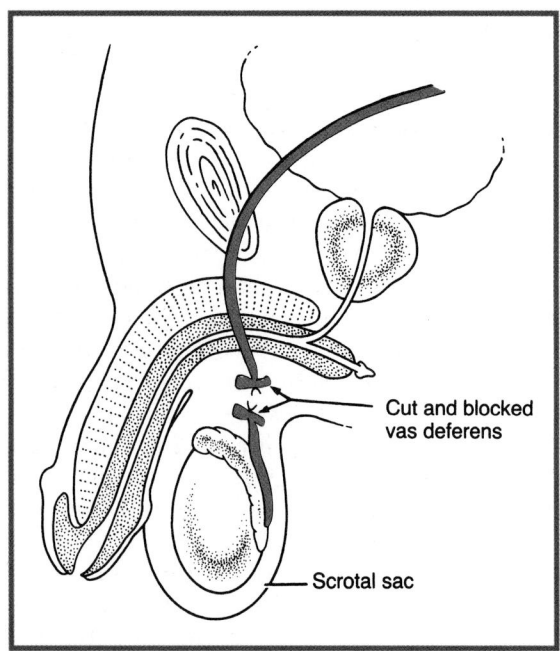

FIGURE 39-17 Vasectomy. (From Chabner DE: *The language of medicine*, ed 7, Philadelphia, 2004, Saunders.)

The procedure can be performed in a physician's office with a local anesthetic agent, such as lidocaine (Xylocaine). With the standard procedure, which takes approximately 30 minutes, the physician makes a small incision on both sides of the scrotum with a scalpel to reach and clip the vas deferens bilaterally, then closes the site by cauterization or with sutures. The no-scalpel vasectomy is a newer technique that takes approximately 10 minutes. The physician palpates and clamps the vas deferens under the scrotal sac, makes a tiny puncture through the skin, pulls the vas deferens out and cuts it, replaces the tube, and seals the site. The procedure is then repeated on the other side. Patients must be aware that sterility is not immediate because sperm may be present in the ducts. It may take as long as 1 month for the semen to be sperm free. Patients should use a backup method of birth control until two sperm counts 4 to 6 weeks apart show no evidence of sperm.

CRITICAL THINKING APPLICATION

Sara routinely assists Dr. Fineman with urologic and male reproductive examinations. She is also responsible for orienting new employees of the practice and helping them learn the procedures that typically occur in the office. Summarize the role of a medical assistant in helping with these examinations.

CLOSING COMMENTS

Patient Education

Most men under the age of 50 have not seen a physician in years. Medical studies reveal that attitude, not biology, has a lot to do with the difference between men's and women's life spans. Men just do not go to the doctor as often as women and tend to ignore indicators of disease. The solution to maintaining good health is preventive care, and the first step is establishing a good rapport with a physician of choice. As a general rule, a man in good health should have three checkups in his twenties, from three to four checkups in his thirties, and a checkup every other year in his forties. After the age of 50 a yearly checkup is recommended. In addition to testing for conditions such as cancer, heart disease, stroke, and diabetes, the entire medical team can empower male patients with the knowledge to make responsible decisions regarding good health.

The American Cancer Society recommends that men 50 years of age and older have an annual fecal occult stool test and a flexible sigmoidoscopy every 5 years; a double contrast barium enema every 5 years; and a colonoscopy every 10 years to screen for colorectal cancer. Prostate screening (DRE and PSA blood test) is also recommended for all men over the age of 50 but should also be done at age 40 in blacks and men with a history of prostate cancer.

Many procedures are required in a urology setting, and there is a strong need for patient education, especially of male patients. A medical assistant should see this need as an opportunity to become a greater asset to the physician-employer, the patient, and the profession. The urinary system remains a very

private, personal part of the patient's body. Patients often feel embarrassed to ask questions about how to obtain the requested urine or semen sample. The medical assistant can provide this information in a sincere, confidential manner to relieve patient anxiety and worry. Using diagrams, models, and handouts helps the patient to understand the disease process and treatment regimen and also encourages patient compliance.

Legal and Ethical Issues

When working in a urology office, a medical assistant must be very careful to ensure that patients have given informed consent for the procedures to be performed. If the patient refuses a procedure, the assistant needs to have the patient sign the appropriate informed refusal forms; these forms are then included in the medical record. All patient education should be done after the physician has completed the explanation and has given the assistant instructions to do so. Never diagnose, prescribe, or offer comment about a patient's condition. Medical assistants who overstep their professional boundaries may place the physician and themselves in legal jeopardy. Remember that the patient who is legally informed and satisfied with the care received is less likely to find the need to take legal action against the physician and the assistant.

The urology practice manages many sensitive patient issues that require strict adherence to confidentiality guidelines. This is especially true for a patient who has a functional disorder with the reproductive system or is diagnosed with an STD. There are special legal guidelines regarding patients diagnosed with HIV that must be strictly followed to avoid litigation.

Health Insurance Portability and Accountability Act Applications

There are major challenges in staying up to date on confidentiality restrictions regarding patient HIV status. Health Insurance Portability and Accountability Act (HIPAA) legislation provides minimum requirements for protection of personal health information, but state laws can override HIPAA regulations if the state law is considered more stringent. In addition, individual healthcare institutions (hospitals, universities, physician practices) may have their own unique policies and procedures for managing HIV and AIDS confidential information. For example, if a physician believes that an HIV-positive individual will not disclose his or her HIV status to significant others, then most states permit the physician to act. First, the physician must attempt to notify the patient that the information is going to be disclosed. Then the physician can inform the spouse, sexual partner(s), child, or needle-sharing partner(s) of the patient who are at risk of being infected with HIV about their risk of exposure. However, the state may limit this disclosure by not permitting the physician to identify the name of the individual who is HIV positive.

- Confidential HIV information includes any records that could reasonably identify the individual as a person who has had an HIV test, is HIV positive, has opportunistic diseases related to HIV, or has AIDS.
- HIPAA protects the patient's confidential *information,* not just the paper or electronic records of that information.

That means verbal disclosure of the individual's HIV and AIDS status is limited to only the personnel who have the right to that information according to individual state laws. For example, if you learn about your neighbor's HIV status at work and you go home and discuss it with your family, your employer is responsible for your disclosure of this information, and both you and your employer may be fined by the state or sued by the patient.

• Disclosure of HIV and AIDS status for treatment, pay-ment, or healthcare operations can be made only with the specific written consent of the affected patient.

• Depending on state laws, written consent may not be needed to release the information if there is a court order for the information; if the case is being reported to state or local vital statistics or public health agencies; or to certain employees of correctional institutions or residential treatment facilities, funeral directors, or emergency personnel.

SUMMARY OF SCENARIO

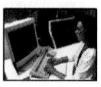

Sara enjoys working with Dr. Fineman and the urologic patients seen in the practice. She recognizes the need to stay current with information regarding disorders of the system and their treatment. Sara continues to learn on the job and through workshops about the urinary system and current therapies. Her expertise is constantly growing, and she uses this knowledge to help with patient education, manage telephone screening, and assist Dr. Fineman with procedures in the office. She is also working on building a database with local resources, support groups, and Internet sites that could be helpful for patients confronted with urologic or male reproductive system problems.

SUMMARY of LEARNING OBJECTIVES

1. Define, spell, and pronounce the terms listed in the vocabulary.
   • Spelling and pronouncing medical terms correctly adds credibility to the medical assistant. Knowing the definition of these terms promotes confidence in communication with patients and co-workers.

2. Describe the organs of the urinary system and their functions.
   • The urinary system is made up of two kidneys, the ureters, the urinary bladder, and the urethra. The functions of the urinary system include removal of waste products; regulating water, electrolytes, and acid-base levels; activating vitamin D; and secreting erythropoietin and renin. The three processes involved in urine formation are filtration, reabsorption, and excretion. The cortex contains the nephron unit where urine is formed, and the medulla is the collection site for urine.

3. Explain the susceptibility of the urinary system to diseases and disorders.
   • The urinary tract is made up of a continuous mucosal lining, which gives organisms that enter the urethra a direct pathway through the system.

4. Identify the primary signs and symptoms of urinary problems.
   • The most common signs and symptoms of urinary problems include changes in the frequency of urination, dysuria, urgency, retention, and incontinence. Abnormal functions of any part of the urinary tract can be determined with urinalysis, BUN levels, and creatinine clearance.

5. Detail common urinary system diagnostic procedures.
   • Diagnostic procedures are summarized in Table 39-1. They include a KUB x-ray examination, renal scanning, cystography or voiding cystography, IVP, renal arteriogram, renal CT, renal ultrasonography, cystoscopy, and retrograde pyelogram.

6. Compare and contrast infections and inflammations of the urinary system.
   • Most UTIs are ascending, starting with pathogens in the perineal area and infecting the continuous mucosa up through the urethra, bladder, and ureters, to the kidneys. Infections and inflammations include urethritis, cystitis, pyelonephritis, and acute or chronic glomerulonephritis.

7. Describe urinary tract disorders and cancers.
   • Renal calculi are created when salts in the urine collect in the kidney or when fluid intake is low. They can block the flow of urine, causing hydronephrosis. Polycystic kidney disease is a genetic disorder that is slowly progressive and irreversible, causing the formation of multiple grapelike cysts in the kidney. Bladder cancer is invasive and can metastasize through the blood or surrounding pelvic lymph nodes. Adenocarcinoma of the kidney is initially asymptomatic, so it frequently has metastasized before being diagnosed. Wilms' tumor is cancer of the kidney in children.

8. Distinguish between the two methods of treating renal failure.
   • Acute renal failure has a sudden, severe onset caused by exposure to toxic chemicals, severe or prolonged circulatory or cardiogenic shock, or acute bilateral kidney infection. Chronic renal failure is a slowly progressive process that is caused by the gradual destruction of the ability of the kidneys to filter waste materials. Dialysis is used to treat acute renal failure until the problem is reversed or for those patients in end-stage renal disease until a transplant can be done. There are two forms of dialysis: hemodialysis and peritoneal dialysis.

Continued

SUMMARY of LEARNING OBJECTIVES

Continued

9. Summarize typical pediatric urologic disorders.
   - Pediatric urologic disorders include enuresis, urine reflux disorder, and cryptorchidism.
10. Illustrate the organs of male reproduction.
    - The male reproductive system is made up of a pair of testes that contain the seminiferous tubule, where spermatozoa are produced and carried to the epididymis for maturation and into the vas deferens for storage. The prostate gland secretes seminal fluid for ejaculation with the sperm by the penis. Testosterone stimulates development of secondary male characteristics and matures sperm.
11. Determine the causes and effects of prostate disorders.
    - Inflammation of the prostate usually develops because of an infection such as an STD. The common symptoms are dysuria, tenderness, and secretion of pus from the tip of the penis. Benign prostatic hyperplasia partially blocks the flow of urine and is diagnosed from patient complaints and with a DRE. Treatment includes the use of medication or surgery. Cancer of the prostate is common in men older than 50 years of age and is the second highest cause of male cancer deaths; complaints include urinary obstruction, UTIs, and nocturia. Prostate cancer is diagnosed by a DRE, elevated PSA, and biopsy; treatment includes radioactive seed implantation, hormone therapy, or prostatectomy.
12. Outline common types of genital pathologic conditions in men.
    - Male genital pathologic conditions include epididymitis, balanitis, prostatitis, and STDs. Testicular tumors usually occur in young men and are generally malignant. ED is typically treated with medication. Male infertility may be caused by cryptorchidism, stricture, varicoceles, low sperm count and motility, and hormonal imbalances.
13. Perform patient education for the testicular self-examination.
    - Patient education for testicular self-examination is summarized in Procedure 39-1. The procedure teaches young men how to palpate for a mass in the testicles. It should be performed monthly, and any masses found should be immediately reported to the physician.
14. Analyze the effects of sexually transmitted diseases in the male patient.
    - Table 39-2 summarizes the signs, symptoms, and treatment of STDs in men. There is no cure for viral STDs, and bacterial causes of infection are becoming increasingly resistant to antibiotic therapy. STDs are frequently asymptomatic and can cause serious health problems. Bacterial STDs include gonorrhea, chlamydia, and syphilis. Viral infections are genital herpes, genital warts, and HIV. Trichomoniasis is a protozoal infection that is asymptomatic.
15. Summarize the characteristics of HIV infection, diagnostic criteria, and treatment protocols.
    - HIV invades CD4 T lymphocytes, destroying their ability to fight infection on the cellular level. Initial exposure may cause flulike symptoms, but after this it could be many years before clinical symptoms of AIDS occur. A patient is considered to be HIV positive when antibodies are detected and to have full-blown AIDS when T-cell counts are below 200 mm^3 and/or opportunistic infections are diagnosed. HIV is transmitted when infected blood or blood products, semen, or vaginal secretions come into contact with the mucous membranes or broken skin of an uninfected person and from infected mother to fetus in utero, during delivery, or by breastfeeding. There are many methods for HIV testing, but all must be confirmed with the Western Blot test. A combination of antiviral drugs is used to control the replication of the virus, but there is no cure for the disease.
16. Describe the medical assistant's role in urologic and male reproductive examinations.
    - The medical assistant's role in a urology practice includes taking a complete patient history, detailing urinary symptoms; patient instruction for diagnostic tests; assisting with a urologic or male reproductive examination, and answering patient questions.

CONNECTIONS

Study Guide Connection: Go to Chapter 39 Study Guide. Read the Case Study and Workplace Applications and complete the assignments. Do online research for answers to the questions in the Internet Activities associated with assisting in urology and male reproduction.

CD Connection: Go to the Medical Assisting Competency Challenge CD and do the training activities under Diagnostic Testing. For a better understanding of the urinary system, view the animation for renal anatomy and function.

evolve   **Evolve Connection:** For more information related to assisting in urology and male reproduction, go to evolve.elsevier.com/kinn and visit related weblinks for Chapter 39. Click on the Medical Assisting Exam Review and do the practice questions to sharpen your test-taking skills.

Assisting in Obstetrics and Gynecology

40

SCENARIO

Betsy Davis, CMA, was recently hired by the University Women's Hospital to work for Dr. Erin Beck, an obstetrician/gynecologist for a busy family-centered care facility in her community. Betsy has worked for a family practice physician for 3 years, but this is her first position in a specialty practice. Betsy is excited about the opportunity to focus on women's health issues and is especially interested in helping in the obstetric area of the practice. Betsy's responsibilities will include understanding current methods of contraception and the patient education factors that are important for each. She also needs to develop expertise in gynecologic diseases and conditions including diagnostic and treatment protocols for cancers of the female system. Medical assistants in the practice are expected to be able to teach breast self-examinations and answer the questions of pregnant patients concerning healthy pregnancy, labor, and delivery.

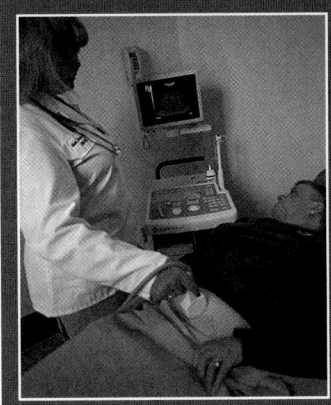

While studying this chapter, think about the following questions:

- What is the basic anatomy and physiology of the female system?
- What should Betsy learn about contraceptives to be able to answer patient questions?
- What gynecological disorders does Betsy need to be familiar with?
- What are the primary malignancies of the female system?
- What should Betsy do when assisting Dr. Beck with a Pap smear?

- How can Betsy teach patients to perform a breast examination?
- What are the stages of pregnancy and birth?
- How can Betsy help patients understand issues surrounding menopause?
- What are the typical diagnostic procedures used in obstetrics and gynecology?

LEARNING OBJECTIVES

1. Define, spell, and pronounce the terms listed in the vocabulary.
2. Identify the major organs of the female reproductive system, and explain the primary function of each.
3. Trace the ovum through the three phases of menstruation.
4. Compare and contrast current contraceptive methods.
5. Summarize menstrual disorders and conditions.
6. Distinguish among different types of gynecologic infections.
7. Differentiate between benign and malignant neoplasms of the female reproductive system.
8. Prepare for and assist with the female examination, including a Papanicolaou (Pap) test.
9. Teach the patient how to perform a breast self-examination.
10. Compare the positional disorders of the pelvic region.

11. Summarize the process of pregnancy and parturition.
12. Describe the common complications of pregnancy.
13. Specify the signs, symptoms, and treatments of conditions related to menopause.
14. Outline the medical assistant's role in gynecologic and reproductive examinations.
15. Demonstrate how to assist with the prenatal examination.
16. Distinguish among diagnostic tests that may be done to evaluate the female reproductive system.
17. Demonstrate patient preparation for a cryosurgery procedure.
18. Determine the estimated delivery date when given the date of the last menstrual period.

National Accreditation Competencies and Content

CAAHEP COMPETENCIES

Clinical

3.b.(4)(e). Prepare patient for and assist with routine and specialty examinations

3.b.(4)(f). Prepare patient for and assist with procedures, treatments, and minor office surgeries

General

3.c.(3)(c). Provide instruction for health maintenance and disease prevention

ABHES COMPETENCIES

Clinical Duties

4.b. Prepare patients for procedures

4.h. Prepare patients for and assist physician with routine and specialty examinations

Instruction

7.c. Teach patients methods of health promotion and disease prevention

VOCABULARY

adnexal (add'-neks-uhl) Pertaining to adjacent or accessory parts.

clitoris (kli'-tuh-ris) Small, elongated erectile body situated above the urinary meatus at the superior point of the labia minora.

coitus Sexual union between male and female; also known as *intercourse.*

colostrum (koh-lahs'-trum) Thin, yellow, milky fluid secreted by the mammary glands a few days before and after delivery.

dilation The opening of the cervix through the process of labor, measured as 0 to 10 cm dilated.

dilatation and curettage The widening of the cervix and scraping of the endometrial wall of the uterus.

dysplasia An alteration in cell growth causing differences in size, shape, and appearance.

effacement The thinning of the cervix during labor, measured in percentages from 0% to 100% effaced.

endocervical curettage The scraping of cells from the wall of the uterus.

fundus The curved, top portion of the uterus; the fundal height can be used as a measurement of fetal growth and estimated gestation.

human chorionic gonadotropin A hormone secreted by the placenta; is found in the urine of pregnant females.

idiopathic Without an apparent or known cause.

lymphedema (limf-uh-de'-muh) Swelling caused by the accumulation of lymph fluid in soft tissues.

mons pubis Fat pad that covers the symphysis pubis.

multiparous Pertaining to women who have had two or more pregnancies.

myelomeningocele A herniation of a portion of the spinal cord and its meninges that protrudes through a congenital opening in the vertebral column.

neural tube defect Any of a group of congenital anomalies involving the brain and spinal column that are caused by failure of the neural tube to close during embryonic development.

nonstress tests (NSTs) Fetal monitoring used in combination with maternal reports of fetal movement to evaluate fetal heart rate response.

parturition (par-too-rih'-shun) Act or process of giving birth to a child.

stereotactic An x-ray procedure to guide the insertion of a needle into a specific area of the breast.

teratogens Substances that result in severe fetal deformities.

vulva The external female genitalia, which begins at the mons pubis and terminates at the anus.

The branch of medicine that deals with pregnancy, labor, and the postnatal period is known as *obstetrics,* and the branch of medicine that deals with diseases of the genital tract in women is called *gynecology.* Frequently, a physician practices both specialties and is known as an *OB/GYN physician.* Assessment of the female reproductive system is an important part of healthcare. Often, patients are hesitant and uncomfortable with talking about sexual matters and wait until symptoms are intolerable or disease is advanced before seeking medical care. In addition to the signs and symptoms of disease, the medical assistant must be aware of the patient's emotional state and must give support when needed.

ANATOMY AND PHYSIOLOGY

The Female Reproductive System

The female reproductive system contains both internal and external organs. The internal organs are located within the pelvis and cannot be seen without special instrumentation, such as a vaginal speculum or a laparoscope. The external organs can be seen during the physical examination.

The primary parts of the female reproductive system are the **vulva,** vagina, uterus, fallopian tubes, and ovaries (Figure 40-1). The vulva includes the **clitoris,** the urethral meatus, and the

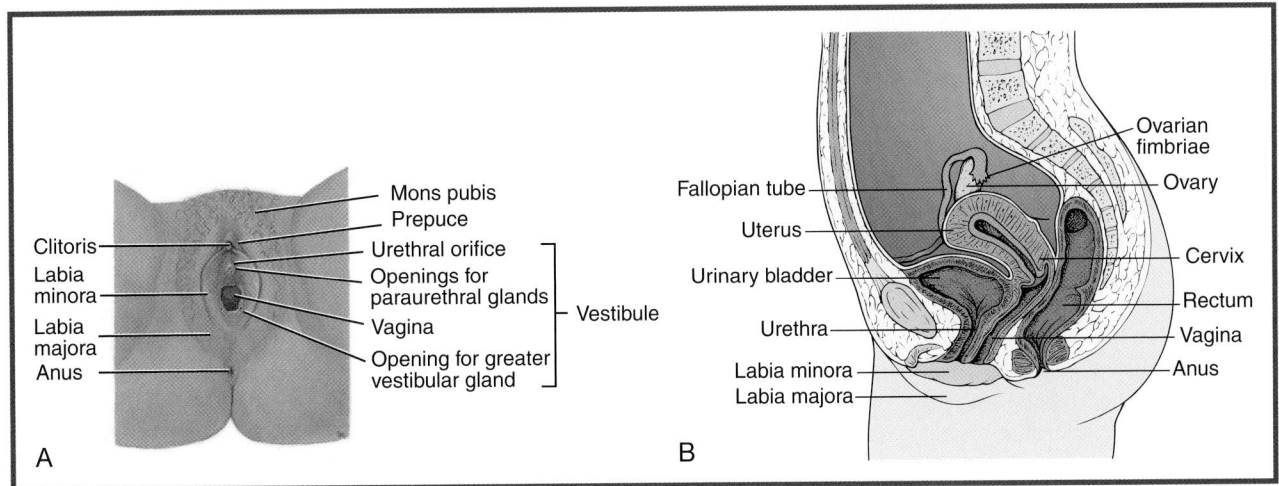

FIGURE 40-1 A, Female external genitalia. **B,** Normal female reproductive system. (*A,* From Applegate EJ: *The anatomy and physiology learning system,* ed 3, Philadelphia, 2006, Saunders; *B,* From Frazier MS, Drzymkowski JA: *Essentials of human diseases and conditions,* ed 3, Philadelphia, 2004, Saunders.)

vaginal orifice. These structures are covered by two sets of lips of tissue. The *labia minora* is a thin layer of skin extending from the top of the clitoris to the base of the vaginal opening. The external set is known as the *labia majora,* and these, along with the **mons pubis,** are covered with hair in the adult.

The vagina is the structure that connects the internal and external organs. This tubelike structure is constructed to receive the penis during **coitus.** It is lubricated by a mucous membrane lining, and its walls are made up of overlapping tissue in the form of *rugae* (overlapping tissue) so that the vagina can expand during the birth of an infant. At the distal end of the vagina is the cervix, often called the *neck of the uterus,* which is approximately 1 to 1½ inches long. The uterus is an upside-down pear-shaped muscular organ with the sole purpose of housing and nourishing the fetus from implantation shortly after conception until **parturition.** The uterine walls have three layers. The inner layer is the *endometrium,* which is rich in blood and changes in consistency during the menstrual cycle. The middle layer, or *myometrium,* is the powerful muscular layer that contracts to make the birth of the baby possible. The outer layer is the *perimetrium,* which protects the structure and attaches to ligaments that support and hold the uterus in place (Figure 40-2).

On both sides of the **fundus** of the uterus are the fallopian tubes, also called the *oviducts.* These tubes extend from the uterus to the ovaries but do not attach to the ovaries. The distal end of the tube opens freely into the abdominopelvic cavity and acts as the passageway for the ovum to the uterus and for the sperm as they search for the ovum. At the distal end of the fallopian tubes are finger-like projections called *fimbriae* which move in a wavelike pattern to draw the released ovum into the tube.

The ovaries are almond-shaped organs that produce and release the egg (ovum) and excrete hormones necessary for the development of secondary sexual characteristics and the maintenance of a pregnancy. The hormones progesterone and estrogen are secreted by the ovaries, and they regulate reproductive function. For pregnancy to occur, the vagina

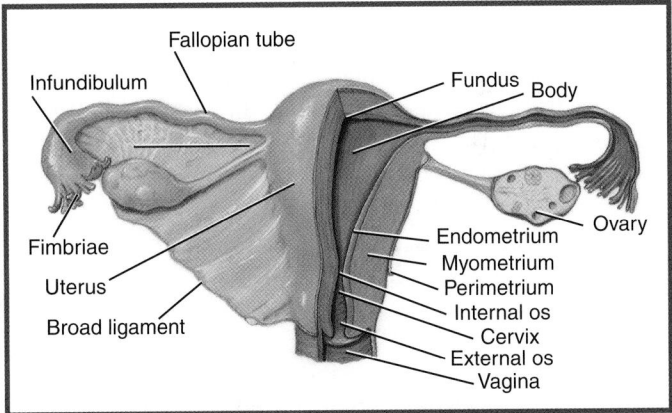

FIGURE 40-2 Uterus and fallopian tubes. (Modified from Applegate EJ: *The anatomy and physiology learning system,* ed 3, Philadelphia, 2006, Saunders.)

receives the sperm from the male; the sperm move up through the opening in the cervix called the *cervical os,* through the uterus, and into the fallopian tubes. As many as 200 to 600 million sperm can be deposited, with about 100,000 surviving the acidic content of the vagina to swim toward the egg.

Fertilization occurs when one sperm cell penetrates and fertilizes an egg. Fertilization usually takes place in the distal third of the fallopian tube. The tiny fertilized ovum, now called a *zygote,* moves by peristalsis and the massaging motion of the cilia that line the fallopian tube into the uterus and implants itself into the uterine wall. After implantation occurs, the placenta forms and will supply the new life with all the nourishment needed for its development. Once pregnancy begins, the serum levels of **human chorionic gonadotropin** (HCG) rise and the hormone spills into the female's urine, where it can be detected with a pregnancy test.

Breast Tissue

Mammary tissue develops from the increased estrogen secretion that occurs during puberty. In the center of each breast is a nipple surrounded by a pigmented region called the *areola.*

Inside the breast are 15 to 20 lobes with their subunits, the lobules of glandular tissue that are separated by connective support tissue and surrounded by adipose tissue. The amount and distribution of adipose tissue determines the size and shape of the breast (Figure 40-3). Breast tissue also contains mammary glands, modified sweat glands that become the organs of milk production, and a system of ducts for the delivery of milk to the nipple. Mammary ducts respond to elevated levels of estrogen and progesterone produced during the menstrual cycle by increasing in size, resulting in premenstrual fullness and tenderness of the breasts.

Four hormones control the mammary glands. *Estrogen* is responsible for the increase in size, *progesterone* stimulates the development of the duct system, *prolactin* stimulates the production of milk, and *oxytocin* causes the ejection of the milk from the glands.

Menstruation

When a girl enters puberty, one of the many changes that will occur is *menarche,* or the beginning of the menstrual cycle. This is a normal body process that occurs in every female and is the physiologic way of ridding her body of the thickened endometrial wall that develops during the 28-day cycle known as *menstruation.* This cycle involves a series of events controlled by hormones from the pituitary gland and ovaries. The 28-day cycle is divided into three phases: follicular phase, luteal phase, and menstrual phase.

Follicular Phase (Proliferative Phase)

The hypothalamus begins the follicular phase by secreting gonadotropin-releasing hormone (GnRH), stimulating the anterior pituitary to release follicle-stimulating hormone (FSH) and luteinizing hormone (LH). These hormones mature a graafian follicle that contains the ovum. The ovarian follicle secretes estrogen, which stimulates the growth of the endometrium. It takes approximately 9 days (to day 14 of the menstrual cycle) for the graafian follicle to ripen and bulge out from the ovarian wall. This wall becomes thinner as the follicle enlarges until it bursts, allowing the ovum to be liberated into the abdominal cavity. The expulsion of the egg ends the follicular phase. The fallopian fimbriae begin their wave-like motion to fan the ovum into the fallopian tube. The rupture spot on the ovary, now called the *corpus luteum,* begins to secrete progesterone. Ovulation causes an increase in body temperature, and some women experience cramping and tenderness in the lower abdominal area at this time as a result of the graafian follicle rupture.

Luteal Phase (Secretory Phase)

Once ovulation is complete, the luteal phase begins (day 15). During this phase, progesterone secreted from the corpus luteum

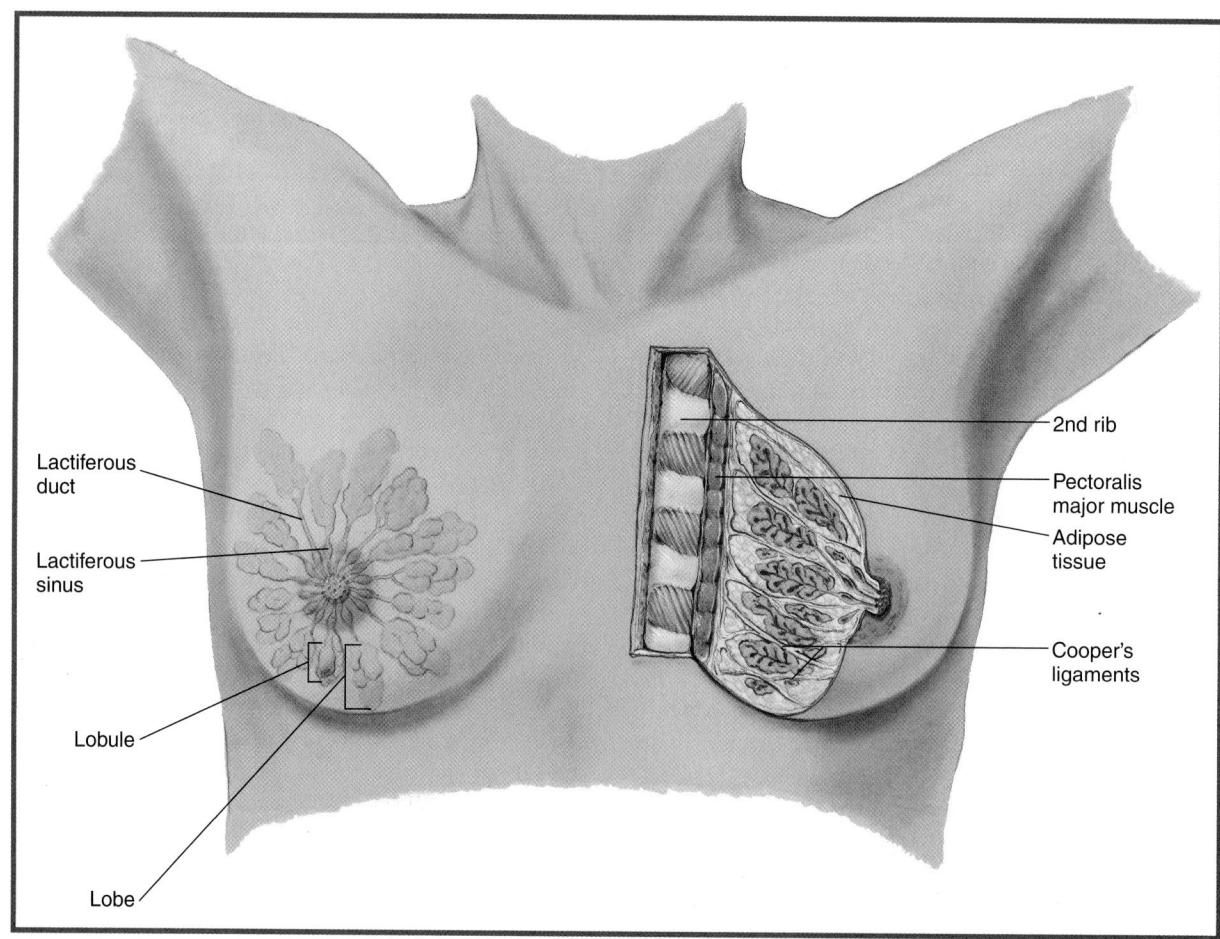

FIGURE 40-3 Normal female breast. (From Jarvis C: *Physical examination and health assessment,* ed 4, Philadelphia, 2004, Saunders.)

causes extensive growth of the endometrium as it prepares for a possible pregnancy. If conception occurs, the corpus luteum will continue to secrete progesterone until the placenta is well established and can secrete progesterone and HCG to maintain the pregnancy. If conception does not occur, HCG is not secreted and the corpus luteum will atrophy. Without increased levels of progesterone and HCG, the endometrium breaks down and menstruation begins.

Menstrual Phase

On day 28, menstruation begins. This discharge is made up of necrotic endometrial tissue, mucus, and the blood that was in the endometrial engorgement. As the uterus contracts to shed the excess tissue, a woman may experience cramping pain and irritability. This phase usually lasts approximately 5 days, then the follicular phase begins again.

Contraception

A woman's choice of a contraceptive method is based on many factors. To help patients make an informed choice, they should know about the risks, benefits, side effects, costs, failure rates, and convenience of each available method. In addition, although condoms are of only moderate success in preventing pregnancy, they should be used consistently to prevent transmission of sexually transmitted diseases (STDs). The medical assistant may help to conduct patient education on contraceptive methods. Table 40-1 summarizes the characteristics of various contraceptive methods.

Barrier Methods

Barrier methods of contraception either kill sperm through the use of a chemical spermicide or prevent their entry into the cervical os. Each method must be used every time intercourse

---

Factors to Consider When Choosing a Contraceptive Method

- Is it effective and safe?
- Does it conveniently match your sexual habits?
- Are you comfortable inserting contraceptive devices into your body?
- Are you at risk for serious side effects?
- Do you smoke?
- Can you afford it?
- Is it reversible?

---

occurs, which means the patient must be motivated to follow through with their use. Barrier methods are relatively inexpensive and include the condom, diaphragm, and cervical cap.

Patient education for the use of a diaphragm includes the following:

- Examine the diaphragm before each use by holding it up to a bright light to check for holes or cracks.
- Place 1 to 2 tablespoons of spermicidal jelly or cream into the diaphragm dome before insertion.
- Leave in place for 6 hours after intercourse; no douching until it is removed.
- Before repeated intercourse, add spermicide to the outside of the diaphragm with an applicator. Do not remove the diaphragm until 6 hours after the last intercourse.
- After removal, wash the diaphragm with soap and water, air dry, and inspect for breaks or holes before storing.
- The diaphragm should be refitted if the patient gains or loses more than 10 to 15 pounds; has a miscarriage, gives birth, or undergoes any type of pelvic surgery; or has

---

TABLE 40-1 Characteristics of Various Contraceptive Methods

TYPE	FAILURE RATE	CHARACTERISTICS	CONTRAINDICATIONS	SIDE EFFECTS
Condom (barrier method)	2%-10%	No prescription or examination needed; easily available; inexpensive	Latex allergy in either partner	Possible allergic response to latex or spermicide
Diaphragm or cervical cap (barrier method)	2%-19%	Must be fitted by clinician; requires instruction on how to insert and remove; spermicide must be used each time; leave in place 6 hr after intercourse (diaphragm)	Latex, rubber, or spermicidal allergy; uterine prolapse; severe cystocele or rectocele	Increased risk for UTI (diaphragm); increased risk abnormal Pap test (cap)
Intrauterine device (IUD)	2%-6%	Causes endometrial inflammation, preventing implantation of a fertilized egg	Cervicitis, vaginitis, endometriosis, pelvic infection, history of STD or ectopic pregnancy	Increased risk of PID; spotting in 10%-15% of users
Depo-Provera (DMPA)	0.5%	Requires 150-mg IM injection q3mo	Intention of becoming pregnant within 1 yr; breast cancer; liver disease	Return of fertility may be delayed 10-18 mo; headache, weight gain, depression possible
Oral contraceptives (OCPs) Hormonal patch Vaginal ring	1%	Suppress ovulation; atrophy the endometrium	Thrombolytic, liver, or coronary artery disease; breast, liver, reproductive tract cancer; smoker over 35; diabetes; sickle cell disease	Nausea, breakthrough bleeding, breast tenderness, fluid retention; hypertension, elevated lipid levels, blood clots, strokes

IM, intramuscular; *PID*, pelvic inflammatory disease; *STD*, sexually transmitted disease; *UTI*, urinary tract infection.

difficulty voiding or moving bowels with the diaphragm in place.

The cervical cap is a thimble-sized, domed barrier method that fits over the end of the cervix and also is used with spermicidal jelly. It is 92% to 96% effective if used properly. One of the advantages of this barrier method is that the cap can be inserted up to 12 hours before intercourse and can stay in place up to 72 hours without affecting effectiveness or safety.

Hormonal Contraceptives

Hormonal contraceptives are a highly effective and reversible form of contraception that work by inhibiting ovulation, changing the cervical mucosa, affecting sperm mobility, and preventing the thickening of the endometrial wall. Hormonal contraceptives include the birth control pill or patch, the vaginal ring, and Depo-Provera injections.

Besides being a highly effective method of birth control, oral contraceptives can be used to treat a wide range of gynecologic conditions, including menstrual irregularities, premenstrual syndrome (PMS) symptoms, anovulation, prevention of ovarian cysts, and may be prescribed to increase bone density. Their effectiveness, however, is based on daily administration. Failure rates are associated with noncompliance and can range from less than 1% in women who are highly compliant to more than 15% in those who do not take the pills as prescribed. Oral contraceptive pills (OCPs) can have serious side effects, so patients should be informed of conditions that require immediate medical attention. These can be remembered with the mnemonic ACHES: abdominal pain (new and severe), chest pain (new and severe), headaches (new or more frequent), eye problems (blurred or vision loss), and severe leg pain. These symptoms may indicate the formation of a blood clot in the abdomen, chest, or leg, or they may be indications of a stroke; blood clot formation and strokes are the most serious complications of taking OCPs.

A type of oral contraception, Seasonale, limits the number of menstrual periods to four per year although patients are more likely to have spotting and breakthrough bleeding with this hormone therapy than with the traditional 28-day birth control pill. It is designed to be taken once a day for 84 days and then an inactive dose for a week during which the woman would menstruate.

The first transdermal hormonal contraceptive patch, Ortho Evra, was introduced in 2001. The patch is a 1¾-inch square that slowly releases estrogen and progestin through the skin and into the bloodstream. It is considered as effective as oral contraceptives in women weighing less than 198 pounds. Women choosing the patch as a birth control method are exposed to 60% more estrogen than those taking OCPs. Because of this, patch users may be at greater risk of side effects. Side effects of the patch are similar to those of birth control pills, but the risk for heart attack, stroke, and blood clots may be slightly greater. Cigarette smoking increases the risk of serious cardiovascular side effects, especially if the patient is over 35. Patients should be told not to apply any creams or oils at the application site, change the patch weekly for 3 consecutive weeks, and go patch-free the fourth week, allowing menstruation to occur. The patch

can be applied to the buttocks, lower abdomen, and upper body but not the breasts. The woman can bathe, shower, and swim while wearing the patch, but if it comes off it should be replaced immediately.

The most recently developed hormonal contraceptive is a vaginal ring (NuvaRing), a device that is made of flexible plastic for insertion into the vagina. The ring slowly releases estrogen and progestin to prevent pregnancy and provide effective contraceptive action for 1 month after insertion. The device is 2 inches in diameter and can be inserted anywhere in the vagina, however, the deeper it is placed the less likely it will be felt after insertion. Side effects of the NuvaRing are similar to those of other hormonal contraceptives, and it may increase the risk of heart attack, stroke, and blood clots. When the patient first starts using the ring, an additional method of birth control must be used for the first week. If the ring falls out, it should be rinsed with warm water and reinserted within 3 hours. If it is out for more than 3 hours, then contraception is not certain and the patient should use another birth control method for 1 week.

Depo-Provera is an injectable contraceptive that contains high doses of progestin. Each dose prevents pregnancy for up to 3 months, but women must be compliant in returning to the healthcare facility for follow-up and repeat doses every 9 to 13 weeks. The first injection should be administered within the first 5 days of the menstrual period for birth control coverage. It is a highly effective method of contraception and is ideal for women who either do not comply with a birth control regimen or do not want to take a pill every day. However, the use of Depo-Provera for 2 years or longer may increase the risk of bone loss and eventual development of osteoporosis. Almost all patients using the injection will experience some menstrual irregularities, but these usually subside after two doses. Women using this form of hormonal contraception are not at risk for the side effects of estrogen exposure, such as an increased risk of blood clots and cardiovascular disease.

Intrauterine Devices

The intrauterine device (IUD) is a T-shaped plastic frame with threads attached that is inserted by the physician into the uterus to prevent pregnancy. Two types of IUDs are currently available: the copper (ParaGard) and the hormonal (Mirena). Both products inhibit fertilization by blocking the sperm's journey to the fallopian tubes, and if fertilization does occur they prevent the embryo from implanting to the uterine wall. In addition, ParaGard releases copper, which acts to slow sperm in the cervix, and Mirena releases progestin, which decreases sperm mobility and prevents the thickening of the endometrial wall during the menstrual cycle. Both types of IUDs are extremely effective— over 99%—in preventing pregnancy; copper types can remain in place as long as 10 years, whereas hormonal IUDs must be replaced every 5 years. The copper IUD may increase vaginal bleeding and menstrual pain, and the hormonal IUD results in both decreased menstrual flow and cramping. Shortly after an IUD is placed there is an increased risk of infection, so the physician may prescribe antibiotics before insertion to reduce this risk. To remove an IUD the physician gently withdraws it by pulling on the IUD string. In rare instances it must be removed surgically.

Permanent Methods

Both male and female patients can undergo surgical procedures that are considered permanent contraceptive methods. Vasectomies in the male were addressed in Chapter 39. For the female a bilateral tubal ligation can be performed in which a portion of both fallopian tubes is excised or ligated. The cost and rate of complications are higher for tubal ligations than for vasectomies. In addition, tubal ligations must be done on an outpatient basis with general anesthesia, so the woman has that additional risk. Both procedures can be reversed, but not always successfully.

CRITICAL THINKING APPLICATION

Dr. Beck's patients often ask questions about birth control methods, including the pros and cons of each. Although Betsy's former employer also prescribed contraceptives, Betsy was not involved in patient education. Dr. Beck expects Betsy to be aware of all birth control options, their characteristics and side effects, and any patient education details that might be requested or appropriate. Betsy has decided to create a reference sheet for herself that includes all these details. What should she include?

GYNECOLOGIC DISEASES AND DISORDERS

Menstrual Disorders and Conditions

Amenorrhea is the absence of menstruation for a minimum of 6 months; with oligomenorrhea, the woman has not experienced a period for 35 days to 6 months. The absence of menstruation outside pregnancy could be a result of a number of factors, including hormonal imbalances, thyroid disease, ovarian failure, or structural defects in the female sex organs. If a patient has established menstruation that stops, it is usually because of either a hypothalamus or a pituitary problem. Suppression of the hypothalamus can occur because of an eating disorder, stress, or extreme exercise resulting in low body-fat content.

Women who do not ovulate and therefore do not go through a monthly shedding of the endometrial wall of the uterus are at greater risk for cancer of the endometrium and the breast. Patients usually are started on oral contraceptives that artificially provide the hormones needed to create a monthly menstrual cycle. These women may experience fertility problems and require further testing and medical intervention to become pregnant.

Abnormal menstrual bleeding is a common cause of OB/GYN visits. *Menorrhagia* is excessive menstrual blood loss, such as a menses lasting longer than 7 days. The physician may ask the patient to count the number of tampons and pads used for several cycles to establish a method for determining an estimate of blood loss. A sign that a woman is losing excessive amounts of blood is iron deficiency anemia. *Metrorrhagia* is spotting or bleeding between menstrual cycles. The physician may prescribe oral contraceptives to atrophy the endometrium and lessen the bleeding. Surgical options for excessive menstrual flow are a **dilatation and curettage** (D&C) or, in extreme cases, a hysterectomy.

Endometriosis

Endometriosis is characterized by the presence of functional endometrial tissue outside the uterus. It is commonly found attached to the ovaries, urinary bladder, fallopian tubes, uterosacral ligaments, intestines, and peritoneum. Many hypotheses have been offered to explain this migration of endometrial tissue, but the most accepted is a retrograde flow during menstruation that causes menstrual fluid and stray endometrial cells to migrate out of the fallopian tubes and implant in the pelvic region. The use of tampons has been suggested as a possible cause. There is also a familial tendency, with 10 times greater risk for developing the disorder if the woman has a first-degree relative affected.

The ectopic endometrial tissue responds to routine hormone changes so that it proliferates, degenerates, and bleeds as the endometrium of the uterus does throughout the menstrual cycle. This causes inflammation at the site of the implantation that recurs with each cycle, ultimately leading to adhesions and obstructions of the affected tissue. The primary symptom of endometriosis is dysmenorrhea (painful menstruation). More than a third of affected patients also report dyspareunia (painful intercourse), and others complain of contact pain in the lower abdomen, pelvis, and back beginning 7 days before menses and lasting 3 days after onset. Other symptoms can include profuse menses, hematuria, rectal bleeding, nausea, vomiting, and abdominal cramps. Infertility is a serious problem for approximately 70% of the women afflicted with endometriosis because of the build up of scar tissue and adhesions in and around the fallopian tubes.

Conservative treatment through the use of hormones is recommended when the woman wants to have children. Treatment may consist of a laparoscopy to remove the ectopic endometrial tissue. Pharmaceutical treatment includes oral contraceptives used continuously to prevent bleeding or Depo-Provera injections. Leuprolide acetate (Lupron) injections may be prescribed intramuscularly every month for 6 months; however, Lupron puts the patient into a state of artificial menopause and can cause menopausal symptoms, including hot flashes, vaginal dryness, and bone density loss. In severe cases a total hysterectomy may be indicated. No cure is available, but pregnancy, nursing an infant, or natural menopause frequently causes remission (Figure 40-4).

CRITICAL THINKING APPLICATION

Melissa Steiner, a 19-year-old patient of Dr. Beck's, was diagnosed with endometriosis when she was 17. She has had two laparotomy procedures and continues to complain of moderate to severe pain before and during menstruation. What can Betsy tell her about the disease to help her understand why she has the pain? Melissa also wants to know about long-term complications, including the impact of the disease on fertility. She asks Betsy to help her understand Dr. Beck's explanation of the disease.

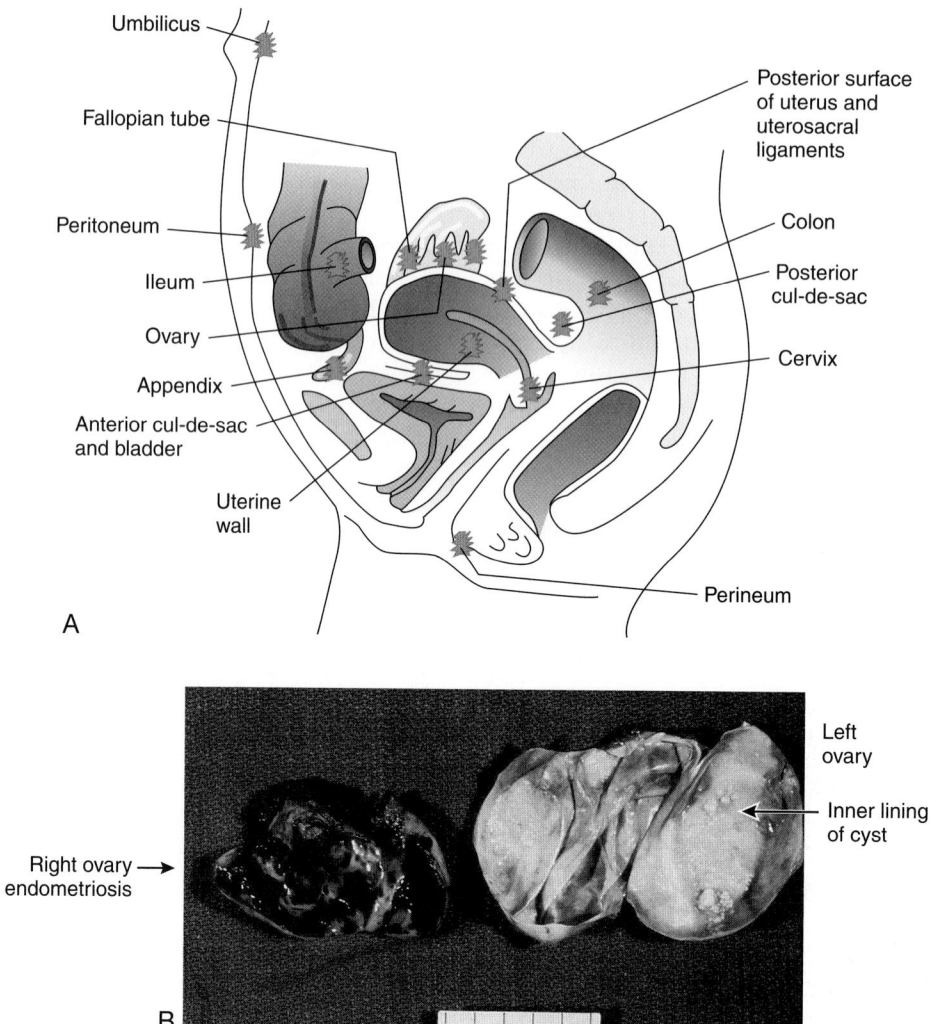

FIGURE 40-4 Endometriosis. **A,** Possible ectopic sites. **B,** Endometriosis involving right ovary (chocolate cyst) and left ovary showing the inner lining of a large cyst with excrescences. (*A,* From Gould BE: *Pathophysiology for the health professions,* ed 3, Philadelphia, 2006, Saunders; *B,* Courtesy RW Shaw, MD, North York General Hospital, Toronto, Ontario, Canada.)

Infections

Candidiasis

Candida albicans is the yeast-like fungus responsible for this infection. *Candida* organisms are commonly part of the normal flora of the mouth, skin, intestinal tract, and vagina. Overgrowth of the organism can be caused by antibiotic use, high estrogen levels, oral contraceptives, diabetes mellitus, and immunosuppression disorders, including acquired immuno-deficiency syndrome (AIDS). Candidiasis also can be spread through sexual contact. Symptoms include vulvovaginal itching; dry, bright-red vaginal tissue; and odorless, white, "cottage cheese" vaginal discharge. This infection is treated with prescription antifungal medications (miconazole or terconazole vaginal suppositories) and over-the-counter medications such as Monistat. A precipitating factor in the development of vaginal candidiasis is antibiotic therapy. To prevent the development of a fungal infection it is helpful for the patient to eat active-culture yogurt as well as drink acidophilus milk.

Bacterial Vaginosis

Bacterial vaginosis (BV) occurs when the normal level of bacteria in the vagina is disrupted and secondary bacteria begin to grow and infect tissue lining. Signs and symptoms include vaginal discharge, odor, pain, pruritus, or burning. Although BV is the most common vaginal infection in women of childbearing age in the United States, it does not usually cause complications. However, an infection of the vagina appears to make women more susceptible to STDs including human immunodeficiency virus (HIV), may lead to pelvic inflammatory disease (PID) if the infection spreads, and in pregnant women is associated with premature or low–birth-weight infants. Because of this, antibiotic therapy is especially important for pregnant women. The antibiotics of choice are either metronidazole or clindamycin.

Cervicitis

Cervicitis is an inflammation of the cervix caused by an invading organism. The main sign is a thick, purulent, whitish discharge with an acrid odor. Dysuria may also be present. Cervicitis can occur after vaginal delivery from an infected cervical laceration. Treatment consists primarily of antibiotics, although cauterization may be indicated when cervical erosion exists.

Pelvic Inflammatory Disease (PID)

PID is any acute or chronic infection of the reproductive system ascending from the vagina (*vaginitis*), cervix (*cervicitis*), uterus (*endometritis*), fallopian tubes (*salpingitis*), and ovaries (*oophoritis*). In these cases the fallopian tubes may contain pus or may be deformed by chronic attacks of inflammation or adhesions. PID is caused by vaginosis, gonorrhea, or chlamydia; or it can develop after pelvic surgery, tubal examinations, and abortion. It accounts for a large percentage of cases of infertility in women, primarily because of the formation of adhesions in the fallopian tubes that prevent the migration of the ovum through the tube. The patient may be asymptomatic or may complain of purulent vaginal discharge, fever, malaise, dysuria, lower abdominal pain, bleeding, nausea, and vomiting. Cultures of cervical discharge are typically done to determine the pathogenic organism. Treatment should include broad-spectrum antibiotic therapy such as Floxin with Flagyl or Rocephin with Vibramycin. If cultures are positive for an STD, treatment of the partner is necessary for the patient to be cured without reinfection.

Sexually Transmitted Diseases

The list of infectious diseases spread by sexual contact continues to grow. These diseases are considered the most common contagious diseases in the United States. All STDs are transmitted from one person to another through body fluids such as blood, semen, and vaginal secretions during vaginal, anal, or oral sex (Figure 40-5). A summary of STDs was included in Chapter 39. In this chapter we focus on the impact of STDs on women.

The human papillomavirus (HPV), which causes genital warts, is of special concern to women. The infection may be asymptomatic up to 2 years after exposure, however, whether the virus causes symptomatic wart development or not, the infection can lead to serious complications in women. HPV is typically first diagnosed by abnormal Pap test results because all 30 of the identified HPV strains can cause Pap test abnormalities. A positive Pap test result is followed up with an HPV DNA test to diagnose the specific strain of HPV that caused the infection. Although the majority of women have healthy immune systems that can successfully clear the virus without developing future health problems, approximately 10 HPV strains are linked to the development of cervical carcinoma. Women diagnosed with one of these carcinogen strains must have regular Pap testing, usually every 3 to 6 months, for early detection and treatment of precancerous and cancerous cells on the cervix.

Trends in Reportable Sexually Transmitted Diseases

- Inflammatory STDs can facilitate the transmission of HIV infection.
- Chlamydia is known as the "silent" STD because 75% of infected women and 50% of infected men are asymptomatic. An estimated 40% of women with untreated chlamydia infections develop PID, with resultant infertility in 20% of those. African American women are diagnosed almost eight times more frequently than white women. The highest rates are seen in 15- to 19-year-olds. The Centers for Disease Control and Prevention (CDC) recommends yearly chlamydia screening for sexually active women under age 26 and those older with risk factors including new or multiple sex partners. Women infected with chlamydia are up to five times more likely to become infected with HIV if exposed. If chlamydia is diagnosed, the patient and partner should abstain from sexual intercourse until treatment is completed, to prevent reinfection.
- Gonorrhea is a major cause of PID. Most affected women are asymptomatic. Transmission can occur during vaginal birth, causing fetal blindness, joint infection, or a life-threatening blood infection. Pregnant women should be treated as soon as gonorrhea is diagnosed to reduce these risks.
- Congenital syphilis can cause stillbirth, neonatal death, physical deformities, and neurologic complications.
- Approximately one out of four women has a genital herpes simplex virus (HSV) infection, which can cause potentially fatal infections in babies. Initial exposure during pregnancy carries a greater risk of fetal transmission.
- At least 50% of sexually active men and women acquire genital human papillomavirus (HPV) infection at some point in their lives. By age 50, at least 80% of women will have acquired genital HPV infection.
- Trichomoniasis is the most common curable STD in young, sexually active women. Symptoms usually appear in women within 5 to 28 days of exposure. Pregnant women with trichomoniasis may have premature or low–birth-weight (less than 5 lb) infants.
- HIV can cross the placenta during pregnancy, infect the baby during birth, and is found in breast milk. Cesarean birth may be recommended to decrease the risk of transmission during the birth process.
- Women who test negative for hepatitis B may receive the hepatitis B vaccine during pregnancy.

A recently developed immunization, Gardasil, is now available to protect women who have not yet been infected by HPV. It is the first vaccine designed to prevent diseases caused by specific strains of HPV, including cervical cancer, precancerous genital lesions, and genital warts. The vaccine is approved for use in females 9 to 26 years of age. It is effective against the two HPV types that cause approximately 70% of cervical cancers and it can prevent 90% of genital warts outbreaks. The vaccine is administered in three separate doses over a 6- month period with a projected cost of $360.

Table 40-2 summarizes the effect of STDs on women. As mentioned in Chapter 39, individuals aged 35 to 39 years

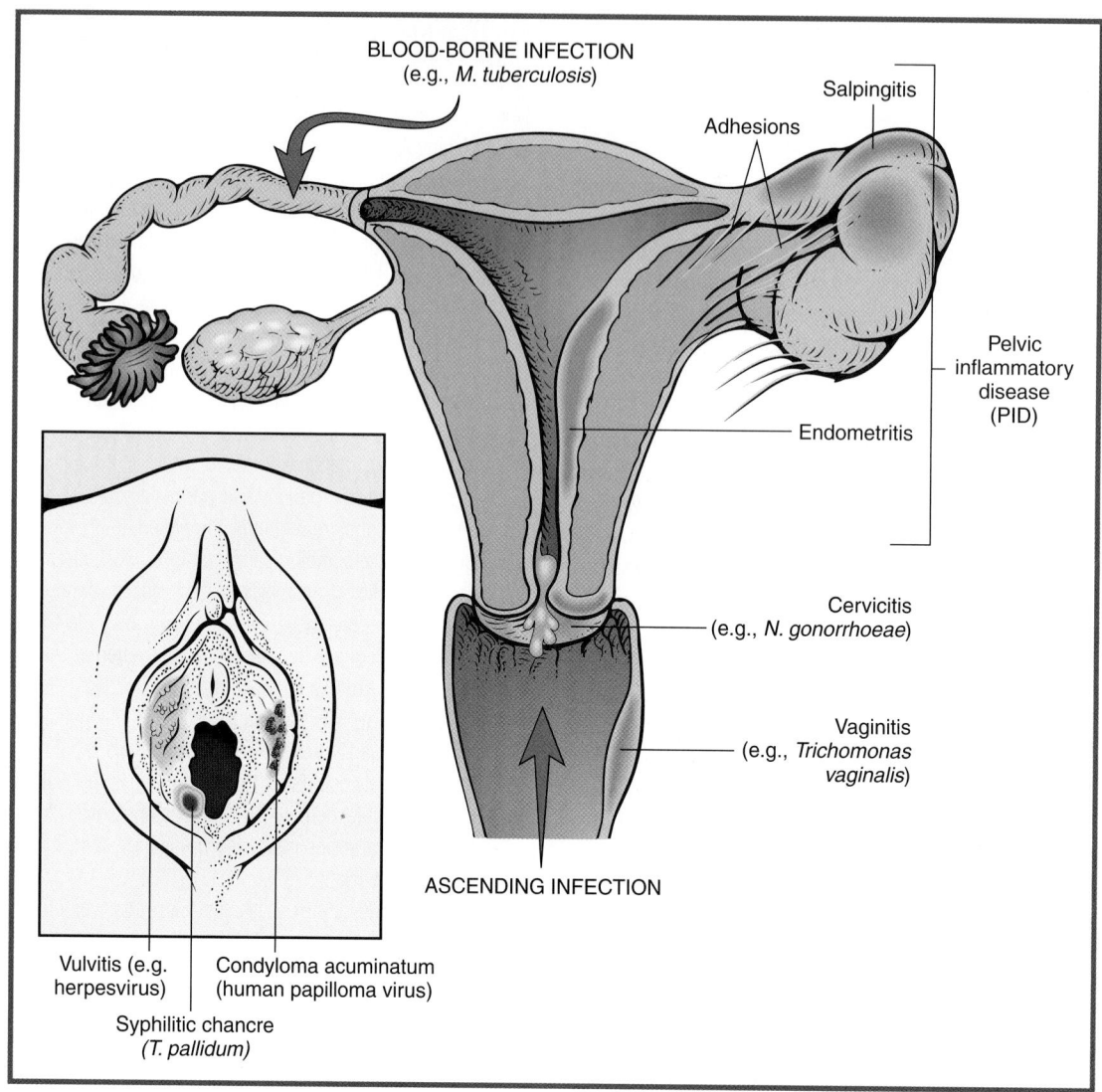

FIGURE 40-5 Ascending infections of the female genital organs are usually caused by sexual contact, pregnancy, or instrumentation. Descending infections usually begin in the blood or lymph nodes. (From Damjanov I: *Pathology for the health-related professions*, ed 3, Philadelphia, 2006, Saunders.)

have the highest reported incidence of HIV and AIDS. The percentage of women and girls with HIV is declining largely because of educational emphasis on the use of condoms; however, heterosexual exposure still accounts for 80% of the HIV cases diagnosed each year. Because HIV can be transmitted through the placenta to the developing fetus, it is crucial that women be diagnosed either before pregnancy or as early in the pregnancy as possible. Treatment of HIV-positive pregnant women with a three-part ZDV (zidovudine, AZT, or Retrovir) regimen decreases the risk of HIV infection in the infant by almost 70%. This treatment protocol recommends that pregnant women start taking ZDV at 14 to 34 weeks, have it administered intravenously during labor and delivery, and have it given to the infant every 6 hours for 6 weeks after birth. Some AIDS drugs are very dangerous for developing infants, so a woman currently receiving treatment may have her medication regimen altered during pregnancy. HIV-positive women should never breastfeed since the virus is present in breast milk.

CRITICAL THINKING APPLICATION

A 28-year-old patient was recently diagnosed with an acute gonorrheal and chlamydial infection. She has had HPV since she was 22. Dr. Beck asks Betsy to give her patient education materials, including potential long-term complications of HPV, and to confirm that she understands the signs and symptoms of STDs in herself and her partner. What should Betsy include in the information?

Benign Tumors

Fibroid Tumors

Uterine fibroid tumors, also called *fibromyomas, leiomyomas,* or *myomas,* are **idiopathic** benign tumors composed mainly of smooth muscle and some fibrous connective tissue. These tumors appear to have a genetic link because they tend to run in families. Fibroids vary in number, size, and location in the uterus and are quite common. Menorrhagia is the primary

TABLE 40-2   Sexually Transmitted Diseases and Women

DISEASE (CAUSATIVE ORGANISM)	SIGNS AND SYMPTOMS	TREATMENT
Chlamydia (*Chlamydia trachomatis*)	Dysuria; urinary frequency; abdominal pain; increased or decreased vaginal discharge. May cause endometritis, PID, and urethritis. Transmission to newborn can occur during vaginal delivery; causes neonatal eye infections and pneumonia.	Curable with antibiotic therapy; azithromycin (Zithromax), tetracycline, or Vibramycin
Genital herpes simplex virus (HSV-2)	Painful genital vesicles and ulcers; erythema and pruritus; tingling or shooting pain 1-2 days before outbreak; cycle through episodes. Viral shedding may occur during asymptomatic periods. Newborns can be infected by active lesions in vagina at birth. Brain damage, blindness, or death of the newborn may occur. Cesarean section if active lesions at time of birth. Increases risk for cervical cancer.	No cure, but antiviral therapy during episodes shortens duration of lesions; acyclovir (Zovirax), famciclovir (Famvir), or valacyclovir (Valtrex)
Genital warts (HPV)	Most prevalent STD; period of communicability is unknown; lesions seen more frequently in women; tend to recur; 25% of women with HPV develop invasive cervical cancer, should be followed with routine (every 3-6 months) Pap smears.	Goal of treatment is to remove symptomatic warts; cryotherapy to lesions; podofilox solution or imiquimod cream to lesions
Gonorrhea (*Neisseria gonorrhoeae*)—bacteria	Dysuria; urinary frequency; abdominal pain; increased or decreased vaginal discharge. May cause endometritis, PID, and urethritis.	Curable with antibiotic therapy; cefixime (Suprax), azithromycin, doxycycline
Syphilis (*Treponema pallidum*)—Spirochete bacteria	Six stages that can affect multiple body systems; 10- to 90-day incubation; initial sign is a painless lesion, or chancre, at the exposure site (vulva or vagina); serous discharge from chancre; lymphadenopathy. If not diagnosed and treated will advance to further stages. Can infect fetus via the placenta, resulting in congenital syphilis.	Penicillin G (Wycillin); if allergic to penicillin, doxycycline or tetracycline
Trichomoniasis (*T. vaginalis*)—protozoa	May be asymptomatic; urinary frequency, urgency, and dysuria; frothy yellow-green vaginal discharge; pruritus.	Metronidazole (Flagyl); need to treat partner

HPV, human papillomavirus; *PID*, pelvic inflammatory disease; *STD*, sexually transmitted disease.

symptom, although the patient may experience bladder or rectal pressure, pelvic pressure, pain, abdominal distortion, and infertility. Fibroid tumors affect premenopausal women because they consist of estrogen-sensitive cells. Fibroid tumors do not recur and do not undergo malignant transformation; therefore patients with fibroid tumors have an excellent prognosis. Treatment depends on the severity of the symptoms and the patient's age, because fibroid tumors tend to become smaller and calcify after menopause. The masses can be removed surgically, or a hysterectomy may be indicated if bleeding is a serious problem (Figure 40-6).

Ovarian Cysts

Ovarian cysts are sacs of fluid or semisolid material that form on or near the ovaries. They can occur in the follicle or the corpus luteum anytime between puberty and menopause. Most cysts are benign, and those that are small and asymptomatic do not require treatment. Large or multiple cysts may cause discomfort, low back pain, nausea, vomiting, and abnormal uterine bleeding. These can be treated with birth control pills over a period of several months to reduce the size of the cysts or prevent the development of new cysts in the future. If pharmaceutical therapy is not sufficient, laparoscopic procedures can be done to

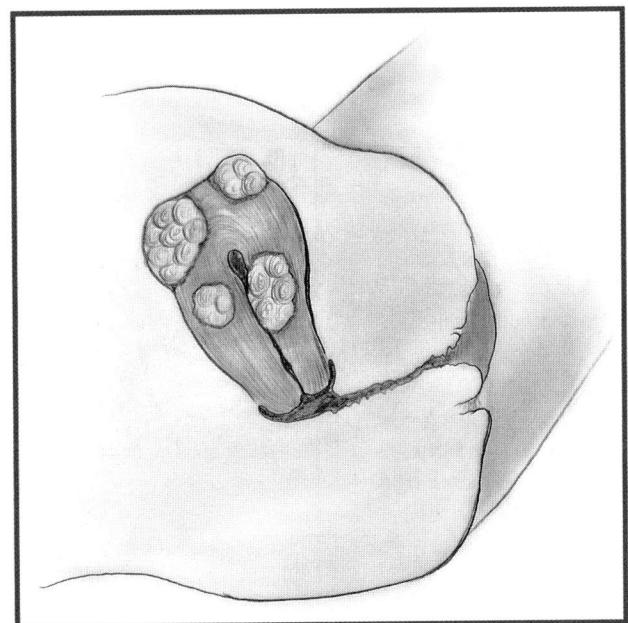

FIGURE 40-6 Uterine fibroid tumors are composed of hormone-sensitive cells. (Redrawn from Jarvis C: *Physical examination and health assessment*, ed 4, Philadelphia, 2004, Saunders.)

drain large cysts or remove them. Surgery may be indicated if a cyst ruptures or if torsion (twisting and cutting off of the blood supply) of the ovary occurs.

A disorder of the ovaries, *polycystic ovary syndrome*, is a hormonal problem that may cause cysts to develop over enlarged ovaries. Diagnosis is dependent on the presence of two or more indicators, including irregular or no menstruation, high testosterone levels, *hirsutism* (excessive body hair in a masculine pattern), acne, and male pattern baldness *(alopecia)*. Women affected by this disorder have unusually high levels of testosterone, estrogen, and LH with decreased amounts of FSH and may be initially diagnosed because of fertility problems. The combination of hormone irregularities causes the symptoms associated with the disorder; however, some women are diagnosed by menstrual irregularity alone. These women are at greater risk for uterine cancer because the endometrium does not slough off on a monthly basis. There appears to be a link with insulin and cholesterol metabolism, so women with this disorder are at greater risk for developing type 2 diabetes mellitus and heart disease. Treatment is with OCPs to stimulate menses artificially, to lower androgen levels, and to reduce masculine-type symptoms if they are present.

Fibrocystic Breast Disease

Fibrocystic breast disease is the presence of multiple palpable nodules in the breasts that are usually associated with pain and tenderness and that fluctuate with the menstrual cycle (Figure 40-7). Over time, the cysts enlarge and the connective tissue of the breast is replaced with fibrous tissue that is dense and firm. The masses may be fibrous tumors that have degenerated or sacs filled with fluid. The cysts feel firm and movable, and the degree of tenderness and size depend on the point in the menstrual cycle, with tenderness peaking just before and during the secretory phase. Several different cellular types of cysts can form, but fibrocystic changes in the breast are not considered precancerous.

Although the risk of breast cancer is not increased with fibrocystic breast disease, the diagnosis of cancerous breast masses

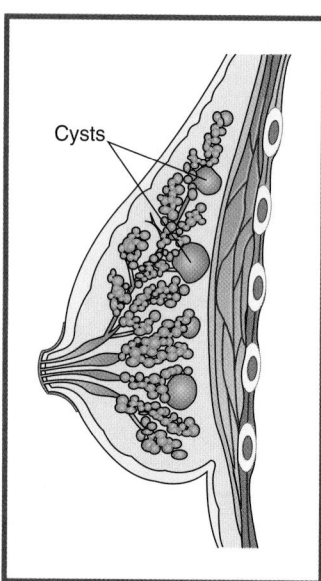

FIGURE 40-7 Fibrocystic breast disease.

Cysts

becomes more complicated. Because the breasts consistently feel lumpy, breast examinations may not isolate a suspicious mass. In addition, accurate mammography screening is complicated by the dense nature of the cysts, making visualization of a cancerous area more difficult. Because caffeine and high-fat diets aggravate the symptoms of fibrocystic breast disease, diet therapy is often recommended. Patients should be encouraged to perform monthly breast self-examination (BSE) and report any changes in the breast immediately.

Malignant Tumors

Most problems encountered with the female reproductive organs are related to abnormal cell growth. Early screening and preventive intervention are essential. Most malignant tumors require surgical removal. Radiation, chemotherapy, and hormone therapy are alternative treatment choices.

Cervical Cancer

It is estimated that half of the cervical cancer cases occurring in women between 35 and 55 years of age are a result of HPV infection. The first stage of cervical cancer is asymptomatic, but early diagnosis of cervical cellular changes is possible with a Papanicolaou (Pap) smear. During the invasive stage the patient will report abnormal vaginal bleeding and persistent discharge as well as bleeding and pain during intercourse. The average age of diagnosis for *carcinoma in situ* (cancerous cells restricted to original site) is currently 35 but continues to drop because of an increasing number of cases occurring in young women. The American Cancer Society recommends that all sexually active women and those over the age of 18 have annual Pap smears (Procedure 40-1). Women with HPV infection may be tested every 3 to 6 months, depending on previous Pap results.

The patient should be informed of factors that can interfere with Pap test results, including menstruation and the use of vaginal creams, spermicidal foams, and douching 2 to 3 days before the examination; the patient should refrain from vaginal intercourse for 24 hours before the examination because it may cause inflammation. The medical assistant should include in the patient history the use of certain medications, such as tetracycline, which may interfere with results; whether the patient has a latex allergy; the date of the last menstrual period (LMP); whether the patient has a history of a bleeding disorder or is taking anticoagulant medications; and whether the patient is pregnant or may be pregnant.

The physician obtains the cervical smear with a Cytobrush or small wooden spatula that is inserted and rotated in the cervical canal to obtain endocervical cells for cytology. The ThinPrep Pap Test is replacing the traditional slide preparation method for analyzing these cells because it is more accurate in diagnosing precancerous and cancerous lesions and rarely has to be repeated because of an inadequate cellular sample. The physician uses the same technique to collect the cellular sample, but instead of fixing it onto a glass slide, the collection device is rinsed into a vial containing a preservative solution. In the laboratory a processor filters the sample and creates a slide with a thin layer of cervical cells that is more uniform and better preserved than is possible with the traditional method.

Prepare Patient for and Assist with Routine and Specialty Examinations: Assist with Examination of the Female Patient and Pap Smear

CAAHEP COMPETENCY: 3.b.(4)(e), 3.b.(4)(f)
ABHES COMPETENCY: 4.b, 4.h

GOAL: *To assist the physician in the examination of a female patient and performance of diagnostic Pap smear.*

EQUIPMENT and SUPPLIES

- Patient gown
- Lubricant
- 4- × 4-inch gauze squares
- Laboratory requisition slips
- Drape sheet
- Examination light
- Cervical spatula and Cytobrush
- ThinPrep container
- Vaginal speculum
- Uterine sponge forceps
- Disposable examination gloves
- Urine specimen container if needed
- Stool for occult blood test if needed
- Biohazard waste container
- Patient record
- Appropriate patient education materials

PROCEDURAL STEPS

1. Assemble the materials needed, and prepare the room. Prepare the equipment and supplies needed for the Pap smear.
2. Wash your hands. Follow standard precautions.
   PURPOSE: Infection control.
3. Identify the patient, and briefly explain the procedure.
   PURPOSE: Explanations gain patient cooperation and alleviate apprehension.
4. Instruct the patient to empty the bladder and collect a urine specimen if needed.
   PURPOSE: Organ palpations are performed on an empty bladder.
5. Instruct the patient to disrobe completely and to put on a gown with the opening in the front.
6. Assist the physician with the breast examination. Patient should start by sitting at the end of the examination table. Drape the patient, and assist the physician with the examination. Provide reassurance to the patient as needed.
7. When the physician is ready to examine the breasts and the abdomen with the patient in the supine position, assist the patient into the supine position and drape as needed.
   PURPOSE: To avoid exposing the patient unnecessarily.
8. When the physician is ready to begin the vaginal examination, assist the patient into the lithotomy position. Have the patient slide down to the end of the table, placing her legs in the stirrups, the knees should be relaxed and rotated outward. Remember always to position the patient while she is underneath the drape.
9. Direct the light source onto the perineal while she is area.
   PURPOSE: Facilitates better viewing of the cervix.
10. Don gloves. Warm the stainless steel vaginal speculum in warm water (physician may prefer disposable plastic speculum). Pass the proper instruments to the physician in proper sequence. Physician will need the Cytobrush for cervical cells and spatula for the cervical sample.
    PURPOSE: Teamwork enhances efficiency.
11. Assist the physician with ThinPrep preparation if desired by swirling the cervical specimen in the preservative solution at least 10 times to ensure that the specimen has been mixed with the preservative solution.
12. Label the specimen container, and place it in a biohazard bag.
13. Apply water-soluble lubricant to the physician's fingers.
    PURPOSE: Facilitates the bimanual examination.
14. Physician may prepare stool for occult blood testing after rectal examination. Have materials ready.
15. Instruct the patient to breathe deeply through the mouth with hands crossed over the chest.
    PURPOSE: Helps relax muscles.
16. Place the soiled instruments in a basin.
    PURPOSE: Helps produce better aesthetic surroundings.
17. Assist the patient off the table and with dressing if needed.
18. While the patient is in the dressing room, clean the room, removing used equipment.
19. Sanitize and sterilize stainless steel equipment. Remove gloves and wash your hands.
    PURPOSE: Infection control.
20. Prepare the Pap smear and other samples for transportation to the laboratory. Complete the requisitions including patient's LMP date and whether she is on hormone therapy.
21. Record all procedures on the patient's medical record.
    PURPOSE: A procedure is not done until it is entered into the patient's record.

See Appendix D for a charting example.

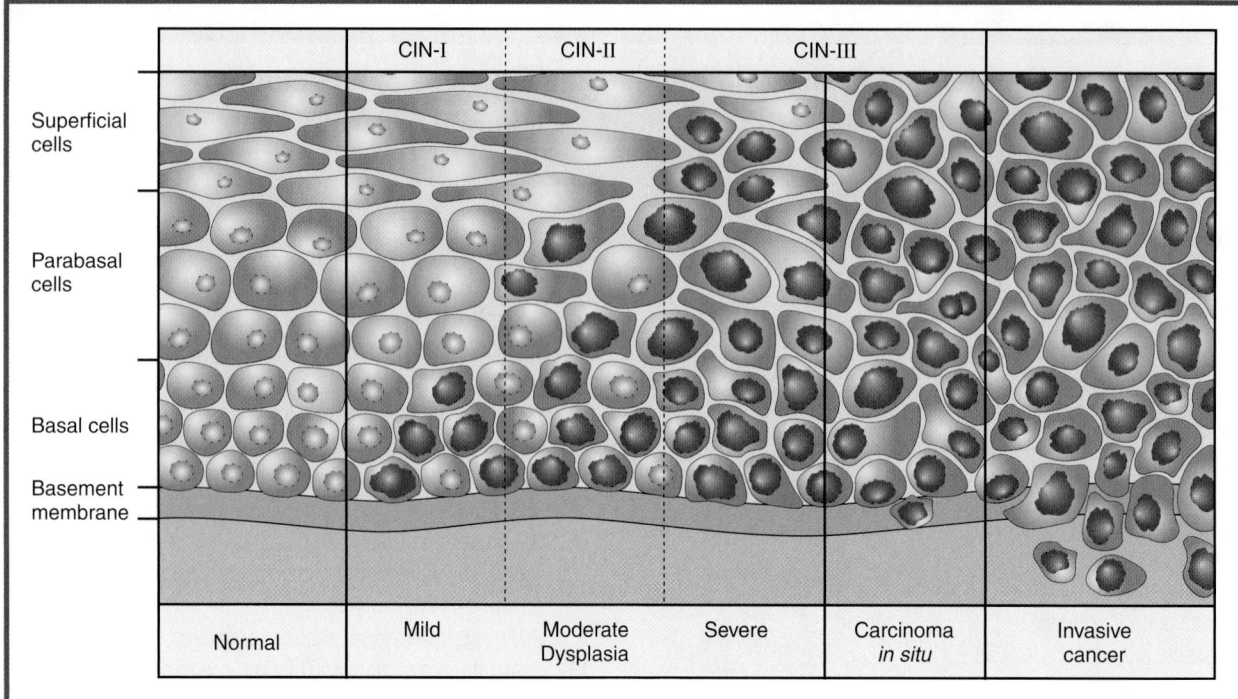

FIGURE 40-8 Carcinoma of the cervix. (From Damjanov I: *Pathology for the health-related professions*, ed 3, Philadelphia, 2006, Saunders.)

The pathologist examines the slide to determine the presence of cellular abnormalities. Results are classified into one of five categories: negative or normal; atypical squamous cells; abnormal with low-grade squamous lesions; abnormal with high-grade lesions (precancerous); or carcinoma cells. Inflammation or STD infection can cause abnormal changes in cervical cells, so the physician will decide how to manage abnormal results based on other diagnostic studies.

If the Pap test indicates abnormal cells, the pathologist can grade cervical changes using a *cervical intraepithelial neoplasia* (CIN) system of I to III, depending on the degree of cellular **dysplasia** (Figure 40-8). CIN I indicates mild-to-moderate dysplasia; CIN II, moderate and moderate-to-severe dysplasia; and CIN III, carcinoma in situ. Patients whose Pap smears indicate dysplasia of any severity should have a colposcopy with biopsy if indicated and possibly an **endocervical curettage** or conization procedure. If adequately diagnosed and treated, carcinoma in situ of the cervix has a 100% survival rate at 5 years.

If the patient is diagnosed with carcinoma of the cervix, it is classified with the following stages:

- Stage 0: Carcinoma in situ
- Stage I: Carcinoma of the cervix with no **adnexal** involvement
- Stage II: Carcinoma of the cervix with minimal adnexal invasion
- Stage III: Carcinoma of the cervix with involvement to the pelvic area
- Stage IV: Carcinoma of the cervix with involvement of structures outside the pelvic area

Colposcopy is the visual examination of the vagina and the cervical surfaces through the use of a colposcope (Figure 40-9). The colposcope is a microscope with a light source and a magnifying lens that can be used during a vaginal examination to locate and evaluate abnormal cells and detect cancer of the cervix in its early stages, examine tissue from which an abnormal Pap smear has been obtained, and monitor areas of the cervix from which malignant lesions have been removed. Colposcopy can also be used to monitor women who are at risk for developing cervical cancer because their mothers were given diethylstilbestrol (DES) during their pregnancy. A cervical biopsy may be performed in conjunction with a colposcopy. One of the major advantages of obtaining a biopsy during a colposcopy is that the instrument permits visualization of the suspicious area so that the biopsy can be taken from the most atypical site.

Colposcopy is a relatively safe and painless procedure that is performed in the physician office setting. Discomfort may

DES

DES is a synthetic estrogen that was prescribed from 1938 to 1971 to pregnant women to prevent miscarriages and premature births. An estimated 5 to10 million pregnant women in the United States and their unborn children were exposed to DES during this time. Subsequent research revealed potential health risks from the DES exposure which include:

- Women prescribed DES while pregnant have an increased risk for breast cancer.
- Women exposed to DES in utero (DES Daughters) have an increased risk of cancer of the vagina and cervix, reproductive tract structural abnormalities, pregnancy complications, and infertility.
- Men exposed to DES in utero have an increased risk for noncancerous cysts in the epididymis.

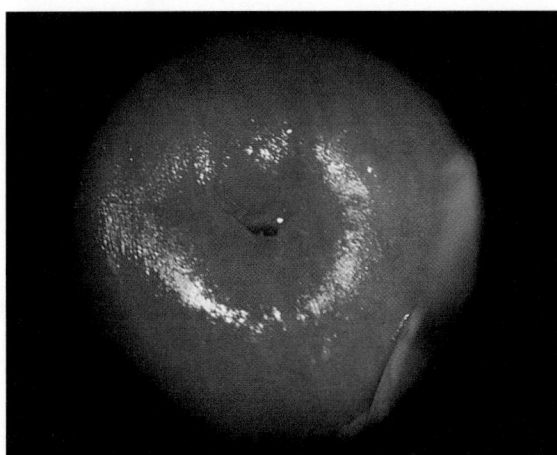

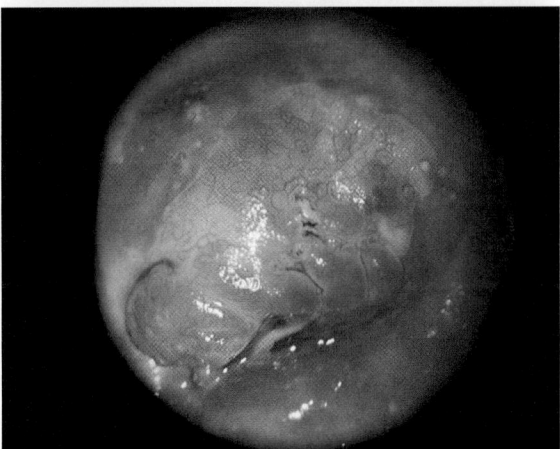

FIGURE 40-9 Colposcopic appearance of normal cervix (top) and abnormal cervix (bottom). (From Damjanov I: *Pathology for the health-related professions*, ed 3, St Louis, 2006, Saunders.)

occur when the speculum is inserted into the vagina to improve visualization of the tissue. Discomfort and bleeding can occur when tissue is taken for biopsy. Depending on the results of a previous biopsy, the patient may need a more extensive procedure or *conization* done, which removes a cone-shaped wedge of cervical tissue for either treatment or further analysis. Some physicians prefer the less invasive *loop electrosurgical excision procedure* (LEEP), which is performed with injection of a local anesthetic to the cervix and insertion of a wire loop into the vagina. A high-frequency electrical current running through the wire is used to remove abnormal tissue from both the cervix and the endocervical canal. Like conization, LEEP can be used as a diagnostic tool to collect biopsy samples and as a treatment to remove abnormal tissue.

Depending on the condition of the cervix, *cryosurgery*, or the application of freezing temperatures, may be used to treat chronic cervicitis and cervical erosion problems. Freezing causes cellular necrosis, and in approximately 1 month the dead cells are replaced with healthy cells. The procedure involves placing a probe against the problem area on the cervix and applying liquid nitrogen to the area for approximately 3 or 4 minutes or until the site is frozen (Procedure 40-2). The patient may experience some pain for 30 minutes or so after the procedure

and a slight watery discharge for up to a week. If any signs of infection, foul discharge, or pain develop, the patient should call the physician's office. She is advised not to engage in sexual intercourse for 1 month and to expect a heavier than usual menstrual flow for the first cycle after the procedure.

Endometrial Cancer

The inner lining of the uterus, the endometrium, is at increased risk for dysplasia in postmenopausal women who never had children and those who experienced early menarche and late menopause. This slow-growing cancer begins with hyperplasia of the endometrial wall, followed by dysplasia. Early signs are irregular vaginal bleeding and leukorrhea (white or yellow) vaginal discharge. Diagnosis usually is made with an endometrial biopsy, and treatment is a complete hysterectomy with radiation and chemotherapy. Because most of these tumors develop after menopause, vaginal bleeding is unusual, which makes it more likely the woman will seek medical attention. Because of this, early diagnosis and treatment lead to almost a 90% survival rate.

Ovarian Cancer

Ovarian neoplasms are the most important pathologic disorder of the ovaries. Ovarian cancer is the second most common gynecologic cancer but is ranked first in gynecologic cancer deaths. In fact, it causes more deaths than all other tumors of the reproductive system combined. Metastasis has occurred in 71% of the cases before the tumor is diagnosed. Symptoms do not appear until the tumor has enlarged enough to exert pressure on nearby structures, with patients presenting with vague abdominal discomfort, bloating, urinary urgency, weight loss, and general malaise.

Researchers are working to perfect a blood test that can be used to screen for ovarian cancer so the disease can be diagnosed in earlier, more treatable stages. Currently, ovarian cancer is diagnosed by a combination of a pelvic examination that indicates a mass in an ovary; a cancer antigen (CA)–125 blood test, which identifies a protein that is found in abnormally high levels in women with ovarian cancer (although there are false-positive and false-negative results with this examination); and a pelvic or transvaginal ultrasound to evaluate the size and shape of the ovaries. The ultimate diagnosis is based on a biopsy to confirm the presence of cancerous cells.

Little is known about how or why ovarian cancer occurs, but pregnancy, breastfeeding, and oral contraceptive use may reduce the risk. Treatment includes a complete hysterectomy (removal of the uterus, fallopian tubes, and ovaries), radiation, and chemotherapy. Ovarian tumors are classified on the basis of their biologic features. About 20% of all ovarian tumors are cancerous, and the recovery rate is linked to the location, stage of the tumor development, and age of the patient.

Breast Cancer

Breast cancer is the second leading cause of cancer deaths in women. According to the American Cancer Society, one in every eight women has a lifetime risk of developing breast cancer and a 1 in 28 risk of dying from the disease. Predisposing factors include family history of breast cancer (especially in

PROCEDURE 40-2

Prepare Patient for and Assist with Procedures, Treatments, and Minor Office Surgeries: Prepare the Patient for Cryosurgery

CAAHEP COMPETENCIES: 3.b.(4)(e), 3.b.(4)(f)
ABHES COMPETENCIES: 4.b, 4.h

GOAL: *To prepare the patient and assist the physician in cryosurgery.*

EQUIPMENT and SUPPLIES

- Cryosurgery machine equipped with liquid nitrogen canister
- Cryoprobe
- Cervical tenaculum
- Cervical ring forceps or disposable cervical swabs
- Vaginal speculum
- 44-inch gauze squares
- Disposable examination gloves
- Gowns and face protection, appropriate PPE
- Specimen containers
- Biohazard waste container
- Cytology request forms
- Patient record

PROCEDURAL STEPS

1. Assemble equipment.
   PURPOSE: Expedite procedure.
2. Wash your hands.
   PURPOSE: Infection control.
3. Take the patient's temperature and blood pressure, and record them on the patient's record.
   PURPOSE: To establish a baseline for vital signs.
4. Drape and assist the patient into the lithotomy position. Don gloves.

5. Assist the physician with the procedure by handing equipment as needed.
6. Encourage the patient to take deep breaths to promote relaxation of the pelvic muscles during the procedure. Observe the patient for any signs of distress.
   PURPOSE: Patient safety.
7. When the procedure is completed, place the patient in a supine position and allow her to rest while you tidy the room and remove the used supplies. Retake temperature and blood pressure.
   PURPOSE: Ensure that vital signs and blood pressure return to baseline levels.
8. Help patient sit up, and assist her in dressing if needed.
   PURPOSE: Patient safety.
9. Remove gloves and wash hands.
   PURPOSE: Infection control.
10. Disinfect and sterilize equipment per manufacturer's directions, and return equipment to the proper storage area.
11. Provide instruction on follow-up care as ordered by the physician.
12. Record procedure and final vital sign measurements on the patient's record.
    PURPOSE: A procedure is not done until it is recorded.

See Appendix D for a charting example.

---

mother or sister), early menarche and late menopause, first pregnancy after the age of 30 years or no pregnancy, prolonged use of estrogen replacement therapy, excess alcohol intake, smoking, and obesity.

Because recent research has failed to link reduced death rates from breast cancer with monthly breast self-examinations (BSE), the American Cancer Society now recommends that women have their physician perform a clinical breast examination (CBE) rather than rely on monthly SBEs for early detection. However, although monthly SBEs are now considered optional, women should still be aware of the normal appearance and texture of the breasts and immediately report any changes or new breast symptoms to their physicians. The medical assistant should be prepared to teach this practice (Procedure 40-3). CBEs should be done every 3 years from age 20 to 39 and annually at age 40 and over. A mammogram should be done annually starting at age 40 and each year after that. If a woman has an increased risk for breast cancer (such as family history) the physician may recommend annual mammogram screening before the age of 40 or other diagnostic procedures such as ultrasound or MRI.

Indications of breast cancer include a palpable breast mass that is firm and immoveable, breast pain, tissue thickening, nipple retraction or dimpling, nipple discharge, and axillary lymphadenopathy. If a breast mass is palpated, a mammogram or ultrasound of the area is ordered and, if indicated, a biopsy is performed. The physician may perform a needle biopsy to remove cells and/or tissue from a palpated mass for evaluation by the pathologist. If a nonpalpable mass is found on a mammogram, a **stereotactic**-guided needle aspiration should be done with possible surgical biopsy as a follow-up. During this procedure the physician uses a mammogram to guide the needle toward the suspicious mass from which a biopsy sample can be taken. If it is not possible to get a tissue sample through a needle, a wire localization may be done to pinpoint the areas of concern from the mammogram. During this diagnostic procedure, a thin wire is passed through the breast to the point of concern (based on mammogram visualization). This wire marking is used during a surgical procedure to pinpoint tissue that was suspicious on the mammogram. If a biopsy shows malignant cells, the physician will order an estrogen and progesterone receptor test

PROCEDURE 40-3

Provide Instruction for Health Maintenance and Disease Prevention:
Teach the Patient Breast Self-Examination

CAAHEP COMPETENCY: 3.c.(3)(c)
ABHES COMPETENCY: 7.c

GOAL: *To teach the patient how to palpate her breast for possible abnormalities.*

EQUIPMENT and SUPPLIES

- Instruction pamphlet
- Teaching model (to use to demonstrate the technique before a return demonstration by the patient)
- Patient record

PROCEDURAL STEPS

1. Assemble equipment.
2. Tell the patient to examine the breasts while bathing or showering in warm water because the fingers will glide over wet tissue easier. The best time to perform this examination is immediately after the menstrual period is completed because at this time there is minimal breast engorgement. Nonmenstruating women should examine breasts the first of the month.
3. Have the patient raise one arm. With her fingers flat, she should press gently in small circles, starting at the outermost top edge of the breast and spiraling in toward the nipple. Touch every part of each breast, including the axillary region, gently feeling for a lump or thickening. Use the right hand to examine the left breast and the left hand for the right breast (Figure 1).
4. After the bath or shower is completed, the patient should continue the examination in front of a mirror with arms at the sides. Then, with the arms raised above the head, look carefully for changes in the size, shape, and contour of each breast. Look for puckering, dimpling, or changes in skin texture (Figure 2).
5. Gently squeeze both nipples and look for discharge (Figure 3).
6. Before dressing, the patient should lie on a bed. Place a towel or pillow under the right shoulder and the right hand behind the head. Examine the right breast using the left hand. Press gently in small circles, starting at the outermost top edge, including the axillary region, and spiraling in toward the nipple. Repeat with left breast (Figure 4).

7. The patient should return the demonstration using the teaching model to confirm understanding.
8. Give the patient an instruction pamphlet to use at home. If you have given her a shower card to follow, show her how it will hang inside the shower on a faucet or the shower nozzle and serve as a quick reference guide.
9. Record all procedures on the patient's medical record.
   PURPOSE: Patient education interventions should always be documented; a procedure is not done until it is entered into the patient's record.

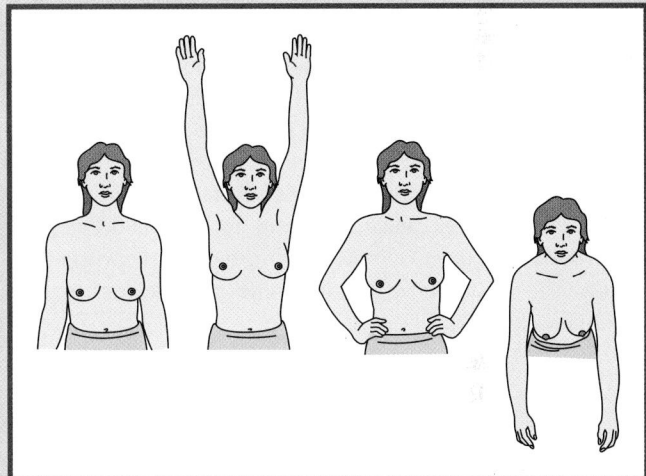

FIGURE 2

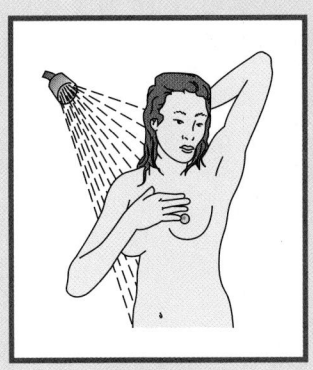

FIGURE 1

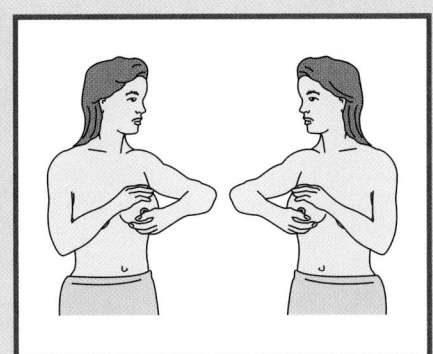

FIGURE 3

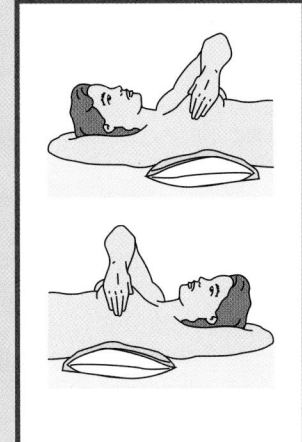

FIGURE 4

to find out if hormones affect the way the cancer grows. If the cancer cells increase growth patterns when exposed to hormone levels, the physician may recommend treatment with a drug such as tamoxifen, which prevents estrogen from binding to these sites.

Treatment of breast cancer is dependent on the type of carcinoma and its staging. Almost always treatment begins with surgery but the type of surgery and extent of tissue removed are dependent on several factors. Breast-saving surgeries include lumpectomy, which removes only the suspicious mass plus a surrounding area of normal tissue and is followed by radiation therapy to destroy any remaining cancerous cells. A partial mastectomy may also be done for more advanced cases; this procedure involves removal of the tumor and tissue surrounding it, part of the chest muscle beneath the mass, and some of the lymph nodes in the axillary region. Complete mastectomies, which include removal of the entire breast, chest muscle, and axillary lymph nodes, may still be indicated if the mass has spread. However, removal of multiple axillary lymph nodes greatly increases the risks of developing subsequent **lymphedema** and recurrent infections in the arm on the affected side. New advances recommend the removal of the *sentinel lymph node,* the first lymph node the cancer is likely to spread to from the tumor. The sentinel node is found by injecting a blue dye near the tumor, the lymph vessels absorb the dye and carry it toward the lymph nodes, and the first node to receive the dye and turn blue is the one that is removed for pathologic testing. If the sentinel node is cancer-free, then there is very little chance the breast tumor has metastasized and no other nodes need to be removed. If cancer cells are evident, then further diagnostic procedures are indicated to determine possible locations of metastatic tumors.

Positional Disorders of the Pelvic Region

The correct anatomic position for the uterus is tipped slightly anteriorly *(anteverted)* and bent over the bladder, with the cervix down and back. However, the uterus may be positioned in various angles because of a congenital anomaly, aging, or the effects of childbirth. With the aging process and/or multiple pregnancies, the muscles and ligaments that support the uterus, bladder, and rectum can stretch or weaken. This weakening of the supportive structures of the pelvic floor can result in multiple structural disorders.

A *cystocele* is a protrusion of the bladder into the anterior wall of the vagina. The bladder becomes angled, and urinary retention is common, along with frequent cystitis. A diagnosis can be made by requesting the patient to bear down as the vaginal opening is examined, allowing the physician to feel the bladder protrusion. A cystocele can result from injury during childbirth, obesity, heavy lifting, chronic coughing, and poor musculature that comes with aging (Figure 40-10).

A *rectocele* is a protrusion of the rectum into the posterior wall of the vagina. Diagnosis can be made by requesting the patient to bear down as the vaginal opening is examined so the physician can palpate the posterior wall. The patient will complain of difficulty with bowel movements and pressure in the pelvic region. Rectoceles are most often seen in postmenopausal women. A rectocele may result from pregnancy, difficult delivery, prolonged labor, obesity, chronic coughing, and lifting heavy objects.

The uterus may also lose supportive structure and drop into the vagina. This structural disorder is called uterine *prolapse.* The prolapse may involve only the descent of the cervix into the vaginal area or may progress to protrusion of both the uterus

Staging of Breast Cancer and Axillary Lymph Nodes

Tumor Staging
- Noninvasive mammary carcinomas are classified as stage TIS (tumor in situ)
- Stage I: Tumor less than 2 cm in diameter, either fixed or not fixed to the pectoral muscle
- Stage II: Tumor 2 to 5 cm in diameter, either fixed or not fixed to the pectoral muscle
- Stage III: Tumor larger than 5 cm in diameter, either fixed or not fixed to the pectoral muscle
- Stage IV: Tumor fixed to chest wall or skin

Lymph Node Staging
Lymph node staging is reported as letters a to d.
- a. N0: No regional lymph node involvement
- b. N1: Palpable, movable nodes
- c. N2: Palpable, fixed nodes
- d. N3: Internal mammary lymph node involvement

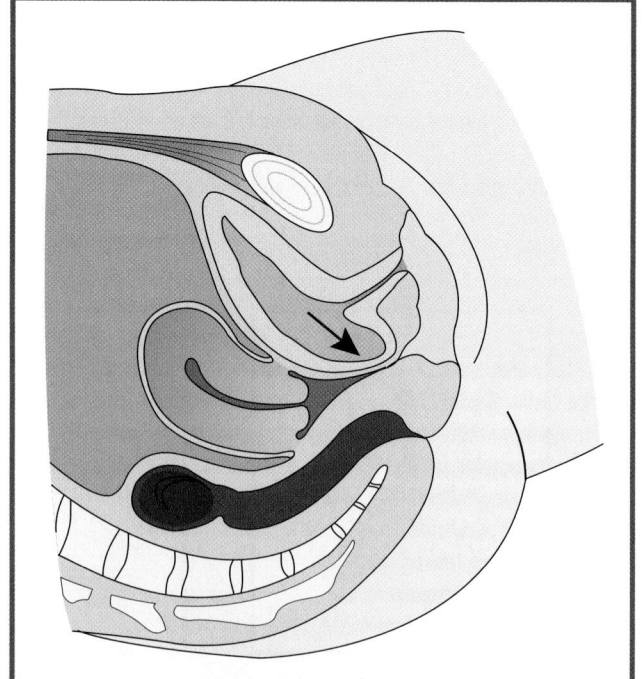

FIGURE 40-10 Cystocele.

and the cervix from the vaginal opening. If severe, all three of these structural abnormalities can be corrected with surgery.

PREGNANCY
Anatomy and Physiology

Fertilization usually takes place in the distal third of the fallopian tube when one sperm cell penetrates and fertilizes an egg, which is then called a *zygote.* The zygote is made up of 23 chromosomes from the ovum and 23 chromosomes from the sperm to form the first complete cell. This cell begins to grow and multiply immediately. The zygote travels down the fallopian tube and reaches the uterus in 5 to 6 days, implanting in the uterine endometrium. Enzymes are secreted by the zygote to aid in the implantation process.

After implantation, the placenta forms within the uterine wall. It is derived from maternal endometrial tissue as well as the *chorion,* which is the outermost membrane that surrounds the developing zygote. The *amnion* is the innermost layer of the membranes, and it holds the fetus suspended in an amniotic cavity surrounded by a fluid called the *amniotic fluid.* The amnion and fluid are sometimes known as the "bag of water." In about 25% of pregnancies, the breaking of the amniotic sac signals the onset of labor.

Within 2 weeks of fertilization the zygote has undergone mitosis and is well established in the uterus. The next stage of development is the *embryonic period,* which includes the third to the twelfth week of the pregnancy (the first trimester). The embryonic period is a crucial time for the developing fetus because this is when all tissues and organs develop. During the second and third trimester periods, the embryo becomes a fetus. This is when cells develop and begin their primary functions, organs mature, and the fetus gains weight and grows in length.

Throughout the pregnancy, maternal and fetal blood never mix. Nutrients and oxygen diffuse from the mother's blood, across the placental membrane, and into the blood vessels of the fetus's umbilical cord. Carbon dioxide and waste materials pass from the umbilical cord, through the placenta, and into the mother's circulatory system for excretion (Figure 40-11).

The placenta also acts as a gland by producing HCG and progesterone to maintain the pregnancy. Low levels of progesterone can lead to spontaneous abortion in pregnant women and menstrual irregularities in nonpregnant women. The average gestation is calculated at 9 calendar months, 10 lunar months, or 266 to 280 days and is divided into first, second, and third trimesters.

First Trimester

The first trimester is the period from the beginning of the last menstrual period (LMP) through the fourteenth week. It is a time of multiple physical and psychologic changes for the woman and is a crucial time for fetal organ development. It is essential that the pregnant woman understand the importance of a nutritious diet and avoidance of potential **teratogens.** The woman may complain of breast tenderness, constipation, headaches, urinary frequency, and nausea and vomiting. Rest, relaxation exercises, plenty of fluids, regular exercise, and small frequent meals will help to relieve these discomforts. It is during this time that the obstetrician obtains a complete health history of the patient, including family, medical, menstrual, and obstetric histories. The obstetric history includes the number of times the patient has been pregnant *(gravida)* and the number of times she has given birth to a live infant *(para).*

Second Trimester

The second trimester extends from the fifteenth through the twenty-eighth week after the LMP. The uterus has enlarged

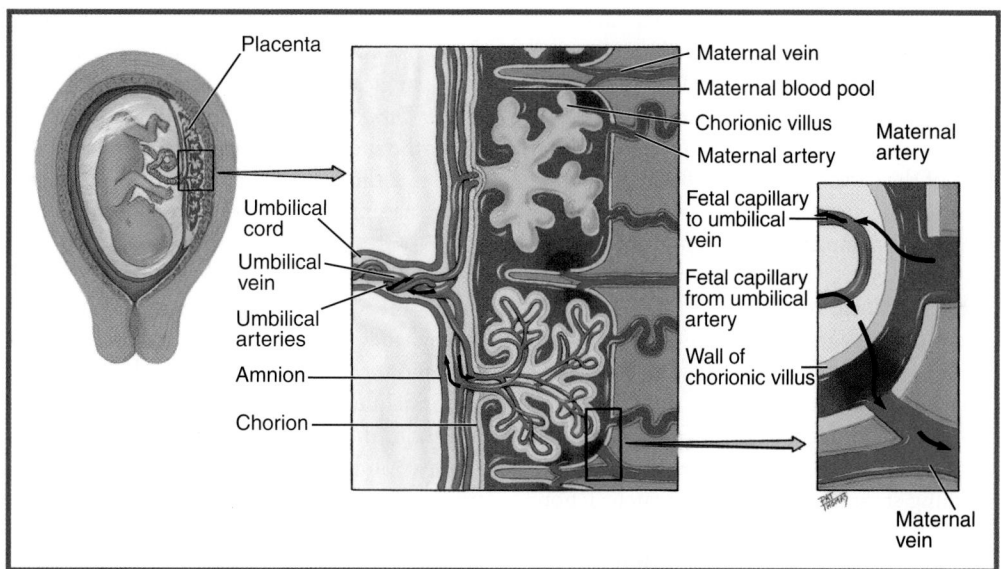

FIGURE 40-11 Structural features of the placenta and exchange of nutrients and wastes between maternal and fetal blood. (From Applegate EJ: *The anatomy and physiology learning system,* ed 3, Philadelphia, 2006, Saunders.)

to above the umbilicus, and the first fetal movements, called *quickening*, are felt by the patient. In addition to the basic health history and physical examination, assessment by abdominal palpation and fetal heart monitoring is conducted. The height of the fundus may be measured in centimeters from the symphysis pubis to the fundus. At each office visit a urine sample is screened with a dipstick to determine the presence of protein or glucose, and her blood pressure is monitored for signs of hypertension. The mother may complain of backache, dizziness, leukorrhea, and leg cramps from the increasing size of the uterus.

Third Trimester

The third trimester begins at the twenty-eighth week and lasts until delivery. This period is marked by rapid fetal growth, with the baby gaining close to 1 pound per week. The patient continues to be closely monitored. Childbirth preparation classes usually begin during this time. The patient experiences noticeable breast enlargement and may experience occasional discharge from the nipples of the clear sticky fluid **colostrum**. The pregnant woman may complain of uterine cramping (Braxton-Hicks contractions), heartburn, edema, and frequent urination. *Lightening*, the dropping of the fetus into the pelvis, may occur a few weeks before birth, especially in *primigravidas* (women with a first pregnancy).

Parturition

Labor is the physiologic process by which the uterus expels the fetus and the placenta (Figure 40-12). For a baby to be born vaginally it must drop down into the pelvic floor and the cervix must efface (thin out) and dilate (open up). **Effacement** is the thinning of the cervix from its prelabor length of 1 to $1\frac{1}{2}$ inches to a completely thin tissue. This occurs when uterine contractions pull cervical tissue upward as labor progresses so that the bottom uterine segment (the cervix) becomes thinner and the top uterine segment (the fundus) becomes thicker. Effacement is measured as a percentage; the cervix is said to be 0% to 100% effaced. **Dilation** (sometimes called *dilatation*) is the opening of the cervix, which allows the infant to pass out of the uterus and into the vaginal birth canal. Dilation is measured in centimeters, which are estimated during vaginal examinations by manual palpation. Labor is divided into three stages:

- Stage I: From the onset of labor through complete dilation and effacement of the cervix (see Figure 40-12, *B*). During this time uterine contractions get longer and stronger and closer together until complete dilation and effacement occur and pushing begins. Stage I is divided into early active (up to 3 cm dilated and 80% to 100% effaced), active (4 to 7 cm dilated and completion of effacement), and transition (8 to 10 cm dilation). The average length of time for primigravidas in stage I is 9 to 11 hours.
- Stage II: From complete dilation and effacement of the cervix through the birth of the fetus (see Figure 40-12, *C*). This is the pushing stage and lasts approximately 1 hour for primigravidas.
- Stage III: From the birth of the fetus through the expulsion of the placenta (see Figure 40-12, *D*); occurs approximately 20 minutes after the birth of the baby.

Pregnancy Complications

Infertility and Abortions

Fertility problems in women can occur for many different reasons, including a history of STDs that have caused scarring or adhesions of the fallopian tubes, failure to ovulate or irregular ovulation, congenital anomalies of the reproductive organs, endometriosis, medications that decrease fertility, and increasing age of the woman.

Problems in becoming pregnant can occur at several points in time, the first being abnormal fertilization. Some couples are unable to have a child because of the inability of the sperm and ovum to unite. Ovarian factors are not totally understood; however, it is known that as women age the ova become less viable. If the couple is able to fertilize an egg, another problem that can occur is improper implantation.

An *ectopic* pregnancy refers to a pregnancy that occurs outside the uterus. Although they can develop on or near the ovary or in the abdominal cavity, most ectopic pregnancies occur in the fallopian tube. As the zygote develops, the cells that form the placenta begin to erode the muscle layer of the tube, bleeding and destruction of the muscular layer occur, and the tube ruptures. Rupture of the fallopian tube containing an ectopic pregnancy is a serious event that requires immediate surgical intervention to prevent fatal hemorrhage.

Once the woman becomes pregnant, there can be problems in carrying the infant to term. An interruption of pregnancy before the term of fetal viability is called an *abortion*, which is identified in lay terms as a miscarriage. There are several different categories of naturally occurring abortions, including the following:

- *Spontaneous*—abortions that do not have an identifiable cause
- *Complete*—complete expulsion of both fetus and placenta without any medical intervention
- *Incomplete*—expulsion of only parts of the fetus and placenta. A D&C must be done to remove the remaining pieces, or the mother will continue to bleed
- *Missed*—the fetus dies in utero and must be removed surgically
- *Threatened*—cervical bleeding but no dilation occurs, and the pregnancy continues uninterrupted

It is estimated that one in three pregnancies will terminate by a naturally occurring abortion, and in most cases the causes are not clear. Chromosomal anomalies are frequently detected in an aborted fetus or placenta and may be the primary reason they occur. Spontaneous abortion is the loss of a pregnancy before the twentieth week of fetal development. Common causes are defective development of the embryo, abnormalities of the placenta, endocrine disorders, malnutrition, infection, drug reaction, blood group incompatibilities, severe trauma, and shock. Symptoms include vaginal bleeding of varying degrees of severity and lower abdominal cramping progressing to cervical dilation with rupture of membranes and complete expulsion of the products of conception. Induced abortions are the evacuation of the uterus at the request of the mother.

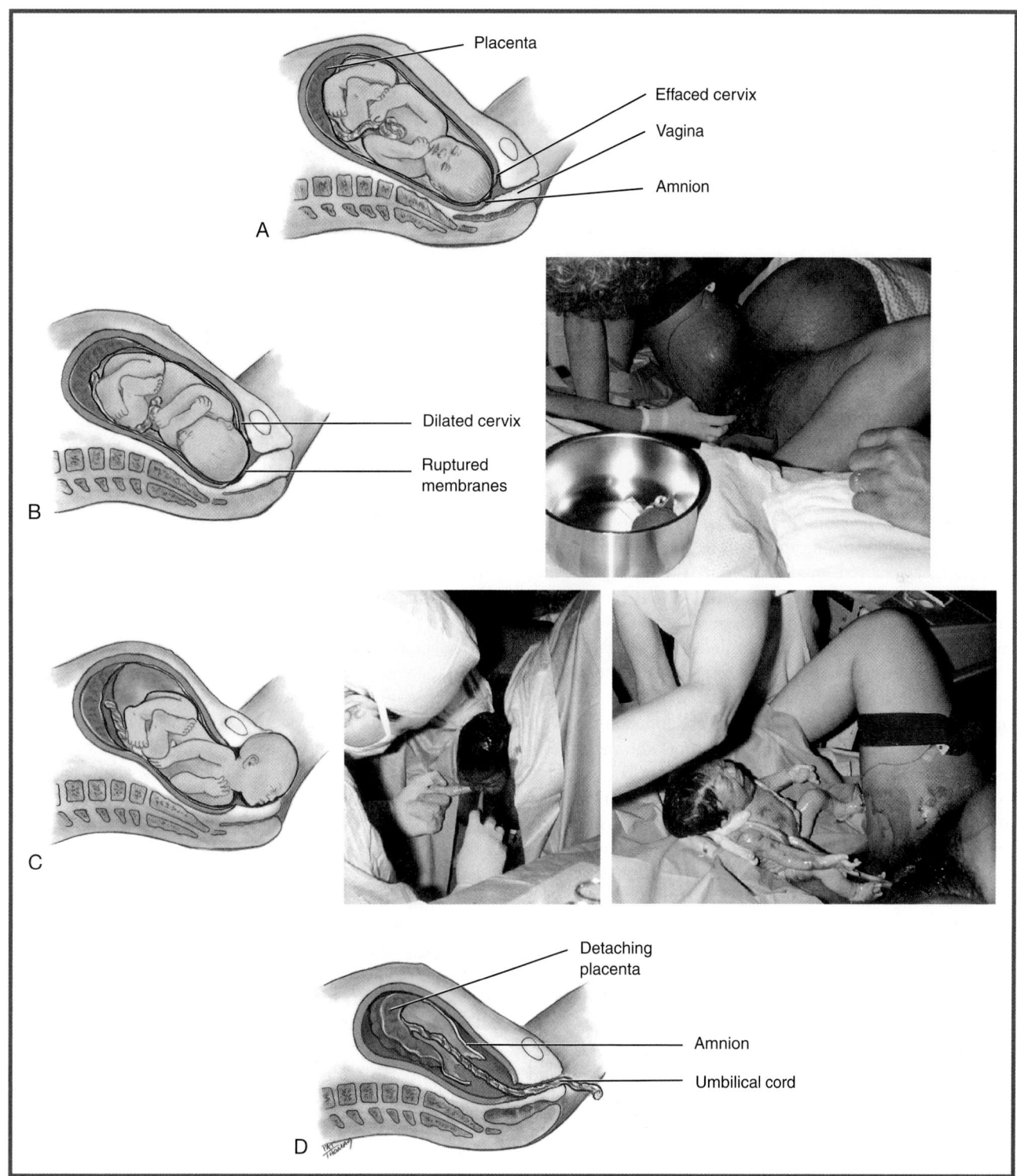

FIGURE 40-12 A, Effaced cervix. **B,** Dilation stage. **C,** Expulsion stage. **D,** Placental stage. (From Applegate EJ: *The anatomy and physiology learning system*, ed 3, Philadelphia, 2006, Saunders.)

Placental Abnormalities

Pregnancy complications can occur because of the site of placental implantation. *Placenta previa* is when the placenta implants in the lower uterine segment. If the condition is diagnosed early in the pregnancy from routine sonograms, it is possible that the placenta will migrate with uterine wall enlargement. If, however, the previa persists throughout the pregnancy and the placenta is implanted on or near the cervix when the mother goes into labor, the dilation and effacement of the cervix can cause the placenta to tear loose (Figure

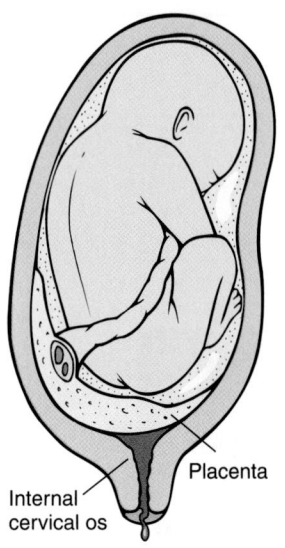

FIGURE 40-13 Placenta previa. (From Frazier MS, Drzymkowski JW: *Essentials of human diseases and conditions,* ed 3, Philadelphia, 2004, Saunders.)

Placenta

Internal cervical os

40-13). It is impossible for complete dilation and effacement to progress without serious oxygen deprivation for the fetus and hemorrhaging in the mother. The signs of placenta previa are painless, bright red vaginal bleeding during or near the last trimester. The diagnosis is confirmed with a sonogram. A cesarean section is done as close to term as possible to prevent complications in both the mother and fetus.

Another placenta problem, *abruptio placentae,* occurs when the placenta detaches from the uterine wall. The pregnant woman reports acute onset of severe abdominal pain with firmness on palpation and hemorrhaging from the vagina. She also exhibits signs of shock, including tachycardia; a thready pulse; hypotension; and clammy, cool skin. The fetus shows signs of distress resulting from lack of oxygen, including decreased fetal heart tones and lack of movement. This is a true obstetric emergency and requires immediate cesarean delivery to save the infant and mother.

Maternal Disorders

Gestational Diabetes. Any degree of impaired glucose tolerance during pregnancy is diagnosed as gestational diabetes mellitus (GDM). Women at greatest risk are those over age 30; those with a family history of diabetes mellitus; those with a body mass index of more than 25 before pregnancy; and certain racial groups, including blacks, Hispanics, and Native Americans.

The most recent recommendations from the American College of Obstetricians and Gynecologists (ACOG) is that all pregnant patients be screened for GDM at 24 to 28 weeks' gestation using a 50-g, 1-hour glucose challenge. The patient is given a concentrated drink equivalent to 50 g of glucose, and blood is drawn 1 hour afterward to measure blood glucose levels. A patient's blood level that is greater than 140 mg/dl is indicative of GDM, but these patients are retested with a 3-hour glucose challenge. Blood is checked every hour for 3 hours after the patient drinks a concentrated glucose solution, and elevations in two of these blood draws is considered positive for GDM.

It is very important that women diagnosed with GDM carefully monitor their blood glucose levels on a regular basis using a glucometer. This requires the patient to place a drop of blood on a machine that will analyze it and report the current blood glucose level. Patients may be able to achieve normal glucose levels with diet therapy and exercise, although some patients will require medication. The majority of women with GDM are prescribed insulin to manage elevated glucose levels; however, the oral hyperglycemic glyburide may also be effective. The mother's problem with glucose metabolism typically goes away after the birth of the infant, but these women are at greater risk for developing type 2 diabetes later in life. Patient education on healthy lifestyles, including the importance of a nutritious diet, weight management, and exercise, is needed to help prevent the occurrence of adult-onset type 2 diabetes.

Medical assistant responsibilities include performing blood tests as ordered, routine urinary dipsticks at each visit, and referral to a dietitian for help with diet therapy management.

Hypertension. Most women who develop hypertension during pregnancy had a normal blood pressure before becoming pregnant and also during early pregnancy but develop hypertension in the second half of the pregnancy. Gestational hypertension (pregnancy-induced hypertension) can be mild to severe and occurs in approximately 10% to 15% of pregnancies.

If hypertension is accompanied by proteinuria after 20 weeks of pregnancy, the patient is diagnosed as having preeclampsia or toxemia, which occurs in approximately 2% to 3% of pregnancies. Preeclampsia usually shows up unexpectedly during a routine prenatal visit. The patient has an elevated blood pressure with protein or albumin in the urine and may also have uremia, altered liver function, and a reduced platelet count. The birth of the baby will cure preeclampsia, with blood pressure returning to normal within a few days of delivery. However, if indicators of preeclampsia occur early in the pregnancy, the physician will attempt to balance the need to prevent premature birth of the infant with what is best for the mother. The baby will be monitored with routine **nonstress tests (NSTs),** sonograms, and maternal reports of fetal movement. If the condition persists, the patient is at risk for severe headaches, vision disturbances, oliguria, and convulsions either before or during labor and may require an emergency cesarean section to prevent serious maternal complications.

The medical assistant is responsible for monitoring the pregnant woman's vital signs at each visit, including any report of a sudden weight gain that may indicate edema, and for performing routine urine dipsticks. Complete and accurate documentation of findings will help alert the physician to possible hypertensive problems.

MENOPAUSE

Menopause is the permanent ending of menstruation because of the cessation of ovarian function. It usually occurs between the ages of 45 and 55 but can occur as early as the 30s and as late as the 60s. Menses may stop suddenly, there may be decreased flow over time, or the time between menses may lengthen until complete cessation occurs. Menopause can be diagnosed only retrospectively. It is only after 12 months of amenorrhea that a woman is said to be in menopause, and the years after this are called *postmenopause.*

Perimenopause begins when hormone-related changes start to appear and lasts until the final menses, for as long as 10 years before menopause. This is the time when women are still ovulating but the uneven rise and fall of estrogen and progesterone may cause symptoms to occur. Some women experience few or no symptoms, whereas others have hot flashes, concentration problems, mood swings, irritability, migraines, vaginal dryness, urinary incontinence, dry skin, and sleep disorders. Treatment focuses on relieving these signs and symptoms. The physician may prescribe low-dose oral contraceptives (Alesse) to balance estrogen and progesterone levels or short-term hormone-replacement therapy (HRT; Premarin or Prempro) to treat symptoms. He or she may also recommend that the patient consume soy products or take soy supplements for a plant source of estrogen. Vitamin E may help to alleviate hot flashes, and vitamin B$_6$ helps to create natural serotonin, a neurotransmitter that affects mood. Other methods that help alleviate symptoms include avoiding caffeine and spicy foods to reduce hot flashes, relaxing to aid with sleep disorders, following a low-fat diet high in calcium, and performing regular weight-bearing exercise to help prevent osteoporosis and heart disease.

Medical treatment of menopause focuses on managing uncomfortable symptoms as well as preventing associated conditions from drops in estrogen blood levels, such as osteoporosis and coronary artery disease. Physicians traditionally treated perimenopause and menopause with long-term HRT for most women; however, recent studies indicate that although HRT does protect the menopausal woman from osteoporosis, hip fractures, and colon cancer, at the same time it increases the risk of heart attacks, strokes, breast cancer, and blood clots. It is now recommended that physicians prescribe HRT to meet individual patient needs short term—no longer than 5 years—rather than as a routine treatment for all menopausal women. Studies show that it is after 5 years that the risk for heart disease and other complications increases. The medical assistant must be aware of the physician's recommendations regarding HRT.

Other medications that may be prescribed include antidepressants, such as venlafaxine (Effexor) or fluoxetine (Prozac, Sarafem) to prevent the occurrence of hot flashes. Gabapentin (Neurontin) and clonidine (Catapres) may also be prescribed to reduce the frequency of hot flashes. Since the development of osteoporosis is of concern in perimenopausal and postmenopausal women, the physician may prescribe alendronate (Fosamax) or risedronate (Actonel) to reduce bone loss and fracture risk. Another drug that may be used to improve postmenopausal bone density is raloxifene (Evista); however, hot flashes are a common side effect of this medication. To treat complaints of vaginal dryness, estrogen can be administered locally by vaginal tablet, ring, or cream or the patient can use K-Y jelly or some other vaginal moisturizer as a lubricant.

CRITICAL THINKING APPLICATION

Rose Conrad, a 53-year-old patient of Dr. Beck's, calls because she read recently that the hormone replacement therapy she has been taking for 3 years may be dangerous. Dr. Beck has reviewed her case and agrees that if she is concerned she can stop taking the medication; however, she recommends that Mrs. Conrad try some alternative therapies. What suggestions might Dr. Beck make for nonpharmaceutical treatment of perimenopausal symptoms?

THE MEDICAL ASSISTANT'S ROLE IN GYNECOLOGIC AND OBSTETRIC PROCEDURES

As the female progresses from menarche through the childbearing years and then into menopause, her medical concerns change and the focal point of the physical examination may change as well. The overall goal of the medical office is to keep her physically and mentally healthy. Being able to assist the physician in identifying possible problems before the problem becomes a threat to the patient's health is a major priority in care. The best way to accomplish this is by listening to the patient. Remember, to the patient there is no such thing as a routine examination.

Examination Preparation

An annual or semiannual examination of the female reproductive system is done to ensure normality of the reproductive organs or to diagnose and treat abnormalities of these organs. Before the physician begins the examination, the medical assistant should obtain a complete gynecologic history. After documentation of the patient's history and chief complaint the medical assistant should prepare the room and the patient for the examination (see Procedure 40-1).

The following should be included when a gynecologic history is taken:

- Age at menarche
- Details regarding the regularity of the menstrual cycle; the amount and duration of the menstrual flow; and a history of menstrual disturbances and their treatment
- Any current indicators of infection including the presence of vaginal discharge, pelvic pain, urinary difficulties, and so on
- Feedback on any breast abnormalities and date of last mammogram
- Date of last Pap test
- Sexual history; STD history
- Number of pregnancies and live births
- Date of LMP
- Lifestyle factors, including diet, exercise, smoking, alcohol use, and so on

The physical examination during a first prenatal visit includes an overall assessment of the woman's health status including vital signs, weight, and urinalysis. The medical assistant must prepare the patient and the supplies and equipment necessary to obtain pelvic measurements, perform serologic tests, and prepare for laboratory tests (Procedure 40-4). The physician will

PROCEDURE 40-4

Prepare Patient for and Assist with Routine and Specialty Examinations: Assist with the Prenatal Examination

<u>CAAHEP COMPETENCIES:</u> 3.b.(4)(e), 3.b.(4)(f)
<u>ABHES COMPETENCIES:</u> 4.b, 4.h

GOAL: *To promote a healthy pregnancy for the mother and fetus and screen for potential problems.*

EQUIPMENT and SUPPLIES

- Scale with height measure
- Sphygmomanometer
- Stethoscope
- Tape measure
- Doppler fetoscope
- Urine specimen container
- Disposable examination gloves, vaginal speculum, and lubricant if vaginal examination conducted
- STD test setups
- Laboratory requisition slips
- Biohazard waste container
- Biohazard bags for specimen transport
- Patient education materials
- Patient chart

PROCEDURAL STEPS

1. Wash your hands, assemble equipment, and identify the patient.
2. Measure and record the patient's weight.
   <u>PURPOSE:</u> The expectant mother's weight reflects maternal nutritional status as well as fetal growth, and an unusual increase in weight may indicate fluid retention.
3. Collect a urine specimen, perform urinalysis, and record urinalysis results to determine the presence of protein, glucose, or ketones in the urine.
   <u>PURPOSE:</u> The presence of these substances in the urine may indicate disease.
4. Measure and record the mother's blood pressure.

5. Instruct the patient to disrobe from the waist down and put on a gown open to the front so the uterine fundal height can be measured.
   <u>PURPOSE:</u> The physician will palpate the abdomen and use the tape measure to assess fundal height as a determinant of fetal growth.
6. Assist the patient onto the examination table if needed and provide a drape for privacy.
7. Assist the physician as needed throughout the examination.
8. After the examination is completed, assist the patient off the examination table, making sure to observe for signs of dizziness or problems with balance.
   <u>PURPOSE:</u> Lying supine or in a lithotomy position places pressure on the aorta, which may result in momentary vertigo when the patient sits or stands.
9. Answer the patient's questions, and provide patient education materials as needed.
   <u>PURPOSE:</u> Take advantage of "teaching moments" to provide information on diet, health habits, and community resources.
10. Collect and package all specimens for transport. Complete labels as needed.
11. Discard supplies and disinfect the equipment according to manufacturer's guidelines. Wear disposable examination gloves and follow OSHA guidelines if handling any contaminated items.
12. Wash your hands.
13. Document pertinent information in the patient chart.

See Appendix D for a charting example.

---

assess heart, lung, and thyroid function and perform a physical examination to rule out any other abnormality. Next, the practitioner will perform an obstetric examination that includes palpation of the mother's abdomen, measurement of the height of the uterus, and an internal or pelvic examination.

A series of blood tests is also performed during the initial prenatal visit. On follow-up prenatal visits, the medical assistant should collect a urine specimen for urinalysis, weigh the patient, measure the blood pressure, and answer questions about diet and health habits. The mother should gain approximately 10 to 12 pounds in the first half of pregnancy and another 15 to 17 pounds during the second half. Experts believe that a healthy weight gain is somewhere between 25 and 35 pounds. The baby's heart tones can be picked up through a specialized method called *Doppler ultrasound* somewhere between 9 and 12

weeks of pregnancy. Once recorded, the fetal heart rate is taken at each subsequent visit.

Prenatal blood and laboratory tests include the following:
- Hematocrit and hemoglobin levels to check for anemia
- Blood type and Rh with antibody screening for possible Rh incompatibility
- Rubella titer to see if the mother is immune to German measles; rubella infection during pregnancy can cause multiple birth defects including deafness, vision disorders, and mental retardation
- Syphilis screening; if result is positive, antibiotic treatment is initiated to protect the fetus from congenital syphilis
- Hepatitis B screening, because this virus can be passed to the fetus in utero
- HIV screening is suggested; if the result is positive,

treatment of the mother will greatly reduce the risk of transmission to the fetus

- Pap smear to check for abnormal cervical cells
- Gonorrhea and chlamydia cultures to prevent infections of the baby at birth
- Urinalysis for presence of protein, white blood cells, or glucose
- Group B streptococcus culture of the lower vagina for strep B infection, performed between the thirty-second and thirty-sixth weeks; if the result is positive, the mother is treated with antibiotics to prevent fetal exposure during vaginal birth
- NST to evaluate fetal heart rate; mother is attached to a fetal monitor, with the goal of seeing accelerations in fetal heart rate with movement
- Stress test or oxytocin challenge test (OCT) if the NST is abnormal; small amount of oxytocin (causes the uterus to contract) is administered intravenously while the mother is attached to a fetal monitor to see how the fetus will respond to the normal stresses of labor

Any concerns of the patient should be noted and reported to the physician. The medical assistant should be prepared to suggest community resources that can provide assistance to new parents such as childbirth and parenting classes; infant cardiopulmonary resuscitation (CPR) courses; nutritional counseling if needed; and contact information for the Special Supplemental Nutrition Program for Women, Infants, and Children (WIC), which helps lower-income expectant mothers get nutritious food.

The examination room needs to be adequately equipped and the surroundings pleasant. A dressing area with an adjacent toilet should be provided. The dressing area should ensure privacy and be equipped with tissues and sanitary protection items as well as disposable examination gowns and drapes. The medical assistant should restock supplies as needed throughout the day.

Assisting with the Examination

This is probably the most emotionally charged medical experience the average female undergoes. Even women with relatively sophisticated attitudes toward their bodies and sexuality may be mortified by the casual, impersonal approach of the medical team during this procedure. Many women fear the physician's findings. Anxieties and fears are best handled through explanations and showing a genuine interest in the patient's concerns.

If the physician is male, the female medical assistant should be present during the examination. The only exception to this rule is when the patient requests that the medical assistant leave the room; if this is done, the request is noted on the patient's medical record. The male medical assistant is usually not in the room during the examination except when it is necessary to assist with a procedure. The physician makes the decision regarding the male assistant's role in the female reproductive system examination. It is the medical assistant's responsibility to support the patient and to assist the physician during the procedure. The procedure should be fully explained to the patient to avoid unnecessary embarrassment and discomfort. During the explanation, the assistant has the opportunity to conduct patient teaching.

The patient should be instructed to void, completely disrobe, and put on an examination gown open to the front. The patient should have been advised at the time the appointment was made not to douche or have sexual intercourse for 24 hours before the examination so that vaginal discharges can be evaluated properly and to ensure accurate results of cytologic studies.

Breast Examination

Begin the examination by assisting the patient into a sitting position and by adjusting the gown so that the breast tissue can be easily exposed. The physician will instruct the patient to place her arms above her head, and the assistant should be present to assist the patient if she has difficulty following these instructions. The physician may prefer to examine the breasts with the patient in the supine position. When the patient is instructed to assume a supine position, help the patient, adjust the gown, and drape as needed for the physician and for the patient's comfort. A small pillow may be placed under the patient's head for comfort. When the examination is completed, the gown is readjusted to cover the breasts. The physician may choose to discuss breast self-examination with the patient at this time or inform the patient that you will be explaining the technique at the end of the examination (see Procedure 40-3).

Abdominal Examination

After examination of the patient's breasts, cover her breasts and position the drape to allow the physician to palpate the abdomen to confirm normal symmetry and detect the presence of possible masses. In the case of pregnancy, the level of the fundus is measured to determine fetal growth. For this examination, the patient's arms should be placed at her sides to achieve better relaxation of the abdominal muscles.

Pelvic Examination

The medical assistant should remain in the examination room to provide reassurance to the patient as well as to offer legal protection to the male physician while the patient's vagina and perineal areas are being examined. Furthermore, the lithotomy position is awkward to assume without assistance and may be embarrassing to the patient. Never position the patient in the lithotomy position until the physician is ready to begin the examination. When you assist the patient into the lithotomy position, always keep the patient totally covered.

The medical assistant should stand at the patient's side to be able to observe the patient and also to be able to move quickly if needed by the physician. First, the physician inspects the external genitalia and palpates the perineal body. The patient may be asked to bear down to show any muscular weaknesses that may be the result of lacerations of the perineal body during childbirth. A third-degree laceration may have involved the rectal sphincter and may cause rectal incontinence.

Next, the vaginal speculum, without lubrication, is inserted for examination of the cervix and the vaginal canal and for obtaining the Pap specimen. The speculum should be preheated with warm water. Have the patient take some deep breaths to help relax the abdominal muscles. The normal cervix points posteriorly and has smooth, pink squamous epithelium. Abnormalities most frequently seen are ulcerations (erosions), Bartholin cysts, and cervical polyps. Because erosions cannot be palpated, inspection is the only method for detecting their presence. Healed lacerations resulting from childbirth are common in the **multiparous** patient. Pregnancy increases the size of the cervix, and hormone deficiency causes it to atrophy. The vaginal wall is reddish pink and has a corrugated appearance from the overlapping tissue (rugae) lining. Vaginal infections change the appearance of the vaginal mucosa. When the Pap specimen is obtained, you may be responsible for labeling the specimen and preparing it for transport to the cytology laboratory. Be sure to follow laboratory instructions during the preparation to avoid having to repeat the examination.

After the vaginal speculum has been removed, the physician does a bimanual examination—that is, two gloved fingers are lubricated with a water-soluble jelly (lubricant) and inserted into the vaginal canal, and the other hand palpates the abdomen over the pelvic organs and the mons pubis (Figure 40-14). The uterus is examined for shape, size, and consistency. The position of the uterus is noted. The normal uterus is freely movable with limited discomfort. A laterally displaced uterus is usually the result of pelvic adhesions or displacement caused by a pelvic tumor. The fallopian tubes and ovaries are evaluated. The normal tubes and ovaries are difficult to palpate. The physician completes the examination by performing a rectovaginal abdominal examination. A stool test for occult blood may be done at this time.

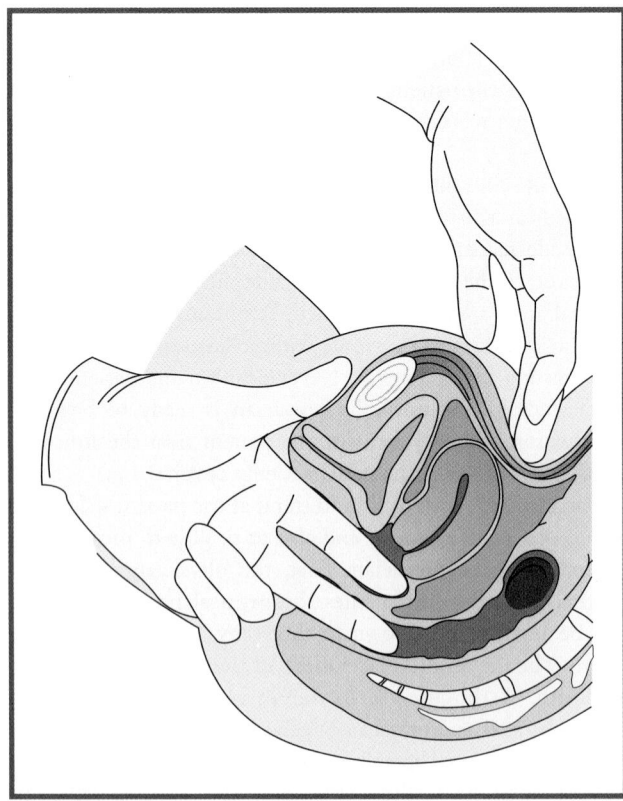

FIGURE 40-14 Bimanual examination.

Postexamination Duties

Once the examination is concluded, help the patient into a sitting position and into the dressing room if needed. Using Occupational Safety and Health Administration (OSHA) standard precautions, remove the examination equipment and supplies while the patient is dressing so that when the physician returns to talk to the patient the room is neat and clean. Once the patient has left, the room should be cleaned and restocked as necessary and made ready for the next patient.

SAFETY ALERT Any instrument that comes in contact with a patient should be disinfected and sterilized before being used for another patient. If the instrument does not penetrate tissue, it can be stored under clean or medically aseptic conditions. Some physicians prefer to use disposable specula for routine pelvic examinations. Instruments that penetrate the tissue must be sterilized and stored under sterile conditions. Examples of such instruments include the uterine biopsy punch, uterine tenaculum, and cervical dilators and sounds.

DIAGNOSTIC TESTING

Sonography

Sonography is a technique that uses high-frequency sound waves to produce images of soft tissues of the body. It can be used to distinguish cysts from tumors and is used during pregnancy to determine the number of fetuses, their age and sex, fetal abnormalities, and the position of the placenta. The skin over the area being studied is coated with conductive gel or lotion, and the transducer is pressed lightly against the area. Sound waves emitted by the transducer bounce off the structure being studied and are converted into electrical impulses that create a picture for analysis. The mother must drink three to four glasses of water 1 hour before the procedure and not void so the full bladder can be used as a reference point.

Sonograph technology is divided into two methods. The grayscale image converts sound wave echoes into graphs or dots that form pictures of organs and blood vessels (Figure 40-15). The Doppler method converts the ultrasound into

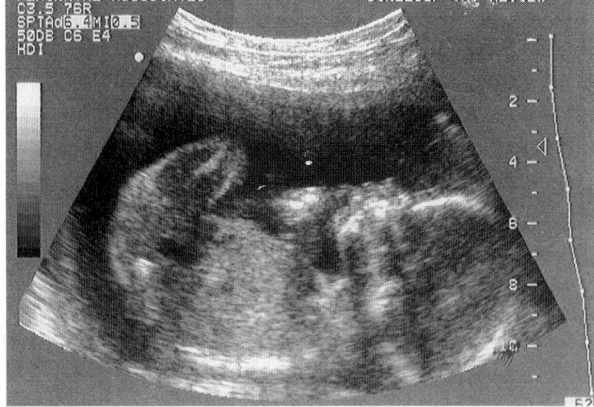

FIGURE 40-15 Sonogram of fetus.

Fetal Diagnostic Tests

- *Chorionic villus sampling: Chorionic villi* are tiny placental projections whose cells have the same genetic material found in fetal cells. A cellular screening performed between 8 and 12 weeks of gestation provides early detection of genetic or chromosomal disorders. Potential complications include accidental abortion, infection, bleeding, and fetal limb deformities. Results are available within several days.
- *Amniocentesis:* Needle aspiration of approximately 2 tablespoons of amniotic fluid after the 14th week of pregnancy to detect genetic and chromosomal abnormalities or inherited metabolic disorders (Figure 40-16). Potential complications include miscarriage, fetal injury, infection, premature labor, and maternal hemorrhage. Results are usually not available for two weeks.
- *Alpha-fetoprotein (AFP):* Maternal blood sample is analyzed between 16 and 18 weeks; elevated level indicates a **neural tube defect** such as a **myelomeningocele**. Levels also increase with multiple pregnancy (twins) or fetal congenital anomalies. The test is controversial because of a high rate of false-positive results.
- *Percutaneous umbilical cord sampling (PUBS):* Under ultrasound guidance a sample of fetal blood is removed from the umbilical cord to detect blood diseases not diagnosed with amniocentesis.

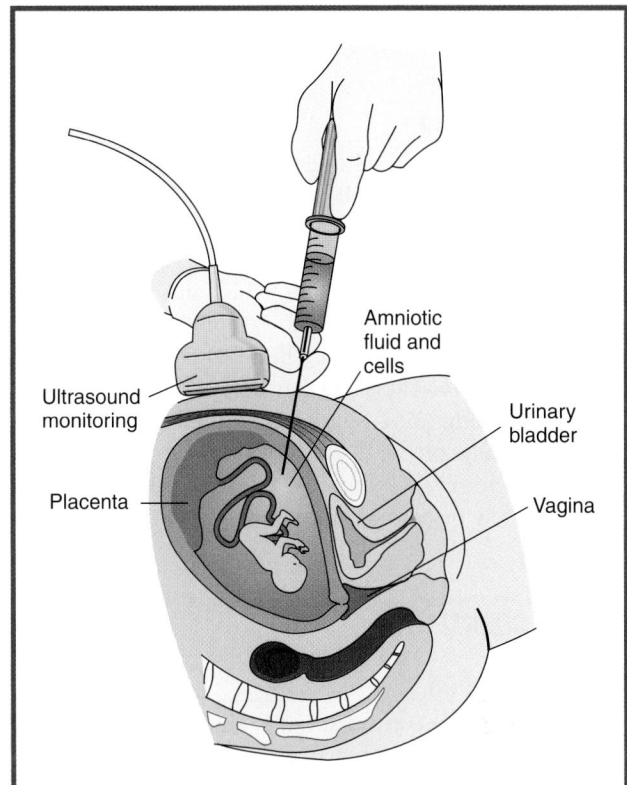

FIGURE 40-16 Amniocentesis.

audible sounds that are heard as pulsations and is used in the obstetrician's office to monitor the heartbeat of the fetus. Color-coded Doppler signals, three-dimensional imaging, and contrast medium enhancement of ultrasound image provide more accurate images and data related to organ structure and function.

Mammography

Mammography is a specialized x-ray technique that provides images of breast tissue and is performed to identify abnormal masses that would otherwise go undetected under a breast palpation examination (Figure 40-17). Special x-ray equipment is used that compresses the breast firmly during each exposure. Compression is essential to provide the high degree of detail needed to visualize the significant, but often subtle, signs of a tumor. This process is not usually painful, but some patients, especially those with fibrocystic breast disease, may find it uncomfortable. If pain persists after the examination, aspirin or ibuprofen is recommended for relief. Women with fibrocystic breast disease may find it helpful to avoid caffeine 24 to 72 hours before the procedure.

In preparation for mammography, patients are instructed not to use underarm deodorant and not to apply powder or lotions on the breasts or axillary areas. These products may contain ingredients that produce artifacts on mammographic images. This is especially true of antiperspirants that contain aluminum salts. When previous mammograms are available, every effort must be made to obtain them, because comparative evaluation is often significant in the radiologic diagnosis.

In addition to routine screening examinations and studies for evaluation of known breast lumps, mammographic techniques

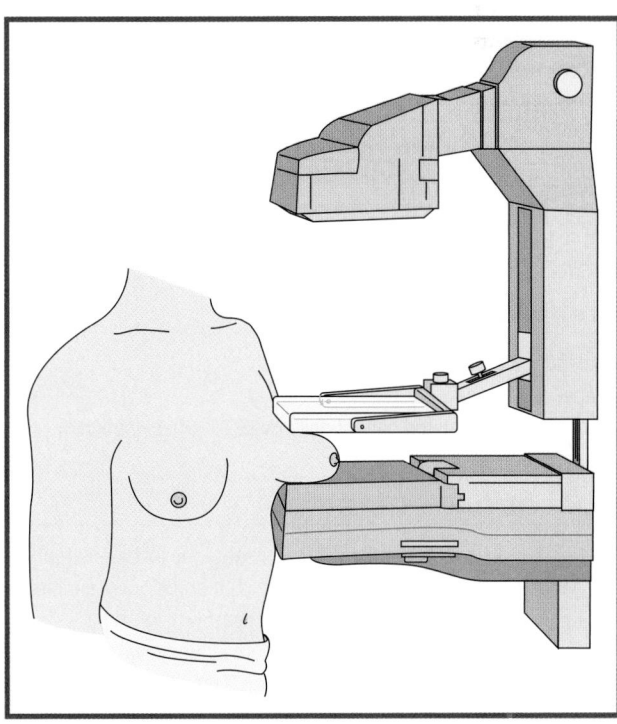

FIGURE 40-17 Proper position of breast for mammogram.

also may be used to localize needle placement for breast biopsies.

Pregnancy Testing

Pregnancy tests are designed to detect HCG, which is secreted after the ovum is fertilized. It appears in the blood and urine of pregnant women as early as 10 days after conception. Once pregnancy is confirmed, the patient undergoes a complete medical and obstetric examination, which includes a number of laboratory tests. The estimated day of delivery (EDD) is also calculated (Procedure 40-5). The EDD is frequently called her *expected due date.* The EDD can be determined by several methods, including using Nägele's rule, the lunar method, or the commercially prepared gestational wheel. Regardless of the method, the EDD is only an educated guess, and most obstetricians rely on sonograms for more reliable data.

CLOSING COMMENTS

Patient Education

The medical assistant can assist the physician by providing information to the patient that promotes sexual health and prevents gynecologic and obstetric disorders throughout the life of the patient.

The woman planning a pregnancy or who has just found out she is pregnant may benefit from some simple guidelines for healthy living. These include the following:

- *Nutrition:* Before pregnancy, emphasize the need for folic acid to prevent neural tube defects. The woman can take a supplement or consume dark green, leafy vegetables.

Many women have iron deficiency anemia, and eating foods high in iron (red meat, spinach, or enriched cereal) is helpful. The pregnant woman is meeting the calcium needs of both herself and her fetus and therefore needs about 1000 mg of calcium per day. Most pregnant women should consume about 2500 calories a day. Women of average weight should gain 25 to 35 pounds, but underweight women should gain 28 to 40 pounds for a healthy infant.

- *Alcohol:* Alcohol passes through the placenta to the fetus and can cause serious problems. No one knows how much is safe, so it is a good idea for pregnant women to avoid alcohol completely.
- *Smoking:* Smoking can cause premature birth and low–birth-weight full-term infants. Smoking is linked to an increased risk of otitis media, heart problems, and upper respiratory infections in infants as well as sudden infant death syndrome (SIDS). Pregnant women should not smoke and should not be exposed to secondhand smoke.
- *Medicine:* All chemicals pass through the placenta; therefore pregnant women should never take any medicine (even over-the-counter drugs) without the knowledge and approval of the obstetrician. If the medical assistant is managing telephone screening, having a list of physician-approved medications next to the phone will help answer patient questions.
- *STD Screening:* STD screening should be done before a woman becomes pregnant. Many STDs are asymptomatic in women but treatable. Infants are at risk for serious health problems if exposed to certain STDs in utero or during the birth process.

PROCEDURE 40-5

Prepare Patient for and Assist with Procedures, Treatments, and Minor Office Surgeries: Establish the Estimated Date of Delivery Using Nägele's Rule and Lunar Method

CAAHEP COMPETENCY: 3.b.(4)(f)
ABHES COMPETENCY: 4.b

GOAL: *To establish the patient's due date.*

EQUIPMENT and SUPPLIES

- Calendar for present and following year
- Paper and pencil
- Commercial estimated date of delivery (EDD) wheel (optional)
- Patient record

PROCEDURAL STEPS

1. Ask the patient for the date of the onset of the last menstrual period (LMP). Be sure that this is the date of the onset and not the date of the termination of the menses.
2. Calculate her EDD using Nägele's method: Begin with the date of the first day of her LMP. Count back 3 months and add 1 year plus 7 days.

EXAMPLE: LMP = June 7, 2002. Count back 3 months: May, April, March 7, 2002. Add 1 year and 7 days = March 14, 2003. Her EDD is March 14, 2003.

3. Using the same LMP, calculate her EDD using the lunar rule: LMP + 9 months + 7 days.
EXAMPLE: LMP = June 7, 2002 + 9 months = March 7, 2003 + 7 days = March 14, 2003.
4. Compare the results for accuracy. Did you obtain the same EDD using both methods?
5. Record the EDD in the patient chart.

Advantages of Breastfeeding

For the Infant
- Breast milk is completely digested by the infant
- Protects against gastrointestinal infection
- Protects against food allergies
- Provides newborn with mother's antibodies to infectious disease
- Associated with higher infant IQ
- Promotes muscular eye and facial development
- Promotes maternal-infant bonding

For the Mother
- Simple, safe, and economical
- Promotes uterine involution, which decreases postpartum bleeding
- Decreases the incidence of breast cancer
- Promotes maternal-infant bonding

Pregnant women are usually searching for information about pregnancy and wellness both during and after the birth. Use the waiting room as an education center with videos, books, and pamphlets on health issues and parenting. Maintaining an up-to-date list of community education and support programs would also be helpful. The obstetric patient who is interested in breastfeeding may need education and support to be successful. The American College of Pediatricians recommends breast milk as the optimal food for newborns. Referral to a breastfeeding support group or lactation consultant will help solve breastfeeding problems and answer maternal questions.

Legal and Ethical Issues

Many ethical and legal issues arise as a result of missed communication. Listen to what every patient reports, and write down any information that will assist the physician in treating the patient. The issue may appear to be an insignificant problem, but to the patient it may be a major concern. Let the physician be the judge of whether the problem is relevant. As the patient's advocate and the physician's assistant, the medical assistant plays an important role in establishing good communication as a vital link in patient care.

Confidentiality is crucial when dealing with obstetric and gynecologic disorders. Only those healthcare professionals who are directly involved in the care of the patient should know the purpose of the patient's visit, diagnosis, or treatment. Maintaining patient confidentiality is not only an ethical responsibility, but in the case of HIV status, it is a legal requirement.

The medical assistant may be in the position to recognize and provide assistance to women who are being mistreated. Battered women seldom come forward and tell healthcare workers they are being abused. If the patient reports such problems to the medical assistant or if it is suspected that an abusive situation exists, the medical assistant should not hesitate to report this information to the physician. The American Medical Association (AMA) has developed guidelines to help caregivers recognize victims of abuse. These include the following:

- Know what to look for: multiple injuries at different sites, especially areas that are normally covered by clothing; the victim may be frightened, anxious, and passive and may have a history of "accidents."
- Know what to ask when collecting a patient history: even patients who exhibit no signs of abuse should be asked if they have ever been in an abusive relationship; if verbal arguments ever become physical; if their partner acts differently when drinking or using drugs; and if their partner is overprotective and jealous.
- Know what to say and do: a battered woman suffers both physical and emotional abuse; she may begin to believe that she deserves to be mistreated and needs unconditional and nonjudgmental emotional support from the healthcare worker. She needs to be treated with warmth and respect and encouraged to develop a plan of action for when the next violent episode occurs. Suggestions include having immediate access to important documents, keys, money, transportation, the address of a safe house, and phone numbers for the police and local domestic violence hotline if available. The National Domestic Violence Hotline can be reached at 1-800-799-SAFE (7233). It provides 24-hour help for victims seeking local shelters.

SUMMARY OF SCENARIO

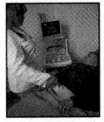

After working with obstetric and gynecologic patients, Betsy has learned that a wide range of disorders and conditions can affect a woman's health and pregnancy. She also has learned how to assist with a number of different diagnostic procedures performed in the ambulatory care setting. One of the integral roles of the medical assistant in the OB/GYN practice is reinforcing the physician's patient education efforts. Betsy enjoys this part of the practice but realizes that it involves extensive reading and discussion with Dr. Beck to determine her preferred method of practice. Betsy stays up to date on current contraceptive practices by attending local AAMA workshops and regional conferences. She has networked with other CMAs to develop a comprehensive community resource guide for obstetric and gynecologic patients in the practice and has created an educational center in the patient waiting room. Betsy recognizes that she must continue to learn about new practices and recent research to help deliver the best possible care to the women in Dr. Beck's practice.

SUMMARY of LEARNING OBJECTIVES

1. Define, spell, and pronounce, the terms listed in the vocabulary.
   - Spelling and pronouncing medical terms correctly adds credibility to the medical assistant. Knowing the definition of these terms promotes confidence in communication with patients and co-workers.
2. Identify the major organs of the female reproductive system, and explain the primary function of each.
   - The female reproductive system is made up of the external genitalia and the internal organs including the vagina; the cervix, which must dilate and efface for the vaginal birth of a child; the uterus; the fallopian tubes; and the ovaries, which mature and excrete ova.
3. Trace the ovum through the three phases of menstruation.
   - The follicular phase matures a graafian follicle so that an ovum can be released while at the same time the endometrial wall is thickening; the luteal phase causes extensive growth of the endometrium; if conception does not occur, the menstrual cycle begins with the breakdown of the endometrium and menstrual flow.
4. Compare and contrast current contraceptive methods.
   - Barrier contraceptive methods include the use of condoms, diaphragm, or cervical cap; all are relatively inexpensive and reversible but must be used with each instance of intercourse. Hormonal contraceptives include Depo-Provera injections, oral and patch contraceptives, and the vaginal ring, which are very effective but have side effects and contraindications, summarized in Table 40-1.
5. Summarize menstrual disorders and conditions.
   - Menstrual disorders include amenorrhea and oligomenorrhea; abnormal menstrual bleeding includes menorrhagia and metrorrhagia; endometriosis is characterized by the presence of functional endometrial tissue outside the uterus.
6. Distinguish among different types of gynecologic infections.
   - Gynecologic infections include candidiasis; BV; cervicitis; PID, which is any acute or chronic infection of the reproductive system ascending from the vagina (vaginitis), cervix (cervicitis), uterus (endometritis), fallopian tubes (salpingitis), and ovaries (oophoritis); and STDs, summarized in Table 40-2.
7. Differentiate between benign and malignant neoplasms of the female reproductive system.
   - Benign tumors of the reproductive system include uterine fibroids; ovarian cysts; the hormonal disease of polycystic ovary syndrome; and fibrocystic breast disease, the presence of multiple palpable nodules in the breasts. Malignant tumors include cervical, endometrial, and ovarian cancers that vary in their diagnostic features and symptoms. Breast cancer can be of multiple origins. Treatment of all forms of reproductive cancer is dependent on the staging and grading of the tumors.
8. Prepare for and assist with the female examination, including a Papanicolaou (Pap) test.
   - Procedure 40-1 explains the steps to assist with the examination of a female patient.

9. Teach the patient how to perform a breast self-examination.
   - Procedure 40-3 explains how to teach breast self-examination.
10. Compare the positional disorders of the pelvic region.
    - Positional disorders of the pelvic region include cystocele or rectocele, which cause the protrusion of the bladder or the rectum into the vaginal wall, and uterine prolapse, in which the cervix or the uterus has dropped into the vaginal area. If severe, all three of these structural abnormalities can be corrected with surgery.
11. Summarize the process of pregnancy and parturition.
    - Pregnancy occurs when the ovum and sperm meet in the fallopian tube and a zygote is formed. The zygote implants in the uterine wall, and the placenta begins to form, which provides hormonal support for the pregnancy. The fetus is surrounded by an amniotic sac and floats in amniotic fluid. Oxygen and nutrients for the fetus pass through the placenta to the umbilical cord. The embryonic period ends at 12 weeks, and by then all tissues and organs have developed. During the remainder of the pregnancy, the organs mature and begin to function, and the fetus grows. Pregnancy is divided into trimesters: the first, second, and third. The first trimester is a crucial time for fetal organ development, the second brings quickening and many physiologic changes in the mother, and the third is when organ systems mature. There are three stages of labor: dilation and effacement of the cervix; birth; and expulsion of the placenta.
12. Describe the common complications of pregnancy.
    - The complications of pregnancy include the potential loss of the pregnancy from different types of abortions (miscarriages). Placental abnormalities include placenta previa, in which the placenta covers the cervical os, and abruptio placentae, in which the placenta breaks away from the uterine wall. Both cause maternal hemorrhage, threaten fetal oxygen supply, and require cesarean birth to protect the fetus and mother. Maternal disorders include GDM, which requires dietary changes and possible insulin therapy; and hypertension, which may progress to toxemia, a life-threatening rise in blood pressure with edema, uremia, and possible seizure activity.
13. Specify the signs, symptoms, and treatments of conditions related to menopause.
    - Menopause is the permanent ending of menstruation because of the cessation of ovarian function. Perimenopause begins when hormone-related changes start to appear and lasts until the final menses. Some women experience few or no symptoms, whereas others have hot flashes, concentration problems, mood swings, irritability, migraines, vaginal dryness, urinary incontinence, dry skin, and sleep disorders. The physician may prescribe low-dose oral contraceptives or HRT, weight-bearing exercise, soy products or vitamin supplements, dietary recommendations, and medication to manage hot flashes, mood swings, and vaginal dryness and prevent osteoporosis.
14. Outline the medical assistant's role in gynecologic and reproductive examinations.

Continued

SUMMARY of LEARNING OBJECTIVES

Continued

- The medical assistant's role in gynecologic and reproductive examinations includes preparing the patient for the examination, equipping the room, making sure supplies are available and properly prepared, assisting with the examination, positioning and draping the patient as needed, assisting with the Pap smear or any other procedures, and providing support and understanding for the patient.

15. Demonstrate how to assist with the prenatal examination.
    - Procedure 40-4 explains how to assist with a prenatal examination.

16. Distinguish among diagnostic tests that may be done to evaluate the female reproductive system.
    - Diagnostic tests for the female reproductive system include sonography during pregnancy to determine the number of fetuses, fetal age and sex, fetal abnormalities, and position

of the placenta; chorionic villi sampling, amniocentesis, or umbilical blood sampling to perform genetic testing; AFP blood tests to diagnose neural tube defects; mammography, which provides an x-ray image of the breast tissue to identify cancerous tumors; colposcopy procedures that permit visualization of abnormal cervical tissue for evaluation or biopsy; and a variety of tests done during pregnancy.

17. Demonstrate patient preparation for a cryosurgery procedure.
    - Procedure 40-2 describes how to prepare a patient for cryosurgery.

18. Determine the estimated delivery date when given the date of the last menstrual period.
    - To determine the estimated delivery date when given the date of the last menstrual period, use the Nägele or lunar method as explained in Procedure 40-5.

CONNECTIONS

 Study Guide Connection: Go to Chapter 40 Study Guide. Read the Case Study and Workplace Applications and complete the assignments. Do online research for answers to the questions in the Internet Activities associated with assisting in obstetrics and gynecology.

 CD Connection: Go to the Medical Assisting Competency Challenge CD and do the training activities under Patient Care and Patient Instruction. View the animations for a better understanding of fetal development in the first, second, and third trimesters.

evolve **Evolve Connection:** For more information related to assisting in obstetrics and gynecology, go to evolve.elsevier.com/kinn and visit related weblinks for Chapter 40. Click on the Medical Assisting Exam Review and do the practice questions to sharpen your test-taking skills.

Assisting in Pediatrics

41

SCENARIO

Susie Kwong, a CMA with 5 years' experience, has been looking for a job and finally decided to accept a position with North Hills Pediatrics, a large, multiphysician practice. Susie's primary responsibility will be to assist in the clinical area, but she will also have to rotate through the telephone triage office as needed. Office policy states that telephone screening employees should manage problems as much as possible, but if patient callbacks are needed they are to be referred to the physician on call that day by noon for morning calls and no later than 5 pm for afternoon calls. Although the physicians in the practice have developed specific guidelines for management of patient problems, Susie is anxious about this responsibility, so she requests that she work with the triage staff for several days before she has to start answering incoming calls.

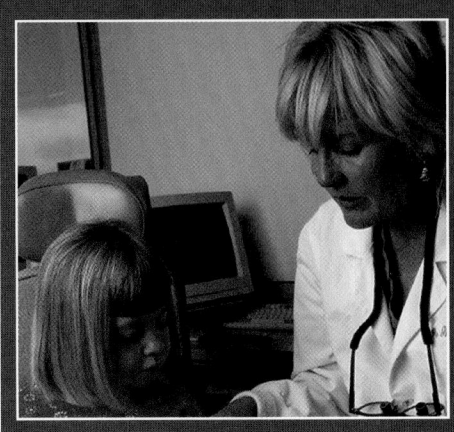

While studying this chapter, think about the following questions:

- What other clinical responsibilities should Susie be prepared to perform?
- Are patient and caregiver health education an important part of delivering high-quality care in a pediatric setting?

- Does Susie need to be clinically competent to perform immunizations and document their administration?
- How can Susie maintain her skill level and continue to learn about patient-centered pediatric care?

LEARNING OBJECTIVES

1. Define, spell, and pronounce, the terms listed in the vocabulary.
2. Describe childhood growth patterns.
3. Summarize the important features of the Denver II Developmental Screening Test.
4. Identify four different growth and development theories.
5. Explain common pediatric gastrointestinal disorders and their signs, symptoms, and treatments.
6. Classify disorders of the respiratory system in children.
7. Distinguish among pediatric infectious diseases.
8. Recognize the etiologic factors and signs and symptoms of the two primary pediatric inherited disorders.
9. Summarize CDC-recommended immunizations for children.
10. Demonstrate how to document and maintain accurate immunization records.

11. Compare and contrast a well-child and a sick-child examination.
12. Outline the medical assistant's role in a pediatric examination.
13. Measure the circumference of an infant's head.
14. Obtain accurate length and weight measurements, and plot growth patterns.
15. Accurately measure pediatric vital signs including vision screening.
16. Correctly apply a pediatric urine collection device.
17. Specify child safety guidelines for injury prevention and management of suspected child abuse.
18. Describe the characteristics and needs of the adolescent patient.

National Accreditation Competencies and Content

CAAHEP COMPETENCIES

Clinical

3.b.(4)(a) Perform telephone and in-person screening
3.b.(4)(b) Obtain vital signs
3.b.(4)(e) Prepare patient for and assist with routine and specialty examinations
3.b.(4)(f) Prepare patient for and assist with procedures, treatments, and minor office surgeries
3.b.(4)(h) Maintain medication and immunization records

ABHES COMPETENCIES

Clinical Duties

4.b. Prepare patients for procedures
4.d. Take vital signs
4.h. Prepare patient for and assist physician with routine and specialty examinations
4.n. Maintain medication and immunization records
4.ff. Perform telephone and in-person screening

VOCABULARY

attenuated (uh-ten-yuh-wat′-ed) Weakened, or changed; refers to the virulence of a pathogenic microorganism.

hydrocephaly (hi-dro-suh′-fuh-le) Enlargement of the cranium caused by abnormal accumulation of cerebrospinal fluid within the cerebral system.

laryngoscopy (lar-uhn-gahs′-kuh-pe) Visual examination of the voice box area through an endoscope equipped with a light and mirrors for illumination.

microcephaly Small size of the head in relationship to the rest of the body.

rhonchi (rahn′-ki) Continuous dry rattling in the throat or bronchial tube as a result of partial obstruction.

serous Thin, watery, serum-like drainage.

stridor Shrill, harsh respiratory sound heard during inhalation in the presence of a laryngeal obstruction.

suppurative Characterized by formation and/or discharge of pus.

Pediatrics is the medical specialty that deals with the development and care of children and with the treatment of childhood diseases. The age range of pediatric patients is from birth to puberty. Some practices continue to see the child until he or she graduates from high school. Subspecialties within pediatrics include surgery, cardiology, and psychiatry.

Approximately 50% of the patients in a pediatric office are there for well-baby or well-child visits. The roles of the pediatrician and the medical office staff are to supervise and help maintain the health of these patients. Parents must be involved in the care and development of their young children for treatment to be a success. The medical assistant can help by encouraging therapeutic communications among the patient, parents, and medical staff. The trust that a child develops in the relationships and consideration received in the physician's office forms the basis of good medical care.

Pediatric care actually starts before the child is born, with the promotion of the mother's good general health before conception and during pregnancy. The confidence and enthusiasm of the parents can have a significant impact on the infant's physical and emotional well-being.

NORMAL GROWTH AND DEVELOPMENT

The terms *growth* and *development* are often used together and refer to the combination of changes that a child goes through as he or she matures. *Growth* refers to measurable changes such as height and weight. The first determinant of these physical characteristics is what we inherit from our parents, but a child's growth can be influenced by many different factors including nutritional status, environmental factors, and the presence of disease. *Development* considers qualitative maturation in motor, mental, social, and language skills. A child's development is determined by a combination of prenatal, environmental, and caregiver factors. Each individual child has his or her own pattern for growth and development. Pediatric assessments need to be individualized for each child according to age, developmental level, health condition, family characteristics, and past experiences with healthcare professionals. The pediatrician looks for indications of growth and development irregularities by comparing a child's physical, intellectual, and social levels with published national standards. This comparison indicates whether the child is at the appropriate stage of growth and development for his or her chronologic age.

Growth Patterns

Physical growth is one of the most visible changes in childhood. The average birth weight is 7 to 7½ pounds, and in 6 months the baby's birth weight doubles. Growth slows down slightly, so that in 1 year, birth weight has tripled and length has increased by 50%. By age 2, the child has reached approximately 50% of his or her adult height. Between ages 1 and 2, the child will gain approximately ½ pound per month. Between ages 2 and 3, weight gain will average 3 to 5 pounds and height will increase

Therapeutic Approaches for Infants (0-12 months)

- Crying is normal; use distraction, but do not overstimulate.
- It is important that the infant be close to his or her caregiver; either have the parent hold the infant or keep the parent in the child's line of vision.
- Involve the parent as much as possible based on the task and the parent's level of comfort.
- Place a familiar object near the infant, and keep frightening ones out of view.
- An infant's negative response to strangers usually develops at approximately 8 months; do not take rejection personally.
- Do not restrain the infant any more than necessary, but be ready to use restraint at times to keep the infant safe (such as when administering injections).
- Encourage the caregiver to cuddle and hug the child after a procedure is completed.
- Unpleasant procedures will be associated with other objects, so do not use play areas for treatment and do not use a favorite toy or object during the procedure; offer it afterward for comfort.

Therapeutic Approaches for Toddlers and Preschoolers (2-6 years)

- Toddlers and preschoolers often fear doctor visits; ignore temper tantrums and negative behavior.
- Praise the child as much as possible.
- Perform unpleasant procedures as quickly as possible; the fear of the procedure is worse than the discomfort experienced.
- Allow the child to keep as much clothing on as possible for security and comfort.
- Use words the child is familiar with, and avoid those that they could misinterpret (e.g., "the test uses dye"—the child may think you mean "die"; "the doctor will put you to sleep so it doesn't hurt"—the family dog may have been put to sleep).
- Explain procedures as the child would sense them—what it will look like, how it will smell, how it will feel, and so on.
- Allow the child to handle equipment when possible.
- Do not use the child's favorite doll or stuffed animal to demonstrate; the child may believe the toy feels pain.
- Explain procedures to the parents away from the child when possible; the child may misinterpret the information.

Therapeutic Approaches for School-Aged Children (7-10 years)

- Allow choices when possible, such as which arm should be used to receive an injection.
- Parent should always be present during examinations.
- Remove only as much clothing as needed for the examination or procedure.
- Explain procedures in concrete terms; use pictures and diagrams when possible.
- Give the child time to ask questions.
- Children in this age group are often curious and cooperative if they know what is expected of them.
- Address the conversation to the child; involve the child in decision making as much as possible.
- Provide privacy.

rate continues through the school-aged period, 6 to 12 years; and as this period of development ends, the child usually is into a growth spurt that indicates impending puberty.

The growth spurt continues for approximately 2 years, then the child reaches adolescence (ages 12 to 18 years). During this period, the adolescent gains almost half of his or her adult weight, and the skeleton and organs double in size. These changes are more noticeable in boys than in girls. Weight will increase in girls by 20 to 25 pounds and in boys by 15 to 20 pounds. Girls will grow 5 to 6 inches, and boys will grow 4 to 5 inches. As the growth spurt is completed, the teenager reaches sexual maturity. In the girl, sexual maturity is signaled by the onset of the menstrual cycle, and in the boy, maturity is determined by the presence of sperm in the semen. Timing of sexual maturity in both sexes varies greatly.

Completion of skeletal growth occurs in girls between 15 and 16 years of age and in boys between ages 17 and 18. Skeletal growth is complete when the growth plates (*epiphyseal* plates) of the long bones of the extremities have completely fused.

Therapeutic Approaches for Adolescents (12-18 years)

- The adolescent is self-conscious and strongly influenced by peers.
- Privacy is very important.
- Address how a procedure might affect appearance.
- Do not be judgmental; listen without condemning.
- Encourage the teen to verbalize concerns and fears.
- The adolescent may regress to more childish behaviors when sick.
- Teens want to be treated like adults; they want to know what is being done and why.
- Encourage the teen to see the physician without the parent present.

2 to $2^1/_2$ inches. Most children slim down during this period, so that by the time the third birthday arrives, the potbellied toddler has become the characteristic preschooler.

During the preschool period, ages 3 to 6 years, weight increases 3 to 5 pounds per year and height increases at a slower but steady rate of $1^1/_2$ to $2^1/_2$ inches per year. By age 4, the child usually doubles his or her birth length. During this time the legs are the fastest growing part, and fatty connective tissue continues to increase slowly until approximately age 7. This same growth

CRITICAL THINKING APPLICATION

Based on what you have learned about therapeutic approaches for the pediatric patient, what would be the best way to deal with the following patient situations?

1. A crying 3-month-old being seen today for a well-child visit
2. A 10-month-old with otitis media
3. A 2-year-old who has to have a dressing changed on an infected wound
4. A 5-year-old who is scheduled for a vision and hearing screening
5. An 8-year-old who has to have a throat culture done to rule out a strep infection
6. A 12-year-old who has to receive a penicillin injection in the dorsogluteal site
7. A 15-year-old female patient with complaints of abdominal pain who is accompanied by her mother

Growth charts that can be used to compare the child's individual growth pattern with national standards have been used since 1977, but in 2000 the Centers for Disease Control and Prevention (CDC) revised the charts to reflect cultural and racial diversity (samples are available at www.cdc.gov/growthcharts). The CDC charts also take into account both formula-fed and breastfed infants because breastfed infants may grow differently in the first year of life.

In addition, the CDC growth charts include information on the average body mass index (BMI) for individuals 2 to 20 years of age, giving pediatricians another weapon in the fight against childhood obesity. BMI was discussed in Chapter 29 as a way of considering the individual's height and weight. BMI conversion charts are typically available, but BMI can be calculated by dividing the child's weight in kilograms by the height in meters squared, or:

$$BMI = \text{weight in kg} \div [\text{height in meters}]^2$$

Denver II Developmental Screening Test

Each child develops individually and will display differences in attaining developmental plateaus. The Denver II Developmental Screening Test is a standardized tool that is given to children between 1 month and 6 years of age to screen healthy infants for developmental delays, to validate concerns about an infant's development, or to monitor high-risk children for potential problems (Figures 41-1 and 41-2). It should be administered to an infant at 3 to 4 months, at 10 months, and again at 3 years of age. Although the test is not difficult to administer, only those trained in the procedure and interpretation of results should administer it. The assessment focuses on four developmental areas:

- *Gross motor skills:* Evaluates the child's ability to control large muscle groups—e.g., standing, kicking, running, and balance.
- *Language:* Assesses the child's verbal comprehension—e.g., word comprehension, following simple commands, use of subjects, and counting.
- *Fine motor skills:* Tests the child's coordination of fine motor muscles—e.g., reaching, grasping, piling blocks, and drawing.
- *Personal skills:* Examines the child's self-confidence and socialization—e.g., playing games, using a fork and spoon, dressing, and brushing teeth.

Once the test is completed, the results are analyzed and determined to be normal, suspect, or the child is determined to be untestable. A child receiving an abnormal finding should be rescreened 1 to 2 weeks later to rule out temporary developmental delays caused by fatigue or anxiety. When the results are not normal, the child may be retested with other developmental tests, either by the pediatrician or by a professional pediatric testing agency.

Developmental Patterns

General patterns of child development occur rapidly during the first year of life as the infant progresses from reflex activities, such as grasping fingers and sucking, to learning to manipulate simple objects, such as pulling open drawers or throwing toys out of the crib. In addition to these motor skills, the child also learns verbal patterns, progressing from cooing and crying for attention to speaking first words.

By age 3, the child is showing increased autonomy. Now the child can walk, is toilet trained, sits at the table and eats with the family, can make simple sentences, understands the word "no," and even imitates the parent by using verbal gestures that he or she has seen used. The child's vocabulary consists of up to 900 words.

During the preschool stage the child becomes increasingly independent and initiates activities. Preschoolers have mastered many gross motor skills and are perfecting their fine motor development. Verbal communication has increased to full simple and even complex sentences but remains quite literal. For example, if you tell a preschool child that you are going to fly to visit Aunt Sue, the child thinks you are going to flap your arms and fly. Nonverbal communication skills are also being mastered. The vocabulary now includes more than 2000 words. During this period, children need to develop social skills, such as sharing and taking part in peer-group activities.

The school-aged child has perfected fine motor skills and can paint, draw, and play an instrument, enjoys team activities, and expands reading and writing skills. His or her intellectual skills are developing, and social skills are going through refinement as a sense of self-achievement and self-worth is developed. It is during this time that the child learns and tests the rules for socializing outside the immediate family as an independent individual.

The adolescent, or transition, stage is when the individual attempts to establish an adult identity. The teenager proceeds by trial and error, experimenting with adult roles and behavior patterns. Traditional values learned in childhood may be questioned, and peer relationships take on new importance. It is during this time that teenagers must develop the emotional maturity and motivation to make beneficial decisions. The family is looked to for encouragement and guidance in making decisions that will help the adolescent develop self-confidence and to become patient and less impulsive and self-centered.

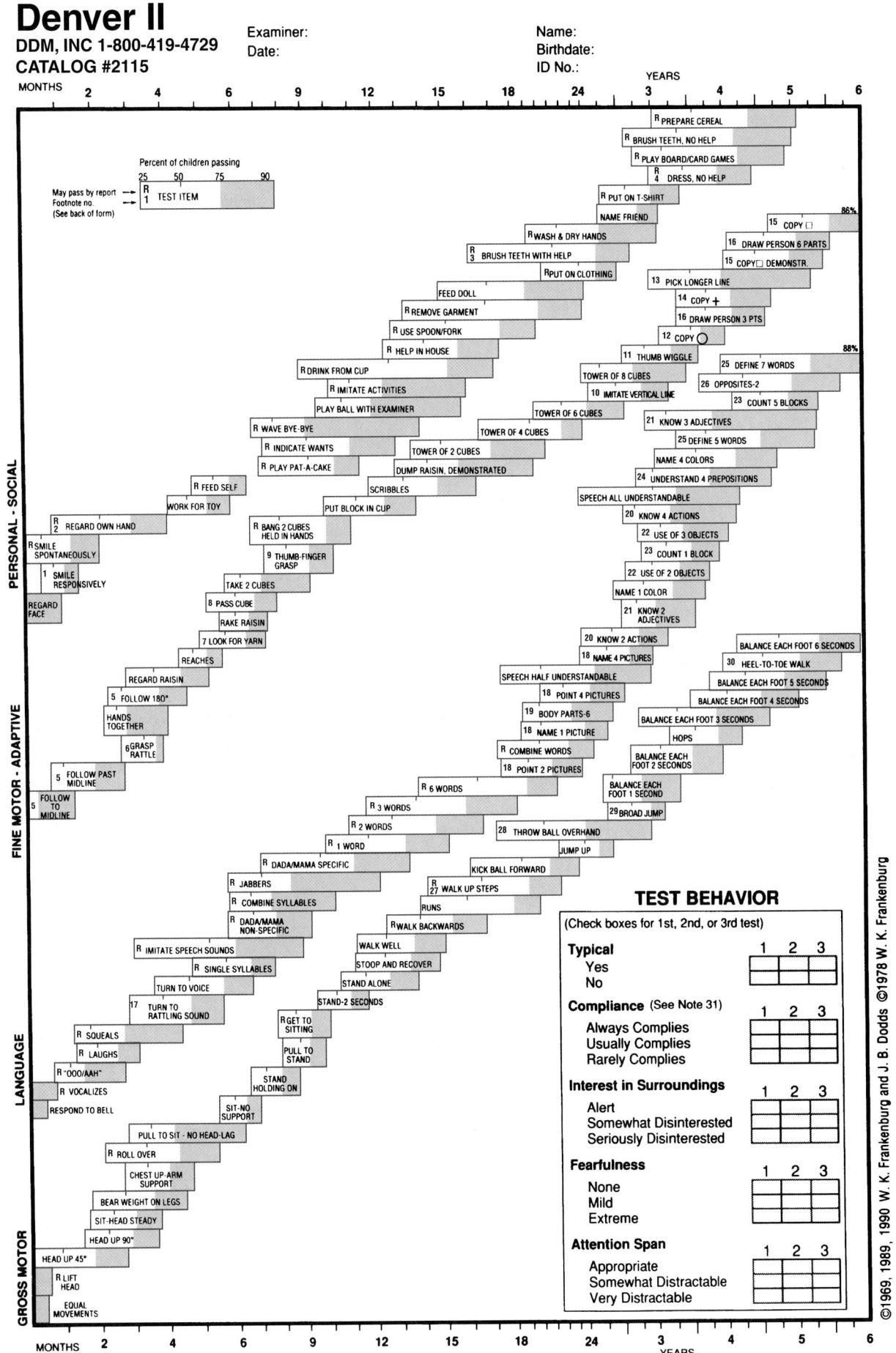

FIGURE 41-1 Denver II Developmental Screening Test (DDST). (©1969, 1989, 1990 W.K. Frankenburg and J.B. Dodds. ©1978 W.K. Frankenburg. Copies can be obtained from Denver Developmental Materials, Inc., (800) 419-4729, www.denverll.com.)

DIRECTIONS FOR ADMINISTRATION

1. Try to get child to smile by smiling, talking or waving. Do not touch him/her.
2. Child must stare at hand several seconds.
3. Parent may help guide toothbrush and put toothpaste on brush.
4. Child does not have to be able to tie shoes or button/zip in the back.
5. Move yarn slowly in an arc from one side to the other, about 8" above child's face.
6. Pass if child grasps rattle when it is touched to the backs or tips of fingers.
7. Pass if child tries to see where yarn went. Yarn should be dropped quickly from sight from tester's hand without arm movement.
8. Child must transfer cube from hand to hand without help of body, mouth, or table.
9. Pass if child picks up raisin with any part of thumb and finger.
10. Line can vary only 30 degrees or less from tester's line. |/
11. Make a fist with thumb pointing upward and wiggle only the thumb. Pass if child imitates and does not move any fingers other than the thumb.

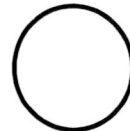 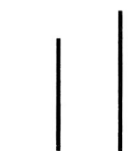 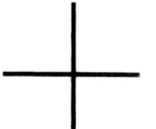 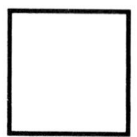

| 12. Pass any enclosed form. Fail continuous round motions. | 13. Which line is longer? (Not bigger.) Turn paper upside down and repeat. (pass 3 of 3 or 5 of 6) | 14. Pass any lines crossing near midpoint. | 15. Have child copy first. If failed, demonstrate. |

When giving items 12, 14, and 15, do not name the forms. Do not demonstrate 12 and 14.

16. When scoring, each pair (2 arms, 2 legs, etc.) counts as one part.
17. Place one cube in cup and shake gently near child's ear, but out of sight. Repeat for other ear.
18. Point to picture and have child name it. (No credit is given for sounds only.)
    If less than 4 pictures are named correctly, have child point to picture as each is named by tester.

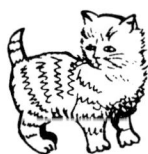 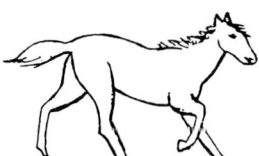 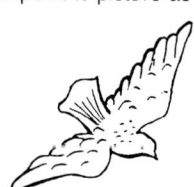 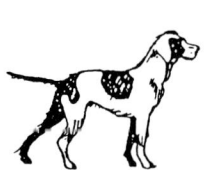 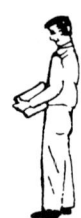

19. Using doll, tell child: Show me the nose, eyes, ears, mouth, hands, feet, tummy, hair. Pass 6 of 8.
20. Using pictures, ask child: Which one flies?... says meow?... talks?... barks?... gallops? Pass 2 of 5, 4 of 5.
21. Ask child: What do you do when you are cold?... tired?... hungry?   Pass 2 of 3, 3 of 3.
22. Ask child: What do you do with a cup? What is a chair used for? What is a pencil used for?
    Action words must be included in answers.
23. Pass if child correctly places <u>and</u> says how many blocks are on paper. (1, 5).
24. Tell child: Put block **on** table; **under** table; **in front of** me, **behind** me. Pass 4 of 4.
    (Do not help child by pointing, moving head or eyes.)
25. Ask child: What is a ball?... lake?... desk?... house?... banana?... curtain?... fence?... ceiling? Pass if defined in terms
    of use, shape, what it is made of, or general category (such as banana is fruit, not just yellow). Pass 5 of 8, 7 of 8.
26. Ask child: If a horse is big, a mouse is __? If fire is hot, ice is __? If the sun shines during the day, the moon shines
    during the __? Pass 2 of 3.
27. Child may use wall or rail only, not person. May not crawl.
28. Child must throw ball overhand 3 feet to within arm's reach of tester.
29. Child must perform standing broad jump over width of test sheet (8 1/2 inches).
30. Tell child to walk forward, ⚬⚬⚬➤ heel within 1 inch of toe. Tester may demonstrate.
    Child must walk 4 consecutive steps.
31. In the second year, half of normal children are non-compliant.

OBSERVATIONS:

FIGURE 41-2 Instructions for DDST. (©1969, 1989, 1990 W.K. Frankenburg and J.B. Dodds. © 1978 W.K. Frankenburg. Copies can be obtained from Denver Developmental Materials, Inc., (800) 419-4729, www.denverll.com.)

CRITICAL THINKING APPLICATION

Susie receives a call from the mother of a 6-month-old child. The mother has concerns about whether her child is meeting his developmental timetable. What type of information regarding the child's growth and development should Susie gather? If Susie is unable to answer the mother's questions, what should she do?

Developmental Theories

Psychologists have been researching and developing theories regarding human behavior since the beginning of the twentieth century. The first of these theorists to gain influence was Sigmund Freud, who believed that the motivating stimulus for human behavior is the libido, which is defined as an individual's pleasure-seeking instincts. Freud's theory describes four major components of the mind: the *unconscious mind*, which cannot be accessed but affects our behavior; the *id*, which focuses on immediate self-gratification; the *ego*, which develops throughout life and balances the immediate desires of the id with the reality of the social world; and the *superego*, the individual's conscience, which helps the child incorporate social expectations and norms. Freud was also the first therapist to identify developmental stages that all individuals must achieve, including the oral, anal, phallic, latency, and genital stages.

The next developmental theory to gain general acceptance was the psychosocial approach of Erik Erikson. Erikson expanded Freud's work to recognize cultural and social influences on individual development. His theory is based on eight stages of development that the individual must pass through and master. Each stage focuses on a developmental crisis, starting in infancy and ending in old age. The stages that children must master include:

- *Trust versus mistrust*—Infants learn to rely on caregivers; mistrust occurs if needs are not met.
- *Autonomy versus shame and doubt*—Toddlers learn language skills and gain independence; may feel shame and doubt if they cannot meet parental expectations or are overprotected.
- *Initiative versus guilt*—Preschoolers actively seek out new experiences; children become hesitant if restrictions or reprimands make them feel guilty or afraid to try more challenging skills.
- *Industry versus inferiority*—School-aged children enjoy finishing projects and receiving recognition; they develop feelings of inferiority if not accepted by peers or if they cannot please their parents.
- *Identity versus role confusion*—Adolescents face many physical and hormonal changes in this stage. Teenagers work at figuring out who they are and where they fit; they are looking for a direction for their lives. If they are unable to establish an identity and sense of direction, they become role confused.

Piaget's developmental theory focuses on intellectual growth, with four stages of cognitive development. From birth to 24 months children progress through the *sensorimotor stage*, where they begin with reflexive behavior and advance to learning by doing. The *preoperational stage* (2 to 7 years) is characterized by language development and using play to understand the world. In the *concrete operational stage* (7 to 11 years) children develop logical thinking and become less egocentric. Finally, the *formal operational stage* (11 years or older) brings abstract thinking and deductive reasoning to establish values and determine the meaning of life.

Kohlberg focuses on moral reasoning with levels that are similar to Piaget's cognitive development theory, while recognizing the influence of culture and interpersonal relationships on the child's moral development. In *preconventional morality* the child's behavior is based on the external control of authority figures. The child perceives the goodness or badness of a behavior based on parental reaction. During the *conventional level* the child wants to follow the rules of the group or society and internalizes the values of others. As the child reaches adolescence, the *postconventional level*, the child develops individual morality and values, with behavior regulated internally rather than externally. Table 41-1 summarizes these growth and development theories.

PEDIATRIC DISEASES AND DISORDERS

The disease process in pediatric patients poses special problems because children are constantly changing physically and functionally. As a child grows and develops, the immune system matures, and with the aid of routine prophylactic immunizations the child is fortified with long-term protection against certain infectious diseases.

Gastrointestinal Disorders

Colic

Colic is usually seen in the newborn period or in early infancy. The problem is intermittent. The classic situation is an infant between 2 weeks and 4 months of age with crying episodes that occur at least three times a week for greater than 3 hours a day and lasting 3 weeks. During an attack the infant draws up the legs, clenches the fists, and cries inconsolably. The abdominal distress of colic usually occurs in the late afternoon and evening. Many theories suggest why infants have colic, but none has been proven correct. If the baby receives infant formula, pediatricians recommend switching formulas—perhaps to a non–cow's milk type—because this may help relieve the infant's discomfort. Treatment consists of determining the cause; however, the child frequently outgrows the condition before the causative agent can be identified. Drugs are not helpful and in some cases may be dangerous for the infant. Parents need reassurance that they are not responsible for the child's discomfort and may find counseling and assistance in developing coping techniques helpful.

Diarrhea

Diarrhea can be caused by a variety of microorganisms, including bacteria, viruses, and parasites. However, children can sometimes have diarrhea without having an infection,

TABLE 41-1 Growth and Development Theories Summarized

AGE GROUP	FREUD PSYCHOSEXUAL THEORY	PIAGET COGNITIVE THEORY	ERIKSON PSYCHOSOCIAL THEORY	KOHLBERG MORAL REASONING
Infant	Oral stage; child operates with the pleasure principle, and the id develops	Sensorimotor level; uses reflexive behavior; has to do things to learn.	Building basic trust vs mistrust; learning drive and hope.	Avoids punishment and obeys for obedience's sake.
Toddler	Passes through oral aggressive stage to anal stage; elimination is used to control and inhibit	Coordinates more than one thought at a time; uses thought to create new solutions.	Autonomy vs shame and doubt; learning self-control and willpower.	Avoids punishment and the power of authority figures.
Preschool to early school years	From phallic stage where the ego (conscious reality) develops to the latent stage where the superego (morality) develops	Intuitive-preoperational; preschoolers are egocentric and have magical thinking. Early school-aged children begin to develop understanding of cause and effect. Child functions symbolically using language; develops understanding of life events and relationships.	Preschool processing initiative vs guilt and attempting to develop direction and purpose. Children mimic others and are more purposeful in establishing goals.	Develops preconventional morality; follows the standards of others to avoid punishment or to earn a reward; recognizes some things are self-satisfying and some are done to satisfy others.
School age	Latent stage continues; superego develops morality or a conscience; represses the sexual drive	Concrete operations: uses mental reasoning to solve problems; attempts to reach logical solutions; tests beliefs to establish values.	Industry vs inferiority; establishing methods for solving problems and a feeling of competence; is mastering tasks and using hands to create things.	Conventional morality; doing what is expected is important. Children need to be good in their own eyes as well as doing what they perceive others expect of them; they want to please others.
Adolescence	Genital stage	Formal operations developing; adolescents are determining values that will guide their lives and religious affiliations; they develop abstract ideas that can be based in reality.	Identity vs role confusion; developing self-identity that will determine devotion and fidelity in future relationships.	Postconventional morality; developing a respect for the laws of society; adolescents are learning to consider the greatest good for the greatest number; values are related to one's group. Behavior is controlled internally.

as when diarrhea is caused by food allergies or as a result of taking medicines such as antibiotics. Diarrhea is diagnosed when the child has two or more watery or apparently abnormal stools within a 24-hour period. The child may not show other signs of illness or may have nausea, vomiting, stomach aches, headache, or fever. If diarrhea continues for more than 2 days, medical intervention is needed because prolonged diarrhea, in which fluid loss becomes excessive, can cause dehydration and electrolyte imbalance. In addition, a resultant diaper rash and excoriation can produce painful stool elimination.

Pediatric diarrhea needs to be followed closely with observation and, in the case of bloody stools, laboratory analysis to determine causative factors. Infants and small children should be followed up by telephone in 12 hours, then daily until diarrhea has stopped. Parents should know the indications of dehydration, including lack of tears when crying; lethargy; fewer wet diapers or decreased urination; dry mouth and lips; and weight loss. The physician may recommend the use of oral rehydration therapy such as Pedialyte or Infalyte with small amounts (approximately 2 tablespoons every 15 minutes) offered at a time to prevent

vomiting. Soft drinks, juices, sport drinks, and tea should be avoided because they lack electrolytes and may lead to even more diarrhea. Parents need to be aware that the child's diarrhea may not stop when the child is given oral rehydration therapy, but it will prevent the child from becoming dehydrated. It is important to continue to feed the child because lack of food can cause damage to the villi in the small intestine. If the infant is being breastfed the baby should continue to nurse, and formula feeding should be continued as well. For older children a diet of bananas, rice, and applesauce (the BRAT diet) or foods high in carbohydrate are most helpful in enhancing fluid and sodium absorption in the child's irritated gastrointestinal tract. The child should not be given over-the-counter antidiarrheal medications such as Pepto-Bismol, Kaopectate, Imodium, or Lomotil because these can cause serious side effects including decreased motility of the bowel, respiratory depression, and drowsiness. The physician may prescribe antibiotics if stool cultures are positive, and children with severe dehydration will require hospitalization with intravenous (IV) hydration to replace electrolytes and fluids.

CRITICAL THINKING APPLICATION

Susie receives a call from the grandmother of a 3-year-old child who has had diarrhea since last night. What are some of the questions Susie should ask to determine the seriousness of the problem? Should the child be seen today, even though appointments are already overbooked?

Failure to Thrive

Failure to thrive is a symptom more than a disease; it is diagnosed in an infant or young child whose weight is consistently below the third percentile on standardized growth charts or one who is 20% below the ideal body weight for length. Physical, mental, and social skills are also delayed in these children; manifestations include failure to roll over, smile, coo, stand, or walk at age appropriate developmental levels. It can be caused by a physiologic factor (such as malabsorption disease or cleft palate), or it may have a nonorganic cause that is associated with the parent-child relationship. The physician needs to have an accurately recorded history of the child's birth weight and subsequent length, weight, and head circumference. A comprehensive family history is important to rule out genetic growth abnormalities or a history of malabsorption problems such as cystic fibrosis or celiac disease.

Children with failure to thrive need more calories than usual to catch up to their target weight, approximately 150% of their normal calorie load. Both medical and social factors must be evaluated when treating children with this problem. Experts believe that infants may suffer from this problem if they are being neglected, but it is also possible to have low weight gains with parents who are extremely attentive and cautious. The family must be considered as a whole to effectively treat nonorganic causes, including the use of support groups and parental counseling.

Obesity

Just as with adult weight patterns, children are assessed according to their BMI. A child's level of body fat varies as he or she grows; for example, it is normal for children to slim down as they reach school age and very often their weight increases as they mature from adolescence to adulthood. In addition, body fat levels vary between boys and girls as they reach puberty. Therefore pediatricians use growth charts that plot the child's BMI-for-age to determine if the child's weight, in comparison with height, is within healthy limits. A child is considered at risk for being overweight if the BMI-for-age is between the 85th and 95th percentiles and is identified as overweight if the BMI is at or greater than the 95th percentile. It is estimated that more than 30% of school-aged children are overweight, and almost 20% are considered obese.

The reasons for childhood obesity vary, including a family history of obesity, inactivity, high-calorie diets, and stress. Rarely, childhood obesity may be caused by metabolic or endocrine disorders. Overweight and obese children are at greater risk for developing serious health conditions including asthma, type 2 diabetes, sleep apnea, and hypercholesterolemia, which increases the risk of cardiovascular disease and hypertension. The psychosocial impact of obesity can be overwhelming for many children, with isolation, loneliness, and self-esteem issues common. Studies have shown that 40% to 80% of overweight teenagers become overweight adults with all of the health risks and psychologic issues that come with weight problems. The pediatrician can provide assistance by recommending a comprehensive diet and exercise program that emphasizes healthy living. You can help by providing educational materials, encouragement for the child and parents, and referral to community education and support programs.

Respiratory Disorders

Common Cold

The common cold, or *infectious rhinitis,* has more than 100 causative pathogens and is highly contagious. It is spread through respiratory droplets from rhinitis, sneezing, or coughing, either from direct contact or from touching contaminated items. The signs include nasal congestion, low-grade fever, and general malaise. Most colds are self-limiting and run their course in about a week. In infants and young children the primary concerns are nasal congestion and loss of appetite. The parent may need to be shown how to use a nasal bulb syringe to suction the nose of an infant (Figure 41-3). Secondary infections in the lower respiratory tract or in the middle ear can occur.

One of the secondary infections that can occur is strep throat, which is caused by group A *Streptococcus* bacteria. It is easily spread when an infected person coughs or sneezes contaminated droplets into the air and another person inhales them. A person can also get infected from touching secretions, then touching his or her mouth or nose. Symptoms of strep throat infections may include severe sore throat, fever, headache, and lymphadenopathy, and the throat appears bright red with pustules possible on the tonsils. If not treated, strep infections can lead to scarlet or rheumatic fever; infections of the skin, bloodstream, or ears; and pneumonia. Scarlet fever is characterized by a bright red, rough-textured rash that spreads all over the child's body. Rheumatic fever is a serious disease that can damage the heart valves.

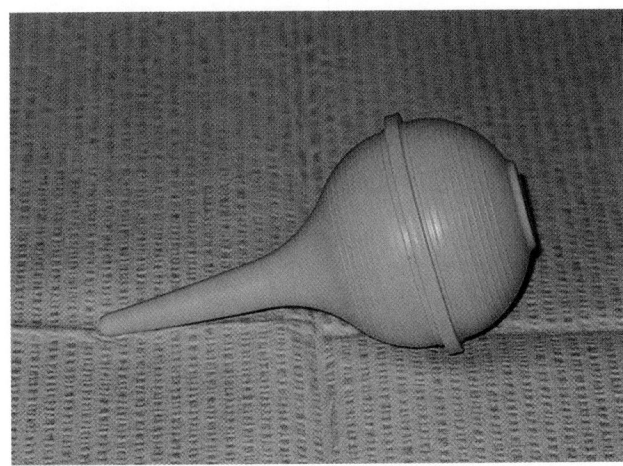

FIGURE 41-3 Nasal bulb syringe.

Otitis Media

Infection or inflammation of the middle ear is usually a side effect of a cold or other upper respiratory tract disorder but can also be caused by allergies. Otitis media usually occurs in children younger than 3 years of age. Signs include inflammation of the middle ear, with fluid building up behind the tympanic membrane. The child may cry persistently, tug at the ear, have a fever, be irritable, and have decreased hearing in the affected ear. These symptoms may sometimes be accompanied by diarrhea, nausea, and vomiting.

Otitis media is classified as either **serous** (Figure 41-4) or **suppurative** (Figure 41-5), depending on the composition of accumulated fluid in the middle ear. It may be caused by a bacteria or virus, so it is difficult to determine the most appropriate treatment. Traditionally children with indications of a middle ear infection were treated with antibiotics; however, if the infection is caused by a virus, antibiotics will not help. Because of concern over the growing problem of antibiotic-resistant strains of bacteria, current recommendations include treatment with acetaminophen or ibuprofen if the child is in pain or has a fever but delay in prescribing antibiotics for 24 hours to give the body a chance to fight the infection by itself. Children 6 to 24 months old who show no improvement in symptoms within 24 hours or children older than 24 months who do not improve in 72 hours should be prescribed antibiotics (typically amoxicillin or Zithromax). The medication is usually ordered for a shorter course—5 days rather than 10 to 14 days—because patients and their parents are more compliant with short-term treatment. However, regardless of how long the medication is prescribed, it is very important that the complete prescription be administered to prevent a relapse.

If fluid in the middle ear persists for longer than 3 months and/or if the child is experiencing hearing loss, the physician may recommend an operation—a myringotomy—in which a small incision is made in the tympanic membrane and a tube is inserted to drain the fluid and balance the pressure between the outer and middle ear. The tube typically stays in the eardrum for 6 to 12 months and falls out as the child grows. While tubes are in place it is important to keep water out of the child's ears and report any drainage to the physician.

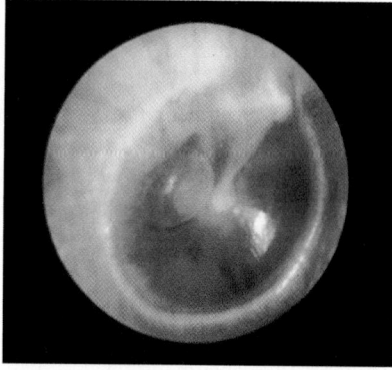

FIGURE 41-4 Serous otitis media. (From Swartz MH: *Textbook of physical diagnosis*, ed 5, Philadelphia, 2006, Saunders.)

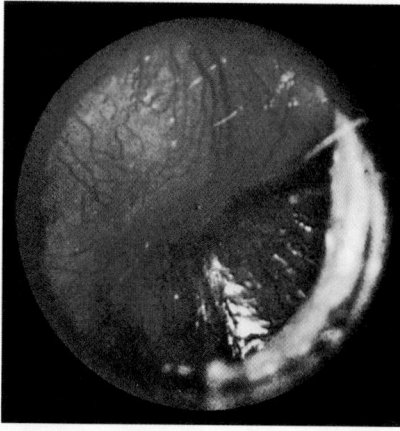

FIGURE 41-5 Suppurative otitis media. (Courtesy Dr. Richard A. Buckingham and Dr. George E. Shambaugh, Jr.)

CRITICAL THINKING APPLICATION

A young mother calls, extremely upset about her 4-year-old son. His symptoms started 3 days ago with a cold, but now the child is complaining of a sore throat and an earache. What questions should Susie ask to determine whether the child should be seen today?

Croup

Croup is a viral inflammation of the larynx and the trachea that causes edema and spasm of the vocal cords. This varying degree of obstruction to the cords produces hoarseness, a harsh barking cough, and **stridor** during inhalation. The episodes usually occur at night, and all symptoms may be gone by morning. The infection is usually self-limiting, and the child typically recovers without treatment. Children with allergies may require medical treatment. If the problem becomes chronic or continues for a period of time, it may become necessary to do a **laryngoscopy** or perform throat cultures to determine the underlying cause.

Bronchiolitis

Bronchiolitis is a viral infection of the small bronchi and bronchioles that usually affects children under 3 years of age. The infection varies in severity and is seen in children with a family history of asthma and children exposed to cigarette smoke. The child typically has a previous history of rhinitis and cough with acute onset of wheezing and dyspnea. Symptoms occur because of inflammation, edema, increased secretions, and bronchospasm in the respiratory pathway. Treatment includes acetaminophen for discomfort and fever as well as a bronchodilator inhaler (albuterol sulfate) or nebulizer treatment for relief of wheezing. Most children fully recover in 2 weeks, but as many as 50% of them will have recurrent wheezing and coughing.

Asthma

Asthma is the most common chronic health problem among children. Asthma is the result of two specific reactions—bronchospasm and inflammation. During an asthma attack the bronchial tubes begin to spasm, thereby decreasing the amount of air that can pass through them, while at the same time tissue lining the bronchioles becomes edematous and secretes mucus. This means that a person having an asthma attack has smaller airways that are filling up with mucus and secretions. Air passing through these secretions is what causes the classic symptom of asthma–wheezing. Asthma has a strong hereditary link. Factors that can trigger an attack include:

- Respiratory infections, including infections caused by common cold viruses
- Exposure to cigarette smoke
- Stress
- Strenuous exercise
- Weather conditions, including cold, windy, or rainy days and extreme humidity
- Allergies to animals, dust, pollen, or mold
- Indoor air pollutants, such as paint, cleaning materials, chemicals, or perfumes
- Outdoor air pollutants, such as ozone

Children with asthma have a nonproductive cough accompanied by an expiratory wheeze and shortness of breath. Shallow breathing makes it difficult for the child to speak more than a few words at a time. The child complains of tightness or pressure in the chest, and the physician will hear **rhonchi** on auscultation. An asthma attack can last minutes to days and may develop into a medical emergency. Each child and each attack needs to be evaluated independently.

The therapeutic plan is determined by the severity and frequency of attacks. Children with mild to moderately persistent disease (from symptoms occurring less than twice a week to daily symptoms) should be referred to a specialist. If they experience symptoms two or more times per week, they should be on daily medication to prevent asthma attacks. These may include inhaled corticosteroids that deliver an antiinflammatory directly to the bronchioles such as Advair Diskus and Flovent (fluticasone); long-acting bronchodilators including salmeterol (Serevent); and oral medications such as montelukast (Singulair) or zafirlukast (Accolate). The child is also prescribed a quick-acting medication, or "rescue inhaler," such as albuterol (Proventil, Ventolin) for acute relief of bronchospasm or exercise-induced asthma; this inhaler should be readily available at all times. Further management of asthma is covered in Chapter 45.

Influenza

Influenza (the "flu") is an acute, highly contagious viral infection of the respiratory tract. Its highest incidence is in school-aged children, but it is most severe in infants and toddlers. It is transmitted by direct contact with moist secretions. Children tend to have high fevers with influenza and are susceptible to pulmonary complications. There is a broad range in the severity of flu cases, from very mild to life-threatening. The virus can destroy the respiratory epithelium, which is one of the body's defense mechanisms against bacterial invasion. With the loss of this protective mechanism, bacteria can invade any part of the respiratory tract and cause pneumonia.

There is no medication that cures influenza. Some drugs can shorten the duration of the disease, but they must be taken at the onset of symptoms to be effective. Examples of these are zanamivir (Relenza), which is inhaled every 12 hours, and oseltamivir (Tamiflu), which is available in pill form. Antibiotics may be prescribed to treat a secondary bacterial infection, such as sinusitis. The usual treatment for influenza is bed rest, increased fluids, and a nonaspirin analgesic to reduce fever and relieve discomfort.

Flu vaccines are available but are beneficial only if the individual is vaccinated before the onset of the disease, and annual vaccines do not provide immunity from all strains of the flu virus. The CDC recommends flu vaccinations for all children 6 months to 2 years of age and their caregivers; children with chronic heart or lung diseases (including asthma); those on long-term aspirin therapy; children with diabetes mellitus or sickle cell anemia; and those with kidney, blood, or suppressed immune system diseases.

Infectious Diseases

Conjunctivitis

Pinkeye, also called *conjunctivitis,* was discussed in Chapter 36. It is a common infection in children and is highly contagious, especially in day care centers and schools. It can be caused by a bacterial or viral infection that produces white or yellowish pus that may cause the eyelids to stick shut in the morning. Health teaching for caregivers of infected children includes the following:

- Use good hand-washing practices and hygiene, including proper use and disposal of paper tissues.
- Do not share towels or any other item that comes into contact with the child's face.
- Disinfect any articles that may have been contaminated.
- Children diagnosed with infectious conjunctivitis should be treated with an antibiotic for at least 24 hours before returning to day care or school.

Tonsillitis

Tonsillitis is caused by many infectious agents, but the most frequent is *Streptococcus* A. The onset is sudden, and the disorder can cause intense pain in a brief period of time, with fever and general malaise. The tonsils appear enlarged and inflamed and may be covered with pustules. A throat culture is usually performed to determine the causative organism. The treatment consists of bed rest, liquid to soft diet, analgesic throat spray, and oral antibiotics if the causative organism is bacterial. The danger is in the secondary problems that can occur, which include rheumatic heart disease and kidney disease.

Fifth Disease

Fifth disease, also called *erythema infectiosum* or *slapped cheek disease,* is an infection caused by parvovirus B19. Outbreaks most often occur in winter and spring, but a person may become ill with fifth disease at any time of the year. Symptoms begin with a mild fever and general malaise. After a few days, the cheeks take on a flushed appearance that looks like the face has been slapped. There may also be a lacy rash on the trunk, arms, and legs. Not all infected persons develop a rash.

Most children who get fifth disease are not very ill and recover without any serious consequences. However, children with sickle cell anemia, chronic anemia, or an impaired immune system may become seriously ill when infected and require medical care. If a pregnant woman becomes infected with parvovirus B19, the fetus may suffer damage, including the possibility of stillbirth. The woman herself may have no symptoms or a mild illness with a rash and/or *arthralgia* (joint pain).

Fifth disease is spread through direct contact or by breathing in respiratory secretions from an infected person. Patients are most contagious before the onset of the rash; once the rash appears they are no longer considered contagious.

Varicella (Chickenpox)

Chickenpox is caused by a member of the herpesvirus group and is transmitted by direct or indirect droplets from the respiratory tract of an infected person. The incubation period is 14 to 21 days. The child usually runs a slight fever for up to 3 days before the skin eruptions occur and is contagious at this time. The skin lesions continue to erupt for 3 to 4 days and cause intense itching. The infection lasts for approximately 2 weeks and, in most cases, leaves the child with lifetime immunity. The disease is so contagious in its early stages that an exposed person who is not immune to the virus has a 70% to 80% chance of contracting the disease.

The varicella virus vaccine, Varivax, is available for protection against chickenpox. Children aged 12 months to 12 years can be immunized with a single injection of the vaccine; two injections 4 to 8 weeks apart are recommended for adolescents and adults who have never had chickenpox. Varivax has proven to be safe and effective and can be administered at the same time as the measles, mumps, and rubella vaccine.

Although chickenpox is not a serious disease for most children, newborns or persons with impaired immune systems (e.g., those who are receiving chemotherapy for cancer, have acquired immunodeficiency syndrome [AIDS], or take steroidal medications, such as prednisone) may have a severe case or can even die. Chickenpox can be very dangerous for pregnant women, causing stillbirths or birth defects, and can be spread to their babies during childbirth. Occasionally chickenpox can cause serious, life-threatening illnesses, such as encephalitis or pneumonia, especially in adults. After infection the virus migrates to a dermatome and may cause "shingles" or herpes zoster (see Chapter 37). An adult with shingles can spread the virus to an adult or child who has not had chickenpox, and the susceptible person can develop the disease.

Meningitis

Meningitis is an inflammation of the membranes that cover the brain and spinal cord. The cause of this inflammation is infection with bacteria, fungi, or viruses. Viral meningitis is usually mild and clears up on its own within 10 days. Fungal meningitis can be quite serious and is typically seen in immunocompromised individuals such as AIDS patients. Meningitis caused by a bacterial infection (sometimes called *spinal meningitis*) is one of the most serious types, sometimes leading to permanent brain damage or even death. Bacterial meningitis is most commonly caused by these bacteria: *Neisseria meningitidis* (meningococcal meningitis), *Streptococcus pneumoniae*,

or *Haemophilus influenzae* serotype b (*H. influenzae* meningitis). These bacteria are carried in the upper back part of the throat (*nasopharynx*) of an infected person and are spread either through the air (when the person coughs or sneezes) or by direct contact with secretions, such as through kissing or sharing eating or drinking utensils. However, transmission usually occurs only after very close contact with the infected person.

Signs and symptoms of bacterial meningitis include sudden onset of fever, headache, neck pain or stiffness, vomiting (often without abdominal complaints), and irritability. These signs and symptoms may quickly progress to a decreased level of consciousness (difficulty in being aroused), convulsions, and death. For this reason, if any child displays symptoms of possible meningitis, he or she should receive medical care immediately.

Meningitis caused by *H. influenzae* serotype b (Hib) can be prevented with Hib vaccine, which is given as part of the routine childhood immunizations. Some cases of meningococcal meningitis can also be prevented by vaccine. However, this vaccine is not used routinely—usually only during outbreaks or in high-risk children. Many states require reporting of bacterial meningitis cases to the health department, which will probably recommend preventive antibiotics for potentially exposed persons.

Hepatitis B

Hepatitis B virus (HBV) infection can lead to serious and chronic infection of the liver. The virus can be transmitted across the placenta or during the birth process if the mother is infected. HBV can also be transmitted sexually, by blood transfusion, or by direct contact. A child can carry the virus for years and only later develop liver failure or liver cancer as a result. Many states now include immunizations for HBV in the recommended immunization schedule, which is usually begun in the newborn nursery.

Reye's Syndrome

The cause of Reye's syndrome is unknown, but it has been linked to the use of aspirin during a viral illness. It is an acute and sometimes fatal illness characterized by fatty invasion of the inner organs, especially the liver, and swelling of the brain. It is most often seen in children from infancy through puberty (age 16). The syndrome moves through five stages, as shown in Table 41-2.

TABLE 41-2 Five Stages of Reye's Syndrome	
STAGE	**SIGNS AND SYMPTOMS**
1	Restlessness, vomiting, liver malfunction
2	Elevated respiratory rate, hyperactive reflexes, increased liver dysfunction
3	Internal organ tissue changes, coma
4	Loss of brain function, deepening coma
5	Seizures, respiratory arrest, death

Prevention is the best treatment, which means children should never be given aspirin. Parents should be advised to use nonsalicylate analgesics and antipyretics, such as ibuprofen and acetaminophen, for fevers or discomfort. Parents should also be warned to read the labels of over-the-counter medication carefully, because cold and flu remedies may contain aspirin.

CRITICAL THINKING APPLICATION

A father of a 10 year-old girl calls this morning, concerned about his daughter's symptoms. She has a sore throat, fever, and bright red cheeks. He wants to give her aspirin for the fever. What advice should Susie give the father? What questions should she ask to determine the seriousness of the child's problem?

Inherited Disorders

Cystic Fibrosis

Cystic fibrosis is an autosomal recessive genetic disorder (i.e., both parents are carriers but do not have the disease) that prevents the normal movement of sodium chloride (salt) into and out of cells. The lungs and pancreas are primarily affected, causing a buildup of abnormally thick secretions in the lungs and blockage of the pancreatic ducts, which prevents the excretion of pancreatic digestive enzymes and results in malabsorption problems in the child. The child is prone to develop an emphysema-like lung condition as a result of the obstruction of air pathways with mucus. There is also an abnormality in the sweat glands, which produce sweat that is very high in sodium chloride.

Signs and symptoms of cystic fibrosis include a salty taste to the skin, which may be noticed when parents kiss the child, *steatorrhea* (large, greasy, foul-smelling stools), abdominal distention, failure to thrive, chronic cough, and frequent respiratory infections.

The primary diagnostic test is the sweat test, which shows an elevated chlorine level. The treatment of the disease is complicated, requiring a multispecialty approach, because there are so many systems involved. The goals of treatment are to prevent bronchial obstruction through routine chest percussion therapy and the use of bronchodilators and antibiotics for signs of infection. The child is also given pancreatic enzymes to improve digestion and absorption of nutrients. Cystic fibrosis is a chronic, progressive disease that has no cure, with a life expectancy of 30 to 35 years. Genetic testing can identify carriers, and its presence can be determined through prenatal genetic testing with either chorionic villi sampling or amniocentesis. Cystic fibrosis usually occurs without any warning (parents have no idea they are carriers), so families need support and understanding to cope with the demands of caring for a child with the disease.

Duchenne's Muscular Dystrophy

Muscular dystrophy is an X-linked genetic disease (passed from mothers to sons) that causes progressive muscle degeneration. The disease usually develops before age 5, with muscular weakness, frequent falls, waddling gait, possible swallowing problems, and difficulty climbing stairs. The disorder is diagnosed with a blood test that shows an elevated creatine phosphokinase (CPK) level, electromyography, and a muscle biopsy. As the disease progresses and the necrotic skeletal muscles are replaced with fat and fibrous connective tissue, muscle function is gradually lost. Respiratory insufficiency and infections are common because of involvement of the muscles used for breathing. The disease has no cure and no specific treatment, except for supportive care. Family counseling is helpful so that family members can learn to cope with the disease. Death usually occurs in the early 20s because of respiratory or cardiac complications.

IMMUNIZATIONS

Over the years immunization has helped dramatically reduce potentially lethal childhood infections. Figure 41-6 summarizes the 2006 immunization recommendations from the CDC, which can be found at www.cdc.gov/nip/recs/child-schedule-image1-ppt.jpg.

This schedule is updated periodically as new vaccines become available and/or research indicates a better method for giving the vaccine. For example, it is now recommended that all children be immunized against Hepatitis A. The CDC recommends immunization against infectious diseases for all children, except those for whom a particular vaccination would pose a risk. However, each state develops its own immunization program and methods for enforcement.

Immunizations consist of a vaccine suspension of **attenuated** organisms or their toxins that is administered to stimulate an active immune response in the child's body, resulting in the production of antibodies against the specific pathogenic organisms. Booster doses are usually equivalent to one single dose of the initial immunization; for some immunizations, such as tetanus, boosters are prescribed at designated intervals to ensure maintenance of immune levels.

Vaccine manufacturers have trade names for each product and have established protocols to ensure potency and stability. All vaccines are tested for safety and effectiveness. In every package of vaccine is an insert that fully describes the vaccine, its use, route of administration, and adverse reactions and signs and symptoms that the parent might observe after immunization that would indicate a potential problem. Untoward responses include high fever, swelling at the site of the injection, urticaria, breathing difficulties, severe headache, and convulsions. Any of these should be reported to the physician immediately. Vaccine storage should follow manufacturer guidelines (e.g., some vaccines must be refrigerated; others must not be exposed to sunlight).

Some vaccines are grown in bird eggs or in a medium made from animal organs, or are weakened with chemicals. Therefore a child who is allergic to eggs cannot receive some of the vaccines, such as those for measles, mumps, and rubella (MMR) and for varicella. It is the medical assistant's responsibility to know potential allergic problems, common symptoms, and adverse reactions to immunizations and to be certain that the parent is informed. Table 41-3 details guidelines for childhood immunizations.

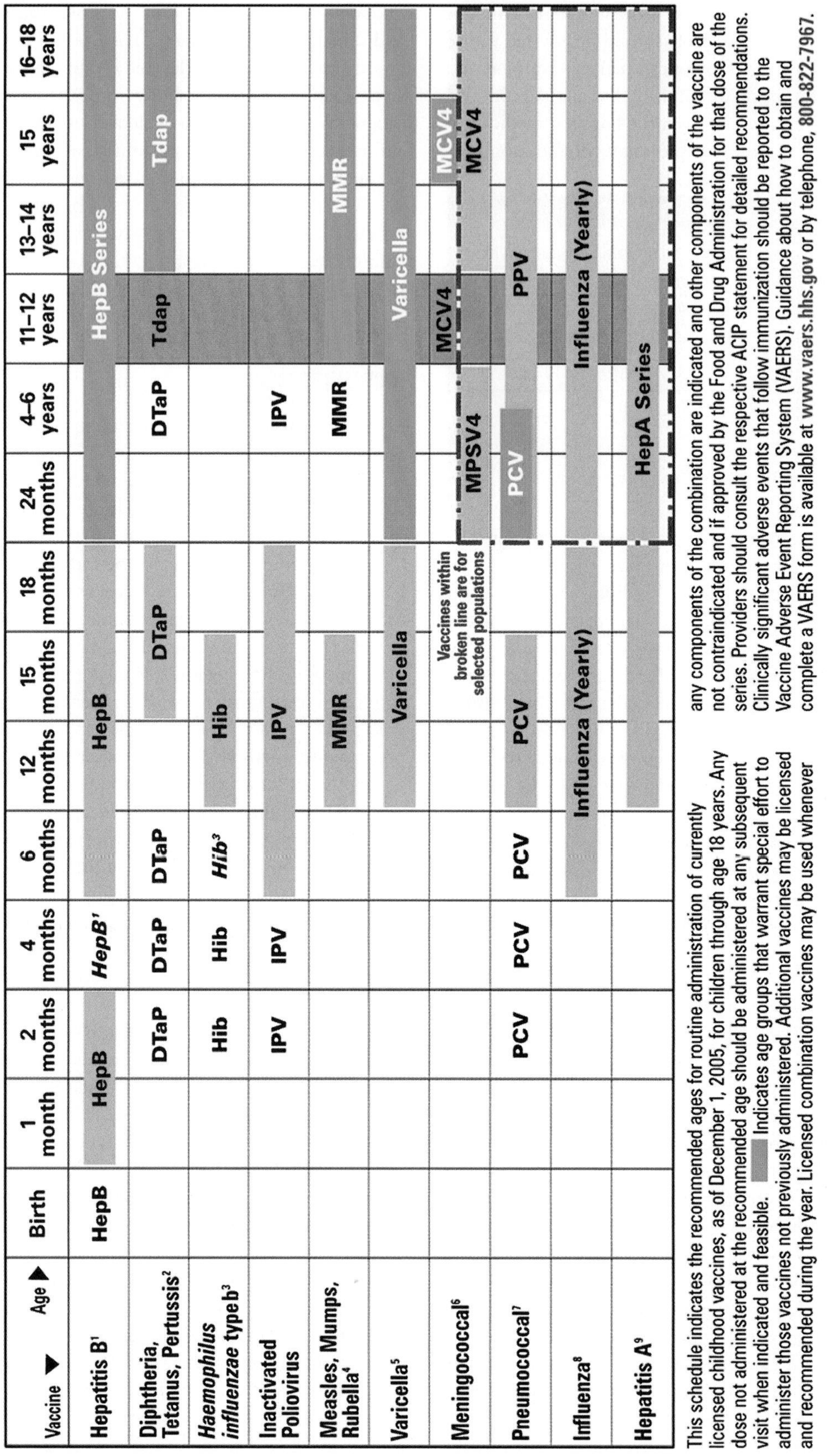

Vaccine ▼ Age ▲	Birth	1 month	2 months	4 months	6 months	12 months	15 months	18 months	24 months	4-6 years	11-12 years	13-14 years	15 years	16-18 years
Hepatitis B[1]	HepB	HepB		HepB[1]		HepB					HepB Series			
Diphtheria, Tetanus, Pertussis[2]			DTaP	DTaP	DTaP		DTaP	DTaP		DTaP	Tdap		Tdap	
Haemophilus influenzae type b[3]			Hib	Hib	Hib[3]	Hib	Hib							
Inactivated Poliovirus			IPV	IPV		IPV	IPV			IPV				
Measles, Mumps, Rubella[4]						MMR	MMR			MMR		MMR		
Varicella[5]						Varicella	Varicella				Varicella			
Meningococcal[6]								Vaccines within broken line are for selected populations	MPSV4	MPSV4	MCV4		MCV4 / MCV4	
Pneumococcal[7]			PCV	PCV	PCV	PCV	PCV		PCV	PCV	PPV	PPV		
Influenza[8]						Influenza (Yearly)				Influenza (Yearly)	Influenza (Yearly)			
Hepatitis A[9]										HepA Series	HepA Series			

Range of recommended ages   Catch-up immunization   11-12 year old assessment

This schedule indicates the recommended ages for routine administration of currently licensed childhood vaccines, as of December 1, 2005, for children through age 18 years. Any dose not administered at the recommended age should be administered at any subsequent visit when indicated and feasible. ▨ Indicates age groups that warrant special effort to administer those vaccines not previously administered. Additional vaccines may be licensed and recommended during the year. Licensed combination vaccines may be used whenever any components of the combination are indicated and other components of the vaccine are not contraindicated and if approved by the Food and Drug Administration for that dose of the series. Providers should consult the respective ACIP statement for detailed recommendations. Clinically significant adverse events that follow immunization should be reported to the Vaccine Adverse Event Reporting System (VAERS). Guidance about how to obtain and complete a VAERS form is available at www.vaers.hhs.gov or by telephone, 800-822-7967.

FIGURE 41-6 Recommended childhood and adolescent immunization schedule. (From U.S. Centers for Disease Control, 2006. Available at: www.immunize.org/catg.d/p2022b.pdf.)

TABLE 41-3 Guidelines for Childhood Immunization

VACCINE AND DISEASE	ROUTE OF ADMINISTRATION	CONTRAINDICATIONS (MILD ILLNESS IS NOT A CONTRAINDICATION)	SIDE EFFECTS
DtaP Diphtheria, tetanus, pertussis (whooping cough)	IM; Td (tetanus and diphtheria) boosters at 11-12 yr if at least 5 yr since last dose; subsequent booster every 10 yr	Moderate or severe acute illness; neurologic problem; complication such as fever or convulsion after previous dose	Mild fever, anorexia, irritability, drowsiness
HBV Hepatitis B (can use either Energix B or Recombivax HB brands)	IM; may give with all other vaccines but at a separate site; requires three injections	Moderate or severe acute illness; yeast allergy; severe cardiovascular disease	Fever, pain at site, headache, malaise, vomiting
Hib Haemophilus influenzae serotype B meningitis	IM; may give with all other vaccines but at a separate site	Not routinely given to children ≥5 yr of age; moderate or severe acute illness	Minimal
IPV Inactive poliovirus for polio	SC or IM; four doses; may give with all other vaccines but at a separate site	Moderate or severe acute illness; egg allergy	Uncommon
MMR Measles, mumps, rubella	SC; may give with all other vaccines but at a separate site	Moderate or severe acute illness; immunocompromised patients (may be given if HIV positive); pregnancy or possible pregnancy in 3 months; egg allergy	Fever
Pneumococcal Pneumococcal pneumonia	IM or SC; all children 2-23 mo of age; administer every 6 yr for high-risk patients		
Varicella Varicella (chickenpox)	SC; may give with all other vaccines but at a separate site; all susceptible children ≥12 mo of age	Confirmed history of chickenpox; pregnancy or possible pregnancy in 1 mo; moderate or severe acute illness; immunocompromised patients; egg allergy	No salicylates for 6 wk after to prevent possible Reye's syndrome

HIV, human immunodeficiency virus; *IM*, intramuscular; *SC*, subcutaneous.

Before a child or adult receives a vaccine the healthcare provider is required by the National Childhood Vaccine Injury Act (NCVIA) to provide a copy of a Vaccine Information Sheet (VIS) to either the adult patient or the child's parent or legal guardian. A VIS provides information that informs caregivers about the risks and benefits of each vaccine. If this is the medical assistant's responsibility, you should do the following (Procedure 41-1):

- Before administering the vaccine, give the parent the most current VIS available for that particular vaccine. Give the individual time to review the material, and answer any questions or refer concerns to the physician before administering the vaccination.
- Document in the child's chart the date the VIS was given and the publication date of the VIS (appears on the bottom of the VIS).

- To make sure the office has the most current VIS forms, either call the state health department or refer to the CDC site at www.cdc.gov/nip/publications/VIS/default. htm. Forms can be printed directly from the site.
- Informed consent must be signed and attached to the child's health record before immunizations are given. Documentation of immunization administration must include the date the vaccine was administered, vaccine manufacturer, manufacturer's lot number, type of vaccine, exact site of administration if an injection is given, any reported or observed side effects, the name and title of the person administering the vaccine, and the address of the medical office where the vaccine was administered.
- An official immunization booklet should be given to the parent and updated as needed to reflect the child's current immunization status. The medical assistant should not

only document the required details in the patient's chart but also complete the parent's immunization booklet each time the child receives another vaccination or booster. These parent records help schools and child care centers determine the child's immunization status. Some states are developing computerized immunization record systems.

CRITICAL THINKING APPLICATION

Susie will be administering pediatric immunizations during well-baby visits scheduled for today. To prepare for this responsibility, Susie looked up the primary vaccinations, their routes of administration, contraindications, and possible side effects. The first child is here for her 4-month checkup. What immunizations should the child receive, and how should they be administered? The baby's father asks if she will get sick from the vaccines. What should Susie tell him? What does Susie need to do to meet the requirements of the National Childhood Vaccine Injury Act?

THE PEDIATRIC PATIENT

A newborn's first physical assessment comes at the time of delivery, when the pediatrician assesses the newborn's ability to thrive outside the uterus. The Apgar score is a system of evaluating the infant's physical condition at 1 and 5 minutes after birth (Table 41-4). Developed by pediatrician Virginia Apgar, the scoring system evaluates the following: *A*ppearance (color); *P*ulse (heart rate); *G*rimace (reflex; response to stimuli); *A*ctivity (muscle tone); and *R*espiration (breathing). These parameters are each rated 0, 1, or 2. The maximum total score is 10. Infants with low scores require immediate medical attention.

Well-Child Visits

The frequency of well-child visits varies with the physician and the community. It may follow this pattern: 2 weeks, 4 weeks, 8 weeks, 4 months, 6 months, 12 months, 18 months, 2 years, 5 years, 10 years, and 15 years. These visits focus on maintaining

PROCEDURE 41-1

Maintain Medication and Immunization Records: Documentation of Immunizations

CAAHEP COMPETENCY: 3.b.(4)(h)
ABHES COMPETENCY: 4.n

GOAL: *To accurately document the administration of a pediatric immunization.*

CASE STUDY

Document the administration of the second dose of the hepatitis B immunization to a 5-week-old infant, Samantha Anderson.

EQUIPMENT and SUPPLIES

- Vaccine immunization administration record (Figure 1)
- Parent immunization booklet
- Patient chart
- VIS form for hepatitis B

PROCEDURAL STEPS

1. Gather forms.
   PURPOSE: Efficiency.
2. Make sure the physician obtained informed consent from the parent, the hepatitis B VIS form was given, and that any parental questions were answered.
   PURPOSE: Risk management practice.
3. After dispensing the vaccine dose and before administration, complete the information required on the Vaccine Administration Record, including the name of the vaccine, the date given, route of administration and site, vaccine lot number and manufacturer, the date on the VIS form, the date it was given to the parent, and your signature or initials.
   PURPOSE: To meet the legal requirements of the National Childhood Vaccine Injury Act.

4. Administer the vaccine intramuscularly as taught in Chapter 34.
5. Record the date of administration, the name and address of the physician practice, and the type of vaccine administered in the parent's immunization booklet.
   PURPOSE: To maintain an accurate and comprehensive parental record of childhood immunizations for school and/or day care purposes.
6. After administration of the hepatitis vaccine, record in the child's chart the following details:
   a. Date the vaccine was administered
   b. Vaccine manufacturer, batch and lot numbers, expiration date
   c. Type of vaccine administered and dose
   d. Route of administration and exact site if an injection is given
   e. Any reported or observed side effects
   f. Publication date of the VIS form given to the parent (on the bottom of the form)
   g. Parent education regarding possible side effects of the vaccination
   h. Name and title of the person administering the vaccine.

See Appendix D for a charting example.

Continued

Vaccine Administration Record for Children and Teens

Patient name: _____

Birthdate: _____

Chart number: _____

Before administering any vaccines, give the parent/guardian all appropriate copies of Vaccine Information Statements (VISs) and make sure they understand the risks and benefits of the vaccine(s). Update the patient's personal record card or provide a new one whenever you administer vaccine.

Vaccine	Type of Vaccine[1] (generic abbreviation)	Date given (mo/day/yr)	Route	Site given (RA, LA, RT, LT)	Vaccine		Vaccine Information Statement		Signature/ initials of vaccinator
					Lot #	Mfr.	Date on VIS[2]	Date given[2]	
Hepatitis B[3] e.g., HepB, Hib-HepB, DTaP-HepB-IPV			IM						
			IM						
			IM						
			IM						
Diphtheria, Tetanus, Pertussis[3] e.g., DTaP, DT, Tdap, DTaP-Hib, DTaP-HepB-IPV, Td			IM						
			IM						
			IM						
			IM						
			IM						
			IM						
			IM						
Haemophilus influenzae type b[3] e.g., Hib, Hib-HepB, DTaP-Hib			IM						
			IM						
			IM						
			IM						
Polio[3] e.g., IPV, DTaP-HepB-IPV			IM•SC						
			IM•SC						
			IM•SC						
			IM•SC						
Pneumococcal PCV (conjugate) PPV (polysaccharide)			IM						
			IM						
			IM						
			IM						
Measles, Mumps, Rubella[3] e.g., MMR, MMRV			SC						
			SC						
Varicella[3] e.g., Var, MMRV			SC						
			SC						
Hepatitis A HepA			IM						
			IM						
Meningococcal[4] MCV4 (conjugate) MPSV4 (polysaccharide)									
Influenza[5] TIV (inactivated) LAIV (live, attenuated)									
Other									

1. Record the generic abbreviation for the type of vaccine given (e.g., DTaP-Hib, PCV), *not* the trade name.
2. Record the publication date of each VIS as well as the date it is given to the patient. According to federal law, VISs must be given to patients (or parent/guardian of a minor child) before administering each dose of DTaP, Td, Hib, polio, MMR, varicella, PCV, or HepB

vaccine, or combinations thereof. Use of the VISs for hepatitis A, influenza, and meningococcal vaccines will become mandatory in later 2005.
3. For combination vaccines, fill in a row for each separate antigen in the combination.
4. Give MCV4 via the IM route and MPSV4 via the SC route.
5. Give TIV via the IM route and LAIV intranasally (IN).

www.immunize.org/catg.d/p2022b.pdf • Item #P2022 (10/05)

Immunization Action Coalition • 1573 Selby Ave. • St. Paul, MN 55104 • (651) 647-9009 • www.immunize.org • www.vaccineinformation.org

TABLE 41-4 The Apgar Scoring System*

	ASSIGNED SCORE		
CLINICAL SIGN	**0**	**1**	**2**
Heart rate	Absent	Under 100	Over 100
Respiratory effort	Absent	Slow and irregular	Good and crying
Muscle tone	Limp	Some flexion of the arms and legs	Active movement
Reflex irritability	No response	Grimace	Coughing and sneezing
Color	Blue and pale	Body pink and extremities blue	Pink all over

*The readings are taken by the pediatrician at 1-minute and 5-minute intervals after birth. At *1 minute*, if the score is 7 or less, some nervous system problems are suspected. If the score is below 4, resuscitation is usually necessary. At *5 minutes*, if the score is at least 8, the child is probably reacting normally.

2006 Immunization Schedule Recommendations from the Centers for Disease Control and Prevention

- All infants should receive the hepatitis B vaccine (HepB) at birth.
- A new tetanus toxoid, reduced diphtheria toxoid, and acellular pertussis vaccine (DTP/DTaP) is recommended for adolescents who completed the recommended childhood DTP/DTaP series but have not received a booster dose; tetanus boosters should be given every 10 years.
- Meningococcal conjugate vaccine (MCV4) should be given to all children at age 11 to 12 years, unvaccinated adolescents at high school entry, and college freshmen living in dormitories.
- Influenza vaccine is recommended for children aged >6 months with certain risk factors.
- Hepatitis A vaccine is recommended for all children at age 1 year (12 to 23 months); two doses administered at least 6 months apart.

the health of the child through basic system examinations, immunizations, and upgrading of the child's medical history record.

The decision about whether the child is to be seen alone or with the parent depends on the pediatrician and on the age of the child. Often the child will look to the parent for approval before answering or performing a skill; for this reason the physician may want to assess the child alone. If this is the case, explain to the parent that the physician wants to evaluate the child's independent abilities and that as soon as testing is completed, the physician will explain the results of the tests.

The medical history is an essential guide to the pediatric examination. With an infant, the physician depends on the caregiver for the history, but as the child gets older, some history may be obtained from the child and clarified or amplified by the parent. Close observation also gives the physician considerable information.

Sick-Child Visits

Sick-child visits occur whenever needed—usually on short notice. For this reason, most pediatric offices keep open appointments in the schedule to accommodate calls for sick child visits. The length and frequency of this type of visit depends entirely on the child and the illness. The medical assistant is frequently the first point of contact for a sick child and his or her caregiver. Determining whether the child should be seen immediately or if the problem can wait for an opening in the schedule is crucial to pediatric care. The medical assistant should follow established office policies, but when in doubt about the seriousness of the problem, he or she should ask the office manager or physician for advice. Usually the physician would prefer to see the child rather than delay seeing a patient with a potentially serious condition. When conducting telephone screening, if the child is young (less than 2 years old) and the parent reports frequent cycles of crying, lethargy, vomiting longer than 24 hours, diarrhea (more than 6 stools in the last 12 hours), or fever of 101° F (38.5° C) or higher, it is best to see the child right away. He or she cannot verbalize associated pain or problems.

Table 41-5 summarizes some of the action principles for telephone screening of an older child who can communicate his or her symptoms. It is important to focus on the *onset* (when symptoms first started), *frequency* (are symptoms constant, or do they cycle through recurrences), and *duration* (how long the episodes last) of the problem as well as attempted treatments and their effectiveness. As with any other patient, all telephone communications should be documented to record the reason for the call, the information gathered, and the action taken, including whether the physician was consulted, any orders given, and if and when an appointment was scheduled.

THE MEDICAL ASSISTANT'S ROLE IN PEDIATRIC PROCEDURES

The medical assistant is responsible for assisting the pediatrician with examinations; upgrading patient histories; performing ordered screening tests such as vision, hearing, urinalysis, and hemoglobin checks; administering immunizations; measuring and weighing children as needed; and providing patient and caregiver support. A medical assistant must develop a relationship with the pediatric patient that encourages cooperation and compliance with tests and treatment plans. If the child becomes upset, everything that needs to be done during that visit will be done under duress, and the chance for future mistrust will intensify.

Interacting with children requires special techniques, depending on the age of the child. To gain cooperation, a calm,

TABLE 41-5 Action Principles for Telephone Screening	
COMPLAINT	**SCREENING QUESTIONS**
Pain	Onset, frequency, duration of pain?
	On a scale of 1-10, how severe is the pain?
	Where is the exact location?
	Was there any accident involved (include details)?
	Has the pain gotten worse over time?
	Has the pain interfered with sleep?
	Is there associated fever, vomiting, diarrhea, or rash?
Gastrointestinal	Onset, duration, frequency of symptoms? Has the child been vomiting longer than 24 hr without improvement?
	Is the child receiving clear liquids only?
	Is the child dehydrated (dry mouth, no urination in 8-10 hr, listless)?
	If diarrhea, were there more than 5-6 watery stools in 12 hr?
	Does the child have other symptoms (vomiting, fever over 103° F [39.4° C], rapid breathing)?
Respiratory	Onset, duration, frequency of symptoms?
	Describe the child's breathing.
	Has the child been diagnosed with a breathing disorder?
	Is a prescribed treatment being used?
	Are there any other signs or symptoms (severe headache, stiff neck, fever, cough)?
	If the child is coughing, what does it sound like?
	Are there signs of a sore throat or earache?

unhurried manner is essential. The tone of voice should be gentle but confident. Using a firm, direct approach about expected behavior is important in gaining the cooperation of older children. Offer reasonable choices when possible, such as, "Would you like your shot in your left or right leg?" not, "Are you ready for your shot now?" Offering sincere praise for the child during the examination or procedures helps decrease anxiety and builds self-esteem. If the child is having an unusually difficult time, try to discover the reason. If the child has a history of a negative healthcare experience, the child may be afraid of what might happen. Each step should be explained in a language the child (and parent) can understand. Children younger than 2 feel better when the parent holds them or remains very close (Figure 41-7). Preschool children enjoy playing, so making a game out of the situation is helpful (Figure 41-8). Whatever the age of the child, the medical assistant should be sensitive to his or her individual needs and adapt the examination and procedures to meet those needs as much as possible.

The sequence of the physician's examination varies and is frequently adapted based on the cooperation of the child. The pediatrician will probably leave procedures and tests that will cause the most objection until the end of the appointment. The physician is constantly evaluating the child's growth and development. A child's alertness and responses tell the physician a considerable amount. In infants and in young children of preschool age, the parent is closely questioned about the child's eating, sleeping, and elimination habits. A school-aged child is usually a little more cooperative during an examination and can answer most questions without parental assistance. Adolescent patients should be given the option of not having parents present during an examination. This may permit teenagers to respond more honestly about lifestyle factors as well as protect their privacy.

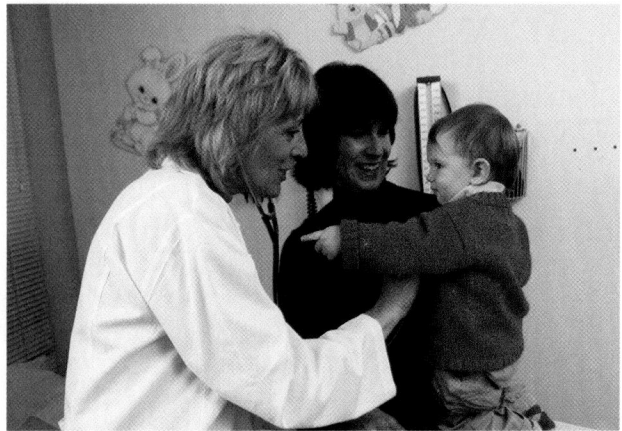

FIGURE 41-7 Sometimes a pediatric patient is more comfortable when held by a parent.

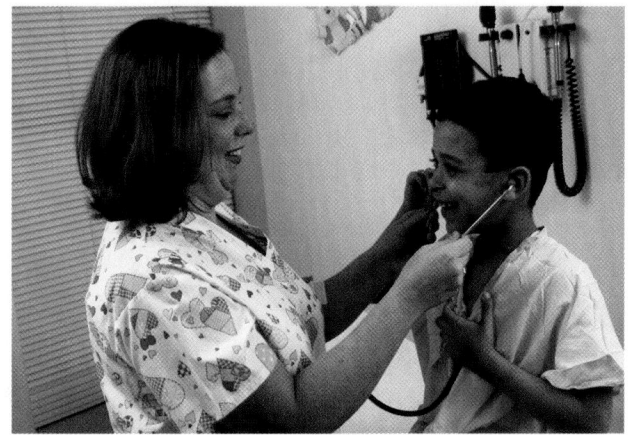

FIGURE 41-8 Making a game out of a procedure.

Measurement

Examination of the child during routine well-child care includes measurement of the circumference of the infant's head to determine normal growth and development (Procedure 41-2). The size of the child's head reflects the growth of the brain. Brain growth is 50% completed by 1 year of age, 75% by age 3, and 90% by age 6. Routine head measurement is recommended in children until 36 months of age and in older children whose head size is not within norms. If the circumference of the head deviates greatly from normal measurements, **hydrocephaly** or **microcephaly** may be suspected. It is important to discover any congenital problem as early as possible so that appropriate treatment measures can be initiated.

The medical assistant should record the child's length or height, weight, and head circumference on growth charts so the physician can compare the child's measurement statistics with national standards (Procedure 41-3). Growth charts consist of a series of percentile curves that illustrate the distribution of selected body measurements.

The revised CDC 2000 growth charts consist of 16 charts (eight for boys and eight for girls). These charts represent re-

visions to the 14 previous charts, as well as the introduction of two BMI-for-age charts for boys and for girls, ages 2 to 20 years (Figures 41-9 and 41-10). BMI is the recommended method for determining whether children or adults are overweight or obese. The BMI growth charts can be used beginning at 2 years of age, when height can be measured accurately.

Assisting with the Examination

The pediatrician will have a designated set of procedures that the medical assistant completes before the physician sees the child (Procedure 41-4, p. 896). Vital signs are measured first (Table 41-6, p. 897). Depending on the age and level of cooperation from the child, the temperature may be obtained by axillary, oral, or tympanic methods; however, it is easiest and quickest to use a tympanic thermometer. It is important to remember that the younger the child, the more immature the ability to regulate body heat. Therefore the temperature of an infant may fluctuate easily and rapidly. The child's pulse rate is affected in a fashion similar to an adult's and can increase through activity, anxiety, illness, and environmental temperature. If the child is younger than 2, the pulse is measured apically by placing the

---

PROCEDURE 41-2

Prepare Patient for and Assist with Routine and Specialty Examinations: Measure the Circumference of an Infant's Head

CAAHEP COMPETENCY: 3.b.(4)(e)
ABHES COMPETENCY: 4.h

GOAL: *To obtain an accurate measurement of the circumference of an infant's head.*

EQUIPMENT and SUPPLIES

- Flexible disposable tape measure
- Age- and sex-specific growth chart
- Patient's chart
- Pen

PROCEDURAL STEPS

1. Wash your hands.
   PURPOSE: Infection control.
2. Identify the patient and gain infant cooperation through conversation.
   PURPOSE: Alleviate anxiety and gain the child's trust.
3. Place the infant in the supine position; an older child may sit on the examination table; alternatively, the infant may be held by the parent.
4. Hold the tape measure with the zero mark against the infant's forehead, slightly above the eyebrows and the top of the ears. Ask the parent for assistance if necessary.
5. Bring the tape measure around the head, just above the ears, until it meet (Figure 1).
6. Read to the nearest 0.01 cm or ¼ inch.
7. Record the measurement on the growth chart and the patient's chart.
   PURPOSE: A procedure is not done until it is recorded.

8. Dispose of the tape measure.
9. Wash your hands.
   PURPOSE: Infection control.

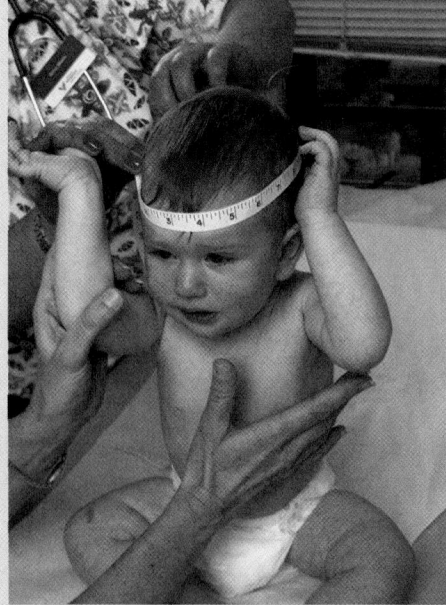

FIGURE 1

PROCEDURE 41-3

Prepare Patient for and Assist with Routine and Specialty Examinations: Measure Infant Length and Weight

CAAHEP COMPETENCY: 3.b.(4)(e)

ABHES COMPETENCY: 4.h

GOAL: *To accurately measure infant length and weight so growth patterns can be monitored and recorded.*

EQUIPMENT and SUPPLIES

- Infant scale with paper cover
- Flexible measuring tape
- Examination table paper
- Pen
- Sex-specific infant growth chart
- Patient's chart
- Biohazard waste container

PROCEDURAL STEPS

MEASURING INFANT LENGTH:

1. Wash your hands, assemble equipment, and explain the procedure to the infant's caregiver.
2. Undress the infant in preparation for measurement of length and weight. You may leave the diaper on while the length measurement is taken, but it must be removed before the infant is weighed.
3. Ask the caregiver to place the infant on his or her back on the examination table, which is covered with paper. If it is a pediatric table with a headboard, ask the caregiver to gently hold the infant's head against the board while you straighten the infant's leg and mark on the paper the location of the heel. If there is no headboard, ask the caregiver to gently hold the infant's head still while you extend the leg for measurement.
4. Measure and record the infant's length with the tape measure.
5. Document the results in either inches or centimeters, depending on office policy, on the infant's growth chart, in the progress notes, and in the caregiver's record if requested. Complete the growth chart graph by connecting the dot from the last visit.

MEASURING INFANT WEIGHT:

6. Wash your hands, assemble equipment, and explain the procedure to the infant's caregiver.
7. Prepare the scale by sliding weights to the left and covering it with disposable paper to reduce the risk of pathogen transmission.
8. Completely undress the infant, including the diaper.
9. Place the infant gently onto the center of the scale, keeping your hand directly above the infant's trunk for safety.
10. Slide the weights across the scale until balance is achieved. Attempt to read the infant's weight while he or she is still.
11. Return the weights to the far left of the scale and remove the baby. The caregiver can apply a diaper while you discard the paper covering the scale. If it has become contaminated during the procedure, follow OSHA guidelines for gloves and disposal of contaminated waste. Disinfect the equipment according to manufacturer guidelines.
12. Wash your hands.
13. Document the results in either pounds or kilograms, depending on office policy, on the infant's growth chart, in the progress notes, and in the caregiver's record if requested. Complete the growth chart graph by connecting the dot from the last visit.

See Appendix D for a charting example.

---

stethoscope on the left side of the chest medial to the nipple. Always count the beats for 1 full minute for accuracy.

An alternative method of obtaining the pulse of a very young child is to use the brachial artery in the upper arm. After 2 years of age, the child's pulse may be taken at the radial pulse site. Anticipate a pulse rate that is higher than adult level; the younger the child, the faster the pulse. The respiratory rate is easily obtained in a child, because the chest can be readily observed. Expect the rate to be increased according to the age (the younger the child, the faster the normal respiratory rate) and health of the child. The ratio of four pulse beats to one respiration should remain constant in a healthy child. Blood pressure measurements are not included in most pediatric examinations. However, if there is a heart or kidney anomaly, a blood pressure reading may be ordered. The cuff must be the appropriate width to obtain an accurate reading, and the bell of the stethoscope must be small enough to seal over the site. It is best to use a pediatric stethoscope with a pediatric bell when obtaining an infant's pressure. Blood pressure readings in a young child will be lower than those in an adult.

To prevent a small child or infant from rolling the head from side to side during the physician's examination, stand at the head of the table and support the child's head between your hands, making certain not to press on the ears or on the anterior or posterior fontanelles. It is not necessary to drape an infant, but privacy is important to an older child. Sincere respect and friendly conversation at the child's level accomplishes a great deal. Always be patient with children. Be certain that they understand what is expected. Always involve the parents or caregivers as much as possible.

Obtaining a Urine Sample

The easiest way to obtain a urine sample from a child older than 2 who is toilet trained is to give the parent the container

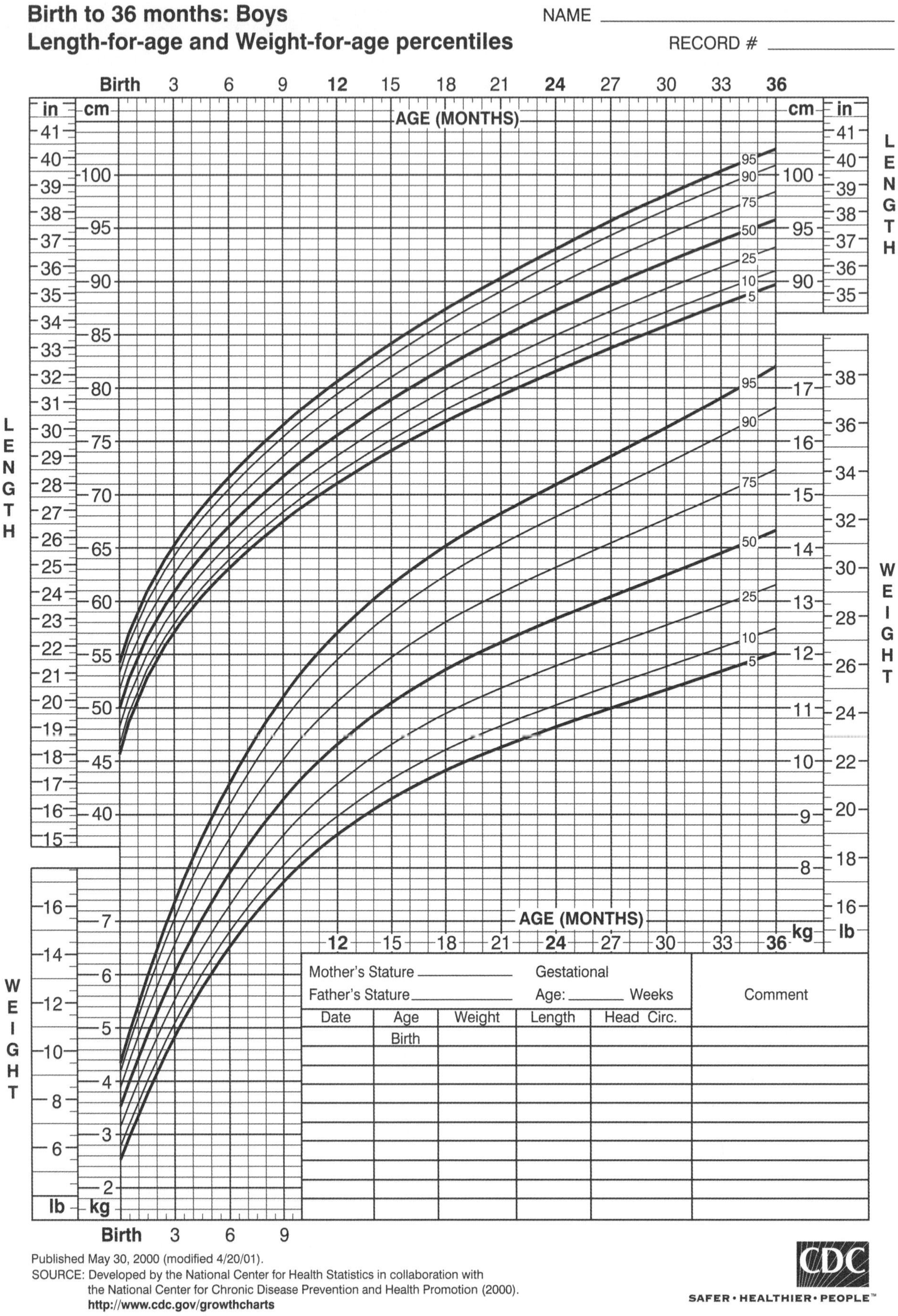
Birth to 36 months: Boys
Length-for-age and Weight-for-age percentiles
NAME
RECORD #
Birth 3 6 9 12 15 18 21 24 27 30 33 36
AGE (MONTHS)
in
cm
LENGTH
WEIGHT
95
90
75
50
25
10
5
kg
lb
Mother's Stature
Father's Stature
Gestational
Age: Weeks
Comment
Date
Age
Weight
Length
Head Circ.
Birth
Published May 30, 2000 (modified 4/20/01).
SOURCE: Developed by the National Center for Health Statistics in collaboration with
the National Center for Chronic Disease Prevention and Health Promotion (2000).
http://www.cdc.gov/growthcharts
CDC
SAFER • HEALTHIER • PEOPLE™

FIGURE 41-9 Growth rate graph: males (birth to 36 months).

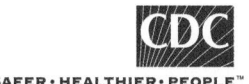

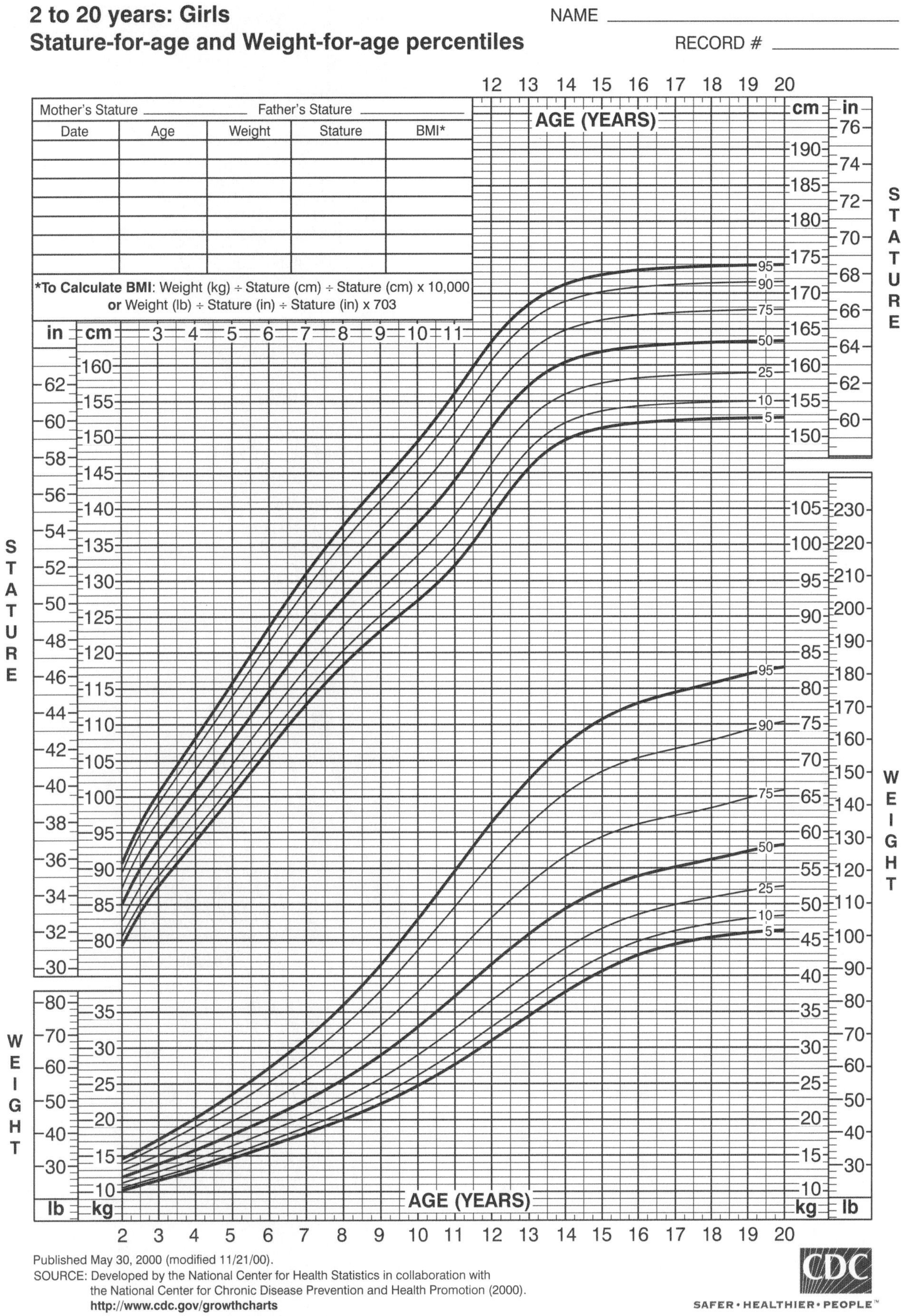
2 to 20 years: Girls
Stature-for-age and Weight-for-age percentiles
NAME
RECORD #
Mother's Stature
Father's Stature
Date
Age
Weight
Stature
BMI*
*To Calculate BMI: Weight (kg) ÷ Stature (cm) ÷ Stature (cm) x 10,000
or Weight (lb) ÷ Stature (in) ÷ Stature (in) x 703
AGE (YEARS)
STATURE
WEIGHT
in
cm
lb
kg
95
90
75
50
25
10
5
2 3 4 5 6 7 8 9 10 11 12 13 14 15 16 17 18 19 20
Published May 30, 2000 (modified 11/21/00).
SOURCE: Developed by the National Center for Health Statistics in collaboration with
the National Center for Chronic Disease Prevention and Health Promotion (2000).
http://www.cdc.gov/growthcharts
CDC
SAFER • HEALTHIER • PEOPLE™

FIGURE 41-10 Growth rate graph: females (2 to 20 years).

PROCEDURE 41-4

Prepare Patient for and Assist with Routine and Specialty Examinations: Obtain Pediatric Vital Signs and Vision Screening

<u>CAAHEP COMPETENCIES:</u> 3.b.(4)(b), 3.b.(4)(e)
<u>ABHES COMPETENCIES:</u> 4.d, 4.h

GOAL: *To accurately obtain vital signs for and assess vision of a pediatric patient.*

EQUIPMENT and SUPPLIES

- Digital or tympanic thermometer
- Pediatric blood pressure cuff
- Wristwatch with sweep second hand
- Weight scale with height bar
- Stethoscope
- Snellen E eye chart and oculator
- Pen
- Patient's chart

PROCEDURAL STEPS

1. Gather equipment.
   <u>PURPOSE:</u> Efficiency.
2. Wash your hands.
   <u>PURPOSE:</u> Infection control.
3. Explain the procedure to the parent, and if you want the parent to help by holding the child, explain the technique you want him or her to employ.
   <u>PURPOSE:</u> Explanations ahead of time save time and enhance cooperation.
4. Help the child stand in the center of the scale, and weigh the child. Ask the child to turn around, and obtain the child's height. Record your findings.
5. Obtain tympanic or axillary temperature using the procedure explained in Chapter 30 (Figure 1).
6. Record the temperature. Indicate the method used: A = axillary, T = tympanic.
   <u>PURPOSE:</u> A procedure is not done until it is recorded in the patient's record.
7. Place the stethoscope on the child's chest at the midpoint between the sternum and the left nipple. Listen for the apical beat (Figure 2).

8. Count the apical beat for 1 full minute.
9. Record the apical pulse. Be sure to place an Ap before the rate to indicate that this is an apical pulse reading.
   <u>PURPOSE:</u> A procedure is not done until it is recorded on the patient's record.
10. Place your flat hand on the child's chest, and count the respirations for 1 full minute.
11. Record the respiration rate.
    <u>PURPOSE:</u> A procedure is not done until it is recorded on the patient's record.
12. Check to be sure that you have the correct-size blood pressure cuff, then proceed with taking the blood pressure. Follow procedure in Chapter 30 (Figure 3).
13. Record the blood pressure.
    <u>PURPOSE:</u> A procedure is not done until it is recorded in the patient's record.
14. If vision screening is to be done, familiarize the child with the E chart by asking him to make an E point the same way as your

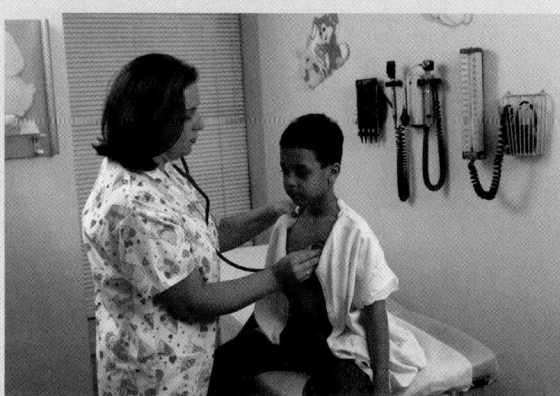

FIGURE 2

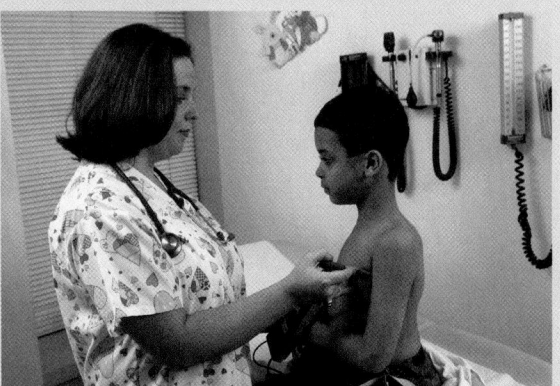

FIGURE 1

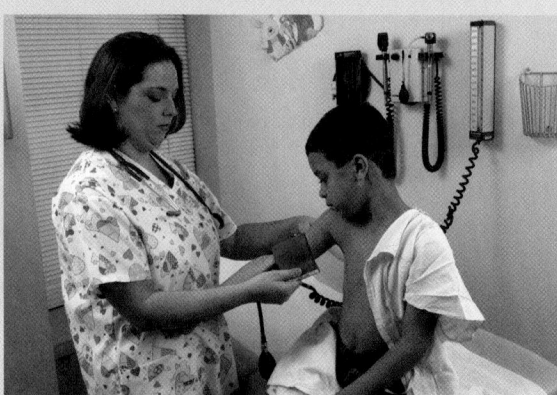

FIGURE 3

Continued

PROCEDURE 41-4—cont'd

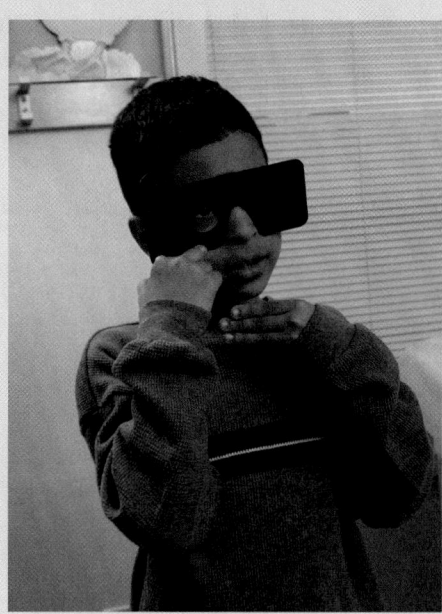

FIGURE 4

E is pointing. Then position the child in front of the pediatric E Snellen chart (Figure 4) and have him match the E sign (using his fingers) with the E on the chart that you are pointing to.

15. Record the vision results: OD = right eye; OS = left eye; OU = both eyes.
    PURPOSE: A procedure is not done until it is recorded in the patient's record.
16. Compliment the child on his or her performance, and if the parent is present, share the praise with the parent.
    PURPOSE: Builds rapport and encourages self-confidence in the child.
17. Wash your hands.
    PURPOSE: Infection control.
18. Perform appropriate disinfection, and return all equipment used to proper storage area.

TABLE 41-6 Reference Ranges for Pediatric Vital Signs	
VITAL SIGN	
Temperature	
Oral	98.6° F or 37° C
Aural	100.4° F or 38° C
Axillary	97.6° F or 36.4° C
Pulse	
Newborn	100-180 beats per minute
3 months-2 years	80-150 beats per minute
2-10 years	65-130 beats per minute
Older than 9 years	60-100 beats per minute
Respirations	
Newborn	30-35 breaths per minute
1-2 years	25-30 breaths per minute
4-6 years	23-25 breaths per minute
Older than 7 years	16-20 breaths per minute
Blood Pressure	
Newborn	Systolic <90, diastolic <70 mm Hg
1-5 years	Systolic <100, diastolic <70 mm Hg
Older than 9 years	Systolic <120, diastolic <84 mm Hg
Older than 13 years	Systolic 100 + age, diastolic 30-40 mm Hg less

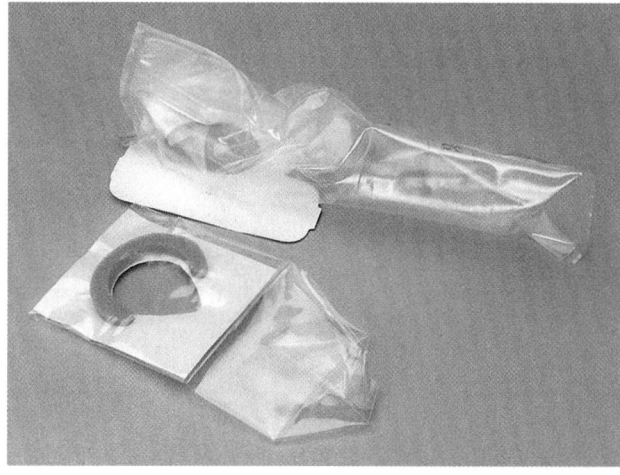

FIGURE 41-11 Urine collection devices.

can be applied to collect the sample (Figure 41-11 and Procedure 41-5). Place this device on the child as soon as the child appears in the office, so that you increase your chances of obtaining the needed sample before the child leaves. Once the device is in place, the child can be diapered to aid in holding the device properly. Be sure that the adhesive sticks tightly so the specimen will collect in the device when the child urinates.

In some cases the child may need to be catheterized to obtain the specimen. Pediatric catheterization kits contain all the supplies needed for this procedure. In getting the kit ready for the pediatrician's use, always remember that this is a sterile procedure. The pediatrician will usually ask the parent to hold the infant's legs apart, and the medical assistant labels and prepares the specimen for the laboratory.

and instructions ahead of time. Then when the child appears at the office for the examination, the sample is available to be tested. If the sample is needed while the child is at the office, consult with the parent for the best method to use. If the child is younger than 2 years old, a pediatric urine collection device

PROCEDURE 41-5

Prepare Patient for and Assist with Procedures, Treatments, and Minor Office Surgeries:
Apply a Urinary Collection Device

<u>CAAHEP COMPETENCY:</u> 3.b.(4)(f)
<u>ABHES COMPETENCY:</u> 4.b

GOAL: *To properly apply a pediatric urinary collection device.*

EQUIPMENT and SUPPLIES

- Pediatric urine collection bag
- Labeled laboratory urinary container
- Laboratory test request form
- Antiseptic wipes
- Biohazard waste container
- Disposable examination gloves

PROCEDURAL STEPS

1. Assemble all needed supplies.
   <u>PURPOSE:</u> Time management.
2. Wash your hands, and don gloves.
   <u>PURPOSE:</u> Infection control.
3. Ask the parent to remove the diaper from the child, or place the child in a supine position on the examination table and remove the diaper.
4. Cleanse the genitalia with antiseptic wipes.
   Male: Cleanse the urinary meatus in a circular motion, starting directly on the meatus, and work in an outward pattern. Repeat with a clean wipe. If the child is not circumcised, retract the foreskin to expose the meatus, and when you have completed cleansing, return the foreskin to its natural position.
   Female: Hold the labia open with your nondominant hand and with your dominant hand, cleanse the inner labia, from the clitoris to the vaginal meatus, in a superior to inferior pattern. Discard the first wipe and repeat with a clean wipe, cleaning both sides of the inner labia.

<u>PURPOSE:</u> To prevent contamination of the urine specimen with surface pathogens.

5. Make sure the area is dry. Unfold the collection device, remove the paper from the upper portion, place this portion over the mons pubis, and press it securely into place. Continue by removing the lower portion of the paper and securing this portion against the perineum. Be sure that the device is attached smoothly and that you have not taped it to part of the infant's thigh.
6. Rediaper the infant, or if the parent is helping, the parent may rediaper the infant at this time. The diaper will help hold the bag in place.
7. Suggest that the parent give the child liquids if allowed, and check the bag for urine at frequent intervals.
   <u>PURPOSE:</u> Increasing intake helps increase output.
8. When there is a noticeable amount of urine in the bag, apply gloves, remove the device, cleanse the skin area that was attached to the device, and rediaper the child.
9. Pour the urine carefully into the laboratory urine container, and handle the sample in a routine manner.
10. Dispose of all used equipment in a biohazard waste container.
11. Remove gloves, dispose of them in a biohazard container, and wash your hands.
12. Record the procedure in the patient's record.
    <u>PURPOSE:</u> A procedure is not done until it is recorded.

See Appendix D for a charting example.

INJURY PREVENTION

Unintentional injuries are the leading cause of death and disability for children in the United States. Injuries cause more childhood deaths than all diseases combined. The primary causes of childhood injuries include motor vehicle accidents, drowning, burns, falls, poisoning, aspiration with airway obstruction, and firearm accidents. Childhood injuries are linked to the child's growth and development level and are usually preventable. Young children are totally dependent on caregivers to keep them safe, so constant supervision and a childproof environment are essential for this age group. Older children need to be aware of health hazards and should be encouraged to protect themselves from injury—for example, by using bike helmets, protective padding when skateboarding, seat belts, and so on. The highest incidence of accidental injuries is in children under 9 years of age, but as children grow older, the percentage of deaths from injuries increases. Healthcare workers play a major role in injury

prevention. It is the medical assistant's responsibility to make sure that the ambulatory care environment is safe and parents are educated about potential hazards.

CRITICAL THINKING APPLICATION

The office manager asked Susie if she would check the entire office for potential child safety issues. After inspecting the facility, Susie is concerned about some safety issues, so she decides to create a checklist for future use. What precautions or safety features should she include?

THE ADOLESCENT PATIENT

The adolescent patient may present the greatest challenge to health education and disease management. Adolescence begins with the onset of puberty, a time when the child's

Child Safety Guidelines

- Position healthy full-term infants on the back or side to sleep.
- Stairs should be carpeted and protected with nonaccordion gates.
- Install and maintain smoke detectors on each floor and near sleeping areas.
- Develop and practice a plan of escape in the event of a fire.
- Put a self-latching lock on basement stairs.
- Store dangerous products out of reach (including medicines and vitamins), in cabinets with locks, and in their original containers.
- Keep potentially harmful plants out of reach.
- Post the numbers of the Poison Control Center and the child's physician by all phones.
- Teach children to call 911 as soon as possible.
- Regularly inspect toys for sharp or removable parts.
- Use an approved car seat that is appropriate for the child's age every time the child is in the car, and make certain it is properly installed.
- Follow guidelines for placing children in the front seat of motor vehicles.
- Parents should use seat belts every time they are in a car to protect themselves and set a good example.
- All children should wear properly fitting, approved helmets when biking and pads when skateboarding or participating in other impact sports.
- If firearms are in the home, store them unloaded, with the ammunition stored separately, and in a locked container.
- If the child has access to a swimming pool, make certain it is fenced, with self-locking gates.
- All adults and older children should learn cardiopulmonary resuscitation (CPR).

SIGNS OF ABUSE

Obvious Signals

Previously filed reports of physical or sexual abuse of child
Documented abuse of other family members
Different stories of how an accident happened between parents and child
Stories of incident and injuries found are suspicious
The cause of the injuries are blamed on other family members
Repeated visits to the emergency room for injuries

Findings on Examination

Trauma to the nervous system
Internal abdominal pain
Discolorations/bruising to the buttocks, back and abdomen
Elbow, wrist, and shoulder dislocations

Changes in Behavior

Too eager to please the parent
Overly passive and too compliant
Aggressive and demanding
Parenting the parent—role reversal
Delays in the normal growth and development patterns
Erratic school attendance

Physical Indicators

Poor hygiene
Malnutrition
Obvious dental neglect
Neglected well-baby procedures such as immunizations

FIGURE 41-12 Signs of abuse.

reproductive system matures, and is marked by rapid changes in the endocrine and musculoskeletal systems. The adolescent undergoes rapid growth spurts and the development of secondary sexual characteristics. Health examinations for patients in this age group should include screenings for height and weight; gathering details regarding diet and exercise routines; sexually transmitted disease (STD) screening and Pap tests if female adolescents are sexually active, especially to screen for human papillomavirus (HPV); review of vaccination history with booster administration as indicated; and assessment of high-risk behaviors such as substance abuse and sexual behavior.

Some of the health problems most frequently seen in adolescent patients include eating disorders (anorexia nervosa and bulimia nervosa), obesity, and injury-related problems. Accidents are the leading cause of death and injury in adolescence, and suicide is the third leading cause of death. All healthcare personnel should be on the alert for indicators of suicide including:

- Signs of depression such as headaches, abdominal discomfort, anorexia, fatigue, aggressiveness, drug or alcohol abuse, and sexual promiscuity
- Verbal statements that hint at the adolescent's intention to commit suicide; talking about dying
- Actions such as giving away prized objects, withdrawing from social groups, sudden changes in normal behavior patterns, or writing a suicide note

CHILD ABUSE

The federal Child Abuse Prevention and Treatment Act states that all threats to a child's physical and/or mental welfare must be reported. This means that every teacher, healthcare worker, and social worker—in fact, every citizen—who suspects that a child is being neglected or abused must report this to the proper authority. The agency must record the report, and after three similar reports, the agency must investigate.

When a suspected abuse is reported, the individual must provide his or her name, but this is considered confidential information and will not be given to the child's parent or guardian, nor is it given to the investigating officer. The individual making the report is also protected under the law from any liability for reporting suspicions of child abuse. Figure 41-12 lists some of the signs of abuse the medical assistant should know.

If the medical assistant suspects that a child is a victim of abuse, he or she should consult with the pediatrician immediately, before the patient is seen. In most states, both the medical assistant and the physician can make separate reports to the authorities. However, state laws vary, so state and local reporting protocols should be outlined in the office procedure manual.

> **PARENT EDUCATION TOPICS**
>
> Normal growth and development
> Child safety
> Pediatric nutrition needs
> Alternative feeding habits
> Immunizations
> Sexual curiosity
> Answering "sex" questions
> Toilet training
> Adolescent behavior
> Adolescent trust vs mistrust
> Common health problems

FIGURE 41-13 Parent education topics.

CLOSING COMMENTS

Patient Education

In a pediatric practice the child is usually joined by one or both parents during visits to the physician. Parents need reinforcement, praise, and understanding in dealing with the health and welfare of their child, and they expect to receive such support from the pediatrician and the office staff. Provide parents with information to help them understand their children's behavior and improve their parenting skills. Understanding normal behavioral characteristics of a particular developmental stage may increase the parents' confidence and reinforce expectations for the child (Figure 41-13).

The waiting room is an ideal place for parent education. Use the space and resources available to provide up-to-date information on child health issues as well as local resources for support and assistance. If the pediatrician has pamphlets available, discuss them with the parents. Answer questions when possible, or alert the physician so that questions can be answered during the office visit. Every opportunity should be taken to teach parents about sound healthcare. Because so many ambulatory care visits involve infectious disorders, educating children and parents on the following infection control measures may help decrease the spread of disease.

- Children should cover their mouths with a disposable tissue when they cough and should blow their noses with disposable tissues.
- Use a tissue only once, then immediately throw it away.
- Do not allow children to share toys that they have put in their mouths.
- After a child has discarded a toy that was in the mouth, it should be placed in a bin for dirty toys that is out of reach of others. Wash and disinfect these toys before allowing children to play with them again.
- Make sure all children and adults use good hand-washing practices.

Legal and Ethical Issues

In the United States children are considered to be persons who are growing and developing physically, emotionally, and mentally. Our laws view children as a distinct group, and there are laws and customs dealing with the protection of children's rights. Occasionally in the pediatric office, legal and ethical issues arise, and the entire office staff may be faced with an ethical situation. If this type of situation occurs, the first option is to talk it over with the pediatrician. It may be necessary to have an office staff meeting to identify the conflict, note pertinent laws and facts, consider possible options and the consequences of each, and decide on a course of action. Facing ethical issues confidently may reduce the risk of liability. If the pediatrician's feelings are different from yours, this might be a totally separate dilemma that you will have to deal with. Always remember that as your employer, the physician makes the final decision, and as long as you work in that office you are required to do things according to that decision.

If something happens that you cannot ethically support, seek the help of the local medical assistant organization. You may find that others have been in similar situations and that they can suggest possible methods to solve the problem.

SUMMARY OF SCENARIO

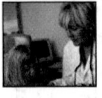

After working with the telephone triage staff, Susie realizes how important it is that she be familiar with childhood diseases and disorders as well as the management policy of the physicians who employ her. Many times Susie has had to refer to the office disease manual to make certain she is asking the right questions and gathering all of the information needed for the physician who will be making daily response calls. When working in the clinical area, Susie has also realized there are actually two groups of patients in a pediatric practice: the child and the caregivers. She must be sensitive to the needs of both groups and develop communication skills that build trust with the child as well as his or her parents. Susie is working on developing a comprehensive education site within the office for interested parents as well as creating a community resource guide for interested caregivers. She recognizes the need to stay up to date on CDC recommendations regarding childhood immunizations and routinely refers to the CDC site to make sure the office has the most recently published VIS forms. Susie regularly attends her local American Association of Medical Assistants (AAMA) chapter meetings to maintain her certification and continue to learn about the specialty pediatric practice.

SUMMARY of LEARNING OBJECTIVES

1. Define, spell, and pronounce the terms listed in the vocabulary.
   - Spelling and pronouncing medical terms correctly adds credibility to the medical assistant. Knowing the definition of these terms promotes confidence in communication with patients and co-workers.

2. Describe childhood growth patterns.
   - By 6 months of age, the child's birth weight has doubled; at 1 year it has tripled, and length has increased by 50%. By age 2 the child has reached approximately 50% of adult height. This same growth rate continues through the school-aged period, 6 to 12 years, which leads into a growth spurt that indicates impending puberty. In adolescence, ages 12 to 18 years, the adolescent gains almost half of his or her adult weight and the skeleton and organs double in size.

3. Summarize the important features of the Denver II Developmental Screening Test.
   - The Denver II Developmental Screening Test is a standardized tool that is given to children between 1 month and 6 years of age to screen healthy infants for developmental delays, to validate concerns about an infant's development, or to monitor high-risk children for potential problems. The assessment focuses on four developmental areas.

4. Identify four different growth and development theories.
   - Table 41-1 summarizes Freud's psychosexual, Piaget's cognitive, Erikson's psychosocial, and Kohlberg's moral reasoning theories.

5. Explain common pediatric gastrointestinal disorders and their signs, symptoms, and treatments.
   - Pediatric gastrointestinal disorders include infant colic; diarrhea, which can be caused by a variety of different microorganisms and is treated medically when it continues for more than 2 days; failure to thrive caused by a physiologic factor (such as malabsorption disease or cleft palate) or a nonorganic cause that is associated with the parent-child relationship; and obesity if the child's BMI is equal to or greater than the 95th percentile.

6. Classify disorders of the respiratory system in children.
   - The common cold may lead to secondary bacterial infections, including strep throat or otitis media; croup, a viral disorder that affects the larynx; bronchiolitis, a viral infection of the bronchioles that causes acute onset of wheezing and dyspnea; asthma, causing bronchospasms and inflammation of the bronchioles; and influenza, an acute, highly contagious viral infection of the respiratory tract.

7. Distinguish among pediatric infectious diseases.
   - Pediatric infectious diseases include conjunctivitis, caused by a bacterial or viral infection; tonsillitis, typically caused by beta-hemolytic Streptococcus; fifth disease, also called erythema infectiosum, a mild infection caused by parvovirus B19; chickenpox, caused by a member of the herpesvirus group; meningitis, an inflammation of the membranes that cover the brain and spinal cord, caused by bacteria or viruses, with bacterial meningitis the more dangerous; HBV, which can lead to serious and chronic infection of the liver and can be transmitted across the placenta; and Reye's syndrome, which is linked with the use of aspirin during a viral illness.

8. Recognize the etiologic factors and signs and symptoms of the two primary pediatric inherited disorders.
   - Pediatric inherited disorders include cystic fibrosis, an autosomal recessive genetic disorder that causes exocrine glands to produce abnormally thick secretions and primarily affects the lungs and pancreas; and Duchenne's muscular dystrophy, an X-linked genetic disease that causes progressive muscle degeneration and subsequent replacement of muscle fibers with fat and fibrous connective tissue.

9. Summarize CDC-recommended immunizations for children.
   - CDC recommendations for childhood immunizations are summarized in Table 41-3. Children should be vaccinated against diphtheria, tetanus, pertussis, hepatitis A and B, influenza, and the viruses that can cause some forms of meningitis, polio, measles, mumps, rubella, pneumonia, and chickenpox.

10. Demonstrate how to document and maintain accurate immunization records.
    - Procedure 41-1 summarizes how to document immunizations on both the official vaccination record and the parent's immunization booklet. Documentation of immunization administration must include the date the vaccine was administered, vaccine manufacturer, manufacturer's lot number, type of vaccine, route of administration and exact site if an injection is given, any reported or observed side effects, the name and title of the person administering the vaccine, and the address of the medical office where the vaccine was administered. The date on the VIS form that was given to the parent must also be included.

11. Compare and contrast a well-child and a sick-child examination.
    - Well-child visits are typically scheduled from 2 weeks of age through 15 years of age to focus on maintaining the health of the child with physical examinations, immunizations, and upgrading of the child's medical history record. Sick-child visits occur whenever the child needs to be seen because of illness or injury. Criteria to consider when conducting telephone screening include the age of the child and severity of symptoms and the onset, frequency, and duration of the problem. Table 41-5 summarizes action principles for telephone screening.

12. Outline the medical assistant's role in a pediatric examination.
    - The medical assistant assists the pediatrician with examinations; maintains patient histories; performs ordered screening tests such as vision, hearing, urinalysis, and hemoglobin checks; administers immunizations; measures and weighs children as needed; and provides patient and caregiver support.

13. Measure the circumference of an infant's head.
    - Procedure 41-2 outlines the steps for measuring an infant's head.

Continued

SUMMARY of LEARNING OBJECTIVES
Continued

14. Obtain accurate length and weight measurements, and plot growth patterns.
    - Procedure 41-3 outlines the steps for measuring infant length and weight.
15. Accurately measure pediatric vital signs including vision screening.
    - Procedure 41-4 summarizes the steps for obtaining accurate pediatric vital signs and performing a vision screening on a child. Tympanic thermometers are the easiest and quickest method for measuring temperature; the apical pulse should be taken for a full minute, respirations observed and recorded, and blood pressures taken with the appropriate sized cuff when indicated. Use the E Snellen chart after patient education to perform vision screening and accurately record results.
16. Correctly apply a pediatric urine collection device.
    - Procedure 41-5 summarizes the steps for application of a urinary collection device. Clean the site carefully according to the sex of the child; apply the sticky portion of the device to the genitalia; encourage the child to drink fluids; remove the device and collect the specimen after the child urinates.

17. Specify child safety guidelines for injury prevention and management of suspected child abuse.
    - The medical assistant should be involved in parent education regarding injury prevention in children. Childhood injuries are linked to the child's growth and development level and are therefore often predictable, and many times preventable. Refer to the box on child safety and Figure 41-12 for indicators of abuse. If child abuse is suspected, all healthcare workers are expected to report this suspicion to the authorities.
18. Describe the characteristics and needs of the adolescent patient.
    - Adolescents are going through extreme physical and emotional changes and require an extra measure of patience and understanding to establish therapeutic interactions. Securing privacy, giving them the option to be seen without parents, and providing pertinent education materials are all important factors in patient-centered adolescent care.

CONNECTIONS

Study Guide Connection: Go to Chapter 41 Study Guide. Read the Case Study and Workplace Applications and complete the assignments. Do online research for answers to the questions in the Internet Activities associated with assisting in pediatrics.

CD Connection: Go to the Medical Assisting Competency Challenge CD and do the training activities under Patient Care.

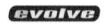

Evolve Connection: For more information related to assisting in pediatrics, go to evolve.elsevier.com/kinn and visit related weblinks for Chapter 41. Click on the Medical Assisting Exam Review and do the practice questions to sharpen your test-taking skills.

Assisting in Orthopedic Medicine 42

SCENARIO

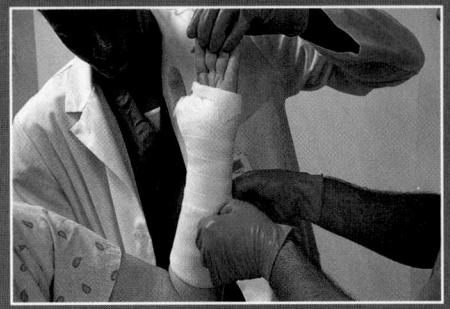

Kaiwan Tillman became interested in orthopedics before he even knew what the word meant. When he was in the sixth grade, he broke his right femur while riding his bicycle. He spent 2 months in traction in the hospital on an orthopedic floor. On graduation from high school, he attended the local community college and enrolled in an associate-degree medical assisting program. Since earning his CMA, Kaiwan has worked in a sports medicine clinic. The clinic staff includes three orthopedic surgeons, two physical therapists, and two massage therapists. Kaiwan is very excited about working in the clinic, although he was initially somewhat intimidated. Dr. Steve Alexander is the team physician for a local professional baseball team, and part of Kaiwan's responsibilities include assisting Dr. Alexander with treating the team.

While studying this chapter, think about the following questions:

- What are the primary medical assisting responsibilities in an orthopedic practice?
- What clinical skills are required in this specialty practice?
- What are the common musculoskeletal injuries and disorders that the CMA should understand?
- What diagnostic and treatment procedures are typically used in an orthopedic practice?

LEARNING OBJECTIVES

1. Define, spell, and pronounce the terms listed in the vocabulary.
2. Describe the principal structures of the musculoskeletal system and their functions.
3. Differentiate among tendons, bursae, and ligaments.
4. Summarize the major muscular disorders.
5. Identify and describe the common types of fractures.
6. Explain the difference between osteomalacia and osteoporosis.
7. Classify typical spinal column disorders.
8. Differentiate among the various joint disorders.
9. Summarize the medical assistant's role in assisting with orthopedic procedures.
10. Explain the common diagnostic procedures used in orthopedics.
11. Compare and contrast therapeutic modalities used in orthopedic medicine.
12. Apply cold therapy to an injury.
13. Assist with hot moist heat application to an orthopedic injury.
14. Properly apply therapeutic ultrasound.
15. Explain the use of common ambulatory devices.
16. Prepare for and assist with cast application.
17. Apply a sling to immobilize an injury.
18. Prepare for and assist with cast removal.
19. Properly fit a patient with crutches, and explain the correct mechanics of crutch walking.

National Accreditation Competencies and Content

CAAHEP COMPETENCIES

Clinical

3.b.(4)(e). Prepare patient for and assist with routine and specialty examinations
3.b.(4)(f). Prepare patient for and assist with procedures, treatments, and minor office surgeries

ABHES COMPETENCIES

Clinical Duties

4.b. Prepare patients for procedures
4.h. Prepare patient for and assist physician with routine and specialty examinations

VOCABULARY

arthritis Inflammation of a joint.

articular (ar-ti'-kyuh-luhr) Pertaining to a joint.

atrophy (a'-truh-fe) Wasting away, decreasing in size.

bursae Fluid-filled, saclike membranes that provide for cushioning and frictionless motion between two tissues.

cartilage Rubbery, smooth, somewhat elastic connective tissue covering the ends of bones.

cervical (ser'-vi-kuhl) Pertaining to the neck region containing seven cervical vertebrae.

corticosteroids Antiinflammatory hormones, natural or synthetic.

crepitation (kre-puh-ta'-shun) Dry, crackling sound or sensation.

diaphysis (di-a'-fuh-suhs) Midportion of a long bone that contains the medullary cavity.

epiphysis (i-pi'-fuh-suhs) End of a long bone.

gait Manner or style of walking.

goniometer Instrument for measuring the degrees of motion in a joint.

inflammation Tissue reaction to trauma or disease that includes redness, heat, swelling, and pain.

kyphotic (ki-fo'-suhs) Relating to normal convex curvature of the thoracic spine region.

ligaments Tough connective tissue bands that hold joints together by attaching to the bones on either side of a joint.

lordotic (lor-do'-tik) Relating to normal concave curvature of the cervical and lumbar spine regions.

lumbar Lower back region containing five lumbar vertebrae.

luxation Dislocation of a bone from its normal anatomic location.

malaise (muh-laz') Indefinite feeling of debility or lack of health, often indicative of or accompanying the onset of an illness.

medullary cavity Inner portion of diaphysis containing bone marrow.

periosteum The thin, highly innervated, membranous covering of a bone.

prosthesis (prahs-the'-suhs) Artificial replacement for a body part.

reduction The return to correct anatomic position, as in reduction of a fracture.

scoliosis Abnormal lateral curvature of the spine.

subluxation Incomplete dislocation of a bone from its normal anatomic location.

synovial fluid Clear fluid found in joint cavities that facilitates smooth movements and nourishes joint structures.

tendons Tough bands of connective tissue connecting muscle to bone.

An *orthopedic physician* diagnoses and treats diseases and disorders of the musculoskeletal system and deals primarily with the bones. *Rheumatologists* are specialists in treating inflammatory joint disorders. *Osteopaths* are doctors of osteopathic medicine (DOs); they treat the body from the viewpoint that the body can heal itself when the skeletal system is in proper alignment. *Chiropractors* are doctors of chiropractic (DC); they use manual adjusting procedures to correct subluxations or misalignments of the spine to allow maximal nerve function, thus facilitating the body's maintenance of homeostasis and prevention of disease.

The musculoskeletal system includes all of the skeletal muscles, bones, joints, and supportive connective tissues **(cartilage**, tendons, and **ligaments)**. The general functions of the musculoskeletal system include the following:

- Protection of internal organs
- Support to stand erect
- Movement
- *Hemopoietic* function (production of blood cells in the red bone marrow)
- Mineral storage in the bones

ANATOMY AND PHYSIOLOGY OF THE MUSCULOSKELETAL SYSTEM

Muscles

There are more than 600 muscles attached to the human skeleton (Figure 42-1). These muscles account for approximately half of a person's weight and contribute to the body's distinct shape. This chapter is concerned with the skeletal muscles that attach to bones and allow movement. There are two other types of muscles in the body: cardiac (in the heart) and smooth muscle (line organs and blood vessel walls). Both of these are involuntary—a person cannot control their function. Skeletal muscles are voluntary and can be controlled when they contract or relax. Special fibers in skeletal muscles allow them to shorten (contract) and lengthen (relax), causing movement (Table 42-1). These muscles are connected to bone with bands of tough, fibrous connective tissues called **tendons.**

Bones

The human skeleton contains more than 200 bones and makes up about one tenth of a person's weight (Figure 42-2, p. 908).

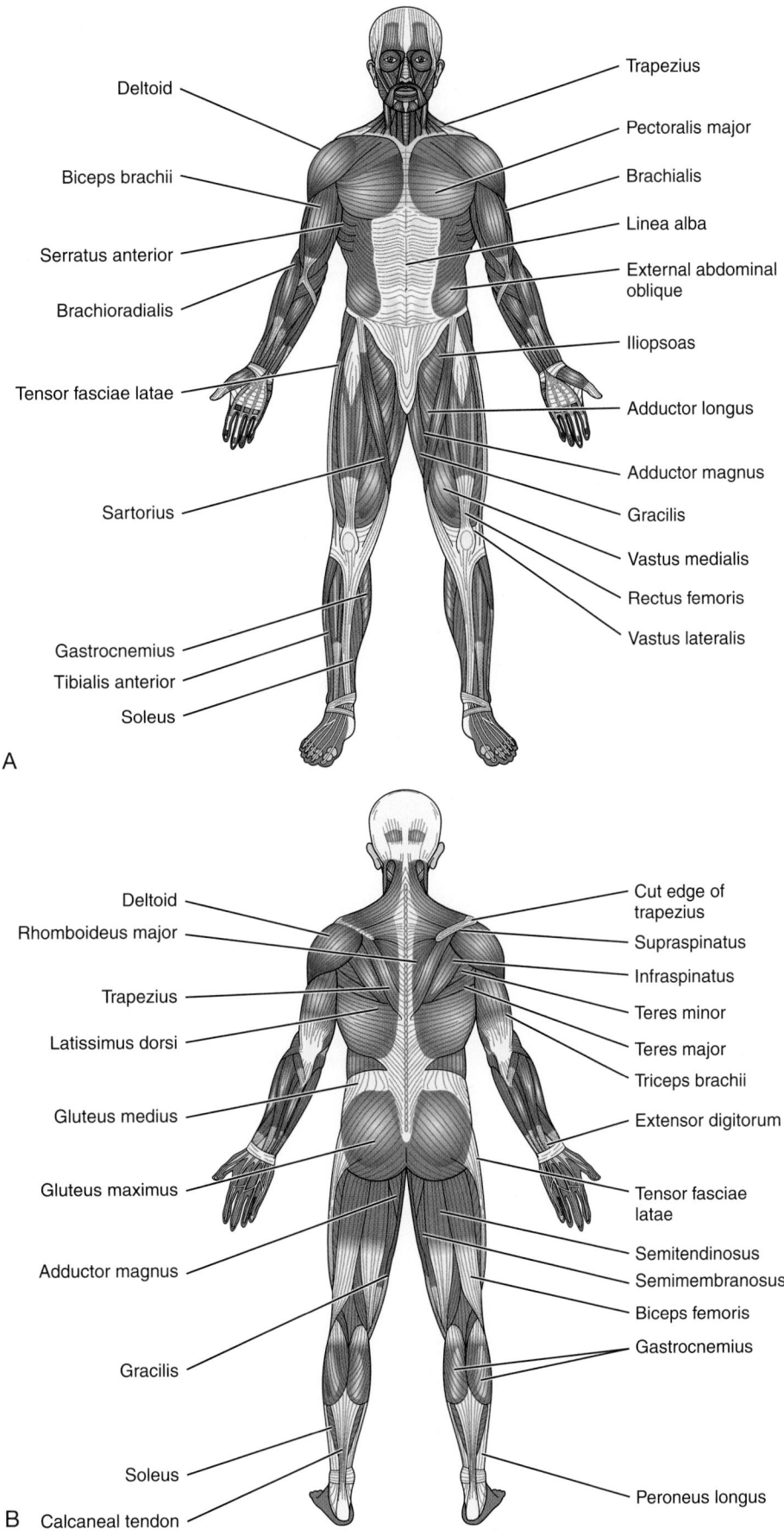

FIGURE 42-1 Muscles of the body. **A,** Anterior view. **B,** Posterior view. (From Chester GA: *Modern medical assisting*, Philadelphia, 1999, Saunders.)

TABLE 42-1 Types of Body Movement

MOVEMENT	DEFINITION OR EXAMPLE	MOVEMENT	DEFINITION OR EXAMPLE
Flexion 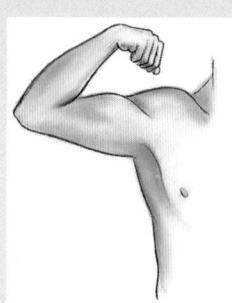	Decreases the angle of the joint and brings the two bones closer together.	Circumduction 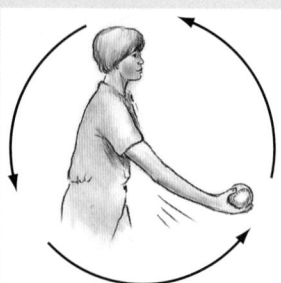	The circular movement of a limb. It is a combination of abduction, adduction, extension, and flexion.
Extension 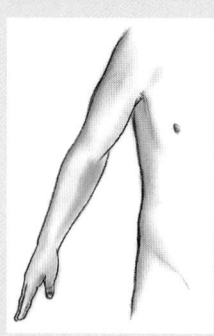	The opposite of flexion; increases the angle or the distance between two bones or parts of the body.	Dorsiflexion 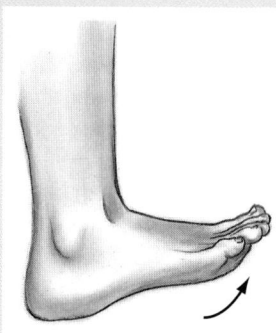	Moving the instep of the foot up and dorsally. It decreases the angle between the foot and the leg.
Hyperextension 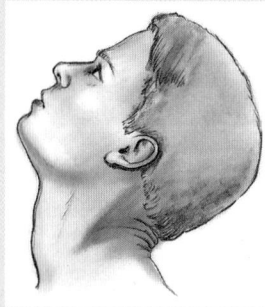	Extension greater than 180 degrees; body part is extended beyond its anatomic position.	Plantar flexion 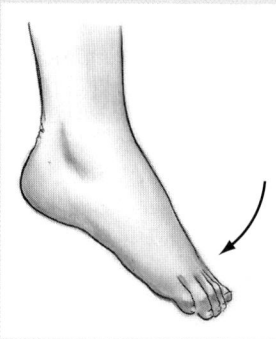	Movement of the ankle joint in which the joint is straightened and the toes are pointed downward
Abduction 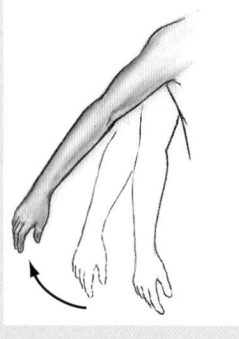	Moving the body part away from the midline or median plane of the body.	Eversion 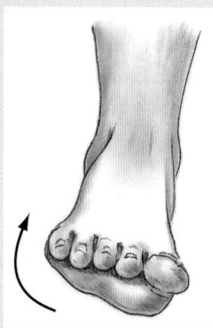	Turning of the sole of the foot laterally or outward.

Continued

TABLE 42-1   Types of Body Movement—*cont'd*

MOVEMENT	DEFINITION OR EXAMPLE	MOVEMENT	DEFINITION OR EXAMPLE
Adduction	The opposite of abduction. It moves the body part toward the midline of the body.	Inversion	The opposite of eversion. It is turning of the sole of the foot medially or inward.
Rotation	The rotation of a bone around its central axis, common in ball-and-socket joints.	Pronation	Rotation of the forearm that turns the palm of the hand backward or posteriorly.
		Supination	The opposite of pronation. It is the rotation of the forearm that turns the palm of the hand forward or anteriorly.

Bones supply a framework that provides protection for vital organs. In general, the size of a bone is related to how much it moves and how much body weight it must carry. Sometimes the size and shape of a bone are more related to its protective function for the underlying organs.

Bones are generally categorized by shape, including long, short, flat, rounded, and irregular. A long bone is made up of a **diaphysis** (shaft) with an expansion at each end called an **epiphysis** (Figure 42-3). The epiphysis is covered with **articular** cartilage and is attached by ligaments to the epiphysis of another bone, forming a joint. Articular cartilage decreases the stress of weight-bearing and the friction of movement. The thickness of the cartilage depends largely on the amount of stress placed on a particular joint. The **medullary cavity** is found within the diaphysis and contains yellow bone marrow.

Bone is living, changing tissue that is constantly being remodeled in response to stress or injury. Bone is also a storage location for minerals including calcium and phosphorus. Red bone marrow produces blood cells and is found in the spongy *(cancellous)* bone of the proximal epiphyses of the humerus and femur, sternum, ribs, and vertebrae of adults. Bones are covered with a thin membranous tissue called **periosteum.** The periosteum contains many sensory nerves.

CRITICAL THINKING APPLICATION

What is the benefit of Kaiwan's knowing the names and locations of the major bones of the extremities? How might this knowledge make his job at Sports Medicine Associates more interesting?

Joints

Bones are connected to each other at junctions called joints. The two main kinds of joints are nonsynovial and *synovial*. In nonsynovial joints the bones are joined with fibrous cartilage and are immovable (e.g., the sutures of the skull) or only slightly moveable (e.g., the vertebrae). Synovial joints are freely moveable because the adjacent ends of two bones are covered with cartilage and are enclosed in a joint cavity that contains a viscous, slippery fluid called **synovial fluid,** which is an excellent lubricant. Synovial joints such as the elbow and knee are basically hinge joints that allow movement in only one plane (Figure 42-4). Other synovial joints, such as the hip and shoulder, allow movement in many planes, thus permitting a wider range of motion (ROM) than a hinge joint.

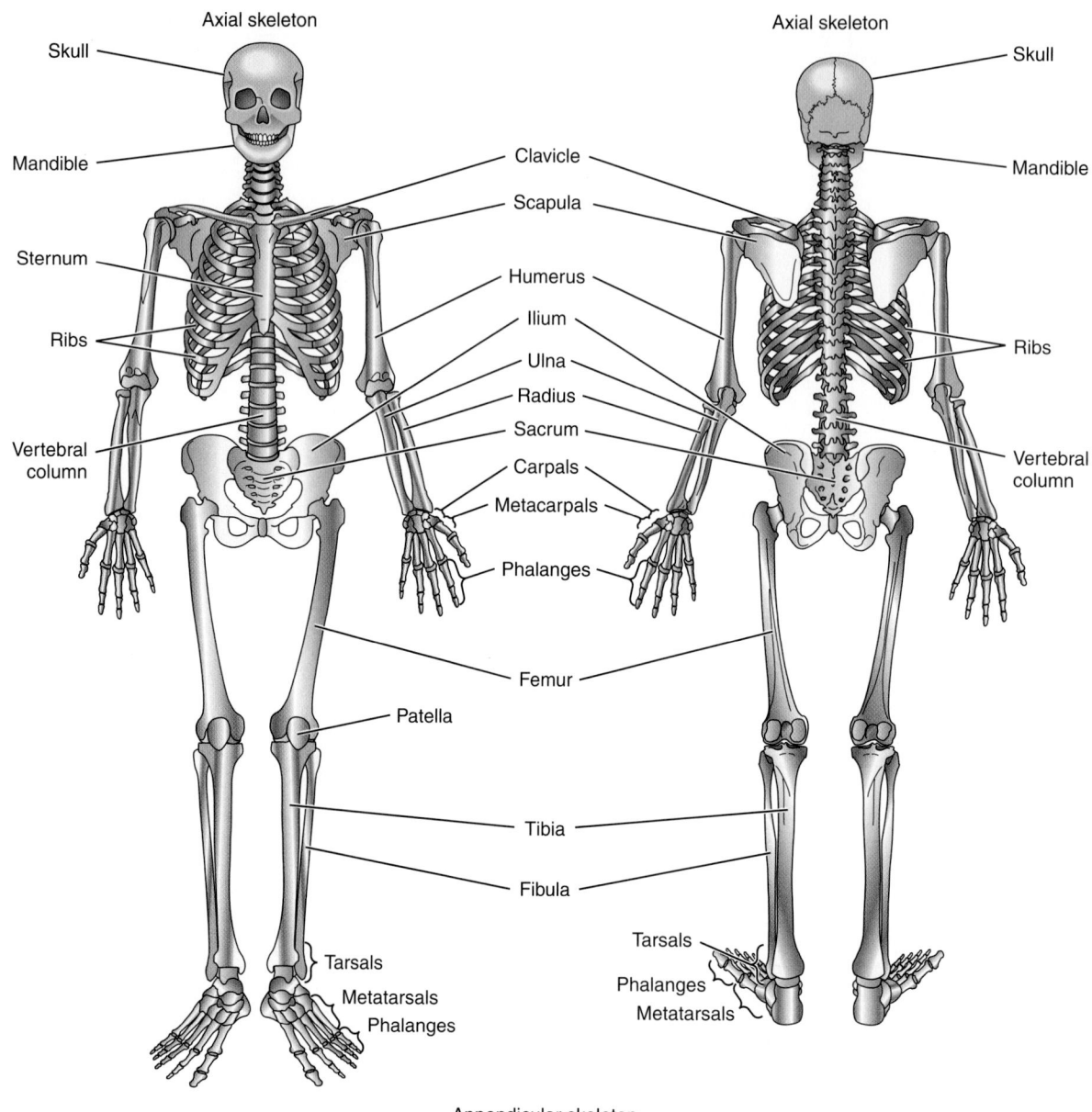

FIGURE 42-2 Axial skeletal bones (listed in outside columns) and appendicular skeletal bones (listed in the middle column). (From Chester GA: *Modern medical assisting*, Philadelphia, 1999, Saunders.)

Types of Joints

Joints are classified by the way they are shaped or by their ability to move. The joints of the skull are known as *sutures*. Sutures permit the skull to grow with the child but have very limited flexibility. The *hinge* joints of the elbow and knee allow for movement in one plane, such as bending up and down. A *gliding* joint, such as those in the wrist and foot, are made up of two flat-surfaced bones that slide over each other, allowing limited movement. Ball-and-socket joints, as in the shoulder and hip, allow for the greatest ROM by permitting the joint to rotate in a complete circle. Artificial ("manmade") joints have been successfully implanted to replace many joints that have been damaged by disease or trauma, including the joints of the hip, knee, ankle, shoulder, elbow, wrist, and finger.

Ligaments, Tendons, and Bursae

Ligaments are powerful, strong, fibrous connective tissue bands that connect *bone to bone* at the joint and encase the joint capsule. Ligaments allow purposeful joint movement and prevent excessive movement in any particular joint. Ligaments may be oblique or parallel to the joint, as in the knee, and may surround the joint, as in the hip.

A tendon is a strong bundle of connective tissue that attaches *muscle to bone*. Tendons can be flat or round and can pass between muscles, between bones, or through specialized openings between bones.

Bursae are fibrous sacs that lie between tendons and bones; they are lined with synovial membranes that secrete synovial

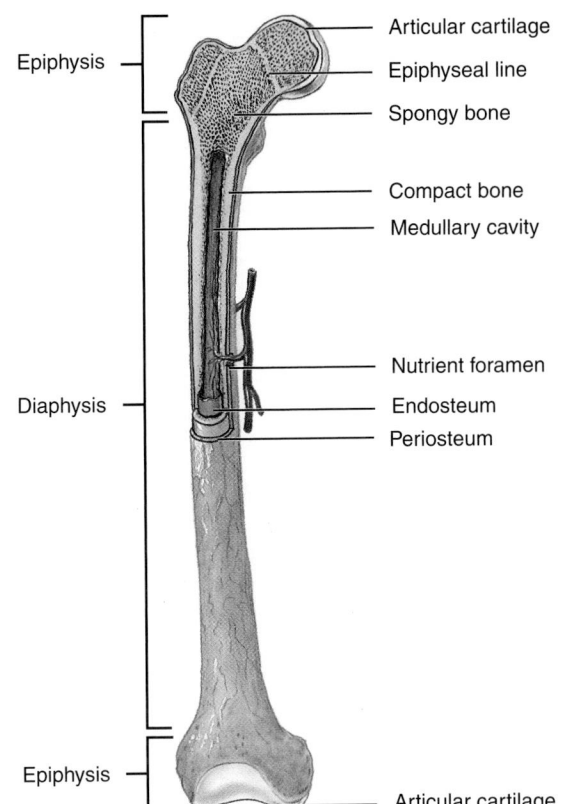

Epiphysis

Articular cartilage

Epiphyseal line

Spongy bone

Compact bone

Medullary cavity

Diaphysis

Nutrient foramen

Endosteum

Periosteum

Epiphysis

Articular cartilage

FIGURE 42-3 Long bone features. (From Applegate EJ: *The anatomy and physiology learning system*, ed 3, St Louis, 2006, Saunders.)

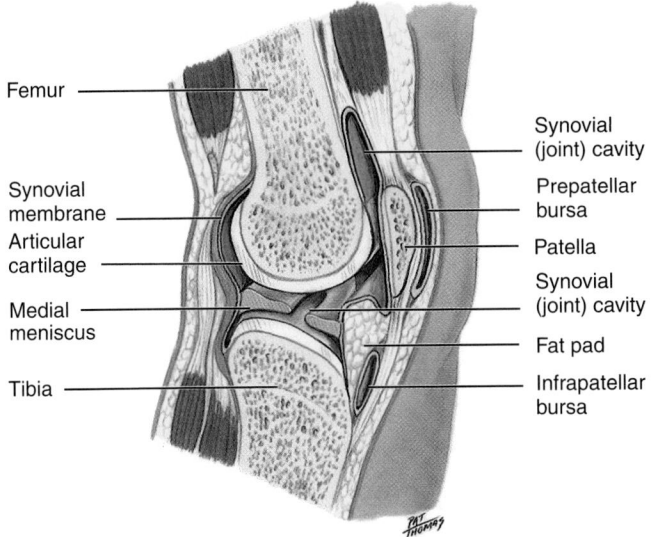

Femur

Synovial (joint) cavity

Prepatellar bursa

Synovial membrane

Articular cartilage

Patella

Synovial (joint) cavity

Medial meniscus

Fat pad

Tibia

Infrapatellar bursa

FIGURE 42-4 Sagittal section of the knee joint. (From Applegate EJ: *The anatomy and physiology learning system*, ed 3, St Louis, 2006, Saunders.)

fluid and act as cushions between a bone and tendon or between a tendon and ligament. Bursae reduce friction and help muscles and tendons glide smoothly over bone.

MUSCULOSKELETAL DISEASES AND DISORDERS

Musculoskeletal diseases and conditions can affect any of the muscles, bones, or joints. These problems are common and have

a tremendous impact on an individual's quality of life. Brittle or deformed bones that are prone to fracture often mark bone disorders such as osteoporosis and osteomalacia. Joint disorders such as osteoarthritis (OA), rheumatoid **arthritis** (RA), and gout can lead to painful, swollen, or inflamed joints. Muscle problems such as sprains and spasms can bring on sudden pain or cause stiffness. Myasthenia gravis, an autoimmune disorder in which there is abnormal transmission of nerve impulses to skeletal muscles, can cause severe muscle weakness (Table 42-2).

Trauma to the musculoskeletal system can quickly lead to **inflammation** in the area of injury. This type of injury is one of the leading causes of time lost from work and for visits to primary care physicians and emergency rooms. As soon as possible after injury, even before a patient is seen by a physician, RICE therapy should be initiated. (RICE stands for *rest, ice, compression,* and *elevation.*) The injured part should not be used, an ice bag should be applied, gentle compression with an elastic bandage should be initiated, and the extremity should be elevated. A combination of these measures will help decrease swelling and inflammation as well as enhance healing.

To maintain musculoskeletal health, it is important to have a significant dietary intake of foods rich in calcium and vitamin D, avoid smoking, and include weight-bearing exercises (such as walking) in your daily routine. In addition to these lifestyle measures, medications are sometimes required for conditions that impair normal functioning of this system. The conditions discussed in the following sections are typically seen in an orthopedic practice.

CRITICAL THINKING APPLICATION

Why is it so important to obtain an accurate history for an injured patient who comes to the office for the first time? What is Kaiwan's responsibility in finding out why a new patient is being seen?

Muscular Disorders

Fibromyalgia

Fibromyalgia is a condition of widespread connective tissue, and muscular pain, and often severe fatigue of unknown origin. A patient with fibromyalgia usually complains of diffuse aches and pains all over the body. It can affect people of all ages and is found more frequently in women than in men. Chronic pain and fatigue are the cardinal signs in the absence of any other known cause. The pain is described variously as burning, shooting, throbbing, aching, piercing, or stabbing. Associated conditions can include sleep disorders, irritable bowel syndrome, chronic

Frozen Pea Ice Bag

A bag of frozen peas (or corn) easily conforms to the shape of a body part and serves as an excellent medium for immediately applying ice to a musculoskeletal injury. The vegetable ice bag should be applied for 20 minutes, put back into the freezer for 30 to 60 minutes, and applied again.

TABLE 42-2 Common Musculoskeletal Conditions

DISEASE	SYMPTOMS AND SIGNS	DIAGNOSTIC PROCEDURES	LABORATORY TESTS	TREATMENT AND MEDICATIONS
Bursitis and tendonitis	Painful joint with decreased ROM	History, physical examination, x-ray studies to rule out fracture	CBC to rule out infectious arthritis	RICE, temporary immobilization, NSAIDs
Carpal tunnel syndrome	Hand and finger pain, numbness, tingling, and difficulty grasping or holding objects, especially in the morning	History, physical examination, compression test	None	Rest, splint, forearm extensor strengthening exercises, surgical decompression in severe cases
Dislocation	Painful joint that is out of place and has severely decreased ROM	History of trauma, physical examination, x-ray studies	None	Reduce and temporarily immobilize joint
Fibromyalgia	Chronic, severe musculoskeletal pain and generalized weakness	History, physical examination to rule out other causative conditions	As appropriate to rule out other conditions	NSAIDs, rest, decrease stress, muscle relaxants (Flexeril) and tricyclics (Elavil and Thorazine), SSRIs
Fractures	Severe pain, swelling, and decreased ROM	History, physical examination, x-ray studies	None	Reduction, immobilization, analgesics, NSAIDs
Gout	Painful, inflamed joint, often affects great toe, very sensitive to touch and movement	History, physical examination, microscopic synovial fluid examination for uric acid crystals	Serum uric acid test	Analgesics, NSAIDs
Herniated disk	Depend on location and severity of herniation, back pain, extremity pain or weakness	History, physical examination, CT, MRI	None	Immobility, physical therapy, traction, muscle relaxants, surgical laminectomy in severe cases
Infectious arthritis	Severely inflamed joint	History, physical examination, microscopic synovial fluid examination for cell count and presence of bacteria	CBC, culture of joint fluid	NSAIDs, corticosteroids, appropriate antibiotic or antiviral agents
Lupus	Widely disparate presentations of symptoms with no known cause; very difficult to diagnose	Very careful history and physical examination to rule out possible causes of presenting symptoms; frequently this is a diagnosis of exclusion	Diagnostic tests as needed to rule out possible symptom causes	Symptomatic relief
Lyme disease	Generalized malaise, fatigue, fever, headaches, myalgias, and polyarthralgias	Careful history and physical examination to look for tick bite location	CBC and perhaps other blood studies	Antibiotics and symptomatic relief
Myasthenia gravis	Profound muscular weakness, frequently starting with facial muscles, can involve any voluntary muscles	History, neurologic examination, EMG	Anti-AchR antibody test	Cholinesterase inhibitors, NSAIDs, steroids, immune inhibitors, thymectomy, plasmapheresis
Osteoarthritis	Gradually increasing joint pain and gradually decreasing ROM in affected joint	History, physical examination, x-ray studies, possible CT scan	RA latex test to rule out rheumatoid arthritis, CBC to rule out infectious arthritis	NSAIDs, physical therapy, analgesics, ambulatory support
Osteomalacia	Fractures, muscle weakness, bone pain	History, physical examination, x-ray studies, bone scan	Serum vitamin D, serum calcium, serum alkaline phosphatase, PTH level, occasionally bone biopsy	Vitamin D and calcium supplementation
Osteoporosis	Frequent fractures, exaggerated thoracic kyphosis, decreased height, back pain	History, physical examination, x-ray studies, bone density studies	DEXA scan, blood calcium level	Weight-bearing exercise, calcium supplementation, and pharmaceutical treatment with alendronate (Fosamax), etidronate (Didronel), or calcitonin-salmon (Miacalcin)

Continued

TABLE 42-2 Common Musculoskeletal Conditions—*cont'd*

DISEASE	SYMPTOMS AND SIGNS	DIAGNOSTIC PROCEDURES	LABORATORY TESTS	TREATMENT AND MEDICATIONS
Rheumatoid arthritis	Severe joint pain and joint deformity	History, physical examination, x-ray studies	RA latex test	NSAIDs, analgesics, joint replacement in severe cases
Scoliosis	Lateral spinal deformity accompanied by back pain	Physical examination, radiographic studies	None	Braces, casts, surgery
Sprain, strain, spasm	Cardinal signs of inflammation, redness, heat, swelling, pain along with decreased ROM	History, physical examination, including active and passive ROM, x-ray studies to rule out fracture	None	RICE and NSAIDs

CBC, complete blood count; *CT,* computed tomography; *DEXA,* dual energy x-ray absorptiometry; *EMG,* electromyography; *MRI,* magnetic resonance imaging; *NSAIDs,* nonsteroidal antiinflammatory drugs; *PTH,* parathyroid hormone; *RA,* rheumatoid arthritis; *RICE,* rest, ice, compression, elevation; *ROM,* range of motion; *SSRIs,* selective serotonin reuptake inhibitors.

headaches, temporomandibular joint (TMJ) problems, increased chemical sensitivity, and other musculoskeletal complaints. Although the cause remains unknown, fibromyalgia can be triggered by automobile accidents or bacterial or viral infection or can follow the diagnosis of other medical conditions, such as RA, lupus, or hypothyroidism. It is aggravated by changes in the weather or temperature, monthly hormonal variations, stress, anxiety, and depression. A diagnosis is made by eliminating any other cause for the symptoms and finding 11 of 18 specific points to be extremely tender to palpation (Figure 42-5). Treatment goals include reducing pain, enhancing sleep, and decreasing anxiety and stress. There is no known cure.

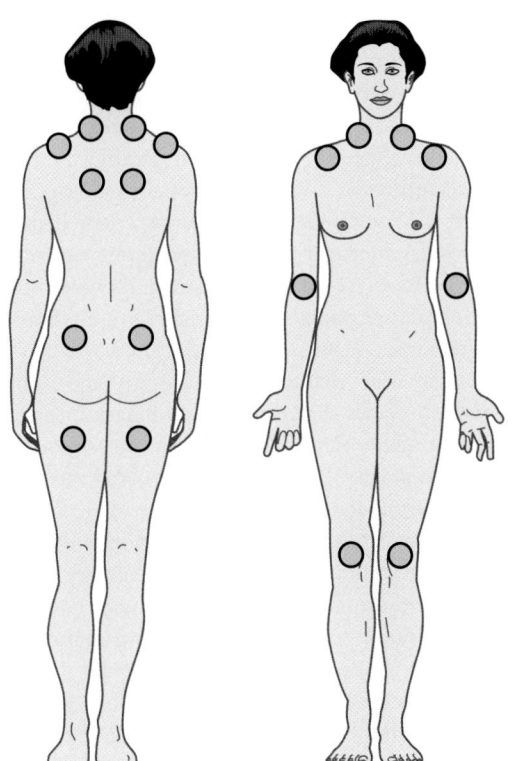

FIGURE 42-5 Fibromyalgia tender points.

Myasthenia Gravis

Myasthenia gravis is a chronic autoimmune neuromuscular disease of unknown origin that affects voluntary muscle contraction and can occur at any age but most frequently affects young adult women (under 40) and older men (over 60). Frequently the patient experiences a sudden onset of weakness in the muscles that control eye and eyelid movement, facial expression, and swallowing. Symptoms vary in type and severity and may include a drooping of one or both eyelids *(ptosis);* blurred or double vision *(diplopia)* resulting from weakness of the muscles that control eye movements; unstable or waddling **gait;** weakness in arms, hands, fingers, legs, and neck; altered facial expressions; difficulty in swallowing; shortness of breath; and impaired speech *(dysarthria).*

Myasthenia gravis is caused by a defect in the transmission of nerve impulses to muscles. It occurs when a nervous stimulus is unable to stimulate a muscle at the *neuromuscular junction*—the place where nerve cells connect with the muscles they control. Normally when impulses travel down the nerve, the nerve endings release acetylcholine (ACh), a neurotransmitter that activates muscular contraction. In myasthenia gravis, antibodies block, alter, or destroy the receptors for ACh at the neuromuscular junction, which prevents the muscle contraction from occurring. The primary treatment involves a medication that inhibits acetylcholinesterase, the enzyme that normally breaks down ACh. This allows ACh to remain at the neuromuscular junction longer than usual so that more of the remaining receptor sites can be activated. Surgical removal of the thymus gland *(thymectomy)* reduces symptoms in most patients and may cure some individuals. Spontaneous improvement and remissions can occur.

Sprains, Strains, and Spasms

A *sprain* is a wrenching or twisting of a joint in an abnormal plane of motion or beyond its normal ROM that results in the stretching and/or tearing of a ligament. There may be concurrent damage to area blood vessels, muscles, tendons, and nerves. Probably the most common sprain is the sprained ankle (Figure 42-6), which can result from stepping off a curb or into a small depression and twisting the ankle. Severe sprains are so

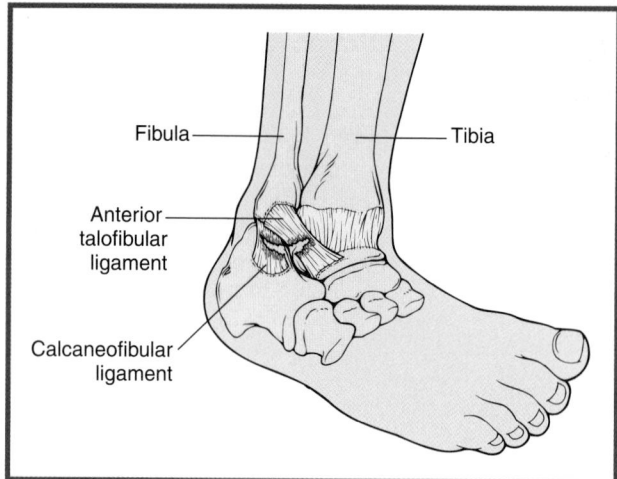

FIGURE 42-6 Ankle sprain. (From Frazier MS, Drzymkowski JW: *Essentials of human diseases and conditions,* ed 3, Philadelphia, 2004, Saunders.)

Telephone Screening

Kaiwan shares the responsibility of answering phones and making appointments for patients. If a patient calls reporting an injury to a joint, these are some of the guidelines he should use when deciding about the need for an appointment.

- Presence of severe pain and inability to put any weight on the injured joint
- Crooked appearance of injured area or unusual lumps and bumps
- Inability to move the injured joint
- Inability to walk more than four steps without significant pain
- Attempts to use the joint cause limb to buckle or give way
- Numbness in any part of the injured area
- Inflammation that spreads out from the injured area
- History of injury to this particular joint
- Pain, swelling, or inflammation over a bony prominence

painful that the joint cannot be used and are accompanied by swelling and reddish to bluish discoloration because of ruptured blood vessels in the area.

A *strain* may be a simple overstretching of a muscle or tendon, or it can be caused by a partial or complete tear of the tissue away from the bone.

The diagnosis of these soft-tissue injuries is made by a comprehensive history and physical examination. Usually x-ray films are obtained to rule out fractures. Treatment includes RICE: rest of the injured joint with no weight-bearing to prevent further damage; cold application for 20 minutes at a time, four to eight times per day, during the first 24 to 48 hours to reduce pain and swelling; compression with an elastic wrap or air cast to reduce swelling; and elevation of the injured part. The physician may also recommend the use of over-the-counter antiinflammatory drugs such as aspirin or ibuprofen to help decrease pain and inflammation at the site. If severe soft-tissue injury occurs, immobilization by casting, surgical repair, or both may be required.

Treatment of a sprain or strain may also include rehabilitation exercises to improve the condition of the injured area and restore its function. The physician typically prescribes an exercise program designed to prevent stiffness, improve the joint's ROM, and restore normal flexibility and strength. Some patients may also be referred to physical therapy for complete return of function after the initial pain and swelling have subsided.

CRITICAL THINKING APPLICATION

A patient comes into the clinic hopping on one foot and holding the other in the air. She says she thinks she broke her ankle when she stepped off the curb wrong and fell. What is the first thing Kaiwan should do for this patient? What test will Dr. Alexander most likely order? Why?

Muscle *spasms* occur spontaneously and may persist for hours. They are typically caused by heavy exercise and muscle fatigue but may be a result of dehydration, hypothyroidism, lack of calcium or magnesium, kidney failure, or alcoholism. Muscle spasms can be quite painful, and treatment can include massage, direct pressure, ultrasound, stress reduction, stretching exercises, and muscle relaxants in some cases.

Skeletal Disorders

Fractures

A fracture is a break or crack in a bone that generally is the result of trauma or disease. Many different types of fractures occur, and each has its own set of problems (Table 42-3). The common symptom of all fractures is pain. Other symptoms may include swelling, bleeding, inability to move, misalignment of the bone, and discoloration of the immediate area.

When a patient with a suspected fracture comes into the office, you should make him or her as comfortable as possible. First aid includes RICE; positioning the patient in a manner that does not put stress on the injured area; elevating the injured extremity if possible; controlling any bleeding but never applying pressure over a suspected fracture. Do not attempt to straighten the fracture or move it in any way. If the patient must be moved, either apply a splint or support the joints above and below the suspected fracture before and while moving the patient. The fracture must be confirmed by x-ray examination as soon as possible.

Treatment includes **reduction** if necessary and immobilization. Reduction places the fractured bone back into its correct anatomic alignment. Reduction may be closed or open. In a *closed* reduction the physician manipulates the bone into its correct position. If this is not possible, or if the fractured bones have pierced the skin, an *open* reduction will be required, which means realigning the bone with surgery. During an open reduction the orthopedic physician may have to install metal pins, plates, or screws to facilitate and maintain correct bone alignment. These metal implants may be temporary or permanent, depending on the extent of injury (Figure 42-7). After the fracture has been reduced, it must be immobilized by splinting or casting to prevent movement of the fracture site and thus facilitate healing. Immobilization can also be accomplished

TABLE 42-3 Types of Fractures

FRACTURE	DEFINITION	FRACTURE	DEFINITION
Closed or simple	Broken bone is contained within intact skin	Pathologic	Results from weakening of bone by disease as in osteoporosis or sarcomas
Open or compound	Skin is broken above the fracture, which is thus open to the external environment, resulting in potential for infection	Nondisplaced	Bone ends remain in alignment
Longitudinal	Fracture extends along the length of the bone	Displaced	Bone ends are out of alignment
Transverse	Produced by direct force applied perpendicular to a bone; fracture runs across the bone	Spiral	Results in long, sharp, pointed bone ends; produced by twisting or rotary forces; suspicious for child abuse injury
Oblique	Produced by a twisting force with an upward thrust; fracture ends are short and run at an oblique angle across the bone	Compression	Produced by transmitted forces that drive bones together

Continued

TABLE 42-3 Types of Fractures—*cont'd*

FRACTURE	DEFINITION	FRACTURE	DEFINITION
Greenstick 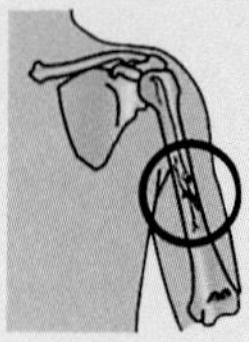	Produced by compression or angulation forces in long bones of children younger than 10; bone is cracked on one side and intact on the other because of softness	Avulsion 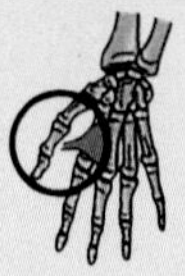	Produced by forceful contraction of a muscle against resistance, with a bone fragment tearing at the site of muscle insertion
Comminuted 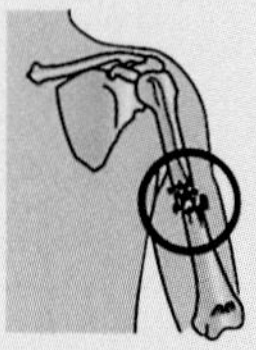	Has multiple fragments and is produced by severe direct violence	Depression 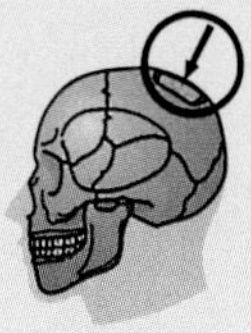	Bone fragments of the skull are driven inward
Impacted 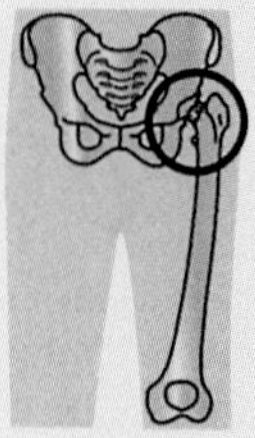	Produced by strong forces that drive bone fragments firmly together		

From Chester GA: *Modern medical assisting*, Philadelphia, 1999, Saunders.

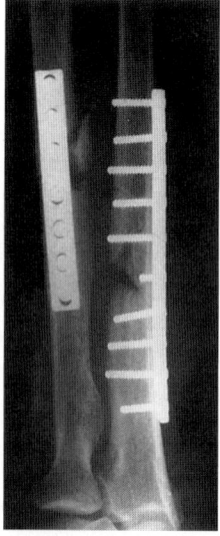

FIGURE 42-7 Orthopedic hardware from open reduction of fractures of the radius and ulna. (From Mettler MA: *Essentials of radiology*, ed 3, Philadelphia, 2004, Saunders.)

by taping or wrapping the area, depending on the location and severity of the injury.

Osteomalacia

Osteomalacia literally means "softening of the bones." This is a metabolic disease in which there is inadequate calcium, phosphorus, or both available for the building of new bone during growth or remodeling. It is caused by a deficiency of vitamin D or problems with the metabolism of this vitamin. The skeleton gradually loses calcium, and the bones soften and become more flexible. Weight-bearing gradually changes the shape of the softened bones. Symptoms can include decreased endurance, easy fatigability, **malaise,** and generalized bone tenderness and pain. Osteomalacia may be caused by a fat absorption problem in the gastrointestinal tract that prevents adequate absorption of dietary fats resulting in *steatorrhea* and vitamin D deficiency. Vitamin D promotes the body's absorption of *calcium*, which is essential for the normal development and maintenance of healthy teeth and bones. It is a nonessential vitamin, because vitamin D can be produced by the body, but production starts with adequate sun exposure. Use of very strong sunscreen, limited exposure of the body to sunlight, short days of sunlight, and smog are factors that decrease formation of vitamin D within the body.

Osteomalacia occurring in children is called *rickets*. A much less common cause of osteomalacia is dietary vitamin D deficiency and consequently inadequate calcium absorption and use. This is quite rare, because when exposed to even small amounts of sunlight, the skin makes vitamin D, and nearly all milk sold in the United States is fortified with vitamin D. However, osteomalacia can occur in individuals who remain indoors and those who avoid milk because of *lactose intolerance*. Treatment is with vitamin D, calcium, and phosphorus supplements.

Osteoporosis

Osteoporosis is a disease in which calcium in the bone gradually decreases and bones become increasingly weak and brittle so that even small stressors such as bending over or coughing can cause fractures. Bone strength is dependent on the size and density of the bone structure and the amount of calcium, phosphorus, and other materials deposited and maintained in the bone. Bones are constantly changing through a process called *remodeling*, or bone turnover. This process allows bones to grow and heal. As we age, remodeling breaks bone down more quickly than it forms new bone. Peak bone mass is reached by the mid 30s, so the risk of developing osteoporosis is dependent on the bone mass collected by the ages of 25 to 35 and how rapidly bone tissue is lost after that. Lack of vitamin D and calcium in the diet results in a lower peak bone mass and a more rapid onset of bone loss later. People over 50 years of age are particularly at risk, and women are four times more likely to develop osteoporosis than men. Osteoporosis is a major public health threat in the United States, affecting more than 40 million individuals.

Osteoporosis is often called the "silent disease," because the progressive loss of bone density occurs without any symptoms. *Osteopenia* refers to mild bone loss that is not severe enough to be called osteoporosis but that increases the risk for osteoporosis. By the time fractures occur, the disease is quite advanced. Patients with osteoporosis complain of back pain because of a fractured or collapsed vertebra; loss of height over time, with stooped posture (kyphosis or the "dowagers hump"); and fractures that typically include those of the vertebrae, wrists, and hips. Risk factors include being a postmenopausal woman over 50 years of age; a slight build with a family history of osteoporosis; history of amenorrhea; low dietary calcium intake; excessive intake of caffeinated soda; inactive lifestyle; smoking; alcohol abuse; hyperthyroidism; decreased lifetime exposure to estrogen; and long-term treatment with certain medications including antiseizure drugs and heparin. Men over 50 years of age with low testosterone levels are also at risk. Osteoporosis occurs in all races but is slightly more common in whites and Asians.

Diagnosis is made by a specialized form of x-ray evaluation that specifically measures bone density. This can diagnose osteoporosis before a fracture occurs and thus allow intervention

to prevent fractures. Readings are repeated annually to determine the rate of bone loss and to monitor treatment effectiveness. Intervention and treatment include increasing dietary intake of calcium and vitamin D; increasing weight-bearing exercise; and pharmaceutical treatment with bisphosphonates (Fosamax, Didronel, and Actonel), raloxifene (Evista), and calcitonin-salmon (Miacalcin). The best screening test is a dual energy x-ray absorptiometry (DEXA) scan, which measures the bone density of the spine, hip, and wrist. Other tests that can accurately measure bone density include ultrasound and quantitative computed tomography (CT) scanning.

The National Osteoporosis Foundation recommends that all women have a bone density test if they are not receiving estrogen replacement therapy and are in any of the following categories:

- Are undergoing long-term treatment with medications that can cause osteoporosis, such as prednisone
- Have type 1 diabetes, liver disease, kidney disease, or a family history of osteoporosis
- Experienced early menopause (in the early 40s)
- Are postmenopausal, are older than 50, and have at least one risk factor for osteoporosis
- Are postmenopausal, are older than 65, and have never had a bone density test

Spinal Column Disorders

Abnormal Spinal Curvatures

When one looks at a patient's back, the spine should be vertically straight. Any abnormal deviation or curvature to the right or left is termed **scoliosis.** Mild scoliosis generally causes no problems and is usually not even noticeable. When scoliosis is severe, it can cause significant back pain and possibly heart or lung problems because of the decreased space in the thoracic cavity on one side.

When the spine is viewed from a lateral position, there are four normal curves present (Figure 42-8). The **cervical** and the **lumbar** regions should have curves toward the front of the body; these are called **lordotic** curves. The normal curves in the thoracic regions of the spine and the sacrum are toward the back and are called **kyphotic** curves. Loss of cervical lordosis is called *military neck*. Excessive lumbar lordosis is called *swayback*. Excessive upper thoracic kyphosis is called *hunchback* (Figure 42-9).

Diagnosis of these conditions is made by inspection and palpation and may be confirmed with x-ray studies. Treatment may include orthopedic devices such as braces, shoe lifts, exercises, and electrical muscle stimulation. In severe cases rigid casting with or without surgery may be necessary.

Herniated Disk

A herniated disk occurs when the soft nucleus of an intervertebral disk protrudes through a tear or weakened area in its tough outer cartilaginous covering (Figure 42-10). This condition occurs most often in the lumbar region, frequently in the cervical region, and rarely in the thoracic region of the spine. In children and young adults, disks have high water content. As people

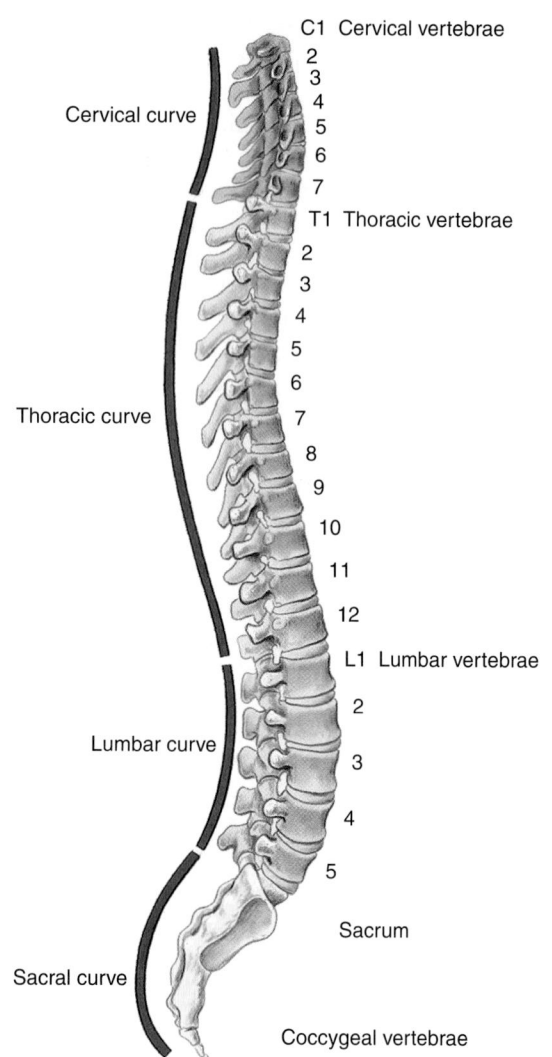

C1 Cervical vertebrae
2
3
Cervical curve
4
5
6
7
T1 Thoracic vertebrae
2
3
4
5
6
Thoracic curve
7
8
9
10
11
12
L1 Lumbar vertebrae
2
Lumbar curve
3
4
5
Sacrum
Sacral curve
Coccygeal vertebrae

FIGURE 42-8 Normal spine curves. (From Applegate EJ: *The anatomy and physiology learning system,* ed 3, St Louis, 2006, Saunders.)

age, the water content in the disks decreases and the structures begin to shrink and become less flexible. This causes the spaces between the vertebrae to get narrower. Factors that can weaken intervertebral disks include improper lifting; smoking; excessive body weight that places added stress on the disks of the lower back; sudden, possible slight pressure; and repetitive strenuous activities. Herniation may also occur gradually over time as a result of a progressive deterioration of the disks.

Symptoms depend on the location and the extent of the protrusion of the nucleus beyond its normal location. If the herniation occurs in the lumbar region, it usually results in severe low back pain that can radiate down the leg and cause difficulty walking. If the herniated disk is in the cervical region, there is usually a burning pain in the neck that can radiate down the arms to the fingers.

Diagnosis is made from a careful history, physical examination, either magnetic resonance imaging (MRI) or CT scans to confirm which disk is injured, or an electromyography (EMG) test that measures the nervous stimulation of affected muscles. Treatment depends on the severity of the herniation and

the symptoms. Conservative treatments include chiropractic adjustments, physical therapy mobilization of the involved area, and applications of cold until muscle spasms stop, then the use of heat. Traction of the affected area, especially of the neck, may help relieve pressure on affected nerves. Muscle relaxants, such as carisoprodol (Soma) and cyclobenzaprine (Flexeril) and/or analgesics may be given. If these measures are ineffective and the patient has recurring pain, numbness, and progressive weakness, surgery may be necessary.

Joint Disorders

Dislocation

Dislocation of a joint is also called a **luxation,** a condition in which two bones of a joint are no longer in approximation (Figure 42-11). A **subluxation** is an incomplete dislocation of a joint, meaning that the bones are only slightly out of proper alignment and location. It is possible to have a congenital dislocation, especially of the hip. Common dislocations occur to the finger, thumb, and shoulder and are usually caused by trauma, frequently while a person is playing sports. Symptoms include pain, swelling, loss of motion, and sometimes temporary paralysis of the affected part. A dislocation requires immediate reduction and immobilization to prevent permanent injury to structures adjacent to the joint, such as nerves and major blood vessels. Occasionally, surgical reduction and repair may be necessary to stabilize the joint.

CRITICAL THINKING APPLICATION

A patient comes into the office from a sandlot softball game. After sliding into home plate he was immediately unable to move his right arm and complained of a great deal of pain in his right shoulder. What steps should Kaiwan take to help this patient?

Gout

Gout, which may also be called *gouty arthritis,* is a metabolic disease in which there is an overproduction or improper elimination of uric acid. Uric acid is a waste product formed from the breakdown of purines, which are found naturally in the body as well as in certain foods including organ meats (liver, brains, and kidney), anchovies, herring, asparagus, mushrooms, cold cuts, sausage, and alcohol. Uric acid should dissolve in the blood so that it can be excreted as it passes through the kidneys. However, with gout, uric acid is not effectively excreted, so needlelike crystals of uric acid collect in the synovial fluid of the affected joint, causing extreme sensitivity to touch, pronounced inflammation, and severe pain. The most frequently affected area is the great toe (Figure 42-12). Risk factors include consumption of alcohol, obesity, untreated hypertension, diabetes, hyper-cholesterolemia, and a family history of the disease. Men are more likely to experience gout than women, but women become increasingly susceptible to gout after menopause.

In general, keeping uric acid levels within a normal range is the key to preventing future episodes of gout. Therefore long-range treatment includes dietary modifications to eliminate purine-containing foods. For treatment of an acute onset of inflam-

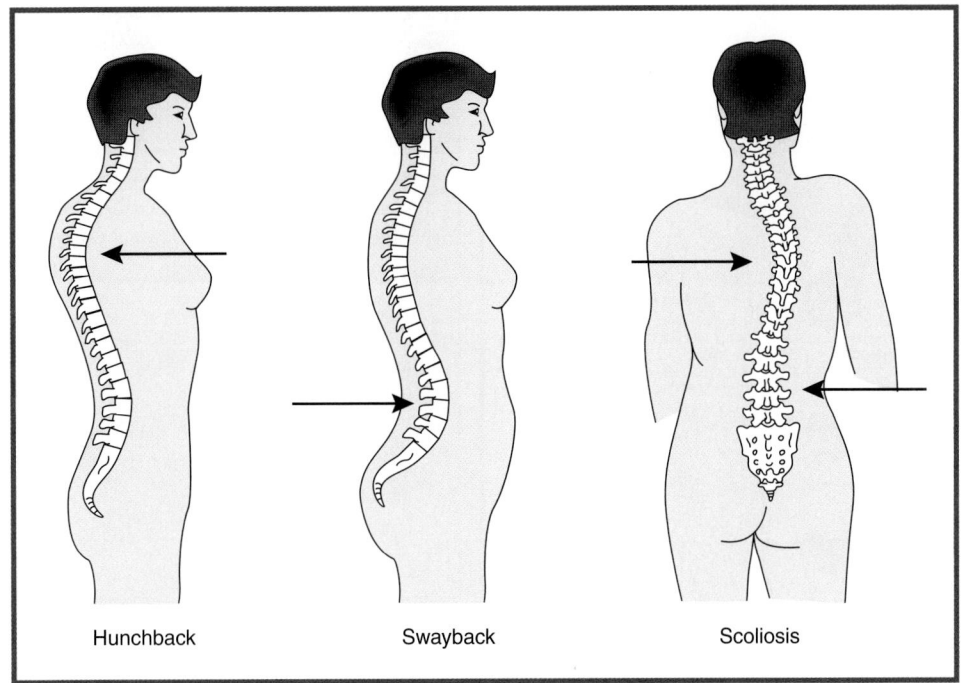

FIGURE 42-9 Spinal curve abnormalities.

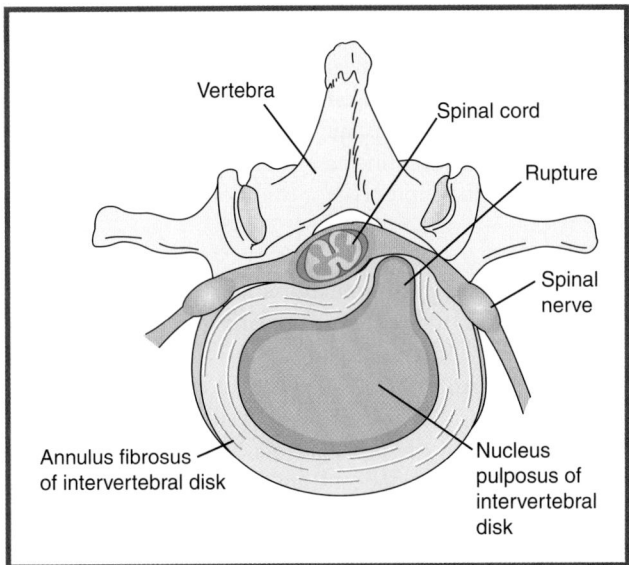

FIGURE 42-10 Herniation of vertebral disk.

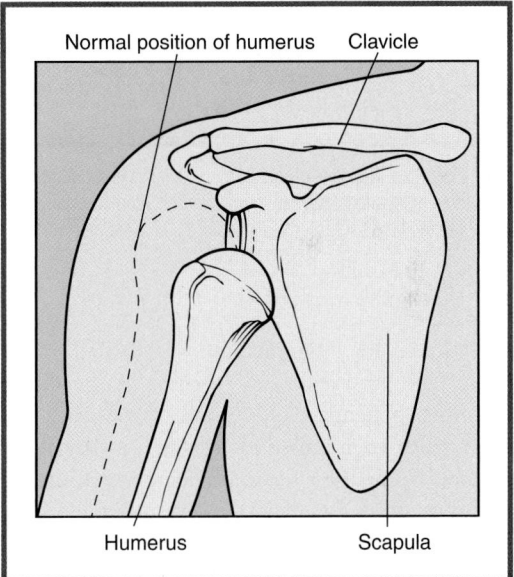

FIGURE 42-11 Luxation or dislocation of the shoulder. (From Frazier MS, Drzymkowski JW: *Essentials of human diseases and conditions*, ed 3, Philadelphia, 2004, Saunders.)

mation the patient may take nonsteroidal antiinflammatory drugs (NSAIDs) such as ibuprofen and Aleve for the pain and joint inflammation, and in severe cases the physician may prescribe prednisone. To reduce the risk or lessen the severity of future episodes, pharmaceutical treatment includes allopurinol (Zyloprim, Aloprim) and probenecid (Benemid). Taken daily they slow the rate of uric acid production and enhance its elimination from the body.

Lupus

The three main types of lupus are systemic lupus erythematosus (SLE), discoid lupus erythematosus, and drug-induced lupus. Of

these, SLE is the most common and serious form of the disease. SLE is an autoimmune disease of unknown cause. It occurs primarily in women 20 to 50 years of age, although it can occur in both younger and older persons as well. Other risk factors include recurrent infections from the Epstein-Barr virus, a family history of the disease, and being an African American.

SLE is difficult to diagnose, and the course is entirely unpredictable. The patient develops autoantibodies (antibodies to self) that can attack any tissue or organ in the body, which

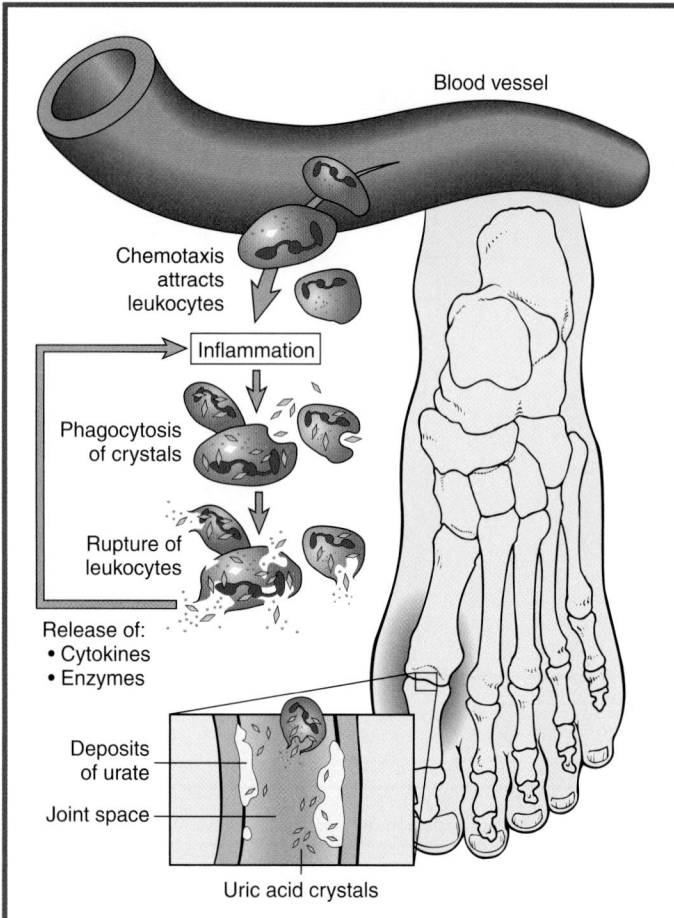

FIGURE 42-12 Gout. Deposits of uric acid crystals in the connective tissue. The inflammation most often affects the joint of the big toe. (From Damjanov I: *Pathology for the health-related professions*, ed 3, St Louis, 2006, Saunders.)

SLE Symptoms

According to the American Rheumatism Association, the diagnosis and classification of lupus require four of the following 10 clinical and laboratory criteria:

- Malar rash—a butterfly-shaped rash that covers the bridge of the nose and spreads across the cheeks
- Discoid rash—raised, scaly patches that may cause scarring
- Marked sensitivity to sunlight
- Oral ulcers
- Arthritis that involves two or more peripheral joints
- Inflammation of the lining of the heart or lung (*serositis*)
- Renal disease
- A neurologic disorder, such as seizures or psychosis
- A hematologic disorder such as anemia, thrombocytopenia, or leukopenia
- Elevated antinuclear antibody blood levels (an indicator of an autoimmune disease)

Infectious Arthritis

Infectious arthritis usually occurs after some type of systemic or local infection in some other part of the body. It can also occur after a joint has been violated by trauma or surgery. Causes can include bacteria, fungi, and viruses. The joint usually exhibits signs of severe inflammation and shows significantly decreased ROM. To determine the diagnosis the physician may order an x-ray evaluation and bone scan and may draw synovial fluid for microscopic examination and culture. Treatment goals are to decrease inflammation, increase ROM, and treat the causative organism with the appropriate medication.

Lyme Disease

Lyme disease is an infection caused by the bacteria *Borrelia burgdorferi* and is transmitted to humans by a bite from ticks of the *Ixodes* family. It is named after Lyme, Connecticut, where it was first identified in 1975 in a cluster of children who showed signs of what was thought to be RA. Eventually epidemiologists traced the cause of the problem to a bacterial infection. Signs and symptoms may include a "bull's-eye lesion" called *erythema migrans* surrounding the area of the tick bite appears within a few days, even up to a month, after exposure. The rash can last from several days to several weeks and occurs in as many as 80% of people infected with Lyme disease. Additional indicators of the disease include flulike symptoms such as fever, chills, fatigue, body aches, and headache. If the infection remains untreated, the patient will complain of multiple joint pain; late-stage Lyme disease symptoms include meningitis, Bell's palsy, numbness or weakness of the limbs, memory loss, difficulty concentrating, and changes in mood or sleep habits.

Diagnosis is made by taking a careful history, including the patient's level of outdoor exposure, locating the tick bite, and ruling out other causes for presenting symptoms. Laboratory tests to identify antibodies to the bacterium are used to help confirm the diagnosis. These tests are most reliable a few weeks after an infection because it takes some time for antibodies to develop. The blood test most often used to screen for Lyme

may result in severe inflammation with tissue changes and destruction. The progresion and severity of the disease vary widely among patients. Furthermore, problems associated with SLE change over time and overlap with those of many other disorders. For these reasons, doctors may not initially consider lupus until the signs and symptoms become more obvious. At times the disease may become severe, and at other times it may subside completely. There is no known cure; the therapeutic goal is to have the patient remain as functional and active as possible. The type of pharmaceutical treatment prescribed depends on which parts of the body are affected by the disease and the severity of symptoms. Some medications used to treat SLE include NSAIDs such as naproxen sodium and ibuprofen to reduce joint pain and inflammation; antimalarials such as hydroxychloroquine (Plaquenil) to treat skin and joint problems and the ulcers that some people develop in the mouth or nose; **corticosteroids** (prednisone) during acute inflammatory processes; and immunosuppressive medications such as azathioprine (Imuran) and cyclophosphamide (Cytoxan) to suppress the immune system. The kidneys may fail even with treatment, which may necessitate either kidney dialysis or a kidney transplant.

Patient Education for Prevention of Lyme Disease

- Wear pants tucked into socks and long-sleeved shirts when walking in wooded or grassy areas.
- Use insect repellents that contain DEET.
- Tick-proof your yard by clearing brush and leaves where ticks live.
- Check yourself, your children, and your pets for ticks; deer ticks are no bigger than the head of a pin or a grain of pepper; shower immediately after being in wooded areas, because ticks can remain on the skin for hours before attaching themselves.
- Do not assume you are immune; Lyme disease can occur in the same person more than once.
- Remove a tick with tweezers by gently grasping it near the head or mouth; do not squeeze or crush the tick, but pull it out carefully and steadily. After removal apply antiseptic to the bite area.
- A vaccine, LYMErix, was available until February 2002, but the vaccine's manufacturer cited poor sales as the reason for pulling the vaccine off the market.

disease is the enzyme-linked immunosorbent assay (ELISA), which detects antibodies to *B. burgdorferi*. If the ELISA test is positive, the Western blot test is performed to confirm the diagnosis. Antibiotics, such as doxycycline (Doryx, Monodox) or amoxicillin (Amoxil, Trimox), are the standard treatment for Lyme disease in its early stages. If the disease has progressed to a later stage the patient may be hospitalized for treatment with intravenous (IV) ceftriaxone (Rocephin).

Osteoarthritis

OA, also called degenerative joint disease (DJD), is marked by significant thinning and degeneration of the articular cartilage of synovial joints. The severity of symptoms depends on the amount of degeneration that has taken place and ranges from mild to severe. As the articular cartilage disintegrates and wears away, the roughened surface of the bone is exposed, leaving bone rubbing against bone, with resultant pain and stiffness of the involved joint. Commonly involved joints include the fingers, the spine, and the weight-bearing joints of the hips, knees, and feet. Diagnosis frequently includes x-ray films, which show degenerative changes in the joint surfaces and asymmetric joint space narrowing.

Treatment goals include relieving pain, maintaining normal motion in the joint, and attempting to prevent crippling deformities. Medications may include analgesics, NSAIDs, and intraarticular steroid injections. Using a walker or cane may be helpful for maintaining mobility. In severe cases surgery to remove the affected joint and replace it with a joint **prosthesis** is necessary.

Rheumatoid Arthritis

RA is an autoimmune inflammatory condition that involves an immune system response to the synovial membranes that results in synovitis. Proteins are released at the site of the joint inflammation, eventually causing thickening of the synovium and damage to the cartilage, bone, tendons, and ligaments

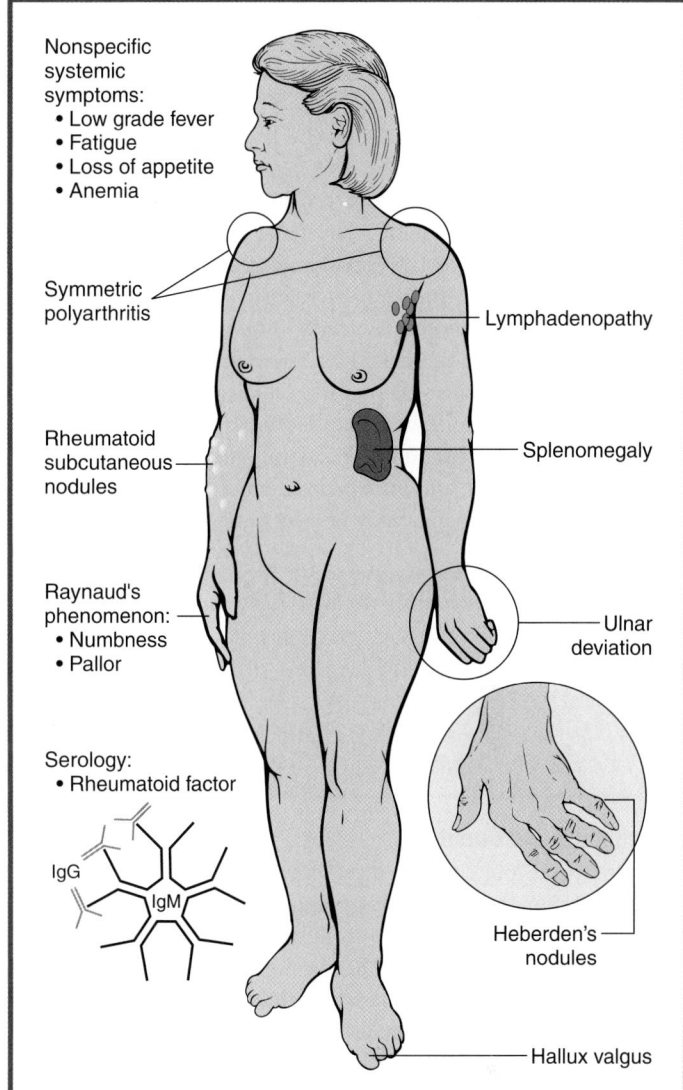

FIGURE 42-13 Signs and symptoms of rheumatoid arthritis. (From Damjanov I: *Pathology for the health-related professions*, ed 3, St Louis, 2006, Saunders.)

of the affected joint. Gradually the joint loses its shape and alignment causing deformity and pain. Researchers suspect RA is triggered by an infection in people with an inherited susceptibility to the disease.

Early symptoms include malaise, fever, weight loss, and morning stiffness of the affected joints. One or more joints may become painful and inflamed. Usually, bouts of arthritis will increase in frequency and severity over time. As this occurs, the joints become damaged and joint swelling and deformity occur. The patient ultimately loses the ability to move the affected joints, and a pronounced loss of strength occurs in the muscles attached to the inflamed joints. Small lumps, called *rheumatoid nodules,* may form at pressure points located in the elbows, hands, feet, Achilles tendons, knees, and posterior scalp, and even in the lungs. Patients with RA may appear undernourished and chronically ill because of the formation of degenerative lesions occurring in the collagen (connective tissues) in the lungs, heart, blood vessels, and pleura (Figure 42-13). Periods of increased disease activity—called *flare-ups*—alternate with periods of relative remission, during which the swelling, pain, difficulty sleeping, and weakness fade or disappear. X-ray findings show uniform joint space narrowing, which is different from the degenerative changes seen in OA.

Rest and exercise seem to be the key elements in treating RA. Therapeutic exercises are designed to prevent and correct deformities, control pain, strengthen weakened muscles, and improve joint function. The most frequently prescribed medications are NSAIDs including aspirin (acetylsalicylic acid), indomethacin (Indocin), diclofenac (Voltaren), naproxen (Naprosyn), and ibuprofen (Motrin). Corticosteroids (prednisone and Medrol) may be prescribed for severe flare-ups. To limit the extent of joint damage early in the disease, the physician will prescribe disease-modifying antirheumatic drugs (DMARDs) such as hydroxychloroquine (Plaquenil), the gold compound auranofin (Ridaura), and infliximab (Remicade). In severe cases surgical joint replacement may be necessary.

CRITICAL THINKING APPLICATION

An 80-year-old male patient with severe arthritis comes into the office complaining of severe joint pain in his knees, hips, and lower back. He cannot possibly get up onto the examination table because of the pain. What should Kaiwan do? Is this patient required to get onto the examination table? Why or why not?

Tendonitis and Bursitis

Tendonitis is one of the most common causes of pain in the shoulder and elbow. Inflammation of tendons may be associated with calcium deposits in the bursae around the joint causing concurrent bursitis. The diagnosis is made if the patient has increased severity of pain when abducting the arm beyond 50 degrees. Treatment includes pain relief and decreasing the localized inflammation to make exercise possible and to prevent shoulder immobility, called *frozen shoulder*. Medications might include analgesics, NSAIDs, and injections of long-acting corticosteroids. Cold applications are helpful in relieving pain, whereas heat applications are contraindicated because they tend to aggravate calcium tendonitis.

Bursitis is a painful inflammation of a joint bursa that most commonly follows a repetitive movement or prolonged pressure on a joint. The pain is increased with movement of the affected joint. It can also occur from staphylococcus or tuberculosis infections and with some joint diseases including gout and arthritis. Treatment includes preventing the activity that caused the bursitis and protecting the affected site from excessive pressure and movement. NSAIDs may provide pain relief, but corticosteroid antiinflammatories may be needed in severe cases. The best prevention is to limit the underlying causes.

THE MEDICAL ASSISTANT'S ROLE IN ASSISTING WITH ORTHOPEDIC PROCEDURES

The role of the medical assistant begins with accurately recording the patient's description of the circumstances surrounding the onset of the problem, what measures were undertaken to alleviate the problem, and the patient's current concerns.

Record the exact location of pain or discomfort, and ask the patient to quantify the intensity of the pain at that time on a scale of 1 to 10. Also record information about any medications taken, including the names of drugs, dose, frequency, and the date and time of the last dose.

Be sure to offer assistance when escorting the patient to the examination room. Use a wheelchair if necessary. Assist the patient to a comfortable position in the examination room by offering a pillow or folded blanket to support the painful or injured body part. The patient may have limited mobility because of pain, so you may need to provide assistance with disrobing and getting into an examination gown. Be sure the patient is warm enough by offering an additional sheet or blanket. Explain clearly what is happening and what the patient can expect. Notify the physician as soon as the patient is ready for the examination.

Assisting with the Examination

The physician may use inspection, palpation, ROM testing, and muscle testing to examine the major skeletal muscles and joints. Much of the examination involves comparing muscles and joints on the affected side with those on the contralateral side for size, position, and strength. When the patient needs to assume a certain position, it may be helpful to demonstrate the position or movement desired. Watch the patient during the manipulative and palpatory portion of the examination for a facial grimace or physical jerk or jump, which may indicate pain.

As a general rule the unaffected side is examined first, then the affected side is examined and compared. You may be responsible for making notes during the examination. Keep the patient properly draped, and assist the physician by handing the equipment to him or her as needed. Most examinations require the use of a measuring tape, **goniometer**, blood pressure cuff, stethoscope, and felt-tipped washable marker. Be alert and ready to prevent the patient from falling during the examination, because some of the requested movements and positions may place the injured patient off balance and at increased risk for falling.

The physician will perform a gait analysis by watching the patient walk in a straight line with or without the patient knowing he or she is being observed. In addition to being associated with disorders of the musculoskeletal system, gait abnormalities may be caused by an associated neurologic condition.

SPECIALIZED DIAGNOSTIC PROCEDURES IN ORTHOPEDICS

Range-of-Motion Evaluation

Often orthopedic injuries severely affect the normal ROM of a joint. Measuring the ROM of specific joints is an objective measure of both the seriousness of an injury and the recovery progress. When evaluating the ROM of a particular joint, usually both active ROM and passive ROM results are measured and recorded.

The joint movement in a single plane is measured with a goniometer. A goniometer has two arms that are fixed together

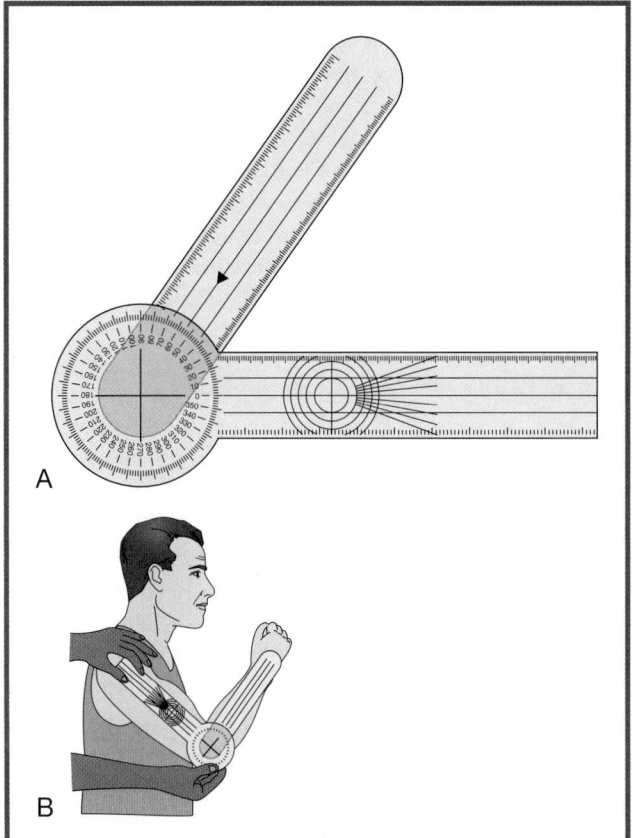

FIGURE 42-14 **A,** Goniometer. **B,** Correct position of goniometer on the arm.

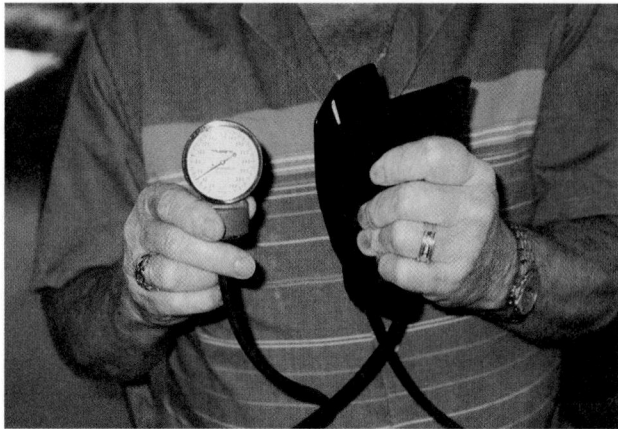

FIGURE 42-15 Assessing strength measurement using a blood pressure cuff.

Assessment of Strength Using a Blood Pressure Cuff

- Roll up an aneroid blood pressure cuff, and have the patient hold it in one hand.
- Inflate the cuff to 20 mm Hg pressure.
- Ask the patient to squeeze the cuff as tightly as possible.
- Note the increase in mm Hg pressure on the dial. A normal grip will be above 150.
- Record the hand tested and the results of the test.
- Repeat on the contralateral side.

with a hinge joint at one end (Figure 42-14). Each of the arms is lined up with a bone on each side of the joint being tested. The degrees of motion are indicated on a scale on the hinged end of the instrument. To determine the active ROM of a joint, the patient is asked to move the joint as far as possible. For evaluation of passive ROM, the patient is asked to relax and the physician moves the joint as far as possible. All ROMs are measured in degrees. During these examinations you may be asked to record the degrees of motion for active and/or passive ROM for specific joints as well as noting pain, tenderness, or **crepitation** experienced by the patient during the examination.

CRITICAL THINKING APPLICATION

How can Kaiwan best assist Dr. Alexander in testing upper extremity ROM in a new patient? What equipment should Kaiwan have ready for the examination? What patient position would best facilitate this examination? Why?

Muscle Strength Evaluation

During the ROM evaluation the physician will also assess each muscle group for strength. Normal muscle strength allows for complete voluntary ROM in the presence of resistance. This resistance can be gravity, as when rising from sitting to a standing position, or physical, as in pulling, pushing, or lifting an object. Muscle strength is bilaterally equal in normal conditions. The evaluation compares like muscles in each hemisphere of the

body, such as comparing the grip of the right hand with the grip of the left hand using a blood pressure cuff (Figure 42-15).

RADIOLOGY

Radiology and diagnostic imaging are frequently used to assist in diagnosing orthopedic conditions (Figure 42-16). Many orthopedic and chiropractic offices have the equipment for taking x-ray films in the office and may employ an x-ray technician. X-ray evaluation is necessary to accurately diagnose fractures, dislocations, and bone and joint diseases. X-ray films can also be used to track the healing of a fracture to determine when it is healed enough to remove a cast.

CRITICAL THINKING APPLICATION

A patient who has just undergone x-ray studies stops Kaiwan and wants to see his x-ray films. How should Kaiwan handle this situation? If a patient is in an examination room with her own x-ray film on the view box and she asks Kaiwan to show her where the break is, how should he respond to this request?

When one of these diagnostic tests is necessary, you should explain the procedure to the patient. Your explanation should include what will be done, how it is done, where it will take place, and approximately how long it will take. Patients will always be concerned about whether the procedure will hurt.

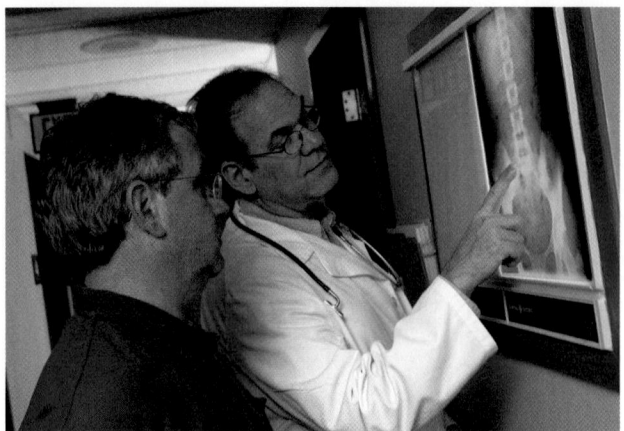

FIGURE 42-16 Reading a lumbar radiograph.

Specialized Imaging Techniques Used in Orthopedics

- Arthrograms: Used to visualize joints
- Myelograms: Used to identify intervertebral disk disorders
- Bone scans: Used to evaluate areas of bone growth, bone density, and bone tumors, as well as other bone disease patterns
- Computed tomography (CT) scans: Used to visualize soft tissue such as tumors, lesions, or some spine injuries
- Electromyography and nerve conduction velocity studies: Used to evaluate muscles
- Biopsies of bone and muscle: Used to identify cancerous tumors and other neoplasms and pathogens

Tell the truth. If the procedure is painful, let the patient know so he or she can prepare for it. Most painful procedures are performed only after the patient has been given a mild sedative. Discuss the procedure in a professional yet empathetic manner. If the patient wishes to talk with the physician about the test, make sure that this happens.

THERAPEUTIC MODALITIES

Physical treatment methods called *modalities* are often used in orthopedic, chiropractic, and physical therapy offices to treat orthopedic conditions. These can include the application of cold, heat, baths, electric currents, therapeutic ultrasonography,

massage, and therapeutic exercises. Cold applications are recommended for the first 48 hours after an injury to assist in controlling pain and swelling. Heat application is used after this to help improve circulation, decrease pain, and maintain muscle and joint function (Table 42-4). *Diathermy* is a technique for creating deep tissue heat through the use of a high-frequency current, ultrasonic waves, or microwave radiation. Like surface heating, deep heat is used to: reduce pain, relieve muscle spasms, resolve inflammation, and promote healing. Deep heat may be used to treat chronic arthritis, bursitis, fractures, and other musculoskeletal problems.

General Principles of Cold Application

Cold applications, such as ice packs and cold compresses, act as vasoconstrictors and also cause contraction of the involuntary muscles of the skin ("goose bumps"). These two actions decrease the blood supply to the area and cause a numbing effect on the sensory nerve endings. Cold applications can help control bleeding, prevent further swelling and inflammation, and decrease pain. For cold application, disposable, reusable, or homemade ice packs are most commonly used (Figure 42-17 and Procedure 42-1).

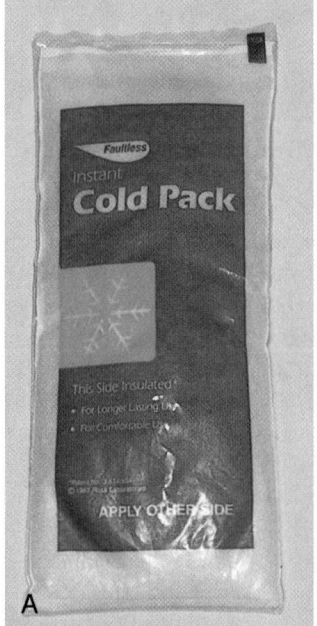 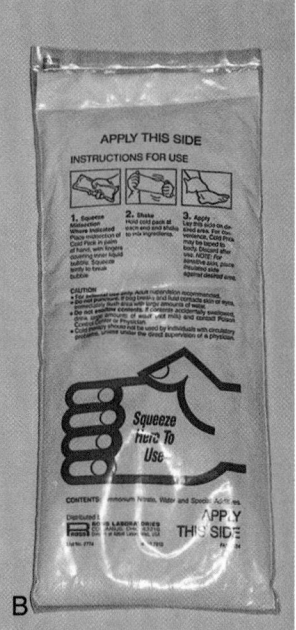

FIGURE 42-17 A, Commercial ice pack. B, Instructions on the back side.

TABLE 42-4 Effects of Heat and Cold Application

APPLICATION	CAUSES	TISSUE RESPONSE	THERAPEUTIC EFFECT
Heat	Vasodilation	Increased blood flow	Increased nutrients to site
	Muscle relaxation	More white blood cells to area	Faster removal of wastes
	Increased metabolism	Reduced muscle spasm	Phagocytosis
	Local warmth	Decreased pain	Faster tissue repair
Cold	Vasoconstriction	Decreased blood flow	Inhibition of swelling
	Numbness of nerve endings	Local anesthesia	Reduced inflammation
	Reduced metabolism	Decreased oxygen need	Decreased pain
	Increased blood viscosity	Faster blood clotting	

PROCEDURE 42-1

Prepare Patient for and Assist with Procedures, Treatments, and Minor Office Surgeries: Assist the Patient with Cold Application

CAAHEP COMPETENCY: 3.b.(4)(f)
ABHES COMPETENCY: 4.b

GOAL: *To apply a cold compress to a body area to decrease pain, prevent further swelling, and/or decrease inflammation.*

EQUIPMENT and SUPPLIES

- Small ice cubes or ice chips
- Ice bag or closeable disposable plastic kitchen food bag
- Towel
- Patient record

PROCEDURAL STEPS

1. Wash your hands.
2. Explain the procedure to the patient, and answer any questions.
3. Check the bag for possible leaks.
4. Fill the bag with small cubes or chips of ice until it is about two thirds full.
   PURPOSE: Small chips conform more easily to the shape of the body.
5. Push down on the top of the bag to expel excess air, and apply the cap.

PURPOSE: To remove as much air as possible from the bag, because air is a poor conductor of cold.
6. Dry the outside, and cover it with one or two towel layers.
7. Help the patient position the ice bag on the injured area.
8. Advise the patient to leave the ice bag in place for about 20 to 30 minutes or until the area feels numb, whichever is first.
9. Check the skin for color, feeling, and pain.
   PURPOSE: If the area being treated becomes very painful, remains numb, or is pale or cyanotic, the ice bag should be removed and the physician notified.
10. Record the procedure in the patient's chart.
    PURPOSE: A procedure is not considered done until it is recorded.

See Appendix D for a charting example.

Heat Modalities

Heat produces local vasodilation, which causes increased circulation. This accelerates the inflammatory process, promotes local drainage, decreases swelling, relaxes muscles, and repairs tissues and cells. The effects of external heat application depend on the type of heat used, the length of time it is applied, the frequency with which it is applied, the general condition of the patient, and the size of the area needing treatment. Heat application is an excellent therapeutic modality, but it must be used with caution to prevent overheating and burning of surface tissues. Special care must be taken in patients who have reduced sensation because they may not sense a burn occurring. Therefore, heat application is contraindicated in the following circumstances:

- In the presence of acute inflammatory conditions, particularly during the first 48 hours
- In persons with severe circulatory problems of any kind
- In persons with decreased or abnormal sensation
- Over areas containing encapsulated pus
- On blisters from previous burns
- Over scar tissue, because it does not have a normal blood supply and easily overheats
- In body areas that contain cancerous tumors
- Over inflamed skin because the initial erythema caused by a burn cannot be detected
- Over any metal jewelry and over any area containing metal implants

Body parts may safely be heated to 110° F (44° C) without any tissue damage. Redness appears, because the skin capillaries

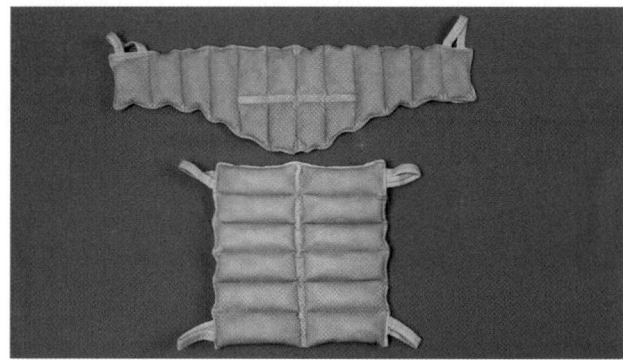

FIGURE 42-18 Commercial hot packs made of canvas that contain a silicone gel.

become congested at the skin's surface. Heat modalities may be either wet or dry and can have either superficial or deep effects. Dry heat therapies include heating pads, infrared radiation lamps, ultraviolet radiation, and hot water bottles. More penetrating methods of dry heat application include diathermy and ultrasound. Moist heat modalities include soaks, whirlpool treatments, hot moist compresses (Figure 42-18), and paraffin baths.

Paraffin Bath

A paraffin bath is especially useful in treating chronic joint inflammation. A mixture of seven parts paraffin and one part mineral oil is melted and heated to approximately 125° F (52° C). The patient's body part, usually a hand, an elbow, or a foot, is dipped into the warm paraffin mixture and removed

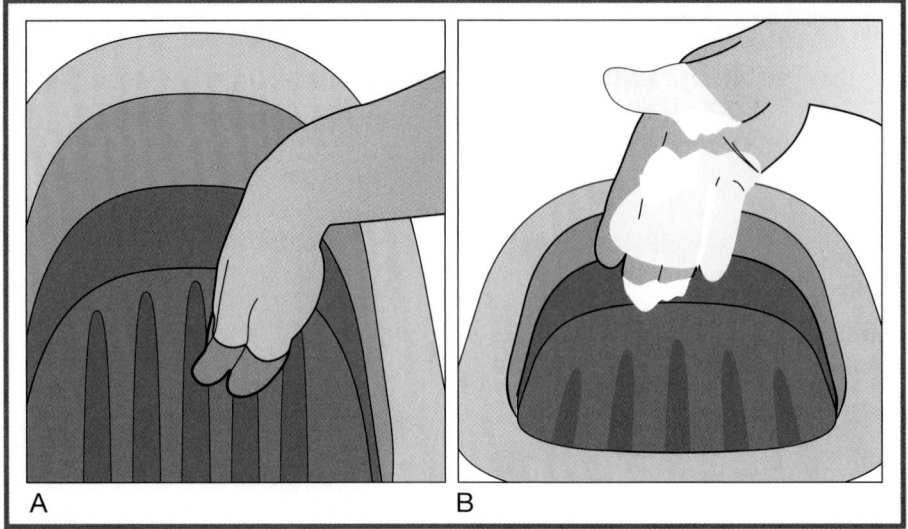

FIGURE 42-19 The paraffin bath is especially helpful for pain relief in patients with arthritis. **A,** The hand is dipped into warm paraffin. **B,** The warm paraffin is left on the hand for about 30 minutes, then is peeled off.

immediately, leaving a thin coating on the skin. This dipping is repeated numerous times until a thick coating of paraffin remains on the body part (Figure 42-19). The part is then wrapped with plastic and a towel to allow the heat to penetrate into the tissues. The paraffin is kept on for 30 minutes then is peeled off. The process leaves the skin soft, warm, moisturized, and pliable, with slight erythema.

CRITICAL THINKING APPLICATION

Kaiwan helps a 56-year-old patient with RA to get a paraffin bath treatment for both hands. He did not check the temperature before having the patient put her hands in the bath. When she puts her hands in the bath, she immediately pulls them out and complains that it is too hot. How should Kaiwan handle this situation? What should he say to the patient? What steps should he take to prevent this from occurring with another patient?

Hot Water Bottle

Hot water bottles are often used at home without any concern for correct technique. Patients should be cautioned to keep the water temperature below 125° F (52° C). The hot water bottle can usually be left in place until it becomes cold. If the patient is a child, the temperature should be kept below 115° F (46° C) to prevent burns. Generally a hot water bottle should not be applied to a child for longer than 15 minutes without a physician's instruction. A hot water bottle that is less than half full conforms better to the body surface and is more comfortable (Procedure 42-2).

SAFETY ALERT ELECTRIC HEATING PADS SHOULD BE LEFT IN PLACE NO LONGER THAN 30 MINUTES TO PREVENT POTENTIAL BURNS.

Patient Instructions for Applying a Hot Compress at Home

1. Moisten a clean hand towel with warm water.
2. Wring it out and fold it to the appropriate size.
3. It should be warm, not hot.
4. Place the folded warm moist compress directly onto the skin.
5. Cover the towel with plastic to keep in the moist heat.
6. Cover the plastic with a dry towel to help maintain the heat.
7. Apply for as long and as often as the physician orders, usually 20 to 30 minutes at a time.

Therapeutic Ultrasonography

Ultrasound is the energy carried by very high-frequency sound waves. Ultrasound works on the same principle as sonar, used in oceanography. The sound that we hear is the result of sound waves vibrating from 100 to 12,000 hertz (Hz; cycles per second). Ultrasonic waves vibrate at a rate up to 1 million Hz and cannot be heard by the human ear. The ultrasound transducer contains a quartz crystal that vibrates very rapidly when an electric current is passed through it. It is placed into contact with the body, and the vibrations are passed into the tissues. These waves do not travel through air; therefore complete contact with the body must be maintained during treatment by using a coupling agent (a water-soluble gel) between the ultrasound transducer and the skin.

The ultrasound waves cause the tissue to vibrate, generating heat as they penetrate superficial tissues, and speeding up circulation to the area. This increases the metabolism in the local area, which has a beneficial effect on the body's healing process. Because ultrasound waves travel best through water, they peetrate deeper into body tissues that have a high water content, such as muscles. Ultrasonography may decrease pain

PROCEDURE 42-2

Prepare Patient for and Assist with Procedures, Treatments, and Minor Office Surgeries: Assist with Hot Moist Heat Application in the Office

<u>CAAHEP COMPETENCY:</u> 3.b.(4)(f)
<u>ABHES COMPETENCY:</u> 4.b

GOAL: *To apply moist heat to a body area to increase circulation, increase metabolism, and relax muscles.*

EQUIPMENT and SUPPLIES

- Commercial hot moist heat packs
- Towel
- Patient record

PROCEDURAL STEPS

1. Wash your hands.
2. Explain the procedure to the patient, and answer any questions.
3. Ask the patient to remove all jewelry from the area to be treated.
4. Place one or two towel layers over the area to be treated.
5. Apply the commercial moist heat packs (Figure 1).
6. Cover with the remaining portion of the towel.
7. Advise the patient to leave the heat pack in place no longer than 20 to 30 minutes, off for the same amount of time, and repeat if needed.
   <u>CAUTION:</u> Monitor the patient for complaints of discomfort or signs of potential burns including erythema and blister formation.

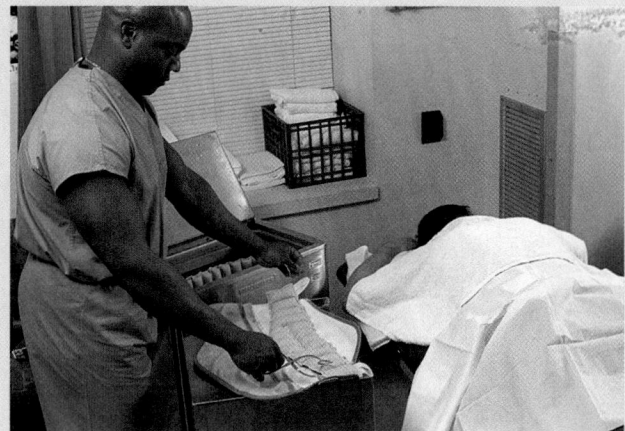

FIGURE 1

See Appendix D for a charting example.

PROCEDURE 42-3

Prepare Patient for and Assist with Procedures, Treatments, and Minor Office Surgeries: Assist with Therapeutic Ultrasonography

<u>CAAHEP COMPETENCY:</u> 3.b.(4)(f)
<u>ABHES COMPETENCY:</u> 4.b

GOAL: *To apply ultra–high-frequency sound waves to a patient's deep tissues for therapy. The medical assistant should perform ultrasound therapy only under the supervision of the physician or a physical therapist.*

EQUIPMENT and SUPPLIES

- Ultrasound machine
- Ultrasound gel or lotion
- Patient record

PROCEDURAL STEPS

1. Prepare the equipment and wash your hands.
2. Confirm the patient's identity.
3. Explain the procedure, and tell the patient to notify you of any discomfort during the procedure.
   <u>PURPOSE:</u> To ensure that the patient does not experience any pain or injury.
4. Ask the patient about the presence of any internal or external metal objects.
   <u>PURPOSE:</u> Metal objects must be avoided during the ultrasound procedure.

5. Position the patient comfortably, with the area to be treated exposed.
6. Apply a warmed ultrasound gel liberally over the area to be treated and to the applicator head.
   <u>PURPOSE:</u> To effectively transmit the sound waves through a water-based medium.
7. Begin the treatment with the intensity control at the lowest setting.
8. Set the timer on the machine to the ordered time.
   <u>PURPOSE:</u> The timer starts the machine.
9. Slowly increase the intensity control to the ordered amount.
10. Hold the applicator with the head firmly and completely against the patient's skin over the area to be treated (Figure 1).
    <u>PURPOSE:</u> To ensure close contact between the applicator head and the patient's skin.

Continued

PROCEDURE 42-3—cont'd

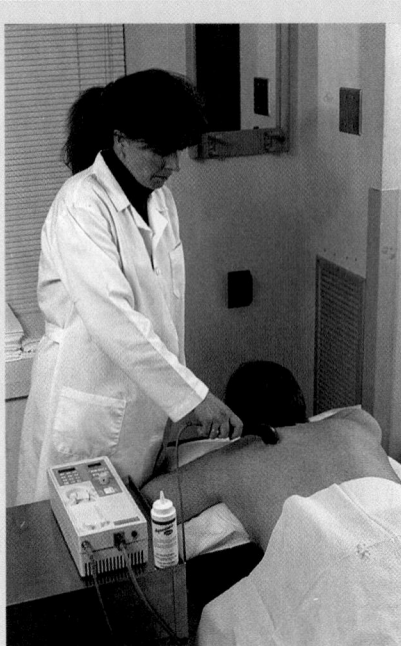

FIGURE 1

11. Work the applicator over the area to be treated by moving it continuously in a circular fashion at a speed of 2 inches per second or as directed by the physician.
12. Keep the applicator head in contact with the patient's skin at all times while the machine is on, and keep it moving continuously during the treatment time.
    PURPOSE: Constant motion prevents hot spots from occurring as a result of the accumulation of excessive ultrasonic waves in one area.
13. When the timer sounds, it shuts off the machine automatically. Then you can safely lift the applicator head away from the patient.
14. Return the intensity control to zero.
15. Remove the ultrasound gel from the patient's skin and from the applicator head with a tissue or paper wipe. Wash your hands.
16. Assist the patient to get dressed if necessary.
17. Record the procedure in the patient's chart, including the date, area treated, intensity setting, duration of treatment, and any unusual reactions that may have occurred during treatment. If none occurred, indicate that also.
    PURPOSE: A procedure is not considered done until it is recorded.

See Appendix D for a charting example.

and increase the rate of collagen synthesis, which promotes healing. Because bone has almost no water content, ultrasonography must be used very carefully around bony areas, because the waves can concentrate and cause damage (Procedure 42-3).

Massage and Exercise

Massage is a form of passive exercise that relieves tension and pain. The systematic, therapeutic stroking or kneading of the body or body part can effectively relieve or significantly reduce both localized and referred pain. You will not usually be asked to apply therapeutic massage to patients, but you should be familiar with the terminology.

A growing branch of healthcare employs exercise to aid muscle relaxation, promote healing, and provide relief from tension and pain resulting from stress or a wide variety of physical disorders. Exercise can also be used to restore mobility, coordination, and strength. If the motion in a joint is restricted

even for a short time, the joint tissues become dense, hard, and shortened. These changes can begin to occur in as little as 4 days. This can be prevented or decreased by the use of active or passive exercises.

In active exercise the patient initiates and controls movements of a particular part of the body. Special equipment may be used, such as stationary bicycles, treadmills, and/or weight machines. In passive exercise the therapist moves the body part without the voluntary action of the patient. Both active and passive exercises can be performed to maintain normal ROM or remedy decreased ROM after an injury.

Electric Muscle Stimulation

An electric stimulation unit is a low-voltage machine creating a controlled electric current that is applied to the patient through disposable gel electrodes. This low-voltage current is useful for stimulating the motor and sensor nerves that supply muscles. Stimulation provides a passive means of exercising a muscle when a patient cannot activate the muscle voluntarily because of injury. Electric muscle stimulation is frequently used to prevent **atrophy** of a normal muscle.

Another means of using electric stimulation in orthopedics is called *transcutaneous electric nerve stimulation* (TENS) (Figure 42-20). A TENS unit sends a controlled electrical current through electrodes attached to the skin to help relieve pain caused by arthritis, back injuries, and sports injuries. Since TENS units operate by electrical stimulation, it is not recommended for patients with heart disease and/or cardiac pacemakers.

Therapeutic Massage Terminology

- Effleurage: A light, gentle, stroking movement
- Friction: Deep stroking that affects the deeper soft tissues, traditionally used for back massage
- Pétrissage: Kneading or rolling with pressing of the muscles
- Tapotement: Rapid, light percussion done with the sides of the hands

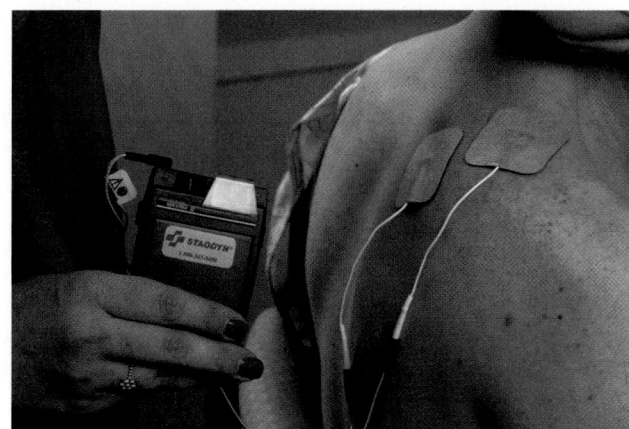

FIGURE 42-20 TENS unit application.

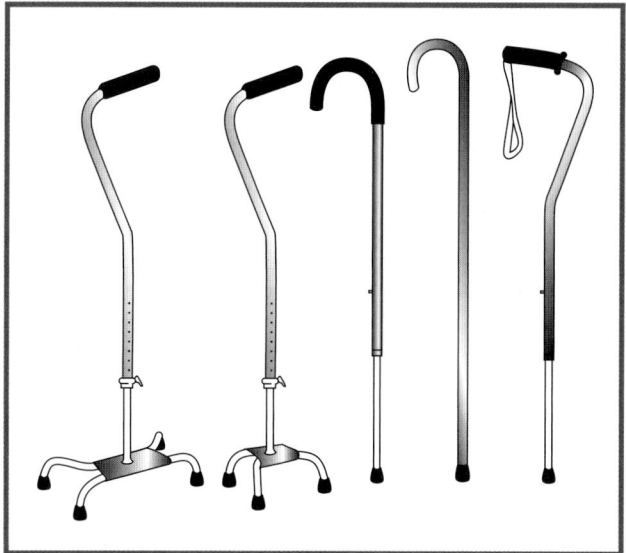

FIGURE 42-22 Types of standard canes.

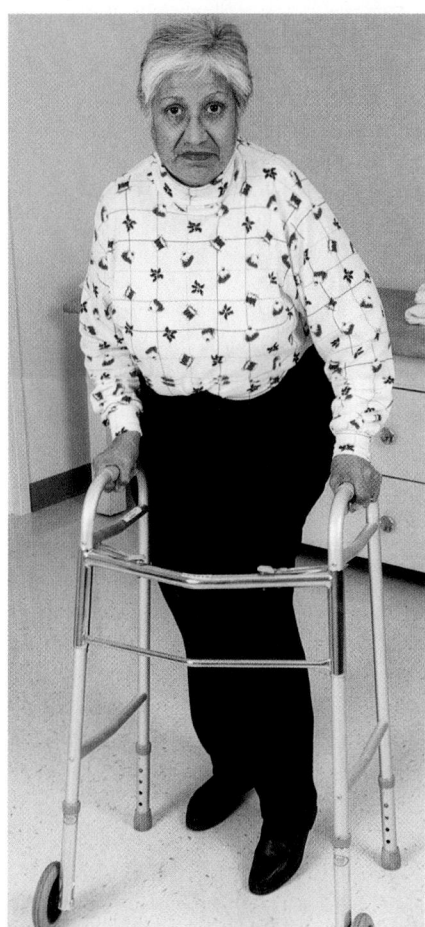

FIGURE 42-21 A properly fitted walker. Note angle of arms and height of walker.

AMBULATORY DEVICES

Walkers

Walkers are usually made of aluminum and can be easily adjusted to fit an individual. They are lightweight, are easily folded for storage and traveling, and can be equipped with a front pack to carry items. They can also be fitted with a fold-down seat. The disadvantage of using a walker is it cannot be used on stairs or in small, cramped quarters.

To adjust the height of a walker, have the patient stand by the examination table. The top of the walker should be just below the patient's waist at the same height as the top of the hip bone. When the walker is correctly adjusted to the patient, the patient's elbows will bend about 30 degrees while he or she uses the walker (Figure 42-21).

Canes

Canes come in a variety of designs (Figure 42-22). The single-tipped cane with a curved handgrip is indicated for individuals who need only minimal assistance with walking. Another type is the legged cane, which has a tripod or quad base. This base provides a greater stability for the patient than a single-tipped cane does. It is heavier and is recommended for patients who need greater support.

To fit a cane properly, have the patient stand up straight and measure the distance from the wrist crease to the floor. If the patient is 70 years of age or older or finds that extra length would feel more comfortable, up to 2 additional inches can be added to the previous measurement. This is the total length of the cane fitted to the patient. The patient's elbow should be bent to approximately 30 degrees when the cane is correctly adjusted to the patient. The patient needs to be taught to strike the ground with the injured leg and the cane at the same time. Start by positioning the cane one small stride ahead and step off with the injured leg, finishing the step with the stronger leg.

Wheelchairs

Wheelchairs provide mobility for patients who cannot walk or who are able to walk only short distances. With a manual wheelchair, the patient uses arm muscles for mobility. Wheelchairs also come with motors that can be controlled by the patient. The patient is referred to an orthopedic appliance store, where the appropriate wheelchair will be fitted to him or her.

SAFETY ALERT ALWAYS SET BRAKES ON THE CHAIR BEFORE THE PATIENT IS TRANSFERRED INTO OR OUT OF THE CHAIR.

ASSISTING WITH CASTING

When a cast is used to immobilize a fracture or sprain, you will need to know what type of cast is to be applied (Procedures 42-4 through 42-6). Casting material possibilities include plaster of paris, fiberglass or plastic, synthetic material, or the air cast. Plaster of paris is the oldest of the casting materials and is formed by briefly soaking rolls of casting material in warm water, then rolling them around the fracture site. It is like a wet bandage and is easily be formed to the extremity; the surface is rubbed smooth, then allowed to dry and harden. This casting material is made of roller gauze that has been impregnated with calcium sulfate, also called plaster of paris. The fiberglass casting material has impregnated fiber or resin in the roller gauze and is

---

PROCEDURE 42-4

Prepare Patient for and Assist with Procedures, Treatments, and Minor Office Surgeries: Assist with Cast Application*

CAAHEP COMPETENCY: 3.b.(4)(f)
ABHES COMPETENCY: 4.b

GOAL: *To assist the physician in applying a fiberglass cast.*

EQUIPMENT and SUPPLIES

- Rolls of fiberglass casting material
- Stockinette
- Sheet wadding and/or spongy padding
- Tape
- Scissors
- Water
- Basin
- Bandage
- Gloves for physician and medical assistant
- Stand to support foot (lower extremity)
- Patient record

PROCEDURAL STEPS

1. Wash your hands.
2. Identify the patient.
3. Explain the procedure for applying a cast, and answer questions before application.
   PURPOSE: Knowing what to expect will reassure the patient about the procedure. Questions regarding the injury should be directed to the physician.
4. Assemble equipment.

5. Seat the patient comfortably, as directed by the physician. If the cast is being applied to the lower extremity, the toes must be supported by a stand.
   PURPOSE: The amount of flexion of the ankle can be controlled by supporting the toes so that the patient can more easily maintain the desired position without fatigue.
6. Clean the area that the cast will cover. Note any objective signs and ask about subjective symptoms (chart them at the end of the procedure).
   PURPOSE: The condition of the area under the cast must be noted before the cast is applied. This will be compared with the site when the cast is removed. Clean the area with a mild soap solution or as directed. Dry thoroughly.
7. Cut stockinette to fit the area the cast will cover.
8. Apply stockinette smoothly to the area that the cast will cover. Leave 1 or 2 inches of excess stockinette above and below the cast area to finish the cast (Figure 1).
9. Excess stockinette may be cut away where wrinkles form (e.g., at the front of the ankle) (Figure 2).

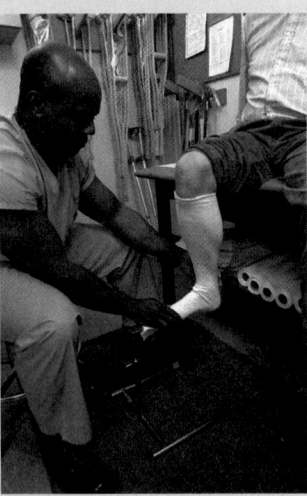

FIGURE 1

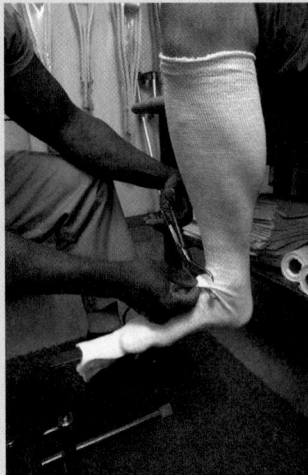

FIGURE 2

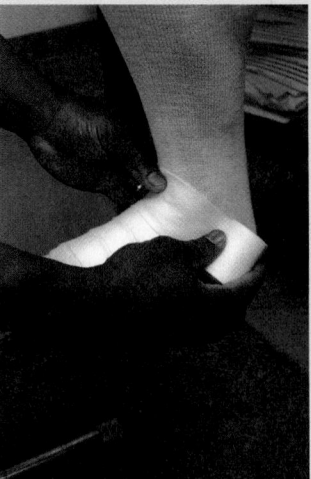

FIGURE 3

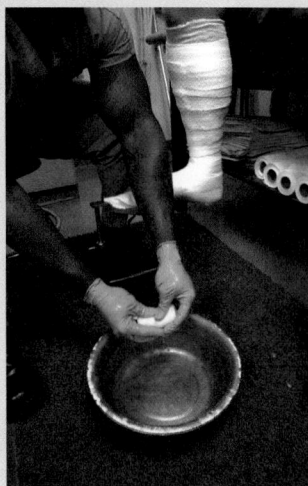

FIGURE 4

Continued

PROCEDURE 42-4—cont'd

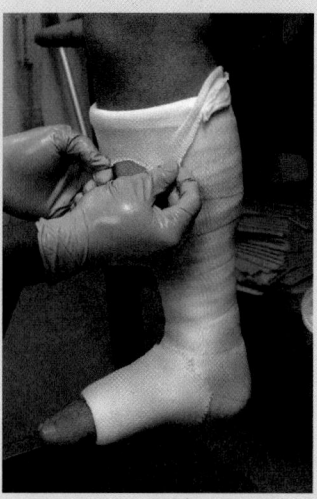

FIGURE 5

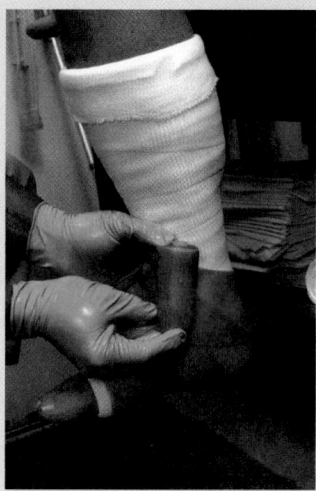

FIGURE 6

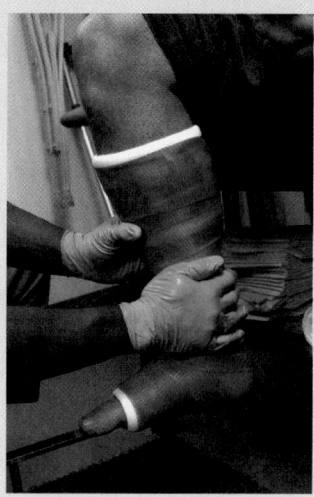

FIGURE 7

PURPOSE: Stockinette must lie smooth and cannot be too bulky or wrinkled, as this may cause a pressure wound.

10. Sheet wadding is applied along the length of the cast using a spiral bandage turn. Extra padding may be used over bony prominences such as the bones of the elbow or ankle (Figure 3).
   PURPOSE: Padding the cast helps reduce pressure against bony prominences, which could cause skin breakdown.

11. Don gloves.

12. With lukewarm water in the basin, wet the fiberglass tape as directed by the physician (Figure 4).
   PURPOSE: Immersing the roll of fiberglass tape in water begins the chemical reaction that will cause the cast to harden. The cast can be shaped while wet and will harden in the shape that is formed.

13. Assist as directed as the physician applies the inner layer of fiberglass tape (shown in the photograph as beige). A length of 1 to 2 inches of stockinette is rolled over the inner layer of the cast to form a smooth edge when the outer layer is applied (Figure 5).

14. Assist as directed by the physician to open and apply an outer layer of fiberglass tape (shown in the photograph as blue) (Figure 6).

15. Assist to shape the cast as directed. All contours must be smooth (Figure 7).
   PURPOSE: If flat or dented areas develop on the cast, they may cause pressure on the skin below.

16. Discard the water and excess materials. Remove gloves, and wash hands.

17. Reassure the patient, review cast care verbally, and provide written instructions.

18. Document observations and procedure in patient record.
   PURPOSE: A procedure is not considered done until it is recorded in the patient's chart.

---

*Procedure adapted and figures taken from Hunt SA: *Saunders fundamentals of medical assisting*, Philadelphia, 2001, Saunders.
See Appendix D for a charting example.

PROCEDURE 42-5

Prepare Patient for and Assist with Procedures, Treatments, and Minor Office Surgeries: Triangular Arm Sling Application

<u>CAAHEP COMPETENCY:</u> 3.b.(4)(f)
<u>ABHES COMPETENCY:</u> 4.b

GOAL: *To properly place a casted arm in a triangular sling.*

EQUIPMENT and SUPPLIES

- Triangular-shaped arm sling
- Large safety pins
- Patient record

PROCEDURAL STEPS

1. Review the physician's order for a triangular arm sling.
2. Wash your hands and obtain the desired sling.
3. Explain the procedure to the patient.

Continued

PROCEDURE 42-5—*cont'd*

PURPOSE: To obtain maximal patient cooperation.

4. Position the patient's injured arm across the chest so that it is parallel to the floor and the patient's waist, with the hand slightly elevated.
   PURPOSE: To help reduce swelling.

5. Carefully slide the triangular sling between the patient's chest and the affected arm.

6. Bring the lower front corner up over the shoulder of the affected side to the neck.

7. Grasp the opposite corner, and tie or pin the ends together at the side of the neck.
   PURPOSE: Tying at the side of the neck helps to avoid the headache and muscle discomfort that might be caused by tying at the back of the neck.

8. Fold in the tail and fasten with a safety pin to secure the elbow (Figure 1).

9. Fold the sling edge to form a smooth edge along the wrist.
   PURPOSE: Patient comfort.

10. Record the procedure in the patient's chart.
    PURPOSE: A procedure is not considered done until it is recorded.
    NOTE: If using a commercial sling, follow the manufacturer's instructions for proper application.

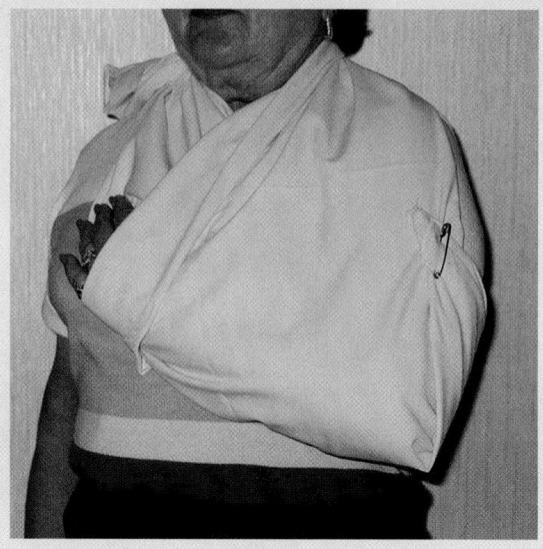

FIGURE 1

PROCEDURE 42-6

Prepare Patient for and Assist with Procedures, Treatments, and Minor Office Surgeries: Assist with Cast Removal

CAAHEP COMPETENCY: 3.b.(4)(f)
ABHES COMPETENCY: 4.b

GOAL: *To remove a cast.*

EQUIPMENT and SUPPLIES

- Cast cutter
- Cast spreader
- Large bandage scissors
- Basin of warm water
- Mild soap
- Towel
- Skin lotion
- Patient record

PROCEDURAL STEPS

1. Explain the procedure to the patient.
   PURPOSE: Allays the patient's fear and anxiety and ensures cooperation.

2. Provide adequate support for the limb throughout the entire procedure.
   PURPOSE: Patient comfort.

3. Make a cut on the medial and lateral sides of the long axis of the cast (Figure 1).

4. Pry the two halves apart using the cast spreader (Figure 2).

5. Carefully remove the two parts of the cast.

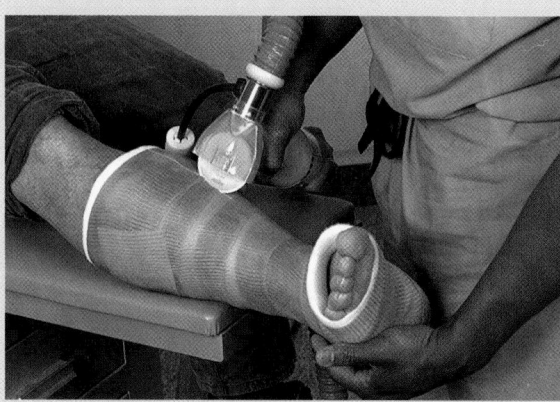

FIGURE 1

Continued

PROCEDURE 42-6—cont'd

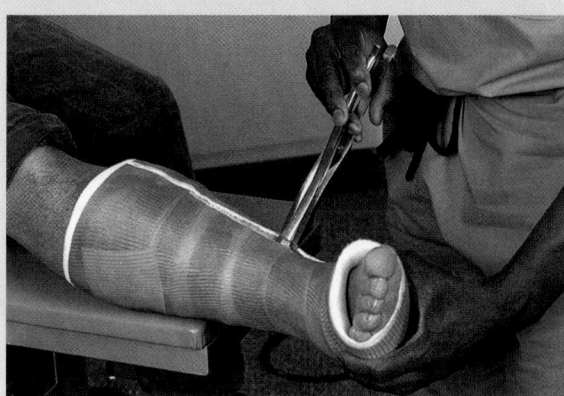

FIGURE 2

6. Use large bandage scissors to cut away the stockinette and padding remaining.
7. Gently wash the area that was covered by the cast with mild soap and warm water.
   PURPOSE: Patient comfort.
8. Dry and apply a gentle skin lotion.
   PURPOSE: Patient comfort.
9. Give the patient appropriate instructions about exercising and using the limb, as directed by the physician.
   PURPOSE: To enhance continuation of healing, restore lost strength, and prevent injury.
10. Record the procedure in the patient's medical record.
    PURPOSE: A procedure is not considered done until it is recorded.

---

applied in a similar fashion. A fiberglass cast is stronger, weighs less, and is relatively waterproof.

Before applying any type of cast, the area is first wrapped with cotton padding to protect the skin. For the injured area to be immobilized, the splint or cast needs to cover the joints above and below the fracture. If the site is edematous, a splint may be used until the swelling subsides, with a full cast applied after the swelling has decreased. In some cases a cast may have to be replaced as the swelling decreases if the patient reports the cast is too big. As a fracture heals, the physician may decide to remove the cast and apply a splint until the fracture is completely mended. A patient may call the office complaining that the splint or cast feels tight. Swelling typically occurs in the first 48 to 72 hours after the injury. The patient should be told to elevate the injured part above the heart to help collected fluid drain from the site; gently move fingers or toes at the affected area to improve circulation; and apply ice around the splint or cast in a plastic bag at the level of the injury to help reduce swelling.

If the patient needs to wear a cast only when using the limb, there are synthetic casts in the shape of a boot or sleeve with Velcro fasteners that fit like a sandwich over the fracture to immobilize the area. An air cast is a temporary cast that is inflated around the limb to immobilize it. The type of cast to be used will depend on the location and severity of the injury, the age and occupation of the patient, and the physician's preference. After cast application the medical assistant may also have the responsibility of instructing the patient on the use of crutches (Procedure 42-7). This may include proper fitting of crutches and teaching the appropriate technique to avoid further injury to the patient.

CRITICAL THINKING APPLICATION

What methods could Kaiwan use to teach a deaf patient how to use crutches?

Warning Signs Following Splint or Cast Application

The patient should be told to contact the physician's office if any of the following occurs after the application of a splint or cast:

- Increased pain and/or a feeling that the splint or cast is too tight
- Numbness and tingling in the affected hand or foot, indicating pressure on the nerves
- Burning and stinging because of pressure on the skin
- Excessive swelling below the cast, which may mean the cast is slowing circulation
- Loss of active movement of toes or fingers; this requires an urgent evaluation by the physician

CRITICAL THINKING APPLICATION

Kaiwan has just finished helping Dr. Alexander put a cast on the arm of a 6-year-old girl who fell out of her neighbor's tree house and fractured her radius. Her mother wants to take her home immediately after the cast is applied. Should the patient be allowed to leave immediately? Why? What could possibly happen if she left immediately?

CLOSING COMMENTS

Patient Education

An informed patient is better prepared to continue with home care when this is required. Musculoskeletal conditions, particularly arthritis, can be so painful and debilitating that these patients may be easy prey for miracle drug promotions. It is important for you to recognize the need for patient education about the condition and to work diligently with the patient and family to encourage participation in effective care programs.

Patient Education for the Care of a Splint or Cast

The American Academy of Orthopaedic Surgeons has the following recommendations for caring for a cast or splint:

- Keep the device dry; moisture weakens the plaster, and damp padding can irritate the skin. Use two layers of plastic or purchase waterproof shields to keep the splint or cast dry while you shower or bathe. The physician can apply a waterproof cast in special circumstances.
- Do not walk on a "walking cast" until it is completely dry and hard; it takes at least 1 hour for fiberglass and 2 to 3 days for plaster to become hard enough to walk on.
- Keep dirt, sand, and powder away from the inside of the splint or cast.
- Do not pull out the padding.
- Do not stick objects such as coat hangers inside the device to scratch itching skin; if itching persists, contact your physician.
- Do not break off rough edges of the cast or trim the cast before asking your physician.
- Inspect the skin around the cast; if it is red or raw around the cast, contact your physician.
- Inspect the cast regularly; let your physician know if it becomes cracked or develops soft spots.

When you work with the physician and the physical therapist in helping the patient, you become an important member of the healthcare team. This type of involvement leads to patient satisfaction as well as personal satisfaction and achievement.

Legal and Ethical Issues

Working with orthopedic patients may involve triage procedures, assisting with assessments, and performing procedures that directly involve the patient's recovery plan. Many of the procedures in this chapter are not the basic procedures that you will be required to perform when you are first hired as a medical assistant. These techniques all involve additional on-the-job training and practice. Before performing any of the described procedures, you should check with your local and state medical assistant organizations regarding the laws in your state. Whenever you perform the procedures and techniques described in this chapter, you are responsible for them. The following steps are all required before you execute any procedure on a patient:

- You must have a written order before doing a procedure.
- You must follow a procedure precisely as it is ordered, without variation.
- Never advise the patient without permission.
- Know what instructions the physician gave the patient.

PROCEDURE 42-7

Prepare Patient for and Assist with Procedures, Treatments, and Minor Office Surgeries: Assist the Patient with Crutch Walking

<u>CAAHEP COMPETENCY:</u> 3.b.(4)(f)
<u>ABHES COMPETENCY:</u> 4.b

GOAL: *To properly fit crutches and teach the patient how to use the crutches properly in three-point walking.*

EQUIPMENT and SUPPLIES

- Crutches with arm pads and foam handgrips
- Patient record

PROCEDURAL STEPS

1. Fit the crutches to the patient so they are 1 to 1½ inches below the armpits while they are standing up straight. The handgrips should be even with the top of the hip line.
2. Be sure that all wingnuts are tight.
3. Make sure the foam pads at the armpits and around the handgrips are comfortable.
4. Instruct the patient to keep the injured leg as relaxed as possible and slightly bent at the knee.
5. The patient's elbow should be bent approximately 30 degrees when holding the handgrip.
6. Place the crutch tips approximately 6 inches away from and parallel to the toes.
7. Ask the patient to push down on the crutches and lift the body slightly, nearly straightening the arms (Figure 1). The patient should hold the top of the crutches tightly to his or her sides and

use the hands to absorb the weight. Do not let the tops of the crutches press into the armpits.
<u>PURPOSE:</u> To prevent injury to the muscles and nerves of the axillary region.
8. Have the patient swing the body forward about 12 inches.
9. Instruct the patient to stand on the good leg, and then move the crutches just ahead of the good foot and repeat.
10. Stairs: To walk up and down stairs with crutches, face the steps, hold the handrail with one hand and tuck both crutches under the armpit on the other side. To go up the steps, start with the uninjured side keeping the injured side raised behind. When going down, hold the injured foot up in front, and hop down each stair on the good foot. If the stairway does not have handrails, use the crutches under both arms and hop up or down each step on the uninjured leg. If necessary the patient can sit on the stairs and move up or down each step.
11. Document the patient education intervention in the patient record.

See Appendix D for a charting example.

Continued

PROCEDURE 42-7—*cont'd*

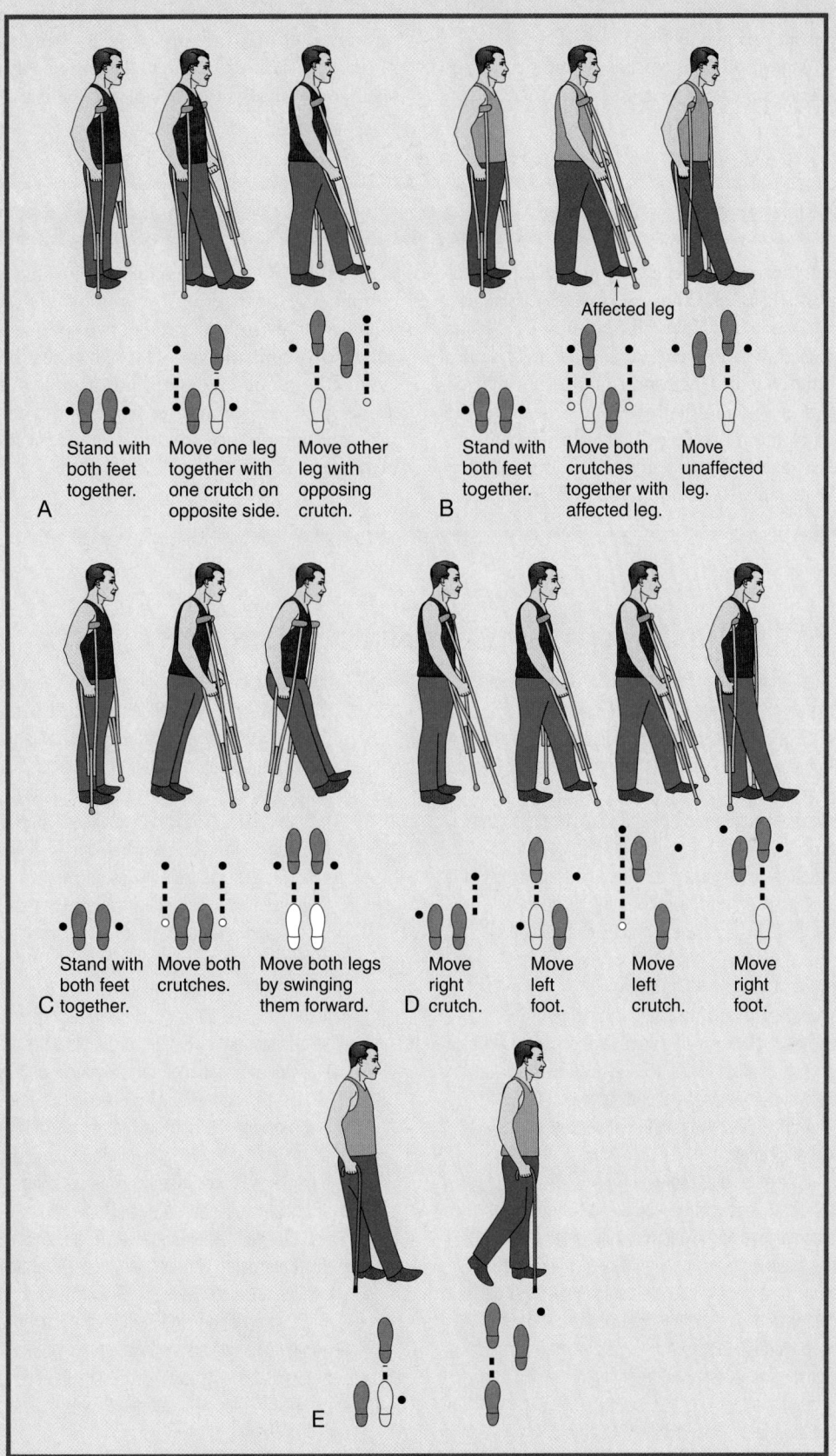

A   Stand with both feet together.   Move one leg together with one crutch on opposite side.   Move other leg with opposing crutch.

B   Stand with both feet together.   Move both crutches together with affected leg.   Move unaffected leg.

Affected leg

C   Stand with both feet together.   Move both crutches.   Move both legs by swinging them forward.

D   Move right crutch.   Move left foot.   Move left crutch.   Move right foot.

E

FIGURE 1

- Reinforce the instructions the physician gave the patient.
- Be sure you are comfortable performing a procedure.
- If you have any concerns about a procedure, discuss them with the physician privately before proceeding.
- Do not perform a procedure if you are uncomfortable; get someone to help you.

Always remember: You are the assistant, and this is the physician's patient. The physician is ultimately responsible for every aspect of the patient's care. If you feel uncertain or unsure of any order that the physician has written for a patient, you must get it clarified before you proceed. Always stay within the legal and ethical guidelines of the medical assisting profession in your state.

SUMMARY OF SCENARIO

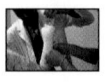

Kaiwan is becoming more and more comfortable in his position as an orthopedic medical assistant at the sports medicine clinic. His enthusiasm is contagious. Patients consistently comment on his positive, upbeat manner. Kaiwan is motivated to learn new things and methods for better assisting the physicians with routine procedures. He always seeks answers to questions that occur with new patients. He has gained a great deal of confidence and now remembers to always check the paraffin bath temperature before starting a treatment. One of the most enjoyable aspects of his job continues to be assisting Dr. Alexander with treating the team members. Kaiwan has attended two sports medicine continuing education seminars with Dr. Alexander. He is now thinking about continuing his education part-time to become an athletic trainer while continuing to work at the clinic. Kaiwan recognizes the importance of continuing education in maintaining orthopedic skills.

SUMMARY of LEARNING OBJECTIVES

1. Define, spell, and pronounce the terms listed in the vocabulary.
   - Spelling and pronouncing medical terms correctly adds credibility to the medical assistant. Knowing the definition of these terms promotes confidence in communication with patients and co-workers.
2. Describe the principal structures of the musculoskeletal system and their functions.
   - The main structures of the musculoskeletal system include the skeletal muscles, which provide movement; tendons, which connect muscles to bones; bones, which provide support, protection, mineral storage, and blood cell development; and ligaments, which connect bone to bone.
3. Differentiate among tendons, bursae, and ligaments.
   - Tendons are the tough bands that connect muscles to bones; ligaments provide support by connecting bone to bone and preventing a joint from moving beyond its normal ROM. Bursae prevent friction between different tissues in the musculoskeletal system.
4. Summarize the major muscular disorders.
   - Fibromyalgia is a condition of unknown origin that causes widespread connective tissue and muscular pain with sleep disorders and extreme fatigue. Myasthenia gravis is an autoimmune disorder that affects the use of ACh at the neuromuscular junction, resulting in muscular weakness, especially in the face and eyes. A sprain is the tearing of ligaments and a strain is the overstretching or tearing of a muscle or tendon.
5. Identify and describe the common types of fractures.
   - The common types of fractures are explained in Table 42-3.

6. Explain the difference between osteomalacia and osteoporosis.
   - Osteomalacia is the softening of bone because of a problem with the metabolism or absorption of vitamin D, calcium, and phosphorus; in children the condition is called *rickets*. Osteoporosis is a decrease in bone density caused by many factors including lack of dietary calcium earlier in life; it leads to brittle bones that easily fracture.
7. Classify typical spinal column disorders.
   - Spinal column disorders are related to the shape of the spine; scoliosis is a lateral deviation, lordosis or swayback is a pronounced curve of the lower back, kyphosis is a pronounced cervical curve or hunchback.
8. Differentiate among the various joint disorders.
   - Joint disorders include dislocations when the two bones of the joint are no longer approximated; gout, which is a form of arthritis caused by a collection of uric acid crystals most commonly in the synovial membrane of the great toe; SLE, which is a widespread autoimmune disorder that can affect any organ system in the body; Lyme disease, a form of infectious arthritis that is caused by bacteria transmitted by a tick bite and that can result in extensive joint and neurologic problems if left untreated; OA, caused by degeneration of the articular cartilage of synovial joints; RA, an autoimmune disorder that causes crippling pain and deformity of the joints; and tendonitis and bursitis, which are inflammatory reactions of supportive tissue that are typically caused by the overuse of a joint.
9. Summarize the medical assistant's role in assisting with orthopedic procedures.
   - The medical assistant is responsible for gathering and

Continued

SUMMARY of LEARNING OBJECTIVES

Continued

recording a detailed history of the patient's presenting problem; providing the patient with assistance as needed; and assisting with the orthopedic examination.

10. Explain the common diagnostic procedures used in orthopedics.
    - Common diagnostic procedures routinely performed in the orthopedic office include ROM evaluation, inspection, palpation, percussion, muscle strength evaluation, and x-ray studies. Other diagnostic tools include arthrograms, myelograms, bone scans, CT, MRI, electromyography, biopsies, and diagnostic ultrasonography.

11. Compare and contrast therapeutic modalities used in orthopedic medicine.
    - Therapeutic modalities include the application of cold and heat; paraffin baths; hot water bottles and moist heat packs; therapeutic ultrasonography; massage and therapeutic exercise; and electric muscle stimulation.

12. Apply cold therapy to an injury.
    - Cold should be used immediately after an injury to help decrease pain and inflammation, to inhibit additional swelling, and to help relieve pain; the ice pack should remain in place for 20 minutes at a time, several times a day, and the area should be checked for feeling and color after each application. Refer to Procedure 42-1.

13. Assist with hot moist heat application to an orthopedic injury.
    - Refer to Procedure 42-2 for application of heat. Heat should be used on injuries after 48 hours to promote circulation and healing, decrease swelling, and cause soft-tissue relaxation in the affected area. Care must be taken to avoid burns.

14. Properly apply therapeutic ultrasound.
    - Therapeutic ultrasound applies deep tissue heat to an injured area. Refer to Procedure 42-3. It is important to constantly keep the applicator head rotating in a circular fashion over the injured site during the treatment.

15. Explain the use of common ambulatory devices.
    - The most common ambulatory assistive devices are crutches, canes, walkers, and wheelchairs. The most important aspects of using these assistive devices in an orthopedic practice are to fit them properly to the patient and to give the patient adequate instruction on how to use the device properly and safely.

16. Prepare for and assist with cast application.
    - To prepare for and assist with cast application, refer to Procedure 42-4. Safeguard the tissue underneath the cast by applying a stockinette and sheet wadding; immerse the casting material in water, and carefully roll it around the limb.

17. Apply a sling to immobilize an injury.
    - To apply a sling to immobilize an injury, refer to Procedure 42-5.

18. Prepare for and assist with cast removal.
    - To prepare for and assist with cast removal, refer to Procedure 42-6.

19. Properly fit a patient with crutches, and explain the correct mechanics of crutch walking.
    - To properly fit a patient with crutches and explain the correct mechanics of crutch walking, refer to Procedure 42-7. The patient's elbows should be bent approximately 30 degrees; while standing on the good leg, the patient should swing the injured leg between the crutches.

CONNECTIONS

 Study Guide Connection: Go to Chapter 42 Study Guide. Read the Case Study and Workplace Applications and complete the assignments. Do online research for answers to the questions in the Internet Activities associated with assisting in orthopedic medicine.

 CD Connection: Go to the Medical Assisting Competency Challenge CD and do the training activities under Diagnostic Testing. For a better understanding of the orthopedics, view the animations for muscle range of motion and spine structure.

 Evolve Connection: For more information related to assisting in orthopedic medicine, go to evolve.elsevier.com/kinn and visit related weblinks for Chapter 42. Click on the Medical Assisting Exam Review and do the practice questions to sharpen your test-taking skills.

Assisting in Neurology and Mental Health

43

SCENARIO

Mai Lee is a CMA who has been working in Dr. Kim Song's neurology practice for 2 years. Dr. Song has always been pleased with Mai's professional behavior and her ability to treat all patients with respect. Mai is conscientious in accurately charting notes for each one of her patients. Dr. Song has just asked Mai to train a new medical assistant in the clinical procedures of the office. He is expanding his clinic hours and wishes to have Mai more involved in assisting him with patients, particularly in the area of patient education. She is excited to have additional responsibilities with Dr. Song's patients, and she is quite happy about the raise in salary that goes along with her new position.

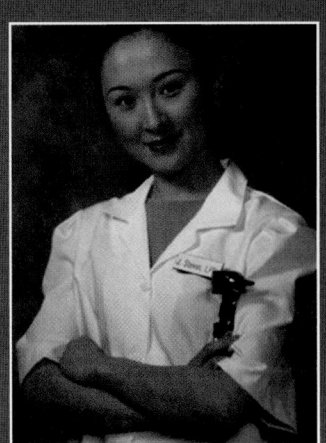

While studying this chapter, think about the following questions:

- What is the basic anatomy and physiology of the neurological system?
- What neurologic disorders should Mai be familiar with?
- What are the diagnostic and treatment procedures for typical nervous system disorders?
- What is the medical assistant's role in the neurologic examination?

- Is patient education a significant factor when working with patients who are diagnosed with either nervous system or mental health disorders?

LEARNING OBJECTIVES

1. Define, spell, and pronounce the terms listed in the vocabulary.
2. Summarize the anatomy and physiology of the nervous system.
3. Differentiate between the central and peripheral nervous systems.
4. Identify the typical symptoms associated with neurologic disorders.
5. Distinguish among common nervous system diseases and conditions.
6. Describe the pathology of cerebrovascular diseases.
7. Identify the various types of epilepsy.
8. Compare and contrast encephalitis and meningitis.

9. Explain the dynamics of head and spinal cord injuries.
10. Summarize the neurologic diseases that affect mobility.
11. Differentiate among common mental health disorders.
12. Analyze the medical assistant's role in the neurologic examination.
13. Explain the common diagnostic procedures for the nervous system.
14. Outline the steps needed to prepare a patient for an EEG test.
15. Describe the procedural steps for preparing a patient for and assisting with a lumbar puncture.

National Accreditation Competencies and Content

CAAHEP COMPETENCIES	ABHES COMPETENCIES
Clinical	**Clinical Duties**
3.b.(4)(e). Prepare patient for and assist with routine and specialty examinations	4.b. Prepare patients for procedures
3.b.(4)(f). Prepare patient for and assist with procedures, treatments, and minor office surgeries	4.h. Prepare patients for and assist physician with routine and specialty examinations

anomalies (uh-noh′-muh-lez) Deformities or deviations from a normal condition, resulting from faulty development of a fetus.

ataxia (uh-taks′-e-uh) Failure or irregularity of muscle actions and coordination.

atrophy Decrease in the size of a normally developed organ.

aura Peculiar sensation preceding the appearance of a more definite disturbance.

benign Not cancerous and not recurring.

blood-brain barrier An anatomic-physiologic structure made up of astrocyte glial cells that prevents or slows the transfer of chemicals into the neurons of the CNS.

coma An unconscious state from which the patient cannot be aroused.

compression The state of being pressed together.

contralateral (kon-trah-la′-tehr-uhl) Pertaining to the opposite side of the body.

cryptogenic (krip-tuh-je′-nik) Having a hidden origin.

embolus Foreign material blocking a blood vessel, frequently a blood clot that has broken away from some other part of the body.

exacerbation Worsening of disease symptoms.

gait How a person walks.

homeostasis (ho-meh-oh-sta′-sis) Maintaining constant internal environmental conditions compatible with life.

idiopathic (i-de-o-path′-ik) Of unknown cause.

ipsilateral (ips-uh-la′-tehr-uhl) Pertaining to the same side of the body.

malignant Cancerous.

myelin sheath Segmented, fatty tissue that wraps around the axon of the nerve cell and acts as an electrical insulator to speed the conduction of nerve impulses.

occlusion Complete blocking off of an opening.

papilledema Swelling of the optic disc from increased intracranial pressure.

paresthesia Abnormal sensation of burning, prickling, or stinging.

paroxysmal (par-ehk-siz′-muhl) Pertaining to a sudden recurrent spasm of symptoms.

plaque Abnormal accumulation of a fatty substance.

radiopaque Substance that can easily be visualized on an x-ray film.

remission Lessening in the severity of a disease or symptoms.

syncope (sin′-kuh-pe) Fainting.

thrombus Blood clot.

transection Cross-section; division made by cutting across.

The human brain weighs about 3 pounds, requires about the same amount of energy that it takes to light a 20-watt light bulb, stores more than 100 trillion bits of information, and works better than any computer. The matter making up the brain is approximately 85% water and therefore has a soft texture. Early scientists believed that the brain's function was to cool the blood. Today's scientists have shown us that even though the brain does receive 20% of the body's blood supply, its function is much more complex than cooling blood.

Neurologists specialize in the diagnosis and treatment of medical disorders and conditions of the nervous system. A *neurosurgeon* provides surgical management and treatment for trauma and other conditions requiring surgery. A *psychiatrist* is a physician who treats behavioral disorders and neurologic conditions that affect behavior.

ANATOMY AND PHYSIOLOGY

The nervous system works with the endocrine system to integrate stimulus from both within the body and the outside environment to regulate body systems so that **homeostasis** can be maintained. It is divided into two major parts: the *central nervous system* (CNS), made up of the brain and spinal cord, and the *peripheral nervous system* (PNS), which includes all of the nervous tissue and neurologic responses found outside of the

CNS. The brain is the "president" or "chief executive officer" of the body. It constantly receives information from the periphery, including all of the organs and systems inside and on the body's surface. This information—stimuli—is carried to the brain by the peripheral nerves along the *afferent* or ascending tract. The brain monitors and interprets the stimuli received from the afferent nerves and sends appropriate responses back along *efferent* pathways to the organs or to the body surface. These responses from the brain cause a specific reaction in the organ, in the glands, or in skeletal muscles. These reactions keep the body running smoothly and allow us to react instantly to both external and internal stimuli.

The functioning cell of the nervous system is the neuron (Figure 43-1). The brain contains billions of individual neurons. The nervous system begins very early in embryonic development in utero—by week 3—as the *neural tube*, which eventually develops into the brain and spinal cord. Each neuron is made up of a main cell body containing the nucleus and a relatively long extension of the cell called the *axon*, which may be covered with a **myelin sheath.** Multiple filaments, called *dendrites,* extend from the neuron body. Dendrites receive the nervous impulse from a preceding neuron and carry it into the cell body. Impulses are carried away from the cell body through the axon to another neuron or to cells in another tissue. This transfer of stimuli begins as an electrical impulse traveling down an axon of one neuron and becomes a chemical impulse while moving across the *synapse* (space between two neurons) to the dendrite of another neuron. The transfer of impulses from the end of one neuron to the dendrites of another is enhanced by the presence of chemical neurotransmitters, which bind to specific receptor sites on the dendrites of the next neuron. If the nerve

When You Accidentally Touch a Hot Iron

1. Impulses travel to the central nervous system (CNS) along an afferent (sensory neuron) nervous pathway, carrying the information "hot."
2. The CNS carries out a hasty analysis and determines that a heat danger is present.
3. The CNS sends a quick and strong message back to skeletal muscles via the efferent (motor neurons) pathway to move the finger immediately.
4. You quickly pull your hand away from the hot iron, preventing a serious burn and maintaining homeostasis.

impulse is traveling to a muscle or to any other organ or tissue instead of another neuron, the chemical neurotransmitters bind to special receptors in the target tissue. Messages move throughout the entire nervous system in this manner. Impulses in the neuron are electrical, the impulses become chemical as a specific neurotransmitter is released at each synapse, and they become electrical again as they are picked up by the subsequent dendrites of another neuron or by the target tissue.

Supportive cells of the nervous system are called glial or *neuroglial* cells. Although these specialized cells perform specific functions within the nervous system—such as Schwann cells, which form the myelin sheath, or astrocytes, which help form the **blood-brain barrier**—they do not carry on any of the functions of the nervous system. The blood-brain barrier closely regulates what substances enter the brain tissue. Oxygen, water, and glucose molecules easily pass into the brain, whereas many chemicals and drugs are prevented from moving into brain tissue. However, brain inflammation can increase the ability of many drugs to cross the blood-brain barrier.

Central Nervous System

The brain and spinal cord together make up the CNS. The brain is in the skull in the cranial cavity. The spinal cord is a bundle of nervous tissue that extends inferiorly from the brain stem at the base of the brain and exits the skull at the foramen magnum. It descends for about 17 inches within the spinal canal, which courses through the vertebrae of the backbone.

Brain

The brain accounts for only about 2% of a person's weight, but it consumes about 20% of the body's oxygen. The brain is divided into three main areas: the cerebrum, cerebellum, and brain stem (Figure 43-2). The *cerebrum* is the largest and uppermost section of the brain and has multiple convolutions along its surface called *gyri* that are formed by the folding in of the cerebral cortex. The gyri are separated by shallow grooves called *sulci*. The

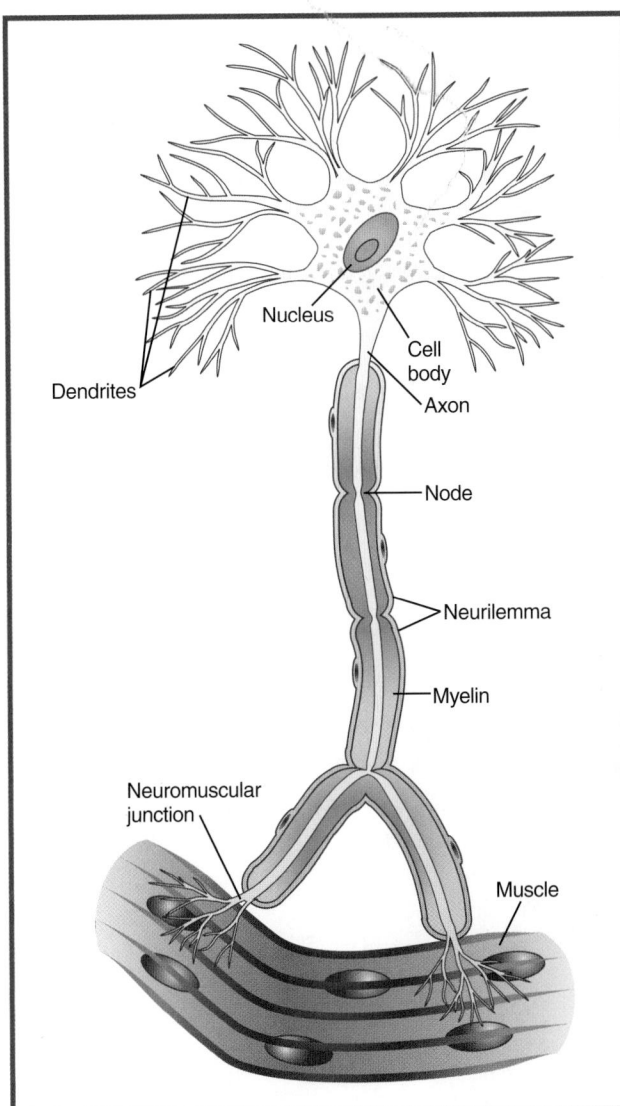

FIGURE 43-1 Neuron.

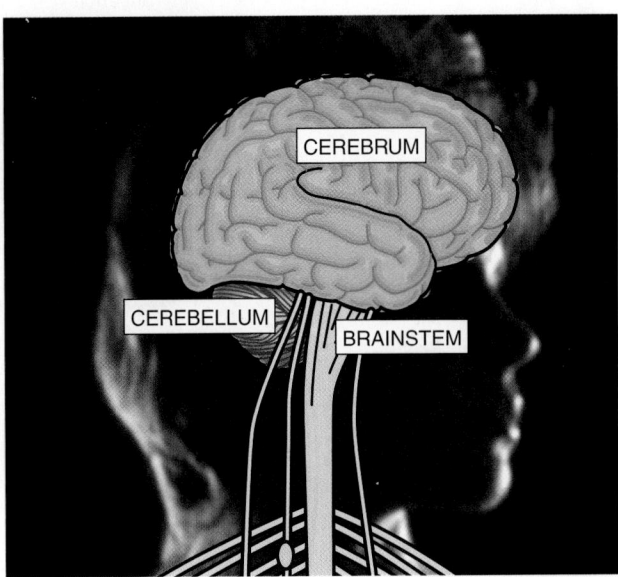

FIGURE 43-2 The brain. (Modified from Chester GA: *Modern medical assisting,* Philadelphia, 1999, Saunders.)

gyri greatly increase the surface area of the cerebrum, thereby maximizing the potential of the CNS neurons in each area. The cerebrum is divided into lobes, which are named after the region of the skull under which they are located. The cerebrum is separated by a longitudinal fissure into left and right *hemispheres.* The right hemisphere usually controls artistic functions like drawing, rhythm, and picture memory. The left hemisphere controls verbal functions, such as reading, writing, speaking, and mathematic calculations. The *diencephalon,* located deep in the center of the cerebrum near the superior portion of the brain stem, is made up of the thalamus and the hypothalamus. The *thalamus* acts as a relay station between sensory neurons and the cerebral cortex. The functions of the *hypothalamus* include controlling the autonomic nervous system, regulating endocrine processes, and managing body temperature, sleep, and appetite to maintain homeostasis. Within the cerebrum are four spaces, called *ventricles,* which contain cerebrospinal fluid (CSF). CSF nourishes, lubricates, and provides some cushioning protection for the brain and the spinal cord.

The *cerebellum* is just inferior to the occipital lobe of the cerebrum and controls balance, equilibrium, posture, and muscle coordination. The *brain stem* controls reflexes and also serves as a sensory relay station for input coming into the brain from the body. The brain stem plays a vital role in vision, hearing, respiration, heart rate, blood pressure, waking, and sleeping.

Spinal Cord

The spinal cord extends from the inferior portion of the brain stem roughly 17 inches to approximately the second lumbar vertebra. Thirty-one pairs of spinal nerves extend from the spinal cord through openings in the vertebrae. Starting just below the first cervical vertebra in the neck, a nerve extends out from the spinal cord on each side; therefore a pair of spinal nerves originates at each level. Each of these pairs of nerves innervates a specific organ or area of the body. The spinal cord carries messages between the spinal nerves and the brain.

Meninges

Because both the brain and spinal cord are of critical importance for life, both are well protected. First, they are both encased in some of the thickest bones in the body; then they are surrounded with three membranes called *meninges;* finally, they are cushioned with CSF (Figure 43-3).

The outer layer of the meninges is called the *dura mater* ("hard mother") because it is a tough membrane, similar to a very strong rubber band. The *subdural space* lies below the dura mater and contains small veins that have little support. Trauma to the head can cause bleeding of these tiny vessels, ultimately leading to the development of a subdural hematoma. Above the dura mater is the *epidural space.* Arterial supply to the meninges comes from blood vessels that line the inner aspect of the skull. If the skull is fractured, these arteries can be damaged, resulting in a collection of blood between the skull and the dura mater called an *epidural hematoma.*

The middle meningeal layer is the *arachnoid,* given the name because of its fine spider-web appearance. Beneath the arachnoid membrane in the *subarachnoid space* is CSF, a clear liquid that contains glucose, protein, and chloride produced by specialized cells in the ventricles (Table 43-1). CSF circulates continuously through the ventricles and around the brain and spinal cord, carrying nutrients and removing wastes.

The innermost layer, which covers the brain and spinal cord, is the delicate *pia mater* ("tender mother"); it is highly vascular and is the thinnest of the three layers. The pia mater provides support for the blood vessels of the brain.

Peripheral Nervous System

The PNS is made up of the nerves that exit the brain or spinal cord. The peripheral nerves exiting the brain directly through

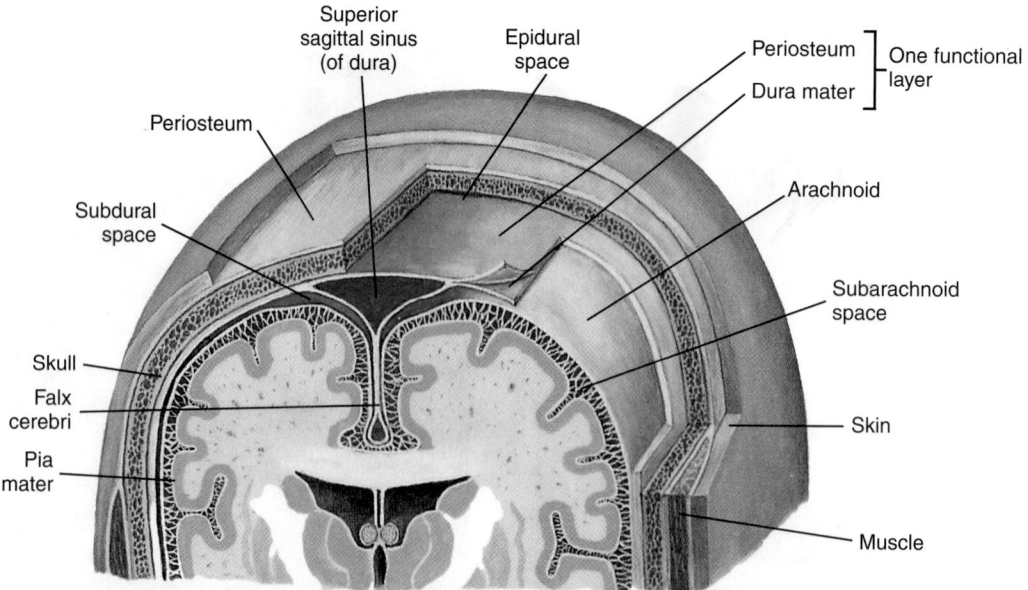

FIGURE 43-3 Protective coverings of the brain. (Thibodeau GA, Patton KT: *Anthony's textbook of anatomy and physiology,* ed 17, St Louis, 2003, Mosby.)

TABLE 43-1 Typical Cerebrospinal Fluid Laboratory Values

CONDITION	PRESSURE (MM)	APPEARANCE	CELLS	PROTEIN (MG/DL)	GLUCOSE (MG/DL)
Normal	50-200	Clear, colorless	0-10 lymphocytes and monocytes	<45	50-80
Acute bacterial meningitis	200-500	Turbid	100-10,000 granulocytic neutrophils	50-500	Absent or low
Subarachnoid hemorrhage	200-500	Bloody	RBCs	50-1000	50-80

RBC, Red blood cells.

Hydrocephalus

Hydrocephalus is the abnormal accumulation of CSF within the ventricles of the brain. It is the result of either overproduction of CSF or failure of the fluid to drain properly. If left untreated, hydrocephalus causes gross enlargement of the skull and severe brain tissue damage from increased intracranial pressure. The only treatment is surgery to place a shunt (tube) from a ventricle in the brain to either the right atrium or the abdominal cavity. This shunt allows the excess CSF to drain away from the brain.

TABLE 43-2 Cranial Nerves and Their Functions

NUMBER	NAME	FUNCTION
I	Olfactory	Smell
II	Optic	Vision
III	Oculomotor	Eye movement Pupillary constriction and accommodation
IV	Trochlear	Eye movement
V	Trigeminal	Muscles of chewing General sensations from anterior half of head including entire face and meninges
VI	Abducent	Eye movement
VII	Facial	Muscles of facial expression Tearing, salivation, and taste
VIII	Vestibulocochlear	Hearing and equilibrium
IX	Glossopharyngeal	Swallowing and taste
X	Vagus	Parasympathetic to thorax and abdomen
XI	Spinal accessory	Shoulder and head movements
XII	Hypoglossal	Tongue movements

the cranium are called *cranial nerves.* The spinal nerves from the spinal cord enter and exit the spinal canal through spaces between the vertebrae. Cranial nerves originate from the underside of the brain and relay information to and from the sensory organs and muscles of the face and neck (Table 43-2).

Spinal nerves carry information to and from the brain through the spinal cord. Sensory fibers in these nerves carry stimuli from the skin and internal organs to the CNS. Motor fibers carry messages from the CNS to skeletal muscles, causing them to contract.

The *autonomic nervous system* (ANS) is part of the PNS. Autonomic nerves control homeostasis, or keep the body running smoothly, much like a thermostat controls the temperature in a room. The ANS is an automatic system that regulates body functions such as breathing, heart rate, sweating, circulation, and digestion. It also controls the actions of muscles in blood vessel walls, organs, and glands. Just as a thermostat can control both heating and cooling in a room to maintain a comfortable temperature, the autonomic system is made up of two divisions, called the *sympathetic* and *parasympathetic* systems. The sympathetic system promotes responses for the protection of the individual ("fight or flight"), generally causing an increasing effect: it speeds up the heart; increases blood glucose levels and blood pressure; decreases peristalsis; and widens the bronchioles, allowing more oxygen to enter the body quickly. The parasympathetic system generally promotes rest or a decreasing effect: it slows the heart rate; constricts the bronchioles; and increases digestive system function (Figure 43-4).

CRITICAL THINKING APPLICATION

Dr. Song mentions a patient's nervous system function to Mai. The patient hears this conversation and asks Mai, "What does my nervous system do?" How should Mai answer this question? What items could she use to help explain the nervous system to the patient?

DISEASES AND DISORDERS OF THE CENTRAL NERVOUS SYSTEM

Because the CNS and PNS are so complex, diseases and conditions affecting them can cause a wide range of signs and symptoms. Causes include trauma, infection, congenital **anomalies,** degeneration, tumors, and vascular disorders (Table 43-3). The medical assistant needs to listen carefully when a patient describes his or her neurologic symptoms. Many different types of symptoms could indicate a serious condition of the nervous system.

Cerebrovascular Disease

Cerebrovascular disease (CVD) continues to be the third leading cause of death and the most frequent cause of crippling disease in the United States. Generally, CVD is related to arteriosclerosis or atherosclerosis of the cerebral arteries but may also be caused by untreated or uncontrolled hypertension, thrombi, or emboli. Arteriosclerosis causes progressive loss of elasticity of the arterial

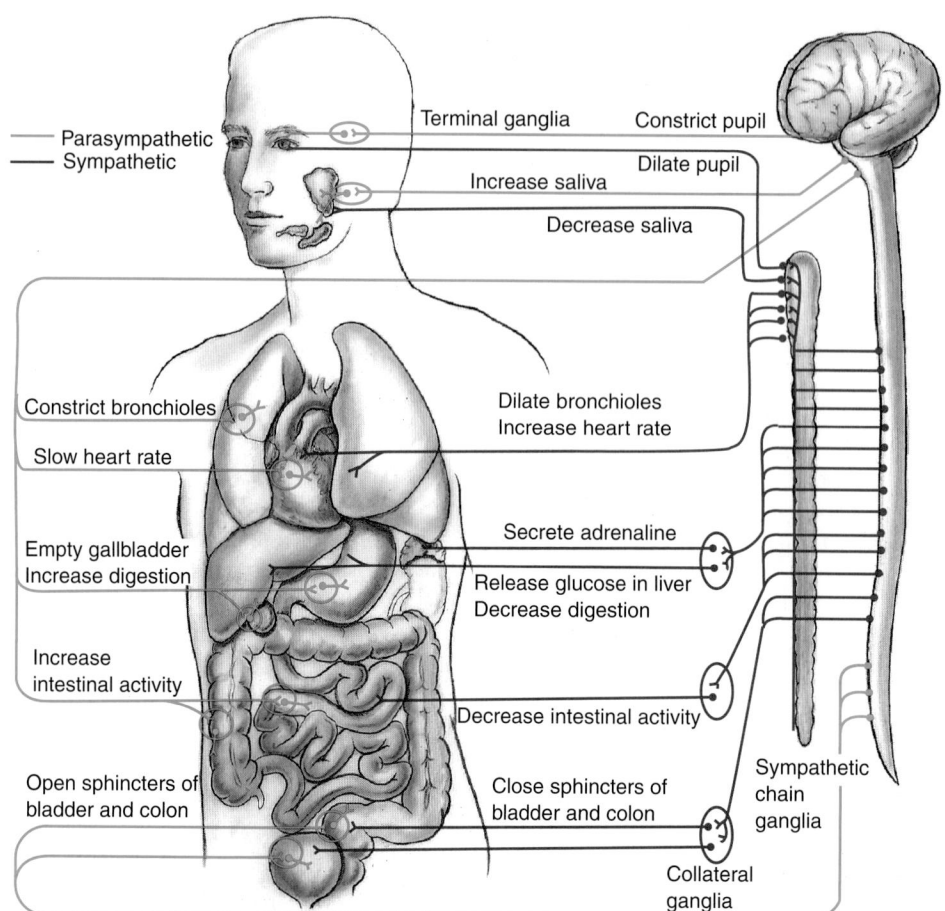

FIGURE 43-4 Structure and function of the autonomic nervous system. (From Applegate E: *The anatomy and physiology learning system*, ed 3, St Louis, 2006, Saunders.)

Polygraph or Lie Detector Test

A polygraph ("many pictures") actually measures several body functions that are strongly influenced by the autonomic nervous system. It simultaneously measures and records blood pressure, heart rate, respiratory rate, and the sweatiness of the fingertips. When the person being given the test is stressed, for example, involuntary changes occur in these functions, and these show up on the graph. This is an example of the autonomic nervous system at work. When the person is asked a question such as, "What day is today?" there is no significant change in any of the measured parameters. Answering this question correctly causes no stress in the individual. Do you think you could beat the polygraph?

Symptoms That Suggest Possible Neurologic Problems

- Recurrent headache
- Periodic memory loss
- Change in sleeping patterns
- Frequently dropping items
- Difficulties with particular speech patterns
- Numbness in a specific body area
- Visual disturbances or abrupt changes in vision
- Loss of consciousness
- Confusion or disorientation as to date, time, and place

wall and is seen in elderly persons with CVD. Atherosclerosis, the deposit of fatty **plaque** on the inside of the arterial wall, can involve any of the major arteries supplying the brain or any of their branches. There also may be sudden narrowing, or **occlusion,** when an artery becomes blocked by a **thrombus** or an **embolus.**

This disorder usually is diagnosed through cerebral arterial angiography, which is done by injecting a **radiopaque** dye into the vessel to be examined, then immediately taking a radiograph. Other confirming tests include magnetic resonance imaging (MRI), computed tomography (CT), and electroencephalography (EEG).

Transient Ischemic Attacks

Transient ischemic attacks (TIAs), also called *ministrokes,* occur when the blood supply to a particular part of the brain is inadequate for a limited period of time, usually seconds to minutes. TIAs occur when brain tissue becomes ischemic for a short time, causing the same symptoms as a stroke. Because the cause of the ischemia is limited, the symptoms dissipate quickly.

TABLE 43-3 Common Nervous System Diseases and Conditions

DISEASE	SIGNS AND SYMPTOMS	DIAGNOSTIC PROCEDURES	LABORATORY TESTS	TREATMENT AND MEDICATIONS
Alzheimer's disease	Short-term memory loss, progressive irreversible confusion and disorientation	History	None specific; ordered to rule out other causes of dementia	Supportive care Cognex and Aricept
Brain tumor	Generally caused by increased intracranial pressure; depend on location	History Neurologic examination Imaging studies	None	Estrogen Surgery Radiation Chemotherapy
CVA	Depend on severity; speech difficulties, hemiplegia, confusion, loss of muscle coordination	History Neurologic examination CT, MRI	Lumbar puncture	Thrombolytics Antiinflammatories Anticoagulants Hyperbaric oxygen Rehabilitation Supportive care
Encephalitis	Increased intracranial pressure, cerebral edema	History Neurologic examination CT, MRI	Lumbar puncture	Antivirals Supportive care
Epilepsy	Grand mal—tonic-clonic muscle contractions; petit mal—momentary absence, stare, amnesia	History Neurologic examination CT, MRI, EEG	Blood work	Anticonvulsants
Closed head injury caused by trauma	Depend on location and severity of injury; headache, increased intracranial pressure	History Neurologic examination CT, MRI	Lumbar puncture	Diuretics Decrease intracranial pressure
Meningitis	Headache, nuchal rigidity	History Neurologic examination Kernig's, Brudzinski's signs	Lumbar puncture	Antibiotics Anticonvulsants Antiinflammatories
Mental illness	Emotional, physical, behavioral, or cognitive symptoms that can affect all areas of one's life	History Neurologic examination occasionally	Blood work occasionally	Medications Psychotherapy
Migraine	Unilateral throbbing sensation, nausea, vomiting, blurred vision	History Neurologic examination	Tests to rule out organic causes for headaches	Vasodilators Vasoconstrictors
Multiple sclerosis	Problems with vision, sensation, motor function, change in emotions	History Neurologic examination MRI	None	Interferon Corticosteroids Antispasmodics Antidepressants
Parkinson's disease	Resting tremor, shuffling gait, masklike face	History Neurologic examination	None	Anticholinergics Dopamine agonists

CT, computed tomography; *CVA*, cerebrovascular accident; *EEG*, electroencephalography; *MRI*, magnetic resonance imaging.

Symptoms can include numbness or weakness in the face, arm, or leg or on one side of the body; confusion or difficulty in talking or understanding speech; vision abnormalities including diplopia; difficulty with walking; and vertigo or loss of balance and coordination.

These episodes may occur in the days, weeks, or months before a stroke. Patients and their families should understand that any strokelike symptom should be taken seriously. Individuals experiencing TIAs should be seen within an hour of the onset of symptoms so they can be evaluated carefully and treated to prevent a possible stroke. Those with atrial fibrillation (an irregular rapid firing of electrical activity in the atria of the heart) may be prescribed anticoagulants (heparin or Coumadin), or they may be put on daily low-dose aspirin or clopidogrel (Plavix) because these individuals are at increased risk for emboli formation. TIAs are important warning signs that the patient is at serious risk for having a debilitating stroke. When TIAs occur, it is time for preventative treatment and patient education including altering and/or treating such factors as hypertension, smoking, heart disease, diabetes, carotid artery disease (carotid artery occlusion with atherosclerotic plaques), and alcohol abuse.

Cerebrovascular Accident

Cerebrovascular accident (CVA) is the most important clinical manifestation of CVD. CVA, commonly referred to as a *stroke*, occurs when a vessel in the brain either ruptures or occludes and the tissue on the other side of the damaged vessel becomes oxygen deprived. Cerebral artery ruptures are caused by uncontrolled hypertension or the hemorrhage of a weakened section of an artery in the brain. The rupture causes the surrounding brain tissue to become filled with blood, thereby damaging and possibly destroying the affected tissue. An occlusion occurs when an embolus or thrombus becomes wedged in an artery and obstructs the flow of blood to an area of the brain (Figure 43-5).

The patient's subsequent symptoms depend on the location of the arterial occlusion or rupture. Some of the most common symptoms include slurred or inaudible speech, unexplained confusion, sudden severe headache, difficulty swallowing, vertigo, diplopia, loss of consciousness, personality change, loss of bowel or bladder control, and paralysis on one side of the body.

Treatment for stroke requires immediate emergency transport to the hospital. Initial emphasis is on minimizing

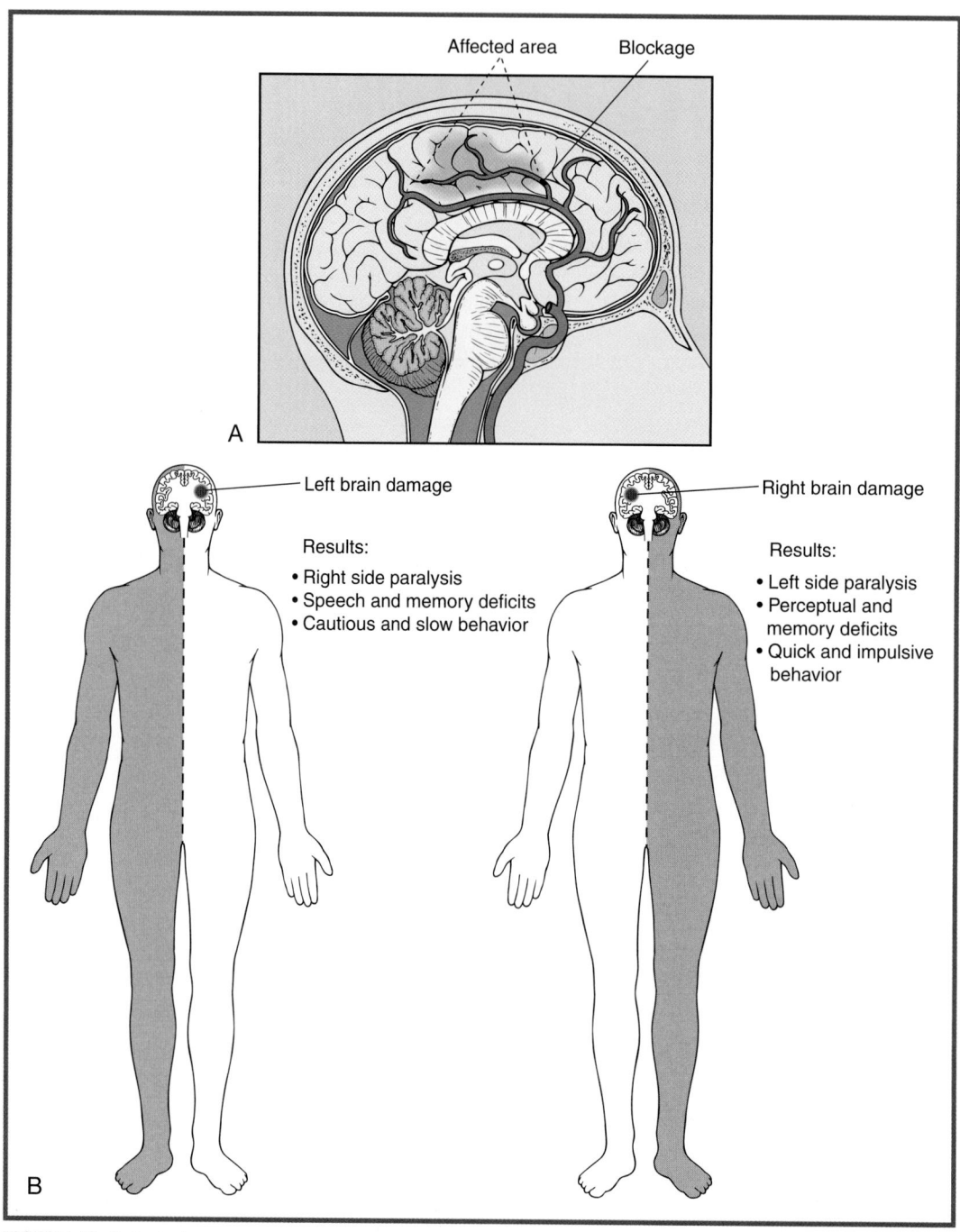

FIGURE 43-5 Cerebral artery occlusion and hemiplegia. (Modified from Frazier MS, Drzymkowski JW: *Essentials of human diseases and conditions*, ed 3, Philadelphia, 2004, Saunders.)

Cerebrovascular Accident Types, Causes, and Risks

Thrombotic stroke: a blood clot (thrombus) forms in a cerebral artery and blocks distal blood flow.

Embolic stroke: a blood clot from somewhere else in the body (such as the lower legs) or a piece of plaque (typically from the carotid arteries) breaks away and flows through the bloodstream to the brain; the embolus blocks a cerebral artery, causing distal ischemia.

Cerebral hemorrhage: an artery in the brain ruptures; may be a result of untreated or uncontrolled hypertension or a congenital aneurysm.

Any of the following factors can increase the risk of a stroke:

- Hypertension
- Diabetes (increases the risk by two to three times)
- Hypercholesterolemia
- Cigarette smoking (increases the risk by 50%)
- Obesity
- Family history of stroke
- Endocarditis (may promote thrombus formation)
- Arteriosclerosis and atherosclerosis
- Heart disease (such as atrial fibrillation, which increases the risk by five times)
- Sleep apnea
- Sickle cell anemia
- Cocaine abuse

Individuals with three or more of the following five health conditions are two times more likely to have a cerebrovascular accident: obesity, low HDL cholesterol levels, high triglyceride levels, a blood pressure of 130/85 or higher, diabetes, and/or prediabetes (fasting blood sugar between 100 and 125).

the long-term disabilities often seen with strokes by applying immediate treatment to salvage as much brain tissue as possible. Thrombolytic drugs to dissolve the clot and anticoagulants may be given if the cause of the stroke was a thrombus or embolus. However, thrombolytic medication can effectively treat resulting ischemia only if it is given within the first 3 to 6 hours after the ischemia began. If cerebral edema is present, the patient is treated with corticosteroids and diuretics to reverse the swelling. Hyperbaric oxygen also can be used to increase oxygenation of the brain. An important part of subsequent recovery is extensive treatment in a stroke rehabilitation program that includes physical, occupational, and speech therapies.

CRITICAL THINKING APPLICATION

Mai answers the phone at the clinic. The caller is an anxious female patient who is desperately trying to say something but appears unable to do so. Mai thinks the patient is trying to say something like "help," although it is not clear. Mai checks the number on the caller ID display, looks it up on the office computer, and learns that it belongs to a 50-year-old patient who came in 2 days earlier because of frequent severe headaches. How should Mai handle this situation? Be sure to think about what she should do, why she should do it, and what might happen if she does nothing.

Migraine Headache

More than 28 million Americans—three times more women than men—suffer from migraine headaches. Migraine headaches are **paroxysmal** attacks of headaches that can be completely incapacitating and frequently are associated with other symptoms, such as nausea, vomiting, visual disturbances, and throbbing pain on one side of the head. The manifestations of migraine headaches differ from one individual to another. The patient may experience a sensory warning sign—an **aura**—before the onset of the headache. An aura often consists of some form of visual disturbance, such as dark lines or spots within the visual field or a flash of light.

Medical science has not yet discovered the underlying cause of migraines. However, some researchers believe they may be caused by a combination of a problem with the trigeminal nerve and an imbalance of chemicals in the brain, especially the neurotransmitter serotonin, which cause cerebral blood vessels to become dilated and inflamed, resulting in the acute onset of a terrible headache. Individuals who suffer with migraine headaches report a number of different triggers including changes in estrogen levels; certain foods, such as alcohol, chocolate, aspartame, caffeine, and monosodium glutamate (MSG); elevated stress levels; bright lights, sun glare, and certain smells; altered sleep patterns; and changes in weather, especially with changing altitude levels and barometric pressures. Diagnosis usually is established from a complete medical history. Additionally, EEG, CT scan, or MRI can be performed as part of the diagnostic process to rule out other possible causes of the headaches.

Drugs used to treat migraines include nonsteroidal anti-inflammatory drugs (NSAIDs) or triptans such as sumatriptan (Imitrex) or rizatriptan (Maxalt), which mimic the effects of serotonin, causing vascular constriction (these drugs must be taken at the onset of the headache to be effective). Other medications recommended for the prevention of migraines include beta-blockers, antiseizure medications, and antidepressants. A new drug, topiramate (Topamax) is showing promise in decreasing the frequency and severity of the headaches. Other treatments include biofeedback techniques and elimination diets to avoid migraine triggers.

Dementia and Alzheimer's Disease

The term *dementia* describes a group of symptoms that are caused by altered brain function. Dementia symptoms may include short-term memory loss; disorientation about person, time, and place; neglect of personal hygiene, nutrition, and safety; personality changes; and the inability to follow simple directions. Dementia can be caused by multiple conditions. Some, like nutrition disorders or disorientation caused by a minor head injury, can be reversed. Others, such as multi-infarct (vascular) dementia and Alzheimer's disease, are irreversible.

Multi-infarct dementia is caused by a series of small strokes that have interfered with the brain's blood supply, resulting in multiple areas of tissue necrosis. The location of the infarcts determines the degree of disability and the dementia symptoms that might arise. Acute onset of dementia symptoms is typically caused by this type of dementia. People with multi-infarct dementia are likely to show signs of improvement or remain stable for long periods of time, then quickly develop new symptoms if more strokes occur. Untreated or uncontrolled hypertension is usually the cause of this type of dementia.

Alzheimer's disease is the most common form of dementia among older people today. It is a devastating, chronic, progressive, and degenerative disease that begins in the parts of the brain that control thought, memory, and language. The patient exhibits slow, increasing loss of recent memory; loss of recognition of people, places, and events; confusion and disorientation; and physical deterioration leading to death. The cause remains unknown, and there is no known cure. Treatment is supportive care only. Alzheimer's disease is addressed in more detail in Chapter 47.

CRITICAL THINKING APPLICATION

Mr. Jackson, a 75-year-old Alzheimer's patient, is coming in for his first visit. He does not respond to verbal commands and is unable to make any intelligible conversation. How can Mai get him into the examination room and into a patient gown while preserving Mr. Jackson's dignity?

Epilepsy

Epilepsy is a chronic brain disorder associated with abnormal electrical impulses generated by some of the neurons in the brain. These errant impulses cause seizures to occur (Figure 43-6). A seizure is characterized by abnormalities in levels of consciousness, sensory disturbances, and impaired motor function. A diagnosis of a seizure disorder is made if the indi-

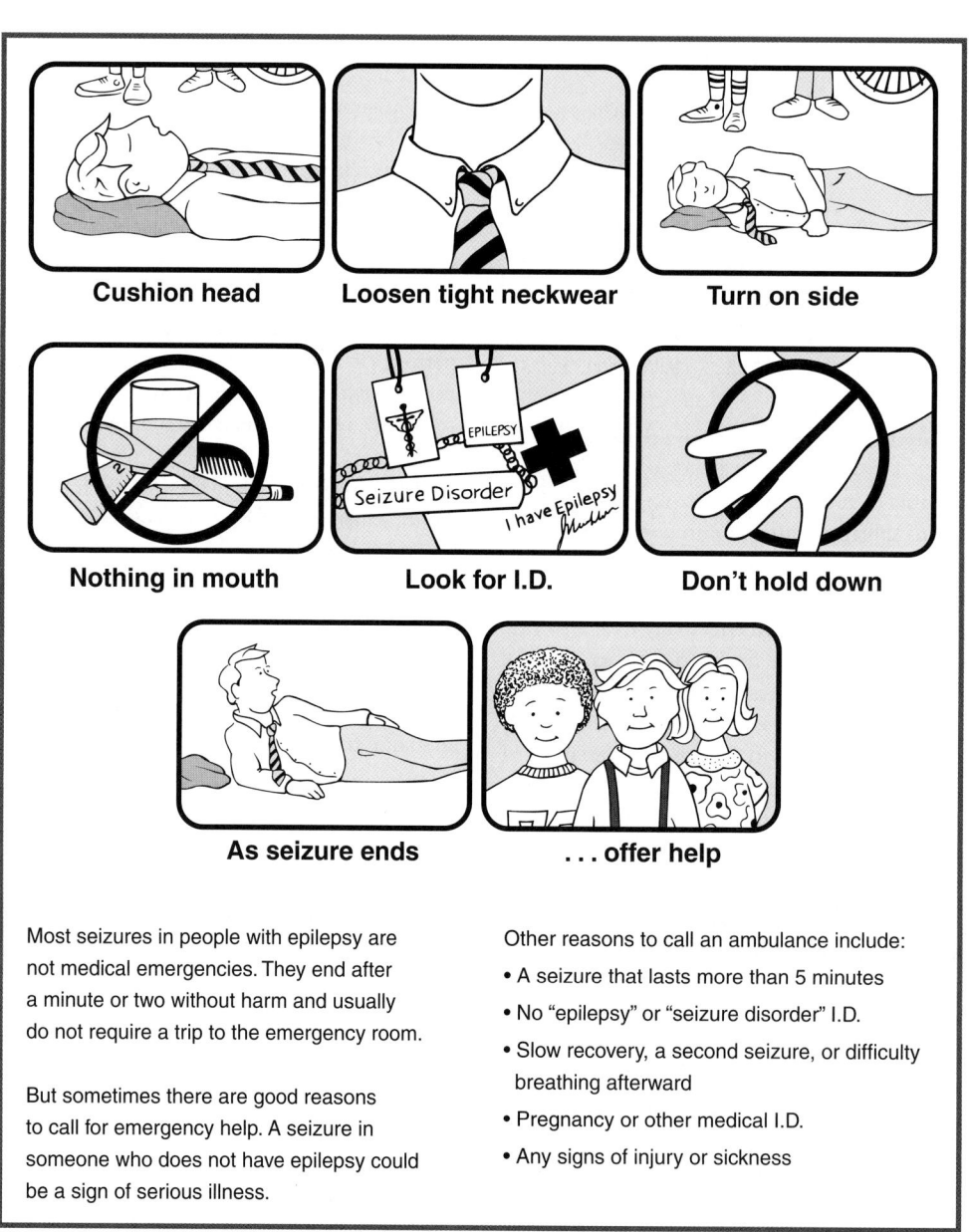

Cushion head **Loosen tight neckwear** **Turn on side**

Nothing in mouth **Look for I.D.** **Don't hold down**

As seizure ends **. . . offer help**

Most seizures in people with epilepsy are not medical emergencies. They end after a minute or two without harm and usually do not require a trip to the emergency room.

But sometimes there are good reasons to call for emergency help. A seizure in someone who does not have epilepsy could be a sign of serious illness.

Other reasons to call an ambulance include:

• A seizure that lasts more than 5 minutes

• No "epilepsy" or "seizure disorder" I.D.

• Slow recovery, a second seizure, or difficulty breathing afterward

• Pregnancy or other medical I.D.

• Any signs of injury or sickness

FIGURE 43-6 First aid for seizures. (From Epilepsy Foundation of America, Landover, Md.)

vidual has two or more seizures. Children may have a single seizure associated with a high fever–febrile seizure–but that alone does not mean that the child has a seizure disorder. However, the majority of individuals with the disorder have an onset of seizures during childhood, although many children grow out of the problem as they age. In many cases the cause is never identified; however, some known causes include brain tumors, CNS infections, anoxia, CVA, and traumatic head injury.

Seizures are classified as either partial or generalized, based on how much of the brain is involved in the abnormal electrical activity. Partial seizures result from abnormal electrical activity in just one part of the brain, whereas generalized seizures involve most or all of the brain. Seizure classifications are divided into more specific categories including *simple partial seizures* that originate in a small localized area of the brain, do not cause loss of consciousness, and are identified by a routine action such as shaking of an arm or a leg or altered speech. *Complex partial seizures* also begin in a small area of the brain but cause staring and repeated movements such as hand rubbing, lip smacking, and swallowing, as well as postseizure confusion or amnesia. Generalized seizures include *petit mal seizures*–brief episodes characterized by staring, subtle body movement, and brief lapses of awareness. Probably the most well known seizure disorder is the generalized tonic-clonic form that causes *grand mal seizures,* with loss of consciousness, tonic (stiffening) muscle contractions, followed by clonic (twitching, jerking) muscle contractions of the limbs, clenched teeth, and/or loss of bowel or bladder control. After the shaking subsides, the individual may fall asleep or appear confused for a few minutes. The patient may experience an aura, usually a sensory warning such as a specific smell or taste, before a grand mal seizure occurs.

Diagnosis is dependent on an accurate seizure history, EEG, and CT or MRI. Seizures cannot be cured but usually can be controlled effectively by pharmaceutical treatment; however, finding the most effective medication at the right dose can be complex. Some individuals with epilepsy require more than one drug or have to try multiple medications until the most effective one is found. Antiseizure (anticonvulsant) medications include phenytoin (Dilantin), carbamazepine (Tegretol), valproic acid (Depakene), gabapentin (Neurontin), phenobarbital, clonazepam (Klonopin), and lamotrigine (Lamictal). It is very important that patients know never to stop taking their seizure medication without physician supervision, because this may trigger more frequent and severe seizure episodes.

Central Nervous System Infections

Encephalitis

Most cases of encephalitis are of viral origin and are transmitted to humans from mosquitoes and ticks or caused by other infections such as herpes infections. Symptoms in a mild case can include headaches, muscle aches, malaise, and general flulike symptoms. More severe cases can include fever, delirium, convulsions, **coma,** and even death.

A quiet, nonstimulating environment is necessary to avoid triggering seizure activity, to relieve headache, and to promote

---

What Is Electroencephalography?

Electroencephalography (EEG) is used to record the brainwave activity of a patient suspected of having a seizure disorder or to determine the effectiveness of pharmaceutical treatment to control the brain's abnormal electrical activity. The particular pattern of brainwave activity helps diagnose the seizure disorder type. Electroencephalograms are also used to help localize the area of the brain that is causing a partial seizure disorder. During an EEG, 32 electrodes are placed on the patient's scalp with either paste or an elastic cap to record the electrical activity of the brain. The patient must remain very still during the examination, even sleep if possible, so that the electrodes can pick up the electrical impulses of the brain without interference. Sedation may be required for pediatric patients (Figure 43-7).

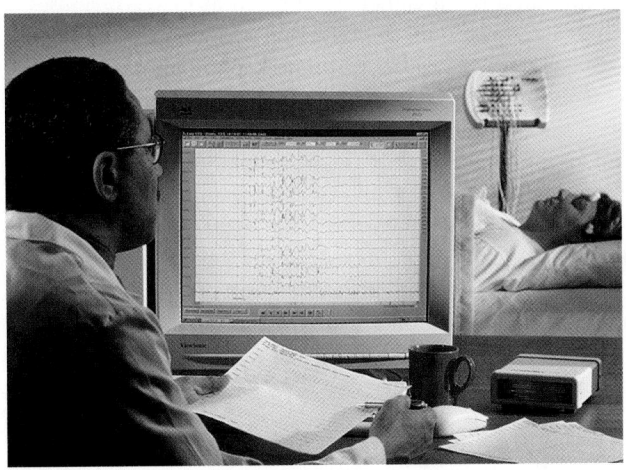

FIGURE 43-7 Patient undergoing an electroencephalogram. (From Linton AD, Maebius NK: *Introduction to medical-surgical nursing,* ed 3, St Louis, 2003, Saunders.)

rest. The patient with cerebral inflammation from encephalitis may suffer from confusion, disorientation, and other behavioral changes. These symptoms are part of the disease and usually disappear when the condition improves.

Patient management treats the symptoms and is aimed at controlling fever and seizure activity as well as constant monitoring of respiratory and urinary functions. In patients with severe CNS damage, recovery usually is prolonged and physical therapy is necessary to overcome the neurologic and musculoskeletal complications. If the encephalitis is caused by the herpes simplex or varicella zoster virus, treatment includes the use of acyclovir (Zovirax) or ganciclovir (Cytovene).

Meningitis

Meningitis is an infection and inflammation of the meninges and CSF of the brain and spinal cord that can be caused by a virus, bacteria, or fungus. Viral meningitis is usually mild, with flulike symptoms that typically resolve in 10 days or less. Fungal meningitis is seen in patients with immune deficiencies, such as acquired immunodeficiency syndrome (AIDS), and can be life-threatening. Acute bacterial meningitis can occur as a

Brudzinski's and Kernig's Signs

Brudzinski's Sign

The patient is placed in the supine position. The head is passively flexed toward the chest. If the patient spontaneously flexes the arm, hip, and knee in response to the neck flexion, Brudzinski's sign is present.

Kernig's Sign

With the patient in a supine position the physician flexes both one hip and the **ipsilateral** knee to 90 degrees, then attempts to completely straighten the leg by straightening the knee. Kernig's sign is present if pain prevents straightening the leg or the patient involuntarily flexes the **contralateral** knee and hip.

Signs of a Concussion

Signs that occur seconds to minutes after a head injury:
- Possible loss of consciousness
- Difficulty focusing, with slowed responses
- Slurred speech
- Nausea and vomiting
- Headache
- Blurred vision
- Confusion and disorientation or amnesia

The patient should be seen immediately if he or she reports any of the following signs and symptoms days or weeks after a head injury:
- Persistent headache
- Vertigo (dizziness)
- Inability to concentrate
- Repeated problems with memory
- Nausea or vomiting (especially if vomiting is projectile)
- Unusual anger, irritability, anxiety, or depression
- Sleep disorders
- Seizures

complication of an earlier infection from the ears, sinuses, or lungs. It can be quite serious, with symptoms that include a high fever, severe headache, stiff neck, photophobia, confusion, seizures, and positive Brudzinski's and Kernig's signs. Lumbar puncture confirms the diagnosis by the presence of cloudy CSF containing large numbers of white blood cells and bacteria. Culturing CSF usually allows identification of the causative organism so the patient can be treated with intravenous antibiotics that are appropriate for the type of bacteria causing the infection. The patient is also treated with analgesics and appropriate medications to decrease cerebral edema. Despite treatment, meningitis can be fatal or cause long-term neurologic damage in some patients.

Brain and Spinal Cord Injuries

Traumatic brain injuries are caused by a blow or jolt to the head and may be limited to a particular section of the brain or may result in generalized neurologic damage. Injuries can range from a mild concussion to severe injury, coma, and death. With a minor concussion there are usually no long-term side effects; however, a moderate to severe brain injury can result in headaches, amnesia, confusion, personality changes, and seizures. Spinal cord injuries usually result from severe, accidental trauma to the back or neck. These injuries are most common in the 16- to 30-year-old age group and are associated with automobile and sports accidents. The higher the damage to the spinal cord, the more serious the injury becomes.

Fortunately, CNS injuries can be prevented with the proper use of child car seats, adult safety belts, and helmets in childhood sports and activities and with the reduction of drinking and driving incidents. However, severe brain injuries continue to affect both the injured people and their families. Several types of brain injuries can occur, depending on the type and amount of force with which the head is struck.

Cerebral Concussion and Contusion

Concussion is the mildest and the most common type of brain injury. Trauma from an impact or a sudden change in motion can cause a concussion with loss of consciousness, which may last from seconds to several minutes and may be followed by a period of disorientation that lasts up to 24 hours (Figure 43-8). A single concussion may disrupt the normal electrical activity in the brain, but the brain usually is not injured permanently. However, research has shown that the damage from multiple concussions may be cumulative, and neurologists recommend that children should be removed from all sporting activities if they have experienced three concussions.

A more serious injury to the brain can cause a contusion or bruised area to form, usually because of a skull fracture. Symptoms can include headache, nausea, vomiting, vision disturbances, and sensitivity to light. Talking with the patient may reveal decreased levels of concentration, irritability, or periods of amnesia. Part of the patient's initial assessment may include an evaluation of consciousness according to the parameters of the Glasgow Coma Scale (Table 43-4).

TABLE 43-4 Glasgow Coma Scale

SCORE	1	2	3	4	5
Eye opening	No response	To pain	To voice	Spontaneously	
Best motor response (movement of arms and legs)	No response	Extension to pain	Flexion to pain	Localizes to pain	Follows commands
Best verbal response	No response	Incomprehensible sounds	Inappropriate words	Disoriented and converses	Oriented and converses

Scoring: 13 to 15, Mild head injury; 9 to 12, moderate head injury; 3 to 8, severe head injury.

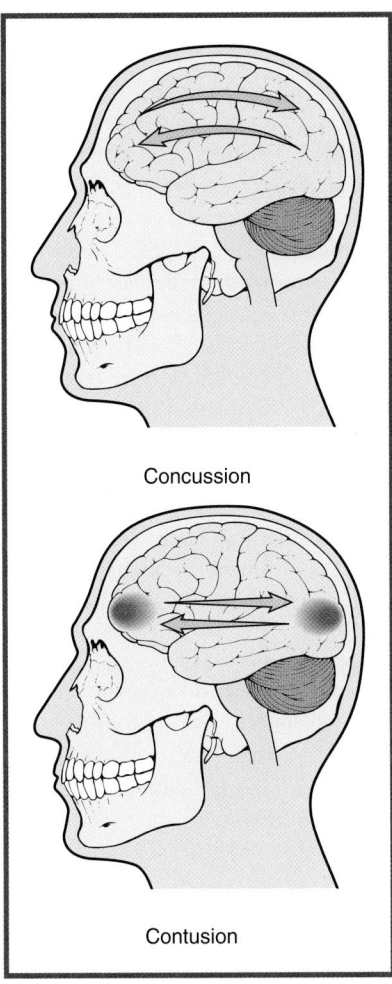

FIGURE 43-8 Brain concussion and contusion. (Modified from Frazier MS, Drzymkowski JW: *Essentials of human diseases and conditions,* ed 3, Philadelphia, 2004, Saunders.)

Concussion

Contusion

CRITICAL THINKING APPLICATION

■ Mai is putting together a head injury information sheet for the family of a patient who recently suffered a minor concussion. What symptoms should the family watch for in this situation? How will the family know if they should seek additional medical care?

■ Dr. Song said he would approve the leaflet after Mai completed it, but he was called away on an emergency before he saw it. A patient sees it behind the desk and asks to take one. Should Mai let him? Why or why not?

Open and Closed Head Injuries

A *closed* head injury occurs when there is a brain injury but the skull is not fractured. A more serious brain injury can occur with an *open* head injury, because the skull is fractured or displaced. When a patient experiences a serious head injury, significant life-threatening damage can occur to the intracerebral structures. *Subarachnoid hemorrhage* may occur when there is a rupture of the delicate meningeal blood vessels, resulting in blood collecting in the subarachnoid space. This causes a rapid increase in intracranial pressure, which may give rise to sudden, severe headache; nausea and severe projectile vomiting; motor disturbances; visual disturbances; and seizures. In addition to

trauma, other predisposing factors that can cause subarachnoid hemorrhage include hypertension, family history, and congenital malformations of cranial blood vessels. Treatment includes decreasing the intracranial pressure, sometimes surgically.

A *subdural hematoma* is a collection of blood in the space between the dura mater and the arachnoid layers of the meninges, usually as a result of trauma to the head that has caused a slow bleed from ruptured blood vessels within the meningeal layers. Symptoms of increased intracranial pressure occur over a period of days as the size of the hematoma increases. Signs and symptoms build over time and include headache, motor disturbances, speech abnormalities, nausea and vomiting, seizures, and a decreased level of consciousness. Treatment requires surgery to stop the bleeding and decrease the pressure inside the skull. People age 75 and older are at greatest risk for developing a subdural hematoma after a minor fall or cranial impact.

Shaken Baby Syndrome

Shaken baby syndrome is the most common cause of serious head injury in infants. It is caused by violently shaking the infant back and forth, forcing the brain against opposite ends of the skull. Shaking is so dangerous for babies because of their small size in comparison to their relatively large head size as well as their undeveloped neck muscles. The typical presentation is a child of approximately 6 months of age who is brought to the clinic or emergency room because of difficulty breathing or marked lethargy. Usually there is little or no external bruising or trauma. Physical findings on examination or autopsy include subdural hematoma and retinal hemorrhages. The history given by the caregiver usually indicates that the baby "fell" from the sofa, coffee table, or bed or was "dropped." Approximately one fourth of these infants die of their injuries.

Spinal Cord Injuries

If a traumatic accident completely transects the spinal cord, all CNS stimulation to nerves distal to the injury stops, resulting in paralysis of the areas below the injury. Paralysis because of cord **transection** is grouped into one of two categories (Figure 43-9). In *paraplegia,* transection occurs below the midpoint of the spinal cord, causing paralysis of both legs and loss of function below the level of injury, including loss of bladder and bowel control as well as sexual dysfunction in males. In *quadriplegia,* transection occurs in the upper thoracic or cervical region of the spinal cord, causing paralysis of all four limbs, respiratory difficulty, and loss of function to all muscles below the injury points. *Hemiplegia* is unrelated to spinal cord injury and occurs when a CVA, vascular injury such as an aneurysm, or tumor occurs on one side of the brain, resulting in paralysis on the opposite side of the body.

No surgery or treatment can successfully restore a transected cord, although this is an area in which much research is currently being done. If the spinal cord is injured but not completely transected, the degree of paralysis will depend on the degree of injury. Such patients usually respond well to physical therapy, and their ability to restore motor function is good, although they may always have some functional limitations.

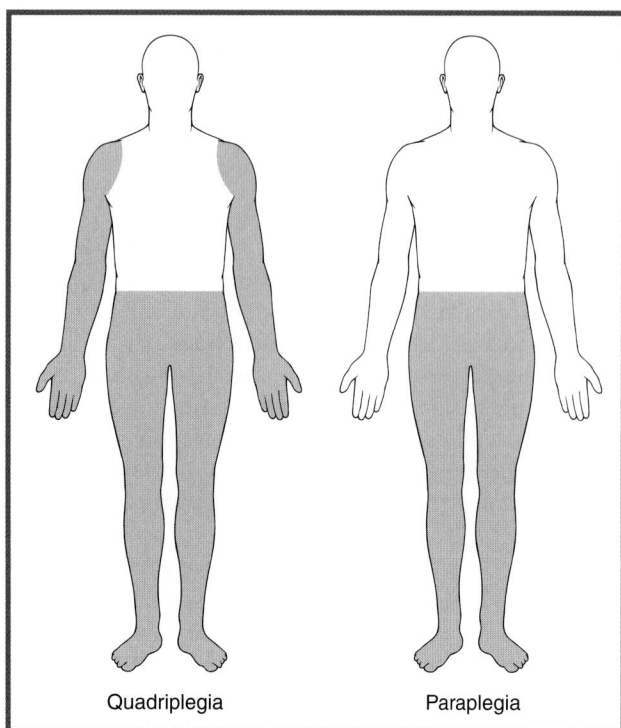

FIGURE 43-9 Types of paralysis: quadriplegia and paraplegia. (Modified from Frazier MS, Drzymkowski JW: *Essentials of human diseases and conditions,* ed 3, Philadelphia, 2004, Saunders.)

Additional Central Nervous System Pathologies

Parkinson's Disease

Parkinson's disease (PD) is a chronic, progressive, debilitating disease that affects about one in every 100 adults over the age of 60 years; more than 60,000 new cases occur annually in the United States. It affects men more frequently than women. The four primary symptoms of PD are tremors of the hands, arms, legs, jaw, and face; rigidity of the limbs and trunk; *bradykinesia,* or slowness of movement; and postural instability with impaired balance and coordination. The typical presentation of PD includes a unilateral pill-rolling tremor, a high-pitched monotone voice, difficulty swallowing, a masklike facial expression, and bowed head and forward-bent posture. Tremors and rigidity increase in severity over time. There are currently no laboratory tests specific for PD; therefore the diagnosis is based on a comprehensive medical history and neurologic examination. The condition is caused by a deficiency of the neurotransmitter dopamine in the brain. There is no known cure for PD, but various medications are prescribed for symptomatic relief including carbidopa-levodopa (Sinemet), which provides the brain with artificial dopamine. Surgical destruction of the most affected area of the brain may produce some relief of symptoms. A recently approved treatment, deep brain stimulation (DBS), uses electrodes that are implanted into the brain and connected to a small electrical device that is externally programmed to help control the tremors and **gait** problems associated with the disease.

Tumors

The symptoms of a brain tumor depend on the type and location of the mass, but generally the initial symptoms are headaches, vomiting, dizziness, diplopia, and alterations in muscle strength and coordination. Changes in personality and mental function, seizures, progressive paralysis, loss of speech, and sensory disorders appear as the tumor enlarges.

CNS tumors can be diagnosed via CT, MRI, EEG, or lumbar puncture. Ophthalmoscopic examination may reveal **papilledema.** Accurate diagnosis of a brain tumor includes determining its precise location in the brain and whether it is **benign** or **malignant.** Approximately half of all brain tumors are metastatic growths from other primary cancer sites within the body. Lung cancer, breast cancer, and melanoma frequently spread to the brain by metastasis. Regardless of whether the mass is benign or malignant, as brain tumors grow, they cause serious problems and complications for the patient because of the limited space inside the skull. Treatment of brain tumors can include surgery, chemotherapy, and radiation in any combination.

CRITICAL THINKING APPLICATION

A 34-year-old man has just found out he has a brain tumor, and Mai has just scheduled him for surgery next week. Before he leaves the office, he wants to talk to Mai "privately." They go into an examination room, and he says to Mai, "Tell me the truth: this is cancer and I'm going to die, right?" How should Mai respond to this frightened patient?

DISEASES OF THE PERIPHERAL NERVOUS SYSTEM

Multiple Sclerosis

The axon of a nerve cell in the PNS is covered with a myelin sheath to protect and insulate electrical stimulation as it is passed to the terminal end of the neuron. Multiple sclerosis (MS) causes progressive inflammation and deterioration *(demyelination)* of the myelin sheath, leaving nerve fibers uncovered and resulting in a scattering of the nervous message as it passes down the axon. Early symptoms may include numbness, **paresthesia,** diplopia, **ataxia,** and bladder control problems. As the disease progresses, patients experience increased spasticity, vertigo, depression, gait problems, joint pain, fatigue, and varying degrees of paralysis. It most commonly begins in women in their early 30s. The cause remains unknown; however, it is more common in Northern climates and is associated with an autoimmune reaction. MS is frequently diagnosed by the **exacerbation** and **remission** of neurologic symptoms that are characteristic of the condition. Patients cycle through remission and relapse with an ever-increasing degree of dysfunction occurring after each episode. An MRI may show plaques on nerve fibers where the myelin sheaths have been destroyed.

There is no cure for MS, so treatment goals focus on alleviating symptoms and delaying the progression of the disease. Medications used to treat the disease include corticosteroids during periods of exacerbation; interferon (Betaseron, Avonex) to reduce the frequency and severity of relapses; and additional medications to treat fatigue, pain, spasticity, and bladder control problems. Some patients may live an essentially normal life with only occasional attacks, whereas other patients experience rapidly progressive incapacitation.

Amyotrophic Lateral Sclerosis

Amyotrophic lateral sclerosis (ALS), or Lou Gehrig's disease, is a rapidly progressive, destructive, ultimately fatal neurologic disease that destroys the motor neurons that are responsible for voluntary muscle control. Without stimulation from motor neurons, muscles cannot function and gradually weaken and **atrophy.** ALS usually begins with small, local, involuntary muscle contractions in the forearms and hands. As ALS progresses, the patient has difficulty with speech, chewing, swallowing, and breathing. In most cases the disease does not affect a person's personality, intelligence, or memory, nor does it affect the ability to see, smell, taste, hear, or recognize touch. The first drug treatment for the disease, recently approved by the U.S. Food and Drug Administration (FDA), is riluzole (Rilutek), which decreases damage to motor neurons and prolongs survival, especially in patients who have difficulty swallowing. Other treatments are palliative in nature—attempts to keep the individual as comfortable as possible and to help with pain, depression, sleep disturbances, and constipation. Death from failure of the respiratory muscles usually occurs within 3 to 5 years after the onset of symptoms. The cause is unknown, but the disease most commonly occurs in males over the age of 50.

Bell's Palsy

Bell's palsy causes temporary facial paralysis because of damage or trauma to the seventh cranial nerve of the face. It occurs suddenly, with symptoms reaching their peak within 48 hours, and usually subsides spontaneously over several weeks to months. Symptoms range in severity from mild weakness to complete paralysis on the affected side, dependant on the degree of nervous involvement. The patient can experience facial twitching, drooping eyelid, excessive tearing of the affected eye, and drooping mouth with drooling of saliva. The patient is unable to completely close the eye on the affected side and may experience taste disturbances. The cause is unknown; however, researchers believe that viral inflammation of the facial nerve may be responsible for the disorder. The antiviral acyclovir may be prescribed, as well as prednisone, to reduce the inflammation and control edema. The physician will recommend an eye patch to protect the exposed eye, especially at night, to prevent corneal abrasions.

Peripheral Neuropathy

Peripheral neuropathy is not a disease in itself but rather a condition of peripheral nerve dysfunction that can have more than 100 different known causes. It can be **cryptogenic** or **idiopathic,** meaning the underlying cause cannot be identified. The following conditions can cause peripheral neuropathies: diabetes mellitus, human immunodeficiency virus (HIV) infection, nutritional deficiencies, and neurologic side effects of some medications. Symptoms usually affect the legs and arms and can include muscular weakness and pain or sensory disturbances such as burning, numbness, and tingling.

Symptoms can vary widely from person to person in both number and severity. Patients often experience extreme frustration when trying to explain to the physician the abnormal sensations they are experiencing. Peripheral neuropathies can result from damage or injury to any portion of the neuron. Peripheral neuropathy treatment is most effective when the causative condition is diagnosed then successfully treated. Encouraging a healthy lifestyle, with weight control, exercise, nutritious diet, and limiting or avoiding alcohol, helps control the physical and emotional effects of peripheral neuropathy.

Carpal Tunnel Syndrome

Carpal tunnel syndrome (CTS) results from **compression** of the median nerve as it passes through the carpal bones of the wrist. The carpal tunnel contains the flexor tendons of the forearm and the median nerve, which runs from the forearm to the hand. Compression of these structures within the carpal tunnel can occur spontaneously but more commonly is the result of repetitive movements. CTS is the most common of the repetitive strain injuries (RSIs). One frequently reported cause is daily use of the computer keyboard for prolonged periods. The symptoms of median nerve compression are pain, weakness, numbness in the hand and wrist that radiates up the arm, and paresthesia of the radial-palmar region of the hand. As symptoms worsen, individuals may experience decreased grip strength, making it difficult to form a fist, grasp small objects, or perform other fine motor tasks.

Treatment includes taking breaks from repetitive hand or wrist activities, wearing a wrist support, taking NSAIDs, applying ice, and undergoing physical therapy. If these treatments do not resolve the problem, surgery may be required to relieve the pressure on the median nerve.

MENTAL HEALTH

Each year more than 44 million Americans are affected with a diagnosable mental condition that adversely affects their work, their relationships with family and friends, and their activities of daily living. Mental health disorders may be caused by any of the following (alone or in combination): changes in brain chemicals, hereditary makeup, psychologic disposition, and life experiences. Emotional and physical symptoms can occur for no apparent reason and can remain quite persistent. Emotional symptoms can include panic, apprehension, fear, anxiety, nightmares, withdrawal, flashbacks, and ritualized repetitive behaviors such as constant hand washing. Physical symptoms can include tachycardia, shortness of breath, sleep disturbances, gastrointestinal upset, muscular tension, and cold, clammy hands. Often patients do not associate these symptoms with a mental health disorder and therefore do not get appropriate diagnosis and treatment.

Depressive Disorders

About 10% of adults in America experience depression each year, with almost twice as many women as men affected by the disorder. Depression interferes with daily activities and causes pain and suffering not only to those who have the disorder, but also to those who care about them. Although multiple medications and psychosocial therapies are available to treat and manage depression, most individuals do not seek treatment. Depressive disorders affect the way a person thinks, feels, eats, and sleeps. People with depression cannot "snap out of it" and without treatment may experience symptoms that persist for weeks, months, or years.

Types of depressive disorders include major depressive, dysthymic, and bipolar disorders. Individuals with *major depression* exhibit a combination of symptoms that interfere with their ability to work, study, sleep, eat, and enjoy activities they once considered pleasurable. *Dysthymic disorders* are a less severe type of depression in which patients experience long-term, chronic symptoms that are not incapacitating but affect their level of performance and daily emotions. Many people with dysthymia also experience major depression at some time in their lives. Individuals with *bipolar disorders*, also called *manic-depression*, cycle through a wide range of moods from extreme highs *(mania)* to extreme lows *(depression)*. When in the depression cycle, they can exhibit any or all of the symptoms of a depressive disorder. When cycling through mania they may make decisions or act in a way that can be both embarrassing and dangerous. Manic individuals are extremely energetic and rarely sleep. If left untreated the disorder can progress to a psychotic state.

Patients need to understand that antidepressant medications take a minimum of 3 to 4 weeks for the full therapeutic effects of the drug to occur. Once they start to feel better, many individuals are tempted to stop taking the medication. *It is important that treatment is maintained for a minimum of 4 to 9 months to prevent a recurrence of the depression.* The patient should never stop taking antidepressant medication suddenly or without the direction of a physician. Individuals with bipolar disorders or chronic major depression may need to be on maintenance therapy indefinitely. Antidepressant medications include amitriptyline (Elavil), imipramine (Tofranil), citalopram (Celexa), and sertraline (Zoloft).

Anxiety Disorders

Anxiety disorders affect approximately 19 million American adults. The primary symptoms are an overwhelming, irrational feeling of anxiety and fear. Anxiety disorders include panic disorder, obsessive-compulsive disorder (OCD), posttraumatic stress disorder, and phobias. Individuals with *panic disorder* report feelings of terror that strike unexpectedly with nausea, chest pain, palpitations, diaphoresis, weakness, vertigo, **syncope,** and a fear of impending doom or loss of control. People with OCD experience anxious thoughts or images *(obsessions)* that they cannot control, so they resort to performing specific rituals *(compulsions)* to try to prevent or dispel the obsession. For example, an individual may be obsessed with germs or dirt, so he or she repeatedly washes the hands, or an individual may have to repeatedly check to see if a door is locked because of fear that it will be left open. Performing the ritual does not bring pleasure, only a temporary relief from the anxiety caused by the

Symptoms of Depression

According to the National Institute of Mental Health (NIMH), the severity of depressive symptoms varies among individuals and also with each episode. A discussion of the following symptoms can be found at www.nimh.nih.gov.

- Persistent sad, anxious, or "empty" feeling
- Feelings of hopelessness, pessimism
- Feelings of guilt, worthlessness, helplessness
- Loss of interest or pleasure in hobbies and activities that were once enjoyed, including sex
- Decreased energy and complaints of fatigue
- Difficulty concentrating, remembering, making decisions
- Insomnia, early-morning awakening, or oversleeping
- Either anorexia and weight loss or overeating and weight gain
- Thoughts of death or suicide with possible suicide attempts
- Restlessness, irritability
- Persistent physical complaints that do not respond to treatment, such as headaches, gastrointestinal disturbances, or chronic pain

obsession, which will grow if the compulsion is not performed. *Posttraumatic stress disorder* can occur after a patient is a part of or witnesses some terrifying, horrendous, or violent physical or emotional event, such as assault, battery, rape, war, natural disasters, acts of terrorism, and serious accidents during which many people are killed or injured. The person who survives the ordeal often has flashbacks; feelings of panic, fear, or guilt; constant replaying of the event in his or her mind; or deep feelings of emotional numbness. Severe depression and inability to function normally in daily activities also may be present. A *phobia* is an intense, irrational fear of something that is of little or no actual danger and may include such things as fear of heights, escalators, tunnels, and water. Although the individual may realize that the fear is unreasonable, just the thought of facing the feared object or situation causes a panic attack or severe anxiety. There are two types of treatment for anxiety disorders: antianxiety medication, such as alprazolam (Xanax) or buspirone (BuSpar), and specific types of psychotherapy.

Schizophrenia

Schizophrenia is a chronic, severe, and disabling brain disorder with symptoms that include hallucinations and delusions; difficulty speaking and expressing emotions; and cognitive deficits such as problems with concentration and memory loss. Schizophrenia cannot be cured, but psychotic episodes can be decreased significantly by long-term and consistent pharmaceutical treatment. However, relapses are not unusual, because most individuals with schizophrenia stop taking their antipsychotic medication periodically because they feel better, don't believe they need the medication, or don't think taking it regularly is important. In addition, the antipsychotic medications that were first developed, such as chlorpromazine (Thorazine) and haloperidol (Haldol), caused disturbing side effects including rigidity, persistent muscle spasms, tremors, and restlessness. Newer drugs have limited side effects and include risperidone (Risperdal) and olanzapine (Zyprexa).

Suicide Facts from the National Institute of Mental Health

- More than 90% of the individuals who commit suicide have a diagnosable mental disorder, typically depression, or are substance abusers.
- The highest suicide rates in the United States are in white men over 85 years of age.
- Although women attempt suicide two to three times more often than men, four times as many men are successful.
- Risk factors vary with age, gender, and ethnic group but include serious depressive disorders; decreased levels of serotonin (a neurotransmitter); a prior suicide attempt; family violence, including physical or sexual abuse; and exposure to the suicidal behavior of others, including family members and peers.

THE MEDICAL ASSISTANT'S ROLE IN THE NEUROLOGIC EXAMINATION

As with other physical examinations, a careful history provides the physician with valuable clues in diagnosing neurologic conditions. These may include a record of seizures, syncope, diplopia, incontinence, or any of the subjective symptoms previously mentioned in this chapter. The patient's general health often complicates a neurologic diagnosis. The purposes of a neurologic examination are to determine whether a nervous system malfunction is present, discover its locations, and identify its type and extent. During the examination the physician may determine the effect of the symptoms on the patient's emotional status, intellectual performance, cognitive ability, and general behavior (Procedure 43-1). The patient's grooming and mannerisms are carefully observed, as is his or her ability to communicate effectively, including the appropriate use of speech, language, and writing skills. The medical assistant should carefully listen for difficulty in putting words together, slurred speech, and whether conversation makes sense. If you notice inappropriate changes in the patient, note them on the patient's record for the physician's attention and evaluation.

Physical examination of the neurologic system includes evaluation of the cranial nerves. You can assist by helping the patient assume the proper position necessary for each test and by having the instruments the physician will need ready for use. For example, cranial nerve I (the olfactory nerve) is tested by determining the patient's ability to identify familiar odors such as coffee, tobacco, or cloves. Cranial nerve V (the trigeminal nerve) is checked by the patient's ability to differentiate between

PROCEDURE 43-1

Prepare Patient for and Assist with Routine and Specialty Examinations: Assist with the Neurologic Examination

CAAHEP COMPETENCY: 3.b.(4)(e)
ABHES COMPETENCY: 4.h

GOAL: To assist the physician in obtaining an accurate neurologic examination of the patient.

EQUIPMENT and SUPPLIES

- Patient gown
- Drape
- Otoscope
- Ophthalmoscope
- Percussion hammer
- Disposable pinwheel
- Penlight
- Tuning fork
- Cotton ball
- Tongue depressor
- Small vials of warm and cold liquids prepared according to the physician's instructions
- Small vials of sweet and salty liquids prepared according to the physician's instructions
- Small vials containing substances with distinct odors, such as instant coffee, cinnamon, and vanilla, prepared according to the physician's instructions
- Patient record

PROCEDURAL STEPS

1. Assemble the materials needed, and prepare the room. Prepare the equipment and supplies needed for the neurologic examination.
2. Wash your hands. Follow standard precautions.
   <u>PURPOSE:</u> Infection control.
3. Identify the patient, and briefly explain the procedure.
   <u>PURPOSE:</u> Explanations gain patient cooperation and alleviate apprehension.
4. Instruct the patient to disrobe as needed for the examination and to put on a gown with the opening in the back.
5. During the examination, be prepared to assist the patient in changing positions as necessary. Have the necessary examination instruments ready for the physician at the appropriate time during the examination. Record all results from the examination as indicated by the physician.
   <u>PURPOSE:</u> To facilitate a thorough and accurate neurologic examination.
6. The neurologic examination will generally follow the following order but can be modified according to physician preference:
   a. Mental status examination
   b. Proprioception and cerebellar function
   c. Cranial nerve assessment
   d. Sensory nerve function
   e. Reflexes
7. Record all procedures on the patient's medical record.
   <u>PURPOSE:</u> A procedure is not completed until it is accurately documented in the patient's medical record.

warm and cold objects held against his or her right and left cheeks.

Peripheral nerve function is evaluated by examining the motor system, including muscular strength, gait, and movements. The diameters of the upper arms and the calves of the legs may be measured and compared to diagnose muscle atrophy. Motor functioning can be assessed through the use of the Romberg test, in which the patient is asked to stand with the feet together,

arms horizontal to the body, and eyes closed. The sensory system is examined by noting the patient's ability to perceive superficial sensations, such as a wisp of cotton brushed on the skin, a light pinprick, or hot and cold touching certain areas. Several deep tendon reflexes (DTRs), such as the patellar and Achilles, are tested (Figure 43-10). Stroking the lateral aspect of the sole of the foot with a dull instrument (such as the handle of a reflex hammer or a tongue blade) checks Babinski's reflex. For

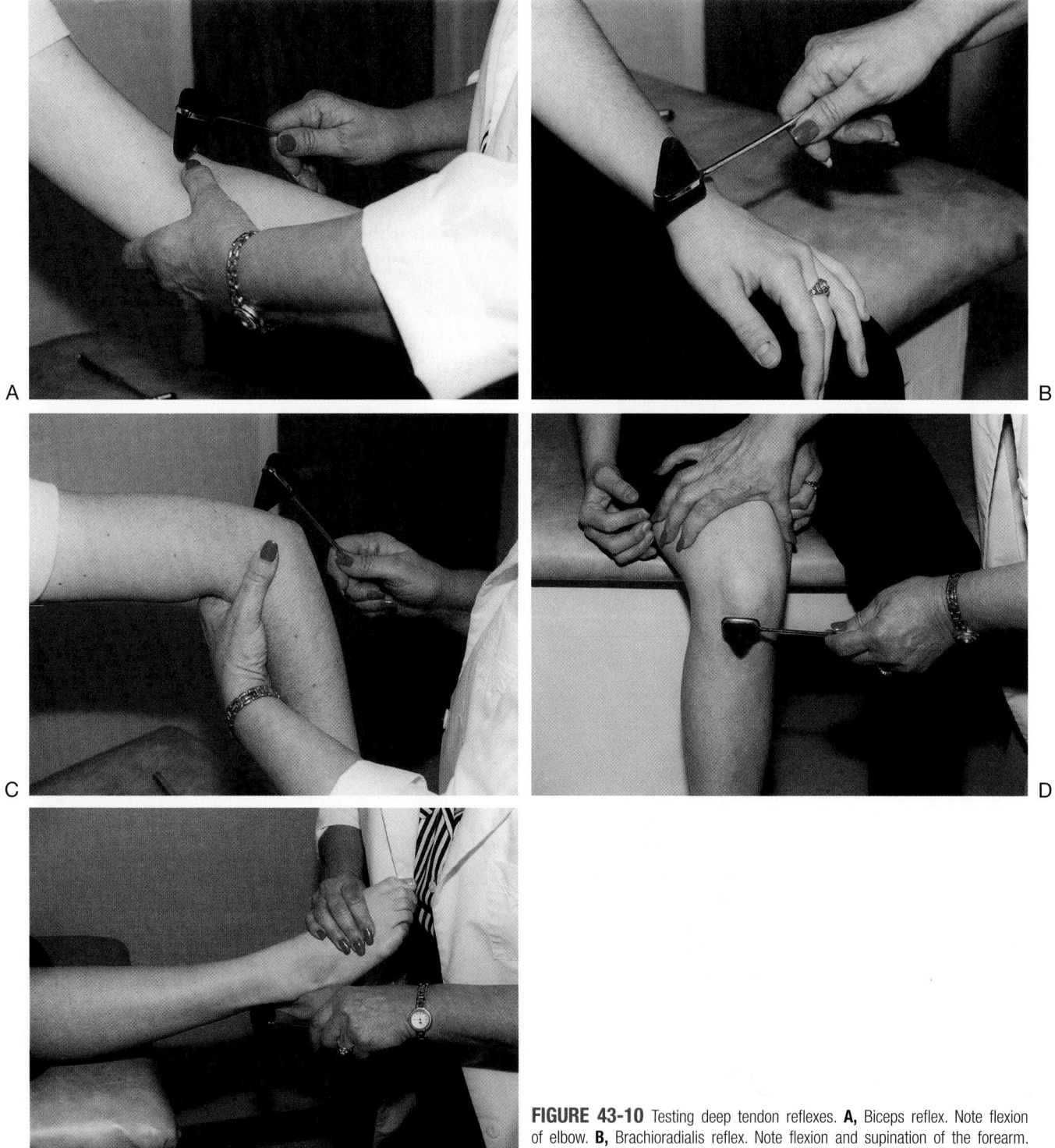

FIGURE 43-10 Testing deep tendon reflexes. **A,** Biceps reflex. Note flexion of elbow. **B,** Brachioradialis reflex. Note flexion and supination of the forearm. **C,** Triceps reflex. Note extension of the arm. **D,** Patellar reflex. Note extension of the leg. **E,** Achilles reflex. Note plantar flexion of the foot.

a positive Babinski test result, the great toe dorsiflexes while the other toes fan out. This may indicate a possible stroke or brain lesion. Other diagnostic tests may include a skull radiograph, carotid arteriogram, myelogram, EEG, MRI, and CT studies.

DIAGNOSTIC TESTING

Several diagnostic tests are used to help the physician accurately diagnose conditions and diseases of the neurologic system. The most common diagnostic procedures include lumbar puncture and various radiographic studies (Table 43-5).

Electroencephalography

EEG is the recording of changes in electrical impulses in various areas of the brain by means of electrodes placed on the scalp. Every individual has a unique EEG pattern. In a healthy brain most of the recorded waves are the occipital alpha waves coming from the back of the head. Irregular slow waves are called *delta waves,* which normally are found in people deeply asleep and in infants and young children. It is abnormal to find a delta wave pattern in an awake adult. Rhythmic slow waves, called *theta waves,* show a decrease in brain activity. Electrical silence (flatline EEG) indicates no evidence of brain activity and is one of the criteria used to determine brain death. EEG is valuable in diagnosing epilepsy, brain tumors, and other brain conditions (Procedure 43-2).

Lumbar Puncture

If the physician suspects that an infection or inflammation of the CNS is present, a lumbar puncture (spinal tap) is ordered to collect a CSF sample for culture, analysis of glucose and protein, or determination of the presence of increased intracranial pressure or an area of intracranial bleeding (Figure 43-11). The patient is placed on the left side in the fetal position; using sterile technique the physician injects the lumbar puncture site with a local anesthetic, and the puncture is performed by inserting a special needle into the subarachnoid space, usually between the L4 and L5 vertebrae. The pressure within the subarachnoid space is recorded and a sample of CSF is collected for laboratory analysis.

After the procedure, the patient must remain flat in bed for approximately 8 hours. Medical practices usually have a specially equipped room where this procedure is performed. If you are working in such an office, you may be responsible for both assisting with the procedure and monitoring the patient after the procedure until he or she is sent home. Watch for side effects such as severe headaches, visual disturbances, and pain.

TABLE 43-5 Diagnostic Tests for the Nervous System

TEST	PROCEDURE AND PATIENT PREPARATION	RESULTS
Arteriography (angiography)	The patient is usually given a sedative. Then, after a local anesthetic is injected, a catheter is threaded into an artery toward the head. Contrast medium is injected, and video fluoroscopic studies are recorded. The patient must remain still during the procedure, which may last up to 1 hr.	Allows visualization of vertebral and carotid arteries, cerebral arterial circulation, leaking vessels, aneurysms, and occluded vessels
CT scan	Patient's head is strapped into a foam block to prevent movement, and patient lies on a moveable table. The table moves into the CT machine, which converts an x-ray study into a visual image of multiple transverse sections of the brain. Procedure lasts for up to 1 hr, and the patient must remain still the entire time.	Allows visualization of multiple, serial, radiographic sections of a structure, differentiating between bone and soft tissues
EEG	Patient relaxes comfortably on a recliner or bed. Electrodes are attached to the head. The examiner may ask the patient questions, give the patient various forms of visual or auditory stimulation, or have the patient sleep.	Recording of electrical activity of the brain to determine cerebral function, determine origin of seizure activity, diagnose sleep disorders, and determine death
Lumbar puncture	With the patient in a side-lying fetal position, a local anesthetic is injected before a needle is inserted into the subarachnoid space between the third and fourth lumbar vertebrae. The procedure normally takes from 5-20 min and the patient must remain very still during the procedure.	Determine CSF pressure, obtain CSF specimens for testing, reduce intracranial pressure, and for injecting contrast medium for radiographic studies
MRI	Patient's head is strapped into a foam block to prevent movement and patient lies on a moveable table. The table moves into the MRI machine that converts electromagnetic energy of the body's cells into a visual image. Procedure lasts for up to 1 hr and the patient must remain still the entire time. Patient should not have metal in body.	Like CT, allows visualization of multiple, serial, radiographic sections of a structure; shows images of brain, spinal cord, and surrounding vascular and soft tissue
PET scan	Radioactive isotope is injected into the patient and the brain is scanned to locate areas where the isotope was concentrated. Procedure lasts for up to 2 hrs and patient must remain still the entire time.	Radionuclide study can identify areas of increased metabolic activity, vascular abnormalities, and space-occupying lesions.
X-ray studies	Patients head is placed in a specific position in front of the x-ray film; patient must remain still for about 1 min while x-ray is taken.	Bone studies to identify fractures and other bone pathologies

CT, Computed tomography; *EEG,* electroencephalography; *CSF,* cerebrospinal fluid; *MRI,* magnetic resonance imaging; *PET,* positron emission tomography.

PROCEDURE 43-2

Prepare Patient for and Assist with Procedures, Treatments, and Minor Office Surgeries: Prepare the Patient for an EEG

CAAHEP COMPETENCY: 3.b.(4)(f)
ABHES COMPETENCY: 4.b

GOAL: *To prepare a patient properly both physically and psychologically to obtain an accurate and useful EEG recording.*

PROCEDURAL STEPS

1. Greet the patient, and introduce yourself. Explain to the patient that you will go over what is going to happen step by step to ensure the best results.

2. Explain to the patient the purpose of the EEG, how the procedure will be carried out, and what will be expected of the patient during the test.

3. Tell the patient that the electrodes pick up tiny electrical signals from the body and that there is no danger of electrical shock.

4. Explain that the test is painless because the electrodes are attached to the scalp with paste.

5. If this is a sleep EEG, suggest that the patient stay up later than usual the night before the test so that it will be easier to fall asleep.
   PURPOSE: The physician prefers not to use sleep medications because they may alter the brainwave pattern.

6. Go over the physical preparation, including the diet to be followed for the 48 hours before the test. This usually includes no stimulants like coffee, chocolate, or sodas, and no meal skipping.

PURPOSE: Meal skipping may cause hypoglycemia, which alters brain function.

7. Tell the patient that a baseline EEG will be taken at the beginning of the test, and during this time the patient will be asked to avoid all movement, even eye and tongue movement.
   PURPOSE: These activities can be very disruptive to the brainwave tracing.

8. If a stimulation examination is ordered, explain that the brain will be stimulated by the patient viewing flickering lights. The EEG will be measuring the brain's response to this stimulation.

9. Ask the patient whether he or she has any questions. If so, answer the questions so that the patient understands the procedure clearly.
   PURPOSE: Patients are more likely to be cooperative it they are informed so they will not be unduly apprehensive before and during the test.

10. Document the procedure in the patient record.

NOTE: Performing EEGs requires advanced training.

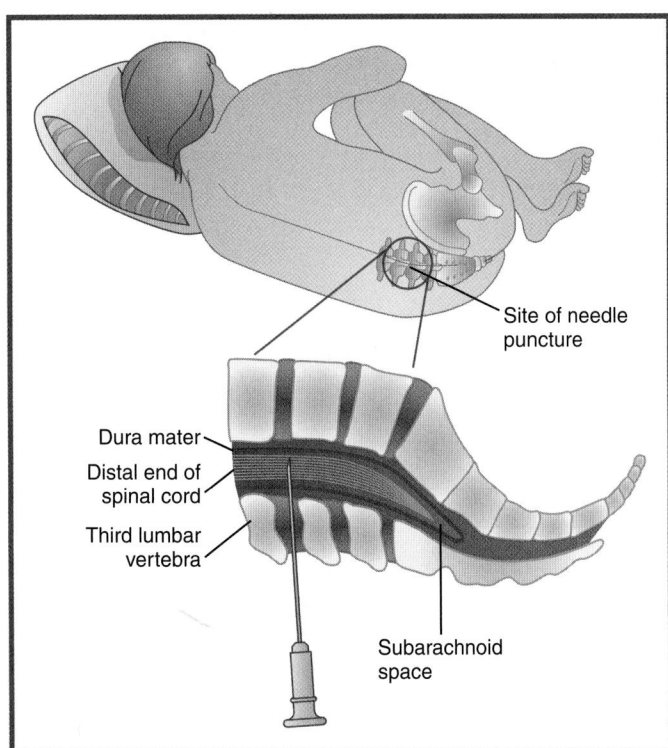

FIGURE 43-11 Lumbar puncture.

Labels: Site of needle puncture; Dura mater; Distal end of spinal cord; Third lumbar vertebra; Subarachnoid space

You will also have particular office protocols to follow regarding the frequency of vital signs, liquid intake, urine output, and visitors. Lumbar puncture is usually performed in hospitals, outpatient clinics, or surgical centers (Procedure 43-3). On discharge, patients should be told to immediately notify the physician if they experience any numbness and tingling of the legs; drainage of blood or liquid from the injection site; inability to urinate; or a persistent headache.

CRITICAL THINKING APPLICATION

Dr. Song is going to perform a lumbar puncture on a 10-year-old girl who he suspects has bacterial meningitis. Her mother agrees to the procedure, but while Mai is preparing the girl for the procedure, the mother changes her mind. She is afraid her daughter will become paralyzed by having a needle put into her spine. What should Mai do in this situation?

CLOSING COMMENTS

Patient Education

The nervous system is the major communication and control system in the human body. It influences and regulates all mental activity, including thought, learning, and memory. It is

PROCEDURE 43-3

Prepare Patient for and Assist with Procedures, Treatments, and Minor Office Surgeries: Prepare the Patient for and Assist with a Lumbar Puncture

<u>CAAHEP COMPETENCY:</u> 3.b.(4)(f)
<u>ABHES COMPETENCY:</u> 4.b

GOAL: *To prepare a patient properly both physically and mentally for a lumbar puncture to obtain a specimen of CSF for testing.*

EQUIPMENT and SUPPLIES

- Patient gown
- Drape
- Local anesthetic
- Sterile, disposable lumbar puncture kit
- Instrument stand
- Sterile gloves
- Permanent marker to label tubes
- Laboratory requisitions as needed
- Biohazard lab transport bag
- Patient record

PROCEDURAL STEPS

1. Assemble the materials needed, and prepare the room. Prepare the equipment and supplies needed for the lumbar puncture.
2. Wash your hands. Follow standard precautions.
   <u>PURPOSE:</u> Infection control.
3. Identify the patient and introduce yourself. Explain to the patient that you will go over what is going to happen step by step to ensure the best results.
4. Have the patient void just before the procedure.
   <u>PURPOSE:</u> To improve the patient's comfort during the procedure.
5. Give the patient a hospital gown, and have him or her put it on with the opening down the back.
6. Place the patient in a left, side-lying fetal position for the lumbar puncture.
   <u>PURPOSE:</u> To give the physician the easiest access to the lumbar region of the spine.
7. Support the patient's head with a pillow as necessary, and provide a pillow for between the knees if needed also.
   <u>PURPOSE:</u> Make the patient as comfortable as possible for the procedure.
8. Perform a sterile skin preparation of the patient's lumbar region in the usual manner.

<u>PURPOSE:</u> To prevent bacterial infection at the puncture site.

9. Place the sterile disposable lumbar puncture kit on an instrument stand and open it, establishing a sterile field. Drape a sterile fenestrated drape over the lumbar region of the patient, so that only the L3-L4 region of the lower spine is exposed.
   <u>PURPOSE:</u> To isolate the area of the procedure in a sterile field.
10. When the physician is ready to do the lumbar puncture, provide the local anesthetic by holding the vial for the physician or pouring it into the sterile medicine cup on the sterile field.
    <u>PURPOSE:</u> To maintain sterile technique and expedite the procedure.
11. Reassure the patient, and help him or her to hold still during the injection of the local anesthetic and the insertion of the spinal needle.
    <u>PURPOSE:</u> To facilitate accurate insertion of the spinal needle by the physician.
12. Using the permanent marker, label the specimens #1, #2, and #3 in the order in which they are collected. This is a critically important step in this procedure.
    <u>PURPOSE:</u> Different tests are done on different tubes. The accuracy of these tests is dependent on the tube on which they are performed.
13. Complete the laboratory requisition form, and prepare the CSF specimens for transport to the laboratory.
    <u>PURPOSE:</u> To ensure that all the necessary tests are ordered correctly.
14. Clean the area by disposing of sharps, biohazard materials, and regular waste in the normal manner.
15. Monitor the patient, and give liquids as directed by the physician.
16. Document the procedure in the patient's chart.

See Appendix D for a charting example.

---

responsible for homeostasis, or maintaining complete balance in the body. Through its many receptors, the nervous system constantly monitors what is going on inside the body and in the environment outside of the body.

When the nervous system becomes damaged or diseased, signs and symptoms can appear in every other body system. Motor activity can become erratic, or activity level can decrease to the point that the person becomes unable to communicate or function normally.

Your main responsibilities as a medical assistant in neurology are to observe, listen, and report any changes in patients. Even signs and symptoms that may seem rather slight may give the physician the one clue needed to put the puzzle together and arrive at a correct diagnosis before proceeding to an appropriate treatment. It is crucial that medical assistants working in a neurology practice recognize the importance and significance of a variety of symptoms. For example, severe headache accompanied by vomiting may indicate a serious intracranial problem that needs immediate attention. The medical assistant in a neuro-logy practice must remain alert to these types of situations at all times because neurologic emergencies can occur quite rapidly.

Legal and Ethical Issues

In neurology you will be faced with a variety of behaviors and personality changes that are frequently a part of neurologic conditions. Often a patient is not aware of these changes and may appear as though nothing is wrong. You must treat this patient with the same dignity and respect as you would all other patients, despite how the patient may be treating you. Some patients are concerned that loved ones have turned against them and are treating them in an abusive manner. A patient's family may be experiencing severe emotional stress in coping with the patient's behavior. You must remember the medical assistant's code of ethics and the need for total confidentiality. Whatever is discussed in the examination room cannot be repeated to other staff members in the office and never discussed outside the office. Confidentiality must be strictly observed.

Health Insurance Portability and Accountability Act Applications

Although patients typically have the right to obtain a copy of their confidential health information, under the Health Insurance Portability and Accountability Act (HIPAA) privacy regulations, patients do not have the right to access their psychotherapy notes. These notes are not suppose to be stored in the patient's general chart and should not be released to third-party payors. Disclosure of psychotherapy notes requires specific patient permission before any documentation can be released to an insurance provider. Under federal law it is up to the therapist to decide if the notes will be released to the patient, and if the therapist decides not to release the information, the patient cannot appeal this decision. However, the final authority rests with individual state laws. If a state law is stricter than the federal mandate or gives the patient greater access to psychotherapy notes, then state law takes precedence over federal law.

SUMMARY OF SCENARIO

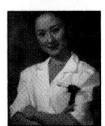

Mai has excelled in her new position as clinical assistant and patient educator. With Dr. Song's approval, she has developed a series of patient information sheets that explain what the nervous system is, what symptoms to watch for after a head injury, the kinds and causes of headaches, and infections of the nervous system. Patients often ask for information sheets for other family members and for their friends and neighbors. She also developed a set of information sheets to explain typical neurologic diagnostic tests and how best to prepare for them. Although the patient receives a copy of the information sheet, Mai still talks with each patient to ensure that he or she understands exactly what is going to happen for the test and to ensure that all questions are completely answered. Mai feels a great deal of personal satisfaction from working with patients and helping them understand their diagnosis and treatment protocols.

SUMMARY of LEARNING OBJECTIVES

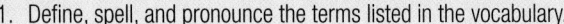

1. Define, spell, and pronounce the terms listed in the vocabulary.
   - Spelling and pronouncing medical terms correctly adds credibility to the medical assistant. Knowing the definition of these terms promotes confidence in communication with patients and co-workers.
2. Summarize the anatomy and physiology of the nervous system.
   - The main function of the nervous system is to control body functions so homeostasis can be maintained. It does this by receiving messages in the CNS from the PNS, then sending a response to the appropriate location in the body, again via the PNS. The neuron is the functional cell of the nervous system, and neuroglial cells support and protect neurons throughout the system. The brain is made up of the cerebrum, cerebellum, and brain stem. The CNS is well protected, first by the skull and then by the dura mater, arachnoid mater, and pia mater meninges.
3. Differentiate between the central and peripheral nervous systems.
   - The nervous system is made up of two parts: the CNS, which includes the brain and spinal cord, and the PNS, which includes all of the nerves outside of the CNS.
4. Identify the typical symptoms associated with neurologic disorders.
   - Symptoms of potentially serious neurologic conditions include headache, nausea and vomiting, change in vision, altered level of consciousness, memory loss, sleep disorders, confusion or disorientation, and problems with mobility.
5. Distinguish among common nervous system diseases and conditions.
   - Table 43-3 summarizes the most common nervous system diseases and conditions.
6. Describe the pathology of cerebrovascular diseases.
   - CVD may be caused by atherosclerosis, hypertension, thrombi, emboli, or aneurysm. A TIA is a temporary limiting of function as a result of short-term ischemia. A CVA occurs when blood supply to a particular part of the brain is cut off by an embolus, a thrombus, or an aneurysm that bursts. Migraine headaches are associated with a disturbance in the blood supply to the brain.
7. Identify the various types of epilepsy.
   - Seizures are classified as either partial or generalized, based

Continued

SUMMARY of LEARNING OBJECTIVES

Continued

on how much of the brain is involved in the abnormal electrical activity. Partial seizures result from abnormal electrical activity in just one part of the brain, whereas generalized seizures involve most or all of the brain. Generalized seizures include petit mal seizures, which are brief episodes characterized by staring, subtle body movement and brief lapses of awareness. Probably the most well known seizure disorder is the generalized tonic-clonic disorder that causes grand mal seizures.

8. Compare and contrast encephalitis and meningitis.
   - Encephalitis is a viral infection of the brain that can cause serious CNS symptoms. Meningitis may be caused by a virus, bacteria, or fungus. Bacterial meningitis is most serious. Viral meningitis usually resolves without treatment or incident.

9. Explain the dynamics of head and spinal cord injuries.
   - Traumatic brain injuries can range from a mild concussion to severe injury, coma, and death. A minor concussion usually causes no long-term side effects; however, a moderate to severe brain injury can result in headaches, amnesia, confusion, personality changes, and seizures. The higher the damage to the spinal cord, the more serious the injury. Head injuries can be either open or closed, with possible serious intracerebral damage and potential complications within the meningeal layers. Shaken baby syndrome is caused by violently shaking an infant back and forth, forcing the brain against opposite ends of the skull.

10. Summarize the neurologic diseases that affect mobility.
   - PD is a chronic, progressive, debilitating neurologic disease that is caused by lack of the neurotransmitter dopamine. MS causes progressive inflammation and demyelination of the axon, resulting in a scattering of the nervous message as it passes down the axon. ALS is a rapidly progressive, destructive, ultimately fatal neurologic disease that destroys the motor neurons responsible for voluntary muscle control. Bell's palsy causes temporary facial paralysis because of damage or trauma to the seventh cranial nerve of the face. Peripheral neuropathies can result from damage or injury to any portion of

the neuron and are typically caused by other system diseases such as diabetes. CTS results from compression of the median nerve as it passes through the carpal bones of the wrist.

11. Differentiate among common mental health disorders.
   - Depressive disorders affect the way a person thinks, feels, eats, and sleeps. People with depression cannot "snap out of it" and without treatment may suffer from symptoms that last for weeks, months, or years. Types of depressive disorders include major depression, dysthymic, and bipolar disorders. Anxiety disorders cause an overwhelming, irrational feeling of anxiety and fear and include panic disorder, OCD, posttraumatic stress disorder, and phobias. Risk factors for suicide include serious depression disorders; decreased serotonin levels; a prior suicide attempt; family violence; and exposure to the suicidal behavior of others. Schizophrenia is a chronic, severe, and disabling brain disorder with symptoms that include hallucinations and delusions; difficulty speaking and expressing emotions; and cognitive deficits.

12. Analyze the medical assistant's role in the neurologic examination.
   - When assisting in neurology, the medical assistant must be particularly careful to recognize signs and symptoms, which frequently are quite subtle but yet can be extremely significant in helping to assess and diagnose the neurologic patient accurately. Refer to Procedure 43-1.

13. Explain the common diagnostic procedures for the nervous system.
   - Neurologic system diagnostic tests are summarized in Table 43-5 and include arteriograms, CT and MRI scans, EEG, lumbar puncture, PET scan, and various x-ray studies.

14. Outline the steps needed to prepare a patient for an EEG test.
   - Procedure 43-2 outlines the steps needed to prepare a patient for an EEG test.

15. Describe the procedural steps for preparing a patient for and assisting with a lumbar puncture.
   - Procedure 43-3 describes the procedural steps for preparing a patient for and assisting with a lumbar puncture.

CONNECTIONS

Study Guide Connection: Go to Chapter 43 Study Guide. Read the Case Study and Workplace Applications and complete the assignments. Do online research for answers to the questions in the Internet Activities associated with assisting in neurology and mental health.

CD Connection: Go to the Medical Assisting Competency Challenge CD and do the training activities under Patient Care. For a better understanding of neurological function, view the animation for brain anatomy.

evolve **Evolve Connection:** For more information related to assisting in neurology and mental health, go to evolve.elsevier.com/kinn and visit related weblinks for Chapter 43. Click on the Medical Assisting Exam Review and do the practice questions to sharpen your test-taking skills

Assisting in Endocrinology

44

SCENARIO

Miguel Vasco has been a CMA for 10 years and has worked for the last 3 years with a multiphysician endocrinology and internal medicine practice. Although he has taken care of patients with many different endocrinologic disorders, the majority of the case load for the practice consists of individuals with type 2 diabetes mellitus. One of Miguel's responsibilities includes teaching newly diagnosed diabetic patients how to monitor their blood glucose levels and maintain healthy lifestyles.

While studying this chapter, think about the following questions:

- What are the primary medical assisting responsibilities in an internal medicine practice?
- What clinical skills are required in this specialty practice?
- What are the common endocrine system diseases and disorders that CMAs working in this field should be able to discuss and explain?
- What diagnostic and treatment procedures are typically used in an endocrinology practice?
- What information should the CMA know about the management of diabetes and the possible complications associated with the disease?

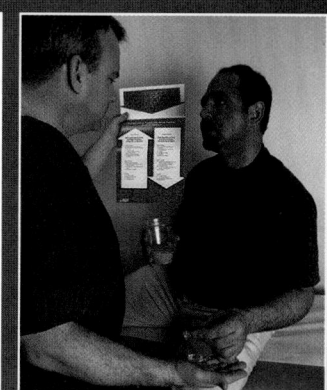

LEARNING OBJECTIVES

1. Define, spell, and pronounce the terms listed in the vocabulary.
2. Summarize the anatomy of the endocrine system.
3. Explain the mechanism of hormone action.
4. Differentiate among common endocrine disorders.
5. Describe the diagnostic criteria for diabetes mellitus.
6. Outline the treatment plan and management of diabetes mellitus.
7. Perform blood glucose screening with a Glucometer.
8. Identify the characteristics of hyperglycemia and hypoglycemia.
9. Compare and contrast type 1, type 2, and gestational diabetes mellitus and prediabetes.
10. Categorize the complications associated with diabetes mellitus.
11. Summarize patient education approaches to diabetes.

National Accreditation Competencies and Content

CAAHEP COMPETENCIES

Clinical

3.b.(4)(f). Prepare patient for and assist with procedures, treatments, and minor office surgeries

General

3.c.(3)(b). Instruct individuals according to their needs
3.c.(3)(c). Provide instruction for health maintenance and disease prevention

ABHES COMPETENCIES

Clinical Duties

4.b. Prepare patients for procedures
4.h. Prepare patient for and assist physician with routine and specialty examinations

Instruction

7.b. Instruct patients with special needs
7.c. Teach patients methods of health promotion and disease prevention

adrenocorticotropic hormone (ACTH) (uh-dren-o-cor-ti-ko-tro′-pik)   A hormone that stimulates the production and secretion of glucocorticoids; released by the anterior pituitary gland.

follicle-stimulating hormone (FSH) A hormone secreted by the anterior pituitary; stimulates oogenesis and spermatogenesis.

gluconeogenesis (glu-kuh-ne-uh-je′-nuh-suhs) The formation of glucose in the liver from proteins and fats.

glycogen   The sugar (starch) formed from glucose and stored mainly in the liver.

glycosuria The abnormal presence of glucose in the urine.

growth hormone (GH) Also called *somatotropic hormone;* stimulates tissue growth and restricts tissue glucose dependence when nutrients are not available.

luteinizing hormone (LH) (lu-te-uh-niz′-ing) Hormone produced by the anterior pituitary gland; promotes ovulation.

nocturia Excessive urination during the night.

polydipsia (pah-le-dip′-se-uh) Excessive thirst.

polyphagia (pah-le-faj′-e-uh) Increased appetite.

polyuria (pah-le-yur′-e-uh) Excessive urine production.

prolactin (PRL) Hormone secreted by the anterior pituitary gland; stimulates the development of the mammary gland.

specific gravity Weight of urine compared with an equal volume of water.

thyroid-stimulating hormone (TSH) A hormone secreted by the anterior pituitary gland that stimulates the secretion of hormones produced by the thyroid gland.

Individuals with endocrine system disorders are usually seen first by the primary care physician (PCP) and may be referred to either an internist or an endocrinologist for specialized care. Patients with certain endocrine disorders, such as diabetes mellitus (DM), may also be seen in clinic settings for follow-up and treatment. The medical assistant can be employed in any of these ambulatory care settings, assisting with diagnostic procedures and specialized examinations as well as patient education. It is important that the medical assistant understand the dynamics behind endocrine system diseases as well as be able to assist patients in understanding how to administer their medication and prevent long-term complications from their disease.

ANATOMY AND PHYSIOLOGY OF THE ENDOCRINE SYSTEM

Both the nervous system and the endocrine system control the body's physiologic responses to internal and external stimuli. The nervous system is electrical in nature and sends immediate messages along a nerve pathway to evoke a response, while the endocrine system relies on the bloodstream to carry hormonal messages to a target cell for action. Through hormonal action, the endocrine system regulates all body functions. *Endocrinology* is the study of hormones, their receptor cells, and the results of hormone action.

The word part *endo-* means in or within; the suffix *-crine* means secrete. The endocrine system consists of glands located throughout the body that produce and secrete chemicals known as *hormones.* Hormones function as the body's chemical messengers, transferring information from one group of cells to another. Hormones control growth, mood, system functions, metabolism, sexual maturity, and reproduction. Hormone levels vary and can be affected by outside factors such as illness and stress.

Basic Anatomy

Glands are identified as either exocrine or endocrine. *Exocrine* glands, such as sweat glands and salivary glands, secrete either through a duct or directly onto the surface of the skin or in the mouth. *Endocrine* glands release hormones directly into the bloodstream, where they are transported to target cells for action.

Figure 44-1 identifies the primary glands of the endocrine system including the hypothalamus, pituitary, thyroid, parathyroids, and adrenals and the reproductive glands—the ovaries and the testes. Some nonendocrine organs, especially the pancreas, can also produce and release hormones. The hypothalamus, located in the inferior midportion of the brain, is the major connection between the nervous and endocrine systems. The hypothalamus controls the action of the pituitary gland, a pea-sized gland located below the hypothalamus. The pituitary gland is often called the "master gland" because it secretes hormones that regulate multiple endocrine glands.

The pituitary gland is separated into two parts: the anterior and posterior lobes. The anterior pituitary, or *adenohypophysis,* regulates the functions of the thyroid, adrenals, and reproductive glands. It produces **growth hormone (GH), thyroid-stimulating hormone (TSH), adrenocorticotropic hormone (ACTH), prolactin (PRL), follicle-stimulating hormone (FSH), and luteinizing hormone (LH).** The posterior lobe of the pituitary, or *neurohypophysis,* excretes *oxytocin,* which stimulates the contractions of the smooth muscle of the uterus that occur during labor and the flow of breast milk toward the nipple when an infant breastfeeds. The posterior pituitary also produces *antidiuretic hormone* (ADH), which helps to control fluid balance by acting on the kidneys to reabsorb fluid as needed to maintain homeostasis (Figure 44-2).

When stimulated by TSH, the thyroid gland produces the thyroid hormones triiodothyronine (T_3) and thyroxine (T_4), which control the body's metabolic rate and are important factors

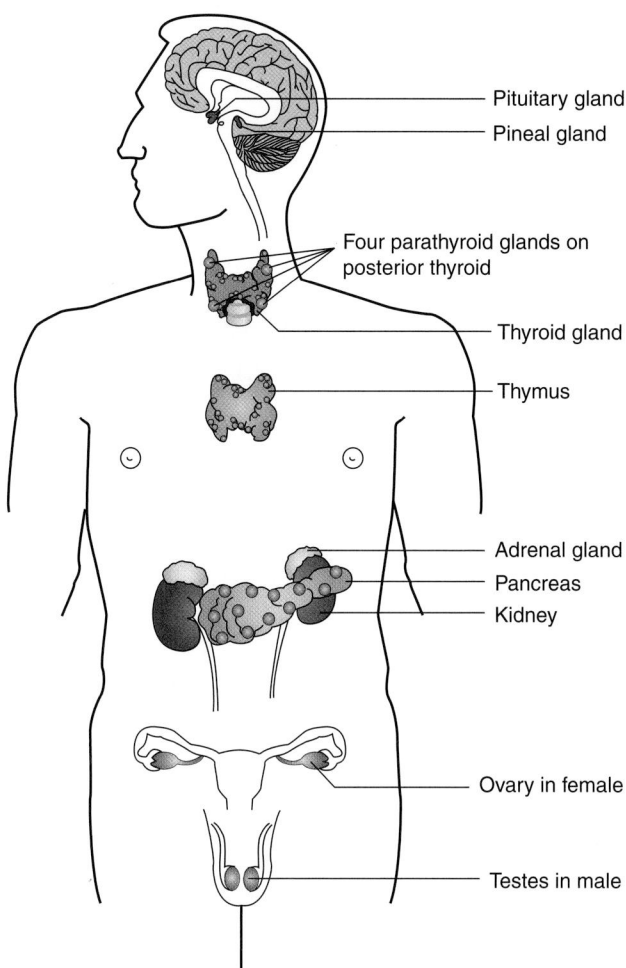

FIGURE 44-1 Location of the endocrine glands. (From Gould: *Pathophysiology for the health professions*, ed 2, Philadelphia, 2002, Saunders.)

Pituitary gland
Pineal gland

Four parathyroid glands on posterior thyroid

Thyroid gland

Thymus

Adrenal gland
Pancreas
Kidney

Ovary in female

Testes in male

in bone growth and nervous system development in children. On the dorsal aspect of the thyroid gland are several small parathyroid glands, which release hormones (parathyroid and calcitonin) that regulate the level of calcium in the blood. The parathyroid hormone (PTH) maintains a constant concentration of calcium in the body by regulating absorption of calcium from the gastrointestinal tract and stimulating reabsorption of calcium stored in the bone as needed to maintain homeostasis. Calcitonin stimulates deposition of calcium into the bone when excess amounts of calcium are available.

On the top of each kidney are the adrenal glands, triangular-shaped glands consisting of an outer layer called the *adrenal cortex* and an inner body called the *adrenal medulla*. The adrenal cortex secretes corticosteroid hormones, including cortisol, aldosterone, and adrenal androgens that influence a wide range of bodily functions. The adrenal medulla produces epinephrine, also called *adrenaline,* which activates the body's reaction to stress.

The gonads produce sex hormones. The male gonads are the testes; they secrete testosterone, which regulates the development of secondary sexual characteristics, such as voice changes and the growth of facial and pubic hair, and promotes the production of sperm. The female gonads, the ovaries,

produce eggs or ova *(oogenesis)* and secrete estrogen and progesterone. The female hormones control the development of breast tissue and other secondary sexual characteristics, regulate menstruation, and play important roles during pregnancy.

The pancreas performs essential endocrine functions by producing insulin and glucagon, which work together to maintain normal blood glucose levels and store glucose for energy.

CRITICAL THINKING APPLICATION

Miguel is asked to order education supplies for patients with endocrine system disorders. Because he thinks it is important for patients to understand their health problems, he wants to order a brochure that clearly depicts and describes the anatomy of the endocrine system. What glands and organs should be included in the handout?

Mechanisms of Hormone Action

The goal of hormone regulation is to maintain homeostasis. Hormone secretion is regulated by a number of mechanisms, including nervous stimulation, endocrine control (a hormone from one gland, such as the anterior pituitary, stimulates the release of a hormone from another gland), and feedback systems. An example of nervous system regulation of endocrine function is the release of adrenaline from the adrenal medulla in response to stimulation from the sympathetic nervous system during a stressful episode. In the most common feedback system, *negative feedback,* an endocrine gland is activated by an imbalance and acts to correct the imbalance by stopping the secretion process. For example, if calcium blood levels fall below normal, the parathyroid glands are stimulated to release PTH. PTH acts to increase blood calcium levels by either stimulating the absorption of calcium from the gut or demineralizing bone to release stored calcium. This change in the blood calcium level is detected by the parathyroid gland, which then stops production of PTH.

Each hormone that is released into the bloodstream has particular *target cells* for action. The target cells have receptors that attract only specific hormones and permit the hormone to pass through the cell membrane and affect cellular action.

DISEASES AND DISORDERS OF THE ENDOCRINE SYSTEM

Faulty secretion of any hormone, whether too much or too little, can cause health problems for patients. The goal of treatment is either to control the hypersecretion of hormones or to replace hormones that are not being secreted at therapeutic levels.

Posterior Pituitary Gland Disorder

Diabetes Insipidus

When ADH (or *vasopressin*) is not produced or released in sufficient amounts, the patient develops a condition called *diabetes insipidus.* ADH increases the permeability of the renal tubules and collecting tubules in the kidneys, permitting fluid to be reabsorbed and causing the urine to become more concentrated. Without the action of ADH, fluid is not reabsorbed

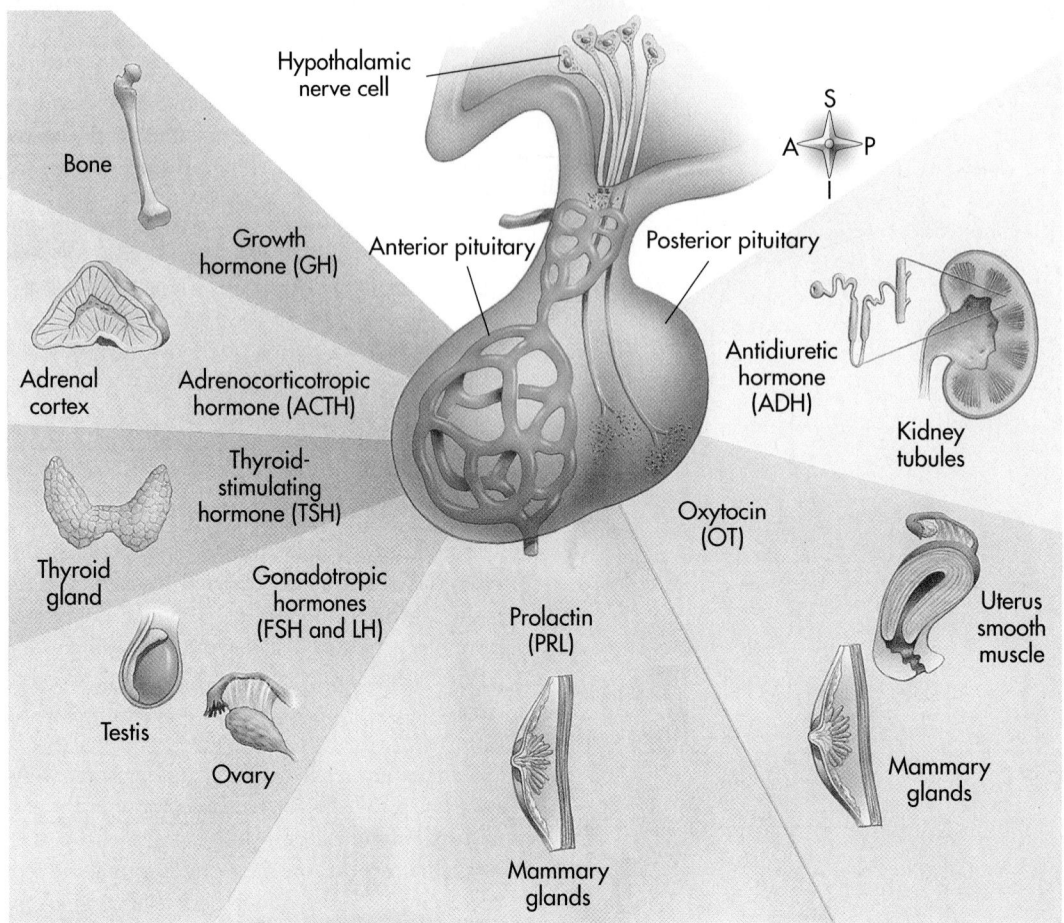

FIGURE 44-2 Pituitary hormones. Principal anterior and posterior pituitary hormones and their target organs. (From Thibodeau GA, Patton KT: *The human body in health and disease*, ed 4, St Louis, 2005, Mosby.)

from the renal tubules, which causes a large amount of fluid to be excreted in the urine, with the potential onset of dehydration in the patient. A lack of ADH results from either a tumor in the hypothalamus or posterior pituitary gland or diabetes insipidus, which may develop because of an inadequate response to ADH in the renal tubules.

Diabetes insipidus usually has an acute onset, with the patient presenting with **polyuria, polydipsia, nocturia,** low urine **specific gravity,** and high blood plasma *osmolality* (concentration). It can result in fatal dehydration if fluid and electrolyte levels cannot be controlled. Replacement therapy with a synthetic vasopressin (desmopressin) nasal spray can be used to treat the disorder.

Diseases of the Anterior Pituitary

Hormones secreted by the anterior pituitary control a number of glandular functions. The effects on the body to altered anterior pituitary gland secretions are dependent on whether the hormones are being produced at an abnormally low level *(hypopituitarism)* or if they are being produced at a very high level *(hyperpituitarism).* If a patient is diagnosed with *panhypopituitarism,* there is a deficiency of all of the hormones produced

by the anterior pituitary; thus symptoms will reflect systemic inactivity of all of the glands stimulated by the anterior pituitary hormones.

Growth Hormone Abnormalities

Hypopituitary dwarfism occurs when the pituitary gland fails to produce normal amounts of GH. The child's height is impaired, but he or she will have a normal size head and trunk. Hypersecretion of GH causes two different disorders, depending on the developmental age of the patient. Oversecretion of GH in childhood before the epiphyseal plates in the long bones have closed will cause the long bones to grow excessively. Those affected may reach 8 feet or taller. Because GH has a secondary effect on the blood glucose level, these persons may develop DM. Slow-growing, benign anterior pituitary adenomas are frequently the cause of gigantism, and treatment consists of removing the tumor if possible, radiation therapy, or drug therapy.

If hypersecretion of GH occurs in adulthood, the disorder is called *acromegaly.* The epiphyseal plates are closed so the long bones cannot grow. Therefore a wide range of manifestations can occur because of the growth of excessive connective tissue and overproduction of bone. Signs and symptoms include arthralgia, an enlarged tongue, overactive sebaceous and sweat glands, coarse skin, excessive body hair, and nerve damage caused by pressure exerted on peripheral nerves by increasing amounts of bone and soft tissue. There is a gradual but noticeable enlargement in the bones of the jaw, face, hands, and feet (Figure 44-3). Advanced acromegaly causes complications such as congestive heart failure, DM, cerebrovascular abnormalities, and neurologic symptoms as the tumor grows within the confined space of the hypothalamus. Treatment of acromegaly requires either surgical removal or irradiation of the pituitary tumor.

CRITICAL THINKING APPLICATION

Many different disorders can occur if there is a problem with the anterior pituitary. Describe two such health problems using your knowledge of target organ action.

Disorders of the Thyroid

Hypothyroidism

Deficient secretion of the thyroid hormones may result from a number of factors. One cause of hypothyroidism is endemic iodine deficiency, a lack of iodine in the diet, resulting in the

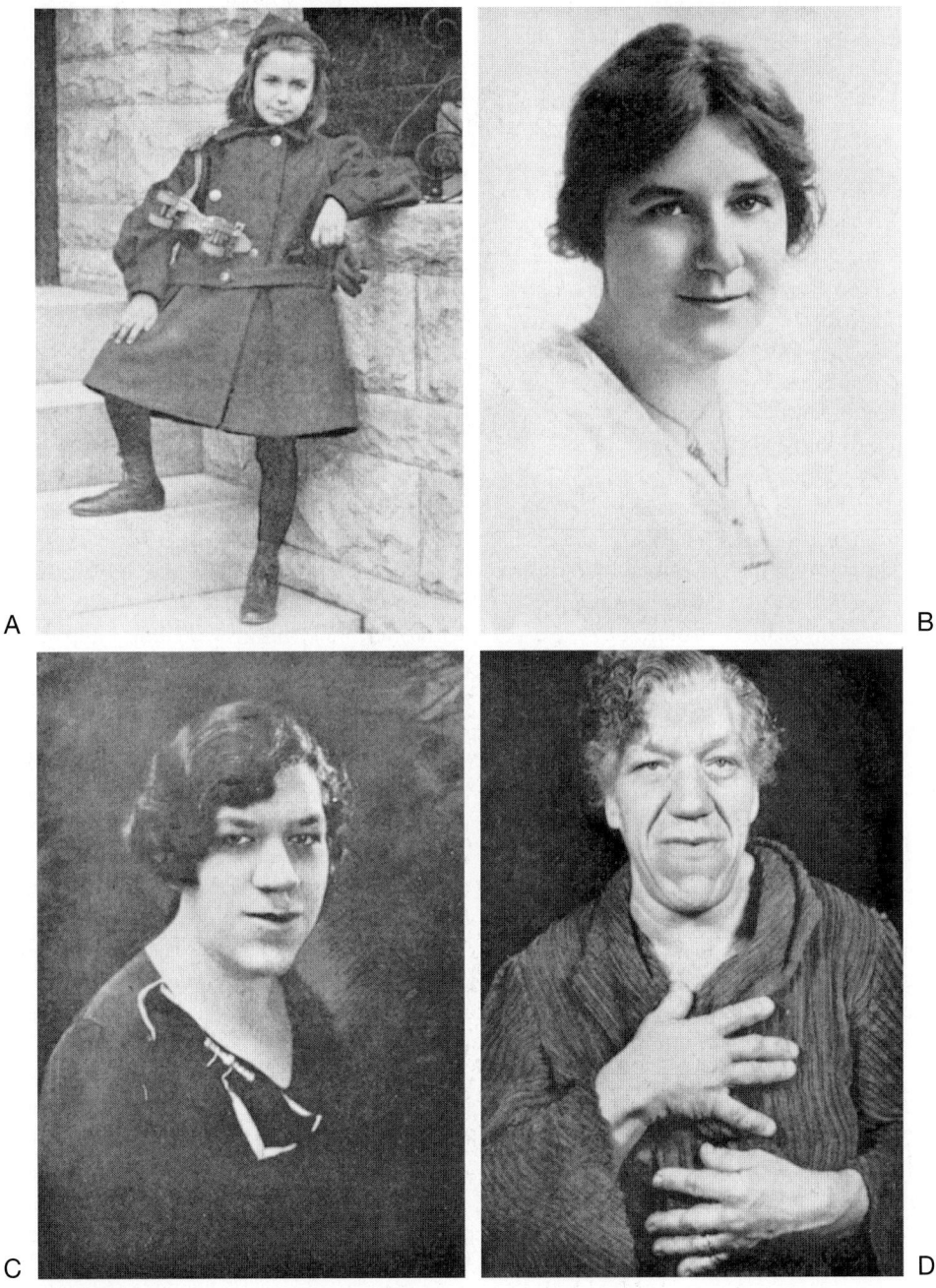

A
B
C
D

FIGURE 44-3 Progression of acromegaly. **A,** Patient at age 9 years. **B,** Patient at age 16 years, with possible early features of acromegaly. **C,** Patient at age 33, with well-established acromegaly. **D,** At age 52, end-stage acromegaly. (From Clinical Pathological Conference, *Am J Med* 20:133, 1956.)

formation of a simple goiter. A *simple goiter* is any thyroid enlargement that has not been caused by an infection or neoplasm. Endemic goiters occur in certain geographic areas. If more than 10% of the children 6 to 12 years of age in a particular area have goiters, that geographic location is defined as endemic for goiters.

T_3 and T_4 are produced in the thyroid gland from iodine and are responsible for the regulation of metabolic activities in all body cells. When the thyroid gland is unable to obtain sufficient amounts of iodine from the circulating blood, it enlarges or *hypertrophies* in an attempt to produce the hormones needed by the body. A decreased amount of thyroid hormones results in a lower metabolic rate, heat loss, and poor mental and physical development. The incidence of iodine deficiency is rare in the United States because of the widespread use of iodized table salt and the distribution of foods from iodine-rich areas. The treatment for a simple goiter is to reduce its size by prescribing dietary supplements of iodine, thyroid hormone replacement, or surgery.

Improper development of the thyroid in an infant or young child is usually congenital. The absence of adequate levels of thyroid hormones results in a condition known as *cretinism*. Newborns exhibit feeding problems, constipation, and a hoarse cry, and they sleep for extreme lengths of time. Symptoms include lethargy, bradycardia, stunted skeletal growth, and varying degrees of mental retardation, depending on the severity and the length of the hypothyroidism.

When severe or chronic hypothyroidism occurs in an adult or older child, the condition is called *myxedema*. The patient exhibits fatigue, weight gain, loss of hair, slower pulse rate, lowered body temperature, muscle cramps, menorrhagia, and thick, dry, puffy skin. Routine tests to diagnose hypothyroidism include radioimmunoassay, a radiologic blood test, for T_3, T_4, and TSH. Adequate doses of thyroxine (Levothroid, Levoxyl, or Synthroid) will restore normal function and appearance. Patients diagnosed with hypothyroidism must take hormone replacement therapy daily for the rest of their lives.

Hyperthyroidism

Thyrotoxicosis, a condition in which the serum levels of thyroid hormones are excessively high, can also be caused by a number of factors. Symptoms include weight loss, tachycardia, palpitations, hypertension, agitation, nervousness, depression, tremor, excessive sweating, goiter, and *exophthalmia* (protruding eyes). Graves' disease, an autoimmune disorder that stimulates overactive thyroid hormone production, is the most common cause of thyrotoxicosis (Figure 44-4). The goal of treatment is to control excessive thyroid hormone production through drug therapy (carbimazole, methimazole, and propylthiouracil), radioactive implants to destroy part of the gland, or surgical removal of a section of the gland. After radiation or surgical removal of part of the thyroid gland, the patient's thyroid hormone levels are evaluated. It is frequently necessary for the patient to receive replacement hormone therapy (Levothroid, Levoxyl, or Synthroid) postoperatively to maintain normal thyroid hormone levels.

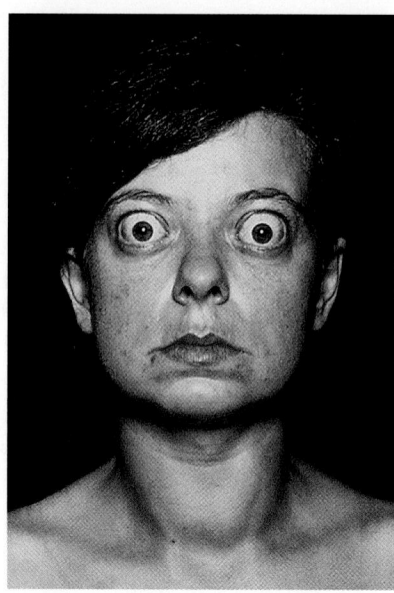

FIGURE 44-4 Exophthalmos in Graves' disease. (From Seidel HM et al: *Mosby's guide to physical examination*, ed 6, St Louis, 2006, Mosby.)

CRITICAL THINKING APPLICATION

One of the internists, Dr. Misha, asks Miguel if he could describe the signs and symptoms a patient with hypothyroidism or hyperthyroidism would exhibit. Summarize his answer.

Disorders of the Adrenal Gland

Adrenal insufficiency is called *Addison's disease*. This condition is relatively rare and is caused by an autoimmune reaction that affects the adrenal cortex, which secretes corticosteroid hormones. Symptoms include hypoglycemia, increased pigmentation of the skin, muscle weakness, gastrointestinal disturbances, and fatigue. Cortisol and aldosterone deficiencies lead to retention of potassium and the excretion of water and sodium in the urine. Severe dehydration, low blood volume, low blood pressure, and circulatory shock can occur. Treatment includes long-term daily administration of glucocorticoids (such as prednisone), an adequate fluid intake, maintaining a balance of sodium and potassium, and a diet high in complex carbohydrates and protein.

Hypersecretion of the adrenal cortex, causing increased levels of cortisol, is known as *Cushing's syndrome*. Usually a pituitary tumor or a tumor of the adrenal cortex causes the release of excessive amounts of ACTH. The tumor may be benign or malignant. Symptoms associated with Cushing's syndrome may be seen in persons who are receiving corticosteroids for medical reasons such as organ transplants, severe asthma, or rheumatoid arthritis. Excessive levels of cortisol cause an accumulation of adipose tissue in the trunk, a round or "moon" face, and fat pads in the cervical spine region, causing the formation of a "buffalo hump" (Figure 44-5). The patient also exhibits glucose intolerance because of insulin resistance at the target cell level.

Additional symptoms include hyperpigmentation, muscle wasting, problems with wound healing, hypertension, kidney

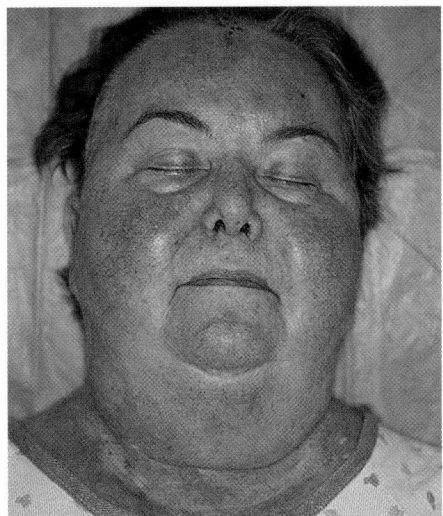

FIGURE 44-5 Cushing's syndrome. (From Seidel HM et al: *Mosby's guide to physical examination*, ed 6, St Louis, 2006, Mosby.)

stones, and osteoporosis. Female patients exhibit menstrual irregularity, and many patients with Cushing's syndrome experience mental disorders such as irritability, depression, or severe psychiatric disorders. Treatment is dependent on the cause of the disorder but includes medication, radiation, and surgery.

Endocrine Dysfunction of the Pancreas: Diabetes Mellitus

DM is a common hormonal imbalance that has reached epidemic proportions in the United States. Approximately 21 million Americans, or 7% of the population, have diabetes, and this number is growing. Diabetes occurs in people of all ages and races but is more common in aging persons as well as African Americans, Latinos, Native Americans, and Asian Americans/Pacific Islanders. DM is characterized by chronic hyperglycemia and problems with carbohydrate metabolism. This problem with glucose management is caused by either a lack of insulin production and/or resistance to insulin at the target cell level. The pancreas contains islets of Langerhans, which produce and secrete the hormones insulin and glucagon. When the blood glucose level is too high, beta islet cells secrete insulin, which is sent through the bloodstream to the target tissue site to conduct glucose into the cell. Glucagon is secreted by the alpha islet cells when blood glucose levels are low, to stimulate the liver to convert **glycogen** (stored glucose) into circulating glucose.

If there is resistance to insulin at the target cell wall or there is not enough insulin to help transport glucose from the blood into the cells, an individual experiences a variety of symptoms including **glycosuria,** polyuria, polydipsia, **polyphagia,** rapid weight loss, drowsiness, fatigue, itching of the skin, visual disturbances, and skin infections. The American Diabetes Association identifies four major types of diabetes: type 1 DM, type 2 DM, gestational diabetes, and prediabetes. If left untreated or managed poorly, DM can have serious, life-threatening consequences such as cardiovascular disease, stroke, hypertension, blindness, kidney disease, nervous system disorders, amputations, pregnancy complications, and diabetic coma. Patient education

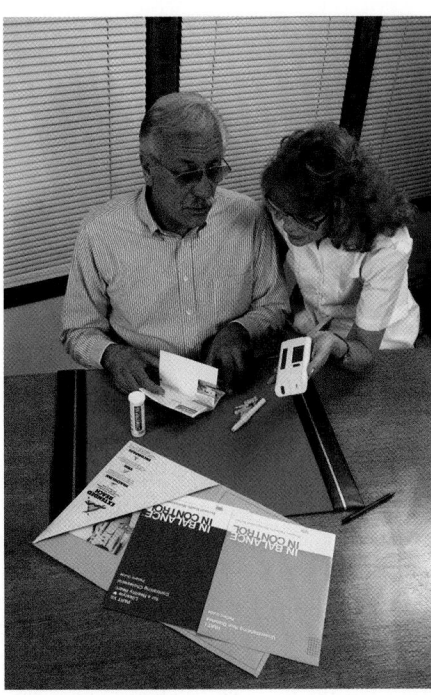

FIGURE 44-6 Educating patients about the risks of diabetes is an important part of the medical assistant's job.

is crucial for compliance with treatment and prevention of life-threatening complications (Figure 44-6).

Prediabetes

Prediabetes is a condition in which an individual has a higher than normal blood glucose level but not high enough for a diagnosis of type 2 diabetes. It is estimated that 41 million people in the United States, ages 40 to 74, have prediabetes. Some of the long-term damage to vascular and cardiac systems may be occurring during prediabetes. Studies indicate that the majority of individuals with prediabetes develop type 2 diabetes within 10 years. However, if patients lower blood glucose levels, they can delay or prevent its onset. Experts recommend that patients with prediabetes lose 5% to 10% of their weight and perform moderate physical activity for 30 minutes daily. A loss of just 10 to 15 pounds can make a huge difference in blood glucose levels.

Two different tests are used to diagnose prediabetes: the fasting plasma glucose test (FPG) or the oral glucose tolerance test (OGTT). A person with prediabetes has a fasting blood glucose level between 100 and 125 mg/dL, and individuals with an FPG of 126 mg/dL or higher are diagnosed as diabetic. A prediabetic would have a 2-hour OGTT of 140 to 199 mg/dL, and diabetes is diagnosed if the OGTT is 200 mg/dL or higher.

Type 1 Diabetes

Type 1 diabetes most often develops in children and young adults and was previously known as either *juvenile-onset diabetes* or *insulin-dependent diabetes*. In type 1 DM the pancreas is unable to produce insulin because of the destruction of the beta islet cells from autoimmune, genetic, or environmental factors. Type 1 diabetes typically has an acute onset and affects 5% to 10% of patients with diabetes. Insulin administration is required for

Diagnostic Criteria for Diabetes Mellitus

- Plasma glucose level of ≥200 mg/dL (norm is 80 to 120 mg/dL) with the classic symptoms of polyuria, polydipsia, and unexplained weight loss
- Fasting plasma glucose level ≥126 mg/dL (norm is 70 to 110 mg/dL) on more than one occasion
- 2-hour oral glucose tolerance test (OGTT) result ≥200 mg/dL
- Urinalysis positive for glucose and possibly ketones
- Glycosylated hemoglobin >7% (normal range is 4% to 6%)

Alternative Insulin Administration Methods

- An insulin pump is a computerized device that administers a constant dose of insulin using a small portable pump. The pump is programmed to deliver a measured dose of insulin by continuous subcutaneous infusion through a catheter. This method more closely resembles the body's normal surge of insulin and is designed to maintain blood glucose levels consistently within normal limits.
- Insulin can be administered through an injector pen that comes in preloaded cartridges for easy use (Figure 44-7). Insulin pens are disposable or refillable and easily portable and so can be used by diabetic patients when they are away from home.
- An inhaled form of insulin, Exubera, was released in 2006. Exubera is a meal-time insulin in powdered form that should be taken 10 minutes before eating. People with type 1 diabetes may use Exubera in place of meal-time injections of rapid-acting insulin but still have to take injections of longer-acting insulin; those with type 2 diabetes may use it as an alternative or in combination with traditional oral medications. Potential side effects include low blood glucose, dry mouth, chest discomfort, and decreased lung capacity.

the treatment of type 1 diabetes. The goal for insulin therapy is to maintain blood glucose levels as close to normal as possible without causing hypoglycemia. Many types and brands of insulin are available, but only genetically engineered human insulin should be used, to prevent allergic reactions. At this time the only method for insulin administration is injection because gastrointestinal processes destroy insulin if it is given by mouth; however, multiple studies are in progress with buccal, inhaled, and patch forms of the hormone. Subcutaneous administration of insulin was presented in Chapter 34. The medical assistant is usually involved in teaching patients how to administer their insulin accurately. Table 44-1 summarizes the various types of insulin. Although insulin should be stored in the refrigerator, injecting the cold solution may be painful for the patient. Therefore the physician may recommend that the patient store the bottle that is in use at room temperature for up to 1 month. Extreme temperatures can damage the drug so it should not be frozen, left in the sunlight, or carried in the glove compartment of a car.

Successful type I diabetic treatment is a complicated combination of insulin injections using various types of insulin in multiple injections (as many as four) throughout the day. The insulin type and dosage are balanced by the patient's typical exercise regimen as well as diet. The patient must monitor blood glucose levels using a glucometer periodically during the day to determine whether they are within the normal range. The physician will typically prescribe glucometer testing in the morning before breakfast, before dinner, and possibly before lunch and at bedtime if the patient is having difficulty keeping

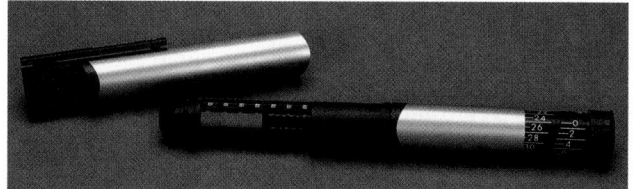

FIGURE 44-7 Nova Pen.

the blood plasma levels stabilized. An important responsibility of the medical assistant is to teach the patient how to perform glucometer screening (Procedure 44-1).

Glucometers are palm sized and use very small amounts of capillary blood from a site in the finger, forearm, upper arm, or abdomen (Figure 44-8). There are many different types of glucometers available, but regardless of the type of machine, test results are displayed within seconds, and the results are stored for future reference. The medical assistant should stress that the accuracy of blood glucose results depends on following the

TABLE 44-1 Insulin Types and Characteristics

INSULIN TYPE	ONSET OF ACTION	PEAK ACTION	DURATION	APPEARANCE
Humalog (Lispro), NovoLog (Aspart)	10-15 min	30-90 min	4 hr	Clear
Regular	30-60 min	2-4 hr	5-7 hr	Clear
NPH	60-120 min	6-14 hr	24 hr	Cloudy
Lente	60-180 min	6-14 hr	24 hr	Clear
Ultralente	6 hr	18-24 hr	36 hr	Clear
Glargine (Lantus)	2-4 hr	Peakless	20-24 hr	Clear
70:30 (70% NPH, 30% Regular)	70%: 60-120 min 30%: 30-60 min	70%: 6-14 hr 30%: 2-4 hr	70%: 24 hr 30%: 5-7 hr	Cloudy Cloudy

PROCEDURE 44-1

Prepare Patient for and Assist with Procedures, Treatments, and Minor Office Surgeries: Perform a Blood Glucose Accu-Chek Test

<u>CAAHEP COMPETENCY:</u> 3.b.(4)(f)
<u>ABHES COMPETENCIES:</u> 4.b, 4.h

GOAL: *To perform accurately a blood test for possible diabetes mellitus.*

EQUIPMENT and SUPPLIES

- Accu-Chek glucose monitor or similar glucose monitoring device
- Accu-Chek glucose testing strip
- Lancet and autoloading finger-puncturing device
- Alcohol preps
- Gauze squares
- Sharps container
- Disposable gloves
- Patient record

PROCEDURAL STEPS

1. Check the physician's order, and collect the necessary equipment and supplies needed to complete the testing procedure. Perform quality-control measures according to manufacturer guidelines and office policy.

2. Wash your hands, and put on gloves.
   <u>PURPOSE:</u> Infection control.

3. Ask the patient to wash his or her hands in warm soapy water, then to rinse them in warm water and dry them completely.
   <u>PURPOSE:</u> Clean the area that will be punctured; warm fingers may increase peripheral blood flow.

4. Check the patient's index and ring fingers, and select the site for puncture.
   <u>PURPOSE:</u> Site of puncture must be free of trauma.

5. Turn on the Accu-Chek monitor by pressing the ON button (Figure 1*).

6. Make sure the code number on the LED display matches the code number on the container of test strips.
   <u>PURPOSE:</u> If code numbers do not match, the device must be reprogrammed with the new code for the test results to be valid.

7. Remove a test strip from the vial, and immediately replace the vial cover.
   <u>PURPOSE:</u> Vial must be closed to protect unused strips from possible contamination.

8. Check the strip for discoloration by comparing the color of the round window on the back of the test strip with the designated "unused" color chart provided on the test strip vial label.
   <u>PURPOSE:</u> This will establish the validity of the testing procedure.

9. Do not touch the yellow test pad or round window on the back of the strip when handling the strip.

10. When the test strip symbol begins flashing in the lower right-hand corner of the display screen, insert the test strip into the designated testing slot until it locks into place. When the test strip is inserted correctly, the arrows on the test strip will be facing up and pointing toward the monitor (Figure 2).

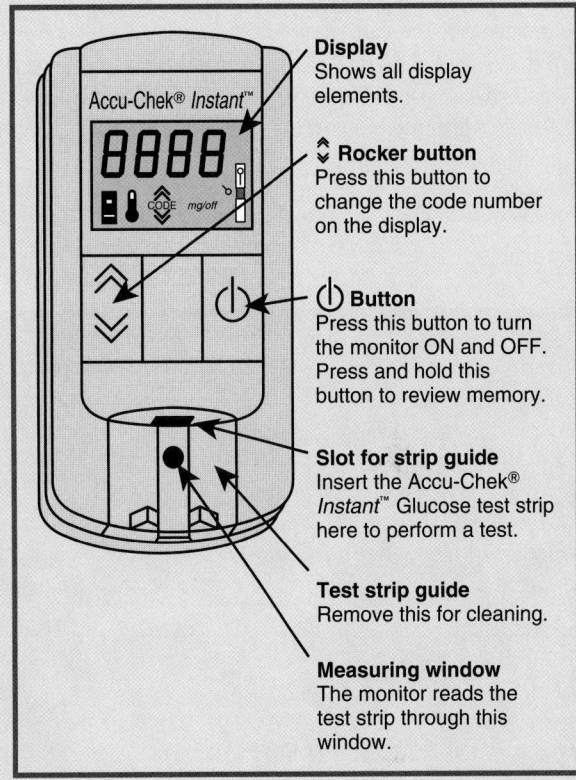

Display
Shows all display elements.

Rocker button
Press this button to change the code number on the display.

Button
Press this button to turn the monitor ON and OFF. Press and hold this button to review memory.

Slot for strip guide
Insert the Accu-Chek® *Instant*™ Glucose test strip here to perform a test.

Test strip guide
Remove this for cleaning.

Measuring window
The monitor reads the test strip through this window.

FIGURE 1

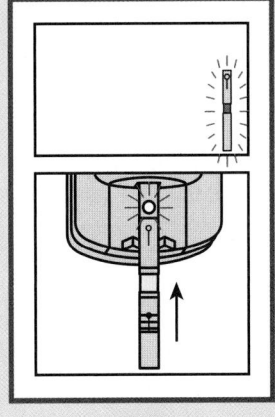

FIGURE 2

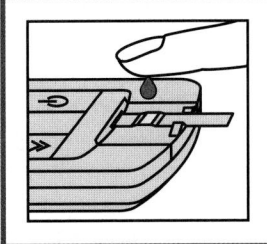

FIGURE 3

11. Cleanse the selected site on the patient's fingertip with the alcohol wipe, and allow the finger to air dry.

12. Perform the finger puncture, and wipe away the first drop of blood.
    <u>PURPOSE:</u> There may be tissue fluid present in the first drop of blood.

Continued

PROCEDURE 44-1—cont'd

13. Apply a large hanging drop of blood to the center of the yellow testing pad (Figure 3).
    a. Do not touch the pad with the patient's finger.
    b. Do not apply a second drop of blood.
    c. Do not smear the blood with your finger.
    d. Be certain the yellow test pad is saturated with blood.
14. Give the patient a gauze square to hold securely over the puncture site.
15. The monitor will automatically begin the measurement process as soon as it senses the drop of blood.
16. Read the test result when it is displayed in the display window in milligrams per deciliter.

17. Turn off the monitor by pressing the "0" button.
18. Discard all biohazard waste into the proper waste containers.
    PURPOSE: Infection control.
19. Clean the glucometer according to manufacturer guidelines, disinfect the work area, remove gloves and dispose of them properly, and wash your hands.
20. Record the testing results in the patient's medical record.
    PURPOSE: A procedure is considered not done until it is recorded.

*Figure from Stepp CA, Woods MA: *Laboratory procedures for medical office personnel,* Philadelphia, 1998, Saunders.
See Appendix D for a charting example.

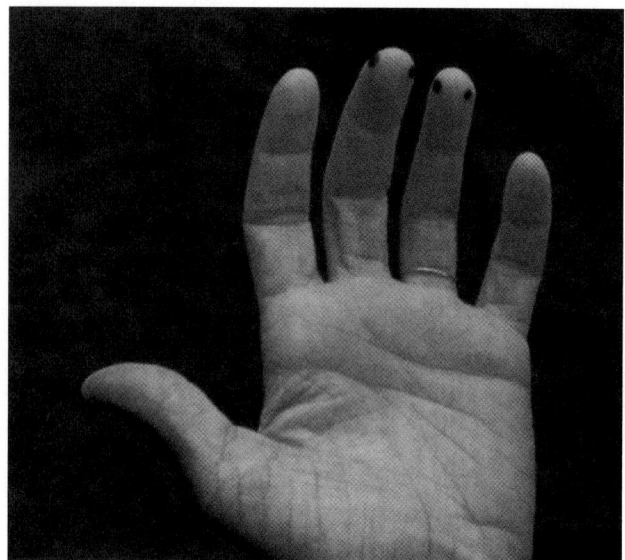

FIGURE 44-8 Capillary puncture sites on fingers.

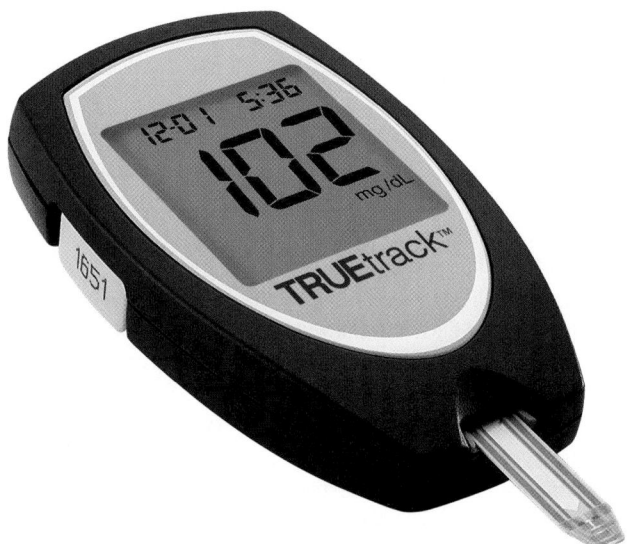

FIGURE 44-9 Blood glucose monitoring device, TrueTrack®. (Courtesy TrueTrack Smart System® by Home Diagnostics, Inc.)

instructions for the particular type of glucometer used by the patient. It is important to use the same machine that the patient will use at home when teaching the patient about glucometer screening and to stress keeping a record of glucometer readings to determine long-term serum glucose control.

The patient education intervention should include not only the steps for successfully checking blood glucose levels but also quality-control mechanisms as suggested by the manufacturer of the machine (Figure 44-9). Some examples of quality controls include the following:

- Correctly follow manufacturer instructions.
- Perform instrument maintenance specified by the manufacturer, including correct cleaning and storage of the instrument.
- Check expiration dates on test strips and solutions, and store these products correctly.
- Match and correctly enter the test strip code into the instrument before use.

- Contact the physician if test results do not match patient symptoms.

Patients with diabetes also need to find the best method for disposal of their syringes and lancets. Local pharmacies or hospitals may offer assistance with disposal of used sharps. If the patient does not have access to a sharps return program, a puncture-resistant container with an opening that can be easily and tightly sealed before disposal is a good choice.

Regardless of the type of diabetes, for treatment to be successful, patients must play an active role in the management of their disease. The medical assistant should consistently encourage patients to be active participants in maintaining blood glucose levels within the normal range and constantly be on alert for possible complications from their disease. The ideal is to maintain blood plasma levels as close to the norm as possible to prevent complications. The American Diabetes Association recommends blood levels between 90 and 130 mg/dL before meals and less than 180 mg/dL 2 hours after starting a meal, with a glycated (glycosylated) hemoglobin level less than 7%.

Type 2 Diabetes

Type 2 DM, once called *adult-onset* or *non–insulin-dependent diabetes*, usually develops in adults but may be seen at any age. Factors that increase the risk of developing type 2 DM include a family history, a history of gestational diabetes, impaired glucose tolerance, physical inactivity, and obesity. In this type of DM the pancreas produces insulin, but not enough, and/or the target cells are resistant to insulin action. Type 2 diabetes is responsible for 90% to 95% of the total cases of diabetes mellitus.

This form of diabetes frequently goes undetected for many years because of the gradual onset of hyperglycemia and the absence of classic diabetic symptoms. However, because of this insidious onset overtime, patients with type 2 diabetes are at even greater risk for developing vascular complications. Insulin resistance at the target cell level may improve with weight reduction and/or pharmacologic treatment.

Treatment for type 2 diabetes includes weight loss, exercise, dietary restrictions, and oral hypoglycemic medications that act to stimulate insulin production and/or improve tissue response to insulin. Some common oral hypoglycemics are Diabinese, Prandin, Glucophage, Avandia, Actose, and Precose. Medications for type 2 diabetes have multiple functions, including stimulation of insulin secretion from pancreatic islet cells in patients with some pancreatic function; decreasing insulin resistance at the cellular level; improving sensitivity to insulin in muscle and adipose tissue; and inhibiting hepatic **gluconeogenesis.**

As with type 1 diabetes, the goal of treatment for type 2 is to maintain blood glucose levels within the normal range. For some patients, exercise, diet, and weight loss are sufficient to control blood glucose levels. Sometimes just the loss of 10 to 20 pounds is enough to bring blood glucose levels under control. Other patients may need medication to maintain normal blood glucose levels; however, levels must be monitored

daily with a glucometer to determine the success of treatment. Over time, the type 2 diabetic may require insulin for control of hyperglycemia. Table 44-2 summarizes the characteristics of hyperglycemia and hypoglycemia.

Injectable Drugs Recently Approved for Type 2 Diabetes

- Pramlintide (Symlin) is a synthetic form of the hormone amylin that works with insulin and glucagon to maintain normal blood glucose levels; injections taken with meals help improve A_{1c} levels; approved for people with type 1 diabetes who are not achieving recommended A_{1c} levels and people with type 2 diabetes who are using insulin but not achieving A_{1c} goals.
- Exenatide (Byetta) lowers blood glucose levels by increasing insulin secretion; injected with meals; helps patients achieve modest weight loss and improved glycemic control.

CRITICAL THINKING APPLICATION

Carlos Vespa is a 47-year-old patient who was recently diagnosed with type 2 DM. He is 52 pounds overweight; eats a high-fat, high-carbohydrate diet; and does not exercise. What health issues should Miguel include in his patient teaching intervention? Mr. Vespa tells Miguel he cannot afford the medication prescribed by the physician or the glucometer needed to monitor his blood glucose levels. Is there anything Miguel can do to help him with these issues?

Gestational Diabetes

A pregnant woman is diagnosed as having gestational diabetes if she has any two of the following:

- A fasting blood sugar (FBS) greater than 105 mg/dL
- During an OGTT, a 1-hour glucose level greater than 190 mg/dL, a 2-hour glucose level greater than 165 mg/dL, or a 3-hour glucose level greater than 145 mg/dL

Gestational diabetes is considered a risk factor for developing type 2 DM later in life and affects about 4% of pregnant women in the United States each year.

TABLE 44-2 Characteristics of Hyperglycemia and Hypoglycemia

DISEASE	CAUSES	ONSET	SIGNS AND SYMPTOMS	TREATMENT
Hyperglycemia: High serum glucose level	Too little insulin Body not able to use insulin properly Too many calories Not enough exercise Illness Stress	Slow	Polyphagia, polyuria, glycosuria, ketonuria, weight loss, pruritus Possible ketoacidosis with shortness of breath, "fruity" breath, dry mouth, nausea and vomiting, lethargy	Exercise if blood glucose level below 240 mg/dL Decrease caloric intake Physician may alter amount and timing of insulin
Hypoglycemia: Low serum glucose level	Too much insulin Not enough calories Overexercise People with type 2 diabetes using insulin-boosting medications	Rapid	Shakiness, vertigo, palpitations, diaphoresis, headache, hunger, pallor, fatigue, confusion, irritability, poor judgment Visual disturbances, seizures, coma	Ingest sugar; glucose tablets recommended Monitor blood levels in 15 minutes If still low and symptoms persist, take another glucose tablet If patient passes out, physician can order injected glucagon; *call for emergency services*

Some factors that increase the risk of developing gestational diabetes are obesity; maternal age over 40 years; history of delivering infants who weigh more than 10 pounds at birth; a family history of diabetes; previous, unexplained stillbirth; previous birth with congenital anomalies; smoking; and belonging to certain ethnic groups, including Hispanics, Native Americans, Asian Americans, and blacks. Some women are asymptomatic, whereas others exhibit classic symptoms of diabetes. Because many pregnant women have gestational diabetes without obvious symptoms, all pregnant women are routinely screened between the twenty-fourth and twenty-eighth weeks.

Gestational diabetes is precipitated by a buildup of insulin resistance at the cellular level, resulting in hyperglycemia. The elevated glucose in the mother's blood passes through the placenta into the baby, causing hyperglycemia with increased insulin production in the fetus. The extra carbohydrate energy is stored in the infant as fat and may result in a *macrosomic* or "fat" baby who is at higher risk for breathing problems at birth, obesity, and type 2 diabetes.

The treatment goal for gestational diabetes is to keep plasma glucose levels equal to those of pregnant women without the disorder. The treatment plan always includes special meal plans and regular physical activity. In obese women a 30% calorie reduction will reduce hyperglycemia. Some women may require insulin to maintain blood glucose levels within therapeutic range and thereby decrease the possible complications for the fetus. Most women return to normal glucose tolerance postpartum. However, two out of three women will experience gestational diabetes in future pregnancies. Because these women are at greater risk for developing type 2 diabetes later in life, patient education should stress weight management, a healthy diet, and regular exercise to maintain normal blood glucose levels.

Complications of Diabetes Mellitus

Acute Complications. Two acute complications can occur in diabetic patients, depending on the level of glucose in their bloodstream. If an adult patient's blood glucose level is below 45 to 60 mg/dL, the exhibited symptoms are caused by hypoglycemia. This reaction is related to insulin treatment and may also be called *insulin shock*. Symptoms are those shown with hypoglycemia in Table 44-2. The goal is to prevent such episodes with adequate patient education and reinforcement of individualized medical management of diabetes as well as frequent blood glucose monitoring. The treatment for hypoglycemia is immediate glucose replacement. The recommended form of sugar supplement is glucose tablets because each tablet contains a known amount of glucose. The patient can use other sugar supplements—such as candy, orange juice with sugar, or nondiet soft drinks—but the quantity of glucose in these items is unknown and the patient may actually become hyperglycemic from the ingestion of too much glucose. After the hypoglycemic crisis has ended, if the next meal is more than 1 hour away the patient should have a mixed protein and carbohydrate snack (peanut butter crackers, cheese crackers) to maintain blood glucose levels until the next meal.

The more serious acute complication is *diabetic ketoacidosis*, or diabetic coma. In this case the person with diabetes is unable

Treating Hypoglycemia: Rule of 15

- Take 15 g of carbohydrate (CHO) if glucometer reading is lower than 80 mg/dL.
- 15 g of CHO equals three glucose tablets, 1/2 cup fruit juice, five or six pieces of hard candy.
- Wait 15 minutes and check glucometer reading again; if level is still low, repeat the treatment.
- After symptoms are relieved, eat regular meal as planned to maintain plasma glucose levels.
- Treat hypoglycemia immediately, because it may cause the patient to faint.
- The physician may order injected glucagon to quickly raise blood plasma levels.

to use glucose for energy because insulin is either absent or insufficient or there is resistance to insulin at the target cell site. Hyperglycemia results, with blood glucose levels rising to 300 to 750 mg/dL. Because cells cannot use carbohydrates for energy, the body begins to burn fat. Ketones are waste materials from fat metabolism that build up in the bloodstream and cause it to become more acidic. Although the development of ketoacidosis takes longer than insulin shock, it can become a medical emergency if the patient does not recognize the signs, monitor his or her blood glucose level, and administer insulin as prescribed by the physician.

CRITICAL THINKING APPLICATION

Mr. Vespa returns to the office one week later and tells Dr. Misha he has not been feeling well. Sometimes he feels very shaky, dizzy, and tired; he has been getting headaches and cannot think straight. Dr. Misha orders a glucometer reading, which shows Mr. Vespa's blood glucose level at 65. Dr. Misha's diagnosis is hypoglycemic episodes, and Dr. Misha asks Miguel to reinforce patient teaching about hypoglycemic and hyperglycemic signs and symptoms as well as treatment. What should Miguel include in the teaching intervention? How can he best reinforce the material so that Mr. Vespa will remember how to manage his disease?

Chronic Complications

Microvascular disease. Arterial changes at the capillary level can occur within 1 to 2 years of the onset of DM. Hyperglycemic episodes combined with the duration of the disease cause degeneration of tissue arterioles, which results in multiple system disorders, including *diabetic retinopathy*. Diabetes is a leading cause of new blindness in people 20 to 74 years of age and is often a result of 8 to 10 years of diabetes. Ninety percent of patients with type 1 diabetes and 65% of patients with type 2 diabetes will develop retinopathy.

Hyperglycemic episodes damage the blood vessels in the retina; therefore close glucose control helps delay the onset of retinopathy and slows its progression. The disturbances of vision occur from vascular changes in the capillaries of the retina. These complications can lead to retinal detachment and blindness. In addition, people with diabetes are at much higher risk for developing glaucoma and cataracts and should receive yearly eye screenings and frequent ophthalmologic examinations during routine office visits for early diagnosis of diabetic retinopathy.

Microvascular disease can also cause *diabetic nephropathy.* Kidney disease is present in 10% to 21% of all diabetic persons and is the most common cause of kidney failure in the United States. Diabetic kidney disease is the greatest threat to life in adults with type 1 diabetes. Diabetes damages the small blood vessels in the kidneys and impairs their ability to filter waste from blood. Degenerative changes cause destruction of the glomerular unit and can lead to renal failure. High blood pressure and smoking often are associated with diabetic nephropathy. Because urinary protein is usually the first sign of kidney damage, frequent testing for albuminuria is suggested. Early treatment reduces the progression of kidney disease. Good glucose control can often reverse the early stages of diabetic nephropathy. With disease progression, renal failure may occur, resulting in the need for dialysis and possible kidney transplant.

Macrovascular disease. Macrovascular disease, in the form of atherosclerosis, is a serious health issue for all diabetic patients, especially those with type 2 DM. Persons who have diabetes are two to four times more likely to have atherosclerotic heart disease or strokes. Coronary artery disease (CAD) is the most common cause of death for those with type 2 diabetes. Patients most affected are women at or before middle age. The longer the patient has had diabetes, the greater the risk for CAD. Cerebrovascular accidents (CVAs, or strokes) occur twice as frequently in diabetic compared with nondiabetic patients. Hypertension is common in diabetic persons and contributes to the CAD and CVA rates.

Peripheral vascular disease (PVD), a disease process in blood vessels outside the heart, is associated with atherosclerotic changes in small arteries and arterioles and contributes to the incidence of gangrene and amputations in diabetic patients. Patients with type 2 diabetes frequently have signs and symptoms of PVD when first diagnosed. Compromised circulation in the lower extremities causes the formation of ulcers, poor wound healing, and possible progression to gangrene. This progression of PVD may result in amputation of the toes, foot, or leg. Blockage of blood vessels can lead to impotence in diabetic men. About 13% of men with type 1 and 8% of men with type 2 diabetes have impotence from diabetic vascular disease.

Diabetic neuropathy. Diabetic neuropathy is the most common complication of diabetes, with 60% to 70% of persons with diabetes experiencing some form of diabetic nerve damage. This type of nerve damage is caused by both vascular changes and hyperglycemia. The chief areas that exhibit pathology are the nerves and blood vessels in the eyes, kidneys, legs, and feet. The first signs of diabetic neuropathy are usually numbness, pain, or tingling in the hands, feet, or legs. The loss of sensation in the extremities is important because it affects the patient's ability to be aware of injuries, especially to the feet. Because of peripheral vascular compromise, foot injuries can develop into ulcers or lesions that can become infected and ultimately lead to gangrene and amputation (Figure 44-10). Even a minor undetected

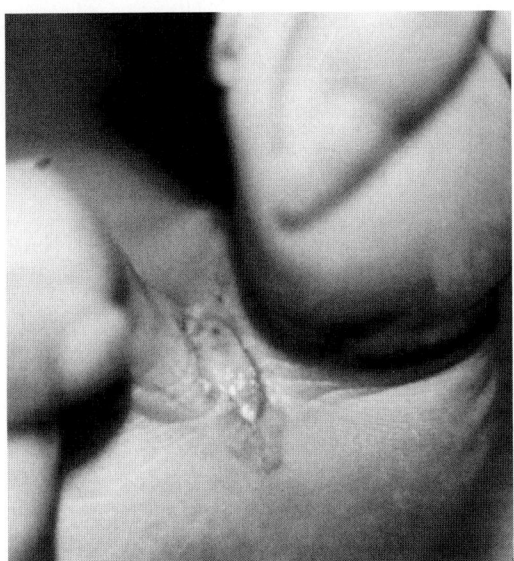

FIGURE 44-10 Ulceration between toes from wearing thong sandals. (From Levin ME: Pathogenesis and general management of foot lesions in the diabetic patient. In Bowker JH, Pfeifer MA, editors: *Levin and O'Neal's the diabetic foot*, ed 6, St Louis, 2001, Mosby.)

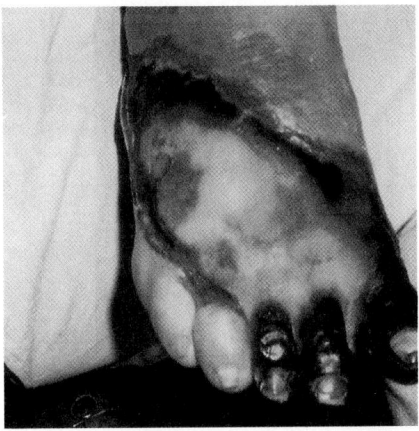

FIGURE 44-11 Diabetic patient with peripheral neuropathy and an insensate foot. Cold packs were applied to the patient's foot for treatment of a sprain. Frostbite developed, and the patient required a transmetatarsal amputation. (From Levin ME: Pathogenesis and general management of foot lesions in the diabetic patient. In Bowker JH, Pfeifer MA, editors: *Levin and O'Neal's the diabetic foot*, ed 6, St. Louis, 2001, Mosby.)

injury, such as a foot blister, can lead to a serious problem for the diabetic patient. Diabetic individuals may also lose temperature sensation and so are more susceptible to heat or cold injuries such as burns and frostbite (Figure 44-11). Diabetic patients should have their feet inspected at every physician office visit to promote early detection and treatment of problems. Healthcare providers should provide verbal and written advice to help prevent or reduce these potentially serious injuries.

Infection. All diabetic patients are at increased risk for infection because of a number of different factors. Those with impaired vision and neuropathies have an increased risk of injury because they may not be able to see or feel potentially dangerous items to prevent injury. Once an injury does occur and the integrity of the skin has been compromised, damaged or atherosclerotic

Questions to Ask When Screening for Diabetic Neuropathy (from the American Diabetes Association)

- Can you feel your feet when walking?
- Have you noticed weakness in the muscles of your feet and legs?
- Do you have problems with balance when standing or walking?
- Do you have trouble feeling heat or cold in your feet or hands?
- Do you have open sores on your feet and legs that heal slowly?
- Have you noticed that your feet have changed shape?
- Do your feet tingle or feel like "pins and needles," or do you have burning or shooting pains in your feet? Do they hurt at night? Are they numb?
- Are your feet very sensitive to touch?
- Do your feet and hands get very cold or very hot?

Diabetic Foot Care

Diabetic patients need instruction about foot hygiene and foot inspection during each visit. Education guidelines should include:

- Wash the feet every day with warm (not hot) water and mild soap.
- Cut nails straight across to avoid ingrown toenails and possible injuries.
- Apply lotion to the feet, especially the heels. If the skin is cracked or red, speak to your doctor.
- Check your feet every day, using a mirror if necessary. Call your doctor at the first sign of redness, swelling, or numbness.
- Speak with your doctor before treatment of corns, calluses, or bunions.
- Do not go barefoot or allow your feet to get too hot or cold.
- Check shoes for foreign objects or rough areas before wearing them.
- Wear comfortable, well-fitting shoes.
- Stop smoking. Smoking causes vasoconstriction, which decreases circulation to the extremities.

blood vessels are unable to deliver the blood needed for healing, and the thickened blood vessel walls impede the release of white blood cells (WBCs) to the area. The WBCs of diabetic patients exhibit reduced phagocytosis, and so their ability to destroy pathogens is limited. In addition, some pathogens multiply rapidly in the glucose-rich environment of diabetic patients. Therefore the best method of controlling infections in diabetic patients is to prevent skin trauma or damage.

CRITICAL THINKING APPLICATION

Mr. Vespa and his wife are scheduled for a long visit today so Dr. Misha can review his treatment plan. Dr. Misha asks Miguel to reinforce the possible complications of DM and criteria for foot care. What should Miguel include in his teaching intervention? How can he make sure Mr. and Mrs. Vespa understand the disease, its management, and possible complications?

DIABETIC PATIENT FOLLOW-UP

Experts agree that the best method for prevention of diabetic complications is to maintain blood glucose levels consistently at near-normal ranges. Several laboratory tests can be ordered to monitor patient blood glucose levels. A test that measures the glucose levels in a blood specimen from a fasting individual is an FBS test. Often the test is referred to as an FPG and requires a 12-hour fast. The normal range established for an FPG is 70 to 110 mg/dL. Even though the physician may order periodic FBS tests, both type 1 and type 2 diabetic patients need to check their blood glucose levels as ordered using home glucometer devices.

A routine test for monitoring long-term diabetes therapy is the glycosylated hemoglobin (HbA_{1c}) test. This test has distinct advantages over routine FBS studies because the FBS reflects glucose levels at a given point in time, whereas the glycosylated hemoglobin test reflects serum glucose control over several months. The test measures glucose levels that have been chemically bound to the hemoglobin molecule on the red blood cell (RBC) over a 120-day period (the lifespan of an RBC). The physician can then assess average daily glucose levels over the preceding 2 to 3 months and therefore assess treatment compliance and results. The patient does not need to restrict food or fluid intake for this test and should continue to take prescribed medication before the blood sample is drawn. The patient's total glycosylated hemoglobin level should be less than 7%. The higher the glycosylated hemoglobin result, the higher the risk that a patient will develop diabetic complications.

Developing a Diabetic Patient Education Plan

Newly diagnosed individuals with diabetes should have their plan of care developed from a holistic point of view. Holistic care means that the diabetic team (including the medical assistant) considers all aspects of the patient's needs, including lifestyle factors such as diet and level of exercise; medications and the education needed to comply with their use; education that includes the details of their disease as well as its possible complications; demonstration and return demonstration as needed until the patient is proficient in glucometer testing and/or insulin administration; family involvement in the treatment process; and the use of community resources such as a diabetic educator, support group, and dietician to assist with management of the disease (Figure 44-12). The equipment and

Correlation between A₁c Levels and the Average Plasma Glucose Levels

A_{1c} (%)	Plasma Glucose (mg/dL)
6	135
7	170
8	205
9	240
10	275

From the American Diabetes Association.

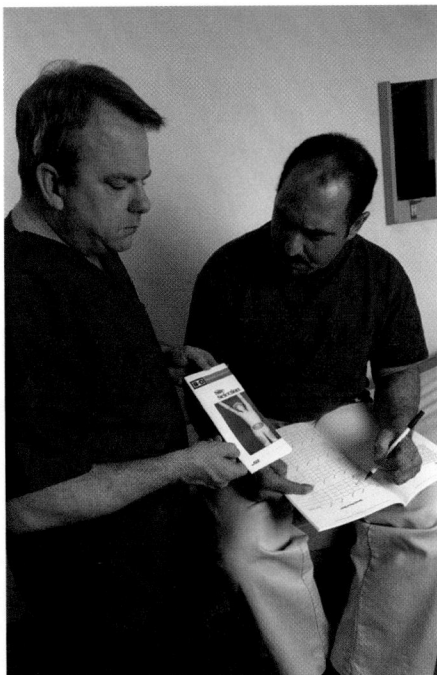

FIGURE 44-12 The medical assistant can use premade education materials to discuss new lifestyle habits with a diabetic patient.

supplies needed to treat diabetes effectively can be extremely expensive, so the medical assistant should investigate alternative methods of getting these materials if the patient is unable to afford them. The need for continuous daily glucose control must be emphasized at each patient visit. The medical assistant can research various websites and suggest that these be explored.

CLOSING COMMENTS

Patient Education

Because management of endocrine disorders can be quite complicated, the medical assistant must be certain the patient understands the proper procedures for at-home treatment. By demonstrating a given procedure in the office, the medical assistant can address any inaccurate information or answer any questions the patient may have. Visual materials, such as brochures and procedure cards, are also helpful because they can be taken from the office and used as a reminder. If the patient is taking medication, the medical assistant should review the dosage schedule with the patient, discuss the purpose of the treatment, and clarify any confusion over the physician's instructions. As always, if the medical assistant is uncertain of any procedures or information, he or she should ask the physician for assistance before explaining anything to the patient.

Legal and Ethical Issues

Pathophysiology of the endocrine system can have wide-reaching effects on the functioning of the affected patient. Patient education interventions should be completely documented to

---

Diabetic Patient Education

- Physical activity (too much or too little), stress, the presence of disease, medication, and diet all combine to affect blood glucose levels; following an effective dietary plan is the first step toward self-management.
- The medical assistant measures the patient's weight and height and should reinforce the physician recommended body mass index (BMI); supply information about basic nutritional requirements needed either to help the individual maintain his or her ideal body weight or to lose weight.
- The goal of a diet plan is to help maintain a homeostatic blood glucose level. If a healthy blood glucose level is maintained, the patient will avoid complications that can develop with hypoglycemia or hyperglycemia. Basic guidelines, according to the person's ethnic influences, age, sex, and physical activity, are used to establish a therapeutic meal plan. (Refer to Chapter 29 for meal planning.) Family members should be involved in dietary health teaching, and appropriate community resources, such as a registered dietician, should be used to assist with patient understanding and compliance.
- Medical management of diabetes can be quite complicated and overwhelming for many patients. People with type 2 diabetes who are prescribed oral hypoglycemics must understand their mechanism of action and accurate dosage. Patients with type 1 and type 2 diabetes who require daily insulin must be able to prepare and administer their medication accurately and understand the connection between glucometer readings and insulin dosage. All diabetic patients must be capable of accurate glucometer use and must be aware of the possible complications of their disease.

---

have legal proof of the information shared with the patient. Never assume that the patient understands the disease process and treatment recommendations. Suggestions that ensure patient welfare and promote risk management include the following:

- Advise patients that a medic alert bracelet with his or her diagnosis and medication information is an important safeguard.
- Patients must take medication as prescribed, following directions for dosage, route of administration, and storage and being alert for possible side effects.
- Newly diagnosed diabetic persons should avoid driving until glycemic control is stabilized and should be warned about possible visual impairment from the disease.
- Remember that you are always representing your profession and employer, and respond to each situation accordingly.
- Ask for assistance or further information if you feel unprepared to perform a procedure or to give accurate information.

SUMMARY OF SCENARIO

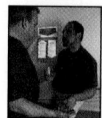

In his interactions with clients, Miguel has learned to pay attention to both verbal and nonverbal messages. He has used this technique consistently when interacting with Mr. Vespa. Miguel recognizes the complexity of endocrine system disorders and the importance of understanding the anatomy and physiology of the system as well as the most frequently seen endocrine

disorders. As a concerned medical assistant, Miguel continues to read professional journals and attend workshops so that he is prepared to answer questions from clients. He is especially interested in DM because there are so many diabetic patients in the practice where he works. Miguel never hesitates to ask the attending physicians questions about the disease and its management.

SUMMARY of LEARNING OBJECTIVES

1. Define, spell, and pronounce the terms listed in the vocabulary.
   - Spelling and pronouncing medical terms correctly adds credibility to the medical assistant. Knowing the definition of these terms promotes confidence in communication with patients and co-workers.

2. Summarize the anatomy of the endocrine system.
   - The endocrine system consists of glands located throughout the body that produce and secrete chemicals known as *hormones*. The primary glands of the endocrine system are the hypothalamus, pituitary, thyroid, parathyroids, and adrenals and the reproductive glands—the ovaries and the testes. Some nonendocrine organs, such as the pancreas, produce and release hormones. Through hormonal action, the endocrine system regulates all body functions.

3. Explain the mechanism of hormone action.
   - Hormones are chemical transmitters produced by glands and transported to target tissue by the bloodstream. Hormone secretion is regulated by a combination of nervous stimulation, endocrine control, and feedback systems. Each hormone that is released into the bloodstream has particular target cells that it acts on.

4. Differentiate among common endocrine disorders.
   - Hypersecretion or hyposecretion of hormones can cause endocrine disorders. When ADH is not produced or is not released in sufficient amounts, the patient develops a condition called diabetes insipidus. Gigantism and acromegaly are both diseases of the pituitary gland involving the GH. When this condition affects children, gigantism is the result; in adults, acromegaly causes excessive growth of the facial area and extremities. Deficient secretion of thyroid hormone may be caused by an endemic iodine deficiency resulting in a simple goiter. Improper development of the thyroid in an infant or young child causes cretinism; in an adult or older child the condition is called myxedema. Hypersecretion of the thyroid gland causes thyrotoxicosis or Graves' disease. Adrenal cortex insufficiency is called Addison's disease. Hypersecretion of the adrenal cortex, causing increased levels of cortisol, is known as Cushing's syndrome.

5. Describe the diagnostic criteria for diabetes mellitus.
   - Diabetes is diagnosed if the patient has a plasma glucose level of ≥200 mg/dL with polyuria, polydipsia, and unexplained

weight loss; an FPG level ≥126 mg/dL on more than one occasion; a 2-hour OGTT ≥200 mg/dL; a urinalysis positive for glucose and possibly ketones; or a glycosylated hemoglobin >7%.

6. Outline the treatment plan and management of diabetes mellitus.
   - All diabetic patients must monitor their blood glucose levels on a regular basis to determine the effectiveness of treatment. The goal of treatment is to maintain plasma glucose levels as close to the normal range as much as possible. Management of DM is a complicated interaction among exercise, therapeutic diet, weight control, and medication. Patients with type 1 diabetes require daily injections of a combination of insulins. Patients with type 2 and gestational diabetes may be prescribed oral hypoglycemics or insulin if needed.

7. Perform blood glucose screening with a glucometer.
   - Procedure 44-1 describes how to accurately perform a plasma glucose screening with a glucometer. There are many different types of glucose meters on the market so it is important that the patient be taught how to perform the skill with the same type of machine that will be used at home.

8. Identify the characteristics of hyperglycemia and hypoglycemia.
   - With hyperglycemia the patient will experience a sudden onset of polyphagia, polyuria, glycosuria, ketonuria, weight loss, pruritus, "fruity" breath, dry mouth, nausea and vomiting, and lethargy owing to an inadequate dosage of insulin, target cell resistance, overeating, lack of exercise, illness, or stress. Hypoglycemia causes shakiness, vertigo, headache, hunger, pallor, fatigue, confusion, irritability, visual disturbances, seizures, and possible coma.

9. Compare and contrast type 1, type 2, gestational, and pre-diabetes mellitus.
   - Prediabetes is a condition in which an individual has a higher than normal blood glucose level but not high enough for a diagnosis of type 2 diabetes. Type 1 diabetes develops in children and young adults and is characterized by a complete absence of insulin production. Patients must receive daily injections of insulin to survive. Type 2 diabetes develops gradually because of an insufficient amount of insulin and/or resistance at the target cell site or both. Weight management, diet therapy, exercise, and medications are used to control glucose levels. Gestational diabetes occurs in

Continued

SUMMARY of LEARNING OBJECTIVES
Continued

some pregnancies but typically resolves itself after the infant is born. Affected women may need insulin therapy for glucose metabolism.

10. Categorize the complications associated with diabetes mellitus.
- Complications of DM include hypoglycemia; hyperglycemia, and diabetic coma; diabetic neuropathy; microvascular diseases, including diabetic retinopathy and nephropathy; macrovascular diseases such as atherosclerosis, CAD, CVA, and PVD; and decreased resistance to infection.

11. Summarize patient education approaches to diabetes.
- Patient education for diabetic patients is an intricate mix of

information on the dynamics of the disease; the importance of exercise, diet, and weight control in preventing disease complications and maintaining health; an understanding of the various types of insulin and when and how they should be administered; knowledge about oral medications for type 2 diabetes, their side effects and dosage; home care management including proper use of glucose meters and insulin administration; prevention of complications through effective control of blood glucose levels; proper foot care; and monitoring for and immediately contacting the physician about infections or other complications.

CONNECTIONS

Study Guide Connection: Go to Chapter 44 Study Guide. Read the Case Study and Workplace Applications and complete the assignments. Do online research for answers to the questions in the Internet Activities associated with assisting in endocrinology.

CD Connection: Go to the Medical Assisting Competency Challenge CD and do the training activities under Diagnostic Testing. For a better understanding of endocrinology, view the animation for adrenal function.

Evolve Connection: For more information related to assisting in endocrinology, go to evolve.elsevier.com/kinn and visit related weblinks for Chapter 44. Click on the Medical Assisting Exam Review and do the practice questions to sharpen your test-taking skills.

Assisting in Pulmonary Medicine

45

SCENARIO

Michael McGuire, CMA, works for a primary care physician, Dr. John Samuelson, in the small town in which he grew up. Dr. Samuelson's practice is open to all patients, but a large number of individuals with respiratory disease seek his help in managing their pulmonary problems. Michael has learned in the 6 months since he started to work in the practice how to assist with pulmonary diagnostic tests and the special needs of patients with respiratory diseases. Michael has become familiar with the diagnosis and treatment of many common pulmonary problems and adept at accurately documenting respiratory system signs and symptoms. Many of the patients in Dr. Samuelson's practice smoke cigarettes, and the main employers in the community are coal mining and construction companies, so many patients are at risk for smoking and occupation-related respiratory problems.

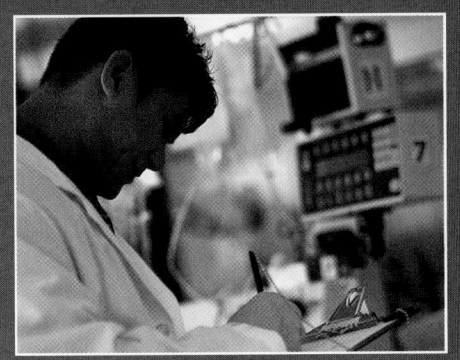

While studying this chapter, think about the following questions:

- What are the common pathologic conditions of the pulmonary system and the terms Michael has learned to use to identify and explain these patient disorders?
- What are the primary medical assisting responsibilities for working with patients who have pulmonary problems?
- What clinical skills are required in this specialty practice?
- What pulmonary complications are associated with smoking and occupational respiratory hazards?
- What diagnostic and treatment procedures are typically used in a pulmonary practice?

LEARNING OBJECTIVES

1. Define, spell, and pronounce the terms listed in the vocabulary.
2. Describe the organs of the respiratory system and their functions.
3. Explain the process of ventilation.
4. Employ correct respiratory system terminology in documentation procedures.
5. Compare and contrast infections and inflammations of the respiratory system.
6. Describe the diagnosis and treatment of tuberculosis.
7. Summarize the disorders associated with chronic obstructive pulmonary disease and their treatments.
8. Teach a patient how to use a peak flow meter.
9. Perform a nebulizer treatment.
10. Detail patient teaching for the use of a metered-dose inhaler.
11. Describe the cancers associated with the respiratory system.
12. Distinguish among common respiratory system diagnostic procedures.
13. Perform a volume capacity spirometric test.
14. Correctly employ a pulse oximeter.
15. Prepare a patient to collect a sputum sample for culture.

National Accreditation Competencies and Content

CAAHEP COMPETENCIES

Clinical
3.b.(4)(f). Prepare patient for and assist with procedures, treatments, and minor office surgeries

General
3.c.(3)(b). Instruct individuals according to their needs
3.c.(3)(c). Provide instruction for health maintenance and disease prevention

ABHES COMPETENCIES

Clinical Duties
4.b. Prepare patients for procedures
4.h. Prepare patient for and assist physician with routine and specialty examinations

Instruction
7.c. Teach patients methods of health promotion and disease prevention

VOCABULARY

bronchiectasis (brong'-ke-ek-tuh-sis) Dilation of the bronchi and bronchioles associated with secondary infection or ciliary dysfunction.

chronic bronchitis Recurrent inflammation of the membranes lining the bronchial tubes.

cilia (sil'-e-uh) Hairlike projections that are capable of movement; in the lungs cilia waves move unwanted substances such as mucus, dust, and pus upward; cilia are destroyed by smoking.

clubbing Abnormal enlargement of the distal phalanges (fingers and toes), associated with cyanotic heart disease or advanced chronic pulmonary disease.

hypercapnia (hi-per-kap'-ne-uh) Excess levels of carbon dioxide in the bloodstream.

pulmonary consolidation Process by which the lungs become solidified as they fill with exudates in pneumonia.

rhinorrhea (ri-no-re'-uh) Discharge of nasal drainage.

tubercle (too'-buhr-kuhl) A nodule produced by the tuberculosis bacillus.

tracheostomy (tra-ke-os'-tuh-me) Surgical opening through the neck into the trachea for breathing.

virulent (vir'-u-lent) Exceedingly pathogenic, noxious, or deadly.

The respiratory system has two primary functions. The first is to exchange oxygen from the atmosphere for carbon dioxide waste. The two types of respiration are *external respiration*, which brings oxygen into the lungs, where carbon dioxide exchange occurs in the blood vessels surrounding the alveoli, and *internal respiration*, in which oxygen is exchanged for carbon dioxide at the cellular level. Cells soon stop functioning and die if they are deprived of oxygen. The second function of the lungs is to maintain acid-base balance within the body. Failure of this function may result in respiratory acidosis or alkalosis. *Respiratory acidosis* occurs if the patient experiences hypoventilation and carbon dioxide levels increase in the body, causing **hypercapnia.** *Respiratory alkalosis* is related to an excess release of carbon dioxide caused by hyperventilation, which may be associated with anxiety or an acute asthma attack. Both conditions can be life-threatening if the underlying causes are not corrected. The respiratory and circulatory systems work together to supply body cells with oxygen and remove metabolic wastes. The ventilation process is controlled by the respiratory center in the central nervous system and assisted by the intercostal muscles and the diaphragm.

THE RESPIRATORY SYSTEM

The *thoracic cage,* sometimes called the *rib cage,* is a bony structure that is narrower at the top and wider at the base. It is held in place by the thoracic vertebrae of the spine in the center of the back and the sternum in the center of the anterior aspect of the body. The first seven ribs attach directly to the sternum and are called the *true ribs.* Ribs 8, 9, and 10 fasten one to another,

Preconditions for Normal Respiration

- An open airway leading to the lungs
- Ability of the lungs to expand rhythmically
- Intact alveolar membranes
- Coordination of the intercostal muscles and the diaphragm
- Proper action of the central nervous system's respiratory control center

forming the false ribs, and ribs 11 and 12 are the "floating" ribs, or half ribs, because their only attachment is to the thoracic vertebrae. At the base or floor of the rib cage is the diaphragm, a musculotendinous membrane that separates the thoracic cavity and the abdominal cavity (Figure 45-1). The respiratory system is divided into two anatomic regions: the upper and lower tracts.

Upper Respiratory Tract

The upper respiratory tract, which transports air from the atmosphere to the lungs, includes the nose, pharynx (throat), and larynx (Figure 45-2). As air enters the nasal cavity, it is cleaned by the **cilia,** warmed by capillary blood vessels, and moistened by mucous membranes. The paranasal sinuses, hollow cavities that are also lined with mucous cells and cilia, open into the nasal cavity. The filtered, warmed, and moistened air moves past the tonsils, which have an immunity function and help defend the body from potential pathogens, and through the pharynx. As the air continues toward the lungs, it passes through the larynx. The opening into the larynx is protected by a moveable piece of cartilage, the epiglottis. The larynx, or voice box, is made up of vocal cords, which vibrate when air is exhaled, creating the sound of the voice. Once the air passes through the larynx, it enters the lower respiratory tract.

Lower Respiratory Tract

The lower respiratory tract consists of the trachea, bronchial tubes, and lungs (see Figure 45-2). These structures are also lined with mucous tissue that is covered with cilia. The collection of dust and foreign particles in the cilia initiates the coughing reflex, aiding in expectorating mucus, which may contain possible pathogens. Without these defense mechanisms, pathogens would remain in the lungs, potentially causing disease. Cigarette smoke and other air pollutants slow down or paralyze the cleansing action of the cilia and damage the mucous membrane lining throughout the respiratory tract.

The trachea (windpipe) is a tube that begins at the larynx and extends into the center of the chest, where it divides or bifurcates into the right and left bronchi. It is about 5 inches long and is surrounded by C-shaped cartilaginous rings. The open area between the edges of the cartilage allows the esophagus to

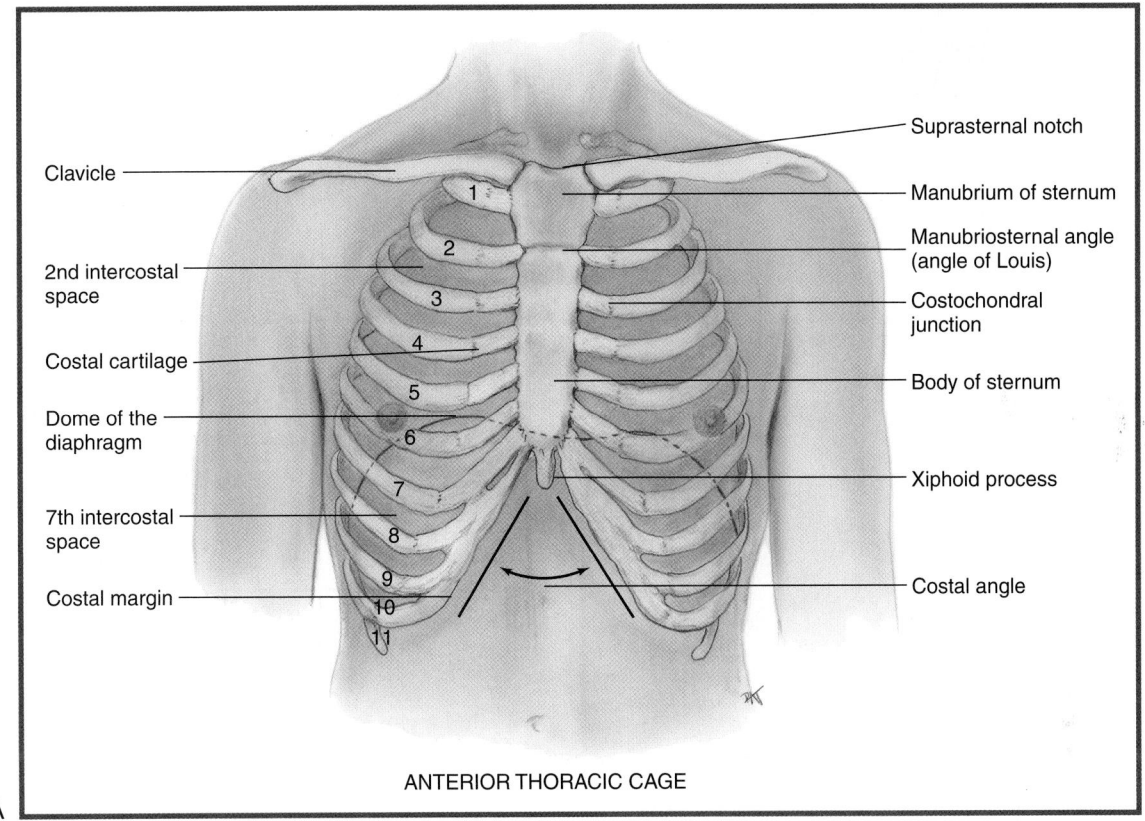

Clavicle

2nd intercostal space

Costal cartilage

Dome of the diaphragm

7th intercostal space

Costal margin

Suprasternal notch

Manubrium of sternum

Manubriosternal angle (angle of Louis)

Costochondral junction

Body of sternum

Xiphoid process

Costal angle

ANTERIOR THORACIC CAGE

A

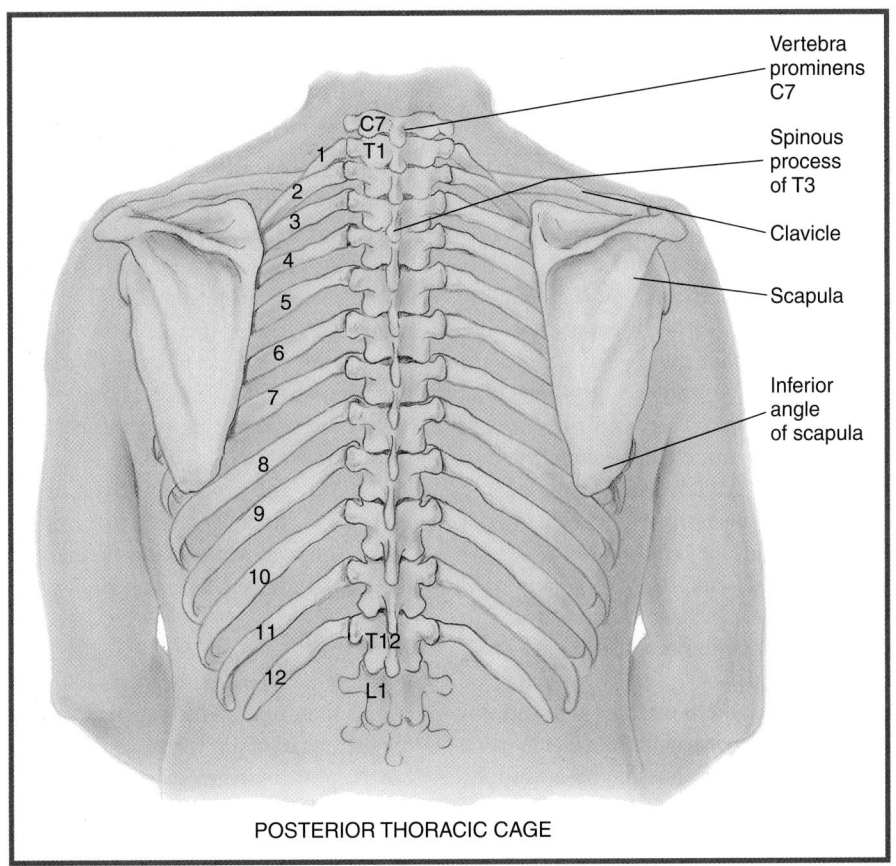

Vertebra prominens C7

Spinous process of T3

Clavicle

Scapula

Inferior angle of scapula

POSTERIOR THORACIC CAGE

B

FIGURE 45-1 A, The anterior thoracic cage. **B,** The posterior thoracic cage. (From Jarvis C: *Physical examination and health assessment*, ed 4, Philadelphia, 2004, Saunders.)

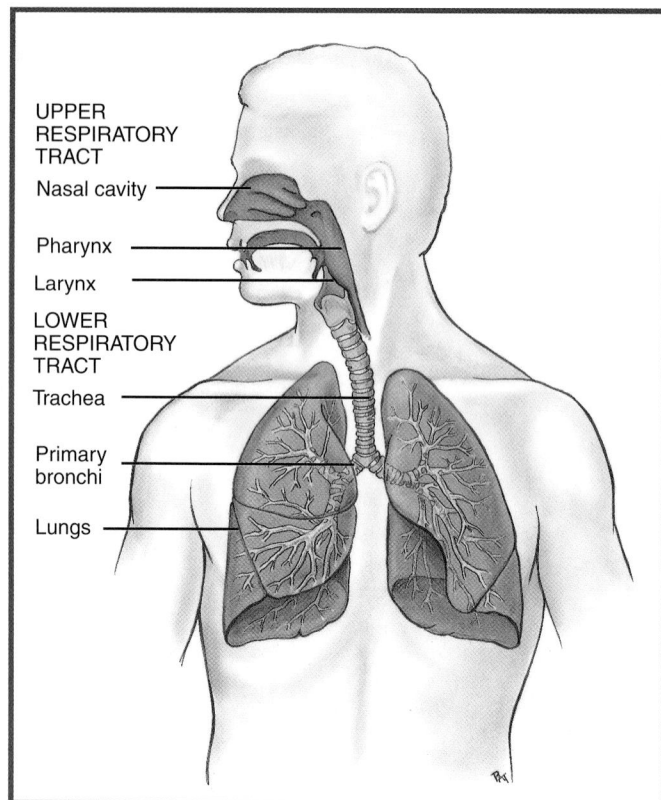

FIGURE 45-2 The upper and lower respiratory tract. (From Applegate EJ: *The anatomy and physiology learning system,* ed 3, Philadelphia, 2006, Saunders.)

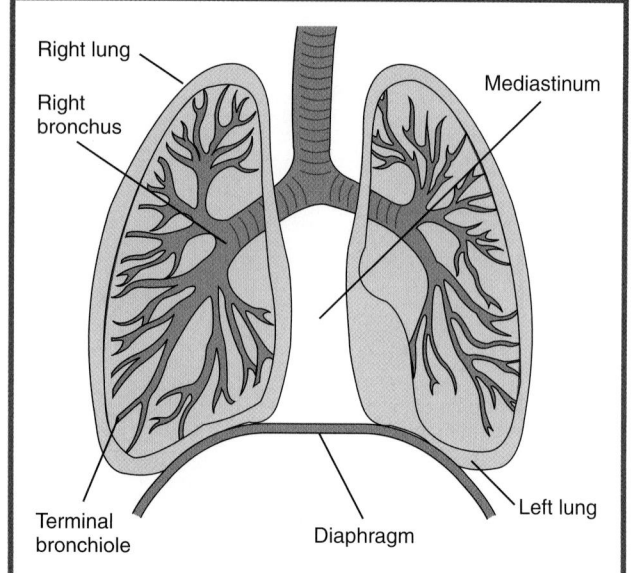

FIGURE 45-3 The bronchial tree.

Each lung is encased in a double-layered sac called the *pleural membrane.* The membrane closest to the lung is called the *visceral pleura,* which doubles back to form the *parietal pleural* membrane. Small amounts of pleural fluid fill the space between the two membranes and provide lubrication for the movement of the lungs during inhalation and exhalation.

VENTILATION

In the very delicate lung tissue the bronchioles deposit oxygenated air into the grapelike structures of the alveoli. Surrounding each alveolus is a network of pulmonary capillaries filled with waste air. The oxygenated air moves through the single-celled walls of the alveoli and into the single-celled walls of the pulmonary capillaries (Figure 45-5). As this is happening the waste air is forced out of the capillaries, into the alveoli, then into the bronchioles. This carbon dioxide–oxygen exchange provides oxygen-rich blood that is returned to the heart for distribution throughout the body; carbon dioxide wastes are excreted with exhalation. The process involved in gaseous exchange is called *ventilation.* The movement of oxygen from the atmosphere into the alveoli is *inspiration,* and the movement of waste gases from the alveoli into the atmosphere is *expiration.*

Inspiration

Inspiration begins with a signal from the medulla oblongata in the brainstem. This signal is carried by the phrenic nerve to the major muscle of inspiration, the diaphragm. When the diaphragm receives the signal, it flattens out and pulls downward. At the same moment the intercostal muscles located between the ribs contract, causing the ribs to move outward and the chest cavity to enlarge. This movement causes the lungs to expand and increase their volume. The more these muscles are contracted, the deeper the inhalation is and the greater the air volume becomes. Respiratory distress occurs when an individual

enlarge when food is swallowed. These rings hold the trachea open regardless of the air pressure changes exerted on it.

When the trachea bifurcates, it forms the right and left bronchi. It is often said that the bronchial tubes look like a tree hanging in the chest (Figure 45-3). The right bronchus is wider than the left to accommodate the right lung lobes, which are also larger. This means that foreign substances are more frequently seen in the right bronchus. Once the bronchi enter the lungs, they branch into smaller and smaller passageways, much as blood vessels do in the circulatory system. This branching continues until it becomes microscopic. These very tiny bronchi are called *bronchioles.* Every tiny bronchiole terminates into microscopic air sacs called *alveoli.* The alveoli are made of thin tissue, only one cell wall thick, which allows the exchange of oxygen and carbon dioxide through the cell wall.

The bronchial tree and alveoli are the major structures housed within the right and left lungs. The lungs are soft and spongy because of the air sacs that comprise most of their mass. They hang in the right and left sides of the chest, separated by the pericardial sac, which contains the heart. The right lung is divided into three lobes and has a greater volume capacity than the left lung. Each lobe has its own bronchus and blood supply, which makes it possible for one lobe to be removed *(lobectomy)* while the rest of the lung sustains little, if any, damage. The left lung is longer and narrower and has a distinct indentation in the center of it, known as the *cardiac notch,* where the left ventricle of the heart is located and an apical pulse is heard. The left lung has only two lobes—the upper and lower sections (Figure 45-4).

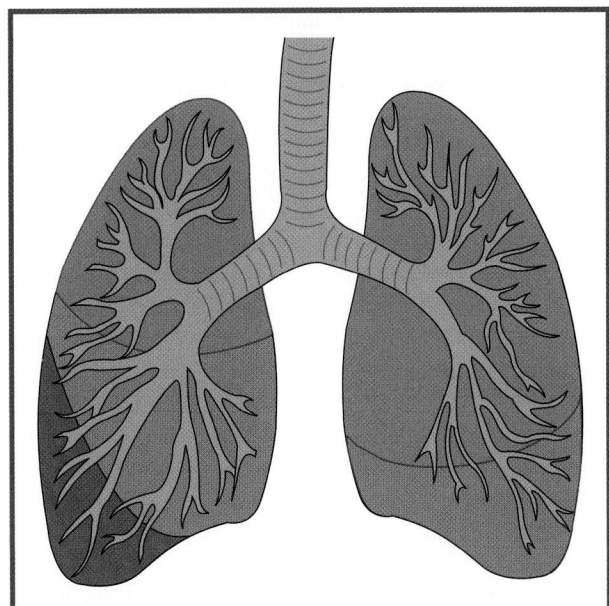

FIGURE 45-4 Lobes of the lungs.

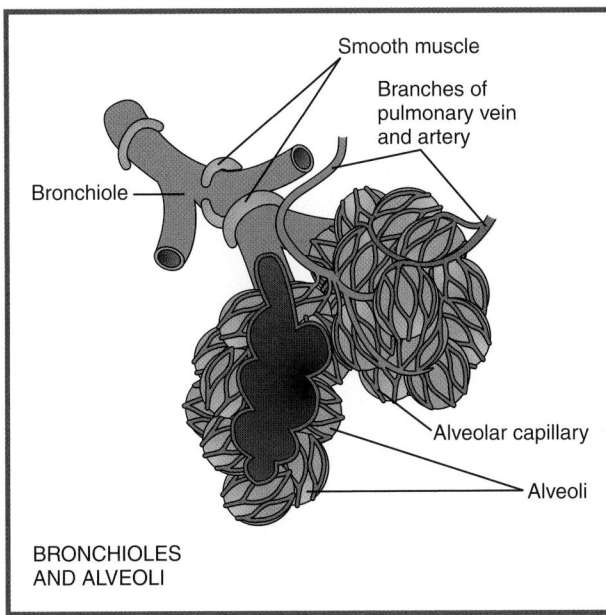

Smooth muscle

Branches of
pulmonary vein
and artery

Bronchiole

Alveolar capillary

Alveoli

BRONCHIOLES
AND ALVEOLI

FIGURE 45-5 Alveoli with capillary network.

is unable to move an adequate amount of air into the lungs, using the diaphragm and intercostal muscles, to meet the body's needs.

Expiration

The second half of ventilation is expiration. Once inspiration is completed, the diaphragm and intercostal muscles relax, causing the diaphragm to move upward into the thoracic cavity and the ribs to move inward causing a decrease in lung capacity. This movement forces the waste air out of the lungs and back into the atmosphere. Expiration requires very little energy and takes place with minimal effort by the body. However, in certain respiratory conditions, such as asthma or emphysema, the person has difficulty getting air out of the lungs, and accessory muscles in the chest and abdomen are needed to assist the intercostal and diaphragm muscles for complete exhalation.

RESPIRATORY SYSTEM DEFENSES

Every part of the respiratory system has a defense mechanism. In the upper respiratory tract, the mucus-covered ciliated surface of the mucous membranes trap particles; through the continuous flow of the mucus back toward the nasopharynx, the particles are either sneezed outward or swallowed.

The lower respiratory tract is sterile, which is phenomenal considering that each day these airways are exposed to approximately 10,000 L of air containing an endless number of microorganisms and foreign material. It is the ever-changing air flow, inspiration to expiration, that creates a turbulence that makes it very difficult for these invading substances to remain in the bronchi. This, combined with coughing, sneezing, and a functioning immune system, protects the respiratory tract and helps the body maintain homeostasis. Disease occurs when something happens to disrupt the normal homeostatic chain of events.

MAJOR DISEASES OF THE RESPIRATORY SYSTEM

Many diseases affect this system; however, the major ones can be divided into infectious diseases, obstructive disorders, and tumors. Respiratory diseases cause common symptoms including sneezing, a productive or nonproductive cough, sore throat or hoarseness, fever, general malaise, altered breath sounds, and changes in breathing patterns. The medical assistant is expected to be familiar with common respiratory terms and use them in documenting patient signs and symptoms. Some common medical terms are defined in Table 45-1.

CRITICAL THINKING APPLICATION

Michael is taking a patient history for a new patient, who reports the following problems: Difficulty breathing; sometimes she has to sit up to breathe comfortably; occasionally she coughs up blood and has excessive nasal drainage. Six months ago she experienced very rapid breathing and a blue color to her skin, so she was admitted to the hospital and diagnosed with blood and fluid around her right lung, which had become infected, causing her lung to collapse. Based on what Michael knows about respiratory system terminology, how should he document this information? Document it below.

_____

_____

_____

_____

Infectious Diseases

Respiratory tract infections fall into two categories depending on where they are located. Diseases of the nose and upper respiratory tract are more common than are diseases of the lower

TABLE 45-1 Respiratory System Terms

MEDICAL TERM	DEFINITION
Apnea	Absence of breathing
Atelectasis	Collapsed lung
Dyspnea	Difficulty breathing
Empyema	Accumulation of pus in the pleural space
Hemoptysis	Expectoration of blood
Hemothorax	Accumulation of blood and fluid in the pleural cavity
Hypercapnia	Greater than normal amounts of carbon dioxide in the blood
Hyperpnea	Deep, rapid, labored respiration that may occur because of exercise or pain and fever
Hypoxemia	Low level of oxygen in the blood
Orthopnea	Person must sit or stand to breathe comfortably
Pleurisy	Inflammation of the parietal pleura causing dyspnea and stabbing pain; friction rub may be auscultated
Pneumothorax	Collection of air or gas in the pleural space causing the lung to collapse
Pyothorax	Collection of pus in the pleural cavity from infection
Rales	A bubbling or popping sound heard on auscultation produced by passage of air through bronchi that are constricted or contain secretions
Rhinoplasty	Plastic surgery to repair or alter the structure of the nose
Rhinorrhea	Excessive drainage from the nose
Rhonchi	A continuous rumbling sound heard on auscultation caused by thick secretions or spasms
Tachypnea	Abnormally rapid rate of breathing
Thoracotomy	Surgical opening into the thoracic cavity

respiratory tract (e.g., pneumonia). Respiratory tract infections account for approximately 75% of all clinically diagnosed infections. Only about 5% of these infections involve the lungs. Most lung infections are seen in hospitalized patients, elderly persons, substance abusers, alcoholics, and patients with acquired immunodeficiency syndrome (AIDS). Pneumonia is the seventh leading cause of death in the United States and is often the cause of death for debilitated people.

Upper Respiratory Tract Infections

Common Cold. The common cold was discussed in Chapter 41 as an acute inflammatory process affecting the mucous membranes that line the nose, pharynx, larynx, and bronchus. Usually the term "cold" is used when only the membranes of the nose and pharynx are affected; however, the same virus can affect the larynx and the lungs. The viral invasion can be followed by bacterial infections of the pharynx, sinuses, and middle ear. Frequently seen signs of an upper respiratory tract infection (*URTI* or *URI*) include nasal congestion and **rhinorrhea**, sneezing, watery eyes, pharyngitis (sore throat), laryngitis (hoarseness), and coughing. Nasal discharge is usually clear and watery in the early stage but can become greenish yellow as the virus becomes more **virulent** or when bacteria

invade. The patient usually complains of headache, low-grade fever, chills, and anorexia.

There is at present no cure for the common cold; the infection usually runs its course in 3 to 5 days. The best way to treat it is by getting plenty of rest and drinking fluids. Taking an over-the-counter cold remedy, cough syrup, and acetaminophen may lessen the discomfort of cold-related symptoms. Antibiotics are prescribed only if evidence of a secondary bacterial infection is present. The physician may recommend the use of echinacea, an herbal remedy, at the first signs of a cold to alleviate symptoms and reduce the duration of a cold or flu. Many herbalists also recommend echinacea to help boost the activity of the immune system and to help the body fight infections.

Sinusitis. The paranasal sinuses are air-filled spaces in the skull located in the brow area over the eyes, inside each cheekbone, behind the bridge of the nose, and behind the eyes. Each sinus has an opening into the nose for the free exchange of air and is lined with a continuous mucous membrane. Healthy sinuses are sterile, but an infection or an allergic reaction can cause one or more of the sinuses to become inflamed or infected. Inflammation causes edema and the collection of mucus within the sinus cavity, creating a feeling of pressure, nasal congestion or rhinorrhea, and classic sinus headaches. The location of sinus pain depends on the sinus cavity involved but can be described as pain in the forehead (frontal sinuses), upper jaw and teeth discomfort (maxillary sinuses), pain between the eyes (ethmoid sinuses), and/or an earache and neck pain (sphenoid sinuses). Treatment is with decongestants, antibiotics for bacterial infections, and analgesics. Sinusitis can be acute, lasting from 2 to 8 weeks, or chronic, with symptoms lingering much longer.

Allergic Rhinitis (Hay Fever). Although not caused by a pathogenic organism, allergic rhinitis is frequently confused with infectious disease. This disorder affects millions of people every year. It is caused by a reaction of the nasal mucosa to an environmental allergen. The most frequent allergen is plant pollen; this is where the term *hay fever* originated. Signs and symptoms include sneezing, nasal congestion, nasal itching, and rhinorrhea. Symptoms can be controlled with either over-the-counter treatments such as Sudafed or Chlor-Trimeton or with prescription antihistamines such as fexofenadine hydrochloride (Allegra), cetirizine hydrochloride (Zyrtec), montelukast (Singulair), and fluticasone (Flonase) and cromolyn sodium (Nasalcrom) nasal sprays. The list of possible allergens is extensive. When this condition is seen in the respiratory practice, the patient is usually referred to an allergist for testing and possible immunotherapy.

Patients may have difficulty determining whether symptoms are caused by a cold or an allergy. The condition is usually an allergy if the eyes, ears, nose, throat, and roof of the mouth (palate) are itchy; the eyes are red and watery; there is a clear, thin nasal discharge; symptoms are seasonal and last for weeks or months; and the patient does not have a fever.

Lower Respiratory Tract Infections

Pneumonia. Pneumonia is both a specific disorder and a general term meaning inflammation of all or part of the lungs

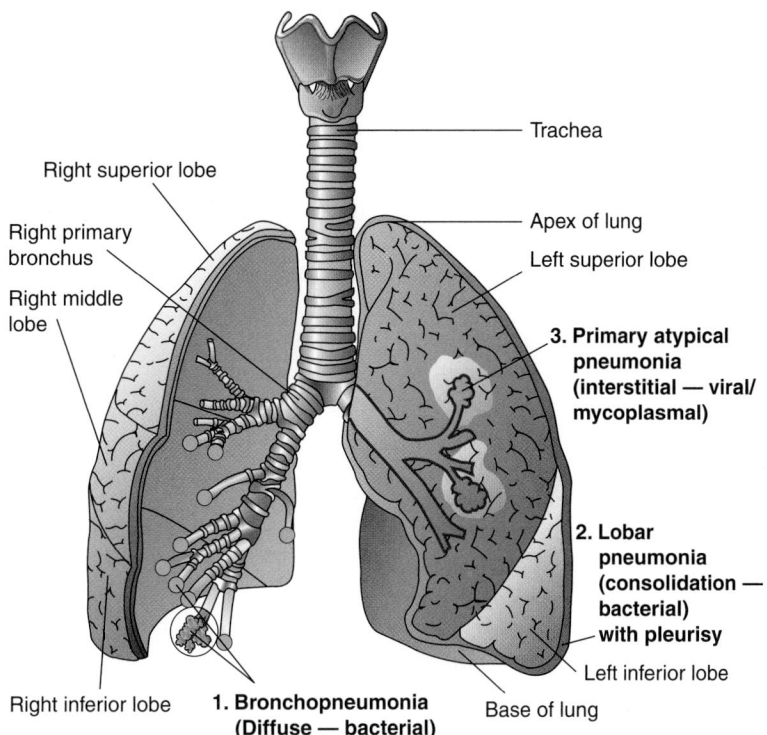

- 3. **Primary atypical pneumonia (interstitial — viral/ mycoplasmal)**
- 2. **Lobar pneumonia (consolidation — bacterial) with pleurisy**
- 1. **Bronchopneumonia (Diffuse — bacterial)**

Trachea
Apex of lung
Left superior lobe
Left inferior lobe
Base of lung
Right superior lobe
Right primary bronchus
Right middle lobe
Right inferior lobe

FIGURE 45-6 Types of pneumonia. (From Gould BE: *Pathophysiology for the health professions*, ed 2, Philadelphia, 2002, Saunders.)

(Figure 45-6). Pneumonia may be caused by bacteria, viruses, or other pathogens (Table 45-2). It can also be caused by inhaling irritants or poisonous gas and by aspirating solids or fluids into the lungs. The most frequently seen causative organisms are staphylococci and streptococci.

Pneumonia can occur in any age group but most often affects preschool-aged children and the elderly (older than 65) and can range from a mild complication to a life-threatening illness. Risk factors include smoking, alcoholism, and immunosuppression caused by diseases or treatment. The patient usually comes to the office with symptoms of high fever, chills, and general malaise. Signs of the illness include dyspnea, tachypnea, chest pain during inspiration, and a relentless cough with possible hemoptysis. Auscultation of the chest reveals rales, rhonchi, and other signs of **pulmonary consolidation.** The infection may spread into the pleural cavity, causing empyema and pleurisy.

Diagnosis is confirmed with a chest x-ray evaluation; sputum culture and sensitivity testing to identify the invading organism and determine appropriate antibiotic therapy; and white blood cell (WBC) count, including a differential count to determine whether the pneumonia is viral or bacterial. If the pneumonia is viral, there is no increase in the number of white cells; but if it is bacterial, the greater the invasion, the higher the WBC count will be. With bacterial pneumonias the differential count shows elevated neutrophil and monocyte levels. Treatment is based on destroying the invading organism. If the organism is bacterial, the treatment of choice is antibiotics and lung function therapy until the patient has recovered. If the organism is viral, the patient is given supportive care, such as antipyretics, fluids, and oxygen until the immune system can control viral spread.

TABLE 45-2 Pathogens Causing Pneumonia	
PATHOGEN	**TYPE OF INFECTION**
Bacteria	*Streptococcus pneumoniae*
	Haemophilus influenzae
	Staphylococcus aureus
	Mycobacteria
Virus	Influenza virus
Fungi	*Aspergillus fumigatus*
	Candida albicans
	Mycoplasma pneumoniae
Parasite	*Pneumocystis carinii* (opportunistic infection, seen in immunosuppressed, debilitated, or terminally ill patients)

Tuberculosis. According to the Centers for Disease Control and Prevention (CDC), approximately one third of the world's population is infected with tuberculosis (TB). TB causes more deaths than any other infectious agent in the world. For more than 50 years the incidence of TB in the United States steadily declined, but from the late 1980s through 1990s there was a resurgence of reported cases. This increase was believed to be the result of increased travel and immigration; the number of AIDS patients, who have little resistance to disease; an increase in the number of homeless and malnourished persons; and the overwhelming proliferation of drug-resistant TB bacilli.

Mycobacterium tuberculosis is the bacterium that causes TB. This organism is covered with a waxy substance that makes it possible for it to survive outside a living host for a long time. It is transmitted by droplets of sputum that are expectorated into the environment by an infected host and inhaled by another person. In the presence of the warm, moist respiratory tract, these organisms can again become active if the individual is susceptible to the disease. TB can also be spread when an infected person coughs or sneezes, releasing airborne infected droplets, which are inhaled and cause an infection if the person is susceptible.

TB develops in two stages. The primary infection occurs when the person is first infected with the bacteria and the lungs become inflamed. Cell-mediated immunity takes place, isolating the bacteria and forming a **tubercle.** At this point a healthy individual can stop the spread of infection, causing the TB bacillus in the tubercle to become inactive. In this case, the person was exposed to the pathogen but never developed active disease so is said to have a *latent* TB infection. Individuals with latent TB are asymptomatic and are not infectious. However, because an exposed individual develops antibodies to the disease, he or she will consistently test positive to TB skin screening tests and, rather than the purified protein derivative (PPD; Mantoux test), should have chest x-ray studies to diagnose active TB.

At any time the bacilli in the tubercles can be reactivated, and secondary or *active* TB can develop. The patient is now actively infected with the disease, which can spread to the bones, brain, and kidneys (Figure 45-7). Some people develop active TB disease soon after becoming infected before their immune systems can fight the TB bacteria, whereas others develop it later in life when their immune systems are weakened for other reasons.

TB is diagnosed most frequently in people living in crowded conditions with poor hygiene, who are malnourished, and who have other chronic conditions. It spreads most rapidly in large cities, in the elderly, alcoholics, and the homeless. Symptoms of an active infection include intermittent fever peaking in the afternoon, night sweats, weight loss, and general malaise. As the infection becomes virulent within the host, there will be a productive cough with thick, dark, frequently blood-tinged mucus expectorated.

The primary diagnosis of TB is established through patient signs and symptoms. The infection is suspected with a positive chest x-ray film but confirmed with a sputum culture. Traditional culture methods originally took 4 to 6 weeks to confirm the diagnosis. This extended period of time allowed a potentially infectious individual to continue to spread the disease; new culture techniques identify the bacterium in as little as 36 to 48 hours. The physician may also order a blood test, the *QuantiFERON-TB Gold* test (QFT), to diagnose TB infection. The QFT measures the response to TB proteins when they are mixed with a small amount of blood.

Once the diagnosis is confirmed, the patient is prescribed long-term treatment with a combination of drugs to completely eradicate the bacilli. If the patient has tested positive for TB but does not have an active infection, the physician will prescribe isoniazid (INH) and rifampin (RIF) for 6 months. If the patient has active pulmonary TB, the CDC recommends a four-drug regimen, including INH, RIF, pyrazinamide, and ethambutol daily for 6 months. The patient is retested, and pharmaceutical

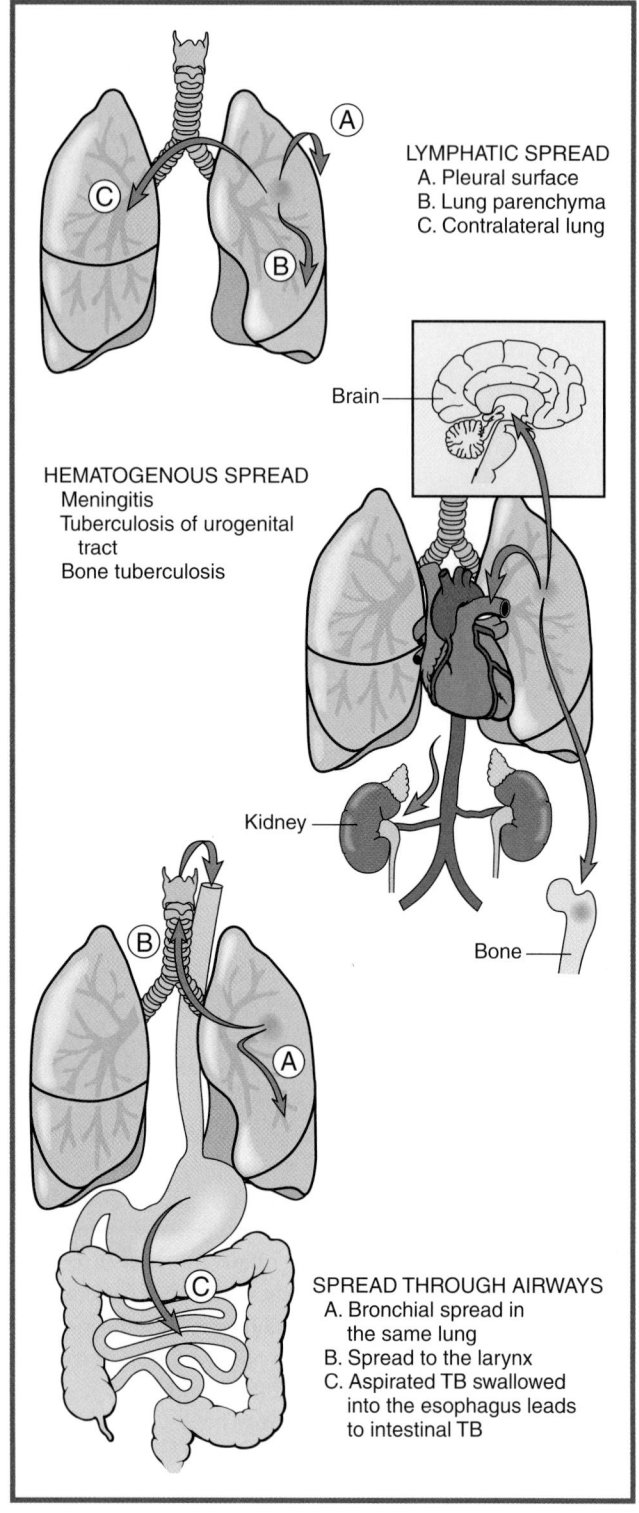

LYMPHATIC SPREAD
A. Pleural surface
B. Lung parenchyma
C. Contralateral lung

Brain

HEMATOGENOUS SPREAD
Meningitis
Tuberculosis of urogenital tract
Bone tuberculosis

Kidney

Bone

SPREAD THROUGH AIRWAYS
A. Bronchial spread in the same lung
B. Spread to the larynx
C. Aspirated TB swallowed into the esophagus leads to intestinal TB

FIGURE 45-7 Spread of tuberculosis. (From Damjanov I: *Pathology for the health-related professions*, ed 3, Philadelphia, 2006, Saunders.)

treatment is continued for 3 months beyond a negative sputum culture. All tuberculin-negative healthcare workers should have a PPD annually; workers who show a positive reaction but are not actively infected with TB should have an annual chest x-ray evaluation to screen for the disease.

Signs and Symptoms of Latent versus Active Tuberculosis According to the Centers for Disease Control and Prevention

Latent Tuberculosis
- Asymptomatic
- Not infectious
- Positive PPD test result
- Positive QuantiFERON-TB Gold blood test result
- Normal chest x-ray studies
- Negative sputum culture

Active Tuberculosis
- Symptoms include cough for 3 weeks or longer, chest pain, hemoptysis, fatigue, weight loss, anorexia, fever with chills, and night sweats.
- Infectious (highest risk of infection is with close family members or associates)
- Positive PPD and QuantiFERON-TB Gold blood tests
- Abnormal chest x-ray studies and/or positive sputum culture

CRITICAL THINKING APPLICATION

Dr. Samuelson is the primary care physician for a nursing home in the area and is concerned because one of the employees has had a positive result to a Mantoux test. What other tests will Dr. Samuelson order to confirm the diagnosis? If those tests come back positive, how will the patient be treated? What about the other employees and residents of the nursing home?

Chronic Obstructive Pulmonary Disease

Chronic obstructive pulmonary disease (COPD) is a group of diseases with the common characteristic of chronic airway obstruction. COPD is the fourth leading cause of death in America, with the majority of deaths related to smoking. Among the diseases included in this group are **chronic bronchitis, bronchiectasis,** and emphysema. Although the mechanism of the obstruction may vary, the patient with COPD is unable to ventilate the lungs freely, resulting in an ineffective exchange of respiratory gases, dyspnea, and productive cough. Over time the patient finds it increasingly difficult to eliminate carbon dioxide from the lungs during expiration.

Asthma

Pediatric asthma was addressed in Chapter 41. Asthma attacks occur in response to a number of triggers that cause inflammation and bronchospasm with resultant airflow obstruction. Asthma can develop into a chronic disease characterized by increased activity or sensitivity of the bronchial tubes to external factors, such as environmental irritants, poor air quality, and allergies, or to internal factors, such as stress, exercise, infection, and allergen inhalation. Asthma also has a strong hereditary factor.

Asthma attacks can be mild to severe and can last minutes to days. Bronchospasms trap air in the lungs while the inflammatory response creates edema and causes secretion of mucus into the constricted bronchioles. An asthmatic patient complains of a nonproductive cough, dyspnea, expiratory wheezing, and chest tightness. Because of difficult breathing, tachycardia, pallor, and diaphoresis may also be present. The patient can speak only a few words at a time, stopping intermittently to regulate his or her air intake. When the chest is auscultated, the physician hears diminished breath sounds with wheezes and rhonchi in the lungs. Spirometry can be used to measure the degree of airflow obstruction. Chest x-ray studies may show changes in the lungs from mucous obstructions. Blood tests include a complete blood cell count with a differential count to determine whether the attack is allergy related.

Asthmatic patients, regardless of their age, should be actively involved in the day-to-day management of their disease. It may be the medical assistant's responsibility to teach the patient how to perform peak flow measurements either daily or at the onset of an attack. Peak flow meters assess the ability of the patient to move air into and out of the lungs. The physician may want the patient to keep a log of daily peak flow results or to use the instrument as an at-home monitoring device when chest tightness and wheezing occur. The meter measures the peak expiratory flow rate, which is the fastest speed at which the patient can blow air out of the lungs after taking in as big a breath as possible (Procedure 45-1). Peak flow readings provide an evaluation of the viability of airways that the patient can perform at home with limited assistance. Readings can help predict an asthma attack if levels are falling; can measure the degree of bronchospasm; and provide the physician with feedback regarding the effectiveness of asthma treatment. The physician uses three zones of measurement to interpret peak flow rates. The green zone is considered normal—the reading is 80% to 100% of normal peak flow rates, indicating the patient's asthma is under control. The yellow zone signals caution—the patient's highest reading is 50% to 80% of normal. The physician will make treatment decisions and recommendations at this point, or the patient may already be instructed on how to manage medications if readings are within these levels. The red zone includes readings that are less than 50% of the normal level, and immediate action must be taken to prevent severe bronchospasms.

If the patient is having an asthma attack, the bronchioles are constricting, becoming edematous, and filling up with mucus, so the patient is unable to exhale strongly enough to raise the indicator to a normal level. If readings are below normal, the physician will prescribe a treatment plan that may include contacting the physician when peak flow levels are below a certain point or starting nebulizer treatments. The physician may recommend an increase in antiinflammatory medication if there is more than a 20% variation in readings from normal. The medication therapy chosen depends on the severity and frequency of acute attacks, but management is necessary to prevent permanent lung damage and emphysema-like changes in the lungs.

Asthma treatment consists of a regimen of medications, including "rescue" inhalers—ipratropium bromide (Atrovent), albuterol (Ventolin), or pirbuterol acetate (MaxAir)—which are used to relieve bronchospasms or for exercise-induced

PROCEDURE 45-1

Prepare Patient for and Assist with Procedures, Treatments, and Minor Office Surgeries: Teach a Patient How to Use a Peak Flow Meter

CAAHEP COMPETENCIES: 3.b.(4)(f), 3.c.(3)(b)
ABHES COMPETENCIES: 4.b, 4.h, 7.c

GOAL: *To instruct the patient in the proper method for performing a peak flow meter test.*

EQUIPMENT and SUPPLIES

- Peak flow meter
- Disposable mouthpiece
- Notebook with pen
- Patient record
- Biohazard waste container

PROCEDURAL STEPS

1. Wash your hands.
2. Place the mouthpiece on the peak flow meter, and slide the marker to the bottom of the scale.
   PURPOSE: The indicator must be at the bottom of the scale for proper measurement of expiratory effort (Figure 1).
3. Introduce yourself, and confirm the identity of the patient.
4. Explain the purpose of the test.
   PURPOSE: To help reassure the patient.
5. Explain the actual maneuver of forced expiration.
   PURPOSE: The patient needs to understand the maneuver so he or she can cooperate fully to obtain the best test results.
6. Be certain the patient is comfortable and in a proper position—either sitting upright or standing (standing is preferred).
   PURPOSE: Proper positioning is necessary to ensure maximum lung expansion and accurate test results.
7. Loosen any tight clothing, such as a necktie, bra, or belt.
   PURPOSE: Tight clothing may restrict breathing capacity.

8. Hold the meter upright, being careful not to block the opening with the fingers (Figure 2).
   PURPOSE: To prevent obstruction of forced exhalation.
9. Instruct the patient to inhale as deeply as possible, place the mouthpiece into the mouth beyond the teeth, and form a tight seal with the lips. Caution the patient not to put the tongue in the mouthpiece when exhaling.
   PURPOSE: To prevent any leakage of air around the mouthpiece and any obstruction of air flow.
10. Instruct the patient to exhale as hard and as fast as possible into the peak flow meter.
11. The forced exhalation will move the marker up the scale and stop at the point of the peak expiratory flow. Record this number, and return the marker to the bottom of the scale.
12. Repeat the procedure two more times, sliding the indicator to the bottom of the scale before each reading, and record each result.
13. Encourage the patient to inhale as deeply as possible and to exhale as fast and as forcefully as possible with each effort.
14. Place the test results on the patient's chart for physician review, noting the time and date of the highest reading.
15. Clean and disinfect the equipment, discarding waste in a biohazard waste container, or give the patient the meter for continued use at home with instructions to follow the manufacturer's cleaning recommendations.

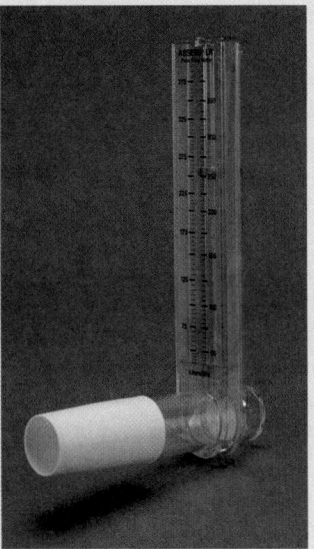

FIGURE 1

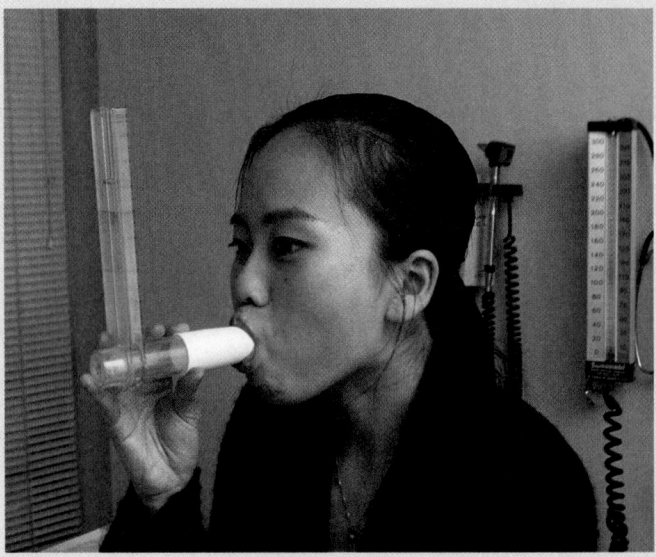

FIGURE 2

Continued

PROCEDURE 45-1—cont'd

16. Wash your hands.
   PURPOSE: Infection control.
17. Record testing information on the patient's chart.
   PURPOSE: Procedures that are not recorded are considered not done.

CAUTIONARY NOTE: Peak flow readings may trigger bronchospasms or severe coughing in patients experiencing an asthma attack. If this occurs, instruct the patient to rest and try again. If the patient is unable to perform three readings because of bronchospasms and/or coughing, follow the physician's guidelines regarding how this should be managed.

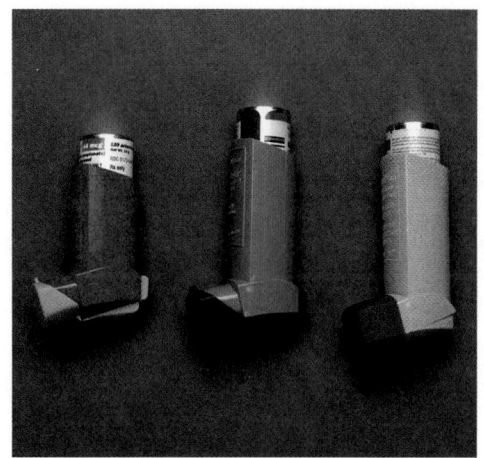
A
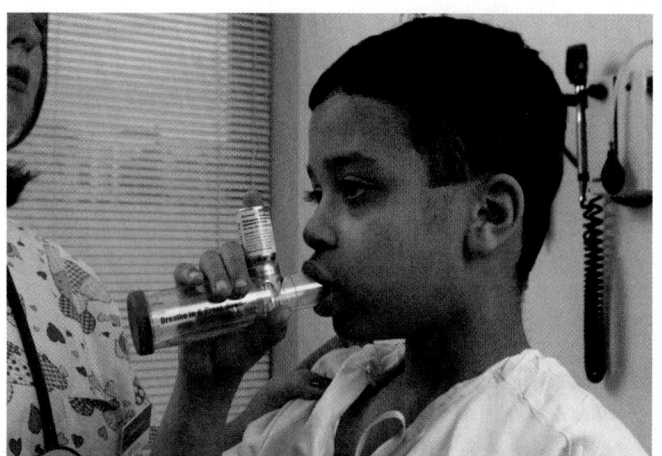
B

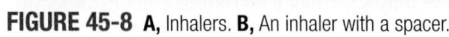

FIGURE 45-8 A, Inhalers. **B,** An inhaler with a spacer.

asthma (Figure 45-8). Tissue inflammation can be treated with steroid inhalers—flunisolide (Aerobid), triamcinolone acetonide (Azmacort), or fluticasone propionate (Flovent)—and/or an oral leukotriene-receptor antagonists such as zafirlukast (Accolate) or montelukast sodium (Singulair) taken on a regular basis. If an attack is severe, it may require injections of epinephrine, oral corticosteroids (Prednisone), and/or nebulizer treatments with a bronchodilator (Procedure 45-2). A nebulizer forces compressed air through a medication chamber that converts liquid medication (albuterol or Pulmicort) into an aerosol or mist form that can be inhaled though a mask or mouthpiece.

The physician prescribes an inhaler dose according to the number of "puffs" of a metered-dose inhaler (MDI) the patient should administer. MDIs consist of a pressurized canister containing medication and a mouthpiece. Most MDIs hold about 200 doses of medication as well as a pressurized gas propellant, which forces the drug out of the canister. When the canister is inverted and depressed, a metered dose (premeasured) is delivered through the mouthpiece in aerosol form. Patient teaching is very important to ensure that the patient operates the device correctly so the medication can be administered

Instructing the Patient in the Use of Metered-Dose Inhalers

1. Shake the canister vigorously and place it into the mouthpiece device.
2. The patient should open his or her mouth and hold the inhaler approximately 1 inch away. (If the patient places the mouthpiece in the mouth, the gas propellant will cause the drug to bounce off the back of the throat, and much of it will be lost around the mouth.)
3. The patient should exhale normally, and while beginning to slowly inhale, he or she should depress the canister, releasing a metered dose of medication.
4. The patient should continue to breathe in until the lungs are full, hold the breath to a count of 10, if possible, then breathe out normally.
5. If a second dose is prescribed, the patient should wait at least 1 minute between puffs.
6. Some inhalers come attached to spacers or can be adapted to meet the needs of children or older patients who have difficulty managing the technique. When the canister is depressed, the medication stays in the spacer, and the patient can take more time to inhale the particles (Figure 45-8, B).

PROCEDURE 45-2

Prepare Patient for and Assist with Procedures, Treatments, and Minor Office Surgeries: Perform a Nebulizer Treatment

CAAHEP COMPETENCY: 3.b.(4)(f)
ABHES COMPETENCY: 4.b

GOAL: *To perform a nebulizer treatment.*

EQUIPMENT and SUPPLIES

- Nebulizer machine
- Disposable connector tubing with medication dispenser
- Disposable mouthpiece or mask as ordered
- Medication as ordered and sterile saline or water (diluent) for mixing
- Patient record and pen
- Biohazard waste container

PROCEDURAL STEPS

1. Plug the nebulizer into a properly grounded electrical outlet.
2. Introduce yourself, and confirm the identity of the patient.
3. Explain the purpose of the treatment.
   PURPOSE: To help reassure the patient.
4. Wash your hands.
5. Measure the prescribed dose of drug and diluent and place the mixture into the nebulizer medication cup (Figure 1).
6. Replace the top of the medication cup, and connect it to the mouthpiece or face mask.
7. Connect the disposable tubing to both the nebulizer and the medication cup.

8. The patient should be sitting upright to allow for total lung expansion.
   PURPOSE: Proper positioning is necessary to ensure adequate dispensing of medication.
9. Turn the nebulizer on (a mist should be visible coming from the back of the tube opposite the mouthpiece or into the face mask).
   PURPOSE: The mist is the medication aerosol.
10. If using a mask, position it comfortably but securely over the patient's mouth and nose.
11. If using a mouthpiece, instruct the patient to hold it between the teeth with the lips pursed around the mouthpiece (Figure 2).
12. Encourage the patient to take slow, deep breaths through the mouth. Hold each breath 2 to 3 seconds to allow the medication to disperse through the lungs.
    PURPOSE: To allow for maximum distribution of medication in the lung tissue.
13. Continue the treatment until aerosol is no longer produced (approximately 10 minutes).
    CAUTION: If the patient is receiving a bronchodilator (albuterol) he or she may experience dizziness, tremors, or tachycardia. Continue the treatment unless otherwise ordered by the physician.
14. Turn the nebulizer off.
15. Encourage the patient to take several deep breaths and cough loosened secretions into disposable tissues.
16. Dispose of the mouthpiece or mask, tubing, and instruct the patient to dispose of the contaminated tissues in a biohazard container.
    PURPOSE: Infection control.

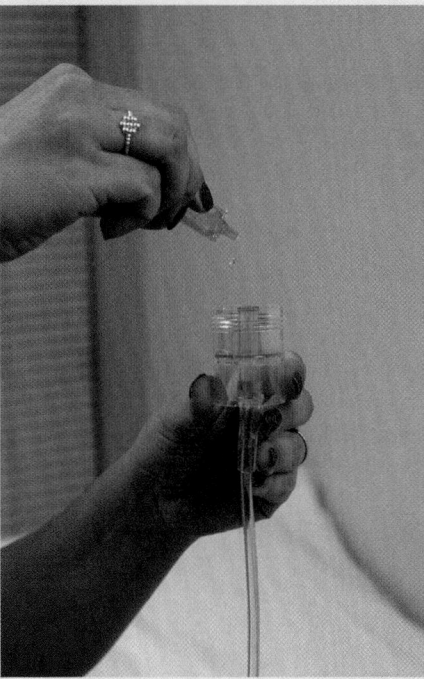

FIGURE 1

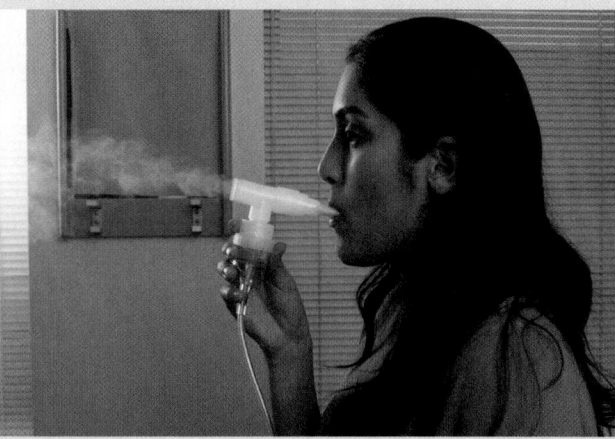

FIGURE 2

Continued

PROCEDURE 45-2—cont'd

17. Wash your hands.
  PURPOSE: Infection control.
18. Record the nebulizer treatment, the patient's response, including the amount of coughing and whether coughing was productive or nonproductive, and any side effects of the medication.
  PURPOSE: Procedures that are not recorded are considered not done.

19. If the patient is to continue home nebulizer treatments, conduct patient education with both the patient and caregivers as appropriate. Make sure they demonstrate the treatment steps to confirm understanding.
  PURPOSE: Feedback through demonstration of technique assures patient follow through.

---

as ordered. If both a steroid and bronchodilator have been prescribed, the bronchodilator should be taken first, because this will open the airways so the steroid can be better distributed throughout the lungs.

Pneumoconioses

Environmental causes of respiratory diseases include inhaled dusts, fumes, and various kinds of organic or inorganic matter. A majority of these respiratory diseases are occupational: they are the consequence of long-term exposure to unsafe air in the workplace. Although the respiratory system is designed to filter and trap air contaminants, the system can become overloaded after intense exposure. Subsequently irritants enter the lungs, with the amount of damage to pulmonary tissue increasing if the particles are very small and can enter the alveoli; if the individual is exposed to a large quantity of contaminants over a long period of time; and when there is the added irritation of cigarette smoking.

Some of the occupations that can cause pneumoconiosis include coal mining *(anthracosis)*; insulation manufacture and shipbuilding *(asbestosis)*; and stonecutting or sandblasting *(silicosis)*. Tissue changes caused by the inhalation of these substances into the lungs are irreversible. Patients develop dyspnea, cough, and emphysema-like changes and have an increased risk for cancer of the lung.

Emphysema

Emphysema causes a loss of elasticity in the walls of the alveoli, eventually leading to the walls stretching and breaking, creating air spaces that are unable to conduct oxygen and carbon dioxide exchange. The remaining alveoli become overinflated, and as time progresses individuals find it very difficult to exhale completely. Emphysema is a progressive obstructive disease of the pulmonary system and is irreversible. Cigarette smoking is the primary contributing factor; however, patients who develop emphysema at an early age may have a genetic predisposition to the disease. Other contributors include exposure to pollutants (pneumoconioses) or chronic respiratory disorders (chronic bronchitis or asthma).

Patients may not exhibit symptoms until irreversible damage has occurred. When signs and symptoms do occur they include dyspnea, shortness of breath (SOB), wheezing, production of thick mucus, restlessness, fatigue, anorexia, persistent cough (productive or nonproductive), and peripheral cyanosis with

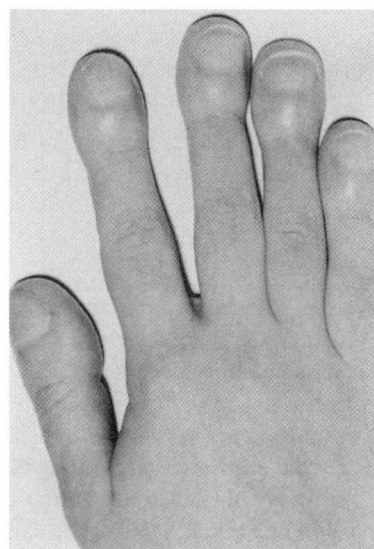

FIGURE 45-9 Clubbing. (From Zitelli BJ, Davis HW: *Atlas of pediatric physical diagnosis*, ed 4, St Louis, 2002, Mosby.)

clubbing (Figure 45-9). The patient is typically diagnosed from presenting signs and symptoms and a chest x-ray examination, as well as a pulmonary function test (PFT) that shows increased residual volume and decreased forced expiratory volume (Table 45-3).

Patients are encouraged to avoid respiratory irritants and individuals with respiratory infections and to stop smoking. Many of these patients require oxygen therapy and benefit from postural drainage and chest percussion to expectorate trapped mucus. Nebulizer treatments may also be prescribed.

Patients with emphysema expend a great deal of energy just to expel air from their lungs, so they should consume a high-calorie, high-fluid diet and perform certain exercises, such as pursed-lip breathing, to help them conserve energy. An emphysema patient requires continuous care and support, therefore, encouraging family involvement in the treatment plan is important. Referral to a pulmonary rehabilitation program or support group is beneficial to both patient and family.

Obstructive Sleep Apnea

Obstructive sleep apnea occurs when the muscles in the posterior pharynx that support the soft palate, uvula, tonsils, and tongue relax during sleep. This relaxation causes the trachea

TABLE 45-3 Pulmonary Function Tests

LUNG FUNCTION	DESCRIPTION	PATIENT INSTRUCTIONS
Tidal volume (TV)	Volume of air inspired and expired during a normal respiration	Patient breathes in and out normally with lips pursed around mouthpiece
Vital capacity (VC)	Maximum amount of air that can be expired after maximum inspiration	Patient takes deep breath and exhales completely (not forcefully)
Inspiratory capacity (IC)	Maximum amount of air that can be inspired after a normal expiration	Patient breathes in and out normally, then forcibly inhales at the end of the TV
Expiratory reserve volume (ERV)	Maximum volume of air that can be exhaled after a normal expiration	Patient breathes in and out normally, then exhales forcibly at the end of the TV
Residual volume (RV)	Volume of air left in lungs after forced expiration	
Functional residual volume (FRV)	Amount of air left in the lungs after a normal expiration	FRV = ERV + RV
Forced vital capacity (FVC)	Amount of air that can be forcefully exhaled from a maximal inhalation	Patient inhales as deeply as possible, then forcibly exhales as much as possible.
Maximal volume ventilation (MVV)	Maximum volume that patient can breathe in and out in 1 minute	Patient breathes in and out as deeply and as frequently as possible for 15 seconds (total volume is multiplied by 4)

to narrow or close with inhalation, momentarily stopping breathing. Blood oxygen levels are lowered, and the brain senses hypoxemia so it stimulates the patient from sleep to reopen the trachea. The patient is awake so briefly he or she is not aware of the arousal, but this occurs repeatedly throughout the night, preventing the person from achieving a deeper, more restful level of sleep. Because of this interrupted sleep the individual frequently complains of sleepiness during the day.

Patients are at greater risk for developing obstructive sleep apnea if they are overweight, because a fat or thick neck may narrow the trachea; if they have enlarged adenoids or tonsils; if they are male, because men develop sleep apnea twice as frequently as women; if they have a family history of sleep apnea; and if they use alcohol or sedatives, because these chemicals relax throat muscles.

Sleep apnea is typically treated with a continuous positive airway pressure (CPAP) machine that delivers air pressure through a mask placed over the mouth and nose. The air pressure created by the machine is greater than that of the surrounding air, forcing the upper airway passages open and preventing tracheal collapse. Although CPAP is the preferred method of treatment, it can be awkward and uncomfortable, making it difficult to sleep. Patients must be encouraged to follow through with the recommended treatment. Individuals with mild obstructive sleep apnea can try alternative treatment with a dental device that opens the throat by bringing the jaw forward. Surgery may also be performed to remove from the nose or throat excess tissue that vibrates during exhalation and/or is blocking the upper respiratory tract.

CRITICAL THINKING APPLICATION

Dr. Samuelson has quite a few patients with either asthma or emphysema. Under the direction of Dr. Samuelson, Michael is expected to reinforce patient education and answer patient and/or

Common Signs and Symptoms of Obstructive Sleep Apnea

- Excessive daytime sleepiness *(hypersomnia)*
- Persistently loud, disruptive snoring
- Snoring, choking, or gasping sounds while asleep
- Episodes of breathing cessation during sleep
- Dry mouth or sore throat on awakening
- Morning headache

family questions. Michael decides to make a file on pertinent health education information and review it with Dr. Samuelson before using it to help coordinate the care of these patients. What information should Michael include in the file? What community resources or groups should be included for patient support?

Pulmonary System Tumors

The most prevalent neoplasms of the respiratory system are lung cancer and carcinoma of the larynx.

Lung Cancer

Lung cancer is the leading cause of cancer-related deaths for both men and women in the United States. It is estimated that 90% of lung tumors are linked to cigarette smoking; other risk factors include chronic exposure to second-hand smoke, carcinogens (such as radon gas and asbestos), and a genetic predisposition. The risk of developing cancer is higher for patients who started to smoke at a young age and who have smoked more than a pack a day for a long period (Figure 45-10). Individuals who quit smoking can significantly lower their risk for lung cancer; after 10 years the risk is reduced by one-third. Female smokers are at greater risk of lung cancer than male smokers.

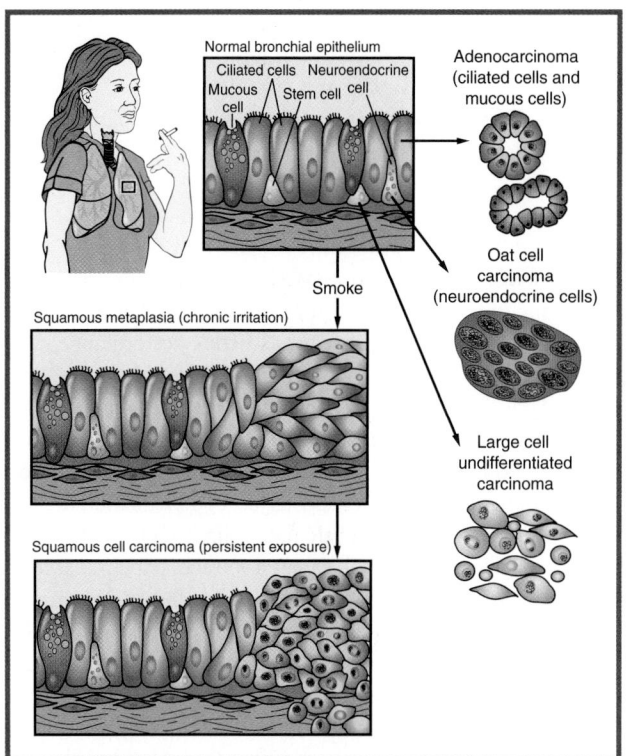

FIGURE 45-10 Classification of lung cancer. (From Damjanov IL: *Pathology for the health-related professions*, ed 3, Philadelphia, 2006, Saunders.)

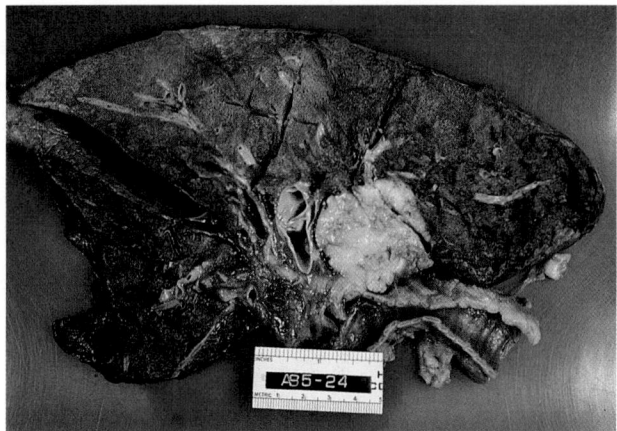

FIGURE 45-11 Lung cancer. (From Damjanov IL: *Pathology for the health-related professions*, ed 3, Philadelphia, 2006, Saunders.)

The lung is a common site for secondary tumors from metastasis as well as primary carcinomas. There are several different cellular types of tumors that can develop in the lungs, but the one seen most frequently is bronchogenic carcinoma, which originates in the epithelial lining of the bronchioles (Figure 45-11). The early symptoms of lung cancer—chronic productive cough, SOB, and chest tightness—are masked by symptoms regularly displayed by habitual smokers. A tumor may be discovered accidentally during a routine chest x-ray evaluation or may not be discovered until metastatic symptoms, such as anemia, weight loss, and fatigue, lead to a diagnosis of

a primary lung tumor. Patients who do show symptoms usually display local effects of a tumor in the chest such as bronchial obstruction, atelectasis, hemoptysis, chest pain, and pleural membrane involvement. Unless the tumor is diagnosed very early, lung cancer has a poor prognosis. Treatment consists of surgery, radiation therapy, and chemotherapy.

Carcinoma of the Larynx

Carcinoma of the larynx is pathologically linked to smoking and chronic alcohol consumption. Ninety percent of the cases of laryngeal cancer occur in men; most of those affected are between 60 and 70 years of age. Patients show early signs of hoarseness, loss of voice, and dysphagia (difficulty swallowing), and occasionally, respiration becomes impaired. Because of these early symptoms, most laryngeal tumors are discovered in their early stages and can be removed, resulting in a very good prognosis. Surgical treatment consists of a partial or total laryngectomy. With a total laryngectomy the voice is permanently lost, and a **tracheostomy** is performed. Patients undergoing such procedures need comprehensive preparation and would benefit from meeting a laryngectomy survivor as well as participating in a support group to deal with postsurgical adjustments.

THE MEDICAL ASSISTANT'S ROLE IN PULMONARY PROCEDURES

Assisting with the Examination

Preparing a patient for a respiratory examination includes having the patient disrobe to the waist and don a gown with the opening in the front. To assess the status of the respiratory system, the physician uses inspection, palpation, percussion, and auscultation on the anterior thorax, then repeats the process on the posterior and lateral thorax. The medical assistant is responsible for assisting the physician throughout the examination, providing the patient privacy and support, and performing diagnostic tests as ordered.

Diagnostic Procedures

Tuberculosis

If the physician orders TB screening, the medical assistant will administer the Mantoux test (see Chapter 34). The test uses an intradermal injection of PPD from a live tuberculin bacillus culture to test for the presence of tuberculin antibodies. A positive Mantoux reaction indicates the possibility of active or latent TB or exposure to the disease. Further testing by sputum culture and chest x-ray examination is required for a definitive diagnosis.

Spirometry

PFTs are performed to diagnose a pulmonary abnormality and/or to determine the extent of a pulmonary disease. Lung function measurements are taken in the physician office setting with a spirometer (Figure 45-12). Table 45-3 summarizes the aspects of pulmonary function that are measured during a PFT. Successful spirometry requires the application of consistent methods for

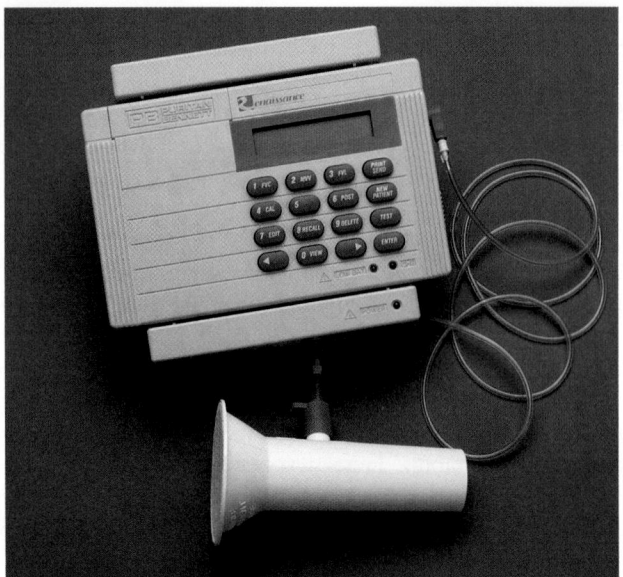

FIGURE 45-12 Spirometer.

preparing the patient, explaining and performing the procedure, and determining the results. Patient preparation begins when the procedure is scheduled. The patient should be instructed not to smoke and to refrain from using bronchodilators and nebulizers for 6 hours before the test.

The medical assistant may be responsible for conducting this test in the ambulatory care setting (Procedure 45-3). Before the patient is scheduled for the procedure the physician will consider certain health problems, such as a pneumothorax, a history of angina or recent myocardial infarction, or the presence of vascular aneurysms that contraindicate the examination. When the patient arrives for testing, the medical assistant should explain the purpose of the test, obtain the patient's vital signs (including height and weight), and explain the maneuver. Spirometry should be described briefly, in simple terms. One statement that works well is, "I am going to have you blow into a machine to see how much air your lungs hold and how fast you can expel it. The test does not hurt, but it does require your cooperation and lots of effort." The patient should be in a comfortable upright position with the legs uncrossed and both feet on the floor. Dentures that fit poorly may be a nuisance and should be removed if they might interfere. The chin should be slightly elevated and the neck slightly extended. This position should be maintained throughout the forced expiratory procedure.

Give specific instructions in simple, direct terms—for example, "I want you to take the deepest breath possible, put the mouthpiece in your mouth and seal your lips tightly around it, and then blow into the tube as hard and as fast as you can in one long, complete breath." One analogy that is sometimes helpful to further explain the maneuver is, "It's like blowing out the candles on a birthday cake when they don't all go out; you need to keep blowing the same breath until they do."

Next, demonstrate the maneuver. Many patients will forget some or all of the instructions they just received, so demonstration

reinforces exactly what to do. Show the patient proper chin and neck position, how to place the mouthpiece at the right time, and how to blow the air out and continue to blow.

When the demonstration is done, remind the patient of the following points:
- Take as deep a breath as possible.
- Blow air out hard.
- Do not stop blowing until you are told to stop.

Use active and forceful coaching while the patient is performing the maneuver. You may need to raise your voice with some urgency to improve the patient's performance, using such phrases as, "Blow, blow, blow!" "Keep blowing, keep blowing!" and "Don't stop blowing!" After the maneuver, give the patient some feedback on the quality of the test and describe what improvements could be made. Continue to repeat efforts until the patient has completed three acceptable maneuvers. The two best efforts are used to calculate pulmonary function. The physician calculates normal values for each patient based on individual age, height, weight, and sex, which are documented as a percentage. If the patient's best efforts are greater than 80% of pretest calculated values, pulmonary function is considered normal. Spirometry tests provide the physician information about the impact of obstruction or pulmonary disease on airflow. If results are less than 60% of the predicted value, the patient may be given bronchodilators and be retested to determine the impact of the inhalant on function.

Test Results. Place the results of the maneuvers with the patient's chart on the physician's desk when the tests are completed. Many physicians rely on the assistant to include comments pertinent to the testing, such as patient condition during the test and compliance with coaching. If any questions arise regarding the quality of the results, ask the patient to wait while the physician reviews the results. If the patient has delayed taking medication, check with the physician as to when the patient should resume taking it.

CRITICAL THINKING APPLICATION

Michael is in the process of orienting Cinda, a new employee, on how to perform a spirometer test. He has summarized the steps of the procedure on a card next to the machine for easy reference. Cinda knows nothing about the procedure. What would be the best way for Michael to teach her about the test? What information should he include?

Acceptable Spirometer Test

An acceptable spirometer test has five characteristics:
- No coughing
- Good start of test
- No early termination
- No variable flows
- Consistency

PROCEDURE 45-3

Prepare Patient for and Assist with Procedures, Treatments, and Minor Office Surgeries: Perform Volume Capacity Spirometric Testing

CAAHEP COMPETENCY: 3.b.(4)(f)
ABHES COMPETENCIES: 4.b, 4.h

GOAL: *To perform volume capacity testing.*

EQUIPMENT and SUPPLIES

- Scale with height measuring device
- Sphygmomanometer and stethoscope
- Spirometer with recording paper in place
- External spirometric tubing
- Disposable mouthpiece
- Nasal clip if needed
- Biohazard waste container
- Patient record

PROCEDURAL STEPS

1. Wash your hands and assemble the spirometer.
2. Introduce yourself, and confirm the identity of the patient. Determine whether any special preparation was needed by this patient and if it was followed.
   PURPOSE: If special procedures were not followed, the test may have to be rescheduled.
3. Explain the purpose of the test.
   PURPOSE: To help reassure the patient.
4. Measure and record the patient's vital signs, height, and weight.
5. Explain the actual maneuver.
   PURPOSE: The patient needs to understand the maneuver so he or she can cooperate fully to obtain best testing results.
6. Be certain the patient is comfortable and in proper sitting or standing position.
   PURPOSE: Proper positioning is necessary to ensure maximum lung expansion and accurate test results.
7. Loosen any tight clothing, such as a necktie, bra, or belt
   PURPOSE: Tight clothing may restrict breathing capacity.
8. Show the patient the proper chin and neck position.
9. Practice the maneuver with the patient before you begin.
   PURPOSE: To relieve apprehension and enhance understanding.
10. Place a soft nose clip on the patient's nose.
    PURPOSE: To prevent the escape of air through the nose during exhalation.
11. Place the mouthpiece in the mouth, and instruct the patient to seal the lips around the piece.
12. The patient should inhale according to instructions.
13. Use active, forceful coaching during exhalation (Figure 1).
    PURPOSE: Coaching improves performance.

14. Give the patient feedback after the maneuver is completed.
    PURPOSE: Positive feedback and explanations of mistakes in the maneuver will help improve patient compliance.
15. Carefully observe the patient for indications of vertigo or dyspnea or any other signs of difficulty. If complications occur, stop the test and inform the physician.
16. Continue testing until three acceptable maneuvers have been performed.
17. Place the test results on the patient's chart for physician review. Dismiss the patient only if results are satisfactory.
18. Clean and disinfect the equipment. Discard waste in a biohazard waste container.
19. Wash your hands.
    PURPOSE: Infection control.
20. Record testing information on the patient's chart.
    PURPOSE: Procedures that are not recorded are considered not done.

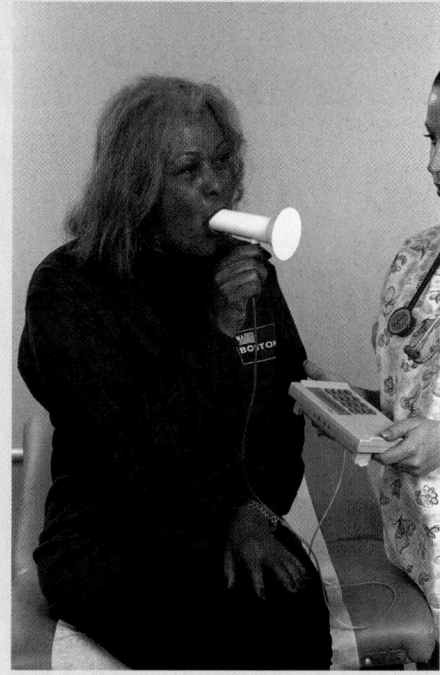

FIGURE 1

Pulse Oximetry

Pulse oximetry is a noninvasive method of evaluating the oxygen saturation of hemoglobin in arterial blood, as well as the pulse rate. It identifies the percentage of hemoglobin that is oxygenated in comparison with the total amount of hemoglobin that is available. Many ambulatory settings have pulse oximeters available to assess a patient's oxygenation status with such disorders as pneumonia, bronchitis, emphysema, or asthma (Figure 45-13, *A*).

To perform the procedure, the medical assistant clips a probe on the patient's earlobe or finger (Figures 45-13, *B* and *C*). Fingernail polish must be removed before the clip is

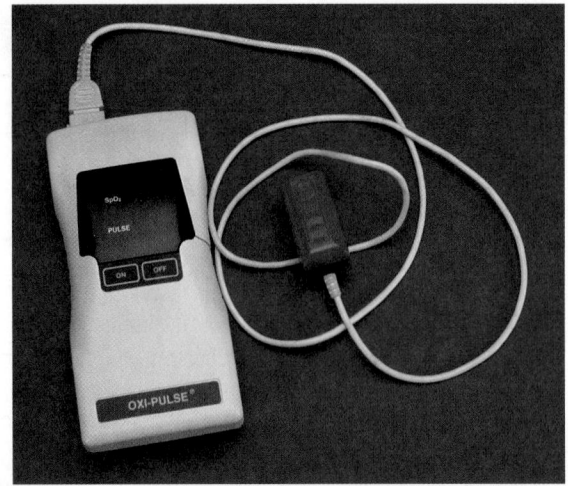

A

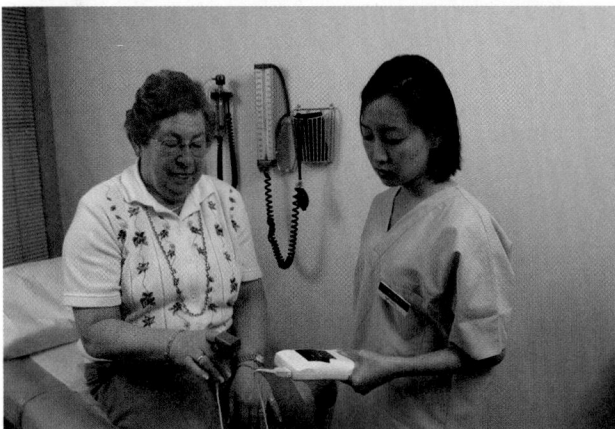

B

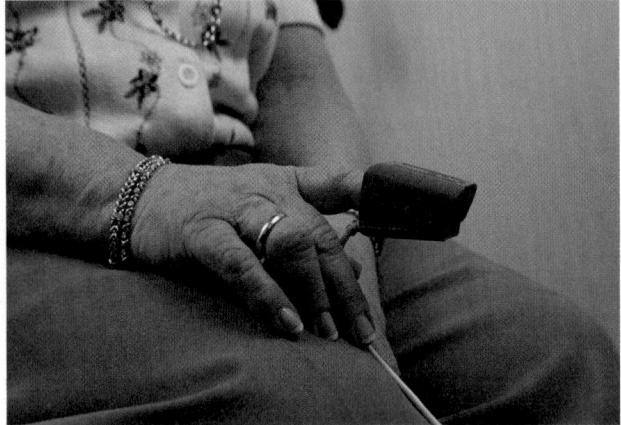

C

FIGURE 45-13 A, BCI 3301 hand-held pulse oximeter. **B,** A pulse oximetry clip. **C,** A patient with a pulse oximeter. (*A* Courtesy of Smiths Medical PM, Inc. Waukesha WI. BCI is a registered trademark of the Smiths Medical family of companies.)

applied. A beam of infrared light passes through the tissue and the machine measures the amount of light absorbed by oxygenated hemoglobin, which is displayed on the digital screen as a percentage. At the same time the light also measures the patient's pulse rate, which is also shown on the screen. A normal pulse oximeter reading is greater than or equal to 95% (meaning 95% of the total available hemoglobin attachments for oxygen are carrying oxygen). Treatment, such as oxygen or

bronchodilator therapies, is usually started when readings are at 90% to 92% or lower.

Obtaining Sputum for Culture

A sputum culture is requested when there are signs and symptoms accompanied by physical evidence of pneumonia, TB, or other infectious diseases of the lower respiratory tract. The sample is sent to a laboratory equipped to handle bacteriologic samples that are potentially infectious. Once the sample arrives at the laboratory, it is cultured and incubated. The pathogenic organism grown in the culture medium is then identified. If possible, the physician will not start antibiotic therapy until the sputum has been collected. The sample may also be sent to the laboratory for cytologic analysis that might suggest a cancerous condition of the lungs or bronchi.

Methods of Collection. In the ambulatory care setting the primary method for collection of a sputum sample is expectoration (Procedure 45-4), but sputum can be collected by tracheal suctioning and bronchoscopy. If the sample is to be collected by expectoration, most physician practices will have the patient perform the procedure at home with instruction. The medical assistant may be responsible for explaining the procedure to the patient or reinforcing physician instructions. The patient should understand that the best time for sputum specimen collection is in the morning when the patient first wakes up, before eating or drinking. The patient can rinse out his or her mouth with water before collecting the sample to decrease contamination from the oropharynx. The sample is collected from sputum coughed up from the lungs, not from saliva, so the patient should be encouraged to cough deeply and forcefully to collect a satisfactory sample. It may help to have the patient take several deep breaths, then cough. At least 1 teaspoon of sputum should be collected in a sterile specimen cup (the patient needs to know how to handle the specimen cup to maintain sterility), which needs to be returned to the office or laboratory as soon as possible after collection.

If the patient is taking antibiotic medications at the time of the specimen collection, this information should be included on the laboratory slip. If the cough does not produce sputum, chest physiotherapy or nebulization may be ordered by the physician to induce it. In some cases the physician may order sputum collection for three consecutive mornings.

CRITICAL THINKING APPLICATION

Tomas Garcia, a 68-year-old patient, has a chronic cough, and Dr. Samuelson orders a sputum culture to rule out an infectious disease. Mr. Garcia is supposed to collect the specimens every morning for the next 3 days, but he is very hard of hearing and does not understand English very well. His daughter is with him at today's visit, and she is bilingual. How should Michael relay the information about how to collect the sputum sample? What important details should be reviewed with Mr. Garcia's daughter?

Bronchoscopy

Bronchoscopy is typically performed in the outpatient clinic or hospital setting. However, the medical assistant should be

PROCEDURE 45-4

Prepare Patient for and Assist with Procedures, Treatments, and Minor Office Surgeries: Obtain a Sputum Sample for Culture

<u>CAAHEP COMPETENCIES:</u> 3.b.(4)(f), 3.b.(1)(e)
<u>ABHES COMPETENCIES:</u> 4.b, 4.r

GOAL: *To collect a sputum sample while observing standard precautions.*

EQUIPMENT and SUPPLIES

- Sterile laboratory specimen cup, accurately labeled
- Biohazard laboratory specimen bag with laboratory requisition
- Disposable examination gloves
- Face shield with goggles
- Impervious gown
- Biohazard waste container
- Cup of water
- Ginger ale or juice
- Patient record

PROCEDURAL STEPS

1. Assemble the equipment, and label the specimen cup.
2. Identify the patient, and explain the procedure.
   <u>PURPOSE:</u> An informed patient is more cooperative.
3. Wash your hands and don gloves, face shield with goggles, and impervious gown.
   <u>PURPOSE:</u> Standard precautions must be followed when collecting potentially infectious materials.
4. Have the patient rinse his or her mouth with water.
   <u>PURPOSE:</u> Any food particles in the mouth will contaminate the specimen.
5. Carefully remove the specimen cup lid, taking care not to touch the inside of the lid or the inside of the container, and place it upside down on a side table.
   <u>PURPOSE:</u> To maintain the sterile environment of the specimen cup.
6. Instruct the patient to take three deep breaths then cough deeply to bring up secretions from the lower respiratory tract.

<u>PURPOSE:</u> The organisms for culture must be from the lung fields in the lower respiratory tract.

7. Tell the patient to spit directly into the specimen container and to avoid getting any sputum on the exterior of the container. Do not touch the inside of the container during the procedure.
   <u>PURPOSE:</u> Sputum on the exterior of the container is considered hazardous. Prevent contamination of the inside of the container.
8. Place the lid on the container securely, taking care not to touch the inside of the lid, then place the container into the plastic specimen bag.
   <u>PURPOSE:</u> Maintain the sterility of the container, and minimize the possibility of spreading the potentially hazardous specimen.
9. Offer the patient a glass of juice or ginger ale.
   <u>PURPOSE:</u> The patient may have a bad taste in his or her mouth after the test, which may cause nausea.
10. If another test is ordered for the next morning, instruct the patient when to come to the office or explain how to complete the procedure at home. Remind him or her to follow the same instructions for preparation. Stress the importance of maintaining the sterility of the container and collecting the specimen first thing in the morning.
11. Clean the work area, and properly dispose of all supplies.
    <u>PURPOSE:</u> Observe standard precautions.
12. Wash your hands.
    <u>PURPOSE:</u> Infection control.
13. Process the specimen immediately to ensure optimal test results.
    <u>PURPOSE:</u> Microorganisms may propagate or die, creating either a false-positive or a false-negative result.
14. Record the procedure in the patient's record.
    <u>PURPOSE:</u> Procedures that are not recorded are considered not done.

---

familiar with the procedure, because he or she will probably schedule the test, instruct the patient on preparation, and help answer patient or family questions. Bronchoscopy provides an endoscopic view of the larynx, trachea, and bronchi. The procedure is performed by a pulmonary specialist or a surgeon with a flexible fiberoptic instrument through which the physician can visualize respiratory tissues and collect biopsy specimens or bronchial washings as needed for cytologic evaluation or culture. Laser therapy to treat endotracheal lesions is also possible through the flexible scope.

The patient should remain on nothing-by-mouth (NPO) status for 4 to 8 hours before the test to reduce the risk of aspiration. The patient should perform good mouth care before

the procedure to reduce the number of bacteria present. Dentures should be removed, and he or she will receive medication before the procedure to aid in relaxation and to dry up oral secretions. The patient should be reassured that the procedure does not interfere with breathing.

Before the instrument is inserted the physician will spray a topical anesthetic (lidocaine) in the mouth and on the back of the throat to help suppress the gag reflex and reduce any discomfort from passage of the instrument. The tube can be inserted through the nose or mouth, and as it reaches the glottis, more lidocaine is sprayed to control the cough reflex. The physician continues to pass the tube through the bronchi and larger bronchioles, collecting biopsy specimens of any suspicious tissue and obtaining cellular washings if indicated. Because the patient is sedated, it is not an uncomfortable procedure, but the patient may complain of a sore throat and experience hemoptysis for several hours after the procedure. Biopsy and culture reports are usually not available for 2 to 7 days.

CLOSING COMMENTS

Patient Education

It is often said that the greatest fear a person has is the fear of the unknown. Often the patient worries about tests that the physician orders. The imagination can create all types of frightening scenarios with even more alarming outcomes. The medical assistant can play a vital role in allaying patient fears by explaining diagnostic tests, making certain the patient understands how to prepare for the examination and what will be expected of him or her during the procedure. Make sure that the patient receives literature that explains the procedure that he or she can review at home. Answer all of the patient's questions, and consult with the physician regarding concerns or questions before the patient leaves the office.

Legal and Ethical Issues

When the respiratory system is mentioned, people generally think of breathing, but this is only one of the activities of the respiratory system. The cells of the body need a continuous supply of oxygen to maintain life. The respiratory system works together with the circulatory system to supply this oxygen and to remove the waste products of metabolism. Too often people take breathing for granted and assume that nothing could possibly happen to their ability to breathe. Sadly, respiratory diseases are the leading cause of death, and that means there are people we know and love who will suffer with and die of some of the diseases discussed in this chapter.

If the pulmonary test ordered is an invasive test, such as bronchoscopy, be certain that a written consent form is obtained from the patient and is in the patient's chart. If the patient is to see another specialist, a consent form must be signed to give permission to copy and forward patient information to the consultant. If oxygen therapy is ordered, the physician must write a prescription that specifies the amount of oxygen to be given and the type of device to be used for delivery. The physician may also write an order for a respiratory care practitioner to follow up on the patient at home.

SUMMARY OF SCENARIO

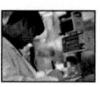

Michael has become very adept at performing respiratory diagnostic procedures and treatments for ambulatory patients. He enjoys interacting with this special group of patients and works at maintaining an up-to-date file on educational and resource assistance in the community. Michael especially enjoys the patient education aspect of caring for persons with respiratory diseases. Many of these patients have chronic diseases that will require long-term physician care, and Michael attempts to use available "teaching moments" to reinforce healthy lifestyle habits and confirm patient understanding of treatments. He continues to take advantage of local American Association of Medical Assistants (AAMA) meetings to keep up with recent practice trends and took a medical terminology refresher course at the local community college to improve his patient interview and charting skills. He is investigating developing a Smoke Stoppers group out of Dr Samuelson's office to encourage patients to develop healthier lifestyles and emphasizes to his patients who are employed in area coal mines and construction businesses the importance of consistently wearing a respirator.

SUMMARY of LEARNING OBJECTIVES

1. Define, spell, and pronounce the terms listed in the vocabulary.
   - Spelling and pronouncing medical terms correctly adds credibility to the medical assistant. Knowing the definition of these terms promotes confidence in communication with patients and co-workers.
2. Describe the organs of the respiratory system and their functions.
   - The respiratory system exchanges oxygen for carbon dioxide waste through external and internal respiration and helps maintain acid-base balance within the body. It works with the circulatory system to supply body cells with oxygen and remove metabolic wastes. The upper respiratory tract transports air through the nose, pharynx, and larynx. The lower respiratory tract consists of the trachea, bronchial tubes, and lungs.
3. Explain the process of ventilation.
   - Ventilation is the process by which the bronchioles deposit oxygenated air into the alveoli; a network of pulmonary capillaries surround the alveoli; oxygenated air moves out of the single-celled walls of the alveoli and into the capillaries; and carbon dioxide is forced out of the capillaries and into the alveoli, then out through the bronchioles. Inspiration is the movement of oxygen from the atmosphere into the alveoli, and the movement of carbon dioxide from the alveoli into the atmosphere is called expiration.

Continued

SUMMARY of LEARNING OBJECTIVES

Continued

4. Employ correct respiratory system terminology in documentation procedures.
   - Table 45-1 defines common respiratory system terms that should be used when charting patient signs and symptoms.
5. Compare and contrast infections and inflammations of the respiratory system.
   - URIs include the common cold, which is caused by a virus; sinusitis, which may be a result of an infection or allergic reaction; allergic rhinitis, which is triggered by multiple factors and causes nasal symptoms; and pneumonia, which is an infection of the lungs that can be caused by multiple pathogens and may range from a minor infection to a life-threatening disease.
6. Describe the diagnosis and treatment of tuberculosis.
   - TB, caused by *M. tuberculosis*, can be either active or latent. Individuals with active TB are infectious and exhibit the symptoms of the disease; those with latent TB have activated tubercles because of a weakened immune system. TB is diagnosed by a combination of PPD testing, chest x-ray studies, blood tests, and sputum cultures. It is treated with multiple medications dependent on the type and stage of the disease.
7. Summarize the disorders associated with chronic obstructive pulmonary disease and their treatments.
   - COPD is a group of diseases with the common characteristic of chronic airway obstruction. They include chronic bronchitis, bronchiectasis, asthma, pneumoconiosis, emphysema, and sleep apnea. The mechanism of obstruction may vary, but patients are unable to ventilate the lungs freely, which results in an ineffective exchange of respiratory gases. Treatments include bronchodilator and corticosteroid inhalers, evaluation of peak flow values, nebulizer treatments, oxygen, chest therapy, and CPAP machines.
8. Teach a patient how to use a peak flow meter.
   - Procedure 45-1 outlines the procedure for teaching a patient how to perform an accurate peak flow reading.
9. Perform a nebulizer treatment.
   - Procedure 45-2 outlines the procedure for performing a nebulizer treatment.

10. Detail patient teaching for the use of a metered-dose inhaler.
    - To accurately use an MDI, first shake the container and place it into the dispenser; open the mouth and while holding the dispenser about 1 inch away push the container down and inhale deeply; hold the breath for the count of 10 and then slowly exhale. The next dose should be administered in no sooner than 1 minute. The patient can use a spacer if needed to administer the dose.
11. Describe the cancers associated with the respiratory system.
    - Lung cancer is the leading cause of cancer-related deaths for both men and women; the lung is a common site for metastatic tumors as well. Prognosis is very poor for lung cancer, because early symptoms mimic chronic conditions present in long-term smokers. Carcinoma of the larynx is linked to smoking and chronic alcohol consumption; most laryngeal tumors are discovered in their early stages and are associated with a good prognosis.
12. Distinguish among common respiratory system diagnostic procedures.
    - Diagnostic procedures include the Mantoux intradermal test for TB; PFTs, which use a spirometer to diagnose pulmonary abnormalities; pulse oximetry, a noninvasive method of evaluating the oxygen saturation of hemoglobin in arterial blood and the pulse rate; cultures performed on expectorated sputum; and bronchoscopy, an endoscopic view of the larynx, trachea, and bronchi that uses a flexible fiberoptic instrument.
13. Perform a volume capacity spirometric test.
    - Procedure 45-3 summarizes the method for performing spirometer testing.
14. Correctly employ a pulse oximeter.
    - For use of a pulse oximeter, the probe is placed on the patient's earlobe or finger. An infrared light passes through the tissue, and the machine measures the amount of light absorbed by oxygenated hemoglobin, which is displayed on the digital screen as a percentage. The patient's pulse rate is also displayed.
15. Prepare a patient to collect a sputum sample for culture.
    - Procedure 45-4 summarizes how to collect a patient sputum specimen.

CONNECTIONS

Study Guide Connection: Go to Chapter 45 Study Guide. Read the Case Study and Workplace Applications and complete the assignments. Do online research for answers to the questions in the Internet Activities associated with assisting in pulmonary medicine.

CD Connection: Go to the Medical Assisting Competency Challenge CD and do the training activities under Diagnostic Testing. For a better understanding of pulmonary function, view the animation for normal cardiopulmonary physiology and inhalation.

Evolve Connection: For more information related to assisting in pulmonary medicine, go to evolve.elsevier.com/kinn and visit related weblinks for Chapter 45. Click on the Medical Assisting Exam Review and do the practice questions to sharpen your test-taking skills.

Assisting in Cardiology

46

SCENARIO

Adam Stern, CMA, has been working for more than 3 years as a medical assistant in a variety of physicians' offices. Adam was recently hired to work at City Hospital in the cardiology department. His job description includes working in the clinical area of the practice as well as assisting attending physicians with patient education and follow-up. Because Adam has never worked for a cardiologist, he is concerned about his knowledge base and competency in cardiac patient care. Part of Adam's responsibilities will be helping investigate patient education materials regarding the warning signs of a heart attack, especially the differences between the symptoms experienced by male versus female patients. In addition, the practice is in the process of updating the policies and procedures manual, and Adam is asked to create scenarios for telephone screening for patients calling in with symptoms of chest pain.

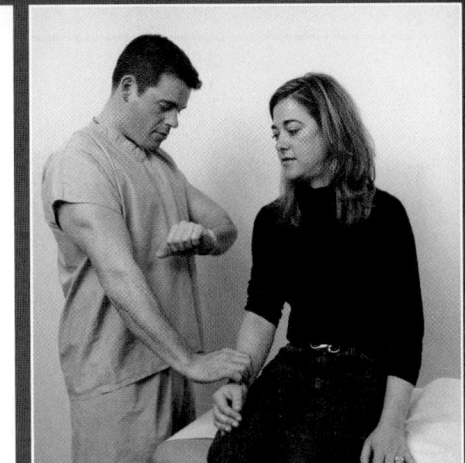

While studying this chapter, think about the following questions:

- Why is it important that Adam understand the normal anatomy and physiology of the cardiovascular system if he is going to work in a cardiologist's practice?
- What are some of the common diseases and disorders of the cardiovascular system with which Adam should be familiar?
- What are the common cardiovascular diagnostic procedures that Adam should be prepared to discuss and explain to patients?
- How should he go about developing these scenarios based on physician preference?

LEARNING OBJECTIVES

1. Define, spell, and pronounce the terms listed in the vocabulary.
2. Illustrate the anatomy and physiology of the heart and its significant structures.
3. Summarize risk factors for the development of cardiovascular disease.
4. Describe the signs, symptoms, and medical procedures employed in the diagnosis and treatment of coronary artery disease and myocardial infarction.
5. Compare and contrast the treatment protocols for hypertension.
6. Outline the causes and results of congestive heart failure.
7. Illustrate the effects of inflammation and valvular disorders on cardiac function.
8. Describe the anatomy and physiology of the vascular system.
9. Differentiate among the various types of shock.
10. Summarize the characteristics of common vascular disorders.
11. Outline typical cardiovascular diagnostic procedures.

National Accreditation Competencies and Content

CAAHEP COMPETENCIES	ABHES COMPETENCIES
Clinical	**Clinical**
3.b.(4)(f). Prepare patient for and assist with procedures, treatments, and minor office surgeries	4.b. Prepare patients for procedures
	4.h. Prepare patient for and assist physician with routine and specialty examinations
General	**Instruction**
3.c.(3)(b). Instruct individuals according to their needs	7.c. Teach patients methods of health promotion and disease prevention
3.c.(3)(c). Provide instruction for health maintenance and disease prevention	

VOCABULARY

bruit Abnormal sound or murmur heard on auscultation of an organ, vessel, or gland.

chordae tendineae (kor'-duh/ten'-din-uh) Tendons that anchor the cusps of the heart valves to the papillary muscles of the myocardium, preventing valvular prolapse.

intermittent claudication Recurring cramping in the calves caused by poor circulation of blood to the muscles of the lower leg.

Marfan syndrome An inherited condition characterized by elongation of the bones, joint hypermobility, abnormalities of the eyes, and development of aortic aneurysm.

scleroderma (skluh-rah-der'-muh) Autoimmune disorder that affects the blood vessels and connective tissue, causing fibrous degeneration of the major organs.

In the past, cardiac disease was frequently seen in men but seldom seen in women. That has changed, and today the most frequent cause of illness and death, regardless of gender, is cardiovascular disease. Medical assistants in all specialties often care for patients with heart disorders. Seldom does the cardiologist discover the heart problem. Most patients who see this specialist have already been diagnosed with a suspected heart disorder and were referred to the cardiologist for verification of the initial diagnosis and specialized treatment.

Because of the overwhelming number of people with cardiovascular problems, all medical assistants need to understand the cardiovascular system, be able to recognize early symptoms of potential disorders, perform basic screening tests when ordered by the physician, and assist the physician in the examination of the heart and blood vessels.

ANATOMY OF THE HEART

The heart is a hollow, muscular organ situated in the thoracic cavity in the mediastinal region, between the right and left pleural spaces. It weighs about 9 ounces and is about the size of a fist, with approximately two thirds of it located to the left of the sternum (Figure 46-1). The heart is a muscular pump that provides the force needed to push blood through all the arteries of the body, thus circulating a continuous supply of oxygen and nutrients to the cells and picking up the metabolic waste products from them. Deprived of these vital functions, the cells will die. At the same time, the heart also pushes deoxygenated blood through the pulmonary artery to the lungs for oxygen saturation and receives oxygenated blood back through the pulmonary veins into the left side of the heart. The average adult heart pumps about 5 L of blood every minute. If the heart loses its pumping action for even a few brief minutes, death or permanent damage can result.

Layers of the Heart

The heart is enclosed in a double-membrane sac called the *pericardium.* The outer layer of the pericardial sac, the *parietal pericardium,* is a tough membrane that connects the heart to the diaphragm and serves as a physical barrier to protect the heart

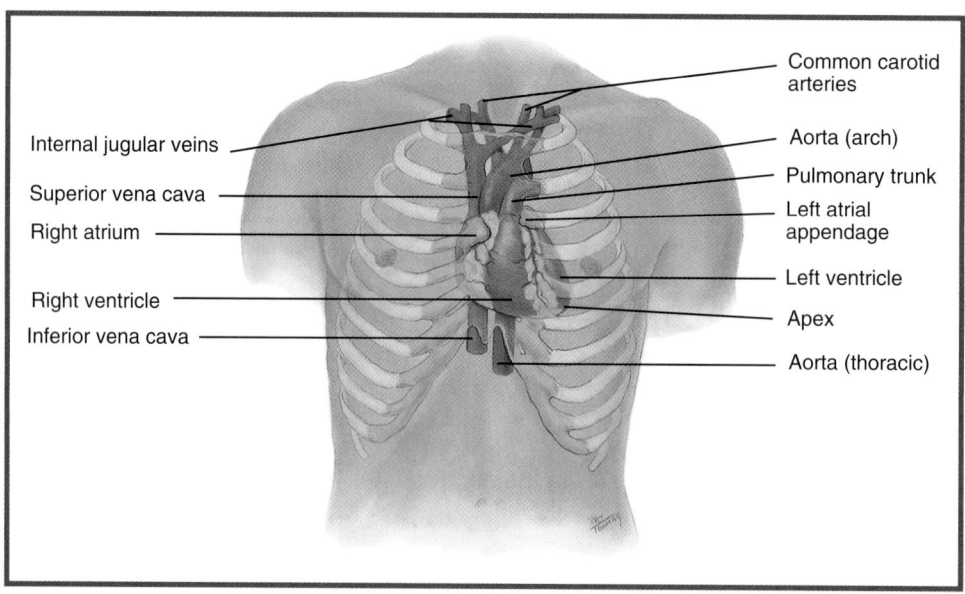

Internal jugular veins
Superior vena cava
Right atrium
Right ventricle
Inferior vena cava

Common carotid arteries
Aorta (arch)
Pulmonary trunk
Left atrial appendage
Left ventricle
Apex
Aorta (thoracic)

FIGURE 46-1 Location of the heart in the thoracic cavity. (From Applegate EJ: *The anatomy and physiology learning system,* ed 3, St Louis, 2006, Saunders.)

against infection or inflammation from the lungs or pleural space. The inner layer, the *visceral pericardium* or *epicardium*, forms the first layer of the heart. Between the two membranes is a small space, the *pericardial cavity*, which contains about 30 mL of *pericardial fluid* that lubricates the internal surfaces of the membranes, enabling them to slide across each other during heart contractions. The middle layer of the heart is the *myocardium*, the muscle layer that constitutes the largest percentage of the heart wall. Contractions of this muscle layer force the blood from the heart into the vessels. The inner layer of the heart is the *endocardium*, which includes the heart valves that separate the chambers of the heart and provide a means of blocking the flow of blood from major blood vessels entering and exiting the heart (Figure 46-2).

Heart Chambers and Arteries

The heart is divided into four chambers (Figure 46-3). The *atria*, the top chambers, receive blood, and the *ventricles*, the bottom chambers, pump the blood out. The blood flow through the heart begins in the right atrium, which receives deoxygenated blood from the inferior and superior *venae cavae*. The atria contract, and blood passes through the tricuspid valve into the

right ventricle; the ventricles contract, and blood passes from the right ventricle to the lungs via the *pulmonary artery* (the only artery in the body that contains deoxygenated blood). Oxygenation occurs in the alveoli of the lungs, and the now-oxygenated blood returns to the left atria through the *pulmonary veins* (the only veins in the body that carry oxygen-rich blood).

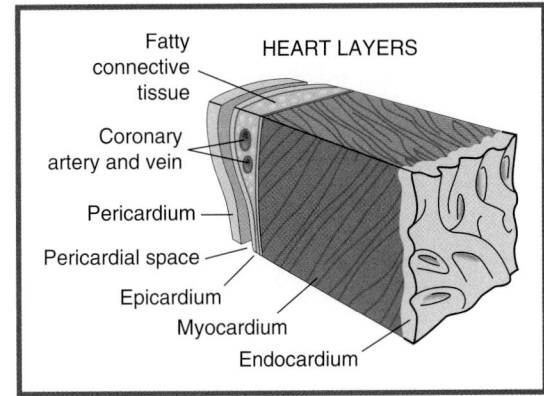

FIGURE 46-2 Layers of the heart. (From Damjanov I: *Pathology for the health-related professions*, ed 3, St Louis, 2006, Saunders.)

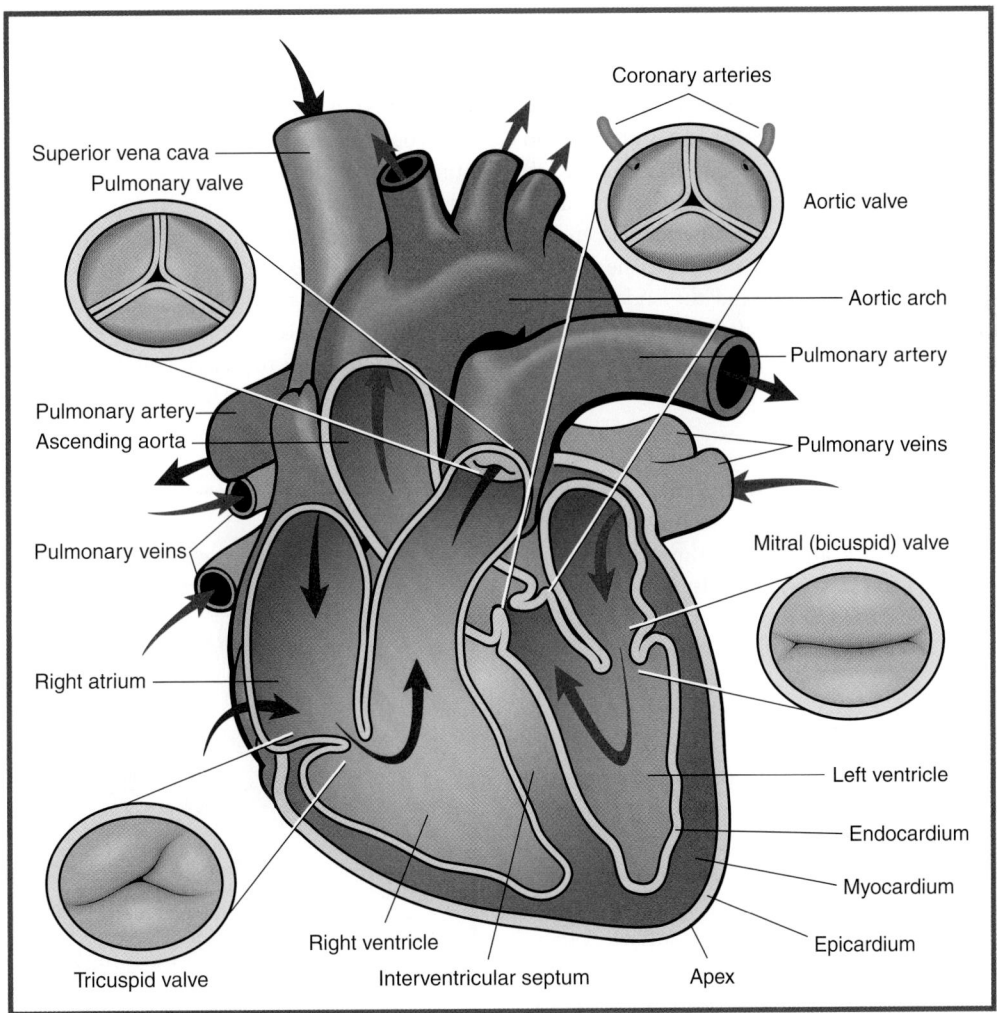

FIGURE 46-3 Chambers of the heart. (From Damjanov I: *Pathology for the health-related professions*, ed 3, St Louis, 2006, Saunders.)

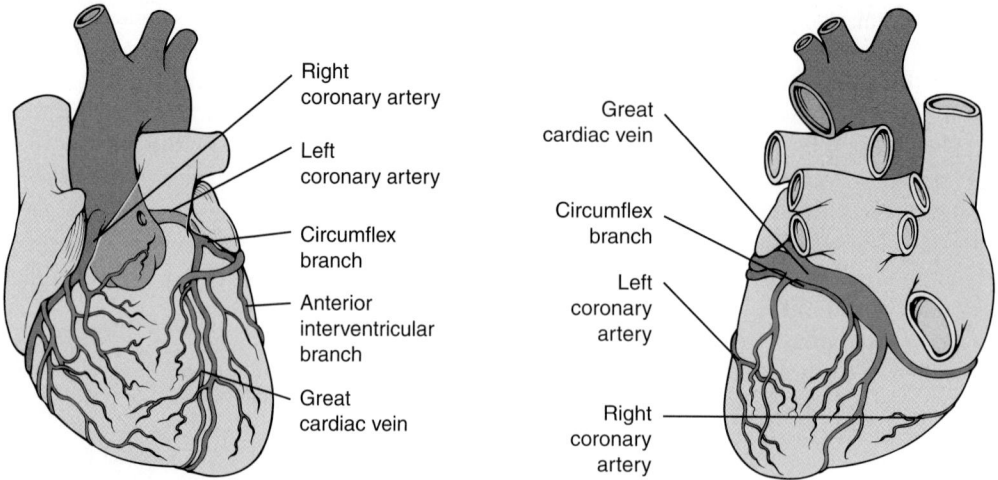

FIGURE 46-4 Coronary arteries. (From Frazier MS, Drzymkowski JW: *Essentials of human diseases and conditions*, ed 3, Philadelphia, 2004, Saunders.)

The atria contract, and blood passes through the mitral (bicuspid) valve into the left ventricle; the ventricles contract, and oxygen-rich blood is sent out to the body through the *aorta* (the largest artery in the body).

The myocardium requires a continuous supply of oxygen and nutrients, which are delivered through two coronary arteries that branch off the aorta above the aortic valve (Figure 46-4). The right coronary artery nourishes the anterior and posterior myocardium on the right side of the heart, and the left coronary artery does the same on the left side. The left coronary artery quickly divides and forms the left anterior descending artery and the left circumflex artery. Smaller branches of the coronary arteries feed the myocardium and the endocardium. Any interference in blood flow in any of the coronary vessels will alter heart action.

Heart Conduction

A sophisticated electrical conduction system operated by specialized cells located at various sites within the myocardium stimulates contractions. These muscle contractions move blood through the chambers of the heart and out through the aorta to the rest of the body. Each electrical impulse passes through the heart muscle in a twisting, spiral motion. These rhythmic waves cause the cardiac cells to beat, which causes the heart to contract.

The cardiac impulse originates in specialized muscle tissue called the *sinoatrial* (SA) node. The SA node rhythmically initiates impulses 70 to 80 times a minute; because it creates the basic rhythm, it is called the *pacemaker* of the heart. It is located in the posterior, superior wall of the right atrium, at the junction of the superior vena cava and the atrium and just above the tricuspid valve. When the SA node discharges its rhythm pattern into the myocardium, it causes both atria to contract, forcing blood through the valves and into the ventricles. The wave then passes through a second area of specialized muscle tissue located on the septal wall between the right atrium and right ventricle, called the *atrioventricular* (AV) node. The AV node

holds the impulse for a fraction of a second to prevent inappropriately high atrial rates as well as to permit the blood to empty from the atria through the tricuspid and mitral valves. The **chordae tendineae,** at this moment, close the valves between the atria and the ventricles tightly. Then the AV node releases the charge, sending it down through the *bundle of His,* located in the septum between the right and left ventricles. This bundle is divided into two main branches—the right bundle, located on the right side of the septum, and the left bundle, located on the left side. From the bundle branches, the transmission of the cardiac wave continues through a mass of cardiac muscle fibers known as the *Purkinje fibers*. The Purkinje fibers totally encase both ventricles, and the cardiac wave causes the ventricles to contract (Figure 46-5).

Contraction of the atria and the ventricles is also called *depolarization*. After the chambers contract, a period of electric

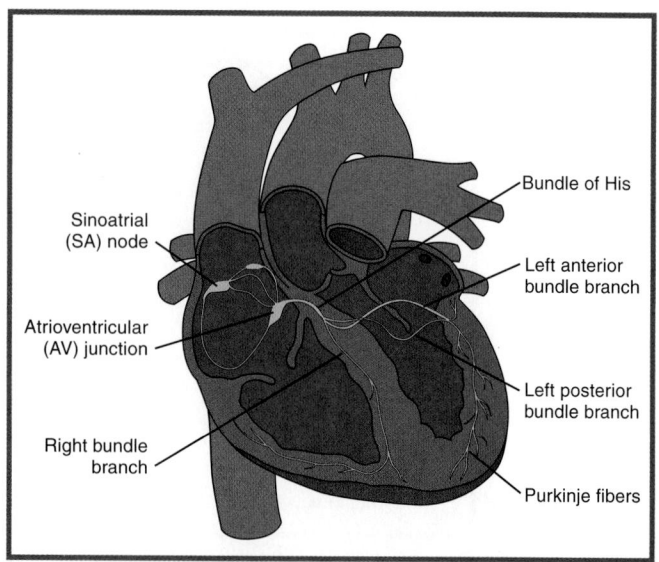

FIGURE 46-5 Cardiac conduction system.

recovery occurs, called *repolarization,* then the heart returns to resting *(polarization),* which starts the entire cycle again. The normal cardiac cycle consists of atrial contraction, ventricular contraction, then recovery and heart rest. This cycle maintains the average range of 60 to 100 beats per minute and a normal heart rhythm. It is this electrical force that is traced and evaluated when an electrocardiogram (ECG) is done. Chapter 48 presents ECGs.

DISEASES AND DISORDERS OF THE HEART

Many diseases and disorders affect the heart and its blood vessels. Disorders that occur when the rhythm of the heart becomes irregular are addressed in Chapter 48. There are multiple risk factors for cardiac disease, some that individuals can change or seek treatment for and others that cannot be changed. The more risk factors the person has, the greater the risk for developing cardiovascular disease.

Coronary Artery Disease and Myocardial Infarction

Coronary artery disease (CAD) causes over 1 million deaths in the United States every year. In CAD the arteries supplying

---

Risk Factors for Heart Disease According to the American Heart Association

Risk Factors That Cannot Be Changed

- Increasing age—the majority of people who die of heart disease are 65 years old or older; older women are more likely to die of myocardial infarctions (MIs) than older men.
- Gender—men are at greater risk for MIs and experience heart attacks earlier in life.
- Heredity and race—children of parents with heart disease are more likely to develop it; African Americans are at greater risk for developing hypertension and heart disease associated with it; Mexican Americans, American Indians, native Hawaiians, and some Asian Americans are also at greater risk.

Lifestyle Risk Factors That Can Be Modified or Treated

- Smoking—smokers develop heart disease two to four times more frequently. Smoking is associated with sudden cardiac death. Exposure to secondhand smoke also increases the risk.
- High blood cholesterol—heart disease risk increases with rising blood cholesterol levels.
- Hypertension—Hypertension increases the amount of work the heart has to do to circulate blood throughout the body.
- Sedentary lifestyle—regular exercise helps prevent cardiovascular disease.
- Obesity and overweight—excess weight, especially increased body fat at the waist, is associated with increased risk of heart disease and stroke; losing as little as 10 pounds can lower the risk.
- Diabetes mellitus—risks are even greater if blood glucose levels are not controlled; almost 75% of people with diabetes die of some form of heart or blood vessel disease.

---

the myocardium become narrowed by atherosclerotic plaques. A plaque originates at the site of a chronic injury to the endothelial lining of the artery caused by risk factors (such as smoking or hypertension) associated with heart disease. Platelets attach to the site of the endothelial injury, and lipids continue to accumulate. Eventually an *atheroma* forms, made up of a tough collagen shell covering a fatty center that extends out into the lumen of the vessel, restricting blood flow past the plaque. Inflammation at the site attracts platelets to the surface of the atheroma, resulting in the formation of a clot *(thrombus)* that can completely occlude the lumen of the vessel, depriving the myocardium of an adequate nutritious blood supply (Figure 46-6). The cardinal symptom of myocardial ischemia (holding back of blood) is angina pectoris. The features of anginal chest pain are pain behind the sternum that is precipitated by exertion but can be relieved by either rest or sublingual nitroglycerin.

Patients may be asymptomatic until the disease becomes fully developed. The first symptom may be angina, followed by pressure or fullness in the chest, syncope, shortness of breath, edema, unexplained coughing spells, and fatigue. A patient reporting any of these symptoms should be seen by the physician immediately.

Over recent years the rate of heart disease has declined in men but not in women. Traditional risk factors negatively affect both genders; however, women are at greater risk if they have *metabolic syndrome* (a combination of hypertension, elevated insulin levels, excess body fat around the waist, and high blood cholesterol levels); if they experience increased levels of stress and/or depression; if they smoke (female smokers are at much greater risk than male smokers); and if they have decreased estrogen production before menopause. The difference in female risks and symptoms is associated with the method of plaque buildup in women–they tend to develop an evenly spread layer of plaque along the entire lumen of blood vessels rather than localized plaque buildup as seen in vessels in men. Women with heart disease typically experience this diffuse atheroma buildup in smaller vessels, which causes more subtle symptoms than the crushing chest pain associated with classic myocardial infarctions (MIs).

The major concern in heart disease is the lack of blood to the myocardium, which occurs when a vessel becomes totally blocked. Ischemia over a prolonged period leads to *necrosis* (death) of a portion of the myocardium, resulting in an MI, or heart attack. Symptoms of MI are similar to those of angina, but MI is identified by pain lasting longer than 30 minutes that is unrelieved by rest or nitroglycerin tablets. An MI is life-threatening; intervention must begin within the first hour, or death may occur.

CRITICAL THINKING APPLICATION

A patient who is scheduled for an appointment in 2 days calls the office and reports that she is not feeling well. She complains that she has a feeling of fullness in the chest, her arms ache, and she is very tired. Although this patient does not have a history of myocardial infarction, what should Adam do?

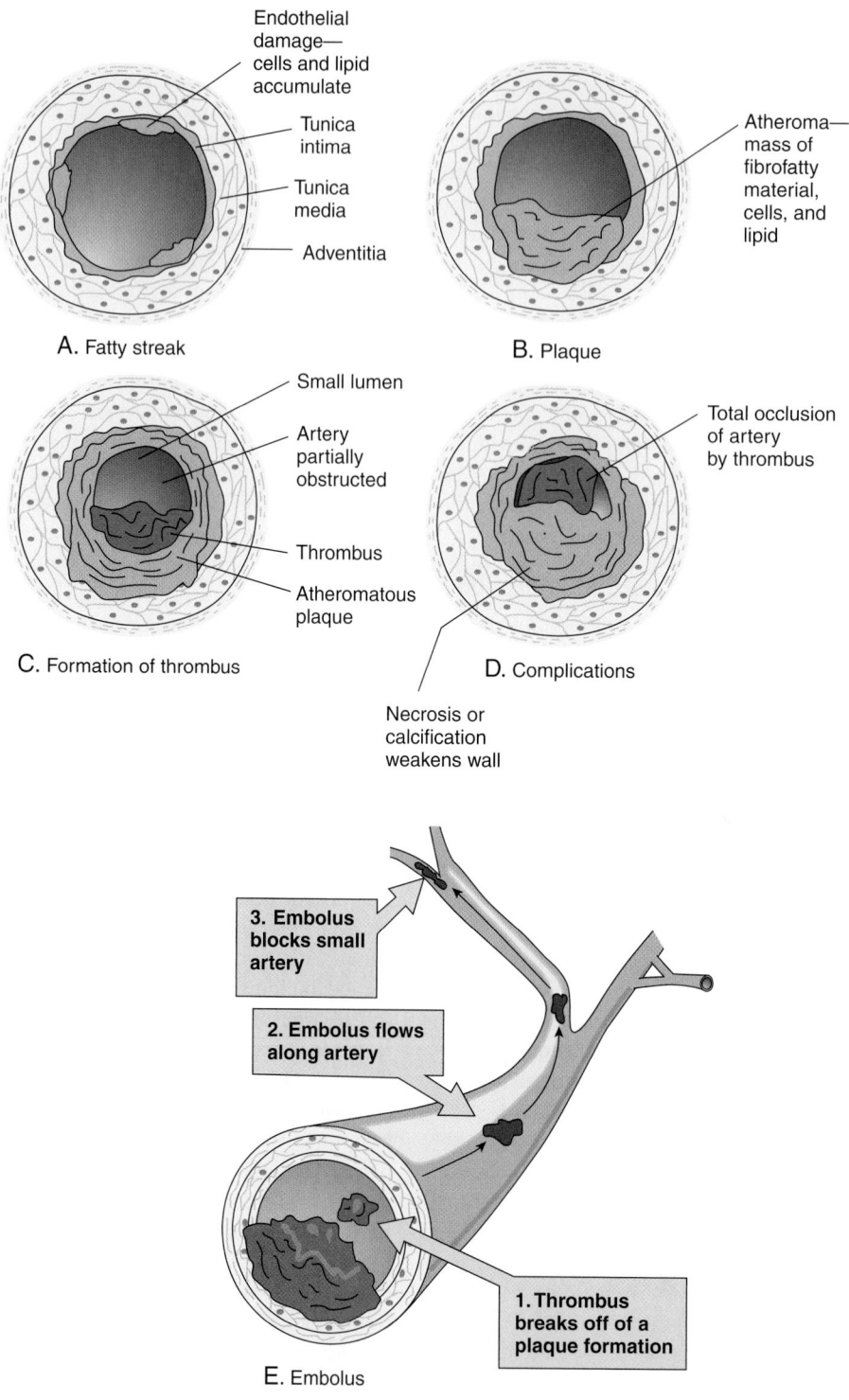

FIGURE 46-6 Development of an atheroma leading to arterial occlusion. (From Gould BA: *Pathophysiology for the health professions*, ed 3, Philadelphia, 2002, Saunders.)

Diagnostic and Therapeutic Procedures

An MI is diagnosed by ECG changes and elevated cardiac enzymes (creatinine phosphokinase [CPK] and lactate dehydrogenase [LDH]) 6 to 12 hours after the episode. These enzymes are released by the necrotic myocardium and may be within normal limits initially but continue to increase for 24 to 49 hours after the MI has occurred. Patients diagnosed with an MI are hospitalized immediately, started on oxygen, and continuously monitored by ECG. Additional diagnostic procedures such as echocardiograms and heart catheterizations are discussed later in this chapter.

Medical treatment includes the use of thrombolytic medications, such as streptokinase, to dissolve the coronary artery blockage; however, this treatment must be started within

Signs and Symptoms of Myocardial Infarction in Women

In addition to angina, the signs and symptoms of heart attack in women include the following:

- Abdominal, neck, shoulder, or upper back pain
- Jaw pain
- Shortness of breath
- Sweating
- Indigestion or nausea and vomiting
- Extreme fatigue
- Aching in both arms

Telephone Screening for Chest Pain

The medical assistant should activate emergency medical services if the patient reports any of the following:

- Current chest pain that is crushing, pressing, or radiating to the arms, upper back, or jaw
- Sweating, difficulty breathing, nausea, indigestion, or dizziness
- A history of coronary artery disease, myocardial infarction, or angina
- A change in the pattern of the angina
- Chest pain that occurs when resting or with minimal exertion

6 hours of the episode and no longer than 24 hours after initial symptoms to be effective in preventing permanent myocardial damage. This timetable makes it extremely important that patients be identified and treatment started as soon as possible. Additional pharmaceutical treatment includes the use of aspirin to prevent blood clotting; nitroglycerin to dilate the coronary arteries so more blood can be delivered to the myocardium; beta-blockers (Tenormin, Lopressor, or Inderal) to slow the heart rate and lower blood pressure; anticoagulants (warfarin [Coumadin]) for 3 to 6 months to prevent thrombus formation; and anticholesterol agents (Lipitor, Mevacor, or Zocor) to lower blood cholesterol levels and prevent subsequent formation of atherosclerotic plaques.

When blockage or occlusion has taken place in the coronary arteries that supply blood to the myocardium, either percutaneous transluminal coronary angioplasty (PTCA) or coronary artery bypass surgery (CABG) may be indicated. These procedures are discussed later in this chapter. After discharge from the hospital, patients with CAD that has resulted in an MI face multiple lifestyle changes to prevent the occurrence of another episode. Recommendations include no smoking; regular light exercise, such as walking up to an hour three times per week; a diet that is low in salt, fat, and cholesterol; and stress reduction. The medical assistant should be prepared to provide encouragement and reinforce the importance of lifestyle changes to prevent future heart problems. If ordered by the physician, professional referrals to a cardiac rehabilitation program and dietitian can also be helpful.

CRITICAL THINKING APPLICATION

Adam receives a telephone call from a patient who complains of nausea, has difficulty taking a deep breath, and feels like he is going to faint. What questions should he ask to determine the seriousness of the problem?

Hypertensive Heart Disease

Chronic elevated blood pressure can result in left ventricular *hypertrophy* (enlargement), angina, MI, or heart failure. Hypertension is also a major cause of stroke and *nephropathy* (kidney disease). Some of the risk factors for developing hypertension include a family history of hypertension or stroke, *hypercholesterolemia* (high blood cholesterol), smoking, high sodium intake, diabetes, excessive alcohol intake, sedentary lifestyle, obesity, aging, prolonged stress, and race (blacks have a higher incidence than whites). Hypertension has an insidious onset, with the patient showing few, if any, signs and symptoms until permanent damage occurs. Initial symptoms may include general malaise and headache; epistaxis (nosebleed), vertigo, nausea, or syncope can occur with prolonged hypertension.

The two types of hypertension are primary and secondary. *Secondary hypertension* occurs because of a disease process in another body system, such as renal disease or an endocrine disorder. Before secondary hypertension can be properly treated, the underlying disease process must be resolved.

Primary, or essential, hypertension is *idiopathic* (of unknown cause) and is diagnosed if the patient's blood pressure is persistently higher than 119 mm Hg systolic and/or 79 mm Hg diastolic at two or more office visits over several weeks or months. If the medical assistant first notes a patient's elevated blood pressure, it is recommended that the blood pressure be checked in both arms with the patient seated and after the patient has been standing for at least 2 minutes with a cuff that is the proper size for the patient's arm. If the pressure readings are different, the physician will use the higher value for diagnostic purposes. The patient's blood pressures should be checked again after at least 2 minutes. All of these readings must be documented in the patient record. Some patients have what is called "white-coat" hypertension, which appears only when they visit the physician. If the patient has a history of this problem, have him or her lie down on the examination table and rest for a few minutes before the blood pressure is taken; this may help to get a more accurate reading (Table 46-1).

The medical assistant can be an interactive part of this therapy by teaching the patient how to take his or her own blood pressure at home, providing literature that reinforces the necessity of monitoring the blood pressure, and helping the patient to understand that this condition cannot be cured but can be controlled for the rest of his or her life. Continued encouragement and support are needed because compliance with the treatment regimen is difficult for a patient who is not exhibiting any symptoms of disease.

TABLE 46-1 Stages of Hypertension and Treatment Recommendations

BLOOD PRESSURE	TREATMENT
Prehypertension (120 to 139/80 to 89 mm Hg)	Lifestyle modification (reduced sodium, low-fat diet; regular aerobic activity; moderate alcohol intake; smoking cessation; weight loss; and stress reduction) Drug therapy in patients with diabetes mellitus or chronic kidney disease
Stage 1 (140 to 159/90 to 99 mm Hg)	Consider coexisting conditions Thiazide-type diuretics (furosemide [Lasix] or Dyazide) for most patients
Stage 2 (≥160/≥100 mm Hg)	Consider coexisting conditions Two-drug combination for most patients

Recommendations by the Joint National Committee on Prevention, Detection, Evaluation, and Treatment of High Blood Pressure.

CRITICAL THINKING APPLICATION

Essential hypertension is a common problem for patients seen in the cardiology department where Adam works. What could Adam do to help patients with primary hypertension? What informational materials or community resources would be helpful in gaining patient compliance with treatment?

Congestive Heart Failure

Congestive heart failure (CHF) occurs when the myocardium is unable to pump an adequate amount of blood to meet the needs of the body. Although the problem can have an acute onset, it typically develops over time because of weakness in the left ventricle from chronic hypertension, MI of the ventricular wall, valvular heart disease, or pulmonary complications. Typically, heart failure initially occurs on one side of the heart, followed by the other side. Left-sided heart failure usually results from essential hypertension or left-ventricular disease, whereas right-sided heart failure can develop from lung disease. Right-sided heart failure that occurs because of pulmonary hypertension associated with chronic obstructive pulmonary disease (COPD) is called *cor pulmonale.*

Left-sided heart failure, in which the left ventricle cannot completely empty, causes a backup of blood in the left atria and ultimately the lungs, resulting in *pulmonary edema,* a collection of fluid in the lungs. Signs and symptoms include dyspnea, orthopnea, nonproductive cough, rales, and tachycardia. *Right-sided heart failure,* when the right ventricle cannot maintain complete output, causes a backup of blood in the right atrium, which prevents complete emptying of the vena cava, resulting in systemic edema, especially in the legs and feet. Both types of heart failure cause fatigue, weakness, exercise intolerance, dyspnea, and sensitivity to cold temperatures.

Nonmedication treatment for CHF includes limiting physical activity so that the heart does not have to work so hard, restricting salt, not smoking, reducing stress, and controlling weight. Patient education for an individual with CHF must stress the importance of monitoring weight gain, because a sudden increase in weight may indicate fluid retention. Patients should weigh themselves one or two times per week and report an increase in weight of more than 3 pounds to the physician.

Drug therapy for CHF begins with diuretics to treat dyspnea and orthopnea and control edema. Other medications may include an angiotensin-converting enzyme (ACE) inhibitor—a type of vasodilator that widens blood vessels to lower blood pressure and decrease the workload on the heart. Examples include enalapril (Vasotec), lisinopril (Prinivil, Zestril) and captopril (Capoten). Digoxin is often prescribed to increase the strength of myocardial contractions, and beta-blockers (carvedilol [Coreg] and metoprolol [Lopressor] are used to slow the heart rate and improve heart function. Because potassium loss is a common side effect of diuretic and digitalis use, patients may also be prescribed a potassium (KCl) supplement. The physician will order routine monitoring of serum electrolytes to determine the need for a potassium supplement so that potential complications can be avoided.

Implantable Cardioverter-Defibrillator

An implantable cardioverter-defibrillator (ICD) is a pager-size device implanted in the chest under the skin and attached to the heart with small wires. It continuously monitors the heart rhythm and is designed to deliver a measured electric shock to the myocardium to correct life-threatening arrhythmias such as ventricular tachycardia or ventricular fibrillation. ICDs have become the standard treatment for anyone with a serious arrhythmia who is at risk for sudden cardiac death.

CRITICAL THINKING APPLICATION

Kate Glasgow, a 76-year-old patient with a history of CHF, is in the office today for a checkup. Miss Glasgow does not understand why she needs to stop using salt and does not weigh herself regularly at home. What can Adam do to help this patient understand the importance of her treatment regimen?

Orthostatic Hypotension

Orthostatic or postural hypotension is diagnosed if the patient experiences a drop in blood pressure when standing, especially when quickly going from a prone or seated position to an upright one. When we stand our blood pressure quickly adapts to the pull of gravity by reflexively increasing the heart rate and constricting systemic arterioles. Patients who experience orthostatic hypotension have blood pressures that adjust either sluggishly or not at all to rapid changes in position. An acute episode of orthostatic hypotension may be caused by blood pooling in the lower extremities, a reaction to antihypertensive or antidepressant medication, or prolonged immobility. It is a common problem in elderly people and may significantly contribute to falls and related injuries. Patients need to be evaluated for secondary causes and encouraged to adjust from a prone position by sitting at the side of the bed before standing.

To evaluate orthostatic hypotension, the physician will request you check the patient's blood pressure while seated, leave the cuff in place, have the patient stand, and immediately check the patient's blood pressure again. Both blood pressure readings should be recorded in the patient's chart for the physician to evaluate. Include in your note any patient complaints after standing including dizziness or a feeling of lightheadedness.

Inflammations and Valvular Disorders

Rheumatic Heart Disease

Rheumatic heart disease develops because of an unusual immune reaction that occurs within 5 weeks after an untreated beta-hemolytic streptococcal infection. The infection starts as "strep" throat or an upper respiratory infection but progresses to the creation of antibodies that react with collagen to cause inflammation in the joints, skin, brain, and heart. During a first rheumatic fever attack, about half of those affected develop heart inflammation, but most have a complete recovery. However, some people experience damage and scar formation of the heart's valves. The disease process in the heart can involve all layers of heart tissue.

Pericarditis, inflammation of the outer layer of the heart, causes reduced cardiac activity and *pericardial effusion* (collection of blood or fluid in the pericardium). *Myocarditis,* inflammation of the muscular lining of the heart, is usually self-limiting but may lead to acute heart failure because of weakening of the myocardial wall. *Endocarditis,* inflammation of the inner lining of the heart and the heart valves, is the most common heart complication. Vegetations form along the outer edges of the valve cusps, causing scarring and stenosis, preventing the damaged heart valve from closing or opening completely. The valvular damage may be asymptomatic at first but can eventually cause serious problems. The mitral valve is affected most frequently, which impacts the ability of the left ventricle to function normally.

Treatment includes the use of antibiotics (penicillin) to eliminate the streptococcal infection completely and anti-inflammatory agents for the inflammatory reaction. Follow-up includes the prompt treatment of strep infections and possible antibiotic prophylaxis prescribed before all invasive procedures (such as dental work) to prevent a recurrence of the immune response and additional damage to the heart valves.

Valvular Disorders

Disorders of the valves of the heart may be caused by a congenital defect or an infection such as endocarditis or rheumatic heart disease. Two specific problems can occur with valve disease. The valve can be *stenosed,* or hardened, which restricts the forward flow of blood, or it can be *incompetent,* meaning that it does not close completely, so blood can leak backward or regurgitate. The most common valve defect is *mitral valve prolapse* (MVP), an incompetence in the mitral valve, because of a congenital defect or vegetation and scarring from endocarditis.

Valve disorders can ultimately lead to ventricular hypertrophy and *cardiomegaly* (enlargement of the heart). Physicians typically prescribe prophylactic amoxicillin, 2 g, 1 hour before an invasive procedure, to prevent further vegetative growth on the valve. Severely damaged valves or serious congenital defects may necessitate surgical replacement of the affected valve.

BLOOD VESSELS

Blood vessels are divided into two systems that begin and end with the heart (Figure 46-7). The pulmonary system carries deoxygenated blood from the right ventricle to the lungs and oxygenated blood back to the left atrium. The systemic system carries blood from the left ventricle throughout the entire body and back to the right atrium. The vessels are classified according to their structure and function as arteries, which carry oxygenated blood away from the heart; capillaries, the microscopic vessels that are responsible for the exchange of oxygen and carbon dioxide in the tissue; and veins, the vessels that carry deoxygenated blood back to the heart.

Arteries

All arteries, except the pulmonary artery, carry oxygenated blood away from the heart to all the cells of the body. The largest of these vessels is the aorta, which starts at the left ventricle and travels through the center of the body into the lower abdomen, where it bifurcates into the right and left femoral arteries with arteries branching off of this system down to the feet. As the aorta passes through the body, arteries branch off from it into smaller and smaller vessels, which ultimately become microscopic. These vessels are referred to as *arterioles* and terminate into tissue *capillaries,* which are the smallest and most plentiful of the blood vessels. Capillaries are a single epithelial cell thick so that nutrients and gases can cross through the wall to be exchanged on the cellular level. Arterioles deliver *erythrocytes* (red blood cells [RBCs]), which carry oxygen attached to hemoglobin molecules to surrounding tissues. When the blood leaves the capillary bed, the oxygen supply has been depleted, and it now begins the return portion of the blood cycle.

Veins

As the blood leaves the capillary beds, it enters the smallest veins, called *venules.* From this point on, the blood will flow into larger and larger veins until it reaches the largest veins in the body, the inferior and superior *venae cavae.* The venae cavae deposit deoxygenated blood into the right atrium, where the blood again begins its trip through the heart, into the pulmonary arteries to the lungs, then through the pulmonary veins, which will bring the extremely rich oxygenated blood back from the lungs to the left atrium.

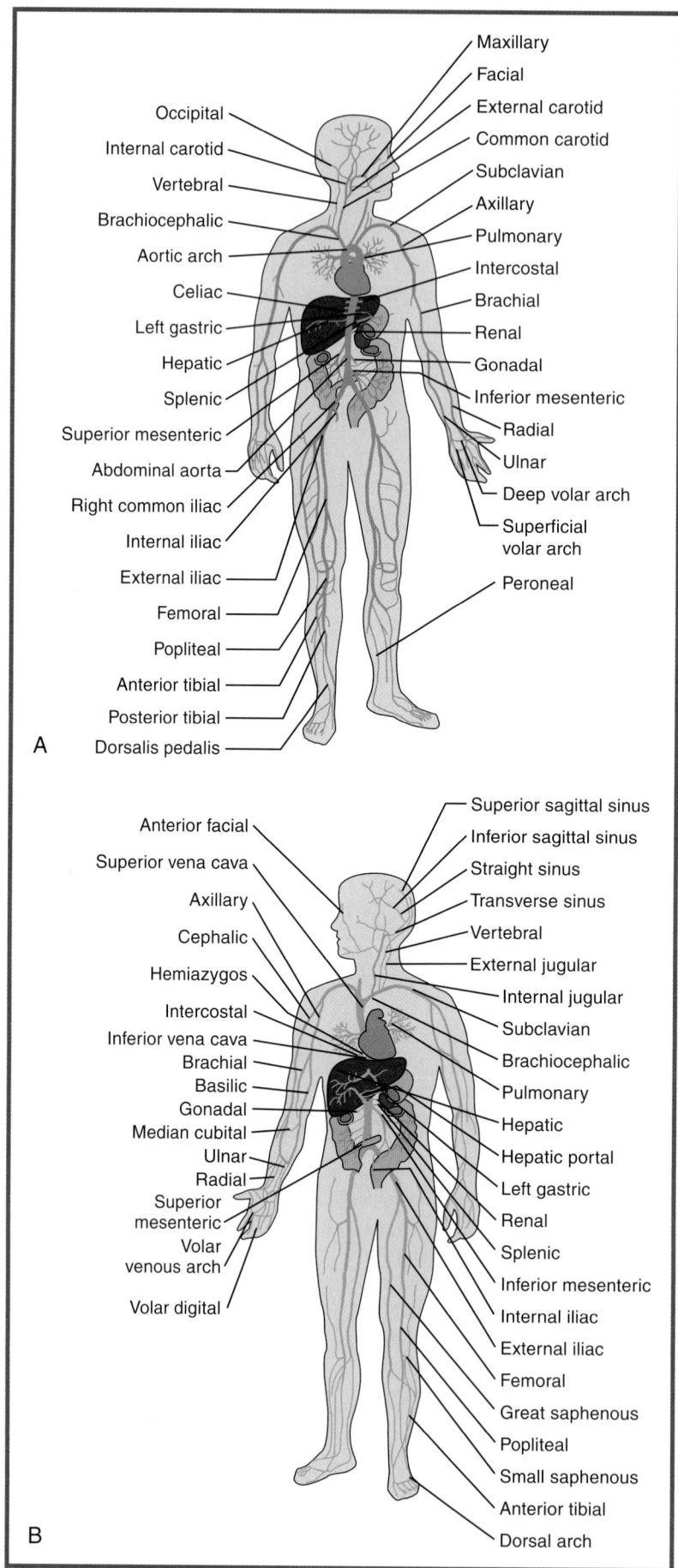

FIGURE 46-7 A, Systemic arteries. **B,** Systemic veins.

The walls of veins are thinner than those of the arteries because they do not contain a muscular lining. Instead, veins have valves that open and close because of the contraction of surrounding muscles to prevent the backflow of blood. These venous valves are especially important in the arms and legs because they prevent pooling of blood in the extremities.

VASCULAR DISORDERS

The vascular system is constantly busy supplying blood that contains oxygen and nutrients to all of our tissues and picking up waste from tissue metabolism. For tissues to receive an adequate amount of oxygen and nutrients, the arterial vessels must maintain elasticity and their linings need to remain smooth to prevent occlusion and decreased blood flow.

Shock

Many different situations cause shock (Table 46-2), but they all result in the same signs and symptoms and possible complications. Shock is the general collapse of the circulatory system, including decreased cardiac output, hypotension, and *hypoxemia* (decreased oxygen in the blood). The initial signs of shock are extreme thirstiness, restlessness, and irritability. The body attempts to compensate for circulatory collapse with constriction of peripheral blood vessels, allowing blood to pool in the vital organs. This vasoconstriction causes a generalized feeling of cool, clammy skin; pallor; tachycardia; and decreased urinary output. Symptoms progress to a rapid, weak, thready pulse; tachypnea; and altered levels of consciousness. If the process is not reversed, the central nervous system becomes depressed and acute renal failure may occur.

The cause of the shock must be treated for the patient to survive. If the medical assistant identifies a patient in shock, emergency treatment should be started at once. Do not wait for the first indicators of shock to worsen before calling for help. If the physician is not available, call 911 for emergency medical care. Place the patient in a supine position, assess vital signs frequently, keep the patient warm, administer oxygen, and elevate the legs (if there is no indication of head or neck trauma) to encourage the flow of blood back to the heart.

Vein Disorders

Varicose Veins

Varicose veins are dilated, tortuous, superficial veins in the legs (Figure 46-8). Varicosities can be caused by congenitally defective valves in the saphenous veins and those veins branching off of them. Other contributing factors are pregnancy, obesity, prolonged standing or sitting, and heavy lifting. Whatever

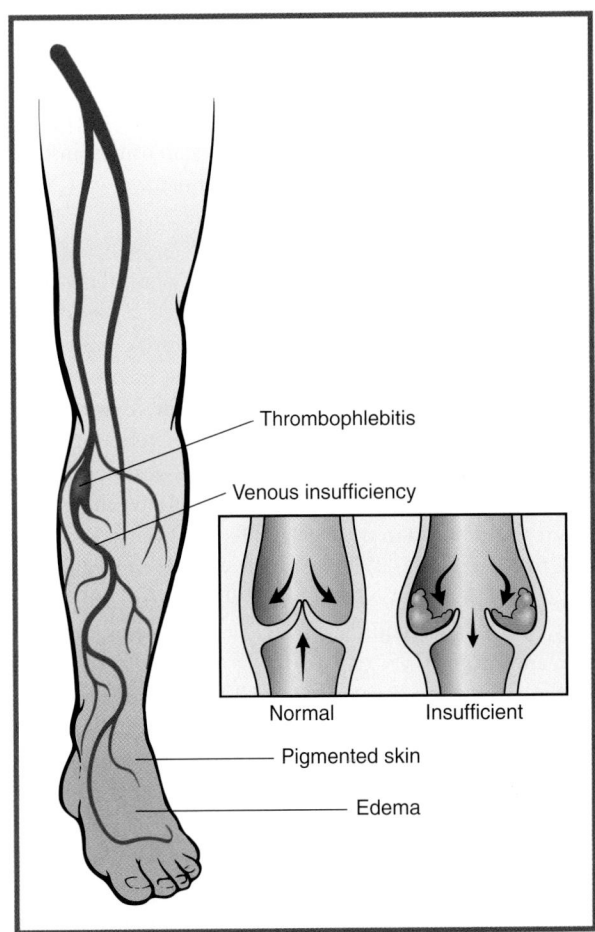

FIGURE 46-8 Varicose veins of the calf. (From Damjanov I: *Pathology for the health-related professions*, ed 3, St Louis, 2006, Saunders.)

TABLE 46-2 Types and Causes of Shock		
TYPE	**DEFINITION**	**CAUSE**
Cardiogenic	Low cardiac output caused by inability of heart to pump	Acute MI, arrhythmias, pulmonary embolism, CHF
Hypovolemic	Excessive loss of blood or body fluids	GI bleeding, internal or external hemorrhage, excessive loss of plasma or body fluids, burns
Neurogenic	Peripheral vascular dilation resulting from neurologic injury or disorder	Spinal cord injury, emotional stress, drug reaction
Anaphylactic	Systemic hypersensitivity to an allergen causing respiratory distress and vascular collapse	Drug, vaccine, shellfish, nuts, insect venom, chemical, allergies
Septic (septicemia)	Systemic vasodilation caused by the release of bacterial endotoxins	Systemic infection or bacteremia

CHF, Congestive heart failure; *GI,* gastrointestinal; *MI,* myocardial infarction.

the cause, the valves do not completely close, allowing blood to flow backward, thus causing the vein to distend from the increased pressure.

Treatment includes consistent aerobic exercise and limiting heavy lifting. The legs should be elevated when possible, and support stockings should be worn by persons who must stand for long periods. Varicose veins may need surgical intervention consisting of laser treatments, saline injections, or surgical ligation and stripping. Although treatment may be successful, varicosities can recur over time. Patients should be warned to investigate insurance coverage of treatment costs because many insurance companies consider treatment of varicose veins cosmetic surgery. However, if the patient has documented proof of a health risk associated with the varicosities, insurance companies are more likely to pay for treatment.

Deep Vein Thrombosis

Phlebitis is an inflammation of a vein, most commonly seen in the lower legs. When a vein becomes inflamed, a blood clot or *thrombus* may develop at the site. A thrombus is a collection of platelets that form a clot that attaches to the interior wall of a vessel. *Deep vein thrombosis* (DVT) is a thrombus with inflammatory changes that has attached to the deep venous system of the lower legs, causing a partial or complete obstruction of the vessel. The most common sites for DVT are the calf veins, but they can also develop in the iliac and femoral veins. Risk factors for the formation of a DVT are recent surgery, immobilization, older age (with increased risk over the age of 50), trauma, obesity, use of oral contraceptives, varicose veins, pancreatic cancer, and pregnancy.

In the early stages approximately 50% of patients with DVTs are asymptomatic. Some patients complain of calf pain and edema of the affected leg, with warmth and erythema at the site. If a thrombus becomes dislodged and begins to circulate through the general circulation, it is then called an *embolus*. *Pulmonary embolism* (PE), a DVT that has become loose and is carried to the lungs, causing blockage of a pulmonary artery, is the most serious complication and may be the first indication that the thrombus was present.

DVTs are typically diagnosed with venous Doppler studies, which use ultrasound to measure the rate of blood flow through the vessel and can accurately detect venous obstruction. Ultrasound can also be used to create an image of the blood flow through the targeted vessel, allowing visualization of the thrombus. *Venography* may also be ordered; in venography a dye is injected into a large vein of the foot or ankle and x-ray films of the veins are taken. Once the diagnosis is confirmed, patients are usually hospitalized for intravenous anticoagulant therapy (heparin). On discharge, oral anticoagulant treatment (warfarin [Coumadin]) is continued for several months. Patients require regular follow-up, including prothrombin time analysis. The medical assistant may perform venipuncture on these patients and, if so, should follow the office policy for blood draws on patients taking anticoagulants. In addition, the medical assistant should reinforce the physician's recommendations regarding prevention of future thrombi and precautions regarding anticoagulant use.

CRITICAL THINKING APPLICATION

Alitza Lincoln is a 43-year-old patient who has large varicose veins in both legs and a history of phlebitis. She is a checkout clerk at the local Wal-Mart, so she stands for extended periods of time. The physician is concerned about the development of a DVT and instructs Adam on the prevention, signs, and symptoms of a thrombus. Alitza asks Adam what she can do to prevent further problems with the veins in her legs. Adam uses a picture to illustrate the valves in the leg veins and explains preventive measures. What measures should Adam include?

Arterial Disorders

Arteriosclerosis and Atherosclerosis

Arteriosclerosis is a general term for the thickening and loss of elasticity of arterial walls that is associated with the aging process. Other conditions that can lead to hardening of the arterial wall are hypertension, **scleroderma,** and diabetes mellitus. Arteriosclerosis can occur in arteries throughout the body and cause systemic ischemia and necrosis over time.

Atherosclerosis is a form of arteriosclerosis in which there is the formation of an atheroma, a buildup of cholesterol, cellular debris, and platelets along the inside vessel wall (Figure 46-9). Cholesterol was discussed in Chapter 29, with recommendations for high-density lipoprotein (HDL) and low-density lipoprotein (LDL) levels. Cholesterol is a nonessential nutrient that can be produced in the liver and forms the base for many of the hormones created in the body. Problems arise from dietary and lifestyle factors that elevate blood cholesterol levels to a dangerous point, causing the formation of atheromas, which ultimately block arteries and cause such disorders as heart attacks and strokes.

Treatment of elevated blood cholesterol levels consists of dietary reductions in saturated fats and foods high in cholesterol as well as aerobic exercise to elevate HDL levels. Patients are encouraged to stop smoking. Statin drugs such as atorvastatin calcium (Lipitor) and simvastatin (Zocor) may be used to control or reverse plaque buildup. The medical assistant can help by educating the patient about risk factors and promoting alterations in lifestyle. Referrals to a dietitian may help patients who are having a difficult time controlling their fat intake.

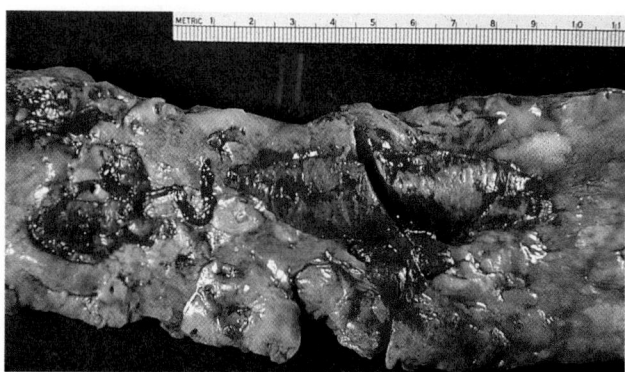

FIGURE 46-9 Atherosclerotic vessel. (From Damjanov I: *Pathology for the health-related professions,* ed 3, St Louis, 2006, Saunders.)

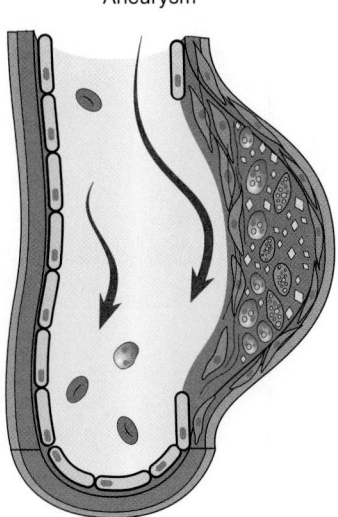

FIGURE 46-10 An aneurysm resulting from weakening of the vessel wall. (From Damjanov I: *Pathology for the health-related professions,* ed 3, St Louis, 2006, Saunders.)

Aneurysm

An aneurysm is a ballooning or dilation of a blood vessel wall (Figure 46-10). The patient may have an inherited factor for the development of aneurysms, such as in **Marfan syndrome,** but a common cause is the buildup of atherosclerotic plaques, which weaken the vessel wall. Aneurysms can occur in any artery but usually develop in either the abdominal aorta or the cerebral arteries. In either case, the patient seldom has any signs or symptoms. Occasionally, the patient describes a pounding or pulsating pain in the area of the aneurysm.

An aneurysm can be diagnosed when auscultation of the affected vessel over the area of the aneurysm reveals turbulent blood flow sounds, or a **bruit.** Radiologic studies, sonography, and computed tomography all help to confirm the diagnosis. Patients are monitored on a routine basis for changes in the size of the aneurysm. Surgical repair is recommended for all aneurysms 6 cm or larger, but smaller ones can also rupture. If an aneurysm is tender and known to be enlarging rapidly, no matter what the size, surgery is essential. If a rupture occurs, immediate lifesaving intervention must be done.

The medical assistant may aid the physician by observing the patient for signs of pain, mental changes, and alterations in pulse and respirations. If any of these signs is observed, the physician must be notified immediately. As with any serious condition, the patient may exhibit a high level of anxiety, and the medical assistant's role is to support the patient and family while encouraging consistent follow-up.

Peripheral Arterial Disease

Peripheral arterial disease develops because of widespread atherosclerotic plaque buildup in the arteries outside of the heart, especially in the legs. Plaque deposits decrease the size of the lumen of the blood vessel, thereby decreasing the amount of oxygenated blood that is delivered to the tissues. This lack of oxygen causes symptoms, most notably leg pain when walking—a condition called **intermittent claudication.** Other signs and symptoms of peripheral arterial disease include leg numbness or weakness; persistently cold extremities; sores of the feet or legs that do not heal; and hair loss on the extremities. The most effective treatments for intermittent claudications are regular exercise and smoking cessation. Bypass surgery or angioplasty may be necessary if exercise does not improve the blood flow to tissues.

DIAGNOSTIC PROCEDURES AND TREATMENTS

The cardiovascular examination begins with the medical assistant obtaining the patient's height and weight, temperature, radial and apical pulses, respirations, and blood pressure in both arms. Most cardiologists will also want a complete list of the prescription and over-the-counter medications that the patient is taking, including the strength and frequency of use for each one. A large portion of the physician's examination focuses on subjective symptoms. The physical examination covers the chest, heart, and vascular systems. General appearance, color of skin, symmetry, clubbing of fingers, jugular vein distention, temperature of extremities, and breathing patterns are a few of the notations that are made by the cardiologist.

Patient support and education are two very strong areas of medical assisting involvement. When patients understand their condition and are encouraged to take an active role in their treatments, they are inclined to comply with the physician's orders in a more precise and orderly fashion. Although cardiovascular diagnostic procedures are not typically done in the ambulatory care setting, the medical assistant should be familiar with the purpose of the tests so patient questions can be answered knowledgeably.

Doppler Studies

Doppler studies can identify occlusions of both veins and arteries from thrombi, emboli, or atherosclerotic plaques. The physician may order arterial Doppler studies for patients with intermittent claudications, lack of a pedal pulse, or leg ulcers that refuse to heal. Venous sonography is ordered to assess patients with pronounced varicosities or those with a swollen painful leg to rule out the possibility of a DVT. For a continuous wave Doppler study, a conductive gel is applied to the skin over the test site. The Doppler transducer is moved over the site, directing an ultrasound beam at the vessel being checked (Figure 46-11). The sonographic beam picks up the speed of RBCs as they travel through the vessel as a "swishing" sound. The physician listens to the change in the pitch of the sound produced by the transducer to evaluate the blood flow through an area that may be blocked or narrowed. Variations in RBC velocity indicate either a partial or complete occlusion of the blood vessel. A two-dimensional image of an artery can be produced with a duplex Doppler scan that directly shows stenosis or occlusion of the artery. These studies are usually conducted in a vascular laboratory but may be done in a vascular surgeon's office as an initial assessment of the patient or follow-up after bypass grafting. The medical assistant working in this type of practice will require additional training to perform this procedure.

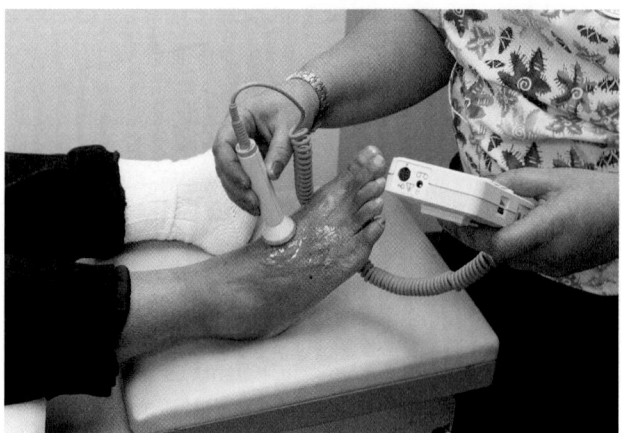

FIGURE 46-11 Doppler study.

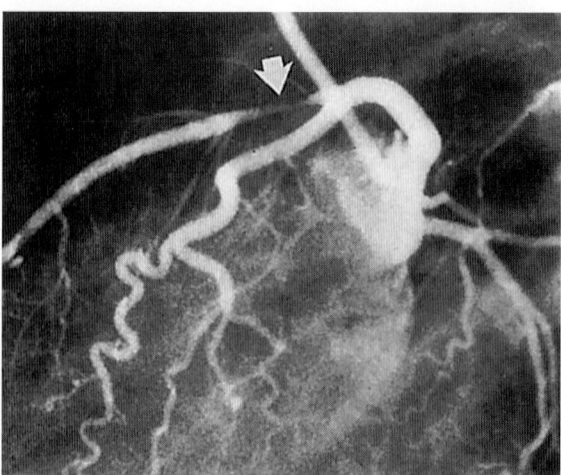

FIGURE 46-12 Coronary angiography shows stenosis (arrow) of the left anterior descending coronary artery. (From Braunwald E: *Heart disease: a textbook of cardiovascular medicine*, ed 4, Philadelphia, 1992, Saunders.)

Angiography

Angiography (arteriography) can be used to evaluate any of the arterial pathways in the body (Figure 46-12). A catheter is placed into a major artery, usually the femoral, and advanced to the artery under study. A radiopaque contrast medium is rapidly injected while x-ray films are taken. The study is used to identify abnormal blood vessels, determine blood flow through the vessel, and diagnose arterial anomalies. Angiography can also be used to identify and locate occlusions of the aorta and arteries of the lower extremities. If the radiopaque substance does not pass through the vessel, or only partially passes through, the distal end of the artery will not be visualized or will be only partially visible on the x-ray films. Arteriosclerotic disease can create a total or partial occlusion; emboli typically cause total occlusion of the artery. The study can also diagnose the dilation of a vessel from an aneurysm.

Echocardiography

Echocardiography is a noninvasive sonographic procedure that assesses the structure and movement of the various parts of the heart. High-frequency sound waves from a transducer that is held against the chest wall penetrate the heart. The sound waves bounce off the heart and echo back through the transducer into the machine, where they are converted into a picture that shows the exact size and movement of the parts of the heart that are being measured. Two-dimensional echocardiography can also be done to provide a spatial picture of the anatomic structures of the heart. Echocardiography usually includes color Doppler studies to show the pattern and velocity of blood flow within the heart and in the great vessels. Backflow of blood, as in a valve that is incompetent, can be identified by changes in color.

A *transesophageal echocardiogram* (TEE) is a type of echocardiogram that uses a long tube with a microphone-like device mounted on one end that the patient swallows into the esophagus. Once in place the device is in very close proximity to the heart, and sound waves emitted by the microphone create high-quality views of the heart and heart valves. Before the patient swallows the device the mouth and throat are sprayed with medication that numbs the area. The patient may be given a sedative to help him or her relax and remain still during the procedure. Echocardiography is used to diagnose pericardial effusion, valvular heart disease, aneurysms, and myocardial wall abnormalities that are seen in CHF or MI.

Cardiac Catheterization and Angioplasty

Cardiac catheterization is used to diagnose or evaluate a variety of heart disorders. Patients who have chronic shortness of breath, vertigo or syncope, chest pain, heart palpitations, arrhythmias, or abnormal stress test or echocardiography results or who have recently experienced an MI are all considered likely candidates for a heart catheterization procedure.

In this procedure a catheter is passed into the heart through a peripheral vein or artery. If the right side of the heart is to be evaluated, the catheter is usually passed through the subclavian, brachial, or femoral vein; the right femoral artery is usually used for left-sided views. As the catheter is passed through the vessels into the heart and coronary arteries, pressures are monitored, oxygen levels are measured, and cardiac output is determined. Once the catheter has reached the desired position, contrast medium is injected and fluoroscopy is used to visualize the heart chambers, valves, and coronary arteries. The cardiologist evaluates the condition of these structures, and any deviation from normal is noted. Cardiac catheterization is performed in a hospital and usually takes 2 to 3 hours to complete. Patients are required to remain immobile and under observation for 4 to 6 hours after the procedure.

During a heart catheterization procedure, if atherosclerotic plaques are discovered occluding the coronary arteries, PTCA may be performed. The goals of angioplasty are to restore blood flow to ischemic myocardial tissue, reduce the need for cardiac medication, and eliminate or reduce the number of episodes of angina. When the plaque area is found, a balloon that surrounds the upper portion of the catheter is inflated and the atherosclerotic material is pressed against the vessel walls, relieving the obstruction. More than one blockage can be treated during a single session, depending on the location of the blockages and the patient's condition. The procedure can take 30 minutes to several hours, depending on the number of blockages being treated.

Lasers may also be used to dissolve the obstruction, or a coronary arterial stent, which is a mesh wire that stretches and molds to the arterial wall, may be inserted and left in place within the vessel to keep the vessel open. If multiple coronary artery occlusions are present, it may be necessary for the patient to have a CABG procedure. This surgery uses either part of the saphenous vein or an artificial Dacron graft to bypass the occluded, diseased section of the coronary artery. The graft creates a bypass for the blood to flow through to bring nourishment to the ischemic myocardium.

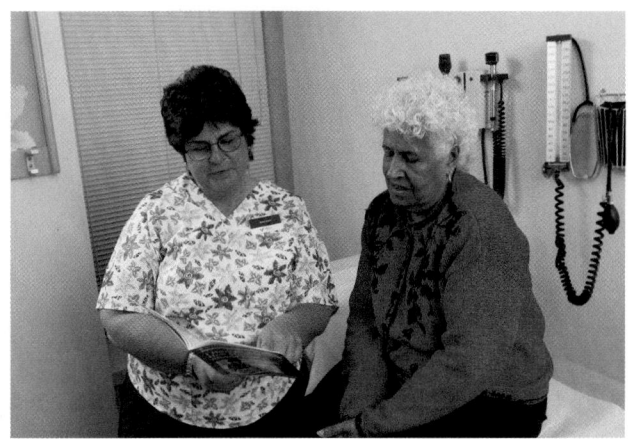

FIGURE 46-13 Patient education.

CLOSING COMMENTS

Patient Education

Heart disease and stroke account for more than one third of all deaths. Familial genetics, predisposition, and lifestyle factors such as smoking, lack of exercise, and poor diet play a significant role in the development of heart disease. Successful management of cardiovascular disease requires major lifestyle revisions for most patients. The medical assistant can help by providing encouragement and support as well as by using community resources to provide assistance for the patient (Figure 46-13).

Sources of information include the American Heart Association, workshops and conferences, professional organizations such as the American Association of Medical Assistants (AAMA), and reputable Internet sites.

Because many patients learn best through visual aids, having pictures, brochures, and pamphlets to give them is an effective method for generating learning. Always document education interventions so that on a return visit the information can be clarified or expanded.

Legal and Ethical Issues

Diagnostic procedures can have a marked effect on the patient's treatment. When entrusted with performing testing procedures, the medical assistant assumes responsibility for accuracy and performing the tests precisely. This is an important role because the results submitted could strongly influence the therapeutic plan of treatment.

SUMMARY OF SCENARIO

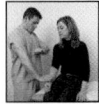

Adam enjoys his new position but recognizes the challenges of interacting with cardiovascular patients. Most individuals seen at the clinic must make considerable lifestyle changes to improve health or to prevent further complications from their diseases. Adam has found it difficult at times to try to help patients who refuse to quit smoking, do not exercise regularly, and continue to eat a diet high in fat. He relies on the hospital dietitian for educational support and encourages MI patients to follow the cardiologist's advice and participate actively in the cardiac rehabilitation program offered by the department. He also works hard to stay up to date on cardiovascular medications and treatments because so many of the department's patients have complicated therapeutic plans. Adam has attended several workshops recently to help him choose patient education materials that meet the needs of clients in his practice. With the approval of practice physicians he has developed a basic policy and procedure manual for managing common telephone scenarios. He recognizes the need to continue his education in the area of cardiology to stay current with the rapid developments in medication and treatments.

SUMMARY of LEARNING OBJECTIVES

1. Define, spell, and pronounce the terms listed in the vocabulary.
   - Spelling and pronouncing medical terms correctly adds credibility to the medical assistant. Knowing the definition of these terms promotes confidence in communication with patients and co-workers.

2. Illustrate the anatomy and physiology of the heart and its significant structures.
   - The heart is a muscular organ that pumps blood through all the arteries of the body. It has three layers of tissue surrounded by a double-membrane sac called the pericardium—the epicardium, or the first layer of the heart; the middle, muscular layer of the heart, the myocardium; and the inner layer, the endocardium, which forms the heart valves. The blood flow through the heart begins in the right atrium, which receives deoxygenated blood from the inferior and superior venae cavae. The atria contract, and blood passes through the tricuspid valve into the right ventricle; the ventricles contract, and the blood passes from the right ventricle to the lungs via the pulmonary artery. Oxygenation occurs in the lungs, and the blood returns to the left atria through the pulmonary veins; the atria contract, and blood passes through the mitral (bicuspid) valve into the left ventricle; the ventricles contract, and oxygen-rich blood is sent out to the body through the aorta.

3. Summarize risk factors for the development of cardiovascular disease.
   - Risk factors for the development of cardiovascular disease that cannot be changed include genetic predisposition and familial history, aging, and race; factors that can be altered are hypertension, diabetes, elevated blood cholesterol levels, smoking, obesity, lack of exercise, and stress.

4. Describe the signs, symptoms, and medical procedures employed in the diagnosis and treatment of coronary artery disease and myocardial infarction.
   - In CAD, the arteries supplying the myocardium become narrowed by atherosclerotic plaque, which causes ischemia of the myocardium. The cardinal symptom is angina pectoris, followed by pressure or fullness in the chest, syncope, unexplained coughing spells, and fatigue; however, women may exhibit a different clinical picture. Ischemia leads to necrosis of a portion of the myocardium, resulting in an MI. An MI is characterized by pain lasting longer than 30 minutes that is unrelieved by rest or nitroglycerin tablets. It is diagnosed by ECG changes and elevated cardiac enzymes 6 to 12 hours after the episode. Medical treatment includes the use of thrombolytic medications, aspirin, beta-blockers, ACE inhibitors, anticoagulants, and anticholesterol agents. When occlusion has taken place either a PTCA or CABG surgery may be indicated.

5. Compare and contrast the treatment protocols for hypertension.
   - The two types of hypertension are primary and secondary. Secondary hypertension occurs because of a disease process in another body system. Primary hypertension is idiopathic and is diagnosed when the patient's blood pressure is consistently above 139 systolic and 89 systolic. Primary hypertension

is classified as either prehypertension (120 to 139/80 to 89 mm Hg), requiring lifestyle modification and drug therapy in selected patients; stage 1 (140 to 159/90 to 99 mm Hg), treated with diuretics; or stage 2 (≥160/≥100 mm Hg), treated with a two-drug regimen. Chronic elevated blood pressure can result in left ventricular hypertrophy, angina, MI, heart failure, cerebrovascular accident, and nephropathy. Some of the risk factors for developing hypertension include a family history of hypertension or stroke, hypercholesterolemia, smoking, high sodium intake, diabetes, excessive alcohol intake, aging, prolonged stress, and race.

6. Outline the causes and results of congestive heart failure.
   - CHF occurs when the myocardium is unable to pump an adequate amount of blood to meet the needs of the body. It typically develops over time and initially involves one side of the heart followed by the other side. Left-sided heart failure causes a backup of blood in the left atria and lungs, resulting in pulmonary edema with dyspnea, orthopnea, nonproductive cough, rales, and tachycardia. Right-sided heart failure causes a backup of blood in the right atrium, preventing emptying of the vena cava, resulting in systemic edema, especially in the legs and feet. Both types of heart failure cause fatigue, weakness, exercise intolerance, dyspnea, and sensitivity to cold temperatures.

7. Illustrate the effects of inflammation and valvular disorders on cardiac function.
   - Rheumatic heart disease develops because of an unusual immune reaction that occurs approximately 2 weeks after an untreated beta-hemolytic streptococcal infection; endocarditis is the most common heart complication, with valvular damage. Disorders of the valves of the heart may be caused by a congenital defect or an infection. Two specific problems can occur with valve disease. The valve can be stenosed, which restricts the forward flow of blood, or it can be incompetent so that blood can leak backward. The most common valve defect is MVP, resulting from a congenital defect or vegetation and scarring from endocarditis.

8. Describe the anatomy and physiology of the vascular system.
   - Blood vessels are divided into two systems that begin and end with the heart. Vessels are classified according to their structure and function as arteries, which carry oxygenated blood away from the heart; capillaries, the microscopic vessels that are responsible for the exchange of oxygen and carbon dioxide in the tissue; and veins, the vessels that carry deoxygenated blood back to the heart.

9. Differentiate among the various types of shock.
   - Table 46-2 outlines the various types of shock. All result in the same signs and symptoms and possible complications. Shock is the general collapse of the circulatory system, including decreased cardiac output, hypotension, and hypoxemia. The body attempts to compensate for the circulatory collapse with vasoconstriction of peripheral blood vessels; as a result, blood can be pooled in the vital organs. Symptoms progress to a

Continued

SUMMARY of LEARNING OBJECTIVES

Continued

rapid, weak, and thready pulse; tachypnea; and altered levels of consciousness. If the process is not reversed, the central nervous system becomes depressed and acute renal failure may occur.

10. Summarize the characteristics of common vascular disorders.
   - Varicose veins are dilated, tortuous, superficial veins in the legs that develop because the valves do not completely close, allowing blood to flow backward, thus causing the vein to distend from the increased pressure. Phlebitis is an inflammation of the veins most commonly seen in the lower legs. DVT is a thrombus with inflammatory changes that has attached to the deep venous system of the lower legs and has caused a partial or complete obstruction of the vessel. If a thrombus becomes dislodged and begins to circulate through the general circulation, it is then called an embolus. Arteriosclerosis is a general term for the thickening and loss

of elasticity of arterial walls; it can occur in arteries throughout the body and cause systemic ischemia and necrosis over time. Atherosclerosis is a form of arteriosclerosis in which the formation of an atheroma occurs. An aneurysm is a ballooning or dilation of the wall of a vessel caused by weakening of the vessel wall. Peripheral arterial disease affects the vessels outside of the heart, especially the legs and feet, in which circulation is decreased and ischemia can occur.

11. Outline typical cardiovascular diagnostic procedures.
   - Cardiovascular diagnostic procedures include Doppler studies of the patency of blood vessels; angiography to show arterial pathways; echocardiography to assess the structure and movement of the parts of the heart, especially the valves; and cardiac catheterization to show the heart chambers, valves, and coronary arteries.

CONNECTIONS

Study Guide Connection: Go to Chapter 46 Study Guide. Read the Case Study and Workplace Applications and complete the assignments. Do online research for answers to the questions in the Internet Activities associated with assisting in cardiology.

CD Connection: Go to the Medical Assisting Competency Challenge CD and do the training activities under Diagnostic Testing. For a better understanding of the function of the heart, view the animation for normal cardiopulmonary physiology.

Evolve Connection: For more information related to assisting in cardiology, go to evolve.elsevier.com/kinn and visit related weblinks for Chapter 46. Click on the Medical Assisting Exam Review and do the practice questions to sharpen your test-taking skills.

Assisting in Geriatrics

47

SCENARIO

Bill Novelli, CMA, works for Dr. Sara Kennedy, a primary care physician in a small town close to where he grew up. Although patients of all ages are seen in the practice, most patients are 65 years of age or older. Bill has learned to recognize the unique communication needs of aging patients and the importance of using family and community resources to maintain optimal health in this special population.

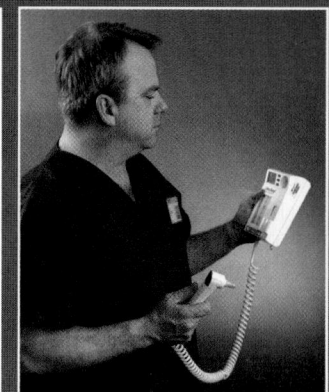

While studying this chapter, think about the following questions:

- Are there myths about aging and stereotypes about aging people that can negatively affect older individuals?
- What are the most common changes that occur in the aging body and what recommendations can be made for health promotion in this age group?
- What suggestions can be made to aging patients and their families to optimize their health and protect them from injury and disease?
- How is Alzheimer's disease diagnosed and what are the stages of its development?
- Why is depression such a common occurrence in aging persons and how is it diagnosed and treated?
- How can the medical assistant most effectively communicate with an older person?
- Why is the utilization of community resources such an important factor in the care of aging people?

LEARNING OBJECTIVES

1. Define, spell, and pronounce the terms listed in the vocabulary.
2. Identify the various impacts of an increasing aging population on society.
3. Role-play the effect of sensorimotor changes of aging.
4. Explain the changes caused by aging in each of the body systems.
5. Summarize the major diseases and disorders faced by older patients.
6. Describe various screening tools for dementia, depression, and malnutrition.
7. Explain the effect of aging on sleep.
8. Differentiate among independent, assisted, and skilled nursing facilities.
9. Summarize the role of the medical assistant in caring for aging patients.
10. Determine the principles for effective communication with older adults.
11. Identify legal and ethical issues regarding aging patients.

National Accreditation Competencies and Content

CAAHEP COMPETENCIES	ABHES COMPETENCIES
Clinical	**Instruction**
3.c.(2)(b). Instruct individuals according to their needs	7.b. Instruct patients with special needs
3.c.(2)(c). Provide instruction for health maintenance and disease prevention	7.c. Teach patients methods of health promotion and disease prevention

VOCABULARY

collagen (kah'-luh-jen) Protein that forms the inelastic fibers of tendons, ligaments, and fascia.

costal Pertaining to the ribs.

decubitus ulcers Sores or ulcers over a bony prominence that are the result of ischemia from prolonged pressure; bedsores.

elastin Essential part of elastic connective tissue that, when moist, is flexible and elastic.

lacrimation (la-krihm-a'-shun) The secretion or discharge of tears.

According to the U.S. Bureau of the Census, the aging population—those 65 years of age and older—numbered almost 36.3 million in 2004 (the last year that data were collected). This represents 12.4% of the total population of the United States, an increase of 3.1 million since the last census in 1994. About one in every eight Americans is older than 65. The "oldest old" (people older than 85) are the most rapidly growing age group. It is projected that people older than 65 will represent 16% of the population in 2020 and increase to 20% by 2030. This means that by the middle of the twenty-first century, over 71 million people will be older than 65 years (Figure 47-1). The average life expectancy of an individual who reaches age 65 is an additional 18.5 years (19.8 years for women and 16.8 years for men). Older women outnumber older men, with 21.1 million women over the age of 65 compared with 15.2 men. About 30% of older persons who reside outside of institutions live alone; half of women over the age of 75 live alone. Almost half a million grandparents over the age of 65 are the primary caregivers for their grandchildren who live with them. Most older persons have at least one chronic medical condition, and many have multiple conditions. The federal government's Administration on Aging cites hypertension, arthritis, heart disease, cancer, and diabetes as the most frequently occurring health problems seen in the elderly.

What does all of this mean to those of us who have chosen careers in healthcare? As the aging population expands, it will affect all aspects of society. One area in particular will be the greater use of health services. To provide better services to the aging consumer, it is necessary to understand the aging process,

which includes the physical and sensory changes encountered by older people (Procedure 47-1). This knowledge enables the healthcare professional to recognize the special needs of the aged and to develop therapeutic management and communication skills to effectively care for the older client. Because of ongoing research and education about the aging process, many of the old stereotypes about aging are disappearing.

Aging is a complex physiologic, psychologic, and social process. Old age is not an illness but a normal life process that individuals experience in different ways. Lack of exercise, poor nutrition, substance abuse, continual stress, and air pollutants are all factors that cause one to show the effects of aging decades earlier than someone who has practiced healthy living habits.

As people age, they experience changes in their physical appearance and abilities as well as sensory changes in vision, hearing, taste, and smell. These changes do not occur at the same time in everyone; however, sensorimotor changes can have a profound effect on the individual's ability to interact with his or her environment.

CRITICAL THINKING APPLICATION

When Bill first started working with aging patients, he believed many of the stereotypes regarding persons over the age of 65. Since working with Dr. Kennedy, he realizes that many of these myths have no foundation in actual practice. Based on the myths mentioned in the text, what do you think about these beliefs on aging?

CHANGES IN ANATOMY AND PHYSIOLOGY

The aging process brings about changes in all of the body systems. Table 47-1 summarizes these changes and what can be done to promote healthy aging.

Cardiovascular System

Cardiovascular disease is the most frequent cause of illness and disability in the aging population; congestive heart failure (CHF) is the most common reason for hospitalization. Changes in the cardiovascular system are age related, but disease and lifestyle habits such as lack of exercise, poor diet, and stress are factors that contribute to these changes. Heart disease is ranked as the leading cause of death among men and women; therefore the proper management of cardiovascular disease can help

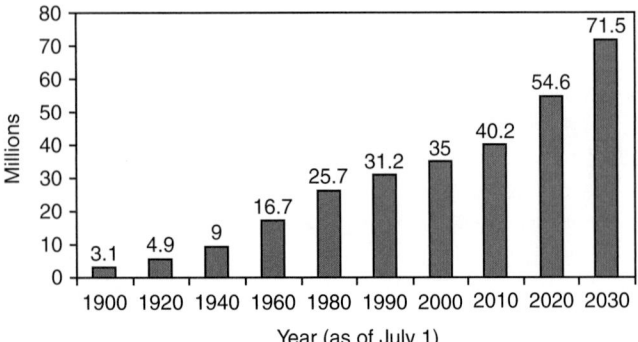

FIGURE 47-1 Older population by age, 1900-2030. (From U.S. Administration on Aging. Available at: www.aoa.gov.)

PROCEDURE 47-1

Instruct Individuals According to Their Needs: Sensorimotor Changes of Aging

CAAHEP COMPETENCIES: 3.c.(2)(b), 3.c.(2)(c)
ABHES COMPETENCIES: 7.b, 7.c

GOAL: *Role-play to better understand the needs of aging persons.*

EQUIPMENT and SUPPLIES

- Yellow tinted glasses, ski goggles, or laboratory goggles
- Pink, white, yellow "pills" (various colors of Tic Tacs work)
- Vaseline
- Cotton balls
- Eye patches
- Tape
- Thick gloves
- Utility glove
- Tongue depressors
- Ace bandages
- Medical forms in small print
- Pennies
- Button shirts
- Walker

PROCEDURAL STEPS

1. Role-play vision and hearing loss:
   - Put two cotton balls in each ear and an eye patch over one eye. Follow your partner's instructions.
   - Partner: Stand out of the line of vision (to prevent lip-reading). Without using gestures or changing voice volume, tell your partner to cross the room and pick up a book.

2. Role-play yellowing of lens:
   - Line up "pills" of different pastel colors.
   - Partner: Pick out the different colors while wearing the yellow tinted glasses.

3. Role-play difficulty with focusing:
   - Put on goggles smeared with Vaseline, and follow your partner's directions.
   - Partner: Stand at least 3 feet in front of your partner and motion for him or her to come to you (your partner is deaf, so talking will not help).

4. Role-play loss of peripheral vision:
   - Put on goggles with black paper taped to sides.
   - Partner: Stand to the side out of the field of vision and motion for your patient to follow you.

5. Role-play aphasia and partial paralysis:
   - You are unable to use your right arm or leg. Place tape over your mouth. Let your partner know you need to go to the bathroom.
   - Partner: Stand at least 3 feet away with your back to your partner and wait for instructions.

6. Role-play problems with dexterity:
   - Put thick gloves on your hands and try to sign your name, button a shirt, tie your shoes, and pick up pennies.

7. Role-play problems with mobility:
   - Use the walker to cross the room.
   - Partner: After your partner starts to use the walker, hand him or her a book to carry.

8. Role-play changes in sensation:
   - Put a rubber utility glove on; turn on hot water; test the difference in temperature between the gloved hand and nongloved hand.

9. Summarize and share with the group your impressions of the effect of age-related sensorimotor changes.

Myths and Stereotypes About Aging

- All aging people become senile.
- Disease is normal and unavoidable.
- Older workers are less productive than younger ones.
- Most older people end up in long-term care facilities.
- Most aging people have no interest in, or capacity for, sexual relations.
- Aging people are resistant to change and cannot learn new things.
- Damage to health because of lifestyle factors is irreversible.

Shingles Risk Reduction

The FDA recently approved a new vaccine, Zostavax, to reduce the risk of shingles in people 60 years of age and older. The varicella-zoster virus causes both shingles and chickenpox. After an active chickenpox infection, the virus lies dormant in a nerve dermatome. As people age, they are at risk of the virus reactivating and causing the formation of blisters and varying degrees of pain along the affected nerve pathway. It is estimated that 2 out of 10 people will develop shingles in their lifetime. Zostavax, a live virus vaccine, boosts immunity against the varicella-zoster virus. The vaccine is administered as a single subcutaneous injection. Studies have shown the vaccine will reduce the number of shingles cases by 50% in individuals over the age of 60 and by 64% in persons ages 60 to 69. Those individuals who develop shingles even though they are immunized experience a shorter length of symptoms. It is recommended that all individuals over the age of 60 receive the Zostavax vaccination.

maintain the health of an aging population as well as reduce mortality rates.

Structural changes occur in the heart as a result of the aging process. Myocardial cells enlarge and there are increased deposits of fat and connective tissue, which combine to make

TABLE 47-1 Health Promotion and Body System Changes Associated with Aging

BODY SYSTEM	AGE-RELATED CHANGES	HEALTH PROMOTION
Cardiovascular	Arteriosclerosis and atherosclerotic plaque buildup reduces blood flow to major organs; hypertension common; CVD number one killer of women and men in their 60s	Exercise regularly; control weight; eat diet rich in fruits, vegetables, and whole grains; monitor cholesterol and blood glucose levels
Central nervous system	Brain shrinks by 10% between ages 30 and 90; takes longer to learn new material; attention span and language remain same; signs and symptoms may be caused by depression, vascular disease, and drug reactions	Aerobic exercise to increase blood flow to CNS and maintain mental activities such as reading and interacting with others
Endocrine	After age 50, women have sharp decline in estrogen and men more gradual decline in testosterone	Possible hormone replacement therapy or natural soy supplements
Gastrointestinal	Decline in gastric juices and enzymes by age 60; decreased peristalsis with increased constipation; some nutrients not absorbed as well	High-fiber adequate fluid intake, regular exercise diet to prevent constipation
Musculoskeletal	Muscle mass decreases; tendency to gain weight; gradual loss of bone density; deterioration of joint cartilage	Strength training to increase muscle mass; stretching to remain limber; exercise; vitamin D and calcium supplements
Pulmonary	At age 55 the lungs become less elastic and the chest wall gradually stiffens, making oxygenation more difficult	Quit smoking and do regular aerobic exercise
Sensory organs	Hearing intact through mid 50s but declines by 25% by age 80; oral problems common; skin thins and loses elasticity with age; presbyopia after age 40; cataracts common after age 60	Avoid exposure to loud noise and use hearing aids; maintain good dental hygiene; avoid sun damage to skin; get annual eye examinations and eat a diet rich in dark green, leafy vegetables to avoid cataracts and macular degeneration
Urinary	Kidneys become less efficient; bladder muscles weaken; one third of seniors experience incontinence; prostate enlargement common	Pelvic exercises, drugs, or surgery for incontinence; annual PSA monitoring for men
Sexuality	Men: Impotence not a symptom of normal aging; men over age 50 may have some altered function Women: Menopause causes vaginal narrowing and dryness, causing painful intercourse	Men: Maintain cardiovascular health with exercise, weight control, no smoking Women: Use vaginal lubricants or estrogen cream

CNS, Central nervous system; *CVD*, cardiovascular disease; *PSA*, prostate-specific antigen.

TABLE 47-2 Normal Changes of Cardiac Output

	BLOOD PUMPED BY RESTING HEART (QUARTS PER MINUTE)	MAXIMUM HEARTBEAT DURING EXERCISE (BEATS PER MINUTE)
Age 30	3.6	200
Age 40	3.4	182
Age 50	3.2	171
Age 60	2.9	159
Age 70	2.6	150

From the American Heart Association.

the myocardial wall stiffer and increase the amount of time needed for the relaxation phase of the cardiac cycle. As a result, cardiac output decreases, making aging persons more susceptible to CHF. This reduction in cardiac output leads to pooling of blood in the legs, cold extremities, and edema (Table 47-2). In addition, the heart cannot respond as quickly, or as forcefully, to an increased workload, so exercise, sudden movements, and changes in position can result in dizziness and loss of balance. Aging also brings with it an increase in blood pressure, requiring the heart to work harder to pump blood into the systemic

circulation. Hypertension increases the workload of the left ventricle, which may result in hypertrophy of the chamber and weakening of the myocardial wall. The valves of the heart tend to thicken and become more rigid, making it more difficult for blood to circulate through the cardiopulmonary vessels. With these cardiovascular problems, arrhythmias become more common.

Aging causes venous walls to weaken and stretch, damaging the valves within these blood vessels, especially in the veins of the legs where the walls are subject to greater pressure as blood struggles to return to the heart against the force of gravity. As a result, edema and varicose veins of the lower extremities are very common in the elderly, increasing the risk of phlebitis and deep vein thrombosis (DVT) formation.

Arteriosclerosis is considered part of the aging process. The vessel walls thicken and become less elastic as a result of the calcification and buildup of connective tissue. In addition, the ability of the arteries to dilate and contract decreases. To maintain an adequate blood supply throughout the body, the heart must work harder to overcome the resistance caused by stiffened vessels. There is also an increased incidence of orthostatic hypotension in older adults. The clinical criterion for alterations in blood pressure from sitting to standing is a drop of more than 20 mm Hg in systolic pressure or a drop of more than 10 mm Hg in diastolic pressure when position is changed. Such a decrease is typically caused by a decrease in the volume of circulating blood and can be an important diagnostic sign for aging patients. The physician may have the medical assistant take orthostatic blood pressures as part of the routine intake protocol for aging patients.

Endocrine System

Hormonal changes that occur with aging are related to a general decrease in hormone production combined with changes in tissue receptor binding. The most common endocrine system disorder seen in aging patients is type 2 diabetes mellitus. As we age, insulin production by the beta cells in the pancreas decreases and insulin resistance at the tissue level increases. According to the National Institutes of Health, more than half of the 16 million Americans diagnosed with diabetes type 2 are over the age of 65. Elderly patients with diabetes are at increased risk for developing vascular disease, including renal disorders, retinopathy, neuropathy, myocardial ischemia, angina, myocardial infarction, cerebrovascular accidents, and peripheral vascular disease, such as lower-extremity ulcers.

Older patients do not always experience classic diabetic symptoms—polyuria, polydipsia, polyphagia—but may display a variety of problems, including unexplained weight loss, slow wound healing, recurrent bacterial or fungal infections, changes in mental state, cataracts, macular disease, muscle weakness and pain, angina, foot ulcers, and uremia. The range of symptoms is largely attributable to the insidious onset of diabetes in older people, who may have gradually developing hyperglycemia for years before diagnosis.

The treatment protocol for aging patients with diabetes is the same as it would be for other age groups; however, special consideration must be given to the ability of the patient to understand and comply with the therapeutic plan. In addition, because the patient may have other existing health problems that are being treated with medications, the newly diagnosed aging diabetic patient may face a complicated treatment regimen that requires explicit instruction and continual follow-up in the ambulatory care setting.

The medical assistant must be aware of any sensory abnormalities, such as decreased vision or fine motor skills, which may interfere with the patient's ability to follow treatment guidelines. Adaptations need to be made in teaching and treatment plans to meet the individual needs of each patient.

Gastrointestinal System

Age-related changes in the gastrointestinal system begin in the mouth with dental problems, a decrease in the number of taste buds and production of saliva, and diminishing sense of smell. Older people generally find eating less pleasurable, have a reduced appetite, and are unable to chew and lubricate their food as well as younger people, making *dysphagia* (difficulty swallowing) a common age-related problem. Aging also brings a decrease in the production of hydrochloric acid, which affects the digestion of calcium and iron. Secretion of intrinsic factor, a protein that allows vitamin B_{12} to be absorbed, also decreases,

---

Factors That Can Affect Diabetes Management in Older People

- Modifying lifestyle risk factors may be more difficult because of poor nutrition, inability to exercise, and long-standing habits such as smoking and diets high in fat and calories.
- Previously diagnosed health conditions, such as hypertension and heart disease, increase the challenge of treating diabetes.
- Older people are more likely to be prescribed multiple medications (*polypharmacy*), which increases the risk of adverse drug interactions.
- Diabetic complications can develop quickly because of a long history of prediabetes before diagnosis.
- Older people may have decreased physical and/or mental abilities that make it difficult for them to understand and adhere to a complicated treatment regimen.
- Older patients may not be able to afford the medications and supplies needed to maintain health.

---

affecting the function of the nervous system and the formation of red blood cells, resulting in excessive fatigue. It is not unusual for aging patients to be seen in the physician's office on a regular basis for vitamin B_{12} injections.

The rate of food passage through the small intestine increases, causing poorer absorption of vitamins and minerals. Peristalsis in the colon decreases, making aging patients more susceptible to constipation and diverticular disease. Poor eating habits, reduced fluid intake, and some medications (such as antidepressants, diuretics, antacids containing aluminum or calcium, and medications for Parkinson's disease) also contribute to constipation. The liver decreases in size and weight after age 70. It is still able to perform vital functions; however, the time needed to metabolize drugs and alcohol is increased. All of these factors combine to increase the potential for adverse drug reactions in older adults.

Aging persons have an increased incidence of several gastrointestinal system diseases, such as gastroesophageal reflux disease (GERD), peptic ulcers, diverticulosis (related to lack of dietary fiber and constipation), cholelithiasis, and colorectal cancer. Dietary counseling and annual screenings should be part of the routine care of aging patients.

Integumentary System

The skin is considered the body's first line of protection against infection and is responsible for preventing the loss of body fluid and regulating body temperature. Changes in the appearance and function of the integumentary system are usually caused by a combination of ordinary age-related changes and environmental factors, especially the amount of sun exposure over time. Exposure to ultraviolet light from the sun is frequently the cause of wrinkles, age spots, blotches, and leathery-dry, loose skin, all of which are associated with aging. Changes caused by the ultraviolet light from the sun or from the normal aging process can affect all three layers of the skin: the epidermis, dermis, and subcutaneous tissue.

The cells in the epidermis reproduce more slowly as people age. This slower regeneration causes the skin to appear thinner. The skin becomes more prone to tearing and blistering. The risk for infections is increased, the healing process takes longer, and older people are more susceptible to bruising. Because the skin can be easily torn, it is important to select an appropriate adhesive when covering a wound or venipuncture site on an older patient. Vitamin D synthesis, which is a major function of the epidermis, significantly decreases in aged skin, and a decrease in the number of melanocytes increases photosensitivity.

The dermis loses 20% of its mass during the aging process, resulting in the paper-thin or transparent skin seen in older adults. The number of **collagen** cells in the dermis also decreases with age, causing the skin to sag and wrinkle. Both sweat and sebaceous glands decrease, making it difficult for aging persons to tolerate higher temperatures because they perspire less. At the same time, the blood supply to the dermis decreases making it difficult to regulate temperature and leading to an increased susceptibility to both hypothermia and heat stroke in aging persons. Any situation in which an older adult is exposed to extremes of cold or heat should be avoided. Make sure there is a blanket available in the examining room if the air conditioning is on. Inquire about whether the patient is too cold or too hot, and take the necessary steps to make the older patient feel more comfortable.

Atrophy of the subcutaneous layer increases the skin's susceptibility to trauma, so patients bruise much more easily. The skin is denied natural lubrication, causing dry skin to be one of the most common complaints among older people. In addition, fat deposits increase in the abdomen of men and in the abdomen and thighs of women as they age.

Pain receptors are distributed throughout the skin. Because of age-related changes in the receptors, older persons experience an increased threshold to pain. They may not notice a cut or burn as quickly as a younger person would; therefore a burn may become more severe before it is noticed. In addition, wound healing becomes a problem because of decreased blood flow to dermal tissues.

Other changes occur in the skin appendages. Hair changes in color, growth, and distribution. Hair grays because of the decreased rate of melanin production and the replacement of pigmented hair with nonpigmented hair. Women lose hair on their trunk and have increased facial hair. Although alopecia (male balding) is caused by an inherited trait, aging also causes hair loss. Hair on the eyebrows, nose, and ears becomes coarser and longer in men. Nails of older people take longer to grow and are more brittle. Nails, particularly toenails, thicken as a result of trauma or nutritional deficiencies. It is not unusual for nails to split, making them more susceptible to fungal infections.

Seborrheic keratoses, usually referred to as "age spots," are one of the most common benign skin disorders found in the aging population. They appear as waxy, greasy papules that vary from a tan to a dark brown color (Figure 47-2). They are typically found in areas of sun exposure, such as the trunk, back, face, neck, extremities, and scalp. They may be removed for cosmetic purposes but are not dangerous.

Suggestions for Helping Older Patients Prevent and Treat Dry Skin

- Humidifier to obtain artificial humidification
- Bathe less frequently, using warm rather than hot water
- Use a mild soap or cleansing cream such as Aveeno, Basis, or Dove
- Wear protective clothing in cold weather
- Moisturize dry skin
- Creams and moisturizers should be applied after getting out of the bathtub or shower to decrease the possibility of falls

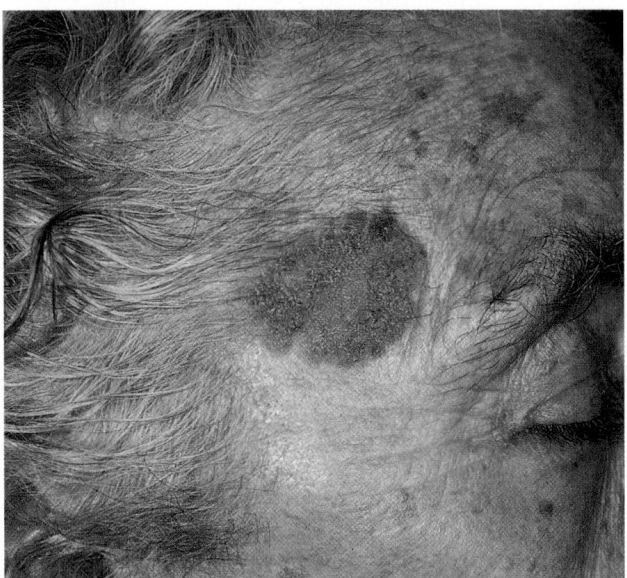

FIGURE 47-2 Seborrheic keratosis. (From Habif TP: *Clinical dermatology: a color guide to diagnosis and therapy,* ed 4, St Louis, 2004, Mosby.)

CRITICAL THINKING APPLICATION

Mrs. Rose DeLuca is a 71-year-old patient of Dr. Kennedy's who is complaining about the changes that have occurred in her skin in the last several years. Based on what Bill knows about the normal changes that occur in the skin as people age, how can he explain these changes to Mrs. DeLuca, and what suggestions can be made to help with dryness and other typical aging changes?

Musculoskeletal System

As the body ages, changes occur in the muscles, bones, and joints that affect the individual's appearance, strength, and mobility. The amount of change depends on diet, exercise, and heredity. Cartilage loss and degeneration, producing osteoarthritis, commonly occur in the weight-bearing joints of older people. Joint range of motion is affected, and the intervertebral disc spaces are decreased, causing a loss of height as we age. A breakdown in joint structures may lead to inflammation, pain, stiffness, and deformity.

Aging brings a decrease in the strength and speed of muscle contractions in the extremities but only a slight decline in overall

---

Suggestions for Helping the Older Adult with Mobility, Dexterity, and Balance

- Use assistive devices such as adaptive silverware, tub seat or shower chair, electric razor, and reaching devices.
- Assist with gripping devices as needed (wait for the patient to place his or her hand around a cup or help him or her with it before letting go).
- Older adults may need more time to complete tasks but prefer to do so independently, so slow down.
- Stroke victims should be supported on the weak side when walking or transferring from chair to examination table.
- Physician may recommend physical therapy for range-of-motion exercises.
- Encourage activity: a lack of activity causes decreased ability to function.

Risk Factors for the Development of Osteoporosis

- Female (women have a five times greater risk than men)
- Small-boned frame, thin
- Family history of osteoporosis
- Estrogen deficiency before age 45 years from either early menopause or oophorectomy
- Estrogen deficiency resulting from an abnormal absence of menses (eating disorders, excessive aerobic exercise, fibrocystic ovaries)
- Racial background—white and Asian women at highest risk
- Aging
- Extended use of anticonvulsant drugs, prednisone, and excessive thyroid hormone medications
- Sedentary lifestyle, smoking, excessive alcohol intake, lack of calcium and vitamin D when growing up

---

muscle endurance. Muscular changes in the aging patient are directly related to the activity level of the individual. Research shows that musculoskeletal disease is not an inevitable result of the aging process; however, 40% to 50% of women over the age of 50 years have a serious problem with bone demineralization. Men also experience bone loss but at a later age and at a much slower rate than women.

Osteoporosis

Osteoporosis (see Chapter 42) is the primary cause of hip fractures, which can lead to a loss of independence and complications that ultimately can end in death. The spinal vertebrae also can collapse, producing the stooped posture associated with "dowager's hump." Sometimes bones break because of the sheer weight of the body on them. Often people say they fell and broke a bone, when in reality the bone fractured, causing them to fall. Multiple factors contribute to the development of osteoporosis, but it is most common in postmenopausal women.

Weight-bearing exercises and calcium and vitamin D supplements are recommended to prevent demineralization of the bones. Medications to prevent and/or treat osteoporosis include Fosamax and Actonel, which decrease the rate of demineralization; Evista, which slows bone thinning and causes some increase in bone thickness; and calcitonin (Calcimar or Miacalcin), which is either injected or inhaled as a nasal spray and results in a decrease in the rate of bone thinning and relieves the pain associated with spinal compression.

Falls

The risk of injuries from falls increases with age, with falls causing the greatest number of injuries in people over the age of 70 years. Some of the reasons aging persons are at greater risk for falling include sensorimotor changes in vision and mobility, osteoporosis, and cerebrovascular accidents. Falls in older patients usually result in fractures because of the presence of osteoporosis in a large percentage of the population. Serious fractures, such as those of the hip, require patients to be

immobile for extended periods and open the door to a wide range of debilitating complications such as **decubitus ulcers,** pneumonia, placement in long-term care facilities, and even death. Falls are largely preventable. The medical assistant can play an active role in helping family members as well as patients be aware of the risk factors for falls as well as understanding measures that can be taken to prevent falls from occurring.

Suggestions for Preventing Falls

- Undergo regular hearing and vision testing to be aware of possible dangers.
- Understand the side effects of medications, especially those that cause vertigo.
- If you experience orthostatic hypotension, rise slowly and stand still for a moment with support before moving.
- Limit the use of alcohol.
- If needed, use assistive devices such as a cane or walker consistently for support.
- Wear low-heeled, rubber-soled shoes with good support.
- Avoid going outside in icy weather.
- Engage in regular weight-bearing exercise for bone strength.
- Keep hallways, stairs, and bathrooms well lit.
- Assess the home for possible danger areas; remove throw rugs; use handrails on steps and grab bars in bathrooms; keep emergency numbers handy.

CRITICAL THINKING APPLICATION

The family of a 73-year-old patient, Mrs. Rita Schaeffer, is concerned about the risk of falls. Mrs. Schaeffer was recently diagnosed with osteoporosis and lives alone. What information should Bill give the family to help them prevent accidents in their mother's home? Her 43-year-old daughter is concerned about developing osteoporosis as well. What methods should the daughter employ to prevent the disease?

Nervous System

Cognitive ability, the ability of a person to think, is influenced by many factors, including a person's general state of health, educational background, and genetic code. The normal process of aging may contribute to a change in the thinking process. The brain begins to get smaller at approximately age 50 years and continues to do so as we age because of a loss of fluid within the neurons and the shrinkage of dendrites. Thinning of the dendrites makes it more difficult for messages to be transmitted from one neuron to the next. These factors combine to produce an aging brain that weighs less, is smaller, and has started to pull away from the sheath or cortical mantle. Older neurons process information more slowly; so the ability to retrieve old information and learn new information takes longer. Reaction time also slows, and aging persons are distracted more easily; however, recent research shows that the loss of brain cells is minimal and that the older brain is still capable of generating new neurons. Researchers believe that continued, moderate physical and mental activity can maintain the cognitive abilities of aging individuals.

Dementia, the severe loss of intellectual ability, is not an inevitable part of aging but rather is the result of an organic disorder. Most men and women remain mentally competent until the end of their lives. Sudden loss of memory, disorientation, and trouble performing the daily tasks of life indicate a problem exists that should be investigated. Many conditions can cause signs and symptoms of dementia, including depression; reactions to prescription and over-the-counter drugs; alcoholism; malnutrition; thyroid, liver, heart, and vascular disorders; and Parkinson's disease. Multiple factors can interfere with mental judgment and motor skills, giving the impression of decreased mental status.

The best way to ensure mental functioning in later life is to remain mentally and physically stimulated. Exercise improves memory and thinking because of its positive effect on vascular health, increasing the amount of oxygen delivered to the aging brain. Other ways to maintain mental function are to be socially active; practice stress-reduction activities; quit smoking; drink alcohol in moderation; use hearing aids and glasses if they are needed to stay in touch with the world; and receive treatment for depression, diabetes, hypertension, and high cholesterol levels.

One of the most frequently used screening tools for dementia is the Mini-Mental Status Examination, a 5-minute test that was designed to evaluate basic mental function in a number of different areas. The test assesses the patient's ability to recall facts, write, and calculate numbers. It provides the physician with a quick way to determine whether more in-depth testing is needed. Each area of the examination is given a score. These scores show whether the person is functioning within the expected range for his or her age (Figure 47-3). The medical assistant may be expected to administer this examination.

Alzheimer's Disease

Alzheimer's disease (AD) is a progressive deterioration of the brain caused by the destruction of CNS neurons, leading to

Risk Factors for Cognitive Decline
• Hypertension, diabetes, heart disease (these decrease blood flow to the brain)
• Environmental exposure to lead
• High stress levels
• Sedentary lifestyle and lack of social interaction
• Low education level
• Smoking and substance abuse

problems with memory, language, thinking, and behavior. Cellular destruction is related to the buildup of amyloid plaques and neurofibrillary tangles within the brain. Patients displaying signs and symptoms of dementia are first evaluated for organic causes, such as systemic disease or depression. There is no definitive diagnostic test for AD because it can be confirmed only through examination of the brain during autopsy. If the patient exhibits a gradual onset of progressive difficulty with memory, functional abilities, and behavior and shows no evidence of other causes for these disturbances, the physician makes the diagnosis of AD.

Researchers believe that as many as 4.5 million Americans suffer from AD. The disease typically begins after age 60, with the risk of developing the disorder increasing with age, although younger people can be diagnosed with AD. An estimated 5% of people age 65 to 74 have AD, and almost half of people age 85 or older are diagnosed with the disease. However, despite these statistics, AD is not considered a normal part of the aging process.

AD is a slowly progressive disease that begins with mild memory problems and ends with severe brain damage. The course the disease takes and how fast changes occur vary among individuals, but on average patients live from 8 to 10 years after they are diagnosed. No treatment can stop the progression of the disease; however, there is a great deal of ongoing research regarding the diagnosis and treatment of AD.

The goal of treatment is to maintain normal activities as long as possible. Patients in the early and middle stages of the disease may be treated with tacrine (Cognex), donepezil (Aricept), rivastigmine (Exelon), or galantamine (Razadyne) to help prevent memory loss from becoming worse for a limited time. Memantine (Namenda) has been approved for treatment of moderate to severe AD, although it also has limited effects. Individuals with AD frequently experience alterations in behavior, so medications may be prescribed to help control sleeplessness, agitation, wandering, anxiety, and depression. Treating these problems helps make the patient more comfortable while easing the burden on caregivers.

Supportive care for family members is absolutely essential because they are faced with caring for a loved one who is suffering progressive memory loss. The medical assistant can be especially helpful in recommending educational workshops, support groups, and stress management skills for caregivers. Multiple resources are available, including online information and support groups that family members may find helpful.

Patient _____ Examiner _____ Date _____

Maximum Score	Score	

Orientation

5 ( ) What is the (year) (season) (date) (day) (month)?
5 ( ) Where are we: (state) (county) (town) (hospital) (floor)

Registration

3 ( ) Name three objects: (Apple, Penny, Table) 1 second to say each. Then ask the patient all three after you have said them. Give 1 point for each correct answer. Then repeat them until he or she learns all three. Count trials and record.

Trials _____

Attention and Calculation

5 ( ) Serial 7's. 1 point for each correct. Stop after five answers. Alternatively spell "world" backwards.

Recall

3 ( ) Ask for the three objects repeated above. Give 1 point for each correct.

Language

9 ( ) Name a pencil, and watch (2 points)
Repeat the following "No ifs, ands, or buts." (1 point)
Follow a three-stage command:
  "Take a paper in your right hand, fold it in half, and put it on the floor." (3 points)
Read and obey the following:
  CLOSE YOUR EYES (1 point)
Write a sentence (1 point)
Copy design (overlapping pentagons) (1 point)
Total Score

Overlapping pentagons

_____ ASSESS level of consciousness along a continuum _____

Alert	Drowsy	Stupor	Coma

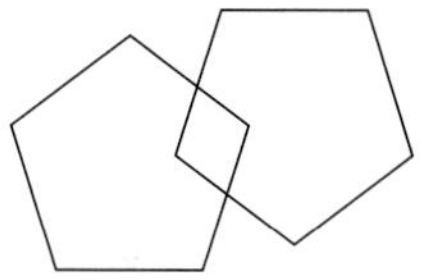

Instructions for Administration of Mini-Mental State Examination

Orientation

(1) Ask for the date. Then ask specifically for parts omitted, e.g., "Can you also tell me what season it is?" One point for each correct.
(2) Ask in turn "Can you tell me the name of this hospital?" (town, country, etc.). One point for each correct.

Registration

Ask the patient if you may test his or her memory. Then say the names of three unrelated objects, clearly and slowly, about 1 second for each. After you have said all three, ask him or her to repeat them. This first repetition determines his or her score (0–3), but keep saying them until he or she can repeat all three, up to six trials. If he or she does not eventually learn all three, recall cannot be meaningfully tested.

Attention and Calculation

Ask the patient to begin with 100 and count backwards by 7. Stop after five subtractions (93, 86, 79, 72, 65). Score the total number of correct answers.
If the patient cannot or will not perform this task, ask him or her to spell the word "world" backwards. The score is the number of letters in correct order, e.g., dlrow = 5, dlorw = 3.

Recall

Ask the patient if he or she can recall the three words you previously asked him or her to remember. Score 0–3.

Language

Naming: Show the patient a wrist watch and ask him or her what it is. Repeat for pencil. Score 0–2.
Repetition: Ask the patient to repeat the sentence after you. Allow only one trial. Score 0 or 1.
Three-stage command: Give the patient a piece of plain blank paper and repeat the command. Score 1 point for each part correctly executed.
Reading: On a blank piece of paper print the sentence "Close your eyes," in letters large enough for the patient to see clearly. Ask him or her to read it and do what it says. Score 1 point only if he or she actually closes his or her eyes.
Writing: Give the patient a blank piece of paper and ask him or her to write a sentence for you. Do not dictate a sentence, it is to be written spontaneously. It must contain a subject and verb and be sensible. Correct grammar and punctuation are not necessary.
Copying: On a clean piece of paper, draw intersecting pentagons, each side about 1 inch, and ask him or her to copy it exactly as it is. All 10 angles must be present, and 2 must intersect to score 1 point. Tremor and rotation are ignored.
Estimate the patient's level of sensorium along a continuum, from alert on the left to coma on the right.

FIGURE 47-3 Mini-Mental Status Examination. (Redrawn from Folstein M, et al: Mini mental state. *J Psychiatr Res* 12:196-198, 1975.)

Stages of Alzheimer's Disease

- First Stage: Occurs during the 2 to 4 years leading up to diagnosis; memory loss affects job performance; confusion and disorientation are common. Patient experiences mood or personality changes, difficulty making decisions and paying bills; gets lost easily; withdraws from others; loses things.
- Second Stage: Lasts 2 to 10 years after diagnosis; increased memory loss and confusion, shorter attention span, restlessness. Patient makes constant repetitive statements; exhibits problems with reading, writing, and numbers; may be irritable or suspicious; experiences motor problems; has difficulty recognizing close friends and family members.
- Terminal Stage: Lasts 1 to 3 years. Patient does not recognize family; experiences weight loss; is unable to care for self; is incontinent of bladder and bowel; requires complete care.

CRITICAL THINKING APPLICATION

Maria Angelone is an 86-year-old patient of Dr. Kennedy's who is in the second stage of AD. Her husband and children are showing signs of stress from the continuous care required by Mrs. Angelone. Her family still does not understand what is happening to her and what to expect in the future. What information can Bill share with them about the disease, and what resources could be helpful to the family in dealing with the stress of caring for a loved one with dementia?

Pulmonary System

Maximum lung function decreases with age. The rate of air flow through the bronchi slowly declines after age 30, and the maximal force one is able to achieve on inspiration and expiration decreases. The lungs lose their elasticity owing to changes in **elastin** and collagen. They become smaller and flabbier. The alveoli enlarge, their walls become thinner, and the number of capillaries is reduced. As a result the effective area for gas exchange in the lungs is reduced. The chest wall may stiffen from osteoporosis of the ribs and vertebrae and calcification of the **costal** cartilage. The respiratory muscles become weaker, making it harder to move air into and out of the lungs. To compensate, older adults rely more on accessory muscles, such as the diaphragm. Weakening of the respiratory muscles and the stiffening of the chest wall make it harder to cough deeply enough to clear mucus from the lungs. Pulmonary

function tests reveal a decrease in vital capacity and an increase in residual volume. The incidence of sleep apnea and sleep disorders increases, causing a potential problem with nocturnal hypoxemia. All of these factors combine to put the older adult at greater risk for pneumonia and aspiration as well as reactivation of tuberculosis.

The larynx also changes with aging, causing a change in the pitch and quality of the voice. The voice sounds quieter and slightly hoarse. The individual's voice may sound weaker but it should not interfere with the ability to communicate effectively.

Sensory Organs

Vision

By the time a person reaches age 50, structural and functional changes in the eye become noticeable (Table 47-3). The eyebrows and eyelashes start to gray. The skin around the eyelids wrinkles, and the loss of orbital fat allows the eye to sink deeper into the orbit. The cornea increases in thickness and has reduced refractive power. A yellow-gray ring *(arcus senilis)* may develop on the periphery of the cornea. The iris loses pigmentation, and as a result most older people appear to have gray eyes.

The lens of the eye continues to grow. As new lens fibers grow, old lens fibers are compressed and pushed to the center, causing the lens to become denser. The lens becomes flatter, thicker, less elastic, and more opaque, progressively yellowing with age. By the age of 70, the lens has tripled in mass. Clouding of the lens causes light rays to scatter, creating glare.

The pupil is designed to adjust to control the amount of light entering the eye. The ciliary muscle that causes the pupil to dilate weakens during the aging processes. As a result a reduction in the size of the pupil occurs, limiting the amount of light available to reach the retina. Tear production normally decreases. Tear glands do not make enough tears, or the tears are of poor quality and do not keep the eyes wet enough. Eye irritation and excessive tearing are a result of decreased **lacrimation.**

During the fourth decade of life, *presbyopia* develops, which makes it difficult to focus on detailed objects close at hand. This requires the use of corrective lenses to accommodate age-related farsightedness. The ability to refocus quickly from far to near or near to far decreases. Also, the ability to follow a moving object is decreased. The yellowing of the lens causes it to act like a filter, making it difficult to distinguish certain color intensities. Blues, greens, and violets are hard to differentiate, whereas yellows,

TABLE 47-3 Age-Related Changes in the Structures of the Eye		
STRUCTURE	**AGE-RELATED CHANGE**	**OUTCOME**
Lens	Thickens, becomes more opaque	Decreased refraction causing blurred vision; decreased color acuity; cataracts
Anterior chamber	Decrease in size and volume	May develop increased intraocular pressure and glaucoma
Ciliary muscles	Affects pupil constriction and dilation	Limits light accommodation
Cornea	Thickens, and curve decreases	Problems with refraction
Retina	Decrease in number of rods and nerves	Decreased clarity; requires increase in minimum amount of light needed to see clearly

reds, and oranges are easier to identify. The loss in the ability to discriminate closely related colors can affect the older person's ability to judge distances or his or her depth perception. This increases an aging person's susceptibility to falls and accidents. Stairs become a potential hazard because the edges of the steps cannot be seen clearly.

Older persons need as much as six times more light to read; however, increasing the level of light does not completely compensate for visual decline, because the elderly also experience an increased sensitivity to glare. Glare is probably one of the most painful experiences for the aging eye. Exposed light bulbs, such as those used in chandeliers, and light from highly reflective surfaces such as glass tables and floors, can produce excessive glare. The eye has a decreased ability to respond to abrupt changes from light to dark or dark to light. Going from a well-lit waiting room into a dim hallway or negotiating the way down dimly lit aisles in a movie theater could be treacherous to an older person.

Cataracts, Glaucoma, and Macular Degeneration. Eye diseases and disorders that occur frequently in older persons are cataracts, glaucoma, and macular degeneration. *Cataracts* are cloudy or opaque areas in the lens that cause blurring of vision; rings or halos around lights and objects; and a blue or yellow tint to the visual field. Surgical lens extraction and implantation with an artificial lens improves vision in 95% of the cases. The procedure is performed in an outpatient facility, either using a small incision to remove the lens, laser therapy, or *phacoemulsification* (ultrasonic vibrations), which breaks up the lens and removes it without the need for an incision. Postoperatively patients must avoid bending or lifting heavy objects for 3 to 4 weeks; wearing an eye shield at night and glasses during the day helps to protect the eye until it heals.

Glaucoma is a result of blockage to the outflow of aqueous humor, which causes an increase in intraocular pressure and damage to the optic nerve. If not treated, glaucoma can cause progressive loss of peripheral vision and ultimately lead to blindness; however, it can be treated with medication.

The macula is the part of the eye responsible for sharp vision and color. The damage or breakdown of the macula is called *macular degeneration*, which causes progressive loss of the central field of vision. Macular degeneration is the leading cause of blindness in aging people, and at this time there is no effective treatment or cure. All three of these eye disorders are discussed in more detail in Chapter 36.

Hearing

Hearing loss can produce a profound psychologic effect on aging persons, causing depression, social withdrawal, and feelings of isolation. Hearing loss occurs gradually over a long period of time and may go undetected by the older person and healthcare providers. Lack of attention when being spoken to, inappropriate responses, asking to have statements repeated, and speaking too loudly or too softly are often signs of hearing loss. Changes in auditory ability begin around age 30, and by age 65, 25% of aging people have a hearing impairment, which increases to 65% of those over the age of 80 years. Age-related hearing loss is usually caused by a dysfunction or loss of cochlear cilia, resulting in an inability to hear high-frequency sounds and difficulty understanding speech. Hearing impairment is compounded by impacted cerumen, otitis media, otosclerosis, Meniere's disease, long-term exposure to intense noise, and certain ototoxic drugs such as aspirin.

Presbycusis, which is explained in Chapter 36, is associated with normal aging and causes a decreased ability to hear high frequencies and to discriminate sounds. Parts of a conversation may be missed because the sound of the word goes above the 2000-cycle frequency. Often words that sound similar are hard to differentiate. Consonants such as *g, f, s, sh, t,* and *z* produce high-pitched sounds that are more difficult to hear and differentiate. Low-frequency pitched sounds, such as the vowels *a, e, i, o,* and *u,* may be more easily heard by people with presbycusis. The inability to hear different frequencies combined with low background noise from groups of people talking, noise from appliances, or busy public places will compromise an older person's ability to hear clearly. Hearing aids, which can be used to amplify speech, also increase background noises, resulting in sensory overload.

Another hearing disorder common among older people is *tinnitus,* a ringing or buzzing in the ear. It can be caused by impacted cerumen, an ear infection, use of antibiotics, a reaction to medication, or a nerve disorder. Tinnitus can cause difficulty in understanding conversational speech and can make sleeping difficult because of the continuous sensation of ringing in the ears.

There is a direct relationship between hearing loss with its resultant isolation and the development of depression in older adults. Treatable depressions are often overlooked in the elderly population because of coexisting physical illnesses that mask the symptoms of depression. The medical assistant may be able to contribute to information about depression in elderly patients through conversations with the individual and family members. The physician may use, or train the medical assistant to use, the Geriatric Depression Scale short form, which questions the patient about daily activities, interests, and feelings to help diagnose depression in the ambulatory setting (Figure 47-4).

Suggestions for Helping the Visually Impaired Older Adult

- When escorting an older person, whether he or she is visually impaired or not, allow the client to place his or her hand above your elbow. It is easier for the person to follow your movements. This method also provides a source of support and security.
- Use high levels of evenly distributed glare-free light.
- Ask the pharmacist to use large lettering when labeling medicine bottles.
- Use paper that has a nonglare finish, and use large print for forms and educational materials.
- Make distinct differences (e.g., size of containers or color-coding with bright primary colors) for pills that are similar in size and color.
- Place all objects within the visual field, and avoid clutter.

GERIATRIC DEPRESSION SCALE (SHORT FORM)

Choose the best answer for how you have felt over the past week:

1. Are you basically satisfied with your life? YES / **NO**
2. Have you dropped many of your activities and interests? **YES** / NO
3. Do you feel that your life is empty? **YES** / NO
4. Do you often get bored? **YES** / NO
5. Are you in good spirits most of the time? YES / **NO**
6. Are you afraid that something bad is going to happen to you? **YES** / NO
7. Do you feel happy most of the time? YES / **NO**
8. Do you often feel helpless? **YES** / NO
9. Do you prefer to stay at home, rather than going out and doing new things? **YES** / NO
10. Do you feel you have more problems with memory than most? **YES** / NO
11. Do you think it is wonderful to be alive now? YES / **NO**
12. Do you feel pretty worthless the way you are now? **YES** / NO
13. Do you feel full of energy? YES / **NO**
14. Do you feel that your situation is hopeless? **YES** / NO
15. Do you think that most people are better off than you are? **YES** / NO

Answers in **bold** indicate depression. Although differing sensitivities and specificities have been obtained across studies, for clinical purposes a score >5 points is suggestive of depression and should warrant a follow-up interview. Scores >10 are almost always depression.

FIGURE 47-4 Geriatric depression scale.

Taste and Smell

During the aging process, there is a subtle decline in the ability to taste and smell. Deterioration and atrophy of the taste buds are part of the aging process. The ability to taste salt and sweet flavors is reduced, whereas the ability to detect bitter and sour flavors remains relatively the same. As a result, food frequently tastes bland and unappetizing. Patients on salt-restricted diets and diabetic patients must be cautioned about the use of excessive amounts of salt and sugar. A decrease in the sense of smell accompanies the decrease in taste. This not only affects the individual's enjoyment of food, but it also exposes the person to environmental dangers such as gas leaks, smoke, and other dangerous odors that may go undetected. Checking for gas leaks around stoves and heaters and using smoke alarms reduce some of the danger. Also, dating food when it is put into the refrigerator is a good idea.

Nutritional Status. Aging persons, because of the many environmental, social, economic, and physical changes of aging, are at greater risk for poor nutrition, which can adversely affect

Suggestions for Helping the Hearing-Impaired Older Adult

- Stand in the patient's direct line of vision, and gently touch the person to get attention.
- Use gestures, pictures, and large, bold print to communicate.
- Talk in short sentences into the ear with better hearing.
- Do not increase the volume of your speech—this also raises the frequency of the voice, which is the hearing most impaired in aging people. Use expanded speech—lower the tone of your voice and talk in distinct syllables.
- Avoid background noise. Give instructions in a quiet room with the door closed. If the patient has a hearing aid, make sure it is on.

their health and energy level. It is estimated that 25% of the aging population suffers from malnutrition. Nutrition screening should be part of routine primary care to identify nutritional deficiencies and correct them before disease process occurs or to assist in the treatment of chronic disease. Patients with chronic conditions, such as cardiovascular disease, hypertension, and diabetes, can benefit from nutrition assessments and interventions. Malnourished older patients get more infections; their injuries take longer to heal; surgery on them is riskier; and their hospital stays are longer and more expensive.

The most effective method of assessing a patient's nutritional status is through a comprehensive patient interview that considers all potential barriers to adequate nutrition. The medical assistant can contribute to determining the nutritional status of older patients by considering the following items when conducting patient interviews.

- Oral health: Does the patient wear dentures, and do they fit properly? Is there mouth pain? Can the patient swallow without difficulty?
- Gastrointestinal complaints: Does the patient have anorexia, nausea, vomiting, diarrhea, or constipation? Is the patient lactose intolerant (incidence increases with age)?
- Sensorimotor changes: Is there loss of vision, hearing, or changes in taste and smell? Can the patient feed herself or himself? Does the patient need adaptive utensils?
- Diet influences: Can the patient shop for, afford, and prepare food? Are there ethnic or religious influences? Are there any disease-related diet restrictions? What is the patient's alcohol consumption?
- Social and mental influences: Is the patient depressed, lonely, or isolated? Are support systems available?

CRITICAL THINKING APPLICATION

Multiple sensory changes occur as people age. Dr. Kennedy asks Bill to develop a handout for patients and family members to help them understand normal, age-related sensorimotor changes as well as adaptations that can be made to improve communication. What information should Bill include?

Urinary System

As the body ages, structural changes in the kidneys cause the urinary system to become less efficient. Between the ages of 40 and 80, the kidney loses about 20% of its mass. The number of functional nephron units decreases. Blood flow to the kidneys is reduced owing to a decrease in cardiovascular efficiency. The reduction of blood flow to the kidneys and the decreased number of nephrons cause the kidneys to be less efficient at filtering waste from the blood. This results in a more-diluted, less-concentrated urine. The kidneys require more water to excrete the same amount of waste. Medication takes longer to be removed from the body. Older adults are at increased risk for toxic levels of medication in the bloodstream because of this reduced filtration rate.

Fibrous connective tissue replaces the smooth muscle and elastic tissue in the bladder. This thickening of the bladder wall decreases the bladder's ability to expand. The bladder's capacity to store fluid comfortably is reduced from 400 to 250 ml. These structural changes in the bladder lead to increased frequency of urination and urinary retention. Older adults are at an increased risk for urinary tract infections because of residual urine. Sleep is interrupted by the need to void during the night. The sensation of bladder fullness is not recognized as quickly by the older brain. Reduced time between awareness of the need to void and involuntary urination can cause anxiety. Often older adults decrease their fluid intake to prevent possible embarrassment. Unfortunately this causes dehydration and an increased risk of urinary tract infections. Another change is loss of muscle tone in the urethra. In addition, the pelvic floor muscles in the aging woman relax as a result of decreased estrogen levels or previous pregnancy and childbirth.

Despite these changes the kidneys have great reserve capacity and are able to continue functioning normally. Urinary incontinence, the involuntary loss of urine, is a significant problem for aging patients but is not a normal part of the aging process. Changes in the urinary system make older persons more vulnerable to incontinence, but factors such as infection, confusion, difficulty with mobility, and side effects from medications contribute to the development of the problem. Incontinence is an emotional as well as a physical problem. To avoid the chance of an embarrassing accident, people with this problem may avoid social occasions or activities they enjoy. Often people are too embarrassed to admit they have this condition, or they believe it is just part of aging. Once the condition is diagnosed by the urologist, pelvic floor muscle exercises, medication, or surgery may be recommended.

Reproductive System

Menopause is discussed in Chapter 40. Aging brings a decrease in circulating levels of the female hormones estrogen and progesterone, while androgen levels increase. The results of this decrease are changes in the genital tract. The vagina diminishes in width and length and becomes less elastic. The cervix, uterus, and ovaries decrease in size. Vaginal secretions decrease; therefore lubrication diminishes, resulting in vaginal dryness. Bacterial or yeast infections may occur because vaginal secretions are less acidic. Estrogen cream applied to vaginal tissue may be prescribed by the physician for help with dryness and thinning of the vaginal tissue. The benefits and risks of estrogen replacement therapy should be discussed by the physician with the patient to determine whether it should be used.

Even though sperm production may decline in those over 50, men remain virile well into old age. However, men do experience a change in hormonal levels of testosterone, and these changes can affect the prostate gland, as discussed in Chapter 39. The prostate enlarges over time and presses down on the urethra, causing difficulty with urination. Surgery may be required to remove excess portions of the gland. Unfortunately, the operation may cause impotence, which can be treated medically with erectile dysfunction medications.

Men experience some changes in sexual functioning as they age. It takes longer for the penis to become erect, longer for an orgasm to occur, and longer to recover. Direct stimulation may be required before an erection occurs, and when it does, it may be less firm when compared with how it was when they were younger.

Some drugs and illnesses can interfere with sexual function. Drugs used to control high blood pressure, antihistamines, antidepressants, and some stomach acid blockers, as well as diabetes, arthritis, and arteriosclerosis, can have an adverse effect on sexual function. Often people who have experienced heart surgery or have had heart attacks are concerned about sexual activity. Patients need to feel comfortable and not embarrassed to discuss their concerns openly with their physicians. It is important for healthcare providers to dismiss myths that older patients have lost the desire for and interest in sexual intercourse.

Sleep Disorders

Complaints of sleeping difficulties increase with age. The amount of time spent sleeping may be slightly longer than in a younger person, but the quality of sleep decreases. Older people are often light sleepers and experience periods of wakefulness in bed. Rapid eye movement (REM) sleep is the stage of sleep when people experience dreaming. Non-REM sleep is the period of deepest sleep. The amount of time spent in the deepest stages of sleep decreases with age. Sleep that is disturbed or that leaves the person feeling tired is not part of the aging process and may indicate some underlying emotional or physical problem. Lack of sleep can result in restlessness, disorientation, "thick" speech, and mispronounced words. Often these symptoms are mistaken as signs of dementia. Other factors that might influence sleep patterns are medications, caffeine, alcohol, depression, and environmental or physical changes.

Common sleep problems in older adults include *dyssomnias*, such as periodic limb movement disorder (PLMD), in which the person experiences periodic jerking of the legs during sleep, and sleep apnea, which is common among overweight persons and can occur frequently during the night, causing sleep interruption. Numerous medical conditions can interfere with sleep, including joint and bone pain; Parkinson's disease (because of difficulty changing positions); CHF; chronic obstructive pulmonary disease; diabetes mellitus, which increases nocturia; depression; and certain medications (e.g., beta-blockers can cause nightmares, antidepressants increase PLMD, and barbiturates may result in nightmares or hallucinations).

It is important to be aware of the effect of sleep problems because often these can be confused with dementia. Patients who are experiencing difficulty with sleeping should be encouraged to document their sleeping patterns, napping patterns, medications, diet, exercise routines, and any events that have resulted in a change of lifestyle. They should discuss this problem with their physician. Simple modification of behavioral patterns may resolve the problem. Taking fewer naps, completing exercise several hours before bedtime, changing eating times, decreasing the amount of alcohol and caffeine ingested, drinking a glass of milk before bedtime, or changing medications or the time they are taken are all suggestions that might alter the factors responsible for sleep disturbances.

If behavioral approaches are not effective, medications may be considered for short-term use only because they have a high incidence of physical and psychologic dependence. The elderly population is especially susceptible to side effects from these drugs, for example, next-day drowsiness and temporary memory loss. Sedatives or hypnotics that may be prescribed include Ambien, Lunesta, Sonata, and Restoril.

Living Arrangements

At any given time only 5% of the elderly population lives in long-term care facilities. According to information published by the National Institute on Aging, most older people live close to their children and are in frequent contact with them. People prefer to age in place or, in other words, live in their own home environment as long as possible. Individuals are admitted to nursing homes because they are no longer able to perform activities of daily living, such as bathing, dressing, eating, walking, and maintaining bladder and bowel continence. They also exhibit difficulty with grocery shopping, housekeeping, and money management. Chronic health conditions and accidents interfere with the older person's ability to perform these tasks.

Many resources are available that enable seniors to maintain their independence. Outreach programs, such as Meals on Wheels, deliver nutritious meals to the homes of older adults. Senior centers serve as a focal point for many activities and a source of information. Transportation services provide rides to doctors' appointments, day care centers, shopping centers, and community events. Home health agencies provide several types of services, which include personal care, shopping, transportation, and meal preparation. Some home health agencies provide a range of activities from patient education to intravenous therapy; medical-social services; physical, speech, and occupational therapies; and nutrition and dietary counseling. Advanced technology allows people to receive services at home that had formerly been provided at a hospital or physician's office only.

Adult day care centers provide socialization, recreation, meals, and, in some centers, physical therapy, occupational therapy, and transportation. These centers provide supervision for older adults who may be taken care of by family members in the evening but need care during the day. They also serve as respite for a caregiver.

Assisted-living facilities can be retirement homes or board and care homes. These facilities are appropriate for older adults who need assistance with some activities of daily living, such as bathing, dressing, and walking. Skilled nursing facilities provide 24-hour medical care and supervision. In addition to medical care, residents receive care that may include physical, occupational, and speech therapies. The objective of treatment is to improve or maintain the person's abilities.

Suggestions for Effective Communication with Aging Patients

- Address the patient by Mr., Mrs., or Miss unless the patient has given permission to use his or her first name.
- All healthcare workers should introduce themselves and their purpose before performing a procedure.
- Face the aging person and softly touch him or her to get attention before beginning to speak.
- Use expanded speech, gestures, demonstrations, or written instructions in block print.
- If the message must be repeated, paraphrase or find other words to say the same thing.
- Observe the patient's nonverbal behaviors for cues to indicate whether he or she understands.
- Provide adequate lighting without glare.
- Allow patients time to process information and take care of themselves unless they ask for assistance.
- Communications should be conducted in a quiet room without distractions.
- Involve family members as needed for continuity of care.
- When leaving a telephone message, remember to speak slowly and clearly and repeat the message in the same manner. It is hard to interpret a message, and even more difficult to write it down, if the message was delivered in a hurried manner.
- Use referrals and community resources for support such as the following:
  - Alzheimer's Association (1-800-272-3900)
  - American Council of the Blind (1-800-424-8666)—provides referrals to state and other organizations that provide services and equipment for the blind
  - American Speech-Language-Hearing Association (1-800-638-8255)—offers information on hearing aids, hearing loss, and communication problems in older people and provides a list of certified audiologist and speech pathologists.
  - Arthritis Foundation Information Line (1-800-283-7800)—makes referrals to local chapters and provides information
  - Eldercare Locator (1-800-677-1116)—run by the National Association of Area Agencies on Aging; help line provides information on contacting local chapters that oversee services to older adults
  - National Institute on Aging Information Center (1-800-222-2225)—provides information on geriatric health issues
  - National Meals-on-Wheels Foundation (1-800-999-6262)
  - Hospice Helpline (1-800-658-8898)—provides information about hospice care and makes referrals to local hospices

THE MEDICAL ASSISTANT'S ROLE IN CARING FOR THE OLDER PATIENT

Elderly patients in the ambulatory care setting present a specific set of needs that require a certain amount of accommodation by the staff. To reinforce independence, aging patients require more time, but staff members may want to hurry them so the schedule can be maintained. In the best interests of the patient, however, he or she should be treated with respect and given whatever time is needed to prepare for examinations, ask questions and receive answers, and have procedures explained. A system that is sensitive to the needs of older patients will schedule longer periods for appointments; have adequate lighting in the waiting room and provide forms in large print; have an examination room that is equipped with furniture, magazines, and treatment folders especially designed for older adults; and invite a professional in the management of older patients for in-service training.

The primary issue in elder care is effective communication. How you communicate with people is often influenced by what you know or do not know about them. Older people are subject to many changes that affect how they are able to interact with their environment. It is important to recognize these changes as well as investigate one's personal perception of older people to break down the barriers that prohibit effective communication.

As people age they frequently experience a loss of control over their lives because of physical disabilities, economic constraints, and institutional living. Part of our job is to help aging people maintain their dignity and independence while they are in the ambulatory care setting. Remember, each patient, regardless of his or her education, socioeconomic status, or age, deserves to be treated with compassion and respect. Ask the patient directly what is wrong rather than discussing the patient with family members. It also is important to listen carefully and to be specific and sincere when responding. When a patient is talking, take time to allow him or her to complete the sentence. Do not finish it for him or her. Give the patient your full attention rather than continuing with other tasks while he or she is speaking. Older people may take a little longer to process information, but they are capable of understanding. Do not hurry through explanations or questions; rather, take time to review a form or give instructions as needed.

Guidelines for Effective Patient Education with Older Adults

- May have short-term memory loss, so need to repeat the information using different words
- Distracted more easily, so learning in a group may be difficult
- Take longer to process information, so teach at a pace that matches patient needs
- Provide large-print, block-letter handouts for reviewing information at home
- Involve family members as needed for continuity of care

CRITICAL THINKING APPLICATION

New staff members in the practice are complaining of having to repeat information to older clients and that these patients do not pay attention when procedures are being explained. Dr. Kennedy has decided to invite a gerontologist from the local university to present an in-service workshop on healthy aging. She asks Bill to coordinate the in-service workshop and prepare materials requested by the guest speaker. What information regarding caring for the ambulatory aging patient should be included in the workshop?

CLOSING COMMENTS

Patient Education

The medical assistant must keep the sensorimotor changes that accompany aging and respectful patient communications in mind when conducting patient education with older clients. Remember, the aging process does not affect a person's ability to learn; it just may take longer to process the information, and the material may need to be repeated for understanding. Exhibiting sensitivity to the needs of aging learners will ensure successful patient education and improve compliance with prescribed treatment plans. The current aging population is generally respectful toward authority; so if the medical assistant cannot gain patient cooperation, the physician may be able to provide authoritative reinforcement of material.

Legal and Ethical Issues

All patients have the right to know about the medications, treatments, and alternatives available to them. The Patient's Bill of Rights (see Chapter 7) informs the patient of his or her rights in a healthcare setting. These rights include the right to privacy about personal and medical information and the right to informed consent, which holds the physician accountable to explain clearly the advantages and risks of any procedures, tests, or treatments. The patient must give permission for medical care and has the right to refuse treatment. The patient has the right to be informed about his or her condition and treatment and the chances of recovery. The patient also has the right to have advance directives explained to him or her.

Consent must be given by the individual undergoing the procedure as long as he or she is judged to be competent, that is, as long as the patient is able to understand the consequences of the procedure. In an emergency situation, or if a court has ruled the patient incompetent, someone else must give consent. This may be a person who was already designated to hold the durable power of attorney, a close family member (spouse, adult child, parent, sibling), or a court-appointed guardian.

Most states have legal documents available, *advance directives* that provide written instructions specifying the type of medical care a person wishes to receive in the event she or he becomes incapacitated. The document designates someone to have a durable power of attorney—an authorization for making medical decisions on a person's behalf if that individual is unable to make his or her own treatment decisions. The document provides a list of specific instructions for the proxy to follow. Various issues may be covered in these documents. Do not resuscitate (DNR) orders allow a patient to refuse attempts to restore heartbeat. The patient may decide to withdraw life-sustaining treatment such as the use of respirators or feeding tubes. A copy of the directive should be kept on file as part of the patient's medical record. It is important to check the laws of the state in which you are practicing about advance directives because these vary among states (Figure 47-5).

Another legal issue surrounding the care of aging patient is the possibility of elder abuse. Mistreatment of aging persons crosses all social, racial, and economic levels. The abuse may

---

Indications of Elder Abuse

- Poor general appearance and poor hygiene
- Pattern of changing doctors and frequent emergency room visits
- Skin lesions, signs of dehydration, bruises (signs of new and old bruising together), abrasions, welts, burns, or pressure sores
- Recurrent injuries caused by accidents
- Signs of malnutrition and weight loss without related illness
- Any injury that does not fit the given history

Directive made this _____ th day of _____ in the year _____ .
      (day)   (month)   (year)

I, _____ , being of sound mind, willfully and voluntarily make known my desire that my life shall not be artificially prolonged under the circumstances set forth in this directive.

If at any time I should have

— an incurable or irreversible condition caused by injury,
— disease,
— or illness certified to be a terminal condition by two physicians

and if the application of life-sustaining procedures would serve only to artificially postpone the moment of my death, and if my attending physician determines that my death is imminent or will result within a relatively short time without the application of life- sustaining procedures. I direct that those procedures be withheld or withdrawn, and that I be permitted to die naturally.

In the absence of my ability to give directions regarding the use of those life-sustaining procedures, it is my intention that this directive be honored by my family and physicians as the final expression of my legal right to refuse medical or surgical treatment and accept the consequences from that refusal.

If I have been diagnosed as pregnant and that diagnosis is known to my physician, this directive has no effect during my pregnancy. This directive is in effect until it is revoked.

I understand the full import of this directive and I am emotionally and mentally competent to make this directive. I understand that I may revoke this directive at any time.

I request that only comfort care be provided to me, no antibiotics, no artificial nutrition, no mechanical ventilation, and no hydration. It is my strong preference to be allowed to die outside of a care facility if possible, even if that preference is determined by my physician to shorten my period of dying. The only condition under which I desire these preferences for end of life care to be altered is in the case of possible organ and tissue donation. I request that any and all organs and tissue that may be salvaged be provided for transplant. My remains may then be cremated.

Signed _____ in the City of _____ etc.

I am not a person designated by the declarant to make a treatment decision. I am not related to the declarant by blood or marriage. I would not be entitled to any portion of the declarant's estate on the declarant's death. I am not the attending physician of the declarant or an employee of the attending physician.

I have no claim in against any portion of the declarant's estate on the declarant's death. Furthermore, if I am an employee of the health care facility in which the declarant is a patient, I am not involved in providing direct patient care to the declarant and am not an officer, director, partner, or business office employee of the heath care facility or of any parent organization of the health care facility.

Witness _____

Witness _____

FIGURE 47-5 Sample Advance Directive.

be physical, mental, sexual, material, or financial; may involve neglect or failure to provide adequate care; or may involve self-neglect when aging persons are unable or refuse to care for themselves. The abuse of elders by their caregivers may be difficult to identify. The aging victim feels embarrassed, guilty, or afraid to report the abuse. If abuse is suspected, interviewing the caregiver and questioning the demands of care and self-reported perceptions of stress levels may help the physician detect the problem. Many states now have laws that require reporting suspected elder abuse. Check your state laws to determine the requirements for healthcare workers.

SUMMARY OF SCENARIO

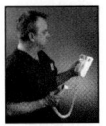

Since working with Dr. Kennedy, Bill has learned to understand the special needs of aging patients. He thought that most older people were chronically sick and would ultimately end up in long-term care facilities. Now he understands that the majority of aging people lead healthy, active lives and that the disorders occurring in later life are usually a result of lifestyle factors such as diet and lack of exercise. Bill has also learned how to communicate effectively with older patients and to conduct patient interviews that investigate their physical, mental, emotional, and nutritional health.

SUMMARY of LEARNING OBJECTIVES

1. Define, spell, and pronounce the terms listed in the vocabulary.
   - Spelling and pronouncing medical terms correctly adds credibility to the medical assistant. Knowing the definition of these terms promotes confidence in communication with patients and co-workers.
2. Identify the various impacts of an increasing aging population on society.
   - Almost 36.3 million Americans are over the age of 65. The "oldest old" (people older than 85) are the most rapidly growing age group. By the middle of the twenty-first century, over 71 million people will be older than 65 years. Most older persons have at least one chronic medical condition, and many have multiple conditions. The aging population will affect all aspects of society. The healthcare professional must recognize the special needs of the aged and develop effective management and communication skills to better service the older client.
3. Role-play the effect of sensorimotor changes of aging.
   - Procedure 47-1 outlines the steps in role-playing the sensorimotor changes that accompany aging.
4. Explain the changes caused by aging in each of the body systems.
   - Table 47-1 summarizes changes associated with aging that occur across all body systems. There are normal age-related changes that can be expected and compensated for, but these intensify with poor health habits and chronic disease. General changes include an increase in arteriosclerosis; a change in cognitive abilities; a sharp decline in estrogen for women and an increased risk of osteoporosis; an increase in malabsorption problems and constipation; a decrease in muscle mass, a tendency to gain weight and deterioration of joint cartilage; decreased elasticity of lung tissue; presbycusis and presbyopia; enlargement of the prostate; and weakening of bladder muscles. Age-related changes can be managed through regular exercise; a healthy diet; avoidance of sun damage; and annual physical examinations with health screening.

5. Summarize the major diseases and disorders faced by older patients.
   - Major health issues of older people are related to an increase in atherosclerosis and potential cardiovascular disease; hypertension; type 2 diabetes mellitus; integumentary system changes; arthritis; osteoporosis; an increased risk of injury from falls; dementia attributable to metabolic or cardiovascular disease or AD; pneumonia, aspiration, and reactivation of tuberculosis; cataracts, glaucoma, and macular degeneration; depression; malnutrition; urinary tract abnormalities; menopausal changes; and sleep disorders.
6. Describe various screening tools for dementia, depression, and malnutrition.
   - A commonly used screening tool for dementia is the Folstein Mini-Mental Status Examination, a 5-minute screening test that is designed to evaluate basic mental function. The physician may use the Geriatric Depression Scale short form, which questions the patient about daily activities, interests, and feelings. Nutritional status can be assessed through a comprehensive patient interview that considers all potential barriers to adequate nutrition.
7. Explain the effect of aging on sleep.
   - Complaints of sleeping difficulties increase with age. The amount of time spent in the deepest stages of sleep decreases with age. Factors that might influence sleep patterns are medications, caffeine, alcohol, depression, and environmental or physical changes. Common sleep problems in older adults include PLMD and sleep apnea.
8. Differentiate among independent, assisted, and skilled nursing facilities.

Continued

SUMMARY of LEARNING OBJECTIVES

Continued

- Aging persons prefer to remain within their home environment for as long as possible. Adult day care centers can provide supervision for older adults who may be taken care of by family members in the evening but need care during the day. Assisted-living facilities are appropriate for older adults who need assistance with some activities of daily living. Skilled nursing facilities provide 24-hour medical care and supervision.

9. Summarize the role of the medical assistant in caring for aging patients.
   - The medical assistant's role in caring for the older patient is to develop effective communication skills that are reflective of age-related sensorimotor changes; to allow time for longer appointments; to provide adequate lighting and forms in large print; and to develop appropriate in-service training as requested by the physician. Examination rooms should have furniture and treatment folders especially designed for the elderly patient. Use referrals and community resources for patient and family support.

10. Determine the principles for effective communication with older adults.
    - Effective communication with aging patients includes addressing the patient with an appropriate title; introducing yourself and the purpose of a procedure before touching the patient; establishing eye contact and getting the patient's attention before beginning to speak; using expanded speech, gestures, demonstrations, or written instructions in block print; repeating the message as needed for understanding; observing the patient's nonverbal behaviors for cues to indicate whether he or she understands; allowing time to process information; avoiding distractions; and involving family members as needed.

11. Identify legal and ethical issues regarding aging patients.
    - Legal and ethical issues associated with aging patients include adequate informed consent, the use of advance directives, and staying alert for signs of possible elder abuse.

CONNECTIONS

Study Guide Connection: Go to Chapter 47 Study Guide. Read the Case Study and Workplace Applications and complete the assignments. Do online research for answers to the questions in the Internet Activities associated with geriatrics.

CD Connection: Go to the Medical Assisting Competency Challenge CD and do the training activities under Patient Care and Patient Instruction.

evolve   **Evolve Connection:** For more information related to geriatrics, go to evolve.elsevier.com/kinn and visit related weblinks for Chapter 47. Click on the Medical Assisting Exam Review and do the practice questions to sharpen your test-taking skills.

Principles of Electrocardiography

48

SCENARIO

Martha Reyes works as a medical assistant in the coronary care unit at the local hospital where she has been employed for almost 4 years. The head cardiologist at the hospital, Dr. Julie Lee, has recognized Martha's abilities and hard work and recently offered her a position in her busy cardiology practice. Martha is very enthusiastic but realizes that she has much more to learn on the job to provide the best patient service possible in Dr. Lee's practice. Although Martha has worked in the cardiology department and is familiar with hospital-based procedures, she will need to be able to understand and perform ambulatory patient procedures, especially electrocardiography.

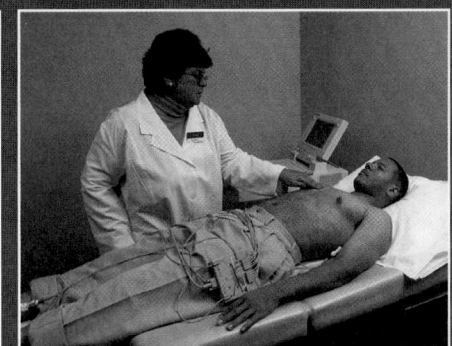

While studying this chapter, think about the following questions:

- To fulfill her job description with Dr. Lee, what does Martha need to know about the electrical conduction system of the heart
- How does an ECG machine work?
- How should a patient be prepared for an electrocardiogram?
- How will Martha perform an ECG diagnostic procedure?
- What is the normal appearance of ECG complexes?
- What are the characteristics of common ECG arrhythmias that Martha must be able to recognize?
- What additional cardiac tests should Martha be prepared to assist with and explain to patients?

LEARNING OBJECTIVES

1. Define, spell, and pronounce the terms listed in the vocabulary.
2. Illustrate the electrical conduction system through the heart.
3. Explain the concepts of cardiac polarization, depolarization, and repolarization.
4. Summarize the properties of the electrocardiograph.
5. Describe the electrical views of the heart recorded by the 12-lead electrocardiograph.
6. Discuss the process of recording an electrocardiogram.
7. Perform an accurate recording of the electrical activity of the heart.
8. Compare and contrast electrocardiograph artifacts and the probable cause of each.
9. Interpret a typical electrocardiograph tracing.
10. Identify common electrocardiograph arrhythmias.
11. Summarize cardiac diagnostic tests.
12. Apply a Holter monitor.

National Accreditation Competencies and Content

CAAHEP COMPETENCIES	ABHES COMPETENCIES
Clinical	**Clinical Duties**
3.b.(3)(a). Perform electrocardiography	4.b. Prepare patients for procedures
3.b.(4)(e). Prepare patient for and assist with routine and specialty examinations	4.h. Prepare patient for and assist physician with routine and specialty examinations

VOCABULARY

arrhythmia (ar-rith′-me-uh) Abnormality or irregularity in the heart rhythm.

atria The two upper chambers of the heart.

atrioventricular (AV) node Part of the cardiac conduction system located between the atria and the ventricles.

bifurcates (bi′-fuhr-kats) (Divides from one into two branches.

bradycardia (bra-de-kar′-de-uh) Heart rate of less than 60 beats per minute.

bundle of His Specialized muscle fibers that conduct electrical impulses from AV node to ventricular myocardium.

cardiac arrest Condition in which cardiac contractions completely stop.

cardioversion Use of electroshock to convert an abnormal cardiac rhythm to a normal one.

defibrillator Machine used to deliver an electroshock to the heart through electrodes placed on the chest wall.

ectopic (ek-tohp′-ik) Originating outside of the normal tissue.

infarction Area of tissue that has died from lack of blood supply.

ischemic (is-ke′-mik) Characterized by temporary interruption in the blood supply to a tissue or an organ.

myocardial (my-oh-kar′-de-uhl) Pertaining to the heart muscle.

myocardium (my-oh-kar′-de-um) Heart muscle.

sinoatrial (SA) node Pacemaker of the heart, located in the right atrium.

tachycardia (tak-eh-kar′-de-uh) Heart rate over 100 beats per minute.

ventricles The two lower chambers of the heart.

vertigo Dizziness.

Electrocardiography is a painless and safe procedure and is the test most frequently used for the diagnosis of heart disease in the ambulatory care setting. In electrocardiography, electrodes are attached to the patient's skin and connected to wires that go to the electrocardiograph. Electrocardiography amplifies the electrical impulses from the beating heart, and a pattern of these impulses is recorded on electrocardiographic paper. This record is called the *electrocardiogram* (ECG). The ECG is read and evaluated by the physician and becomes a part of the patient's chart (Figure 48-1).

For the ECG to accurately represent the true cardiac activity of a patient, it must be performed with a high degree of accuracy and skill. A medical assistant must have an understanding of normal cardiac function and the relationship of the ECG recordings to normal function. It is the medical assistant's responsibility to ensure that the patient has been prepared mentally and physically and that the equipment is set up properly. When performing electrocardiography, a medical assistant must be able to recognize problems with the recording and make appropriate corrections so the physician has a clear record of the patient's cardiac activity. The goal is to obtain the most accurate ECG possible.

History of Electrocardiography

Dutch physiologist Willem Einthoven developed techniques to record the electrical activity of the heart in the late 1800s. He called this recording an *Electro Kardio Gramm*; hence the acronym *EKG*. Many physicians and other health care providers still call the recording an EKG, although the newer, preferred term is *ECG* for *electrocardiogram*.

THE ELECTRICAL CONDUCTION SYSTEM OF THE HEART

The Cardiac Cycle

The cardiac cycle includes all of the events occurring in the heart during one single heartbeat. Each chamber of the heart goes through two phases during the cardiac cycle: *systole* and *diastole*. Systole is when both the **atria** and **ventricles** contract and empty of blood. Diastole is the relaxation phase of the heart during which the chambers are refilling with blood. Venous blood from the inferior and superior vena cava empties into the right atrium during atrial diastole. As the right atrium fills, increased pressure in the chamber causes the tricuspid valve to open, and the right ventricle begins to fill. At the same time, blood returning from the lungs via the pulmonary veins fills the left atrium, causing the mitral valve to open, emptying blood into the left ventricle. Before systole occurs the ventricles are already 70% filled. The cardiac cycle for a healthy adult lasts approximately 0.8 seconds. However, the amount of time it takes for the heart to empty and refill is dependent on many factors including the condition of the **myocardium** and the heart's electrical system.

The electrocardiograph records both the intensity and the actual time it takes for each part of the cardiac cycle to occur. It measures the electrical conductive impulses of the heart muscle and therefore allows the physician to see any disturbances or disruptions in normal heart activity. In addition to being recorded as an ECG, the cardiac cycle can also appear as a continuously moving pattern on a monitor screen, accompanied by a sound for each beat. On televised programs, one frequently sees and hears electrocardiographic activities.

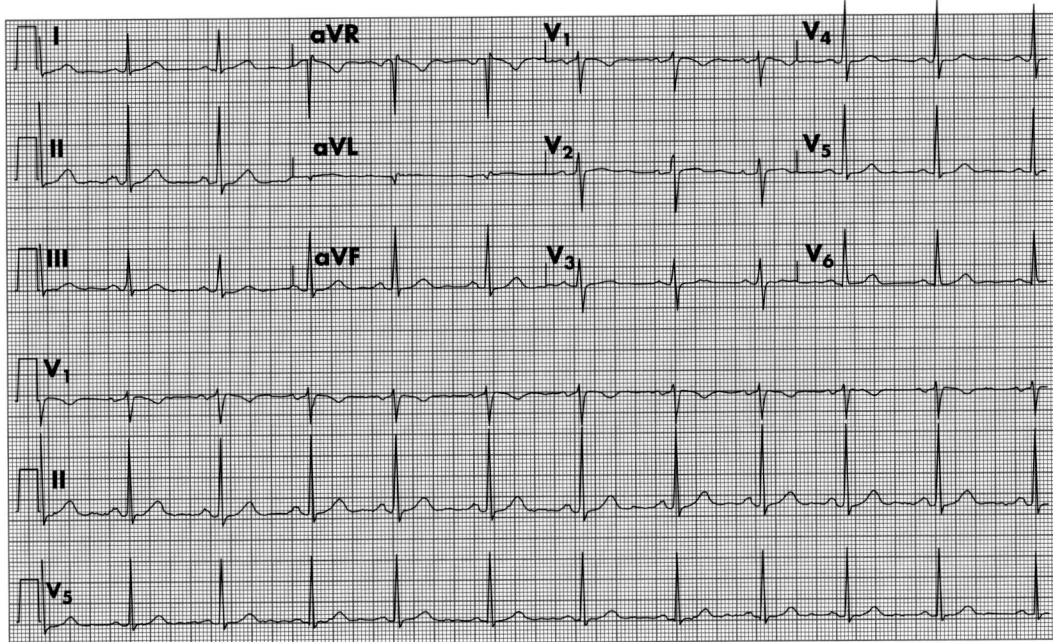

FIGURE 48-1 An example of a 12-lead ECG. (From Aehlert B: *ECGs made easy*, ed 3, St Louis, 2006, Mosby.)

The specialized electrical conduction system of the heart (Figure 48-2) initiates each heartbeat. The main part of this system is the **sinoatrial (SA) node,** which is located in the upper back wall of the right atrium at the junction of the superior vena cava and the right atrium. The SA node controls the rate of heart contraction by initiating electrical impulses 60 to 100 times per minute. Each cardiac cycle or heartbeat starts with the SA node generating an electrical impulse that travels in a wavelike pattern across the cardiac muscle of the atria, causing them to contract almost simultaneously. This electrical impulse then stimulates the **atrioventricular (AV) node,** which is located in the posterior, superior portion of the right atrial septal wall, directly behind the tricuspid valve. A slight delay in conduction at this point allows the atria to empty completely. The electrical impulse is then transmitted to a special group of conduction fibers, the **bundle of His,** which is located in the upper part of the interventricular septal wall. The bundle of His divides into two branches; the right bundle branch carries electrical impulses to the right ventricle, and the left bundle branch carries impulses to the left ventricle. The right and left bundle branches divide into smaller and smaller branches, ending in the Purkinje fibers, which spread across the apex of the heart and through the myocardium, stimulating ventricular contraction. The ventricles contract in a twisting sort of action, forcing the blood out of the chambers and into the pulmonary artery on the right side of the heart and the aorta on the left side.

Normal sinus rhythm (NSR) refers to a regular heart rate that falls within the average range of 60 to 80 beats per minute (beats/min). Sinus **bradycardia** is a heart rate less than 60 beats/min, whereas a rate of greater than 100 beats/min is called sinus **tachycardia.** In both of these conditions the rhythm remains even, but the rate is pathologic. An irregular cardiac rhythm is called an **arrhythmia.** Conditions that interrupt the conduction

pathway, SA node to AV node to bundle of His to right and left bundle branches, can cause arrhythmias.

Polarization, Depolarization, and Repolarization

Polarization is the resting state of the myocardial wall when there is no electrical activity in the heart and is recorded on the ECG strip as a flatline. In this state the myocardial cells are ready for stimulation. When the electrical system of the heart stimulates a myocardial cell, *depolarization* occurs, resulting in the contraction of the stimulated heart muscle. After depolarization the heart muscle cells must return to a resting state before they can be electrically stimulated again. The process of reaching this resting state is called *repolarization.*

The electrocardiograph records a series of waves, or deflections, above or below a baseline on the ECG paper. Each deflection corresponds to a particular part of the cardiac cycle (Table 48-1). The normal ECG cycle consists of waveforms that are labeled the P wave, the Q wave, the R wave, the S wave, and the T wave. The Q, R, and S waves are usually grouped together and called the *QRS complex.* One entire cardiac cycle can be called the *PQRST complex.* In the next section, each part of the ECG is discussed in more detail.

PQRST Complex

The *P wave* occurs during the contraction of the atria and shows the beginning of cardiac depolarization. The P wave is the first deflection from the baseline, is typically smooth and rounded, and should occur before each QRS complex. Atrial repolarization is not recorded on the ECG strip because its electrical impulse is small and is hidden in the QRS complex. The *PR segment* is the return to baseline after atrial contraction. The *PR interval* is the time from the beginning of atrial contraction to the beginning of ventricular contraction. It contains the P wave

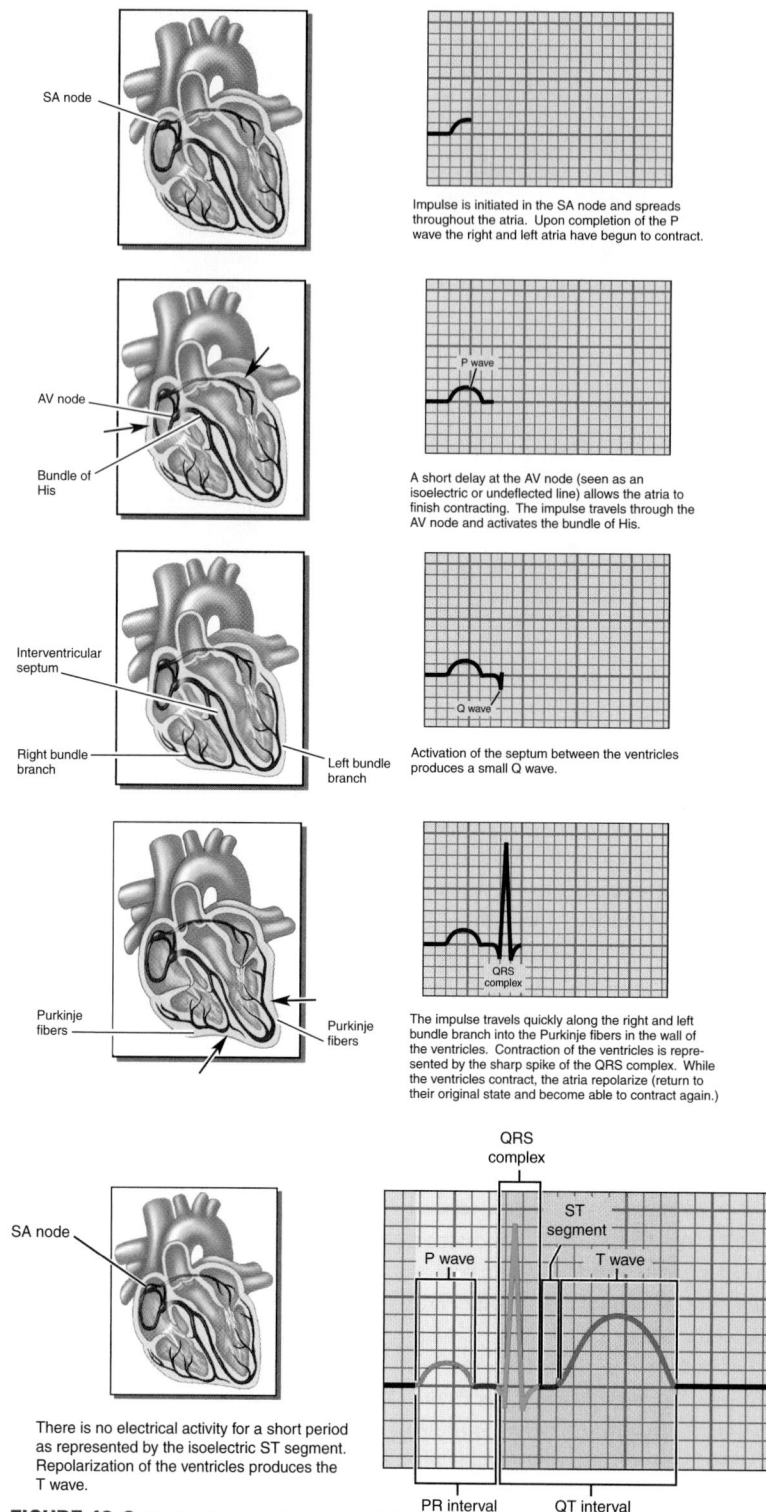

FIGURE 48-2 Electrical conduction system of the heart. (From Hunt SA: *Saunders fundamentals of medical assisting*, Philadelphia, 2002, Saunders.)

(depolarization of the atria) and the spread of the electrical impulse through the AV node, bundle of His, right and left bundle branches, and Purkinje fibers. As the heart rate increases, the PR interval typically shortens. The *QRS complex* shows the contraction of both ventricles and also reflects the completion of cardiac depolarization. Repolarization of the atria also occurs during this time, but it cannot be seen on the ECG because the recording of the much stronger QRS activity overshadows it. Depolarization of the ventricles results in the contraction of a much larger muscle mass than does depolarization of the atria. Therefore the QRS complex is recorded as a much more significant electrical activity than the P wave. The *ST segment* reflects the time between the end of ventricular contraction and the beginning of ventricular recovery. The *T wave* represents

TABLE 48-1 The Cardiac Cycle

STAGE	HEART ACTIVITY	ELECTRIC CURRENT
P wave*	Atrial contraction	Atrial depolarization
PR segment†	Contraction traversing the atrioventricular node	Depolarization traversing the atrioventricular node
QRS complex‡	Ventricular contraction	Ventricular depolarization
ST segment	Time interval between ventricular contraction and the beginning of ventricular recovery	Time interval between ventricular depolarization and ventricular repolarization
T wave	Ventricular contraction subsides	Ventricular repolarization (electric recovery)
U wave (not always present)	Associated with further ventricular relaxation	Associated with further ventricular repolarization
Baseline§	The heart at rest	Polarization
PR interval‖	Time interval between atrial contraction and ventricular contraction	Time interval between atrial depolarization and ventricular depolarization
QT interval	Time interval between the beginning of ventricular contraction and the subsiding of ventricular contraction	Time interval between the beginning of ventricular depolarization and ventricular repolarization (electric recovery)

*Wave: A uniformly advancing deflection (upward or downward) from a baseline on a recording.
†Segment: A portion of an ECG recording between two consecutive waves. Represents the time needed for an electric current to move on.
‡Complex: The portion of the ECG tracing that represents the sum of three waves (contraction of the ventricles).
§Baseline: A neutral line against which waves are valued as they deflect upward (positive) or downward (negative) from the line.
‖Interval: The lapse of time between two different electrocardiographic events.

How Did We Get "PQRST"?

Mr. Einthoven was also responsible for naming the wave in the PQRST fashion. The letters ABCDE were already used to describe the unprocessed waves of electrical activity from the heart, so they could not be used. Moving on in the alphabet, N and O had other distinct usages in mathematics, so the next available letter that began an available sequence was P, which began the second half of the alphabet. Therefore he named the processed waves PQRST, and the term is used to this day.

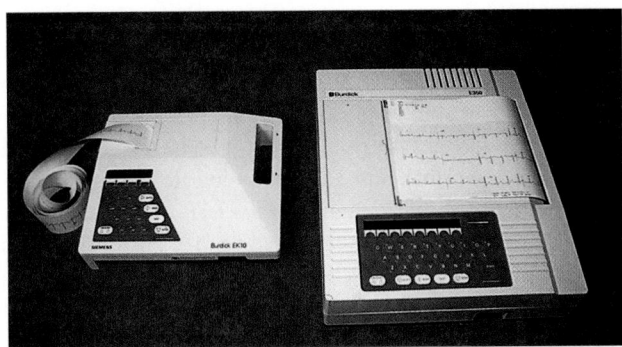

FIGURE 48-3 There is a wide variety of ECG machines, ranging from single to multichannel. (From Chester GA: *Modern medical assisting*, Philadelphia, 1999, Saunders.)

ventricular recovery or repolarization of the ventricles. After the T wave there is a time period of complete heart rest, also called *polarization,* which is indicated on the ECG as a straight line. The *QT interval* is the time between the beginning of the QRS complex through the T wave. During this time the ventricles contract and relax. A *U wave* can occasionally be seen as a small waveform just after the T wave in patients who have a low serum potassium level or other metabolic disorders.

By measuring the actual configuration and location of each wave in relation to the other waves and to the baseline as well as the intervals between waves and segments, the physician is able to detect rhythmic disturbances of the heart and to identify different types of cardiac disorders.

THE ELECTROCARDIOGRAPH

Most physicians are now using an electrocardiograph (Figure 48-3) that can record six leads simultaneously and are called *six-channel ECG machines.* Limb and chest leads must be placed on the patient at specific anatomic locations before the recording starts. When the ECG is started, the machine records all 12 leads

automatically and marks each lead with identifying letters. These multichannel ECG tracings take seconds to perform and can be placed into the patient's chart without mounting. Older electrocardiographs are single channel and record each of the 12 leads one at a time. These strips must then be cut apart, and each lead's recording is mounted onto the adhesive area of a mounting card before placement in the patient's chart.

CRITICAL THINKING APPLICATION

Martha has not been taught how to use the six-channel ECG machine in Dr. Lee's office. What steps should she take to learn how to use this machine and feel comfortable and confident using it to obtain ECGs?

Electrocardiograph Paper

Electrocardiograph paper is heat sensitive and pressure sensitive, which means either heat or pressure can cause a mark to appear. The stylus on an ECG machine makes the image on the ECG paper. When the machine is on, the stylus becomes hot and burns a marking on the paper as the paper moves horizontally past the stylus. Because the paper is pressure sensitive, it must be handled carefully to avoid making any additional markings that would blemish the tracing.

ECG paper is graph paper that has horizontal and vertical lines at 1-mm intervals. This is an agreed-on international standard that allows physicians anywhere in the world to interpret a patient's ECG in the same manner. A medical assistant needs to know both the size and the meaning of each square on ECG paper to understand its significance.

The horizontal axis of the paper represents time, and the vertical axis represents amplitude. Each small square measures 1 mm on each side. Every fifth line, both vertically and horizontally, is darker than the other lines and creates a larger square measuring 5 mm on each side. When the electrocardiograph runs at normal speed, one small 1-mm square passes the stylus every 0.04 second, which means that one large 5-mm square passes the stylus every 0.2 second. Continuing this logic, in 1 second, five large squares pass the stylus. When examining an ECG, five sequential large squares will show the record of what occurred with the heart during a time span of 1 second (5 large squares × 0.2 seconds = 1 second). Another way to say this is that at normal speed the ECG paper travels past the stylus at a rate of 25 mm per second (Figure 48-4).

The voltage or strength of the heartbeat is also recorded on the paper. Voltage can be displayed as either a positive or a negative deflection. One millivolt (mV) of electrical activity moves the stylus upward over 10 mm (two large squares). This is the standard normally used for obtaining an ECG and can be adjusted to match the strength of the electrical activity of the heart. The machine must be calibrated so that 1 mV of electrical activity will produce a deflection that is 10 mm either above or below the baseline. When properly calibrated the ECG records both the strength of the electrical activity of the heartbeat in mV and the speed of the heartbeat over time.

Electrodes and Leads

Ten sensors called *electrodes* are placed on the patient's arms (two), legs (two), and chest (six) to pick up the electrical activity of the heart. Electrodes must be applied to specific locations to record the heart's electrical activity from different angles and planes. Ten color-coded and labeled *lead wires* ending in a small metal clip are attached to the electrodes. The lead wires carry the signal of the heart's electrical activity to the ECG machine. Most offices use single-use, self-stick, disposable electrodes that are packaged with conductive jelly in the center. Some older ECG machines have only five leads, requiring the single chest lead to be moved to a different chest-wall location to obtain each one of the chest (V) recordings. Other older machines may have metal disks as electrodes that are attached by rubber bands to the extremities with metal suction cups that are placed on the chest. These types of electrodes require the application of conductive jelly to the patient's skin at the location of electrode placement to improve the transfer of the heart's electrical activity into the ECG machine.

The *leads* to the electrocardiograph carry the cardiac electrical impulses into the machine, where they are magnified by an amplifier. These amplified impulses are then converted into mechanical action that is recorded on the ECG paper by the stylus and/or shown on a monitor. A single lead records the electrical activity of the heart between two different electrodes, one positive and one negative. The placement of the positive electrode determines the particular view of the heart that is recorded. If depolarization occurs towards the positive electrode, the deflection is upright, and if it moves toward the negative electrode, the waveform is deflected downward. Each lead records the average electrical flow at a specific time in a specific location of the heart. The ECG records views of the heart on both a frontal and a transverse plane. The frontal leads include leads I, II, III, aV_R, aV_L, and aV_F. Horizontal plane leads include the six *precordial* or chest leads.

Lead Placement

The standard ECG consists of 12 separate leads, or recordings of the electrical activity of the heart, from different angles.

Standard Leads

The first three leads recorded are called the *standard* or *bipolar* leads because they each use two limb electrodes to record the heart's electrical activity (Figure 48-5, *A*). The right arm electrode

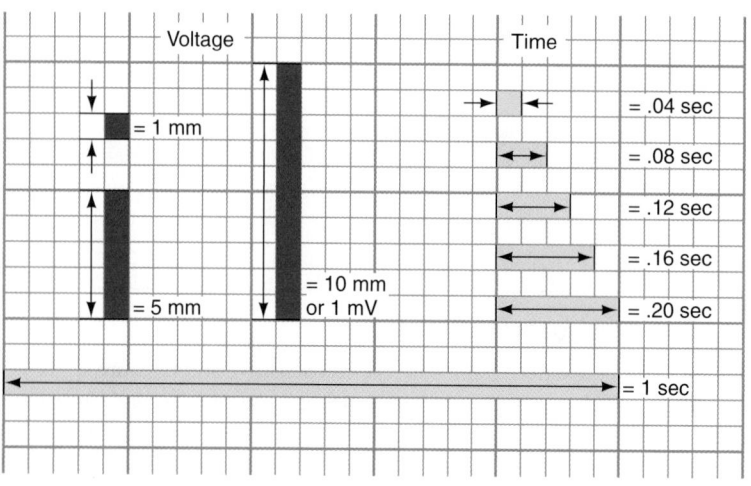

FIGURE 48-4 ECG paper. (From Chester GA: *Modern medical assisting*, Philadelphia, 1999, Saunders.)

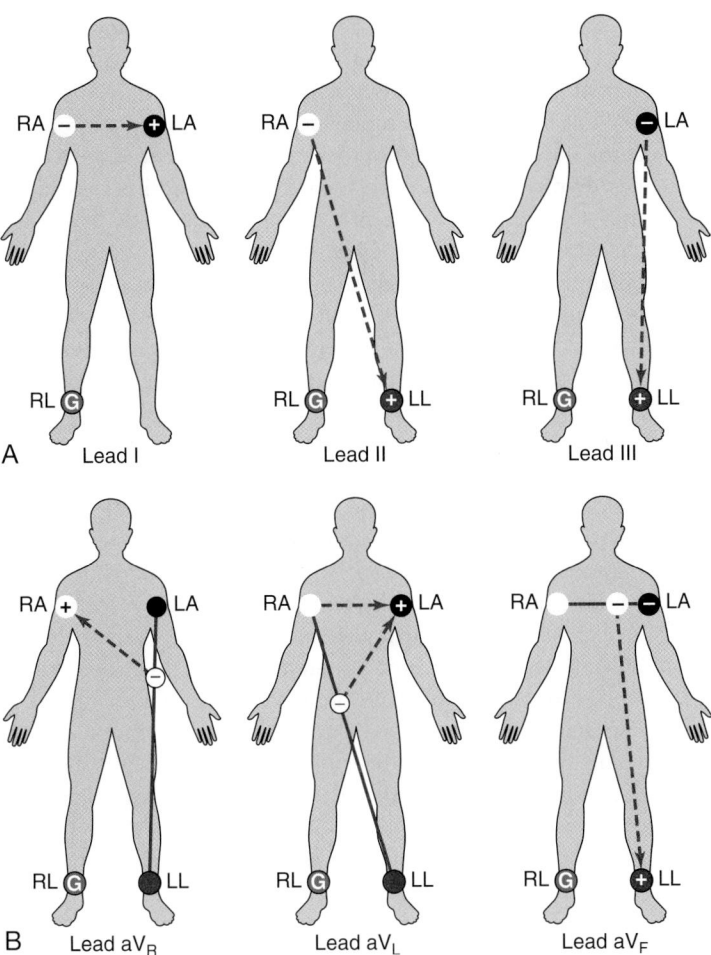

FIGURE 48-5 Standard **(A)** and augmented **(B)** limb leads. (From Chester GA: *Modern medical assisting*, Philadelphia, 1999, Saunders.)

is the negative pole, and the left leg or left arm electrodes are the positive poles. Roman numerals I, II, and III are used to designate these leads.

- Lead I records tracings between the right arm and left arm, recording the electrical activity of the lateral part of the left ventricle.
- Lead II records tracings between the right arm and left leg, recording the electrical activity of the inferior surface of the left ventricle; this is the lead recorded on a cardiac monitor or on the rhythm strip at the bottom of the 12-lead ECG.
- Lead III records tracings between the left arm and left leg and records the electrical activity of the inferior surface of the left ventricle.

Augmented Leads

The next three leads are the augmented or combined leads (Figure 48-5, *B*). These are designated augmented voltage right arm (aV$_R$), augmented voltage left arm (aV$_L$), and augmented voltage left leg (aV$_F$). The electrical activity recorded by these leads is relatively small, and therefore the ECG machine amplifies (or augments) the electrical potential when recorded. These are all unipolar leads with a single positive electrode that uses the right leg for grounding.

- aV$_R$ records the electrical activity of the atria from the

right shoulder; P waves and QRS complexes are deflected below the baseline.
- aV$_L$ records the electrical activity of the lateral wall of the left ventricle from the left shoulder.
- aV$_F$ records the electrical activity of the inferior surface of the left ventricle from the left leg.

Precordial Leads

The *precordial* or chest leads are unipolar and provide a transverse plane view of the heart. They are designated V$_1$, V$_2$, V$_3$, V$_4$, V$_5$, and V$_6$. The V means chest, and each of the numbers represents a specific location on the chest. The QRS complex shows as a negative deflection in V$_1$ and V$_2$, views with each subsequent lead becoming more positive. Precordial leads measure the electrical activity among six specific points on the chest wall and a point within the heart (Figure 48-6). It is important to avoid electrode placement directly over a bony prominence.

- V$_1$–the electrode is placed in the fourth intercostal space, just to the right of the sternum
- V$_2$–the electrode is placed in the fourth intercostal space, just to the left of the sternum
- V$_3$–the electrode is placed midway between V$_2$ and V$_4$
- V$_4$–the electrode is placed in the fifth intercostal space, at the left midclavicular line

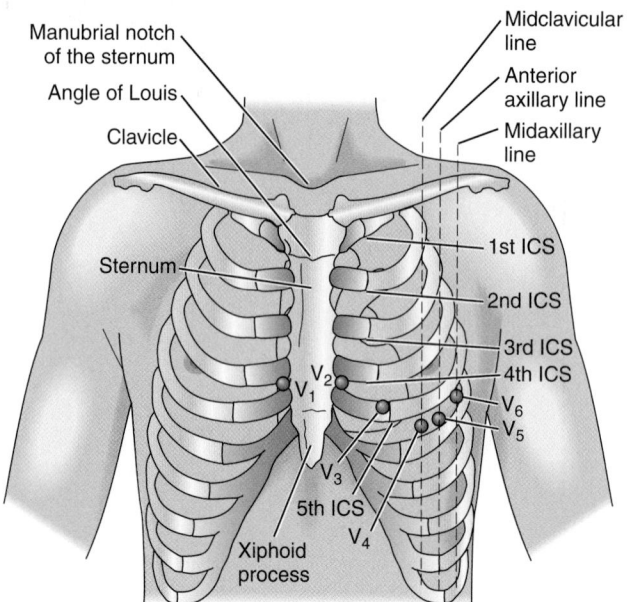

FIGURE 48-6 Chest leads. (From Chester GA: *Modern medical assisting*, Philadelphia, 1999, Saunders.)

- V_5–the electrode is placed horizontal to V_4 in the left anterior axillary line
- V_6–the electrode is placed horizontal to V_4 in the left midaxillary line.

CRITICAL THINKING APPLICATION

Dr. Lee has asked Martha to perform her first ECG on a patient who just came into the office. Martha is not confident that she knows how to properly place the chest leads in the correct location. How should she handle this situation? Should she perform the ECG procedure "the best that she can"? Why or why not?

PERFORMING ELECTROCARDIOGRAPHY

Preparation of the Room and Patient

The room should be in the quietest location in the office and should be as far away as possible from all other electrical equipment, including x-ray machines, diathermy devices, laboratory equipment, centrifuges, fans, refrigerators, and air conditioners. The room should be warm and have adjustable lighting.

The treatment table should be comfortable and wide enough to provide full support for the patient. The table should be wood or have an electrically insulated surface. Position the table so you can work from the side of the patient that is most comfortable for you. Electrocardiographers most often work on the patient's left side, but as long as the electrodes are placed in the proper position, it really makes no difference which side you work from.

Small pillows are helpful for relaxing the patient and providing maximum comfort during the procedure. Offer a pillow for the head and one for under the knees. If a head pillow is used, it should not elevate the patient's shoulders.

The patient should disrobe to the waist and be gowned with the opening down the front; there must be easy access to the patient's extremities. Pantyhose must be removed.

Place the patient in a supine position, with arms comfortably at the sides and the legs not touching one another. If the patient has dyspnea or orthopnea, semi-Fowler's position should be used, or alternatively the patient can be seated on a wooden chair. However, make sure you check with the physician before obtaining an ECG in an alternative position. If a seated position is being used, the patient's feet must rest comfortably on the floor or on a footstool. The legs should not be dangling, nor should there be any pressure on the back of the lower thighs. Note any alternative position on the ECG recording.

The patient should empty the bladder, then rest for at least 10 minutes before the ECG recording is made. Check to see if the patient followed all of the instructions in Figure 48-7. Record the patient's vital signs and current medications on the patient's chart. This information can be programmed into some ECG machines and automatically printed on the ECG recording.

Explain to the patient the nature and the purpose of the ECG. Attempt to answer all questions and make the patient as comfortable as possible during the procedure. Stress the importance of not moving during the entire procedure, and assure the patient that there is no danger of being shocked. Soften the lighting in the room to obtain maximal patient comfort. When you tell the patient to lie still, observe that he or she is breathing normally. Patients often hold their breath when asked to lie still.

Applying Leads to the Patient

Disposable, single-use electrodes are placed on the patient's limbs and chest in very specific locations (Figure 48-8). The lead wires from the machine are then connected to the electrodes. Making the proper connections is facilitated by specific lead markings or color-coding on the end of each lead wire (Figure 48-9).

- RA lead is attached to the electrode on the patient's right arm.
- LA lead is attached to the electrode on the patient's left arm.
- RL lead is attached to the electrode on the patient's right leg.
- LL lead is attached to the electrode on the patient's left leg.
- The labeled lead wires are then placed on each precordial electrode.

CRITICAL THINKING APPLICATION

Two weeks later, after Martha feels much more confident in her skills at electrode placement and in taking an ECG, a new patient, Mr. Sonderford, comes to the office complaining of mild chest pain that he noted when he got out of bed this morning. What concerns might Martha have about Mr. Sonderford? His vital signs are P: 104 beats/min, weak and irregular; R: 24 breaths/min and quite shallow. Mr. Sonderford is sweating quite profusely. What should Martha do? Why?

INSTRUCTIONS FOR PATIENT BEFORE AN ELECTROCARDIOGRAM

Name: _____

Your cardiogram appointment is _____ , _____ at _____ AM / PM
                                          Day   Date   Time

These instructions are simple, but it is important that you follow them. Please call us if you are unable to follow these instructions or keep your appointment so we may make another appointment.

1. There is no discomfort or sensation in having an electrocardiogram. No electricity is put into the patient in any way. Small disposable electrodes are placed on the calf of each leg and on each arm and at different places on the chest. The minute impulse generated by your heart is simply picked up by these electrodes and recorded by the machine.

2. You will be asked to lie down on a comfortable table while the test is being performed by the technician.

3. For your convenience, it is best to wear loose clothing. You will be asked to disrobe to your waist to expose the chest. It will also be necessary to expose your lower legs from the knees down and the upper arms just below the shoulders.

4. The actual test only takes about 5 minutes, but you will be asked to rest for about one-half hour before the test. It is best you do not have a heavy meal for about 2 hours before the test. You should not consume any cold drinks or ice cream or smoke just before the test. It is also advisable to refrain from excessive exercise just before the test. Do not take any medications without the physician's usual instructions and knowledge.

5. During the test, you will be asked to lie absolutely still and relax, because the slightest movement interferes with an accurate tracing. Do not talk.

6. The skin on the legs, arms, and chest must be free from skin ointments, oils, and medications.

7. The technician taking the test is specially trained to perform the test but is unable to tell you the results of the test, because he or she is neither trained nor authorized to make any interpretations of the cardiogram. This is the task of the physician.

FIGURE 48-7 ECG patient instructions.

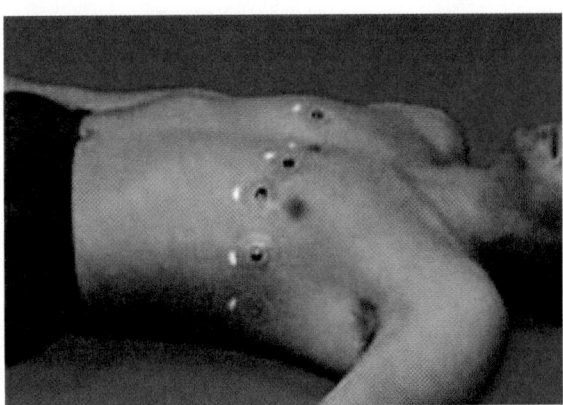

FIGURE 48-8 Chest lead locations. (From Aehlert B: *ECGs made easy*, ed 3, St Louis, 2006, Mosby.)

Recording the Electrocardiogram

Procedure 48-1 explains how to record an ECG. It is important that you are familiar with the type of machine used in your practice. Machines vary according to the age and make of the model but the majority of electrocardiographs being used today perform standardization functions and labeling automatically. You may have the option to enter specific information about the patient such as patient age, sex, prescriptions, and so on. Follow office protocol when performing the procedure. After the machine is programmed, remind the patient to lie still, and press the appropriate key to run the ECG strip. Six-channel machines will print and label all 12 leads with a rhythm strip across the bottom of the paper in lead II in a matter of seconds. Review the printout for clarity, and, if acceptable, give the recording to the physician for review. Once approved, remove the leads and electrodes from the patient, assist him or her into a sitting position, and provide assistance in getting off the table and dressing if necessary.

Standardization, Sensitivity, and Speed

Standardization has been determined by international agreement so that an ECG can be interpreted in the same way anywhere in the world. This requires the electrocardiograph to be calibrated according to universal measurements. Each time you take a patient's ECG, you must make certain that the machine is correctly standardized.

When a machine is in standard or set at 1 STD, 1 mV of electricity causes the stylus to move vertically 10 mm, or two large squares. When the machine is properly set in this way, it is possible to calculate electrical voltages by measuring the vertical movement of the stylus on the paper. The stylus should deflect exactly 10 mm when the standardization button is depressed with a quick pecking motion. The recording of the standardization would be 2 mm wide and rectangular. Each manufacturer's manual explains the exact method of adjustment to obtain a perfect standardization.

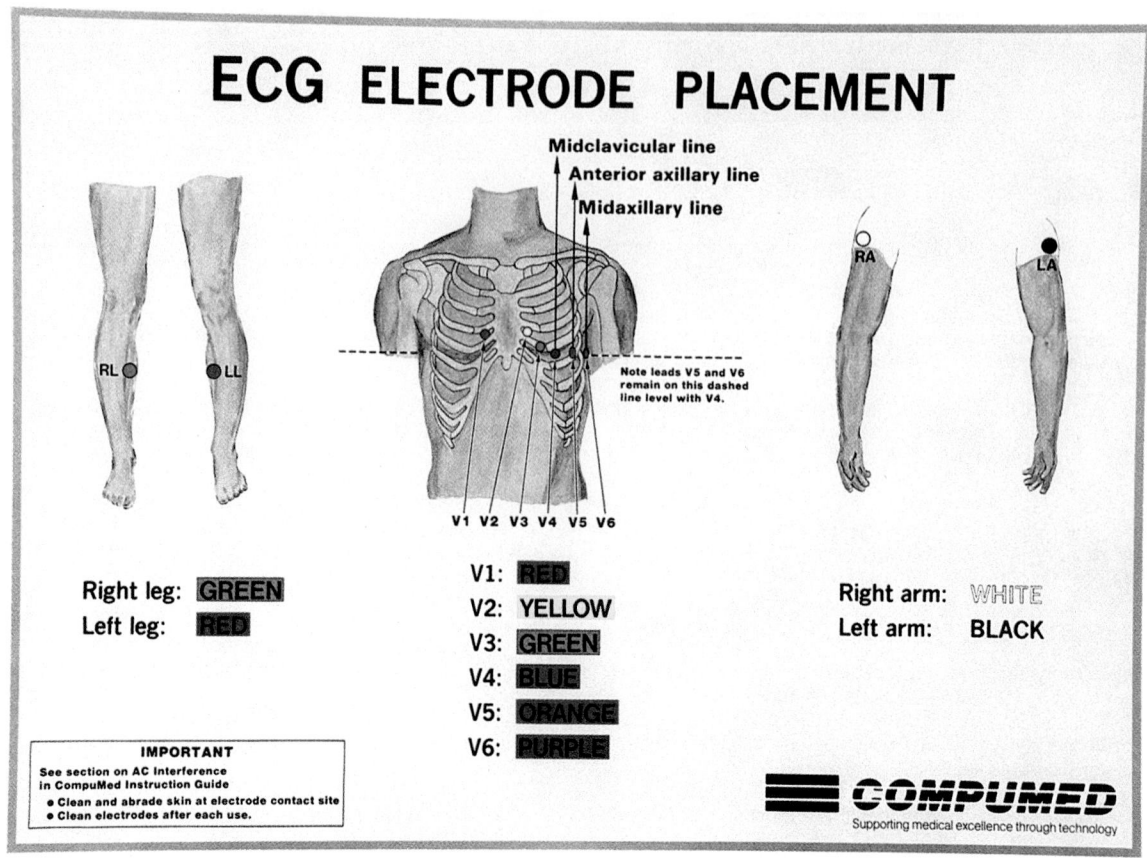

FIGURE 48-9 Color codes. (Courtesy CompuMed, San Diego, Calif.)

At a minimum, standardization must be performed before recording the first lead. Some physicians require a separate standardization in each one of the individual 12 leads.

Most machines have three sensitivity standards that can be selected: $^1/_2$ STD, which deflects the stylus 5 mm or one large square; 1 STD, which deflects the stylus 10 mm or two large squares; and 2 STD, which deflects the stylus 20 mm or four squares. The appropriate standard is selected in the following manner. If the QRS complex is too tall and is causing the stylus to move off the paper, the STD should be set to $^1/_2$ STD. If the QRS complex is too short, the STD should be set to 2 STD. Figure 48-10 shows what the three sensitivity standards look like when recorded on the ECG paper.

The usual speed for an ECG recording is 25 mm/sec. If the patient's heart rate is very rapid or if certain parts of the complex are too close together, it may be necessary to adjust the paper to run at double speed, or 50 mm/sec. This will extend the recording to twice the normal length. Any change in the speed must be noted on the ECG.

Mounting an Electrocardiographic Tracing

Newer ECG machines do not require that the recording be mounted. However, if working with an older machine, your office will select the mount that is best suited to the type of ECG equipment used in that particular office. It is advisable to select a mount that allows reading of all 12 leads together on one page. The most commonly used mounts are self-adhesive

mounting pages that are designed so that an entire test is placed on one side of one page (Figure 48-11). Tracings are usually retained in records for many years, so a mount must last for a long time.

Paper clips and staples are never used, because they will scratch and mark a tracing. Clear tape should not be used, because it can become sticky or yellow with age. A single photocopy of the ECG can be made without damaging the original. Many offices routinely put a photocopy in the patient's chart because it is thinner than the mounted ECG and less likely to be damaged by handling.

Regardless of the particular method used, each ECG should be carefully and neatly mounted, with complete information recorded on each one. This must include the following:
- Patient's full name
- Sex
- Age
- Date and time of ECG
- List of all medications and/or supplements the patient takes
- Variations from normal sensitivity and normal speed

Additional notations should be recorded for any variation from the routine, such as the following:
- A very nervous or anxious patient
- Lack of rest before the test
- Smoking immediately before the test
- Failure to follow any pretest instructions

PROCEDURE 48-1

Perform Electrocardiography: Obtain a 12-Lead ECG

<u>CAAHEP COMPETENCIES:</u> 3.b.(3)(a), 3.b.(4)(e)
<u>ABHES COMPETENCIES:</u> 4.b, 4.h

GOAL: *To obtain an accurate, artifact-free recording of the electrical activity of the heart.*

EQUIPMENT and SUPPLIES

- ECG machine with patient lead cable
- 10 disposable, self-adhesive electrodes
- Patient gown and drape
- ECG mounting card if necessary
- Patient record

PROCEDURAL STEPS

1. Wash your hands.
   <u>PURPOSE:</u> Infection control.
2. Explain the procedure to the patient.
   <u>PURPOSE:</u> To alleviate apprehension and gain patient cooperation.
3. Ask the patient to disrobe to the waist (including the female patient's bra), and remove socks, stockings, or pantyhose as necessary.
   <u>PURPOSE:</u> Electrodes must be applied to bare skin and without interference from clothing.
4. Position the patient prone on the examination table, and drape appropriately.
   <u>PURPOSE:</u> To ensure the modesty and comfort of the patient.
5. Turn on the machine to allow the stylus to warm up (may not be necessary in newer machines).
   <u>PURPOSE:</u> To ensure proper machine performance.
6. Label the beginning of the tracing paper with the patient's name, date, time, and current cardiovascular medications, or input this information into the machine.
   <u>PURPOSE:</u> To properly identify the ECG recording.

7. At each location you are going to place an electrode, clean the skin with an alcohol wipe (Figure 1).
   <u>PURPOSE:</u> To obtain good electrode adhesion to the skin.
8. Apply the self-adhesive electrodes to clean, dry, fleshy areas of the extremities (Figure 2). It may be necessary to shave extremely hairy areas to achieve adequate electrode attachment or to place a piece of tape over the electrode to make sure it is secure.
9. Apply the self-adhesive electrodes to clean areas on the chest (Figure 3).
10. Carefully connect the lead wires to the correct electrode with the alligator clips on the end of each lead. Make sure the lead wires are not crossed.
    <u>PURPOSE:</u> To prevent artifacts.
11. Press the AUTO button on the machine, and run the ECG tracing. The machine will automatically place the standardization at the beginning, then the 12 leads will follow in the three-channel matrix with a lead II rhythm strip across the bottom of the page.
12. Watch for artifacts during the recording. If artifacts are present, make appropriate corrections, and repeat the recording to get a clean reading.
13. Remove the lead wires from the electrodes, then remove the electrodes from the patient.
14. Assist the patient with getting dressed as needed. Clean and return the ECG machine to its storage area.
15. Mount the ECG, or give the unmounted ECG recording to the physician as directed.
16. Wash your hands.

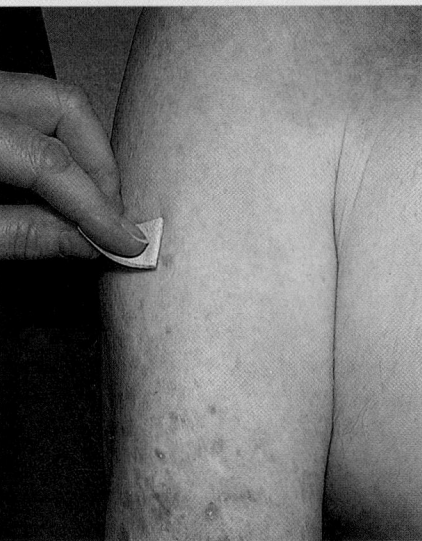

FIGURE 1

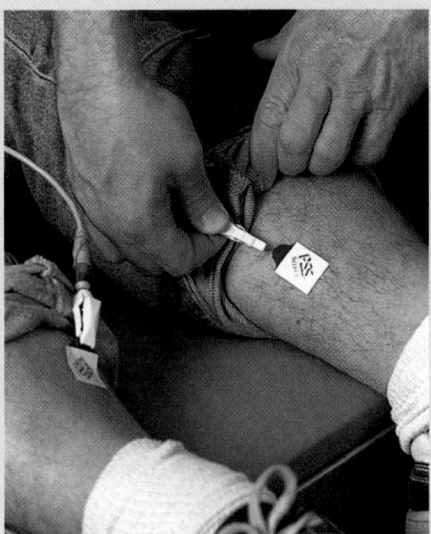

FIGURE 2

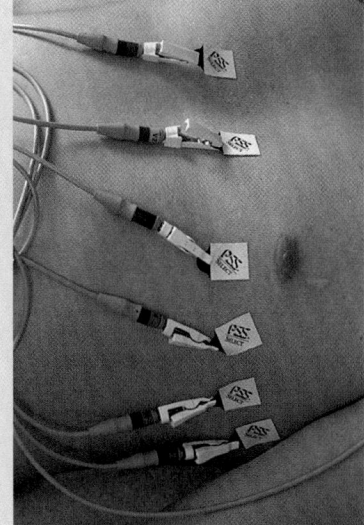

FIGURE 3

Continued

PROCEDURE 48-1—*cont'd*

17. Document the procedure in the patient's chart.
<u>PURPOSE:</u> Procedures are not considered done until they are documented in the patient's medical record.

See Appendix D for a charting example.

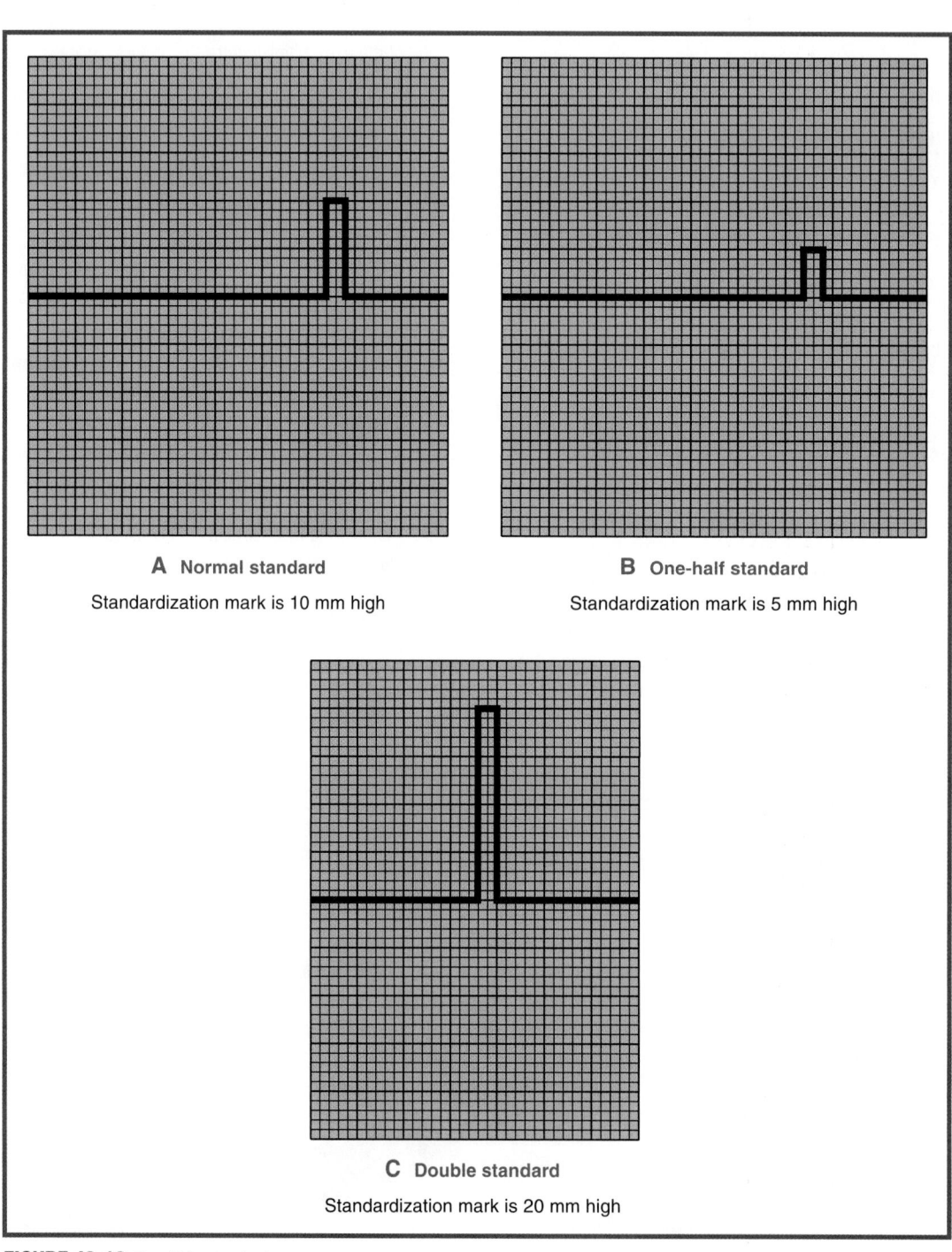

A Normal standard

Standardization mark is 10 mm high

B One-half standard

Standardization mark is 5 mm high

C Double standard

Standardization mark is 20 mm high

FIGURE 48-10 Sensitivity standards.

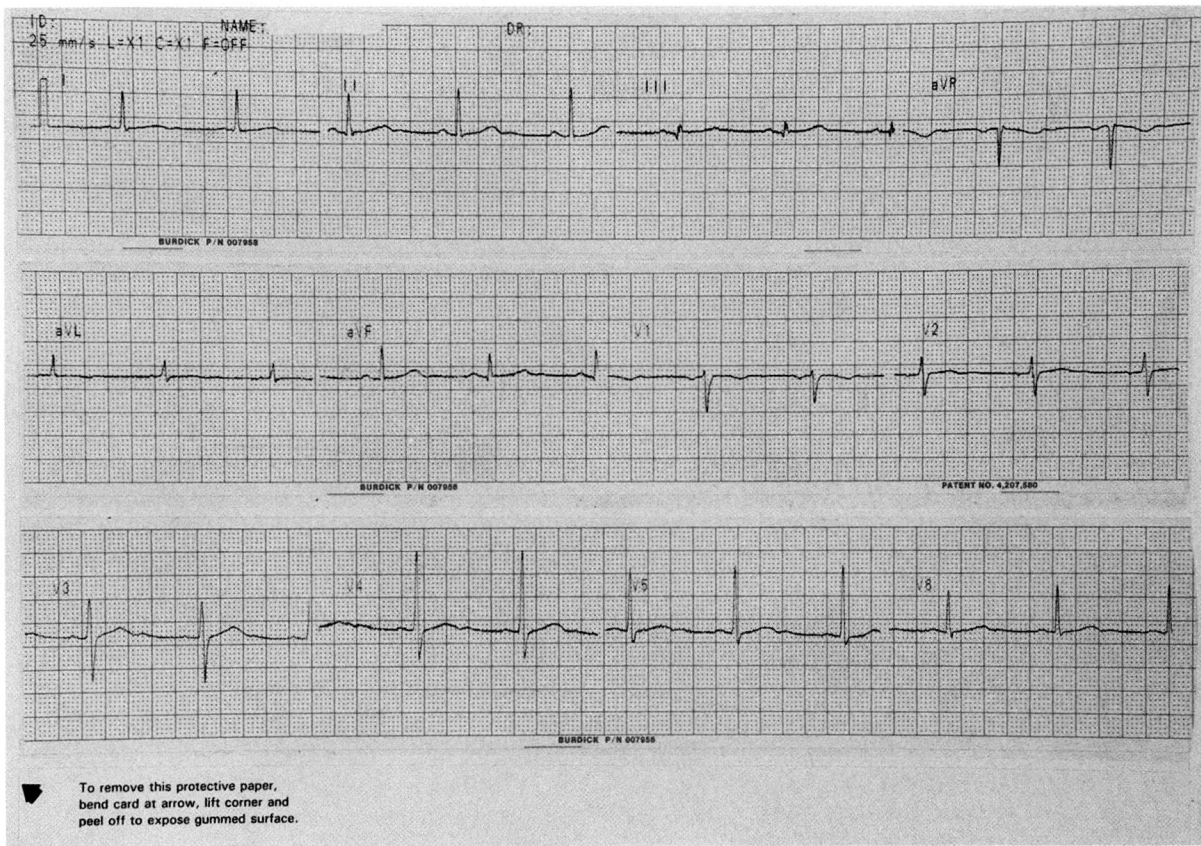

FIGURE 48-11 ECG mount. (Courtesy Burdick Corporation, Melton, Wisc.)

Care must be taken when mounting an ECG. Most tracings are easily scratched or marked, so be careful not to accidentally damage the tracing with watches, rings, fingernails, or clothing buttons. Do not stack other items on top of the open-faced type of mount.

Note: If trimming the strip is required for mounting, do not cut off the label that identifies the lead recording. Some mounts place the precordial leads in horizontal rows, whereas others place them in vertical columns. Take great care not to mount a lead upside down. If you have been requested to show the STD in a lead, be sure to include it where requested. Do not cover the tips of the QRS complexes with the sides of the slotted-type mount. Place the mounted ECG tracing on the physician's desk for evaluation with the patient's medical record and any previous ECG tracings. Physicians nearly always wish to compare the newest ECG with previous ECGs.

Some physicians will wish to see the entire strip before it is mounted and may even choose which sections to mount. If this is the case, be careful to mount the sections indicated by the physician.

Telephone Transmission

An electrocardiograph with phone transmission capabilities can transmit a recording over a telephone to an ECG data interpretation center. The machine is equipped with a direct ECG fax transmitter. The recording is interpreted by a computer at the data center and verified by a cardiologist. Patient information that may be important to the interpretation such as medications and vital signs is also sent with the ECG data. A printout with the computer-assisted interpretations is returned to the sender by fax or email.

Interpretive Electrocardiographs

Interpretive electrocardiographs are equipped with a computer that analyzes the recording as it is being run. With this capability, immediate information on the heart's activity is available, which can be valuable for reaching an early diagnosis and initiating immediate treatment. Patient baseline data must be entered into the computer before the ECG is recorded. The computer analysis of the ECG and the reason for each interpretation are then printed on the top of the recording.

Artifacts

An artifact is unwanted, erratic movement of the stylus on the paper resulting from outside interference. The electrocardiograph is extremely sensitive to any kind of nearby electrical activity. Electrical artifacts on the tracing make it difficult to accurately interpret the ECG. The medical assistant should have a thorough understanding of the causes of and remedies for these artifacts. The main types of artifacts include wandering baseline, somatic tremor, alternating current (AC), and interrupted baseline.

Wandering Baseline

With the wandering baseline the stylus gradually shifts away from the center of the paper. This usually results from slight movement of the patient during the tracing or poor electrode attachment (Figure 48-12). A wandering baseline is resolved by reminding the patient to remain as still as possible and can be facilitated by maintaining patient comfort. Metal electrodes can be a major cause of this phenomenon; using disposable, stick-on electrodes should eliminate this cause.

Somatic Tremor

Somatic tremor means muscle movement. Any muscle movement, including movement of skeletal muscle, produces a measurable electrical impulse. This additional input causes unwanted stylus movement during the tracing that shows up on the recording as jagged peaks of irregular height and spacing with a shifting baseline (Figure 48-13). The most common causes include patient discomfort, apprehension, movement, talking, or having a condition that causes uncontrollable body tremors. The patient with uncontrolled tremors needs to be as calm and comfortable as possible to minimize the somatic tremor artifact. The other causes can all be resolved after they have been correctly identified.

Alternating Current (AC) Interference

AC interference appears as a series of uniform small spikes on the paper (Figure 48-14). Electrical currents that are present in nearby equipment or wiring can leak small amounts of electrical energy into the area in which the ECG is located. The very sensitive electrocardiograph can easily pick up this additional electrical energy signal. This can be minimized by making certain the ECG is plugged into a three-pronged, grounded outlet; keeping lead wires uncrossed; unplugging other electrical appliances in the room; moving the table away from the wall;

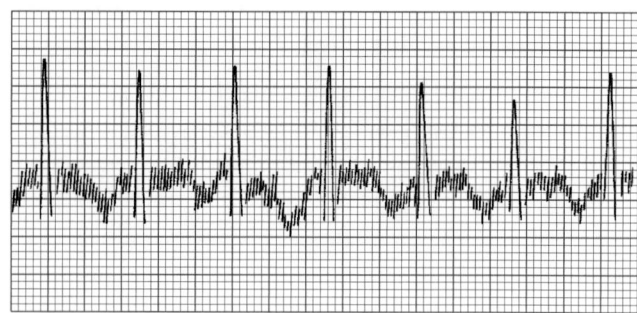

FIGURE 48-14 Sixty-cycle interference. (From Aehlert B: *ECGs made easy*, ed 3, St Louis, 2006, Mosby.)

and perhaps even turning off overhead fluorescent lights. If all of these measures fail, you may need to move to another examination room for the procedure. The last step is to call the manufacturer or your local service representative.

Interrupted Baseline

Baseline interruption occurs when the electric connection has been interrupted. The stylus moves onto the margin of the paper erratically (Figure 48-15). The stylus moves violently up and down across the paper, or it may record a straight line across the top or the bottom of the paper. Noticeable patient movement that dislodges the electrodes causes most baseline interruption. This cause is virtually eliminated by using disposable, stick-on electrodes. Other causes include a broken wire in the patient cable and cable tips that are attached too loosely to the electrodes.

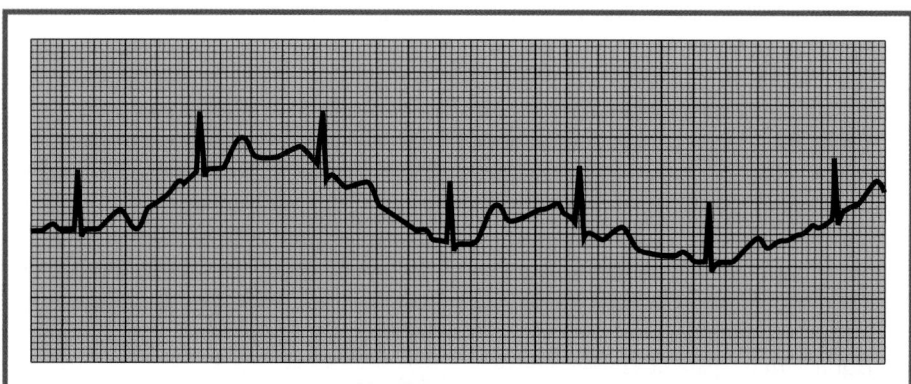

FIGURE 48-12 Wandering baseline.

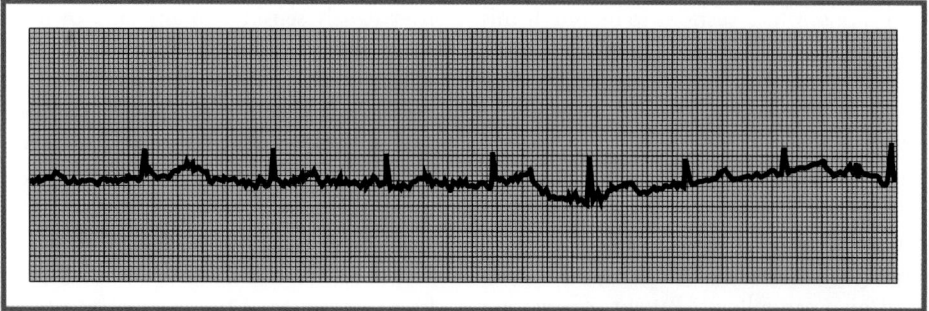

FIGURE 48-13 Somatic tremor.

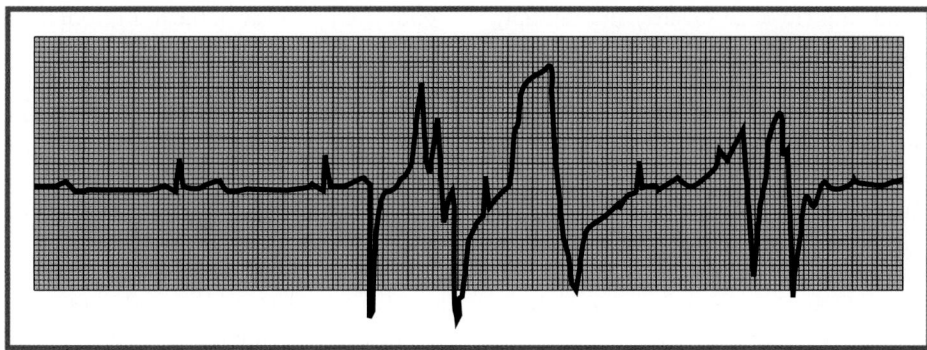

FIGURE 48-15 Interrupted baseline.

TABLE 48-2 Normal Appearances of ECG Waveforms and Complexes

WAVE OR COMPLEX	DURATION (IN SECONDS OR AMPLITUDE)	CHARACTERISTICS TO EXAMINE
P wave	0.06-0.11	Are P waves present? Normal shape (not notched or peaked)? Normal size (<3 mm)? Do all deflect upward (positive)? Is there one for each QRS? Evenly spaced from QRS?
PR interval	0.12-0.20	Is it constant?
QRS complex	0.08-0.12	Evenly spaced from T waves? Do all point in same direction? Do all QRS complexes appear the same?
ST segment	On baseline (isoelectric line)	Is it on baseline? Is it constant?
T Wave	5 mm or less in leads I, II, III 10 mm or less in V_1-V_6	Is T wave present? Are all the same? Do all show upward deflection (positive)?
QT interval	Should not be more than half the RR interval if patient has regular rhythm	Is it constant?
U Wave	Rounded, upright deflection	Is it present?

CRITICAL THINKING APPLICATION

Dr. Lee asks Martha to explain to her the causes of artifacts and the methods for correcting ECG recordings that show outside interference. Based on what you have learned about ECG artifacts, what are the typical causes, and how would you recommend correcting each?

INTERPRETING AN ECG STRIP

The medical assistant working in the cardiovascular practice needs to be able to recognize rhythm abnormalities that may appear on the tracing. Alerting the physician to the presence of an arrhythmia while the patient is still connected to the machine may give the physician the opportunity to observe the patient while the machine is running or immediately institute some type of therapeutic or prophylactic intervention.

The physician can determine two important heart functions when interpreting the ECG: heart rate and heart rhythm.

Normal Appearances of ECG Complexes

When examining the ECG recording, first look at the characteristics of each of the waves in the recording (Table 48-2). Are the P waves, QRS complexes, and T waves clearly present? Do they have a consistent appearance and do they occur at regular intervals? Are any odd beats present that do not fit in with the others? Is the rate normal, fast, or slow? Is the rhythm regular or irregular?

In NSR (see Figure 48-1), each beat of the heart is initiated with an impulse from the SA node that then travels, without interruption, along the normal conduction pathway of the heart. In NSR each beat on the ECG shows a P wave followed by a QRS complex.

Rate

To calculate the heart rate from the ECG recording, count the number of P waves in a 6-second strip (30 large squares) and multiply by 10. In the same manner, you can count the number of P waves in a 3-second strip (15 large squares) and multiply by 20. To get the ventricular contraction rate, you can count the number of complete QRS complexes that occur within 6 seconds and multiply that number by 10 to get the number of ventricular contractions in 1 minute.

Heart rate can also be calculated by counting the number of small squares between two R waves. Then divide that number into 1500; 1 minute on an ECG strip passes 1500 small boxes. When the number of boxes from one cardiac event to the next same event is divided into 1500 the result is the patient's heart rate. You can practice these by using the ECGs in Figures 48-1 and 48-11.

Rhythm

The rhythm of the patient's heartbeat indicates whether it is regular or not. You may pick up an irregular heartbeat when taking the patient's pulse. This same patient will show an irregularity—a difference in the length of time between cardiac cycles—when an ECG is recorded. If the patient's heart is beating in a regular rhythm, each cardiac cycle occurs within the same time frame, and individual cardiac cycles occur exactly the same length of time apart. To check for ventricular rhythm you can measure the distance between two consecutive RR intervals. Atrial rhythm is determined by measuring the distance between two consecutive PP intervals. If the heart rhythm is regular, each of these interval measurements will be the same.

TYPICAL ECG RHYTHM ABNORMALITIES

Abnormalities in cardiac rhythm are termed *arrhythmias*. These can result from disturbances anywhere along the electrical

---

Calculating a Patient's Heart Rate

To calculate the patient's heart rate from an ECG strip, remember the following:
- 5 large boxes on the graph paper = 1 second
- 15 large boxes = 3 seconds
- 30 large boxes = 6 seconds

Method for Analyzing an ECG Strip

The ECG rhythm strip (lead II view) is evaluated from left to right. Each strip should be assessed for the following:
- Rate
- Rhythm
- P waves—one P wave before each QRS complex; each is a positive deflection and similar in size and shape
- Intervals—for duration and distance
- Appearance of the segments and wave forms—Are there rhythmic PQRST cycles? Do you notice any abnormalities such as more than one P wave, QRS segments without a previous P wave, or an elevated ST segment? All of these abnormalities should be brought to the physician's attention immediately

---

conduction pathway in the heart from the SA node through the right and left bundle branches. The best way to determine if an arrhythmia is present is to know what the NSR looks like on an ECG. Study the NSRs present in the mounted ECGs in Figures 48-1 and 48-11. NSR is a heart rate between 60 and 100 beats/min. Any deviations from this should be recognized during the ECG recording, and the medical assistant should immediately notify the physician.

Cardiac arrhythmias commonly fall into one of the following broad categories: sinus arrhythmias, atrial arrhythmias, ventricular arrhythmias, and biochemical arrhythmias. The characteristics of several arrhythmias in each of these categories are compared in Table 48-3.

Sinus Arrhythmias

Sinus rhythm is considered normal—the heart's electrical activity begins in the SA node and follows through the electrical system, ending in atrial and ventricular depolarization. In sinus arrhythmias the pathway of the electrical charge is normal but the rate or rhythm of the heartbeat is altered. Sinus arrhythmias may be caused by the SA node firing too slowly or too quickly. In sinus bradycardia the heart rate is less than 60 beats/min. This can be a normal heart rate in well-conditioned athletes but is abnormal in other individuals. In sinus tachycardia the heart rate is more than 100 beats/min. This can be a normal heart rate in a person who is doing aerobic exercise but can be abnormal in the resting individual (Figure 48-16).

Atrial Arrhythmias

Problems with the electrical discharge of the atria are caused by faulty electrical impulse formation or conduction defects within the atria. *Premature atrial contraction* (PAC) occurs when the atria contract before they should for the next cardiac cycle. This can appear on the ECG as an abnormally shaped P wave or an extra P wave. PACs can be seen in smokers and people who consume large amounts of caffeine. Occasional PACs are not abnormal but are of medical concern if they regularly occur more than six times per minute. In this situation, the PACs can indicate developing cardiac abnormalities.

Atrial flutter occurs when the atria beat at an extremely rapid rate that can be up to 300 beats/min. In atrial flutter the impulses come from many **ectopic** atrial locations but are blocked at the AV node, which prevents ventricular fibrillation. Atrial flutter is reversed with medication to slow the heart or with **cardioversion** (electrical shock).

Ventricular Arrhythmias

Premature ventricular contractions (PVCs) occur when the ventricles contract before they should for the next cardiac cycle—in other words, a QRS complex appears before a P wave. They occur when there is an electrical charge originating in either ventricle. This can appear on the ECG as an absent P wave, an abnormally shaped T wave, and a widened QRS complex. This is followed by a pause before the initiation of the next cardiac cycle. PVCs can result from use of tobacco, alcohol, medications containing

TABLE 48-3 Characteristics of Arrhythmias

NAME	SIGNS AND SYMPTOMS	CAUSE	ECG CHANGES
Sinus Arrhythmias			
Bradycardia	<60 beats/min	Vagal nerve stimulation; sleep; SA node ischemia; digitalis toxicity; drugs Can be normal in athletes	Essentially "normal" appearing, but slow
Tachycardia	Nonpathologic; heart rate >100 beats/min pathologic	Increased demand for cardiac output; ectopic pacemaker	P wave can be obscured by the ST segment (increasing the ECG speed can reduce this problem)
Atrial Arrhythmias			
PAC	Not pathologic if only several per minute	Increased SA node excitability, causing premature beats of atria Can be caused by nicotine or caffeine	"Extra" P waves
Flutter	200-350 beats/min	Many ectopic atrial pacemakers, normally unstable and will progress to atrial fibrillation if not corrected	Multiple, sawtooth-appearing P waves before essentially normal-appearing QRS complexes
Ventricular Arrhythmias (see Figure 48-20)			
PVC	Generally none	Ectopic pacemakers originating in ventricles from electrolyte imbalance, hypoxia, acute MI	Widened QRS complex
V-tach	Heart rate >100 beats/min, always pathologic	Damaged tissue around one of the "bundles" causing a difference in conduction speed between the two branches or ectopic pacemaker cells	Rapid rate, irregular pattern that includes "extra" or erratic, irregular, or wide QRS complexes
V-fib*	Shock, unconsciousness, no pulse	Complete loss of synchronization of conduction system	Erratic deflections on the ECG (can be either coarse or fine) No identifiable ECG waves present
Asystole	<5 beats/min	Death imminent	Flatline
Biochemical Arrhythmias			
Digitalis toxicity	Abnormal bradycardia, abnormal tachycardia	Digitalis dose is too high	"Swooping" ST segment depression and/or extended PR intervals
Hypokalemia	Malaise, fatigue, weakness, muscle cramps	Potassium too low, usually from unsupplemented diuresis, from IV fluid administration, or from excessive vomiting	Prominent U waves, T wave and U wave together look like a two-humped camel
Hyperkalemia†	May have none	Potassium too high, usually from IV supplementation	Peaked T wave (can be as tall as R wave) with widening of all wave forms

IV, Intravenous; *MI*, myocardial infarction; *PAC*, premature atrial contraction; *PVC*, premature ventricular contraction; *SA*, sinoatrial.
*Most life-threatening arrhythmia; frequently precedes asystole if not reversed.
†Life-threatening situation that must be corrected immediately.

epinephrine, and occasionally from anxiety. Infrequent PVCs are not abnormal but are of medical concern if they regularly occur more than six times per minute. Pathologic PVCs occur in patients with hypertension, coronary artery disease, and lung disease.

Ventricular tachycardia (commonly referred to as *V-tach*) is diagnosed when the ventricles beat at extremely rapid rates. It may be seen when multiple PVCs occur in a row, as a short run of fast beats, or persist longer than 30 seconds. The patient's heart rate may range from 101 to 250 beats/min. V-tach can precede ventricular fibrillation if not reversed with drugs and/or cardioversion. V-tach always reflects a pathologic state.

Ventricular fibrillation (commonly referred to as *V-fib*) is the most critical, life-threatening arrhythmia and will result in death quickly if not effectively treated. It is estimated that V-fib precedes 85% of cases of **cardiac arrest** in adults. In V-fib the electrical conduction system of the heart is in total dysfunction. The heart muscle is quivering uncontrollably and is essentially ineffective in pumping any blood; therefore there is no pulse, and the patient is unresponsive and not breathing. Cardioversion with a **defibrillator** is necessary to restore normal electrical conduction system function.

Asystole is the result of no heartbeat or cardiac cessation and results in a flatline on the ECG (Figure 48-17).

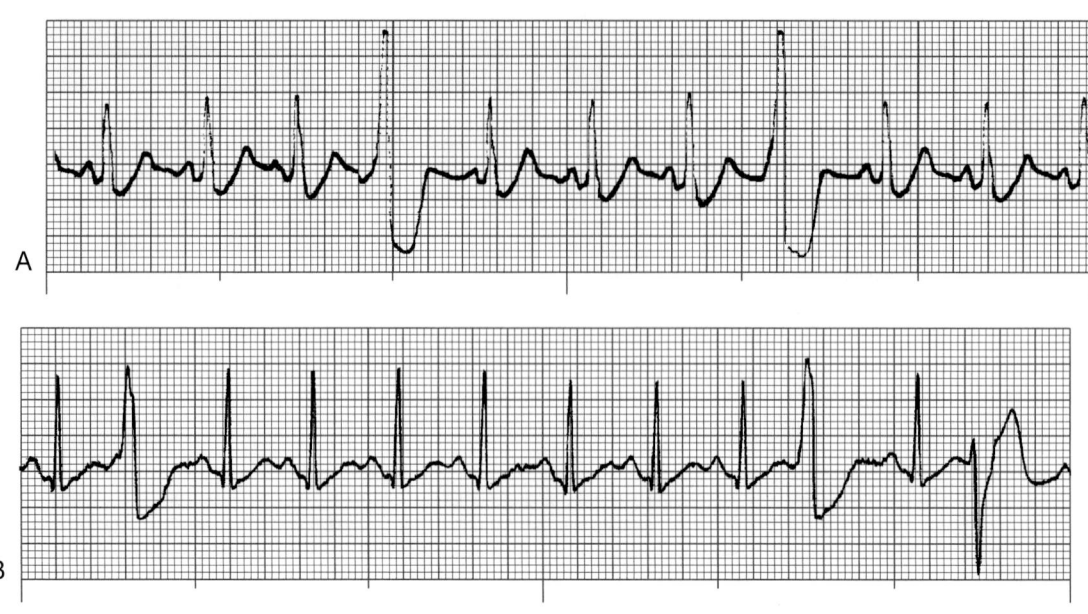

FIGURE 48-16 Sinus tachycardia, **A,** with frequent uniform PVCs; **B,** with multiform PVCs. (From Aehlert B: *ECGs made easy*, ed 3, St Louis, 2006, Mosby.)

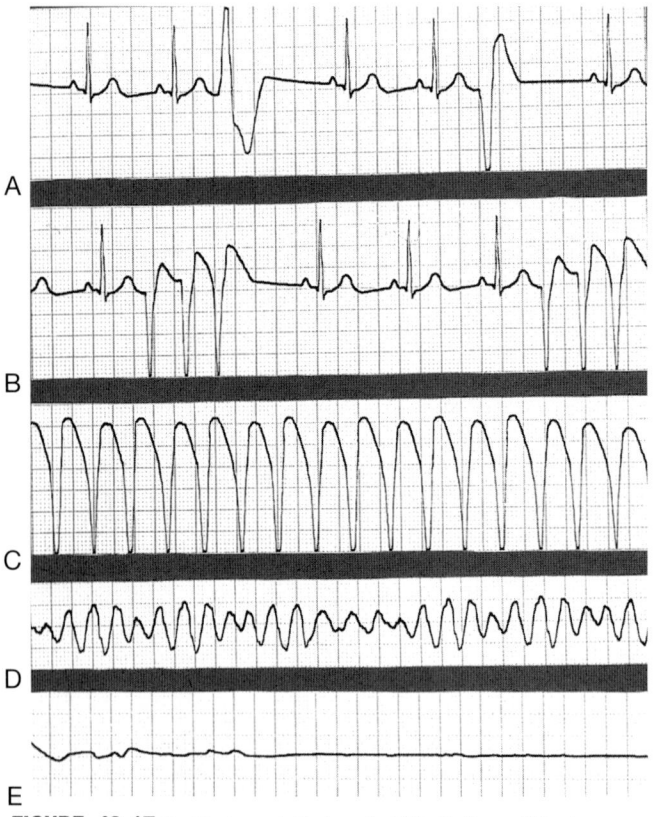

FIGURE 48-17 Ventricular arrhythmias. **A,** PVC. **B,** Three PVCs in a row. **C,** V-tach. **D,** V-fib. **E,** Asystole. (From Chester GA: *Modern medical assisting*, Philadelphia, 1999, Saunders.)

Biochemical Arrhythmias

Digitalis, frequently called *dig* (pronounced *dij*), is a common cardiac drug that is used to slow and strengthen the heartbeat. The heart is quite sensitive to digitalis, and too much can prove toxic and cause changes in the ECG (Figure 48-18). This condition reverses after reduction in the dosage of digoxin or digitoxin (both forms of digitalis).

Potassium is a critical mineral for normal cardiac function. Too much potassium in the blood *(hyperkalemia)* or too little potassium in the blood *(hypokalemia)* can both cause life-threatening arrhythmias that must be quickly corrected. Giving intravenous potassium can reverse hypokalemia. Giving a diuretic that does not effectively spare potassium can reverse hyperkalemia.

Pacemaker Rhythms

The implantation of a pacemaker into a patient sometimes corrects cardiac conduction system abnormalities. Electrodes extend from the pacemaker to the cardiac myocardium. The pacemaker contains a battery that produces small electrical charges that cause the heart to beat. A pacemaker can be used to stimulate regular contraction of just the atria, just the ventricles, or the entire heart. Pacemakers cause wide variations in the appearance of the ECG, and the firing of the pacemaker or pacing spikes may or may not be visible. Demand pacemakers automatically turn off when the heart beats above a certain rate and turn back on when the rate falls below a certain rate. The surgeon sets these rates before the pacemaker is implanted into the patient.

Automatic Implanted Cardioverter Defibrillator

The automatic implanted cardioverter defibrillator, more commonly known as an AICD, monitors the heart rhythm and delivers a shock to the heart if it detects a dangerous tachycardia. It is a small, battery-operated device that is implanted under the skin in the chest or abdomen. An AICD can be used to reverse V-tach and V-fib, especially after the patient has previously had a myocardial **infarction** (MI), or heart attack. The generator

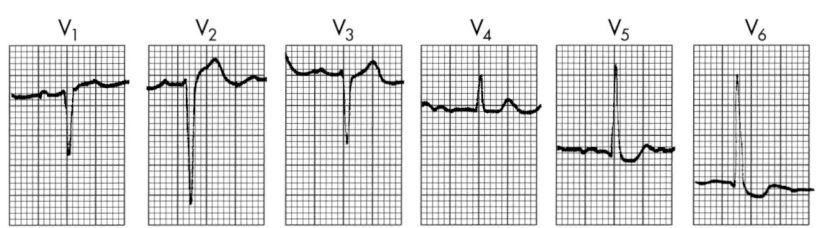

FIGURE 48-18 ECG shows effects of digitalis. Note the "scooping" of the ST segment as seen in leads V5 and V6. (From Aehlert B: *ECGs made easy*, ed 3, St Louis, 2006, Mosby.)

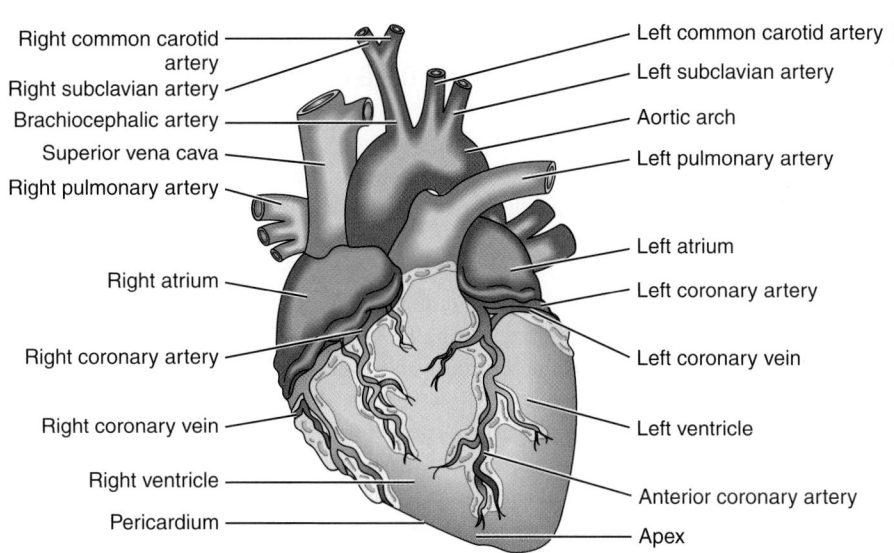

FIGURE 48-19 Coronary vessels. (From Chester GA: *Modern medical assisting*, Philadelphia, 1999, Saunders.)

TABLE 48-4 Phases of Myocardial Infarction with Changes Seen on Electrocardiogram

PHASE	WHEN ECG CHANGES APPEAR	SPECIFIC CHANGES SEEN ON ECG
I. Hyperacute	Occurs in first few hours	ST segment elevation from baseline (this is the earliest indication on ECG); peaked "hyperacute" T waves
II. Fully evolved	After hours or days	Deep T waves; pathologic Q waves appear (negative deflection)
III. Resolution	Days to weeks	ST segment returns to normal position; T waves return to normal
IV. Stabilized chronic	Permanent	Negative Q wave deflection remains

is programmed specifically to treat the patient's particular or potential cardiac arrhythmia.

Myocardial Infarction

Sudden heart attack, or MI, occurs in over 1 million Americans each year according to the American Heart Association. Approximately 20% of these patients die before reaching the hospital, and approximately 30% die within 30 days of their heart attack. An MI occurs when a portion of the heart muscle becomes **ischemic** because the blood supply to that area is interrupted. Ischemia eventually leads to tissue necrosis or infarction.

The heart muscle, the myocardium, receives its oxygen supply from a network of coronary arteries (Figure 48-19) located on the heart surface. The right coronary artery supplies much of the right side of the heart. The left coronary artery **bifurcates** into two main branches: the left circumflex artery, which supplies blood principally to the left lateral and posterior walls of the left ventricle, and the left anterior descending coronary artery, which

supplies principally the anterior wall of the left ventricle and the interventricular septum. The left anterior descending coronary artery is sometimes called the "sudden death artery" because it feeds such a large portion of the left ventricle.

MI causes specific, recognizable changes on the ECG recording. These changes are related to which one of the four phases (Table 48-4) of the MI the patient is in when the ECG is recorded. The three most common changes are elevated ST segments, inverted (upside-down) T waves, and abnormal (pathologic) Q waves.

The sooner treatment is initiated after the patient's first awareness of a heart attack, the more effective it becomes. Immediate therapy for MI includes administration of nasal oxygen (to increase available oxygen), sublingual nitroglycerin (to dilate coronary arteries), a narcotic analgesic (to eliminate pain), aspirin (to reduce inflammation and decrease clotting time), and possibly a thrombolytic agent to dissolve the clot that is causing the coronary arterial obstruction. Early administration of thrombolytic agents enhances the likelihood of restoring

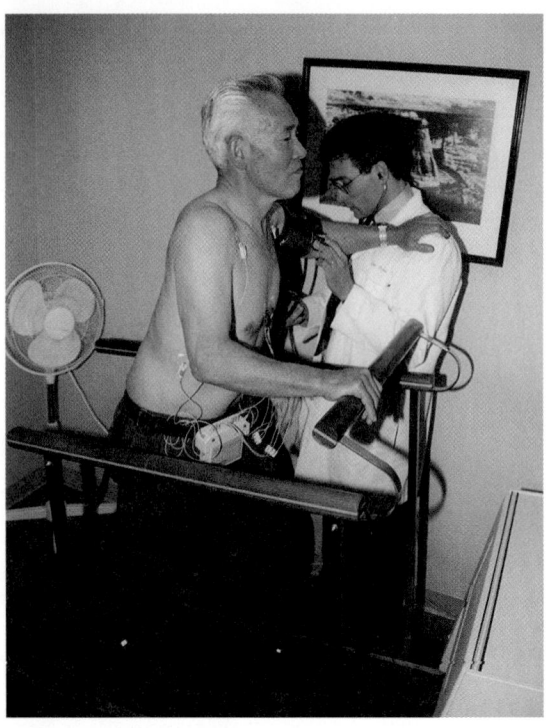

FIGURE 48-20 Cardiac stress test.

circulation to the myocardium distal to the occluding thrombus (blood clot). After discharge from the hospital, the patient should quit smoking, modify the diet as instructed by a nutritionist, and enter a cardiac rehabilitation program to improve cardiac strength and recovery by exercise.

Complications of acute MI include a sudden episode of atrial fibrillation, V-fib, or bradycardia that may necessitate implantation of a pacemaker.

RELATED CARDIAC DIAGNOSTIC TESTS

Stress Test

Cardiac stress testing is conducted to observe and record the patient's cardiovascular response to measured exercise challenges (Figure 48-20). Stress testing is performed to accomplish the following:

- To diagnose cardiac disease that cannot be detected by a standard, resting ECG
- To determine an individual's energy performance capacity
- To prescribe a specially designed exercise plan

The stress test is performed while the patient is exercising on either a bicycle or a treadmill, under careful supervision. The patient must be given the appropriate information explaining the purpose, preparation, and procedure for the test (Figure 48-21).

Cardiac Stress Test

Cardiac stress testing (also known as an exercise tolerance test or treadmill test) is a means of observing, evaluating, and recording your heart's response during a measured exercise test. This test determines your capacity to adapt to physical stress.

There are various reasons that your physician may suggest this test for you:

1. To aid in determining the presence of suspected coronary heart disease.
2. To aid in the selection of therapy.
   a. For angina pectoris (tightness or pain in the chest).
   b. Following a myocardial infarction (heart attack).
   c. Following coronary bypass surgery (open heart surgery).
3. To determine your physical work capacity.
4. To authorize participation in a physical exercise program.

Preparation for the Test

1. Avoid eating a heavy meal within 2 hours of your appointment.
2. Take your medications as you usually do, unless your doctor advises you not to take them.
3. Wear a shirt or blouse that buttons down the front with slacks, a skirt, jogging pants, or shorts.
4. Do not wear one-piece undergarments, jumpsuits, or dresses.
5. Tennis shoes are ideal if you have them. Otherwise, wear comfortable flat or low-heeled shoes. Do not wear clogs, sling-backs, crepe soles, boots, or high heels, as they make walking on the treadmill more difficult.

The Procedure

When you arrive in the Cardiology Department, areas of your chest may be shaved (men only) to allow the electrodes to adhere tightly to your chest. A blood pressure cuff will be wrapped around your arm, and an electrocardiogram (ECG) is taken while you are at rest. The technician will then demonstrate how to walk on the treadmill and will answer any questions you may have.

You will then perform a graded exercise test on a motor-driven treadmill. You will begin walking very gradually at a rate you can easily accomplish.

Progressively throughout the test, the speed and grade of the treadmill will be increased, and you will be walking at a faster pace up a slight incline. At no time will you be asked to jog or run, nor will you be asked to exercise beyond your capabilities.

At all times during the test, trained personnel are in the room with you, monitoring your heart rate and blood pressure and observing you for signs of fatigue or discomfort. We do not wish to exercise you to a level that is medically unsafe or physically distressing.

An ECG is taken again when you finish walking. Your cardiologist will immediately interpret the results of the test and explain his or her findings to you. If necessary, medications or treatment will be discussed. A letter with the results of the stress test will be sent to your referring physician.

The entire procedure will take 1 to 1 1/2 hours. If you have any questions regarding the cardiac stress test or any problems with your appointment, please contact us.

FIGURE 48-21 Patient information for a cardiac stress test.

A serious risk of a cardiac stress test is possible cardiac arrest. The medical assistant must be able to recognize symptoms of dyspnea, **vertigo,** extreme fatigue, severe arrhythmia, and other abnormal ECG readings that may develop during the stress test or immediately after the test during the rest period. All members of a cardiac stress testing team must be prepared to terminate testing immediately if the patient is unable to continue or when abnormalities appear on the monitor. Therefore cardiac stress testing team members need to be certified in cardiopulmonary resuscitation (CPR) and emergency intervention. The physician must always be present in the office during this procedure. In addition to the routine monitoring equipment, oxygen, defibrillator, endotracheal intubation tray, artificial breathing bag, and emergency cardiac medications must be available in case of cardiac crisis.

CRITICAL THINKING APPLICATION

Mr. Sonderford actually had an MI when he was previously at Dr. Lee's office. He has now completed cardiac rehabilitation and is at the office for a checkup. Dr. Lee wants him to be scheduled for a stress test. Mr. Sonderford has never had one before. He confides to Martha that he is afraid if he takes the test, he will die from another heart attack. How should Martha handle this situation?

Holter Monitor

A Holter monitor is a portable system for recording the cardiac activity of a patient over a 24-hour period or longer (Figure 48-22 and Procedure 48-2). It is a small, lightweight device that is worn while the patient carries out his or her usual daily activities. The Holter monitor can be programmed to record cardiac information continuously or periodically, when activated by the patient when symptoms occur, or during periods of stress.

The patient must keep a journal of all stressful events and activities (as well as of specific details regarding activities when any cardiologic symptoms occur) during the entire time the monitor is worn. Journal entries include the time, duration, and specific activity during the cardiac event such as rush hour traffic, bowel movements, intercourse, climbing stairs, and periods of anger or emotional distress. Some monitors can even record the patient's voice describing a symptom or event so that it can later be correlated with the ECG recording in the same time frame.

Many cardiologists routinely use Holter monitors in their practices. A medical assistant is often responsible for applying and removing the monitor. The patient must have a full understanding of what is required during monitoring, particularly how to use the event marker in case a significant symptom is experienced. When this marker is used, the patient must also know how to record the event in a written diary. The patient may only take sponge baths during the 24 hours of the test. The number of electrodes and leads varies with the number of channels on the particular monitor. Electrode placement is determined by the physician or manufacturer guidelines and should be followed precisely. The skin may need to be shaved so that electrodes can be firmly attached. The wires are attached to the electrodes and to the Holter. It is worn on a belt or in a pouch slung over the shoulder or worn around the waist.

At the end of the monitoring period the patient returns to the office; the monitor is disconnected, and the electrodes are removed. The recording is placed into a Holter scanner or computer and the results are analyzed. Any portion of the tape can be printed for further study.

CRITICAL THINKING APPLICATION

Mrs. Jamison was fitted with a Holter monitor at the office yesterday at 4 pm. When Martha arrived at the office at 8 o'clock this morning, she found Mrs. Jamison had left a message with the answering service to call her as soon as possible. When Martha returned the call, she told her she took a shower last night, and she noticed when she got up to go to the bathroom that the "light is not on" on the monitor. How should Martha handle this situation?

Cardiac Event Monitor

The cardiac event monitor is a small recording device that can be worn up to 30 days to catch events that are difficult to record in a 24-hour Holter monitor period including vertigo, weakness, and palpitations. Patients are instructed to trigger the recording when they feel any indication of a cardiac event. Based on the information gathered during the recording period the physician is able to diagnose heart abnormalities and design the most effective treatment. The monitor needs to be removed during bathing so the patient must be taught how to remove and reapply the electrodes throughout the test period. Patient education for the use of the event monitor includes the following:

- Protect the monitor from damage and wear it all times except when bathing
- Do not alter lifestyle; regular activities need to be maintained to reflect the cause of cardiac symptoms
- Trigger the recording by pushing the event monitor when symptoms occur
- Use the diary to record activities when events occur

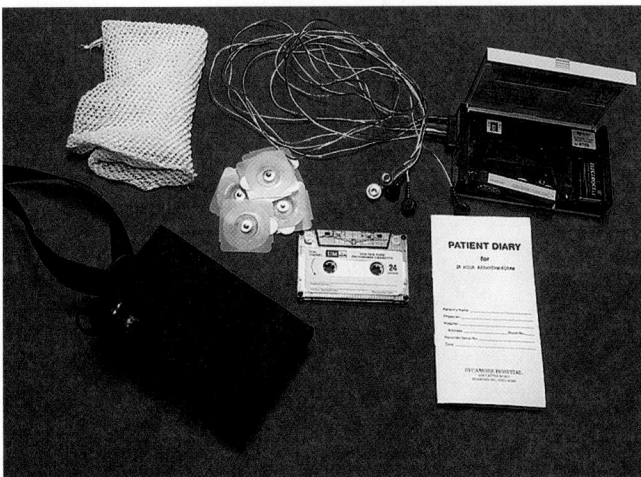

FIGURE 48-22 Holter monitor. (From Chester GA: *Modern medical assisting,* Philadelphia, 1999, Saunders.)

PROCEDURE 48-2

Prepare Patient for and Assist with Routine and Specialty Examinations: Apply a Holter Monitor

CAAHEP COMPETENCY: 3.b.(4)(e)
ABHES COMPETENCY: 4.h

GOAL: *To establish a possible correlation between coronary disorders and the patient's 24-hour daily activities.*

EQUIPMENT and SUPPLIES

- Holter monitor with new battery and blank recording tape
- Disposable electrodes
- Razor
- Gauze pads or abrasive tool as needed
- Activity diary
- Carrying case with belt or shoulder strap
- Alcohol swabs
- Cloth tape (nonallergenic)
- Patient record

PROCEDURAL STEPS

1. Wash your hands.
   PURPOSE: Infection control.
2. Assemble equipment needed.
3. Install a new battery or fully charged rechargeable battery into the monitor (Figure 1*).
   PURPOSE: A new or fully charged battery ensures accurate monitor function for a 24-hour period.
4. Greet the patient, and explain the procedure.
   PURPOSE: An informed patient helps ensure testing accuracy.
5. Ask the patient to disrobe to the waist and to sit at the end of the examination table or lie down.
   PURPOSE: This places the patient at the best working level for the medical assistant.
6. Clean each electrode application site with the alcohol swab, and allow the sites to air dry.
   PURPOSE: To remove all surface skin oil to ensure maximal electrode adherence. Clean before shaving to prevent irritation and patient discomfort.
7. If the patient has a hairy chest, dry shave the area at each of the electrode sites.
   PURPOSE: Skin must be hairless to provide maximal electrode adherence.

8. Fold a gauze pad over your index finger and briskly rub the sites or use an abrasive tool as indicated (Figure 2).
   PURPOSE: Will help electrodes to stick more tightly to the skin.
9. Apply the electrodes to the sites recommended by the manufacturer, making sure to use enough pressure that they adhere completely to the skin (Figure 3). Rub the edges of each electrode a second time to make certain that the electrode will stay in place.
   PURPOSE: Secure attachment of the electrodes is absolutely necessary to produce an accurate tracing.
10. Attach the lead wires to the electrodes, and connect the end terminal to the patient cable.
11. Place a strip of cloth tape over each electrode.
    PURPOSE: Aids in securing electrode placement if any pulling of the wires occurs during the testing period.

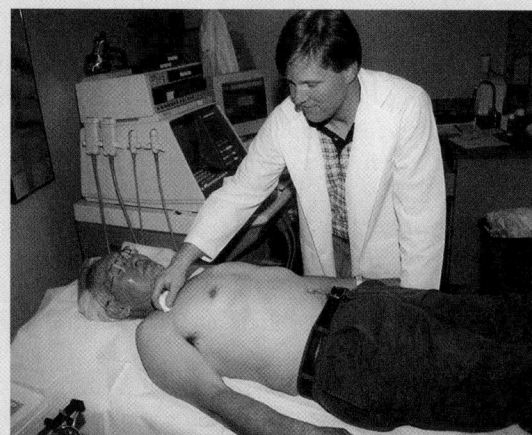

FIGURE 2

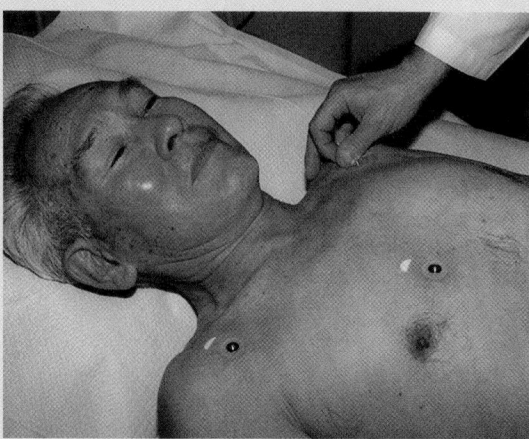

FIGURE 3

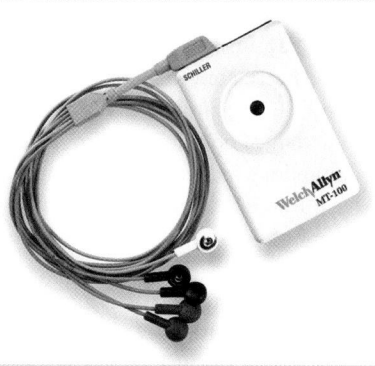

FIGURE 1

Continued

PROCEDURE 48-2—cont'd

12. Attach the test cable to the monitor and plug it into the electrocardiograph. Run a baseline test tracing as directed by manufacturer guidelines.
PURPOSE: To ensure proper connections of the electrodes and running of the monitor.

13. Help the patient get dressed without disturbing the connected electrodes. Be certain that the cable extends through the buttoned front or out the bottom of the shirt or blouse (Figure 4).

14. Place the monitor in the carrying case, and attach it to the patient's belt or place it over the shoulder. Be sure the wires are not being pulled or bent in half.
PURPOSE: Taut or badly bent wires may loosen or malfunction.

15. Plug the electrode cable into the monitor.

16. Record the patient's name, date of birth, and starting date and time in the patient's activity diary.
PURPOSE: To establish the starting time of the test and cardiac activity.

17. Give the patient the activity diary, and advise him or her to begin by writing in his or her present activity (Figure 5). Include patient education information on the importance of continually recording activities in the diary; using the event marker on the monitor if he or she experiences any symptoms; and correlating the event with a recording in the diary including the time and details regarding the related activity before or during the event.
PURPOSE: Diary must correlate patient's activity with cardiac activity.

18. Schedule the patient for a return appointment in 24 hours.

19. Wash your hands.
PURPOSE: Infection control.

20. Record the procedure in patient's chart.
PURPOSE: A procedure is not considered done until it is recorded in the patient's medical record.

*Figure 1 photo courtesy Welch Allyn, Skaneateles Falls, NY.
See Appendix D for a charting example.

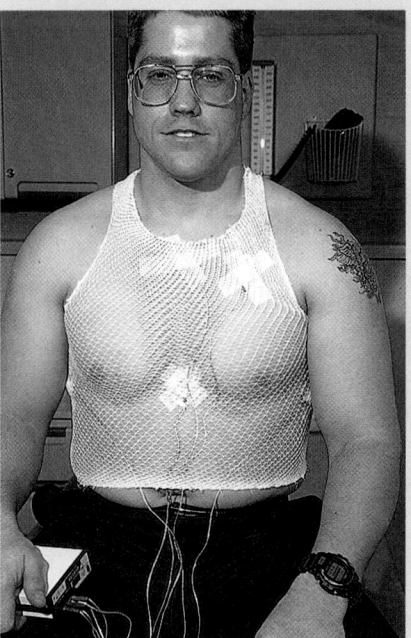

FIGURE 4

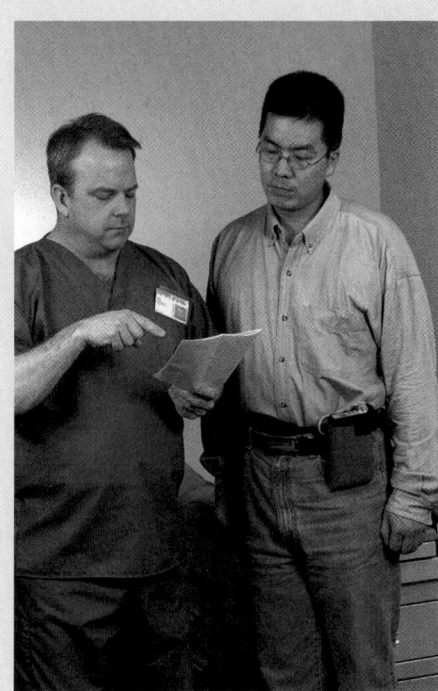

FIGURE 5

- Change the electrodes daily and the batteries at the same time each day
- To prevent skin irritation do not apply replacement electrodes at the same spot
- Apply electrodes on the rib cage under the left breast and in the midaxillary region under the right shoulder
- Most event monitor recordings can be transmitted via phone; if using this type provide instructions on how to transmit recordings

- Provide contact information for the patient if there are any questions

Heart Scan

A noninvasive method of assessing possible cardiac risk is a specialized computed tomography (CT) called an *electron beam tomography* (EBT) heart scan (also called an *ultrafast CT*). The heart scan takes less than 5 minutes and does not require any needles or injections. It is a screening tool that allows physicians to see the amount of plaque that is present in the coronary arteries by showing the presence of calcium deposits. Calcium makes up approximately 20% of arterial plaque deposits. The EBT heart scan is read, and the physician assigns the patient a calcium score that can be a predictor of future cardiac problems.

CLOSING COMMENTS

Patient Education

Heart disease and stroke account for more than one third of all deaths. Genetic predisposition and detrimental lifestyle habits, such as smoking, lack of exercise, high-fat diets, and obesity, play a significant role in the development of heart disease. Talk to the patient about factors that could be changed or modified, and give him or her encouragement for any attempt at complying with these suggestions.

Before you can successfully counsel a patient in changing a habit, you will need to obtain background knowledge in possible techniques to use. Places to obtain this information include the American Heart Association and reputable Internet sites.

Many patients like visual aids in learning, and brochures with pictures or posters in the office are effective methods for initiating both patient learning and patient questions. Make a note in the chart regarding what educational items you give the patient on each visit. On a subsequent visit, ask about the helpfulness of the information, whether the patient tried any modifications, and what the results were. Ask for any suggestions that might help another patient in a similar situation.

Legal and Ethical Issues

An ECG is a valuable diagnostic tool that continues to be one of the most common procedures used in the diagnosis of cardiac diseases and conditions. The cardiologist measures the patient's heart activity and compares the results with known values by analyzing the ECG tracing. Comparing an ECG tracing with previous tracings can identify changes in the condition of the patient's heart.

The physician must be able to accurately interpret the ECG tracing and establish its value in correctly diagnosing the patient's condition; therefore the medical assistant has the ethical obligation to complete the task as accurately and carefully as possible. Diagnostic procedures have a profound effect on a patient's subsequent treatment. When you are entrusted with performing testing procedures, you assume full responsibility for the accuracy and precision of each test you perform. This is a critical role in the medical assisting profession. The results you submit will strongly influence each patient's therapeutic treatment plan. No test is ever just routine.

SUMMARY OF SCENARIO

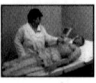

Martha has now worked at Dr. Lee's office for almost 8 months. She has become quite confident in her ability to quickly and accurately perform electrocardiography. She also has learned a great deal about how to effectively communicate with patients regarding their fears and concerns about various cardiac diagnostic tests. She never forgets to tell a patient the importance of not taking a shower during the 24-hour Holter monitoring period. In 2 months she and Dr. Lee are going to attend a national meeting of cardiologists in Chicago. There will be 2 days of continuing education classes for medical assistants who work in cardiology. Martha is very excited to be able to continue learning and to sharpen her skills as a cardiology medical assistant.

SUMMARY of LEARNING OBJECTIVES

1. Define, spell, and pronounce the terms listed in the vocabulary.
   - Spelling and pronouncing medical terms correctly adds credibility to the medical assistant. Knowing the definition of these terms promotes confidence in communication with patients and co-workers.
2. Illustrate the electrical conduction system through the heart.
   - The heart beats in response to an electrical signal that originates in the SA node in the right atrium, spreads over the atria, and causes atrial contraction. This impulse continues to the AV node, through the bundle of His, through the right and left bundle branches, and into the Purkinje fibers, eventually causing ventricular contraction.

3. Explain the concepts of cardiac polarization, depolarization, and repolarization.
   - Polarization is the resting state of the myocardial wall when there is no electrical activity in the heart. When the electrical system of the heart stimulates a myocardial cell, depolarization occurs, resulting in the contraction of the stimulated heart muscle. The heart muscle cells must then return to a resting state; the process of reaching this resting state is called repolarization.
4. Summarize the properties of the electrocardiograph.
   - A six-channel ECG machine records all 12 leads simultaneously within seconds. Limb and chest electrodes

Continued

SUMMARY of LEARNING OBJECTIVES

Continued

with leads must be placed on the patient at specific anatomic locations before the recording starts. ECG paper is standardized to represent amplitude and time. The horizontal lines permit the determination of the intensity of the electrical activity, and the vertical lines represent time; each of the large squares represents 0.2 seconds; five of them equal 1 second.

5. Describe the electrical views of the heart recorded by the 12-lead electrocardiograph.
   - Lead I records the electrical activity of the lateral part of the left ventricle, and leads II and III that of the inferior surface of the left ventricle. The augmented lead aV_R records the electrical activity of the atria with negative deflection of the P waves and QRS complexes, aV_L records the electrical activity of the lateral wall of the left ventricle, and aV_F records the electrical activity of the inferior surface of the left ventricle. The precordial leads provide a transverse plane view of the heart. They include V_1, V_2, V_3, V_4, V_5, and V_6, with each of the numbers representing a specific location on the chest. The QRS complex is a negative deflection in V_1 and V_2 views, with each subsequent lead becoming more positive.

6. Discuss the process of recording an electrocardiogram.
   - Recording an ECG requires knowledge of where to place electrodes and connect leads to obtain the most accurate recording possible; ability to recognize and correct the most common types of artifacts on the ECG recording; and proper use of the machine available. The patient must lie still during the procedure. Six-channel machines print and label all 12 leads with a rhythm strip across the bottom of the paper in lead II in a matter of seconds. Review the printout for clarity, and give the recording to the physician for review.

7. Perform an accurate recording of the electrical activity of the heart.
   - Procedure 48-1 outlines the steps for performing a 12-lead ECG recording.

8. Compare and contrast electrocardiographic artifacts and the probable cause of each.
   - An artifact is unwanted, erratic movement of the stylus on the paper resulting from outside interference. The main types include wandering baseline artifacts, in which the stylus gradually shifts away from the center of the paper because of slight movement or poor electrode attachment. Somatic tremor artifacts are a result of patient muscle movements that cause jagged peaks of irregular height and spacing and

a shifting baseline. AC interference causes a series of uniform small spikes on the paper because of electrical energy in the area. Interrupted baseline artifacts occur when the electric connection between the electrode and the lead is interrupted.

9. Interpret a typical electrocardiographic tracing.
   - Table 48-2 summarizes the normal appearance of ECG waveforms and complexes. The ECG tracing is made up of repeated cardiac cycle (PQRST) recordings. To calculate the heart rate from the ECG recording, count the number of P waves in a 6-second strip (30 large squares) and multiply by 10. To get the ventricular contraction rate, count the number of complete QRS complexes within 6 seconds and multiply by 10 to get the number of ventricular contractions in 1 minute. The rhythm of the patient's heartbeat indicates whether it is regular or not. If the patient's heart is beating at a regular rhythm, each cardiac cycle occurs within the same time frame and individual cardiac cycles occur exactly the same length of time apart.

10. Identify common electrocardiographic arrhythmias.
    - Sinus rhythm is when the heart's electrical activity begins in the SA node and follows through the electrical system, ending in atrial and ventricular depolarization. In sinus bradycardia the heart rate is less than 60 beats/min; in sinus tachycardia the rate is more than 100 beats/min. A PAC occurs when the atria contract before they should for the next cardiac cycle. Atrial flutter occurs when the atria beat at an extremely rapid rate—up to 300 beats/min. PVCs occur when the ventricles contract before they should for the next cardiac cycle. V-tach causes the ventricles to beat at extremely rapid rates, from 101 to 250 beats/min. V-fib is the most critical, life-threatening arrhythmia and will result in death if not effectively treated. Asystole is the result of no heartbeat. There can also be arrhythmias because of biochemical systemic problems.

11. Summarize cardiac diagnostic tests.
    - Cardiac diagnostic tests include ECG; a stress test to determine the patient's cardiac response to exercise; the use of a 24-hour Holter monitor to pick up abnormalities during the patient's routine day; a 30-day event monitor to record infrequent cardiac symptoms; and a heart scan to provide noninvasive diagnostic information.

12. Apply a Holter monitor.
    - Procedure 48-2 explains how to apply a Holter monitor.

CONNECTIONS

Study Guide Connection: Go to Chapter 48 Study Guide. Read the Case Study and Workplace Applications and complete the assignments. Do online research for answers to the questions in the Internet Activities associated with principles of electrocardiography.

CD Connection: Go to the Medical Assisting Competency Challenge CD and do the training activities under Diagnostic Testing. For a better understanding of the principles of electrocardiography, view the animations for sinus tachycardia, sinus bradycardia, and normal sinus rhythm.

Evolve Connection: For more information related to principles of electrocardiography, go to evolve.elsevier.com/kinn and visit related weblinks for Chapter 48. Click on the Medical Assisting Exam Review and do the practice questions to sharpen your test-taking skills.

Assisting with Diagnostic Imaging 49

SCENARIO

Sara Elwood, CMA, is employed by Metro Urgicenter, an urgent care clinic in an urban setting. Metro is staffed around the clock and sees patients with urgent problems that are not immediately life-threatening. Facilities at the center include an x-ray department where films of the spine and the extremities are taken to evaluate injuries for possible fractures and chest films are taken to aid in the diagnosis of patients with respiratory complaints. The center's staff physicians read the x-ray films as they are taken. Afterward, the films are sent to a local hospital for formal interpretation by a radiologist. Sara often assists David Swain, the radiographer, by preparing patients for x-ray examinations and processing the films. Sometimes it is her responsibility to send the films to the hospital for interpretation and to file them when they are returned. When patients are sent to other facilities for special imaging studies, it is Sara's duty to make the arrangements and provide preliminary explanations of the procedures to the patients.

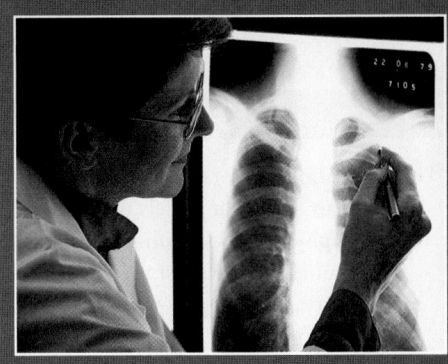

While studying this chapter, think about the following questions:

- To fulfill her job description at the Urgicenter, what does Sara need to know about preparing patients for routine x-ray examinations?
- How should a film be processed so there are no handling artifacts?
- What should Sara know about various diagnostic procedures so she can effectively supplement patient education and scheduling questions?

LEARNING OBJECTIVES

1. Define, spell, and pronounce the terms listed in the vocabulary.
2. Identify the principal components of an x-ray machine.
3. Describe the cassette and film image receptor system, and explain its function in radiography.
4. Recognize the precautions to be taken when unloading, loading, and processing radiograph film and cassettes.
5. Distinguish among the three body planes, and use these terms correctly when discussing radiographic positions.
6. Identify anteroposterior (AP), posteroanterior (PA), lateral, oblique, and axial radiographic projections.
7. Compare and contrast radiography and fluoroscopy, and give examples of appropriate applications of each.
8. List and describe imaging modalities that do not involve x-rays.
9. Explain patient preparation guidelines for typical diagnostic imaging examinations.
10. Outline the general procedure for assisting with an x-ray examination.
11. Summarize guidelines for scheduling multiple diagnostic procedures.
12. Apply patient education principles when providing instructions for preparation for diagnostic procedures.
13. Describe the health risks associated with low doses of x-ray exposure such as those used in radiography.
14. Summarize the steps to ensure that patients receive the least possible exposure during x-ray procedures.
15. Describe precautions to ensure the safety of equipment operators and staff during x-ray procedures.
16. Explain the legal responsibilities associated with x-ray procedures and the administrative management of diagnostic images.

National Accreditation Competencies and Content

CAAHEP COMPETENCIES	ABHES COMPETENCIES
Clinical	**Clinical Duties**
3.b.(4)(e). Prepare patient for and assist with routine and specialty examinations	4.b. Prepare patients for procedures
	4.h. Prepare patient for and assist physician with routine and specialty examinations

VOCABULARY

angiocardiography (an-je-o-kahr-de-og′-ruh-fe) Radiography of the heart and great vessels using an iodine contrast medium.

angiography (an-je-og′-ruh-fe) Radiography of blood vessels using an iodine contrast medium.

angioplasty (an′-je-o-plas-te) Interventional technique using a catheter to open or widen a blood vessel to improve circulation.

anteroposterior (AP) (an-tuhr-o-pos-ter′-e-ohr) Frontal projection in which the patient is supine or facing the x-ray tube.

aortogram (a-or′-ti-gram) Radiography of the aorta using an iodine contrast medium.

arteriography (ahr-ter-e-og′-ruh-fe) Radiography of arteries using an iodine contrast medium.

arthrogram (ahr′-thro-gram) Fluoroscopic examination of the soft-tissue components of joints with direct injection of a contrast medium into the joint capsule.

axial projections Radiographs taken with a longitudinal angulation of the x-ray beam; sometimes referred to as semiaxial projections.

bucky Moving grid device that prevents scatter radiation from fogging the film.

cathartics Laxative preparations.

computed tomography (CT) Computerized x-ray imaging modality providing axial and three-dimensional scans.

contrast media Radiopaque substances used to enhance visibility of soft tissues in imaging studies.

coronal plane Plane that divides the body into anterior and posterior parts.

coulombs per kilogram (C/kg) International unit of radiation exposure.

dosimeter Badge for monitoring radiation exposure of personnel.

embolization Interventional technique using a catheter to block off a blood vessel to prevent hemorrhage.

fluoroscopy (floo-ros′-kuh-pe) Direct observation of the x-ray image in motion.

frontal projection Radiographic view in which the coronal plane of the body or body part is parallel to the film plane; AP or PA.

gantry Doughnut-shaped portion of a scanner that surrounds the patient and functions, at least in part, to gather imaging data.

Gray (Gy) International unit of radiation dose.

intravenous urogram (IVU) Radiographic examination of the urinary tract using intravenous injection of an iodine contrast medium.

latent image Invisible changes in exposed film that will become an image when the film is processed.

lateral projections Radiographic views in which the sagittal plane of the body or body part is parallel to the film.

limited radiography Limited-scope radiography practice, usually in an outpatient setting, that does not require the same credentials needed for professional radiologic technology; also called *practical radiography.*

lower gastrointestinal series Fluoroscopic examination of the colon, usually employing rectal administration of barium sulfate as a contrast medium; also called a *barium enema.*

magnetic resonance imaging (MRI) Imaging modality that uses a magnetic field and radiofrequency pulses to create computer images of both bones and soft tissues in multiple planes.

myelography (mi-uh-log′-ruh-fe) Fluoroscopic examination of the spinal canal with spinal injection of an iodine contrast medium.

NPO Nothing by mouth, from the Latin *nil per os.*

nuclear medicine Imaging modality that uses radioactive materials injected or ingested into the body to provide information about the function of organs and tissues.

oblique projections Radiographic views in which the body or part is rotated so that the projection is neither frontal nor lateral.

phosphors (fos′-fors) Fluorescent crystals that give off light when exposed to x-rays.

posteroanterior (PA) Frontal projection in which the patient is prone or facing the x-ray film or image receptor.

rad Conventional unit of radiation dose.

radiograph An x-ray image.

radiographer Person qualified to perform radiographic examinations.

radiography Making diagnostic images using x-rays.

radiologist Physician specialist in medical imaging or therapeutic applications of radiation.

radiolucent (ra-de-o-loo′-suhnt) Describing a substance that is

List continued from previous page

easily penetrated by x-rays; these substances appear dark on radiographs.

radiopaque (ra-de-o-pak′) Describing a substance that is not easily penetrated by x-rays; these substances appear light on radiographs.

rem Convention unit of radiation dose equivalent.

roentgen (R) (rent′-gen) Conventional unit of radiation exposure.

sagittal plane Plane that divides the body into right and left parts.

Sievert (Sv) (se′-vuhrt) International unit of radiation dose equivalent.

sonography (suh-nog′-ruh-fe) Imaging modality that uses sound waves to produce images of soft tissues; also called *diagnostic ultrasound.*

tracers Radioactive substances administered to patients for nuclear medicine imaging procedures.

transducer Part of the sonography machine that is in contact with the patient; the transducer sends high-frequency sound waves and receives the sound echoes that return from the patient's body.

transverse plane Plane that divides the body into superior and inferior parts.

upper gastrointestinal (UGI) series Fluoroscopic examination of the esophagus, stomach, and duodenum using oral administration of barium sulfate as a contrast medium.

For more than 100 years physicians have been using x-ray images to examine the internal structures of the body. The fascinating field of medical imaging now includes a wide variety of diagnostic imaging methods. This chapter provides an overview of imaging modalities and introduces you to **radiography.** Emphasis is placed on x-ray examinations because these are the procedures most commonly performed in the medical assistant's practice setting.

BASIC PRINCIPLES OF RADIOGRAPHY

Radiography

Radiography refers to the making of x-ray images called **radiographs.** X-rays are produced in a vacuum tube when electrons traveling at high speed strike certain materials, such as tungsten. When the x-rays are emitted from the tube, they diverge into space, forming the cone-shaped x-ray beam. The cross section of the x-ray beam at the point of use is called the *radiation field* (Figure 49-1). The patient or part to be x-rayed is placed in the radiation field, between the x-ray tube and the image receptor or film.

X-rays can penetrate most substances to some degree, but some substances such as metals and bones are more difficult to penetrate and are said to be **radiopaque.** Air, gases, and soft tissues such as fat, skin, and lungs are much easier to penetrate than bone and are said to be **radiolucent.** During the exposure, x-rays from the tube pass through the patient. Some of the x-rays are absorbed by the patient and others are not, resulting in a pattern of varying intensity in the x-ray beam that exits on the opposite side of the patient and exposes the film. The film

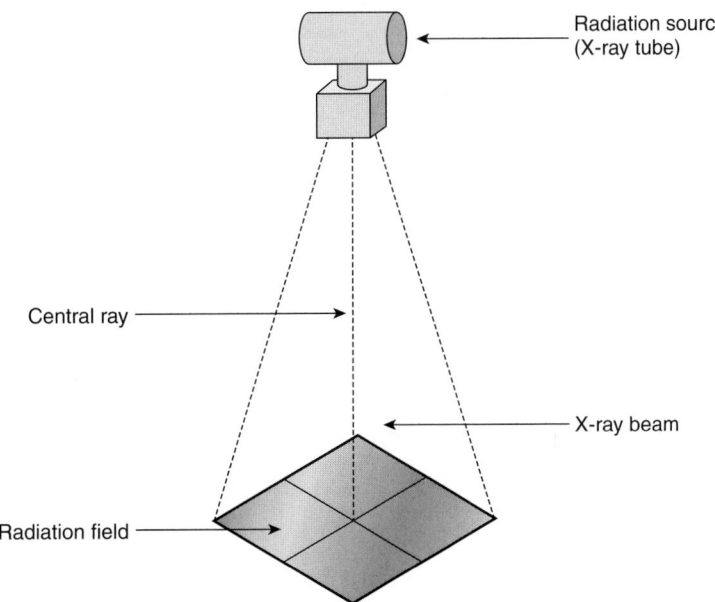

FIGURE 49-1 The primary x-ray beam leaves the x-ray tube and diverges into space. The center of the beam is called the *central ray*, and the cross-section of the beam at the point of use is called the radiation field. (From Hunkele MM: *Radiography essentials for limited practice,* ed 2, Philadelphia, 2006, Saunders.)

then has a pattern of exposure, a **latent image,** and must be processed to develop the latent image into one that is visible. On the finished radiograph, radiopaque objects appear light and radiolucent objects appear dark or black (Figure 49-2).

Routine plain films are simple radiographs taken of specific body structures such as the chest or the bones of the extremities or spine. These are the examinations most often performed in physicians' offices and most likely to be performed by medical assistants who are qualified to practice radiography.

X-Ray Exposure

Prime Factors

The **radiographer** must take a number of factors into consideration in determining the proper technique and exposure factors for an x-ray examination. The four principal exposure factors are called the *prime factors of exposure.* The interaction of these factors determines the level of x-ray production and ultimately the amount of exposure to the patient. Prime factors include the following:

- *Milliamperage* (mA)–the electrical control setting that determines how rapidly the radiation is produced; the higher the mA setting, the greater the quantity of x-rays produced per second.
- *Exposure time* (seconds)–the duration of the patient's x-ray exposure; most exposures are less than 1 second, so the total amount of time that a patient is exposed to the x-ray is measured in milliseconds. The amount of x-rays produced is dependent on the length of exposure.
- *Kilovoltage* (kVp)–the electrical control setting that determines the penetrating power of the x-ray beam; voltage controls the speed and power of x-ray beams; the higher the voltage, the shorter the x-ray wavelengths, and the greater the energy of the x-ray beam.
- *Source-to-image distance* (SID)–the distance between the x-ray tube and the film or other image receptor; the greater

the distance, the more widely the x-ray beam will spread, and the lower the intensity of the beam.

The total quantity of radiation in an exposure is indicated by the milliampere-seconds (mAs), which is determined by multiplying the rate of x-ray current flow (milliamperage) by the exposure time. The total amount of x-ray exposure used to conduct a particular diagnostic study is a combination of kilovoltage, milliamperage, exposure time, and source-to-image distance.

Technique Charts

A technique chart located near the control console provides the radiographer with a listing of recommended milliampere-seconds, kilovoltage, and source-to-image distance settings for x-ray studies of various body parts in patients of different sizes. The radiographer must refer to technique charts before performing the ordered radiographic procedure. Some control consoles have computerized units that are preprogrammed with the required exposure settings for the selected body part and size.

Radiographic Equipment

The X-Ray Tube and Housing

The x-ray tube is where the x-rays form and is surrounded by a lead-lined protective housing (Figure 49-3). The housing absorbs any radiation that is not part of the x-ray beam. The housing protects and insulates the x-ray tube itself while providing a base for attachments that allow the radiographer to manipulate the x-ray tube and to control the size and shape of the x-ray beam.

The principal attachment to the tube housing is the collimator, a box-like device mounted beneath the opening of the housing. Collimators allow the radiographer to vary the size of the radiation field and to indicate with a light beam the size, location, and center of the field. There is usually a centering light that helps align the cassette tray as well (Figure 49-4).

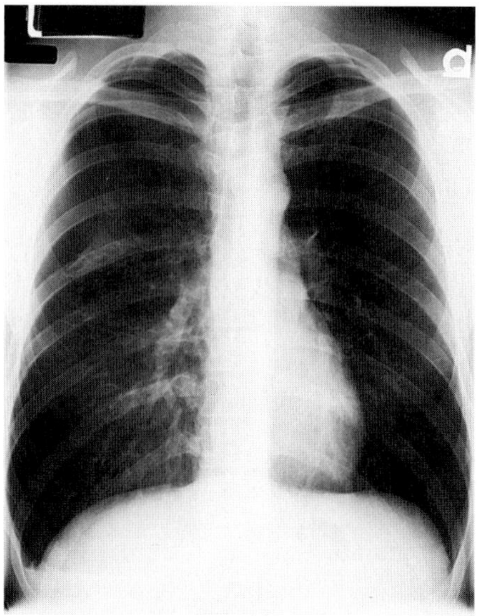

FIGURE 49-2 A chest radiograph demonstrates dark, radiolucent lungs with a light, radiopaque shadow of the spine and heart in the center. (From Hunkele MM: *Radiography essentials for limited practice,* ed 2, Philadelphia, 2006, Saunders.)

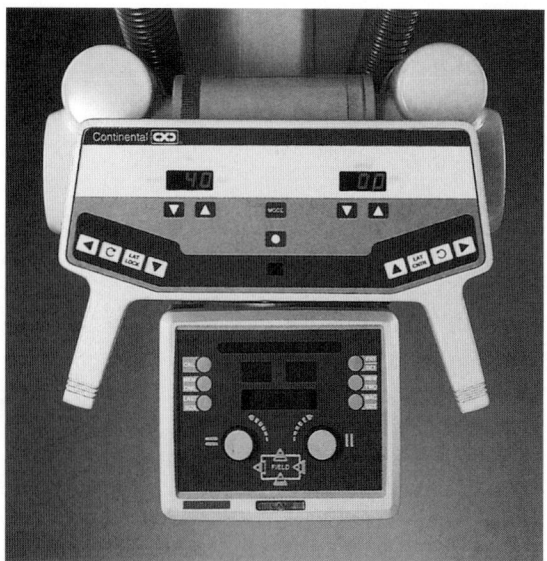

FIGURE 49-3 X-ray tube housing and collimator. (From Hunkele MM: *Radiography essentials for limited practice,* ed 2, Philadelphia, 2006, Saunders.)

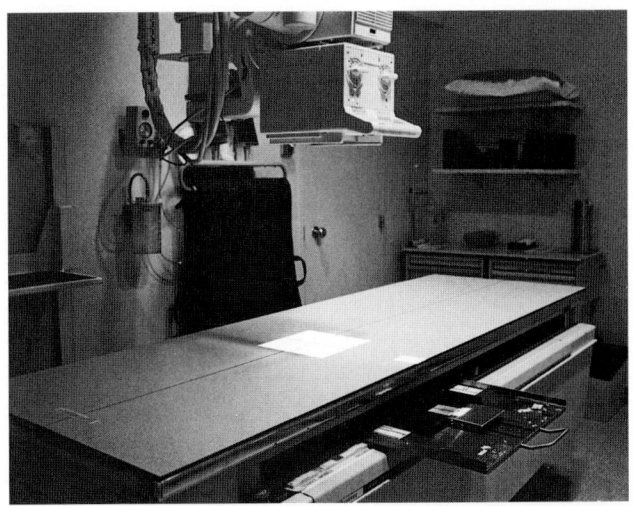

FIGURE 49-4 Collimator light beam demonstrates the radiation field and aids in aligning the cassette tray. (From Hunkele MM: *Radiography essentials for limited practice*, ed 2, Philadelphia, 2006, Saunders.)

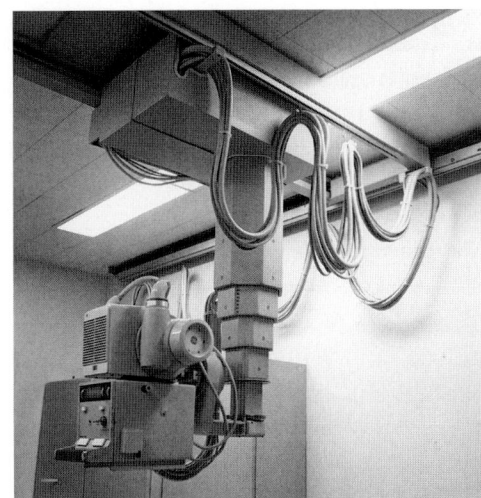

FIGURE 49-5 Ceiling-mount tube support. (From Hunkele MM: *Radiography essentials for limited practice*, ed 2, Philadelphia, 2006, Saunders.)

X-Ray Tube Support

The tube housing may be attached to a ceiling mount or a tube stand. Both types of mountings provide support and mobility for the heavy tube. The ceiling mount (Figure 49-5) moves on a system of tracks to allow positioning of the tube at locations throughout the room. This type of tube mount facilitates positioning the tube over a stretcher or placement in various locations. A tube stand (Figure 49-6) is a vertical support with a horizontal arm that suspends the tube over the radiographic table. The tube stand rolls along a track that is secured to the floor (and sometimes also the ceiling), allowing horizontal motion. Outpatient x-ray departments are more likely to have a tube stand.

A system of electric locks holds the tube in position. The control system for all, or most, of these locks is an attachment on the front of the tube housing. To move the tube in any direction, the locking device must be released. Moving the tube without first releasing the lock may damage the lock, making it impossible to secure the tube in position. Typical tube motions include the following:

- Longitudinal movement—motion along the long axis of the table
- Transverse movement—motion across the table, at right angles to longitudinal movement
- Vertical movement—up and down, increasing or decreasing the distance between the tube and the table
- Roll (tilt, angle)—allows the tube to be angled according to the anatomic part being examined and the type of x-ray ordered
- Rotation—allows the entire tube support to turn on its axis, changing the direction in which the tube arm is extended

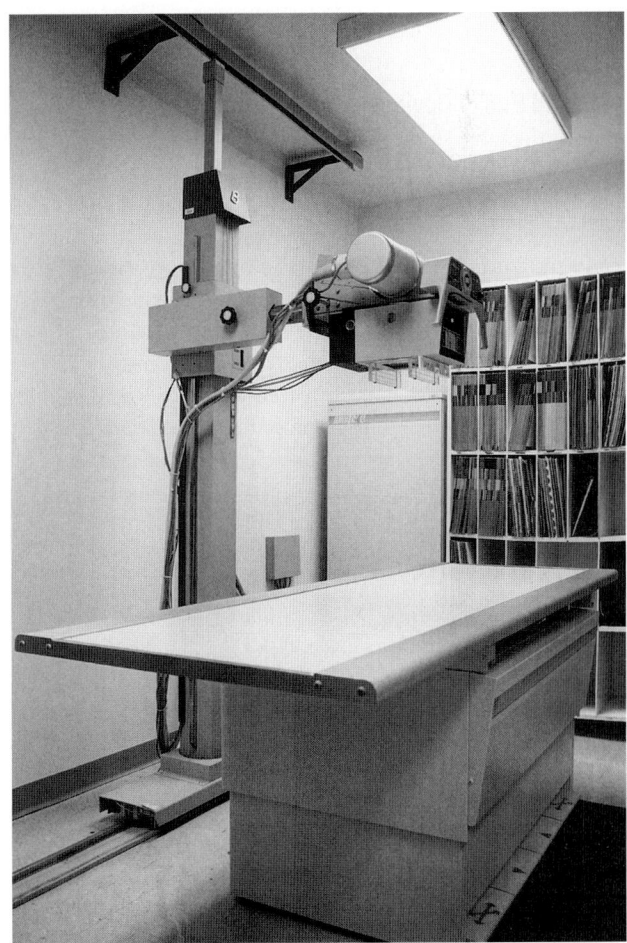

FIGURE 49-6 Tube stand. (From Hunkele MM: *Radiography essentials for limited practice*, ed 2, Philadelphia, 2006, Saunders.)

Radiographic Table

The radiographic table is a specialized unit that is more than just a support for the patient. Some tables are adjustable in height for easy patient access, and some are designed to tilt into upright and Trendelenburg positions. A floating tabletop is a feature that assists in aligning the patient to the tube and film. Using the table to move the patient allows for x-ray imaging in a variety of angles and positions.

Scatter Radiation

- Radiation that is scattered or created as a result of the interaction of the primary x-ray beam with the patient or other matter in its path.
- Scatter radiation travels in all directions from the scattering medium and is very difficult to control. Generally, it has less energy than the primary beam.

Safety Precautions When Moving X-ray Equipment

- Be sure that footboard and shoulder guards are secure before tilting a table holding a patient.
- Check that no equipment is under the table before tilting it.
- Release the locks before attempting to move the x-ray tube.
- Move the x-ray tube out of the way before assisting a patient to or from the table to avoid injuring the patient.
- Be sure that equipment is in a safe position before shutting off power to the locks.

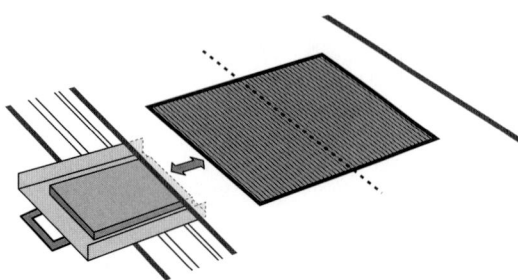

FIGURE 49-7 A bucky grid is under the surface of the x-ray table. (From Hunkele MM: *Radiography essentials for limited practice*, ed 2, Philadelphia, 2006, Saunders.)

Grids and Bucky Devices

Beneath the table surface is a moving grid device called a **bucky** (Figure 49-7). X-ray film is placed in a cassette tray, then into a bucky device that is under the radiographic table. The cassette that holds the film can then be moved up and down the table inside the bucky to a point directly under the area that is to be x-rayed. The grid is situated between the tabletop and the film inside the cassette. It is a plate made of tissue-thin lead strips, mounted on edge to protect the film from being fogged by scatter radiation that is displaced when the x-ray study is performed. Because the strips must be carefully aligned with the path of the x-ray beam, precise alignment of the x-ray tube in relationship to the bucky is essential. When the x-ray image is actually taken, the bucky device will automatically move the grid so that it is not visible on the radiograph. Bucky grids are generally used only for body parts that measure more than 10 to 12 cm in thickness (the average adult's neck or knee measures 12 cm). When a grid is not needed, the cassette is placed on the tabletop.

Upright Cassette Holder

The upright cassette holder, as its name implies, is a device to hold the film in the upright position for radiography. It is usually placed against a wall, and its height is adjustable. It may incorporate a bucky or stationary grid. When a grid is included, the unit may be referred to as a *grid cabinet* or *upright bucky.* When the patient is sitting or standing at the upright cassette holder for radiography, the tube is angled to face the wall and cassette holder. The distance from the tube to the film may be adjusted to 40 inches or to 72 inches, depending on the requirements of the procedure.

Control Console

The control console, located in the control booth, is the access point for the radiographer to determine exposure factors and

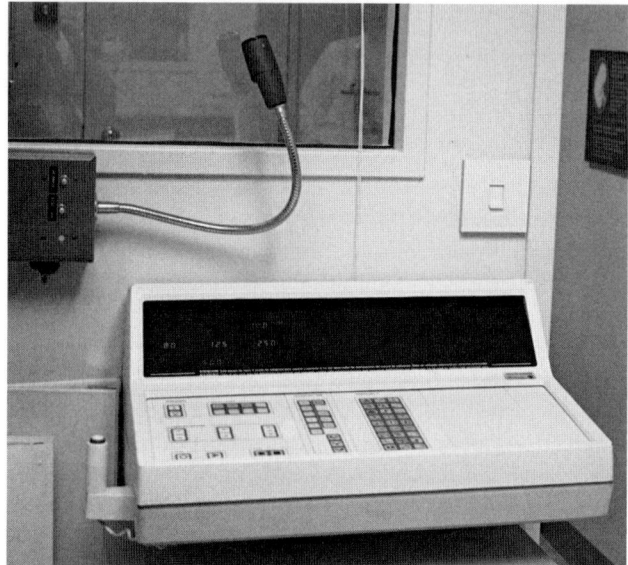

FIGURE 49-8 X-ray control console. (From Hunkele MM: *Radiography essentials for limited practice*, ed 2, Philadelphia, 2006, Saunders.)

to take the x-ray image (Figure 49-8). Radiographic control consoles have buttons, switches, dials, or digital readouts for some or all of the following functions:

- Off/On—controls the power to the control panel
- mA—allows the operator to set the milliamperage (mA), the rate at which the x-rays are produced
- kVp—controls the kilovoltage (kVp), determining the penetrating power of the x-ray beam
- Timer—controls the duration of the exposure
- mAs—some units have an mAs control instead of mA and time settings
- Bucky—activates the motor control of the bucky device so that the grid will move during the exposure
- Automatic exposure controls—special settings available on certain units that allow termination of exposure when a certain quantity of radiation has reached the film
- Meters or digital readouts—to indicate the status of the settings
- Prep (ready or rotor) switch—prepares the tube for exposure
- Exposure switch—initiates the exposure and must be continuously activated until the exposure is complete

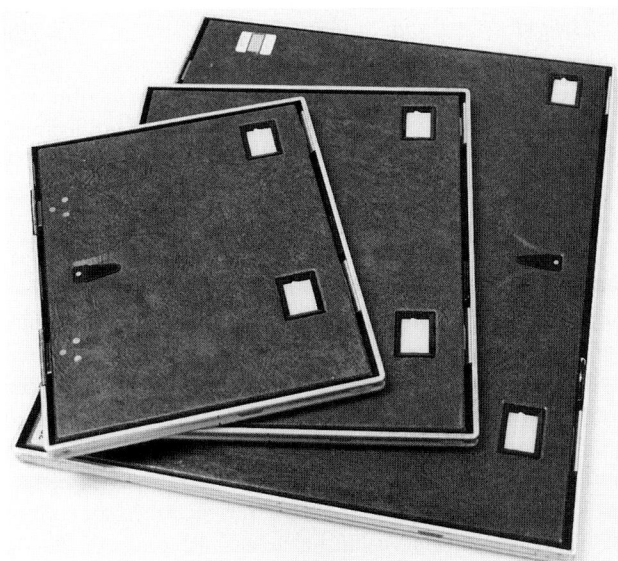

FIGURE 49-9 X-ray cassettes. (From Hunkele MM: *Radiography essentials for limited practice*, ed 2, Philadelphia, 2006, Saunders.)

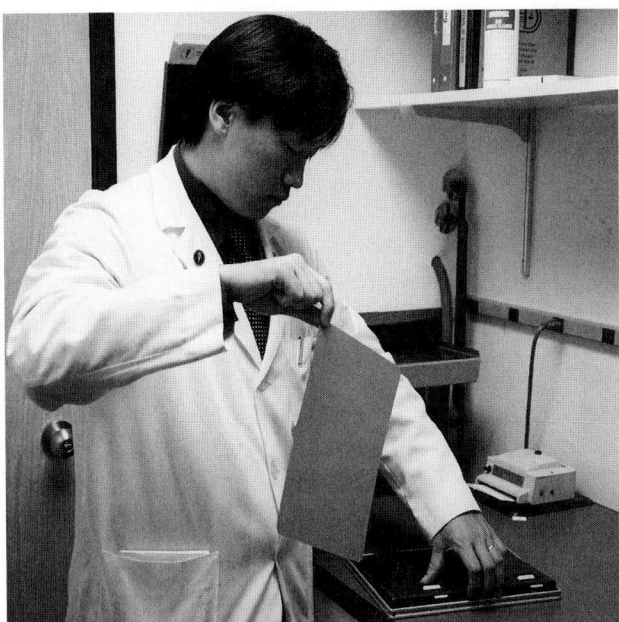

FIGURE 49-10 When holding film with one hand, let it hang vertically. (From Hunkele MM: *Radiography essentials for limited practice*, ed 2, Philadelphia, 2006, Saunders.)

Image Receptor Systems

Cassettes and Intensifying Screens

The cassette (Figure 49-9) serves as the film holder during the x-ray procedure. It provides a light-tight, rigid structure to protect the film and also houses *intensifying screens.* Most cassettes contain two intensifying screens, one front and one back, with the film sandwiched between them. Intensifying screens are plates coated with **phosphors** (fluorescent crystals) that give off light when exposed to x-rays. Their purpose is to reduce the amount of exposure required. Without intensifying screens, as much as 50 to 100 times more exposure would be needed. Intensifying screens greatly reduce the exposure of a patient to radiation during an x-ray procedure.

Each cassette has a small area where there is no intensifying screen and where exposure is blocked from the film by lead foil. This area is reserved for the photographic imprint of the patient identification. Its location is indicated on the front of the cassette by the position of the identifying label.

Intensifying screens are expensive and easily damaged. Damaged areas, dirt, or stains on the screens prevent light from exposing the film and result in artifacts on the image. For these reasons, it is important to avoid touching the screens and to keep the film processing area free of dust and dirt.

Film

Radiographic film is manufactured with a particular sensitivity to the light emitted by intensifying screens. Green-sensitive film is used with screens that emit green light, and blue-sensitive film is matched with blue-emitting screens. Film for routine radiography is coated on both sides so that the film responds to light from both intensifying screens. This double-emulsion system decreases the exposure required by half. Because both sides of the film are identical, there is no "right" or "wrong" side to a sheet of double-emulsion film.

Film and cassettes come in standard sizes. You will work more effectively in the clinical area when you have learned to recognize them at a glance. The most common sizes are as follows:

- 8 × 10 inches (20 × 25 cm)
- 9 × 9 inches (23 × 23 cm)
- 10 × 12 inches (25 × 30 cm)
- 11 × 14 inches (28 × 35 cm)
- 7 × 17 inches (18 × 43 cm)
- 14 × 14 inches (36 × 36 cm)
- 14 × 17 inches (36 × 43 cm)

Film Care and Handling. Film must be stored correctly to avoid fog, a generalized exposure that reduces image quality. A good storage area is clean, cool, and dry and is protected from radiation and processing chemical fumes. Film boxes should stand on edge with the expiration date visible. This date is checked to ensure that older film is used before its expiration date.

To avoid artifacts from improper film handling, be sure your hands are clean and dry, and touch only the corner of the film when removing it from the cassette. Avoid bending and crimping or scraping the film by allowing it to hang vertically when holding it with only one hand (Figure 49-10). To place it horizontally, use both hands and hold by opposite corners.

Film Processing. A comprehensive darkroom orientation is needed before you try to develop patient films. It is especially important to know how to turn on the processor properly and to know when it has warmed up sufficiently for correct processing.

The exposed cassette is taken to the darkroom for processing under safelight conditions. Safelights provide a red or orange light that is quite dim but provides just enough illumination for you to see where things are located. Make sure the darkroom door is locked so that no one will open it while you are processing the film.

Film identification is essential for knowing the identity of the patient represented in the image and the date and location of the examination. Serious errors in diagnosis and treatment might occur if films are not correctly identified. The identification information is typed on a card that is inserted into the photographic printer in the darkroom. The printer is used to stamp the information on the film after it is removed from the cassette and before it is processed (Figure 49-11).

The film is then fed into the automatic processor. The cassette is reloaded with a single sheet of fresh film (Figure 49-12) from the film bin, a storage unit located under the counter. A tone or a red light on the processor will indicate when it is safe to feed another film or to turn on the lights.

The reloaded cassette should be immediately returned to the proper place so that it is ready for use. Correct locations for cassettes are essential because it is not possible to determine by looking at the cassette whether the film is exposed. Only by following established routines and facility policies can you be confident that a cassette is unexposed and ready for use.

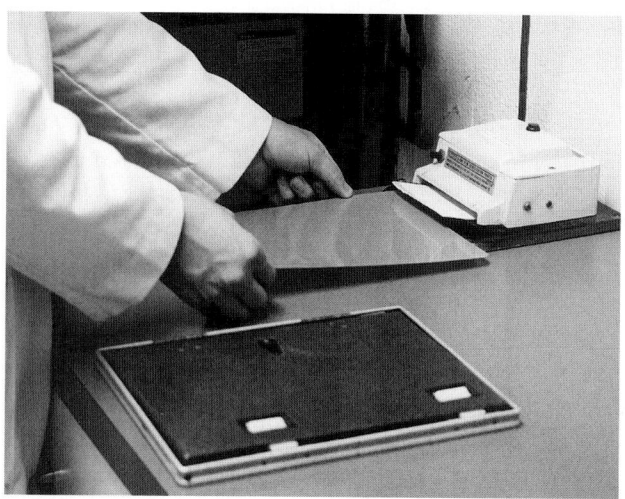

FIGURE 49-11 Film is inserted into printer to stamp it with identification from the printer card. (From Hunkele MM: *Radiography essentials for limited practice*, ed 2, Philadelphia, 2006, Saunders.)

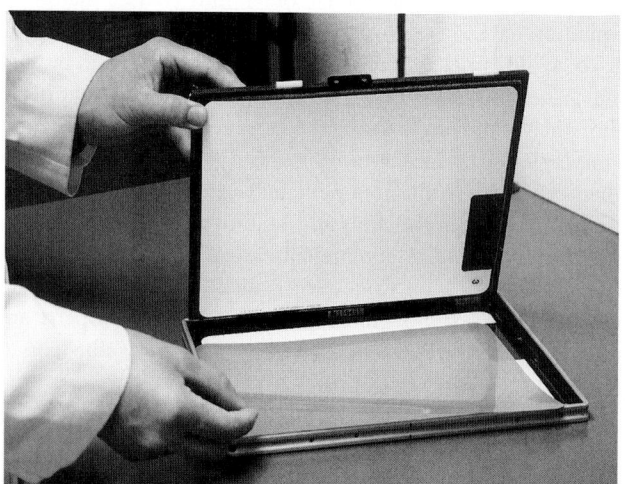

FIGURE 49-12 Reload cassette promptly with a fresh film. Make certain the film is properly situated, and secure both latches. (From Hunkele MM: *Radiography essentials for limited practice*, ed 2, Philadelphia, 2006, Saunders.)

Daylight Processing. Some departments have a "daylight" system to process film without a darkroom. These systems include a special film processor and a daylight film identification camera that uses special cassettes. Films can be identified while still in the cassette, then the entire cassette is fed into the processor. The processor automatically removes and processes the film then reloads the cassette with fresh film.

Computed and Digital Radiography

Computed radiography (CR) is a radiographic imaging system that does not use film. An image receptor, similar to an intensifying screen, is exposed in a special cassette using conventional x-ray equipment. The radiographer inserts the exposed cassette into a special processor and selects the type of examination from a menu so that the image will be processed correctly. A small beam from a high-intensity laser in the processor converts the latent image to a visible image that is converted into an electronic signal and stored in a computer. The image can then be displayed on a high-resolution monitor. Hard copies can be produced using a laser film printer.

Digital radiography is another type of filmless imaging system. Special radiographic tables and upright cabinets contain digital receptors that react to the pattern of the radiation from the patient and transmit a digital signal directly to the computer system. No cassettes and no processing are involved. Although digital radiography has for some time been used for special applications such as **fluoroscopy** and **angiography,** technical limitations and cost factors have prevented widespread adoption of digital systems for general radiography.

Once stored in the computer system, digital images from either computed or digital radiography are organized and cataloged and can be accessed on screen from multiple locations connected to the system network. These digital images can be manipulated electronically to enhance visibility. Conventional radiographs can be added to the system by scanning them with a laser device called a *film digitizer.*

The computer hardware and software technology used to manage digital images in hospitals and large health care systems is called a *picture archiving and communication system* (PACS). These systems provide image storage, connect images with patient database information, facilitate laser printing of images, and display both images and information at workstations throughout the network as needed. PACS may include transmission equipment for teleradiology, allowing images to be viewed in remote locations such as a physician's home and receiving images from remote locations such as outlying clinics. PACS technology can transmit images directly over telephone lines and via the Internet. These advanced technologies will become more commonplace as computerized medical record systems become more widespread.

RADIOGRAPHIC POSITIONING

The medical assistant may be involved in either explaining x-ray positions to a patient or actually helping the patient into various positions, so it is important that you are familiar with commonly used terms. Terms that indicate the surfaces,

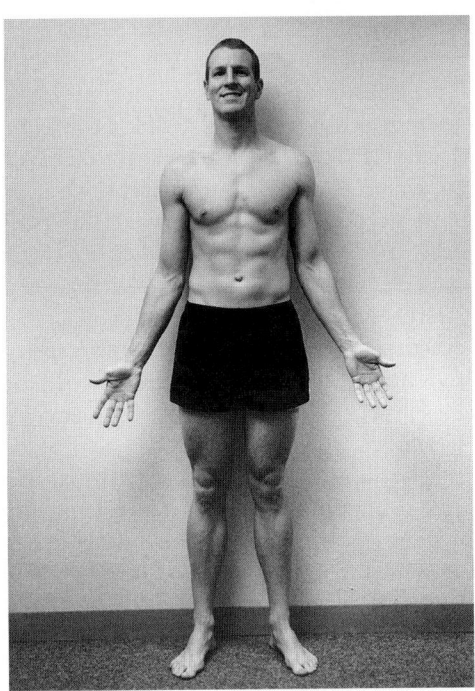

FIGURE 49-13 Anatomic position. (From Hunkele MM: *Radiography essentials for limited practice*, ed 2, Philadelphia, 2006, Saunders.)

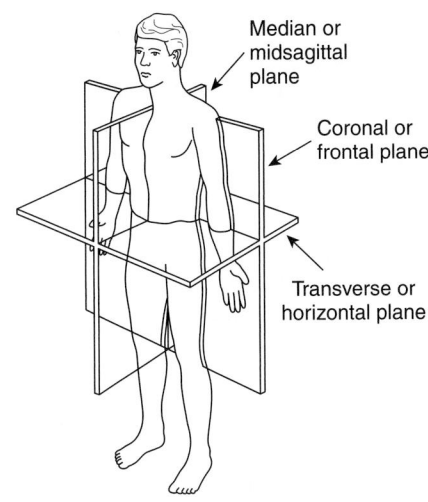

FIGURE 49-14 Body planes. (From Hunkele MM: *Radiography essentials for limited practice*, ed 2, Philadelphia, 2006, Saunders.)

directions, and planes of various body locations are based on the anatomic position.

As shown in Figure 49-13, *anatomic position* is a view of the body in which the individual is standing, facing the observer, with the palms of the hands forward. Terms that describe locations on and within the body include the following:

- Anterior: Forward or front portion of the body or body part.
- Cephalic: Pertaining to the head; toward the head.
- Caudal: Toward the tail or end of the body; away from the head; the opposite of cephalic.
- Distal: Away from the source or point of origin. For example, the wrist is distal to the elbow, the elbow distal to the shoulder.
- External: To the outside, at or near the surface of the body or a body part.
- Inferior: Below, farther from the head. For example, the diaphragm is inferior to the lungs.
- Internal: Deep, near the center of the body or a part; the opposite of external.
- Lateral: Referring to the side, away from the center to the left or right.
- Medial: Toward the center of the body or body part; the opposite of lateral.
- Palmar: Referring to the palm (anterior surface) of the hand.
- Plantar: Referring to the sole of the foot.
- Posterior: Backward or back portion of the body or body part; the opposite of anterior.
- Proximal: Toward the source or point of origin; the opposite of distal. For example, the part of the femur that

is attached at the hip is the proximal end of the femur, and the part of the bone that is located at the knee is the distal end of the femur.

- Superior: Above, toward the head; the opposite of inferior. For example, the esophagus is superior to the stomach.

Besides anatomic positional terms, procedures for radiographic positioning are also described using the planes of the body (Figure 49-14). The **sagittal plane** divides the body into right and left parts, and the midsagittal plane divides the body into equal right and left parts. The **coronal plane** divides the body into anterior and posterior parts. The midcoronal or midfrontal plane divides the body into relatively equal parts; it passes through the external auditory meatus (the opening of the ear), the center of the shoulder, the greater trochanter (the bony prominence in the lateral hip area), and the lateral malleolus (the bony prominence on the lateral surface of the ankle). The **transverse plane** divides the body into superior and inferior portions. It may be drawn at any level.

The medical assistant may assist with radiographic procedures by helping position the patient for a particular x-ray view. These positions can be used as follows in x-ray positioning:

- Prone: Lying face down
- Recumbent: Lying down; the position may be further described by adding the name of the body surface on which the patient is lying:
  - Dorsal recumbent: lying on the back (supine) with the knees bent and the feet flat on the table
  - Lateral recumbent: lying on the side
  - Ventral recumbent: lying face down, prone
- Supine: lying on the back face up
- Upright: standing or seated

Projections

A radiographic projection indicates the relative positions of the body part that is meant to be x-rayed, the film, and the placement of the x-ray tube.

For a **frontal projection,** the coronal plane of the body or body part is parallel to the film plane and the central ray is perpendicular to both. If the patient is supine, or facing the x-ray tube, the projection is said to be **anteroposterior (AP)** (Figure 49-15). If the patient is prone, or facing the film, the projection is said to be **posteroanterior (PA)** (Figure 49-16). Note that these

terms indicate the direction of the x-ray beam, from front to back or back to front.

Lateral projections are those in which the sagittal plane of the body or body part is parallel to the film. Lateral projections are always named for the side of the patient that is nearest the film—that is, either left or right lateral (Figure 49-17).

Oblique projections are those in which the body or part is rotated so that the projection is neither frontal nor lateral. Oblique projections are also named for the part of the body that is nearest the film. For example, in a right anterior oblique (RAO) projection, the patient's right, anterior aspect is closest to the film. Figure 49-18 illustrates all four oblique projections: RAO, right posterior oblique (RPO), left anterior oblique (LAO), and left posterior oblique (LPO).

Axial projections, sometimes referred to as *semiaxial projections,* are radiographs taken with a longitudinal angulation of the x-ray beam. The x-ray beam is projected at an angle, either cephalad (toward the head) or caudad (away from the head) (Figure 49-19).

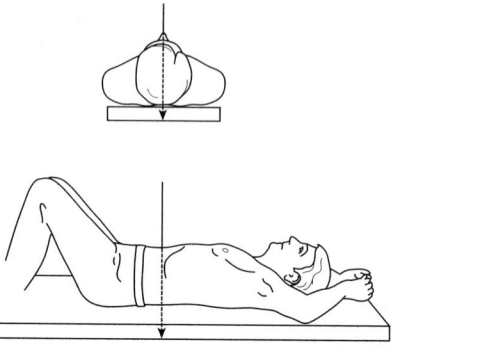

FIGURE 49-15 Anteroposterior (AP) projection. (From Hunkele MM: *Radiography essentials for limited practice,* ed 2, Philadelphia, 2006, Saunders.)

DIAGNOSTIC IMAGING MODALITIES

Fluoroscopy and Contrast Media

Fluoroscopy
Fluoroscopy is a technique using special equipment that permits the **radiologist** to view x-ray images in motion. Fluoroscopy also permits the physician to survey an area quickly, without the delay involved in taking and processing films. Most fluoroscopic units are properly called *radiographic/fluoroscopic* (R/F) units because they are designed to take both x-ray images and

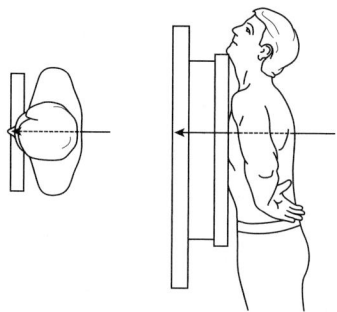

FIGURE 49-16 Posteroanterior (PA) projection. (From Hunkele MM: *Radiography essentials for limited practice,* ed 2, Philadelphia, 2006, Saunders.)

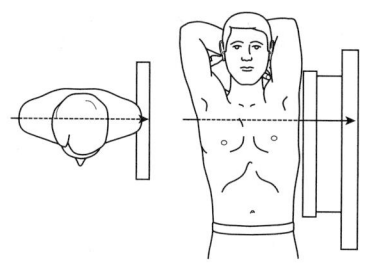
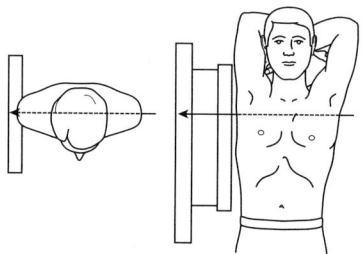

Left lateral   Right lateral

FIGURE 49-17 Lateral projections are named for the side of the body nearer the film. (From Hunkele MM: *Radiography essentials for limited practice,* ed 2, Philadelphia, 2006, Saunders.)

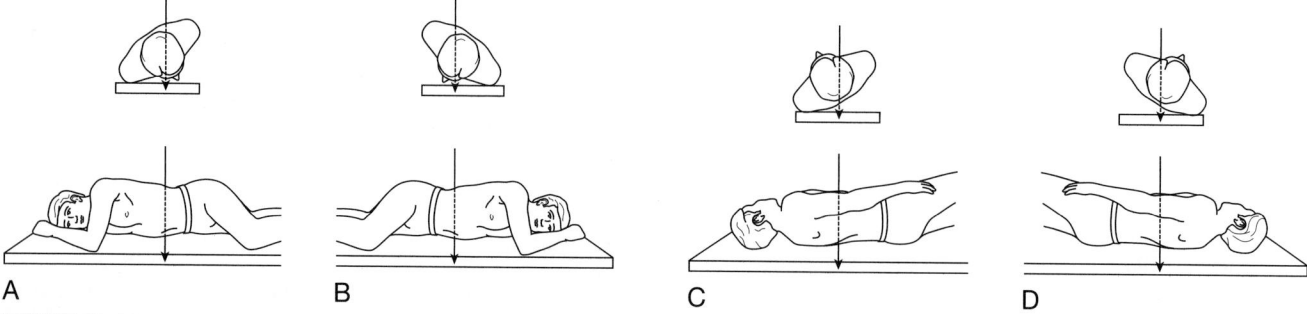

A   B   C   D

FIGURE 49-18 Oblique projections. **A,** Right anterior oblique (RAO). **B,** Left anterior oblique (LAO). **C,** Left posterior oblique (LPO). **D,** Right posterior oblique (RPO). (From Hunkele MM: *Radiography essentials for limited practice,* ed 2, Philadelphia, 2006, Saunders.)

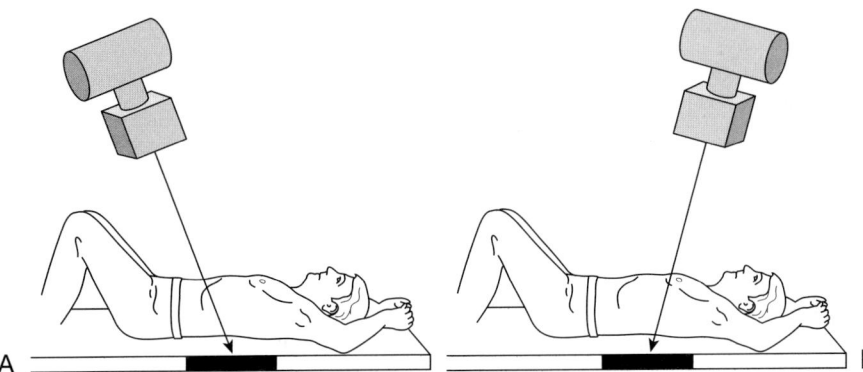

FIGURE 49-19 Axial projections use angulation of the x-ray tube to direct the central ray along the long axis of the body or part. **A,** Cephalad angulation. **B,** Caudad angulation. (From Hunkele MM: *Radiography essentials for limited practice*, ed 2, Philadelphia, 2006, Saunders.)

fluoroscopic views. The x-ray films taken during a fluoroscopic procedure are called *"spot films"* and record the image as seen on the fluoroscope; sometimes the entire fluoroscopic examination is recorded digitally, on videotape, or on cine (movie) film. After the fluoroscopic portion of the study is completed, larger radiographs are usually taken for comprehensive visualization of the entire anatomic region.

An example of a fluoroscopic diagnostic procedure is a barium swallow. If the physician suspects that the patient has difficulty swallowing, a fluoroscope is used to visualize the actual movement of the substance down the esophagus and into the stomach while the patient is in the act of swallowing. Fluoroscopic procedures typically require the use of **contrast media** such as barium.

X-Ray Studies Using Contrast Media

Although the lungs and bony structures of the body produce clear x-ray images on plain film radiographs, internal organs such as the stomach and the kidneys are difficult to see because they absorb radiation to the same degree as the tissues that surround them. To enhance visibility of these structures, special agents called *contrast media* can be used to fill hollow organs and demonstrate their inner contours. Although gases such as air and carbon dioxide are sometimes used as contrast media, it is far more common to use radiopaque substances such as barium sulfate or iodine compounds. The agent and the technique vary with the structures to be viewed.

Among the most common fluoroscopic examinations are studies of the upper and lower gastrointestinal (GI) tract using barium sulfate as a contrast medium. Both require careful patient instruction and advance preparation for a successful study. An **upper gastrointestinal (UGI)** series (Figure 49-20) uses oral administration of a barium sulfate suspension to diagnose ulcers, tumors, and other abnormalities of the esophagus, stomach, and duodenum.

A **lower gastrointestinal series** (Figure 49-21) involves a barium enema that fills the colon and helps visualize its inner surfaces. This procedure is especially useful in the diagnosis of polyps, tumors, and diverticulosis. For this examination the inner lining of the large intestine must be clean and free of all fecal matter. The preparation may be complex, taking place over several days. Commercial bowel preparation kits are usually made available by the radiology department to ensure complete

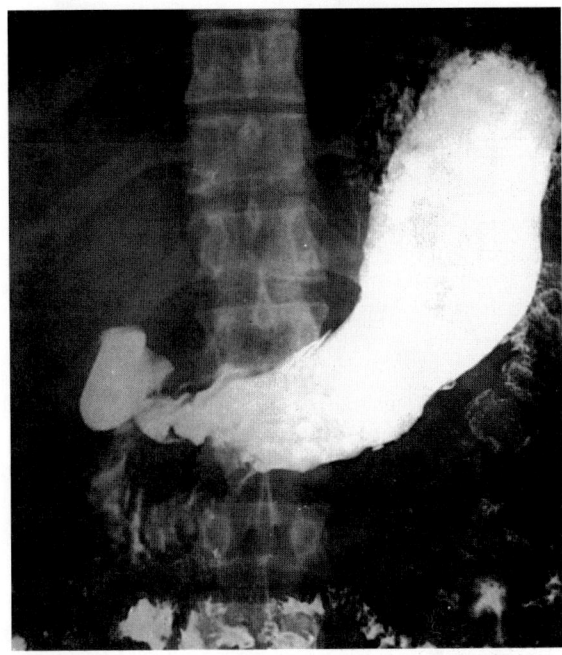

FIGURE 49-20 Radiographic image of the stomach, part of an upper gastrointestinal (UGI) series using oral administration of barium sulfate to provide contrast. (From Ballinger PW, Frank ED: *Merrill's atlas of radiographic positions and radiologic procedures*, ed 10, vol 2, St Louis, 2003, Mosby.)

emptying of the large intestine. If preparation is not adequate then the examination will have to be rescheduled.

Water-soluble iodine compounds are used as contrast media for a wide variety of applications. When injected intravenously, the contrast agent circulates in the blood and is excreted by the kidneys, causing the urine to become radiopaque. Radiography of the kidneys, ureters, and bladder after intravenous (IV) contrast injection is called an **intravenous urogram (IVU)** and is useful in identifying kidney stones, tumors, and other abnormalities of the urinary tract. Preparation for an IVU involves fasting and bowel cleansing, although the preparation is usually less rigorous than for a lower GI series.

Iodine contrast agents can also be injected into joint capsules to produce an **arthrogram,** an image of the soft-tissue components of joints, especially the knee and the shoulder. **Myelography** involves injection of iodine compounds into the spinal canal to demonstrate spinal pathology such as tumors and

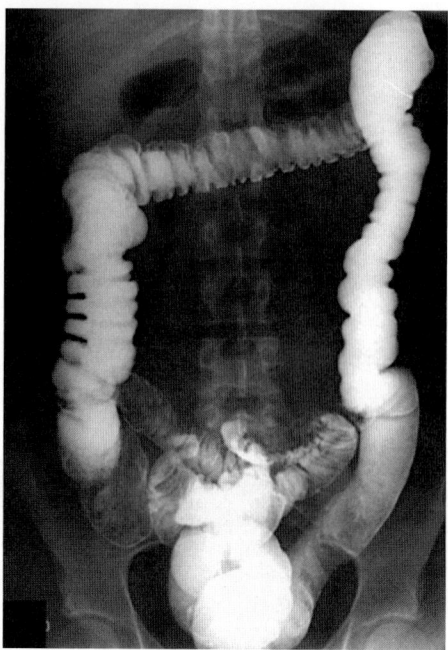

FIGURE 49-21 Lower gastrointestinal (GI) series. Radiograph of the colon filled with barium sulfate administered by way of a barium enema. (From Ballinger PW, Frank ED: *Merrill's atlas of radiographic positions and radiologic procedures,* ed 10, vol 2, St Louis, 2003, Mosby.)

herniated intervertebral disks. Table 49-1 lists some common radiographic examinations using contrast media, together with the route of contrast administration and the structures that are visualized. Part of the screening process for diagnostic procedures that use iodine contrast injections is carefully questioning the patient regarding a history of iodine allergy. All patients who are allergic to shellfish will also be allergic to iodine dye and are at risk for a serious anaphylactic reaction if the contrast agent is injected. The medical assistant is responsible for clarifying allergies with the patient and/or family members and alerting

the diagnostic facility if the patient does have an iodine allergy. In addition, patients need to understand that it is normal to feel flushed or a heat rush when the dye is injected and that some patients initially experience waves of nausea. However, both of these sensations pass quickly.

Cardiovascular and Interventional Radiography

The highly specialized radiographic procedures that display blood vessels are collectively known as angiography. A cerebral angiogram, for example, demonstrates the vessels of the brain (Figure 49-22), and renal angiograms show the arteries and veins of the kidneys. An **angiocardiogram** is a contrast study that shows the interior of the heart chambers and the great vessels that enter and exit the heart, and an **aortogram** demonstrates the aorta. Selective **angiocardiography,** or cardiac catheterization, is used to display the coronary arteries. **Arteriograms** are pictures of specific arteries, and **venograms** are studies of veins.

For all these examinations, iodine compounds are injected for radiographic contrast and a rapid series of films is taken or fluoroscopy is used to show the area of concern. Direct injection may be used for some angiographic studies, such as those of the extremities, but the preferred injection method for angiocardiography, aortography, and most **arteriography** is to use a special catheter. A large artery, usually the femoral or brachial, is entered with a large-bore needle, and a guidewire is threaded through the needle and into the artery under fluoroscopic control. The needle is then removed, the guidewire is left in the vessel, and the catheter is threaded over the wire. The wire is then removed, and the catheter remains in the artery for the duration of the examination. Further manipulation of the catheter may be needed to ensure correct placement in the vessel before injection. For selective catheterization of smaller vessels, the catheter tip is maneuvered into the root of the vessel of interest, such as the coronary, celiac, renal, or carotid artery.

A timed sequence of images is taken during and after injection of the contrast medium, usually with the aid of an

TABLE 49-1 Radiographic Procedures Using Contrast Media

EXAMINATION	CONTRAST MEDIUM	ROUTE OF ADMINISTRATION	STRUCTURES SHOWN
Angiocardiography	Iodine compounds	Intraarterial injection via femoral or brachial catheter	Heart and large vessels
Angiography	Iodine compounds	Intraarterial or intravenous injection	Blood vessels
Arteriography	Iodine compounds	Intraarterial injection via catheter	Arteries
Arthrography	Iodine compounds	Direct injection into joint capsule	Joints, especially knee, shoulder, and ankle
Barium swallow	Barium sulfate suspension	Oral	Esophagus
Hysterosalpingography	Iodine compounds	Direct injection via cannula	Uterus and fallopian tubes
Intravenous urography	Iodine compounds	Intravenous injection	Kidneys, ureters, and urinary bladder
Lower GI series (barium enema)	Barium sulfate suspension, sometimes also with air	Rectal catheter	Colon
Lymphangiography	Iodine compounds	Direct injection to lymphatic vessels in the feet	Lymphatic vessels and lymph nodes
Myelography	Iodine compounds	Intrathecal injection (spinal tap)	Spinal canal
Upper GI Series	Barium sulfate suspension	Oral	Esophagus, stomach, and duodenum

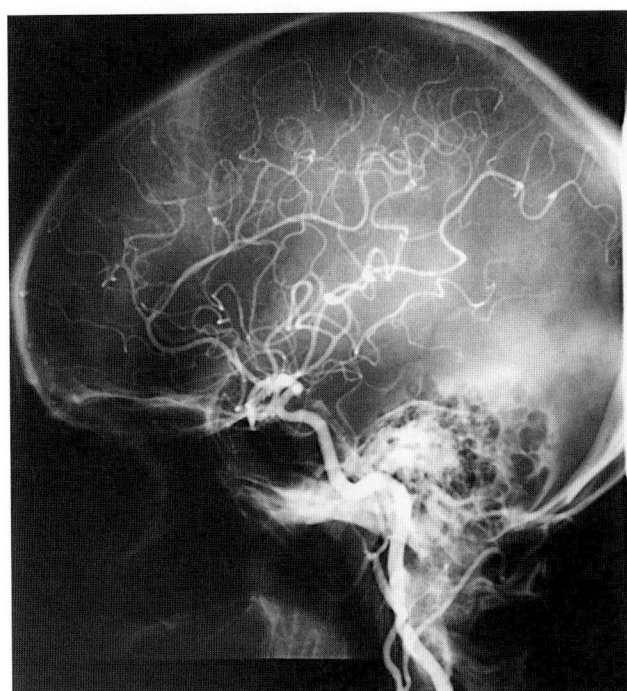

FIGURE 49-22 Cerebral angiogram shows the circulation of the brain enhanced by iodine contrast medium. (From Ballinger PW, Frank ED: *Merrill's atlas of radiographic positions and radiologic procedures,* ed 10, vol 2, St Louis, 2003, Mosby.)

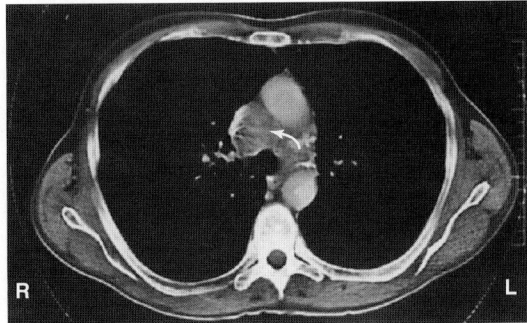

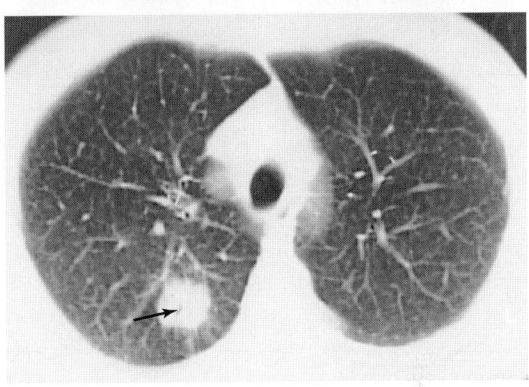

FIGURE 49-23 Two computed tomography windows demonstrate structures of the chest from the same image. **A,** Mediastinal structures are demonstrated in the center of the field, but the lungs are not well seen. **B,** "Lung window" demonstrates the blood vessels of the lungs and a lung tumor *(arrow).* (From Seeram E: Computed tomography, ed 2, Philadelphia, 2001, Saunders.)

automatic power injector that is electronically coordinated with a programmable film changer and automated exposure control. Digital receptors are replacing film and film changers in some imaging centers, and for some studies, such as angiocardiograms, digital fluoroscopy equipment may be used to record the images.

Because these procedures are expensive and involve a relatively high degree of risk, angiography has been replaced somewhat by technologic advances in other imaging modalities discussed in this chapter, particularly Doppler ultrasound, **nuclear medicine,** magnetic resonance angiography (MRA), and computed tomography angiography (CTA).

Despite these advances, angiography continues to be used extensively because it provides the best anatomic view of structures within the circulatory system and also offers the opportunity for immediate therapeutic interventions to treat vascular problems as they are identified. Specialized catheter techniques are used for vessel repair, called **angioplasty,** to widen or open arteries that are narrowed or occluded. **Embolization** refers to therapeutic intervention techniques that decrease or stop blood flow to control hemorrhage, cut off blood supply to a tumor, or reduce blood loss during surgery.

Computed Tomography

Computed tomography (CT), formerly called *computerized axial tomography (CAT)* scanning, uses a special x-ray scanner to produce detailed pictures of a cross-section of tissue. The x-ray studies are taken in the transverse plane and can be "reconstructed" by the computer to display anatomic structures in other planes as well. The images are viewed in a variety of formats, called *"windows,"* which are designed to enhance

the views of specific tissues (Figure 49-23). Multiple levels of pictures can be taken in a very short period of time, with up to 25 continuous images recorded in the time it takes the patient to hold a single breath. Most CT examinations are noninvasive, are painless, and do not require any special patient preparation. However, the equipment may cause apprehension because standard machines require the patient enter a tube for the procedure. Careful explanations are necessary to achieve patient cooperation and a satisfactory outcome of the study.

The CT scanner (Figure 49-24) consists of a movable table with remote control, a circular **gantry** structure that supports the x-ray tube and detectors, an operator console with a monitor, and a supporting computer system. The CT unit also includes both hardware and software to archive and manage data and produce hard copies of images. During a scan the x-ray tube rotates around the patient to collect data. In conventional CT units the tube makes a complete rotation to gather data for each slice. The table then moves, and the tube rotates again to obtain the next slice. A newer generation of scanners, designated as *spiral* or *helical,* scans a spiral path around the patient and can collect data on a larger volume of tissue. These scanners can reconstruct views to create three-dimensional images.

The versatility of CT is illustrated by its wide range of applications, including studies of the brain, spine, abdomen, pelvis, chest, neck, and paranasal sinuses. CT is a valuable tool for emergency use, especially in the detection of intracerebral or intraabdominal hemorrhage. It is also used for orthopedic examinations of the extremities and for contrast-enhanced

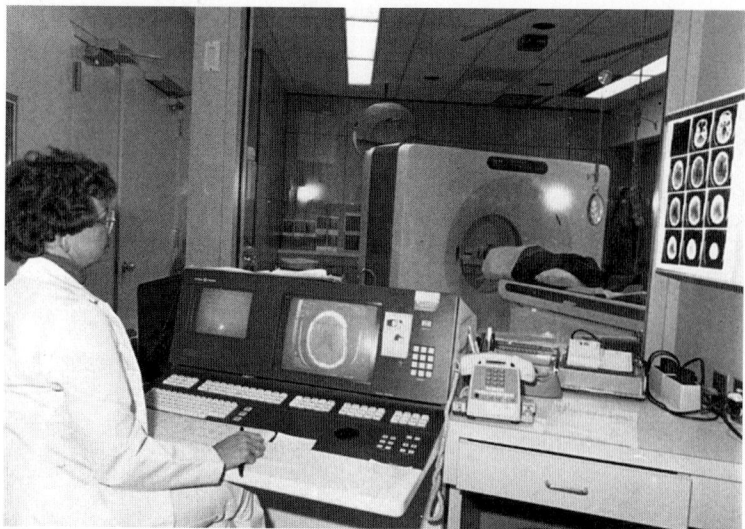

FIGURE 49-24 Computed tomography (CT) technologist monitors the patient while performing a CT scan of the brain. (From Ehrlich RA, McCloskey ED, Daly JA: *Patient care in radiography*, ed 6, St Louis, 2004, Mosby.)

vascular studies. CT is useful in localizing both lesions and needle position during needle-aspiration biopsy, a nonsurgical method of obtaining cells for laboratory examination, and is often used with myelography to expand the range of information available.

Although many CT examinations do not require contrast media, the use of contrast agents vastly increases the scope of CT imaging. Studies of the abdomen usually use oral contrast media to help differentiate the GI tract from the surrounding tissues. A special barium compound or an oral iodine preparation is ingested by the patient over a specified period before the study. The amount of contrast medium and the time period vary depending on whether the examination includes only the upper abdomen or the entire abdomen and pelvis. For these studies, the patient is instructed to not eat for 12 hours and to report to the facility early to drink the contrast preparation before the procedure is scheduled. Some departments have the patient take the contrast medium home with instructions to drink it before reporting for the appointment.

IV injection of an iodine contrast medium may also be employed to increase the contrast level of the patient's tissues. This is advantageous for studies of the chest, abdomen, and soft tissues of the neck because it highlights blood vessels and enhances visibility of vascular organs such as the liver and spleen. The contrast defines the internal structures of the kidneys, ureters, and bladder as the agent is excreted in the urine (Figure 49-25). In selected cases IV contrast agents are employed in CT scans of the head to demonstrate brain lesions.

Magnetic Resonance Imaging

Magnetic resonance imaging (MRI) is a noninvasive diagnostic modality that allows visualization of anatomic structures without the use of radioactive x-rays. A powerful magnetic field and radiofrequency pulses are combined to produce a radio signal in the body that can be detected and processed electronically to provide images on a computer monitor. The images can be managed in a computer database and can also be stored on magnetic tape and photographed with a special camera to produce film copies that appear similar to x-ray images.

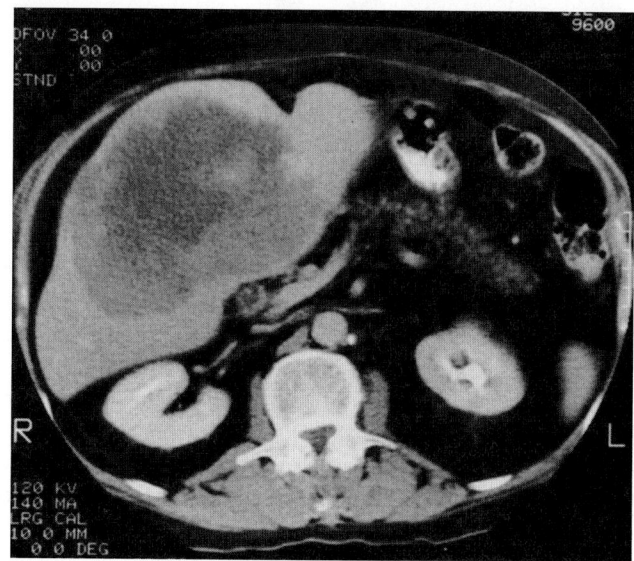

FIGURE 49-25 Axial computed tomography "slice" of the abdomen demonstrates contrast-enhanced liver, kidney, and intestinal structures. (From Ehrlich RA, McCloskey ED, Daly JA: *Patient care in radiography*, ed 6, St Louis, 2004, Mosby.)

The MRI gantry houses the magnet and the main radiofrequency coil. Conventional gantries are tubular, are 5 to 8 feet long, and typically require the body part being studied to be placed in the tube during the scanning process. An open gantry design, the open MRI, provides better accommodation for large or claustrophobic patients, but it does not always provide image quality equal to that produced by conventional units.

MRI provides excellent imaging of the soft tissues of the nervous system (Figure 49-26) and is useful in the diagnosis of many types of pathology, including brain and spinal cord tumors and diseases such as multiple sclerosis. MRI is also used for the diagnosis of herniated intervertebral disks and to obtain images of the soft-tissue components of joints, particularly the knee, shoulder, and temporomandibular joint. A more recent advance in MRI is MRA, which uses magnetic resonance technology to study the cardiovascular system. MRA aids in the

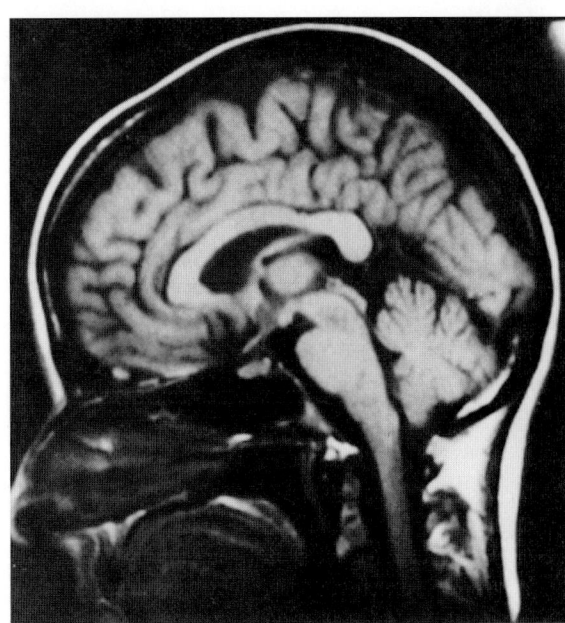

FIGURE 49-26 Midsagittal magnetic resonance image of the brain. (From Ehrlich RA, McCloskey ED, Daly JA: *Patient care in radiography*, ed 6, St Louis, 2004, Mosby.)

diagnosis and treatment of heart disorders, stroke, and blood vessel diseases.

Typical scan time for a series of slicelike images ranges from 1 to 10 minutes, and several series demonstrating different body planes and using a variety of radiofrequency pulse sequences may be included in an examination. It is critically important that the patient remain still during a scan series and that the initial position be maintained throughout the study.

Although contrast media are not required for most MRI studies, special paramagnetic agents are sometimes injected intravenously. These agents provide contrast enhancement of certain lesions, particularly brain and spinal cord tumors, and aid in differentiating disk material from scar tissue in postoperative spinal examinations. Contrast injections are also used in MRA studies.

The unique MRI environment requires special safety precautions. Conditions affecting patient safety involve both the powerful magnetic field within the gantry and the thermal effects of radiofrequency pulses on certain materials that could overheat and possibly burn the patient. The principal means of ensuring patient safety during an MRI is careful patient screening before the procedure. Although extensive patient interviews are conducted in the magnetic resonance department, preliminary screening of patients should be conducted by the medical assistant before the appointment is made. The magnetic field or the rapid radiofrequency pulses may be hazardous for patients with artificial heart valves, aneurysm clips, neurostimulators, middle ear prostheses, or intrauterine devices. Cardiac pacemakers are a particular hazard, and patients with pacemakers cannot have MRI examinations. Fatalities have resulted from overheating of these implanted devices when patients with pacemakers were scanned. Other conditions that merit assessment before the patient enters the magnetic field

include hemolytic anemia, orthopedic pins and screws, and metal fragments or shrapnel in the soft tissues. Most orthopedic hardware is safe in the magnet, although it may compromise image quality in the surrounding area.

Metalworkers who might have steel slivers in their tissues must have a screening x-ray or CT head examination to detect fragments that could damage their eyes or brain because the pull of the magnetic field is so strong that it could cause the fragments to move. Although the energies involved in MRI have not been demonstrated to cause complications with pregnancy, the current philosophy is to avoid examination of pregnant patients except in urgent cases, especially during the first trimester.

Patients should be assured that everything possible will be done to provide assistance in dealing with both physical and emotional discomfort. Few people are completely comfortable for any length of time in a tightly enclosed space. Even patients with no history of claustrophobia may feel anxious when entering a conventional tubular MRI gantry. Occasionally, this anxiety is so severe that it creates panic, preventing the patient from continuing the examination.

Patients may be reassured if they know what to expect in advance. The procedure requires that the patient lie down on the MRI table, which will then automatically move into the gantry. Plenty of air is available, and there is no physical discomfort except for the need to lie still. The machine will make a loud "knocking" noise during the scanning process (similar to a hammer tapping metal). Earplugs or earphones with recorded music may be offered. Patients can communicate with the technologist through an intercom, and the technologist will be watching and listening from an adjacent area throughout the procedure. Because no radiation danger exists, a friend or family member can sit in the room if the patient feels more comfortable with company. Severely claustrophobic patients may be scheduled at a facility with an open-gantry MRI or may be given an antianxiety medication before the procedure. Analgesic medications may be administered to patients whose pain makes it impossible to lie still for the duration of the study.

Sonography

Diagnostic medical **sonography** is a noninvasive procedure that is considered to be very safe for the patient. Sonography was introduced in Chapter 40 because it is used extensively for fetal imaging. This imaging modality, often referred to as *diagnostic ultrasound*, uses high-frequency sound waves to produce echoes within the body. As the echoes return to the sending point, or **transducer,** their strength and timing are interpreted by a computer to produce a map or graphic image of the echo distribution.

The transducer is covered with a lubricant and is moved over the surface of the body so the image can be viewed in real time on a computer monitor. Special transducer probes can be inserted into body cavities such as the rectum and the vagina to obtain more detailed examinations of the prostate gland and the uterus. Any interface between substances or tissues of varying density produces an ultrasound echo, making sonography an

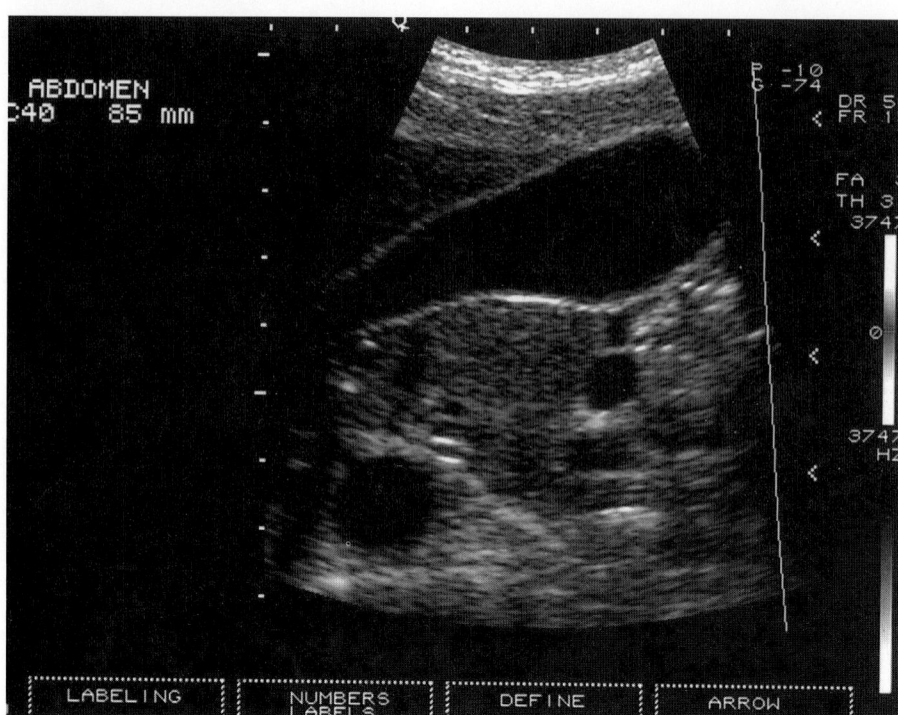

FIGURE 49-27 Abdominal sonogram. (From Ballinger PW, Frank ED: *Merrill's atlas of radiographic positions and radiologic procedures*, ed 10, vol 2, St Louis, 2003, Mosby.)

effective technique to show the shape, size, and condition of organs such as the heart, spleen, gallbladder, breast, and pancreas (Figure 49-27). Sonography can also be used to detect the presence of an abscess, cyst, or tumor in adipose tissue. Recent advances in ultrasound technology include computer integration of data to produce three-dimensional images. In addition, Doppler ultrasound is used to detect vascular disease, such as atherosclerosis in the carotid arteries and venous thrombosis of the lower extremities.

Nuclear Medicine

Nuclear medicine images are created by scanning the patient after special radioactive materials called **tracers** have been swallowed or injected intravenously. Tracers are similar to substances that are commonly used by the body, so they enter into the same chemical reactions and are metabolized in a similar way. They are taken up in the target organ or tissue over a period of time that may vary from half an hour to several days. The tracer can then be detected and its location recorded by a special nuclear medicine scanner called a *gamma camera*. Two types of tracers used in diagnostic studies are radioactive iodine and radioactive carbon.

Nuclear medicine scans do not provide clear images of anatomic structures. They are used to obtain information about the function of organs and tissues. Abnormal tissues are demonstrated on the image because the tracer is metabolized at a different rate, at a different location, or to a greater or lesser extent than in normal tissue.

Figure 49-28 is an example of a nuclear medicine bone scan. The tracer is absorbed by the bones and appears in greater or lesser amounts depending on the level of metabolic activity within the bone. In this scan the region of the right shoulder shows a high level of radioactivity that indicates an

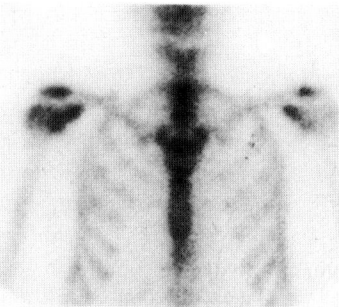

FIGURE 49-28 Bone scan showing increased tracer uptake in right shoulder region resulting from inflammation.

inflammatory process. Tumors of the bone can be diagnosed by "hot spots" in the x-ray image that show up much brighter because of rapid cellular division, resulting in a higher level of metabolic activity.

Structures that are visualized using nuclear medicine techniques include the thyroid gland, liver, lungs, brain, skeletal system, kidneys, heart, and blood vessels. Thallium stress studies of the heart are nuclear medicine examinations that permit the physician to view the coronary arteries to diagnose or rule out blockage. Incomplete visualization of the myocardium after administration of a nuclear tracer indicates lack of blood supply to the area and damage to the muscle of the heart. Table 49-2 lists some common nuclear medicine procedures and their purposes.

The radioisotopes used in nuclear medicine decay within a short time, from a few hours to a few days, and are eliminated in the urine or feces. They have a very low level of radioactivity and produce less exposure to the patient than most x-ray examinations. Positron emission tomography (PET) and single

TABLE 49-2 Common Nuclear Medicine Procedures

PROCEDURE	PURPOSE
Bone scan	Helps to detect fractures, tumors, and inflammation; used to determine bone growth
Brain scan	Often used together with other imaging methods to detect tumors and vascular problems
Liver scan	Useful in diagnosing cirrhosis and hepatitis and in detecting tumors and liver abscesses
Lung scan	Often done to detect emboli, blood clots that have traveled through the bloodstream to the lungs
Thallium stress test	Used for evaluation of cardiac condition and response to stress
Thyroid scan	The rate of uptake is an indicator of thyroid function and is also useful in detection of tumors

photon emission computed tomography (SPECT) are highly specialized nuclear medicine techniques that use different types of tracers and scanners than conventional nuclear medicine, but the basic principle is the same. Radioactive substances from within the body are detected and mapped by specialized equipment to obtain information about the function of organs, tissues, or systems. These newer modalities acquire digital images that can be reconstructed by the computer to render images in multiple planes and dimensions.

BASIC RADIOGRAPHIC PROCEDURE

Patient Preparation and Explanation

Before a patient undergoes x-ray studies, a physician examines the patient and orders one or more specific x-ray procedures to help diagnose the patient's problem or to follow up on a previously diagnosed condition. The physician is responsible for getting the patient's informed consent for any procedure but may ask the medical assistant to make sure the consent form is signed. For diagnostic studies that are not invasive the patient may not have to sign a consent form, because acceptance of the procedure is adequate evidence of consent. In some facilities, however, patients may be asked to sign a consent form regardless of the type of radiographic procedure. If it is your duty to answer patient questions about the procedure or assist with obtaining consent, be certain that you are prepared to do so.

Patients often express concerns about radiation exposure. You can assure them with confidence that the risks are extremely small and outweigh the health risks of treatment without the information that the examination will provide. It may help to point out that the radiographer is well trained in radiation safety and that the equipment is designed to provide good images with the least possible exposure. You can explain that the amount of radiation involved in the procedure is less than the exposure to natural background radiation that the population receives every year.

Patient preparation for routine radiography involves removing outer clothing from the area to be radiographed and providing a gown if appropriate. Underwear is usually not a problem. No metal objects should be included in the radiation field because these items will appear as artifacts on the images. This includes jewelry; zippers, snaps, and other clothing fasteners; underwire bras; and the contents of pockets. Nonmetal objects

that are thick or heavy should also be removed. Buttons and the heavy seams in jeans are examples of other clothing items that can cause artifacts on radiographs if they are in the imaging field. Metal items that are not in the radiation field are not a problem, so there is no reason for patients to remove jewelry or clothing that will not be included in the radiograph. When the patient is ready, the next step in the radiographic procedure is to assist the patient into the general position required for the x-ray examination (Figure 49-29). For example, if a hand is to be imaged, the patient can be seated at the end of the x-ray examination table (Figure 49-29, A). If a chest examination is ordered, the patient will stand at an upright film holder (Figure 49-29, C). For a spine examination the patient may need to lie on the table (Figure 4-29, B).

The radiographer then selects the correct cassette, places a lead marker on it to identify the patient's right or left side, and places the cassette in position for the exposure (Figure 49-30). Next, the patient is positioned precisely and the x-ray tube is aligned with the body part and the film at a specific distance (Figure 49-31). The body part must be measured to determine the proper exposure factors according to a technique chart. At this point, lead shields are positioned for radiation protection. The radiographer then goes to the control booth, consults the technique chart, and sets the x-ray control panel to the desired exposure. Final instructions are given to the patient (typically that the patient must remain still during the x-ray procedure) and the exposure is made. If more than one exposure is needed, the film is changed, the patient is repositioned, and the steps are repeated until the examination is complete (Procedure 49-1).

After ensuring that the patient is safe and comfortable, the film is taken to the darkroom for processing. Film processing usually requires less than 10 minutes before the film can be evaluated. If the film is satisfactory and no further exposures are needed, the patient is returned to an examination room or dressing room. The radiographer or the medical assistant then readies the x-ray room for the next examination and prepares the films for interpretation.

The films are kept together and given to the physician with the appropriate paperwork. Films are kept in large file envelopes that may contain more than one set of films for the same patient. These envelopes must be accurately identified for proper filing. When images are added to the file, notations are often added to the envelope. After the films have been read,

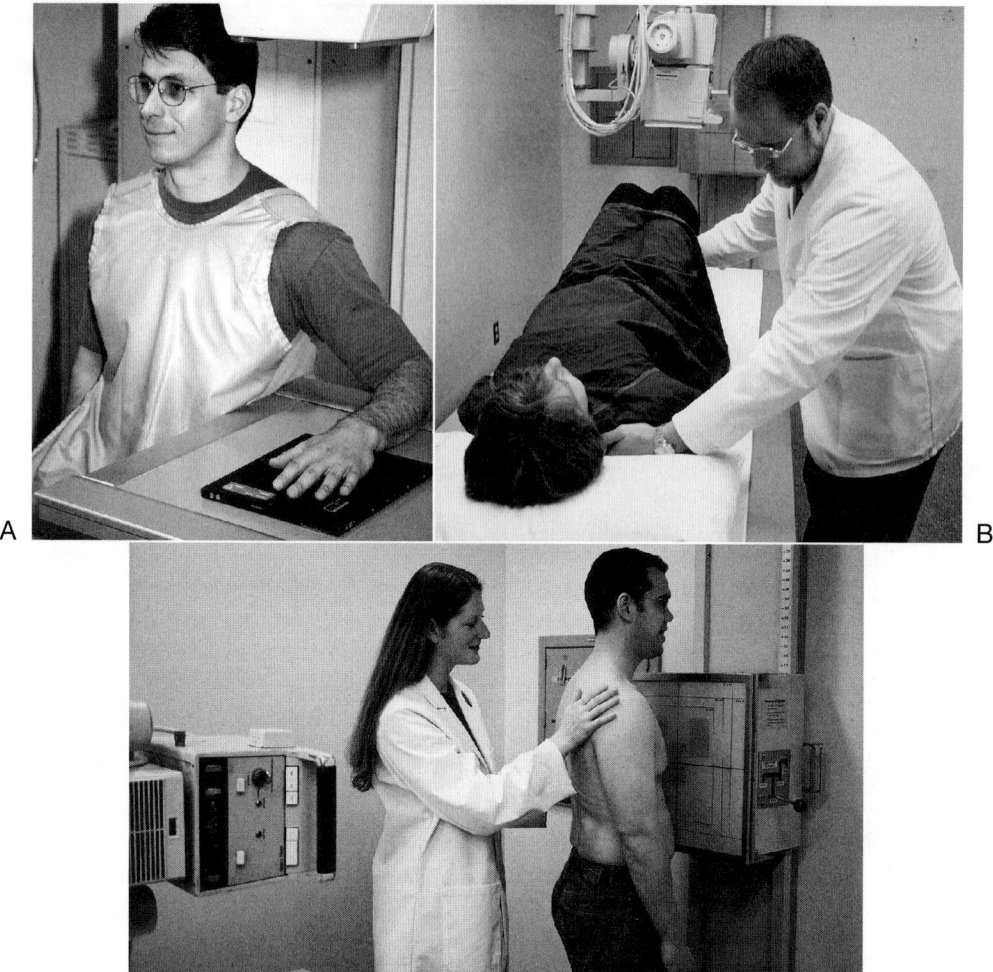

FIGURE 49-29 General positions for radiography. **A,** Patient may be seated at the x-ray table for some upper-extremity examinations. **B,** Radiographer assists patient to lie down for spine radiography. **C,** Radiographer assists patient into position at upright bucky for chest radiographs. (From Hunkele MM: *Radiography essentials for limited practice*, ed 2, Philadelphia, 2006, Saunders.)

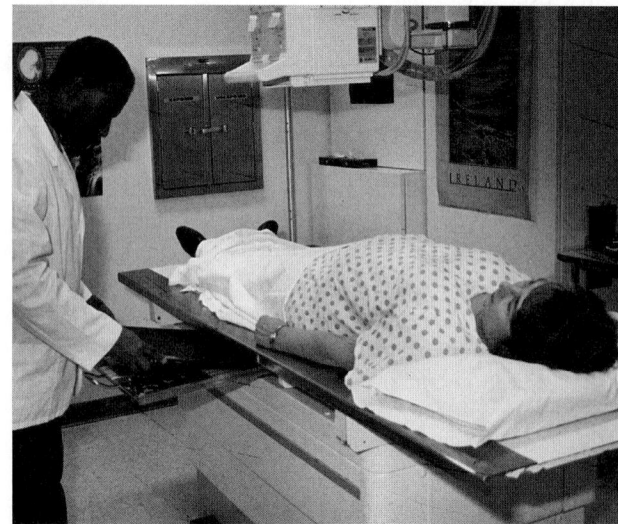

FIGURE 49-30 The cassette must be latched securely in the bucky tray and the tray aligned to the anatomy of interest. (From Ehrlich RA, McCloskey ED, Daly JA: *Patient care in radiography*, ed 6, St Louis, 2004, Mosby.)

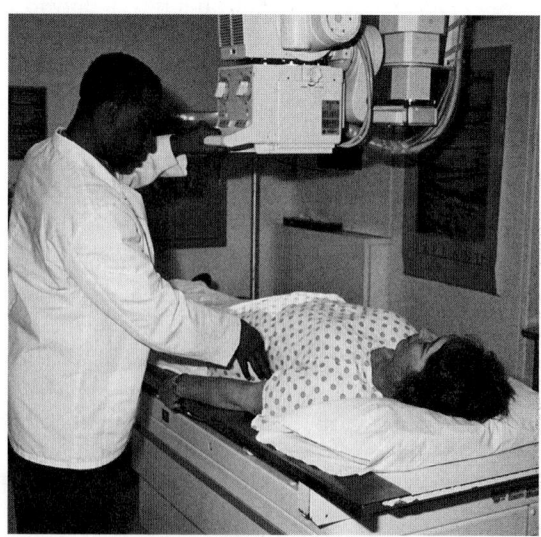

FIGURE 49-31 The x-ray tube must be aligned with the patient and cassette at the proper distance. (From Ehrlich RA, McCloskey ED, Daly JA: *Patient care in radiography*, ed 6, St Louis, 2004, Mosby.)

PROCEDURE 49-1

Prepare Patient for and Assist with Routine and Specialty Examinations: General Procedure for X-Ray Examination

<u>CAAHEP COMPETENCY:</u> 3.b.(4)(e)
<u>ABHES COMPETENCIES:</u> 4.b, 4.h

GOAL: *To assist with an x-ray examination under the supervision of a physician.*

EQUIPMENT and SUPPLIES

- Physician's order for an x-ray examination
- Patient identification card to imprint radiographs
- X-ray machine
- X-ray cassettes, loaded with film
- Appropriate accessory items for patient comfort and shielding
- X-ray darkroom with automatic processor
- Patient record

PROCEDURAL STEPS

1. Check order and equipment needed. Ascertain whether any special preparations are needed.
2. Introduce yourself, and confirm the identity of the patient. Ascertain whether any necessary preparations were implemented.
   <u>PURPOSE:</u> If special preparations were not followed, the examination may need to be rescheduled.
3. Explain the procedure to the patient, and respond appropriately to any questions or concerns.
   <u>PURPOSE:</u> Helps to reassure the patient and alleviates fear and anxiety.
4. Ask childbearing women if pregnancy is possible, and confirm that the patient does not have allergies to iodine dye and/or shellfish if iodine dye will be used.
   <u>PURPOSE:</u> To prevent possible injury to developing fetus if the woman is pregnant and complications from allergic reaction to dye.
5. Place the x-ray cassette correctly (Figure 1).
6. Check to make certain that the patient has removed all metal objects from the area to be examined.
   <u>PURPOSE:</u> Metal objects appear on the film and may obscure important diagnostic information (Figure 2).

7. Position the patient properly, and immobilize the part, if necessary (Figure 3).
   <u>PURPOSE:</u> Proper positioning and complete stillness are necessary to achieve a clear, readable radiograph.
8. Drape the patient as necessary, and shield the gonads if appropriate (Figure 4).

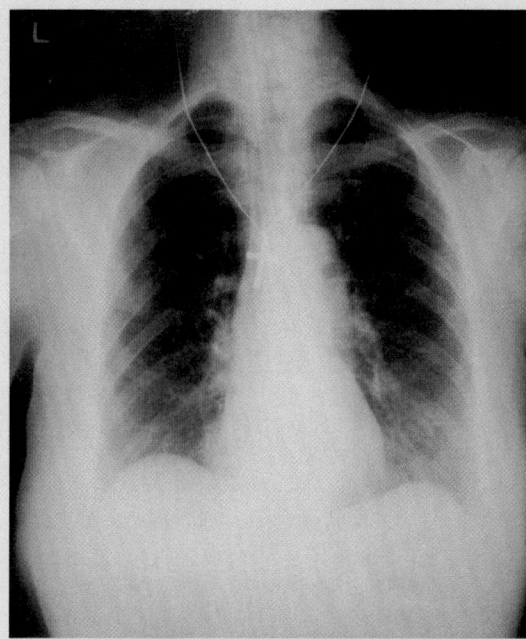

FIGURE 2

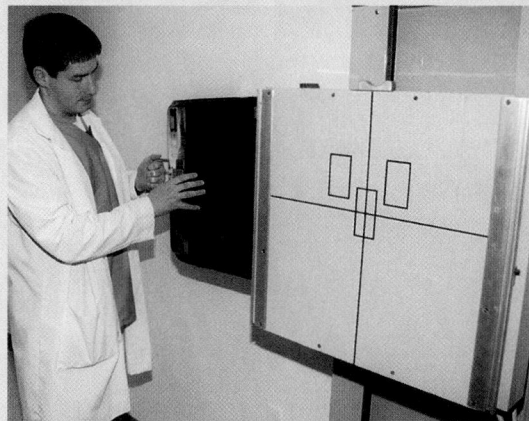

FIGURE 1

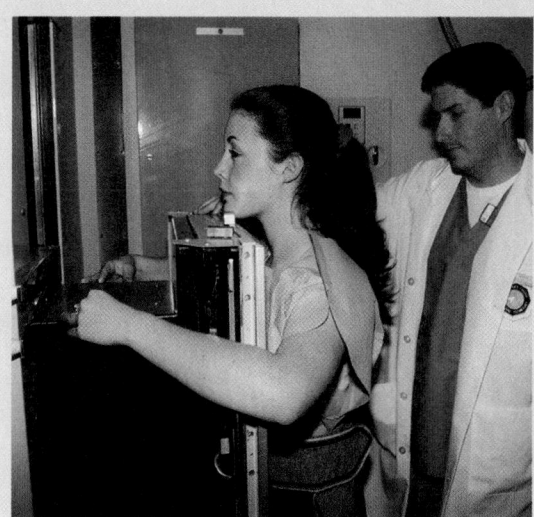

FIGURE 3

Continued

PROCEDURE 49-1—*cont'd*

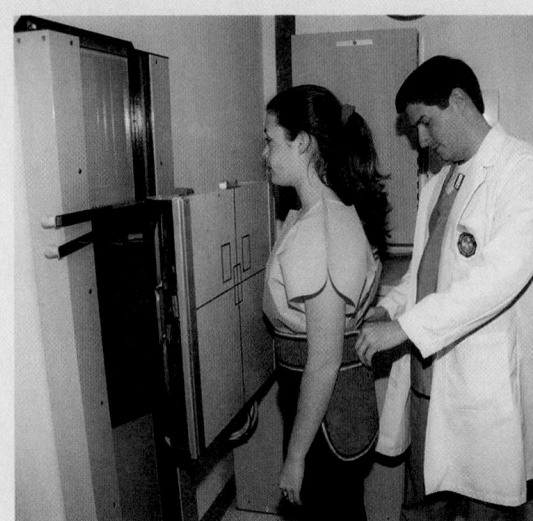

FIGURE 4

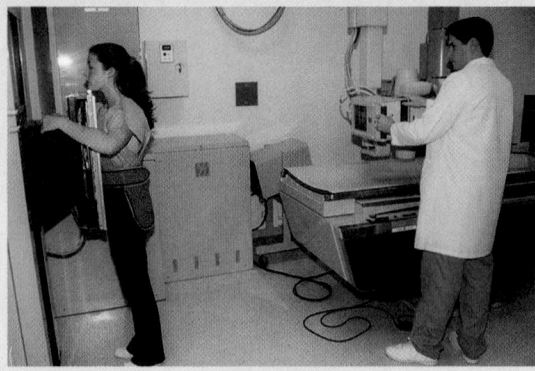

FIGURE 5

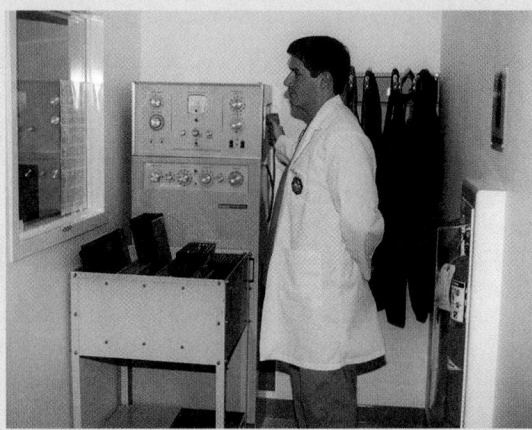

FIGURE 6

<u>PURPOSE:</u> Drapes provide warmth and protect patient's modesty; shields are required to minimize potential genetic radiation effects.

9. Align the x-ray tube with the cassette at the proper distance (Figure 5).

10. Measure the patient's thickness through the path of the central ray, and set the control panel for the correct exposure.
    <u>PURPOSE:</u> The measurement is needed to calculate the proper exposure from the technique chart. If the exposure is not correct the image will not be readable.

11. Stand behind a lead shield during the exposure (Figure 6).
    <u>PURPOSE:</u> Lead shields provide protection from scattered radiation.

12. Ask the patient to assume a comfortable position after the examination is completed, and wait until the films are processed.
    <u>PURPOSE:</u> In the event that it is necessary to take additional films, the patient will be readily accessible.

13. In the darkroom, remove the film from the cassette, identify the film, and process the film in the automatic processor (Figure 7).

14. Dismiss the patient when all films are satisfactory.

15. Place the finished radiograph(s) in a properly labeled envelope, and present it to the physician for interpretation. When it has been read, file it according to the policies of the office.

16. Record the x-ray examination on the patient's chart, along with the final written x-ray findings.
    <u>PURPOSE:</u> A procedure is not complete until it has been recorded.

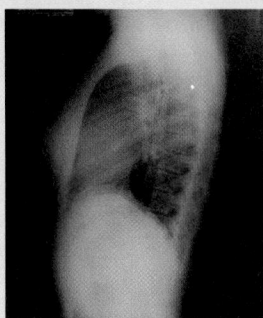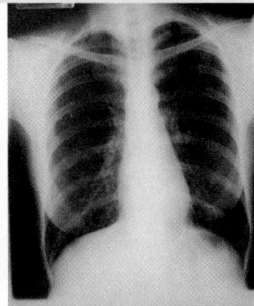

FIGURE 7

they are promptly filed so that they can be retrieved quickly when needed for future reference. Radiology reports must also be filed. Usually the original is filed in the patient's chart; copies may be filed separately or with the films.

SCHEDULING AND SEQUENCING DIAGNOSTIC IMAGING PROCEDURES

One of the most important communications between medical assistants and imaging departments involves the scheduling of multiple diagnostic procedures that may all be ordered at one time by the physician. Consultation is often needed to decide how many procedures can be done in one day and to sequence them in such a way that they will not interfere with one another. For example, a UGI series usually results in barium sulfate scattered throughout the intestinal tract for several days. Even tiny amounts of residual barium cause complications in radiographic examinations of the urinary tract and biliary system, where tiny opacifications are diagnostically significant. Residual barium in the digestive tract also causes unacceptable artifacts on abdominal CT scans. For this reason, barium studies are scheduled last in any series of procedures.

Some imaging departments will schedule a series of several examinations in one day for patients who are able to tolerate this approach. Radiologists prefer various scheduling practices. For example, some departments schedule gallbladder and upper and lower GI studies on the same day. Others may insist on 2 or 3 days for the completion of the same examinations. You should become familiar with the practice in the institution where you usually schedule patients.

Scheduling several examinations on the same day may be less stressful for the patient resulting in a single bowel preparation, a single period of fasting, and a single trip to the imaging center. However, the number of examinations that an individual patient can tolerate varies a great deal, especially if that patient is elderly or ill. Make sure that you discuss scheduling options with the patient and/or family before planning more than one examination per day.

When fiberoptic studies, such as gastroscopy or sigmoidoscopy, are ordered in conjunction with radiographic examinations requiring barium as a contrast medium, fiberoptic studies are usually done first. This avoids the possibility that the barium will interfere with visual assessment during the fiberoptic examination. Patients undergoing gastroscopy usually receive sedation and a muscle relaxant before the physician inserts the gastroscope. When a UGI series is to follow, it should be delayed to allow sufficient time for the patient to become responsive and alert before the UGI series because oral administration of barium to a sedated patient increases the risk that the patient may choke on the barium.

Another study to be considered when sequencing diagnostic procedures is any thyroid assessment test that involves iodine uptake. Because the administration of contrast media containing iodine causes inaccurate results in such tests for at least 3 weeks, thyroid assessment tests (T_3 or T_4) or nuclear medicine thyroid scans must be performed before any contrast medium with iodine is administered.

SEQUENCING ORDER FOR DIAGNOSTIC STUDIES
1. All x-ray examinations not requiring contrast media
2. Any laboratory studies or nuclear medicine procedures involving iodine uptake
3. CT studies with IV contrast any time after iodine uptake blood studies
4. Radiographic examinations of the urinary tract
5. Radiographic examinations of the biliary system
6. Fiberoptic studies (gastroscopy, endoscopy, sigmoidoscopy, colonoscopy, etc.)
7. CT studies of the abdomen or pelvis should be done before barium studies
8. Lower GI series (barium enema)
9. UGI series (barium swallow)
CT, Computed tomography; *GI*, gastrointestinal; *IV*, intravenous; *UGI*, upper gastrointestinal.

An additional consideration in patient scheduling involves deciding which patients will need early morning appointments and which can be scheduled later in the day. Imaging departments always begin the daily routine with patients who must fast in preparation for examination so that they will not have to go without food for too long. When scheduling, request early priority for pediatric and geriatric patients because they have the most difficulty maintaining nothing-by-mouth (**NPO**) status for long periods, and extended fasting may actually interfere with their recovery. Diabetic patients who must postpone their insulin until their morning meal also need priority in scheduling. Diabetic outpatients should be reminded to postpone their morning insulin until the examination is complete, even if they have been scheduled for an early appointment. If an emergency should cause a delay, the patient who has had insulin may suffer a reaction. Paperwork done in the office for diagnostic studies needs to include information about patients with diabetes so that the radiology staff is aware of their status.

CRITICAL THINKING APPLICATION

Mrs. Pellegrini, a 62-year-old diabetic patient, calls Metro Urgicenter at 8:30 am to confirm her 10:00 am appointment for an outpatient imaging procedure that requires fasting. On speaking with her, Sara discovers Mrs. Pellegrini has already taken her morning insulin. What should Sara tell Mrs. Pellegrini and David, the radiographer? Should Mrs. Pellegrini keep her appointment or be rescheduled? Why or why not?

When instructing the patient regarding preparation for an examination, it is important to have printed instructions prepared in advance. If more than one alternative is printed on any given paper, be certain to indicate, both orally and in writing, which instructions are to be followed. Review the sheet with the patient slowly, explaining any words or procedures that may not be familiar. Have the patient explain back to you what is to be done (remember the importance of feedback in establishing whether the patient understands). If the patient is too young, too ill, confused, or incapable of understanding and following the instructions, give the instructions (oral and written) to the person who will be responsible for assisting the patient. Be sure to include the telephone numbers of your clinical facility and of the imaging department so that the patient or the patient's family may call if any questions arise after the patient leaves the office.

In preparation for a UGI series, the patient must fast, avoiding water, smoking, and chewing gum. The NPO order is instituted for a limited period, usually 8 to 12 hours, before the procedure. This ensures that the stomach will be empty at the time of examination so that an accurate radiographic image of its inner surfaces can be produced. Chewing gum and smoking are avoided because they tend to increase gastric secretions.

The preparation for a barium enema involves the use of a bowel cleansing kit. These kits usually contain one or more types of **cathartics,** a suppository, a low-volume enema, and illustrated instructions in several languages. Research has demonstrated that increased fluid intake enhances the effectiveness of cathartics and aids in minimizing patient discomfort. For this reason, instructions for cathartics are accompanied by a fluid intake schedule that suggests at least 8 ounces of water or clear liquid every 2 hours between noon and midnight on the day preceding the examination. The medical assistant should emphasize the importance of fluid intake. The required doses of cathartics have a strong, thorough action that occasionally causes patients to experience painful spasms of the bowel and irritation of the intestinal lining. Persistent diarrhea may last through the night, preventing sleep. Although patients may find this preparation uncomfortable and inconvenient, its effectiveness in cleansing the bowel usually outweighs these considerations. Caution must be exercised in implementing an aggressive preparation for elderly or frail patients who are likely to be adversely affected. A gentler alternative should be available for these debilitated patients. Those with chronic or acute diarrhea may require a lower dose or less active preparation than is usually given. When decreasing the routine strength or amount of cathartics, several days of a low-residue diet and increased fluid intake become critically important to the success of the preparation. Patients should always be advised of the nature of the action expected from the cathartic when it is given. Table 49-3 summarizes common diagnostic procedures and the patient preparation required for each.

CRITICAL THINKING APPLICATION

Dr. Roberts, a physician at Metro Urgicenter, has scheduled Mr. Tillman for a barium enema, and David asks Sara to provide preparation instructions for the procedure to Mr. Tillman. What information should Sara obtain from Mr. Tillman to determine whether the usual bowel preparation is appropriate? If Sara thinks the usual preparation might be too harsh for Mr. Tillman, how should she explain her concern to David and Dr. Roberts? Who should decide whether to implement a variation in protocol—Sara, David, or someone else?

RADIATION SAFETY

Radiation Units

Two systems are used to measure radiation and radiation dose: the conventional (British) system and the international system (Système International [SI]) established in 1981. The conventional system is still the most commonly used in the United States. Table 49-4 lists the units used in both systems. The reason for the measurement determines which unit is most appropriate.

The **roentgen (R)** is the conventional unit of radiation exposure. It represents a measurement of radiation intensity and is determined by the interaction of the x-ray beam with air. For example, an x-ray machine might produce 0.01 R during the exposure for a chest radiograph. The corresponding SI unit is **coulombs per kilogram (C/kg),** specifying the electrical charge in coulombs produced by the exposure of 1 kg of dry air.

The roentgen is not a useful dose unit because dose varies with the depth of measurement and the quantity of radiation energy absorbed in the tissue that is exposed. To measure both therapeutic radiation doses and specific tissue doses received in diagnostic applications, the conventional unit is the **rad,** which stands for *radiation absorbed dose*. It is usually qualified by the specific body part to which it applies. For example, a radiation oncologist may prescribe a treatment involving 150 rad to the pelvis. Examples of patient dose received in typical radiographic examinations are provided in Table 49-5. The SI unit for dose measurement is the **Gray (Gy).**

The biologic effect of radiation exposure varies according to the type of radiation involved and its energy; equal doses of various types of radiation will not necessarily result in equal biologic effects. To measure occupational dose or other exposure that may involve more than one type of radiation, the dose equivalent unit used is the **rem,** which stands for roentgen equivalent in man. Dose equivalents are usually assumed to represent whole-body dose or the dose to unspecified tissues. The SI unit for dose equivalent is the **Sievert (Sv).**

Because the radiation quantities involved in diagnostic radiology are so small, units may be used that represent $1/_{1000}$ of the common units: milliroentgen (mR), millirad (mrad), and millirem (mrem). It may be confusing to determine which units should be used in a given situation. This is made more difficult by the tendency of many radiographers to use the traditional roentgen, rad, and rem units interchangeably. This practice does not cause serious inaccuracy when speaking only of diagnostic x-ray studies because exposure to 1 roentgen of x-ray energy will result in approximately 1 rad of absorbed dose, which is equal to a dose equivalent of 1 rem.

Effects of Low-Dose Radiation Exposure

Cellular Response to Exposure

Most cellular effects of radiation exposure are extremely short-lived because chemical alterations within the cells are quickly repaired. Even if a cell dies, cell death is an insignificant injury unless the number of cells involved is massive. Some cells may sustain damage that requires several days for the body to repair.

TABLE 49-3 Diagnostic Procedures and Patient Preparation

DIAGNOSTIC STUDY	DIAGNOSTIC PURPOSE	PROCEDURE	PATIENT PREPARATION
Arteriogram	Diagnosis of arterial occlusion, aneurysm, hemorrhage, abnormal vessels, and transient ischemic attacks	Catheter inserted into femoral or brachial artery; advanced under fluoroscopy to site; dye injected; x-ray images taken	Clear liquids 24 hr before test; NPO 8 hr before test; if abdominal vasculature is to be imaged, patient may need laxative and enemas
Arthrogram	Detect damage to joint connective tissue and structures	Fluoroscopic and radiographic examination of a joint after injection of air or contrast dye	NPO 8 hr
Barium enema	Bowel obstruction, celiac sprue, colon cancer, polyps, diverticulitis, irritable bowel syndrome	Fluoroscopic and radiographic examination of colon after barium enema to find internal structural abnormalities; takes approximately 1 hr	Bowel must be emptied before procedure; clear liquid diet 24 hr before test; laxatives day before test; enemas morning of test
Barium swallow	Detect dysphagia, esophageal varices, hiatal hernia, pyloric stenosis, stomach cancer, ulcers	Fluoroscopic and radiographic examination as barium is swallowed to detect abnormalities of the pharynx, esophagus, and stomach; takes about 15 min	NPO 8 hr
Bone scan	Detect cancer of bone; bone infection; osteoarthritis; osteomyelitis	Nuclear medicine; radioactive isotope injected IV; body scanned and levels of isotope recorded on film; areas of high metabolism show up as "hot spots"; scan done 1-3 hr after isotope injection	NPO 4 hr; must void before scan; radioactive material is excreted in urine within 48 hr and is not harmful to others
Computed tomography (CT)	Provides detailed, cross-sectional views of all types of tissue; one of the best tools for studying the chest and abdomen	Uses special x-ray equipment and computers to obtain image data from different angles around the body; produces multiple cross-sectional views (tomographs)	NPO after midnight if IV contrast medium used; no metal objects; must lie very still; advise of confined space and possible claustrophobia
Intravenous urogram (IVU) or intravenous pyelogram (IVP)	Evaluates structure and function of kidneys, ureters, bladder	Contrast medium injected IV, and x-ray films taken of renal structures	Bowel cleansing 24 hours before with laxatives and enema important to prevent obstruction of views; NPO 8 hr
Magnetic resonance imaging (MRI)	Diagnosis of intracranial and spinal lesions; aneurysms; heart defects; multiple sclerosis; and soft-tissue abnormalities throughout the body	Magnetic field and radiofrequency energy are transmitted to a computer, which produces cross-sectional images of soft tissue; may eliminate need for arthrography and myelography; patient lies on a flat table that moves into a tunnel-shaped scanner; no radiation exposure; takes 45-90 min	May have fluid restriction; radioactive contrast dye may be used; must remove all metal; any metallic implants with iron (pacemakers, artificial heart valves, aneurysm clips, material associated with metal-related occupation, etc.) are contraindications; patient will hear loud tapping noise during test and must remain still
Myelogram	Diagnosis of spinal lesions, ruptured disk, spinal stenosis	Fluoroscopic and radiographic examination of spinal column after injection of contrast medium into the subarachnoid space; takes about 1 hr	NPO 8 hr

IV, Intravenous; *NPO,* nothing by mouth.

TABLE 49-4 Radiation Units

	CONVENTIONAL UNITS	SI UNITS
Units of exposure	Roentgen (R)	Coulombs per kilogram (C/kg)
Units of dose	rad (radiation absorbed dose)	Gray (Gy) 1 Gy = 100 rad
Dose equivalent units	rem (roentgen equivalent in man)	Sievert (Sv) 1 Sv = 100 rem

The body produces special enzymes that function to repair DNA protein molecules. Sometimes a cell may be damaged in such a way that its DNA "programming" is changed and the cell no longer behaves normally. This type of injury may eventually result in the runaway production of new, abnormal cells, causing a tumor or malignant blood disease.

The relative sensitivity of different types of cells is summarized in the laws of Bergonié and Tribondeau, which state that cell sensitivity to radiation exposure depends on four characteristics of the cell:

- *Age:* Younger cells are more sensitive than older ones.
- *Differentiation:* Simple cells are more sensitive than highly complex ones.

TABLE 49-5 Typical Doses for Radiographic Examinations

EXAMINATION	ENTRANCE SKIN EXPOSURE (MRAD)	MEAN MARROW DOSE(MRAD)	GONAD DOSE (MRAD)
Skull	200	10	<1
Chest	10	2	<1
Cervical spine	150	10	<1
Lumbar spine	300	60	225
Abdomen	400	30	125
Pelvis	150	20	150
Extremity	50	2	<1

- *Metabolic rate:* Cells that use energy rapidly are more sensitive than those that have a slower metabolism.
- *Mitotic rate:* Cells that divide and multiply rapidly are more sensitive than those that replicate slowly.

According to these laws, blood cells and blood-producing cells are very sensitive. Cells that are in contact with the environment are quite simple, have relatively short lives, and are quite sensitive. These include the cells of the skin and the mucosal lining of the mouth, nose, and GI tract. Some glandular tissue is also particularly sensitive, especially that of the thyroid gland and the female breast. The tissues of embryos, fetuses, infants, children, and adolescents tend to be more sensitive than those of adults because of their young age and higher metabolic and mitotic rates. Nerve cells, which have a long life and are quite complex, are much less vulnerable to radiation injury.

Somatic Effects

Radiation effects may be classified as somatic or genetic. *Somatic* effects are those that occur to the body of the person who is irradiated. Whereas the effects of relatively high doses of radiation are immediate and predictable, the effects of the very low doses associated with radiography produce long-term effects. They are not easily identified as a result of radiation exposure because they occur 3 to 30 years after treatment and because the same problems can occur in the absence of radiation exposure. Only extensive research with large populations and computer analysis can demonstrate the role of radiation in causing these effects. In other words, radiation causes increased risk for health problems, but the complications cannot be predicted with respect to any one individual. Although the individual risk is extremely small, increasing exposure to the entire population poses public health risks that require the attention and concern of everyone involved in applying ionizing radiation to human beings.

The documented latent effects of low doses of ionizing radiation include the following:

- *Cataract formation:* This is a risk for radiologists and radiographers who work extensively in fluoroscopy and those who perform other work that involves repeated exposure to the eyes.
- *Carcinogenesis:* Increased risk of malignant disease, particularly cancer of the skin, thyroid, breast, and leukemia.

- *Life-span shortening*: A study of the life span of radiologists who died before 1945 showed that they had shorter life spans than physicians who did not use radiation in their practices. This group included radiologists who had used radiation since the early days of x-ray science. More recent studies show that occupational exposure no longer has a measurable effect on the life span of radiologists. Nevertheless, because radiation exposure has been linked to life-span shortening, it is a public health concern and another reason to practice a high level of radiation safety.

Radiation and Pregnancy

Radiation exposure poses risks to the developing embryo or fetus. Research has demonstrated that excessive radiation during pregnancy may result in spontaneous abortion, congenital defects in the child, growth retardation, increased risk of cancer and leukemia in childhood, and an increase in significant genetic abnormalities in the children of parents who were exposed in utero. Studies of women exposed to radiation as a result of diagnostic and therapeutic procedures confirm that radiation in excess of 5 rad to the uterus is cause for concern. This is more exposure than is received with most x-ray examinations, but these levels may be encountered with direct exposure to the pelvis, especially with CT examinations or fluoroscopic studies.

Genetic Effects

Genetic effects in the form of changes or mutations to the hereditary material of reproductive cells may be caused if the ovaries or testes are exposed to radiation. In the female, all the ova cells that the individual will ever produce are present at birth. Because no new egg cells are created as the individual ages, the effect of radiation exposure to the ovaries accumulates over time. In addition, the genetic effects of radiation to the testes may cause damage to stem cells that produce sperm, resulting in production of sperm with a genetic mutation. Most genetic mutations threaten the survival of an individual. Even when these changes are recessive (not apparent in the offspring), they may be passed on to future generations.

Guidelines for Pediatric X-ray Examinations

- Provide age-appropriate explanations about the procedure and instructions for patient compliance.
- Inform parents about the procedure, and answer questions.
- Give patient or parents written information when needed about preparation for the examination.
- Explain that permitting parents in the x-ray room will be up to the facility.
- Use commercial immobilization devices (restraint board with Velcro closures, papoose board, positioning chair, and so on [Figure 49-32]) when possible to position the child.
- A parent should help the child maintain a particular position when immobilization devices are not available or are ineffective. The parent must wear appropriate lead shield equipment.

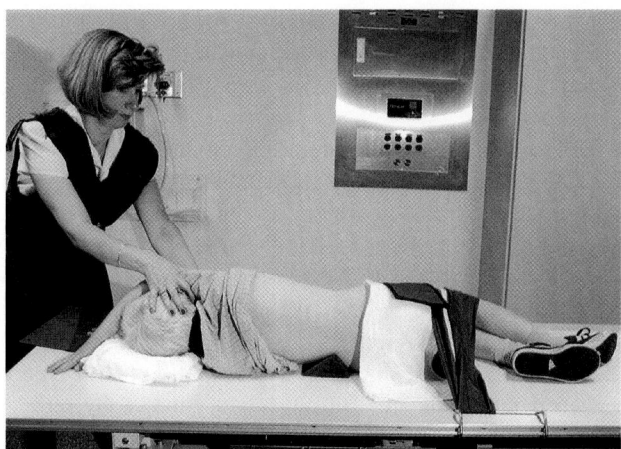

FIGURE 49-33 When holding a child for a radiographic procedure, wear a lead apron and stay as far from the primary x-ray beam as possible. (From Ballinger PW, Frank ED: *Merrill's atlas of radiographic positions and radiologic procedures*, ed 10, vol 2, St Louis, 2003, Mosby.)

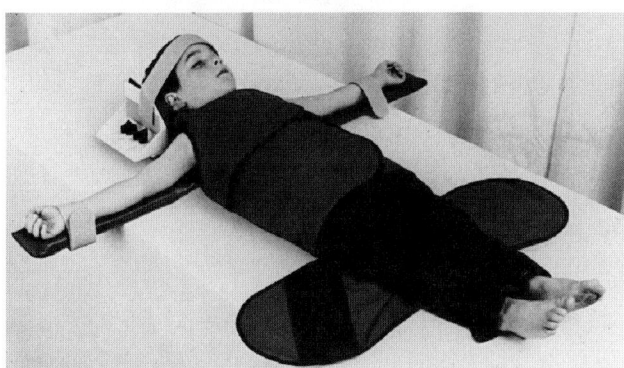

FIGURE 49-32 Immobilization device for pediatric patient. (From Long B, Frank E, Ehrlich RA: *Radiography essentials for limited practice*, St Louis, 2005, Saunders.)

Radiation Protection

Clearly, exposure to x-rays creates some risk for both patients and radiographers; therefore it is essential that those performing radiographic studies are knowledgeable about and diligently practice radiation safety. All unnecessary radiation exposure to patients, co-workers, and self must be prevented.

Personnel Safety

In diagnostic x-ray departments, radiation hazards exist from exposure to the primary x-ray beam as well as to *scatter radiation* caused by an interaction between the primary beam and the patient or other material in its path. Scatter radiation is present throughout the x-ray room during an exposure. X-rays travel at the speed of light. They do not linger in the room after the exposure, and they are not capable of making the objects in the room radioactive. Therefore the only time a radiation hazard exists is during the x-ray exposure itself.

Because radiographers are considered to be "occupationally exposed individuals," they are prohibited from activities that would result in direct exposure to the primary x-ray beam. This means that they are not allowed to hold patients or cassettes during x-ray exposures and must stand clear of the path of the primary x-ray beam during fluoroscopic and mobile

radiographic examinations. Whenever possible, patients should be immobilized without the need for someone to hold them. When infants or children must be held, a parent (as long as the parent is not pregnant) is usually the appropriate person to perform this duty, with required lead covering.

Medical assistants may or may not be considered occupationally exposed persons, depending on their work assignments and the frequency with which they are involved with radiation use. Medical assistants who are not routinely exposed may occasionally assist with procedures by holding patients or cassettes. When this is the case, the medical assistant should wear a lead apron and should avoid direct exposure from the primary x-ray beam, if possible (Figure 49-33). If the hands will be in the primary beam, lead gloves should also be worn.

Personnel are not exposed to any significant amount of radiation when standing well behind the protective lead barrier of the control booth. X-rays travel in straight lines and do not turn corners. Scatter radiation is not powerful enough to generate additional radiation of concern when it interacts with matter, so it is not necessary for the control booth to be sealed.

Occupational exposure increases when assisting with fluoroscopic procedures or using mobile x-ray equipment. The three principal methods used to protect personnel from unnecessary radiation exposure are time, distance, and shielding.

Because the amount of exposure received is directly proportional to the time spent in a radiation area, dose is

Preexposure Safety Check

Before making an exposure, be certain of the following:
- The x-ray room door is closed; a closed door indicates an exposure is in progress, so do not go into the room if the door is closed.
- No nonessential persons are in the x-ray room; all essential persons outside of the lead barrier are appropriately shielded.
- All persons in the control booth are completely behind the lead barrier.
- No cassettes are in the room except the one in use.

decreased when this time is minimized. For example, you might shorten the time of exposure by stepping into the control booth during fluoroscopic procedures when not required to be near the patient.

The second method involves using distance. Increasing the distance between yourself and a radiation source decreases your exposure in proportion to the square of the distance, so small increases in distance have a relatively large effect. Mobile x-ray units have long cords on the exposure switches, enabling the radiographer to get as far from the radiation source as possible while making an exposure.

The third method, shielding, is the most common type of personnel protection used in outpatient radiography settings. The lead wall of the control booth provides a radiation safety barrier and is the principal defense for personnel. Other types of shielding include lead aprons, gloves, goggles, and thyroid shields. These types of shielding are worn during fluoroscopic procedures and mobile radiographic examinations.

Personnel Monitoring

A device for monitoring radiation exposure to personnel is called a **dosimeter.** Dosimeters should be worn in the region of the collar and should be outside a lead apron if it is used. There are three basic types of dosimeters used: film badges, thermoluminescent dosimeters (TLDs), and optically stimulated luminescence dosimeters (OSLs). A film badge consists of one or two pieces of dental film, paper-wrapped and enclosed in a badgelike holder that incorporates several filters. The disadvantage of this type of dosimeter is that the dental film is subject to fog when exposed to heat or fumes, and this exposure could result in a false reading. TLD badges contain one or more lithium fluoride crystals that absorb radiation energy then emit the energy in the form of light when heated. They are more durable than film badges and respond only to ionizing radiation exposure. OSLs are the most recently developed monitoring dosimeter (Figure 49-34) and use aluminum oxide as the radiation detector. OSLs provide greater stability and precision plus the ability to reanalyze and confirm results.

Your facility will contract with a radiation monitor badge service laboratory to provide badges, processing services, and reports. The laboratory is also responsible for maintaining permanent records of the radiation exposure of each person monitored. Depending on facility policy, badges are sent for evaluation of radiation exposure on a weekly, monthly, or quarterly basis. Personnel who receive relatively high doses of occupational exposure change their badges most frequently. Occupationally exposed personnel who are always or nearly always in a control booth during exposures are usually best monitored with quarterly service. Monthly service is a better choice for those who work in fluoroscopy or use mobile x-ray equipment.

Service companies provide an extra badge in every batch that is marked "CONTROL." This badge's purpose is to measure any radiation exposure to the entire batch while in transit. Any amount of exposure measured from the control badge will be subtracted from the amounts measured from the other badges in the batch. The control badge should be kept in a safe place, away

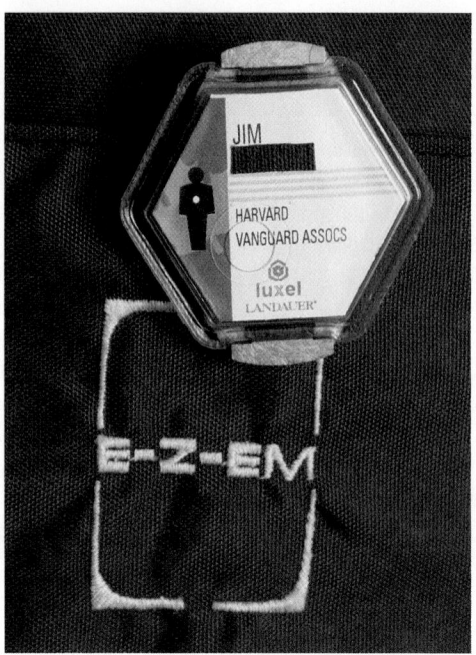

FIGURE 49-34 Optically stimulated luminescence (OSL) dosimeter.

from anywhere that x-ray exposure could occur. *It should never be used to measure occupational dose or for any other purpose.*

Exposure reports are sent to the facility for each batch with an annual summary of personnel exposure. The report sent by the laboratory that processes the personnel dosimeters will report occupational dose in rem. Personnel should be advised of the radiation exposure reported from their badges and should be provided with copies of the annual reports for their own records. Employers are required to provide a complete record of radiation exposure history to all employees who have radiation exposure records before the employees leave the employment of that facility.

Effective Dose Equivalent Limits

The ALARA principle is the guiding philosophy associated with all radiation use that involves exposure to humans, both patients and workers. It states that all radiation exposure to humans should be limited to levels that are *As Low As Reasonably Achievable.*

The effective dose equivalent (EDE) limiting system is used to calculate the upper limit of occupational exposure that is permitted. For occupationally exposed personnel, the EDE limit is 5 rem (50 mSv) per year. This applies to workers over the age of 18 who are not pregnant and is assumed to be a whole-body dose. These limits apply to occupational exposure only and do not include diagnostic imaging exposure that the worker may receive as a result of tests related to their own healthcare.

The established EDE limits ensure that the safety of radiation workers is comparable with that of workers in other, safe occupations. The allowable exposure is considered to be so low as to pose an insignificant risk. The occupational exposure received by radiographers is usually well below the established limit.

Occupational Precautions During Pregnancy

Radiation exposure during pregnancy must be closely monitored because of possible complications for the developing fetus. The EDE limit of whole-body radiation for the pregnant worker is 0.5 rem over the 9-month course of the pregnancy. The worker must first submit a written document to her employer declaring the pregnancy. The employer is then responsible for providing fetal radiation monitoring and for ensuring that the occupational dose does not exceed the EDE limit for pregnant workers. Here again, the ALARA principle is important. Every effort should be made to minimize exposure, keeping the dose as far below the limit as possible.

For a pregnant radiographer, the safest work assignment would be one in which a permanent lead barrier (control booth) always shields the worker during exposures. Pregnant radiographers, or those of childbearing age who may be pregnant, should pay particular attention to personal safety measures when assisting with fluoroscopy or using mobile x-ray equipment.

Patient Protection

Patients must be consistently protected from unnecessary radiation exposure. The following methods are employed to minimize radiation dose to patients:

- Avoid errors. Double-check requisitions and patient identification so that the right patient gets the right examination.
- Establish good routine procedures and follow them strictly so that careless errors do not necessitate repeat exposures.
- Collimate. Use the smallest radiation field needed to fulfill the physician's order. The size of the radiation field should always be less than the size of the film.
- Use the highest kVp that is consistent with acceptable film quality. This permits using the least possible mAs to obtain an acceptable exposure.
- Use at least 40 inches SID. This practice limits patient exposure from tube housing leakage and collimator scatter.
- Use the fastest films and screens consistent with the necessary film quality.
- Provide shielding for gonads, eyes, breasts, and thyroid, as appropriate.

Gonad Shielding

Lead shields that prevent unnecessary radiation exposure to the reproductive organs are required when the patient is of reproductive age or younger, whenever the gonads are within the primary radiation field, and when the shield will not interfere with the examination. This applies to most patients under the age of 55 years. A shield device consisting of at least a 0.5-mm lead or equivalent is placed between the x-ray tube and the patient. Shields attached to the collimator (shadow shields) may be positioned by viewing their shadows within the collimator light field. Shields placed on or near the patient's body are referred to as *contact shields* and are somewhat more effective than shadow shields. Both types meet the legal requirements for gonad shielding. The female shield is placed with its lower

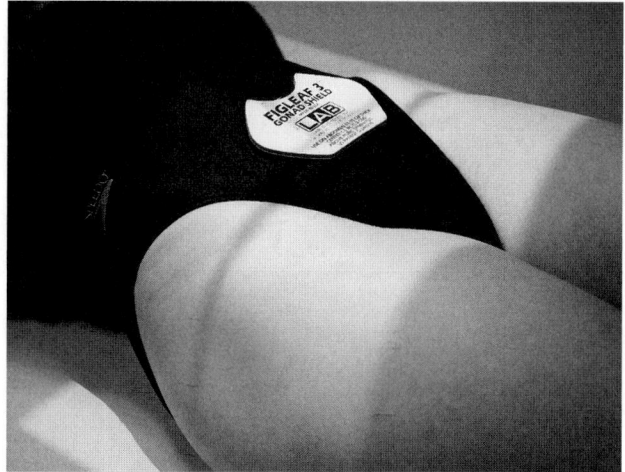

A

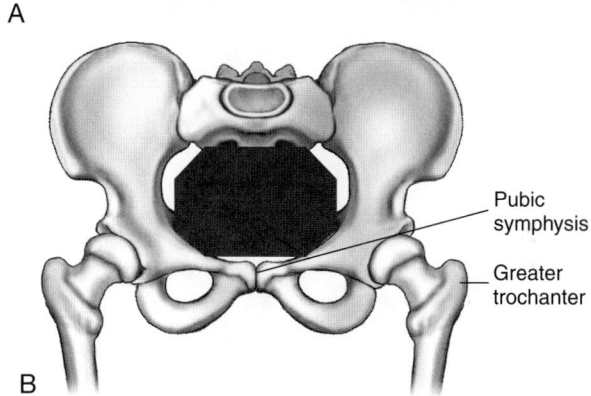

B

Pubic symphysis

Greater trochanter

FIGURE 49-35 When precise gonad shielding is required for female patients, place the lower margin of the shield on the upper margin of the pubic symphysis. (From Hunkele MM: *Radiography essentials for limited practice*, ed 2, Philadelphia, 2006, Saunders.)

margin at the level of the pubic symphysis (Figure 49-35). The male shield is positioned with its upper margin about 1 inch below the pubic symphysis (Figure 49-36). It is helpful to note that the pubic symphysis is at about the same level as the greater trochanter of the femur, avoiding the necessity of palpating the pubic symphysis for proper shield placement.

Pregnant or Potentially Pregnant Patients

The greatest risks for spontaneous abortion, fetal death, and significant birth defects exist when significant levels of exposure occur during the first trimester of pregnancy. The embryo is most vulnerable to radiation insult while tissues are in the process of differentiation. Unfortunately, this creates the greatest hazard at a time when a woman may not yet be aware she is pregnant.

The public is generally aware that x-rays should be avoided during pregnancy, and this may lead to irrational fears on the part of pregnant women or their families. The chance is extremely remote that a routine x-ray examination of the chest or an extremity would harm the developing child. On the other hand, examinations requiring direct radiation to the pelvis, especially relatively high-dose fluoroscopy studies or CT scans of the abdomen or lumbar spine, may be cause for concern.

Radiation-control regulations require that female patients of childbearing age be advised of potential radiation hazards

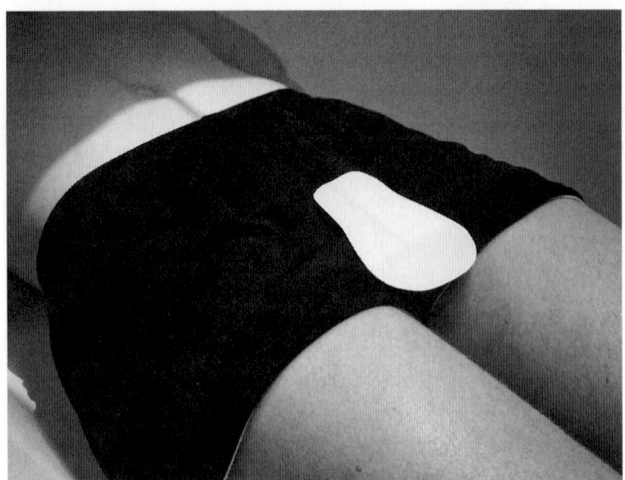

A

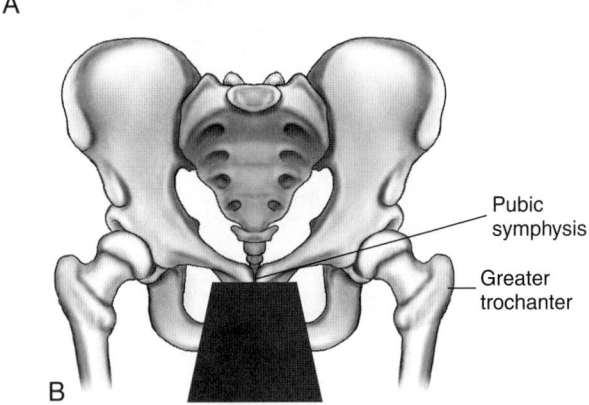

Pubic
symphysis

Greater
trochanter

B

FIGURE 49-36 When precise gonad shielding is required for male patients, place the upper margin of the shield 1 inch below the pubic symphysis. (From Hunkele MM: *Radiography essentials for limited practice*, ed 2, Philadelphia, 2006, Saunders.)

before an x-ray examination. This requirement is usually met by posting signs in the radiology department advising women to tell the radiographer before the examination if they may be pregnant. These signs should be written in all languages commonly used in the community.

The medical assistant should ask specific questions to rule out pregnancy when taking a medical history. If pregnancy is a possibility, an early pregnancy test should be done to rule out the possibility. If the patient is pregnant and the proposed x-ray examination involves direct pelvic radiation, the physician must weigh the potential risks and benefits of the examination and discuss them with the patient before proceeding with the study. In the case of minor or chronic complaints, typically the examination is delayed until after the child is born. In practice, however, the possibility of pregnancy may not even be considered. This is especially true with accident or injury, when the patient is being cared for by unfamiliar physicians in an emergency situation. For this reason it is essential to consider the possibility of pregnancy in any female of childbearing age and to ask specific questions to determine whether the physician has addressed the issue of pregnancy before proceeding with scheduling or assisting with an x-ray examination.

If an x-ray examination of a pregnant patient must be done, modifications in procedure can help to minimize the dose

to the embryo or fetus. If the part to be examined is not the abdomen or pelvis, this area can be shielded with a lead apron. If the abdomen or pelvis is to be evaluated, the number of views or the size of the radiation field may be minimized, resulting in less radiation exposure than that required for a routine procedure.

CRITICAL THINKING APPLICATION

Ingrid White is gowned and ready for a lumbar spine x-ray examination and Sara asks Ingrid whether there is any possibility that she might be pregnant. Ingrid confides that she and her husband have been trying to conceive for several months, and she is not sure whether she is currently pregnant. What should Sara do?

THE ROLE OF THE MEDICAL ASSISTANT

Depending on your location, you may or may not be legally permitted to take x-ray films. Most states require some sort of license or permit to practice radiography. Some, such as New York and New Jersey, grant licenses only to professional radiologic technologists who have completed at least a 2-year education program and obtained certification in radiography from the American Registry of Radiologic Technologists (ARRT).

Limited radiography, sometimes called *practical radiography,* is practiced primarily in clinics and physicians' offices. This field developed as nurses, medical assistants, chiropractic assistants, and other health care office personnel were trained to perform basic x-ray procedures in addition to their primary duties. It is called *limited* because the scope of practice is restricted compared with that of registered radiologic technologists. Limited practice does not usually involve the use of contrast media, and additional restrictions may be applied depending on the scope of practice permitted in the states where limited radiography can be legally practiced.

However, even if you are not qualified as a radiographer, it may be helpful to understand the general procedures involved in performing an x-ray examination and to identify areas where the medical assistant might be of help to the patient and/or radiographer. The exact nature of your duties will vary with your qualifications, your place of employment, the size of the staff, and the equipment available.

In summary, the process of radiography involves validation of orders, patient preparation, proper selection of cassettes and film, correct positioning of patient and equipment, measurement of the part to be examined, protective shielding, correct setting of the exposure controls, and identification and processing of the film. These basic procedures vary considerably depending on the body part to be examined.

LEGAL AND ETHICAL ISSUES

Only licensed health practitioners are permitted to order x-ray examinations. The interpretation of diagnostic images is part of the professional practice of making a diagnosis and is solely the privilege of physicians. Although you may learn to recognize certain conditions represented in diagnostic images, you must never discuss your observations with the patient.

In most states, x-ray machines are required to be licensed and personnel operating this equipment must have a current license or permit. In all states that regulate radiography, the practice is defined as more than simply pushing the exposure button. If you position the x-ray equipment, position the patient, or set the exposure controls, even though you do not make the exposure, you are probably practicing radiography as defined by law. Practicing without a valid license or permit or practicing outside the scope of one's credentials may result in fines, imprisonment, or both. Employers may also be penalized if their employees practice radiography in violation of regulations. Everyone who practices radiography must be aware of the legal standards that apply to them and take care that their practice conforms to these standards. Even if you work in a state that currently has no requirements for practicing radiography, you should be aware that the safe practice of radiography requires additional education and experience beyond that provided in this chapter.

X-ray films and other diagnostic images are the property of the institution or facility where they are taken. Even though the patient may pay for the procedure, this does not mean that the patient owns the films. They are considered a part of the medical record and are subject to the same kinds of requirements with respect to confidentiality, retention, and availability to the patient. Retention periods vary from state to state and are usually 5 to 7 years. Images may be loaned or transferred to other healthcare providers to assist in the patient's care. The patient should sign a release when images or copies of images are to be sent to another healthcare provider, and a record of the date and the name and address of the borrower must be kept when original images are loaned to another facility. The patient may deliver the films when referred to another physician but it is preferable to send the films directly to the provider. When the patient must carry the films, it is best that the physician review the films with the patient in advance so that the patient does not misinterpret the images and reach an incorrect conclusion.

CRITICAL THINKING APPLICATION

One of the new medical assistants at Metro Urgicenter, Carla O'Neal, tells Sara she is not qualified to practice radiography in the office's jurisdiction. David has instructed her to position a patient and set up the equipment for an x-ray examination. When Carla stated that she was not yet qualified to practice radiography, David replied, "Don't worry. I'll come by in a few minutes and make the exposure." What should Sara tell Carla, and what should Carla say to David? Should Sara tell someone else at the clinic?

SUMMARY OF SCENARIO

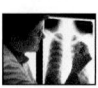

David Swain and the physicians at Metro Urgicenter depend on Sara's assistance to keep the x-ray department running smoothly. Today, for example, she instructed four patients to gown and prepare for routine x-ray examinations. Greg Nolan had PA and lateral views of the chest because of a persistent cough and fever, Margaret and Jeff Barge both needed spine x-ray studies to rule out possible fractures resulting from a car accident, and Dr. Farnsworth ordered AP and lateral views of Ella Jackson's left hip. Sara processed the films and was proud to see that there were no handling artifacts. This afternoon, Sara made an appointment for Cecile Marsden to have a bone scan at University Imaging Center. She was able to describe the procedure for Cecile so that she would know exactly what to expect. Sara recognizes that she must remain up to date with current radiologic diagnostic procedures to provide assistance when needed and to field patient questions as they arise. Sara enjoys her work in the x-ray department and is attending evening classes to become certified as a limited radiographer.

SUMMARY of LEARNING OBJECTIVES

1. Define, spell, and pronounce the terms listed in the vocabulary.
   - Spelling and pronouncing medical terms correctly adds credibility to the medical assistant. Knowing the definition of these terms promotes confidence in communication with patients and co-workers.
2. Identify the principal components of an x-ray machine.
   - The principal component of the x-ray machine is the tube in its barrel-shaped tube housing. The collimator is mounted on the tube housing. The tube housing with its attachments is mounted on the tube support, which may be suspended from the ceiling or attached to a tube stand that runs in a track on the floor. The radiographic table and an upright cassette holder provide support for the patient and the film and incorporate a grid device. The control console is where the operator selects the exposure settings and makes the exposure. It is located in the control booth.
3. Describe the cassette/film image receptor system and explain its function in radiography.
   - The image receptor system for radiography usually consists of a cassette with two intensifying screens that give off light when stimulated by x-ray energy and double-emulsion film that lies between the intensifying screens. The film is exposed on both

Continued

SUMMARY of LEARNING OBJECTIVES

Continued

sides, principally by the light emitted from the screens. This system greatly reduces the amount of radiation and exposure time involved compared with direct exposure of film by x-rays.

4. Recognize precautions to be taken when unloading, loading, and processing radiographic film and cassettes.
   - Cassettes are unloaded and reloaded in the darkroom under safelight illumination only. Precautions include ensuring that the door is locked; that your hands are clean and dry; and that the film is not creased, bent, or scraped in the process of loading and unloading. Take care that the cassette is reloaded with only one fresh film and latched securely. Keep the loading bench clean to prevent dirt from getting into the cassette.

5. Distinguish among the three body planes and use these terms correctly when discussing radiographic positions.
   - The three body planes are the sagittal plane, which divides the body into right and left parts, the coronal plane, which divides the body into anterior and posterior parts, and the transverse plane, which divides the body into superior and inferior parts. For a frontal projection (AP or PA), the coronal plane is parallel to the film and the sagittal plane is perpendicular to it. For a lateral projection, the sagittal plane is parallel to the film and the coronal plane is perpendicular to it. Neither the sagittal plane nor the coronal plane is parallel to the film on an oblique projection.

6. Identify anteroposterior (AP), posteroanterior (PA), lateral, oblique, and axial radiographic projections.
   - The patient is supine and facing the x-ray tube in the AP projection; facing the film in a PA projection, and with the coronal plane parallel to the film. Lateral projections require the coronal plane to be perpendicular to the film. For an oblique projection, neither the coronal nor the sagittal plane is parallel to the film. For an axial or semiaxial projection, the x-ray beam is angled toward the patient's head or the feet along the long axis of the body.

7. Compare and contrast radiography and fluoroscopy and give examples of appropriate applications of each.
   - Radiography and fluoroscopy are both x-ray imaging procedures with a wide variety of applications. Radiography produces still images, usually on photographic film, and fluoroscopy enables the radiologist to view the x-ray image directly and to observe motion.

8. List and describe imaging modalities that do not involve x-rays.
   - MRI uses a strong magnetic field and radiofrequency pulses to produce images of all parts of the body, including bone, soft tissue, and blood vessels. Nuclear medicine studies demonstrate the function of organs and tissues by mapping the radiation given off within the body when radioactive tracers have been ingested or injected into the patient. Sonography is a very safe imaging method that demonstrates soft tissues using high-frequency sound waves.

9. Explain patient preparation guidelines for typical diagnostic imaging examinations.

   - Chest radiography involves undressing to the waist and donning a gown. For a UGI series the patient must fast and avoid water, chewing gum, and smoking for at least 8 hours before the examination. Preparation for a lower GI series is an extensive bowel-cleansing regimen that may involve a low residue or clear liquid diet, forced fluids, cathartics, a suppository, and a low-volume enema. An IVU requires some bowel preparation, such as a cathartic on the previous evening and NPO orders for a period before the examination. A CT examination of the abdomen with an oral contrast medium requires, the patient to fast and arrive at the imaging center 1 to 2 hours in advance to drink the oral contrast medium. Table 49-3 summarizes patient preparation for various diagnostic procedures.

10. Outline the general procedure for assisting with an x-ray examination.
    - Confirm that the patient followed preparation guidelines. If iodine contrast medium will be used, make sure the patient does not have a history of allergies to the dye and/or shellfish. Explain the procedure to the patient, and answer questions. Confirm that women of childbearing age are not pregnant. Check to make sure the patient has removed all metal objects in the radiation field and is gowned appropriately. Position the patient as called for using a shield as needed. Set the control panel, step behind the lead shield, and wait with the patient until the films are processed to make sure the x-ray studies are acceptable. Document the procedure in the medical record, and file the film according to office policy.

11. Summarize the guidelines for scheduling multiple diagnostic procedures.
    - When possible, schedule several examinations on the same day if the patient is strong enough. Diagnostic imaging that does not require contrast media or nuclear medicine should be scheduled first. Next are examinations of the urinary tract and biliary system. Fiberoptic studies (for example, colonoscopy) and CT studies of the abdomen and pelvis should be scheduled before any GI studies that require barium. CT and MRI can be scheduled anytime unless they require IV contrast; if iodine dye is needed, then schedule the procedure after examinations that do not require visualization. Barium studies are always scheduled last, with a UGI series (barium swallow) done as the final procedure.

12. Apply patient education principles when providing instructions for preparation for diagnostic procedures.
    - Table 49-3 summarizes patient preparation guidelines for diagnostic imaging procedures. The patient must be informed of the purpose of the study, how the procedure will be performed, and any important patient preparation steps needed to make sure the examination can be completed successfully. The healthcare facility should have instruction sheets ready to distribute to patients scheduled for diagnostic studies. The medical assistant must understand diagnostic procedures so

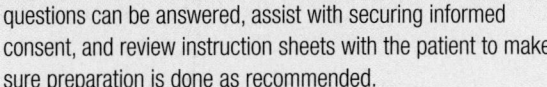

SUMMARY of LEARNING OBJECTIVES
Continued

questions can be answered, assist with securing informed consent, and review instruction sheets with the patient to make sure preparation is done as recommended.

13. Describe the health risks associated with low doses of x-ray exposure like those that are used in radiography.
   - The health risks associated with radiography are extremely small and consist of a slightly increased likelihood of developing cataracts, cancer, or leukemia. The potential also exists for minimal decrease in life span and for a negative outcome when exposure occurs to the abdominal area during pregnancy. Exposure to the reproductive organs may cause genetic changes that can be passed on to future generations.

14. Summarize the steps to ensure that patients receive the least possible exposure during x-ray procedures.
   - To ensure that patients receive the least possible exposure during x-ray procedures, avoid errors that could require repeat exposures; establish good routine procedures and follow them strictly; collimate to the smallest radiation field; use the highest kVp possible; use an SID of at least 40 inches; use the fastest films and screens consistent with the necessary film quality; and shield the reproductive organs and other sensitive organs (such as the eyes, thyroid, and breasts).

15. Describe precautions to ensure the safety of equipment operators and staff during x-ray procedures.
   - The principal safety precaution for x-ray equipment operators and staff is to stay completely behind the lead barrier of the control booth during exposures. Occupationally exposed persons must not hold patients or cassettes during exposures. Any staff required to be in the x-ray room during an exposure should be shielded by a lead apron, should stay as far from radiation sources as possible, and should minimize the time spent in the room during exposures.

16. Explain the legal responsibilities associated with x-ray procedures and the administrative management of diagnostic images.
   - Diagnostic images are the property of the facility in which they are made. They are part of the medical record and must be retained and accessible for a period specified by state law. Images may be loaned or transferred to other healthcare providers to assist in the patient's care, in which case the patient should sign a release, the images should be sent directly to the borrowing provider if possible, and a record must be kept of the loan. Only licensed healthcare practitioners are permitted to order x-ray examinations and/or to interpret x-ray images.

CONNECTIONS

 Study Guide Connection: Go to Chapter 49 Study Guide. Read the Case Study and Workplace Applications and complete the assignments. Do online research for answers to the questions in the Internet Activities associated with assisting with diagnostic imaging.

 CD Connection: Go to the Medical Assisting Competency Challenge CD and do the training activities under Diagnostic Testing.

 Evolve Connection: For more information related to assisting with diagnostic imaging, go to evolve.elsevier.com/kinn and visit related weblinks for Chapter 49. Click on the Medical Assisting Exam Review and do the practice questions to sharpen your test-taking skills.

Assisting in the Clinical Laboratory

50

Robin R. Patterson

SCENARIO

Marsha Rollins has been employed for 3 years as a certified medical assistant in a medical practice. The physicians have an active medical laboratory on site and Marsha has become experienced in collecting specimens, performing laboratory tests, and reporting results. Recently she was offered a position in a smaller practice closer to home; she has accepted the position, knowing that her experience will benefit the practice because the physicians would like to expand their on-site medical laboratory testing and Marsha will be required to equip the lab.

While studying this chapter, think about the following questions:

- What agencies will assist Marsha as she researches the feasibility of setting up a laboratory in the physicians' office?
- What regulations will guide the testing that will be performed in the lab?
- What equipment will she need, and how will she ensure that it remains in good working order?

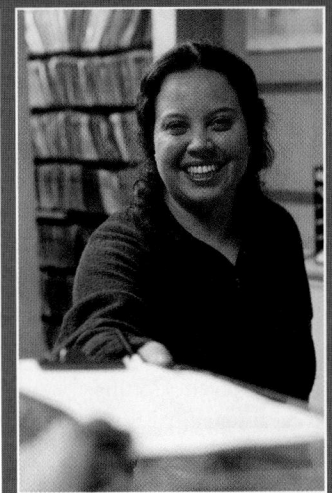

LEARNING OBJECTIVES

1. Define, spell, and pronounce the terms listed in the vocabulary.
2. Discuss the role of the clinical laboratory in patient care and the medical assistant's role in coordinating laboratory tests and results.
3. Describe the divisions of the clinical laboratory, and give an example of a test performed in each division.
4. Describe the Clinical Laboratory Improvement Amendments (CLIA) and how they influence laboratory testing.
5. Differentiate between the three CLIA regulatory categories.
6. Compare and contrast the agencies that govern or influence practice in the clinical laboratory, including the CDC, OSHA, EPA, CLSI, and CAP.
7. List techniques to minimize physical, chemical, and biologic risks in the clinical laboratory.
8. Describe the essential elements of a laboratory requisition.
9. Explain chain of custody, and illustrate why it is important.
10. Explain the differences and similarities between quality assurance and quality control.
11. Convert between Greenwich time and military time.
12. Name the Fahrenheit temperature and Celsius temperature of three important pieces of laboratory equipment.
13. Name the metric units used for measuring liquid volume, distance, and mass.
14. Describe the proper use of pipets.
15. Explain how dilutions are prepared.
16. Name the parts of a microscope, and describe their functions.
17. Describe the safe use of a centrifuge.
18. List quality-control measures necessary to ensure sterilization with an autoclave.
19. Demonstrate the proper use of the microscope.

National Accreditation Competencies and Content

CAAHEP COMPETENCIES

General

3.c.(2)(a). Identify and respond to issues of confidentiality
3.c.(2)(b). Perform within legal and ethical boundaries
3.c.(2)(c). Establish and maintain the medical record
3.c.(2)(d). Document appropriately
3.c.(2)(e). Demonstrate knowledge of federal and state health care legislation and regulations
3.c.(4)(d). Use methods of quality control

ABHES COMPETENCIES

Clinical Duties

4.i. Use quality control

Legal Concepts

5.a. Determine needs for documentation and reporting
5.b. Document accurately
5.c. Use appropriate guidelines when releasing records or information
5.f. Maintain licenses and accreditation
5.g. Monitor legislation related to current healthcare issues and practices

VOCABULARY

aliquot (a'-luh-kwaht) A portion of a well-mixed sample removed for testing.

analyte The substance or chemical being analyzed or detected in a specimen.

anticoagulants Chemicals added to the blood after collection to prevent clotting.

carcinogenic Known to cause cancer.

caustic (kos'-tik) Capable of burning, corroding, or damaging tissue by chemical action.

cerebrospinal fluid Fluid within the subarachnoid space, the central canal of the spinal cord, and the four ventricles of the brain.

cytology (si-tah'-luh-je) The study of cells using microscopic methods.

diluent (dil-yuh'-wunt) A liquid used to dilute a specimen or reagent.

exudates (ek'-syu-dats) Fluids with high concentration of protein and cellular debris that have escaped from the blood vessels and have been deposited in tissues or on tissue surfaces.

hematoma A sac filled with blood that may be the result of trauma.

hemolyzed A term used to describe a blood sample in which the red blood cells have ruptured.

pipets Cylindric glass or plastic tubes used to deliver fluids.

preservatives Substances added to a specimen to prevent deterioration of cells or chemicals.

referral laboratory A private or hospital-based laboratory that performs a wide variety of tests, many of them specialized; physicians often send specimens collected in the office to referral laboratories for testing.

resolution The ability of the eye to distinguish two objects that are very close together; the sharpness of an image.

specimen A sample of body fluid, waste product, or tissue that is collected for analysis.

stat A direction that an action is to be taken quickly (from the Latin word *statin*, meaning "at once"); an order found on a laboratory requisition indicating that the test must be done immediately.

teratogenic (te-rah'-tuh-jen-ik) Known to cause birth defects.

THE ROLE OF THE CLINICAL LABORATORY IN PATIENT CARE

Laboratory medicine or clinical pathology is the medical discipline that applies clinical laboratory science and technology to the care of patients. The laboratory is the place in which a collected **specimen** is analyzed and evaluated. Tests are performed manually (by hand) or through automation (by using specialized instruments).

Personnel in the Clinical Laboratory

Medical laboratories are located either in hospitals or in nonhospital facilities such as physicians' offices, clinics, public health departments, health maintenance organizations, and private referral laboratories. The director of a laboratory facility may be a pathologist, a physician specially trained in the nature and cause of disease, or a clinical laboratory scientist with a doctorate. The laboratory is staffed by various professionally trained personnel, including certified medical technologists (MTs), who have earned a baccalaureate degree, have had additional formal training, and have passed a national certification examination. Other personnel include certified medical laboratory technicians (MLTs) or medical laboratory assistants (MLAs) and certified medical assistants (CMAs). These personnel have completed a specialized training program that is 1 or 2 years in length and have passed a registry examination. One may also find laboratory assistants and phlebotomists, individuals who have received specialized training in the collection and preparation of laboratory specimens.

TABLE 50-1 Certifying Agencies for Laboratory Personnel

CERTIFYING AGENCY	TITLE	POSITION
American Society for Clinical Pathologists	MT(ASCP) MLT(ASCP) MLT-AD(ASCP)	Medical technologist Medical laboratory technician—certificate Medical laboratory technician—associate's degree
American Medical Technologists	MT(AMT) MLT(AMT)	Medical technologist Medical laboratory technician
Department of Health and Human Services	CLT(HHS)	Clinical laboratory technologist
National Certification Agency for Medical Laboratory Personnel	CLS(NCA) CLT(NCA)	Certified laboratory scientist Certified laboratory technician
International Society for Clinical Laboratory Technology	RMT(ISCLT) RLT(ISCLT)	Registered medical technologist Registered laboratory technician
American Association of Medical Assistants (AAMA)	CMA	Certified medical assistant
Accrediting Bureau of Health Education Schools	RMA	Registered medical assistant (ABHES)
California Certifying Board for Medical Assistants	CCMA-C(CCBMA)	California certified medical assistant-clinical
National Healthcareer Association (NHA)	CCMA CPT CML	Certified clinical medical assistant Certified phlebotomy technician Certified medical laboratory assistant

The agencies granting certifications and titles are described in Table 50-1.

The medical assistant is a multiskilled professional who is trained to perform administrative and clinical procedures, including basic laboratory testing. Laboratory tests are an essential part of a medical diagnosis, and aid in treatment. They may also be performed to monitor or prescribe medication. Only a physician may request laboratory testing for a patient. The medical assistant may be responsible for a number of these testing procedures. To assume this responsibility, the medical assistant must know proper patient preparation, the procedures for each test, and the normal range of results for these tests. The medical assistant must carefully follow all laboratory instructions in obtaining and labeling the specimens and sending them to the laboratory. Good communication among the patient, the office staff, and the laboratory personnel is important. The medical assistant should make the patient feel more at ease with these procedures and thus gain the patient's cooperation.

Clinical Laboratory Testing

Clinical laboratory testing is used in conjunction with a thorough health history and physical examination to provide essential data needed for the diagnosis and management of a patient's condition. The body is considered to be healthy when a state of equilibrium in the internal environment exists. In this state, termed *homeostasis,* the physical and chemical characteristics of body substances (e.g., fluids, secretions, and excretions) will be within a certain acceptable range known as the *normal* or *reference range.* A change in homeostasis results in abnormal test values, outside of the reference range. Abnormal values for a particular test may be seen with more than one pathologic condition. For example, a decrease in hemoglobin levels in red blood cells (RBCs) is seen in iron-deficiency anemia, and it is also noted in

hyperthyroidism and cirrhosis of the liver. Thus the physician cannot rely solely on laboratory tests to make a diagnosis but must instead rely on the combination of data obtained from health history, physical examination, and a number of diagnostic and laboratory results.

Tests performed in a clinical laboratory range from simple screening tests to complex profile testing. A screening test is one that examines a particular specimen for the presence of a substance that may indicate a disease state. A screening test is not diagnostic for any particular disease but will indicate that the disease state may exist. Screening tests are often done routinely on patients, based on their age, history, or gender. Screening tests are often qualitative in that they do not have a numeric value attached to the result; results may simply be reported as positive or negative. The occult blood test for blood in the stool is an example of a screening test. Blood is not normally found in the stool, and its presence may indicate the presence of cancerous lesions. A positive test result indicates that blood is present, but additional testing is required to determine the source of the blood. For example, further testing or examination may reveal that the patient had her menstrual period at the time of collection of the specimen or that she had bleeding hemorrhoids.

A quantitative test will have units attached to numeric values. These values often are represented as the amount of **analyte** per given volume of specimen, and it is essential that the results be reported with the units. For example, in a complete blood cell count for a healthy adult, the RBCs will number 5 million per cubic millimeter ($5 \times 10^6/mm^3$), the hemoglobin value will be 15 g per deciliter (15 g/dL), and the hematocrit will be 45%. Generally the units are printed on the laboratory report, but the medical assistant must always ensure that the values are consistent with the testing being performed.

CRITICAL THINKING APPLICATION

The **referral laboratory** telephones to report the values on several tests performed on the urine of a client, Cecelia Roberts. Marsha jots down the following: Total protein, 0.12; Occult blood, positive; Albumin, 50; Glucose, 120. What is wrong with the notations she has just made? Are these tests qualitative or quantitative?

The Clinical Laboratory Improvement Amendments

In 1988 Congress passed the Clinical Laboratory Improvement Amendments (CLIA), establishing quality standards for all laboratory testing to ensure the accuracy, reliability, and timeliness of patient test results regardless of where the test was performed. A laboratory is defined as any facility that performs laboratory testing on specimens derived from humans for the purpose of providing information regarding the diagnosis, prevention, and treatment of disease, or impairment of or assessment of health. The CLIA program is user-fee funded; therefore all costs of administering the program must be covered by the regulated facilities. CLIA requires all entities that perform even one test, including waived tests, to meet certain federal requirements and register as a laboratory. An application must be submitted that reports information about a laboratory's operation. From this information the type of certificate to be issued and the fees to be assessed will be determined.

The CLIA categorization of commercially marketed in vitro diagnostic tests is now the responsibility of the Food and Drug Administration (FDA). The FDA has assumed primary responsibility for performing the CLIA complexity categorization functions, which include the process of assigning commercially marketed in vitro diagnostic test systems to one of three CLIA regulatory categories based on their potential risk to public health: (1) waived tests, (2) moderate-complexity tests, and (3) high-complexity tests.

Waived Tests

Waived tests include the following:

"laboratory examinations and procedures that have been approved by the Food and Drug Administration for home use or that, as determined by the Secretary, are simple laboratory examinations and procedures that have an insignificant risk of an erroneous result, including those that

(A) employ methodologies that are so simple and accurate to render the likelihood of erroneous results by the user negligible, or

(B) the Secretary has determined pose no unreasonable risk of harm to the patient if performed incorrectly"

A CLIA database is available to the public on the Internet. This database contains the commercially marketed in vitro test systems categorized by the FDA since January 31, 2000 and tests categorized by the Centers for Disease Control and Prevention (CDC) before that date. The records can be searched by test system name, specialty or subspecialty, analyte, document number, qualifier, effective date, and complexity.

Moderate- and High-Complexity Tests

The CLIA program oversees the quality of nearly 200,000 different laboratory procedures. An estimated 10,000 different laboratory tests are performed in the United States every day; 75% of them are categorized as moderate-complexity tests by the FDA. Some of these tests are performed in physician's office laboratories (POLs), including hematology and chemistry testing done on an automated analyzer, Gram staining, and microscopic analysis of urine sediment. High-complexity tests usually are not performed in a POL and include Papanicolaou (Pap) smear analysis, blood typing and cross-matching, and cytologic testing.

Laboratories that perform moderate- to high-complexity testing must meet CLIA regulations and are subject to unannounced inspections every 2 years. Each laboratory performing these tests must establish a system to maintain the integrity and identification of patient specimens throughout the testing process and ensure the accurate reporting of results. The laboratory also must have established and must follow written quality-control (QC) and quality-assurance (QA) procedures and must participate in proficiency testing, a form of external quality control. Three times a year the laboratory must test samples provided by an approved proficiency-testing agency using the same tests that they would use to test a patient's sample. Finally, CLIA regulations specify qualifications and responsibilities for personnel in laboratories, from directors to testing personnel. Personnel requirements are most stringent for high-complexity testing.

Medical assistants may perform all CLIA-waived tests and some moderately complex tests, depending on the certification

---

Examples of CLIA-Waived Tests

1. Dipstick or tablet reagent urinalysis (nonautomated) for the following:
   - Bilirubin
   - Glucose
   - Hemoglobin
   - Ketone
   - Leukocytes
   - Nitrite
   - pH
   - Protein
   - Specific gravity
   - Urobilinogen
2. Fecal occult blood
3. Ovulation tests: visual color comparison tests for luteinizing hormone
4. Urine pregnancy tests: visual color comparison tests
5. Erythrocyte sedimentation rate: nonautomated
6. Hemoglobin-copper sulfate: nonautomated
7. Blood glucose by glucose monitoring devices cleared by the FDA specifically for home use
8. Spun microhematocrit
9. Hemoglobin and hemoglobin A_{1c} by single analyte instruments with self-contained or component features to perform specimen-reagent interaction, providing direct measurement and readout

of the laboratory or POL in which they are employed. While medical assistants may not perform high-complexity testing, they often are involved in collection of the specimens required, in the preparation of the patient for testing, and in the recording of the results on a patient's chart.

DIVISIONS OF THE CLINICAL LABORATORY

The laboratory is divided into various departments, which may include hematology, chemistry, microbiology, specimen collection and processing, blood bank, coagulation, serology, histology, **cytology,** toxicology, urinalysis, and special chemistry. The laboratory in the physician's office usually performs procedures in urinalysis, hematology, chemistry, and microbiology.

Urinalysis

Urinalysis includes the physical, chemical, and microscopic examination of urine. In the physical examination the color, clarity, and specific gravity are noted. Chemical analysis is performed to measure levels of such analytes as glucose, protein, ketones, blood, bilirubin, urobilinogen, nitrites, and pH. Microscopically the urine is examined for the presence of red, white, and epithelial cells, mucus, casts, crystals, yeasts, parasites, and bacteria. Additional quantitative tests may also be performed in the urinalysis department to confirm routine screening tests.

Hematology

Tests performed in the hematology division may be qualitative or quantitative. Blood cell counts determine the exact number of RBCs or erythrocytes, white blood cells (WBCs or leukocytes), or platelets (thrombocytes) either by manual counting or by automated counting. Qualitative tests determine the characteristics of cells, such as size, shape, and maturity. In addition, the hematology department will perform tests to determine the coagulating ability of blood components.

Chemistry

The clinical chemistry department analyzes blood, **cerebrospinal fluid** (CSF), urine, and joint fluid (synovial fluid). Procedures may include single tests or profiles, which include tests for a number of related analytes. Lipid profiles, for example, will include assessments of total cholesterol, triglyceride, and high-density lipoprotein (HDL) cholesterol.

Microbiology

Microbiology involves the study of bacteria, fungi, yeasts, parasites, and viruses. In the microbiology laboratory, microorganisms are grown (cultured) from blood, urine, sputum, CSF, and wound specimens and are identified. Susceptibility testing is then performed on these organisms to determine proper antibiotic therapy. Specimens for the microbiology must be collected aseptically in sterile containers.

CRITICAL THINKING APPLICATION

Dr. Watkins has ordered a routine urinalysis (UA), a urine culture and sensitivity (C&S) test, a blood glucose test, and a complete blood count (CBC) for his patient. What division of the laboratory will be responsible for analyzing the specimens for each test?

LABORATORY SAFETY

The importance of safety in the laboratory cannot be overemphasized. Most laboratory accidents are preventable by exercising proper techniques and by using common sense. Using safe practices in the laboratory requires a personal commitment and concern for others; an unsafe act may harm an innocent bystander without harming the person who performs the act.

Safety Standards and Governing Agencies

Safety standards for laboratories are initiated, governed, and reviewed by several agencies or committees including the U.S. Department of Labor's Occupational Safety and Health Administration (OSHA); a nonprofit educational organization known as the Clinical and Laboratory Standards Institute (CLSI–formerly the National Committee for Clinical Laboratory Standards, NCCLS), which provides a forum for development, promotion, and use of national and international standards; the CDC, which is a government agency under the U.S. Department of Health and Human Services; the College of American Pathologists (CAP), a leader in providing laboratory quality-improvement programs; and the Environmental Protection Agency (EPA), a government agency whose mission it is to protect human health and to safeguard the natural environment.

Through OSHA the government has created a system of safeguards and regulations under the Occupational Safety and Health Act of 1970. This system affects nearly every worker in the United States because the regulations apply to all businesses with one or more employees. The regulations are discussed in detail in Chapter 26. Two programs have been mandated by OSHA to ensure the safety of personnel working in clinical laboratories. One covers occupational exposure to chemical hazards; the other covers exposure to blood-borne pathogens. Both of these programs, as they relate to safety in the medical laboratory setting, are discussed later in this chapter.

CRITICAL THINKING APPLICATION

The physicians for whom Marsha works would like to expand the laboratory testing done on site. They ask her to assess the space available and make suggestions for necessary improvements based on requirements by governing agencies. What should she do? Which agency or agencies would be most helpful in providing suggestions?

LABORATORY HAZARDS

Physical Hazards

Physical hazards in the laboratory can be classified as electrical, fire, and mechanical. Electric shock is a threat when any electrical equipment is in use. It is imperative to keep all electrical equipment in proper repair and always to follow manufacturers' instructions.

Use surge protectors, inspect all cords and plugs frequently, never use extension cords, and avoid overloading circuits. Before servicing, unplug the electrical device, and never operate electrical instruments with wet hands. If there is a sink nearby, ensure that electric cords do not come into contact with the water supply. Signs and labels, such as those shown in Figure 50-1, should be placed on specific electrical hazards.

Open flames are rarely used in a laboratory, but the potential for fire still exists. Fires may be ignited by smoking, heating elements, and sparks. Flammable materials should not be stored near any source of ignition. All laboratory personnel should be familiar with the location of fire extinguishers and fire safety blankets. Fire extinguishers should be of the carbon dioxide (CO_2), dry chemical, or halon type—known as the ABC type of extinguisher. The ABC extinguisher can be used on all types of fires. These extinguishers should be inspected by a licensed inspector on a regular basis and replaced or recharged if used. The medical assistant may be responsible for maintaining records on the care and maintenance of fire extinguishers.

Fire safety blankets should be used to smother flames on burning clothing. However, one should avoid wrapping a victim in a fire blanket, because this may intensify burns. Instead, the flames should be patted out or the victim directed to roll on the blanket.

Emergency phone numbers should be posted on the wall near the telephone, and all personnel should know the location of fire alarms, the fire escape routes, and procedures to follow if exits are blocked. Periodic fire drills should be conducted, and hallways and exits should be kept free of clutter.

Mechanical hazards arise from the use of laboratory equipment. Special care should be exercised when using equipment with moving parts, such as centrifuges, and those that rely on pressure, including autoclaves. Centrifuges, devices that separate liquids from solids, present a hazard not only from moving parts but also from glassware that might break during centrifugation and from aerosols that might be created if tubes are not capped tightly. Pressurized equipment, such as autoclaves used in sterilization, presents dangers if opened prematurely. Although centrifuges and autoclaves often have built-in safeguards, such as locks that prevent entry until the environment is safe, improper care of the equipment can result in failure of the safety measures.

Chemical Hazards

The clinical laboratory is home to chemicals that are flammable, **caustic,** poisonous, **carcinogenic,** and/or **teratogenic.** Exposure to these dangers can be through inhalation, direct absorption through the skin, ingestion, entry through a mucous membrane, or entry through a break in the skin. OSHA is involved in regulating the standards directed at minimizing occupational exposure to hazardous chemicals in laboratories. The OSHA hazard communication standard (known as the employee "right to know" rule) became law in 1991 and ensures that laboratory workers are fully aware of the hazards associated with their workplace. The law necessitates the development of a comprehensive plan to implement safe practice throughout the laboratory insofar as chemicals are concerned. This chemical hygiene plan must outline the specific work practices and procedures that are needed to protect workers from any health hazards that may arise from working with in-stock chemicals. Information and training must be provided to all workers. There must be a Material Safety Data Sheet (MSDS) on file for all chemicals in use in the laboratory. OSHA requires the manufacturer of the chemical to make the sheets available, usually as a package insert.

Each MSDS contains the basic information about the specific chemical or product. This includes the trade name, chemical name and synonyms, chemical family, manufacturer's name and address, emergency telephone number, hazardous ingredients, physical data, fire and explosion data, and health hazard and protection information (Figure 50-2).

Following principles of proper handling will reduce your risks of harmful effects. Harmful exposure can be reduced by using proper devices for pipetting; never pipet by mouth. If a chemical produces toxic or flammable vapors, work under a fume hood that exhausts air to the outside. In case of accidental exposure to the skin, rinse the affected area under running water for at least 5 minutes. Remove any clothing that is contaminated. If chemicals are splashed in the eyes, flush the eyes with water from an eyewash station for a minimum of 15 minutes. Prompt medical attention must be given to victims of chemical exposure.

Chemicals should be tightly sealed and properly labeled. A hazard identification system was developed by the National Fire Protection Association that provides, at a glance, information on the potential health, flammability, and chemical reactivity hazards of materials. This identification system consists of four small, colored, diamond-shaped symbols grouped into a larger diamond shape. The top diamond is red and indicates flammability hazard. The diamond on the left is blue and indicates hazards to health. The bottom diamond is white and

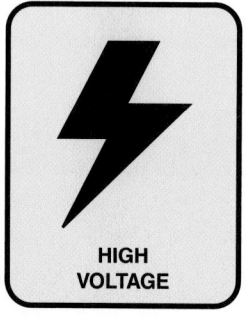
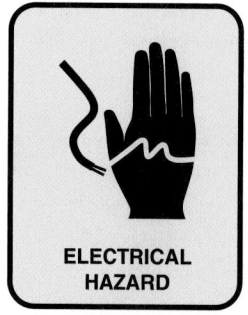

HIGH VOLTAGE   **ELECTRICAL HAZARD**

FIGURE 50-1 High-voltage and electrical hazard labels. (From Stepp CA, Woods MA: *Laboratory procedures for medical office personnel,* Philadelphia, 1998, Saunders.)

MATERIAL SAFETY DATA SHEET

MSDS NO. 396
PAGE 1

SECTION 1 IDENTIFICATION

MANUFACTURER'S NAME: Corelis Corporation
ADDRESS: P.O. Box 93
Camden, NJ 08106

EMERGENCY TELEPHONE NUMBER: 1 (800) 733-8690

TELEPHONE NUMBER FOR INFORMATION: 1 (800) 331-0766

ISSUED: 10/99

IDENTITY: 2% Aqueous Glutaraldehyde Solution

PREPARED BY: Regulatory Affairs

PRODUCT CODE: 3345

TRADE NAME: Aldecyde

SYNONYMS: None

CHEMICAL FAMILY: Aldehydes

MOLECULAR FORMULA: $OHCC_3H_6CHO$ (Active)

RTECS #: MA 2450000 (Active)

MOLECULAR WEIGHT: 100

HAZARD RATING – HEALTH: 3 (Serious Hazard)   FLAMMABILITY: 0   REACTIVITY:0   SPECIFIC: NONE

SECTION 2 HAZARDOUS INGREDIENTS/IDENTITY INFORMATION

COMPONENTS (SPECIFIC CHEMICAL IDENTITY)	CAS #	%	OSHA PEL	ACGIH TLV	OSHA 1910.1200
Glutaraldehyde (active)	111-30-8	2	0.2ppm, C	0.2ppm, C	n/a
Inert buffer salts	n/a		None	None	Nonhazardous
Water	7732-18-5	98	None	None	Nonhazardous

SECTION 3 PHYSICAL/CHEMICAL CHARACTERISTICS

APPEARANCE AND ODOR: 2 components: colorless fluid and liquid salts; turns green when activated. Sharp odor masked with peppermint fragrance.

BOILING POINT: 212°F

SPECIFIC GRAVITY (H_2O=1): 1.003 g/cc

VAPOR PRESSURE (mm Hg): same as water

MELTING POINT: n/a

VAPOR DENSITY (AIR=1): same as water

EVAPORATION RATE (H_2O=1): 0.98

SOLUBILITY IN WATER: complete

pH: 8

FREEZING POINT: same as water

ODOR THRESHOLD: .04 ppm, detectable. (ACGIH)

SECTION 4 FIRE AND EXPLOSION HAZARD DATA

FLASH POINT (METHOD USED): None   FLAMMABLE LIMITS – LEL: nd   UEL: nd

EXTINGUISHING MEDIA: If water is evaporated, material can burn. Use carbon dioxide or dry chemical for small fires. Use foam (alcohol, polymer or ordinary) or water fog for large fires.

SPECIAL FIRE FIGHTING PROCEDURES: Self-contained breathing apparatus and protective clothing should be available to fireman.

UNUSUAL FIRE AND EXPLOSION HAZARDS: None

TOXIC GASES PRODUCED: None

SECTION 5 REACTIVITY DATA

STABILITY: 212°F

CONDITIONS TO AVOID: None

INCOMPATIBILITY (MATERIALS TO AVOID): None

HAZARDOUS DECOMPOSITION OR BYPRODUCTS: None

HAZARDOUS POLYMERIZATION: Will not occur

FIGURE 50-2 Material safety data sheet (MSDS). (From Bonewit-West K: *Clinical procedures for medical assistants*, ed 6, Philadelphia, 2004, Saunders.) *Continued*

MATERIAL SAFETY DATA SHEET

MSDS NO. 396
PAGE 2

SECTION 6   HEALTH HAZARD DATA

ROUTE(S) OF ENTRY – INHALATION: yes   SKIN: yes   INGESTION: yes   EYE: yes

SIGNS AND SYMPTOMS OF EXPOSURE:

EYES: Contact with eyes causes damage.

SKIN: Can cause skin sensitization. Avoid skin contact.

INHALATION: Vapors may be irritating and cause headache, chest discomfort, symptoms of bronchitis.

INGESTION: May cause nausea, vomiting and general systemic illness.

EMERGENCY AND FIRST AID PROCEDURE:

EYES: Flush thoroughly with water. Get medical attention.

SKIN: Flush thoroughly with water. If irritation persists, get medical attention.

INHALATION: Remove to fresh air. If symptoms persist, get medical attention.

INGESTION: Do not induce vomiting. Drink copious amount of milk. Get medical attention.

HEALTH HAZARDS (ACUTE AND CHRONIC):
  Acute: As listed above under Signs and Symptoms of Exposure
  Chronic: None known from currently available information.

MEDICAL CONDITIONS GENERALLY AGGRAVATED BY EXPOSURE: None known from currently available information.

LISTED AS CARCINOGEN BY –   NTP: yes   IARC MONOGRAPHS: no   OSHA: no

TOXICITY: ORAL LD50 (Rat)   Toxicity Rating 1: 500-5000 mg/kg.
            OCULAR (Rabbit)   Toxicity Rating 2: Irritating or moderately persisting more than seven days with.
            DERMAL LD50 (Rabbit)   None by dermal route.
            INHALATION LC50 (Rabbit)   Irritating but non-toxic at highest concentration achieved (2.89 ppm).

SECTION 7   PRECAUTIONS FOR SAFE HANDLING AND USE

STEPS TO BE TAKE IN CASE MATERIAL IS RELEASED OR SPILLED: For LARGE spills, use ammonium carbonate to "neutralize" glutaraldehyde odor. Collect liquid and discard it. For SMALL spills, wipe with sponge or mop down area with an equal mixture of household ammonia and water. Flush with large quantities of water.

WASTE DISPOSAL METHOD: Triple rinse empty container with water and dispose in an incinerator or landfill approved for pesticide containers. Discard solution with large quantities of water.

EPA HAZARDOUS WASTE NUMBER: n/a

PRECAUTIONS TO BE TAKEN IN HANDLING AND STORING: Use normal storage and handling requirements.

SECTION 8   TRANSPORTATION DATA AND ADDITIONAL INFORMATION

DOMESTIC (D.O.T.): Aldehydes, N.O.S.   INTERNATIONAL (I.M.O.): Aldehydes, N.O.S.

PROPER SHIPPING NAME: Glutaraldehyde   PROPER SHIPPING NAME: Glutaraldehyde

HAZARD CLASS: None   HAZARD CLASS: None

LABELS: None Needed   LABELS: None Needed

REPORTABLE QUANTITY: None   UN/NA: 1989

FIGURE 50-2, *cont'd*

provides special hazard information including radioactivity, special biohazards, and other dangerous situations. Finally, the diamond on the right is yellow and indicates reactivity or stability hazard. The system indicates the severity of the hazard by using numbers imprinted in the diamonds from 0 to 4, with 4 being extremely hazardous to 0 being no hazard (Figure 50-3).

Biologic Hazards and Infection Control

Biologic hazards, or biohazards, are materials or situations that present a risk or potential risk of infection. Infection with biohazardous material can occur during specimen collection, handling, transporting, or testing the specimen. Potentially

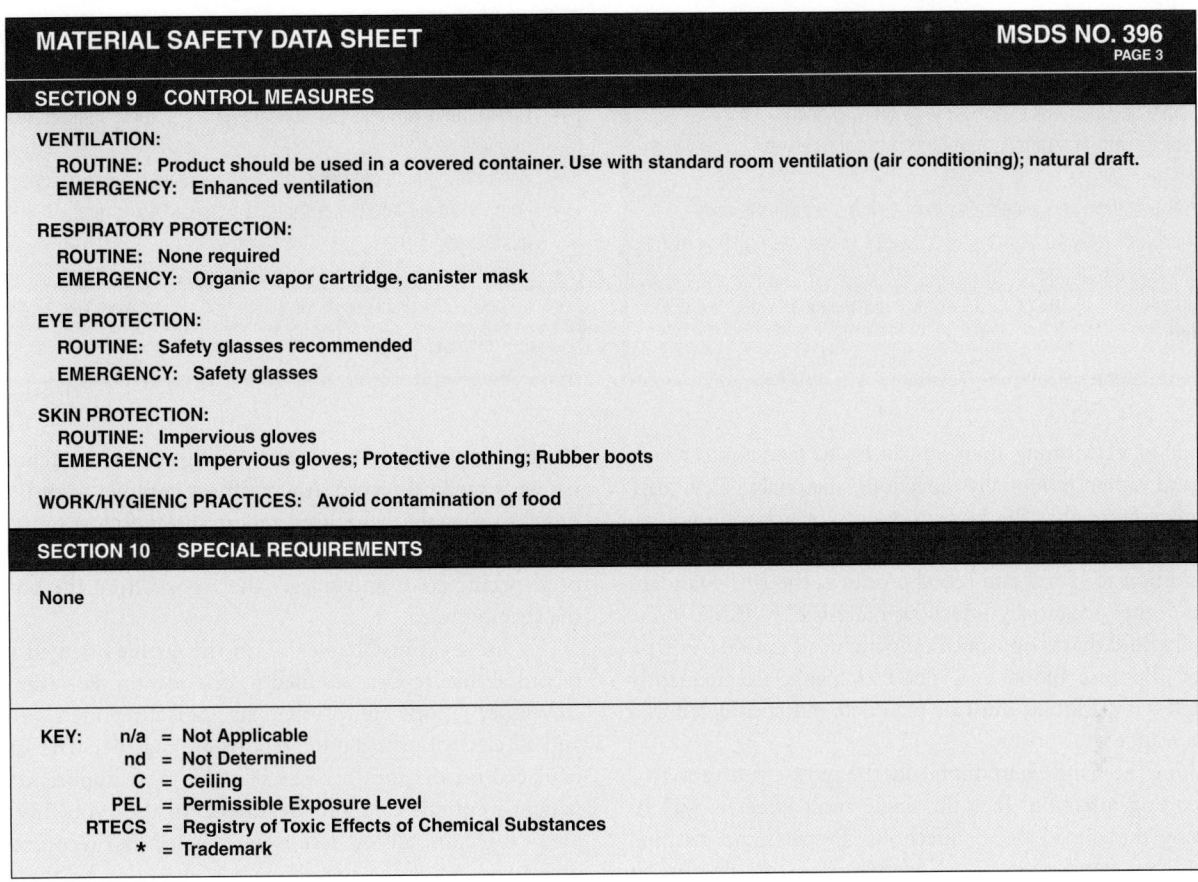

FIGURE 50-2, *cont'd.*

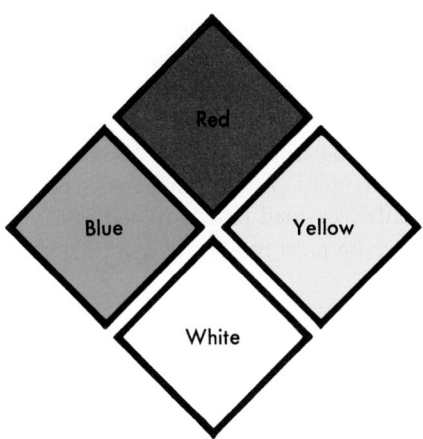

FIGURE 50-3 Identification system of the National Fire Protection Association.

infective specimens include blood, body tissue biopsy specimens, urine, **exudates,** and bacterial cultures and smears. Infection can occur through aspiration of a pathogen, accidental inoculation by a needlestick, aerosols created by uncapping specimen tubes, centrifuge accidents, and entry of pathogens through cuts and scratches.

One of the most important OSHA regulations covers exposure to biologic hazards. The OSHA-mandated program, Occupational Exposure to Bloodborne Pathogens, must be in place and has been law since 1992 as part of a general

infection control policy. In addition, the CDC recommends safety precautions regarding handling of all patient specimens. Previously known as *universal precautions,* they are now referred to as *standard precautions* and are published on the organization's web page and in the publication *Morbidity and Mortality Weekly Report.* Chapter 24 covers the specifics of the OSHA-mandated programs.

The recommendations from the CDC include an infection control plan, engineering and work practice controls, personal protective clothing and equipment, sufficient training and education, provision of hepatitis B vaccination, and medical intervention after exposure incidents. The CLSI also has guidelines for the laboratory worker with regard to protection from blood-borne illness caused by contact with patient specimens. The CAP offers a voluntary accreditation program for clinical laboratories that includes biosafety measures. One important precaution that can be taken is labeling of potentially biohazardous material, as described in Chapter 26.

Standard Precautions

Hepatitis B and the human immunodeficiency virus (HIV) are a constant threat to the health and safety of clinical laboratory personnel. Hepatitis B and HIV are both transmitted through exposure to blood and body fluids. Blood and body fluids are the primary substances handled in the laboratory. OSHA mandated the Bloodborne Pathogens (BBP) Standard, which covers all employees who could be "reasonably anticipated as

Exposure Control Plan Requirements
• Identification of tasks, procedures, and job classification where possible occupational exposure to blood may occur
• Establishment of methods that protect employees and comply with OSHA regulations
• Implementation of a vaccination program for hepatitis B virus
• Provision of training in the proper use of protective equipment for blood-borne pathogens
• Maintenance of records to show compliance with the BBP Standard

Safety Guidelines for Other Potentially Infectious Materials
• Handle and process all specimens as if they contain infectious material.
• Wipe the outside of specimen containers with a germicide.
• Dispose of all infectious materials according to state and federal guidelines.
• Clean up spills using a disinfectant (see Chapter 26).
• Immediately dispose of any chipped or broken glassware in a special disposable container.

the result of performing their job duties to face contact with blood and other potentially infectious materials." The BBP Standard requires that the laboratory employer have a written exposure control plan.

In addition to blood and blood products, the BBP Standard includes "other potentially infectious materials" (OPIM). Urine is the only fluid that is not specifically included in OSHA's BBP Standard. Because blood and blood elements are frequently associated with urine, it must be included and considered as a possible source of exposure.

Washing the hands is undoubtedly the most effective means of preventing infection. It is the single most effective way of preventing the spread of all infections. Proper hand washing protects you, your patient, and your co-workers because it removes organisms. In the laboratory area it is absolutely required to wash your hands in the following situations:

- When you enter and before leaving the area
- Before and after every patient procedure
- After contact with body fluid even if gloves were worn
- Before and after eating
- Before and after using the rest room

Every laboratory should have a safety manual that covers all safety practices and precautions. The manual should clearly explain procedures to be followed in the event of an accident. A section of the manual should prominently list emergency numbers for ambulance, fire, police, and other security services as well as plans for evacuation. Emergency numbers should also be posted near the telephone, and plans for evacuation must be posted. Second, the manual should give instructions for reporting and documenting accidents, and contain an accident log to record the names and persons involved, the type of accident, and the date it occurred. Copies of this incident report form should be in the manual along with an example of a properly completed form. It is important to note that such a form not only documents the accident but also the steps taken to prevent such an accident from recurring.

SPECIMEN COLLECTION, PROCESSING, AND STORAGE

Laboratory Requisitions and Reports

A patient's medical record should be maintained in an organized manner to promote easy access to the desired information.

Various methods are used when filing laboratory reports in a patient's medical record. Many offices compile records in a set order so that the laboratory report sheets follow entry A and precede entry B. Another method is to use standard-sized sheets of a specific color and stagger the reports from the bottom of the sheet upward.

As discussed in Chapter 27, in the source-oriented medical record all like reports are filed in one section. For example, all laboratory reports are together, all surgical reports are together, and all electrocardiographic reports are together. The latest test is placed on the top, because it is the most important for the patient's current care and treatment. In the problem-oriented medical record, all test results are entered and recorded in the objective part of the progress notes, preceded by the number and title of the particular problem.

The medical assistant's responsibility is to make sure that all reports are received for diagnostic tests performed on the patient outside the physician's office. Only after the physician reviews the test results should they be filed into the patient's record.

When the physician requests laboratory testing that must be done outside of the office, a written requisition for the work must be sent to the laboratory with the patient or with the specimen (Figure 50-4). These forms are preprinted, with the most commonly requested tests indicated in logical sequence. Patient information must be complete, accurate, and legible.

Specimen Collection

The medical assistant is responsible for the collection of many different types of specimens. It is important to recognize that all clinical laboratory results are only as good as the specimen received. The importance of specimen collection cannot be overemphasized. If the test results are to be accurate indicators of the patient's state of health, it is imperative that the concepts of specimen collection be understood and followed exactly. The most common specimens are blood, urine, and swab samples collected from wounds or mucous membranes. Less often, feces, gastric contents, CSF, tissue samples, semen, and aspirates, such as synovial fluid or amniotic fluid, are submitted for testing. These specimens are analyzed for levels of many chemicals and drugs, types and numbers of cells present, and the presence of microorganisms.

Initial identification of the patient is essential, as is collection of the specimen in an appropriate collection container. For example, blood may be collected using a vacuum tube system. These tubes are available in a variety of sizes, with and without **preservatives** and **anticoagulants.** The tubes are color-coded so that the color of the stopper denotes which, if any, additive is present (Figure 50-5). Collection in an incorrect tube will result in an unacceptable specimen, and recollection will be necessary. If the specimen is to be tested for the presence of microorganisms, a sterile container must be used. If the patient is to collect the specimen at home, he or she should be provided with the appropriate container and complete instructions for collection.

The medical assistant should always check the laboratory's specimen requirements manual for any unfamiliar tests. The manual lists all specimen-collection information. Any unanswered questions should be resolved by calling the laboratory before collecting the specimen. The container must be labeled properly at the time of collection; unlabeled containers should never be accepted for laboratory testing. Labels should include the patient's full name and the date; for some specimens the time of collection and the type of specimen should also be included on the label.

If the specimen is to be mailed, it must be carefully packaged to prevent breakage, damage, or contamination by all persons handling it. Containers of liquid specimens may be wrapped in absorbent material and inserted in unbreakable tubes with

Example of Information Usually Required When Specimens Are Sent to the Laboratory

- Physician's name, account number, address, and phone number
- Patient's full name, surname first
- Patient's address
- Patient's insurance information
- Patient's age, date of birth, and gender
- Source of specimen
- Date and time of collection
- Specific test (or tests) requested
- Medications the patient is taking
- Possible diagnosis
- Indication of whether test is to be performed **stat**

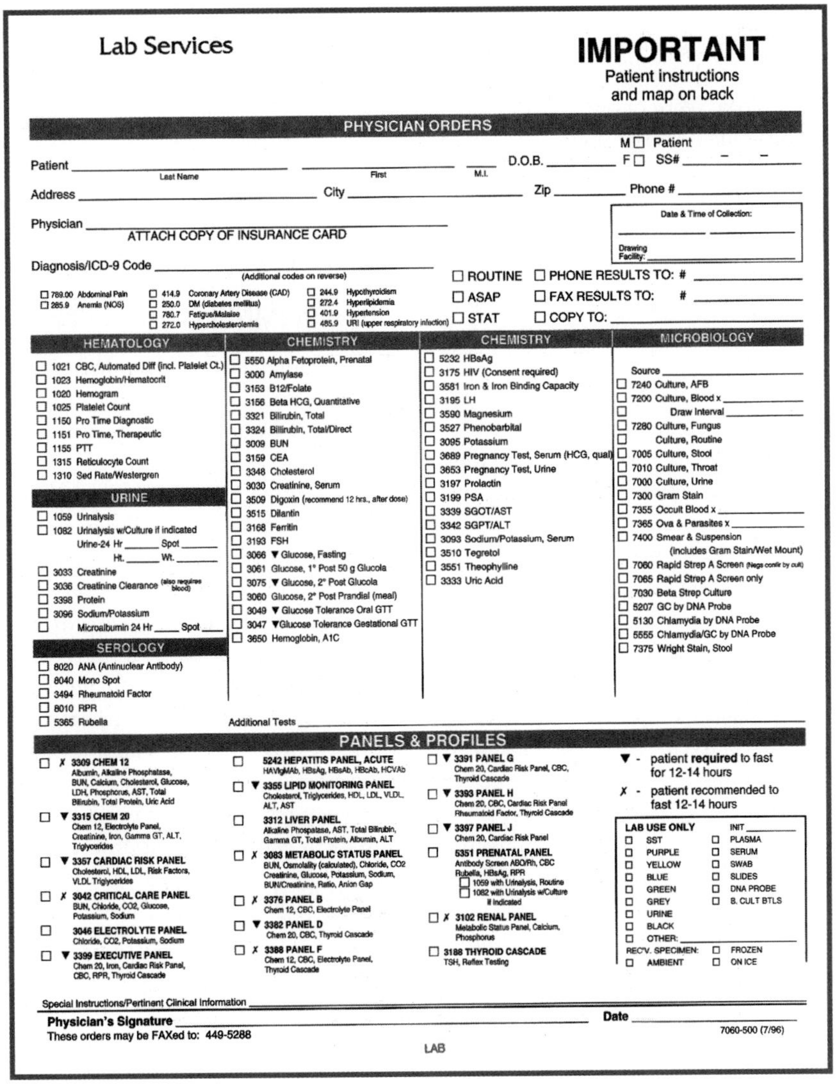

Lab Services

IMPORTANT
Patient instructions and map on back

PHYSICIAN ORDERS

Patient ______ (Last Name) ______ (First) ___ (M.I.) D.O.B. ______ M ☐ F ☐ Patient SS# ___ - ___ - ___
Address ______ City ______ Zip ______ Phone # ______
Physician ______
ATTACH COPY OF INSURANCE CARD
Date & Time of Collection: ______ ______
Drawing Facility: ______
Diagnosis/ICD-9 Code ______ (Additional codes on reverse)
☐ 789.00 Abdominal Pain
☐ 285.9 Anemia (NOS)
☐ 414.9 Coronary Artery Disease (CAD)
☐ 250.0 DM (diabetes mellitus)
☐ 780.7 Fatigue/Malaise
☐ 272.0 Hypercholesterolemia
☐ 244.9 Hypothyroidism
☐ 272.4 Hyperlipidemia
☐ 401.9 Hypertension
☐ 485.9 URI (upper respiratory infection)
☐ ROUTINE ☐ PHONE RESULTS TO: # ______
☐ ASAP ☐ FAX RESULTS TO: # ______
☐ STAT ☐ COPY TO: ______

HEMATOLOGY
☐ 1021 CBC, Automated Diff (incl. Platelet Ct.)
☐ 1023 Hemoglobin/Hematocrit
☐ 1020 Hemogram
☐ 1025 Platelet Count
☐ 1150 Pro Time Diagnostic
☐ 1151 Pro Time, Therapeutic
☐ 1155 PTT
☐ 1315 Reticulocyte Count
☐ 1310 Sed Rate/Westergren

URINE
☐ 1059 Urinalysis
☐ 1082 Urinalysis w/Culture if indicated
Urine-24 Hr ______ Spot ______
Ht. ______ Wt. ______
☐ 3033 Creatinine
☐ 3036 Creatinine Clearance (also requires blood)
☐ 3398 Protein
☐ 3096 Sodium/Potassium
☐ Microalbumin 24 Hr ____ Spot ____

SEROLOGY
☐ 8020 ANA (Antinuclear Antibody)
☐ 8040 Mono Spot
☐ 3494 Rheumatoid Factor
☐ 8010 RPR
☐ 5365 Rubella

CHEMISTRY
☐ 5550 Alpha Fetoprotein, Prenatal
☐ 3000 Amylase
☐ 3153 B12/Folate
☐ 3156 Beta HCG, Quantitative
☐ 3321 Bilirubin, Total
☐ 3324 Billirubin, Total/Direct
☐ 3009 BUN
☐ 3159 CEA
☐ 3348 Cholesterol
☐ 3030 Creatinine, Serum
☐ 3509 Digoxin (recommend 12 hrs., after dose)
☐ 3515 Dilantin
☐ 3168 Ferritin
☐ 3193 FSH
☐ 3066 ▼ Glucose, Fasting
☐ 3061 Glucose, 1° Post 50 g Glucola
☐ 3075 ▼ Glucose, 2° Post Glucola
☐ 3060 Glucose, 2° Post Prandial (meal)
☐ 3049 ▼ Glucose Tolerance Oral GTT
☐ 3047 ▼Glucose Tolerance Gestational GTT
☐ 3650 Hemoglobin, A1C

CHEMISTRY
☐ 5232 HBsAg
☐ 3175 HIV (Consent required)
☐ 3581 Iron & Iron Binding Capacity
☐ 3195 LH
☐ 3590 Magnesium
☐ 3527 Phenobarbital
☐ 3095 Potassium
☐ 3689 Pregnancy Test, Serum (HCG, qual)
☐ 3653 Pregnancy Test, Urine
☐ 3197 Prolactin
☐ 3199 PSA
☐ 3339 SGOT/AST
☐ 3342 SGPT/ALT
☐ 3093 Sodium/Potassium, Serum
☐ 3510 Tegretol
☐ 3551 Theophylline
☐ 3333 Uric Acid

MICROBIOLOGY
Source ______
☐ 7240 Culture, AFB
☐ 7200 Culture, Blood x ______
☐ Draw Interval ______
☐ 7280 Culture, Fungus
☐ Culture, Routine
☐ 7005 Culture, Stool
☐ 7010 Culture, Throat
☐ 7000 Culture, Urine
☐ 7300 Gram Stain
☐ 7355 Occult Blood x ______
☐ 7365 Ova & Parasites x ______
☐ 7400 Smear & Suspension (includes Gram Stain/Wet Mount)
☐ 7060 Rapid Strep A Screen (Negs confir by cult)
☐ 7065 Rapid Strep A Screen only
☐ 7030 Beta Strep Culture
☐ 5207 GC by DNA Probe
☐ 5130 Chlamydia by DNA Probe
☐ 5555 Chlamydia/GC by DNA Probe
☐ 7375 Wright Stain, Stool

Additional Tests ______

PANELS & PROFILES
☐ ✗ 3309 CHEM 12 — Albumin, Alkaline Phosphatase, BUN, Calcium, Cholesterol, Glucose, LDH, Phosphorus, AST, Total Bilirubin, Total Protein, Uric Acid
☐ ▼ 3315 CHEM 20 — Chem 12, Electrolyte Panel, Creatinine, Iron, Gamma GT, ALT, Triglycerides
☐ ▼ 3357 CARDIAC RISK PANEL — Cholesterol, HDL, LDL, Risk Factors, VLDL Triglycerides
☐ ✗ 3042 CRITICAL CARE PANEL — BUN, Chloride, CO2, Glucose, Potassium, Sodium
☐ 3046 ELECTROLYTE PANEL — Chloride, CO2, Potassium, Sodium
☐ ▼ 3399 EXECUTIVE PANEL — Chem 20, Iron, Cardiac Risk Panel, CBC, RPR, Thyroid Cascade
☐ 5242 HEPATITIS PANEL, ACUTE — HAVIgMAb, HBsAg, HBsAb, HBcAb, HCVAb
☐ ▼ 3355 LIPID MONITORING PANEL — Cholesterol, Triglycerides, HDL, LDL, VLDL, ALT, AST
☐ 3312 LIVER PANEL — Alkaline Phospatase, AST, Total Bilirubin, Gamma GT, Total Protein, Albumin, ALT
☐ ✗ 3083 METABOLIC STATUS PANEL — BUN, Osmolality (calculated), Chloride, CO2 Creatinine, Glucose, Potassium, Sodium, BUN/Creatinine, Ratio, Anion Gap
☐ ✗ 3376 PANEL B — Chem 12, CBC, Electrolyte Panel
☐ ▼ 3382 PANEL D — Chem 20, CBC, Thyroid Cascade
☐ ✗ 3388 PANEL F — Chem 12, CBC, Electrolyte Panel, Thyroid Cascade
☐ ▼ 3391 PANEL G — Chem 20, Cardiac Risk Panel, CBC, Thyroid Cascade
☐ ▼ 3393 PANEL H — Chem 20, CBC, Cardiac Risk Panel Rheumatoid Factor, Thyroid Cascade
☐ ▼ 3397 PANEL J — Chem 20, Cardiac Risk Panel
☐ 5351 PRENATAL PANEL — Antibody Screen ABO/Rh, CBC Rubella, HBsAg, RPR
☐ 1059 with Urinalysis, Routine
☐ 1082 with Urinalysis w/Culture if Indicated
☐ ✗ 3102 RENAL PANEL — Metabolic Status Panel, Calcium, Phosphorus
☐ 3188 THYROID CASCADE — TSH, Reflex Testing

▼ - patient **required** to fast for 12-14 hours
✗ - patient recommended to fast 12-14 hours

LAB USE ONLY INIT ______
☐ SST ☐ PLASMA
☐ PURPLE ☐ SERUM
☐ YELLOW ☐ SWAB
☐ BLUE ☐ SLIDES
☐ GREEN ☐ DNA PROBE
☐ GREY ☐ B. CULT BTLS
☐ URINE
☐ BLACK
☐ OTHER: ______
REC'V. SPECIMEN: ☐ FROZEN
☐ AMBIENT ☐ ON ICE

Special Instructions/Pertinent Clinical Information ______
Physician's Signature ______ **Date** ______
These orders may be FAXed to: 449-5288
7060-500 (7/96)
LAB

FIGURE 50-4 Laboratory requisition form.

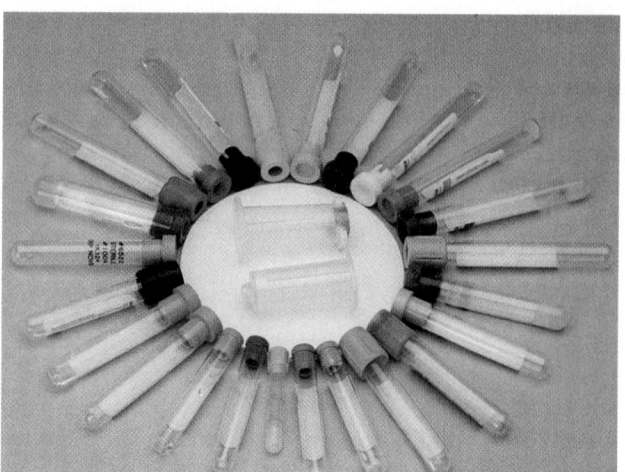

FIGURE 50-5 Vacutainer tubes. Note color-coded tops.

safe-top lids. The lids are taped shut so that no leakage occurs if the specimen container breaks. Place all specimens in a second container, such as an impervious bag, for transport. The completed requisition goes inside the outermost wrap. Usually, Styrofoam mailers (Figure 50-6) are used because they cushion the sample and also provide insulation. Styrofoam inserts can be shaped to fit around the specimen container. A warning label specifying the etiologic agent or biologic specimen is affixed to the outside of the container. The specimen should be given to the laboratory courier or mailed at a post office immediately so that it is not exposed to temperature extremes. Instructions for properly obtaining, processing, and preparing a specimen for transport are usually supplied to the POL by the testing laboratory. If the instructions are not clear or if you have a question regarding a particular collection, the laboratory will answer your question over the phone.

Avoiding Contamination

A medical assistant must take care to avoid contaminating the specimen as well as himself or herself. Expiration dates on swabs, tubes, transport media, and other collection containers should be checked before these items are used. An improperly handled specimen may become contaminated or may contaminate the surrounding environment. Standard precautions should be followed. All blood and other body fluids from all patients should be considered infective.

Sufficient samples should be collected for the tests requested by the physician. Amounts may vary based on the methods used. If a report is returned from the laboratory marked QNS (quantity not sufficient), it indicates a request for an additional specimen. Be certain to clarify any questions concerning the previous specimen by calling the laboratory before collecting a new one.

The specimen collected must be a true representative sample. A swab for a wound culture collected from the surface of the wound generally does not yield the same results as one taken from the depths of the wound. A **hemolyzed** blood specimen or one taken from an atypical area, such as a **hematoma** or the area above or below an intravenous drip, shows marked

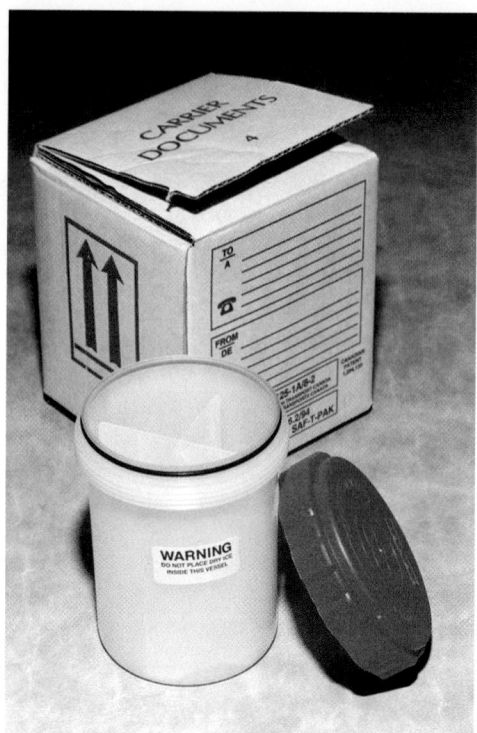

FIGURE 50-6 Specimen mailers.

differences in many tests. If a large volume of specimen is collected, such as a 24-hour urine or fecal fat specimen, the total volume or weight must be carefully measured and recorded. The specimen must be well mixed before an **aliquot** is removed and submitted for testing.

PROPER HANDLING, PROCESSING, AND STORAGE

The specimen must be handled, processed, and stored according to the instructions to avoid causing any alterations that would affect test results. The medical assistant should determine whether the specimen needs to be kept warm or cool. Specimens such as urine require chilling if testing is not going to be performed immediately. Some cultures or specimens need to be kept at body temperature after collection. Samples for gonorrhea cultures and semen analysis are two such examples, because cooling kills the microorganisms and sperm. When required, serum must be separated from the cells as soon as possible after the specimen has clotted to prevent alterations caused by the metabolism of the cells. Specimens for bilirubin testing must be protected from light. Some specimens need to be frozen to prevent chemical constituents from changing. Laboratory specimen requirements should be consulted to ensure that each specimen is handled and processed properly.

Chain of Custody

When a specimen may be needed as evidence in a court case, certain procedures must be followed for collection and handling of the specimen. Forensic or medicolegal implications require that any results of the testing of a specimen be obtained in such a fashion that they are recognized by a court of law. Specimen processing must be documented meticulously, ensuring that there was no tampering of evidence. *Chain of custody* refers to the stepwise method used to collect, process, and test a specimen. The documentation must be signed by every person who has contact with the specimen, from collection to final reporting of results. Blood alcohol level testing often requires chain-of-custody handling. Everything needed for collection of the specimen is provided in a kit–even the latex gloves, the vacuum tube, and the needle to collect the blood specimen. Documentation is included and must be signed by all personnel. Medical assistants and phlebotomists have been subpoenaed to testify in court regarding specimens they have collected; therefore it is in your best interest to follow chain-of-custody procedures rigorously.

QUALITY ASSURANCE AND QUALITY CONTROL

Quality-Assurance Guidelines

QA is the pledge of healthcare professionals to work to achieve the highest degree of excellence in the health care given every patient. QA encompasses a comprehensive set of policies and procedures developed to ensure the reliability of laboratory testing. It includes QC, personnel orientation, laboratory documentation, knowledge of laboratory instrumentation, and enrollment in a proficiency testing program. QA focuses on establishing a series of operating procedures to produce reliable laboratory results for the benefit of the patient, the physician, and the medical assistant who does the laboratory testing.

These policies benefit the physician by reducing the liability for inaccurate reporting of test results. When a physician uses a laboratory test in diagnosing, the results must be compared with reference values. Reference values are also useful in assessing the efficacy of a patient's course of treatment. The QA system enables the laboratory to assess, verify, and document the quality of the test results. This documentation is a way of comparing "what is" with "what should be." QC is covered in *Subpart K* of the February 28, 1992 CLIA regulations published in the *Federal Register*. It is required that POLs have a procedure manual describing the processes for testing and reporting patients' results. Personnel are required to calibrate laboratory instruments and verify the calibrations at least every 6 months. In addition, they must run two levels of control material each day of testing on appropriate tests and document the results, and they must perform and document remedial action when errors or problems are identified. Finally, preventative maintenance schedules must be documented and followed.

Quality-Control Guidelines

The objective of QC in the laboratory is to ensure the accuracy and reliability of test results while detecting and eliminating error. *Accuracy* refers to how close the obtained value is to the real, true value, and *reliability* refers to the reproducibility of the test procedure. POLs play a vital part in QC, because patient treatment is often based on or reinforced by results of laboratory tests. Mandated by law, QC programs monitor all aspects of laboratory activity, from specimen collection through the processing, testing, and reporting steps. Programs check supplies, reagents, machinery, personnel, and actual test performance. Without a QC program, laboratory error is difficult to detect unless the physician would notice test results inconsistent with a patient's history. Undetected laboratory errors may result in harm to the patient.

Specially prepared QC samples are tested daily along with patient samples. The results of testing performed on the QC samples must be within a preestablished range before the patient results can be reported. The QC samples, called *controls*, are usually supplied with prepackaged kits intended for use in the small laboratory. The controls should be analyzed at specified intervals. For example, positive and negative controls supplied with pregnancy test kits should be performed with each patient specimen. Urinalysis dipsticks (used for chemical examination of urine) should be checked daily and each time a new container is opened. Controls for automated chemistry analyses should be performed at specified intervals during the day. Consistent results of controls ensure constant conditions throughout the testing sequence.

Laboratory instrument standardization is important to ensure proper operation and accurate test results. Standardization involves testing samples with specific, known values and adjusting the instrumentation until it displays that value. These samples are known as standards. Preventive maintenance prolongs the life of your equipment and reduces breakdowns; it includes daily cleaning as well as adjustment and replacement of parts when necessary. Each instrument should have a log or worksheet to record all changes, including daily maintenance.

Accurate record keeping is one of the key responsibilities of a medical assistant. Various forms are available to assist in recording laboratory information. The primary record is the laboratory master logbook, in which each procedure performed in the POL is entered with dates clearly shown. Every day that

---

CRITICAL THINKING APPLICATION

As part of her daily routine, Marsha performs quality control on the lab's glucometer before patient testing. The value of the control sample should be 160 mg/dL ± 3 mg/dL, according to the package insert. She performs the test, and the glucometer reads 140 mg/dL. She repeats the test three more times, obtaining values of 141, 140, and 139 mg/dL. Is the instrument accurate? Is the instrument reliable? Can she proceed with the day's testing? If not, what should she do?

Guidelines for a Preventive Maintenance Program

- Follow the manufacturer's instructions for calibration of instruments.
- Read and understand instructions for routine instrument care.
- Perform all preventive maintenance provided by manufacturer's instructions.
- Keep all spare parts available for immediate use.
- Record the name, address, and phone number of a contact person for maintenance or repair.
- Create a maintenance form, or use the one provided.

patient tests are performed, QC tests must also be performed. The results of standardization tests and dates when new control vials are begun must be entered, along with the expiration dates of the controls. The records must be retained for a period of years, the exact number determined by state laws and CLIA mandates. Employee records must be kept confidential and maintained for 30 years.

Example of What to Include in an Employee Record

- Employee name and Social Security number
- Hepatitis B virus immunization status
- Copy of all results of examinations, medical testing, and follow-up necessitated by an exposure incident
- Employer's copy of the examining healthcare professional's opinion with regard to the exposure

CRITICAL THINKING APPLICATION

Marsha is performing a blood urea nitrogen (BUN) test on a sample using an automated BUN analyzer. First she standardizes the instrument, then she runs high, low, and normal controls. Finally she tests the patient's sample and records the value. Explain why she standardized the instrument before she ran the controls, why she ran three controls, and why the patient sample was the last to be tested.

LABORATORY MATHEMATICS AND MEASUREMENT

All laboratory testing, from specimen collection through reporting of results, relies on accurate use of values and measurements. Values are used, for example, for reporting the time of collection of the sample, the quantity of analyte found in a specimen, the volume of the specimen, and dilutions used in sample preparation and for recording QC results.

Measuring Time

Time of day is often a critical factor in patient care. Medications must be administered, diets must be followed, and specimens must be collected on a particular time schedule. Many clinical laboratories use the 24-hour clock when recording time; this method avoids the confusion that comes with the Greenwich clock, which uses the AM (morning) or PM (afternoon) designations.

The 24-hour clock system is also known as *military time* and is expressed with four digits in terms of "hundred hours." Noon is referred to as 1200 ("twelve-hundred") hours; midnight is 0000 ("zero-hundred") hours. The military clock is based on a 60-minute hour, just as the Greenwich clock is; therefore 5:35 PM is expressed as 1735 ("seventeen thirty-five") hours.

Measuring Temperature

Two scales for measuring temperature are currently used; each is divided into units called *degrees*. The Fahrenheit scale is considered to be part of the English system of measurement and

is the scale most commonly used in the United States. The Celsius scale, formerly called the *Centigrade scale,* is used in countries that apply the metric system. On the Celsius (C) scale, water freezes at 0° C and boils at 100° C. On the Fahrenheit (F) scale, water freezes at 32° F and boils at 212° F.

Table 50-2 has common laboratory temperatures. The method for converting temperatures from one form of measurement to another is found in Chapter 30.

Units of Measurement

The units of measurement that we commonly use in the United States differ from those used in the clinical laboratory. In everyday life we use the English system of measurement, in which weight is measured in ounces and pounds, length is measured in inches and feet, and volume is measured in cups and quarts. In the laboratory the metric system and the International System of Units (SI) are used. It is important that the medical assistant memorize and practice these systems so that he or she can communicate professionally.

The metric system is based on a decimal system, in which there are basic units and prefixes that indicate a system of division in multiples of ten. The basic units of the metric system are the gram (g) for weight, the meter (m) for length, and the liter (L) for volume. Prefixes are added to each symbol to reduce or enlarge them by units of ten. This information is included in Chapter 33. The most common metric units used in the laboratory are millimeters (mm), centimeters (cm), micrograms (mcg), milligrams (mg), grams (g), microliters (µL), milliliters (mL), liters (L), and cubic centimeters (cc). The cubic centimeter and milliliter are used interchangeably in the clinical laboratory.

Quantitative test results are reported using the appropriate units of measurement. Some commonly used designations for reporting analytes are mg, µ, g, dL, and L. Blood glucose, for example, is reported in milligrams per deciliter (mg/dL); hemoglobin levels are reported as grams per deciliter (g/dL).

The International System of Units (Système Internationale or SI units) is a system of reporting numbers that are recognized by international organizations such as the World Health Organization (WHO). Many countries have adopted its use; the United States has not completely converted to the SI system.

The SI is an adaptation of the metric system that uses several of the basic units, although many are different for reporting results. For example, blood glucose is reported in millimoles per liter (mmol/L), and hemoglobin is reported in

TABLE 50-2 Common Laboratory Temperatures		
	FAHRENHEIT	**CELSIUS**
Refrigerator temperature	35°-46°	2°-8°
Freezer temperature	32°	0°
Room temperature	59°-86°	15°-30°
Incubator temperature	98.6°	37°
Body temperature	98.6°	37°
Autoclave temperature	254°	121°

grams per liter (g/L). Therefore it is very important to include units of measurement when reporting testing values, double-checking the standard for the laboratory.

Measuring Liquid Volume

Vessels to measure volume in the laboratory can be glass or plastic and may be reusable or disposable. Beakers are wide, straight-sided cylindric vessels that are used for mixing or reagent preparation. They are not calibrated to hold an exact volume but can be used for estimating volume. Erlenmeyer flasks are used for reagent preparation and have a narrower mouth than a beaker. Like beakers, they are not calibrated.

Test tubes come in many sizes and are often disposable. Test tubes may be sterile, and some may be calibrated. Graduated cylinders are used for measuring exact amounts of a liquid. The size of the cylinder should be matched as closely as possible to the volume of liquid being measured to obtain the most accurate reading. In other words, a 50-mL graduated cylinder should not be used to measure 10 mL—a 10-mL cylinder should be used. For the most accurate measurement, a volumetric flask

is used. Volumetric glassware, including flasks and pipets, must go through rigorous calibration to ensure the accuracy of the measurement. They are calibrated to single, specific amounts, such as 100 mL or 500 mL, and cannot be used to measure volumes other than those indicated. Figure 50-7 depicts the glassware described.

Pipets (Figure 50-8) are also used extensively in the laboratory. These long glass, cylindric, calibrated tubes are used to deliver or transfer specified volumes of liquid. Drawing liquid into the pipet requires a bulb or a vacuum pump-type device; mouth-pipetting is forbidden. For most general laboratory procedures, two main types of manual pipets are used: the volumetric pipet, used for transferring, and the graduated pipet, used for measuring. The latter type is classified according to whether it contains or delivers the amount specified. A "to deliver" (TD) pipet will deliver the specified volume by drawing the liquid up to the calibration mark and then allowing it to drain out vertically, unassisted. A small amount of liquid will always remain in the tip of the pipet. A "to contain" (TC) pipet must be emptied completely to deliver the specified amount. When mouth pipetting was routinely being practiced, it was said that these pipets were to be "blown out," meaning that all of the liquid was to be forcibly expelled from the pipet.

A serologic pipet is much like the graduated pipet in appearance. The tip opening, however, is large, which permits a fast flow of liquid but less accuracy. The pipet is also calibrated into the tip. Serologic pipets are used to prepare dilutions of serum but should not be used in preparation of reagents.

When measuring liquid in a narrow vessel, such as a pipet or a graduated cylinder, you will notice that the liquid has a curvature at the surface. This is called the meniscus and should be adjusted so that at eye level the bottom of the curve is at the calibration line (Figure 50-9).

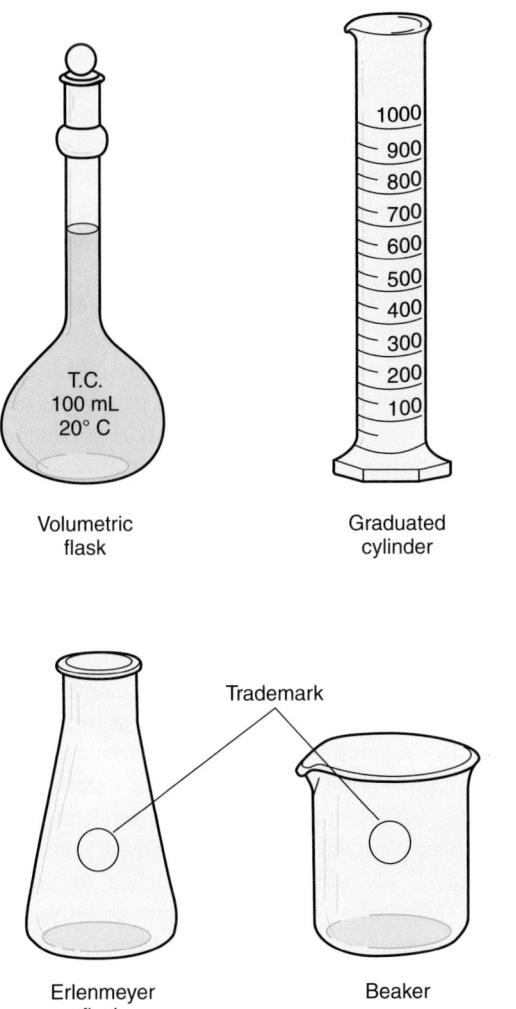

FIGURE 50-7 Laboratory glassware. *T.C.,* To contain. (Redrawn from Linne JJ, Ringsrud KM: *Clinical laboratory science: the basics and routine techniques,* ed 4, St Louis, 1999, Mosby.)

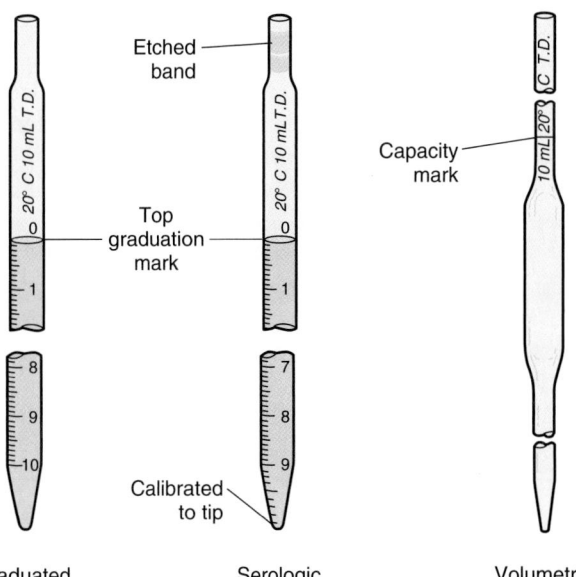

FIGURE 50-8 Types of manual pipets. (Redrawn from Linne JJ, Ringsrud KM: *Clinical laboratory science: the basics and routine techniques,* ed 4, St Louis, 1999, Mosby.)

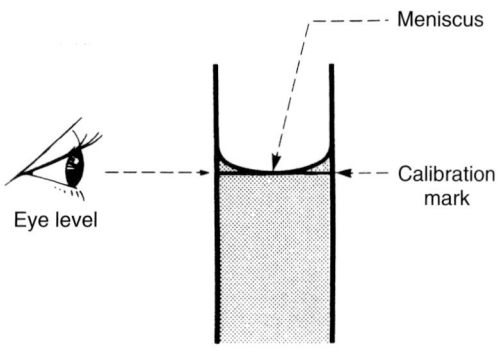

FIGURE 50-9 Reading the meniscus. (From Linne JJ, Ringsrud KM: *Clinical laboratory science: the basics and routine techniques*, ed 4, St Louis, 1999, Mosby.)

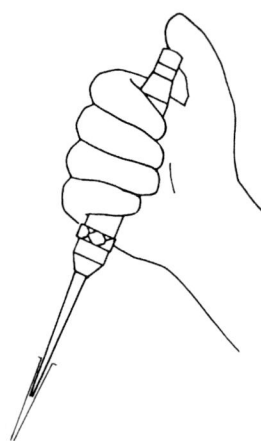

FIGURE 50-10 Piston-type automatic micropipettor. (Modified from Linne JJ, Ringsrud KM: *Clinical laboratory science: the basics and routine techniques*, ed 4, St Louis, 1999, Mosby.)

Micropipettors (Figure 50-10) are used to deliver very small quantities of liquid–from 1 to 1000 microliters (μL). It is important to follow the manufacturer's instructions for the device, because each may be slightly different. These pipetting devices must be fitted with an appropriate disposable tip. These tips may be sterile, depending on their use. The device is fitted with a piston at the top, which must be depressed before the pipet is filled and when the pipet is drained.

CRITICAL THINKING APPLICATION

Marsha is preparing a solution and is required to measure a 6-mL volume of saline solution. She has a 10-mL TD pipet. The pipetting device provided by the laboratory uses vacuum to draw up the liquid and forced air to expel it. Marsha knows that she should allow the pipet to drain with the force of gravity, yet she is required to use a pipetting device. How will she accurately deliver 6 mL?

Preparing Dilutions

When the medical assistant performs laboratory tests, he or she may find it necessary to dilute a body fluid sample with a **diluent,** such as water, saline solution, or a buffer. For example, dilutions must be made when testing for the presence and

strength of antibodies in serum, or when a patient's analyte level is grossly elevated and cannot be read by the instrument.

The term *dilution* refers to parts in total volume; it is a statement of relative concentration and represents expressions of concentration, not expressions of volume. For example, a 1:10 dilution can be prepared by measuring 1 mL of sample and diluting it with diluent to 10 mL. This means adding 9 mL of diluent. The same 1:10 dilution can be prepared by mixing 2 mL of sample and 18 mL of diluent or 0.5 mL of sample and 4.5 mL of diluent. Note that the final volume is not the same in each of the above examples, yet each is a 1:10 dilution. Any volume of a dilution can be made as long as the relative amounts of the components remain the same.

CLINICAL LABORATORY EQUIPMENT

Microscope

Nearly every medical laboratory is equipped with a microscope. This indispensable instrument is used to view objects too small to be seen with the naked eye (Figure 50-11). The microscope is used to evaluate stained blood smears, urine sediment, vaginal secretions, and smears made from body fluids or microbiologic cultures. Laboratories with a CLIA Provider Performed Microscopy Procedure (PPMP) certificate or a Certificate of Waiver (COW) perform tests using a microscope during the course of a patient visit on specimens that are not easily transportable. There typically are no QC procedures for these tests (Table 50-3). PPMP laboratories must meet the same quality standards as a laboratory performing moderate-complexity tests; those laboratories that perform only CLIA-waived tests may perform certain microscopic tests through a COW. In a POL with a COW, only a physician, physician's assistant, dentist, or other highly trained personnel can perform microscopic analysis. If the laboratory is CLIA certified to perform moderate-complexity testing, personnel other than physicians can perform microscopic analysis provided that they are trained and supervised by a qualified individual and the laboratory maintains its CLIA certification.

Microscopes have three components: the magnification system, the illumination system, and the framework, which includes all components responsible for positioning the slide and focusing. The magnification system of the microscope includes the ocular and the objective lenses. Microscopes are either monocular or binocular. A monocular microscope has one eyepiece for viewing, and a binocular has two. The eyepiece, or ocular, is located at the top of the microscope and contains a lens to magnify what is being seen. The usual magnification is 10 times (10×). Compound microscopes have, in addition to the ocular, objective lenses that increase magnification of the specimen. The objectives are attached to the revolving nosepiece. Most microscopes have four objectives; each has a different magnifying power. The shortest objective has the lowest power (4×) and is called the *scanning lens*. This lens is used to scan the field of interest, then focus on a particular object. Greater detail is observed with the next longest objective, which is low power (10×). The high or high dry objective usually has a magnification of 40× or 45×, and the longest objective, oil

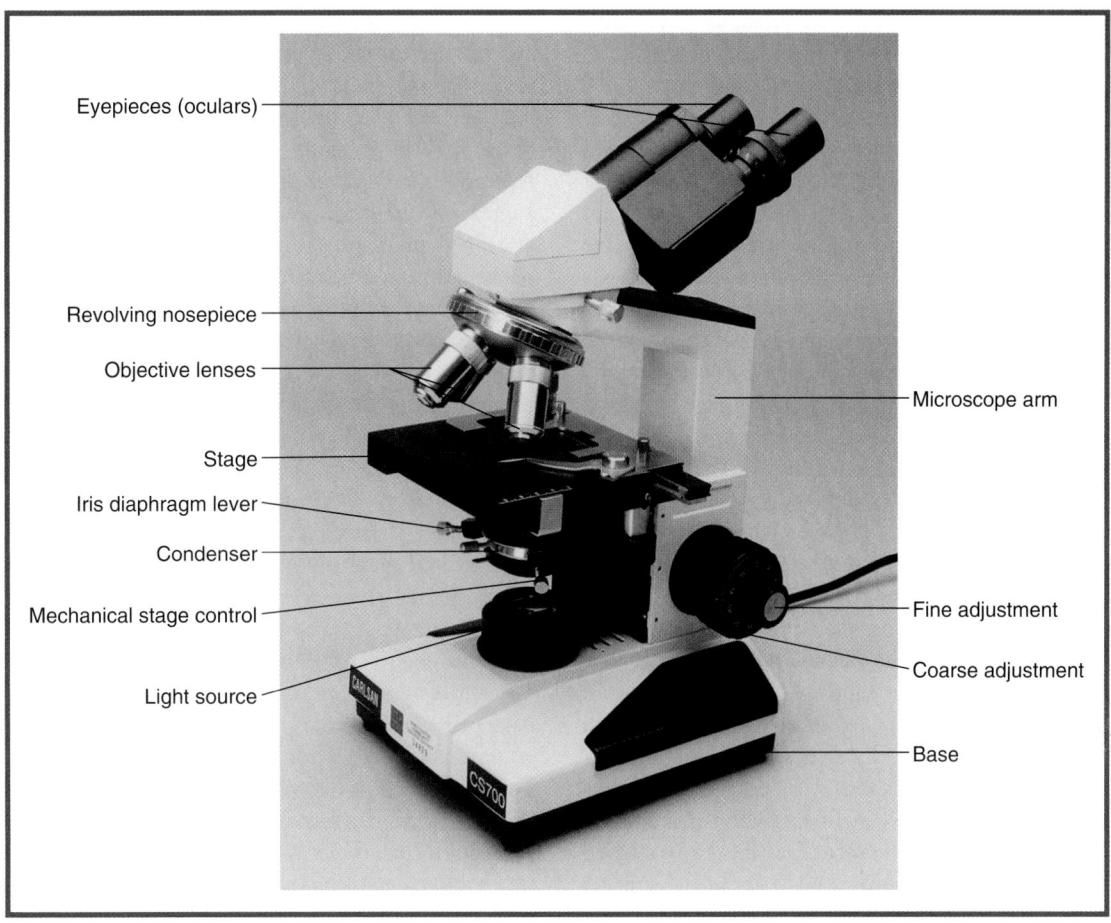

FIGURE 50-11 Parts of a microscope. (Courtesy Cynmar Corporation, Carlinville, Ill.)

TABLE 50-3 Selected Provider-Performed Microscopy Procedure Tests		
TEST NAME	**DESCRIPTION**	**EXAMPLE**
Direct wet mount	Examination of specimens for presence or absence of bacteria, fungi, parasites, and human cellular elements	Observing vaginal secretions for presence of yeast to assist with diagnosis of vulvovaginal candidiasis
KOH preparation	Any preparation using potassium hydroxide	Observing skin scrapings for the presence of fungi
Fecal leukocyte examination	Simple stain of fecal specimen; assists in diagnosis of diarrheal disease	Leukocytes are found in stool in antibiotic-associated colitis, ulcerative colitis, shigellosis, and salmonellosis
Pinworm examination	Preparations are observed for the presence or absence of *Enterobius vermicularis* eggs	See Procedure 54-8, Perform a Cellulose Tape Collection for Pinworms
Postcoital direct, qualitative examinations	Vaginal or cervical mucus is examined 4-10 hr after intercourse for presence of live, motile sperm	Assists in the diagnosis of infertility
Qualitative semen analysis	Semen is examined for the presence or absence of spermatozoa; motility of the sperm is noted	Assists in postvasectomy semen analysis and in the diagnosis of infertility
Urine sediment examination	Urine sediment is examined for presence or absence of formed elements	Part of a routine Urinalysis. See Procedure 51-5, Prepare Urine Specimen for Microscopic Examination

immersion (100×), allows for the finest focusing of the object and requires the use of a special oil that is placed directly on the slide. This special oil, called *immersion oil*, prevents refraction of the light and improves the **resolution** (clarity) of the image that is magnified. Oil immersion is used to view cells and materials that are extremely small, such as bacteria and platelets.

In order to determine the total magnification of the specimen being observed, multiply the magnification of the objective lens by 10 (the magnification of the ocular). Thus, if you have the 10× objective in place when you are observing blood cells, you are magnifying the image 100 times.

The arm of the microscope connects the objectives and

oculars to the base, which supports the microscope and contains its light source. The stage of the microscope holds the slide to be viewed. Together, the light source, the condenser, and the iris diaphragm compose the illumination system. The condenser directs light up through the stage, and the iris diaphragm regulates the amount of light passing through the specimen. Just above the base are the focusing knobs. The coarse adjustment is used only with scanning and low-power lenses, and the fine adjustment is used with high-power and oil immersion lenses.

Microscopes are very precise and expensive instruments that require careful handling. The amount of routine maintenance required depends on the amount of daily use. Dirt is the enemy of the microscope, which must be kept scrupulously clean at all times. Oil, makeup, dust, and eye secretions all can obstruct vision through the lens and cause the possible transmission of infection. The microscope should always be stored in a plastic dust cover when not in use. Lenses should be cleaned before and after each use with lens paper and lens cleaner. Any other type of tissue scratches the lenses or leaves lint residue behind. The routine use of solvent cleaners, such as xylene, is not recommended, because these cleaners may loosen lenses. However, xylene can be used to remove oil that has dried on the lenses. The body of the microscope should be dusted with a soft cloth.

The microscope should be placed in a permanent location in the laboratory on a sturdy table in an area where it cannot be bumped. If a microscope must be moved, it should be carried securely, with one hand supporting the base and the other holding the arm. When the microscope is stored, it should be left covered, with the low-power objective in the lowest position. The stage should be centered.

Using a microscope involves focusing and illumination (Procedure 50-1). The image is focused by moving the objective closer to the specimen, and illumination is accomplished by raising or lowering the condenser and by moving the specimen closer or farther away from the objective.

Focusing the microscope is done through movement of the objective or stage, which is controlled by round knobs located on both sides of the microscope. Proper focusing of the microscope begins with the lowest power objective. The coarse adjustment moves the objective very quickly. This knob is used first to bring the specimen into approximate focus. The fine adjustment focus knob then brings the specimen into precise focus. The fine focus moves the objective more slowly to allow the viewer to zero in on the specimen with greater accuracy.

If the microscope is a binocular model, the viewer may find it necessary to adjust the eyepieces to accommodate the distance between the pupils and the individual's point of greatest visual acuity. A gentle push inward or pull outward will adjust the distance between the eyepieces.

Centrifuge

Centrifugation, which is used when separation of solids from liquids is necessary, involves the application of increased gravitational force achieved by rapid spinning. Centrifugation is used to separate blood cells from serum, and solid materials such as cells and crystals from urine, and is employed in many areas of the clinical laboratory.

Centrifuges (Figure 50-12) are designed for specific uses. They may be bench-top or floor models; some may be refrigerated. Some may have rotors or heads that are interchangeable. A typical clinical centrifuge may have a rotor that is at a fixed angle, in which the specimen cups are held in a rigid position at a fixed angle; one that has a horizontal head with swinging buckets that swing out horizontally during centrifugation; and a third used for centrifuging capillary tubes for microhematocrit determination (see Chapter 52). Centrifuges may also be equipped with timers to automatically stop centrifugation at a set time.

Directions for the use of a centrifuge are usually given in terms of revolutions per minute (rpm). Spinning generates centrifugal force. General laboratory centrifuges operate at up to 6000 rpm, generating relative centrifugal force up to 7300 times the force of gravity (G). Conventional horizontal centrifuges attain speeds of up to 3000 rpm; angle-head centrifuges can attain higher speeds (up to 7000 rpm).

Centrifuges can be dangerous devices if not used correctly. The most important rule is to ensure that the centrifuge is balanced so that tubes of equal size and containing equal volume are directly across from one another in the rotor holders. Therefore, there will always be an even number of specimens in the centrifuge. If a second specimen of the same volume in the same-sized tube is not available for balance, a tube of water may be used to balance the load. Tubes being centrifuged should also be capped to avoid emission of aerosols. Rubber cups should be placed in the bottom of the carrier cups to avoid breakage of glass tubes.

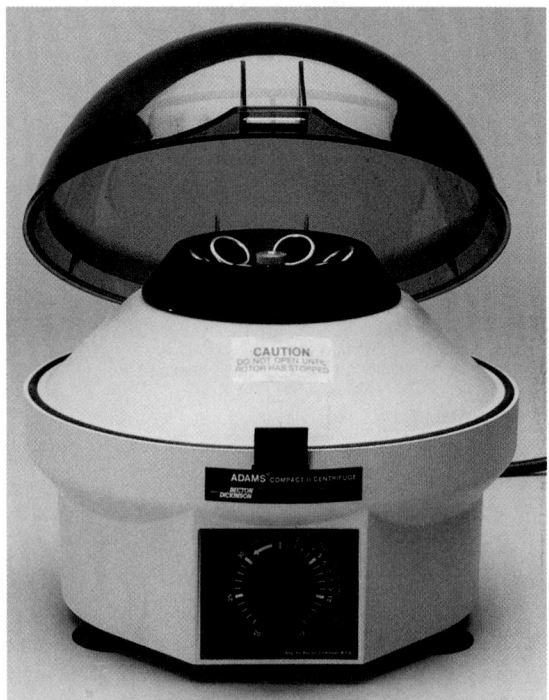

FIGURE 50-12 Centrifuge.

PROCEDURE 50-1

Use the Microscope

GOAL: *To focus the microscope properly, using a prepared slide, under low power, high power, and oil immersion.*

EQUIPMENT and SUPPLIES

- Microscope
- Lens cleaner
- Lens tissue
- Slide containing specimen

PROCEDURAL STEPS

1. Wash your hands.
2. Gather the materials needed.
3. Clean the lenses with lens tissue and lens cleaner.
   PURPOSE: Dust on lenses can obscure elements in the microscopic field.
4. Adjust seating to a comfortable height.
5. Plug the microscope into an electric outlet, and turn on the light switch.
6. Place the slide specimen on the stage and secure it.
7. Turn the revolving nosepiece to engage the 4× or 10× lens.
   PURPOSE: Always begin microscopic observations at low power.
8. Carefully raise the stage while observing with the naked eye from the side.
9. Focus the specimen, using the coarse adjustment knob.
   PURPOSE: The coarse adjustment knob will quickly bring the specimen into focus.
10. Adjust the amount of light by closing the iris diaphragm or adjusting the light from the source.
    PURPOSE: Too much light when using the low-power objective can be irritating to the microscopist's eyes.
11. Switch to the 40× lens. Use the fine adjustment knob to focus the specimen in detail.
12. Turn the revolving nosepiece to the area between the high-power objective and oil immersion.

13. Place a small drop of oil on the slide.
    PURPOSE: Immersion oil has nearly the same refractive index as glass and will prevent refraction of the light, thus improving resolution.
14. Carefully rotate the oil immersion objective into place. The objective will be immersed in the oil.
15. Adjust the focus with the fine adjustment knob.
    PURPOSE: The fine adjustment knob will slowly move the objective, preventing damage to the microscope and the slide.
16. Increase the light by opening the iris diaphragm and raising the condenser.
    PURPOSE: Lighting is crucial to microscopy; the higher the magnification, the more light that is needed.
17. Identify the specimen.
18. Return to low power but do not drag the 40× lens through the oil.
19. Remove the slide.
20. Lower the stage.
21. Center the stage.
    PURPOSE: Returning the microscope to this position will protect it during storage.
22. Switch off the light, and unplug the microscope.
23. Clean the lenses with lens tissue, and remove oil with lens cleaner.
    PURPOSE: Dust and oil must be removed from the lenses after a procedure.
24. Wipe the microscope with a cloth.
25. Cover the microscope.
26. Clean the work area.
27. Wash your hands.

Centrifuges should never be opened while they are in operation, nor should you attempt to slow a centrifuge with your hands. Most models are equipped with a brake, which should only be used in an emergency, the most common of which is a broken glass tube. In this case, wait until the centrifuge comes to a complete stop and follow the manufacturer's instructions for disinfecting the unit.

Centrifuges should be checked, cleaned, and lubricated regularly to ensure proper operation. A photoelectric device or a strobe tachometer must be used by a certified technician to ensure centrifuge speed to comply with QA guidelines set forth by CAP.

Incubator

Incubators are cabinets that maintain constant temperatures. Generally used in the microbiology laboratory, they maintain a constant temperature of 35° to 37° C, although other temperatures may also be appropriate. Some incubator interiors may be enriched with carbon dioxide (CO_2) gas to enhance the growth of pathogenic bacteria; a pressurized tank of CO_2 gas is attached to the cabinet, and the concentration is maintained at 10%. Incubators may have warning alarms if the temperature exceeds or falls below a specified range. The temperature should be checked daily and the cabinets should be cleaned regularly with a disinfectant approved by the manufacturer.

Autoclave

The autoclave is an instrument that uses steam under pressure to sterilize materials that can withstand high temperatures. The principles of operation are explained in Chapter 54.

It is essential that strict QA methods be followed when an autoclave is used. A certified technician should regularly examine the autoclave, and biologic and chemical indicators should be checked on a daily basis. Biologic indicators include spore preparations that are included in the autoclave load. At the end of the sterilization period, they are incubated and checked for germination. If the spores fail to germinate, the autoclave reached the appropriate temperature. Chemical methods include a special tape that changes color to show the word *autoclaved* when the temperature of the autoclave reaches 121° C.

The autoclave is used in the medical laboratory to sterilize specimens or objects before disposal. For example, throat culture collection devices, contaminated latex gloves, or tubes of blood may require sterilization before disposal. These items are placed in an orange biohazard bag, which is sealed and marked with autoclave tape before autoclaving.

CLOSING COMMENTS

Patient Education

Many testing procedures require that patients be given a specific set of instructions to follow. For example, patients may be required to fast 8 to 12 hours before the collection of blood and urine. They may need to follow a high-carbohydrate diet for several days before a glucose tolerance test (GTT). The consumption of some foods and medication must be discontinued. The physician will discuss medication alternatives with the patient. Sometimes it might not be medically advisable to discontinue the medication; this must be noted on the laboratory requisition. The laboratory will then be alerted to the possible drug interferences, and it may be able to use an alternative test method.

Often it is the medical assistant's responsibility to explain to the patient the measures that are to be taken before laboratory testing. Be sure that you have interpreted the physician's orders correctly before explaining the procedure to the patient. Giving the patient written instructions is recommended, with a phone number included on the instruction sheet so that the patient can call if he or she has questions.

Legal and Ethical Issues

If disease did not exist, there would be little need for clinical laboratories. The fact that the human body is susceptible to disease necessitates the existence of laboratory testing. One cannot anticipate or prevent every health and safety risk, but the risks are greatly reduced when everyone who works in the laboratory setting is conscious of safety guidelines.

Use common sense and document everything. If you are in doubt about the safety of a procedure, ask your supervisor. If you are aware of a potential safety problem, report it to the person in charge. Your welfare, the welfare of the patient, and the welfare of your co-workers may depend on your commitment to safety.

SUMMARY OF SCENARIO

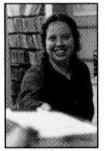

Marsha's experience in clinical laboratory testing made her a valuable asset to her new employer. A thorough understanding of government rules and regulations, including the CLIA, and the guidelines published by the CDC, the EPA, and OSHA helped Marsha to implement laboratory testing in the clinic, including urinalysis with a chemical reagent strip, hemoglobin and hematocrit testing, pregnancy testing, and hemoglobin A$_{1c}$ monitoring. Marsha helped the physicians design a safe, efficient laboratory space with a refrigerator, centrifuge, and biohazard waste station. She developed a rigorous QA program and is now training other medical assistants to perform CLIA-waived testing.

Marsha found it most challenging to determine how to comply with proper medical waste disposal issues. It required her to make several phone calls to state environmental protection agencies, but her diligence was rewarded when the laboratory received certification. Marsha pays close attention to CLIA regulations and receives regular updates of the tests that can be performed in a POL. She is currently determining the feasibility of performing drug screenings for local businesses. Her employers are pleased with her efforts, and the patients appreciate the convenience of on-site testing.

SUMMARY of LEARNING OBJECTIVES

1. Define, spell, and pronounce the terms listed in the vocabulary.
   - Spelling and pronouncing medical terms correctly adds credibility to the medical assistant. Knowing the definition of these terms promotes confidence in communication with patients and co-workers.

2. Discuss the role of the clinical laboratory in patient care and the medical assistant's role in coordinating laboratory tests and results.
   - The clinical laboratory is responsible for analysis of blood and body fluids, providing the physician with test results that become part of the essential data needed to diagnose and manage a patient's condition. Medical assistants are responsible for collecting specimens, instructing patients, and performing CLIA-waived and some moderately complex testing.

3. Describe the divisions of the clinical laboratory, and give an example of a test performed in each division.
   - Most physicians' offices that perform laboratory testing will do so in the areas of urinalysis, hematology, chemistry, and microbiology. Routine urinalysis, complete blood counts, pregnancy testing, and throat cultures are some of the tests that might be performed in a POL.

4. Describe the Clinical Laboratory Improvement Amendments (CLIA) and how they influence laboratory testing.
   - CLIA established the standards of quality for laboratory testing. Medical assistants can perform all CLIA-waived and some CLIA moderate-complexity laboratory procedures.

5. Differentiate between the three CLIA regulatory categories.
   - A CLIA-waived test is one that is approved by the FDA for over-the-counter sales or one that has been determined to pose no unreasonable risk or harm if performed incorrectly. Other levels of tests require more training or education to perform and can be performed only in CLIA-certified laboratories.

6. Compare and contrast the agencies that govern or influence practice in the clinical laboratory, including the CDC, OSHA, EPA, CLSI, and CAP.
   - Federal agencies that regulate the laboratory include the U.S. Department of Labor, the U.S. Department of Health and Human Services, and the EPA. Professional agencies that provide guidelines include CLSI and CAP. Although all of the agencies provide recommendations for operation procedures in the clinical laboratory, not all have the power to enforce them. The Department of Labor and the EPA can impose significant fines for failing to follow regulations, but the standard precautions set forth by the CDC are recommended but not enforceable.

7. List techniques to minimize physical, chemical, and biologic risks in the clinical laboratory.
   - Risks can be minimized in all areas of the laboratory by using common sense and by having a formal safety training program and an up-to-date safety manual. Safety equipment such as fire blankets, fire extinguishers, and eye wash stations should be accessible to employees. Chemicals should be clearly marked with the National Fire Protection Association diamond, and MSDSs should be bound in an accessible manual. Standard precautions should be observed when handling any biologic material.

8. Describe the essential elements of a laboratory requisition.
   - The laboratory requisition must have all information needed to identify the patient, the ordering physician, the test ordered, and the specific details regarding the collection (such as time and source) of the specimen.

9. Explain chain of custody, and illustrate why it is important.
   - Chain of custody is a method used to ensure that a specimen provided by a patient who may be involved in a legal matter is handled in a fashion that will not compromise the test results. All individuals who handle or test the specimen must be identified in writing and provide a signature.

10. Explain the differences and similarities between quality assurance and quality control.
    - QA involves procedures undertaken to ensure that each patient is provided excellent care. QC—ensuring that laboratory testing is accurate and reliable—is part of a QA program.

11. Convert between Greenwich time and military time.
    - Greenwich time uses the designations am and pm, whereas military time uses the 24-hour clock: 3:15 pm is equivalent to 1515 hours.

12. Name the Fahrenheit temperature and Celsius temperature of three important pieces of laboratory equipment.
    - Although the Celsius (Centigrade) thermometer is used in the clinical laboratory, in everyday life we commonly use the Fahrenheit system. The incubator is usually set at 37° C (98° F), the autoclave sterilizes at 121° C (254° F), and refrigerator temperature is 2° to 8° C (35° to 46° F).

13. Name the metric units used for measuring liquid volume, distance, and mass.
    - Liquid volume is measured in liters, distance is measured in meters, and mass is measured in grams. Prefixes commonly used in the clinical laboratory include *milli-* (0.001), *centi-* (0.01), *micro-* (0.000001), *deci-* (0.1), and *kilo-* (1000).

14. Describe the proper use of pipets.
    - Pipets must be chosen according to the job they are to perform. A pipetting device, such as a bulb or pump, should be attached, and particular attention must be given to the emptying of the pipet. The mouth should never be used in pipetting.

15. Explain how dilutions are prepared.
    - Dilutions are prepared by mixing volumes of sample, such as blood, body fluids, or reagents, and volumes of diluent, such as water, saline solution, or buffer. The term *dilution* refers to parts in total volume and is an expression of concentration.

16. Name the parts of a microscope, and describe their functions.
    - The parts of the microscope can be divided into the illumination system (light source, condenser, and iris diaphragm lever), the frame (base, adjustment knobs, arm, stage, stage control), and the magnification system (objective lenses on the revolving nosepiece, oculars). The illumination system

SUMMARY of LEARNING OBJECTIVES
Continued

controls the light that passes through the specimen to the eye, the frame provides the structure for the instrument and the components that allow for the adjustment of the sample, and the magnification system provides the ground glass lenses that magnify the specimen.

17. Describe the safe use of a centrifuge.
   - For safe use of a centrifuge, the proper tube must be used and it must be protected from breakage. Centrifuge loads must be carefully balanced. Specimens must be capped to prevent aerosols. Under no circumstances should centrifuges be opened while they are in operation.

18. List quality-control measures necessary to ensure sterilization with an autoclave.
   - Autoclaves provide sterilization by exposing materials to steam under pressure. The steam must reach a temperature of 121° C. Specialized tape or spore strips must be used to ensure that the proper temperature has been reached.

19. Demonstrate the proper use of the microscope.
   - Procedure 50-1 outlines the steps for using a microscope.

CONNECTIONS

Study Guide Connection: Go to Chapter 50 Study Guide. Read the Case Study and Workplace Applications and complete the assignments. Do online research for answers to the questions in the Internet Activities associated with assisting in the clinical laboratory.

CD Connection: Go to the Medical Assisting Competency Challenge CD and do the training activities under Diagnostic Testing.

Evolve Connection: For more information related to assisting in the clinical laboratory, go to evolve.elsevier.com/kinn and visit related weblinks for Chapter 50. Click on the Medical Assisting Exam Review and do the practice questions to sharpen your test-taking skills.

Assisting in the Analysis of Urine

51

Robin R. Patterson

SCENARIO

As part of her duties as a CMA, Rosa Gonzales performs tests on urine. Urinalysis, she knows, is a very important part of patient care, and a number of tests are performed on urine in the laboratory in Dr. Ronald Hill's busy practice. Dr. Hill most commonly orders routine urinalysis testing, but Rosa also performs some specialized tests.

While studying this chapter, think about the following questions:

- What is involved in a routine urinalysis?
- How are pregnancy and drug testing performed on urine?
- How will Rosa instruct the patients in the collection of urine for a routine urinalysis, a urine culture, and other specialized tests such as pregnancy tests and drug tests?
- What quality assurance measures will she take when performing laboratory tests on urine?

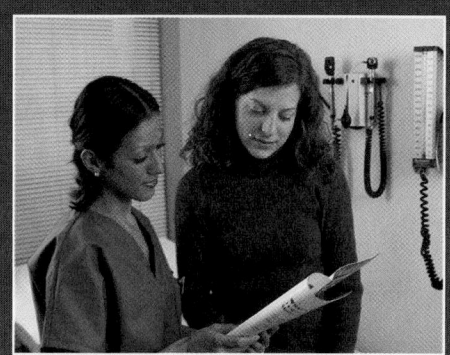

LEARNING OBJECTIVES

1. Define, spell, and pronounce the terms listed in the vocabulary.
2. Understand the purpose of routine urinalysis.
3. Describe the physiology of urine formation.
4. Explain the various means and methods used for collection of urine specimens.
5. Describe the components of the physical and chemical examination of urine.
6. Recognize and correctly identify the formed elements found in urine sediment.
7. Instruct a patient in the collection of a timed urine specimen.
8. Instruct a patient in the collection of a clean-catch midstream urine specimen.
9. Perform a complete urinalysis.
10. Demonstrate the proper use and care of testing equipment.
11. Describe glucose testing using the Clinitest method.
12. Explain the principle of lateral flow technology used in pregnancy testing.
13. Perform pregnancy testing.
14. Explain the principle of lateral flow technology in drug testing on urine.
15. Demonstrate a method of drug testing on a urine specimen.
16. List means by which urine could be adulterated before drug testing.
17. Demonstrate a method of detecting the presence of adulterating substances in a urine sample for drug testing.
18. Describe methods for determining fertility and menopause using CLIA-waived urine tests.

National Accreditation Competencies and Content

CAAHEP COMPETENCIES

Clinical Clinical Duties
3.b.(1)(a).   Perform hand washing
3.b.(3)(c)(i). CLIA waived test: Perform urinalysis
3.b.(4)(i).   Screen and follow up test results

General
3.c.(3)(b).   Instruct individuals according to their needs
3.c.(4)(b).   Perform routine maintenance of administrative and clinical equipment
3.c.(4)(d).   Use methods of quality control

ABHES COMPETENCIES

4.b. Prepare patients for procedures
4.c. Apply principles of aseptic techniques and infection control
4.i.   Use quality control
4.j.   Collect and process specimens
4.k. Perform selected CLIA-waived tests that assist with diagnosis and treatment
4.q. Dispose of biohazardous materials
4.r. Practice Standard Precautions
4.w. Instruct patients in the collection of a clean-catch midstream urine specimen
4.y. Perform urinalysis

Instruction
7.c. Teach patients methods of health promotion and disease prevention.

VOCABULARY

amorphous (a-mohr′-fuhs) Lacking a defined shape.

bilirubinuria (bi-li-roo′-bin-yuhr-e-uh) Presence of bilirubin in the urine.

casts Tubular structures found in urine composed mainly of mucoprotein secreted by certain cells of the kidney.

colony-forming units (CFU) Term used when reporting bacteriuria; one CFU represents one bacterium present in the urine sample.

crenate Forming notches or leaflike scalloped edges on an object.

culture and sensitivity (C&S) A procedure performed in the microbiology laboratory in which a specimen is cultured on artificial media to detect bacterial or fungal growth, followed by appropriate screening for antibiotic sensitivity.

cystoscopy A telescopic examination of the urinary bladder.

enzymatic reaction Chemical reaction controlled by an enzyme.

filtrate Fluid that remains after a liquid is passed through a membranous filter.

glycosuria (gly-koh-suhr′-e-uh) Presence of glucose in the urine.

gold standard A paragon of excellence; the one to which all others are compared.

ischemia Decreased blood flow to a body part or organ, caused by constriction or plugging of the supplying artery.

metabolite The product of the metabolism of a substance such as a drug.

mononuclear white blood cells Leukocytes having an unsegmented nucleus; monocytes and lymphocytes in particular.

myoglobinuria Abnormal presence of a hemoglobin-like chemical of muscle tissue in urine that is the result of muscle deterioration.

phenylalanine (fe-nehl-ah′-luh-nen) Essential amino acid found in milk, eggs, and other foods.

polymorphonuclear white blood cells Leukocytes having a segmented nucleus. Also known as *polymorphonuclear neutrophils* (PMNs) or *segmented neutrophils.*

refractile (re-frak′-tuhl) Causing light to refract, thus creating a sharp boundary or image.

renal thresholds Levels above which substances cannot be reabsorbed by the renal tubules and are therefore excreted in the urine.

supravital Of, relating to, or capable of staining living cells after their removal from a living or recently dead organism.

voided Urinated.

A routine urinalysis (UA) is one of the more common laboratory examinations used in the diagnosis and treatment of disease. It can be easily and quickly performed, and invasive techniques are generally not needed to collect the specimen. The results of a routine UA can reveal diseases of the bladder or kidneys; systemic metabolic or endocrine disorders, such as diabetes; and diseases of the liver, such as hepatitis or cirrhosis, or obstruction of the bile ducts. UA is routinely performed on all patients undergoing physical examinations and on those entering the hospital for treatment.

PHYSIOLOGY OF URINE FORMATION

It has been known for centuries that abnormalities in the urine may be indicators of disruption of homeostasis. One of the earliest known tests of the urine was to pour it on the ground and see if it attracted insects. Such attraction indicated "honey urine," which was known to be excreted by persons with skin eruptions. Today urine is still checked for sugar as a means to detect diabetes.

Historically, examination of the urine became a game for quacks and charlatans. Paintings from the Middle Ages show physicians peering into round-bottomed flasks of urine, claiming not only to be able to diagnose disease, but to see into the future by simply looking at the fluid. These charlatans became known as "Pisse Prophets." During the twentieth century, UA became a practical laboratory procedure, and today urine is the most commonly analyzed body fluid in the clinical laboratory.

Urine is analyzed for two reasons. The first is to detect extrinsic conditions—those in which the kidney is functioning normally, but abnormal end-products of metabolism are excreted as a result of an imbalance in homeostasis. The second is to detect intrinsic pathologic conditions that involve the kidneys or urinary tract themselves.

Anatomy of the Urinary Tract

Medical assistants must have a basic knowledge of kidney structure and urine formation to understand the results of a UA. The urinary tract consists of two kidneys, two ureters, one bladder, and one urethra. The functional unit of the kidney is the nephron. There are more than 1 million nephrons per kidney, and each nephron is composed of five distinct areas, each playing a role in urine formation (Figure 51-1). Each nephron consists of a glomerulus, which acts in filtering, and a

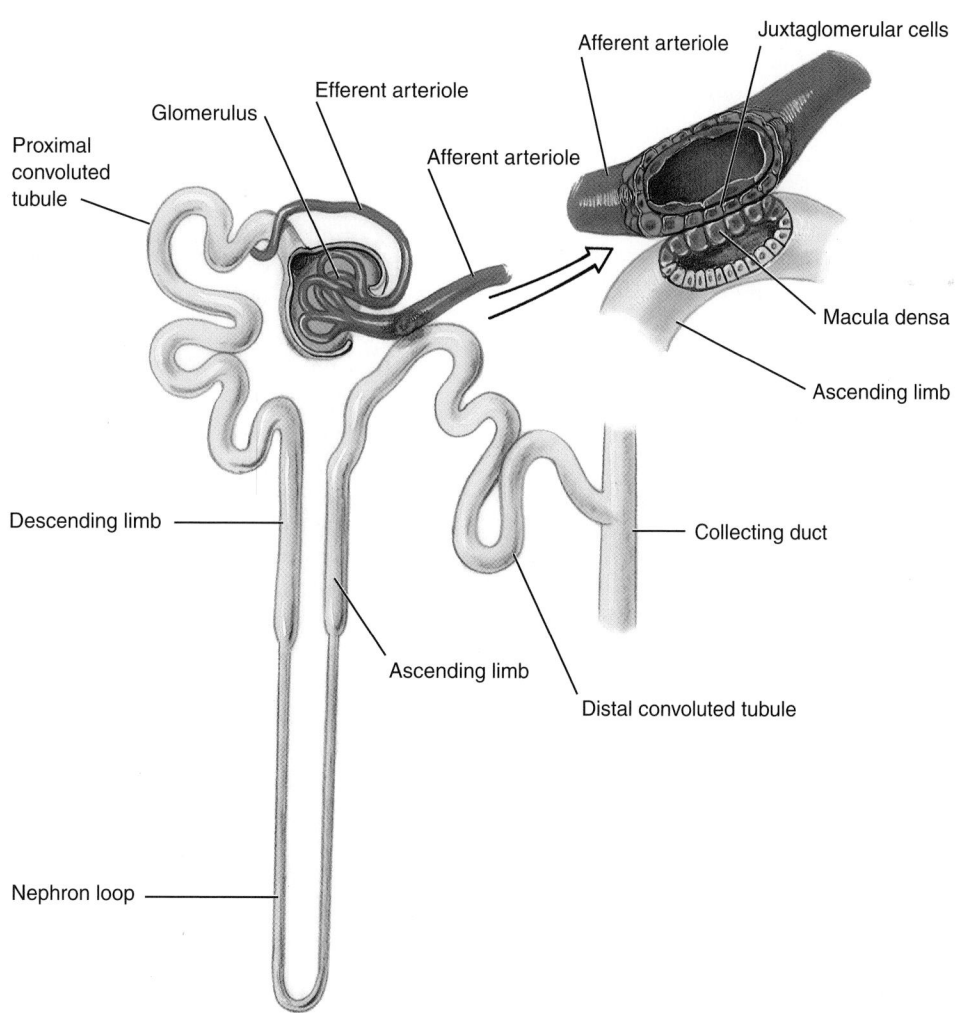

FIGURE 51-1   A nephron. (From Applegate EJ: *The anatomy and physiology learning system*, ed 3, Philadelphia, 2006, Saunders.)

tubule, through which the **filtrate** passes. As the filtrate passes through, various changes occur. Certain solutes are reabsorbed, and others are secreted into the kidney for eventual excretion. Nearly all of the water that passes through the glomeruli is reabsorbed.

The glomerulus is composed of a network of capillaries surrounded by a membrane called *Bowman's capsule.* The afferent arteriole carries blood from the renal artery into the glomerulus, where it then divides to form a capillary network. Where they reunite, the capillaries form the efferent arteriole, through which blood will exit the glomerulus.

The tubular portion of the nephron is composed of the proximal convoluted tubule, the thin-walled segment, and the distal convoluted tubule. The thin-walled descending portion forms a loop known as the *loop of Henle.* Filtrate from several nephrons drains into a collecting tubule, a number of which join to form a collecting duct. The collecting ducts join to form the papillary ducts, which empty at the tips of the papillae into the calyces. The filtrate then drains into the renal pelvis and is now called *urine.* Urine passes from the pelvis of the kidney down the ureter and into the bladder, where it remains until it is **voided** through the urethra.

Formation of Urine

The kidney selectively excretes or retains substances according to body needs and **renal thresholds.** Approximately 1200 mL of blood flow through the kidneys each minute. The blood enters the glomerulus through the afferent arteriole. The capillary walls of the glomerulus are highly permeable to water and the low–molecular-weight solutes of the plasma, and they filter through into Bowman's space then into the tubules. Many components of the filtrate, including glucose, water, and amino acids, are partially or completely reabsorbed by the capillaries surrounding the proximal tubules. More water is absorbed, and hydrogen and potassium ions are secreted in the distal tubules. Urine is concentrated in the system of collecting tubules and the loop of Henle. The kidneys convert nearly 180,000 mL of filtered plasma per day into a final urine volume of 750 to 2000 mL–approximately 1% of the filtered plasma volume. The largest component of urine is water; the majority of the solutes are urea, chloride, sodium, potassium, phosphate, sulfate, creatinine, and uric acid.

COLLECTING A URINE SPECIMEN

Containers

The most important requirement for a collection container is that it be scrupulously clean. The physician's office laboratory should provide a container; patients should not use jars from home. Disposable, nonsterile, plastic, or coated paper containers are the most common and are available in many sizes with tight-fitting lids. Special pliable polyethylene bags with adhesive, described in Chapter 41, are used for collection of urine from infants and children who are not toilet-trained. For specimens that must be collected over a period of time, large, wide-mouthed plastic containers with screw-cap tops are

used. Most routine UA testing, pregnancy testing, and testing for abnormal analytes are performed on urine collected in nonsterile containers.

When urine is to be cultured for bacteria, it is essential that it be collected in a sterile container. Such containers will be recognizable by an intact paper seal over the cap.

It is important to properly label all specimens with name, date, and time of collection and type of collection. Always don gloves before handling filled specimen containers.

CRITICAL THINKING APPLICATION

It is 9 AM, and Rosa has received three urine specimens in the laboratory. She prepares to perform the ordered tests. One of these specimens is collected in a cup with a paper tab, indicating the container was sterile, and the other two are collected in nonsterile containers. What procedures do you think she might do on the urine collected in the sterile container? What might she do with the other urine specimens? What information should she look for on the label of each specimen?

Methods of Specimen Collection

Most analyses are performed on freshly voided urine collected in clean containers. This is called a *random specimen.* If the specimen is ordered to be collected when the patient arises in the morning, it is called a *first morning specimen.* These specimens are most concentrated and are best for nitrite and protein determination, bacterial culture, pregnancy testing, and microscopic examination. Two-hour postprandial urine specimens, collected 2 hours after a meal, are used in diabetic screening and for home diabetic-testing programs. Twenty-four–hour urine specimens are collected over 24 hours to give quantitative chemical analysis, such as hormone levels and creatinine clearance rates (a procedure for evaluating the glomerular filtration rate of the kidneys) (Figure 51-2).

A second-voided specimen is usually collected to determine glucose levels; the first void of the morning is discarded, and the second void of the day is collected. A catheterized specimen requires the physician, physician's assistant, or nurse to insert a catheter into the bladder, and a suprapubic specimen is collected with a needle inserted directly into the bladder.

The minimum volume for a routine UA is usually 12 mL, but 50 mL is preferred. For any type of collection it is imperative that the patient receive adequate verbal and/or written instructions. Asking a patient to half-fill the container is acceptable; it is best to have some room at the top of the container because the urine will need to be mixed before analysis. Never haphazardly ask a patient to "fill the cup."

A clean-catch midstream specimen (CCMS) may be ordered when the urine is to be cultured or examined for microorganisms. The clean-catch technique is used to remove microorganisms from the urinary meatus by thoroughly cleansing the area around the meatus and to flush out the distal portion of the urethra. Because the specimen is collected in the medical office by the patient, the medical assistant needs to give complete, understandable instructions to the patient on the method of collection (Procedure 51-1). Failure to do so may mean that the

PROCEDURE 51-1

Instruct Individuals According to Their Needs: Instruct a Patient in the Collection of a Clean-Catch Midstream Urine Specimen

<u>CAAHEP COMPETENCY:</u> 3.c.(3)(b)
<u>ABHES COMPETENCIES:</u> 4.b, 4.j, 4.w, 7.c

GOAL: *To collect a contaminant-free urine sample for culture or analysis using the clean-catch midstream specimen (CCMS) technique.*

EQUIPMENT and SUPPLIES

- Sterile container with lid and label
- Antiseptic towelettes

PROCEDURAL STEPS

1. Label the container and give the patient the supplies (Figure 1).
   <u>PURPOSE:</u> Labeling the container avoids possible mix-up of specimens.
2. Explain the following instructions to adult patients or to the guardians of child patients.

OBTAINING A CLEAN-CATCH MIDSTREAM SPECIMEN (FEMALE PATIENT)

1. Wash your hands, and remove your underclothing.
2. Expose the urinary meatus by spreading apart the labia with one hand (Figure 2, *A*).
3. Cleanse each side of the urinary meatus with a front-to-back motion, from the pubis to the anus. Use a separate antiseptic wipe to cleanse each side of the meatus.
4. Cleanse directly across the meatus, front-to-back, using a third cotton ball or antiseptic wipe (see Figure 2, *A*).
5. Hold the labia apart throughout this procedure.
6. Void a small amount of urine into the toilet (Figure 2, *B*).
7. Move the specimen container into position and void the next portion of urine into it. Remember, this is a sterile container. Do not put your fingers on the inside of the container.

8. Remove the cup, and void the last amount of urine into the toilet. (This means that the first part and the last part of the urinary flow have been excluded from the specimen. Only the middle portion of the flow is included.)
9. Wipe in your usual manner, redress, and return the sterile specimen to the place designated by the medical facility

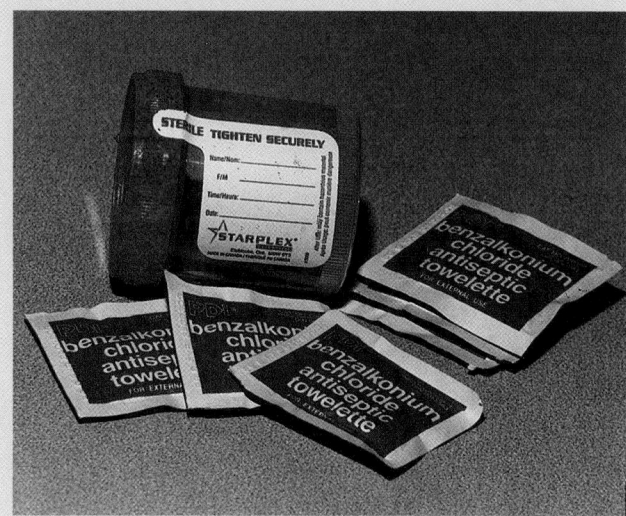

FIGURE 1

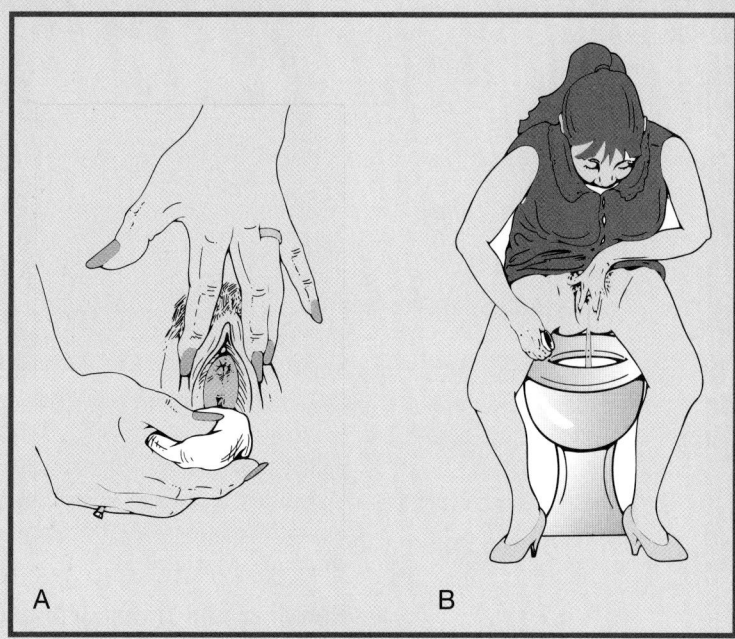

A

B

FIGURE 2

PROCEDURE 51-1—cont'd

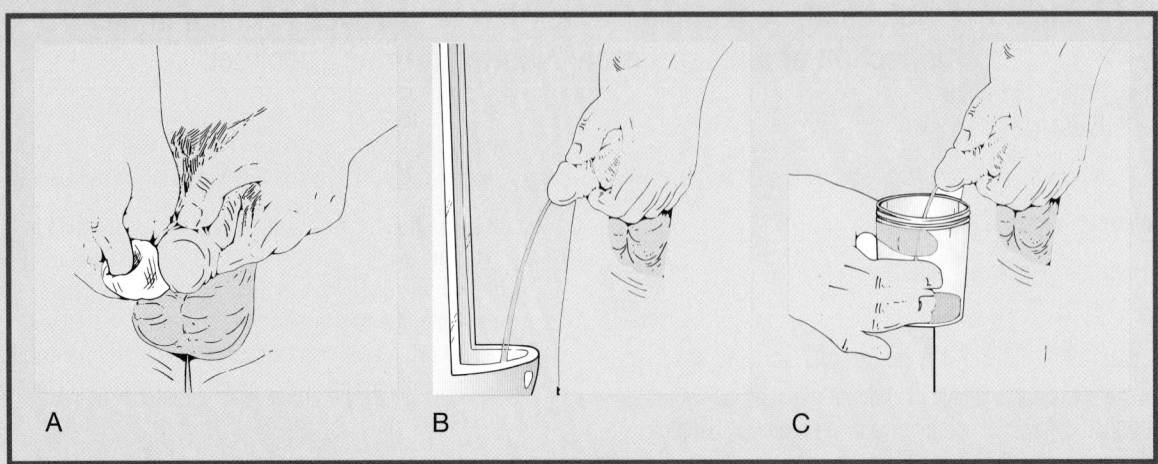

FIGURE 3

OBTAINING A CLEAN-CATCH MIDSTREAM SPECIMEN (MALE PATIENT)

1. Wash your hands, and expose the penis.
2. Retract the foreskin of the penis (if not circumcised).
3. Cleanse the area around the glans penis (meatus) and the urethral opening by washing each side of the glans with a separate antiseptic wipe (Figure 3, *A*).
4. Cleanse directly across the urethral opening using a third cotton ball or antiseptic wipe.
5. Void a small amount of urine into the toilet or urinal (Figure 3, *B*).

6. Collect the next portion of the urine in the sterile container without touching the inside of the container with hands or penis (Figure 3, *C*).
7. Void the last amount of urine into the toilet or urinal.
8. Wipe and redress.
9. Return the specimen to the designated area provided.
   <u>PURPOSE:</u> Instructions must be understood if they are to be followed correctly. By talking to the patient, you can determine whether the patient understands or has any questions.

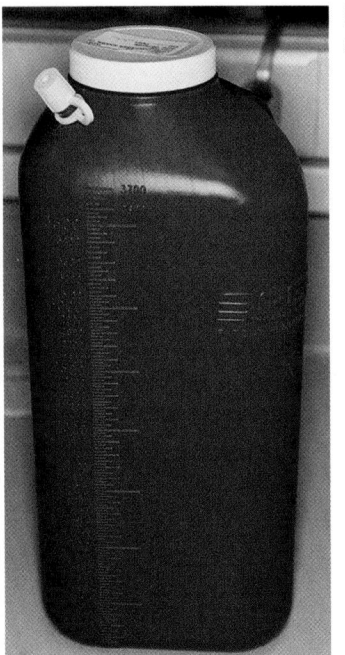

FIGURE 51-2 A 24-hour specimen container.

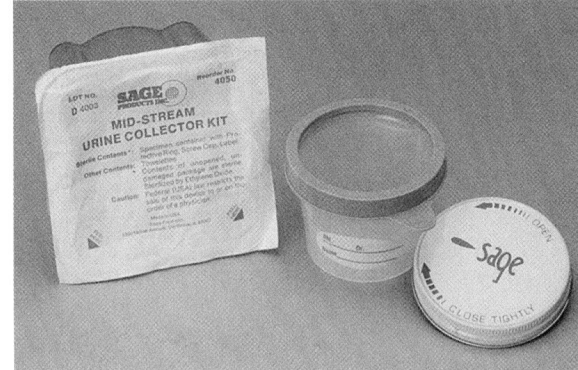

FIGURE 51-3 A sterile container for a midstream specimen.

patient will have to return to the office to allow the collection of another specimen. For culturing, urine should be collected by catheterization or the clean-catch method into a sterile container (Figure 51-3).

Handling and Transporting a Specimen

Proper handling of specimens is essential. The chemical and cellular components of urine change if the urine is allowed to

TABLE 51-1 Changes in Urine at Room Temperature

CONSTITUENT	CHANGE
Clarity	Becomes cloudy as crystals precipitate and bacteria multiply
Color	May change if pH becomes alkaline
pH	Becomes alkaline as bacteria form ammonia from urea
Glucose	Decreases as bacteria metabolize it
Ketones	Decrease because of evaporation
Bilirubin and urobilinogen	Undergo degradation in light
Blood	May hemolyze; false-positive results possible because of bacterial peroxidase
Nitrite	May become positive as bacteria multiply and reduce nitrate
Casts	Lyse or dissolve in alkaline urine
Cells	Lyse or dissolve in alkaline urine
Bacteria	Multiply twofold approximately every 20 minutes
Yeast	Multiply
Crystals	Precipitate as urine cools; may dissolve if pH changes

stand at room temperature (Table 51-1). Urine specimens should be kept refrigerated and should be processed within 2 hours of collection, however, refrigeration can cause precipitation of **amorphous** urates or phosphates, which interfere with the microscopic evaluation.

In the event that refrigeration is not feasible or if the specimen must be transported to a referral laboratory, evacuated transport tubes, which contain preservatives and look much like blood collection tubes, are available (Figure 51-4). The vacuum in the tube allows for the delivery of 7 to 8 mL of urine, using a transfer straw or a urine collection cup with an integrated sampling device. Alternately, the urine can be poured into the tube after the stopper is removed. The preservatives in the BD Vacutainer cherry red/yellow-stoppered tube, chlorhexidine, ethylparaben,

and sodium propionate, will prevent the overgrowth of bacteria and inhibit changes in the urine that can affect the results. Chemical reagent strip testing can be performed on preserved specimens; it should be performed within 72 hours. Tubes may be held at room temperature during this time.

For preservation of urine specimens slated for culture, it is necessary to use a different preservative. The BD Vacutainer preservatives sodium formate and boric acid in the gray-stoppered tube help to preserve the level of bacteria present at the time of the collection. This transport system should be used only for urine specimens that will be cultured. Results on the chemical reagent strip may be altered by these preservatives. **Culture and sensitivity (C&S)** testing should be performed within 72 hours. Tubes may be held at room temperature.

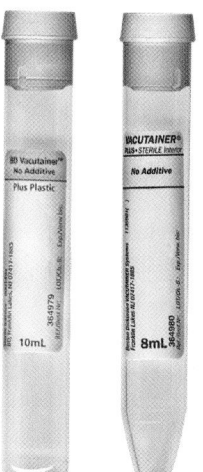

FIGURE 51-4 BD Vacutainer urine preservation tubes. (Courtesy Becton, Dickinson, and Company, Franklin Lakes, NJ.)

Guidelines for Caring for a Urine Specimen Obtained at Home

- Do not put anything but your urine into the bottle.
- Do not pour out any liquid or powdered preservative from the container.
- If you accidentally spill some of the preservative on yourself, immediately wash with water and call the testing center or designated laboratory.
- Always keep the collection bottle cool. Refrigerate or keep the bottle in an ice-filled cooler or pail.
- Keep the cap on the container.
- You may find it more convenient to urinate into the smaller container provided then pour the urine into the larger collection bottle.

CRITICAL THINKING APPLICATION

Dr. Hill has ordered a UA on the specimen from Mr. Parks, a UA and pregnancy test on the specimen from Mrs. Carpenter, and a UA and C&S on the specimen from Ms. Winfrey. After reviewing the requisitions and entering the patient information into the daily logbook, Rosa notes that Mrs. Carpenter's specimen was collected at 6 AM— 3 hours ago. Is this acceptable? Explain your answer. Rosa also notes that the specimen collected in the sterile container from Ms. Winfrey is marked "CCMS." Why is this important?

THE ROUTINE URINALYSIS

Physical Examination of Urine

The first part of a complete UA is assessment of the physical properties and measurement of selected chemical constituents that are of diagnostic importance (Table 51-2, Procedure 51-2).

Appearance

Color. Normal urine color is a shade of yellow, ranging from pale straw to yellow to amber. Color depends on the concentration of the pigment urochrome and the amount

TABLE 51-2 Components of the Macroscopic Urinalysis	
Physical properties	Color
	Clarity
	Specific gravity
	Volume*
	Odor*
	Foam*
Chemical properties	Protein
	Glucose
	Ketones
	Bilirubin
	Blood
	Nitrite
	pH
	Urobilinogen
	Leukocyte esterase

*Not always assessed.

of water in the specimen. A dilute specimen should be pale, and a more concentrated specimen should be a darker yellow. Variations in color may be caused by diet, medication, and disease. Abnormal colors may be related to pathologic or nonpathologic factors (Table 51-3).

PROCEDURE 51-2

Perform Urinalysis: Assess Urine for Color and Turbidity—the Physical Test

CAAHEP COMPETENCY: 3.b.(3)(c)(i)
ABHES COMPETENCIES: 4.j, 4.k, 4.q, 4.r, 4.y

GOAL: *To assess and record the color and clarity of a urine specimen.*

EQUIPMENT and SUPPLIES

- Urine specimen
- Centrifuge tube

   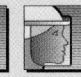

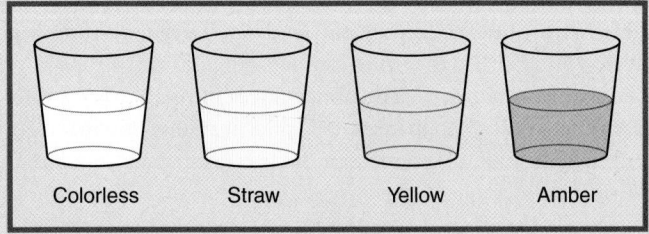

| Colorless | Straw | Yellow | Amber |

FIGURE 1

PROCEDURAL STEPS

1. Wash and dry your hands, and apply gloves.
2. Mix the urine by swirling.
   PURPOSE: Suspended substances settle when urine stands. If urine is not mixed before assessment of appearance, the finding will be incorrect.
3. Label a centrifuge tube if a complete urinalysis is being done.
   PURPOSE: If a complete urinalysis is being done, a portion of the specimen will be centrifuged for microscopic examination. The centrifuged specimen must be labeled to avoid specimen confusion.
4. Pour the specimen into a standard-size centrifuge tube.
   PURPOSE: Standard-size containers are better for assessing color and clarity results.

5. Assess and record the color (Figure 1):
   - Pale straw
   - Yellow
   - Dark yellow
   - Amber
6. Assess the clarity:
   - Clear—no cloudiness
   - Slightly turbid—can see light print through tube
   - Moderately turbid—can see only dark print through tube
   - Very turbid—cannot see through tube.
7. Clean the work area, remove gloves, and wash your hands.
   PURPOSE: Infection control.
8. Record the results in the patient's record.
   PURPOSE: A procedure is considered not done until it is recorded.

TABLE 51-3 Urine Colors

COLOR	PATHOLOGIC CAUSE	NONPATHOLOGIC CAUSE
Straw	Diabetes	Diuretics; high fluid intake (coffee, beer)
Amber	Dehydration	Excessive sweating; low fluid intake
Bright yellow		Carotene, vitamins
Red	Blood, porphyrins	Beets, drugs, dyes
Orange-yellow	Bile, hepatitis	Pyridium (phenazopyridine hydrochloride), dyes, drugs
Greenish yellow	Bile, hepatitis	Senna, cascara, rhubarb
Reddish brown	Old blood, methemoglobin	
Brownish black	Methemoglobin, melanin	Levodopa
Salmon pink		Amorphous urates
White (milky)	Fats, pus	Amorphous phosphates
Blue-green	Biliverdin, infection with *Pseudomonas*	Vitamin B, drugs, dyes

Turbidity. Both normal and abnormal urine specimens may range in appearance from clear to very cloudy. Cloudiness may be caused by cells, bacteria, yeast, vaginal contaminants, or crystals. Often a urine specimen that was clear when voided will become cloudy as it cools, as crystals form and precipitate.

Volume

The amount of urine is rarely measured on a random specimen. With a timed specimen, volume is measured by pouring the entire collection into a large, graduated cylinder. Generally, it is not accurate enough to use the markings on the side of the collection container. Once the volume is measured and recorded, a portion of well-mixed specimen, called an *aliquot*, is removed for testing. The remainder is discarded or stored, depending on the preference of the laboratory.

The normal volume of urine produced every 24 hours varies according to the age of the individual. Infants and children produce smaller volumes than adults. The normal adult volume is 750 to 2000 mL in 24 hours, with an average of about 1500 mL. Excessive production of urine is called *polyuria*. This is common in diabetes and certain kidney disorders. Oliguria is insufficient production of urine and can be caused by dehydration, decreased fluid intake, shock, or renal disease. The absence of urine production, anuria, occurs in renal obstruction and renal failure.

Foam

Normally the presence of foam is not recorded, but careful observation of this property can be a significant clue to an abnormality. Foam is the presence of small bubbles that persist for a long time after the specimen has been shaken; they must not be confused with any bubbles that rapidly disperse. White foam can indicate the presence of increased protein (Figure 51-5). Greenish-yellow foam can mean **bilirubinuria.** Caution should be taken in handling such urines, because the color of the foam may indicate that the patient has viral hepatitis.

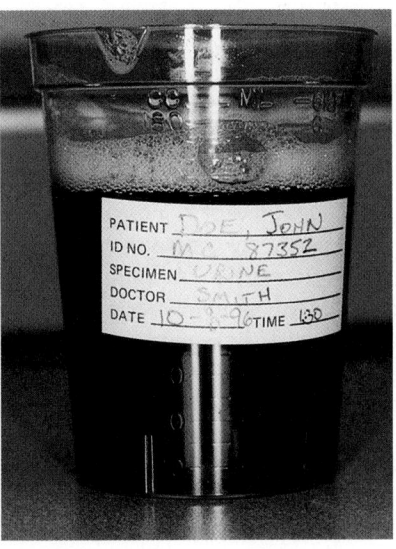

FIGURE 51-5 Dark amber urine with foam indicates possible increased protein and possible hematuria.

Odor

As with foam, odor is not normally recorded but can be an important clue to metabolic disorders. Normal urine odor is said to be aromatic. Changes in the odor of urine may be caused by disease, the presence of bacteria, or diet. The odor of the urine of a patient with uncontrolled diabetes is described as fruity because of the presence of ketones, which are the products of fat metabolism. An ammonia or putrid smell in the urine can be caused by an infection or may be noted in urine that has been allowed to stand before being tested. The bacteria break down the urea in the urine to form ammonia. Foods such as asparagus and garlic can also produce an abnormal odor in the urine. Urine from a child with phenylketonuria (PKU) is said to smell "mousy." PKU is a rare hereditary condition in which the amino acid **phenylalanine** is not properly metabolized, leading to severe mental retardation. Accumulation of phenylalanine in the blood and urine gives body fluids an odor like wet fur. Blood sampling for PKU is discussed in Chapter 52.

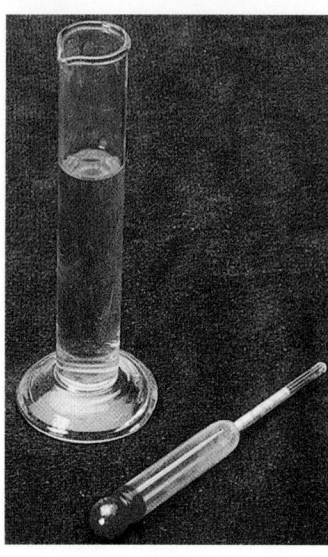

FIGURE 51-6 A urine-filled cylinder and urinometer.

Specific Gravity

Specific gravity is the weight of a substance compared with the weight of an equal volume of distilled water. In UA, it is the rough measurement of the concentration, or amount, of substances dissolved in urine. The specific gravity of distilled water is 1.000. Normal specific gravity of urine ranges from 1.005 to 1.030, depending on the patient's fluid intake. Most samples fall between 1.010 and 1.025. Urine specific gravity indicates whether the kidneys are able to concentrate the urine and is one of the first indications of kidney disease. The presence of glucose, protein, or an x-ray contrast medium used in diagnostic studies may also increase the specific gravity of urine. To measure the specific gravity of urine, laboratories may use a urinometer , a refractometer, or a chemical reagent strip

The urinometer is a sealed glass float with a calibrated paper scale in its stem (Figure 51-6). With a slight spinning motion, it is placed into a cylinder containing a urine sample, and the value is read at the meniscus of the urine. It requires a quantity of urine sufficient to freely suspend the float, usually approximately 20 to 25 mL. If the sample is insufficient to float the urinometer, use a refractometer or record as "QNS" (quantity not sufficient).

A urinometer is fragile, and jarring can cause the paper scale in the stem to shift, resulting in erroneous readings. Occasionally, a damaged urinometer loses its calibration; therefore the calibration of the urinometer should be checked daily with distilled water. The specific gravity of the distilled water should calibrate at 1.000 at 20° C (68° F; room temperature). For example, if the urinometer reads 1.002 in distilled water, 0.002 must be subtracted from the urine readings. However, it is better to replace the instrument. For each 3° C (37.4° F) that the water temperature measures above 20° C (68° F), 0.001 must be added to the reading. For each 3° C (37.4° F) that the water temperature measures below 20° C (68° F), 0.001 must be subtracted from the reading. Use a laboratory thermometer to determine the water temperature. The urinometer method, although considered the **gold standard** of specific gravity testing, uses a large volume of urine and results in contamination of several pieces of glassware. For these reasons, it is rarely used in modern laboratories.

A refractometer measures the refraction of light through solids in a liquid. The result is called the *refractive index*, which for our purposes is the same as specific gravity (Figure 51-7). The refractometer is both faster and easier to use than the urinometer and requires only a drop of urine. One drop of well-mixed urine is placed under the hinged cover of the instrument, and the value is read directly from a scale viewed through an ocular. The refractometer must be calibrated daily with distilled water, which will read 1.000 (Procedure 51-3). Note that the measurement of specific gravity carries no unit of measure after the number.

The reagent strip (dipstick) test is the most commonly used method in the physician's office laboratory (POL), and it is considered a Clinical Laboratory Improvement Act (CLIA)–waived test. The pad on the strip contains a chemical that is sensitive to positively charged ions, such as sodium (Na^+) and potassium (K^+). The strip will detect specific gravity in the range of 1.005 to 1.030.

FIGURE 51-7 A refractometer. (From Stepp CA, Woods MA: *Laboratory procedures for medical office personnel*, Philadelphia, 1998, Saunders.)

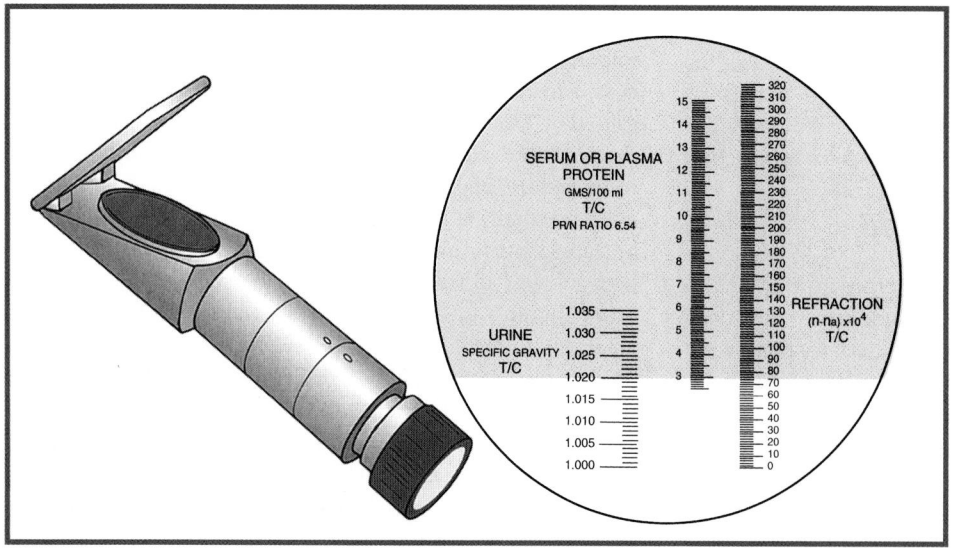

PROCEDURE 51-3

Perform Routine Maintenance of Administrative and Clinical Equipment: Measure Urine Specific Gravity with a Refractometer

CAAHEP COMPETENCIES: 3.b.(3)(c)(i), 3.c.(4)(b)
ABHES COMPETENCIES: 4.i, 4.k, 4.y

GOAL: *To calibrate a refractometer and measure the refractive index of urine. A refractometer is also known as a total solids (TS) meter.*

EQUIPMENT and SUPPLIES

- Urinary refractometer
- Disposable pipet
- Distilled water
- Biohazard waste container

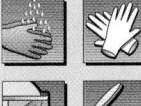
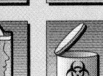

PROCEDURAL STEPS

1. Wash your hands and assemble equipment while the urine specimen reaches room temperature.
   PURPOSE: Measuring specific gravity of cold or warm urine may alter the results.

2. Apply gloves and mix the urine specimen in the collection container.
   PURPOSE: Mixing the urine resuspends solids that have settled during storage.

3. Using a disposable pipet, apply a drop of water to the prism of the refractometer (see Figure 51-7) by lifting the plastic cover. Close the cover and point the device toward a light source such as a window or lamp. Look into the refractometer and rotate the eyepiece so the scale can be clearly read. The scale reads from 1.000 to 1.035 in increments of 0.001.

4. Calibrate the refractometer by inserting the small screwdriver provided by the manufacturer in the screw on the underside of the instrument. Turn the screw so that the line is positioned over 1.000 (see Figure 1*).
   PURPOSE: This step ensures that the refractometer is calibrated properly and must be performed daily.

5. Wipe the prism with a soft, lint-free tissue, and apply a drop of mixed urine. Close the cover, point the device at a light source, and read the specific gravity on the scale Discard the pipet in a biohazard waste container. The value for specific gravity shown in Figure 51-7 is 1.020. Note that specific gravity has no units following the value.
   PURPOSE: A soft cloth should be used to prevent scratching the glass prism.

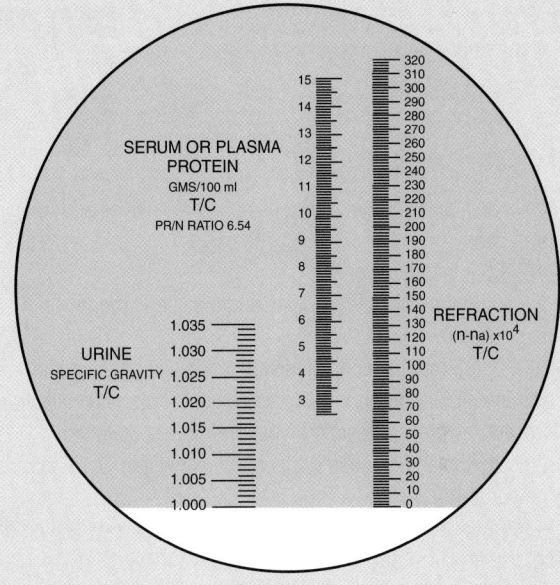

FIGURE 1

6. Wipe the urine from the prism with a disposable, soft, lint-free tissue between samples. When finished, clean with tissue moistened with alcohol or with a disposable alcohol wipe. Discard these tissues in a biohazard waste container.
   PURPOSE: Urine, a biohazardous material, must be removed from the prism. The prism must be decontaminated after use.

7. Record the results, and discard the urine sample.
   PURPOSE: A procedure is not considered finished until it is recorded.
   Remove and discard gloves, and wash your hands.

---

*Figure from Stepp CA, Woods MA: *Laboratory procedures for medical office personnel*, Philadelphia, 1998, Saunders.
See Appendix D for a charting example.

CRITICAL THINKING APPLICATION

■ The requisitions accompanying the urine specimens indicate that all three will require a UA. Rosa performs the physical analysis and notes that Mrs. Carpenter's urine, requiring the pregnancy test, is amber, whereas the other two specimens are pale yellow. Propose possible explanations for Rosa's observations. Should Rosa be concerned about the darker color of Mrs. Carpenter's urine?

■ Ms. Winfrey's urine is turbid, whereas Mr. Parks' urine is clear. What might be causing the cloudiness in Ms. Winfrey's urine? Is a cloudy urine cause for concern?

Chemical Examination of Urine

Tests can be performed on urine to detect the presence of certain chemicals, which can provide valuable information to the physician. In certain situations, these chemical test results can be critical to the diagnosis.

Reagent strips are the most widely employed technique for detecting chemicals in the urine (Procedure 51-4); these strips are available in a variety of types (Figure 51-8). Generally, they are plastic strips to which one or more pads containing chemicals are attached. Tests are available for pH, specific gravity, vitamin C, leukocyte esterase, protein, ketones,

PROCEDURE 51-4

Perform Urinalysis: Test Urine with Chemical Reagent Strips—the Chemical Urinalysis

CAAHEP COMPETENCY: 3.c.(3)(b)
ABHES COMPETENCIES: 4.b, 4.j, 4.w, 7.c

GOAL: *To perform chemical testing on a urine sample.*

EQUIPMENT and SUPPLIES

- Urine specimen
- Reagent strips
- Timer

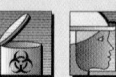

PROCEDURAL STEPS

1. Wash and dry your hands. Put on nonsterile gloves and eye protection.
   PURPOSE: Infection control.
2. Check the time of collection, the container, and the mode of preservation.
   PURPOSE: Proper specimen identification and screening of specimens for appropriate collection containers and collection procedures prevent testing of inappropriate specimens.
3. If the specimen has been refrigerated, allow it to warm to room temperature.
   PURPOSE: Certain tests are temperature dependent. Testing of cold specimens may cause false-negative results.
4. Check the reagent strip container for expiration date.
   PURPOSE: Do not use expired reagents.
5. Remove the reagent strip from the container. Hold it in your hand, or place it on a clean paper towel. Recap the container tightly.
   PURPOSE: Test strips are sensitive to moisture and light and must be stored in tightly sealed containers. Contamination from chemical residues on countertops can affect results.
6. Compare nonreactive test pads with the negative color blocks on the color chart on the container.
   PURPOSE: Discolored pads indicate that the product has not been properly stored and must not be used for testing.
7. Thoroughly mix the specimen by swirling.
   PURPOSE: If settling occurs, certain elements may not be detected.
8. Following manufacturer's directions, note the time and dip the strip into the urine, then remove.
   PURPOSE: Tests are time dependent. Some pads will darken over time.

9. Quickly remove the excess urine from the strip by touching the side of the strip to a paper towel or the side of the urine container.
   PURPOSE: Excess urine on the strip or prolonged dipping time affects test results.
10. Hold the strip horizontally. At the required time, compare the strip with the appropriate color chart on the reagent container (Figure 1). Alternately, the strip can be placed on a paper towel.
    PURPOSE: Holding the strip horizontally prevents runover from one test pad to another and prevents interference from the mixing of chemicals in the test pads.
11. Read the concentration by comparing the strip to the color chart on the side of the bottle. *Do not touch the strip to the bottle.*
    PURPOSE: Timing is critical. Allowing the strip to come into contact with the bottle will contaminate the bottle.
12. Clean the work area, remove your gloves, and wash your hands. If a paper towel was used, dispose of it in the biohazard container.
    PURPOSE: Infection control.
13. Record the results in the patient's record.
    PURPOSE: A procedure is considered not done until it is recorded.

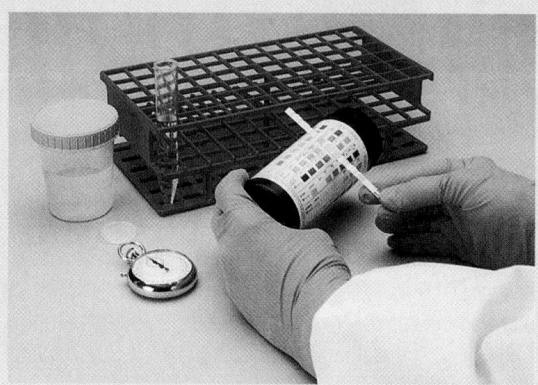

FIGURE 1

glucose, blood, bilirubin, nitrite, urobilinogen, phenylketones, and other chemicals. The presence or absence of these chemicals in the urine provides information on the status of carbohydrate metabolism, liver and kidney function, and the patient's acid-base balance.

Reagent strips are designed to be used once then discarded. The directions for each strip are located in the package, and these instructions must be followed exactly to obtain accurate results. A color-comparison chart is located on the label of the

container. In addition to reagent strips, various tablet tests are available.

All strips and tablets must be kept in tightly closed containers in a cool, dry area and should be removed only immediately before testing. Never touch a strip that has been exposed to urine to the color-comparison chart. If both a UA and a C&S are ordered for a specimen, ensure that the urine has been cultured before beginning the UA. Introducing a reagent strip into the urine will contaminate it.

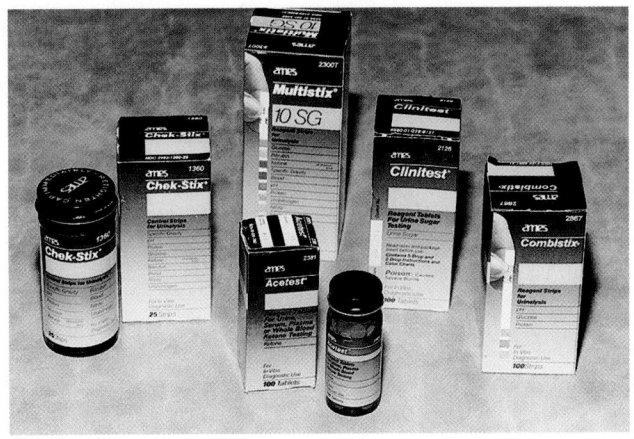

FIGURE 51-8 Examples of reagent strips.

pH

The pH is a measurement of the degree of acidity or alkalinity of the urine. A urine specimen with a pH of 7 is neutral (Figure 51-9). A value less than 7 indicates acidity, and greater than 7 indicates alkalinity. Normal, freshly voided urine may have a pH range of 5.5 to 8. Urinary pH varies with an individual's metabolic status, diet, drug therapy, and disease. In the case of gross bacteriuria, urine pH is alkaline as a result of bacterial conversion of urea to ammonia. Knowing the pH of the urine will also assist in the identification of crystals if they are found in the urine sediment.

Glucose

Glucose is filtered at the glomerulus, but under normal conditions most of it is reabsorbed by the tubules. The minute quantities normally present in the urine are not detected by reagent strips and tablets. Detectable **glycosuria** occurs whenever the renal tubules cannot reabsorb the filtered glucose load. A positive glucose finding is common in urine from diabetic patients and may be the first indication of the disease. The reagent-strip glucose testing method is based on an **enzymatic reaction.** It detects only glucose; in other words, it is specific for glucose.

Protein

Protein in the urine in detectable amounts is called *proteinuria* and is one of the first signs of renal disease. We normally excrete a small amount of protein every day; proteinuria may be light to heavy, constant, or sporadic. It may be affected by posture: in orthostatic proteinuria, protein is excreted only when the patient is in an upright position. Generally, first morning specimens from these patients are negative, but protein is found in urine passed throughout the day. Proteinuria is a common finding in pregnancy. It is also almost always present after heavy exercise. The reagent strip is highly sensitive to urinary albumin and less sensitive to hemoglobin, immunoglobulin, and mucoproteins.

Ketones

Ketones are the end-product of fat metabolism in the body. Acetoacetate, acetone, and beta-hydroxybutyric acid are collectively called *ketone bodies*, or *ketones*. Ketonuria is common in the presence of starvation, low-carbohydrate diets, excessive vomiting, and diabetes mellitus. Because ketones evaporate at room temperature, urine should be tested immediately, or the specimen should be tightly covered and refrigerated. The reagent strip detects only acetoacetate. The Acetest, discussed later in this chapter, can be used to detect both acetone and acetoacetate.

Blood

The presence of blood in the urine may indicate infection or trauma to the urinary tract or bleeding in the kidneys. The blood test pad on the reagent strip reacts with three different blood constituents: intact red blood cells, hemoglobin from red blood cells, and myoglobin, a hemoglobin-like molecule that transports oxygen in muscle tissue.

Hematuria is the presence of intact red blood cells in urine. The color reaction on the reagent strip ranges from yellow through green to dark green when hematuria is present, revealing a speckled appearance. Hematuria can be caused by irritation of the ureters, bladder, or urethra. It is also a common finding in cystitis and in persons passing kidney stones. A random

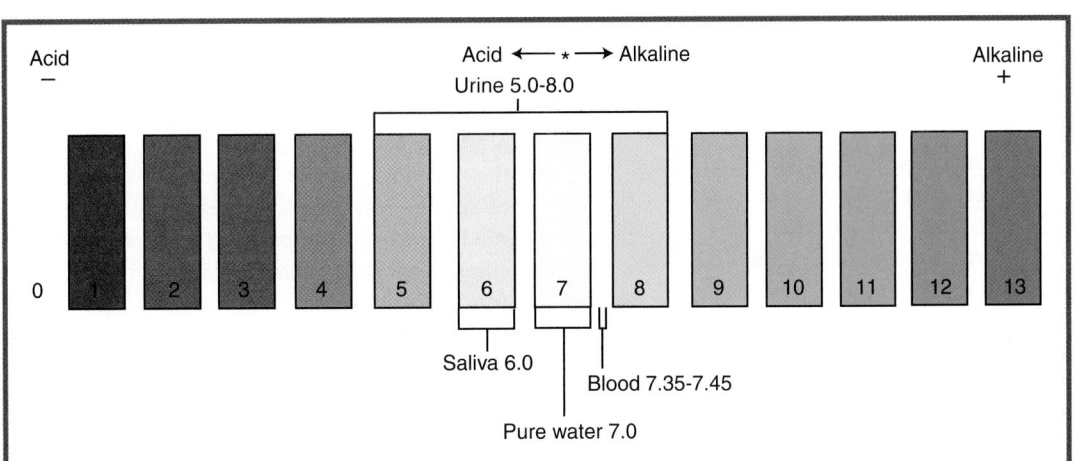

FIGURE 51-9 The pH scale. (From Stepp CA, Woods MA: *Laboratory procedures for medical office personnel*, Philadelphia, 1998, Saunders.)

specimen may contain blood from vaginal contamination if the woman is menstruating.

Hemoglobinuria is the presence of hemolyzed red blood cells. True hemoglobinuria is rare. It occurs as a result of intravascular red blood cell destruction and can be caused by transfusion reactions, malaria, drug reactions, snake bites, and severe burns. **Myoglobinuria** occurs when muscle tissue is damaged or injured, such as in crushing injuries, myocardial infarctions, and contact sports. Muscular dystrophy patients often exhibit myoglobinuria. Hemoglobinuria cannot be distinguished from myoglobinuria by reagent strip testing; both will cause a uniform change of color from light green to dark green on the strip.

Bilirubin and Urobilinogen

Bilirubin is a product of the breakdown of hemoglobin. Hemoglobin is released from old red blood cells and is gradually converted to bilirubin in the liver, then further to urobilinogen in the intestines. Bilirubin is a bile pigment not normally found in urine. Its presence in urine is one of the first signs of liver disease or other disease in which the liver may be involved, such as infectious mononucleosis.

Bilirubinuria can occur even before jaundice or other symptoms of liver disease are evident. It is the result of liver cell damage or obstruction of the common bile duct by stones or neoplasms (tumors). Excessive bilirubin colors the urine yellow-brown to greenish-orange. Because direct light causes decomposition of bilirubin, urine samples must be protected from light until testing is complete.

Urobilinogen is normally present in urine in small amounts. Increases are seen when there is increased red blood cell destruction and in liver disease. When there is total obstruction of the bile duct, no urobilinogen is formed in the intestines, none is reabsorbed into the circulation, and therefore none is present in the urine. Reagent strip methods cannot detect a decrease in urobilinogen.

Nitrite

Nitrite occurs in urine when bacteria break down nitrate, a common component of urine. A positive nitrite test result may indicate the presence of a urinary tract infection (UTI). However, not all bacteria are able to reduce nitrate to nitrite. Negative nitrite tests can also occur when bacteria are insufficient or when the urine has not incubated in the bladder long enough for the reaction to occur. *Escherichia coli*, the organism that causes the majority of UTIs, reduces nitrate to nitrite. False-positive results can occur if a specimen is allowed to sit at room temperature and contaminating bacteria multiply. False-negative results may occur if the bacteria further metabolize the nitrite they have produced to ammonia.

Leukocyte Esterase

Leukocytes (white blood cells) occur in urine in infections of the urinary tract. They can also be contaminants from the vagina. The leukocyte esterase test on reagent strips detects intact and lysed **polymorphonuclear white blood cells.** However, it does not detect **mononuclear white blood cells,** which are

TABLE 51-4 Normal Urine Reference Ranges

REFERENCE	RANGE
Color	Pale yellow to straw
Clarity	Clear to slightly turbid
Specific gravity	1.001-1.035
pH	4.6-8
Protein (mg/dl)	NEG
Glucose (mg/dl)	NEG
Ketone (mg/dl)	NEG
Bilirubin (mg/dl)	NEG
Blood (mg/dl)	NEG
Nitrite (mg/dl)	NEG
Urobilinogen (Ehrlich units)	0.1-1
White blood cells	NEG

occasionally present during infections. The test does not react with the small numbers of white blood cells found in normal urine.

Limitations of Reagent Strip Testing

The reagent strip is a reliable method for chemical analysis of urine if used properly. The normal urine reference ranges using a reagent strip can be found in Table 51-4. A number of sources of error exist; if the strip is soaked excessively in the specimen, chemicals in the pads may be diluted. If the strip is not held horizontally while being read, colors from one pad may bleed onto another. Finally, certain chemicals, such as ascorbic acid, may affect results of nitrite, glucose, bilirubin, and occult blood tests. Normal levels of vitamin C will not interfere, but if a person consumes large quantities of the vitamin, a special strip can be used to detect interfering levels of vitamin C. If an elevated level is found, the patient should be instructed to discontinue vitamin C intake for 24 hours, then another urine specimen should be collected for testing.

Visual interpretation of color on the reagent strip pads is likely to vary among individuals, and some laboratories use automated instruments to read the strips. Several companies manufacture instruments that employ the principle of reflectance photometry in the analysis of reagent strip color. Once the strip has been placed in the instrument, a microprocessor controls the movement of the strip into the reflectometer. There, light of specific wavelengths is beamed onto the strip. Some light will be absorbed, and some light will scatter or be reflected. The amount of light reflected is analyzed by the microprocessor and converted into a digital reading, and the result is printed out (Figure 51-10).

The advantage of this method is that timing and color interpretation are consistent. The disadvantage is that the instrument is not able to identify and compensate for urines that are highly pigmented, leading to false-positive results. The medical assistant should be aware of this and manually test urine specimens that are darkly pigmented.

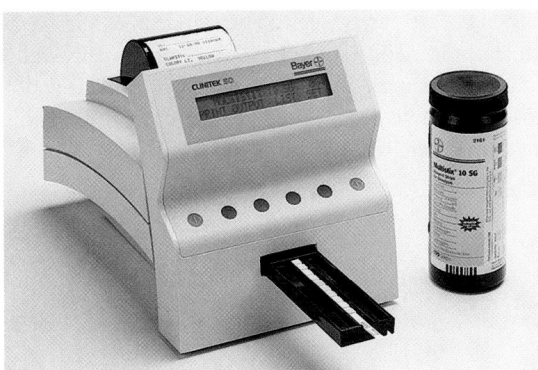

FIGURE 51-10 Clinitek urine analyzer. (From Bonewit-West K: *Clinical procedures for medical assistants*, ed 6, Philadelphia, 2004, Saunders.)

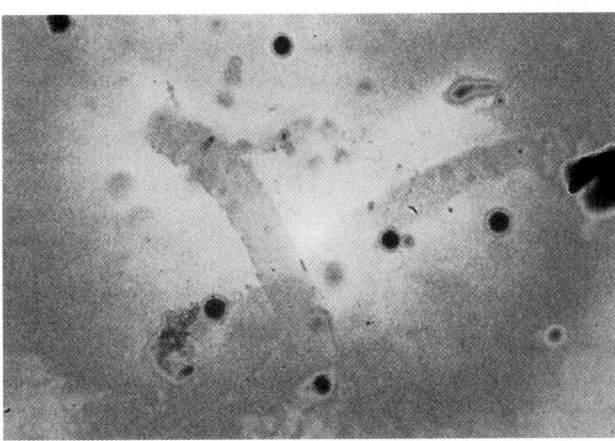

FIGURE 51-11 Hyaline casts. (Sedi-Stain, 400×.) (From Ringsrud KM, Linne JJ: *Urinalysis and body fluids: a color text and atlas*, St Louis, 1995, Mosby.)

CRITICAL THINKING APPLICATION

- Rosa prepares to do the chemical examination of the three urine specimens. Dr. Hill has ordered a UA on the specimen from Mr. Parks, a UA and pregnancy test on the specimen from Mrs. Carpenter, and a UA and C&S on the specimen from Ms. Winfrey. Should she proceed with the chemical analysis of each specimen in exactly the same manner? Explain your answer.
- On completing the chemical analysis of the three specimens, Rosa notes several differences among the samples. Mrs. Carpenter's sample has a high specific gravity. Ms. Winfrey's sample reveals an elevated nitrite, a pH of 8, and an elevated leukocyte esterase. Mr. Parks' test results reveal elevated glucose and ketone levels and a specific gravity of 1.035. Based on this information, what are the probable reasons each of these patients visited Dr. Hill today?

Microscopic Examination of Urine Sediment

The microscopic examination of urine (see Procedure 51-5) consists of categorizing and counting cells, **casts,** crystals, and miscellaneous constituents of the sediment obtained when a measured portion of urine is centrifuged. The test is not categorized as CLIA-waived, and this would not be performed by a medical assistant without additional training and rigid compliance with CLIA quality-assurance protocols for the laboratory, including periodic proficiency testing. The medical assistant, however, should be familiar with preparing the urine for this test and with the possible results. The clear upper portion of the specimen is called the *supernatant.* It is poured off, and a drop of the well-mixed sediment is examined under a microscope. The sediment may be stained with a **supravital** sediment stain to give greater contrast to the formed elements. The most commonly used stain is the Sternheimer-Malbin stain, which consists of crystal violet and safranin. This stain assists in the identification of formed elements by enhancing the detail of internal cellular structure.

Microscopic observation is accomplished most popularly with a bright field, phase-contrast, or polarizing microscope. With a traditional bright field microscope, correct light adjustment is essential. The light must be reduced by closing the condenser iris diaphragm to increase the contrast. The condenser should be lowered slightly. Bright field microscopy is enhanced by the use of stains. Phase contrast microscopy converts variations in refractive index into variations in contrast by fitting a bright field microscope with a special device known as an *annular ring,* which enhances contrast in living cells and low refractive index components. The polarizing microscope is used most commonly in the UA laboratory to confirm the presence of fat, specifically cholesterol, and for identifying crystals.

Many formed elements are found in the urine. Some are significant; others are not. Most important, the microscopic examination should correlate with the physical and chemical analyses. For example, if the presence of red blood cells is confirmed on the reagent strip, red blood cells should be visible on the microscopic examination, and the urine may appear pink or red-tinged.

Casts

Casts are formed when protein accumulates and precipitates in the kidney tubules and is washed into the urine. The protein takes on the size and shape of the tubules—hence the term *casts.* Casts are cylindric, with flat or rounded ends, and are classified according to the substances observed in them. Certain types of casts are associated with renal pathologic conditions; others are physiologic and are generally caused by strenuous exercise.

Casts are counted and reported under low-power magnification, but occasionally high-power magnification is needed to identify the type. Because casts tend to migrate to the edges of the coverslip, this area should be examined closely. Casts dissolve in alkaline urine on standing; therefore examination of a fresh urine specimen is very important.

Hyaline casts are pale, transparent, cylindric structures that have rounded ends and parallel sides (Figure 51-11). Hyaline casts will be missed entirely if the light is not reduced at the condenser. They are formed when urine flow through individual nephrons is diminished. They can be found in persons with kidney disease but can also be found in urine specimens of normal subjects who have exercised heavily. Occasionally, hyaline casts have granular or cellular inclusions.

White blood cell casts are hyaline casts that contain leukocytes. White blood cells usually have a multilobed nucleus, which differentiates them from renal tubular epithelial cells, which have single, round nuclei. White blood cell casts are seen in pyelonephritis (Figure 51-12).

Finely and coarsely granular casts may be caused by exercise but when present in increased numbers may indicate renal disease. On close examination, granular casts show a hyaline matrix with coarse or fine granular inclusions. The granules are thought to be caused by protein aggregation or degeneration of cellular inclusions (Figure 51-13).

Red blood cell casts always indicate a pathologic condition and are highly diagnostic. Red blood cell casts occur in glomerulonephritis. They are hyaline casts with embedded red cells, and their presence indicates damage to the glomerular membrane. They may appear brown as a result of the color of the red blood cells present (Figure 51-14).

Renal tubular epithelial cell casts contain embedded renal tubular epithelial cells. These casts are easily confused with white blood cell casts, particularly if the cells have started to degenerate. Renal tubular epithelial cell casts are found when excessive damage has occurred. Causes are shock, renal **ischemia,** heavy-metal poisoning, certain allergic reactions, and nephrotoxic drugs (Figure 51-15).

Waxy casts are rarely seen. They appear as glassy, brittle, smooth, homogeneous structures. They are usually yellowish, have cracks or fissures, and have squared or broken ends. They are considered to be degenerated cellular casts and are found in persons with severe renal disease (Figure 51-16).

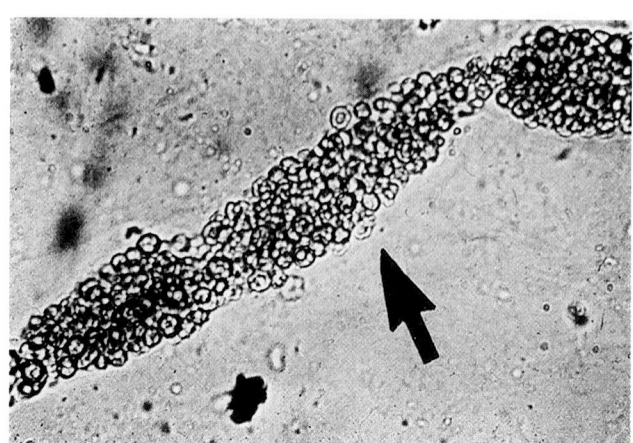

FIGURE 51-14 Red blood cell casts. (From Stepp CA, Woods MA: *Laboratory procedures for medical office personnel*, Philadelphia, 1998, Saunders.)

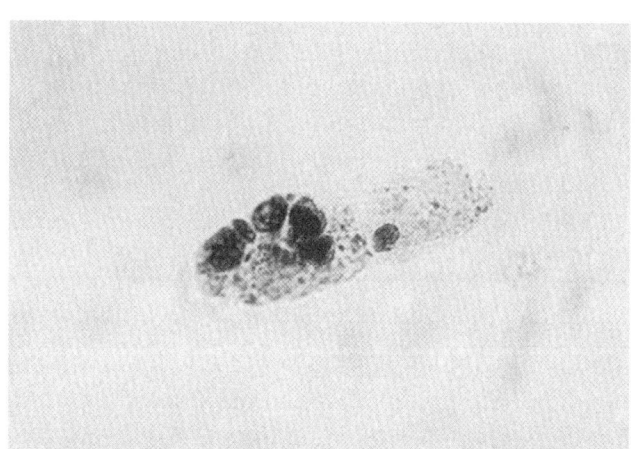

FIGURE 51-15 A renal tubular cell cast, seen with bright field microscopy. (Sedi-Stain, 400×.) (From Brunzel NA: *Fundamentals of urine and body fluid analysis*, Philadelphia, 1994, Saunders.)

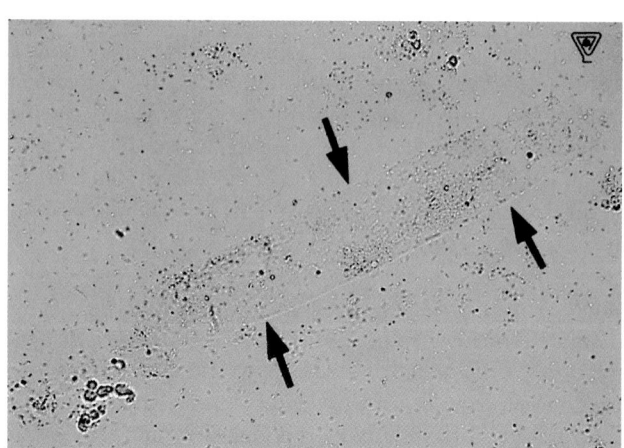

FIGURE 51-12 Hyaline casts. (From Stepp CA, Woods MA: *Laboratory procedures for medical office personnel*, Philadelphia, 1998, Saunders.)

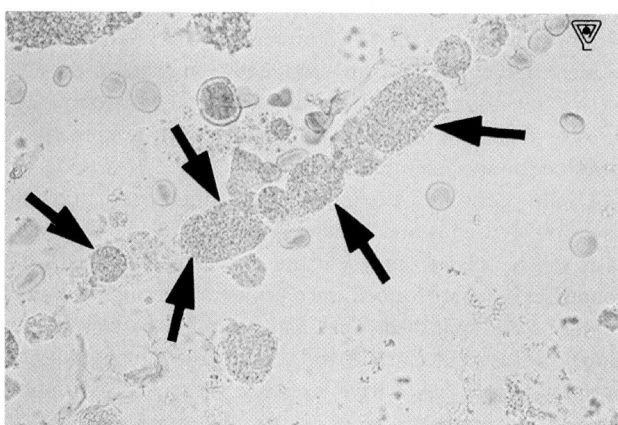

FIGURE 51-13 Granular casts. (From Stepp CA, Woods MA: *Laboratory procedures for medical office personnel*, Philadelphia, 1998, Saunders.)

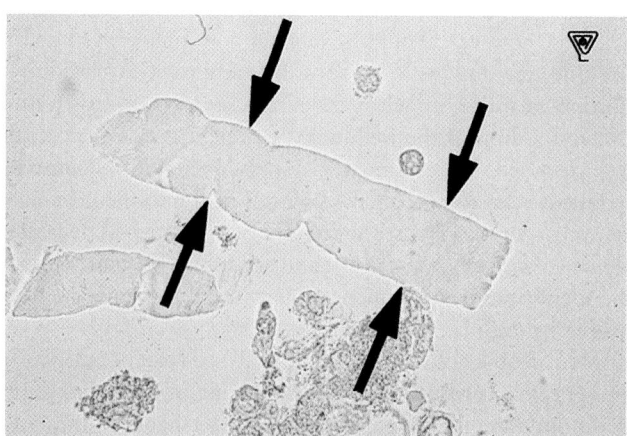

FIGURE 51-16 Waxy casts. (From Stepp CA, Woods MA: *Laboratory procedures for medical office personnel*, Philadelphia, 1998, Saunders.)

Occasionally more than one type of cell will be found in a single cast. Mixed cellular casts have been reported. Absolute identification of the cell types present may be difficult.

Cells

Cells that are found in urine include epithelial cells, which are derived from the lining of the genitourinary tract. Other cells in urine include red blood cells and white blood cells from the bloodstream. Cells are classified and counted under high-power magnification.

Red blood cells may enter the urinary tract at any point at which there is inflammation or injury. They may be found in normal urine in small numbers, usually less than one to two per high-power field. Persistent hematuria should be investigated. Red blood cells are pale, round, nongranular, and flat or biconcave (Figure 51-17). They are smaller than white blood cells and have no nucleus. In hypotonic (dilute) urine, they swell and burst. In hypertonic (concentrated) urine, they may **crenate** and wrinkle. When they crenate, they can be mistaken for white blood cells, because the wrinkled surface makes them appear granular. They are often confused with yeast (see Figure 51-24), oil droplets, and droplets of lens cleaner.

White blood cells, also called *leukocytes,* may occasionally be found in normal urine, but increased numbers (usually greater than five cells per high-power field) are associated with inflammation or contamination of the specimen during collection. White blood cells are larger than red blood cells, have a granular appearance, and usually contain a multilobed nucleus, although nuclear detail may not be evident. Most white blood cells in the urine are neutrophils (Figure 51-18).

Renal tubular or round epithelial cells are somewhat larger than white blood cells, are round to oval, and have a nucleus that is single, large, oval, and sometimes eccentric. A few may be found in normal urine specimens, but their presence in increased numbers indicates tubular damage (Figure 51-19).

Transitional epithelial cells line the urinary tract from the renal pelvis to the upper portion of the urethra. They vary from slightly larger than a round epithelial cell to smaller than a squamous epithelial cell. They are round to oval and may have a tail. Occa-

sionally, two nuclei are seen. When transitional cells are present in large numbers, a pathologic condition may exist (Figure 51-20).

Squamous epithelial cells line the lower portion of the genitourinary tract. When present in large numbers in female patients, they usually indicate vaginal contamination. Squamous

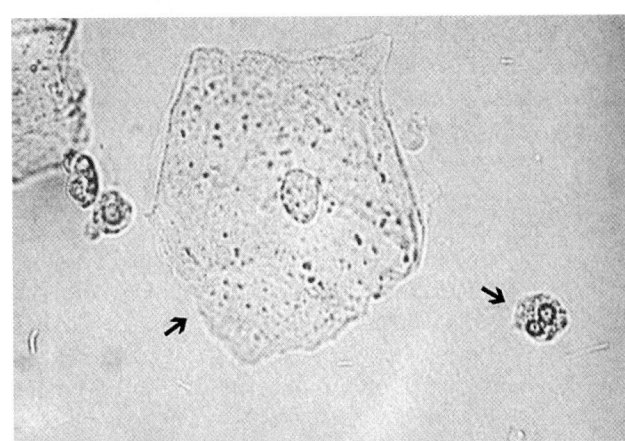

FIGURE 51-18 A, A white blood cell. **B,** A squamous epithelial cell. (Unstained, 640×.) (From Ringsrud KM, Linne JJ: *Urinalysis and body fluids: a color text and atlas,* St Louis, 1995, Mosby.)

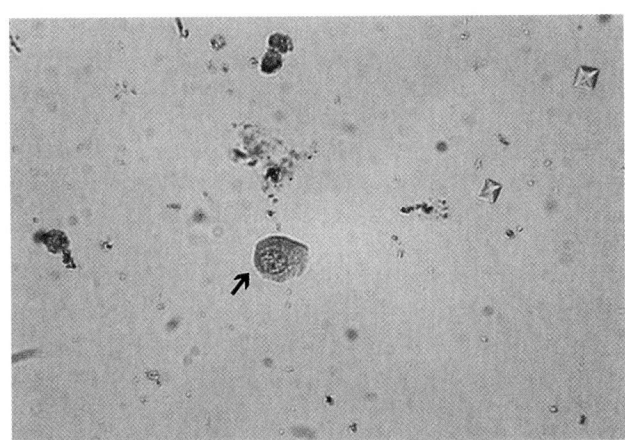

FIGURE 51-19 Renal epithelial cell *(arrow).* (Sedi-Stain, 400×.) (From Ringsrud KM, Linne JJ: *Urinalysis and body fluids: a color text and atlas,* St Louis, 1995, Mosby.)

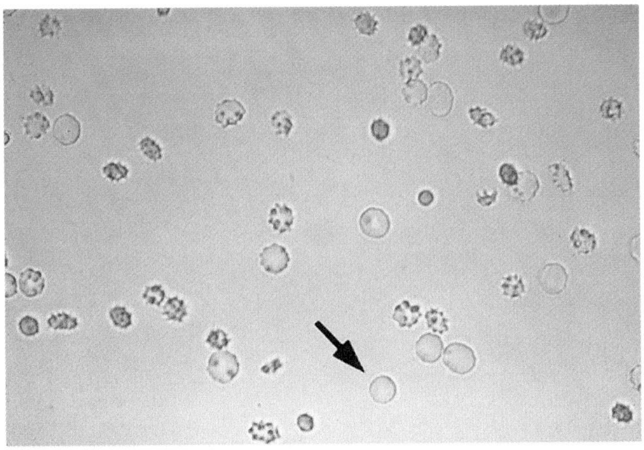

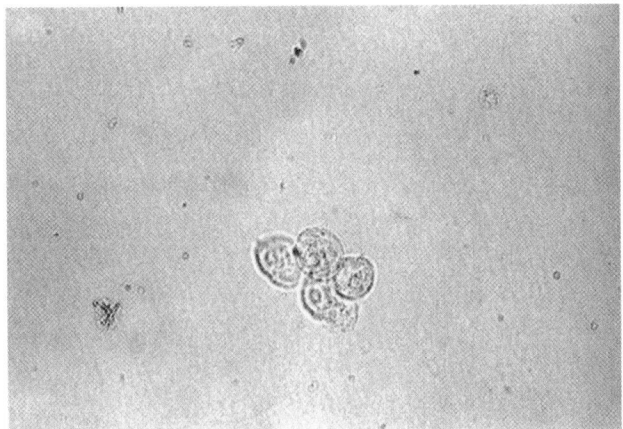

FIGURE 51-17 Red blood cells in urine. (From Stepp CA, Woods MA: *Laboratory procedures for medical office personnel,* Philadelphia, 1998, Saunders.)

FIGURE 51-20 Cluster of small unstained transitional epithelial cells. (400×.) (From Ringsrud KM, Linne JJ: *Urinalysis and body fluids: a color text and atlas,* St Louis, 1995, Mosby.)

epithelial cells are large, flat, irregular cells and are easily recognized under low-power magnification. They have a single, small, round, centrally located nucleus and often occur in sheets or clumps. Because of their flat nature, the edges of the cells are often rolled or folded (see Figure 51-20).

In identifying epithelial cells, it is helpful to remember the appearance of eggs; round epithelial cells resemble hard-boiled eggs that have been cut in half. Transitional forms resemble poached eggs, and squamous cells resemble fried eggs with large, runny whites.

Crystals

Crystals are common in urine specimens, particularly if they have been allowed to cool. Cooling causes the solid crystals to precipitate out of the urine. The presence of most crystals is not clinically significant, unless they are found in large numbers. With only very rare exceptions, abnormal crystals are seen in acidic urine. Abnormal crystals may be of metabolic origin and are present because of certain disease states or an inherited metabolic condition, or they may be of iatrogenic origin and are present as a result of medication or treatment. Identification of crystals begins with the determination of the pH of the urine to ascertain whether the sample is acidic or alkaline. Next, one looks at color, shape, and refractivity. Viewing with a polarized or phase microscope or using a supravital stain can assist in identification. Often a history of medication intake and recent diagnostic testing is helpful.

Identification of crystals is done with the low-power and high-power lenses, and their presence is reported as few, moderate, or many per high-power field. At times crystals can be amorphous. Amorphous urates (Figure 51-21) are salts of uric acid and are seen as shapeless granulation in acidic urine. Amorphous phosphates (Figure 51-22) are found in alkaline urine and are seen as fluffy white precipitate. Amorphous crystals are often so profuse they obscure other formed elements in the sediment. It is not always possible to identify crystals without additional chemical testing, which includes solubility testing in acid and base. A sample of crystals found in urine sediment is shown in Table 51-5.

Miscellaneous Findings

Oval fat bodies are formed when renal tubular epithelial cells or macrophages absorb fats. The fat droplets contained in the cells vary in size and are quite **refractile.** Oval fat bodies are characteristic of the nephrotic syndrome and are best distinguished by using Sudan III stain, because they are easily confused with other elements (Figure 51-23).

Yeast in urine may indicate vaginal contamination or infection of the urine with yeast (Figure 51-24). It is common in the urine of diabetic patients. Yeasts are easily confused with red blood cells, are usually oval, may show budding, and are more refractile. To differentiate yeast from red blood cells, a drop of sediment is placed on the blood test pad of a reagent strip. Yeast does not react, but red blood cells do. Red blood cells dissolve when a drop of dilute acetic acid (regular white vinegar) is added to the sediment, but the yeast will remain intact.

A few bacteria may be found in normal urine specimens. Heavy bacterial concentrations in the absence of white blood cells may indicate that the specimen was allowed to sit at room temperature and the bacteria multiplied. Urine specimens with a putrid odor, numerous white blood cells, and bacteria (Figure

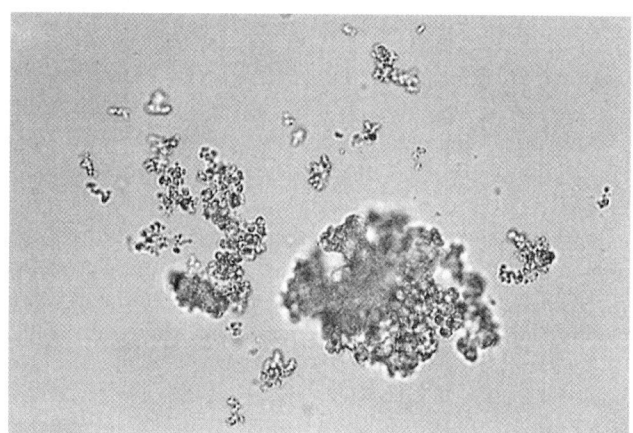

FIGURE 51-22 Amorphous phosphates. (400×.) (From Ringsrud KM, Linne JJ: *Urinalysis and body fluids: a color text and atlas*, St Louis, 1995, Mosby.)

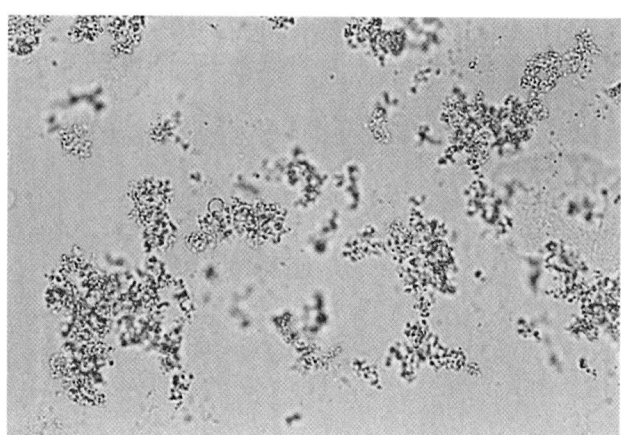

FIGURE 51-21 Amorphous urates. (400×.) (From Ringsrud KM, Linne JJ: *Urinalysis and body fluids: a color text and atlas*, St Louis, 1995, Mosby.)

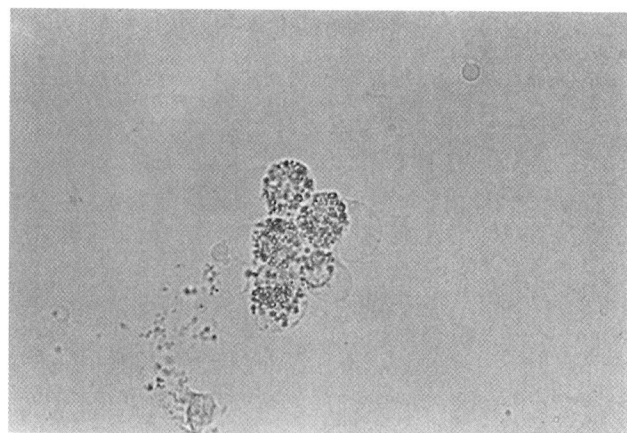

FIGURE 51-23 A small cluster of oval fat bodies. (Unstained, 400×.) (From Ringsrud KM, Linne JJ: *Urinalysis and body fluids: a color text and atlas*, St Louis, 1995, Mosby.)

TABLE 51-5 Crystals

NORMAL CRYSTALS (ACID URINE)	NORMAL CRYSTALS (ALKALINE URINE)	ABNORMAL CRYSTAL

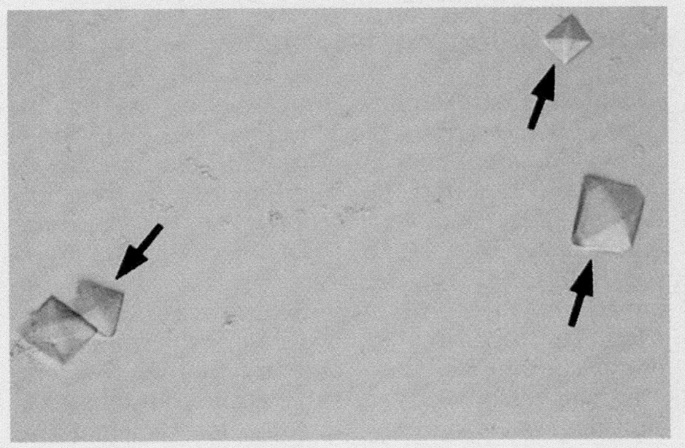

Calcium Oxalate*

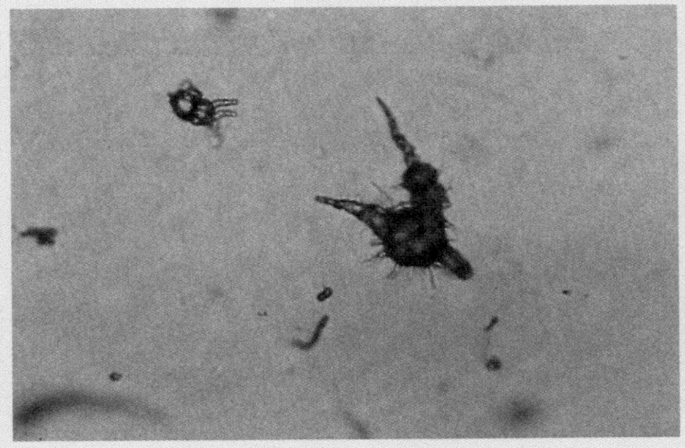

Ammonium biurate†

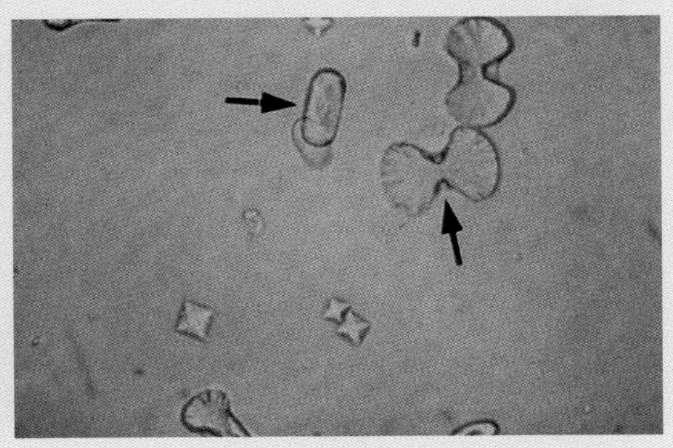

Sulfonamide

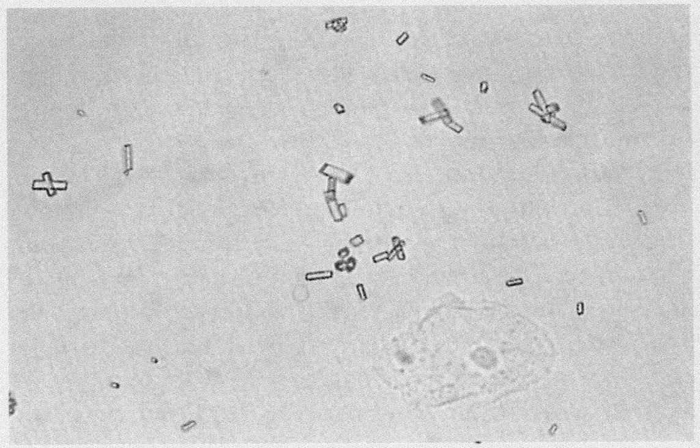

Uric acid†

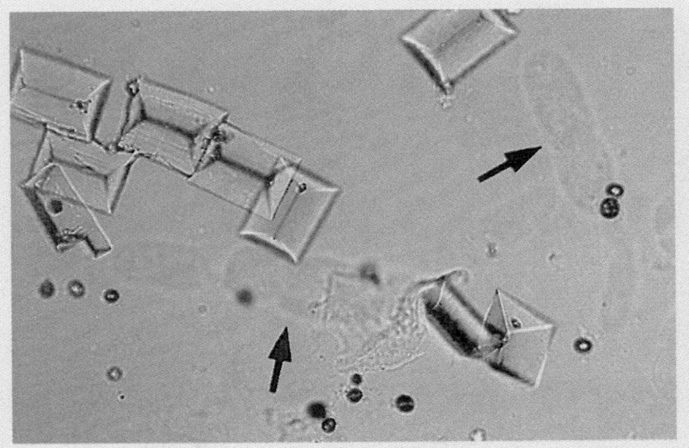

Triple phosphate*

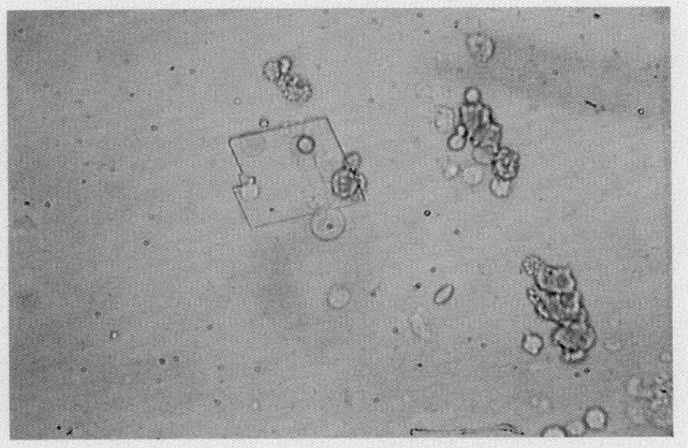

Cholesterol*

*From Stepp CA, Woods MA: *Laboratory procedures for medical office personnel,* Philadelphia, 1998, Saunders.
†From Ringsrud KM, Linne JJ: *Urinalysis and body fluids: a color text and atlas,* St Louis, 1995, Mosby.

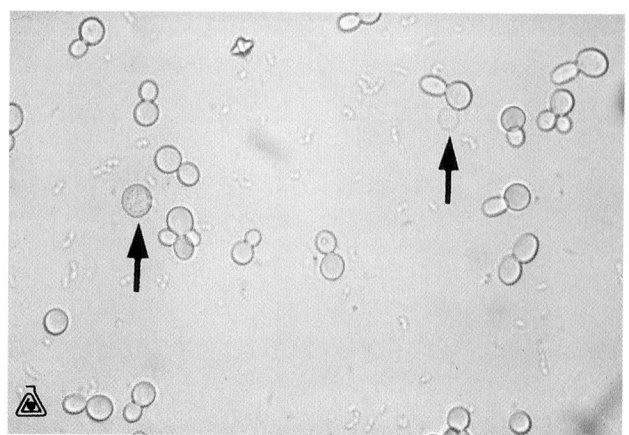

FIGURE 51-24   Yeast in urine. (From Stepp CA, Woods MA: *Laboratory procedures for medical office personnel*, Philadelphia, 1998, Saunders.)

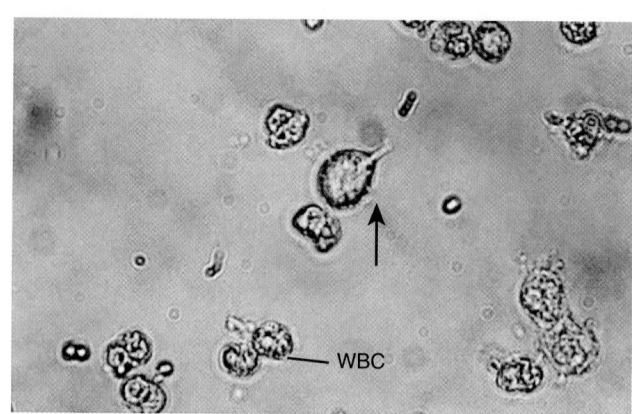

FIGURE 51-26   *Trichomonas* (arrow) in urine. (From Stepp CA, Woods MA: *Laboratory procedures for medical office personnel*, Philadelphia, 1998, Saunders.)

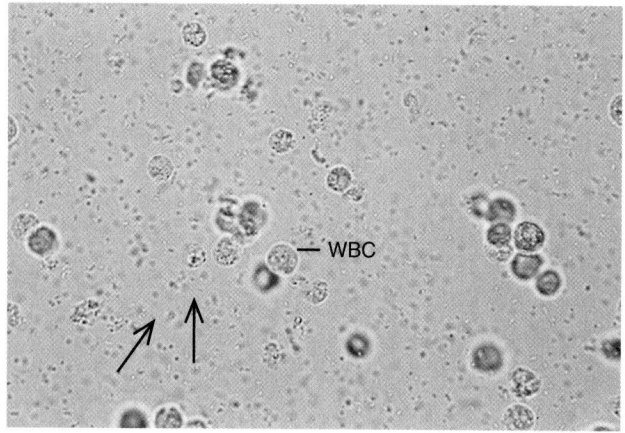

FIGURE 51-25   Many small rod-shaped bacteria (arrows) appearing like possible cocci and white cells. (Unstained, 400×.) (From Ringsrud KM, Linne JJ: *Urinalysis and body fluids: a color text and atlas*, St Louis, 1995, Mosby.)

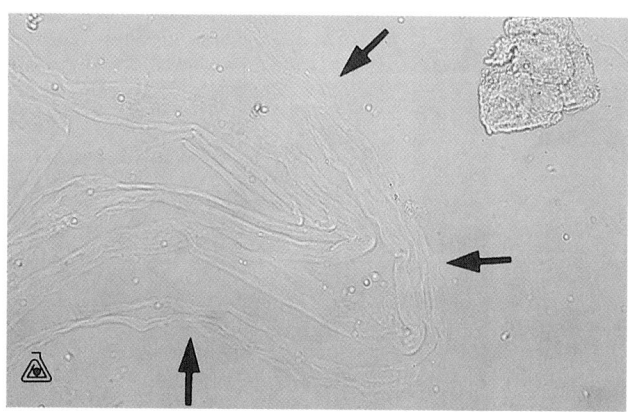

FIGURE 51-27   Mucous threads in urine. (From Stepp CA, Woods MA: *Laboratory procedures for medical office personnel*, Philadelphia, 1998, Saunders.)

51-25) are common in UTIs. Bacteria may be bacilli (rod-shaped) or cocci (spheric) and are identified under high-power magnification. They are often motile.

Spermatozoa can be found in the urine specimens of both male and female patients. In the latter, their presence represents vaginal contamination of the specimen. Sperm usually have pointed, oval heads and long threadlike tails. They may be motile in fresh urine.

The most commonly encountered parasite in urine is *Trichomonas vaginalis* (Figure 51-26). It is usually a vaginal contaminant but may also be found in urine specimens from male patients. When urine is fresh and warm, the *Trichomonas* organisms may be motile and will be darting about rapidly. *Trichomonas* organisms are pear-shaped protozoa with four flagella. They are larger than round epithelial cells but smaller than squamous cells. *Trichomonas* organisms die when the specimen is cooled.

Mucous threads can be found in most urine specimens. They appear as pale, irregular, threadlike structures with tapered ends. Beginners often confuse hyaline casts with mucous threads. Increased numbers are seen in inflammation and when there has been contamination of the specimen with vaginal secretions (Figure 51-27).

Artifacts and contaminants are often found in urine sediment; training is required to distinguish them and to learn to ignore them. As a rule, structures that are apparent when you first view the sediment are unimportant. Starch granules are common artifacts simply because of the extensive use of powdered gloves in the laboratory. The granules are highly refractile and dimpled, resembling a pillow with a center button. Fibers are common in the sediment as well and come from clothing, diapers, or digested plant material. Clothing fibers are often long and twisted and are sometimes colored. Diaper fibers can be confused with casts (Figure 51-28). Plant fibers appear in the urine as a result of fecal contamination (Figure 51-29). Hair is distinguishable not only because of the visible rough and fragmented cuticle but also because of the size (Figure 51-30). Finally, air bubbles are common if the coverslip was improperly placed over the sediment. Air bubbles are structureless and refractile, with a dark outline (Figure 51-31).

Interpretation of the Microscopic Examination

The medical assistant should understand how the findings of a microscopic examination of the sediment are reported. The sediment is first examined under the low-power objective

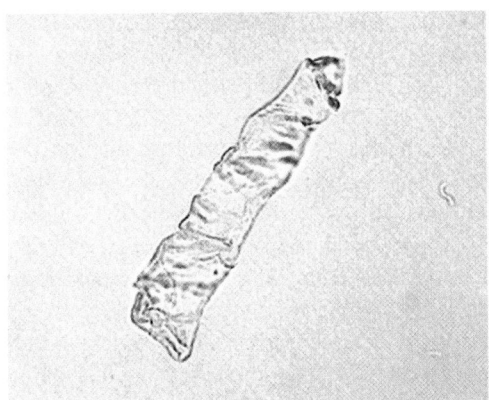

FIGURE 51-28 Diaper fibers. (From Ringsrud KM, Linne JJ: *Urinalysis and body fluids: a color text and atlas*, St Louis, 1995, Mosby.)

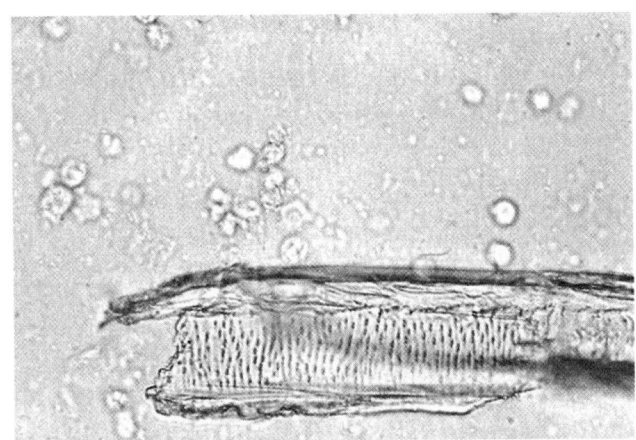

A

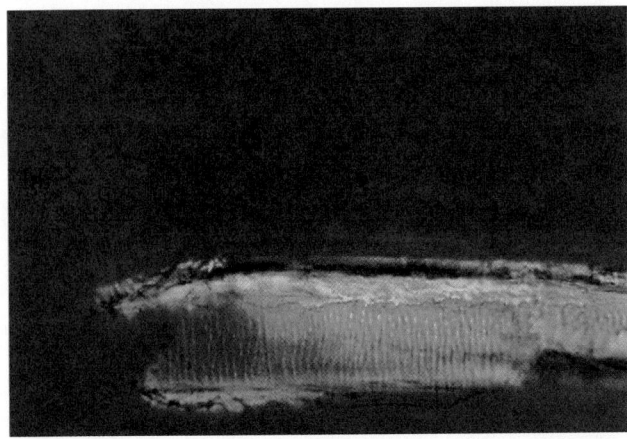

B

FIGURE 51-29 Plant fiber, from fecal contamination. Cells and bacteria are also present. (400×.) **A,** Bright field. **B,** Compensated polarized light showing birefringence. (From Ringsrud KM, Linne JJ: *Urinalysis and body fluids: a color text and atlas*, St Louis, 1995, Mosby.)

and low light to locate casts, which generally will be found around the edges of the coverslip. Ten to 15 low-power fields are scanned, and the number of casts is counted and reported. The high-power objective and increased light are then used to identify red and white blood cells, epithelial cells, yeasts, bacteria, and crystals. Ten to 15 high-powered fields should be scanned, and the number counted, averaged, and reported. The method of counting varies considerably among laboratories.

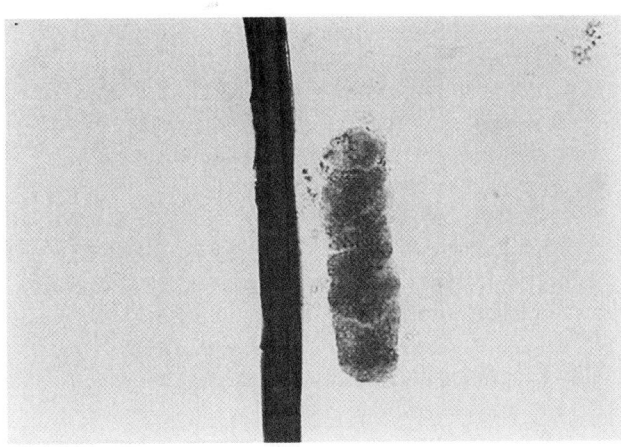

FIGURE 51-30 Fiber, probably hair *(left)*; a waxy cast *(right)*. (Sedi-Stain, 400×.) (From Ringsrud KM, Linne JJ: *Urinalysis and body fluids: a color text and atlas*, St Louis, 1995, Mosby.)

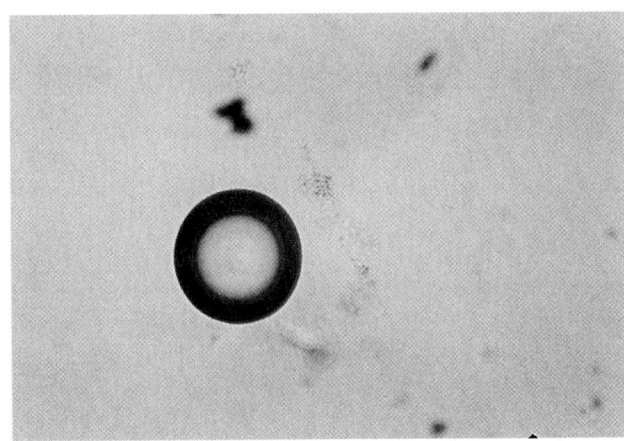

FIGURE 51-31 A large air bubble. (400×.) (From Ringsrud KM, Linne JJ: *Urinalysis and body fluids: a color text and atlas*, St Louis, 1995, Mosby.)

It is important that all workers in the same laboratory use the same counting and reporting systems. Report the results of the microscopic examination as follows:

1. Separately total the numbers for each element counted, then average. (Casts, white blood cells, red blood cells, and the three categories of epithelial cells are counted, totaled, and averaged.) Casts, white blood cells, and red blood cells are reported using numeric ranges based on the average:

   0
   0-1
   1-2
   2-5
   5-10
   10-20 and so forth

   Epithelial cells are reported as occasional, few, moderate, or many, according to the following:

   0
   0-3 = Occasional
   3-6 = Few
   6-12 = Moderate
   12   = Many

2. Estimate the remaining elements as occasional, few, moderate, or many, according to the following:
   Occasional–not seen in every field
   Few–covers less than a quarter of the field
   Moderate–covers approximately half of the field
   Many–covers the entire field
   Do not report fibers, hair, talc granules, oil droplets, and other artifacts.

Table 51-6 shows an example of the way in which a microscopic UA would be calculated and reported.

Quality Assurance and Quality Control in Urinalysis

The FDA categorizes the chemical analysis of urine as a waived test performed by an instrument or reagent strip. The chemical analysis includes the reagent strip (dipstick) tests for bilirubin, glucose, hemoglobin or blood, ketones, leukocyte esterase, nitrite, pH, protein, specific gravity, and urobilinogen. To perform a microscopic UA procedure, a laboratory must be certified to perform moderate-complexity tests. Such a laboratory can also perform waived tests if they meet those qualifications (Procedure 51-5).

To determine the reliability of the reagent strip used in chemical analysis, a commercially available control strip should be employed. One such strip is the Chek-Stix (Bayer, Tarrytown, N.Y.). The plastic control strip has seven pads affixed to it (Figure 51-32). Each of these pads contains synthetic ingredients that mimic human urine when reconstituted in water. After reconstitution, a reagent strip is immersed in the solution, and the results are compared with a chart that accompanies the Chek-Stix. Both positive and negative Chek-Stix are available (Procedure 51-6).

Quality control is as important in the microscopic examination as it is in the chemical analysis of urine. To ensure consistency, standardized commercially available systems can be used such as the KOVA System (HYCOR Biomedical, Garden Grove, Calif.) or the UriSystem (Fisher Scientific, Hampton, N.H.). These systems may include specially designed graduated centrifuge tubes with devices or pipets that allow for easy decanting of supernatant and retention of an exact amount of sediment. They also employ specially designed plastic slides with wells or coverslips that accept only a given amount of sediment. Whatever system is used, the Clinical and Laboratory Standards Institute (CLSI) recommends the following:

- The urine volume should be 12 mL.
- The specimen should be centrifuged for 5 minutes at a relative centrifugal force of 400 g (i.e., 400 times normal gravity).
- A standardized slide should be used to view the sediment.
- A consistent reporting format should be employed.

Additional Tests Performed on Urine

Clinitest

The glucose test on the reagent strip will detect only glucose, which is the most common sugar found in the urine. Sugars other than glucose can appear in the urine as well. Certain metabolic disorders can result in the excretion of sugars such as galactose, fructose, lactose, maltose, or pentoses. Galactosemia, a rare pathologic condition, is a congenital deficiency in the body's ability to metabolize galactose to glucose; galactosemia results in excretion of galactose in the urine. Seen in infants, it results in failure to thrive, vomiting, and diarrhea. If detected

---

TABLE 51-6 Calculating a Microscopic Urinalysis

| | PER LOW-POWER FIELD | | | | | PER HIGH-POWER FIELD | | | | |
FIELD	CASTS	MUCUS	SQUAMOUS EPITHELIAL	WBC	RBC	TRANSITIONAL EPITHELIAL	ROUND EPITHELIAL	BACTERIA	CRYSTALS	OTHER
1	0	Few	1	16	1	0	0	Moderate (rods)	Calcium oxalate—few Uric acid—few	—
2	1 hyaline	Few	3	32	0	0	0	Many	Calcium oxalate— few	Yeast
3	1 coarse granular	Moderate	3	21	2	0	0	Many	Calcium oxalate—few	Yeast
4	1 coarse granular	Few	5	12	1	0	1	Moderate	Uric acid—few	—
5	0	Few	4	25	0	0	0	Many	—	—
Total	1 hyaline 2 coarse granular	Few	16	106	4	0	1	Many	Calcium oxalate—few Uric acid—few	Yeast
Average	0.2 hyaline 0.4 coarse granular	Few	3.2	21.2	0.8	0	0.2	Many	Calcium oxalate—few Uric acid—few	Yeast
Report	**0-1 hyaline 0-1 coarse granular**	**Few**	**Few**	**20-30**	**0-1**	**0**	**Occasionally**	**Many (rods)**	**Calcium oxalate—few Uric acid—few**	**Yeast**

PROCEDURE 51-5

Perfom Urinalysis: Prepare Urine Specimen for Microscopic Examination

CAAHEP COMPETENCY: 3.b.(3)(c)(i)
ABHES COMPETENCIES: 4.c, 4.j, 4.q, 4.r

GOAL: *To perform a microscopic examination of urine to determine the presence of normal and abnormal elements.*

EQUIPMENT and SUPPLIES

- Urine specimen
- Centrifuge tube
- Centrifuge
- Disposable pipet
- Microscope slide and coverslip
- Microscope
- Permanent marker

PROCEDURAL STEPS

1. Wash and dry your hands. Don nonsterile gloves and face protection.
   PURPOSE: Infection control.
2. Gently mix the urine specimen.
   PURPOSE: If the urine is not well mixed, elements that have settled to the bottom of the specimen container will be missed.
3. Pour 10 mL of urine into a labeled centrifuge tube, and cap the tube.
4. Place the tube in the centrifuge (Figure 1).
5. Place another tube containing 10 mL of water in the opposite cup.
   PURPOSE: For proper operation, centrifuges must be carefully balanced. If not properly balanced, damage to the instrument can occur.
6. Secure the lid, and centrifuge for 5 minutes or for the time specified for your instrument.
   PURPOSE: Timing varies based on the speed and the size of the centrifuge head.
7. Remove the tube from the centrifuge after the instrument has come to a full stop.
8. Pour off the clear supernatant from the top of the specimen by inverting the centrifuge tube over the sink drain. Do not turn the tube upright until the supernatant is fully decanted (Figure 2*).
9. Prevent the loss of sediment down the drain.

PURPOSE: The sediment is what will be examined under the microscope.

10. Thoroughly mix the sediment by grasping the tube near the top and rapidly flicking it with the fingers of the other hand until all sediment is thoroughly resuspended (Figure 3*).
    PURPOSE: Elements centrifuge at different rates. Failure to completely mix the entire sediment will cause errors in quantification.
11. Transfer one drop of sediment to a clean, labeled slide using a clean disposable transfer pipet (Figure 4*).

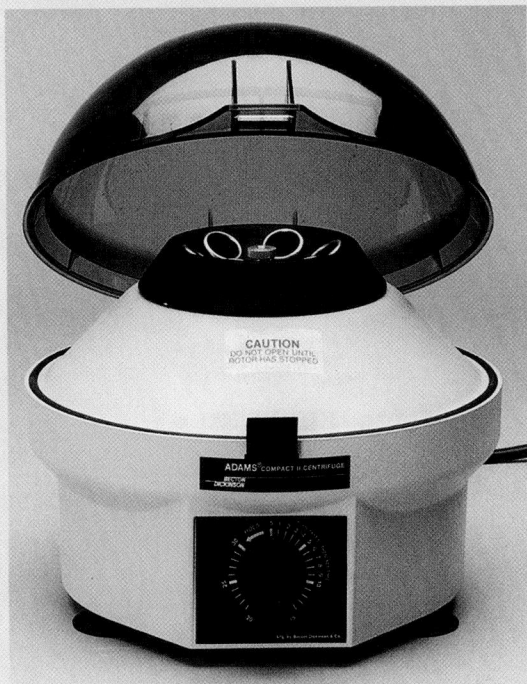

FIGURE 1

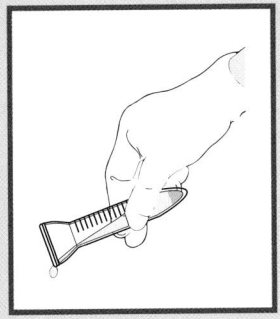

FIGURE 2

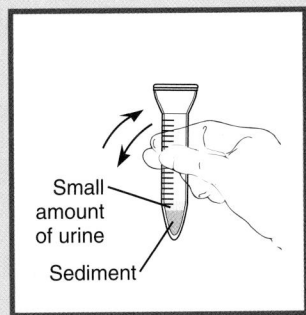

Small amount of urine

Sediment

FIGURE 3

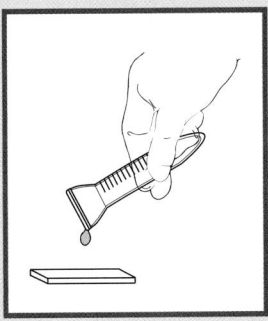

FIGURE 4

Continued

PROCEDURE 51-5—cont'd

12. Place a clean coverslip over the drop, and place the slide on the microscope stage. Remove face protection.

13. Focus under low power, and reduce the light.
    PURPOSE: Mucus and casts are easily missed if reduced light is not used. Constant focusing helps locate them.

14. First, scan the entire coverslip for abnormal findings.
    PURPOSE: Casts tend to migrate to the edges of the coverslips.

15. Examine five low-power fields. Count and classify each type of cast seen, if any, and note mucus if present.
    PURPOSE: Choose five fields so that one is selected from each corner of the coverslip and the last one is chosen from the middle of the coverslip. If you move to an area and there is nothing there, record a zero.

16. Switch to high-power magnification, and adjust the light.
    PURPOSE: As magnification increases, more light is needed.

17. In five high-power fields, count the following elements: red blood cells, white blood cells, and round, transitional, and squamous epithelial cells.

18. In the same five fields, report the following as few, moderate, or many: crystals (identify and report each type seen separately), bacteria (identify as rods or cocci), sperm, yeast, and parasites.
    PURPOSE: These three terms are more easily and universally understood than are exact numbers.

19. Average the five fields, and report the results.
    NOTE: Steps 13 to 19 will be performed only by qualified personnel.

20. Clean up the work area, remove gloves, and wash your hands.

*Figures from Stepp CA, Woods MA: *Laboratory procedures for medical office personnel,* Philadelphia, 1998, Saunders.

PROCEDURE 51-6

Use Methods of Quality Control: Determine the Reliability of Chemical Reagent Strips

CAAHEP COMPETENCY: 3.c.(4)(d)
ABHES COMPETENCY: 4.i

GOAL: *To reconstitute a control sample and to test the reliability of the urinalysis chemical testing strip.*

EQUIPMENT and SUPPLIES

- Chek-Stix Control Strips for Urinalysis (Bayer)
- Distilled water
- Capped tube with milliliter markings
- Test tube rack
- Forceps
- Timer
- Chemical strips for urine testing
- Color chart for chemical strips

PROCEDURAL STEPS

1. Assemble equipment and supplies. Record lot number and the expiration date of the Chek-Stix.
   PURPOSE: Chek-Stix cannot be used if they are expired. Recording lot number and expiration date is an important part of quality assurance.

2. Wash and dry your hands, and put on nonsterile gloves.
   PURPOSE: Infection control.

3. Place a conical tube in the rack and remove the cap.

4. Pour 15 mL of distilled water into the tube.

5. Using forceps, remove one strip from the bottle. Inspect the strips for mottling or discoloration.
   PURPOSE: Mottling or discoloration may mean that the strips

have been exposed to moisture, light, or solvents. Improperly stored control strips should not be used.

6. Place the strip in the water, and tightly cap the tube.

7. Invert the tube for 2 minutes.
   PURPOSE: Chemicals embedded in the pads must be thoroughly dissolved in the water.

8. Allow the tube to sit in the rack for 30 minutes.

9. Invert the tube one time, and remove the strip with forceps.

10. Discard the strip in a biohazard waste container. Once reconstituted, the control solution is stable for 8 hours at room temperature.
    PURPOSE: Infection control.

11. Perform quality control of the chemical reagent strip by dipping it into the control solution according to Procedure 51-4.

12. Read and record the results.

13. Compare the results to the Chek-Stix package insert or chart on the bottle provided by the manufacturer.
    PURPOSE: Results should fall within a given range provided by the manufacturer. If they do not, the chemical reagent strips cannot be used to test patient urine.

14. Discard the chemical reagent strip and the urine control in the biohazard container.

15. Clean up the work area, remove gloves, and wash your hands.
    PURPOSE: Infection control.

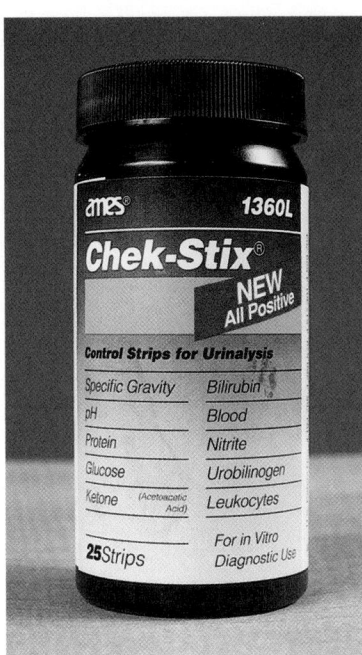

FIGURE 51-32 Chek-Stix control strips. (From Bonewit-West K: *Clinical procedures for medical assistants*, ed 6, Philadelphia, 2004, Saunders.)

early, galactose can be eliminated from the diet and the child will develop normally. Lactose may be found in the urine of pregnant women or premature infants. Rarely, urine may contain fructose or pentoses (such as xylose or arabinose) as a result of excessive consumption of honey or fruit. Maltose may be excreted in diabetes. Of the many sugars, only the presence of glucose or galactose signifies a pathologic condition.

The Clinitest (Bayer), based on the chemical reduction of copper, is commonly used to screen and confirm glycosuria and is used to detect other sugars present in urine (Procedure 51-7). Copper reduction tests are based on the principle that reducing substances are able to chemically convert cupric sulfate to cuprous oxide, resulting in a color change. A sugar's reducing ability is determined by the presence of a "chemical reducing group" present in all monosaccharides. The Clinitest tablet is dropped directly into a test tube containing diluted urine. A heat-releasing reaction occurs, and after the boiling stops, the color of the tube's contents is compared with a chart provided by the manufacturer.

Acetest

Acetest reagent tablets provide an alternative to strip testing when the urine must be tested for the presence of ketones. Ketonuria results when the body metabolizes stored fat because of inadequate cellular uptake of carbohydrates. This is common in the presence of diabetes, starvation, and excessive vomiting. The Acetest tablet test (Bayer) is based on the same chemical reaction as the reagent strip test, but its advantage lies in the fact that the tablet can be used with specimens other than urine and it detects both acetone and acetoacetate.

Urine Pregnancy Testing

The phrase "the rabbit died" came to be a euphemism for a positive pregnancy test in the late 1920s and early 1930s. In about 1927 it was discovered that if the urine of a pregnant

woman was injected into a rabbit, there would be hemorrhaging in the ovaries of the rabbit. These bulging masses could not be seen without killing the rabbit to inspect the ovaries, so invariably, every rabbit died, even if the woman was not pregnant. All pregnancy tests detect the presence of human chorionic gonadotropin (hCG), a hormone produced by the placenta and present in urine during pregnancy. After implantation of the fertilized egg in the uterus, the hCG levels in serum double every few days. This rapid rise occurs for approximately 7 weeks, then begins to decline. Within 72 hours of delivery, the hormone disappears.

Today no rabbits are needed to confirm a pregnancy. The most common type of test for pregnancy is the lateral flow immunoassay test. Many brands are available for laboratory use and are also available over the counter. These tests can be sensitive enough to detect the presence of hCG as early as 1 week after implantation or 4 to 5 days before a missed menstrual period. These tests can be performed in as little as 5 minutes, and the results are easy to interpret, usually as easy as reading a color change. For optimal results, the test should be performed on a first-morning voided specimen. The test is based on reactions that occur between antibodies and antigens. Antibodies are proteins formed in response to antigens. When they are in contact with one another, the antibody binds to the antigen as long as the two are present in sufficient quantity and the antibody is specific for the antigen, like a lock and key.

The pregnancy test cartridge contains a membrane with an absorbent pad overlapping a strip of fiberglass paper that is impregnated with a freeze-dried conjugate of gold particles and antibodies to hCG (Figure 51-33, p. 1144). The urine sample is introduced into the device, and it wicks through the absorbent pad, reaching a chromatographic membrane (reservoir pad). As it contacts the membrane, the urine dissolves the freeze-dried conjugate. In a positive sample the hCG antigen will attach to the antibodies in the colloidal solution. As the conjugate moves forward on the membrane, anti-hCG monoclonal antibodies affixed on the test zone ("T") will bind the hCG-gold conjugate complex, where the gold particles accumulate, forming a pink line. All samples will cause the "C" line to turn pink. The "C" line contains antibodies that will bind to the colloidal gold conjugate regardless of whether they have bound to hCG or not. Presence of this line indicates that the test has been carried out correctly. The QuickVue test is a lateral flow pregnancy test that can be performed on urine (Procedure 51-8). It is used routinely in many physicians' office laboratories.

CRITICAL THINKING APPLICATION

Dr. Hill has ordered a routine UA with a C&S test and a pregnancy test for his patient, and Rosa has instructed the patient in the collection of the specimen. Which laboratory division (or divisions) will be responsible for the testing? Must a separate specimen be collected for each test?

Ovulation Testing

CLIA-waived lateral flow urine tests are available to assist in the prediction of ovulation for women attempting to conceive

PROCEDURE 51-7

Perform Urinalysis: Test Urine for Glucose with the Clinitest Method

CAAHEP COMPETENCIES: 3.b.(3)(c)(i), 3.b.(4)(i)
ABHES COMPETENCIES: 4.j, 4.k, 4.q, 4.r, 4.y

GOAL: *To perform confirmatory testing for glucose in the urine using the Clinitest procedure for reducing substances.*

EQUIPMENT and SUPPLIES

- Urine specimen
- Clinitest tablet, tube, and dropper
- Distilled water
- Test tube rack
- Color chart
- Timer

PROCEDURAL STEPS

1. Wash and dry your hands, and apply nonsterile gloves and eye protection.
2. Holding a Clinitest dropper vertically, add 10 drops of distilled water then five drops of urine to a Clinitest tube.
   PURPOSE: Holding the dropper vertically prevents altering the size of the drops.
3. Place the prepared tube into the rack (Figure 1).
   PURPOSE: The tube will become too hot to hold when the tablet is placed into the tube.
4. With dry hands, remove a Clinitest tablet from the bottle by shaking a tablet into the bottle cap.
   PURPOSE: Clinitest tablets react with moisture and became caustic. Handling tablets with moist hands could result in hydroxide burns.
5. Tap the tablet into the test tube, and recap the container.
6. Observe the entire reaction to detect the rapid pass-through phenomenon, which indicates that the glucose level in the urine is very high. (See step 9).

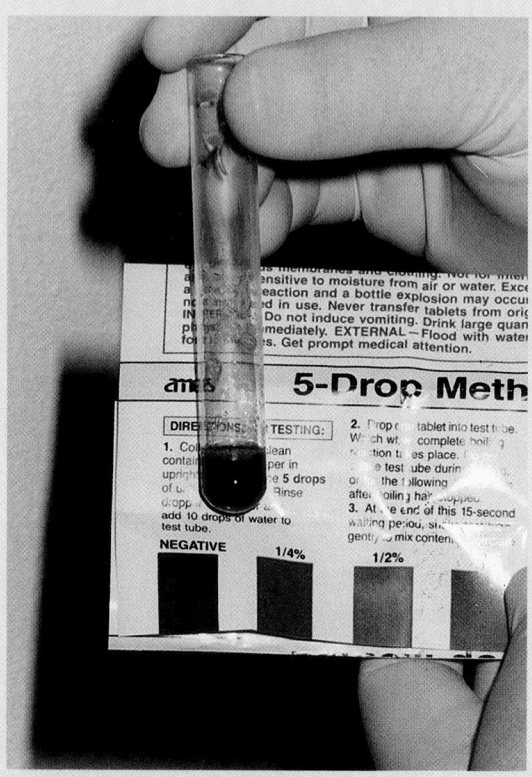

FIGURE 2

PURPOSE: If pass-through occurs but is not detected, the reading will be falsely low.

7. When boiling ceases, time exactly 15 seconds then gently shake the tube to mix the entire contents.
8. Immediately compare the color of the specimen with the five-drop color chart, and record your findings (Figure 2).
   PURPOSE: Color darkens with time. For accurate results, time carefully.
9. If an orange color briefly develops during the reaction, rapid pass-through has occurred, and the test must be repeated using the two-drop color chart.
10. Record results.

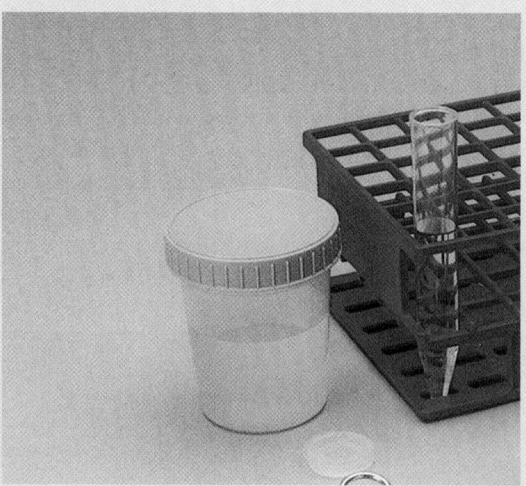

FIGURE 1

PROCEDURE 51-8

Perform Urinalysis: Perform a Pregnancy Test

CAAHEP COMPETENCIES: 3.b.(3)(c)(i), 3.b.(4)(i), 3.c.(4)(d)
ABHES COMPETENCIES: 4.b, 4.c, 4.i, 4.j, 4.k, 4.q, 4.r, 4.y

GOAL: *To perform a pregnancy testing of urine using the QuickVue (Quidel, San Diego, Calif.) pregnancy test method.*

EQUIPMENT and SUPPLIES

- Urine specimen
- QuickVue test kit

PROCEDURAL STEPS

1. Wash and dry your hands. Put on nonsterile gloves.
2. Prepare the testing equipment (Figure 1*).
3. Collect the needed specimen.
4. Remove the test cassette from the foil pouch.
5. Add three drops of urine using the dropper that accompanies the kit (Figure 2*). Dispose of the dropper in a biohazard bag.
   <u>PURPOSE:</u> To ensure accurate test results, specimen amount must be exact.
6. Wait 3 minutes and read the test results.
   <u>PURPOSE:</u> To ensure accurate test results, timing must be exact.
7. Interpret the results (Figure 3*).
   - Negative: A blue control line next to the letter C will be present. No line will be present next to the letter T.
   - Positive: A blue control line next to the letter C will appear along with a pink line next to the letter T.
8. If a blue line does not appear in the C area, the test is invalid and the specimen must be retested using another kit. Check the expiration date of the kit before proceeding.

9. Discard the cassette in a biohazard waste container, remove the gloves, and wash the hands.
   <u>PURPOSE:</u> Infection control.
10. Record the results as either positive or negative.
    <u>PURPOSE:</u> A procedure is not considered finished until it is recorded.

---

*Figures from Bonewit-West K: *Clinical procedures for medical assistants*, ed 6, Philadelphia, 2003, Saunders.
See Appendix D for a charting example.

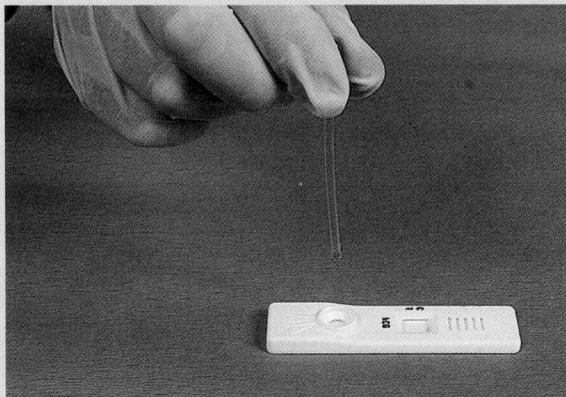

FIGURE 2

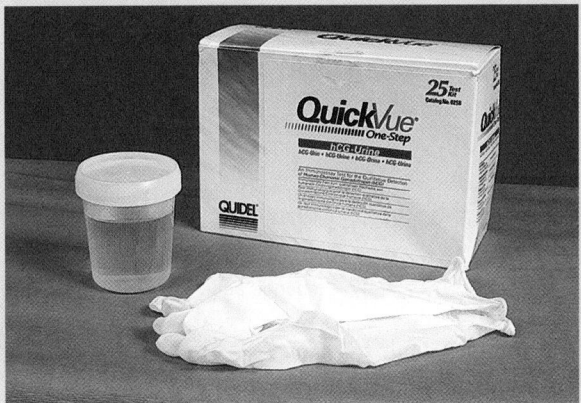

FIGURE 1

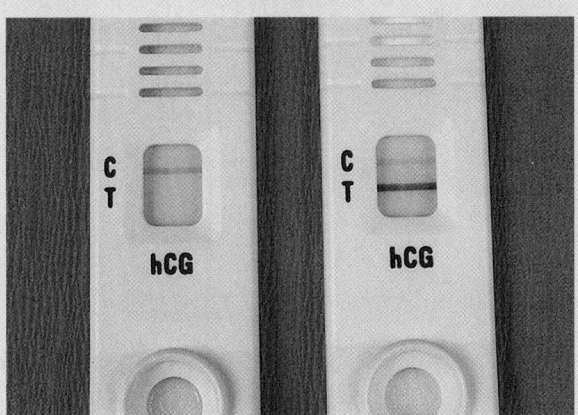

FIGURE 3

either naturally or using artificial insemination. During the menstrual cycle, human luteinizing hormone (LH) remains at a relatively stable level. Approximately 14 days before menstruation the body experiences the "LH surge," a brief, rapid increase in LH. This surge triggers the release of the ovum from the ovary. Two to 3 days after the surge, the LH level returns to the basal level. Conception is most likely to occur within 36 hours after the LH surge. The principle of this test is similar to that of the pregnancy test; the reservoir pad contains anti-LH antibodies conjugated to colloidal gold. A positive test result indicates urine levels of LH of 20 mIU/mL or greater. Testing is usually performed for 5 consecutive days in the middle of the cycle. Once the surge is detected, ovulation can be expected within 2 to 3 days.

Menopause Testing

A woman is said to have reached menopause when menstruation has not occurred for at least 12 months. The time before menopause is called *perimenopause* and can last for years, bringing with it uncomfortable symptoms such as irregular periods, hot flashes, vaginal dryness, or sleep problems. Follicle-stimulating hormone (FSH) is a hormone produced by the pituitary gland. FSH levels increase temporarily each month to stimulate the ovaries. When a woman enters menopause, the ovaries stop producing eggs and the levels of FSH increase. CLIA-waived lateral flow tests detect FSH in the urine. A positive test result indicates that a woman may be in a stage of menopause; a negative test, along with symptoms of menopause, may indicate a woman is in perimenopause. The qualitative lateral flow test should never be used to direct a woman to stop using birth control methods if she does not want to conceive, as pregnancy during perimenopause is still possible.

Bladder Tumor–Associated Antigen Testing

The most reliable test for identifying bladder cancer is **cystoscopy,** but it is invasive. Urine cytology is noninvasive and accurate in detecting high-grade bladder cancer and carcinoma in situ, but

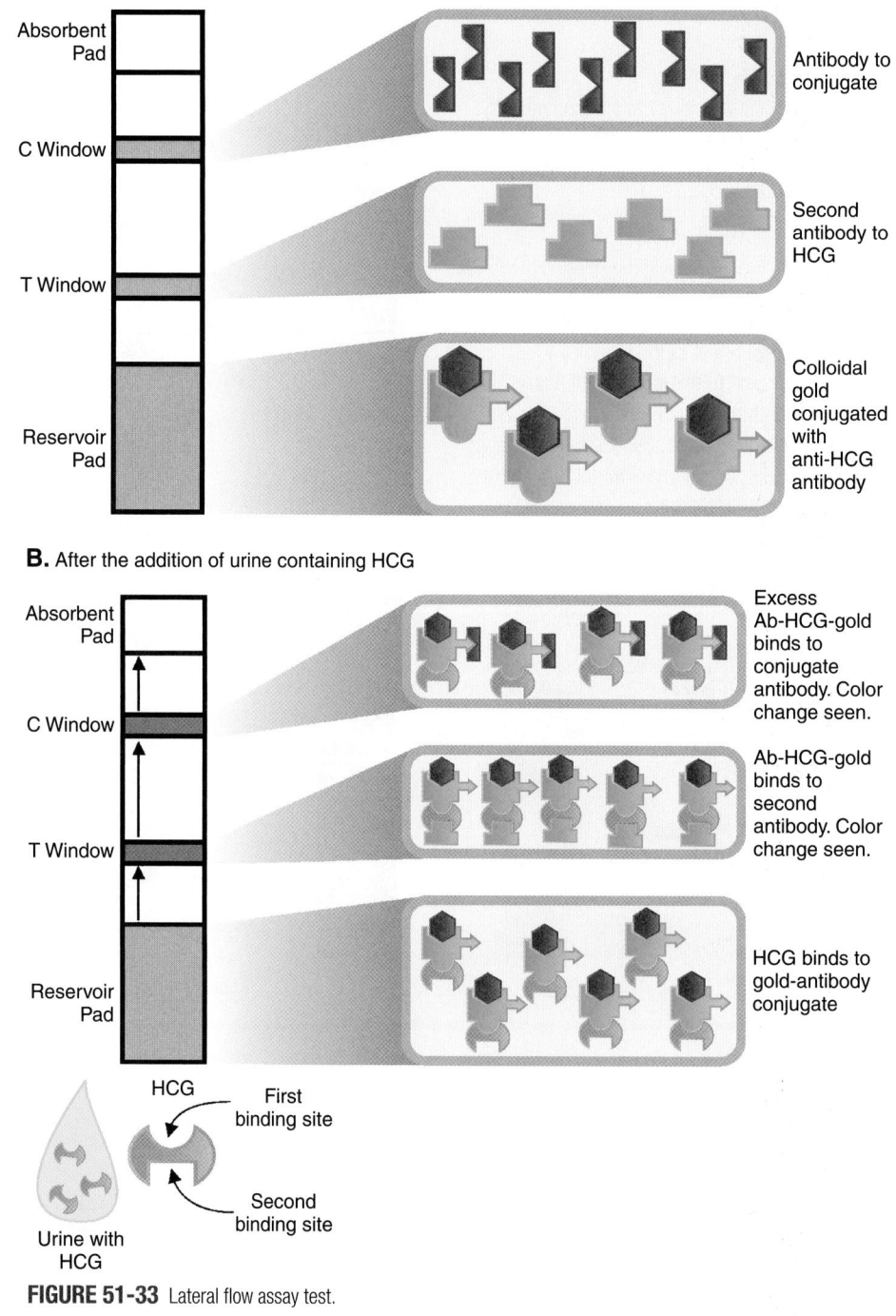

A. Before the addition of urine

Absorbent Pad

C Window — Antibody to conjugate

T Window — Second antibody to HCG

Reservoir Pad — Colloidal gold conjugated with anti-HCG antibody

B. After the addition of urine containing HCG

Absorbent Pad — Excess Ab-HCG-gold binds to conjugate antibody. Color change seen.

C Window — Ab-HCG-gold binds to second antibody. Color change seen.

T Window — HCG binds to gold-antibody conjugate

Reservoir Pad

HCG — First binding site — Second binding site

Urine with HCG

FIGURE 51-33 Lateral flow assay test.

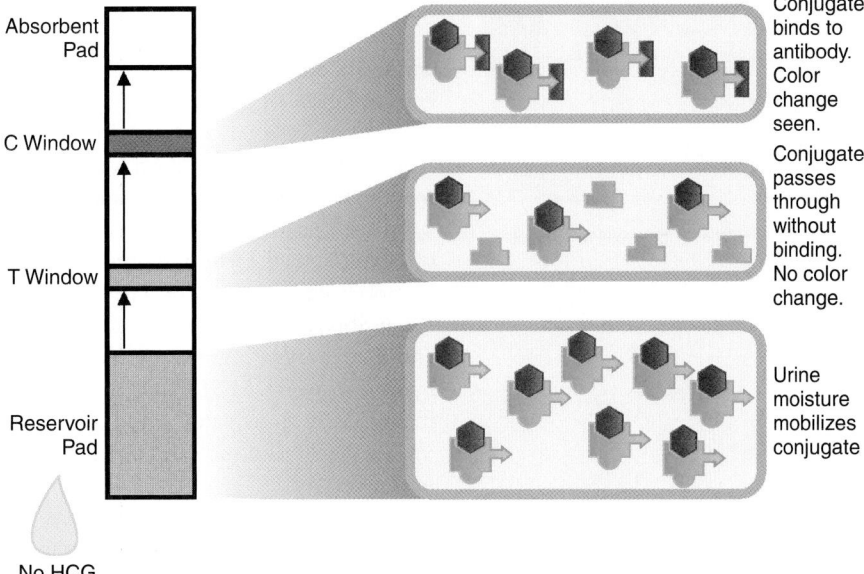

C. After the addition of urine without HCG

Absorbent Pad

C Window

T Window

Reservoir Pad

No HCG

Conjugate binds to antibody. Color change seen.

Conjugate passes through without binding. No color change.

Urine moisture mobilizes conjugate

FIGURE 51-33, *cont'd.*

its ability to detect low-grade cancer is limited. Therefore urine-based marker tests have been developed. These new tests are noninvasive and accurate in detecting low-grade bladder cancer. In addition, they are useful in monitoring for recurring bladder cancer.

The BTA Stat Test (Bion Diagnostics, Woburn, Mass) is a rapid, single-step immunoassay. The disposable test device, which looks much like the device used for pregnancy testing, contains two monoclonal antibodies that detect the presence of human complement factor H–related protein (hCFHrp), shed by cancerous bladder cells but not by normal bladder epithelial cells. When using the BTA Stat Test, freshly voided urine is placed into the sample well of the test device, and positive or negative results are provided in 5 minutes. Bladder cancer is one of the most common forms of cancer in the United States. About 53,000 Americans are diagnosed with bladder cancer each year, and approximately 500,000 people are routinely monitored for the disease. The cancer is most common among people over the age of 50, smokers, and workers exposed to chemicals in the rubber, leather tanning, metal, and dye industries.

CRITICAL THINKING APPLICATION

After centrifugation of the three urine specimens, Rosa prepares to view the sediment. She knows she must correlate the findings from the visual and chemical examination she has already performed on these specimens. She reviews the results and notes that Mr. Parks' and Mrs. Carpenter's specimens were clear, but Ms. Winfrey's specimen was turbid. Given the results of the chemical analysis during which Rosa noted an alkaline pH, an elevated nitrite level, and an elevated leukocyte esterase reading, what might be found when Ms. Winfrey's specimen is observed microscopically?

URINE TOXICOLOGY

Toxicology is the study of poisonous substances and their effects on the body. The clinical laboratory performs testing on body fluids and tissues to monitor use of therapeutic drugs such as digoxin (a cardiac medication) and theophylline (an asthma medication) or to detect poisonings by herbicides, metals, animal toxins, and poisonous gases (such as carbon monoxide).

Laboratory testing for illegal drugs or alcohol is also done. It is most commonly done as an employment, insurance, or legal requirement. Although serum (blood) testing is a more accurate test for determining current impairment or time of ingestion, urine is the specimen of choice for most routine screening. For routine screening, a random specimen is usually collected. Often, there are safeguards to ensure that a specimen is fresh and truly from the patient. Water may be temporarily unavailable in the restroom, bluing agents may be added to the toilets, a container with a temperature sensitive strip may be provided, and someone may accompany the patient into the restroom. In some cases a strict chain of custody is required. The substance being tested for, or its **metabolite,** often remains in urine much longer than the impairment or intoxication lasts. This is one reason that urine screening is favored over serum or blood screening. Some common drug screening tests along with their "maximum detection times" are listed in Table 51-7.

As a medical assistant, you may be responsible for the collection of specimens for toxicology tests and for performing certain tests. Rapid drug-screening devices resemble a credit card in size and shape (Figure 51-34). The device is dipped into a urine sample, or urine is directly applied to the device. The results are read according to the manufacturer's instructions in just minutes. "Negative" results indicate that none of the

TABLE 51-7 Commonly Abused Drugs and Body Retention Times

DRUG	RETENTION TIME
Alcohol	2-10 hours
Amphetamine	24-48 hours
Barbiturates	
Phenobarbital	2-6 weeks
Secobarbital	24 hours
Benzodiazepines (valium class drugs)	3 days to 6 weeks (depends on usage)
Cocaine, cocaine metabolites	1 hr to 4 days
Opiates, heroin, morphine	1-2 days
Methadone	2-3 days
Methaqualone	8 days
Phencyclidine (PCP)	1-8 days
Propoxyphene metabolites	6-48 hours
Tetrahydrocannabinol metabolites (THC)	2 days to 11 weeks

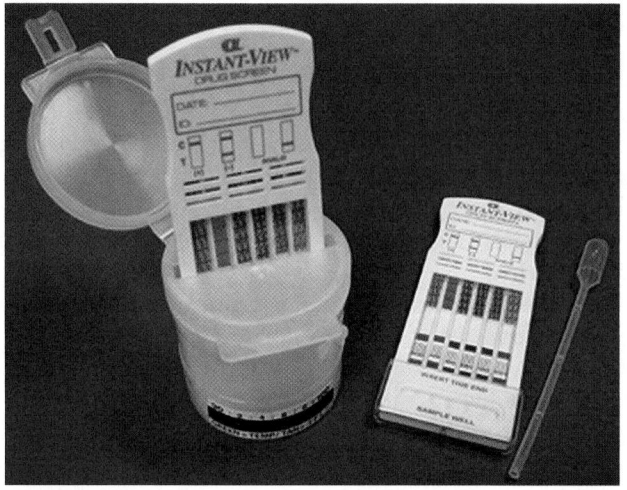

FIGURE 51-34 Instant-View Drug Test (Courtesy Alfa Scientific, Poway, Calif.)

specific to different drug classes, the test permits independent, simultaneous detection of up to six drugs from a single sample in 5 minutes.

In the procedure, urine mixes with labeled antibody-dye conjugate and migrates along a porous membrane. When the concentration of a given drug is below the detection limit of the test, antibody-dye conjugate that did not bind to a drug metabolite binds to antigen conjugate immobilized on the membrane, producing a rose-pink color band in the appropriate band for that drug. If the level of the drug in the urine is at or above the detection limit, free drug competes with the immobilized antigen conjugate on the membrane by binding to antibody-dye conjugate, forming an antigen- antibody complex, preventing the development of a rose-pink color band (Procedure 51-9). Note that, unlike the lateral flow test for pregnancy, ovulation, and menopause, appearance of a line in the T band indicates a negative test result with the drug screen.

Drug testing has legal ramifications, and therefore it is often necessary to perform additional testing to ensure that samples have not been adulterated (Procedure 51-10). Adulteration is the intentional manipulation of a urine sample to falsely pass a drug screening test. It may involve using urine from another person or animal, diluting with water, or adding substances such as bleach, vinegar, eye drops, baking soda, drain openers, soft drinks, or hydrogen peroxide. Urine collection cups with built-in thermometer panels are often used to ensure that urine has been freshly voided from the bladder. A temperature of 90° F to 100° F (32.2° C to 37.7° C) within 4 minutes of collection is expected. Test strips that detect human immunoglobulins (antibodies) in urine can determine if the specimen is human in origin and if it is naturally dilute or has been diluted. Human immunoglobulin G (IgG) is exclusive to humans and will always be found at certain levels in urine, even if it is dilute. In addition, if chemicals have been added to the urine, the reaction on the test strip will be prevented.

Other test strips are available that detect creatinine, nitrite, pH, specific gravity, glutaraldehyde, and oxidants. Creatinine is always present in normal urine because it is excreted from the body at a constant rate. Low or absent levels indicate diluted or substituted nonhuman samples. Dilution of the urine may have resulted from consuming abnormally large quantities of water before testing or from adding water or another liquid to the sample. Creatinine levels are usually checked in conjunction with specific gravity to screen for dilution or substitution adulteration. Specific gravity levels will also determine if substances such as table salt have been added to the urine.

Nitrites are oxidizing substances that react with the drug or drug metabolite molecules in the urine. Nitrites primarily interfere with antibody binding in lateral flow tests. Nitrates must be added to the urine after voiding. Commercial adulterants such as Whizzies, Klear, and UrineLuck are tablets or powders that can be added to voided urine. They do not change the color or temperature of the urine. The level of nitrites found in urine with gross bacteriuria or from therapeutic drug metabolites (e.g., nitroglycerine) is below the cutoff for adulteration screening tests.

targeted drugs was detected in the urine sample at specified cutoff levels; "inconclusive" results indicate that the device reacted with something in the urine and confirmation testing is required.

The Instant-View Multi-Drug Screen (Alfa Scientific, Poway, Calif) urine test is a lateral flow chromatographic immunoassay that tests for urine metabolites of a variety of drugs including amphetamines, barbiturates, benzodiazepines, cocaine, morphine, methadone, phenylcyclidine (PCP), tricyclics, marijuana, Ecstasy, and methamphetamines. Available in cartridges that test from two to six drugs, the test is a competitive binding immunoassay in which drug and drug metabolites in a urine sample compete with immobilized drug conjugate for limited labeled antibody binding sites. By using antibodies that are

PROCEDURE 51-9

Perform Urinalysis: Perform a Multidrug Screen Urine Test

CAAHEP COMPETENCY: 3.b.(3)(c)(i)
ABHES COMPETENCIES: 4.c, 4.i, 4.j, 4.q, 4.r, 4.y

GOAL: *To screen a urine specimen for drugs or drug metabolites at their specified cutoff levels.*

EQUIPMENT and SUPPLIES

- Instant-View Multi-Drug Screen Urine Test in a sealed pouch
- Freshly voided urine sample
- Timer
- Biohazard container

PROCEDURAL STEPS

1. Wash your hands, and assemble the equipment and specimen. Check the expiration date on the test kit.
   PURPOSE: An expired test strip may yield inaccurate results.
2. Determine urine temperature (within 4 minutes of voiding). Temperature should be between 90° F and 100° F (32.2° C and 37.7° C).
   PURPOSE: If the urine temperature is below or above this range, the sample may have been adulterated. Once it is determined that the sample is at the correct temperature, it may be stored at room temperature for 8 hours or in the refrigerator for up to 3 days before testing.
3. Bring specimen and the testing device to room temperature.
   PURPOSE: Both the specimen and device must be at room temperature to ensure accurate results.
4. Remove the device from the foil pouch, and label it with specimen identification.

DIP METHOD

5. Remove the cap of the specimen and dip the device into the specimen for 10 seconds. The surface of the urine must be above the sample well and below the arrowheads in the window (Figure 1*).
   PURPOSE: The pads must be saturated with urine.

ALTERNATE METHOD

6. Remove the pipet from the pouch, and fill the pipet to the line on the barrel with urine. Dispense the entire volume onto the sample well on the testing device (Figure 2*).
   PURPOSE: If there is insufficient urine in the cup to use the dip method, this method applies urine to the device.
7. Recap the urine specimen.
8. Set the timer for 4 to 7 minutes. Do not read results after 7 minutes.
   PURPOSE: Correct timing is essential for reliable, accurate results.
9. Interpret results (Figure 3):
   - Positive—If the C line appears and there is no T line, the test indicates a positive result for that drug.
   - Negative—If the C line and the T line both appear, the test indicates that the level for the drug or its metabolites is below the cutoff level.
   - Invalid—If no C line develops within 5 minutes on any test strip, the assay is invalid. Ensure that the urine has not been

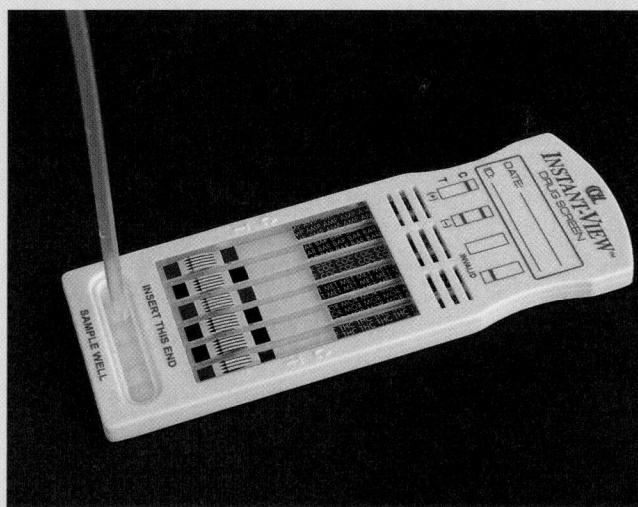

FIGURE 2

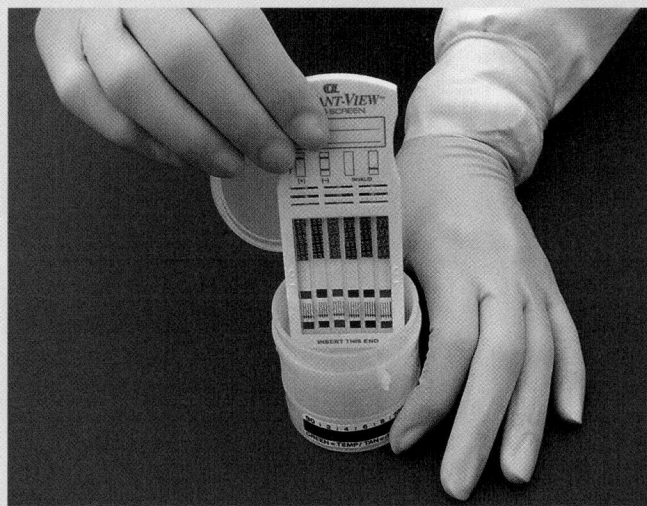

FIGURE 1

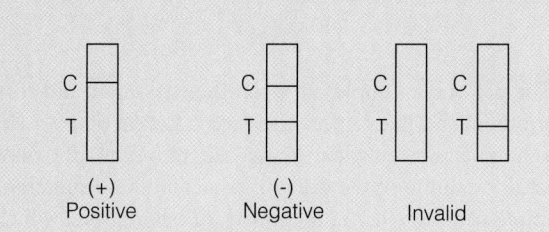

C	C	C	C
T	T	T	T
(+) Positive	(−) Negative	Invalid	

FIGURE 3

Continued

PROCEDURE 51-9—cont'd

adulterated (see Procedure 51-10) and/or repeat the assay with a new test device.

10. Record the results.
    PURPOSE: A procedure is not considered complete until it is recorded.
11. Color photocopying will provide a permanent record of results, but the copy must be made within 7 minutes of adding the urine.

Ensure that the photocopier does not become contaminated; wipe the glass with alcohol or another manufacturer-approved disinfectant after making the copy.

12. Discard urine and device in biohazard container.
13. Remove gloves and wash hands.
    PURPOSE: Infection control.

*(Figures 1 and 2 courtesy of Alfa Scientific, Poway, Calif.)

PROCEDURE 51-10

Perform Urinalysis: Assess a Urine Specimen for Adulteration Before Drug Testing

CAAHEP COMPETENCIES: 3.b.(3)(c)(i), 3.b.(4)(i)
ABHES COMPETENCIES: 4.c, 4.i, 4.j, 4.k, 4.q, 4.r, 4.y

GOAL: To assess a urine specimen for additive adulteration.

EQUIPMENT and SUPPLIES

- Quik Test Adulterant Strips (Quik Test USA, Boca Raton, Fla.)
- Urine sample (freshly voided; urine should be stored at room temperature for no longer than 2 hours or at refrigerator temperature for longer than 4 hours before testing)
- Paper towels
- Timer
- Biohazard waste container

PROCEDURAL STEPS

1. Wash your hands, assemble equipment and specimen. Check the expiration date on the test kit.
   PURPOSE: An expired test strip may yield inaccurate results.
2. Remove one strip from the container, and recap tightly.
3. Dip test strip briefly into the urine, and remove.
4. Blot the strip by touching the side of the strip to paper toweling.
   PURPOSE: Oversaturated strips may not react consistently.
5. Read results within 1 minute by comparing each pad to the color strips on the canister (Figure 1*).
   PURPOSE: Exceeding allotted time may result in error.
6. Dispose of paper towels and strip in the biohazard container.

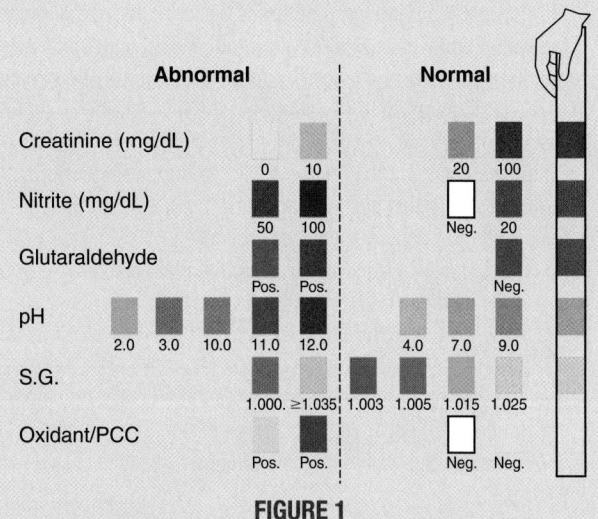

FIGURE 1

7. Remove gloves and wash hands.
   PURPOSE: Infection control.
8. Record results.

*Results for Quik Test Urine Drug Adulteration. Because monitor color may vary, please refer to product package for accurate color reference.

The pH of the sample can affect the enzymatic and antibody reactions in the lateral flow drug tests. Levels of >9.5 or <3.0 may hamper the enzymatic rate. Alteration of pH may also affect the stability of the drug or its metabolite. Adulteration of a sample with bleach, drain cleaners, or baking soda will change the pH, which can be detected by an adulteration strip test.

Glutaraldehyde can mask the presence of illegal drugs. Commercially available products such as UrinAid and Clear Choice contain glutaraldehyde intended to adulterate urine. In addition, a 10% solution of glutaraldehyde is sold over the counter for treatment of warts. The chemical prevents the enzymes in lateral flow tests from reacting properly.

Sensitivity limits for drug screening are set by the U.S. Substance Abuse and Mental Health Services Administration (SAMHSA), the National Institute on Drug Abuse (NIDA), and the U.S. Department of Health and Human Services.

Positive results of tests of urine samples for substances should be confirmed by more specific chemical methods, which include gas chromatography (GC), mass spectrometry (MS), and enzyme multiplied immunoassay (EMIT).

Alcohol Testing

Alcohol testing is not performed on urine, but CLIA-waived tests are available to detect alcohol using saliva. Saliva-based tests have a high degree of correlation to blood alcohol analysis. The saliva alcohol test manufactured by STC Technologies (Bethlehem, Pa.) uses a Dacron swab saturated with saliva to detect ethanol. The test is used primarily for workplace testing, including the federally mandated testing of transportation workers, but also in private company "drug-free workplace" programs and by emergency departments.

CULTURING THE URINE

Urine cultures are performed to assist in the diagnosis of a UTI and to assess the effectiveness of certain antibiotics in the treatment of the infection. Rapid detection systems and culturing of specimens using Petri dishes are addressed in Chapter 52.

CLOSING COMMENTS

Patient Education

Frequently a medical assistant is called on to explain collection techniques to the patient. Patients want to do the procedure correctly but often lack the knowledge of urinary terminology and are embarrassed to or do not know how to ask questions regarding the cleaning of the genital area. When explaining a urinary collection procedure, use pictures and words that the patient will understand. As you explain the procedure in terms

that the patient knows, he or she will also feel comfortable in telling you or asking you pertinent details that may have a definite impact on the treatment of the problem. Providing the patient with a clearly written instruction sheet is also helpful. The instruction sheet should be personalized with his or her name, the time to begin collection or testing (if applicable), what supplies should be used, and a phone number to call if questions arise.

Drug testing may require adherence to certain procedures such as remaining in the restroom while the patient provides the sample, checking the sample immediately for its temperature, and ensuring that the patient does not have adulterating materials on his or her person. Being prepared to firmly explain the regulations to the patient can prevent misunderstandings and unexpected behaviors.

Legal and Ethical Issues

Like all other procedures, the test is only as valid as the specimen and the procedure performed on that specimen. You, as the physician's agent, are responsible for that validity when you instruct the patient and when you perform the test.

A medical assistant who is responsible for office laboratory testing must clearly understand the basic concepts of laboratory medicine. To do this, you must stay current with the rapid technologic advances in laboratory medicine and assist in establishing a protocol of the tests best suited to your physician-employer.

You have the responsibility for properly collecting specimens and accurately testing them. In addition, you are responsible for strict adherence to protocol when collecting and testing specimens when there are legal ramifications to the test results. Patient confidentiality is paramount when performing drug testing, as is rigid conformation to all established rules and regulations.

SUMMARY OF SCENARIO

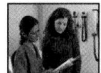

Rosa's capabilities in the laboratory analysis of urine are highly valued by Dr. Hill. Because tests can be performed in the office laboratory, Dr. Hill has the results immediately. Dr. Hill's patients also appreciate the convenience of office laboratory testing, in which physical and chemical microscopic analysis is performed by Rosa and other medical assistants, and microscopic UA is performed by Dr. Hill. Mrs. Carpenter knows the results of her pregnancy test

on her first-morning urine without waiting for a call from the laboratory, and urinalysis of Ms. Winfrey's CCMS urine sample will give clues to Dr. Hill so that he can diagnose a UTI within minutes. Rosa knows that the laboratory services and quality control measures she takes when performing the complete UA or lateral flow tests are an integral part of the excellent patient care provided by Dr. Hill.

SUMMARY of LEARNING OBJECTIVES

1. Define, spell, and pronounce the terms listed in the vocabulary.
   - Spelling and pronouncing medical terms correctly adds credibility to the medical assistant. Knowing the definition of these terms promotes confidence in communication with patients and co-workers.
2. Understand the purpose of routine urinalysis.
   - Routine UA is performed primarily as a screening test to detect metabolic and physiologic disorders. Urine is easily obtained, making it an ideal specimen for testing. Urine is analyzed to detect extrinsic and intrinsic pathologic conditions.
3. Describe the physiology of urine formation.
   - Urine is formed through a filtration mechanism in the kidney via the nephrons. As the filtrate passes through the tubules, various changes occur. Urine is stored in the bladder and voided through the urethra.
4. Explain the various means and methods used for collection of urine specimens.
   - Some urine collections, such as the 2-hour postprandial specimen, must be timed around meals or fasts. Routine UA requires no special preparation, whereas a CCMS requires cleansing of the external genitalia. Only urine that will be cultured must be collected in a sterile container. Urine to be sent to a referral laboratory may require the addition of preservatives.
5. Describe the components of the physical and chemical examination of urine.
   - The physical examination of the urine involves determination of color, turbidity, and specific gravity. Odor and foam color may be noted. The chemical examination of urine involves determination of levels of glucose, pH, protein, ketones, blood, bilirubin, urobilinogen, nitrite, specific gravity, and leukocyte esterase by using a reagent strip.
6. Recognize and correctly identify the formed elements found in urine sediment.
   - Formed elements in the urine sediment include casts, cells, and crystals. Artifacts may be present, but they are not reported.
7. Instruct a patient in the collection of a timed urine specimen.
   - Timed urine specimens are collected to determine the amount of a particular analyte in the urine during a given time frame. Proper patient instruction is necessary to obtain an acceptable specimen.
8. Instruct a patient in the collection of a clean-catch midstream urine specimen.
   - Proper patient instruction is necessary for an acceptable CCMS. Both men and women are given instructions in cleaning the external genitalia to avoid contaminating the urine. Urine must be collected in a sterile container and refrigerated if it cannot be tested within 1 hour.
9. Perform a complete urinalysis.
   - A complete UA involves physical, chemical, and microscopic assessment. The three must correlate with one another. Most testing of urine requires reagent strips or tablets. It is essential that these supplies be stored in dark, cool, moisture-free areas.
10. Demonstrate the proper use and care of testing equipment.
    - See Procedure 51-3.
11. Describe glucose testing using the Clinitest method.
    - The Clinitest detects reducing sugars, including glucose and galactose, in the urine. It is superior to the reagent strip test because it detects sugars other than glucose.
12. Explain the principle of using lateral flow technology in pregnancy testing.
    - Pregnancy tests detect hCG, a hormone produced by the placenta. Anti-hCG antibodies embedded in test cartridges bind to hCG and initiate color changes in test areas. Urine moves through lateral flow devices by capillary action.
13. Perform pregnancy testing.
    - Procedure 51-8 outlines the steps for performing a pregnancy test.
14. Explain the principle of lateral flow technology in drug testing on urine.
    - Drug testing with lateral flow technology is similar to that for pregnancy testing except it uses a competitive binding principle. A line in the "T" region indicates a negative test, unlike the pregnancy test.
15. Demonstrate a method of drug testing on a urine specimen.
    - Refer to Procedure 51-9.
16. List means by which urine could be adulterated before drug testing.
    - Consuming excessive water before urinating, adding water to a urine specimen, and adding chemicals or products sold specifically to adulterate urine all could render a drug test invalid. Adulteration test strips can detect most methods of adulteration.
17. Demonstrate a method of detecting the presence of adulterating substances in a urine sample for drug testing.
    - Refer to Procedure 51-10.
18. Describe methods for determining fertility and menopause using CLIA-waived urine tests.
    - Fertility can be assessed using lateral flow tests that detect LH, a hormone that increases in concentration in the urine shortly before ovulation. Menopause can be assessed using lateral flow tests that detect FSH, which increases as menopause approaches.

CONNECTIONS

 Study Guide Connection: Go to Chapter 51 Study Guide. Read the Case Study and Workplace Applications and complete the assignments. Do online research for answers to the questions in the Internet Activities associated with assisting in the analysis of urine.

 CD Connection: Go to the Medical Assisting Competency Challenge CD and do the training activities under Diagnostic Testing, Patient Instruction, and Operational Functions. For a better understanding of assisting in the analysis of urine, view the animation for renal anatomy and function, urine formation, and kidney infection.

Evolve Connection: For more information related to assisting in the analysis of urine, go to evolve.com/kinn and visit related weblinks for Chapter 51. Click on the Medical Assisting Exam Review and do the practice questions to sharpen your test-taking skills.

Assisting in Phlebotomy

Robin R. Patterson

52

SCENARIO

Leah Barney, a recent graduate of a CMA program, is a new employee at the Health Alliance Medical Clinic. The class on medical laboratory procedures was Leah's favorite in her medical assisting program at the community college; in this class she learned the principles of phlebotomy and even got to perform several venipunctures and capillary punctures. Her instructor said she was a "natural," but she has not had any experience outside the classroom. Her employer has arranged for extensive training with an experienced phlebotomist so that she may assist with phlebotomy duties for the clinic in the future. Nervous, but excited, she begins her training.

As you are studying this chapter, think about the following questions:

- How will Leah know which tubes or the size of needle to use?
- How will Leah approach phlebotomy on a child or an elderly person?
- What conditions will require a capillary puncture?
- How can Leah make the clinic patients comfortable and at ease?
- How will Leah handle a difficult "stick"?

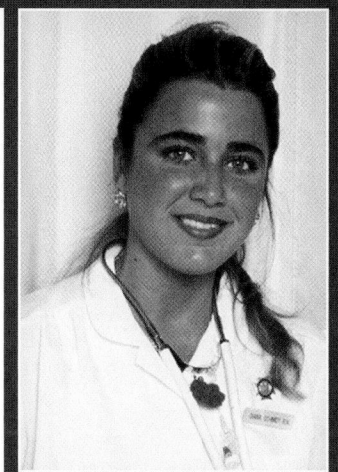

LEARNING OBJECTIVES

1. Define, spell, and pronounce the terms listed in the vocabulary.
2. List the equipment needed for venipuncture.
3. Explain the purpose of a tourniquet.
4. Explain how to apply a tourniquet and three consequences of improper application.
5. Describe the types of sharps used in phlebotomy.
6. Discuss the use of sharps with engineered sharps injury protection.
7. Explain why one chooses a syringe for blood collection rather than an evacuated tube.
8. Explain why the stopper colors on evacuated tubes differ.
9. State the correct order in which various types of tubes should be collected.
10. Describe how to insert a needle properly into the vein and how it should be removed.
11. List, in order, the steps of a routine venipuncture.
12. Describe and name the veins that may be used for blood collection.
13. Explain the reasoning behind choosing a winged infusion set (butterfly) over an evacuated tube.
14. Perform a venipuncture using a winged infusion set.
15. List situations in which capillary puncture would be preferred over venipuncture.
16. Discuss proper dermal puncture sites.
17. Describe dermal puncture devices, and discuss safety features they may have.
18. Describe containers that may be used to collect capillary blood.
19. List the steps for capillary puncture.
20. Explain why the first drop of blood is wiped away when a capillary puncture is performed.
21. Perform a capillary puncture.
22. Collect a capillary sample in a microhematocrit tube and in a capillary tube.
23. Explain the consequences of an accidental needlestick.
24. Describe a plan of action after an accidental sharps exposure.
25. Differentiate whole blood, serum, and plasma, and give an example of a test performed with each.
26. Describe handling and transport methods for blood after collection.

National Accreditation Competencies and Content

CAAHEP COMPETENCIES

Clinical
3.b.(1)(d). Dispose of biohazardous materials
3.b.(1)(e). Practice Standard Precautions
3.b.(2)(a). Perform venipuncture
3.b.(2)(b). Perform capillary puncture

General
3.c.(3)(b). Instruct individuals according to their needs
3.c.(4)(b). Perform routine maintenance of administrative and clinical equipment

ABHES COMPETENCIES

Professionalism
1.i. Conduct work within scope of education, training, and ability

Communication
2.a. Be attentive, listen, and learn
2.b. Be impartial and show empathy when dealing with patients
2.c. Adapt what is said to the recipient's level of comprehension
2.i. Recognize and respond to verbal and nonverbal communication

Clinical Duties
4.b. Prepare patients for procedures
4.j. Collect and process specimens
4.l. Screen and follow up patient test results
4.q. Dispose of biohazardous materials
4.r. Practice standard precautions
4.s. Perform venipuncture
4.t. Perform capillary puncture

Legal Concepts
5.b. Document accurately

VOCABULARY

antiseptic An agent that inhibits bacterial growth that can be used on human tissue.

bifurcation (bi-fuhr-ka′-shun) The point of forking or separating into two branches.

hematocrit (hi-ma′-tuh-krit) The percentage by volume of packed red blood cells in a given sample of blood after centrifugation.

hemoconcentration A situation in which the concentration of blood cells is increased in proportion to the plasma.

hemolysis (hi-muh′-luh-sis) The destruction or dissolution of red blood cells, with subsequent release of hemoglobin.

plasma The liquid portion of whole blood that contains active clotting agents.

serum The liquid portion of whole blood that remains after the blood has clotted.

stat With no delay; at once.

syncope Fainting.

thixotropic gel A material that appears to be a solid until subjected to a disturbance, such as centrifugation, upon which it becomes a liquid.

Phlebotomy, the practice of drawing blood, has its roots in the ancient practice of restoring the four body humors: blood, phlegm, yellow bile, and black bile. The foundation of all medical treatment was to keep these humors in balance by purging, starving, vomiting, or bloodletting. The art of bloodletting was flourishing by the Middle Ages, and both barbers and surgeons performed the art. Barbers advertised with a red (representing blood) and white (representing the tourniquet) striped pole. The pole itself represented the stick the patient squeezed during the procedure. Typically, 16 to 30 ounces (1 to 4 pints) of blood were drained to treat an illness.

When the patient became faint, the "treatment" was stopped. Often, bleeding over large areas of the body was accomplished by multiple incisions. George Washington is reported to have died in 1799 after being drained of 9 pints of blood within 24 hours to cure a throat infection. In Washington's day, it was believed that the blood was a carrier of the impurities of disease, and with bleeding, new and healthy blood would replace what was lost. By the end of the nineteenth century, bloodletting was declared quackery.

Today phlebotomy is performed primarily for diagnosis and monitoring of a patient's condition. According to the American

Society of Clinical Pathologists (ASCP), nearly 80% of physician's decisions are based on laboratory tests, most of which are blood tests. Phlebotomy involves highly developed procedures and equipment to ensure the comfort and safety of the patient. The high standards necessary for the proper practice of phlebotomy led to the creation of different organizations that develop standards for training. Medical assistants are trained to perform phlebotomy, but their training does not certify or license them as phlebotomists. To be certified or licensed, one must complete course work and training at an accredited institution, then pass a national examination. Certifying agencies include ASCP, the International Academy of Phlebotomy Sciences, the National Certification Agency (NCA), and the National Phlebotomy Association (NPA). Continuing education is often required to maintain certification. California and Louisiana were the first states to create state certification requirements.

The most common method of obtaining blood is by venipuncture. In a venipuncture the blood is taken directly from a superficial vein. The vein is punctured with a needle, and the blood is collected in either a syringe or a stoppered tube. The procedure is safe when performed by a trained professional, but it must be performed with care. Much practice is required to become skilled and confident in the technique of venipuncture.

VENIPUNCTURE EQUIPMENT

Proper collection of blood requires specialized equipment. A complete list of materials used in routine venipuncture is shown below. Phlebotomists generally carry the equipment in a portable tray (Figure 52-1). In a physician's office laboratory there will probably be a permanent location where venipuncture is performed. In such cases you will likely seat patients in a venipuncture chair, which has an adjustable locking armrest to protect the patient in the event of fainting.

Equipment Used In Routine Venipuncture

- Double-pointed safety needles
- Evacuated, stoppered tubes
- Needle holder
- Sharps container
- Syringes
- Winged infusion sets (butterfly needles)
- Tourniquet
- Marking pen
- Alcohol swabs
- Gauze pads
- Bandages
- Gloves
- Smelling salts

Reference for postexposure prophylaxis information: Centers for Disease Control and Prevention: Public health service guidelines for the management of health care workers exposures to HIV and recommendations for postexposure prophylaxis, *MMWR Morb Mortal Wkly Rep* 47(RR-7):1:37, 1998.

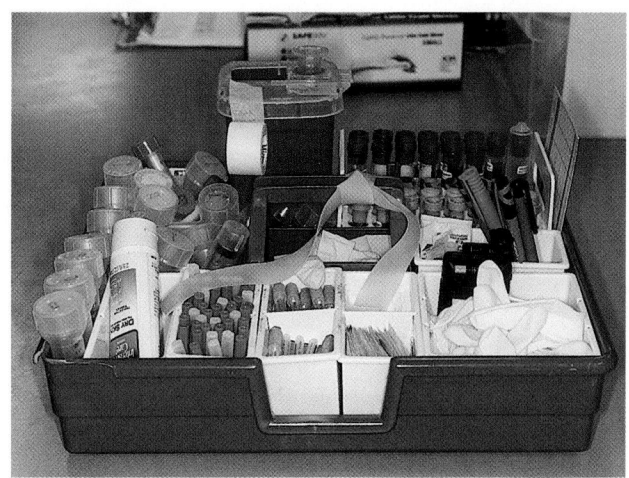

FIGURE 52-1 A fully stocked venipuncture tray. (From Stepp CA, Woods MA: *Laboratory procedures for medical office personnel*, Philadelphia, 1998, Saunders.)

Gloves

Employers must provide gloves, including hypoallergenic gloves, powderless gloves, or glove liners to employees. Glove use during venipuncture is mandated by the Occupational Safety and Health Administration (OSHA), but the agency does not mandate when during the course of the venipuncture the gloves must be put on. Because veins can be difficult to locate with gloved fingertips, the site may be palpated before the gloves are donned. The Clinical and Laboratory Standards Institute (CLSI) standard procedure for venipuncture directs the application of gloves after vein palpation but before preparation of the site. Those who need the final assurance of one last palpation before the needle is inserted must be reminded that touching the prepared site, even with gloves, contaminates the area. To help you find the vein after cleansing the area, make note of certain skin markers such as creases, freckles, or scars. If the area is touched, it must be cleansed again. Keep in mind that the tourniquet should be tied for no longer than 1 minute.

Tourniquets

Before blood can be drawn, a vein must be located. Application of a tourniquet is the most common way to do this and works by preventing venous flow out of the site, causing the veins to bulge. Various types of tourniquets are shown in Figure 52-2. The tourniquet, usually a thin strip of latex rubber, is tied around the upper arm so that it is tight but not uncomfortable and can be released easily with one hand. Latex tourniquets are inexpensive, but they may become contaminated and some patients are allergic to latex. Other tourniquets with Velcro closures are available and may be more comfortable for the patient, but they have the disadvantage of being difficult to release. Single-use, nonlatex tourniquets are available and are suggested for reducing cross-contamination between patients and health care workers, preventing nosocomial infection, and minimizing latex exposure.

Tourniquets are tied 3 to 4 inches above the elbow immediately before the venipuncture procedure begins. Because it impedes blood flow, leaving a tourniquet on for longer than 1 minute

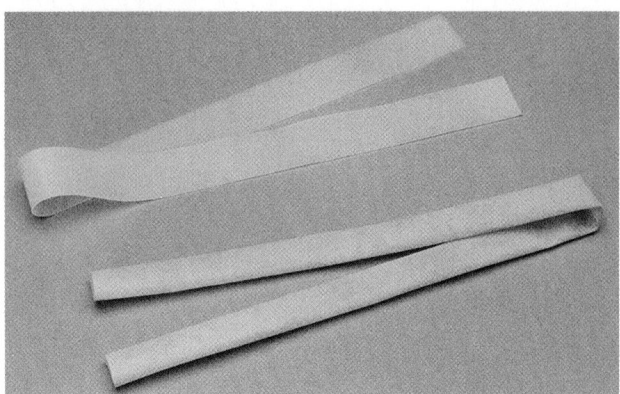

A

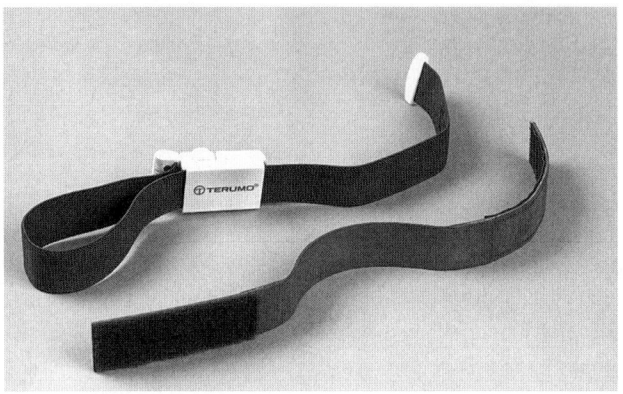

B

FIGURE 52-2 Examples of tourniquets. (*B* From Flynn JC Jr: *Procedures in phlebotomy*, ed 3, Philadelphia, 2005, Saunders.)

greatly increases the possibility of **hemoconcentration** and altered test results. Alternately a blood pressure cuff can be used during a multitube draw and can be released and reinflated as needed to prevent hemoconcentration. The tourniquet should not be tied so tightly as to impede arterial blood flow. This will restrict venous blood return, resulting in poor venous distention. Checking the pulse at the wrist will ensure that arterial flow is not restricted. Tourniquets are also used when drawing blood from hand and foot veins and are tied on the wrist or ankle, respectively.

Tourniquets can be uncomfortable to patients, especially those with heavyset or hairy upper arms, if they are not applied correctly. Be sure that the tourniquet is flat against the skin, and if necessary tie it over the clothing if it is causing the patient discomfort. When reusable tourniquets are used, they should be cleaned regularly with soap and hot water and can be easily cleaned between uses with disposable **antiseptic** towelettes containing benzalkonium chloride.

Antiseptics

To prevent infection, a venipuncture site must be cleansed with an antiseptic. The most commonly used is 70% isopropyl alcohol, also known as *rubbing alcohol.* Prepackaged alcohol "prep pads" are the most commonly used product. The square prep pad is rubbed on the skin in a circular motion, and the alcohol is allowed to dry. Alcohol does not sterilize the skin; it

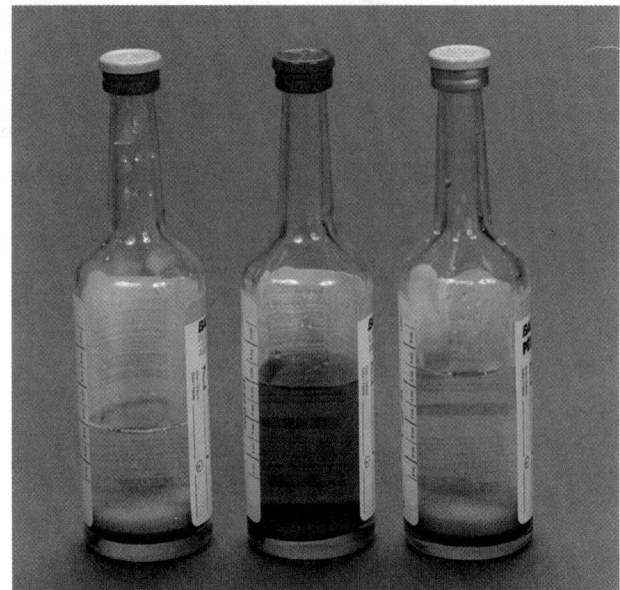

FIGURE 52-3 Bactec blood culture bottles.

inhibits the reproduction of bacteria that might contaminate the sample. To be most effective the alcohol should remain on the skin 30 to 60 seconds. Isopropyl alcohol cannot be used when drawing a blood alcohol test. Sterile soap pads, benzalkonium chloride, or povidone-iodine can be used.

If a blood culture is ordered, additional preparation is needed at the venipuncture site to eliminate contaminating bacteria. Povidone-iodine solution (Betadine) is commonly used. For patients allergic to iodine, chlorhexidine gluconate or benzalkonium chloride can be used. Cleansing the area before a blood culture collection requires more vigorous cleansing than a routine venipuncture. Blood cultures must be drawn into a sterile tube or a bottle specifically designed for the test (Figure 52-3).

Evacuated Collection Tubes

The evacuated tube (Vacutainer) system is the most common collection system in use. It consists of evacuated tubes of various sizes, with color-coded tops indicating tube contents (Table 52-1). Tubes are available in both glass and shatter-resistant glass. The tube contents include anticoagulants, clot activators, and/or **thixotropic gel.** The vacuum in each tube is such that a measured amount of blood is drawn into the tube. Tube volumes range from 2 to 15 mL. Be sure to match the needle gauge to the size of the tube; the larger the tube, the greater the vacuum and the more likely blood will hemolyze if a high-gauge, small–lumen-sized needle is used.

The size of the tube to be used depends on several factors. Each test performed in the laboratory requires a specific amount of blood. Consult the manual provided by the laboratory to ensure that you are drawing the right amount of blood for the test. Tests can often be combined, reducing the number of tubes that must be drawn. For example, both a complete blood count and an erythrocyte sedimentation rate (discussed in Chapter 53) are performed on a lavender-topped tube. It is not necessary to draw two tubes because the 7-mL volume is sufficient for

TABLE 52-1 List of Common Stoppers, Additives, and Their Laboratory Uses

VACUTAINER COLOR*	COLOR	HEMOGARD COLOR†	ADDITIVE AND ADDITIVE FUNCTION§	LABORATORY USE§	OPTIMUM VOLUME/ MINIMUM VOLUME
Adult Tubes					
Yellow		Yellow	Sodium polyanetholsulfonate (SPS); prevents blood from clotting and stabilizes bacterial growth	Blood or body fluid cultures	5 mL/NA
Red		Red	None	Serum testing; chemistry studies, blood bank, serology	10 mL/NA
Red-gray (marbled)		Gold	None, but contains silica particles to enhance clot formation	Serum testing	10 mL/NA
Light blue		Light blue	Sodium citrate; removes calcium to prevent blood from clotting	Coagulation testing	4.5 mL/4.5 mL
Green		Green	Heparin (sodium/lithium/ammonium); inhibits thrombin formation to prevent clotting	Chemistry testing	10 mL/3.5 mL
Green-gray (marbled)		Light green	Lithium heparin and gel for plasma separation	Plasma determinations in chemistry studies	2 mL/2 mL
Yellow-gray (marbled)		Orange	Thrombin	Stat serum demonstrations in chemistry studies	2 mL/2 mL
Lavender		Lavender	Ethylenediaminetetraacetic acid (EDTA); removes calcium to prevent blood from clotting	Hematology testing	7 mL/2 mL
Gray		Gray	Potassium oxalate and sodium fluoride; removes calcium to prevent blood from clotting; fluoride inhibits glycolysis	Chemistry testing, especially glucose and alcohol levels	10 mL/10 mL
Royal blue		Royal blue	Sodium heparin (also sodium EDTA); inhibits thrombin formation to prevent clotting	Chemistry trace elements	7 mL
Pediatric Tubes					
Red		Red			2 mL/NA; 3 mL/NA; 4 mL/NA
Lavender		Lavender			2 mL/0.6 mL 3 mL/0.9 mL 4 mL/1 mL
Green		Green			2 mL/2 mL
Light blue		Light blue			2.7 mL/2.7 mL

Modified from Rodak BF: *Diagnostic hematology*, Philadelphia, 1995, Saunders.
*Stopper colors are based on Becton-Dickinson Vacutainer tubes.
†Hemogard closures provide a protective plastic cover over the rubber stopper as an additional safety feature.
§Additives, additive functions, and laboratory uses are the same for both pediatric and adult tubes.

both tests. When in doubt, call the laboratory. Keep in mind that blood is approximately half cells and half liquid. If a test requires 3 mL of **serum,** 6 mL of blood must be collected.

Patients often express great concern when several tubes of blood must be drawn. You can allay their fears by explaining that the average adult has a little less than 10 pints of blood (5 L). Most adults can relate to donating a unit of blood, which is around a pint (400 to 500 mL). Because the red-topped tube contains 10 mL, you would have to draw 40 to 50 tubes before you have removed a pint.

Tube Additives

All tubes, with the exception of the red-topped tube, contain an additive. Anticoagulants are added to prevent blood from clotting. Tubes may be glass or plastic. The additive may be a powder, a liquid visible in the tube, or a liquid sprayed inside the tube by the manufacturer and allowed to dry. The choice of anticoagulant depends on the test to be done.

Ethylenediaminetetraacetic acid (EDTA) found in the lavender-topped tube prevents platelet clumping and preserves the appearance of blood cells for microscopic examination, but it is incompatible with the testing reagents used in coagulation studies. Consult the manual provided by the laboratory before obtaining a specimen from the patient.

Clot activators promote clotting of blood. Silica particles enhance clotting, for example, by providing a surface for platelet activation. Thrombin quickly promotes clotting and is used in tubes drawn for **stat** chemistry testing or in the event a sample is needed from a patient who is taking a prescribed anticoagulant such as heparin.

Anticoagulants prevent blood from clotting, which allows the contents of the tube to be used in two ways. First, the sample can be used as whole blood; second, the sample can be centrifuged, and the liquid portion, called **plasma**, can be retrieved. Whole blood is used for tests such as complete blood counts and blood typing, whereas plasma is used for stat chemistry testing and coagulation studies.

If blood is allowed to clot then is centrifuged, the liquid portion is referred to as *serum*. Without a clot activator, blood will clot in 30 to 60 minutes, after which it must be centrifuged. The serum must be quickly separated from the cells because cells may continue to metabolize substances such as glucose or may release metabolites that interfere with testing. Thixotropic gel can be found in some tubes, including the SST red-gray and the PST green-gray marbled-topped tubes by Becton-Dickinson. This synthetic gel has a density between that of red cells and plasma or serum, and it settles between the two during centrifugation, forming a barrier. This barrier facilitates retrieval of the liquid portion without cellular contamination.

It is important to mix the tube well after collection by inverting it several times (do not shake the tube) and also to avoid a short draw, a tube that is not completely filled. Having the proper ratio of blood to additive is crucial. The effects of a short draw are described in Table 52-2. Always be sure to check the tube for an expiration date. Outdated tubes may have diminished vacuum, or the additive may have degraded.

CRITICAL THINKING APPLICATION

- Melissa Machen has been assigned to orient Leah to the clinic and her duties as a certified medical assistant. Melissa takes Leah to the laboratory in the clinic. There is a small room with a blood collection chair and a table. What supplies should be on the table to perform venipuncture?
- What else might Leah find in this room?

Order of Collection

In the event that more than one tube must be drawn during a venipuncture, a specified order must be followed so that material from a previous tube is not transferred to the next tube. Carryover of additives from one tube to the next could cause

TABLE 52-2 Effects of Underfilling

STOPPER COLOR	EFFECT
Yellow	Decreases possibility of bacterial recovery
Red	Insufficient sample
Red-gray	Poor barrier formation; insufficient sample
Light blue	Coagulation test results are falsely prolonged
Green	False results because of excess heparin
Green-gray	False results because of excess heparin
Lavender	Falsely low blood cell counts and hematocrits; morphologic changes to red blood cells, staining alteration
Yellow-gray	False results
Gray	False results
Royal blue	False results

sample alteration and erroneous results. The CLSI (formerly the National Committee for Clinical Laboratory Standards [NCCLS]) developed a set of standards outlining the order of draw for a multitube draw. The same order applies to the filling of tubes when blood is collected in a syringe and takes into account the use of newer plastic tubes.

1. Blood culture tubes are filled first because they are sterile.
2. Light blue–topped tubes with sodium citrate are next because other anticoagulants might contaminate the sample collected for coagulation studies. If no blood culture is ordered, CLSI recommends that blood for the light blue–topped tube should be drawn first if routine coagulation testing (prothrombin time [PT] and activated partial thromboplastin time [APTT]–see Chapter 53) has been ordered. For testing other than routine PT and APTT, a red-topped "waste" tube may be filled. When using a winged infusion set, the CLSI currently recommends the drawing of blood into a red-topped tube even if the order does not call for it. This is done to fill the tubing's dead space with blood and to prevent any thromboplastin released during venipuncture from contaminating the blue-topped tube and interfering with coagulation testing. It is not necessary to fill the tube to be discarded.
3. Serum tubes without clot-activator (red stopper) or with clot-activator (red-gold or speckled stopper) are filled next. Although CLSI notes that glass, nonadditive serum tubes can be drawn before the light-blue stoppered tubes, they have simplified the order to function for all serum tubes, regardless of their composition.
4. Green-topped tubes are next because heparin is less likely to interfere with EDTA than vice versa.
5. Lavender-topped tubes follow. Because EDTA binds with calcium, blood for this tube is drawn near the end.
6. The gray-topped tube is last because the contents can elevate electrolyte levels or damage cells if passed into another tube (Table 52-3).

TABLE 52-3 Stopper Color	
STOPPER COLOR	**MIX BY INVERSION**
Yellow	8-10 times
Light blue	3-4 times
Red or red speckled	5 times
Green	8-10 times
Lavender	8-10 times
Gray	8-10 times

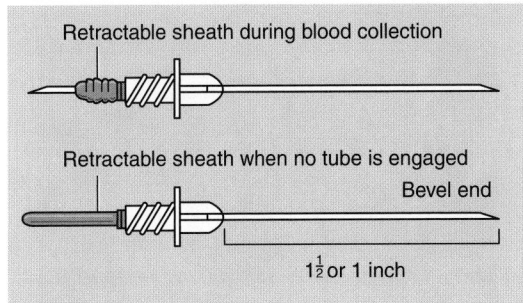

FIGURE 52-4 Multisample needles.

Needles

A critical part of phlebotomy is the knowledge of which needle and which tube or syringe to use in each situation. All needles used in phlebotomy are sterile, disposable, and used only once. Each is housed in a cover, which should be inspected before use to ensure that sterility has not been compromised (i.e., the seal should be intact) and also to ensure that it has no manufacturing defects such as burrs or nicks. Needles have two parts: the hub and the shaft. Shafts differ in length, ranging from $^3/_4$ to $1^1/_2$ inches. The length of the shaft has no bearing on the venipuncture procedure, but some prefer a longer needle because it is less likely to slip out of the vein, whereas others prefer a shorter needle because it makes patients less uneasy. One end of the shaft is cut at an angle and forms the bevel, which creates a very sharp point. The hole in the bevel is called the *lumen.*

Lumen size is important in venipuncture and is referred to as the *gauge.* Gauge is designated by a numeric value; the higher the number, the smaller the lumen. The blood bank uses a 16-gauge needle to collect pints of blood for transfusions because the lumen is wide, which reduces the chance of **hemolysis.** The smallest gauge needles (23-gauge) are used to collect blood from small or fragile veins, such as those of elderly and very young patients. Routine adult venipuncture requires a 20- to 21-gauge needle. Finally, the hub is the point where the needle attaches to the syringe or the needle holder.

Multisample Needles

Multisample needles are commonly used in routine adult venipuncture. They are so called because they are used when several tubes are to be drawn during a single venipuncture. These needles are double-pointed (Figure 52-4). One point enters the patient's vein while the other punctures the rubber stopper of the collection tube. The point that enters the tube is sheathed with a retractable rubber sleeve that allows tubes to be changed without blood leaking into the needle holder or tube holder.

Syringes

Syringes are used when there is concern that the strong vacuum in a stoppered tube will collapse the vein. The syringe needle fits on the end of the barrel and comes in different gauges. The amount of blood drawn into the barrel depends on how much is to be transferred to stoppered tubes When blood is drawn into a syringe, it must be transferred immediately to another tube because the blood will clot in the syringe barrel. In these

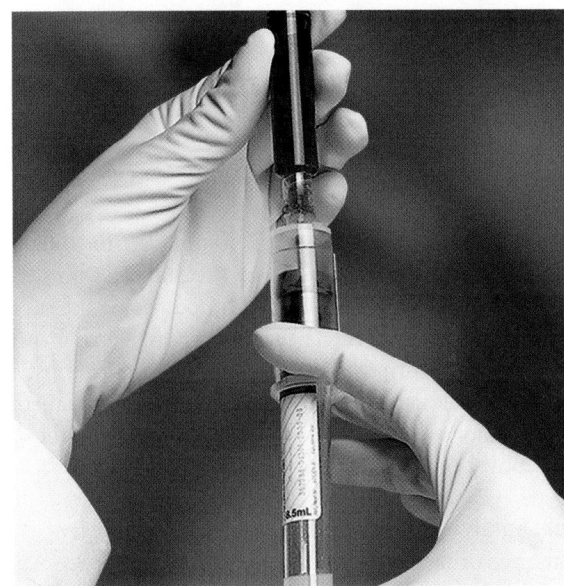

FIGURE 52-5 BD Vacutainer blood transfer device. (Courtesy Becton and Dickinson and Co., Franklin Lakes, N.J.)

situations a syringe with an engineered sharps injury prevention feature and safe work practices should be used. Transfer of the blood from the syringe to the test tube must be done using a needleless blood transfer device, as mandated by OSHA. A special transfer tube adapter is used to transfer the blood to the Vacutainer tube. The adapter connects to the top of the syringe once the needle is capped and removed. The adapter contains an enclosed needle that punctures and delivers the blood into the Vacutainer tube (Figure 52-5).

Winged Infusion Sets (Butterfly Needles)

Butterfly needles (Figure 52-6) are designed for use on small veins such as those in the hand or in pediatric patients. The most common needle size is 23 gauge, and the needle is $^1/_2$ to $^3/_4$ inch long with a plastic, flexible butterfly-shaped grip attached to a short length of tubing. One end is fitted into the syringe or the vacuum tube adapter. Often a syringe is used because the vacuum can be controlled more easily. Smaller evacuated tubes, with a less powerful vacuum, are preferable when using a butterfly set.

Needle Holders

Double-pointed needles must be firmly placed into a needle adapter or tube holder. Usually they are translucent cylinders,

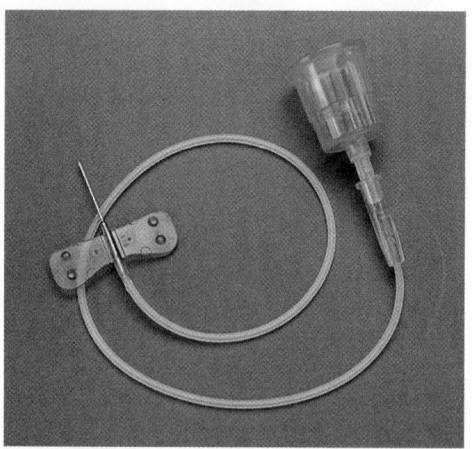

FIGURE 52-6 Winged infusion set attached to an evacuated tube holder with a Luer needle holder. (From Sommer SR, Warekois RS: *Phlebotomy: worktext and procedures manual*, Philadelphia, 2002, Saunders.)

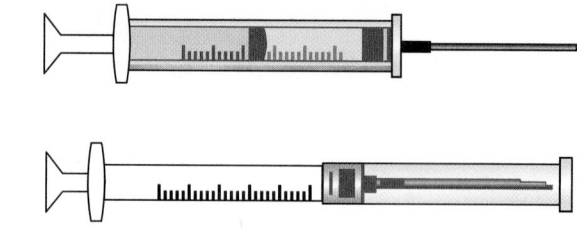

FIGURE 52-7 Self-sheathing device.

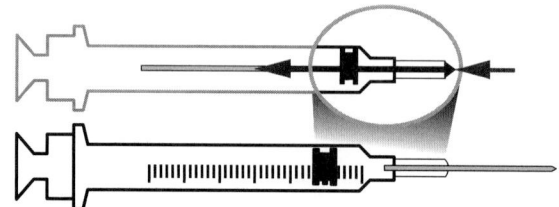

FIGURE 52-8 Retractable safety device.

and they come in different sizes to accommodate the tube being used. The cylinders often have a ring that indicates how far the tube can be pushed onto the needle without losing the vacuum. In order to prevent accidental needlesticks, OSHA has mandated needle holders be disposed of after a single use. In most cases the entire needle and holder are disposed of simultaneously; needles are not removed from the needle holder, and the safety feature must be activated before disposal.

Needle Safety

Healthcare workers (HCWs) who use or may be exposed to needles are at increased risk for needlestick injury. Such injuries can lead to serious or fatal infections with blood-borne pathogens such as hepatitis B virus (HBV), hepatitis C virus (HCV), or human immunodeficiency virus (HIV). An estimated 800,000 needlestick injuries occur each year, with nursing staff being most frequently injured. Needlestick injuries account for up to 80% of accidental exposures to blood. Recapping needles has been the most common practice that leads to injury. Recapping of needles is permitted by OSHA but only under certain conditions. First, the employer must prove there is no other way to dispose of the needle and must justify the practice in writing in the facilities exposure control plan. Reliable evidence must be cited. Recapping can be accomplished only by mechanical means or by using a one-handed technique.

OSHA recently issued a safety and health information bulletin outlining its policy on the disposal of contaminated needles and blood tube holders after phlebotomy. The bulletin is not a standard or regulation creating legal obligations; it is advisory in nature and intends to assist employers in providing a safe workplace.

OSHA has concluded that the best practice for prevention of needlestick injuries after phlebotomy is the use of a "sharp with engineered sharps injury protection" (SESIP) attached to a needle holder. SESIPs, or safety needles, eliminate the need for removal of the needle from the needle holder and in some way shield the needle immediately after use. The *Food and Drug Administration (FDA)* is responsible for approving medical devices marketed and sold in the United States. It recommends devices that provide a barrier between the hands and the needle after use in which the phlebotomist's hands remain behind the needle at all times. Safety shields should also be an integral part of the device that can be activated before or immediately after removal of the needle from the vein and remain in effect after disposal. Finally, these devices should be as simple as possible, requiring little or no training to use. Some examples of SESIPs include the following:

- *Self-sheathing safety devices* (Figure 52-7): These devices have sliding needle shields attached to disposable syringes and vacuum tube holders. Before activation, the sleeve is positioned over the barrel of the syringe. After the procedure, the phlebotomist slides the sleeve forward over the needle, where it locks into place, protecting the needle.
- *Retractable safety devices* (Figure 52-8): After the needle is used and removed from the vein, pushing a plunger retracts the needle into the syringe or needle holder. The entire unit is disposed of in the sharps container.
- *Needle-blunting safety mechanisms* (Figures 52-9 and 52-10): After the venipuncture a blunt tube is moved through the needle, covering the sharp point. With the needle in the needle holder, the vacuum tube is removed then pushed forward again while the needle is still in the vein. This moves the blunt-tip needle forward through the needle, past the sharp needle point. The blunt point tip of the needle can be activated before it is removed from the patient.

  When the butterfly set is used, a third "wing" is rotated after collection and before removal of the needle from the vein. As the third wing is rotated, it moves the blunt needle down the shaft before it is removed from the patient.
- *Hinged or sliding safety mechanisms* (Figure 52-11): These devices, attached to the phlebotomy needle or a winged infusion needle, are manually engaged after the needle is removed from the vein. The plastic sheath covers the

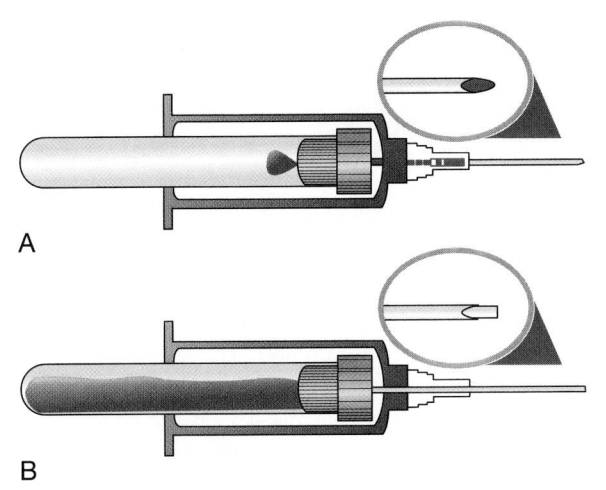

FIGURE 52-9 Needle blunting SESIP for the needle holder. **A,** Needle while collecting specimen before activation. **B,** Needle with blunting device activated.

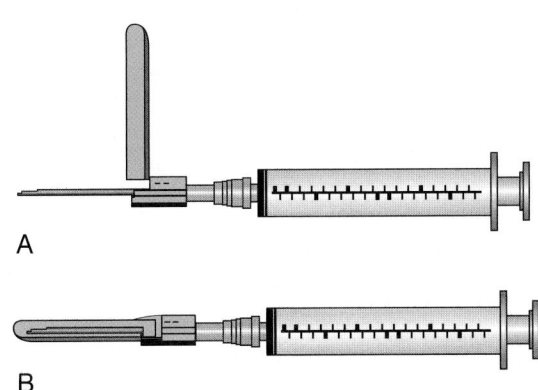

FIGURE 52-11 Hinged or sliding SESIP. **A,** Before venipuncture. **B,** After activation.

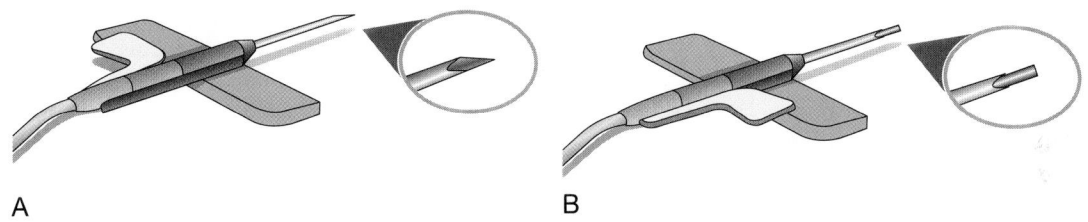

FIGURE 52-10 Needle blunting SESIP for winged infusion sets. **A,** Before activation, with needle in vein. **B,** After activation.

needle, and the entire unit is disposed of in the sharps container.

All HCWs should take the following steps to protect themselves and their fellow workers from needlestick injuries:

- Avoid the use of needles where safe and effective alternatives are available.
- Help your employer select and evaluate devices with safety features.
- Use devices with safety features provided by your employer.
- Do not recap a needle.
- Plan for safe handling and disposal before beginning any procedure using needles.
- Dispose of used needles promptly in appropriate sharps disposal containers.
- Report all needlestick and other sharps-related injuries promptly to ensure that you receive appropriate follow-up care.
- Tell your employer about hazards from needles that you observe in your work environment.
- Participate in blood-borne pathogen training, and follow recommended infection prevention practices, including hepatitis B vaccination.

OSHA mandates that employers establish and maintain a sharps injury log for the recording of injuries from contaminated sharps. This log should contain information about the device involved in the incident, the department or work area where the incident occurred, and an explanation of the incident. Employee confidentiality must be maintained.

Postexposure Management of Needlesticks

An accidental exposure to a contaminated sharp is a terrifying experience, one that more than 800,000 HCWs in the United States face every year. After exposure they must make decisions regarding treatment and prophylaxis, and often there is no single recommended course of action because so many variables surround the exposure. The Centers for Disease Control and Prevention's (CDC's) *Morbidity and Mortality Weekly Report* published a guide with a well-designed process for evaluating exposures as well as recommendations for postexposure management. Although the guide concentrates on exposure to HIV, it outlines a rational postexposure plan (PEP) for all accidental needlesticks. The infectious agents of concern include HBV and HCV in addition to HIV.

An accidental needlestick is a medical emergency. Immediate access to health providers is necessary to evaluate the severity and risk factors of the exposure and to manage an appropriate response. In some cases, preventative medicines must be administered immediately, ideally within 2 hours of the exposure. Effective management of an accidental sharps exposure is as follows.

Care of the Exposure Site. Immediately after injury the wound should be induced to bleed if possible. It should then be inspected for foreign material, which should be removed. The site should be washed for 10 minutes with an antimicrobial soap, 10% iodine solution, or chlorine-based antiseptics. Undiluted bleach should never be used.

Evaluation of the Exposure. In order to make the best postexposure decisions, it is important to establish whether or not an exchange of blood could have transpired. Healthcare providers should consider the severity of the exposure, the route of entry, the amount of blood involved, and the likelihood that the person was exposed to a blood-borne pathogen such as HBV, HCV, or HIV. Those professionals best equipped to conduct the evaluation are the infection control or occupational health nurse and an infectious diseases physician. The CDC has developed an algorithm to determine the level of risk and the protocol for postexposure prophylaxis. In general, it states that an HCW who has been immunized with the HBV vaccine is not at risk for acquiring HBV and no source testing is needed. In the event that the HCW who has sustained the needlestick injury has not been immunized, source testing for infection with HBV is recommended if the source is known and can be located. If the source patient tests positive for HBV, the HCW should receive HBV immune globulin (HBIG) and the series of HBV immunizations should be initiated. If the source tests negative, no treatment of the HCW is indicated. If the source patient cannot be tested, the HCW should be treated as if the source patient were positive for HBV.

Postexposure treatment for HCV also necessitates testing of the source, if possible. If positive the HCW should be monitored for signs and symptoms of hepatitis for 6 months. No postexposure prophylaxis is recommended for HCV infection.

Managing possible HIV infection is complex. Employers of HCWs are required to have a PEP. For HIV exposure, the PEP usually includes a 4-week regimen of antiretroviral drugs. Because this therapy is aggressive and lengthy and HCWs could suffer potentially debilitating side effects, evaluating risk of exposure to HIV is critical. In order to best protect the victim, antiretroviral therapy should be administered within hours of exposure. Therefore, unless the source's HIV status can be ascertained within hours of exposure, the HCW should be prepared to make a decision regarding antiretroviral therapy, weighing the consequences of action and inaction carefully. If the source can be tested and is found to be negative, antiretroviral therapy can be discontinued.

Follow-up Care and Testing. Baseline testing for HBV, HCV, and HIV is recommended when indicated. Interim testing may be performed if the HCW experiences symptoms of acute retroviral syndrome or hepatitis. For HIV, antibody testing should be repeated at 6 weeks, 12 weeks, and 6 months if either the source was HIV positive or the source's status remains unknown. HCWs who acquire HBV, HIV, or HCV through accidental exposure are potentially infectious to others and must work closely with occupational health professionals to determine the best measures to use to prevent subsequent transmission. Follow-up care must also include provisions for emotional support and counseling for both the HCW and the source.

CRITICAL THINKING APPLICATION

- During her lunch break, Leah meets some of her co-workers. The conversation in the lunchroom involves an accident that occurred
  Continued
- several years ago when a former employee was performing venipuncture on a recovering intravenous drug addict and was accidentally stuck with the needle. Describe the actions a HCW must take to report and follow up on an accidental needlestick incident.
- What measures are available to prevent accidental needlesticks?

ROUTINE VENIPUNCTURE

Your appearance and actions reflect your laboratory or facility. A patient's first impression of the facility often comes from you. Clean lab coats or scrubs tell the patient the facility is clean, wearing gloves tells the patient you will treat him or her with care, and speaking knowledgeably provides the impression that the facility is staffed with professionals.

Performing venipuncture involves several important steps with which you must be thoroughly familiar before attempting the procedure. The first step is to select the proper method for venipuncture (syringe or evacuated tube). Next, the patient must be prepared for the procedure. Patient preparation is followed by the actual venipuncture and specimen collection. The final step is care of the puncture site before the patient is discharged.

Patient Preparation

All blood collections begin with a requisition, a form from the patient's physician requesting a test. Requisitions may be computer generated or handwritten and at a minimum must have the following information:

- Patient name
- Date of birth
- Identification number
- Name of physician making the request
- Type of test requested
- Test status (timed, fasting, stat, and so forth)

Venipuncture begins with greeting and identifying the patient. According to the CLSI, proper identification includes asking outpatients to provide full name, address, and an identification number or birth date. This information must be compared with the written information on the requisition. For inpatients the CLSI recommends asking for the same information and comparing it with the information on the requisition and the identification bracelet. If the patient speaks a different language, has limited language skills (such as a child) or is otherwise unable to communicate, a family member or caregiver must provide the information. The name of this person should be documented.

Introduce yourself, and explain briefly the purpose and procedure of the venipuncture. If the patient has questions regarding the tests that have been ordered, request politely that the patient speak to his or her physician and ask whether he or she would like to do so before you collect the sample. Obtain verbal consent for performing the procedure simply by asking if you have permission to take some blood from their arm. Always ask the patient if he or she has experienced problems during routine venipuncture in the past, and take steps to prevent such problems. Your self-confidence in the procedure will be evident to the patient and will help to allay any fears.

Instilling confidence in your patients means acting and speaking professionally. Refer to the patient as "sir" or "ma'am" or "Mr. Jones" or "Ms. Smith," not "honey", "sweetie," Bill, or Margaret. Being friendly is important, but make sure your patients feel respected and understand that you take your role in their care seriously.

Preparing for the Venipuncture

Seat the patient in a chair and ask the patient to extend his or her arm. Inspect both arms, and ask whether the patient has a preference. Generally, veins in the forearm or the elbow (antecubital area) are used for venipuncture (Figure 52-12). The puncture site should be carefully selected after both arms have been inspected. Alternative sites may be indicated if the area is cyanotic, scarred, bruised, edematous, or burned. You may use veins on the lower forearm, the back of the hand, or the wrist. Use foot or ankle veins only if the patient has good circulation in the legs and you have received permission from your supervisor or the physician. Never draw blood from this area if the patient is diabetic.

Apply the tourniquet, request that the patient make a fist, and palpate for an acceptable vein using your ungloved index finger. A thorough survey of both arms should be undertaken before the venipuncture site is chosen. Veins will bounce lightly when palpated. The medial veins generally run parallel or at a slight angle to the fold in the antecubital area, whereas the cephalic veins run lateral or to the outside of the antecubital area. These veins are the veins of choice. The basilic vein, which lies on the inside part of the antecubital area, is very close to the brachial artery and median nerves and should be used only if the medial or cephalic veins are inaccessible. The most common injury patients suffer from phlebotomy is nerve injury. If the patient complains of tingling, numbness, or a shooting pain, discontinue the procedure and choose another site before continuing. Do not probe with the needle under this condition; any attempt at relocating the needle under these conditions puts the patient at great risk of nerve injury.

Performing the Venipuncture

When you have located a vein, remove the tourniquet. A tourniquet can remain in place for 1 minute. After it is removed the phlebotomist must wait 2 minutes before reapplying it. Assemble the appropriate equipment, ensuring that everything is within easy reach, that the sterile packets are torn open, and that the contents are easily accessible. Wash your hands.

Reapply the tourniquet and quickly relocate the vein. Apply your gloves, and cleanse the antecubital area with the alcohol, working outward in a circular motion. Do not touch this area after cleansing. Request that the patient clench his or her hand into a fist. Do not ask the patient to pump the fist, as this may temporarily increase the level of potassium and ionized calcium in the blood. Anchor the vein by stretching the skin downward below the collection site with the thumb of the nondominant hand, and swiftly insert the needle into the vein at a 20- to 30-degree angle. The bevel should be facing up. If the needle is inserted at an angle of greater than 30 degrees, it quickly penetrates the other side of the vein and enters other structures such as nerves or the brachial artery and very likely will cause a hematoma or injury. Pull back on the syringe plunger or push the evacuated tube onto the double-pointed needle. When blood enters the tube or barrel, request that the patient unclench the fist.

Completing the Venipuncture Procedure

Continue to draw the specimen, checking periodically on the patient's condition. As you remove each tube from the needle holder, gently invert it before you place it in the rack. Tubes with clot activator should be inverted five times, light-blue–stoppered tubes for coagulation studies should be inverted three or four times, and all other anticoagulant tubes should be inverted 8 to 10 times. Failure to invert the tubes immediately after collection can lead to small clots forming in the specimen. When you near the end of the draw and the last tube to be collected fills, carefully release the tourniquet without jarring the needle. Remove the needle quickly, then apply the gauze with pressure to the puncture site. Ask the patient to apply direct pressure to the gauze but not to bend the arm. Immediately activate the safety device to cover the needle, and dispose of the entire assembly into a sharps container. Before applying the bandage, conduct a two-point check to be sure the vein is not leaking. Observe the site for 5 to 10 seconds after releasing pressure and removing the gauze. If visible bleeding occurs or if the tissue around the puncture site raises, continue applying pressure until the bleeding has stopped. Apply a bandage, and dispose of the gauze in a biohazard waste container. Clean gauze, not a cotton ball, can be taped over the site in lieu of a bandage. Label all tubes by the patient's side. Never leave the room or release an outpatient until the tubes are labeled. Assess the patient's status one last time, then dismiss the patient or leave the room.

Procedures 52-1 to 52-3 outline the proper procedures for venipuncture using a syringe, the evacuated tube method, and a winged infusion set (butterfly needle).

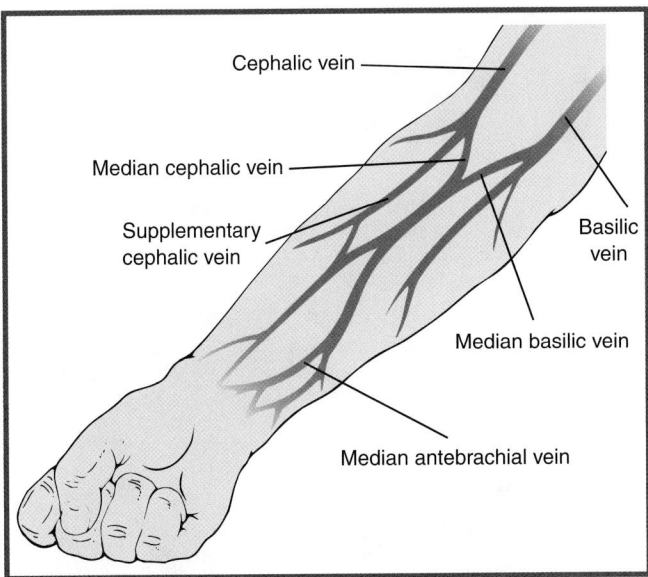

FIGURE 52-12 Veins of the forearm. (From Stepp CA, Woods MA: *Laboratory procedures for medical office personnel*, Philadelphia, 1998, Saunders.)

PROCEDURE 52-1

Perform Venipuncture: Collect a Venous Blood Sample Using the Syringe Method

CAAHEP COMPETENCIES: 3.b.(1)(d), 3.b.(1)(e), 3.b.(2)(a), 3.c.(3)(b), 3.c.(4)(b)
ABHES COMPETENCIES: 1.i, 2.a, 2.b, 2.c, 2.i, 4.b, 4.j, 4.q, 4.r, 4.s, 5.b

GOAL: *To collect a venous blood specimen.*

EQUIPMENT and SUPPLIES

- Needle, syringe with 21- or 22-gauge safety needle
- Vacutainer tubes appropriate for tests ordered
- 70% isopropyl alcohol
- Sterile gauze pads
- Tourniquet
- Syringe adapter for transfer to Vacutainer tubes
- Nonallergenic tape or bandage
- Permanent marking pen
- Biohazard bag or disposal container

PROCEDURAL STEPS

1. Check the requisition form to determine the tests ordered. Gather the correct tubes and supplies you will need.
   PURPOSE: Allows for proper specimen collection.

2. Wash and dry your hands, and put on nonsterile gloves.
   PURPOSE: Infection control.

3. Identify the patient, explain the procedure, and obtain permission to perform the venipuncture.
   PURPOSE: Ascertain patient identity; explanations help to gain the patient's cooperation.

4. Assist the patient to sit with the arm well supported in a slightly downward position.
   PURPOSE: Veins of the antecubital fossa are more easily located when the elbow is straight.

5. Assemble equipment. Choice of syringe barrel size and needle size depends on your inspection of the patient's veins and the amount of blood required for the ordered tests. Attach the needle to the syringe. Pull and depress the plunger several times to loosen it in the barrel. Keep the cover on the needle.
   PURPOSE: Using the smallest syringe possible minimizes the chance of hemolysis. Engaging the plunger ensures that you will

not have to use as much force to pull the blood into the barrel, thereby minimizing the chance of hemolysis.

6. Apply the tourniquet around the patient's arm 3 to 4 inches above the elbow. The tourniquet should never be tied so tightly that it restricts blood flow in the artery (Figure 1*). The tourniquet should remain in place no longer than 1 minute.
   PURPOSE: The tourniquet is used to make the veins more prominent. A quick check of the radial pulse will ensure the tourniquet is not applied too tightly.

7. Ask the patient to make a fist.
   PURPOSE: Clenching the fist produces engorgement of the vein.

8. Select the venipuncture site by palpating the antecubital space, and use your index finger to trace the path of the vein and to judge its depth. The vein most often used is the median cephalic, which lies in the middle of the elbow (Figure 2*).
   PURPOSE: The index finger is most sensitive for palpating. Do not use the thumb because it has a pulse of its own, which may confuse you.

9. Cleanse the site, starting in the center of the area and working outward in a circular pattern with the alcohol pad (Figure 3*) Allow the area to dry before proceeding.

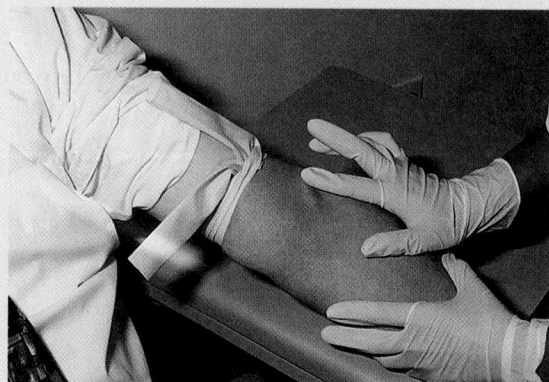

FIGURE 2

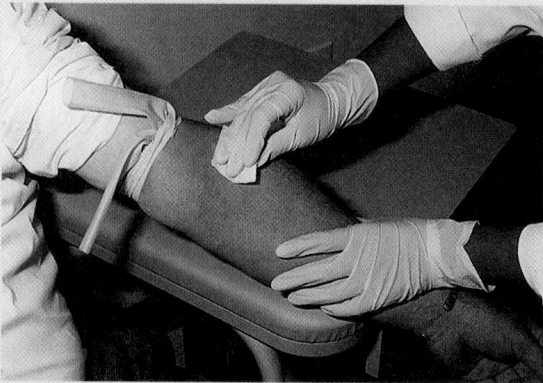

FIGURE 3

FIGURE 1

Continued

PROCEDURE 52-1—cont'd

PURPOSE: The circular pattern helps avoid recontamination of the area. Puncturing a wet area stings and can cause hemolysis of the sample.

10. Hold the syringe in your dominant hand. Your thumb should be on top and your fingers underneath. Remove the needle sheath.

11. Grasp the patient's arm with the nondominant hand while using your thumb and forefinger to draw the skin taut over the site to anchor the vein.
    PURPOSE: Failure to anchor the vein makes puncturing more difficult and painful and may result in a missed vein.

12. Insert the needle through the skin and into the vein with the bevel of the needle up, aligned parallel to the vein, at a 15-degree angle, rapidly, and smoothly (Figure 4*). Observe for a "flash" of blood in the hub of the syringe. Request that the patient release his or her fist.
    PURPOSE: The sharpest point of the needle is inserted first. The angle ensures that the needle does not penetrate through the vein. The appearance ("flash") of blood in the hub ensures that the needle is in the vein.

13. Slowly pull back the plunger of the syringe with the nondominant hand. Do not allow more than 1 mL of headspace between the blood and the top of the plunger. Make sure that you do not move the needle after entering the vein. Fill the barrel to the needed volume (Figure 5*).

14. Release the tourniquet when venipuncture is complete. It must be released before the needle is removed from the arm (Figure 6*).
    PURPOSE: Removal of the tourniquet releases pressure on the vein and helps prevent blood from getting into adjacent tissues and causing a hematoma.

15. Place sterile gauze over the puncture site at the time of needle withdrawal (Figure 7*). Immediately activate the needle safety device.

16. Instruct the patient to apply direct pressure on the puncture site with sterile gauze. The patient may elevate the arm, but it should not be bent.
    PURPOSE: Direct pressure is the best method to stop bleeding. Elevating the arm above the heart also stops bleeding.

17. Transfer the blood immediately to the required tube or tubes using a syringe adapter. Do not push on the plunger during transfer. Discard the entire unit when transfer is complete. Invert tubes after addition of blood, and label with the necessary patient information.
    PURPOSE: The syringe adapter protects against accidental needlesticks and allows the correct amount of blood to be delivered into the tube by vacuum. Pushing the plunger will hemolyze the blood. Blood will begin to clot shortly after collection, so it must be transferred into the vacuum tube and

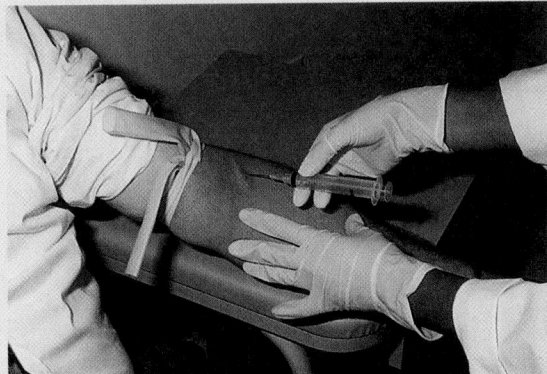

FIGURE 4

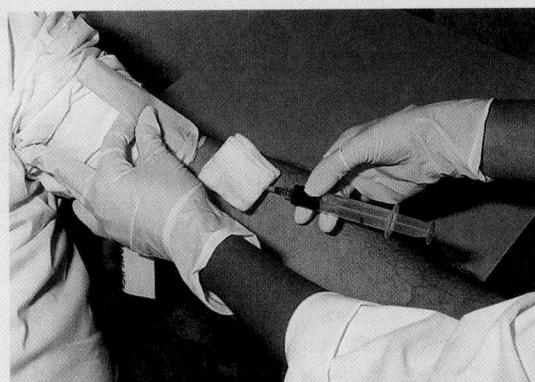

FIGURE 6

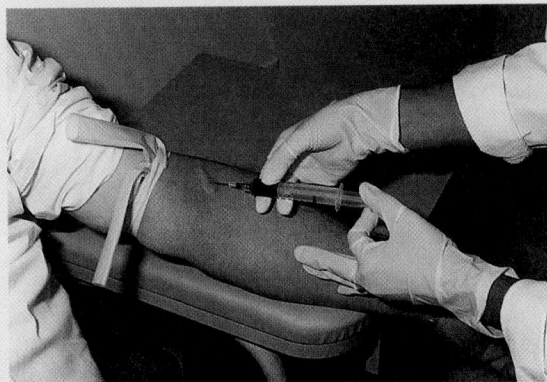

FIGURE 5

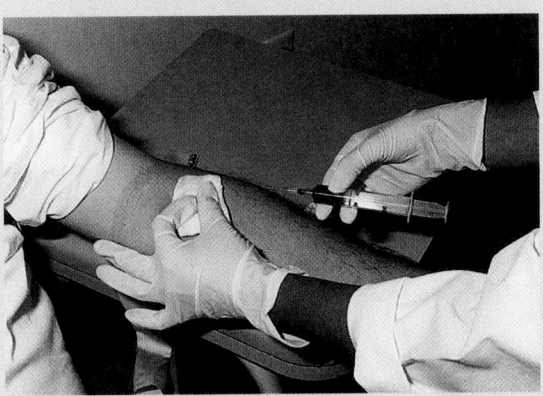

FIGURE 7

Continued

PROCEDURE 52-1—*cont'd*

mixed with anticoagulant immediately after collection. Inverting the tubes ensures anticoagulation.

18. Inspect the puncture site for bleeding or hematoma.
19. Apply a hypoallergenic bandage (Figure 8*).
20. Clean the work area, remove gloves, and wash your hands. Clean the tourniquet with soapy water if it is to be used again. Dispose of any blood contaminated materials such as gauze in a biohazard container.
    <u>PURPOSE:</u> Infection control.
21. Complete the laboratory requisition form, and route the specimen to the proper place. Record the procedure in the patient's record.
    <u>PURPOSE:</u> A procedure is not considered complete until it is recorded.

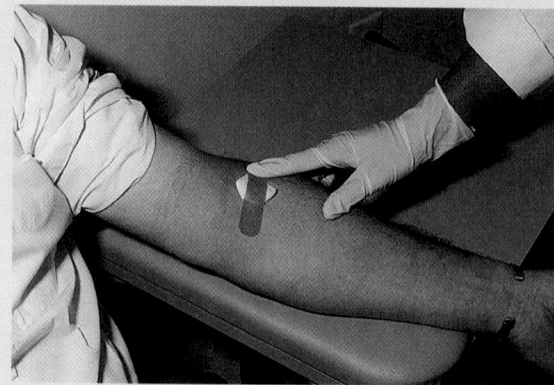

FIGURE 8

PROCEDURE 52-2

Perform Venipuncture: Collect a Venous Blood Sample Using the Evacuated Tube Method

<u>CAAHEP COMPETENCIES:</u> 3.b.(1)(d), 3.b.(1)(e), 3.b.(2)(a), 3.c.(3)(b), 3.c.(4)(b)
<u>ABHES COMPETENCIES:</u> 1.i, 2.a, 2.b, 2.c, 2.i, 4.b, 4.j, 4.q, 4.r, 4.s, 5.b

GOAL: *To collect a venous blood specimen.*

EQUIPMENT and SUPPLIES

- Vacutainer needle, needle holder, and proper tubes for requested tests
- 70% isopropyl alcohol
- Gauze pads
- Tourniquet
- Nonallergenic tape or bandage
- Permanent marking pen
- Biohazard bag or disposal container

PROCEDURAL STEPS

1. Check the requisition form to determine the tests ordered. Gather the correct tubes and supplies that you will need.
   <u>PURPOSE:</u> Allows for proper specimen collection.
2. Wash and dry your hands, and put on nonsterile gloves.
   <u>PURPOSE:</u> Infection control.
3. Identify the patient, explain the procedure, and obtain permission for the venipuncture.
   <u>PURPOSE:</u> Ascertains patient identity, and explanations help gain the patient's cooperation.
4. Assist the patient to sit with the arm well supported in a slightly downward position.
   <u>PURPOSE:</u> Veins of the antecubital fossa are more easily located when the elbow is straight.
5. Assemble equipment. Choice of needle size depends on your inspection of the patient's veins. Attach the needle firmly to the Vacutainer holder. Keep the cover on the needle.
   <u>PURPOSE:</u> A loose needle will cause air to enter the tube, causing frothing and subsequent hemolysis.

6. Apply the tourniquet around the patient's arm 3 to 4 inches above the elbow. The tourniquet should never be tied so tightly that it restricts blood flow in the artery (Figure 1). Tourniquets should remain in place no longer than 60 seconds.
   <u>PURPOSE:</u> The tourniquet is used to make the veins more prominent. A quick check of the radial pulse will ensure the tourniquet is not applied too tightly.
7. Ask the patient to make a fist.
   <u>PURPOSE:</u> Clenching the fist produces engorgement of the vein.

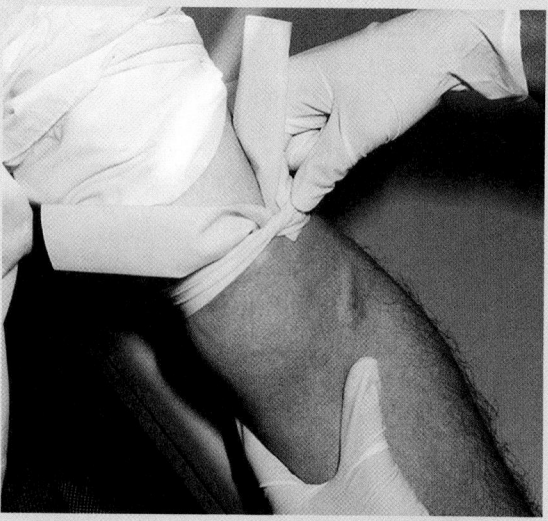

FIGURE 1

Continued

PROCEDURE 52-2—cont'd

Do not ask the patient to pump the fist, as this may disrupt the blood's electrolyte balance.

8. Select the venipuncture site by palpating the antecubital space, and use your index finger to trace the path of the vein and to judge its depth. The vein most often used is the median cephalic, which lies in the middle of the elbow (Figure 2).
PURPOSE: The index finger is most sensitive for palpating. Do not use the thumb, because it has a pulse of its own, which may confuse you.

9. Cleanse the site, starting in the center of the area and working outward in a circular pattern with the alcohol pad (Figure 3).

10. Dry the site with a gauze pad.
PURPOSE: The circular pattern helps avoid recontamination of the area. Puncturing a wet area stings and can cause hemolysis of the sample.

11. Hold the Vacutainer assembly in your dominant hand. Your thumb should be on top and your fingers underneath. You may wish to position the first tube to be drawn in the needle holder, but do not push it onto the double pointed needle past the marking on the holder. Remove the needle sheath.
PURPOSE: Positioning the hand in this manner provides the best visibility of the needle entering the site. Pushing the tube onto the double-pointed needle will cause air to rush into the tube, destroying the vacuum.

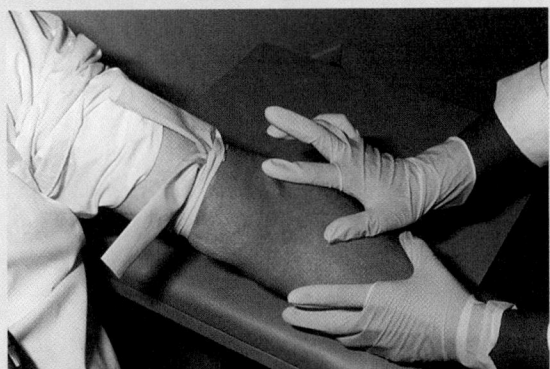

FIGURE 2

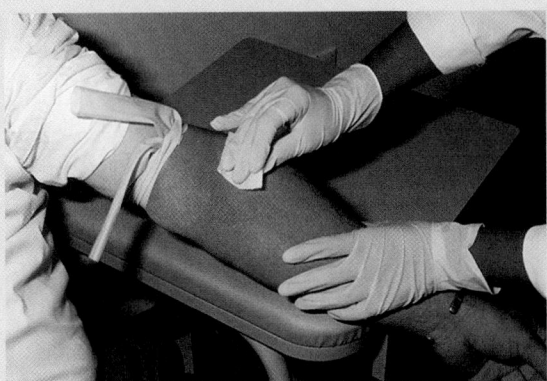

FIGURE 3

12. Grasp the patient's arm with the nondominant hand while using your thumb and forefinger to draw the skin taut over the site, to anchor the vein.
PURPOSE: Failure to anchor the vein makes puncturing more difficult and painful and may result in a missed vein.

13. Insert the needle through the skin and into the vein with the bevel of the needle up, aligned parallel to the vein, at a 15-degree angle, rapidly, and smoothly (Figure 4).
PURPOSE: The sharpest point of the needle is inserted first. Inserting the needle quickly minimizes pain.

14. Place two fingers on the flanges of the needle holder and, with the thumb, push the tube onto the double-pointed needle. Make sure that you do not change the needle's position in the vein. When blood begins to flow into the tube, ask the patient to release the fist.
PURPOSE: The thumb has the strength necessary to push the needle swiftly through the stopper. If you are not careful, however, it is easy to push the needle further into the site when pushing the tube.

15. Allow the tube to fill to maximum capacity. Remove the tube by curling the fingers underneath and pushing on the needle holder with the thumb. Take care not to move the needle when removing the tube.
PURPOSE: Tubes must be full to ensure proper anticoagulant-to-blood ratio. Moving the needle may result in inadvertent penetration of the other side of the vein or slipping of the needle out of the vein.

16. Insert the second tube into the needle holder, following the instructions in the previous steps. Continue filling tubes until the order on the requisition is filled. Gently invert each tube immediately after removing from the needle holder to mix anticoagulants and blood. As the last tube is filling, release the tourniquet.
PURPOSE: The tourniquet should remain in place for no longer than 1 minute to prevent hemoconcentration. Gentle inversion prevents clotting of blood. Vigorous mixing may cause hemolysis.

17. Remove the last tube from the holder. Place gauze over the puncture site (Figure 5), and quickly remove the needle,

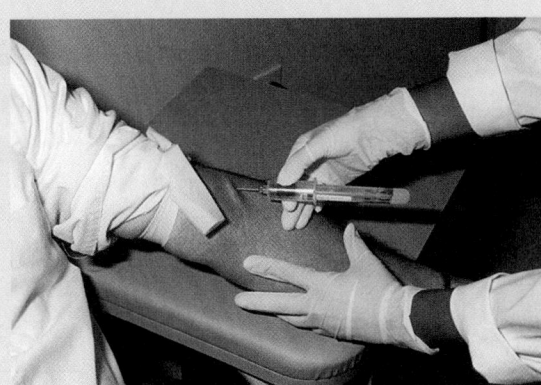

FIGURE 4

Continued

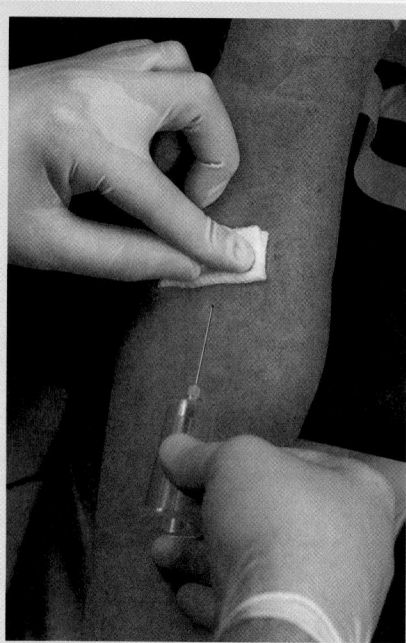

FIGURE 5

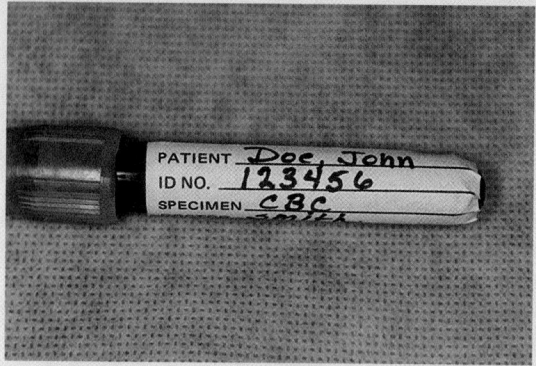

FIGURE 6

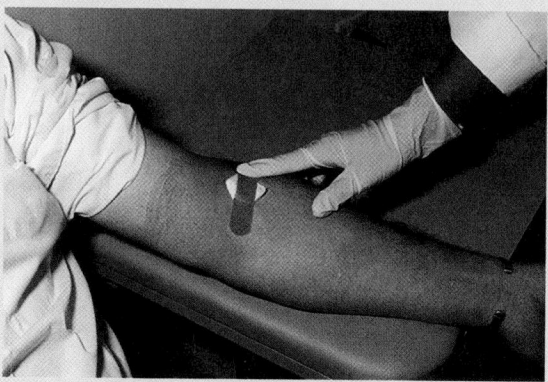

FIGURE 7

engaging the safety device. Dispose of the entire unit in the sharps container.
PURPOSE: Infection control.

18. Apply pressure to the gauze, or instruct the patient to do so. The patient may elevate the arm but should not bend it.
PURPOSE: Direct pressure is the best method to stop bleeding. Elevating the arm above the heart also stops bleeding.

19. Label tubes with the patient's name, the date, and the time (Figure 6).

20. Check the puncture site for bleeding and hematoma formation.

21. Apply a hypoallergenic bandage (Figure 7).

22. Clean the work area, remove gloves, and wash your hands. Clean the tourniquet with soapy water if it is to be used again. Dispose of any blood contaminated materials such as gauze in a biohazard container.
PURPOSE: Infection control.

23. Complete the laboratory requisition, and route to the proper place. Record the procedure in the patient's record.
PURPOSE: A procedure is considered not done until it is recorded.

See Appendix D for a charting example.

PROCEDURE 52-3

Perform Venipuncture : Perform Venipuncture with a Winged Infusion Set (Butterfly Needle)
CAAHEP COMPETENCIES: 3.b.(1)(d), 3.b.(1)(e), 3.b.(2)(a), 3.c.(3)(b), 3.c.(4)(b)
ABHES COMPETENCIES: 1.i, 2.a, 2.b, 2.c, 2.i, 4.b, 4.j, 4.q, 4.r, 4.s, 5.b

GOAL: *To obtain the venous sample accurately from a hand vein using a winged infusion set.*

EQUIPMENT and SUPPLIES

- Tourniquet
- Alcohol pads or other antiseptic preps
- Gauze pads
- Winged infusion ("butterfly") needle set

- Appropriate tubes with a needle and needle adapter
- Syringe with needle
- Sharps disposal container
- Nonallergenic bandage
- Permanent marking pen
- Biohazard bag or disposal container

Continued

PROCEDURE 52-3—cont'd

PROCEDURAL STEPS

1. Check the requisition, and gather the appropriate tubes for the needed tests. Assemble the balance of your supplies.
   PURPOSE: Efficiency in preparation.
2. Wash your hands, and put on gloves.
   PURPOSE: Infection control.
3. Identify the patient, and explain the procedure.
   PURPOSE: Ascertain patient's identity; explanations help to gain the patient's cooperation.
4. Remove the butterfly device from the package, and stretch the tubing slightly. Take care not to accidentally activate the needle-retracting safety device.
   PURPOSE: To keep the tube from recoiling.
5. Attach the butterfly device to the syringe (Figure 1) or needle holder (Figure 2). Figure 2 shows a pediatric tube with a pediatric tube adapter.
6. Seat the first tube into the evacuated tube holder, and place the unit carefully in a place where it will not roll away.
7. Apply a tourniquet to the patient's wrist, just proximal to the wrist bone. Do not apply the tourniquet so tightly that blood flow in the arteries is impeded.
8. Hold the patient's hand in your nondominant hand, with the fingers lower than the wrist.
   PURPOSE: This position helps in identifying the veins and draw site.

9. Select a vein, and cleanse the site at the **bifurcation** (forking) of the veins.
10. Using your thumb, pull the patient's skin taut over the knuckles.
    PURPOSE: Stretching the skin prevents the veins from rolling underneath.
11. With the needle at a 10- to 15-degree angle, bevel up, align it with the vein (Figure 3).
12. Insert the needle by holding the wings or the rear of the set. After insertion the wings are never to be touched again. Ensure that the safety device is not activated.
    PURPOSE: Inserting the needle by holding the wings gives a greater sense of control. If the sides are held, the safety shield will slide forward over the needle when the point of the needle makes contact with the skin.
13. Draw blood into the syringe (Figure 4) or push the blood-collecting tube onto the end of the holder (Figure 5). Note the position of the hands while drawing the blood. When drawing blood into the syringe, ensure that the vacuum you create is slow and steady and that no more than 1 mL of head space

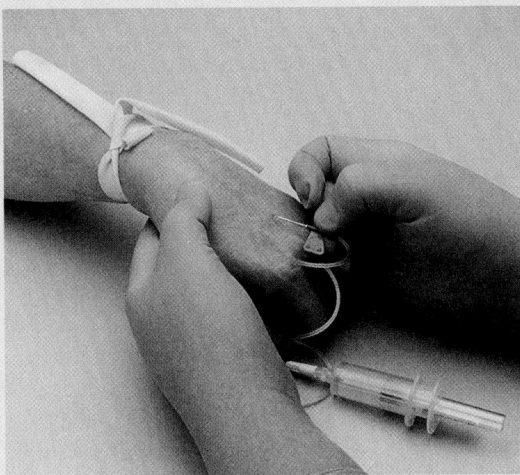

FIGURE 3

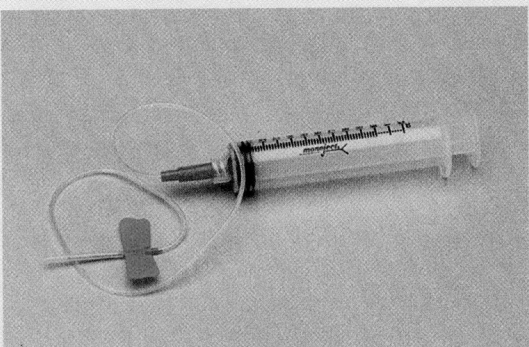

FIGURE 1

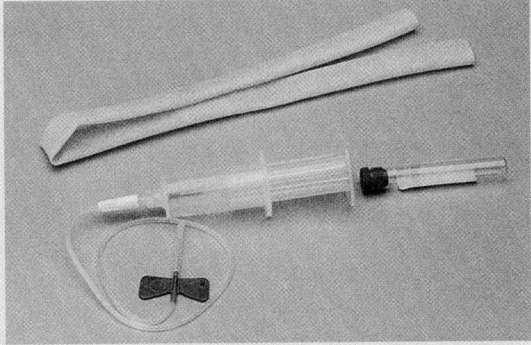

FIGURE 2

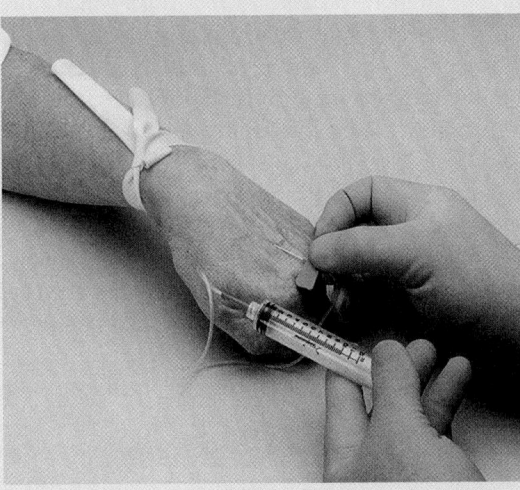

FIGURE 4

Continued

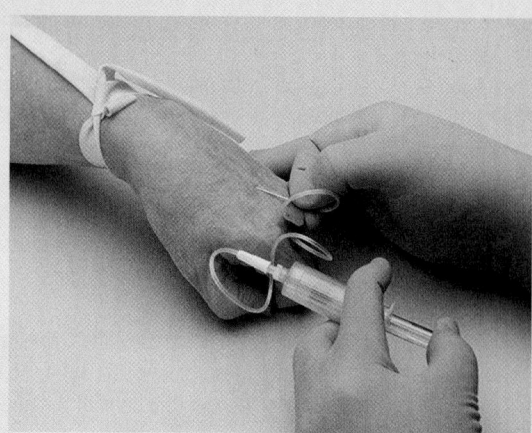

FIGURE 5

between the blood and the plunger is seen.

<u>PURPOSE:</u> Drawing blood too forcefully into the syringe may collapse the vein or hemolyze the blood.

14. Release the tourniquet when the blood appears in the tube or a "flash" of blood is seen in the hub of the syringe.

<u>PURPOSE:</u> The tourniquet should remain in place for no longer than one minute to prevent hemoconcentration.

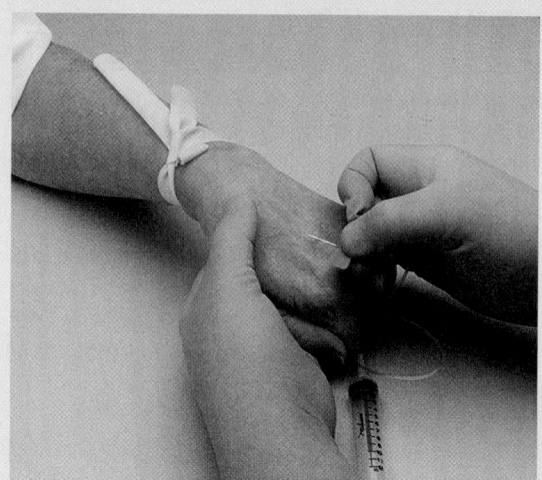

FIGURE 6

15. Always keep the tube and the holder in a downward position so that the tube will fill from the bottom up.

16. Place a gauze pad over the puncture site, and gently remove the needle (Figure 6).

17. Complete the procedure as you would for an antecubital draw (see Procedure 52-2, steps 19 through 23).

PROBLEMS ASSOCIATED WITH VENIPUNCTURE

Failure to obtain blood can be the result of a number of factors. Determining the cause of the problem may help you to decide whether you will be successful on the second attempt. The first issue before you is to remain calm so that you can think clearly, systematically determining the possible cause of the problem.

A hematoma is a large, painful bruised area at the puncture site caused by blood leaking into the tissue, which causes the tissue around the puncture site to swell. The most frequent causes of hematoma formation during the draw are excessive probing to locate the vein, failure to insert the needle far enough into the vein, and the needle going through the vein. A hematoma can form after a draw if you fail to remove the tourniquet before removing the needle or fail to apply adequate pressure on the puncture site or if the elbow is bent while pressure is applied. If a hematoma forms, discontinue the procedure stat, apply pressure to the area for a minimum of 3 minutes, then apply an ice pack to the area. Notify the physician, and observe the site to determine whether the bleeding has stopped. An incident report will need to be completed and recorded in the patient's record.

Fainting, or **syncope**, can have serious consequences, and the phlebotomist must always be prepared. Securing a patient in a blood collection chair will prevent bodily injury to the patient should he or she faint. Constant conversation with the patient during the procedure can identify an impending episode, as can observing the patient's face and breathing rate.

Should the patient begin to faint, quickly remove the tourniquet and needle from the arm and get the needle out of harm's way to prevent an accidental exposure. An ammonium carbonate, or smelling salts, capsule can revive the patient. The capsule should be held away from the face as it is crushed between the fingers, then it should be held approximately 4 inches away from the nostrils until the patient regains consciousness. The ammonia fumes irritate the membranes of the nose and lungs, which in turn triggers a reflex that causes the muscles that control breathing to work faster. Do not allow the contents of the capsule to drip onto the skin or into the mouth, nose, or eyes of the patient, as it can cause caustic burns.

Nerve damage can be a consequence, albeit unlikely, of venipuncture. Preventive measures include avoiding the basilic vein and refraining from blind probing if the vein is missed.

Table 52-4 lists some probable solutions to complications. As a general rule it is wise to limit yourself to two attempts to obtain blood from any one patient. If you fail on the second attempt, ask the patient whether he or she would prefer having someone else try or whether it would be better to come back at another time. This maneuver lets the patient feel that he or she is in control of the situation. At one time or another everyone is unsuccessful at obtaining a needed blood sample, so do not feel that you are a failure.

TABLE 52-4 Managing Blood Draw Complications

POSSIBLE COMPLICATION	STRATEGIES
Burned area	Choose another site because these areas are prone to infection.
Convulsions	Stay calm. Remove the needle, then help guide the patient to the floor, protecting him or her from injury. Call for help.
Damaged or scarred veins or infected areas	Look for an alternative site; do not draw blood from scarred or infected areas.
Edema	Avoid the area; look for an alternative site.
Hematoma	Adjust the depth of the needle or remove the needle and apply pressure.
Intravenous (IV) therapy or blood transfusion sites	Blood samples should not be drawn from an arm that is also the site for IV infusion or blood transfusion owing to the dilution factor.
Mastectomy	Do not draw blood from the site of the mastectomy, because mastectomy surgery causes lymphostasis, which may produce false results.
Nausea	Place a cold cloth on the patient's forehead, give the patient a basin in case of vomiting, and instruct him or her to take deep breaths. Alert the physician.
No blood	Manipulate the needle slightly, or remove the Vacutainer and perform the blood draw again using a syringe or butterfly setup.
Petechiae	Loosen the tourniquet, because this complication usually results from the tourniquet being in place for longer than 2 minutes.
Syncope (fainting)	Position the patient's head between the knees (if in a sitting position). Check and record the patient's pulse, blood pressure, and respiration rate, and continue to observe the patient. Never leave the patient unattended. Breaking an ammonia capsule and passing it briefly under the nostrils may revive the patient.

CRITICAL THINKING APPLICATION

During her second week at the clinic, Leah is confident that she can perform phlebotomy on her own. Melissa has been a good mentor, and Leah has done quite a few successful "sticks" without any problems. Today, however, she is just having a bad day. Mr. Godfrey Lawrence has come to the clinic with numerous problems, and Dr. Gupta has ordered several blood tests. Mr. Lawrence is uncooperative when he sees that Leah must draw four tubes of blood. He angrily tells her that she cannot take that much blood out of him; she is a vampire and she will drain him. How should Leah deal with this problem?

SPECIMEN RECOLLECTION

Sometimes problems with a sample cannot be determined until the specimen is analyzed in the laboratory. Rejected specimens must be recollected. The laboratory may reject a specimen for reasons that include the following:

- Unlabeled or mislabeled specimen
- Quantity not sufficient
- Defective tube
- Incorrect tube used for test ordered
- Hemolysis
- Clotted blood in an anticoagulated specimen
- Improper handling

Hemolysis is the major cause of specimen rejection. Because it cannot be detected until the blood cells separate from the plasma or serum, it is crucial that steps be taken to prevent red cell damage during collection. Hemolyzed serum or plasma will appear rosy to bright red in color owing to the release of hemoglobin from the cells. Some of the more routine tests that are adversely affected by hemolysis are chemistry tests for electrolytes (such as potassium and sodium), bilirubin, total protein, and numerous liver enzymes (such as alkaline phosphatase and gamma glutamyl transferase). Table 52-5 reviews the major causes of hemolysis during collection.

CRITICAL THINKING APPLICATION

- Leah next must draw a sample from Ms. Danielle Rollins. Ms. Rollins indicates that she has a history of bruising after venipuncture, and sure enough a hematoma begins to rise shortly after Leah inserts the needle. She then notices that Ms. Rollins has become pale and is perspiring. What should Leah do first?
- What other steps should Leah take? Can she still obtain the sample?

CAPILLARY PUNCTURE

Capillaries are small blood vessels that connect small arterioles to small venules. The capillary, or dermal, puncture is an efficient means of collecting a blood specimen when only a small amount of blood is required or when a patient's condition makes venipuncture difficult. Because the requisition will not indicate that the collection is to be made in this manner, you must be familiar with the advantages, limitations, and appropriate uses of this technique. Capillary puncture is warranted in the following situations:

TABLE 52-5 Major Causes of Hemolysis during Collection

CAUSE OF HEMOLYSIS	EXPLANATION	PREVENTION
Alcohol preparation	Transfer of alcohol into the specimen causes hemolysis.	Allow venipuncture site to dry completely.
Incorrect needle size	A high-gauge needle will cause the blood to be forced through a small lumen with great force, shearing the cell membranes; a very low-gauge needle will allow a large amount of blood to suddenly enter the tube with great force, causing frothing.	Choose the correct needle for the job, aiming for a 19- to 23-gauge needle.
Loose connections on the vacuum tube assembly	If the connection between the needle holder and the double-pointed needle or the syringe and needle is loose, air can enter the sample and cause frothing.	Ensure that all connections are tight before beginning the venipuncture.
Removing the needle from the vein with the tube intact	Remaining vacuum in the tube can cause air to be drawn forcefully into the tube, causing frothing.	Remove the final tube from the needle holder before withdrawing the needle from the patient's vein.
Underfilled tubes	Underfilling tubes leads to an improper blood/additive ratio. Certain additives, such as sodium fluoride, in disproportionate amounts can cause hemolysis.	Permit blood to flow into the tubes until no more movement can be seen.
Syringe collections	Pulling back forcibly on the plunger draws blood too quickly through the needle, shearing cell membranes; transferring blood into a vacuum tube further traumatizes red blood cells.	Pump plunger several times before use to loosen it within the barrel. Use the smallest syringe possible. Pace the aspiration rate so that there is no more than 1 mL of air space at any time. Transfer blood into vacuum tube immediately, preferably using a transfer device. *Never* push on the plunger when transferring to a vacuum tube. Angle the syringe so the blood runs gently down the side of the tube, preventing the cells from hitting the bottom of the tube with force.
Mixing tubes too vigorously	All tubes except the red-stoppered tube must be mixed. Anything other than gentle inversion (e.g., shaking) can hemolyze cells.	Gently invert tubes immediately after the draw.
Temperature and transport problems	Trauma and temperature extremes can damage cells. Freezing will cause ice crystals that puncture cell membranes.	Tubes should be transported in the upright position with as little trauma as possible. Temperature should be controlled—not too hot or too cold.
Separation of plasma or serum from red cells	Removing the serum or plasma from the cells minimizes the risk of contaminating the specimen with red cell contents.	Blood samples should be centrifuged, when applicable, as soon as possible, and serum or plasma removed from the cells.
Prolonged tourniquet time	While the tourniquet restricts blood flow, interstitial fluid can leak into the veins and hemolyze red cells.	Adhere to the 1-minute rule for tourniquet application.
Poor collection: blood flowing too slowly into the tube	The lumen of the needle may be blocked because it is too close to the inner wall of the vein.	Withdraw the needle slightly to center it in the vein.

- Older patients
- Pediatric patients (especially under the age of 2 years)
- Patients who require frequent glucose monitoring
- Patients with burns or scars in venipuncture sites
- Obese patients
- Patients receiving intravenous therapy
- Patients who have had a mastectomy
- Patients at risk for venous thrombosis
- Patients who are severely dehydrated
- Tests that require a small volume of blood
- When venous blood and capillary blood are not identical

Capillaries are bridges between arteries and veins, and therefore capillary blood is a mixture of the two. Small amounts of tissue fluid are also present in capillary blood, especially in the first drop. Analyte levels are usually the same in capillary and venous blood, with a few exceptions. Hemoglobin and glucose values will be higher in capillary blood; potassium, calcium, and total protein will be higher in venous blood.

Equipment

Skin Puncture Devices

The device used to perform dermal puncture is the lancet. The devices deliver a quick puncture to a predetermined depth (Figure 52-13). OSHA directs that lancets have retractable blades and/or locks that prevent accidental puncture after use and prevent the device from being reused (Table 52-6). Skin puncture devices should always be discarded in a sharps container.

TABLE 52-6 Lancet Blade Recommendations

DEVICE DEPTH AND DIMENSION	BLOOD VOLUME	APPLICATION
2.25-mm, 28-gauge needle	Single drop	Fingersticks
2.25-mm, 23-gauge needle	Single drop	Fingersticks, glucose testing
1-mm × 1.5-mm blade	Low blood flow	Fingersticks, microhematocrit tube, or drop of blood for glucose or cholesterol testing
1.5-mm × 1.5-mm blade	Medium blood flow	Fingersticks, to fill a single Microtainer tube
2-mm × 1.5-mm blade	High blood flow	Fingersticks, to fill multiple Microtainer tubes

Adapted from www.bd.com/vacutainer/faqs/#urine_faq. Accessed September 2006.

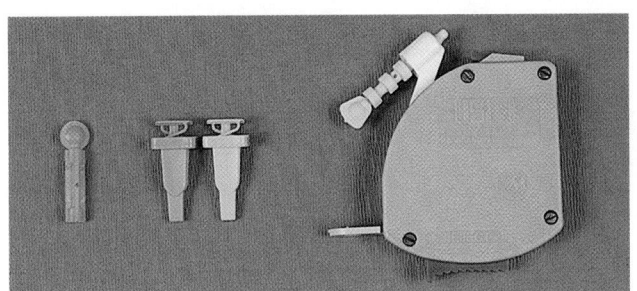

FIGURE 52-13 Skin puncture devices include simple lancets and automated devices that control the depth and width of the incision. (From Bonewit-West K: *Clinical procedures for medical assistants*, ed 6, Philadelphia, 2004, Saunders.)

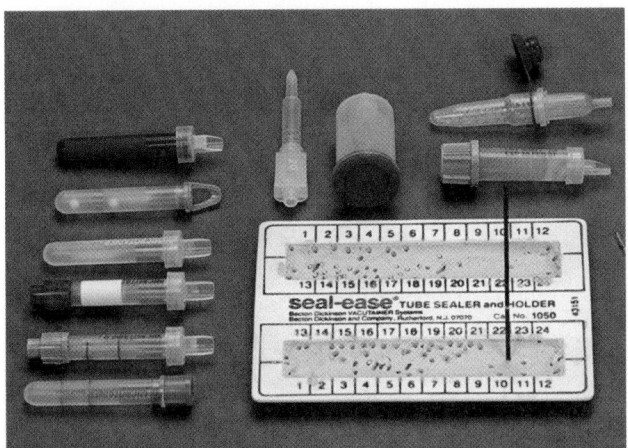

FIGURE 52-14 Microsample containers: Microtainer tubes, capillary tube in sealing clay, and Unopette System.

Collection Containers

Depending on the test to be performed, different types of collection devices and containers are available (Figure 52-14). Microcollection or Microtainer tubes hold up to 750 μl (0.75 mL) of blood and are available with a variety of anticoagulants and additives. The tops are color-coded in the same fashion as evacuated tubes. Blood is collected dropwise into these tubes through a funnel-like device. Capillary tubes are another way to collect blood from a dermal puncture. These are glass or plastic tubes that draw blood by capillary action—that is, the blood fills into these narrow tubes without the need for suction. If the capillary tube is coated with the anticoagulant heparin, a red band will be seen at the top. A common, heparin-coated capillary tube is the microhematocrit tube used for determining the percentage of packed red blood cells in the microhematocrit test (Chapter 53).

The Unopette system (Becton, Dickinson and Company, Franklin Lakes, NJ) is a micropipet and dilution system used for performing manual blood counts. The system includes a reservoir with diluting fluid and a calibrated micropipet.

Manufacturers also provide various collection devices designed to obtain small quantities of blood for "point of care" testing for such analytes as glucose, hemoglobin A_{1c}, and cholesterol (see Chapter 53). The blood is either pulled into the collecting device by capillary action after puncture, or it is dropped onto a reagent strip, which is inserted into the instrument to be analyzed.

Finally, blood from a capillary puncture can be deposited onto paper cards. One such card, known as a *Guthrie card*, is used to test neonates for certain metabolic disorders such as phenylketonuria (PKU). Blood is deposited into circles on biologically inactive filter paper and sent to a referral laboratory for analysis within 24 hours of sampling. Federal postal regulations regarding the mailing of biohazardous material must be followed (Figure 52-15).

Routine Capillary Puncture

Site Selection

In adults and children, the usual puncture site is the ring finger, but capillary blood can be obtained from the middle finger or heel (Figure 52-16). The thumb is usually too callused, and the index finger has extra nerve endings that make the puncture more painful. The fifth finger has too little tissue for a successful puncture. The puncture is made at the tip and slightly to the side of the finger. Be sure to puncture a fleshy area closer to the center of the finger to prevent damage to underlying bone. Avoid areas that are callused, scarred, burned, infected, cyanotic, or edematous.

For children younger than 1 year, dermal puncture is performed on the medial and lateral surfaces of the plantar (bottom) of the heel. Areas other than these are unsafe and may cause bone or nerve damage to an infant. Blood flow from an infant's heel can be increased as much as sevenfold by applying a warm, moist towel (or other warming device) at a temperature no higher than 42° C (108° F) for 3 to 5 minutes. Never place bandages on the heel or anywhere on infants under the age of 2 years. They may peel off and become a choking hazard.

A

FIGURE 52-15 **A,** A Guthrie card used in neonatal screening. (From Sommer SR, Warekois RS: *Phlebotomy: worktext and procedures manual*, Philadelphia, 2002, Saunders. A, Modified from Bonewit-West K: Clinical procedures for medical assistants, ed 6, Philadelphia, 2004, Saunders.)

Correct

Incorrect

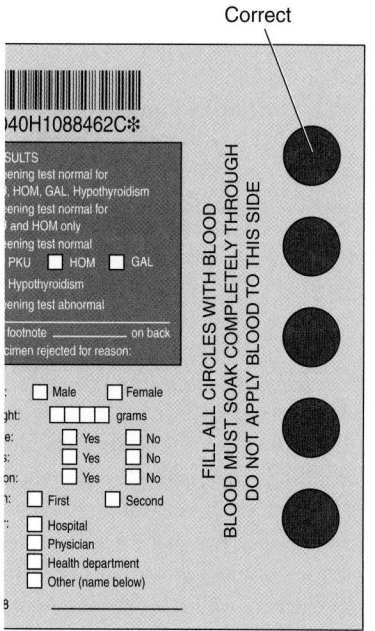
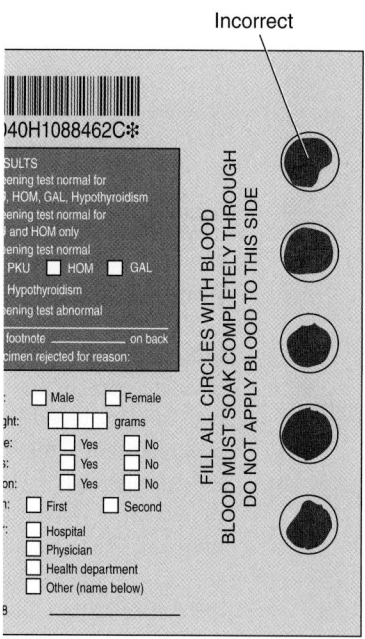

FIGURE 52-15, *cont'd* **B,** Correct and incorrect ways to fill in the circles. (From Sommer SR, Warekois RS: *Phlebotomy: worktext and procedures manual*, Philadelphia, 2002, Saunders.)

B

Patient Preparation

Preparation for a capillary puncture is similar to that for venipuncture. Cleanse the finger well with an alcohol prep pad. If the patient's hands are excessively soiled, request that he or she wash them before the procedure. If the patient's hands are cold, warm them in warm water, drying thoroughly, or ask him or her to rub or shake them vigorously.

Generally, you must work very efficiently when performing a capillary puncture because blood flow stops quickly. Be sure to have your supplies organized and within easy reach. Grasp the finger firmly, applying gentle intermittent pressure, but do not squeeze or "milk" it. Press the puncture device firmly against the skin, and quickly depress the plunger.

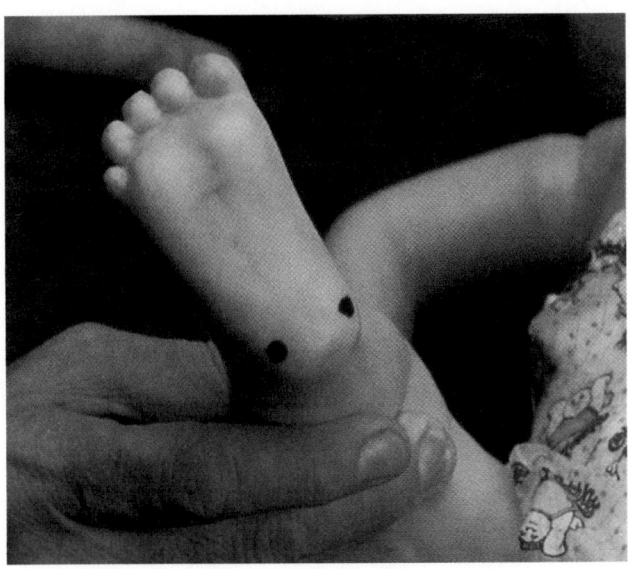
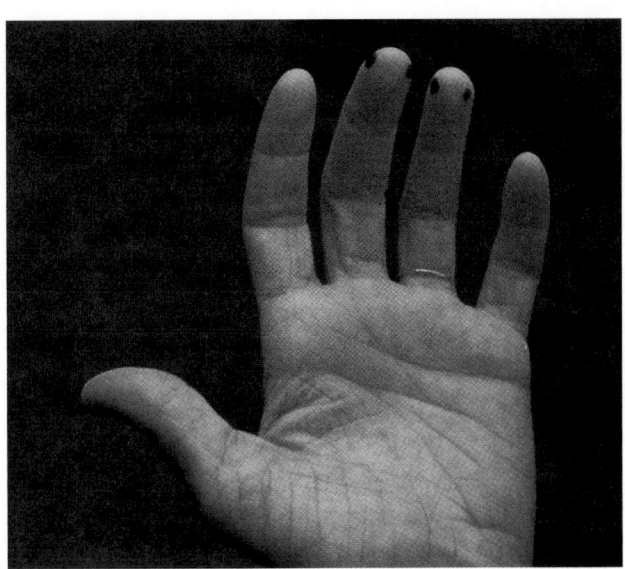

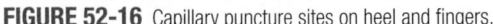

FIGURE 52-16 Capillary puncture sites on heel and fingers.

Collecting the Specimen

After puncturing the dermis, it is important to wipe away the first drop of blood with gauze. This drop contains tissue fluid that could interfere with test results. Fill the sampling containers according to the manufacturer's directions. Touch the container to the drop of blood as it is released from the puncture site, but do not touch the skin. If blood flow stops, wiping the site with clean gauze may reinitiate flow. Be prepared for blood to contaminate your gloves or surfaces by having spare gloves, extra gauze pads, and disinfectant nearby. After the containers are filled, ask the patient to apply pressure to the gauze you have placed over the puncture site if he or she is able. Seal containers as recommended by the manufacturer if necessary.

Specimen Handling

Capillary collection containers are often too small to apply a label. The most efficient way to transport capillary tubes is to remove the stopper from a red-topped tube, insert the capillary tubes, sealed-end down, replace the stopper, and label the tube. Microtainer tubes have plastic plugs that fit over the top. They may be placed in either a labeled tube or a labeled zipper-lock bag for transport. Always decontaminate collection containers before delivering them to the laboratory if blood was deposited on the surface during collection. The procedure for routine capillary collection is outlined in Procedure 52-4.

CRITICAL THINKING APPLICATION

- Melissa calls the first patient into the room. Mrs. Cara Miata is visiting the doctor today to have coagulation studies done. She is a pleasant, talkative woman, 88 years of age. Melissa begins to organize her supplies. She examines Mrs. Miata's arms and decides that it would be best to draw from the hand. Why do you think she makes this decision?
- What supplies will she need to draw from the hand? What tubes will she collect?

PEDIATRIC PHLEBOTOMY

Obtaining blood from children and infants may be difficult and potentially hazardous. The procedure should be performed only by personnel trained in the techniques for pediatric phlebotomy. Successfully obtaining blood from children requires skill and an understanding of pediatric psychologic development as well as appropriate communication skills. The phlebotomist must gain the confidence of the child and must often gain the confidence of the parent as well. Parents often ask the phlebotomist to explain what tests are being done and why. You should be very careful when divulging information in this case; never tell the parents what disease or condition a specific blood test detects. Defer questions to the child's physician. A parent or guardian may or may not be an asset during the procedure. Ask the parent about the child's previous phlebotomy experiences, and ask how cooperative the child is likely to be. Tactfully determine if the parent is comfortable with assisting in restraining an uncooperative child. Parental behavior greatly influences the child's behavior during the procedure. Children should never be restrained as to cause physical injury. If the parent is unable or unwilling to assist with necessary restraint, always refer to the office or laboratory policy on restraints and procedural holds. Table 52-7 (p. 1178) provides information on typical fears and concerns of children during the procedure and suggested parental involvement.

Removing large quantities of blood, especially from premature infants, may result in anemia (Table 52-8, p. 1178). The amount of blood withdrawn must be recorded in the child's chart. Puncturing deep veins in children may result in cardiac arrest, hemorrhage, venous thrombosis, damage to surrounding tissues, or infection. In addition, harm could come to the child during forceful restraint. To prevent these occurrences, blood should be collected only by dermal puncture from children under the age of 2, unless the procedure warrants venous collection (lead levels or blood culture). Venipuncture on children under 2 years of age

PROCEDURE 52-4

Perform Capillary Puncture

<u>CAAHEP COMPETENCIES:</u> 3.b.(1)(d), 3.b.(1)(e), 3.b.(2)(b), 3.c.(3)(b), 3.c.(4)(b)
<u>ABHES COMPETENCIES:</u> 1.i, 2.a, 2.b, 2.c, 2.i, 4.b, 4.j, 4.q, 4.r, 4.s, 5.b

GOAL: *To collect a capillary blood specimen suitable for testing, using fingertip puncture technique.*

EQUIPMENT and SUPPLIES

- Sterile disposable safety lancet
- 70% alcohol prep pads
- Gauze pads
- Nonallergenic tape
- Appropriate collection containers such as capillary tubes or Microtainer devices
- Sealing clay or caps for capillary tubes
- Permanent marking pen
- Biohazard bag or disposal container

PROCEDURAL STEPS

1. Read requisition, and gather all needed supplies.
   <u>PURPOSE:</u> Efficiency.
2. Wash and dry your hands. Put on nonsterile gloves.
3. Identify the patient, and explain the procedure.
   <u>PURPOSE:</u> Ascertain patient identity; explanations help to gain the patient's cooperation.
4. Assemble the needed materials based on the physician's requisition.
   <u>PURPOSE:</u> Once the skin has been punctured, the collection must proceed as rapidly as possible so the blood does not clot before the entire specimen has been collected.
5. Select a puncture site depending on the age of the patient and the sample to be obtained (side of middle or ring finger of nondominant hand, medial or lateral curved surface of the heel, or the great toe for an infant).
   <u>PURPOSE:</u> The nondominant hand may have fewer calluses. The side of the finger is less sensitive, and the skin is usually not as thick. Use great caution when performing capillary puncture on infants.
6. Gently rub the finger along the sides.
   <u>PURPOSE:</u> This promotes circulation. If the finger is very cold, you may immerse it in warm water or moisten it with warm towels.

7. Clean the site with alcohol, and dry it with sterile gauze (Figure 1).
   <u>PURPOSE:</u> Puncturing skin wet with alcohol is painful and can hemolyze the specimen.
8. Grasp the patient's finger on the sides near the puncture site with your nondominant forefinger and thumb.
   <u>PURPOSE:</u> Firmly holding the site allows control of the puncture.
9. Hold the lancet at a right angle to the patient's finger, and make a rapid, deep puncture on the patient's fingertip (Figure 2).
   <u>PURPOSE:</u> Lancets are designed to puncture at specific depths that will permit the free flow of blood.
10. Wipe away the first drop of blood with clean gauze (Figure 3). Dispose of the lancet in the sharps container.
    <u>PURPOSE:</u> The first drop of blood contains tissue fluid.
11. Apply gentle pressure to cause the blood to flow freely.
    <u>PURPOSE:</u> Forceful squeezing liberates fluid that dilutes the blood and causes inaccurate results.
12. Collect blood samples.
    a. Express a large drop of blood, touch the end of the tube to the drop of blood (not the finger), fill capillary tubes

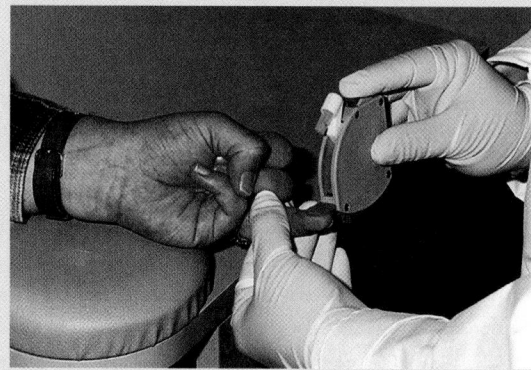

FIGURE 2

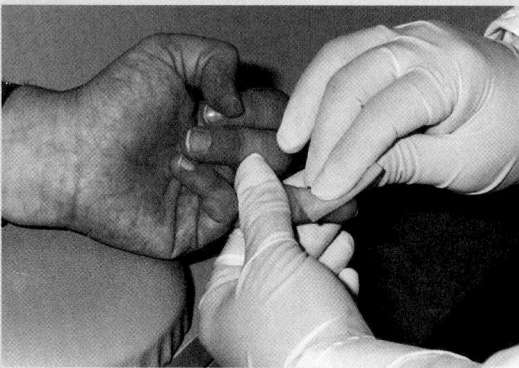

FIGURE 1

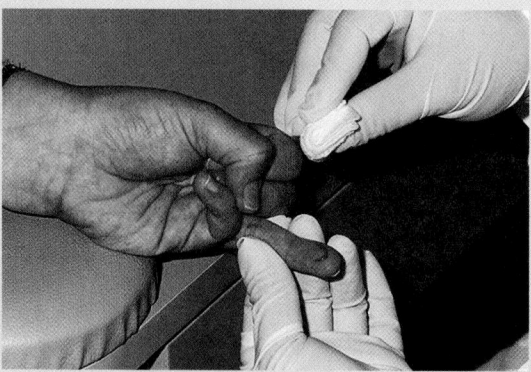

FIGURE 3

Continued

PROCEDURE 52-4—cont'd

(Figure 4, A), place the finger over the blood-free end of the tube, and seal the other end of the tube by inserting it into the sealing clay (Figure 4, B). The tube should be approximately three quarters full before it is sealed.

PURPOSE: Placing the finger over the capillary tube prevents the blood from dripping onto the sealing clay.

b. Wipe the finger with a clean sterile gauze pad, express another large drop of blood, and fill a Microtainer (Figure 5). Do not touch the container to the finger. If more blood is needed, wipe the puncture with clean gauze and gently squeeze another drop. Cap the tube when the collection is complete.

PURPOSE: Touching the container to the finger irritates the puncture site and may cause infection.

13. Apply pressure to the site with clean sterile gauze (Figure 6) when collection is complete. The patient may be able to assist with this step.

14. Select an appropriate means for labeling the containers. Capillary tubes can be placed in a red-topped tube, which is subsequently labeled. Microtainers can be placed in zipper-lock bags that are subsequently labeled.

15. Check the patient for bleeding, clean the site if traces of blood are visible, and apply a nonallergenic bandage if indicated.

16. Dispose of used materials in proper containers.

17. Clean the work area. Remove gloves. Wash your hands. Clean the tourniquet with soapy water if it is to be used again. Dispose of any blood-contaminated materials such as gauze in a biohazard container.

PURPOSE: Infection control.

18. Record the procedure in the patient's record.

PURPOSE: A procedure is considered not done until it is recorded.

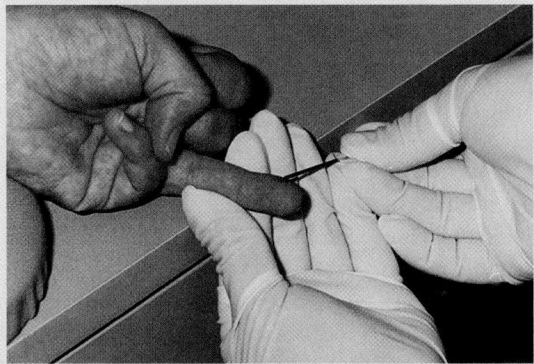

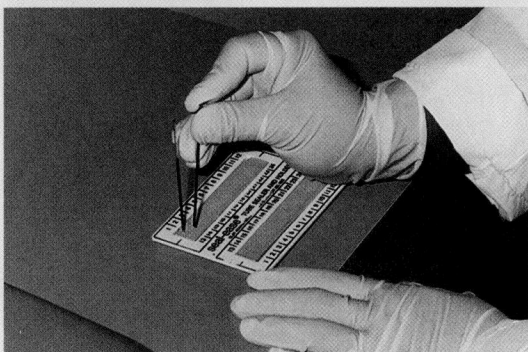

FIGURE 4

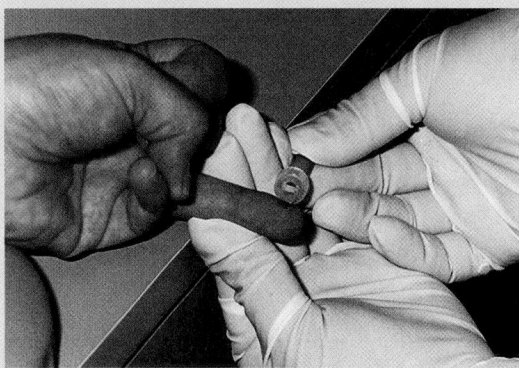

FIGURE 5

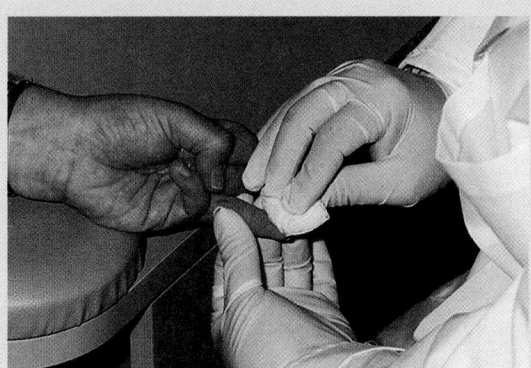

FIGURE 6

should be performed only on superficial veins, including the dorsal hand vein, using a 23-gauge winged infusion set coupled to a syringe or a pediatric vacuum tube collection set.

When required to perform pediatric phlebotomy, wearing a colorful smock, being truthful about the discomfort the child will feel, and providing tokens and praise for bravery will go a long way toward allaying a child's fears. Topical anesthetic creams and disks may be prescribed to lessen pain at the puncture site, but they must be applied at least 1 hour in advance of the procedure. In most cases a calm, professional phlebotomist who

understands the developmental needs of the child and relates to the child on that level can gain the acceptance necessary to perform a successful venipuncture or dermal puncture with a minimum of restraint and frustration.

Postcollection Specimen Handling

It has been said that the results of laboratory testing are only as good as the specimen sent for testing. Specimens that are handled improperly after collection may provide erroneous results, causing unnecessary compromise to the patient's health.

TABLE 52-7 Childhood Behavior and Parental Involvement During Phlebotomy

AGE	TYPICAL MENTAL STATE	SUGGESTED PARENTAL INVOLVEMENT
Newborns (0-12 months)	Trust that adults will respond to their needs.	Parent should assist by cradling and comforting child.
Infants and toddlers (1-3 years)	Minimal fear of danger but fear of separation. Limited language and understanding of procedure.	Parent should assist by holding the child providing emotional support.
Preschoolers (3-6 years)	Fearful of injury to body; still dependent on parent.	Parent may be present to provide emotional support and to assist in obtaining child's cooperation.
School-aged children (7-12 years)	Less dependent on parent and more willing to cooperate. Fear loss of self-control (crying).	Child may not want parent present.
Teenagers (13-18 years)	Fully engaged in the process. Embarrassed to show fear and may exhibit hostility to cover emotions.	Teen may not want parent present.

TABLE 52-8 General Guidelines for Pediatric Venipuncture

WEIGHT (LB)	LIMIT DURING A SINGLE DRAW
8-10	3.5 mL
10-15	5 mL
16-40	10 mL
41-60	20 mL
61-65	25 mL
66-80	30 mL

Indeed, from the moment the specimen is collected, analytes in the blood begin to decay, and it is a race against time to provide results that accurately represent a patient's condition at the time of the blood collection. After collection, it may be necessary to process blood before sending the sample to its final destination. For most samples, this involves the separation of the plasma or serum from the red cells. If the tube contains no anticoagulant, blood will begin to clot once it comes into contact with the glass tube. Plastic tubes require the addition of a clot activator, and the SST speckled-top tube has silica additives to accelerate clotting. "Clot" tubes should be allowed to sit upright in a rack for 30 to 60 minutes at room temperature while a solid clot forms. Tubes with clot accelerator should form a dense clot within 30 minutes. The presence of anticoagulants, such as warfarin (Coumadin) or heparin, in the blood may delay clotting. Once the clot has formed, every effort should be made to remove the clot from the serum within 2 hours.

Removal of the clot from the serum requires centrifugation. In order for the thixotropic gel to form the barrier between the clot and the serum, certain g-force, time, and temperature requirements must be met. A minimum g-force of $1000\,g$ must be achieved by centrifugation, the gel must be at 25° C, and the tube must be centrifuged for 10 to 15 minutes. There is no need to remove the serum from the tube after centrifugation, because the gel has formed a barrier over the red blood cells. Once a tube with thixotropic gel has been centrifuged, it cannot be centrifuged again. The serum, however, can be decanted and centrifuged in another tube.

Tests that require plasma dictate that the plasma be removed from the cells as soon as possible. This can be accomplished with centrifugation followed by aspiration of the plasma and transfer to another tube using a disposable pipet. The green-gray marbled-topped tube, with lithium heparin anticoagulant, has a thixotropic gel, which will form the necessary barrier when centrifuged as described previously. Serum is often refrigerated or frozen if testing cannot be performed immediately.

Certain blood tests, such as the complete blood count, require whole blood. It is wise to check the requirements of the laboratory that will perform the testing as to how the specimen should be transported and stored. The College of American Pathologists recommends that whole blood for automated blood counts be refrigerated and tested within 72 hours.

Often specimens must be transported by courier to other facilities. The Department of Transportation (DOT) Hazardous Materials Shipping Regulations apply to anyone packaging or shipping hazardous materials by ground transportation. Those who ship human specimens must be trained in all aspects of handling, packing, and shipping of biohazardous materials.

CHAIN OF CUSTODY

Blood samples may be collected as evidence in legal proceedings. Blood may be drawn for drug and alcohol testing, DNA analysis, or parentage testing. These samples must be handled according to special procedures to prevent tampering, misidentification, or interference with the test results.

Chain of custody is a legal term that refers to the ability to guarantee the identity and integrity of the specimen from collection to reporting of the test results. It is a process used to maintain and document the chronologic history of a specimen. (Documents should include name or initials of the individual collecting the specimen, each person or entity subsequently having custody of it, the date the specimen was collected or transferred, employer or agency, specimen number, patient's or employee's name, and a brief description of the specimen.)

Collection kits are available and will contain everything needed for the venipuncture, including the tube, the needle, the chain of custody forms and seals, the antiseptic, and even the tourniquet. Familiarize yourself with these kits before you are required to use them. You may be required to testify at a legal proceeding if you are involved in the collection or testing of a sample involved in a legal proceeding.

CLOSING COMMENTS

Patient Education

When working as a phlebotomist, the medical assistant must maintain a professional attitude and still be sympathetic to the fears and apprehensions of the patient. By establishing an environment that encourages the patient to relax, the amount of pain and discomfort experienced by the patient during the procedure are kept to a minimum.

If the patient has a positive attitude, you need to provide little explanation about the procedure. Often, the patient can help you by telling from which site the last blood sample was successfully drawn. It is wise to follow the patient's suggestion in choosing the site for the removal of a blood specimen. When a patient is allowed to become an active participant in the procedure, he or she remains more relaxed, talkative, and confident in your expertise as a phlebotomist.

This atmosphere can change dramatically when the patient has had an unpleasant experience and associates pain and discomfort with venipuncture. Such a patient usually is ill at ease, nervous, and apprehensive. When confronted with this scenario, you need to make every effort to perform the procedure quickly, efficiently, and effectively. Once the blood has been drawn and the patient has relaxed, you then will have an opportunity to help the patient develop a positive attitude.

If your patient has a history of syncope when blood is drawn, or if you suspect that this patient may faint during the procedure, have the patient lie down. Assemble your equipment and alert the physician before beginning the procedure. This type of professional care may help the patient get through the procedure without a traumatic effect.

Always remember to identify your patient and explain what you are going to do. Answer any questions the patient may have, and perform the procedure skillfully before anxiety is allowed to set in.

CRITICAL THINKING APPLICATION

- As much as Leah likes children, performing capillary puncture on little fingers is not one of her favorite things to do. Mrs. Spix brings her son Garrett in for a hemoglobin and hematocrit test. Garrett is 3 years old. Mrs. Spix nervously asks Leah about the procedure and the tests that Garrett must have. How can Leah adequately answer Mrs. Spix's questions and make Garrett and his mother feel at ease about this procedure?
- What supplies will she need? Explain how she will perform the capillary puncture.

Legal and Ethical Issues

Venipuncture and microcapillary blood collection are invasive procedures in which a sterile needle or a lancet is inserted through the skin. Because the skin is penetrated, drawing blood becomes a surgical procedure and is subject to the laws and regulations of surgery. When venipuncture is performed, the rules and regulations must be enforced with no deviations from them. Be sure to follow the procedures as written, and also become familiar with the regulations and standards established by local and state agencies as well as Clinical Laboratory Standards Institute and OSHA. Deviations leave the medical assistant open to accusations of malpractice. Document any situations that arise in which observation of the standard of care comes into question.

On rare occasions patients who have scarred veins from intravenous drug use may request that they be allowed to draw their own blood. You should never permit this and should always take precautions that your supplies are protected.

SUMMARY OF SCENARIO

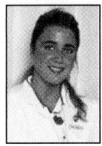

Leah has learned that phlebotomy is truly an art. Although she was nervous at first, she has become quite proficient with this new skill. She discovered that her nervousness was "contagious" and that if she remains calm and organized, her patient is more likely to feel at ease with the procedure. She has learned that it is necessary to talk with the patients before drawing the blood, not only to allay their fears, but also to get clues regarding past problems or the best site for the draw. She has learned that it is her responsibility to explain the tests that are ordered and how much blood she will draw, but that it is not her responsibility to explain why the tests are being done. Effective communication, she has learned, is the most important aspect of phlebotomy.

Through practice and careful attention, Leah has learned the proper equipment to use in phlebotomy and never hesitates to call the referral laboratory used by her employer if she has a question regarding proper collection of a specimen. She has also learned that communicating with children and adults is as different as the equipment she uses for venipuncture; the small veins of children or the elderly require special care, and she has learned to use winged infusion sets and syringes to prevent collapse of the veins. Leah is well aware of the dangers of phlebotomy, and through education and the use of approved safety devices Leah is confident that she can provide excellent care for her patients at the Health Alliance Medical Clinic.

SUMMARY of LEARNING OBJECTIVES

1. Define, spell, and pronounce the terms listed in the vocabulary.
   - Spelling and pronouncing medical terms correctly adds credibility to the medical assistant. Knowing the definition of these terms promotes confidence in communication with patients and co-workers.

2. List the equipment needed for venipuncture.
   - Venipuncture requires the following equipment: a double-pointed safety needle, evacuated collection tubes, a needle holder or a syringe fitted with a safety needle, a tourniquet, an alcohol prep pad, gauze or cotton, a sterile bandage, latex gloves, and a biohazard disposal container.

3. Explain the purpose of a tourniquet.
   - The tourniquet is used to prevent venous flow out of the site, causing the veins to bulge. The tourniquet makes veins easier to locate and puncture.

4. Explain how to apply a tourniquet and three consequences of improper application.
   - Tourniquets are snugly applied around the upper arm (or wrist for a hand draw) in a fashion that permits easy release. Leaving the tourniquet on for a prolonged period results in hemoconcentration; applying the tourniquet too tightly results in unnecessary discomfort to the patient and in release of tissue fluid into the blood.

5. Describe the types of sharps used in phlebotomy.
   - The venipuncture needle has a shaft with one end cut at an angle (bevel). The other end attaches to the syringe or to a needle holder and is called the hub. The opening in the tip is called the lumen and is measured in gauge numbers. Double pointed needles are used with the evacuated tube method. Needles with special adapters are used with disposable syringes. Lancets are used for dermal puncture.

6. Discuss the use of sharps with engineered sharps injury protection.
   - OSHA mandates that all sharps used for phlebotomy are engineered with safety devices. Safety devices include retractable needles, self-sheathing needles, and blunting devices. Needles should never be recapped, and in most cases they are not removed from the venipuncture unit. All sharps must be disposed of in an approved sharps container.

7. Explain why one chooses a syringe for blood collection rather than an evacuated tube.
   - Syringes are more commonly used for blood collection from elderly patients, whose veins tend to be more fragile; from children, whose veins tend to be small; and from obese patients, whose veins tend to be deep. Using a syringe allows a more controlled draw. Syringes are commonly used with winged-infusion sets.

8. Explain why the stopper colors on evacuated tubes differ.
   - Vacuum tubes have various colored stoppers that indicate the contents of the tube. Certain additives are compatible with certain laboratory tests. The phlebotomist must be knowledgeable about blood tests and the type of tube needed. Consulting manufacturer-provided literature will ensure the proper choice of the collection tube.

9. State the correct order in which various types of tubes should be collected.
   - Blood for the various types of tubes should be collected in the following order: (1) Sterile or SPS, (2) light blue, (3) red or red-speckled, (4) green, (5) lavender, and (6) gray. Evacuated tubes should be collected in a specific order to prevent carryover of tube additives.

10. Describe how to insert a needle properly into the vein and how it should be removed.
    - Needles are inserted into the vein at a 15- to 30-degree angle. Do not probe excessively if you are unsuccessful, because probing can lead to a hematoma or nerve damage. Before the needle is removed, the tourniquet should be released. Immediately after removal, the safety device should be activated and the unit should be placed in the sharps container.

11. List, in order, the steps of a routine venipuncture.
    - A routine venipuncture begins with greeting and identifying the patient. The medical assistant then assembles the equipment, locates the vein, draws the blood, removes and properly disposes of the needle, tends to the puncture site, labels the tubes, and delivers them to the laboratory. The medical assistant observes standard precautions during the procedure.

12. Describe and name the veins that may be used for blood collection.
    - The median cephalic vein is the vein of choice for phlebotomy, but blood can be drawn from the cephalic vein and the median basilic vein. Avoid the basilic vein if possible. The dorsal vein on the hand may be used.

13. Explain the reasoning behind choosing why one chooses a winged infusion set (butterfly) over an evacuated tube.
    - A winged infusion set (butterfly) is used on blood draws from the hand and from children. The needle is shorter, and the wings assist with holding and guiding the needle. The tubing minimizes the vacuum and prevents collapse of fragile veins. Using a syringe can control the vacuum to a greater extent than using vacuum tubes.

14. Perform a venipuncture using a winged infusion set.
    - Refer to Procedure 52-3.

15. List situations in which capillary puncture would be preferred over venipuncture.
    - Capillary puncture is preferred over venipuncture for certain tests, such as **hematocrit** or hemoglobin analysis. Capillary puncture is routinely performed on children under the age of 2 years.

16. Discuss proper dermal puncture sites.
    - The middle two fingers (the lateral sides of each) are generally used for capillary puncture. For infants the heel is the site of choice. The center of the heel must be avoided.

17. Describe dermal puncture devices, and discuss safety features they may have.
    - Dermal puncture devices are made of sharp sterile metal. The size of the needle or blade must be chosen based on the amount of blood that is needed for the test. All dermal puncture

Continued

SUMMARY of LEARNING OBJECTIVES
Continued

devices must have internal safety devices that retract the blade after use.

18. Describe containers that may be used to collect capillary blood.
    - Capillary blood can be collected in Microtainer devices, in capillary tubes, or on paper test cards. The Microtainer devices may contain anticoagulants and will have stopper colors consistent with vacuum tubes.

19. List the steps for capillary puncture.
    - Capillary puncture is performed much like venipuncture. No tourniquet is used, however. The site is prepared and punctured; the first drop of blood is wiped away; the containers are filled with drops of blood expressed from the site; and bleeding is stopped by pressure to the site with gauze.

20. Explain why the first drop of blood is wiped away when a capillary puncture is performed.
    - The first drop of blood contains tissue fluid which could affect test results.

21. Perform a capillary puncture.
    - Refer to Procedure 52-4.

22. Collect a capillary sample in a microhematocrit tube and in a capillary tube.
    - Refer to Procedure 52-4.

23. Explain the consequences of an accidental needlestick.
    - Percutaneous puncture with a contaminated sharp brings with it the possibility of infection. The infectious agents of major concern include HBV, HCV, and HIV.

24. Describe a plan of action after an accidental sharps exposure.
    - OSHA requires that employers have a PEP in place for accidental sharps exposures. Plans generally include means to cleanse the wound with an appropriate antiseptic cleanser; evaluate the exposure to determine whether the HCW is at risk for contracting HBV, HCV, or HIV, depending on the circumstance of the injury and information gathered about the source of the blood involved; provide prophylactic care if necessary; provide counseling and advice for the injured and the source; and follow up on the exposure.

25. Differentiate whole blood, serum, and plasma, and give an example of a test performed with each.
    - Whole blood will coagulate unless mixed with an anticoagulant. Many anticoagulants are available; the anticoagulant must be matched with the test so as not to interfere with results. Whole blood is required for the complete blood count and differential. When clotted blood is centrifuged, the cells and liquid separate and the liquid portion is referred to as serum. Most chemistry and serology testing is performed on serum. When anticoagulated blood is centrifuged, the liquid that remains is referred to as plasma. Plasma may be used for coagulation studies and blood glucose testing.

26. Describe handling and transport methods for blood after collection.
    - Blood cells can easily hemolyze and alter test results; therefore serum or plasma should be separated from the cells as soon as possible after collection. This is achieved by centrifugation. Blood samples that are to be transported must be securely packaged and sent according to regulations set forth by governmental agencies.

CONNECTIONS

 Study Guide Connection: Go to Chapter 52 Study Guide. Read the Case Study and Workplace Applications and complete the assignments. Do online research for answers to the questions in the Internet Activities associated with assisting in phlebotomy.

 CD Connection: Go to the Medical Assisting Competency Challenge CD and do the training activities under Diagnostic Testing and Patient Instruction. For a better understanding of assisting in phlebotomy, view the animation for normal blood clotting.

 Evolve Connection: For more information related to assisting in phlebotomy, go to evolve.elsevier.com/kinn and visit related weblinks for Chapter 52. Click on the Medical Assisting Exam Review and do the practice questions to sharpen your test-taking skills.

Assisting in the Analysis of Blood

Robin R. Patterson

53

SCENARIO

Dana Cummings is a certified medical assistant working in the Westhills Family Practice Center. She is preparing to collect blood from Mr. Corrigan, who has had a renal transplant as a result of complications from type 1 diabetes; he is here today for a routine examination. Dr. Fischbach suspects that Mr. Corrigan is anemic and orders an anemia panel in addition to a renal panel; a hemoglobin A_{1c} level; a complete blood count including hemoglobin, hematocrit, and differential; PT; and ALT/AST testing.

While studying this chapter, think about the following questions:

- Why are so many tests being performed?
- Which of these tests will likely be completed today in the office laboratory?

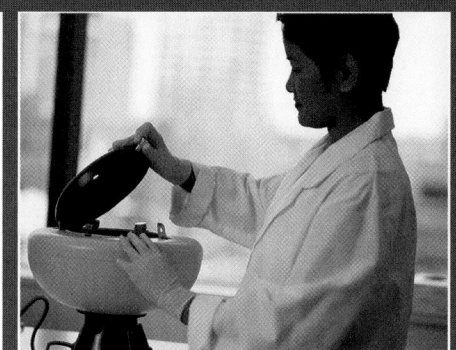

LEARNING OBJECTIVES

1. Define, spell, and pronounce the terms listed in the vocabulary.
2. Name three main functions of blood.
3. Describe the role of the hematology laboratory in patient care.
4. Describe the appearance and function of the erythrocyte.
5. Describe the appearance and function of the granular and the agranular leukocyte.
6. Differentiate between T cells and B cells.
7. Describe the appearance and function of the thrombocyte.
8. Explain the process of clot formation.
9. Identify the anticoagulant of choice for hematology testing.
10. Explain the purpose of a microhematocrit.
11. Accurately perform a microhematocrit.
12. Explain the role of hemoglobin in the body.
13. Determine the level of hemoglobin present in a given blood sample.
14. Identify the tests included in a CBC.
15. Explain the principle behind automated blood cell counting.
16. Describe the RBC indices and how they are calculated.
17. Explain the reasons for performing a differential.
18. Describe the appearance of the five different types of leukocytes seen in a normal Wright-stained differential.
19. Describe the appearance of the normal erythrocyte.
20. Prepare and stain a blood smear using Wright's stain, completing each step in proper sequence.

21. Observe a differential smear, and identify various blood cells from a prepared slide.
22. Cite the reasons for performing an erythrocyte sedimentation rate test.
23. Describe the sources of error for the erythrocyte sedimentation rate test.
24. Determine an erythrocyte sedimentation rate.
25. Describe the tests performed to assess coagulation.
26. Differentiate between the ABO blood groupings and the Rh blood groupings.
27. Discuss rare blood types and the implication of having a rare blood type when transfusion is necessary.
28. Secure a capillary blood sample, and determine the ABO and Rh grouping of the sample.
29. Describe the methodology behind the clinical chemistry testing methods used in the physician's office laboratory.
30. Explain the reasons for testing blood glucose, blood cholesterol, hemoglobin A_{1c}, thyroid hormone levels, and liver enzymes.
31. Perform a glucose test using a U.S. Food and Drug Administration (FDA)–approved glucose monitor.
32. Perform a cholesterol test using an FDA-approved cholesterol monitor.
33. List five typical chemistry panels, the reason for performing each panel, and the individual tests performed in those panels.

National Accreditation Competencies and Content

CAAHEP COMPETENCIES

Clinical

3.b.(1)(d).   Dispose of biohazardous materials
3.b.(1)(e).   Practice Standard Precautions
3.b.(3)(c)(ii).   CLIA waived test: Perform hematology testing
3.b.(3)(c)(iii).   CLIA waived test: Perform chemistry testing

General

3.c.(4)(b).   Perform routine maintenance of administrative and clinical equipment

ABHES COMPETENCIES

Office Management

6.b.   Operate and maintain facilities and perform routine maintenance of administrative and clinical equipment safely

Clinical Duties

4.q.   Dispose of biohazardous materials
4.r.   Practice standard precautions
4.z.   Perform hematology
4.aa.   Perform chemistry testing
4.bb.   Perform immunology testing

VOCABULARY

anemia A condition marked by deficiency of RBCs.

artifacts Structures or features not normally present but visible as a result of an external agent or action, such as one seen in a microscopic specimen after fixation or in an image produced by radiology or electrocardiography.

centrifuge (sen′-truh-fuhj) An apparatus consisting essentially of a compartment spun about a central axis to separate contained materials of different specific gravities or to separate colloidal particles suspended in a liquid.

enzymes Complex proteins that are produced by cells and act as catalysts in specific biochemical reactions.

hormones Substances produced by one tissue and conveyed by the bloodstream to another to effect physiologic activity, such as growth or metabolism.

polycythemia vera (pah-le-si-the′-me-uh/veh′-rah) A condition marked by an abnormally large number of RBCs in the circulatory system.

toxemia An abnormal condition of pregnancy characterized by hypertension, edema, and protein in the urine.

type and cross-match Tests performed to assess the compatibility of blood to be transfused.

urea The major nitrogenous end product of protein metabolism and the chief nitrogenous component of the urine.

urease (yoo′-re-az) An enzyme that catalyzes the hydrolysis of urea to form ammonium carbonate.

The average body holds 10 to 12 pints of blood. The heart circulates the blood through the circulatory system more than 1000 times every day. More than 70,000 miles of passageways, most of which are narrower than a human hair, carry blood throughout the body. The blood is contained in a closed system of vessels, of which the largest is the aorta and the smallest are the capillaries. The capillaries are only one cell layer thick, and these thin, permeable walls allow certain substances to move back and forth between the blood vessels and the surrounding tissue. The circulating blood contains more than 25 trillion cells, and every second the body replaces eight million old red blood cells (RBCs) with eight million new RBCs.

Besides supplying body cells with their needed nutrients and oxygen, the blood also carries away carbon dioxide and **urea,** which are the waste products of normal cell activity. If the blood did not carry away the carbon dioxide and urea, these wastes would accumulate and cause cell damage and possibly **toxemia.** Carbon dioxide is carried in the blood to the lungs, where it is exhaled as part of normal breathing. The blood carries urea to the kidneys where, along with other body wastes, it is excreted in the urine. The blood also distributes **enzymes, hormones,** and other chemicals that the body needs for control and regulation of body activities. In addition, the blood functions to maintain the body at a uniform temperature, to keep other body fluids in a state of pH balance, and to carry the hormones from the secreting gland to the tissues where they are needed.

Blood is the second most common body fluid analyzed in the clinical laboratory. Blood testing is done routinely in the hematology, immunology (serology), immunohematology (blood banking), and chemistry sections of the laboratory. The degree of blood testing performed by medical assistants depends on the level of service of the physician's office and the Clinical Laboratories Improvement Act (CLIA) regulations. As a medical assistant, you will not perform all of the procedures described in this chapter. Some have been replaced with automated procedures, and others are considered highly complex according to the CLIA standards and therefore are not to be performed by a medical assistant. Nevertheless, these procedures are explained in this text because they provide critical background information necessary to understand the analysis of blood, from the collection of the specimen, to testing, and to the recording of the results.

HEMATOLOGY

The hematology section of a laboratory deals with the counting of RBCs, white blood cells (WBCs), and platelets; differentiating WBCs on stained blood smears; measuring the percentage of RBCs in blood (hematocrit); and determining the oxygen-carrying capacity of the blood (hemoglobin).

The complete blood cell count (CBC) is the most frequent laboratory procedure ordered on blood. It gives a fairly complete look at the components of blood and can provide a wealth of information concerning a patient's condition. The CBC routinely includes several tests.

CRITICAL THINKING APPLICATION

- Dana will collect the specimen for Mr. Corrigan's CBC. What tests are included in the CBC? Can any of these tests be performed by capillary puncture? Explain.
- Which vacuum tube will Dana use to collect the CBC?

Whole blood is composed of formed elements suspended in a clear yellow liquid portion called *plasma*. Plasma makes up approximately 55% of blood by volume. The remaining 45% consists of formed cellular elements—the erythrocytes (RBCs), leukocytes (WBCs), and thrombocytes (platelets). These cellular elements all have special functions.

Erythrocytes

RBCs, or erythrocytes, are formed in the red bone marrow of the ribs, sternum, pelvis, and skull and in the ends of long bones in the adult. The immature form of the RBC has a nucleus that disintegrates as the cell matures. Loss of the nucleus results in the familiar shape of the RBC: the biconcave disk, thicker at the rim than in the middle. Erythrocytes transport oxygen from the lungs to the body cells and carry carbon dioxide away from cells, back to the lungs to be exhaled. The main constituent is the red pigment hemoglobin, which is composed of iron and protein. Hemoglobin actually carries oxygen and some carbon dioxide throughout the body.

The life span of an erythrocyte is approximately 120 days. As the cell nears the end of its life, it becomes more fragile and eventually ruptures and breaks. The iron is reused for new RBC formation, and the protein is converted into a bile pigment.

Complete Blood Cell Count Procedures

- Red blood cell count
- White blood cell count
- Hemoglobin determination
- Hematocrit determination
- Differential white blood cell count
- Estimation of platelet numbers
- Red cell indices

Leukocytes

Leukocytes, or WBCs, contain a nucleus and are larger than erythrocytes. The prime function of the leukocyte is to protect the body against infection and disease. The five types of leukocytes are classified into granular and agranular groups. The granular leukocytes are called *polymorphonuclear leukocytes* and include the neutrophils, eosinophils, and basophils. They are characterized by their heavily granulated cytoplasm and segmented nuclei. The agranular leukocytes are the lymphocytes and monocytes, both of which have clear cytoplasm and a solid nucleus.

Granular leukocytes are phagocytic and engulf invading bacteria and viruses. Unlike erythrocytes, leukocytes function in the tissues. During inflammation, the blood carries the WBCs through dilated vessels to the site of injury. Capillary walls become more permeable, and granular cells squeeze through by ameboid motion. Once at the site of infection or injury, the cells engulf the invading microorganism. Pus contains dead leukocytes, bacteria, and tissue cells.

Agranular leukocytes are responsible for the production of antibodies. Agranular leukocytes include the lymphocytes, which are classified into T cells and B cells based on their functional characteristics.

T cells

T cells make up about 65% to 80% of circulating lymphocytes and have a life span of months to years. This is important in conferring long-lasting immunity to microbial infections. T cells are responsible for immune responses to intracellular parasites, viruses, fungi, and bacteria. Delayed hypersensitivity reactions, such as the response to poison ivy, are controlled by T-cell defenses, as is organ transplant rejection. There are several types of T cells, based on function:

- Cytotoxic or killer T cells—kill foreign, virus infected, and tumor cells. They produce proteins called perforans that induce cell death by punching holes in the cell membrane.
- Helper T cells—most numerous type of T cell. They stimulate the activity of other T cells.
- Suppressor T cells—inhibit the activity of other T cells.
- Memory T cells—respond quickly to the presentation of the same antigen at a later date. They have a long life span.
- Natural killer cells—kill cells infected with viruses and tumor cells without prior sensitization.

B cells

B cells are formed in bone marrow then migrate to other lymph organs, where they multiply and reside. When stimulated, B cells differentiate into plasma cells that produce specific antibodies against an antigen. Antibodies circulate in the plasma or are present in secretions. Some antibodies cause cells to clump and precipitate, whereas others activate the complement system. The complement system is a series of reactions between plasma proteins that amplifies the immunologic response to foreign molecules. Activation of the complement system leads to the lysis of microorganisms or their phagocytosis by neutrophils.

Antibodies are protein molecules that attach to antigens. Very small antigens, such as toxins and viruses, can be directly neutralized by antibodies; larger antigens, such as bacteria, require the help of agranular leukocytes. Destroying these pathogens requires three steps:

1. Antigen processing–When a macrophage phagocytizes bacteria, proteins (antigens) from the bacteria are broken down into smaller molecules that are then "displayed" on the macrophage surface attached to special molecules called *major histocompatibility complex class II* (MHC II) molecules. Bacterial proteins are similarly processed and displayed on MHC II molecules on the surface of B lymphocytes.

2. Lymphocyte stimulation–When a T lymphocyte "sees" the same peptide on the macrophage and on the B cell, the T cell stimulates the B cell to turn on antibody production.

3. Antibody production–The stimulated B cell undergoes repeated cell divisions, enlargement, and differentiation to form a clone of antibody-secreting plasma cells. Hence, through specific antigen recognition of the invader, clonal expansion, and B-cell differentiation, an effective number of plasma cells is acquired, all secreting the same needed antibody. That antibody then binds to the bacteria, making them easier to ingest by white cells. Antibody combined with a plasma component called *complement* may also kill the bacteria directly.

Thrombocytes

Thrombocytes are not true cells but rather cytoplasmic fragments of a large cell in the bone marrow, the megakaryocyte. They are the smallest formed elements of the blood. The typical shape is discoid, but when they are activated they become globular and form finger-like cytoplasmic extensions called *pseudopodia*.

Clot Formation

In minor injuries, thrombocytes tend to collect and form plugs in blood vessel openings. To control bleeding from vessels larger than capillaries, a clot must form at the point of injury. The coagulation of the blood is also initiated by blood platelets. The platelets produce a substance that combines with calcium ions in the blood to form thromboplastin, which in turn converts the protein prothrombin into thrombin in a complex series of reactions. Thrombin, an enzyme, converts fibrinogen, a protein substance, into fibrin, an insoluble protein that forms an intricate network of minute threadlike structures called *fibrils,* and causes the blood plasma to gel. The blood cells and plasma are enmeshed in the network of fibrils to form a clot.

Blood clotting can be initiated by the extrinsic mechanism, in which substances from damaged tissues are mixed with the blood, or by the intrinsic mechanism, in which the blood itself is traumatized. More than 30 substances in blood have been found to affect clotting; whether or not blood will coagulate depends on a balance between those substances that promote coagulation (procoagulants) and those that inhibit it (anticoagulants). The coagulation of blood within blood vessels in the absence of injury can cause serious illness or death, especially when a clot forms in the coronary arteries (thrombosis) or cerebral arteries (stroke).

Hemophilia, a bleeding disorder, occurs when a person has a mutation in one of the clotting factor genes. It is a hereditary, sex-linked disorder that affects males of all races and ethnic groups. The mutated gene is on the X chromosome inherited from the mother. Approximately one in 4000 males is born with the disorder; it is rare, but possible, for a female to have hemophilia. People with hemophilia inject themselves with purified clotting factor to prevent bleeding episodes. Internal bleeding, particularly in the joints, is a problem despite treatment and leads to painful arthritis.

Plasma

Plasma is a highly complex liquid that is the carrier for the formed elements and other substances such as proteins, carbohydrates, fats, hormones, enzymes, mineral salts, gases, and waste products. Plasma is composed of approximately 90% water, 9% protein, and 1% various other chemical substances. When plasma proteins and other components are used up during the clotting process, the remaining liquid is called *serum.*

COLLECTION OF BLOOD SPECIMENS

For most hematology tests an adequate blood sample can be obtained from capillaries by finger puncture. If a larger sample is required, blood can be obtained from a vein by venipuncture. To perform a complete blood cell count, venous blood is collected in a tube containing an anticoagulant that prevents clotting. Ethylenediamine tetraacetic acid (EDTA) is the anticoagulant of choice for hematology testing. It is important that blood is not hemolyzed during collection for hematology testing.

Hematocrit

The hematocrit is a measurement of the percentage of packed RBCs in a volume of blood. The spun microhematocrit test is based on the principle of separating the cellular elements from plasma by centrifugation (Procedures 53-1 and 53-2). Two or three drops of blood are collected from a capillary puncture in two capillary tubes and are placed in a specially designed microhematocrit **centrifuge** (Figure 53-1). Alternately, the capillary tubes can be filled with EDTA-anticoagulated blood from a lavender-topped vacuum tube. Capillary tubes can either be preplugged or open and may be made of glass or plastic. If the tube is not plugged, it must be sealed with a special clay before centrifugation.

After centrifugation, RBCs will be at the bottom of the tube, WBCs and platelets in the center, and plasma on top (Figure 53-2). From this separation the microhematocrit is determined by comparing the concentration of RBCs to the total volume of the whole blood sample. The percentage is read by placing the tubes on a special microhematocrit reader. Some microhematocrit centrifuges have a built-in reading scale that reads calibrated capillary tubes. Microhematocrits should be performed in duplicate, and the average of the two results reported.

PROCEDURE 53-1

Perform Hematology Testing: Perform a Microhematocrit

<u>CAAHEP COMPETENCIES:</u> 3.b.(1)(d), 3.b.(1)(e), 3.b.(3)(c)(ii)
<u>ABHES COMPETENCIES:</u> 4.q, 4.r, 4.z

GOAL: *To perform a microhematocrit accurately.*

EQUIPMENT and SUPPLIES

- Fresh sample of blood collected in a tube containing EDTA anticoagulant
- Capillary tubes
- Sealing clay
- Centrifuge

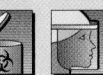

PROCEDURAL STEPS

1. Wash and dry your hands. Put on nonsterile gloves.
   <u>PURPOSE:</u> Infection control.

2. Assemble the materials needed.

3. Fill two plain (blue-tipped) capillary tubes two thirds to three fourths full with well-mixed blood by tipping the blood tube slightly and touching the capillary tube end opposite the blue band to the blood. If the capillary tube and the blood tube are held almost parallel to the table, the capillary tube will fill easily by capillary action.
   <u>PURPOSE:</u> Duplicates should always be done as a means of quality control. Tubes are not filled completely, to provide space for the sealing clay.

4. Wipe the outside of a tube with clean gauze without touching the wet open end of the tube.
   <u>PURPOSE:</u> Wiping the capillary tube removes any blood. Touching the blood with absorbent material removes more plasma than blood cells and can alter the hematocrit.

5. Tip the tube until the blood runs toward the end with the colored band.
   <u>PURPOSE:</u> This prevents blood from accidentally being removed from the tube.

6. Seal the end with the blue band with sealing clay by holding the tube horizontally and inserting the tube. Insert the tube as many times as needed to achieve a plug up to the blue band (Figure 1).

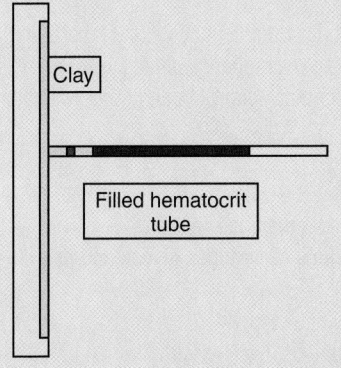

Clay

Filled hematocrit tube

Table top

FIGURE 1

<u>PURPOSE:</u> This prevents the clay from becoming contaminated with blood, helps prevent leakage of blood, and keeps the gasket in the centrifuge from being cut by the capillary tubes.

7. Place the tubes opposite each other in the centrifuge, with sealed ends securely against the gasket. Note the tube arrangement in Figure 53-1.
   <u>PURPOSE:</u> The centrifuge must always be balanced to avoid damage. If the clay ends of the capillary tubes are not outermost against the gasket, the sample will spin out of the tubes, contaminating the centrifuge

8. Note the numbers on the centrifuge slots, and record them.
   <u>PURPOSE:</u> The sample must be identified throughout the entire procedure.

9. Secure the locking top, fasten the lid down, and lock.
   <u>PURPOSE:</u> If the locking top is not firmly in place during the spinning cycle, the tubes will come out of their slots and break. The lid is always locked during centrifugation for safety purposes—that is, to avoid aerosols or broken glass from being ejected.

10. Set the timer, and adjust the speed as needed.
    <u>PURPOSE:</u> The prescribed time is between 3 and 5 minutes at 11,000 to 12,000 rpm. Check the manufacturer's instructions for time and speed.

11. Allow the centrifuge to come to a complete stop. Unlock the lids.
    <u>PURPOSE:</u> Opening the centrifuge before it has stopped could cause harm to the user.

12. Remove the tubes immediately, and read the results. If this is not possible, store the tubes in an upright position.
    <u>PURPOSE:</u> Tubes left in the centrifuge will show altered results, as the RBC layer spreads horizontally.

13. Determine the microhematocrit values using one of the following methods:
    a. Centrifuge with built-in reader using calibrated capillary tubes.
       - Position the tubes as directed by manufacturer's instructions.
       - Read both tubes.
       - The average of the two results is reported.
       - The two values should not vary by more than 2%.
    b. Centrifuge without built-in reader.
       - Carefully remove the tubes from the centrifuge.
       - Place a tube on the microhematocrit reader.
       - Align the clay-RBC junction with the zero line on the reader. Align the plasma meniscus with the 100% line. The value is read at the junction of the red cell layer and the buffy coat. The buffy coat is not included in the reading (Figure 2*).

Continued

PROCEDURE 53-1—cont'd

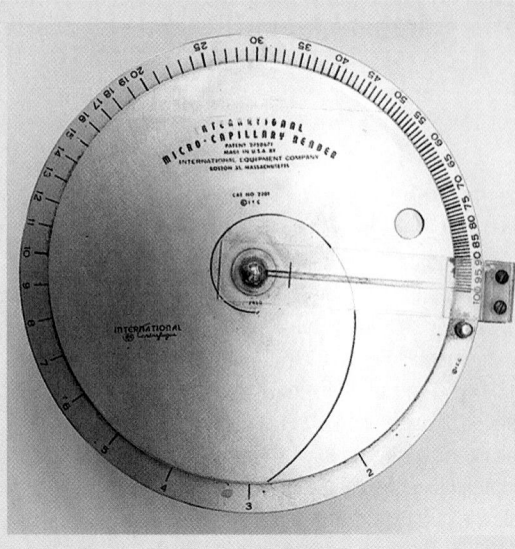

FIGURE 2

- Read both tubes.
- The average of the two results is reported.
- The two values should not vary by more than 2%.

14. Dispose of the capillary tubes in a sharps container.
15. Clean the work area, and properly dispose of all biohazard materials. Remove gloves, and wash your hands.
    PURPOSE: Infection control.
16. Record the results in the patient's medical record.
    PURPOSE: A procedure is not considered done until it is charted.

See Appendix D for a charting example.
*Figure from Stepp CA, Woods MA: *Laboratory procedures for medical office personnel*, Philadelphia, 1998, Saunders.

PROCEDURE 53-2

Perform Routine Maintenance of Clinical Equipment: Preventative Maintenance for the Microhematocrit Centrifuge

CAAHEP COMPETENCY: 3.c.(4)(b)
ABHES COMPETENCY: 6.b

GOAL: *To perform daily, monthly, and quarterly quality control on a microhematocrit centrifuge.*

EQUIPMENT and SUPPLIES

- Microhematocrit centrifuge
- Quality-control logbook
- High-, normal-, and low-quality control samples

PROCEDURAL STEPS

Note: These are generic recommendations. Always check manufacturer's guidelines for specific instructions. Always unplug the power cord before cleaning or servicing the centrifuge. Wear protective gloves and clothing.

DAILY MAINTENANCE

1. Clean the inside of the centrifuge and the gasket with a disinfectant recommended by the manufacturer. Plastic and nonmetal parts may be cleaned with a fresh solution of 5% sodium hypochlorite (bleach) mixed 1:10 with water (one part bleach plus nine parts water).
   PURPOSE: To remove any dried blood or shattered glass. Do not use bleach on the gasket, as it may harden the rubber.

MONTHLY MAINTENANCE

1. Check the reading device. Misuse and zeroing of the reading devices can promote considerable error. Always use a second,

simple reading device as a cross-check. Use a ruler or a flat plastic card especially made for this purpose. These cards are used by laying the spun hematocrit tube on the card and aligning the red cells with a line on the card to obtain the reading.
2. Check the rotor for cracks or corrosion, and check the interior for signs of white powder.
   PURPOSE: Cracks, corrosion, or powder may indicate impending rotor failure and require the immediate attention of a service technician.
3. Record all preventative maintenance in the laboratory logbook.
   PURPOSE: Recording maintenance is necessary to maintain warranties and to comply with CLIA and other regulatory agencies.

SEMIANNUAL MAINTENANCE

1. Check the gasket for cuts and breaks.
   PURPOSE: Cut gaskets allow tubes to leak and need to be replaced.
2. Check the timer with a stopwatch.
3. Perform a maximum cell pack to verify the time required for complete packing by reading a sample after centrifugation then recentrifuging for 1 minute. The results should be the same. If they are not, perform preventive maintenance and/or call the service technician.

Continued

PROCEDURE 53-2—*cont'd*

<u>PURPOSE:</u> If the cells compact further during recentrifugation, the centrifuge is not rotating at the proper speed, and hematocrit results will be falsely elevated.

4. Record all preventative measures in the laboratory logbook.

<u>PURPOSE:</u> Recording maintenance is necessary to maintain warranties and to comply with CLIA and other regulatory agencies.

ANNUAL MAINTENANCE (OR MAINTENANCE PERFORMED AS NEEDED)

1. The centrifuge functions, and maintenance verification should be performed by qualified personnel. This would include checking the centrifuge mechanism, rotors, timer, speed, and electrical leads.

2. Record all professional service calls in the laboratory logbook.

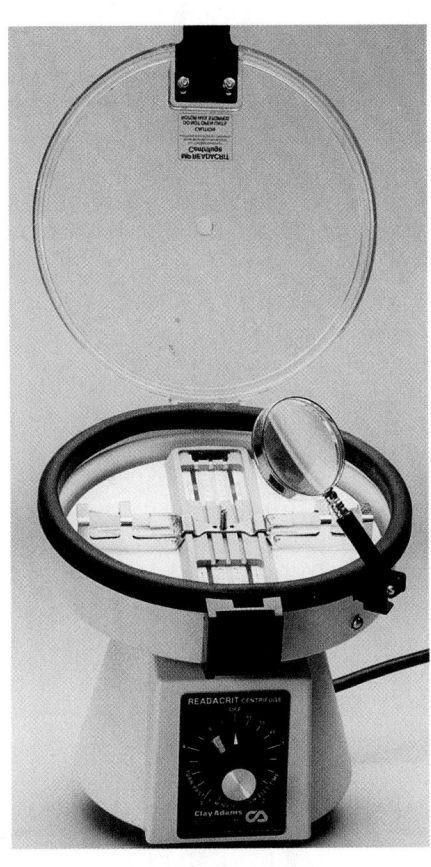

FIGURE 53-1 Centrifuge with capillary tube placement indications.

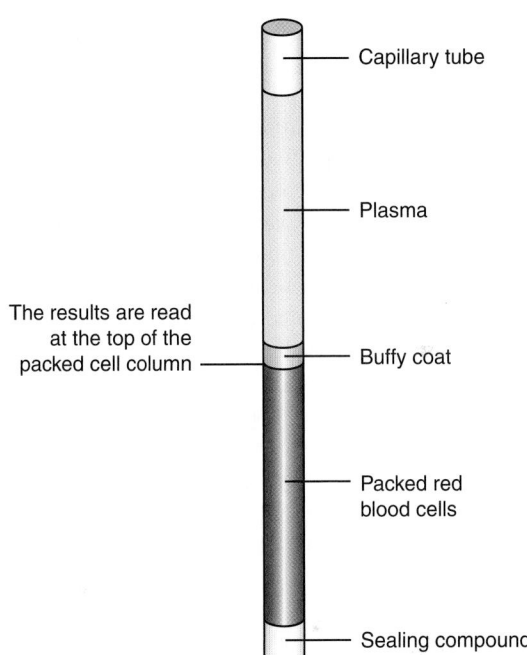

The results are read at the top of the packed cell column

- Capillary tube
- Plasma
- Buffy coat
- Packed red blood cells
- Sealing compound

FIGURE 53-2 Hematocrit test results. Cellular elements are separated from plasma by centrifuging an anticoagulated blood specimen, and the results are read at the top of the packed cell column. (From Bonewit-West K: *Clinical procedures for medical assistants*, ed 6, Philadelphia, 2004, Saunders.)

Inverness Medical Professional Diagnostics (formerly Wampole, Princeton, NJ) manufactures a CLIA-waived instrument that uses electrical conductivity to determine the hematocrit. The STAT-CRIT hct is a self-contained, portable unit that determines hematocrit in 30 seconds. The testing methodology is based on the principle that blood is a conducting medium in which RBCs act as resistors. The plasma conducts electricity based on temperature. The greater the number of erythrocytes in a sample, the more resistance will be recorded. A blood sample is introduced into the sample carrier, which has a thin plastic membrane that permits rapid equilibration of the temperature of the blood and the measuring port. This instrument is best used with fresh blood obtained from a fingerstick; anticoagulants can interfere with conductivity, and heparin, not EDTA, is the anticoagulant of choice.

Hematocrit can also be calculated using the RBC count and RBC size values from an automated cell counter.

The normal values vary with the gender and age of the patient (Table 53-1). The values range from a low of 36% in women to a high of 52% in men. Low microhematocrit values can indicate **anemia** or the presence of bleeding in a patient; high values may be caused by dehydration or a condition such as **polycythemia vera.** Values can be influenced by physiologic or pathologic factors, as well as by collection techniques.

The microhematocrit is a commonly performed test requested by physicians separately or as part of the CBC. Because it is a simple procedure requiring only a small amount of blood, it is an ideal screening test and is often part of a routine physical examination.

HEMOGLOBIN

The hemoglobin determination is a rough measure of the oxygen-carrying capacity of blood. Determining hemoglobin concentration can be performed as part of the CBC or as an

TABLE 53-1 Hematocrit Reference Values	
AGE AND/OR GENDER	**HCT VALUE (%)**
Neonate	44-64
Infant	
1 mo of age	35-49
6 mo of age	30-40
Child, 1-10 yr of age	35-41
Adult	
Men	42-52
Women	36-45

From Stepp CA, Woods MA: *Laboratory procedures for medical office personnel,* Philadelphia, 1998, Saunders.
Hct, Hematocrit.

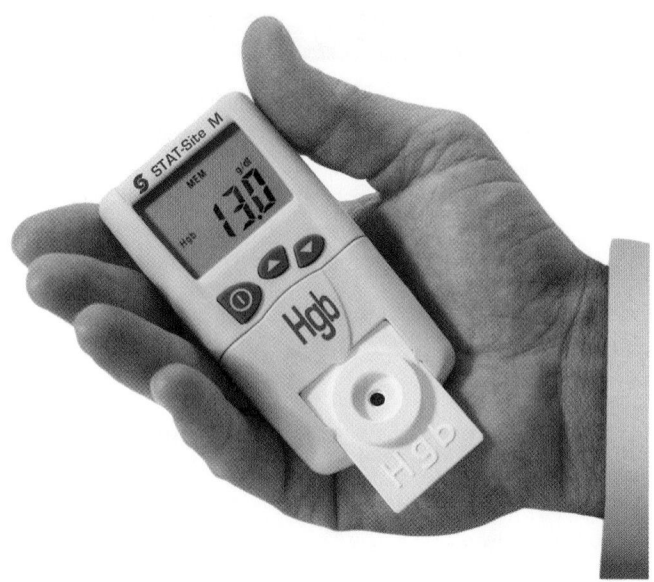

FIGURE 53-3 Hand-held instruments such as the Stat-Site system can analyze hemoglobin quickly and accurately. (Courtesy of Stanbio Laboratory, Boerne, Tex.)

individual test. Many methods of determining hemoglobin concentration have been used over the years. The earliest measures simply involved comparing the color of a drop of blood to a chart. Blood that is dark red has more hemoglobin than pale red blood. The international reference or "gold standard" methodology for hemoglobin determination is the hemiglobincyanide or cyanmethemoglobin (HiCN) method. A sample of whole blood is diluted in Drabkin's reagent, which contains cyanide. The RBCs lyse, releasing hemoglobin, which reacts with cyanide to form hemiglobincyanide. The sample is then placed in a colorimeter, and the amount of light that is absorbed by the sample at a 540-nm wavelength is determined.

A hemoglobinometer is a colorimeter that determines hemoglobin by measuring the amount of light that is absorbed by a sample of blood in which the hemoglobin has been released and chemically modified.

CLIA-waived methods include the STAT-Site® M Hgb (Stanbio Laboratory, Boerne, Tex.), a completely portable, battery-operated, hemoglobin analyzer that fits in the palm of the hand (Figure 53-3) and the HemoCue (Angelgolm, Sweden) (Procedure 53-3). The HemoCue uses plastic cuvettes that contain sodium deoxycholate, sodium nitrite, and sodium azide. The sodium deoxycholate lyses the erythrocytes in the sample to release the hemoglobin, which then reacts with sodium nitrite to form methemoglobin. The methemoglobin reacts with the sodium azide to form azidemethemoglobin, which can be detected at two different wavelengths—570 and 880 nm. Two wavelengths are used in the determination to compensate for possible turbidity in the sample. Capillary, venous, or arterial blood can be used in the cuvette, and cuvettes have a long shelf life.

The copper sulfate method is a CLIA-waived manual method for hemoglobin determination that is often used to screen blood donors. It is based on the principle of specific gravity; when a drop of blood from a patient with normal hemoglobin values is dropped into a copper sulfate solution, it falls rapidly to the bottom (Figure 53-4). If the drop falls slowly or not at all, hemoglobin levels are below reference range.

Normal hemoglobin values vary throughout life. Values are normally quite high at birth, decline during childhood, then increase through the teens until adult levels are reached

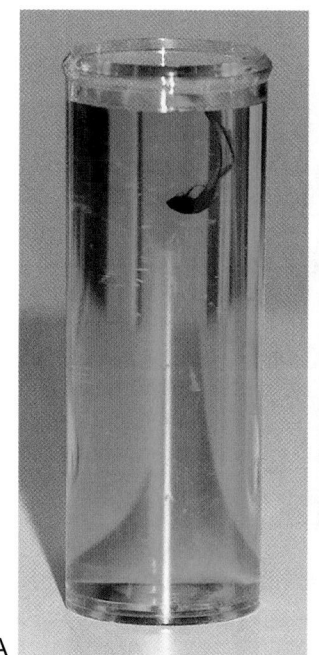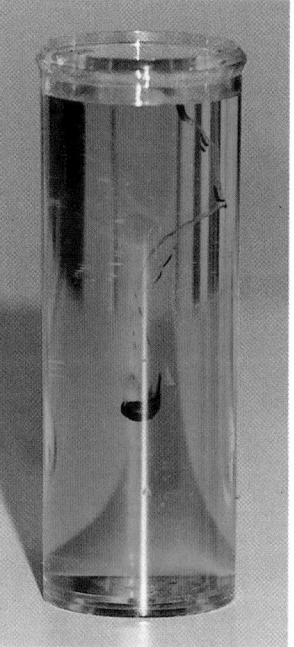

A   B

FIGURE 53-4 Copper sulfate specific gravity method for determining hemoglobin values. **A,** A drop of the patient's blood is placed in copper sulfate. The rate and distance it drops determine the level of hemoglobin present. **B,** The level indicates that this patient's hemoglobin is within reference range. (From Stepp CA, Woods MA: *Laboratory procedures for medical office personnel,* Philadelphia, 1998, Saunders.)

(Table 53-2). Values range from a low of 12 g/dL in women to a high of 17.5 g/dL in men. The various factors that affect the hemoglobin level include age, gender, diet, altitude, and disease.

Hemoglobin and hematocrit are often performed together and are referred to as an "H&H." A quick mental calculation should always be done before reporting out H&H results; hemoglobin value × 3 ± 3 should equal the hematocrit value.

PROCEDURE 53-3

Perform Hematology Testing: Perform a Hemoglobin Test

CAAHEP COMPETENCIES: 3.b.(1)(d), 3.b.(1)(e), 3.b.(3)(c)(ii)
ABHES COMPETENCIES: 4.q, 4.r, 4.z

GOAL: *To determine accurately the level of hemoglobin present in a blood sample using the HemoCue B-Hemoglobin System.*

EQUIPMENT and SUPPLIES

- HemoCue (HemoCue, Lake Forest, Calif.)
- HemoCue cuvette
- Autolet or blood lancet
- Alcohol prep pads
- Gauze squares

 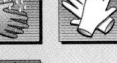

PROCEDURAL STEPS

1. Perform instrument quality control by inserting the control cuvette into the instrument. Ensure that the reading is within acceptable limits before proceeding.
   PURPOSE: Only instruments that record values within the acceptable control limits can be used for patient testing. If the value is out of control, refer to the troubleshooting guide for the instrument, or contact the manufacturer.
2. Wash and dry hands.
   PURPOSE: Infection control.
3. Collect and assemble all equipment and supplies needed.
4. Explain the procedure to the patient.
5. Put on gloves.
6. Examine the fingers, and choose the site to be used to obtain the blood sample.
   PURPOSE: The site to be used must be free of trauma, calluses, and scarring.

7. Clean the site with alcohol or other recommended antiseptic preparation.
8. Perform a capillary puncture, and obtain the blood sample.
9. Wipe away the first drop of blood.
   PURPOSE: This drop may contain tissue fluid.
10. Touch the microcuvette to the drop of blood. Do not touch the finger. The correct volume will be drawn into the cuvette by capillary action. Wipe off any excess blood from the sides of the cuvette (Figures 1 and 2).
    PURPOSE: Blood on the cuvette may alter the readings or contaminate the instrument.
11. Place the cuvette in the cuvette holder, and insert it into the instrument (Figure 3).
12. Read the result, and record it on the patient's medical record.
    PURPOSE: A procedure is not completed until the results are recorded.
13. Dispose of the biohazard waste in correct containers, and properly clean the work area. Turn the instrument off, and return it to the proper storage location.
14. Remove gloves and wash hands.
    PURPOSE: Infection control.

See Appendix D for a charting example.

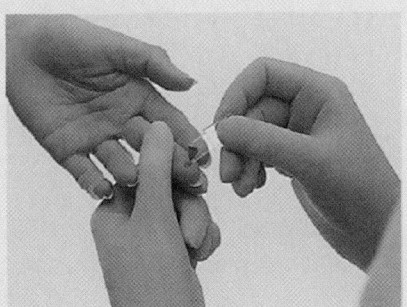

FIGURE 1

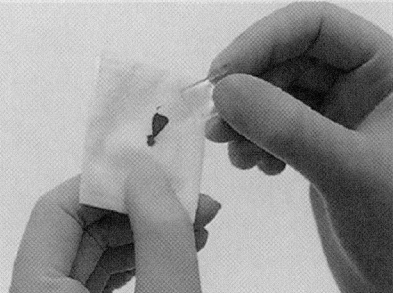

FIGURE 2

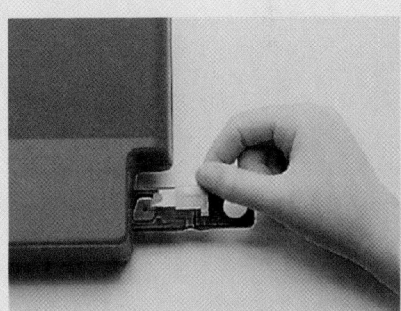

FIGURE 3

For example, if the hemoglobin is 15 g/dL, the hematocrit should be between 42% and 48%.

CRITICAL THINKING APPLICATION

Mr. Corrigan's hematocrit value is 37%. What does Dana calculate as the expected hemoglobin value? Does this test confirm the doctor's suspicions of anemia?

RED BLOOD CELL COUNT

The RBC count is a commonly performed procedure and is part of the CBC (Table 53-3). It approximates the number of circulating RBCs. The function of RBCs is to transport oxygen to tissues. The condition where the oxygen-carrying capacity of blood is below normal is called *anemia*. The RBC count is often decreased in anemia. Increases are found in people with dehydration, polycythemia vera, or severe burns and in people

TABLE 53-2 Hemoglobin (Hgb) Reference Values

AGE AND/OR GENDER	HGB LEVEL (G/DL)
Neonate	17-23
Infant (2 mo of age)	9-14
Child	11-16
Female	12-16
Male	15-17

From Stepp CA, Woods MA: *Laboratory procedures for medical office personnel*, Philadelphia, 1998, Saunders.
Hct, Hematocrit.

who live at high altitudes, as an adaptation to the lower oxygen content of the air.

Normal RBC values range from four million to six million cells/mm^3. RBC counts are usually higher in males than in females.

WHITE BLOOD CELL COUNT

The WBC count gives an approximation of the total number of leukocytes in circulating blood. The count is performed to aid the physician in determining whether an infection is present or to aid in the diagnosis of leukemia. It may also be used to follow the course of a disease and to determine if the patient is responding to treatment.

The normal WBC count varies with age. It is higher in newborns and decreases throughout life. The average adult range is between 4000 and 11,000 cells/mm^3. Many factors affect the WBC count. Elevation of WBCs is called *leukocytosis*.

Physiologic increases in the WBC count are seen with pregnancy, stress, anesthesia, exercise, and exposure to temperature extremes and after treatment with corticosteroids. Pathologic causes of leukocytosis include many bacterial infections, leukemia, appendicitis, and pneumonia. A decrease in the WBC count is called *leukopenia*. This condition may be caused by viral infections or by exposure to radiation, certain chemicals, and drugs.

Determining the Red Blood Cell and White Blood Cell Counts

In the past, blood counts were performed by diluting the blood with special pipets and diluting fluid, placing the sample on a counting slide called a *hemacytometer*, and manually counting the cells using a microscope. The method was time consuming and often inconsistent, and therefore it has largely been replaced by automated cell counting.

Current availability of many different types of cell counters has made it possible for the physician's office to become fully automated. Modern instruments range from relatively simple, inexpensive counters to very complex and expensive instruments. Automation improves the accuracy of cell counting and results in greater efficiency. In addition, automation reduces

TABLE 53-3 Reference Ranges for a Complete Blood Count

TEST	NEONATES	INFANTS (6 MO)	CHILDREN	ADULTS MEN	ADULTS WOMEN
RBCs	4.8-7.1 million/mm^3	3.8-5.5 million/mm^3	4.5-4.8 million/mm^3	4.5-6 million/mm^3	4-5.5 million/mm^3
Hematocrit (Hct)	44%-64%	30%-40%	35%-41%	42%-52%	36%-45%
Hemoglobin (Hgb)	17-23 g/dL	9-14 g/dL	11-16 g/dL	15-17 g/dL	12-16 g/dL
WBCs	9000-30,000/mm^3	6000-16,000/mm^3	5000-13,000/mm^3	4000-11,000/mm^3	
RBC Indices					
MCV	96-108 fL			82-99 fL	
MCH	32-34 pg			26-34 pg	
MCHC	31-33 g/dL			31-37 g/dL	
WBC Differential					
Neutrophils	≥45% by 1 wk of age	32%	60% for children 2 yr of age and older	50%-65%	
Bands	—	—	—	0%-7%	
Eosinophils	—	—	0-3%	1%-3%	
Basophils	—	—	1-3%	0%-1%	
Monocytes	—	—	4-9%	3%-9%	
Lymphocytes	≥41% by 1 wk of age	61%	59% for children 2 yr of age or older	25%-40%	
Platelets	140,000-300,000/mm^3	200,000-473,000/mm^3	150,000-450,000/mm^3	150,000-400,000/mm^3	

From Stepp CA, Woods MA: *Laboratory procedures for medical office personnel*, Philadelphia, 1998, Saunders.
MCH, mean corpuscular hemoglobin; *MCHC*, mean corpuscular hemoglobin concentration; *MCV*, mean corpuscular volume; *RBC*, red blood cell; *WBC*, white blood cell.

the frequency of handling the individual blood specimen and decreases the risk of exposure to blood-borne pathogens. Operation of typical counters used in a physician's office laboratory is considered to be moderately complex by CLIA standards. It is essential that strict standardization procedures and quality-control methods are followed when using automated instruments to perform blood cell counts.

Most automated cell counters operate by first diluting the cells in a fluid that conducts an electrical current. Then these diluted cells pass through a special narrow opening in the instrument. The passing cells interrupt the flow of current, and each interruption is counted. Some instruments use a laser beam instead of an electric current (Figure 53-5). Red cells and white cells are counted in separate diluting chambers or channels. In the white cell counting area the red cells are first lysed, usually with acetic acid, to make the white cells easier to count. Platelets are usually counted in the same channel as the red cells, and the cells are differentiated by size. All cells are reported in units per volume of whole blood.

In addition to counting RBCs, WBCs, and platelets, the instruments also analyze hemoglobin, hematocrit, and the size and shape of the RBCs. Hemoglobin is usually determined using the cyanmethemoglobin method, and the hematocrit is determined mathematically using red cell counts and red cell volumes. With this information, an on-board computer determines certain parameters, known as *red cell indices*, which are included on the printout of the patient's results. Altogether these results make up the CBC.

RED CELL INDICES

A variety of calculations can be performed using the information from the CBC to produce indices that provide information about RBC disorders. Opinions vary regarding the clinical value of red cell indices. They are used to classify anemias and to select additional tests to determine the cause of anemia. They also may be used to monitor treatment of anemia, as they may change in response to treatment. The standard indices are as follows.

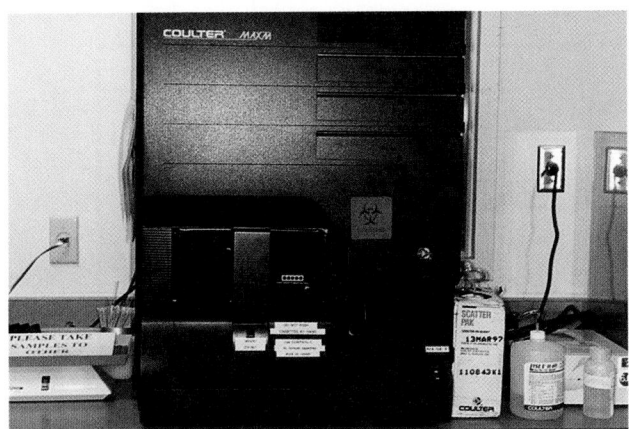

FIGURE 53-5 Automated cell counter. (Courtesy Coulter Corp, Los Angeles, Calif.)

- Mean corpuscular volume (MCV)—MCV is computed using the measurements of each red cell on automated cell counters. With manual methods, it is calculated by dividing the hematocrit by the red cell count and multiplying by 10; the unit of measurement is a femtoliter. MCV measures the size of RBCs and is the most important index for classification of anemias into macrocytic, with higher than normal MCV, and microcytic, with low MCV. The normal reference range is 82 to 108 femtoliters.
- Mean corpuscular hemoglobin (MCH)—MCH = Hemoglobin ÷ RBC count. MCH is calculated to give the average weight of hemoglobin in an individual RBC; the unit is a *picogram*. The reference range is 26-34 picograms.
- MCH concentration or content (MCHC). MCHC = Hemoglobin ÷ Hematocrit. The MCHC indicates the average weight of hemoglobin as compared with the cell size. It is traditionally a calculated value, but some instruments may measure the density of the cells as they are counted and compare this value with the calculated value. The reference range is 32 to 37 g/dL. A decreased MCHC means the RBCs will appear pale, or hypochromic, on observation in a stained blood smear. An increased MCHC is rarely a true value and probably represents an error in the measurement of the hemoglobin or hematocrit.
- Red cell distribution width (RDW). RDW = the degree of red cell size variation or how much difference exists between the largest and smallest red cells. RDW is calculated to provide a measure of the anisocytosis, or variation in size of the RBCs. RDW reference range is 9 to 14.5.

DIFFERENTIAL CELL COUNT

The purpose of the differential, or "diff," is to analyze and quantitate the types of WBCs found in a sample of blood. The differential can be performed manually using a stained blood smear and a microscope or by an automated instrument. A number of automated cell counters have integrated differential analyzers that use high-frequency conductivity to gather information about cell size, internal structure, and density and helium-neon lasers coupled with multiple-angle light scatter that provide information about a cell's internal structure, granulation, and surface characteristics.

Preparation of Blood Smears for the Differential

A blood smear enables you to view the cellular components of blood in as natural a state as possible. The morphology of leukocytes, erythrocytes, and platelets can be studied. Their size, shape, and maturity can be evaluated.

A blood smear is prepared by spreading a drop of blood on a clean glass slide. The slide must be free of dust and grease. The best specimen for a blood smear is capillary blood that has no anticoagulant added. EDTA-anticoagulated blood can be used, provided the smear is made within 2 hours of collection.

The three kinds of blood smears are the coverglass smear, the spun smear, and the wedge smear. The coverglass smear is often used for bone marrow aspirations and involves placing a drop of blood between two coverslips and pulling them quickly apart. The spun smear uses a centrifuge to distribute the blood on a slide and often has the advantage of being a closed system in that the blood tube is punctured by the instrument and does not have to be handled by the technician. The wedge smear involves placing a small drop of blood $1/2$ inch from the right end of a glass slide. The end of a second glass spreader slide is placed in front of the drop of blood at an angle of 30 to 35 degrees. The spreader slide is brought back into the drop until the blood spreads along the edge of the spreader slide. This is done with a quick but smooth gliding motion. The spreader slide is then pushed to the left with a quick, steady motion, spreading the blood across the slide.

A good smear should cover one half to three fourths of the slide. It should show a gradual transition from a thick to a thin end with a feathered edge. It should have a smooth appearance with no ridges, holes, lines, streaks, or clumps (Figure 53-6). The cells should be distributed evenly on microscopic examination.

After the smear has been made, it should be allowed to dry. The slide should be propped up to dry with the thick end (heel) down. Do not blow on the slide to dry it. This can cause **artifacts** in the RBCs from the moisture in your breath.

Once dry, the slide is labeled in the thick portion of the smear by writing the patient's name in the dried blood film. If slides with frosted ends are used, the label can be written on the frosted end with pencil or marker.

After labeling, the slide is fixed in methanol, a fixative that preserves and prevents changes or deterioration of the cellular components. Many of the quick stains available on the market contain the fixative in the stain.

Staining of Blood Smears

Stains commonly used for examination of blood cells are described as *polychromatic* because they contain dyes that will stain various cell components different colors. These stains usually contain methylene blue, a blue stain, and eosin, a red-orange stain. These stains are attracted to different parts of the cell; thus the cells and their structures are more easily seen and differentiated. The most commonly used differential blood stain is Wright's stain. The traditional Wright's stain dates from the early 1890's and was an alcoholic solution of methylene blue and eosin Y. The traditional stain must be diluted 1:2 with buffer before use and this dilution generally was done by flooding the slide with Wright's stain, applying the buffer with a dropper, and blowing on the slide to mix. Since then, there have been many modifications, most involving chemical modification to the methylene blue to improve polychroming. Most Wright's stains today contain mixtures of methylene blue, azure A, thionin, and eosin Y. The quick stain (Procedure 53-4) contains the buffer already dissolved in the stain.

Identification of Normal Blood Cells

Much useful information can be gathered from microscopic identification and evaluation of blood cells in a stained smear. A great deal more information can be acquired from observation of these blood cells than from actual cell counts.

The features of blood cells that the medical assistant may observe and evaluate are cell size, nuclear appearance, and cytoplasmic characteristics. The results of observing these three features will allow for cell identification, although much practice is required to be able to recognize and classify all the blood cells that may be seen in various disease states. A medical assistant might perform the differential analysis if employed in a laboratory that complies with certain CLIA regulations and he or she is specifically trained to perform the analysis.

Cells are examined using the oil-immersion objective of the microscope. The light should be bright to facilitate the visualization of colors and small structures. The slide is examined near the feathered end of the smear, where cells are barely touching one another and are easiest to identify.

RBCs are the most numerous of the cellular elements. They are biconcave disks that have no nuclei. The red cells should appear pinkish tan as a result of the staining of the hemoglobin within the cells (Figure 53-7).

Thrombocytes, or platelets, are the smallest of the cellular elements. They may be round or oval. No nucleus is present because the platelet is just a fragment of cytoplasm from a large bone marrow cell. They stain blue.

Leukocytes are the largest of the normal circulating blood cells (Table 53-4). Each of the five types has a characteristic appearance. The granulocytes include neutrophils, eosinophils,

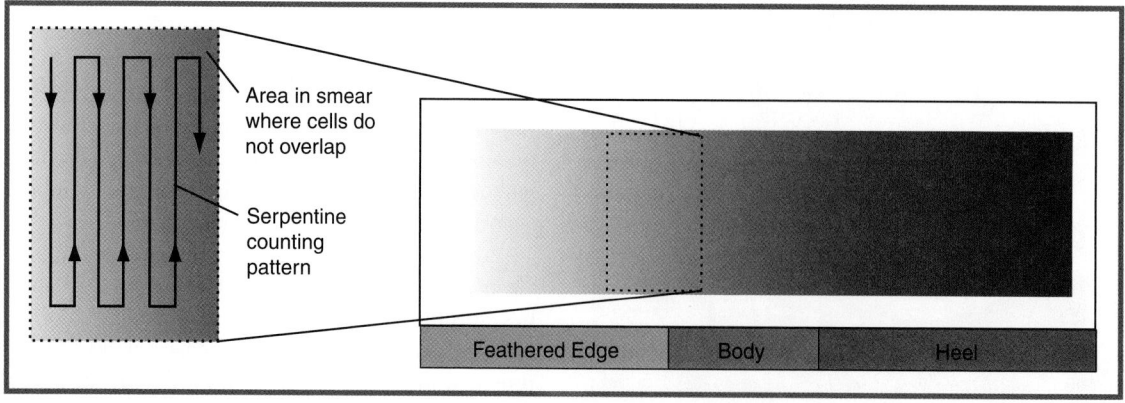

FIGURE 53-6 Appearance of a properly prepared wedge smear and serpentine (winding) pattern used to count cells. (From Stepp CA, Woods MA: *Laboratory procedures for medical office personnel*, Philadelphia, 1998, Saunders.)

Area in smear where cells do not overlap

Serpentine counting pattern

Feathered Edge   Body   Heel

PROCEDURE 53-4

Perform Hematology Testing: Prepare a Blood Smear Stained with Wright's Stain

<u>CAAHEP COMPETENCIES:</u> 3.b.(1)(d), 3.b.(1)(e), 3.b.(3)(c)(ii)
<u>ABHES COMPETENCIES:</u> 4.q, 4.r, 4.z

GOAL: *To prepare and stain a slide that meets the criteria for the performance of a differential examination.*

EQUIPMENT and SUPPLIES

- Clean glass slides
- Transfer pipette or capillary tube
- Wright's stain materials
- EDTA-anticoagulated blood specimen
- Diff-Safe blood dispenser (Alpha Scientific, Malvern, Pa.)

PROCEDURAL STEPS

1. Wash and dry your hands. Put on nonsterile gloves.
   <u>PURPOSE:</u> Infection control.
2. Assemble the materials needed.
3. Mix the blood specimen by gentle inversion.
4. Insert a Diff-Safe blood dispenser into the top of the vacuum tube. Invert the tube, and dispense a drop of blood onto a slide about 1/2 to 3/4 inch from the right end by pressing on the tube (Figure 1).
5. Hold one side of this slide with your nondominant hand.
6. Place the spreader slide in front of the drop of blood at an angle of 30 to 35 degrees. Use your dominant hand (Figure 2).

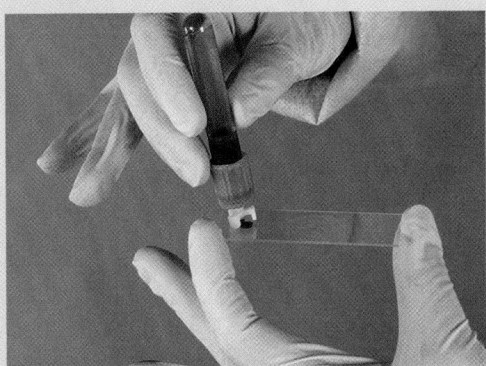

FIGURE 1

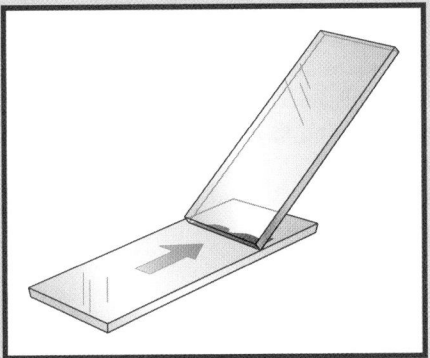

FIGURE 2

<u>PURPOSE:</u> An angle of 30 to 35 degrees makes a smear with a good feathered edge.

7. Pull back the spreader slide into the drop of blood, and allow the blood to spread to the edges of the slide (Figure 3).
8. Push the spreader slide forward with a quick smooth motion, maintaining the same angle throughout (Figure 4).
   <u>PURPOSE:</u> If the motion is not smooth, ridges will occur in the smear.
9. Rapidly but gently wave the slide to accelerate the drying process.
10. Stand the slide with the thick end down, and allow the slide to complete drying (Figure 5).

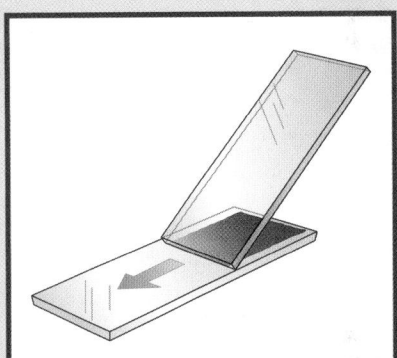

FIGURE 3

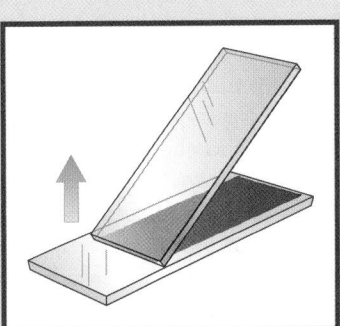

FIGURE 4

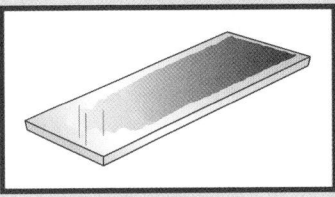

FIGURE 5

Continued

PROCEDURE 53-4—*cont'd*

<u>PURPOSE:</u> If the thick end is up, the undried portion of the blood may run down into the dry thin area and ruin the smear.

11. Label the slide when it is dry. Use a pencil, and write the name in the thick end of the smear or on the frosted area.

<u>PURPOSE:</u> Pencil will scratch the name into the smear and will not wash off in the staining process.

12. Stain according to method used.
   - Two-step method:
      a. Place the smear on a staining rack, with the blood side up.
      b. Flood the smear with Wright's stain.
      c. Wait for 1 to 3 minutes.
      d. Add an equal amount of buffer, drop by drop, on top of the Wright stain.
      e. Blow gently, and mix the two solutions until a green metallic sheen appears. This should appear within 2 to 4 minutes.
      f. Rinse thoroughly with distilled water.
      g. Drain water from the slide.
      h. Wipe the back of the smear with gauze.
      i. Stand the smear to dry.
   - Quick stain:
      a. Place the smear into solutions according to the manufacturer's instructions.
      b. Proceed with steps f through i as listed for the two-step method.

13. Clean the work area. Properly dispose of all biohazard materials. Remove gloves, and wash your hands.

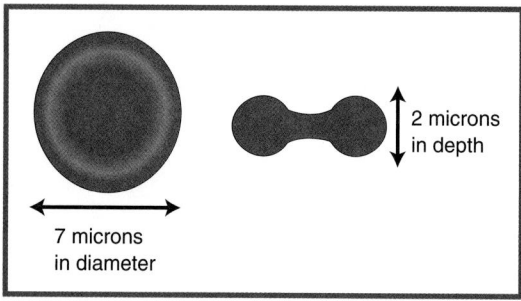

FIGURE 53-7 Red blood cell morphology. (From Stepp CA, Woods MA: *Laboratory procedures for medical office personnel*, Philadelphia, 1998, Saunders.)

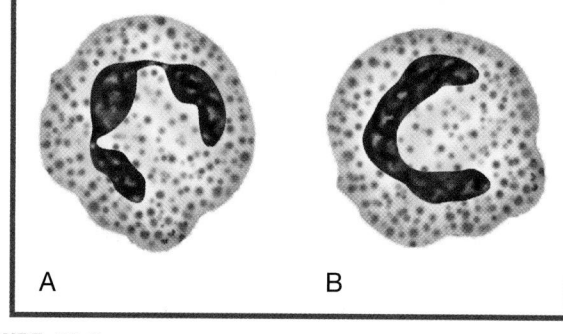

FIGURE 53-8 Neutrophilic cells. **A,** Segmented. **B,** Band. (From Stepp CA, Woods MA: *Laboratory procedures for medical office personnel*, Philadelphia, 1998, Saunders.)

and basophils. Granulocytes contain distinctive granules in their cytoplasm and may have segmented nuclei. The agranulocytes include lymphocytes and monocytes. They have few, if any, granules and nonsegmented nuclei. The nuclei of the leukocytes should appear purple, and their cytoplasm may vary from pink to blue or blue-gray. Neutrophils are known by a variety of names, including polymorphonuclear neutrophils (PMNs), segmented neutrophils, "polys," and "segs" (Figure 53-8). They are the most numerous WBCs in circulation in adults. They are produced in bone marrow, are released into circulation, and eventually enter tissue to fight off invading microorganisms by engulfing them (phagocytosis). Many types of bacterial infections stimulate increased production of neutrophils.

The segmented neutrophil nucleus is segmented into two to five lobes that are connected by a strand. The nucleus stains a dark purple. The cytoplasm is pale pink and contains fine pink or lilac granules.

An immature form of a neutrophil is called a *band* or *stab*. Instead of having a segmented nucleus in which the lobes are separated by a thin filament, the band has an unsegmented nucleus shaped like a horseshoe or a banana. The staining is the same as in the segmented neutrophil. An increase in bands is termed a *shift to the left* and is seen in infections such as bacterial

meningitis, pneumonia, appendicitis, strep throat, and abscesses and in chronic granulocytic leukemia.

The nucleus of an eosinophil is divided into two or three lobes that stain purple. The cytoplasm stains pink and contains large round or oval red-orange granules. Eosinophils are phagocytic and are associated closely with allergies such as hay fever and with asthma as well as with certain parasitic infestations such as tapeworm and amoebic dysentery.

The nucleus of a basophil is segmented and stains light purple. The large, dark, blue-black granules contain histamine, heparin, and other compounds that are a part of the allergic response. Basophils are associated with the immediate immune response to external antigens, such as in asthma, hay fever, and anaphylaxis.

Lymphocytes are the second most numerous type of WBC in adults. In children they are usually the most numerous. Their purple-staining nucleus is usually large, oval or round, and smooth. The cytoplasm stains blue. "Lymphs," as they are commonly called, are responsible for the recognition of foreign antigens and the production of circulating antibodies for immunity to disease. Increased numbers of lymphocytes are found with most viral diseases; with some bacterial infections

TABLE 53-4 Characteristics of Leukocytes

	GRANULOCYTES				AGRANULOCYTES	
	NEUTROPHIL SEGMENTED (MATURE)	NEUTROPHIL BAND (IMMATURE)	EOSINOPHIL	BASOPHIL	LYMPHOCYTE	MONOCYTE
Cell size	10-15 μm	10-15 μm	10-15 μm	10-15 μm	6-15 μm	12-20 μm
Nucleus shape	Two to five lobes connected by threadlike filaments	Band or U-shaped	Bilobed or band	Slightly segmented, granular, or band	Round or oval	Round, indented, or super-imposed lobes
Nucleus structure	Coarse	Coarse	Coarse	Obscured by granules	Smudged, lumpy, or clumped	Brainlike convolutions or folded
Cytoplasm amount	Abundant	Abundant	Abundant	Abundant	Scant	Abundant
Cytoplasm color	Colorless to light pink	Colorless to light pink	Colorless to light pink	Colorless to light pink	Sky blue to dark blue	Dull gray to blue-gray
Cytoplasm inclusions	Many tiny tan, pink, or red-purple granules	Many tiny tan, pink with increased red-purple granules	Large, rounder oval red to red-orange granule	Large, coarse blue-black granules	None to few round red-purple granules	Ground glass appearance, fine red-purple granules, rare blue granules

From Stepp CA, Woods MA: *Laboratory procedures for medical office personnel*, Philadelphia, 1998, Saunders.

such as syphilis and tuberculosis; with leukemias; and in young children who are actively making antibodies. In many viral infections, stimulated or reactive lymphocytes, called *atypical lymphocytes*, are found. These are common in infectious mononucleosis.

Monocytes are the largest type of WBC in circulation. The nucleus may be oval, indented, or horseshoe shaped. The cytoplasm stains a dull gray-blue and may contain vacuoles, which appear as clear spaces in the cytoplasm filled with fluid or air. Monocytes are called *macrophages* when they enter tissues and ingest bacteria and debris of cellular breakdown. They are increased in patients with certain viral infections, such as hepatitis and mumps; rickettsial infections, such as Rocky Mountain spotted fever; and bacterial infections, such as tuberculosis and typhoid fever.

Differential Examination

A specific area of a stained smear must be examined microscopically when the differential count is done. This area must be where RBCs are touching but are not clumped when viewed microscopically. For manually prepared smears this area would be the feathered edge. The entire slide is acceptable for viewing when the smear is prepared by automation. After you have located an appropriate area under low power of the microscope, focus using the oil immersion lens. The differential examination consists of counting and classifying 100 consecutive WBCs while moving in a specific winding pattern through the smear

(see Figure 53-6). This pattern must be followed to avoid counting the same cells twice. A tally of the cells observed is kept on a differential cell counter or a computer (Figure 53-9).

Normal values for a differential vary with age. The reference range for the adult is as follows:

- Neutrophils: 40% to 60%
- Lymphocytes: 20% to 40%
- Monocytes: 2% to 8%
- Eosinophils: 1% to 4%
- Basophils: 0.5% to 1%
- Band: 0% to 3%

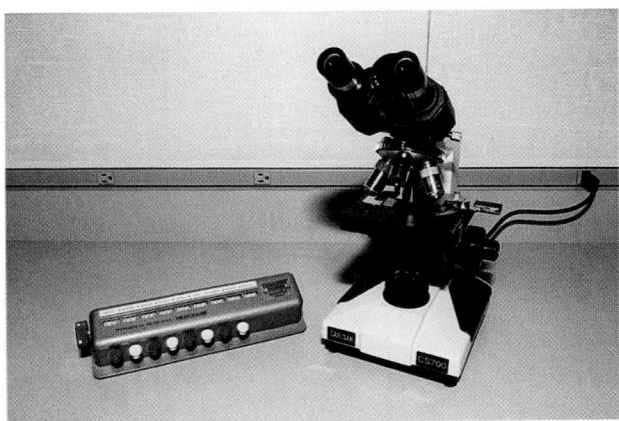

FIGURE 53-9 Microscope with differential cell counter. (Courtesy Cynmar Corporation, Carlinville, Ill.)

Many disease states alter the ratios of the different types of leukocytes, and the differential can be very useful in assisting with the physician's diagnosis (Procedure 53-5).

Red Blood Cell Morphology

After determining the differential cell count, the RBCs are observed and evaluated. Normally, stained RBCs are the same size and shape and are well filled with hemoglobin. Any variations from the normal state are reported (Figure 53-10). Appearance of the RBCs should correlate with the RBC indices.

Size

Normal-sized RBCs are said to be *normocytic*. If the cells are larger than normal, they are *macrocytic;* if smaller, they are *microcytic*. The condition in which different sizes of RBCs are present is called *anisocytosis*.

Shape

Normal RBCs are round or slightly oval. Cells may be shaped like sickles, targets, crescents, or burrs. Poikilocytosis is a significant variation in the shape of RBCs.

Content

An RBC with a normal amount of hemoglobin is said to be *normochromic*. Pale-staining cells are *hypochromic* and have less hemoglobin than normal. Any inclusions in red cells should be reported.

Platelet Analysis

On a stained smear the morphology of platelets is observed for any abnormalities. They are small and irregularly shaped and may vary considerably in size. The average number of platelets seen in 10 to 15 fields is reported. The normal platelet count is 150,000 to 400,000/mm^3. An increase in platelets is called *thrombocytosis*, and a decrease is called *thrombocytopenia*. Excessive clumping of platelets is reported.

In the last 10 years the hematology laboratory has seen great advancements in the use of automation, and many procedures have become "closed-tube" operations. Not only are cell counts performed by instruments that sample the tube without opening it, but slide preparation and staining can be performed by instruments that sample the specimen and make thin, consistent films or smears without ever opening the tube.

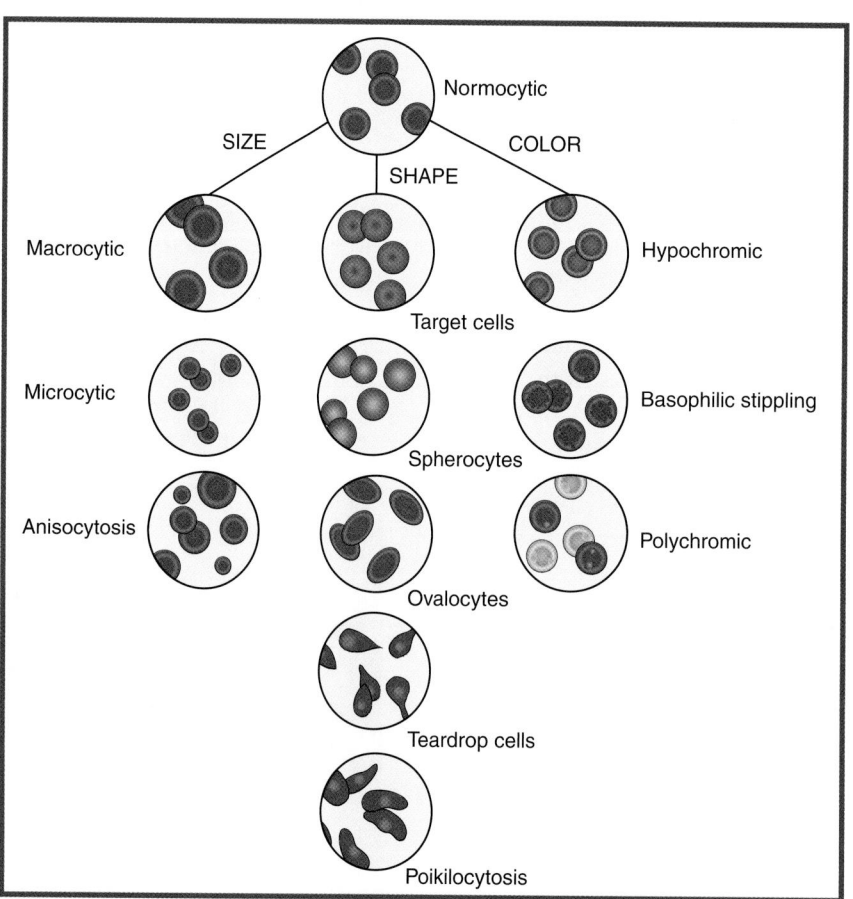

FIGURE 53-10 Abnormal erythrocytes. (Modified from Stepp CA, Woods MA: *Laboratory procedures for medical office personnel*, Philadelphia, 1998, Saunders.)

PROCEDURE 53-5

Perform a Differential Examination of a Smear Stained with Wright's Stain

<u>CAAHEP COMPETENCIES:</u> 3.b.(1)(d), 3.b.(1)(e)
<u>ABHES COMPETENCIES:</u> 4.q, 4.r, 4.z

GOAL: *To perform a differential cell count, evaluate RBC morphology, and estimate the number of platelets.*

EQUIPMENT and SUPPLIES

- Microscope
- Immersion oil
- Lens tissue
- Lens cleaner

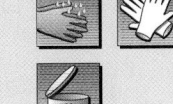

PROCEDURAL STEPS

1. Wash and dry your hands.
   <u>PURPOSE:</u> Infection control.
2. Assemble the materials needed.
3. Clean the microscope with lens tissue and lens cleaner.
   <u>PURPOSE:</u> Dirty optical surfaces interfere with viewing.
4. Place the slide on the stage, with the smear facing up. Position the feathered edge of the smear over the stage aperture.
   <u>PURPOSE:</u> If the slide is face down, you will not be able to focus under oil immersion. Positioning the feathered edge over the aperture brings you closer to the area you will be viewing.
5. Locate an area of the smear where the RBCs barely touch one another or slightly overlap, using the low-power objective.
   <u>PURPOSE:</u> If the slide is too thick, the cells will be crowded, small, and difficult to evaluate. If the slide is too thin, the cells will be very far apart and will show the effects of excessive flattening.
6. Rotate the objective to high power and refocus. Apply a drop of immersion oil to the slide, and rotate the oil immersion lens into place. Increase the light as needed using the iris diaphragm.
7. Count 100 consecutive WBCs in as many viewing fields as necessary using a winding pattern, identifying each cell encountered (Figure 1*).

8. Record each white cell on the differential cell counter by depressing the appropriate key for each cell.
   <u>PURPOSE:</u> The differential examination must proceed systematically, to avoid missing cells or counting any cell twice.
9. Evaluate the RBCs observed in 10 fields. Record any variations in the following:
   - Size—microcytosis, macrocytosis, anisocytosis
   - Shape—poikilocytosis, ovalocytosis, target cells, sickle cells, and so forth
   - Content—normochromic or hypochromic
   <u>PURPOSE:</u> The RBC evaluation gives the physician important information about the RBC population and is an important tool in the assessment of anemias and RBC diseases.
10. Count the platelets in 10 fields, calculate an average, and multiply that average by 15,000 to give an estimate of the platelet count. The normal platelet count is 150,000 to 400,000/mm^3. Report the count as normal, decreased, or increased.
    <u>PURPOSE:</u> Platelet numbers can be a clue to bleeding disorders.
11. Clean the microscope with lens tissue and lens cleaner, paying special attention to removing the oil from the 100× objective.
12. Clean the work area and properly dispose of all materials.
13. Record the testing results in the patient's record.
    <u>PURPOSE:</u> A procedure is considered not done until it is recorded.

---

*Figure from Stepp CA, Woods MA: *Laboratory procedures for medical office personnel,* Philadelphia, 1998, Saunders.

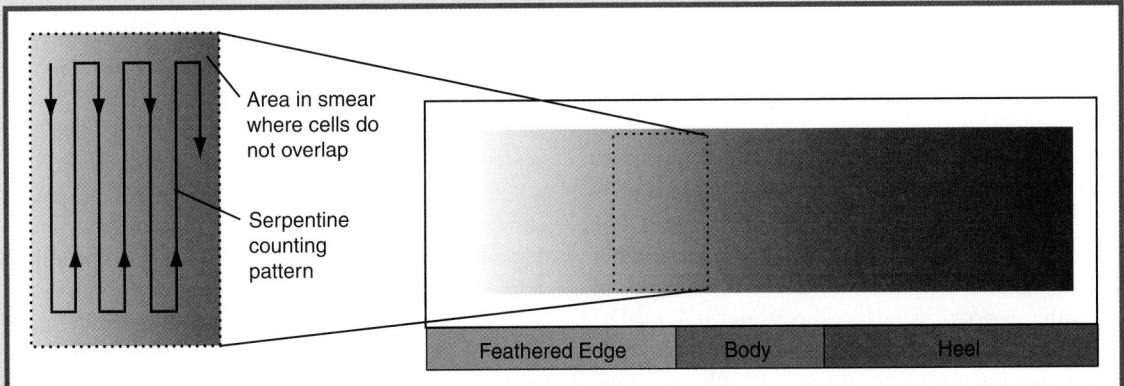

FIGURE 1

TABLE 53-5 Erythrocyte Sedimentation Rate Reference Values

	WINTROBE METHOD (MM/HR)	WESTERGREN METHOD (MM/HR)
Men	0-10	≤50 yr of age: 0-15 >50 yr of age: 0-20
Women	1-20	≤50 yr of age: 0-20 >50 yr of age: 0-30

From Stepp CA, Woods MA: *Laboratory procedures for medical office personnel*, Philadelphia, 1998, Saunders.

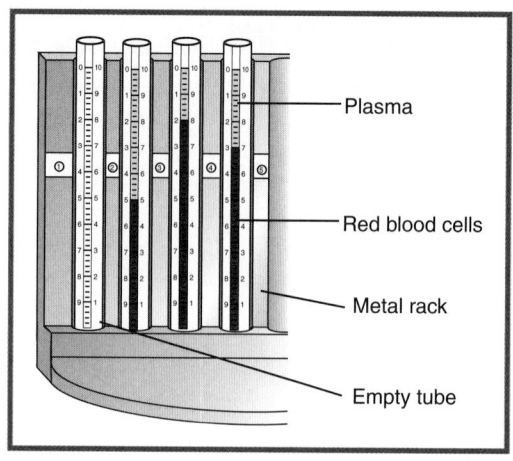

FIGURE 53-11 Wintrobe sedimentation rate system. (From Stepp CA, Woods MA: *Laboratory procedures for medical office personnel*, Philadelphia, 1998, Saunders.)

These instruments are so sensitive that they can adjust the film preparation based on the calculated hematocrit of the CBC. The advantages are many; closed-tube systems are safer for personnel, and results are more consistent. Still, laboratory personnel must watch closely for "flagged," or inconsistent values, and they must be prepared to perform backup tests to verify the results of the automated tests.

ERYTHROCYTE SEDIMENTATION RATE

The erythrocyte sedimentation rate (ESR) is a laboratory test that measures the rate at which erythrocytes gradually separate from plasma and settle to the bottom of a specially calibrated tube in an hour. The test is not specific for a particular disease but is used as a general indication of inflammation. Increases are found in such conditions as acute and chronic infections, rheumatoid arthritis, tuberculosis, hepatitis, cancer, multiple myeloma, rheumatic fever, and lupus erythematosus.

Normal values vary slightly with age and gender (Table 53-5). Only increased ESR rates are significant.

Several methods of measuring ESR are used, including the Wintrobe (Figure 53-11), Westergren (Procedure 53-6), and Landau-Adams methods. All these methods are based on the same principle and differ only in the amounts of blood needed and the tube size and calibration used.

The International Committee for Standardization in Hematology has selected Westergren's method as the recommended method. A straight glass tube 30 cm in length and 2.55 mm (±0.15 mm) in diameter with a bore uniform to 0.05 mm throughout is used. Blood is obtained by clean venipuncture in an EDTA tube and diluted accurately with one volume of 109 mmol/L trisodium citrate to four volumes of blood. The test should be performed within 2 hours of collection, or within 6 hours if the blood is stored at 4° C. The diluted blood sample is drawn to the 200-mm mark in the tube by means of mechanical device or aspiration bulb. The tube is placed vertically in a vibration- and draft-free environment away from direct sunlight. After 1 hour the ESR is measured in millimeters as the height of clear plasma above the column of sedimented cells.

Variations on the standard method have been developed using plastic and disposable glass tubes and capillary tubes for infants. One such method is the Sediplast (Polymedco, Redmond, Wash.). This closed system incorporates a pierceable stopper that, when pierced by a pipette, ensures a leakproof seal. An automatic self-zeroing cap and reservoir accurately bring the blood level to the zero-mark and protect from overfilling. A prefilled vial of sodium citrate diluent is provided for dilution of blood before testing (see Procedure 53-6).

Rapid, automated systems have also been developed. Strek Laboratories (LaVista, Nebr.) manufactures the ESR-10, a nonautomated, CLIA-waived test using ESR-vacuum tubes. The tubes automatically draw the correct amount of sample, then are placed in the rack for 30 minutes. Although not CLIA-waived, analyzers that force readings are also manufactured by Strek Laboratories and allow results in as little as 10 minutes.

Becton-Dickinson has introduced the Seditainer, an ESR tube that fits the Vacutainer system. This self-contained tube contains a buffered sodium citrate solution, providing a proper dilution of buffer to blood when the tube is filled from the venipuncture. There is no need to transfer the specimen to another tube for analysis. The Seditainer is placed in a calibrated stand from which the ESR is read after 60 minutes. The Seditainer tube has a black stopper, and it should be filled after the light-blue–topped and red-topped tubes along with any other additive tubes. It should be inverted 8 times after filling.

Many factors can affect the ESR. The tube must be totally filled with blood and must not contain air bubbles. The tube must be allowed to sit in a vertical position undisturbed for a full hour. Minor degrees of tilting may increase the sedimentation rate; careful timing is important. Jarring or vibrations from nearby machinery will falsely increase the ESR. If testing cannot be performed immediately, blood should be stored at room temperature and testing must be performed within 62 hours.

PROCEDURE 53-6

Perform Hematology Testing: Determine Erythrocyte Sedimentation Rate Using a Modified Westergren Method

CAAHEP COMPETENCIES: 3.b.(1)(d), 3.b.(1)(e), 3.b.(3)(c)(ii)
ABHES COMPETENCIES: 4.q, 4.r, 4.z

GOAL: *To fill a Westergren tube properly and to observe and record an erythrocyte sedimentation rate (ESR) obtained by using the Westergren method.*

EQUIPMENT and SUPPLIES

- EDTA-anticoagulated blood specimen
- Safety tube decapper
- Sediplast ESR system
- Sediplast rack
- Timer

PROCEDURAL STEPS

1. Wash and dry your hands. Put on face protection and nonsterile gloves.
   PURPOSE: Infection control.
2. Assemble the materials needed.
3. Check the leveling bubble of the Sediplast rack.
   PURPOSE: The rack must be horizontal on the table or bench to ensure that the tube is vertical.
4. Bring the blood sample to room temperature if it has been refrigerated, and mix the sample well by inverting the tube gently several times.
   PURPOSE: Cells settle when the specimen stands, and blood must always be well mixed before sampling. Test results will be altered if refrigerated blood is used.
5. Remove the stopper on the blood sample using a tube decapper and on the prefilled Sediplast vial.
   PURPOSE: Removing the cap with a protective device blocks blood splashes and helps to prevent aerosolization of the specimen.

6. Fill the vial to the indicated line, replace the stopper on the prefilled vial, and invert several times to mix. Recap the blood collection tube (Figure 1).
   PURPOSE: This dilutes the blood in accordance with the Westergren procedure.
7. Insert the Sediplast pipette through the pierceable stopper on the vial, and push down until the pipette touches the bottom of the vial. The pipette will automatically draw the blood up to the zero mark.
8. Insert the pipette and the vial into the rack, ensuring that it is vertical (Figure 2*).
   PURPOSE: A pipette that is not vertical will produce erroneous results.
9. Allow the tube to stand undisturbed for 60 minutes.
   PURPOSE: Jarring will increase the sedimentation rate.
10. Measure the distance the erythrocytes have fallen. The scale reads in millimeters, and each line is 1 mm.
11. Clean the work area, and properly dispose of all biohazard materials. Remove face protection and gloves, and wash your hands. Dispose of the pipette in a biohazard container.
12. Record the findings in the patient's medical record.
    REMEMBER: The Westergren ESR is reported in millimeters per hour.
    PURPOSE: A procedure is considered not done until it is recorded.

*Figure 2 courtesy Polymedco, Inc.

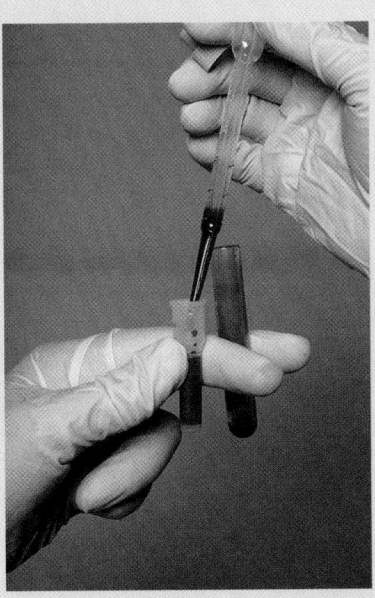

FIGURE 1

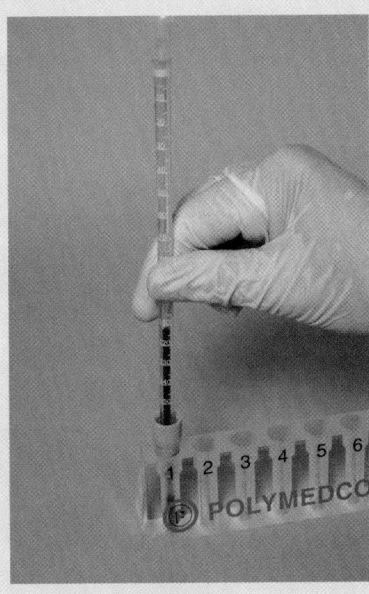

FIGURE 2

COAGULATION TESTING

Coagulation testing is usually performed in the hematology laboratory. The medical assistant may be asked to perform a test to determine prothrombin time (PT) using a hand-held, CLIA-waived instrument that uses whole blood or citrated plasma. The PT is a method of measuring how well the blood clots. Generally, PT is considered to be prolonged if it is more than 1.2 times the control time. Patients who have problems with delayed blood clotting are given a number of tests to determine the cause of the problem. The prothrombin test specifically evaluates the presence of factors VIIa, V, and X, prothrombin, and fibrinogen. Prothrombin is a protein in the liquid part of blood (plasma) that is converted to thrombin as part of the clotting process. Fibrinogen is a type of blood protein called a globulin; it is converted to fibrin during the clotting process. A drop in concentration of any of these factors will cause the blood to take longer to clot.

The PT is used in combination with the partial thromboplastin time (PTT) to screen for hemophilia and other hereditary clotting disorders. PT is also used to monitor the condition of patients who are taking warfarin (Coumadin). Warfarin is a drug that is given to prevent clots in the deep veins of the legs and to treat pulmonary embolism. It interferes with blood clotting by lowering the liver's production of certain clotting factors.

The ProTime Microcoagulation system (ITC, Edison, NJ) measures the PT based on the time it takes the blood to form a fibrin clot. A precise amount of blood is drawn from the fingerstick into channels in the testing strip, where they mix with a thromboplastin reagent (Figure 53-12). The blood is pumped back and forth in the channel, and a series of light-emitting diodes (LEDs) detect the formation of the clot when the movement of the blood stops.

PT test results are reported as the number of seconds the blood takes to clot when mixed with a thromboplastin reagent. The International Normalized Ratio (INR) was created by the World Health Organization because PT test results can vary depending on the thromboplastin reagent used. The INR is a conversion unit that takes into account the different sensitivities of available reagents. The INR is widely accepted as the standard unit for reporting PT results rather than the time in seconds. Normal PT values are 10 to 13 seconds or an INR value of 1 to 1.4. The warfarin (Coumadin) dosage in people being treated to prevent the formation of blood clots or in those who have artificial heart valves is usually adjusted so that the PT is about 1.5 to 2.5 times the normal value (or INR values 2 to 3).

IMMUNOHEMATOLOGY

Formerly called the *blood bank*, the immunohematology division of the laboratory is responsible for blood typing. The major reason for performing immunohematologic tests is to prevent problems caused by incompatibility of blood types. Compatibility testing (cross-matching) is performed to prevent transfusion reactions in patients who are receiving blood transfusions and to identify potential Rh-incompatibility problems in expectant mothers. Rh incompatibility between an expectant mother and the unborn child may result in hemolytic disease of the newborn.

Blood Grouping

There are two major blood antigen systems: the ABO (or Landsteiner) system and the Rh system. In the ABO system there are four major blood groups: A, B, O, and AB. A person is either Rh positive or Rh negative. Certain blood types are more common in certain countries. In China more than 99% of the population has Rh-positive blood. In the United States, about 85% of the population is Rh positive. Blood type is inherited, like eye color. There are racial and ethnic differences in blood type and composition owing to inheritance and populations that have migrated and mixed over time. Different kinds of animals have different kinds of blood as well. Dogs have four blood types; cats have 11; cows have about 800. Table 53-6 shows the distribution of blood types of the peoples of the United States for which data are available.

Determination of ABO Blood Group

The determination of ABO blood groups is a simple test that can easily be performed (Procedure 53-7), but because of the implications of performing the test incorrectly, blood typing is not CLIA-waived. The test detects the presence of A or B antigens on RBCs based on the presence or absence of agglutination with a known antiserum

When the antigen on a patient's RBCs corresponds to the test antibody, agglutination occurs. If the corresponding antigen is not present on the cells, no agglutination will occur.

In addition to the blood antigens found on RBCs, naturally occurring antibodies are found in plasma. These antibodies appear shortly after birth, and the body never produces an antibody that can combine with its own blood antigen. The blood group antibodies require that blood transfusions are specific; type A blood should ideally receive type A blood in a transfusion. In emergencies, there may not be time for the

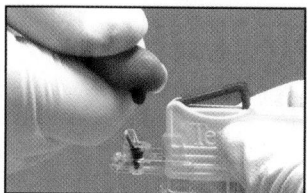

1. Collect sample

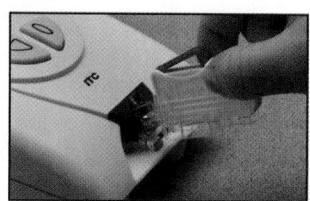

2. Attach Tenderlett Plus

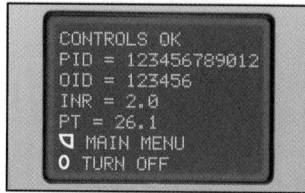

3. Read results

FIGURE 53-12 ProTime microcoagulation system.

TABLE 53-6 Blood Type Distribution in the United States

TYPE	WHITE	AFRICAN AMERICAN	HISPANIC	ASIAN
O+	37%	47%	53%	39%
O−	8%	4%	4%	1%
A+	33%	24%	29%	27%
A−	7%	2%	2%	0.5%
B+	9%	18%	9%	25%
B−	2%	1%	1%	0.4%
AB+	3%	4%	2%	7%
AB−	1%	0.3%	0.2%	0.1%

Data from the American Red Cross.

laboratory to perform a **type and cross-match;** therefore type O negative blood is administered. Type O negative is referred to as the "universal donor" because there are no circulating antibodies to the ABO antigen, nor are there Rh antigens that might sensitize an Rh-negative recipient. Table 53-7 illustrates the compatibility among blood types for transfusion.

Determination of Rh Factor

The determination of Rh type is also a simple (although not CLIA-waived) test that can be performed with a minimum amount of equipment (Procedure 53-8). The Rh factor is so called because it was first discovered in rhesus monkeys. Later this same protein was found on the RBCs of some humans. This test detects the presence of proteins (D antigens) on the surface

TABLE 53-7 Blood Compatibility

RECIPIENT BLOOD*		COMPATIBLE WITH
RBC ANTIGEN	PLASMA ANTIBODIES	DONOR TYPES†
Type O (no antigens)	Anti-A and anti-B	O
Type A (type A antigen)	Anti-B	O and A
Type B (type B antigen)	Anti-A	O and B
Type AB (type AB antigen)	None	O, A, B, and AB

From Stepp CA, Woods MA: *Laboratory procedures for medical office personnel,* Philadelphia, 1998, Saunders.
RBC, Red blood cell.
*Patients with type AB blood are considered to be universal recipients.
†Patients with type O blood are considered to be universal donors.

Examples of Blood Agglutination

- Type A blood will agglutinate in the presence of anti-A antiserum but will not agglutinate in the presence of anti-B antiserum.
- Type B blood will agglutinate in the presence of anti-B antiserum but not in the presence of anti-A antiserum.
- Type O blood will not agglutinate in the presence of anti-A antiserum or anti-B antiserum.
- Type AB blood will agglutinate in the presence of both anti-A antiserum and anti-B antiserum.

of RBCs based on the presence or absence of agglutination with anti-D antiserum. When the D antigen is present, agglutination occurs when the anti-D antiserum is mixed with RBCs. If the D antigen is not present, no agglutination will occur. Rh-positive blood will agglutinate in the presence of anti-D antiserum but not in the presence of the Rh control. Rh-negative blood will not agglutinate in the presence of anti-D antiserum, nor will it agglutinate in the presence of the Rh control.

There are no naturally occurring antibodies to the Rh factor as there are to the A and B antigens. One will develop antibodies to the D antigen only in the event of exposure to the antigen. This is possible if an incompatible transfusion is administered or if an Rh-negative mother is exposed to the Rh-positive blood of her infant during pregnancy, a miscarriage, abortion, or delivery. When this occurs, a mother may develop antibodies against the D antigen. This usually does not cause a problem during the first pregnancy.

In the event of a subsequent pregnancy with an Rh-positive fetus, the woman's immune system will begin to produce more antibodies because she was sensitized during the first pregnancy. These antibodies cross the placenta and destroy the RBCs of the fetus, which can lead to anemia, heart failure, or brain damage in the infant and may even cause death. These events are collectively called *hemolytic disease of the newborn* (HDN). The disease is sometimes also called *hydrops* or *blue baby syndrome.*

Until 1968 there was no preventative measure that could be taken. Exchange transfusion, in which all of the infant's blood is replaced, was the only option. Today, however, this can be prevented by the administration of Rh immune globulin products.

Rho(D) immune globulin is a protein solution containing large amounts of Rh(D) antibodies. It is given to the Rh-negative mother by injection after a miscarriage or abortion or after the delivery of an Rh-positive baby. In most cases it is now also given during pregnancy. The immune globulin prevents the infant's Rh-positive cells from stimulating the mother's immune system, thus preventing HDN.

The source of Rho(D) immune globulin is plasma from women who have had children affected by HDN or from Rh-negative men who are voluntarily injected with Rh-positive RBCs.

PROCEDURE 53-7

Determine ABO Group Using a Slide Test

<u>CAAHEP COMPETENCIES:</u> 3.b.(1)(d), 3.b.(1)(e)
<u>ABHES COMPETENCIES:</u> 4.q, 4.r, 4.z, 4.bb

GOAL: *To determine a patient's ABO group accurately using the slide test technique.*

EQUIPMENT and SUPPLIES

- Glass slides with frosted ends
- Anti-A and anti-B serum (Figure 1*)
- Applicator sticks
- Lancet and automatic finger puncture device
- Alcohol preps
- Sterile gauze squares
- Laboratory marking pen or pencil

PROCEDURAL STEPS

1. Assemble all of the supplies and equipment needed to complete the testing procedure.
2. Wash your hands, and put on face protection and gloves.
   <u>PURPOSE:</u> Infection control.
3. Explain the procedure to the patient.
4. Label the slides in the frosted area with the patient's name.
   <u>PURPOSE:</u> To ensure proper identification of testing results.
5. Place one drop of anti-A serum on slide 1, one drop of anti-B serum on slide 2, and one drop of anti-A and anti-B serum on slide 3.
6. Select the puncture site, and perform a finger puncture procedure.
7. Wipe away the first drop of blood.
   <u>PURPOSE:</u> The first drop of blood may contain tissue fluid.

8. Place one large drop of blood on each of the three prepared slides, close to but not touching the drop of antiserum.
9. Cover the puncture site with a sterile gauze square, and instruct the patient to apply gentle pressure to the site.
10. Mix the antiserum and blood thoroughly, using a clean applicator stick for each slide. The mixture should be spread over an area measuring approximately 20 × 40 mm.
11. Read and interpret the results of the reaction for all slides (Figure 2).
12. Ensure the patient has stopped bleeding, and apply a bandage to the puncture site if necessary.
13. Discard all biohazard testing waste in the appropriate container.
    <u>PURPOSE:</u> Infection control.
14. Clean the testing area.
15. Record the testing results.
    <u>PURPOSE:</u> A procedure is not considered done until it is recorded.
    <u>NOTE:</u> Because of the serious implications of incorrect blood typing, ABO and Rh typing are not routinely performed in a physician's office laboratory. Instead, these tests are performed in a hospital or blood banking facility.

*Figure from Stepp CA, Woods MA: *Laboratory procedures for medical office personnel,* Philadelphia, 1998, Saunders.

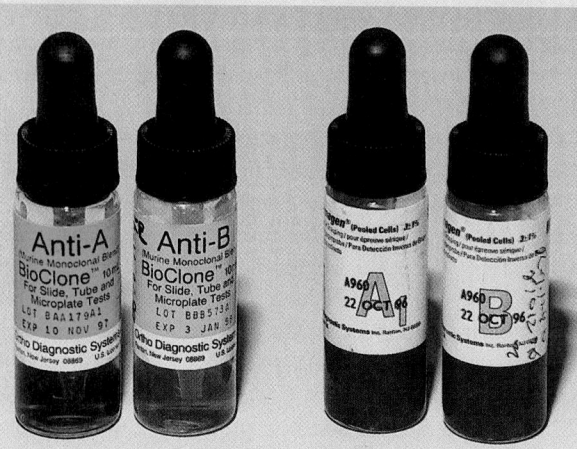

FIGURE 1

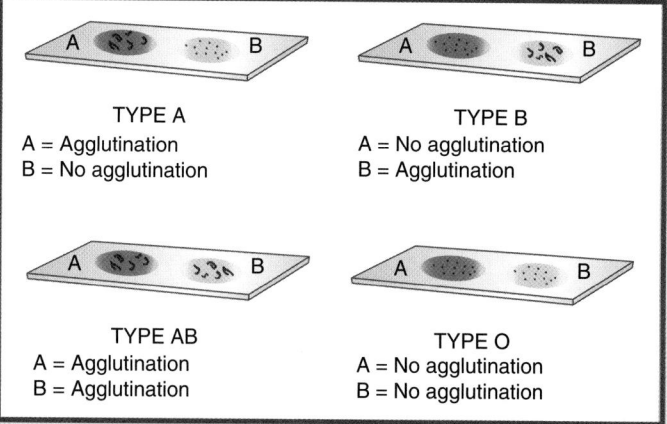

FIGURE 2

PROCEDURE 53-8

Determine Rh Factor Using the Slide Method

<u>CAAHEP COMPETENCIES:</u> 3.b.(1)(d), 3.b.(1)(e)
<u>ABHES COMPETENCIES:</u> 4.q, 4.r, 4.z, 4.bb

GOAL: *To determine accurately the presence or absence of anti-D agglutinations.*

EQUIPMENT and SUPPLIES

- Two glass slides with frosted ends
- Anti-D serum (Figure 1*)
- Applicator sticks
- Lancet and automatic finger puncture device
- Alcohol preps
- Sterile gauze squares
- Laboratory marker or pencil

PROCEDURAL STEPS

1. Assemble all the equipment and supplies needed to complete the testing procedure.
2. Wash your hands, and put on face protection and gloves.
   <u>PURPOSE:</u> Infection control.

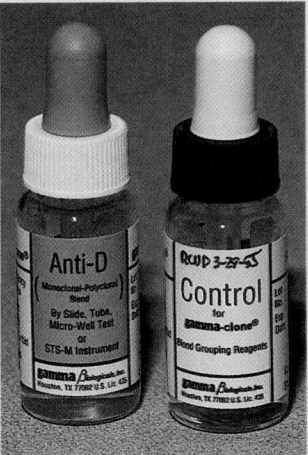

FIGURE 1

3. Label one slide "D" and one slide "C."
   <u>PURPOSE:</u> To differentiate between the anti-D slide and the control slide.
4. Place one drop of anti-D serum on the D slide.
5. Place one drop of the appropriate control reagent on the C slide.
6. Perform a capillary puncture to secure a blood specimen.
7. To each slide, add one large drop of the patient's blood, close to but not touching the antiserum.
8. Thoroughly mix the blood with the anti-D serum and the control, using a clean applicator stick for each slide, and spread the reaction mixture over an area measuring approximately 20 × 40 mm on each slide.
9. Place the slide on an Rh viewbox.
   <u>PURPOSE:</u> The viewbox provides warmth, which promotes agglutination, and also provides extra illumination for viewing.
10. Read the results immediately.
    <u>PURPOSE:</u> Drying of the reaction mixture must not be confused with agglutination.
11. Discard all disposable equipment in the proper biohazardous waste containers.
12. Clean area. Remove gloves and face protection, and wash your hands.
    <u>PURPOSE:</u> Infection control.
13. Record the testing results.
    <u>PURPOSE:</u> A procedure is not considered done until it is recorded.
    <u>NOTE:</u> Because of the serious implications of incorrect blood typing, ABO and Rh typing are not routinely performed in a physician's office laboratory. Instead, these tests are performed in a hospital or blood banking facility.

*Figure from Stepp CA, Woods MA: *Laboratory procedures for medical office personnel,* Philadelphia, 1998, Saunders.

Other Blood Types

In addition to the A and B antigens that characterize the ABO blood grouping, there are more than 600 known antigens and more than 20 other blood type systems. Many are named after the person or family in which the blood type system was discovered. Table 53-8 describes other blood systems. The letters and symbols used in describing a blood type can be confusing. Generally, an abbreviation is followed by a negative (–) or positive (+) symbol; the (–) indicated that the antigen represented by the letters is lacking whereas a (+) indicates that the antigen is present on the RBCs. For example AB+ indicates

that the red cells have the A and B antigens and the Rh (D) antigen, whereas the blood type O–K–Fy+ lacks the A, B, Rh, and K (Kell) antigens, and has the Fy (Duffy) antigen.

Rare Blood types

Approximately one person in 1000 has a rare blood type. Because blood types are inherited, certain rare blood types are more common among certain ethnic groups. Finding compatible blood for life-saving transfusions can become more difficult for those with a rare blood type. Of particular significance is the Duffy system. The Duffy antigens are represented as Fy(a) and Fy(b). The blood types Fy(a–b+), Fy(a+b+), and Fy(a–b+) are

TABLE 53-8 Other Blood Typing Systems

SYSTEM	REMARKS
Diego	Found only among East Asians and Native Americans.
MNS	Useful in maternity and paternity testing.
Duffy	The malarial parasite requires the Duffy antigen to enter the red blood cells. Lacking the antigens confers resistance to malaria. Duffy-negative blood is found only in the descendants of African populations.
Lewis	Antigens are soluble in blood rather than attached to the red blood cells. These are the only blood group antibodies that never have been implicated in hemolytic disease of the newborn.

Other blood group systems include Colton, M, Kell, Kidd, Lewis, Landsteiner-Wiener, P, Yt or Cartwright, XG, Scianna, Dombrock, Chido/Rodgers, Kx, Gerbich, Cromer, Knops, Indian, Ok, Raph, and JMH.

very common among the U.S. Caucasian population. Fy(a–b–) is very rare in the Caucasian population but is present in 68% of the African American population in the United States.

These blood type systems are generally not significant for blood donations but can be troublesome for individuals who have had numerous transfusions and may have developed atypical antibodies, making future cross-matching more of a challenge. The American Red Cross, in collaboration with the American Association of Blood Banks (AABB), maintains a rare donor database as part of the American Rare Donor Program. When a need for a rare type of blood arises, those in the registry can be contacted to make a donation. In addition, blood of a rare type can be frozen to ensure availability when needed.

CRITICAL THINKING APPLICATION

Before Mr. Corrigan's kidney transplant, he had a type and cross-match and was determined to be type O+. Explain how the test was performed and what the technician observed with the anti-A, anti-B, and anti-D antisera.

CLINICAL CHEMISTRY

Most clinical chemistry methods are classified as moderately complex according to CLIA guidelines, and only people with documented training in the method would be permitted to perform testing under the supervision of the physician office laboratory director. Increasingly, however, clinical chemistry tests are being granted CLIA-waived status.

Nearly all of the CLIA-waived chemistry analyzers used in the physician's office use lateral flow immunoassay (described in Chapter 51), reflectance photometry, amperometry (electrochemistry), or chemiluminescence. In reflectance photometry blood is applied to a reagent pad or a reagent area, where it reacts with certain chemicals, including enzymes, causing a color change to take place. A light source, such as an LED, directs light onto the test strip after the chemical reaction takes place. The colored pad on the test strip will absorb the wavelengths of that color and reflect the other wavelengths. The more light that is absorbed by the pad, the less that is reflected, permitting quantitation of the analyte. A detector captures the reflected light, converts it to an electronic signal, and translates that signal into concentration of analyte in the sample.

Amperometry also relies on an enzyme-mediated reaction between the analyte and the reagents in the test system, but in this case electrons are generated by the chemical reactions as opposed to a color change taking place. Electrochemistry quantifies the number of electrons that are generated by capturing them on a mediator and subsequently applying a voltage. This transfers the electrons to an electrode, where the resulting current is converted to an electronic signal that corresponds to the glucose concentration.

Chemiluminescence is the emission of light without heat as a product of a chemical reaction. As a result of the chemical reaction, electrons are in an excited state and they are ejected from the luminescing compound on the test strip. As the electrons move from this excited, more energetic state back to their natural or ground state, they release their excess energy in the form of a light flash. This flash can be detected, measured, and quantified.

In the physician's office laboratory, clinical chemistry tests commonly performed by medical assistants include tests for glucose, cholesterol, triglycerides, hemoglobin A_{1c}, thyroid hormones, and liver enzymes (alanine aminotransferase [ALT]).

BLOOD GLUCOSE TESTING

Glucose is used as a fuel by many cells within the body; under normal circumstances, it is the only substance used to nourish brain cells. Maintenance of blood glucose levels within a normal range is vitally important to homeostasis of the human body. Understanding the importance of glucose helps in understanding the reason why glucose is the most frequently tested analyte.

Elevated blood glucose levels are most often associated with diabetes mellitus but may also indicate pancreatitis, endocrine disorders, or chronic renal failure. Diabetes mellitus is a disorder of carbohydrate metabolism that results in elevated blood and urine glucose levels secondary to the inability of the pancreas to produce sufficient insulin. Diabetes is discussed in Chapter 44.

To check a patient for possible diabetes mellitus, the physician may request a blood glucose tolerance test. For this test the fasting patient receives an adequate carbohydrate meal of 100 g of glucose by mouth. This is usually given to the patient as a drink that is similar to a sweet fruit punch. The amount may be adjusted according to the patient's weight. If the glucose level does not exceed 100 g/dL at onset of the testing period or 180 g/dL 1 hour after ingestion of the glucose drink, the patient is believed to have a normal glucose level. If the blood glucose level exceeds 200 g/dL, glucose will escape into the urine because the renal tubules are no longer able to absorb the excessive amount present in the glomerulus.

Self-monitoring of blood glucose levels has become an important part of treating diabetes. Testing methodologies have evolved over the past 20 years. The earliest test methods available were urine reagent strips (see Chapter 51) that detected glucose and ketones. Although simple to use, they lacked the precision to be useful for adjusting insulin dosage. In the 1970s similar strips for testing glucose levels in the blood were introduced. A drop of blood from a capillary puncture was applied to the strip, and the excess was wiped away. After careful timing, the color of the pad on the reagent strip was compared with a chart. The results were highly dependent on the user.

The first hand-held devices were marketed shortly after this and were designed to read the test strips electronically rather than visually using reflectance photometry. Although such technology still required wiping and timing, the devices were precise enough to monitor blood glucose and assist with insulin adjustment.

In the 1980s blood glucose monitors using electrochemistry and devices that used reflectance photometry joined the market. The need for wiping and timing was eliminated. These technologies use an enzyme to convert glucose to measurable products. Enzymes commonly used are glucose oxidase, glucose dehydrogenase, and hexokinase.

The medical assistant can perform glucose testing using a glucose-monitoring device cleared by the U.S. Food and Drug Administration (FDA) for home use (Procedure 53-9). Blood glucose is routinely monitored by patients with both type 1 (insulin-dependent) and type 2 (non–insulin-dependent) diabetes. Glucose levels may also be monitored by women experiencing gestational diabetes, a condition seen during pregnancy in which the effect of insulin is partially blocked by a variety of other hormones made in the placenta.

CHOLESTEROL TESTING

Cholesterol is a fatlike substance (lipid) that is present in cell membranes. It is also needed to form bile acids and steroid hormones. Cholesterol travels in the blood in distinct particles containing both lipid and proteins. These particles are called *lipoproteins*. The cholesterol level in the blood is determined partly by inheritance and partly by acquired factors such as diet, calorie balance, and level of physical activity.

Patients are often confused by cholesterol testing. The confusion is caused partly by the way some people use the term *cholesterol*, which is often a catchall term for both the cholesterol you eat and the cholesterol that is maintained in the body. A high level of low-density lipoprotein, or LDL cholesterol, reflects an increased risk of heart disease, which is why LDL cholesterol is often called "bad" cholesterol. Lower levels of LDL cholesterol reflect a lower risk of heart disease. When too much LDL cholesterol circulates in the blood, it can slowly build up in the walls of arteries that feed the heart and brain.

Together with other substances, it can form plaque, a thick, hard deposit that can clog those arteries. This condition is known as *atherosclerosis*. If a clot (thrombus) forms where a plaque is, the blood flow can be blocked to part of the heart muscle, causing a heart attack. If a clot blocks blood flow to part of the brain, a stroke results.

About one third to one fourth of blood cholesterol is carried by high-density lipoprotein (HDL). HDL cholesterol is known as the "good" cholesterol because a high level of HDL cholesterol seems to protect against heart attack. Medical experts think that HDL tends to carry cholesterol away from the arteries and back to the liver, where it is passed from the body. Some experts believe that excess cholesterol is removed from atherosclerotic plaque by HDL, thus slowing the buildup; however, low HDL cholesterol levels (i.e., lower than 35 mg/dL) may result in a greater risk for heart disease.

It is recommended that adults over the age of 20 have a cholesterol test at least once every 5 years. Total cholesterol, the combination of HDL and LDL, is typically measured (Procedure 53-10); however, the physician may order an HDL determination separately. Both tests are considered screening tests, and elevated results always require additional testing before a diagnosis can be made. In general, total cholesterol levels under 200 mg/dL are considered normal. Results over 240 mg/dL are considered elevated and, based on confirmed testing, place a person in the high-risk category for coronary heart disease. An HDL cholesterol level of 35 mg/dL is considered acceptable. Values below 35 mg/dL place one in a high-risk category.

The total cholesterol and HDL cholesterol are not significantly affected by food consumption, so fasting is not necessary before testing. The physician, however, may request fasting in preparation. If the total cholesterol is elevated, the physician is likely to order a lipid profile—a series of tests that measures total cholesterol, triglycerides, and HDL and LDL cholesterol levels. Triglyceride levels are affected by food consumption, and the patient must be instructed to fast before the test.

CLIA-waived cholesterol monitors can measure HDL cholesterol, total cholesterol, and triglycerides. The Cholestech LDX analyzer (Hayward, Calif.), uses enzymatic reactions to produce products that are quantified by reflectance photometry using blood from a fingerstick.

Hemoglobin A₁c Testing

During the last two decades diabetes researchers have developed several new laboratory tests that help in the evaluation of blood glucose levels. These tests measure glycohemoglobin, fructosamine, and glycosylated protein. These tests are not substitutes for monitoring blood glucose levels. Instead, they give different information about the diabetic's health and add a new dimension to the evaluation of diabetes.

The glycohemoglobin test was developed in the late 1970s. Other names that have been used to describe the same test are glycosylated hemoglobin and hemoglobin A₁c. This test gives information about the average blood sugar level during the past 2 or 3 months. In the blood, glucose binds irreversibly to hemoglobin molecules within RBCs. The amount of glucose

PROCEDURE 53-9

Perform Chemistry Testing: Perform a Blood Glucose Accu-Chek Test

<u>CAAHEP COMPETENCIES:</u> 3.b.(1)(d), 3.b.(1)(e), 3.b.(3)(c)(iii)
<u>ABHES COMPETENCIES:</u> 4.q, 4.r, 4.aa

GOAL: *To accurately perform a blood test to detect elevated blood glucose.*

EQUIPMENT and SUPPLIES

- Accu-Chek glucose monitor or similar glucose monitoring device
- Accu-Chek glucose testing strip
- Lancet and autoloading finger-puncturing device
- Alcohol preps
- Gauze squares
- Sharps container
- Disposable gloves
- Patient record

  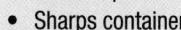 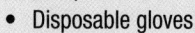 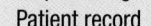

PROCEDURAL STEPS

1. Check the physician's order, and collect the necessary equipment and supplies needed to complete the testing procedure. Perform quality-control measures according to manufacturer guidelines and office policy.
2. Wash your hands, and put on gloves.
   <u>PURPOSE:</u> Infection control.
3. Ask the patient to wash his or her hands in warm soapy water, then to rinse them in warm water and dry them completely.
   <u>PURPOSE:</u> Clean the area that will be punctured; warm fingers may increase peripheral blood flow.
4. Check the patient's index and ring fingers, and select the site for puncture.
   <u>PURPOSE:</u> Site of puncture must be free of trauma.
5. Turn on the Accu-Chek monitor by pressing the ON button (Figure 1*).
6. Make sure the code number on the LED display matches the code number on the container of test strips.
   <u>PURPOSE:</u> If code numbers do not match, the device must be reprogrammed with the new code for the test results to be valid.
7. Remove a test strip from the vial, and immediately replace the vial cover.
   <u>PURPOSE:</u> Vial must be closed to protect unused strips from possible contamination.
8. Check the strip for discoloration by comparing the color of the round window on the back of the test strip with the designated "unused" color chart provided on the test strip vial label.
   <u>PURPOSE:</u> This will establish the validity of the testing procedure.
9. Do not touch the yellow test pad or round window on the back of the strip when handling the strip.
10. When the test strip symbol begins flashing in the lower right-hand corner of the display screen, insert the test strip into the designated testing slot until it locks into place. When the test strip is inserted correctly, the arrows on the test strip will be facing up and pointing toward the monitor (Figure 2).
11. Cleanse the selected site on the patient's fingertip with the alcohol wipe, and allow the finger to air dry.
12. Perform the finger puncture, and wipe away the first drop of blood.

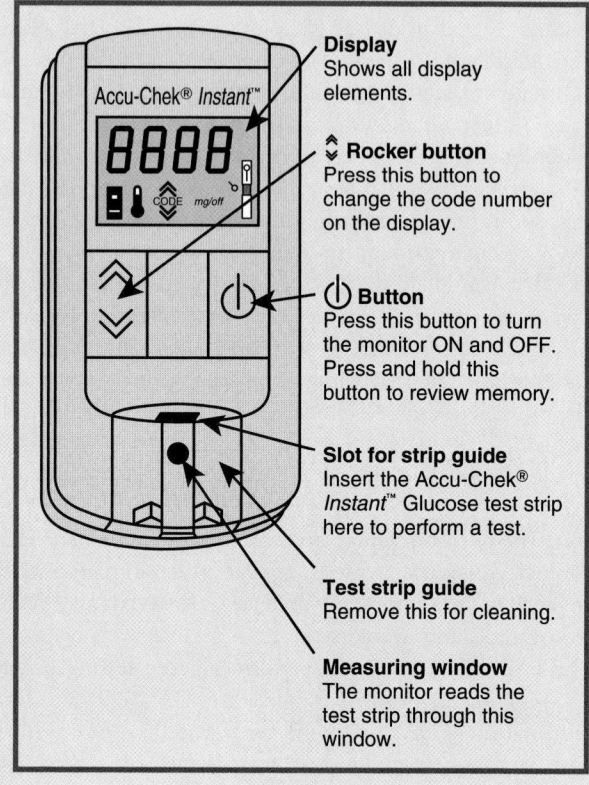

Display
Shows all display elements.

Rocker button
Press this button to change the code number on the display.

Button
Press this button to turn the monitor ON and OFF. Press and hold this button to review memory.

Slot for strip guide
Insert the Accu-Chek® *Instant*™ Glucose test strip here to perform a test.

Test strip guide
Remove this for cleaning.

Measuring window
The monitor reads the test strip through this window.

FIGURE 1

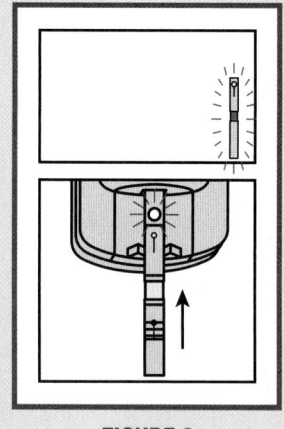 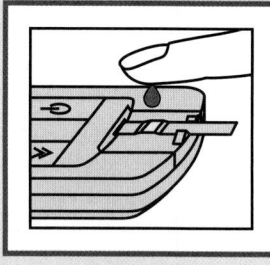

FIGURE 2   **FIGURE 3**

<u>PURPOSE:</u> There may be tissue fluid present in the first drop of blood.

13. Apply a large hanging drop of blood to the center of the yellow testing pad (Figure 3).
    a. Do not touch the pad with the patient's finger.
    b. Do not apply a second drop of blood.

Continued

PROCEDURE 53-9—*cont'd*

c. Do not smear the blood with your finger.

d. Be certain the yellow test pad is saturated with blood.

14. Give the patient a gauze square to hold securely over the puncture site.

15. The monitor will automatically begin the measurement process as soon as it senses the drop of blood.

16. Read the test result when it is displayed in the display window in milligrams per deciliter.

17. Turn off the monitor by pressing the "O" button.

18. Discard all biohazard waste into the proper waste containers.
    <u>PURPOSE:</u> Infection control.

19. Clean the glucometer according to manufacturer guidelines, disinfect the work area, remove gloves and dispose of them properly, and wash your hands.

20. Record the testing results in the patient's medical record.
    <u>PURPOSE:</u> A procedure is considered not done until it is recorded.

Figure from Stepp CA, Woods MA: Laboratory procedures for medical office personnel, Philadelphia, 1998, Saunders.
See Appendix D for a charting example.

PROCEDURE 53-10

Perform Chemistry Testing: Determine Cholesterol Level Using a ProAct Testing Device

<u>CAAHEP COMPETENCIES:</u> 3.b.(1)(d), 3.b.(1)(e), 3.b.(3)(c)(iii)
<u>ABHES COMPETENCIES:</u> 4.q, 4.r, 4.aa

GOAL: *To perform a ProAct test for total cholesterol level and accurately report the results.*

EQUIPMENT and SUPPLIES

- ProAct testing device
- Lithium heparin capillary tube and capillary pipette
- Lancets and lancet device

- Sterile gauze
- Alcohol preps
- Biohazard waste container
- Biohazard sharps container

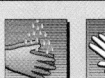

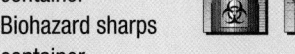

PROCEDURAL STEPS

1. Reread the physician's order, and assemble all the supplies and equipment needed to complete the test.

2. Wash your hands, and put on gloves.
   <u>PURPOSE:</u> Infection control.

3. Explain the procedure to the patient.

4. Load the lancet device with a sterile lancet.

5. Examine the patient's index and ring fingers, and pick a puncture site.
   <u>PURPOSE:</u> Puncture site must be free of trauma.

6. Cleanse the chosen puncture site with alcohol, and allow the site to air dry.

7. Puncture the site, and wipe away the first drop of blood with a sterile gauze square.

<u>PURPOSE:</u> The first drop of blood may contain tissue fluid.

8. Hold the capillary tube horizontally by the colored end of the tube, and allow the tube to fill. Do not allow air bubbles to enter the tube; if this occurs, discard the capillary tube and continue drawing the sample with a new tube.
   <u>PURPOSE:</u> Air bubbles may cause erroneous test results.

9. Give the patient a clean gauze square, and ask the patient to apply pressure to the puncture site.

10. Remove a cholesterol testing strip from the container, and close the container immediately (Figure 1*).
    <u>PURPOSE:</u> Closing the container will avoid possible exposure of the unused strips.

11. Remove the foil protecting the test area of the strip, and place the strip on a dry, hard, flat surface (Figure 2).

12. Attach the capillary tube filled with blood to the pipette.

13. Squeeze the plunger of the pipette completely to allow a drop of blood to form at the end of the capillary tube.

14. Allow the drop of blood to fall onto the center of the red mesh application zone. Make sure that the tip of the capillary tube does not touch the test strip and that all blood is dispensed (Figure 3).

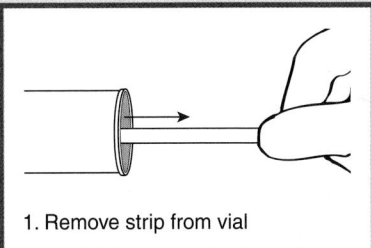

1. Remove strip from vial

FIGURE 1

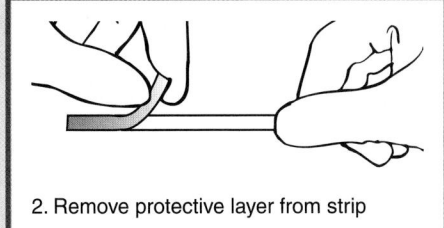

2. Remove protective layer from strip

FIGURE 2

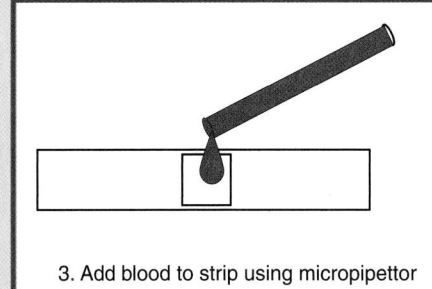

3. Add blood to strip using micropipettor

FIGURE 3

Continued

<u>PURPOSE:</u> Strip must be saturated with blood for best testing results to be obtained.

15. Allow the sample to soak into the red mesh for 3 to 15 seconds.
16. Insert the cholesterol strip into the test port. The ProAct device will count down approximately 160 seconds (Figure 4).
17. Remove the capillary tube from the pipette, and discard it in a biohazard container.
    <u>PURPOSE:</u> Infection control.
18. When the measurement time is completed, REMOVE STRIP will appear in the LED display window. Remove the used test strip, and the test result will appear on the display (Figure 5).
19. Examine the test area of the used testing strip for uneven color development before discarding it into the biohazard waste container.

<u>PURPOSE:</u> If the color appears mottled, the test may not be valid and it is advisable that you repeat the entire testing process.

20. Discard all biohazard testing waste in appropriate containers, clean the testing area, remove gloves, and wash your hands.
    <u>PURPOSE:</u> Infection control.
21. Record the test results in the patient's medical record.
    <u>PURPOSE:</u> A procedure is not considered done until it is recorded.

*Figure from Stepp CA, Woods MA: *Laboratory procedures for medical office personnel*, Philadelphia, 1998, Saunders.

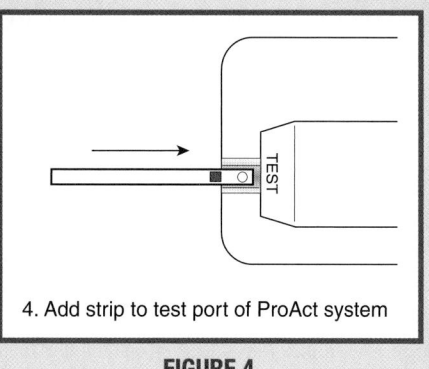

4. Add strip to test port of ProAct system

FIGURE 4

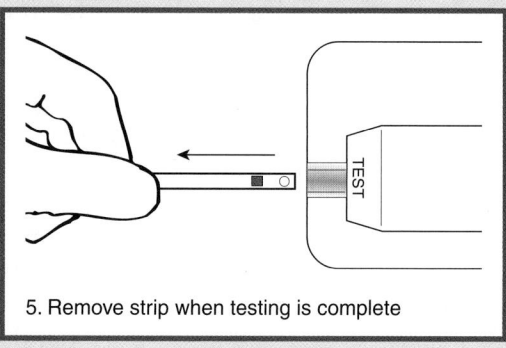

5. Remove strip when testing is complete

FIGURE 5

that is bound to hemoglobin is directly tied to the concentration of glucose in the blood.

Because RBCs have a life span of approximately 90 days, measuring the amount of glucose bound to hemoglobin can provide an assessment of average blood sugar control during the 60 to 90 days preceding the test. This is the purpose of the glycohemoglobin tests, most commonly the hemoglobin A_{1c} (HbA_{1c}) measurement. Because the test results give feedback on the previous 2 to 3 months, performance of an HbA_{1c} test every 3 months will provide data on the average blood glucose level. If the glycohemoglobin value is higher than the normal range, then the average blood sugar has been elevated during the past 2 months.

There are several methods of performing an HbA_{1c} measurement, and the medical assistant can perform HbA_{1c} testing using several CLIA-waived devices. The DCA 2000, made by Bayer Diagnostics (Tarrytown, N.Y.), provides HbA_{1c} values in 6 minutes from one drop of capillary blood obtained via a fingerstick. Patients can also perform HbA_{1c} testing at home using FDA-approved instrumentation including the A1CNow by Metrika (Sunnyvale, Calif.) and the Micromat II from Bio-Rad (Hercules, Calif.).

The fructosamine test was developed more recently. *Fructosamine* is a term that refers to the linking of blood sugar onto protein molecules in the bloodstream. Fructosamine levels change more rapidly than glycohemoglobin does. The fructosamine value depends on the average blood sugar level during the past 3 weeks. Therefore it might be able to detect changes in diabetic control earlier than the glycohemoglobin. The fructosamine test could be viewed as complementary to the glycohemoglobin because the two tests are different reflections of diabetes control: glycohemoglobin looks back approximately 8 weeks, and the fructosamine test looks back approximately 3 weeks.

Other tests similar to the fructosamine test have been proposed; the glycosylated protein test is an example of another test that was suggested. Unfortunately, these newer tests are less reliable than originally hoped, and it seems unlikely that either the fructosamine test or the glycosylated protein test will ever become as widely used for monitoring diabetes as the glycohemoglobin level test.

CRITICAL THINKING APPLICATION

Mr. Corrigan routinely monitors his blood sugar. Why is Dr. Fischbach also interested in his hemoglobin A_{1c} levels? What complications of diabetes led to Mr. Corrigan's need for a transplant?

Thyroid Hormone Testing

The thyroid gland is located anterior to the trachea in the throat. It produces the hormones triiodothyronine (T_3) and thyroxine (T_4). These hormones are essential for life and have many effects on body metabolism, growth, and development. The thyroid gland is influenced by hormones produced by two other organs found in the brain, the pituitary gland and the hypothalamus. The pituitary gland produces thyroid-stimulating hormone (TSH), and the hypothalamus produces thyrotropin-releasing hormone (TRH). Regulation of thyroid hormone production and thyroid disorders are discussed in Chapter 44.

CLIA-waived rapid diagnostic tests to qualitatively measure TSH are available for point-of-care testing. Using whole blood from a fingerstick, these tests screen patients for hypothyroidism by detecting elevated levels of TSH, which constitutes a sign of hypothyroidism. The tests use lateral flow chromatographic immunoassay technology housed in a plastic cassette similar to the pregnancy test discussed in Chapter 51. One such commercially available test is the ThyroTest from ThyroTek (Honeybrook, Pa.).

Alanine Aminotransferase and Aspartate Aminotransferase Testing

Certain drugs can impair liver function and require monitoring of liver enzymes. These drugs include statins and fibrates, pharmaceutical agents used to lower blood cholesterol, and certain antidiabetic and antihypertensive drugs. It is necessary to monitor liver function during therapy with drugs that have a potential for causing liver malfunction. Two liver enzymes, aspartate aminotransferase (AST) and alanine aminotransferase (ALT) can be useful in monitoring homeostasis during drug therapy. The first liver enzyme testing to be CLIA-waived was the Cholestech ALT/AST test, which is performed on the Cholestech L-D-X System (Cholestech, Hayward, Calif.). This system also analyzes glucose, total cholesterol, HDL, and triglycerides, using a combination of enzymatic reactions and reflectance photometry to detect the resulting color changes.

CRITICAL THINKING APPLICATION

For what reason might Dr. Fischbach want to evaluate Mr. Corrigan's liver enzymes? What clinical chemistry tests might he order from the referral laboratory? What Vacutainer tube would be necessary for these tests? What tests for liver enzymes might Dana be able to perform in the physician's office laboratory? What sample will she need for those tests?

Chemistry Panels

Automated blood chemistry analyzers are often used to perform blood chemistry testing. It is not uncommon for several analytes to be detected at once. A physician may order a chemistry panel, such as a renal or liver panel, that will determine the levels of several related analytes (Figure 53-13). Analytes commonly detected in the chemistry laboratory are listed in Table 53-9. Generally, serum is needed for these tests. Typical panels are shown in Table 53-10 (p. 1214).

TABLE 53-9 Blood Chemistry Tests

TEST	ABBREVIATION	NORMAL VALUES	DESCRIPTION	PURPOSE
Alanine aminotransferase	ALT (SGPT)	<45 U/L	Enzyme found predominately in liver but also in kidney	To detect liver disease
Albumin		3.5-5 g/dL	Protein	To assess water
Alkaline phosphatase	ALP	20-70 U/L	Enzyme found in several tissues	To detect liver and bone disease
Aspartate aminotransferase	AST (SGOT)	<40 U/L	Enzyme found in several tissues	To detect tissue damage
Blood urea nitrogen	BUN	7-18 mg/dL; 2.5-6.4 mmol/L	Metabolic products of protein catabolism	To detect renal disease
Calcium	CA	8.4-10.2 mg/dL; 2.1-2.6 mmol/L	Mineral	To assess parathyroid function and calcium metabolism
Chloride	Cl	98-106 mmol/L	Electrolyte	To determine acid-base and water balance
Cholesterol	CH, Chol	Total: <200 mg/dL; <5.18 mmol/L LDL: <130 mg/dL; <3.37 mmol/L HDL: >35 mg/dL; >0.91 mmol/L	Lipid	Screening for atherosclerosis related to heart disease
Creatine phosphokinase	CPK	Specific to testing method used	Enzyme found in several tissues	To assess the source of muscle damage (myocardial infarct)

Continued

TABLE 53-9 Blood Chemistry Tests—*cont'd*

TEST	ABBREVIATION	NORMAL VALUES	DESCRIPTION	PURPOSE
Creatinine	creat	0.2-0.8 mg/dL	Metabolic product of protein catabolism	Screening for renal function
Ferritin		20-50 ng/mL	Iron-carrying protein	To detect the amount of iron stored in the body
Gamma glutamyltransferase	GGT	0-45 U/L	Enzyme found mainly in liver cells	To detect liver disease
Globulin	glob, lg	Varies according to type	Protein	To detect abnormalities in protein synthesis and removal
Glucose fasting blood sugar	FBS	70-100 mg/dL; 3.9-6.1 mmol/L	Carbohydrate	To detect disorders of glucose metabolism (diabetes)
Glucose tolerance test	GTT	Varies with time	Carbohydrate	To detect disorders of glucose metabolism (diabetes)
Iron	Fe	35-140 mcg/dL	Mineral	To assist in diagnosis of anemia
Lactate dehydrogenase	LDH	<240 U/L	Enzyme found in several tissues	To assist in the confirmation of myocardial or pulmonary infarct
pH	pH	7.35-7.45		To assess acid
Phosphorus	P	3-4.5 mg/dL; 0.97-1.45 mmol/L	Mineral	To assist in the proper evaluation of calcium levels and to detect disorders of the endocrine system
Potassium	K	3.5-5.1 mmol/L	Mineral	To assist in diagnosis of acid-base and water balance
Sodium	Na	135-146 mmol/L	Mineral	To assist in diagnosis of acid-base and water balance
Total bilirubin	TB	0.2-1 mg/dL; 3.4-17.1 mmol/L	Metabolic product of hemoglobin catabolism	To evaluate liver function and to aid in diagnosis of anemia
Total iron-binding capacity	TIBC	245-400 µg/dL		A measure of the potential to transport iron
Total protein	TP	6-8 g/dL; 60-80 g/L		To assess the state of hydration; to screen for diseases that alter protein balance
Troponin I and T		<0.4	A cardiac-specific protein only found in heart muscle damage	To aid in diagnosis of myocardial infarct
Thyroid-stimulating hormone (thyrotropin)	TSH	5-6 milliU/L	Hormone produced by the pituitary	To assess thyroid and pituitary gland function
Thyroxine	T_4	5-12 mcg/dL; 64-155 mmol/L	Hormone produced by the thyroid gland	To assess thyroid function
Triglycerides	Trig	30-190 mg/dL; 0.34-2.15 mmol/L		Screening for atherosclerosis related to heart disease
Triiodothyronine	T_3	27%-47%	Hormone produced by the thyroid gland	To assess thyroid function
Uric acid	UA	Male: 3.4-7 mg/dL; 202-416 µmol/L Female: 2.4-6 mg/dL; 143-357 µmol/L	Metabolic product of protein catabolism	To evaluate renal failure, gout, and leukemia

CRITICAL THINKING APPLICATION

What tests are routinely done as part of the renal panel? What information will these tests give Dr. Fischbach regarding the status of Mr. Corrigan's kidney?

CLOSING COMMENTS

Legal and Ethical Issues

In 1991 many states adopted the Blood Safety Act, which requires physicians to provide patients with information concerning blood transfusion options. This information is given

PHYSICIAN'S MEDICAL CENTER
77332 E. CAPITAL DRIVE
ANYTOWN, USA 11123

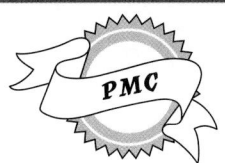

Ronald J. Haldor M.D.
Kaye M. Jones M.D.
Nicholas C. Stepp M.D.

PATIENT – PLEASE NOTE

☐

If this box is checked, don't eat or drink anything, except water, for 14 hours before going to the lab.

PATIENT NAME _____
LAST _____ FIRST _____ M.I. _____

ADDRESS _____ DOB _____

CITY _____ STATE _____ ZIP_____ SEX: M F

TELEPHONE # _____ SOCIAL SECURITY # _____ – _____ – _____

ORDERING PHYSICIAN _____ DATE _____

BILLING: ☐ HMO ☐ MEDICARE ☐ MEDI-CAL ☐ OTHER # _____
(Please attach copy of eligibilty card.)
GUARANTOR (If other than patient) _____

☐ PHONE RESULTS TO _____

☐ SEND ADDITIONAL COPIES OF REPORT TO _____

Patient Diagnosis _____

☐ 906 ARTERIAL BLOOD GASES
ROOM AIR _____
RESP. ASSIST _____
☐ 105 BLOOD CELL PROFILE (Hgb + Hct)
☐ 862 BILIRUBIN (NEONATAL)
☐ 868 BILIRUBIN (TOTAL & DIRECT)
☐ 100 CBC (Complete Blood Count & Diff)
☐ 3000 ELECTROLYTES
☐ (NA, K, CO_2, Cl)
☐ FANA
☐ GLUCOSE
☐ 915 GLUCOSE, PRE-NATAL DIABETIC SCR.
(1 Hour Post-Glucola)
☐ GLUCOSE TOLERANCE TEST
OF HOURS _____ DOSE _____
☐ 3398 HEPATITIS PANEL
(B-Surf Ag/Ab, B-Core Ab, A-Ab)
☐ 988 LIPID PROFILE
(Chol, Trig, HDL, LDL, Cardiac Risk)
☐ 3380 LIVER PANEL
(Alk Phos, Bili, TP, Alb, GGT, SGOT (AST)
SGPT (ALT), & Consult)
☐ 3006 METABOLIC 7
(Na, K, CO_2, Cl, Glu, Mg)

☐ 3035 PANEL 17
(Panel 13 + Na + K + Cl + CO2)
☐ 3020 METABOLIC 10
(Na, K, CO2, Cl, Glu, BUN, Creat)
☐ 3015 METABOLIC 11
(Met 10 & Phos)
☐ 3160 OBSTETRICAL PANEL 1
(CBC, UA, ABO/Rh, Antibody Screen,
Rubella, RPR)
☐ 3172 OBSTETRICAL PANEL 3
(CBC, ABO/Rh, Antibody Screen,
Rubella, RPR)
☐ 3445 OBSTETRICAL PANEL 7
(ABO/Rh, Antibody Screen, Rubella,
RPR)
☐ 3447 OBSTETRICAL PANEL 7A
(ABO/Rh, Antibody Screen, Rubella,
RPR, Hepatitis B Surt Ag)
☐ 3025 PANEL 13
(Glu, BUN, Creat, Uric Acid, Ca, Tp,
Alb, Bili, Chol, Alk, Phos, SGOT (AST),
LDH, Phos)
☐ 3030 PANEL 15
(Panel 13 + Na + K)

☐ 3010 METABOLIC 8
(Na, K, CO2, Cl, Glu, BUN)
☐ 3040 PANEL 20 - SMAC
(Panel 17 + SGPT (ALT) + GGT +
Osmolality)
☐ 3043 S-1 Panel (Panel 20 + Triglyceride)
☐ 500 PROTHROMBIN TIME (PT)
☐ 505 Partial Thromboplastin Time (PPT)
☐ 7500 RPR
☐ 7515 RUBELLA
☐ 2030 THYROID SCREEN
(T4, T3, Uptake, Adj T4)
☐ 704 URINALYSIS

BACTERIOLOGY

SPECIMEN SOURCE **(REQUIRED)**

COLLECTION DATE _____
☐ _____ ROUTINE CULTURE
☐ 8919 AFB CULTURE
☐ 8921 FUNGAL CULTURE

ADDITIONAL LABORATORY TESTS:

LABORATORY OUTPATIENT REQUEST

2804 (4/93)

OFFICE USE ONLY
Telephone Order per _____
Order Received by _____

FIGURE 53-13 Panel request form. (From Stepp CA, Woods MA: *Laboratory procedures for medical office personnel*, Philadelphia, 1998, Saunders.)

TABLE 53-10 Typical Chemistry Panels

PANEL	COMPONENT	PANEL	COMPONENT
Liver	Alkaline phosphatase (ALP) Gamma glutamyltransferase (GGT) Aspartate aminotransferase (AST) Alanine aminotransferase (ALT) Lactate dehydrogenase (LDH)	Cardiac	Creatinine phosphokinase (CPK) Troponin I Troponin T
Anemia	Iron Total iron-binding capacity Ferritin Transferrin	Electrolyte	Sodium Potassium Chloride
Thyroid	Thyroid-stimulating hormone (TSH) Thyroxine (T$_4$) Triiodothyronine (T$_3$)	Renal	Creatinine Blood urea nitrogen Uric acid Glucose

before surgery and before any medical procedure in which the possibility exists that blood transfusion may be necessary. Physicians are also required to note on each patient's medical record that a written summary was given to the patient. As the physician's agent, you share this responsibility. If this is

needed for a particular patient, it is the responsibility of every member of the healthcare team to ensure that this information is supplied to the patient, noted on the chart, and initialed. The written summary has been formally prepared, and copies of it can be requested from the state department of health services.

SUMMARY OF SCENARIO

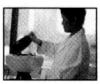

Dana knows the important role laboratory analysis of blood plays in patient care. Often many different tests are needed to assess a patient's health. Mr. Corrigan appreciates that he can have many of these tests done during his routine visits with a simple fingerstick, such as the hemoglobin A$_{1c}$ level, the hemoglobin and hematocrit, the PT test, and ALT and AST testing. The anemia panel, CBC and

differential, and hemoglobin and hematocrit will provide Dr. Fischbach with essential information to diagnose anemia, and the hemoglobin A$_{1c}$ level will be used to monitor Mr. Corrigan's diabetes. The PT test will monitor coagulation and liver enzyme testing and will assure Dr. Fischbach that Mr. Corrigan's liver is functioning properly while he is taking medication to treat the diabetes and to manage the transplant.

SUMMARY of LEARNING OBJECTIVES

1. Define, spell, and pronounce the terms listed in the vocabulary.
   - Spelling and pronouncing medical terms correctly adds credibility to the medical assistant. Knowing the definition of these terms promotes confidence in communication with patients and co-workers.
2. Name three main functions of blood.
   - Blood supplies cells with needed nutrients, delivers oxygen to tissues via hemoglobin, and removes waste.
3. Describe the role of the hematology laboratory in patient care.
   - In the hematology laboratory, blood cells are enumerated, WBCs are differentiated, and the oxygen-carrying capacity of blood is determined. Hematology testing provides an excellent overview of homeostasis.
4. Describe the appearance and function of the erythrocyte.
   - RBCs are also known as erythrocytes because of their red color, which comes from hemoglobin. The biconcave disks lack

a nucleus and are responsible for transporting oxygen and carbon dioxide to and from tissues.
5. Describe the appearance and function of the granular and the agranular leukocyte.
   - WBCs are also known as leukocytes. Agranular leukocytes lack granules in the cytoplasm, and granular leukocytes have granules. All leukocytes function in fighting infection.
6. Differentiate between T cells and B cells.
   - T lymphocytes are important in immunity and play roles in killing foreign, virus-infected, and tumor cells; assist in antibody production; and keep the immune system in check. B cells are responsible for antibody production.
7. Describe the appearance and function of the thrombocyte.
   - The thrombocyte, also known as a platelet, is a fragment of a larger cell, called a megakaryocyte, which is found in the bone

Continued

marrow. Thrombocytes play an important role in clot formation, both physically and chemically.

8. Explain the process of clot formation.
   - Clot formation begins with the aggregation of thrombocytes, which release a substance that initiates the clotting cascade, resulting in a network of minute threads that trap plasma and blood cells.

9. Identify the anticoagulant of choice for hematology testing.
   - The anticoagulant required for most hematology testing is ethylenediamine tetraacetic acid (EDTA). The lavender-topped vacuum tube used in phlebotomy contains this anticoagulant.

10. Explain the purpose of a microhematocrit.
    - The microhematocrit (or hematocrit) test is performed to assess the volume of erythrocytes in relationship to total blood volume by centrifuging a small amount of whole blood in a capillary tube. Whole blood normally consists of slightly less than 50% RBCs. Hematocrit is reported as a percentage and is roughly three times that of hemoglobin.

11. Accurately perform a microhematocrit.
    - Refer to Procedure 53-1.

12. Explain the role of hemoglobin in the body.
    - Hemoglobin is the RBC protein responsible for oxygen transport from the lungs to the tissues. It gives the blood its red color.

13. Determine the level of hemoglobin present in a given blood sample.
    - Refer to Procedure 53-3.

14. Identify the tests included in a CBC.
    - The CBC involves an erythrocyte count, a leukocyte count, a thrombocyte count, a hemoglobin and hematocrit determination, a differential examination of leukocytes, and calculation of red cell indices.

15. Explain the principle behind automated blood cell counting.
    - Blood is first diluted in a fluid that conducts an electrical current. The diluted sample passes through a narrow opening in the blood counting instrument, interrupting the flow of electrical current, and each interruption is counted.

16. Describe the RBC indices and how they are calculated.
    - RBC indices are calculated using values obtained from the CBC, namely the RBC count, hemoglobin, and hematocrit. They assist the physician in diagnosing blood disorders such as anemia.

17. Explain the reasons for performing a differential.
    - A differential WBC count is performed to assess the numbers and types of WBCs in the blood. A thin smear of whole blood is stained, typically with Wright's stain, and examined microscopically. In addition the red cells and platelets are examined for distribution and abnormalities.

18. Describe the appearance of the five different types of leukocytes seen in a normal Wright-stained differential.
    - Typical leukocytes seen in the differential examination include the following: the segmented neutrophil, which has a segmented blue nucleus and lavender granules in the cytoplasm; the eosinophil, which resembles the neutrophil but has orange granules; the basophil, which resembles the neutrophil but has blue-black granules; the lymphocyte, which is a smaller cell with a light-blue cytoplasm and large dark-blue nucleus; the monocyte, the largest cell, which has a cerebriform blue nucleus and a light-blue cytoplasm that appears to have bubble-like inclusions.

19. Describe the appearance of the normal erythrocyte.
    - A normal erythrocyte is circular, evenly stained red-purple, and appears to have a hole or depression in the center.

20. Prepare and stain a blood smear using Wright's stain, completing each step in proper sequence.
    - Refer to Procedure 53-4.

21. Observe a differential smear, and identify various blood cells from a prepared slide.
    - Refer to Procedure 53-5.

22. Cite the reasons for performing an ESR test.
    - An ESR test is performed to assess inflammation and is often used to monitor rheumatoid arthritis. This test measures the rate at which RBCs fall in a calibrated tube in a 60-minute period.

23. Describe the sources of error for the erythrocyte sedimentation rate test.
    - All of the following can affect an ESR: a tube that is not vertically standing in the rack; bubbles in the Westergren or Wintrobe tube; incorrect dilutions; vibrations or jarring; blood at a temperature other than room temperature; and hemolyzed blood.

24. Determine an erythrocyte sedimentation rate.
    - Refer to Procedure 53-6.

25. Describe the tests performed to assess coagulation.
    - PT and PTT are the most commonly performed tests to assess coagulation capacity. The PT test is also routinely performed to assess a patient's response to anticlotting drugs such as warfarin (Coumadin).

26. Differentiate between the ABO blood groupings and the Rh blood grouping.
    - Both the ABO blood type and the Rh type result from antigens on the surfaces of RBCs, and both groups are crucial when it comes to transfusion. There are four different ABO types (A, AB, B, and O), but only two Rh types (positive and negative). Corresponding antibodies are present in the blood for the ABO type (anti-A antibody is found in type B and type O blood, for example); corresponding antibodies are not normally found in the Rh system.

27. Discuss rare blood types and the implication of having a rare blood type when transfusion is necessary.
    - A rare blood type is one in which the blood group antigen (or lack thereof) is not common in a population. More than 20 blood types other than the ABO and Rh systems exist. Persons with rare blood types are at risk for developing atypical antibodies when transfused with incompatible blood.

SUMMARY of LEARNING OBJECTIVES
Continued

These atypical antibodies make future cross-matching more challenging.

28. Secure a capillary blood sample, and determine the ABO and Rh grouping of the sample.
    - Refer to Procedures 53-7 and 53-8.

29. Describe the methodology behind the clinical chemistry testing methods used in the physician's office laboratory.
    - Four methods are generally employed in physician's office laboratory testing:
        - Lateral flow immunoassay: antigen-antibody reactions result in the deposition of a colored molecule or particle on a solid-phase membrane.
        - Reflectance photometry: a chemical reaction produces a colored product whose absorbed wavelength is detected by an instrument.
        - Amperometry (electrochemistry): the number of electrons generated by a chemical reaction is detected by an instrument.
        - Chemiluminescence: electrons generated from a chemical reaction react with a luminescing compound on a test strip. The resulting flash of light is detected by an instrument.

30. Explain the reasons for testing blood glucose, blood cholesterol, hemoglobin A_{1c}, thyroid hormone levels, and liver enzymes.
    - Blood glucose is monitored routinely in both patients with type 1 and those with type 2 diabetes and also in women who are experiencing gestational diabetes during pregnancy.

Cholesterol testing generally refers to assessing levels of HDL cholesterol and LDL cholesterol; it is done to assist in determining susceptibility to coronary artery disease. Hemoglobin A_{1c} levels are tested to determine average blood glucose level during a 2- to 3-month period before the test is done; this test assists in management of diabetes. Thyroid testing is performed in the physician's office laboratory to detect elevated TSH levels to assist with the diagnosis of hypothyroidism. Liver enzyme (ALT and AST) testing is performed in the physician's office laboratory primarily to monitor the side effects of certain therapeutic drugs such as those used to treat elevated cholesterol and diabetes.

31. Perform a glucose test using a U.S. Food and Drug Administration (FDA)–approved glucose monitor.
    - Refer to Procedure 53-9.

32. Perform a cholesterol test using an FDA-approved cholesterol monitor.
    - Refer to Procedure 53-10.

33. List five typical chemistry panels, the reason for performing each panel, and the individual tests performed in those panels.
    - Often clinical chemistry tests are performed in groups called *panels*. Certain tests that provide information about a disease or syndrome are grouped together. A liver panel, for example, detects abnormalities in a number of different liver enzymes.

CONNECTIONS

Study Guide Connection: Go to Chapter 53 Study Guide. Read the Case Study and Workplace Applications and complete the assignments. Do online research for answers to the questions in the Internet Activities associated with assisting in the analysis of blood.

CD Connection: Go to the Medical Assisting Competency Challenge CD and do the training activities under Diagnostic Testing and Patient Instruction. For a better understanding of assisting in the analysis of blood, view the animation for normal blood clotting.

Evolve Connection: For more information related to assisting in the analysis of blood, go to evolve.elsevier.com/kinn and visit related weblinks for Chapter 53. Click on the Medical Assisting Exam Review and do the practice questions to sharpen your test-taking skills.

Assisting in Microbiology and Immunology

Robin R. Patterson

54

SCENARIO

Infectious diseases are a continuing threat for everyone. Anna McIntyre, a medical assistant, knows that some diseases have been effectively controlled with the help of modern technology, but new diseases—such as SARS and West Nile virus infection—are constantly appearing. Other familiar infectious diseases, such as malaria, tuberculosis, and bacterial pneumonias, are now appearing in forms that are resistant to drug treatments. Anna knows that it is important to quickly identify pathogens so that the proper treatment can begin. The identification of pathogens, she has discovered, can involve many different types of tests, many of which can be performed in the POL where she works.

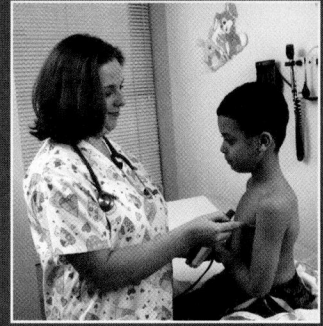

While studying this chapter, think about the following questions:

- How can Anna protect herself and other patients in the practice from infectious microorganisms?
- How can body fluids or other samples be tested for the presence of pathogenic organisms?
- How are pathogenic organisms differentiated from normal, non-pathogenic species?
- What is the role of the laboratory in identifying and treating infections caused by microorganisms?

LEARNING OBJECTIVES

1. Define, spell, and pronounce the terms listed in the vocabulary.
2. Cite the protocols for specimen collection.
3. Identify the elements needed for microbial growth.
4. Describe the bacterial structures used in identification.
5. Compare bacteria with viruses.
6. Compare bacteria with fungi, parasites, and protozoa.
7. Describe the unusual characteristics of chlamydia, rickettsia, and mycoplasma.
8. Describe the collection of a stool specimen for ova and parasite testing.
9. Describe various bacterial morphologies.
10. Describe the equipment needed in a microbiology laboratory.
11. Describe the different growth media used for culturing.
12. Describe the preparation of a bacterial smear.
13. List the steps of the Gram stain.
14. Compare and contrast the throat culture for *Streptococcus pyogenes* with the rapid strep test.
15. Describe the method used for antimicrobial susceptibility testing.
16. Describe three microbiology tests that use a rapid identification technique.
17. Explain how pinworm testing is done and when it must be performed.
18. Discuss the purpose of immunology testing.
19. Describe three rapid immunology tests that could be done in the POL.
20. Discuss legal and ethical issues in laboratory testing.

National Accreditation Competencies and Content

CAAHEP COMPETENCIES

Clinical

3.b.(2)(c).   Obtain specimens for microbiological testing
3.b.(2)(e).   Instruct patients in the collection of fecal specimens
3.b.(3)(c)(iv). CLIA-waived test: Perform immunology testing
3.b.(3)(c)(v). CLIA-waived test: Perform microbiology testing
3.b.(4)(i).   Screen and follow-up test result

General

3.c.(3)(b).   Instruct individuals according to their needs
3.c.(4)(d).   Use methods of quality control

ABHES COMPETENCIES

Clinical Duties

4.c.   Apply principles of aseptic techniques and infection control
4.i.   Use quality control
4.j.   Collect and process specimens
4.k.   Perform selected CLIA-waived tests that assist with diagnosis and treatment
4.q.   Dispose of biohazardous materials
4.r.   Practice Standard Precautions
4.x.   Instruct patient in the collection of fecal specimen
4.bb. Perform immunology testing
4.cc. Perform microbiology testing

VOCABULARY

antimicrobial agents Drugs used to treat infection.

arthropods (ahr′-throh-pod) Members of a class of invertebrate animals that includes the insects, crustaceans, and arachnids.

asepsis The process of removing pathogenic microorganisms or protecting against infection by such organisms.

broad-spectrum antimicrobial agents Drugs used to treat a broad range of infections.

cysts Small capsule-like sacs that enclose certain organisms in their dormant or larval stage.

eukaryotes (yoo-kar′-e-oht) Single-celled or multicellular organisms whose cells contain a distinct membrane-bound nucleus.

fastidious Requiring specialized media or growth factors to grow.

interferon Glycoproteins produced by cells infected with a virus or another intracellular parasite that can be used medically as antiviral or anticancer therapeutics.

interleukin (in-tehr-loo′-kin) A protein produced by certain white blood cells that regulates immune responses by activating lymphocytes and initiating fever.

in vitro Refers to conditions outside of a living body.

macromolecules The molecules needed for metabolism: carbohydrates, lipids, proteins, and nucleic acids.

microorganisms Organisms of microscopic or submicroscopic size.

molecules Groups of like or different atoms held together by chemical forces.

nanometer One billionth (10^{-9}) of a meter.

nosocomial (noh-so-koh′-me-uhl) Pertaining to or originating in the hospital; said of an infection not present or incubating before admittance to the hospital.

organelles (or-guh-nel′) Differentiated structures within a cell, such as mitochondrion, vacuoles, and chloroplasts, which perform a specific function.

pathogens Agents that cause disease, especially living microorganisms such as a bacteria or fungi.

prokaryote (pro-kar′-e-oht) A unicellular organism having cells that lack a membrane-bound nucleus.

prostaglandins (prahs-tih-glan′-dins) Chemicals released from cells that cause smooth muscle contraction and pain.

pure culture A bacterial or fungal culture that contains a single organism.

specimen A sample, as of tissue, blood, or urine, used for analysis and diagnosis.

tissue culture The technique or process of keeping tissue alive and growing in a culture medium.

transport medium A medium used to keep an organism alive during transport to the laboratory.

viable Capable of living, developing, or germinating under favorable conditions.

wet mount A slide preparation in which a drop of liquid specimen or the like is covered with a coverslip and observed with a microscope.

Microorganisms get a lot of publicity. Bioterrorism became a reality in the United States in the fall of 2001 when *Bacillus anthracis* spores sent through the mail caused anthrax, killing three people. Products line our grocery store shelves declaring their ability to keep us germ free. The evening news reports on the latest outbreaks of "flesh-eating bacteria," contaminated water supplies, and antibiotic-resistant microbes. No wonder most people have the impression that all microorganisms are harmful. In reality, however, fewer than 1% of known microorganisms are **pathogens.** In fact, without microorganisms, we could not survive.

Microorganisms are responsible for decomposition of waste and natural recycling. Our normal microbiota, those organisms present on and in our bodies, ensure that our food is digested, that our blood clots properly as a result of vitamin K production by the organisms inhabiting our intestines, and that pathogens are prohibited from invading our skin, mucous membranes, and gastrointestinal and genitourinary tracts. When the normal microbiota are disrupted because of antibiotic use or hormonal changes, for example, certain organisms that are present normally in low numbers will overgrow, causing a superinfection. Vulvovaginal candidiasis, a yeast infection of the vaginal tract, is common in women who are taking **broad-spectrum antimicrobial agents.**

The study of immunology, or the immune system, is closely tied to microbiology. Microorganisms induce an immune response, leading to the production of a variety of **molecules** that come to our defense. These molecules include antibodies and mediators of inflammation such as **interleukin, prostaglandins,** and **interferon.** Often it is necessary to diagnose a bacterial or viral infection indirectly by testing for antibodies to the infectious agent rather than isolating the pathogen itself.

As a medical assistant, you will need to understand the role of microorganisms in both health and disease. The main objective of microbiology procedures is to identify the organisms responsible for illness so that the physician can properly treat the patient. In addition, responsibilities include preventing **nosocomial** infections and assisting with infection control in the physician's office laboratory (POL) and in the society the POL serves. Microbiology procedures may be performed in the POL or in the microbiology department of a medical referral laboratory.

Chapter 26 discussed the chain of infection and how it can be broken using infection control procedures such as proper hand-washing techniques, antiseptics and disinfectants, and sterilization methods. This chapter covers cultivation of microorganisms, detection of infecting organisms by microscopy, detection of specific products of infecting organisms using chemical, immunologic, or molecular techniques, and detection of antibodies produced by the patient in response to an infecting organism (immunodiagnosis).

SPECIMEN COLLECTION AND TRANSPORT

Specimen collection and handling are among the most critical considerations in patient care because any results the laboratory generates are directly dependent on the quality of the specimen and its condition on arrival in the laboratory. Specimens for microbiology testing must be collected in such a way as to prevent the introduction of any contaminating microorganisms. This means not only using special sterile collection and transport devices and taking steps to prevent environmental contamination but also making efforts to eliminate or limit normal microbiota from the patient. Such steps include use of antiseptics on the skin before blood or cerebrospinal fluid collection, instructing a patient in the collection of a urine sample using the clean-catch midstream (CCMS) technique (see Chapter 51), or a process as simple as avoiding the teeth and tongue when collecting a throat culture swab.

When collecting specimens for microbiologic analysis, the medical assistant should always ask herself or himself two questions: "In what ways can I prevent extraneous microorganisms from contaminating this sample?" and "What can I do to prevent myself from becoming infected while I collect this sample?" Answers to the first question include cleansing the area to be sampled with an antiseptic, opening sterile containers only when necessary, and never touching a sterile swab or collection device to a nonsterile surface. Answers to the second question include wearing a disposable surgical mask while collecting a throat or sputum culture, wearing gloves when receiving a urine specimen from a patient who has just voided, and working with collected specimens in an approved biologic hood or cabinet (discussed in Chapter 50).

Ideally, specimens should be collected during the acute phase of an illness and before antibiotics are prescribed. Many types of samples can be collected. Physicians and physician assistants may collect tissue samples or body fluids by needle aspiration. Sterile swabs can be used to collect samples from wounds, the genital tract, and the upper respiratory tract, for example. Serum or whole blood can be used in indirect detection of infectious organisms. Urine and feces can be collected in containers by patients at home. The commonality among all specimens collected for microbiology testing is clear instructions for collection. The referral laboratory is responsible for providing a manual of written instructions to the POL, and the POL is responsible for providing clear instructions (preferably written) to the patient, especially if the patient will be collecting the sample in privacy or at home.

Transport of specimens is also crucial. Many different types of transport devices exist, and close attention must be given to their proper use. Microorganisms are living organisms and must be provided with conditions that permit their survival but do not permit their multiplication. If microorganisms are allowed to multiply after their collection, the culture results will not reflect the true disease state. Specialized transport media, such as modified Stuart's medium or Amie's medium, are often used in the swabbing devices used for specimen collection (Figure 54-1). These collection devices are typically made of a plastic tube that encases a sterile Dacron swab and a sealed vial of **transport medium.** After the specimen is obtained on the swab, it is placed in the plastic tube and the transport medium is released, usually by crushing the internal vial. It is essential that the manufacturer's directions be followed to avoid drying of the swab and specimen.

Ideally a specimen should be transported to the laboratory and cultured immediately after collection. In most situations, however, this is not possible, and the transport device must be handled by a courier en route to a referral laboratory or held in the POL until it can be cultured. For specimens that will be transported by a courier, ensure that the specimens are safely packaged in leakproof containers marked with warning labels (Figure 54-2). Proper temperature and time of storage are crucial. Most pathogenic organisms prefer temperatures around 37° C and will remain **viable** for up to 72 hours if held at room temperature or refrigerator temperature (4° C). Some organisms, however, will die if exposed to cold temperatures. Cultures for gonorrhea and strep throat should never be refrigerated if they cannot be plated immediately. Always refer to the referral laboratory's procedure manual for directions regarding length and temperature of storage before plating. Likewise, microorganisms have oxygen requirements; some, called *aerobes,* require oxygen to stay alive; others, called anaerobes, will die if exposed to oxygen. Collection devices are available for both aerobic and anaerobic collection. Table 54-1 lists the collection, transport, and storage of specimens commonly collected or handled by medical assistants. Figure 54-3 shows some commonly used collection devices.

CRITICAL THINKING APPLICATION

■ Aaron Mitchell, age 9, was brought into the clinic this morning at 9 o'clock with scabbing sores on his upper lip. Dr. Chowdry suspects impetigo and orders a wound culture. How will Anna collect this culture? What device might she use? How should she store this specimen until the courier, who does not come until 3:00 pm, arrives? Anna knows that impetigo is highly contagious. How can she protect herself from becoming infected?

CLASSIFICATION OF MICROORGANISMS

Once the specimen reaches the microbiology laboratory, it will be analyzed for the presence of infectious microorganisms or their components. Although the medical assistant will not be responsible for identifying microorganisms, a working knowledge of the terminology used in classification of microorganisms is essential.

Most cultures handled by the medical assistant have been ordered to diagnose bacterial infections. Bacteria are one type of microorganism; other microorganisms include fungi and protozoa. Parasitic worms are studied in the microbiology

FIGURE 54-1 Culturette collection and transport system. (From Bonewit-West K: *Clinical procedures for medical assistants,* ed 6, Philadelphia, 2004, Saunders.)

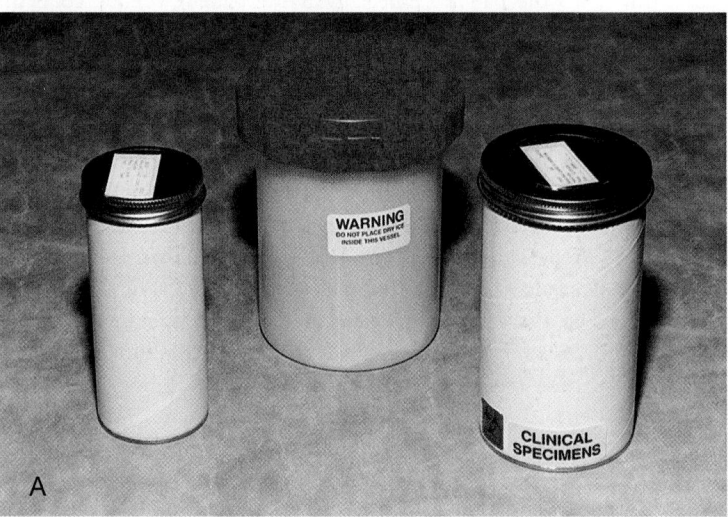

Cap/swab unit   Ampule   Transport medium

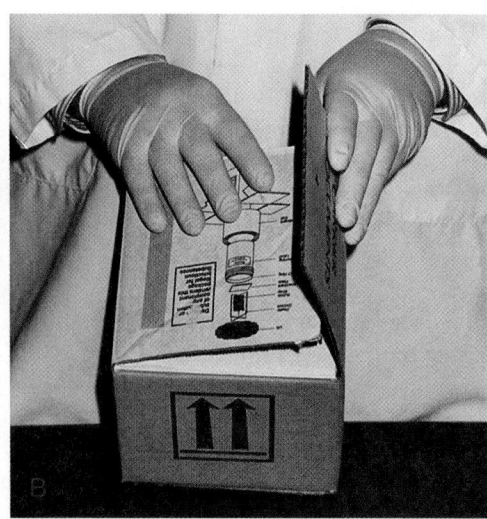

FIGURE 54-2 A, Appropriate containers for transport. **B,** Appropriate packaging for transport.

TABLE 54-1 Collection, Transport, and Processing of Specimens Commonly Submitted to the Physician's Office Laboratory

SPECIMEN	CONTAINER	PATIENT PREPARATION	SPECIAL INSTRUCTIONS	STORAGE BEFORE PROCESSING
Blood	Blood culture media set or Vacutainer brand blood culture tube with SPS	Disinfect venipuncture site with alcohol swab and Betadine	Draw blood during febrile episodes; draw two sets from right and left arms	Deliver to laboratory within 2 hours; incubate at 37° C on receipt in the laboratory
Body fluids (peritoneal, synovial, pleural, etc.)	Sterile, screw-cap container or anaerobic transporter	Disinfect aspiration site with alcohol swab and Betadine	Needle aspirations are preferable to swab collections	Transport immediately, and plate specimen immediately on receipt in the laboratory
Eye	Aerobic transport swab		Moisten swab with Amie's or Stuart's medium before collection	May be stored up to 24 hours at room temperature
Stool	Clean, leakproof container		Transport to laboratory within 24 hours if storing at 4° C	Plate within 72 hours if storing at 4° C
Rectal swab	Swab placed directly in enteric transport medium		Insert swab approximately 2.5 cm past anal sphincter	Store at 4° C, transport within 24 hours to laboratory and plate within 72 hours
Gonorrhea culture	Jembec transport system or transport device with Stuart's or Amie's medium	Wipe away exudate before obtaining culture specimen, obtain culture specimen with swab	Do not refrigerate	Transport to laboratory within 2 hours
Chlamydia culture	Specialized Chlamydia transport medium containing antibiotics	Urogenital swabs preferred; necessary to obtain epithelial cells, not exudate	Transport immediately on ice to laboratory	Store up to 24 hours at 4° C; inoculate cultures within 15 minutes of collection if swab is not on ice
Skin scraping (fungal culture)	Clean, screw-top tube	Wipe skin with alcohol prep pad	Scrape skin at leading edge of lesion	Can be held indefinitely at room temperature but best to process within 72 hours of collection
Sputum	Sterile, screw-cap container	Patient should rinse or gargle with mouthwash before collection	Have patient collect from deep cough; do not collect saliva	Store at 4° C, plate within 24 hours
Throat	Transport swab	Moisten swab with Stuart's or Amie's transport medium	Swab pharynx and tonsils, not mouth, tongue, or teeth	Transport and plate within 24 hours; room temperature storage
Ova and parasite (O&P)	O&P transport device (with formalin and PVA)	Three specimens collected every other day at a minimum for outpatients	Wait 7-10 days if patient has been taking Pepto-Bismol, Kaopectate, or Milk of Magnesia	Store at room temperature and deliver to laboratory within 24 hours
Urine	Sterile, screw-cap container	Instruct patient on clean-catch midstream collection	Hold at 4° C and deliver to laboratory within 24 hours	Hold at 4° C and plate within 24 hours
Superficial wound	Aerobic transport swab	Wipe area with sterile saline or alcohol prep pad before collection	Moisten swab with Amie's or Stuart's medium before collection	Transport and plate within 24 hours; room temperature storage
Deep wound or abscess	Anaerobic transport device	Wipe area with sterile saline or alcohol prep pad before collection	Aspirate material, excise tissue, or insert swab deep into wound	Transport and plate within 24 hours; room temperature storage

Modified from Forbes BA, Sahm DF, Weissfeld AS: *Bailey and Scott's diagnostic microbiology*, ed 11, St Louis, 2002, Mosby.

laboratory but are not considered microorganisms. Viruses, discussed in Chapter 26, are not considered by many microbiologists to be microorganisms simply because they are not, by definition, alive. Viruses consist of a core of either RNA or DNA covered by a protein shell. Alone, they neither metabolize nor reproduce; however, once inside a host cell, viruses use the host cell's **organelles** and **macromolecules** to multiply. Because of this absolute need for a host cell for replication, viruses are called *obligate intracellular parasites*, and they cannot be cultured on artificial media like those used to culture bacteria.

Culturing of viruses must be done in fertilized eggs or in **tissue culture** and will be done by referral or hospital

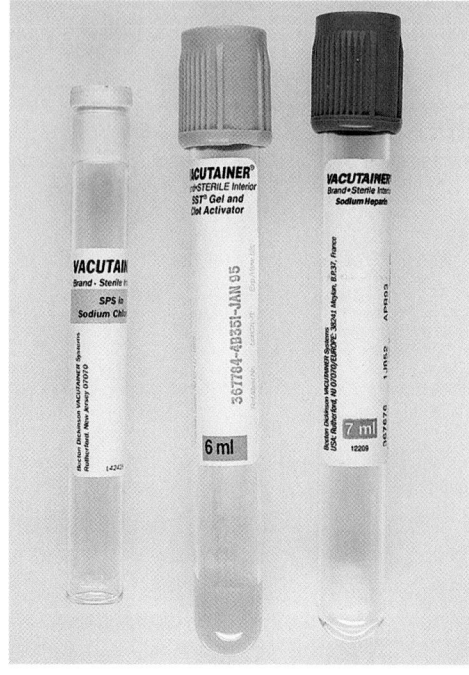

A

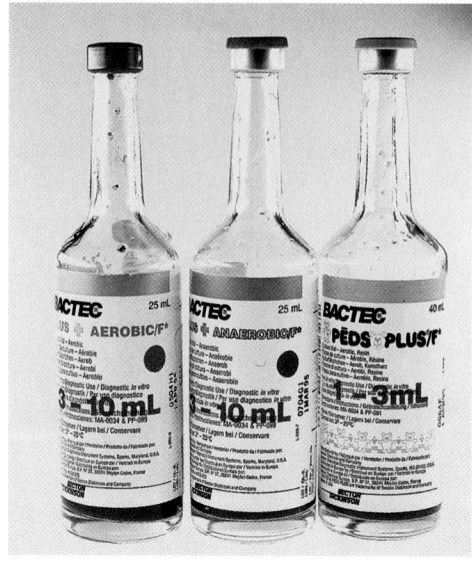

B

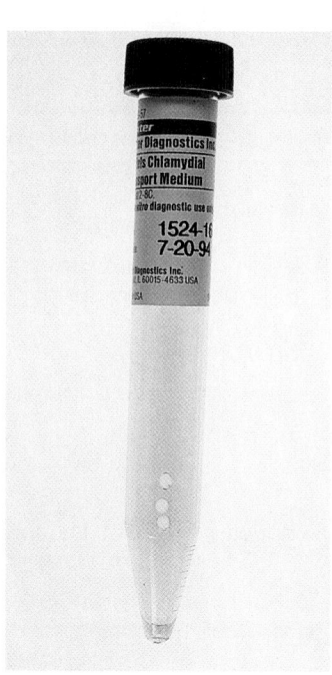

D

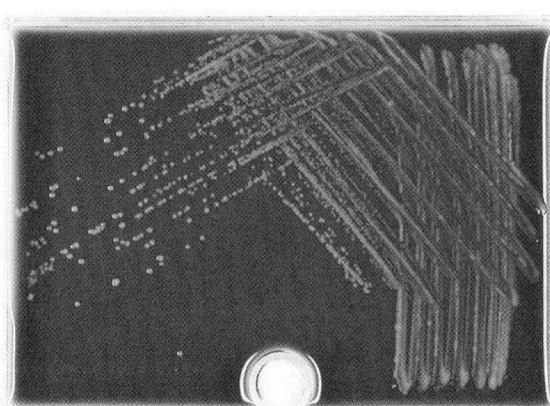

C

FIGURE 54-3 A, Blood collection Vacutainer tubes. **B,** Bactec blood culture bottles. **C,** Jembec plate. **D,** Viral-chlamydial transport medium. (From De la Maza LM, Pezzlo MT, Baron EJ: *Color atlas of diagnostic microbiology*, St Louis, 1997, Mosby; *A* and *B* from Becton, Dickinson and Company, Franklin Lakes, NJ; *C* from BBL Microbiology Systems, a division of Becton, Dickinson and Company, Franklin Lakes, NJ; *D* from Baxter Diagnostics, a division of Baxter Healthcare, Deerfield, Ill.)

laboratories. Often, instead of culturing a specimen for a virus, antigenic products of the virus or antibodies made by a patient to a virus are detected. For example, in the diagnosis of hepatitis B virus infection, the serum is tested for the presence of hepatitis B surface antigen (HBsAg), a protein found in the shell of the virus. Table 54-2 lists common diseases caused by viruses.

Naming of Microorganisms

Scientists have used the binomial system of nomenclature developed by Swedish botanist Carl von Linné to name all living organisms: animals, plants, fungi, protozoa, and bacteria. This binomial system assigns two names; the first name is the genus, and the second is the species. Both names are either italicized or underlined when written. The genus begins with a capital letter, the species with a lowercase letter. Often the name reveals some characteristic about the organism. *Neisseria gonorrhoeae*, for example, is a bacterium that was studied extensively by Albert Neisser, and it causes the sexually transmitted disease gonorrhea.

When reporting culture results, it is essential that both the genus and species names be recorded. Different species may cause different symptoms or require different antibiotic treatment. For example, *N. gonorrhoeae* causes disease, whereas *N. sicca* colonizes the mouth and does not, under normal conditions, cause disease.

The genus name of the organism may be represented by a single letter after the organism's full genus and species name is written once in a report. For example, it is common to refer to *Escherichia coli* as *E. coli*.

CRITICAL THINKING APPLICATION

■ While preparing to collect the specimen from Aaron, Anna receives a telephone call from BioStatLab, the referral laboratory the clinic uses. The results from Ms. Tina Walker's urine culture and from Mr. Robert Livore's abscess culture are complete.

Continued

TABLE 54-2 Common Viral Diseases

DISEASE	VIRUS	TRANSMISSION	SYMPTOMS	TESTS	PREVENTIONS
Smallpox	Variola major	Direct contact; fomites	Vesicles on entire body, including soles and palms		Eradicated (vaccine is still available)
Infectious mononucleosis	Epstein-Barr virus	Direct and airborne	Sore throat, fever, malaise, lymph gland involvement; hepatitis, enlarged spleen	Serology testing for heterophile antibodies; CBC	Avoid direct contact with known cases
Influenza	Myxovirus— influenza A and B	Droplet and fomites	Fever, body aches, cough	Nasopharyngeal swab, nasal wash	Immunization for the old, young, and debilitated
Warts (verucca)	Human papillomavirus	Direct and indirect contact	Circumscribed outgrowths on skin; most common on hands and feet		
Rabies	Rhabdovirus	Contact with saliva of infected animal (dog, cat, skunk, fox, bat are usual)	Fever, uncontrollable excitement, spasms of the throat, profuse salivation	DFA from brain or hair follicle tissue	Vaccine available; vaccinate pets
Mumps	Paramyxovirus — mumpsvirus	Direct contact	Pain, swelling of salivary glands; fever	Acute and convalescent titers	MMR vaccine
Measles	Paramyxovirus — measlesvirus	Direct contact; droplets	Fever, nasal discharge, red eyes; Koplik's spots, rash	Serologic titer	MMR vaccine
Rubella (German measles)		Direct contact; droplets; congenital	Rash, swollen lymph glands; causes severe birth defects	Serologic titer	MMR vaccine
Common cold	Rhinovirus and many other	Direct; droplets; fomites	Headache, fever, runny nose, congestion		Good hygiene (hand washing)
Polio	Poliovirus	Direct contact; carriers enter via mouth	Fever, headache, stiff neck and back, paralysis of muscles		Trivalent oral polio vaccine (TOPV)
Molluscum contagiosum warts	Molluscipoxvirus	Direct contact with infected individual	Small pink or white domes found in clusters	Microscopic evaluation	Avoid contact with infected individual; have existing warts removed

Courtesy Kathleen Moody.
CBC, complete blood count; *DFA*, direct fluorescent antibody; *MMR*, measles, mumps, rubella.

- Anna listens carefully to the technician from the referral laboratory regarding Mr. Livore's abscess culture and jots down *"Staphylococcus"* on the reporting form. She pauses when the technician stops and asks what species of "staph." Why is this important? What species would be considered normal microbiota, and what species is considered pathogenic?
- The technician also reports Ms. Walker's test results, indicating that the organism causing her urinary tract infection was identified as *Escherichia coli*. What shape is *E. coli*? How could *E. coli* have infected the urinary tract?

Typical Pathogenic Bacteria

Bacteria are single-celled **prokaryote** organisms that reproduce by binary fission, a process that involves duplication of the chromosome and subsequent fission (splitting in half) of the cell. This process of asexual reproduction results in tremendous numbers of bacteria from a single cell and explains why bacterial infections can quickly overwhelm a person's immune system and cause an infection. Some bacteria reproduce in as little as 14 minutes, whereas others take days to divide. A single *Escherichia coli* cell, which has a reproduction time of about 30 minutes, will theoretically produce 351,843,724,088,831 offspring in a 24-hour period if it has the opportunity to enter the urinary bladder.

Bacteria are often classified according to their shape, their staining characteristics, and the environmental conditions in which they thrive. Both shape and staining characteristics are direct results of the cell wall composition. Three types of cell wall structures exist among pathogenic bacteria: gram positive, gram negative, and acid fast. These designations are based on reactions in specialized stains used to see the bacteria under the microscope. The bacterial cell wall is composed of peptidoglycan (PG), a molecule composed of carbohydrate and protein. The gram-positive cell has a thick layer of PG with no lipid layer surrounding it, the gram-negative cell has a thin layer of PG with a lipid layer surrounding it, and the acid-fast cell has a thin layer of PG surrounded by a thick layer of waxlike lipids. Acid-fast bacteria will not stain well in Gram stain, and gram-positive and gram-negative bacteria alike stain negative in the acid-fast stain. After staining in Gram stain, gram-positive

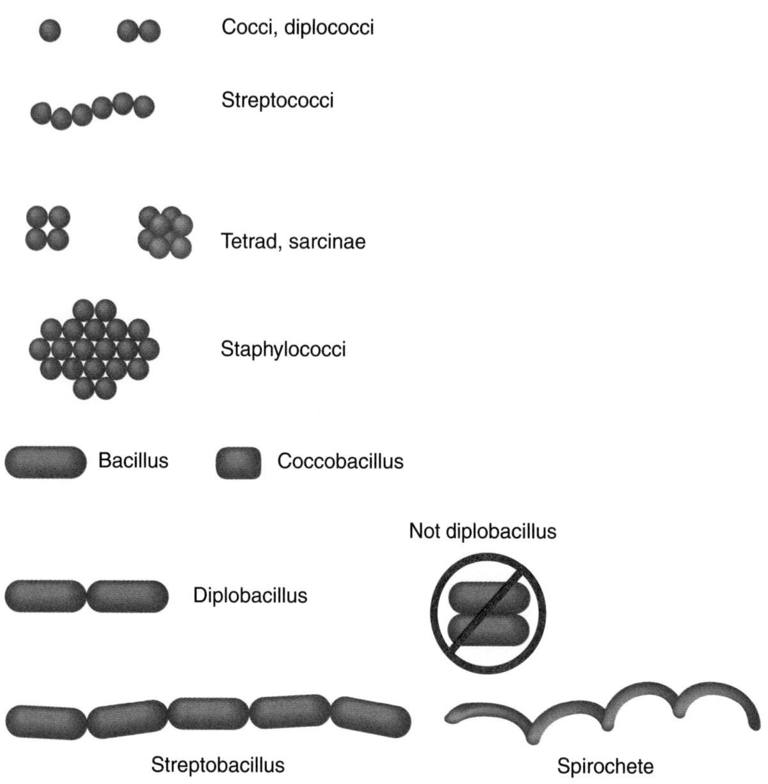

FIGURE 54-4 Typical morphologic arrangements of bacteria.

bacteria stain purple and gram-negative stain pink. After staining in the acid-fast stain, acid-fast–positive bacteria (AFB) stain pink and acid-fast–negative bacteria stain blue.

Bacterial Shapes

Pathogenic bacteria assume three different morphologic shapes. Spheric bacteria are termed *cocci* (singular, *coccus*), rod-shaped bacteria are termed *bacilli* (singular, *bacillus*), and spiral bacteria are termed *spirilla* (singular, *spirillum*). Tightly coiled spirilla are called *spirochetes*. Certain arrangements are also seen in different genera and species. When bacteria are in chains, the prefix *strepto-* is used. When bacteria are found in pairs, the prefix *diplo-* is used, and when they are found in grape-like clusters, the prefix *staphylo-* is used. Cocci in packets of four are called *tetrads* and in packets of 8 or 16 are called *sarcinae* (Figure 54-4).

CRITICAL THINKING APPLICATION

Anna knows that impetigo is caused by *Staphylococcus aureus*. Without using a microscope, she knows what the organism will look like. How does she know?

Bacterial Oxygen Requirements

Bacteria are also classified according to oxygen requirements. Those that require oxygen to live are called *aerobes;* those that will die in the presence of oxygen are called *anaerobes*. Some bacteria are flexible concerning oxygen requirements and, although they are anaerobes, can survive in the presence of oxygen. These organisms are termed *facultative anaerobes*. *Mycobacterium tuberculosis*, an AFB, thrives in white blood cells in the lungs, causing tuberculosis. It is an aerobe. On the other

hand, *Bacteroides fragilis* is the predominant bacterium found in the intestines. This gram-negative bacillus is an anaerobe. *E. coli*, also an inhabitant of the intestines and the most common cause of urinary tract infections, is a facultative anaerobe.

Bacterial Physical Structures

Bacteria can be classified and identified according to physical structures. Some bacteria have thin, long structures called *flagella* that aid in propulsion. *Proteus vulgaris* is a gram-negative bacillus with many flagella surrounding the cell. It is capable of propelling itself into the bladder and is the primary cause of nosocomial urinary tract infections. Second, some bacteria may have thick gelatinous coats surrounding the cell wall called *capsules*. *Streptococcus pneumoniae* is nonpathogenic if it is not producing a capsule, but it is the most common cause of pneumonia in older adults when it is encapsulated. The Pneumovax vaccine, which is given to older patients to prevent pneumonia, is composed of highly purified capsular polysaccharides from 23 strains of *S. pneumoniae*. Last, certain bacteria are able to form intracellular structures called *endospores* that allow the cell to remain viable when environmental conditions are not favorable. *B. anthracis*, mentioned in the chapter's opening paragraph, produces such spores. *Clostridium tetani* is also a spore former. If spores of *C. tetani* enter a wound and germinate, they cause the disease known as *tetanus*. Tables 54-3 to 54-5 list some important infectious diseases caused by typical pathogenic bacteria.

Unusual Pathogenic Bacteria: *Chlamydia, Mycoplasma,* and *Rickettsia*

In the small scale used to measure microorganisms, viruses range between 10 and 100 **nanometers** (nm). Typical pathogenic

TABLE 54-3 Common Diseases Caused by Bacilli

DISEASE	ORGANISM	DESCRIPTION	TRANSMISSION	SYMPTOMS	TESTS AND SPECIMENS	PREVENTION AND IMMUNIZATION
Tuberculosis	*Mycobacterium tuberculosis*	Acid-fast branching bacilli	Inhalation	Pulmonary: cough, hemoptysis, sweats, weight loss. May affect other systems	Sputum for culture; x-ray; skin tests	BCG vaccine (not routinely given in the United States)
Urinary tract infections	*Escherichia coli, Proteus* species, *Klebsiella* species, *Pseudomonas aeruginosa*	Gram-negative bacilli, many flagellated	Ascends urethra; catheterization	Cystitis: frequency, burning bloody urine. Pyelonephritis: flank pain, fever	Clean-catch urine for culture and analysis	Good personal hygiene; always wipe from front to back
Legionnaires' disease	*Legionella pneumophila*	Gram-negative bacillus (stains poorly with usual methods)	Grows freely in water (air conditioning systems)	Pneumonia-like symptoms	Sputum; blood	Avoid smoking
Tetanus (lockjaw)	*Clostridium tetani*	Gram-positive spore-forming bacilli, anaerobic	Open wounds, fractures, punctures	Toxin affects motor nerves; muscle spasms, convulsions, rigidity	Blood	DTaP in childhood; T or Td every 10 years
Gas gangrene	*Clostridium perfringens*	Gram-positive spore-forming bacilli, anaerobic	Wounds	Gas and watery exudate in infected wound	Swab, aspirate of wound for culture	Proper wound care
Botulism	*Clostridium botulinum*	Gram-positive spore-forming bacilli, anaerobic	Improperly cooked canned foods	Neurotoxin affects speech, swallowing, vision; paralysis of respiratory muscles, death	Contaminated food; blood	Botulinus antitoxin; boil canned goods 20 minutes before tasting or eating
Diphtheria respiratory secretions	*Corynebacterium diphtheriae*	Gram-positive bacilli, club-shaped		Sore throat, fever, headache, gray membrane in throat	Swabs; Gram stain, culture; Schick test for immunity	DTaP in childhood
Whooping cough	*Bordetella pertussis*	Gram-negative bacilli	Respiratory secretions	Upper respiratory tract symptoms; high-pitched crowing whoop	Swabs for culture	DTaP in childhood
Plague	*Yersinia pestis*	Gram-negative bacilli	Via flea bite from infected rodents	Fever and chills, delirium, enlarged, painful lymph nodes	Sputum for culture; blood	Vaccine available; rodent control

Courtesy Kathleen Moody.
BCG, Bacille Calmette-Guérin vaccine; *DTaP,* diphtheria-tetanus-acellular pertussis vaccine; *T,* tetanus (toxoid); *Td,* tetanus and diphtheria (toxoids).

TABLE 54-4 Common Diseases Caused by Cocci

DISEASE	ORGANISM	DESCRIPTION	TRANSMISSION	SYMPTOMS	SPECIMENS	TESTS	PREVENTION
Pneumonia	*Streptococcus pneumoniae*	Gram-positive encapsulated cocci in pairs	Direct contact, droplets	Productive cough, fever, chest pain	Sputum; bronchoscopy secretions	Culture, Gram stain	Vaccine
Strep throat	*Streptococcus pyogenes* (group A streptococcus)	Gram-positive cocci in chains	Direct contact, droplets, fomites	Severe sore throat, fever, malaise	Direct swab	Rapid strep test, throat culture	Good personal hygiene
Wound infection, abscesses, boils	*Staphylococcus aureus*	Gram-positive cocci in clusters	Direct contact, fomites, carriers; poor hand washing	Area red, warm, swollen; pus; pain; ulceration or sinus formation	Deep swab; aspirate of drainage	Culture and sensitivity (aerobic and anaerobic)	Good personal hygiene
Staphylococcal food poisoning	*Staphylococcus aureus*	Gram-positive cocci in clusters	Poor hygiene and improper refrigeration of foods	Vomiting, abdominal cramps, diarrhea	Suspected food, stool	Culture of food (organism will not be found in stool)	Refrigerate food to prevent toxin production
Toxic shock	*Staphylococcus aureus*	Gram-positive cocci in clusters	Use of absorbent packing materials (e.g., tampons, nasal packs)	Fever, headache, nausea, vomiting, delirium, low blood pressure	Swab, blood	Culture and serology	Change tampon, packing material often
Gonorrhea	*Neisseria gonorrhoeae*	Gram-negative cocci in pairs; intracellular in WBCs	Sexually transmitted	Females: pelvic pain, discharge; may be asymptomatic Males: urethral drip, pain on urination	Swab of cervix, urethra; rectal and pharyngeal swabs in homosexual men	Gram stain; culture	Avoid unprotected sex
Meningococcal meningitis	*Neisseria meningitidis*	Gram-negative diplococci	Respiratory tract secretions	High fever, headache, projectile vomiting, delirium, neck and back rigidity, convulsions, petechial rash	Nasopharyngeal swabs, cerebrospinal fluid, blood	Gram stain; culture; cell counts and chemistries	Vaccine; prophylactic antibiotics

Courtesy Kathleen Moody.
WBCs, White blood cells.

TABLE 54-5   Common Diseases Caused by Spirilla

DISEASE	ORGANISM	DESCRIPTION	TRANSMISSION	SYMPTOMS	TESTS AND SPECIMENS	PREVENTION AND IMMUNIZATION
Syphilis	*Treponema pallidum*	Spirochete	Sexually; congenitally	Primary: painless sore (chancre) Secondary: generalized rash involving palms and soles of feet Congenital: birth defects	Blood for serologic tests: VDRL, RPR, FTA-ABS	Avoid unprotected sex
Lyme disease	*Borrelia burgdorferi*	Spirochete	Tick bite	Fever, joint pain, red bull's-eye rash	Blood	Avoiding tick-infested areas
Pyloric ulcers	*Helicobacter pylori*	Gram-negative, spiral-shaped	Unknown; possibly food and water	Burning pain in stomach, especially between meals	Stomach biopsy for staining and culture; stool for EIA testing	None known
Food poisoning (most common cause in United States)	*Campylobacter jejuni*	Paired gram-negative curved rods forming a seagull shape	Contaminated food, water, and milk	Bloody or watery diarrhea	Stool for darkfield microscopy and culture	Sanitary food preparation and control of water and milk supplies

Courtesy Kathleen Moody.

EIA, Enzyme immunoassays; *FTA-ABS*, fluorescent treponemal antibody absorption (test); *RPR*, rapid plasma reagin (test); *VDRL*, Venereal Disease Research Laboratory.

TABLE 54-6   Diseases Caused by *Rickettsia*, *Chlamydia*, and *Mycoplasma*

DISEASE	ORGANISM	TRANSMISSION	SYMPTOMS	TESTS AND SPECIMENS
Rocky Mountain spotted fever	*Rickettsia rickettsii*	Tick bite	Headache, chills, fever, characteristic rash on extremities and trunk	Blood for serologic tests; skin biopsy for direct fluorescent microscopy
Typhus	*Rickettsia prowazekii*	Tick bite	Fever, rash, confusion	Blood for serology
Atypical (walking) pneumonia	*Mycoplasma pneumoniae*	Respiratory secretions	Fever, cough, chest pain	Blood, sputum for culture
Nongonococcal urethritis and vaginitis	*Chlamydia trachomatis*	Sexual	May be asymptomatic	Swabs for DNA probe and serologic testing
Inclusion conjunctivitis, pneumonia	*Chlamydia trachomatis*	During birth	Severe conjunctivitis in newborns Afebrile pneumonia in newborns	Swabs for DNA probe and serologic testing

Courtesy Kathleen Moody.

bacteria measure between 1000 and 5000 nm. There are tiny, unusual bacteria that fall between the size range of viruses and typical pathogenic bacteria in the genera *Chlamydia*, *Mycoplasma*, and *Rickettsia*. Classification of these organisms has posed a challenge to microbiologists.

The rickettsiae are tiny gram-negative bacteria that are transmitted by blood-sucking **arthropods.** They cannot multiply outside of a host cell, and once inside the host cell, they are able to perform only some of the life-sustaining metabolic reactions on their own. Chlamydiae are also tiny bacteria that require host cells for growth and once were considered viruses. Chlamydiae, unlike rickettsiae, are not transmitted by arthropod vectors.

Mycoplasma are unusual in that they have no PG in the cell wall, but they are not obligate parasites like rickettsia and chlamydia organisms. Rickettsiae and chlamydiae will not grow on artificial media in the laboratory, and tissue culture or serologic testing is required for their identification. Mycoplasma can be cultivated from a patient specimen in the laboratory (Table 54-6).

Fungi

Mycology is the study of fungi and the diseases they cause. Fungi (singular, fungus) are **eukaryotes,** are larger than bacteria, and include the unicellular yeasts and the multicellular molds. Fungi are present in the soil, air, and water, but only a few species cause disease. They are transmitted by direct contact with infected persons, by prolonged exposure to a moist environment, and by inhalation of contaminated dust or soil. Fungal infections may be superficial, affecting only the skin, hair, or nails. Some fungi, however, can penetrate the tissues of the internal body structures and produce serious diseases of the mucous membranes, heart, lungs, and other organs. Fungal

TABLE 54-7 Common Diseases Caused by Fungi

DISEASE	ORGANISM	PREDISPOSING CONDITIONS AND TRANSMISSION	SYMPTOMS	TESTS AND SPECIMENS
Thrush (oral yeast), vulvovaginal candidiasis, or monilia (vaginal yeast)	*Candida* species (yeast)	Oral: during birth Other: following antibiotic therapy, oral birth control, severe diabetes	White, cheesy growth	Swab for KOH prep, culture
Athlete's foot, jock itch, ringworm (tinea)	*Trichophyton* species, *Microsporum* species, and others (skin fungi)	Opportunist; direct contact; clothing; prolonged exposure to moist environment	Hair loss, thickening of skin, nails; itching; red, scaly patches	Skin scraping for KOH prep; skin, hair for culture
Histoplasmosis	*Histoplasma capsulatum*	Inhalation of dust contaminated with bird or bat droppings	Mild, flulike to systemic	Serologic; culture of biopsy material
Cryptococcosis	*Cryptococcus neoformans*	Contact with poultry droppings	Cough, fever, malaise; can become systemic	Sputum culture; cerebrospinal fluid culture, India ink direct examination
Sporotrichosis	*Sporothrix schenckii*	Farmers, florists, people exposed to soil	Skin lesions that spread along lymphatics; can become systemic	Skin scraping for KOH prep; serologic
Pneumocystis pneumonia	*Pneumocystis carinii*	Widely prevalent in animals; occurs in debilitated persons, immunosuppressed persons; common in AIDS patients	Pneumonia-like	Biopsy of lung tissue with microscopic examination

Courtesy Kathleen Moody.
AIDS, Acquired immunodeficiency syndrome; *KOH*, potassium hydroxide.

infections are resistant to antibiotics used in the treatment of bacterial infections and must be treated with drugs active against the unusual cell walls of this organism.

A superficial fungal infection is often referred to as a *tinea* (Latin for "ringworm"). Tinea pedis, for example, is athlete's foot; tinea barbae is a fungal infection of the facial hair follicles. The term *ringworm* arose because the infected area is often circular and appears wrinkled in the center as a result of the healing process. Diagnosis of fungal infections can be tedious and time-consuming and is usually based on culturing or microscopic observation of skin scrapings, hair samples, or samples of sputum or mucous membranes. Usually, the samples are treated with potassium hydroxide before microscopic observation to dissolve away nonfungal material, making the fungal elements easier to observe (Table 54-7).

CRITICAL THINKING APPLICATION

- Anna notes that it has been 2 weeks since Mr. Livore's culture was sent to the referral laboratory. When the technician tells her that in addition to *Staphylococcus epidermidis*, the culture was positive for the fungus *Sporothrix schenckii*, she understands why it has taken so long. Explain why Anna knows this.
- As Anna records the culture results, she realizes the technician does not provide a list of antimicrobial agents that would be acceptable to treat the infection, as she usually does. Anna is not concerned. Why not? Why would the physician not treat the *S. epidermidis* in Mr. Livore's abscess?

Parasites

Parasitology includes the study of all parasitic organisms that live on or in the human body. In parasitic relationships the host is harmed as the parasite thrives. Parasites are transmitted by ingestion during the infective stage, direct penetration of the skin by infective larvae, and inoculation by an arthropod vector. It is not possible to identify a parasite accurately on the basis of a single test or specimen. Most parasites are identified in urine, sputum, tissue fluids, or tissue biopsy samples (Table 54-8).

Helminths

Helminths are eukaryote parasites called *worms*. Helminths live on or within another living organism and nourish themselves at the expense of the host organism. They can live in animals or humans and are usually transmitted through the soil, by infected clothing or fingernails, or through contact with infected persons or contaminated food or water. Helminths go through the same life cycle as other worms. The adult worm lays eggs (ova). The ova develop into larvae. Larvae grow into adult worms, which lay eggs, and the cycle begins again. Diagnosis is usually based on microscopic examination of feces for ova and parasites and on the patient's signs and symptoms (Figure 54-5).

Protozoa

Protozoa (singular, protozoon) are single-celled parasitic eukaryotes ranging in size from microscopic to macroscopic (visible to the naked eye). They are present in moist environments and in bodies of water such as lakes and ponds. Protozoa are

TABLE 54-8 Common Protozoan and Parasitic Diseases

DISEASE	ORGANISM	TRANSMISSION	SYMPTOMS	TESTS AND SPECIMENS
Malaria	*Plasmodium* species (protozoa)	Bite of the *Anopheles* mosquito	Chills, fever (cyclic)	Blood: examination of stained blood for parasites
Toxoplasmosis	*Toxoplasma gondii* (protozoa)	Fecal contamination (cat litter); congenitally	Febrile illness, rash; congenital: jaundice, enlarged liver and spleen, brain abnormalities	Skin test for screening blood, fluid, or tissue for confirmation
Amebic dysentery	*Entamoeba histolytica* (protozoa)	Fecal contamination of food and water	Bloody diarrhea, cramping, fever	Stool for O&P
Giardiasis	*Giardia lamblia* (protozoa)	Common in intestinal tract, opportunist; contaminated surface water	Asymptomatic to severe diarrhea and abdominal discomfort	Stool for O&P; intestinal biopsy
Trichinosis	*Trichinella spiralis* (roundworm)	Ingestion of undercooked pork, bear meat	Nausea, fever, diarrhea, muscle pain and swelling, edema of face	Biopsy; blood tests
Tapeworm	*Taenia* species	Undercooked meats (beef and pork)	Abdominal discomfort, diarrhea, weight loss	Stool for O&P
	Diphyllobothrium latum	Undercooked fish; common among Norwegians, Japanese	As above, may become anemic	Stool for O&P
Pinworm	*Enterobius vermicularis* (roundworm)	Fecal-oral	Severe rectal itching, restlessness, insomnia	Scotch tape applied to perianal region for ova
Scabies	*Sarcoptes scabiei:* Itch mite	Direct contact; clothing, bedding	Nocturnal itching; skin burrows	Skin scrapings for parasites
Lice	*Pediculus humanus;* *Pthirus pubis* (crabs)	Direct contact; clothing, bedding, furniture (can transmit other diseases via bite)	Intense itching; skin lesions	Finding adult lice or eggs (nits) on body or hair

Courtesy Kathleen Moody.
O&P, Ova and parasites.

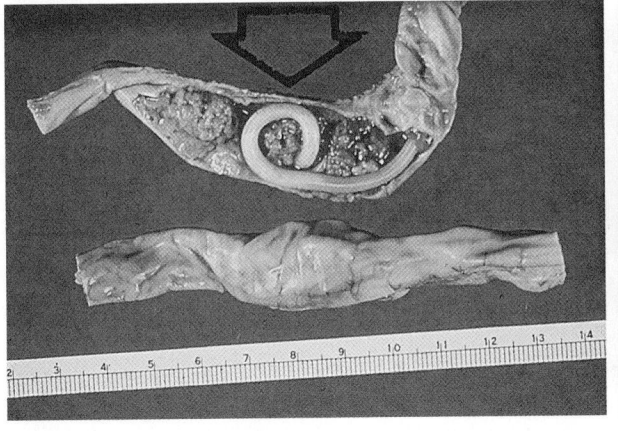
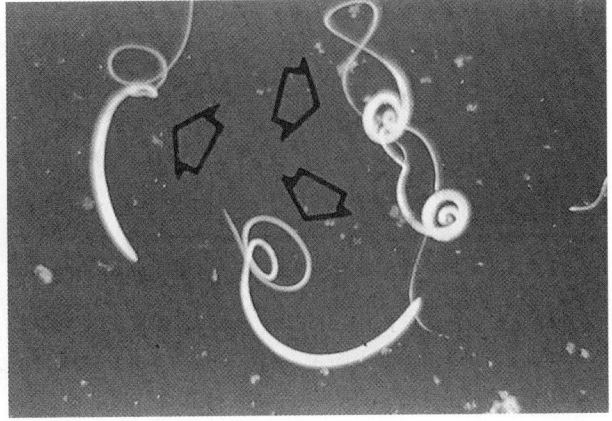

A   B

FIGURE 54-5 A, Roundworms. **B,** Whipworms. (From Stepp CA, Woods MA: *Laboratory procedures for medical office personnel*, Philadelphia, 1998, Saunders.)

transmitted through contaminated feces, food, and drink. Some pathogenic protozoa inhabit the bloodstream, whereas others inhabit the intestines and genital tract. Diagnosis is usually based on the patient's signs and symptoms and on microscopic examination of stool and blood (see Table 54-8).

Stool specimens are commonly examined for parasitic protozoa and helminths. The stool specimen is collected and placed into two vials, each with a preservative. Most commonly, sodium acetate acetic acid formalin (SAF) and polyvinyl alcohol (PVA) are used. From these preparations, a **wet mount** is made to observe motile organisms, a stained smear is made to provide contrast to the existing debris in the stool, and the specimen is concentrated either by sedimentation or flotation to allow recovery of protozoan **cysts** and helminth eggs. The medical assistant should always consult the procedure manual provided by the referral laboratory when an O&P (ova and parasites

PROCEDURE 54-1

Instruct Patients in the Collection of Fecal Specimens to Be Tested for Ova and Parasites

CAAHEP COMPETENCIES: 3.b.(2)(c), 3.b.(2)(e), 3.c.(3)(b)
ABHES COMPETENCIES: 4.c, 4.j, 4.x

GOAL: *To instruct a patient in the proper collection of stool for an ova and parasite microscopic examination.*

EQUIPMENT and SUPPLIES

- Clean, dry container for stool collection
- Parasitology collection vials*
- Plastic zipper-lock bag

PROCEDURAL STEPS

1. Ensure the patient has not taken any antacids, laxatives, or stool softeners before collection.
   PURPOSE: Laxatives increase fecal transit time and may result in a false-negative test result.
2. Instruct the patient to urinate before collecting the specimen.
   PURPOSE: This will eliminate the possibility of contaminating the stool with urine.
3. Collect the specimen.
   a. From adults: Instruct the patient to defecate into the container. Stool cannot be retrieved from the toilet bowl.
   b. From children: Loosely drape the toilet rim with plastic wrap and lower the seat. Instruct the child to defecate into the toilet, onto the wrap. Remove the stool using a disposable plastic spoon.
      PURPOSE: The stool cannot be contaminated or diluted with water.
   c. From infants: Fasten a "diaper" made of plastic wrap over the child using tape or diaper pins. Remove the plastic wrap immediately after defecation, and remove the stool using a plastic spoon. *Never leave the child unattended with the plastic wrap in place, as it could cause suffocation should it be removed.*
      PURPOSE: Stool cannot be collected in a diaper.
4. Instruct the patient to add stool to the collection container.
   a. If the stool is formed, use the scoop on the lid of the container to add large jelly-bean sized piece of stool to the liquid in the containers (Figure 1*).
   b. If the stool is liquid, pour it into the container until the preservative in the vial reaches the indicated level in the containers.

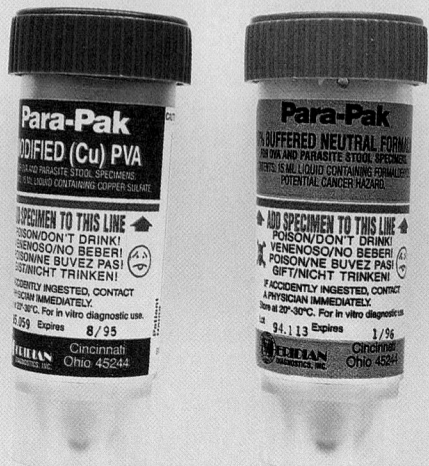

FIGURE 1

5. Instruct the patient to tighten the caps completely and wipe the outside of the vials with rubbing alcohol or wash carefully with soap and water.
   PURPOSE: Infection control.
6. The vials should be labeled and transported to the laboratory immediately if possible. Do not refrigerate the vials.
7. Instruct the patient to wash his or her hands after the procedure.
   PURPOSE: Infection control.

*Several types of preservatives are available. Check with the referral laboratory to ensure that the proper vials are given to the patient for collection. Preservatives include low-viscosity polyvinyl alcohol (LV-PVA), zinc sulfite polyvinyl alcohol (ZN-PVA), sodium acetate acetic acid formalin (SAF), and 10% neutral buffered formalin. (From Meridian Bioscience, Inc., Cincinnati, Ohio.)

---

stool examination) is ordered to ensure proper collection and transport of the specimen (Procedure 54-1).

THE MICROBIOLOGY LABORATORY

The equipment and supplies you will find in a microbiology laboratory vary with the size of the facility. Most laboratories will have a refrigerator, autoclave, safety cabinet, microscope, and incubator (discussed in Chapter 50). In addition, you are likely to find the following equipment and supplies.

Inoculating Equipment

Cultivation and identification of microbes require the use of certain tools. Inoculating loops and needles (Figure 54-6) are needed to transfer samples or microbes to growth media or to slides for staining. Loops and needles may be disposable and presterilized, or they may be made of wire and can be heat-sterilized before and after use. An inoculating loop is shaped like a bubble-wand, and a thin film of liquid will adhere to the loop. The amount of fluid held by the loop can be calibrated; a urine culture requires that a 1-μL sample be applied to the

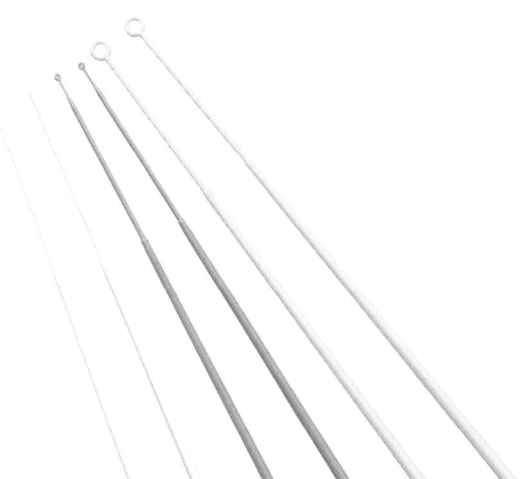

FIGURE 54-6 Inoculating loop and needle. (Courtesy Simport Plastics, Beloeil, Quebec, Canada.)

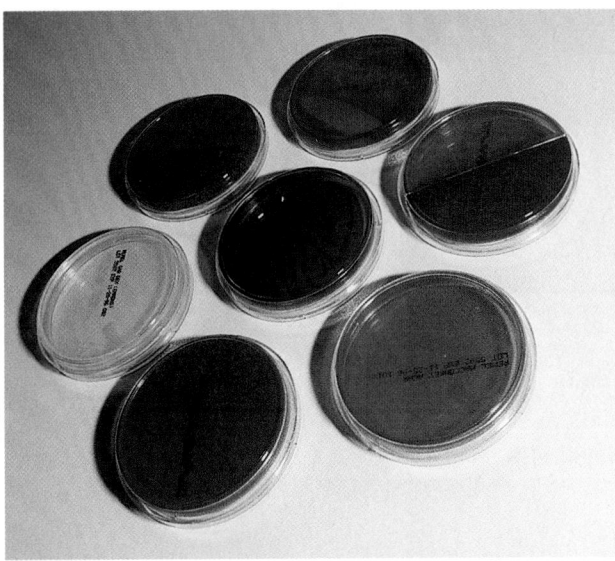

FIGURE 54-8 Media used in cultures. (From Stepp CA, Woods MA: *Laboratory procedures for medical office personnel,* Philadelphia, 1998, Saunders.)

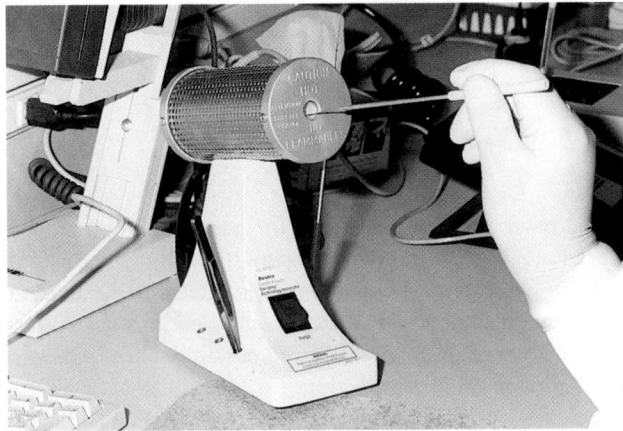

FIGURE 54-7 Loop incinerator. (From Stepp CA, Woods MA: *Laboratory procedures for medical office personnel,* Philadelphia, 1998, Saunders.)

culture medium, and special loops are available that deliver this amount. An inoculating needle is thin and pointed and is ideal for sampling single colonies.

Incineration Equipment

Incineration is the fastest way to sterilize reusable equipment such as wire loops and needles and metal forceps that must be sterilized before and after use. Some laboratories will use a Bunsen burner connected to a natural gas supply, but most use an electric incinerator because of the reduced fire hazard (Figure 54-7). An incinerator can also be used to heat-fix smears when doing a bacterial stain.

Culture Media

Once a specimen has been properly collected, it must be inoculated onto an appropriate medium (Figure 54-8). Under the proper incubation conditions, the bacteria or fungi in the sample will metabolize and reproduce using the nutrients in the medium and become visible as colonies. Media can be solid, liquid, or semisolid. A liquid medium is called a *broth.* The addition of a powdered extract of seaweed called *agar* to a

Four Types of Media

- **All-purpose or nutritive.** All-purpose media are used to support the growth of a wide variety of bacteria but will not support the growth of **fastidious** bacteria.
- **Selective.** Selective media support the growth of one type of organism while inhibiting the growth of others through the addition of a salt, dye, antibiotic, or chemical. Phenyl ethanol agar contains alcohol, which inhibits the growth of gram-negative bacteria and permits gram-positive bacteria to flourish.
- **Differential.** Differential media contain chemicals or dyes that alter the appearance of certain bacterial types. Many differential media are also selective. Mannitol salt agar contains an increased level (7.5%) of sodium chloride (salt), which selects for staphylococci. It also contains mannitol, a carbohydrate that can be fermented to an acid endproduct by *Staphylococcus aureus* but not by *Staphylococcus epidermidis*. The medium contains a pH indicator that turns yellow in the presence of acid. Therefore, if the colony is yellow on the agar medium, it is presumptively *S. aureus*. Differential media are used in biochemical testing.
- **Enriched.** An enriched medium contains complex organic materials that certain fastidious species must have in order to multiply. Blood agar, needed for the growth of *Streptococcus pyogenes*, is made by adding sterile sheep blood to an all-purpose medium. It is widely used in clinical microbiology to cultivate pathogens.

boiling liquid medium allows it to solidify and remain solid at 37° C. The molten medium can be poured into Petri dishes (a plastic dish with a lid) or into tubes.

All media should be inspected for contamination before use. New batches of media should be inoculated with control microorganisms to ensure quality. The manufacturer will provide a list of organisms that can be used.

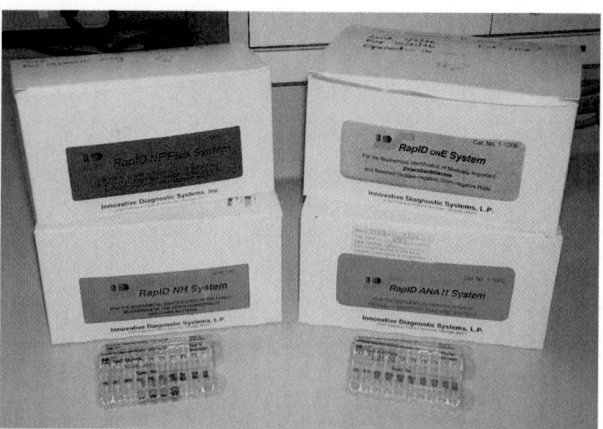

FIGURE 54-9 Rapid biochemical test kits. (From Stepp CA, Woods MA: *Laboratory procedures for medical office personnel*, Philadelphia, 1998, Saunders.)

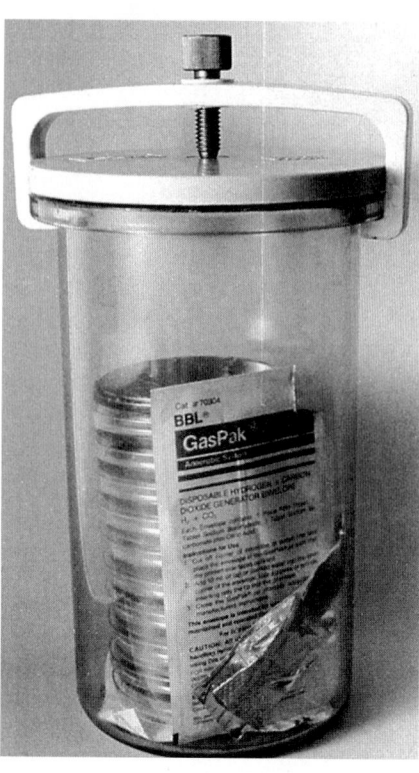

FIGURE 54-10 GasPak anaerobe jar. (Courtesy Becton, Dickinson and Company, Franklin Lakes, NJ.)

Inoculation of Media

Once the specimen has been collected, it must be "plated" or inoculated onto the appropriate medium. If the specimen has been taken on a swab, the swab is rolled onto a portion of the agar medium in a Petri dish, and a sterile inoculating loop is used to spread the sample. If the sample is liquid, such as sputum or urine, a sterile inoculating loop is used to spread the sample.

Several different techniques can be used to spread the sample. The quadrant streak is done with a loop to spread the sample thinly over the agar medium in several directions. This effectively separates the bacteria so that they may grow in individual colonies (Figure 54-9). Another technique, used when assessing antibiotic effectiveness or counting colonies, is the lawn or spread streak. This involves spreading the sample with a swab or loop continuously over the entire plate.

Once the sample is inoculated onto the plate, the plates are incubated in an inverted position so that any condensation that will accumulate on the underside of the lid does not fall down onto the growth. The temperature and conditions of incubation depend on the source of the specimen and the suspected pathogens. Most cultures are incubated in an aerobic atmosphere enriched with 5% carbon dioxide at 37° C. Cultures for fungi are incubated both at room temperature and at 37° C to promote dimorphism, a characteristic of some fungi in which they appear as a budding yeast at 37° C and as a filamentous mold at room temperature.

Cultures for anaerobes must be incubated in an atmosphere devoid of oxygen. Special jars called *anaerobe jars* chemically remove oxygen from the environment and are small enough to place in an incubator (Figure 54-10).

IDENTIFICATION OF PATHOGENS IN THE MICROBIOLOGY LABORATORY

Assessing a Culture

Once the original culture (the primary culture) has incubated at the appropriate temperature for 18 to 24 hours, it is examined for evidence of pathogens. Because there are often plentiful normal microbiota in addition to the pathogens in samples, it takes a trained eye to spot those organisms that might be causing infection. Suspicious colonies will be subcultured onto the appropriate medium in order to isolate them in **pure culture.** When the organism is in pure culture, staining and additional biochemical testing can be done to identify it at the genus and species level. Culturing of throat swabbings and urine are procedures that may be performed in POLs that have achieved certification to perform moderately complex testing.

Throat culture

Streptococcus pyogenes, also known as group A beta-hemolytic *Streptococcus,* causes septic sore throat ("strep throat"). This organism is capable of producing severe complications if not diagnosed and treated promptly, including scarlet fever, rheumatic fever, and glomerulonephritis. A swab of the throat is streaked on a sheep blood agar plate, after which a differentiation disk is placed on the most heavily streaked first quadrant. This disk contains an antibiotic (bacitracin), which inhibits the growth of *S. pyogenes* and is used for differential diagnosis. Complete clearing of the agar around the colonies indicates beta-hemolysis as a result of a toxin produced by the organism that lyses the sheep red blood cells (RBCs) in the agar—hence the name beta-hemolytic "strep" (Figure 54-11 and Procedure 54-2). The presence of beta-hemolytic colonies and a zone of no growth around the disk provides a presumptive diagnosis of strep throat. Additional testing may be needed to confirm the identity of the organism.

Urine Cultures

Urine cultures require a procedure that will permit quantitation of the sample. Most laboratories use a variety of differential and

PROCEDURE 54-2

Inoculate a Blood Agar Plate for Culture of *Streptococcus pyogenes*

<u>ABHES COMPETENCY:</u> 4.j

GOAL: *To inoculate a blood agar plate for the detection of the etiologic agent of "strep throat."*

EQUIPMENT and SUPPLIES

- Blood agar plate
- Bacitracin disk or strep A disk
- Incinerator
- Inoculating loop
- Permanent marker
- Swab from patient's throat (see Procedure 36-8)
- Forceps

PROCEDURAL STEPS

1. Wash and dry your hands. Apply face protection, and put on gloves.
   <u>PURPOSE:</u> Infection control.
2. Remove the swab from the transport device. Grasp the plate by the bottom (media side), and lift the base from the cover, or lift the cover while the plate is on the table.
   <u>PURPOSE:</u> To make handling the plate easier and to prevent contamination of the plate.
3. Roll the swab down the middle of the top half of the plate, then use the swab to streak back and forth on the same half of the plate. Dispose of the swab properly (Figure 1*).
   <u>PURPOSE:</u> Rolling the swab ensures contact with the surface of the agar.
4. Sterilize the loop in the Bacti-cinerator, and allow it to cool (Figure 2).
   <u>PURPOSE:</u> Loops must be sterilized before and after use, to prevent cross-contamination of specimens.
5. Streak for isolation of colonies in the second, third, and fourth quadrants, using the loop. Pull the loop over the surface of the agar, pulling some of the inoculum into the uninoculated portion of the plate, and spread it around. Flame the loop again, and pull some of the inoculum from the second area into the third area, etc. (Figure 3).

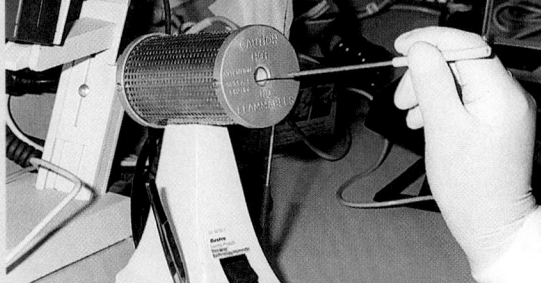

FIGURE 2

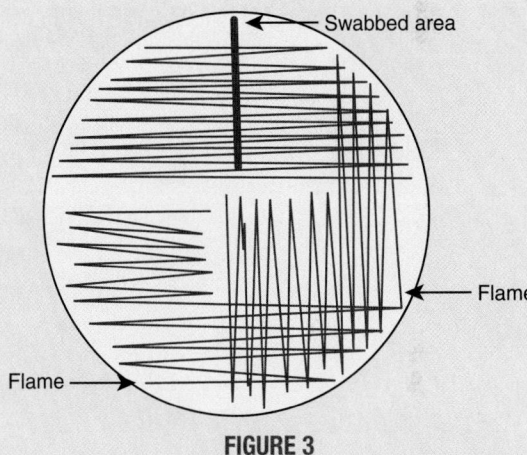

Swabbed area

Flame

Flame

FIGURE 3

6. Use the loop to make three slices approximately 1 cm long in the agar in the area of heavy inoculum–swabbed area. Sterilize the loop (see Figure 3).
   <u>PURPOSE:</u> Isolated colonies are needed for observation of colony morphology. The agar is sliced to allow for detection of subsurface hemolysis.
7. Sterilize the forceps, and remove one disk from the vial. Place the disk on the agar in the first quadrant. Sterilize the forceps.
   <u>PURPOSE:</u> Group A beta-hemolytic streptococci are presumptively identified by their sensitivity to the bacitracin.
8. With permanent marker, label the agar side of the plate with the patient's name and identification number and the date.
   <u>PURPOSE:</u> Labeling the agar side of dish as opposed to the lid prevents mixing up of specimens.
9. Place the plate in the incubator in an inverted position.
   <u>PURPOSE:</u> Placing the plate with the agar side up prevents accumulation of moisture on the surface of the agar.

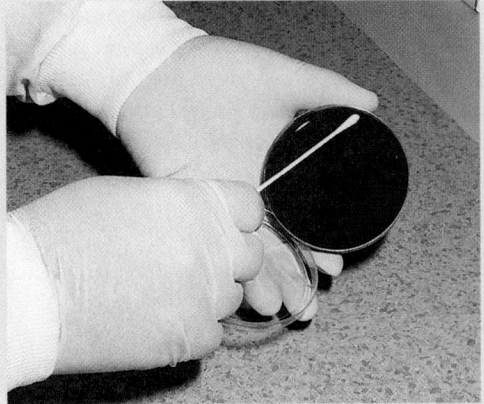

FIGURE 1

Continued

PROCEDURE 54-2—*cont'd*

10. Incubate for 24 hours. Figure 4 shows beta-hemolytic colonies.

11. Incubate negative cultures for an additional 24 hours.
<u>PURPOSE:</u> Some hemolysis patterns are not well defined after 24 hours of growth.

12. Clean the work area, and properly dispose of all biohazard waste.

13. Remove your gloves, and wash your hands.

*Figure from Stepp CA, Woods MA: *Laboratory procedures for medical office personnel*, Philadelphia, 1998, Saunders.

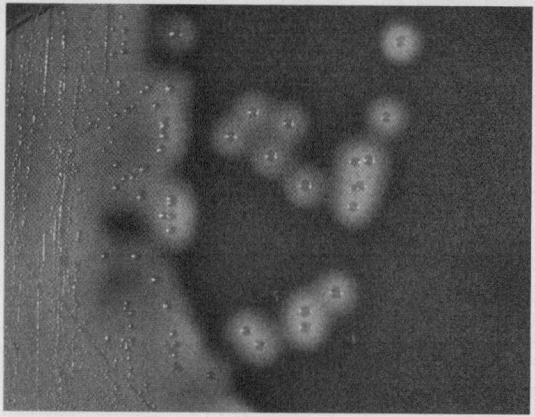

FIGURE 4

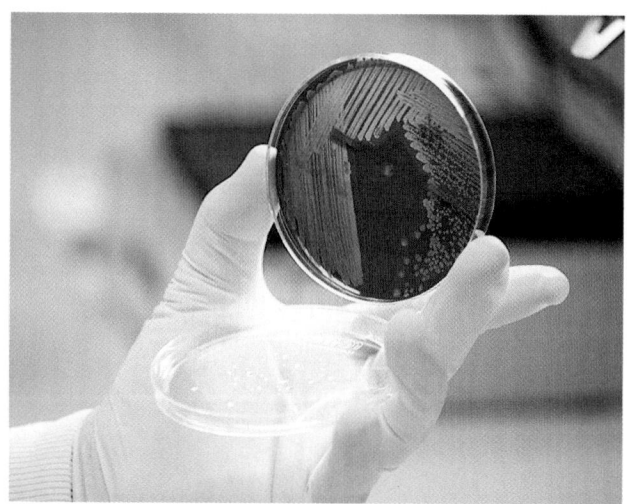

FIGURE 54-11 Beta hemolysis seen as a clear area around the streptococcus colonies. (From Stepp CA, Woods MA: *Laboratory procedures for medical office personnel*, Philadelphia, 1998, Saunders.)

selective media along with an all-purpose medium to which 1 μL ($^1/_{1000}$ mL) of urine is applied to perform this CLIA moderately complex test. A calibrated inoculating loop is dipped into a well-mixed urine sample that has been collected by the CCMS method (described in Chapter 51) or by catheterization. The urine from the loop is spread on the medium and incubated for 18 to 24 hours at 37° C. Each colony that grows on the plate then represents 1000 colony-forming units per milliliter. A system of numeric values has been devised to assess the possibility of a urinary tract infection (Procedure 54-3).

Several self-contained, convenient culture systems for urine are available. These systems are ideal for the smaller laboratory that does not want to purchase plate media and has achieved a certificate to perform moderately complex tests. Examples of these systems include the Diaslide (Diatech Diagnostics,

Boston, Mass.), Bacturcult (Carter-Wallace, Wampole Division, Cranbury, NJ), and Uri-Kit (Culture Kits, Norwich, NY). These devices contain culture media either on a paddle or on the walls of a container. The paddle is dipped into the urine, or the urine is poured into the container, swirled, and discarded. The device is then incubated (often at room temperature), and the number of colonies that form on the media are compared with a colony density chart to determine the level of bacteriuria (Procedure 54-4).

Staining

Pathogenic microorganisms are generally colorless, and a microscope is needed to see them. Special differential stains, such as the Gram stain and acid-fast stain, are often used to differentiate bacteria based on biochemical differences. As discussed previously, the Gram stain differentiates bacteria into two categories according to cell wall thickness, and the acid-fast stain differentiates bacteria into two categories based on the presence or absence of a waxy lipid in the cell wall.

Before a stain can be done, the bacteria must be applied to a labeled slide. A direct smear from a swab can be made, or a culture can be stained. Individual colonies growing on the culture medium can be spread into a drop of sterile saline on a glass slide, or material directly from the site of infection can be spread on the slide from the swab used to collect it. The slide is then air dried and fixed. Either heat or methanol can be used to fix the slide, which results in the material adhering to the slide. Both heat, from either a Bunsen burner or an incinerator, and methanol will cause protein in the sample to denature and stick to the slide, much as egg white sticks to a hot frying pan (Procedure 54-5).

Gram Stain

The Gram stain, developed by Dr. Hans Christian Gram more than 100 years ago, is still the most common stain used in

PROCEDURE 54-3

Perform a Urine Culture

ABHES COMPETENCIES: 4.j, 4.r, 4.cc

GOAL: *To inoculate three plates with 1 μL of urine in order to quantitate the number of bacteria and aid in the diagnosis of a urinary tract infection.*

EQUIPMENT and SUPPLIES

- Urine specimen, collected CCMS in a sterile container
- Bacti-Cinerator
- 1- μl calibrated inoculating loop
- Blood agar plate, MacConkey agar plate, and Columbia nutrient agar plate (or an appropriate selection of all-purpose, differential, and selective media)

PROCEDURAL STEPS

1. Wash and dry your hands. Apply face protection, and put on gloves.
   PURPOSE: Infection control.
2. With the screw-cap lid in place, mix the urine specimen thoroughly by swirling.
   PURPOSE: Microorganisms settle to the bottom of the specimen when the specimen is allowed to stand.
3. Sterilize the calibrated loop, cool, and dip the tip into the specimen.
   PURPOSE: The loop must be allowed to cool, or the heat will destroy the microorganisms as the loop comes into contact with the urine specimen, resulting in falsely low colony counts on the culture. Urine on the shaft of the loop will run down the shaft and increase the size of the specimen deposited on the plate, resulting in a falsely elevated colony count on the culture.
4. Spread the urine on the plate by "painting" the specimen down the center of the plate then streaking thoroughly at right angles to the inoculum (Figure 1).
   PURPOSE: Careful streaking of the plates is necessary for an accurate count of the organisms present.
5. Inoculate the second and third plates in the same manner.
6. Label the bottom of the plates with the patient's name and identification number and the date.
   PURPOSE: Labeling the bottom of the plates prevents mixing up of the specimens.
7. Record all information in the patient's medical record.

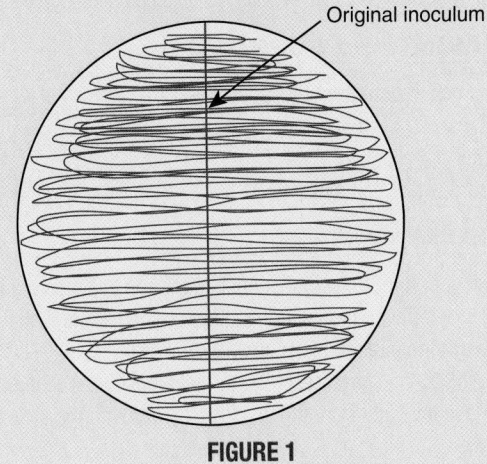

Original inoculum

FIGURE 1

8. Place the plates in the incubator, with the agar sides of the plates facing up.
9. Incubate for 24 hours, then count the colonies on the all-purpose medium.
10. The results will be interpreted by a physician or medical technologist as follows:
    - >100 colonies = >100,000 colony-forming units (cfu)/mL of urine; indicates a urinary tract infection.
    - 10 to 100 colonies = 10,000 to 100,000 cfu/mL of urine; indicates suspicion. The urine may have been allowed to stand at room temperature, which facilitated overgrowth of bacteria, or the patient may have a subclinical infection. Recollection of the specimen is recommended.
    - <10 colonies = 10,000 cfu/mL of urine; indicates normal urethral microbiota.
    PURPOSE: Because the urine was collected by passing through the urethra, some normal bacteria should be present. This system of quantitation accounts for the presence of normal microbiota.
11. Clean the work area, dispose of all biohazard waste, remove gloves, and wash your hands.

---

the microbiology laboratory. It involves applying a sequence of primary dye, mordant, decolorizer, and counterstain to the slide. The dyes are taken up differently according to the chemical composition of the cell walls (Procedure 54-6, p. 1239). Bacteria react best in the Gram stain when they are 24 hours old or less. Gram-positive bacteria stain purple, and gram-negative bacteria stain pink or red (Figure 54-12, p. 1238). Gram staining is considered to be a CLIA moderately complex test; it is useful

for the medical assistant to understand the procedures and the microscopic results that are obtained.

Acid-Fast Stain

The acid-fast stain is used in the identification protocol for *Mycobacterium* species. *M. tuberculosis* and *M. avium* complex (MAC) are two important species of mycobacteria. The former causes tuberculosis and can be isolated from sputum samples

PROCEDURE 54-4

Perform Microbiology Testing: Perform a Screening Urine Culture Test

<u>CAAHEP COMPETENCIES:</u> 3.b.(3)(c)(v), 3.b.(4)(i)
<u>ABHES COMPETENCIES:</u> 4.c, 4.j, 4.k, 4.q, 4.r, 4.cc

GOAL: *To assess the level of bacteriuria using a dip and count method in order to aid in diagnosis of urinary tract infections.*

EQUIPMENT and SUPPLIES

- Clean-catch midstream urine specimen
- Uricult test kit
- Incubator
- Biohazard waste container

PROCEDURAL STEPS

1. Wash your hands, assemble equipment and specimen, and put on gloves. Check the expiration date on the test kit. Label the vial with the patient information (Figure 1*).
   <u>PURPOSE:</u> An expired test kit may yield inaccurate test results.
2. Remove the slide from the test kit. Do not touch the slide or lay it down.
   <u>PURPOSE:</u> Touching the slide or laying it down will contaminate the slide.
3. Dip the slide into the urine specimen, tipping the cup carefully if necessary. Alternately, the urine may be poured over the slide, catching it in another container (Figure 2*).
   <u>PURPOSE:</u> The entire slide must be covered with urine for accurate results.
4. Allow excess urine to drain, then replace the slide in the protective vial. Screw the cap on loosely.
   <u>PURPOSE:</u> The cap must be loose to allow gas exchange in the tube.
5. Incubate the vial upright in a 35° to 37° C (90° to 98.6° F) incubator for 18 to 24 hours.
   <u>PURPOSE:</u> Incubation for less or more time may produce erroneous results. Disease-causing bacteria will grow best at body temperature, which is 35° to 37° C (90° to 98.6° F).
6. After incubation, the test results will be interpreted by removing the slide from its protective vial, assessing bacterial colony density, and comparing the density on the slide with the density chart provided. No actual colony counting is necessary (Figure 3*).

7. The results are interpreted as follows:
   - Normal: Less than 10,000 colony-forming units (cfu)/mL of urine; no urinary tract infection (UTI) is present.
   - Borderline: 10,000 to 100,000 cfu/mL of urine; a chronic or relapsing infection may be present, and the test should be repeated.
   - Positive: More than 100,000 cfu/mL of urine; a UTI is likely.
8. Return the vial to the protective case, and replace the cap.

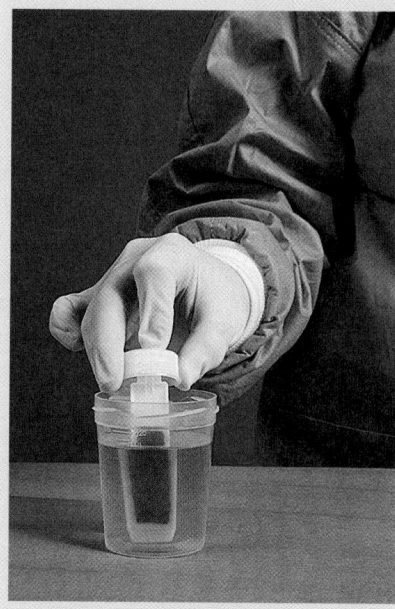

FIGURE 2

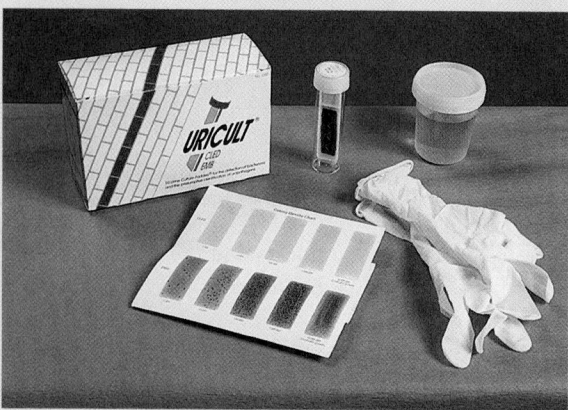

FIGURE 1

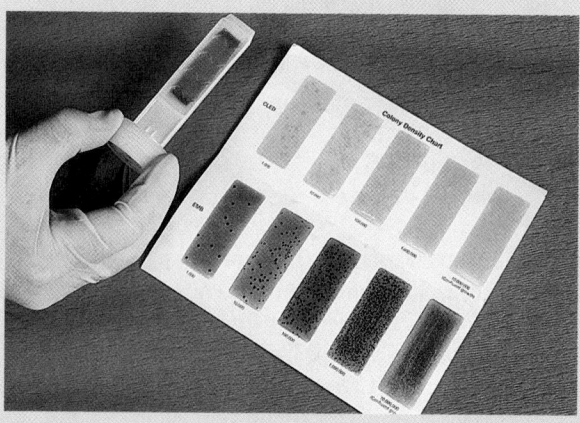

FIGURE 3

Continued

PROCEDURE 54-4—cont'd

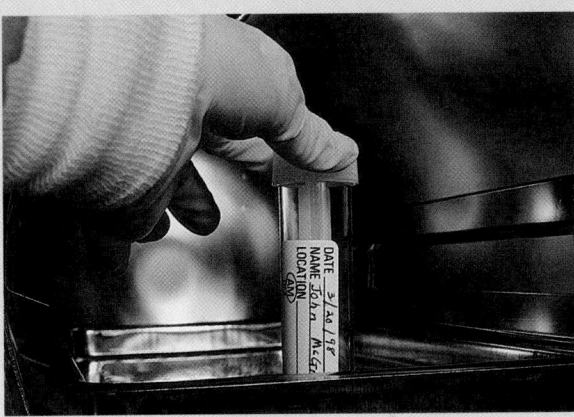

FIGURE 4

9. Dispose of the test in a biohazard waste container (Figure 4*).
   UNDERLINE PURPOSE: The slide is contaminated. Alternately, the protective case may be filled with a disinfectant. such as 1:10 chlorine bleach before the slide is reinserted.
10. Remove gloves, and wash your hands.
   PURPOSE: Infection control.
11. Record the results.
   PURPOSE: A procedure is not considered done until it is recorded.

*Figures from Bonewit-West K: *Clinical procedures for medical assistants*, ed 5, Philadelphia, 2000, Saunders.

PROCEDURE 54-5

Prepare a Direct Smear or Culture Smear for Staining

ABHES COMPETENCIES: 4.j, 4.cc

GOAL: *To prepare a smear for staining from a clinical specimen or from a culture medium.*

EQUIPMENT and SUPPLIES

- Clean glass slides
- Permanent marker
- Incinerator
- Normal saline solution
- Specimen collected on a smear
- 24-hour culture on agar

PROCEDURAL STEPS
DIRECT SMEAR

1. Wash and dry your hands. Put on face protection and gloves.
2. Label the slide with a permanent marking pen.
   PURPOSE: Other labels are destroyed in the staining process.
3. Prepare a thin smear by rolling the swab on the slide. Make certain that all areas of the swab touch the slide (Figure 1).
   PURPOSE: Rolling the swab ensures that all parts of the swab

come in contact with the slide so that the organisms collected are deposited on the slide. Thin smears are needed for evaluation.

4. Allow the smear to air dry. Do not wave it or heat dry it.
   PURPOSE: Waving the slide spreads pathogens. Overheating organisms distorts them.
5. Hold the slide with the smear up. Heat-fix the slide using an incinerator. Check the heating process by touching the slide to the back of the hand (Figure 2). The slide should feel warm, not hot. Check it often by touching the back of the slide to the back of the hand. Cool the slide.
   PURPOSE: Heat-fixing causes materials to adhere to the slide.

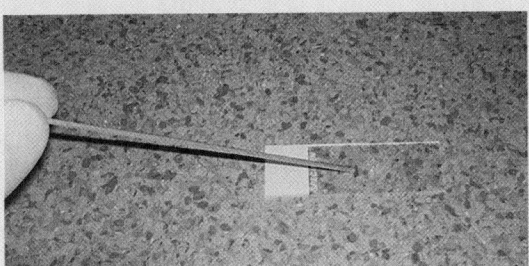

FIGURE 1

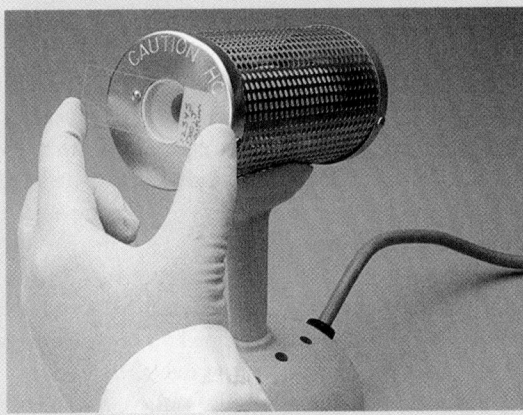

FIGURE 2

Continued

PROCEDURE 54-5—*cont'd*

CULTURE SMEAR

1. Wash and dry your hands. Don face protection and gloves.
2. Identify the colonies to be stained by circling them on the back of the plate and numbering them with a permanent marker. Label the slide accordingly.
   <u>PURPOSE:</u> This allows accurate identification of colonies.
3. Apply a small drop of saline solution to the slide, using a loop.
   <u>PURPOSE:</u> Liquid is needed to emulsify the colony. Large drops require a longer drying time.

4. Touch, with a sterile loop, only the top of the colony chosen. Transfer the material picked up to the appropriate area of the slide, and spread it in a circular motion to the size of a dime. Repeat for each colony chosen using a separate slide.
   <u>PURPOSE:</u> Only a small amount of colony is needed for staining.
5. Allow the smear to air dry.
6. Heat-fix the smear as described for a direct smear.
7. Properly dispose of all biohazard materials, and clean the work area.
8. Remove gloves, and wash your hands.

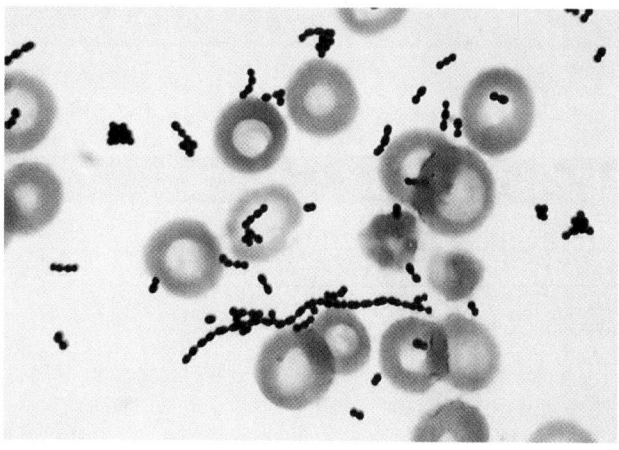

A

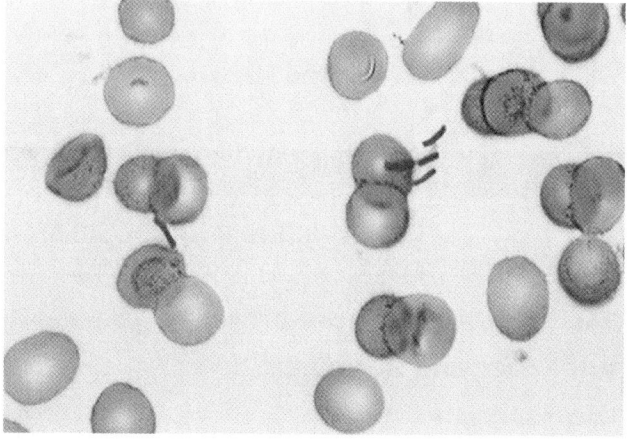

B

FIGURE 54-12 The Gram stain. **A,** Red blood cells (RBCs) and gram-positive cocci. **B,** RBCs with gram-negative bacilli. (From De la Maza LM, Pezzlo MT, Baron EJ: *Color atlas of diagnostic microbiology,* St Louis, 1997, Mosby.)

or tissue samples in infected patients; the latter is a common soil organism that enters through the respiratory tract and disseminates throughout the body. MAC is the third most common cause of death among acquired immunodeficiency syndrome (AIDS) patients. The acid-fast stain involves applying a sequence of primary dye (carbolfuchsin), decolorizer (acid-alcohol), and counterstain (methylene blue). Two procedures can be used, both of which assist in disruption of the waxy cell wall to facilitate staining. In the Ziehl-Neelsen protocol, the primary dye is applied in the presence of heat; in the Kinyoun protocol, the primary dye is mixed with a detergent. Acid-fast-positive bacilli are often referred to as *AFB* (Figure 54-13).

Biochemical Testing

Once a suspected pathogen is isolated and is in pure culture, biochemical testing must be performed to identify the genus and species. Some of these tests, such as a catalase rapid enzyme test or an oxidase test, take only a few minutes to perform. Others, such as fermentation testing using various carbohydrates, take up to 24 hours to perform. Hundreds of tests are available to identify an organism biochemically, and

manufacturers have developed miniaturized multitest systems that speed inoculation and identification (Figure 54-14).

Rapid Identification Methods

POLs with appropriate CLIA certifications are permitted to perform many rapid culture and identification tests. The tests used in a particular laboratory depend on the number of tests performed per month and the amount of refrigerator space available for storage. Dry media tests have a long shelf life, do not require refrigeration, and occupy little incubator space. The rapid culture methods offer presumptive identification of most organisms. Further specialization and sensitivity testing require additional materials, equipment, and procedures. Rapid tests are designed to give the physician a positive indication of the problem so that treatment can be initiated. For a differential or a specific diagnosis, the physician may need additional test results. Some of the rapid tests available determine the presence of *Neisseria* species, *Haemophilus* species, and anaerobes. CLIA-waived tests include rapid detection tests for the presence of *S. pyogenes* (group A beta-hemolytic streptococcus), influenza A and B, and respiratory syncytial virus (RSV) in clinical samples.

PROCEDURE 54-6

Stain a Smear with Gram Stain

<u>ABHES COMPETENCY:</u> 4.cc

GOAL: *To stain a slide, using the Gram stain, so that the organisms present are colored appropriately.*

EQUIPMENT and SUPPLIES

- Gram stain reagents
- Staining rack
- Forceps
- Wash bottle of water
- Prepared smear for staining
- Absorbent paper

PROCEDURAL STEPS

1. Wash and dry your hands.
   <u>PURPOSE:</u> Infection control.
2. Place the slide face up on a level staining rack.
   <u>PURPOSE:</u> If the slide is face down, the organisms will not be stained. If the rack is uneven, the stain will run off the slide surface.
3. Flood the slide with crystal violet. Time for 30 seconds. Figure 1* shows the entire staining process.
   <u>PURPOSE:</u> Crystal violet is the primary stain and colors all cells purple.

4. Flood the stain off with a sharp stream of water from the wash bottle. With forceps, tip the slide to drain the water.
   <u>PURPOSE:</u> Using forceps keeps your fingers clean.
5. Flood the slide with Gram iodine (mordant). Time for 30 seconds.
   <u>PURPOSE:</u> Gram iodine causes the crystal violet stain to set in the organisms that are gram-positive.
6. Flood the iodine off with water. Grasp the slide with forceps, and hold it nearly vertical to assist with draining.
7. Decolorize by running the decolorizer (alcohol) down the slide until the smear stops giving off purple stain in all but the thickest portions (about 10 seconds).
   <u>PURPOSE:</u> This is the critical step. The decolorizer removes stain from the organisms that are gram-negative.
8. Rinse the slide with water, and return it to the staining rack.
9. Flood the slide with safranin, and time for 30 seconds.
   <u>PURPOSE:</u> Safranin is the counterstain and stains red all cells that have decolorized.
10. Rinse the slide well with water.
11. Wipe off the back of the slide with an alcohol tissue.

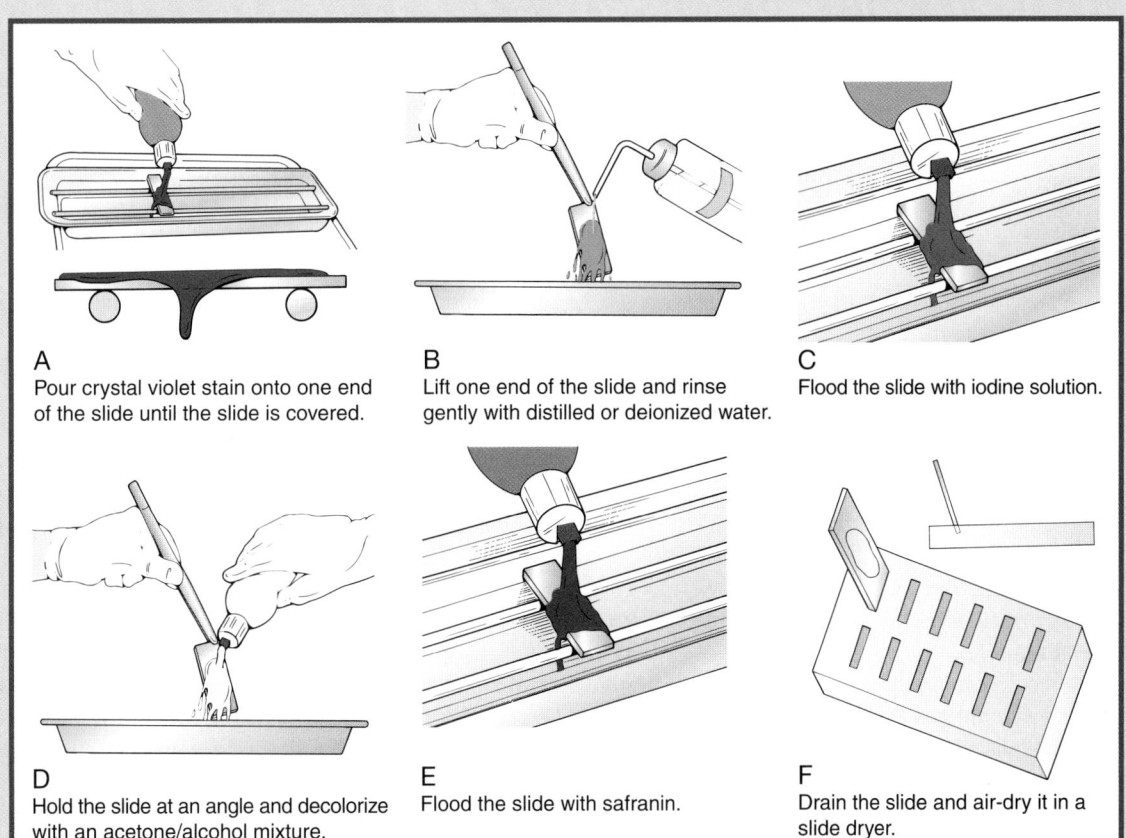

A
Pour crystal violet stain onto one end of the slide until the slide is covered.

B
Lift one end of the slide and rinse gently with distilled or deionized water.

C
Flood the slide with iodine solution.

D
Hold the slide at an angle and decolorize with an acetone/alcohol mixture.

E
Flood the slide with safranin.

F
Drain the slide and air-dry it in a slide dryer.

FIGURE 1

Continued

<u>PURPOSE:</u> The back of the slide is cleaned to remove traces of stain, which make examination of the smear difficult.

12. Blot the slide dry between sheets of absorbent paper.

13. Clean the work area. Remove gloves, and wash your hands.

14. Record the procedure in the patient's record.
<u>PURPOSE:</u> A procedure is not considered done until it is properly recorded.

*Figure from Stepp CA, Woods MA: *Laboratory procedures for medical office personnel,* Philadelphia, 1998, Saunders.

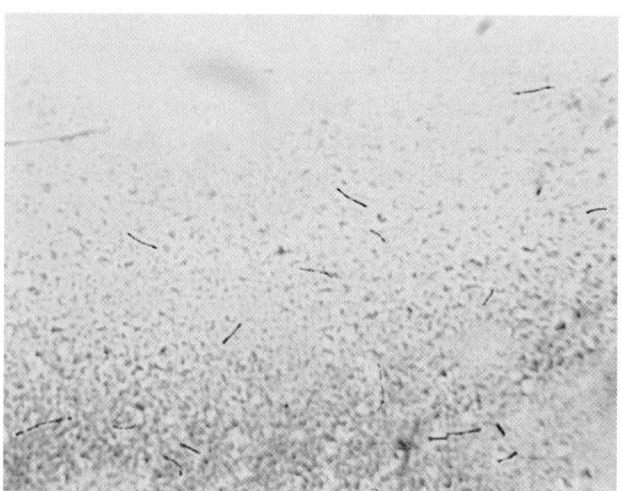

FIGURE 54-13 The acid-fast stain. Pink acid-fast bacilli (AFB) are seen in this smear. (From De la Maza LM, Pezzlo MT, Baron EJ: *Color atlas of diagnostic microbiology,* St Louis, 1997, Mosby.)

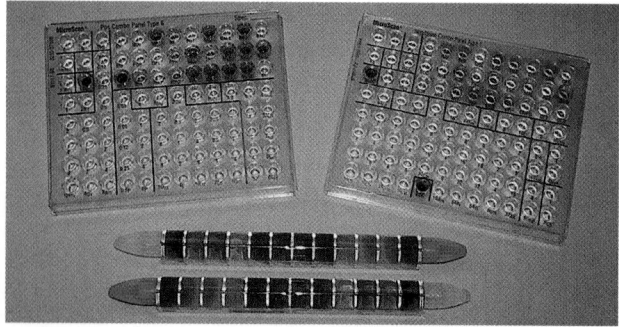

FIGURE 54-14 Enterotube II and Microscan identification tests. (From Stepp CA, Woods MA: *Laboratory procedures for medical office personnel,* Philadelphia, 1998, Saunders.)

Rapid Strep Testing

Rapid strep testing is commonly performed in the POL and can be performed while the patient waits. The patient's throat is swabbed, the swab is placed in an extraction tube, and the extract is tested for the presence of proteins found on the surface of *S. pyogenes* (Procedure 54-7) using an immunochromatographic assay. Negative test results should be confirmed with a throat culture; the rapid strep tests are highly specific but not as highly sensitive. This means that if the test results are positive, there is a high degree of confidence that *S. pyogenes* is in the sample;

if the test results are negative, the organism may not have been present in great enough quantity to be detected.

Influenza A and B Testing

Influenza virus causes influenza, or "the flu," a highly contagious acute viral infection of the respiratory tract. The infection is highly communicable through the respiratory route, and outbreaks are typically seen in the fall and winter. Type A viruses are usually more prevalent than type B viruses; type A viruses typically are associated with epidemics, and type B viruses cause a milder infection. Rapid diagnosis of influenza can assist with decisions to administer antiviral medications, which must be given early in the course of the infection if they are to be effective. CLIA-waived rapid immunochromatographic assays detect the presence of both influenza A and influenza B antigens from nasopharyngeal swabs or nasal washes. If a swab is used, the sample must be eluted from the swab using saline, transport media, or a solution provided by the manufacturer. Nasal washings can be used directly in the test kit.

Respiratory Syncytial Virus Testing

RSV is a major cause of upper and lower respiratory tract infections and the major cause of bronchiolitis and pneumonia in children and infants. Outbreaks typically occur yearly in the fall, winter, and spring and can be severe for very young children. The CLIA-waived rapid immunochromatographic assay for RSV uses a nasopharyngeal swab specimen or nasal washings to detect the presence of a protein that the virus uses to fuse to human cells. Because of the availability of antiviral agents to treat RSV infection, rapid diagnosis can lead to reduced hospital stays, reduced need for antibiotic therapy to treat secondary bacterial infection, and reduction in the cost of hospital care. The tests are intended for children under the age of 5.

ANTIMICROBIAL SUSCEPTIBILITY TESTING

Isolating the infectious agent from a patient is only the first step in successful treatment. When a physician wants to determine the appropriate antibiotic through laboratory testing, he or she will order a "culture and sensitivity" test. The "culture" refers to cultivating the organisms, and the "sensitivity" refers to a test to determine the organism's susceptibility to certain antibiotics. Most bacteria exhibit resistance to antimicrobial agents. These patterns of resistance are continuously changing; therefore they cannot be predicted.

PROCEDURE 54-7

Screen and Follow up Test Results: Perform a Rapid Strep Test

CAAHEP COMPETENCIES: 3.b.(3)(c)(v), 3.b.(4)(i)
ABHES COMPETENCIES: 4.c, 4.j, 4.k, 4.q, 4.r, 4.cc

GOAL: *To perform a rapid strep screening test to assist in the diagnosis of strep throat and to follow up negative results by performing a throat culture collection.*

EQUIPMENT and SUPPLIES

- Directigen Strep A test kit
- Timer or wristwatch with sweep second hand
- Throat swab specimen (see Procedure 36-8)

PROCEDURAL STEPS

1. Collect all supplies and equipment needed to perform the test. Bring all reagents and reaction disks to room temperature (minimum of 30 minutes).
2. Wash and dry your hands. Put on gloves and face protection.
   PURPOSE: Infection control.
3. Position all bottles vertically, and dispense reagents slowly as free-falling drops. Avoid reagent contact with your eyes because the reagent is an irritant (Figure 1).

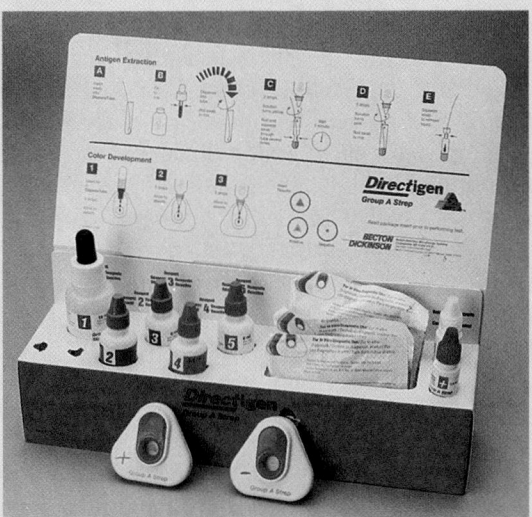

FIGURE 1

4. Add three drops of reagent 1 to an extraction tube. This solution is pink.
5. Add three drops of reagent 2 to the same tube. The solution should turn yellow.
6. Place the specimen swab in the tube, twirling the swab in the mix.
7. Let stand for exactly 1 minute.
8. Add three drops of reagent 3 to the same tube, again twirling the swab in the tube to mix. This solution should be pink.
9. Express the liquid from the swab by squeezing the tube with the thumb and forefinger and rotating the swab as it is withdrawn. The liquid must be thoroughly removed from the swab. Best results are achieved when the liquid reaches or exceeds the line on the tube.
10. Discard the swab in a biohazard waste container.
11. Remove the reaction disk from the pouch, and place it on a dry, flat surface.
12. Pour the entire contents of the tube into the reaction disk.
13. Read the test results when the entire end of assay window turns red (5 to 10 minutes).
14. Properly dispose of all contaminated waste.
    PURPOSE: Items that come in contact with samples are considered potentially infectious.
15. Clean work area, remove gloves, and wash your hands.
    PURPOSE: Infection control.
16. Record the test results in the patient's medical record.
    PURPOSE: A procedure is considered not done until it is properly recorded.
17. If the test results are negative, a second throat swab should be obtained and a throat culture should be performed. Often two swabs are used simultaneously when the sample is collected from the throat so as to avoid recollecting a specimen.
    PURPOSE: Negative rapid strep test results should be confirmed with a throat culture.

Shifting patterns of resistance require testing of individual bacteria against the appropriate antimicrobial agent.

CRITICAL THINKING APPLICATION

The technician from the referral laboratory indicated that Ms. Walker had a urinary tract infection. Anna recorded the results ">100,000 cfu/mL" on the chart. What does this number mean?

How to Assess an Appropriate Antimicrobial Agent

- Demonstrates the most activity against the infectious agent
- Has the least toxicity to the patient
- Has the least impact on the normal microbiota of the body
- Has the desired pharmacologic characteristics
- Is the most economic

The clinical microbiology laboratory can recommend antimicrobial agents based only on their **in vitro** activity. The final therapeutic outcome is the decision of the physician. The physician bases this decision on numerous factors, including the test results, the physical examination, and the knowledge of the patient. The expertise of a pharmacologist can be helpful in choosing the most effective antimicrobial agent for the patient.

Whenever you are inoculating specimens, **asepsis** must be strictly observed to ensure safety and good results. The organism being tested must also be isolated in pure culture before the test. The test, often referred to as the *Kirby-Bauer Antimicrobial Susceptibility Test,* is performed by inoculating sterile water with the pure culture of bacteria to a specified degree of turbidity. This suspension is then spread with a swab in a lawn on the surface of the appropriate agar medium. Disks, each containing an antimicrobic agent such as penicillin or tetracycline, are placed on the agar with forceps or an automatic dispenser. After incubation, the zone of inhibition (area of no growth) around each disk is measured in millimeters and compared with values provided by the manufacturer of the disks (Figure 54-15). Three determinations are possible: S, R, or I. S refers to "susceptible," meaning that the antibiotic is effective against the organism in that particular concentration in vitro; R means that the organism is "resistant" to the antibiotic. The designation I means "intermediate"–additional testing must be performed to determine the dosage of antimicrobial necessary for therapeutic treatment.

CRITICAL THINKING APPLICATION

Anna has recorded the results of Ms. Walker's urine culture and notes that 10 antimicrobial agents had been tested, but the *Escherichia coli* was susceptible to only five of them. How will Dr. Ling determine which of these five antibiotics would be best for Ms. Walker?

MISCELLANEOUS MICROBIOLOGY TESTING

Testing for Pinworms

Enterobius vermicularis, commonly called the pinworm, is a species of parasite that infests primarily young children. Humans are infected by the ingestion of mature eggs via hand-to-mouth transfers, feces-contaminated fingers, or feces-contaminated foods or liquids or by the inhalation of eggs in air currents from infected areas. The eggs hatch in the small intestine, with the females migrating out of the anus, usually at night, to deposit the eggs. The eggs adhere to the skin, perianal hairs, sleeping garments, and other clothing items. This results in itching of the anal area, whereby the eggs come in contact with the hands and fingernails of the host.

In children, specimens are best collected late at night or early in the morning before a bowel movement, urination, or bathing. Petroleum jelly-impregnated paraffin swabs or cellulose tape may be used to collect the eggs deposited by the adult worm during the night. Diagnosis is based on laboratory detection of the eggs in fecal smears. If the parent does not feel comfortable about obtaining the needed specimen, instruct the parent to bring the child to the office as soon as he or she awakens in the morning. Advise the parent to not change the child's clothing or change the child's diaper before coming to the office but to bring the child immediately on waking. When the child arrives, have all the needed supplies ready to use, and do the procedure immediately (Procedure 54-8).

Immunology Testing

Immunology testing provides information about past or present infections with bacteria or viruses and also is done to detect certain types of cancers. Testing done in the immunology laboratory is designed to demonstrate the reaction between antigen and antibody. Antibodies are formed when the body encounters a foreign agent. In the acute phase of a disease the antibody level is high; during the convalescent stage the antibody level decreases. Once an antigen has been recognized by the immune system and antibodies have been made, the level of antibody to that particular antigen remains at a low but detectable level indefinitely. The amount of antibody at any given time can be measured with serologic testing and is referred to as the *titer.* Generally, a titer is performed by preparing serial dilutions of serum or plasma; if the 1:100 dilution of a sample is the last dilution to show a reaction between antigen and antibody, for example, the titer is reported as 100.

The reaction between antigen and antibody can be demonstrated in vitro through several means, most commonly agglutination, precipitation, and immunochromatographic assay. In agglutination and precipitation reactions, latex beads or RBCs from an animal such as a rabbit are needed. The antigen or antibody is chemically bound to the bead or cell by the manufacturer. When the corresponding antibody or antigen molecule comes into contact with the bead or cell, they link together and clump (agglutinate). If this reaction occurs in a test tube, the clumps precipitate to the bottom of the tube. If the reaction occurs on a glass or paper surface, such as a slide, the clumps are visible to the naked eye. Antigen and antibody must be present in roughly equal proportions for clumping to occur because the linking is much like lattice-work. If there is markedly more antigen than antibody, or vice versa, the lattice cannot form properly. This is a false-negative reaction and is termed the *prozone reaction.*

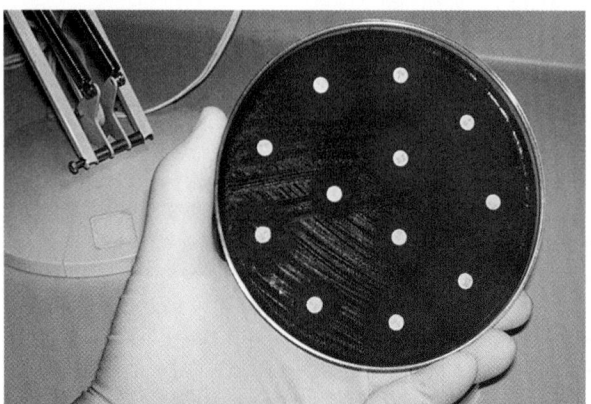

FIGURE 54-15 Antimicrobial susceptibility test. Note the zones of inhibition around 11 of the 12 disks.

PROCEDURE 54-8

Obtain a Specimen for Microbiological Testing: Perform a Cellulose Tape Collection for Pinworms

CAAHEP COMPETENCIES: 3.b.(2)(c), 3.c.(3)(b)
ABHES COMPETENCIES: 4.j

GOAL: *To obtain a rectal sample using cellulose tape for the purpose of testing for pinworm eggs.*

EQUIPMENT and SUPPLIES

- Glass slide
- Clear cellulose tape
- Wooden tongue depressor
- Toluene
- Microscope
- Gauze or cotton balls

PROCEDURAL STEPS

1. Ask the patient to assist you with this procedure.
2. Gather and prepare supplies and equipment needed for obtaining the specimen.
3. Place a strip of cellulose tape on a glass slide, starting $1/2$ inch from one end and running toward the same end. Continue around this end lengthwise. Tear off the strip so that it is even with the other end (Figure 1*).
   NOTE: Do not use Magic transparent tape; use regular clear cellulose tape.
4. Place a strip of paper measuring $1/2 \times 1$ inch between the slide and the tape at the end where the tape is torn flush. This will be the specimen-labeling area. As soon as the child arrives, place the child with the attending parent in the prepared examination room.

5. Wash hands, put on gloves, and apply face protection.
   PURPOSE: Infection control.
6. Remove the clothing and diaper from the child and lay the child in a prone position, over the parent's lap, with the buttocks in a superior plane.
7. To obtain the perianal sample, first peel back the tape on the slide by gripping the label (Figure 2). With the tape looped (adhesive side outward) over a wooden tongue depressor that is held against the slide and extended about 1 inch beyond it, press the tape firmly against the right and left anal folds (Figure 3).
8. Spread the tape back on the slide, adhesive side down (Figure 4).
9. Smooth the tape using a cotton ball or gauze square (Figure 5).
10. Write the patient's name and date on the slide label.
11. Advise the parent that the child can be dressed, or assist with dressing the child if needed.

TESTING THE SAMPLE

12. Lift one side of the tape, and apply one drop of toluene before pressing the tape back down on the glass slide.
    PURPOSE: This will clear the specimen so that any eggs will be visible.

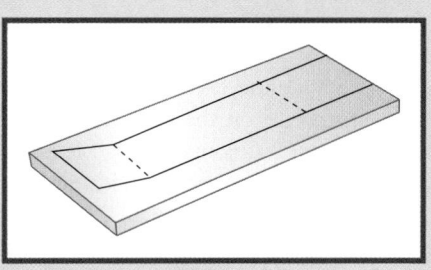

FIGURE 1

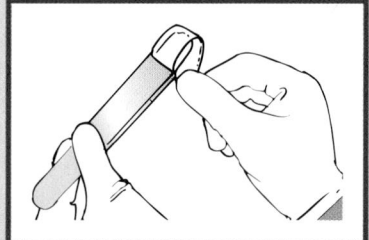

FIGURE 2

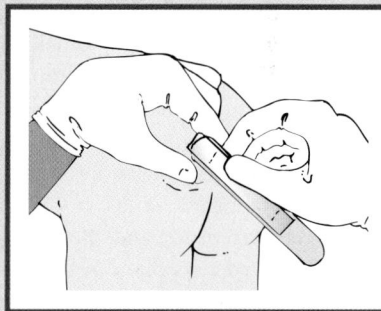

FIGURE 3

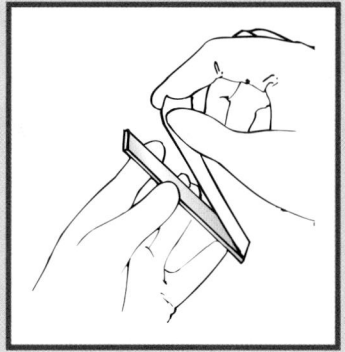

FIGURE 4

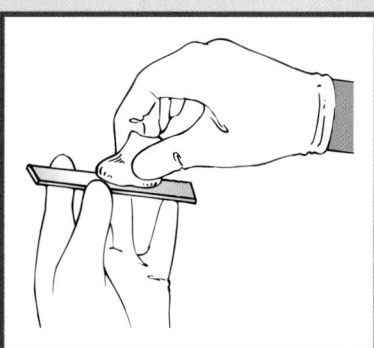

FIGURE 5

Continued

PROCEDURE 54-8—cont'd

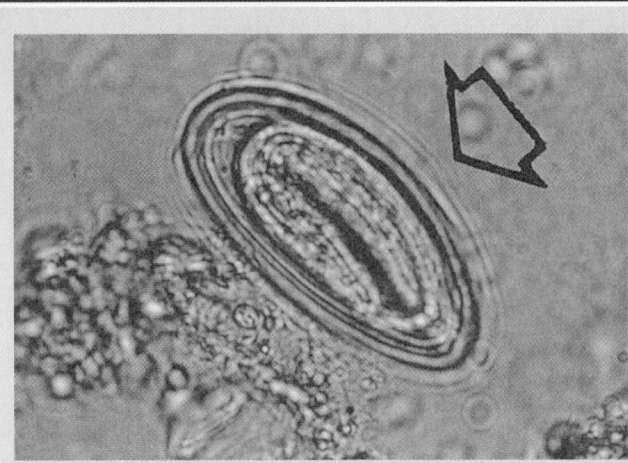

FIGURE 6

13. Place the prepared slide under the microscope's low-power objective for examination by a physician or medical technologist under low illumination (Figure 6).
14. Dispose of all biohazard waste, clean the work area, remove gloves, and wash your hands.

*Figure from Stepp CA, Woods MA: *Laboratory procedures for medical office personnel*, Philadelphia, 1998, Saunders.

Immunochromatographic assays are replacing many of the precipitation and agglutination tests in the serology laboratory because of their enhanced specificity and sensitivity. Solid-phase immunoassay, described in Chapter 51, involves the immobilization (attachment) of antigens or antibodies on solid surfaces such as beads, wells in plastic dishes, or plastic cartridges. Generally, when an antigen-antibody reaction occurs, a color change is visible. With some tests, the more intense the color, the higher the concentration of the substance being measured.

Most serologic testing done in the physician's office is done with individual testing kits. When a serologic test is performed, the first step is to review the package insert provided by the manufacturer. This review will provide valuable information about the test, the principle on which the test is based, the reagents and equipment required, proper specimen collection techniques, preparation requirements, test procedures, and any precautions or warnings that pertain to the procedure. In addition, the inserts provide information regarding quality control, interpretation of results, limitations of the procedure performance characteristics, and references.

The CLIA-waived tests that can be performed by a medical assistant that detect antibody to a pathogen include those for infectious mononucleosis, *Helicobacter pylori*, human immunodeficiency virus (HIV), and Lyme disease.

Infectious Mononucleosis Testing

Infectious mononucleosis, also called "mono" or the "kissing disease," is an acute infectious disease caused by the Epstein-Barr virus (EBV). EBV is one of the most common human viruses. The virus occurs worldwide; it is especially common in teenagers and occasionally in adults, but it is found most frequently in people between the ages of 10 and 25. Most people have been infected with EBV sometime during their lives. In the United States, as many as 95% of adults between 35 and 40 years of age have already been infected.

In children the infection may pass unrecognized or result in a trivial illness lasting only a few days, with sore throat, fever, and swollen tonsils and lymph nodes in the neck. These signs and symptoms can be indistinguishable from other mild illnesses of childhood. In young people, some of the most common complications include the abrupt onset of fatigue, headaches, aching muscles, faint rash, fever, very swollen tonsils, enlarged lymph glands, and loss of appetite often associated with nausea. There may be a short or prolonged period (days or weeks) after the initial illness when the fatigue continues and the patient may feel dispirited and depressed. Occasionally, complications occur, including the development of a swollen spleen or liver. Heart problems or any involvement of the central nervous system (CNS) occurs rarely, and infectious mononucleosis is almost never fatal.

Testing for mononucleosis involves a complete blood count (CBC) and serologic tests. A CBC will reveal an increased number of lymphocytes that appear atypical on the differential examination. The infected lymphocytes undergo a cellular transformation, causing them to take on the appearance similar to a monocyte (hence the name mononucleosis). Most patients exposed to EBV develop a nonspecific antibody response to the virus and produce heterophile antibodies. The antibodies react with surface antigens of horse erythrocytes, causing agglutination (clumping) that is visible on the test slide (Procedure 54-9). Solid-phase immunochromatographic assay tests that use whole blood are also available for the detection of heterophile antibodies.

CRITICAL THINKING APPLICATION

Tiffany Warhola, a seventh grade student, visits Dr. Chowdry complaining of extreme fatigue and sore throat. Dr. Chowdry orders a rapid strep test and a mononucleosis test. What sample will Anna need for the rapid strep test? What sample will she need for the mononucleosis test? How will Anna perform these tests? On completion of the tests, the results of both are negative. What do you think Dr. Chowdry will do next?

PROCEDURE 54-9

Perform Immunology Testing: Perform the Mono-Test for Infectious Mononucleosis

CAAHEP COMPETENCIES: 3.b.(3)(c)(iv), 3.c.(4)(d)
ABHES COMPETENCIES: 4.c, 4.i, 4.j, 4.k, 4.q, 4.r, 4.cc

GOAL: *To perform and interpret a slide test for infectious mononucleosis.*

EQUIPMENT and SUPPLIES

- Mono-Test kit
- Blood specimen (serum or plasma)

PROCEDURAL STEPS

1. Remove the test kit from the refrigerator, and allow the reagents to warm to room temperature. Check the expiration date of the kit.
   PURPOSE: Outdated or cold reagents do not react as expected.

2. Wash and dry your hands. Put on face protection and gloves.
   PURPOSE: Infection control

3. Fill a disposable capillary tube to the calibration mark with serum or plasma (see Chapter 52 for collection of blood). Using the rubber bulb included in the kit, deposit the specimen in the first circle of the clean glass or paper slide also provided in the kit (Figure 1).
   PURPOSE: The capillary tube measures the exact amount of sample for accurate testing.

4. Place one drop of negative control in the second circle and one drop of positive control in the third circle (Figure 2).
   PURPOSE: Known controls ensure that reagents are functioning properly.

5. Thoroughly mix the Mono-Test reagent by rolling the bottle gently between the palms of the hands. Squeeze the enclosed dropper to mix all the contents of the bottle.
   PURPOSE: Reagent RBCs settle on standing and must be mixed before use.

6. Hold the dropper in a vertical position, and add one drop of Mono-Test reagent to each area of the slide. Do not touch the dropper to the slide.
   PURPOSE: Holding a dropper vertically ensures delivery of the same size drop. If the dropper touches other materials, it becomes contaminated, and results will be inaccurate.

7. Using separate stirrers, quickly and thoroughly mix each area, spreading each area out to 1 inch in diameter.
   PURPOSE: Failure to use a clean stirrer for each area would invalidate the test because of cross-contamination.

8. Rock the slide gently for exactly 2 minutes; observe immediately for agglutination. A dark background is best for viewing.
   PURPOSE: Timing is always important.

9. Interpret the test results, and record them. Agglutination is positive, and no agglutination is negative.

10. Clean the work area. Remove gloves, and wash your hands.

11. Record the test results in the patient's medical record.
   PURPOSE: A procedure is not considered done until it is properly recorded.

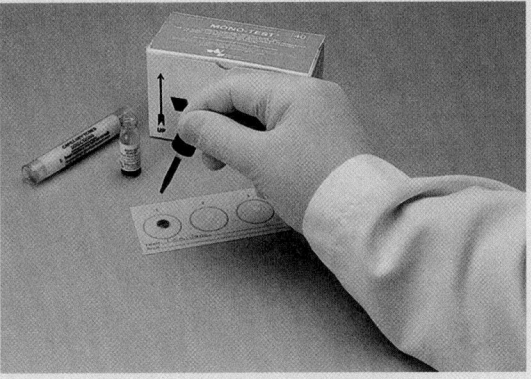

FIGURE 1

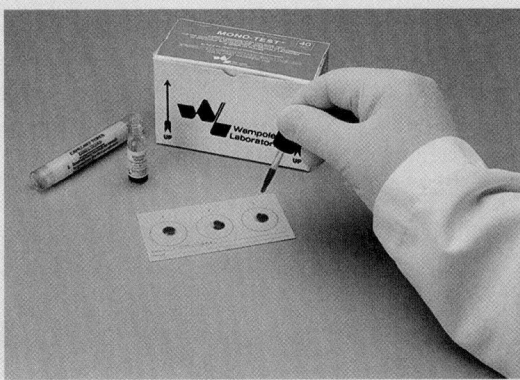

FIGURE 2

Helicobacter pylori Antibody Testing

H. pylori is a spiral-shaped bacterium that can infect the gastric mucous layer or adhere to the epithelial lining of the stomach. *H. pylori* causes more than 90% of duodenal ulcers and more than 80% of gastric ulcers (see Chapter 38). Several methods may be used to diagnose *H. pylori* infection. Serologic tests that measure specific *H. pylori* IgG antibodies can determine whether a person has been infected. CLIA-waived rapid qualitative immunochromatographic assay tests use whole blood applied to a well in a test cartridge. After the blood migrates through the cartridge, lines appear in the window, indicating the presence of antibodies to the pathogen.

Human Immunodeficiency Virus Antibody Testing

The OraQuick Advance Rapid HIV-1/2 Antibody Test (Ora-Sure Laboratories, Bethlehem, Pa.) is a single-use, qualitative immunochromatographic assay to detect antibodies to HIV type 1 (HIV-1) and type 2 (HIV-2) in oral fluid and whole blood. It is a CLIA-waived screening test for HIV-1, the virus that causes AIDS, discussed in Chapter 39. This two-step immunochromatographic assay detects antibodies to HIV-1 and HIV-2. This test will not detect HIV-1 infection in people who contracted the virus within 3 months (approximately) before taking the test. This is because it can take that long for detectable antibodies to HIV-1 to appear in the blood. As this is a screening test, the results must be confirmed by additional, more specific tests. All individuals taking this test must receive the "Subject Information" pamphlet before specimen collection and counseling after receiving their test results.

The test kit (Figure 54-16) includes a testing device with a flat pad that is rubbed once over the upper and lower gums. It is then inserted into the test vial, which is placed into a plastic stand that holds the device at the proper angle. The test results are read in 20 minutes. If whole blood is used, it can be obtained from a fingerstick or venipuncture. A specimen loop is dipped into the drop of blood obtained by fingerstick or into the venipuncture tube. The blood is mixed into the collection vial, and the testing device is inserted. Results are read in 20 minutes. The test includes an internal control band that verifies that specimen has been added and that the test has been run correctly.

Lyme Disease Antibody Testing

Lyme disease is the most common insect-borne infectious disease in North America and is a significant public health concern. The spirochete bacterium, *Borrelia burgdorferi*, is the causative agent of Lyme disease.

The disease is contracted via the bite from an infected tick whose saliva contains the bacteria. These ticks are typically found on deer, mice, dogs, horses, and birds. Infection occurs after the bacteria enter the wound and a characteristic bull's-eye rash, known as *erythema migrans* (EM), may develop at the bite site in 60% to 80% of patients. Lyme disease progresses in three stages, which have unclear transition and overlapping symptoms. As the disease progresses, the spirochete bacterium invades the skin, joints, CNS, heart, eyes, bones, spleen, and kidneys. Arthritic or CNS syndromes often accompany late-stage disease and may be the only clinical, symptomatic indications of infection.

Early detection of Lyme disease can be accomplished using a CLIA-waived test such as the Wampole PreVue B. *burgdorferi* test (MedPointe Co, Princeton, NJ). This immunochromatographic assay tests for the presence of IgG and IgM antibodies in whole blood. A sample of blood is applied to a test cartridge, followed by the addition of a diluent, and results are read in 20 minutes. As per current recommendations, positive results should be followed by confirmatory testing.

CLOSING COMMENTS

Patient Education

Microorganisms such as bacteria, viruses, fungi, and parasites are responsible for most human diseases. Patient education plays an important role in helping the patient and the patient's family to control the spread of infection. The following is a list of teaching topics that will help you in educating the patient in infection control:

- An explanation of the patient's type of infection—bacterial, viral, fungal, or parasitic
- How infection spreads
- Normal barriers to infection
- Risk factors for infection
- Patient preparation for cultures and serologic, hematologic, and imaging tests, as necessary
- The patient's role in specimen collection
- Hand washing, proper storage and cleaning of personal items, and disposal of contaminated supplies

Explain to the patient that infection does not always occur at the entry site; for example, measles can be transmitted through the respiratory tract or through the conjunctivae by touching an affected patient and then rubbing the eye. Reinforce the need for strict adherence to the prescribed antimicrobial therapy by pointing out the possible complications of noncompliance, such as relapse or systemic involvement. Explain to the patient that inadequate drug therapy (not taking the medication as prescribed) may cause the infection to worsen and spread.

Above all, always listen to the patient; be sure that the questions asked are answered. Do not try to answer questions that you are unsure of. Notify the physician of the patient's concerns so that the doctor can include the answers and explanations in the patient's consultation.

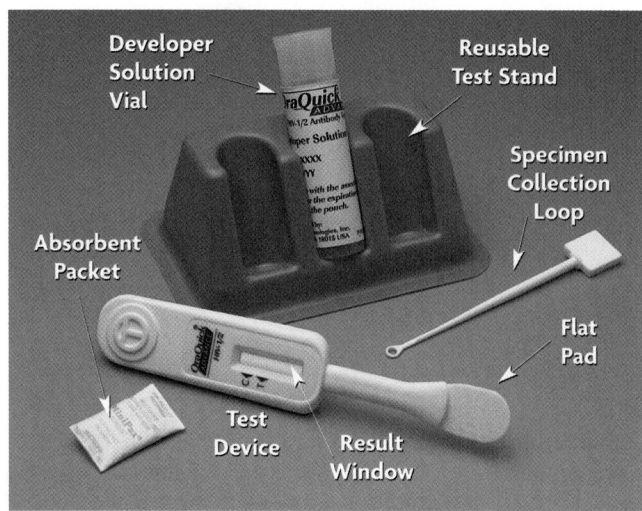

FIGURE 54-16 HIV test kit. (Courtesy OraSure Technologies, Inc.)

CRITICAL THINKING APPLICATION

Aaron's culture was confirmed as *Staphylococcus aureus*. What advice can Anna give to Aaron and his mother concerning contagion of this infection?

Legal and Ethical Issues

Maintaining a laboratory in the office increases the physician's liability. By testing patients' specimens in the office, the physician assumes responsibility for the interpretation and accuracy of the results. As the person in the office who runs the tests and notes the results on the patient's chart, it is your responsibility to maintain optimal accuracy in the testing results. A quality-assurance (QA) program for POLs may reduce the risks involved and still allow the patient to benefit from the convenience of office testing.

Strict confidentiality is essential. Never release information to anyone other than the patient or legal guardian; however, certain infectious diseases must be reported to the Centers for Disease Control and Prevention (CDC) or local board of health. POLs that have established QA programs, with written policies and procedures that govern their laboratory testing and ensure that these policies are implemented, are in compliance with CLIA regulations. If the office where you are employed does not have laboratory guidelines, suggest that testing guidelines be developed.

SUMMARY OF SCENARIO

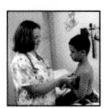

It seems Anna sees something new about harmful bacteria on the television or in the newspaper every day. Outbreaks on cruise ships, biowarfare, and smallpox vaccinations have become common topics, yet Anna knows that most bacteria are harmless. We can protect ourselves from infection by using a few simple techniques such as hand washing and keeping the hands away from the face. Anna makes a point of explaining this to the patients she sees at the family clinic and has developed a program on hand washing that she presents to schools and daycare facilities. Prevention, she knows, is the key to controlling infection.

Anna realizes that the POL can play a vital role in the diagnosis and treatment of infectious disease. She knows that proper specimen collection is of the utmost importance in microbiology testing and that contamination could mean vital time lost in identifying pathogens. Rapid testing allows for quick diagnosis, important when dealing with infectious organisms that reproduce so quickly. Anna has learned that

certain microbiology tests are CLIA-waived, whereas others can be performed in a POL that has obtained a certificate for CLIA moderately complex testing. As a CMA she is qualified to perform waived testing, and with the appropriate documented training she may perform moderately complex tests. Testing, she has discovered, may not always involve detection of the pathogen itself. Culturing on artificial media may be performed on urine, wound, or throat specimens, and sometimes the pathogen is detected by demonstrating its presence using a rapid identification test such as the rapid strep test. At other times, however, it is necessary to detect antibodies made in response to the pathogen in order to diagnose the disease, such as with the mononucleosis test.

Anna knows that the technology for rapid testing is quickly evolving, and she is aware that she can easily check the Food and Drug Administration's website for new tests that could be performed in the POL.

SUMMARY of LEARNING OBJECTIVES

1. Define, spell, and pronounce the terms listed in the vocabulary.
   - Spelling and pronouncing medical terms correctly adds credibility to the medical assistant. Knowing the definition of these terms promotes confidence in communication with patients and co-workers.
2. Cite the protocols for specimen collection.
   - Specimens for the microbiology laboratory must be collected in sterile containers.
   - Transport systems are available if the specimen cannot be plated immediately. These systems often contain a transport medium that keeps the organisms alive but does not let them multiply.
3. Identify the elements needed for microbial growth.
   - All microbes require nutrients and water to stay alive. Aerobes require oxygen; anaerobes die in the presence of oxygen.
   - Most pathogens prefer an incubation temperature of 37° C and a pH of 7.

4. Describe the bacterial structures used in identification.
   - Some bacteria have flagella protruding from the cell wall. These structures aid in propulsion.
   - Some bacteria produce gelatinous capsules that enhance their virulence.
   - Bacteria in the genera *Bacillus* and *Clostridium* produce endospores that allow them to survive harsh conditions.
5. Compare bacteria with viruses.
   - Viruses differ from bacteria in that they are not cells.
   - Viruses have a core of nucleic acid surrounded by a protein coat.
   - Unlike bacteria, viruses do not metabolize, and they cannot replicate on their own.
6. Compare bacteria with fungi, parasites, and protozoa.
   - Bacteria are prokaryotic; fungi, protozoa, and parasites are eukaryotic.
   - Bacteria, fungi, and protozoa must be observed

Continued

SUMMARY of LEARNING OBJECTIVES

Continued

microscopically; helminths, or worms, can be seen with the naked eye.

7. Describe the unusual characteristics of chlamydia, rickettsia, and mycoplasma.
   - Chlamydia and rickettsia organisms are tiny bacteria, but unlike most bacteria they require a host cell for replication.
   - Rickettsia are transmitted by arthropods.
   - Mycoplasma are bacteria without cell walls.

8. Describe the collection of a stool specimen for ova and parasite testing.
   - Stool is collected in special transport devices that contain preservatives and fixatives that will assist in the microscopic examination of the specimen.
   - Explicit instructions must be given to the patient to ensure proper collection.

9. Describe various bacterial morphologies.
   - Identification of bacteria begins with the observation of their morphology.
   - Cocci are spheric organisms, bacilli are rod-shaped organisms, and spirilla are spiral-shaped organisms.
   - Staphylococci are cocci in clusters; streptococci and streptobacilli are organisms arranged in chains, and diplococci and diplobacilli are organisms arranged in pairs.

10. Describe the equipment needed in a microbiology laboratory.
    - Cultivation equipment includes inoculating loops and needles, Petri dishes with agar media, and incubators.
    - Viewing equipment includes slides, stains, and microscopes.
    - Sterilizing equipment includes incinerators and autoclaves.

11. Describe the different growth media used for culturing.
    - Growth media consists of nutrients selected for certain species.
    - Media can be liquid or can be made solid by the addition of agar.
    - Solid media can be prepared as Petri plates or as tube media.
    - Media can be all purpose and support the growth of many species. It can be selective, permitting only a certain type of microbe to grow.
    - Media can also be differential, allowing differentiation of species based on color changes caused by different biochemical reactions.
    - Enriched media support the growth of fastidious bacteria.

12. Describe the preparation of a bacterial smear.
    - Smears can be prepared directly from swabs or from growth on solid media.
    - If a smear is made from a bacterial colony, a small amount of water or saline must be placed on the slide first.
    - Smears must be air dried and heat-fixed before staining.

13. List the steps of the Gram stain.
    - The four steps involve the addition of the primary stain, crystal violet; the mordant, iodine; the decolorizer, alcohol; and the counterstain, safranin.
    - Gram-positive bacteria stain purple, and gram-negative bacteria stain pink or red.

14. Compare and contrast the throat culture for *S. pyogenes* with the rapid strep test.
    - The throat culture involves obtaining a swabbing of the throat and culturing it on a sheep blood agar plate.
    - The throat culture is observed for beta hemolysis and susceptibility to bacitracin, both of which indicate the presence of group A beta-hemolytic streptococci.
    - The rapid strep test does not involve culturing but is an immunochromatographic assay that assesses the presence of Streptococcus antigen in the sample.
    - A negative rapid strep test should be confirmed with a throat culture.

15. Describe the method used for antimicrobial susceptibility testing.
    - Antimicrobial susceptibility testing uses disks impregnated with antimicrobial agents dropped onto the surface of an agar plate inoculated with a pathogen.
    - The pathogen will display susceptibility, resistance, or an intermediate reaction to the antimicrobial agent.
    - These determinations are made by measuring the zone of inhibition around each disk and comparing with a chart provided by the manufacturer.

16. Describe three microbiology tests that use a rapid identification technique.
    - The rapid strep test detects *S. pyogenes* and is used in the diagnosis of streptococcal pharyngitis.
    - The influenza A and B rapid tests detect surface antigens of the virus that causes influenza.
    - The RSV rapid test detects antigens from RSV, which causes pneumonia and bronchiolitis in young children.

17. Explain how pinworm testing is done and when it must be performed.
    - Pinworm testing detects the presence of the eggs of the pinworm, *E. vermicularis.*
    - The worm deposits eggs in the anal folds at night. The eggs can be retrieved by using a sticky collection device either late in the evening or in the morning before a bowel movement.
    - Diagnosis is made on finding the presence of the eggs microscopically.

18. Discuss the purpose of immunology testing.
    - Often cultivation of a pathogen is difficult, or it is difficult to demonstrate the presence of the pathogen with antigen testing.
    - Immunology testing detects the presence of antibodies to a pathogen.

19. Describe three rapid immunology tests that could be done in the POL.
    - Mononucleosis testing detects the presence of heterophile antibodies made in reaction to infection with the Epstein-Barr virus. Serum, plasma, or whole blood can be used, depending on the test.
    - *H. pylori* testing detects antibodies to the bacterium that is a common cause of stomach ulcers. Whole blood is used for the test.

Continued

SUMMARY of LEARNING OBJECTIVES

Continued

- Rapid HIV testing detects the two viruses, HIV-1 and HIV-2, which cause AIDS. Either oral swabbings or whole blood can be used.

20. Discuss legal and ethical issues in laboratory testing.
- The medical assistant must be aware that patient

confidentiality is of utmost importance, but certain infections, such as sexually transmitted diseases and tuberculosis, must be reported to the CDC and to the local board of health.

CONNECTIONS

 Study Guide Connection: Go to Chapter 54 Study Guide. Read the Case Study and Workplace Applications and complete the assignments. Do online research for answers to the questions in the Internet Activities associated with assisting in microbiology and immunology.

 CD Connection: Go to the Medical Assisting Competency Challenge CD and do the training activities under Infection Control and Diagnostic Testing. For a better understanding of the inflammatory response and controlling infection, view the animations for antibiotics and phagocytosis.

evolve **Evolve Connection:** For more information related to assisting in microbiology and immunology, go to evolve.elsevier. com/kinn and visit related weblinks for Chapter 54. Click on the Medical Assisting Exam Review and do the practice questions to sharpen your test-taking skills.

Surgical Supplies and Instruments 55

SCENARIO

Tom Anderson, CMA, works for Dr. Sheila Samanski, a dermatologist who frequently performs minor surgical procedures in the office. Tom assists Dr. Samanski with procedures and is also responsible for maintaining stock supplies in the minor surgery room, including solutions and medications, as well as cleaning, maintaining, and inspecting the surgical instruments. Because no procedures are scheduled for today, Tom is planning to compile an inventory of supplies and equipment and to perform routine maintenance activities.

While studying this chapter, think about the following questions:

- What solutions and medications should be available in the surgical area of a medical office?
- What are the typical instruments used in minor surgical procedures?
- How are surgical instruments identified and classified?
- How should surgical instruments be cared for and handled before, during, and after a surgical procedure?
- What are the types of sutures and needles that are used in minor surgical procedures?

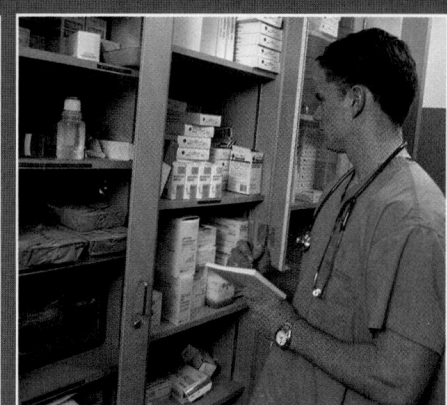

LEARNING OBJECTIVES

1. Define, spell, and pronounce the terms listed in the vocabulary.
2. Describe typical solutions and medications used in minor surgical procedures.
3. Summarize methods for identifying surgical instruments used in minor office surgery.
4. Outline the general classifications of surgical instruments.
5. Describe the care of surgical instruments.
6. Identify types of sutures and surgical needles.

National Accreditation Competencies and Content

CAAHEP COMPETENCIES	ABHES COMPETENCIES
Clinical 3.b.(4)(f). Prepare patients for and assist with procedures, treatments, and minor office surgeries	**Clinical Duties** 4.b. Prepare patients for procedures 4.h. Prepare patients for and assist physician with routine and specialty examinations
General 3.c.(4)(b). Perform routine maintenance of administrative and clinical equipment	**Office Management** 6.b. Operate and maintain facilities and perform routine maintenance of administrative and clinical equipment safely

abscesses Localized collections of pus that may be under the skin or deep within the body and that cause tissue destruction.

cannula (kan'-yoo-lah) Rigid tube that surrounds a blunt trocar or a sharp, pointed trocar inserted into the body; when withdrawn, fluid may escape from the body through the cannula, depending on where it is inserted.

curettage (kyur'-eh-tahjz) Act of scraping a body cavity with a surgical instrument, such as a curette.

dilatation Opening or widening the circumference of a body orifice with a dilating instrument.

dissect To cut or separate tissue with a cutting instrument or scissors.

fascia Sheet or band of fibrous tissue located deep in the skin that covers muscles and body organs.

fistula Abnormal, tubelike passage between internal organs or from an internal organ to the body surface.

lumen Open space, such as within a blood vessel, the intestine, the inside of a needle, or an examining instrument.

obturator Metal rod with a smooth, rounded tip that is placed into hollow instruments to decrease injury to body tissues during insertion.

patency Open condition of a body cavity or canal.

polyps Tumors with stems, frequently found on mucous membranes.

stylus Metal probe that is inserted into or passed through a catheter, needle, or tube used for clearing purposes or to facilitate passage into a body orifice.

Office surgery is restricted to the management of minor problems and injuries. The medical assistant is expected to prepare the patient and the sterile field, assist the physician as needed, take care of the patient after the procedure, properly disinfect the area, and document as needed. Some medical assistants are employed in outpatient surgical facilities and are expected to assist with procedures that were once performed in the hospital. Although these more difficult operations may involve complete gowning and gloving with surgical masks and caps, the two surgical chapters in this text limit discussion and descriptions to the routines necessary to prepare for and assist in minor surgery only. This chapter includes a discussion of surgical supplies and instruments, the care and handling of instruments, and the different types of surgical sutures and needles. It prepares you for Chapter 56, which presents sterilization, preparation of the sterile field, specific minor surgical procedures, and care of the patient.

MINOR SURGERY ROOM

When minor surgery is routinely performed, the medical office is designed to include a changing room and a minor surgery room that are separate from the other examining rooms. The larger surgery centers have recovery rooms and family waiting areas. The minor surgery room in the physician office setting should be near a workroom with a sink and an autoclave if the room does not have its own. It should be easy to disinfect and uncluttered to allow easy movement and minimal dust collection. In addition to the operating table, equipment should include a clock with a second hand, an operating light, sitting stools, and Mayo stands (Figure 55-1). Cabinets with countertops are necessary to serve as a side or back table during the surgery. All surgical supplies are stored in these cabinets. Supplies used in this room should not be used elsewhere, and supplies used elsewhere should not be brought into this room.

SURGICAL SOLUTIONS AND MEDICATIONS

Treatment room supplies include standard solutions and medications that are used in minor surgery and dressing changes. Although the solutions and medications listed here are basic, every physician office practice has preferred items and methods of applying them. The medical assistant uses many of these items; some items are used only by the physician, but the medical assistant is responsible for their care and supply.

Sterile water is kept in two forms. Multiple-dose vials are used as a diluent for medications; larger containers of sterile water are for rinsing instruments that have been in a chemical disinfectant solution.

Sterile physiologic saline solution (0.9%) is also stocked in two sizes. The small multiple-dose vial is used for injection. A larger-size container of sterile saline is used for rinsing and irrigating wounds. These commercially prepared products are ordered from a medical supply company.

The patient's surgical site must be prepared preoperatively with an antiseptic skin cleansing preparation to reduce the number of pathogens. Although it is not possible to remove all microorganisms from the skin, it is important to prepare the surgical site to remove transient and pathogenic microorganisms on the skin surface and to reduce resident flora. In addition, the surgeon's hands and those of the medical assistant require disinfection to reduce the chances of wound contamination even though hands will be covered with sterile gloves. Surgical scrub preparations should have a broad antimicrobial action that is effective against bacterial spores, works rapidly to decrease transient bacteria, shows evidence of persistent activity on the skin, and works despite the presence of organic matter such as blood or wound drainage. Research indicates that chlorhexidine (Hibiscrub or Hibiclens) and povidone iodine (Betadine) are safe and effective antiseptics.

Even minor surgical procedures require the use of anesthetics, which either are injected locally at the site of the procedure

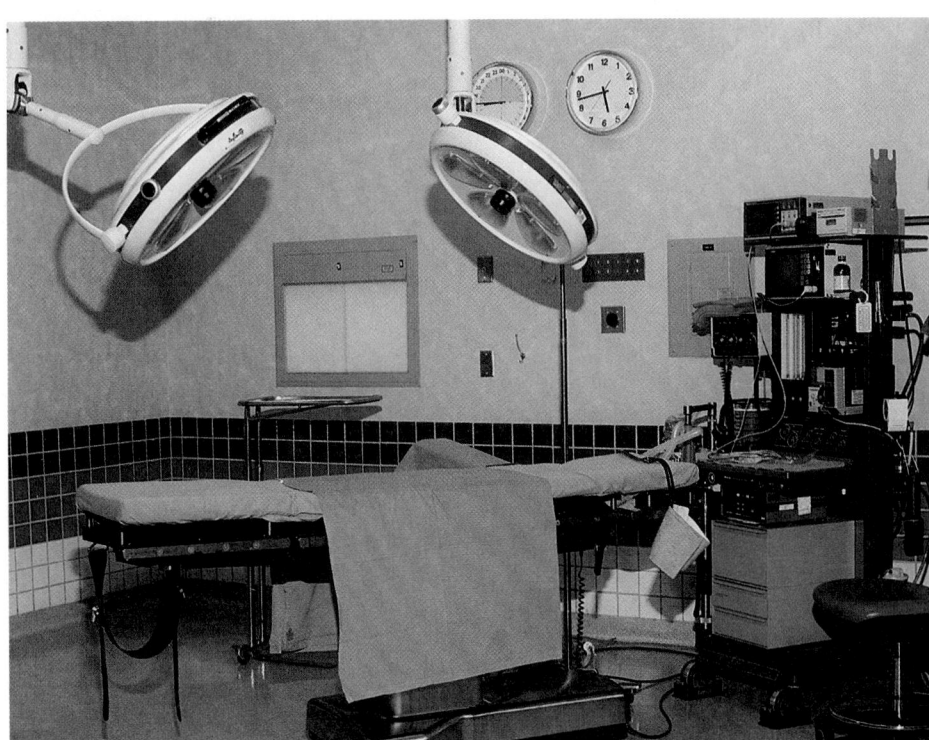

FIGURE 55-1 Operating room and equipment. (Courtesy Fresno Surgery Center, Fresno, Calif.)

or may be sprayed on the skin as a preinjection anesthetic. For patients who find injections of local anesthesia painful or traumatic, the physician may first spray the injection area with a topical anesthetic, such as Fluori-Methane 15%, which is supplied in 3.5-ounce amber glass bottles for either fine or medium spray. Immediately after spraying the site, the physician makes a series of injections around the area with a local anesthetic.

Another topical anesthetic spray is ethyl chloride, a vapocoolant that controls pain associated with minor surgical procedures such as lancing boils or incision and drainage of small **abscesses** by causing localized freezing of the affected area. Because ethyl chloride is highly flammable, it should never be used in the presence of electrical cauterizing equipment, and it requires the application of petroleum jelly to surrounding areas to protect them from the cooling action of the spray. It has a short duration, so all equipment must be prepared and the physician ready to perform the procedure before it is applied.

Local anesthetics are injected into the subcutaneous tissue and result in temporary cessation of feeling at the site of injection by blocking the generation and conduction of nerve impulses. There are many different types of local anesthetics, but all share the same suffix of *-caine*. Those used most frequently include lidocaine (Xylocaine), Nesacaine, and Sensorcaine. Local anesthetics are purchased in multiple-dose vials of 30 to 50 mL and in varying strengths such as 0.5%, 1%, and 2%. They begin acting relatively quickly, within 5 to 15 minutes; the duration of action depends on the type of anesthetic used, but they usually last from 1 to 3 hours. When highly vascular areas are involved, local anesthetics containing epinephrine may be used. Epinephrine causes vasoconstriction at the site, which keeps the anesthetic in the tissues longer, prolonging its effect.

It also minimizes local bleeding. However, epinephrine is not used in areas where decreased circulation may cause problems with healing, such as fingertips or toes.

All tissues removed, or biopsied, from the patient are sent to the pathology laboratory for analysis. A 10% formalin solution is typically used to preserve excised tissue for specimens. Specimen bottles are purchased with preservatives included and should be part of the supplies prepared for a surgical procedure if a biopsy is to be done. The physician will place the specimen in the container, and the medical assistant is responsible for accurately labeling the container with the patient's name, date of collection, and type of specimen.

Sometimes the physician may want to use topical silver nitrate ($AgNO_3$) solution or coated applicator sticks to stop localized bleeding, such as with epistaxis (nosebleed) or capillary bleeding at the site of a wound. The applicators must be kept

---

Additional Surgical Supplies

- Wound drains (Penrose drains): rubber drains placed in a wound at the end of a surgical procedure to drain excess fluid
- Sterilized gauze squares or strips saturated with Vaseline (petroleum jelly or petrolatum): used for packing wounds
- Sterilized iodoform gauze strips: $1/4$ to 2 inches wide, impregnated with iodoform iodine; used to pack abscesses, acting as a wick to draw out the infection and as a local antibacterial agent (Figure 55-2)
- Surgical sponges: used to absorb blood and protect tissues during surgery
- Syringes and needles: used to inject local anesthetics and irrigate wounds

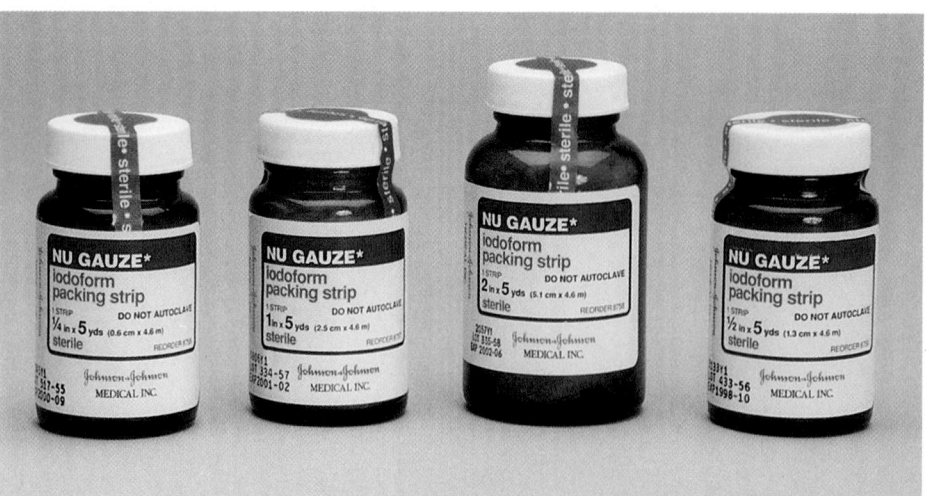

FIGURE 55-2 Iodoform gauze. (Courtesy Johnson & Johnson Medical, Arlington, Tex.)

in lightproof brown containers, and the most commonly used strength is 20%. The applicator sticks are convenient for use in the mouth or nose.

CRITICAL THINKING APPLICATION

Tom is ready to do an inventory of supplies in the minor surgery room. What solutions, medications, and miscellaneous supplies should he make sure are on hand for the busy surgical schedule planned for next week?

SURGICAL INSTRUMENTS

The medical assistant must know which instruments are used for each procedure and should be able to identify and understand the function of the surgical instruments preferred by the physician. Instruments have clearly identifiable parts and can be visually differentiated from one another (Procedure 55-1). The basic components are the handle, the closing mechanism, and the part that comes into contact with the patient, commonly called the *jaws*. Many instruments can be ordered with either straight or curved tips, depending on the operator's preference and the task to be performed.

Instruments have either ring handles (finger rings) or spring handles (sometimes called *thumb-handled* or *thumb grasp* instruments). Scissors are an example of a ring-handled instrument; tweezers are spring-handled. Some instruments have a hinge type of mechanism called a *box lock*. A ring-handled forceps is shown in Figure 55-3, *A;* a box-lock mechanism is shown in Figure 55-3, *B;* and a spring-handled thumb forceps is shown in Figure 55-3, *C.*

Ratchets resemble gears and are located just below the ring handles. They are used to lock an instrument into position. Most ratchets can be closed at three or more positions, depending on the thickness of the tissue or materials being grasped. Figure 55-3, *A* and *B* show ratchet-closing mechanisms.

The inner surfaces of the jaws on some instruments have ridged teeth called *serrations,* and both ring-handled and thumb-type instruments may have them. These serrations may be crisscross, horizontal, or lengthwise (Figure 55-4). Serrations prevent small blood vessels and tissue from slipping out of the jaws of the instrument.

Instrument tips or jaws may be plain tipped or mouse toothed (Figure 55-5, *A*). If the tooth is large, the tip is called rat toothed (Figure 55-5, *B*) rather than mouse toothed. Tissue forceps are usually toothed instruments and are identified by the number of intermeshing teeth (e.g., 12, 23, 34). Figure 55-5, *C* shows Allis tissue forceps. Because Allis forceps are used to grasp delicate soft tissues, the teeth are finer, shallower, and more rounded; others are sharper and deeper. Still others have sharp hooklike single or double teeth, such as a tenaculum or vulsellum. Usually, the tenaculum has a single sharp hook on each jaw. The vulsellum has a double hook that resembles the fangs of a snake. Toothed instruments commonly have ratchets for locking into towels or human tissues. Instrument tips may also be either straight or curved, depending on their use.

An instrument is usually named for its use (e.g., splinter forceps, for removing splinters) or after the person(s) who developed it (e.g., Mayo-Hegar needle holder). Many general instruments are identified by the part of the body on which they are used (e.g., rectal speculum and nasal speculum).

There are thousands of surgical instruments with multiple name variations. The same instrument may carry two or three different names, depending on the physician identifying it or the part of the country in which the practice is located. A physician may ask for a clamp or forceps when a Kelly hemostat is wanted. It is important to learn the physician's preference in terminology. Learn to recognize the distinctive parts of instruments and the reasons for each part, and you will quickly build a working knowledge of hundreds of instruments.

CLASSIFICATIONS OF SURGICAL INSTRUMENTS

Surgical instruments are generally classified according to their use, and most belong to one of four groups:

- Cutting
- Grasping

PROCEDURE 55-1

Identify Surgical Instruments

GOAL: *To identify, correctly spell the names of, and determine the use(s) of standard office instruments or those selected by your instructor.*

EQUIPMENT and SUPPLIES

- Curved hemostat
- Straight hemostat
- Dressing (thumb) forceps
- Paper and pen
- Disposable scalpel and blade
- Dissecting scissors
- Towel clamp
- Vaginal speculum
- Bandage scissors
- Allis tissue forceps

PROCEDURAL STEPS

1. Look for the following parts that determine usage: box-lock, serrations, finger rings, cutting edge, noncutting edge, thumb type, teeth ratchets, and electric attachments.
   PURPOSE: To determine the combination of features and parts for each instrument.
2. Consider the general classification of the instrument: cutting and dissection, grasping and clamping, retracting, or probing and dilating.

PURPOSE: The clue to the name of the instrument may be found by determining the classification.

3. Carefully examine the teeth and serrations.
   PURPOSE: The clue to the name of the instrument may be found by determining its distinctive parts.
4. Look at the length of the instrument to determine the area of the body for which it is used.
   PURPOSE: The clue to the name of the instrument may be found by determining where it can reach.
5. Try to remember whether the instrument was named for a famous physician, university, or clinic.
   PURPOSE: Many instruments are named for the inventor.
6. If the instrument is a pair of scissors, look at the points and determine whether the tips are sharp-sharp, sharp-blunt, or blunt-blunt.
7. Carefully compare the instrument with similar instruments that you know to determine whether it is in the same category or has the same name.
   PURPOSE: The clue to the name of an instrument may be found with the knowledge you already have.
8. Write, with correct spelling, the complete name of each instrument, including its category and use.

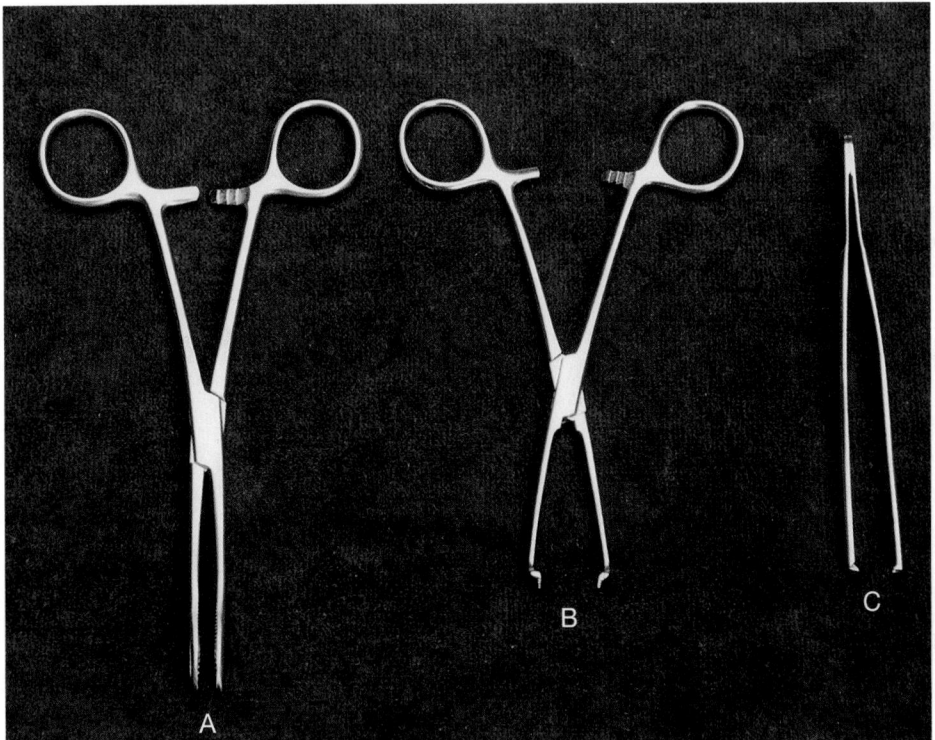

FIGURE 55-3 A, Ring-handle forceps. **B,** Box-lock hinge forceps. **C,** Spring-handle thumb forceps.

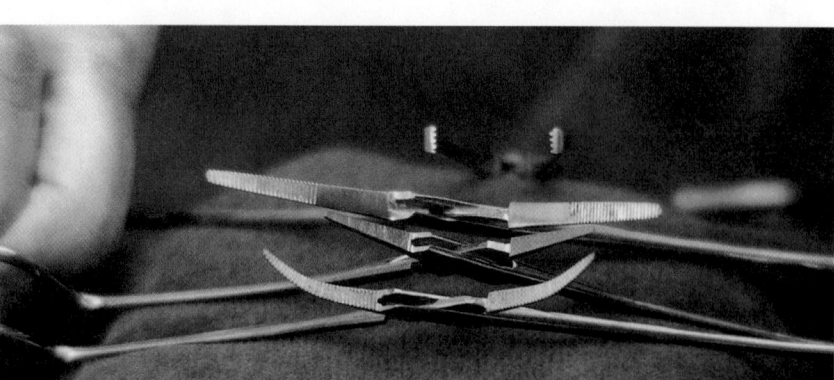

FIGURE 55-4 Instruments with serrations.

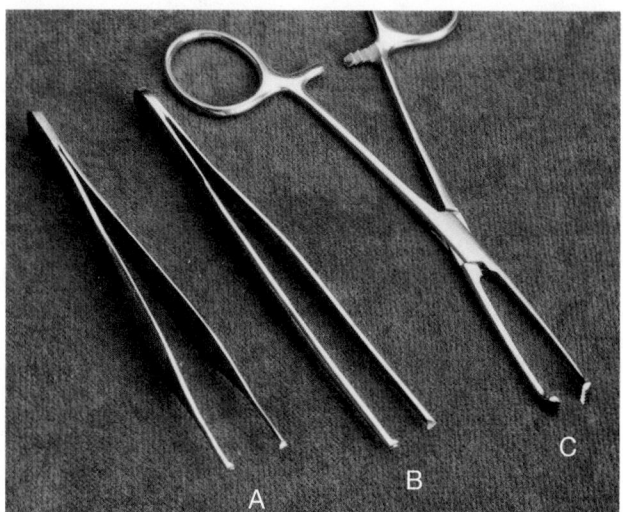

FIGURE 55-5 A, Mouse-toothed jaws. **B,** Rat-toothed jaws. **C,** Teeth of Allis tissue forceps.

- Retracting
- Probing and dilating

Cutting and Dissecting Instruments

These are cutting, incising, scraping, punching, and puncturing instruments. Included are scissors, scalpels, chisels, elevators, curettes, punches, drills, and needles. Instruments with a sharp blade or surface can cut, scrape, or **dissect.**

Bandage Scissors (Figure 55-6, *A*)
- Probe tip is blunt
- Easily inserted under bandages with relative safety
- Used to remove bandages and dressings

Operating (Surgical) Scissors
Metzenbaum (Metz) scissors (Figure 55-6, *B*)
- Most frequently used length is 5$\frac{1}{4}$ inches
- Used to cut and dissect tissue

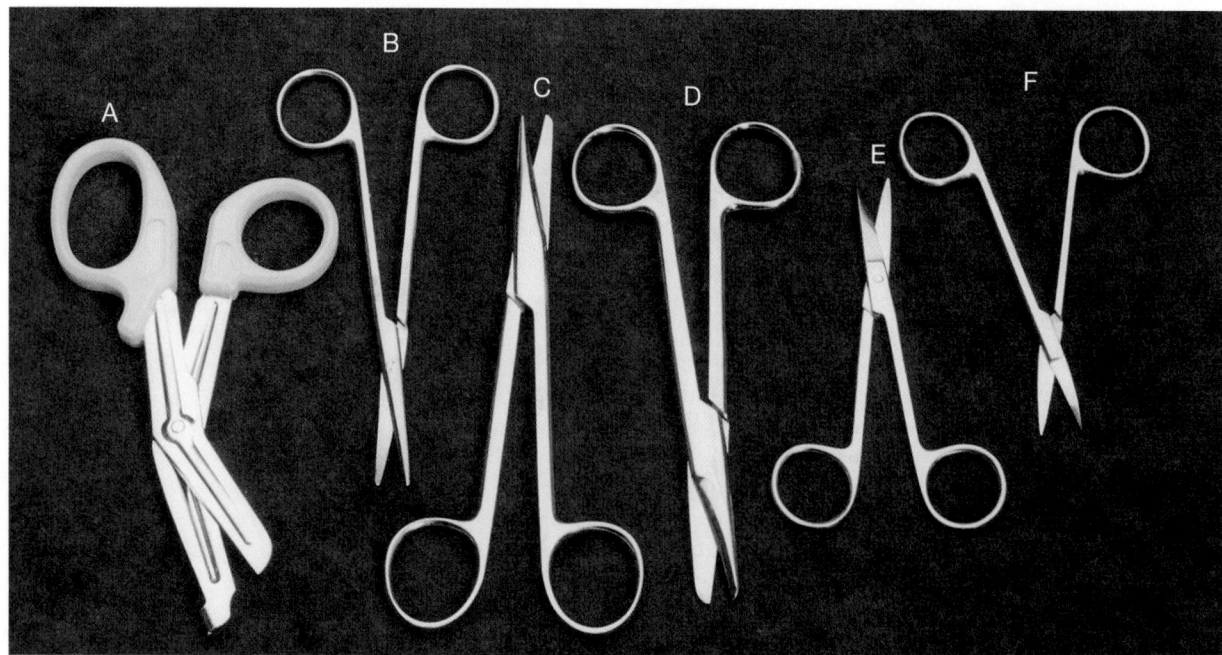

FIGURE 55-6 Operating scissors. **A,** Bandage scissors. **B,** Metzenbaum ("Metz") scissors. **C,** Curved Mayo scissors. **D,** Straight Mayo scissors. **E,** Straight iris scissors. **F,** Curved iris scissors.

Mayo Scissors (Figure 55-6, *C* and *D*)
- Have curved or straight blade tips
- Used to cut and dissect **fascia** and muscle
- Straight Mayo scissors can be used as suture scissors

Iris Scissors (Figure 55-6, *E* and *F*)
- Usual length is 4 inches
- Have curved or straight blade tips
- Straight tips usually used for suture removal

Littauer Stitch or Suture Scissors
- Blade has beak or hook to slide under sutures
- Used to remove sutures

Disposable Scalpels (Figure 55-7)
- Handles: No. 3 is the standard handle; No. 3L and No. 7 are used in deeper cavities
- Blades: No. 15 is commonly used; Nos. 10, 11, and 12 are used for specialty incisions

Grasping and Clamping Instruments

Clamping instruments are used for many different tasks. Many have a sharp tooth or teeth and are used to retract, hold, and manipulate human fascia. The most common clamping instru-

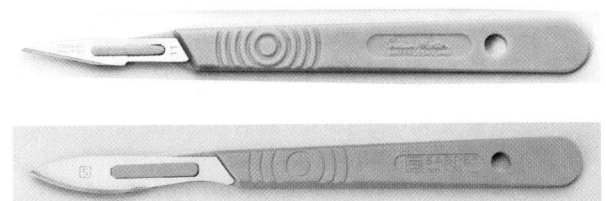

FIGURE 55-7 Disposable scalpels.

ments are hemostats, which were originally designed to stop bleeding or to clamp severed blood vessels. Some clamping instruments are used to grasp other instruments or sterilized materials. Sometimes hemostats and other clamping instruments are used interchangeably.

Hemostat Forceps (Figure 55-8, *A* and *B*)
- Jaws may be fully or partially serrated, without teeth
- May be curved or straight
- Used to clamp small vessels or hold tissue
- Mosquito forceps (4 inches) are smaller and used for very small vessels
- Crile forceps (5 inches) are medium sized
- Kelly forceps (6 to 7 inches) are larger

Needle Holders (Figure 55-8, *C* and *D*)
- Jaws are shorter and stronger than hemostat jaws
- Jaws may be serrated or may have a groove in the center
- Are 4 to 7 inches in size
- Used to grasp a suture needle firmly

Splinter Forceps (Figure 55-9, *A*)
- Design and construction vary
- Fine tip for foreign object retrieval

Smooth Adson Forceps (Figure 55-9, *B*)
- Same use as the Adson thumb forceps

Plain Thumb (Dressing) Forceps (Figure 55-9, *C* and *D*)
- Manufactured in lengths from 4 to 12 inches
- Have varying types of serrated jaws but no teeth
- Used to insert packing into or remove objects from deep cavities

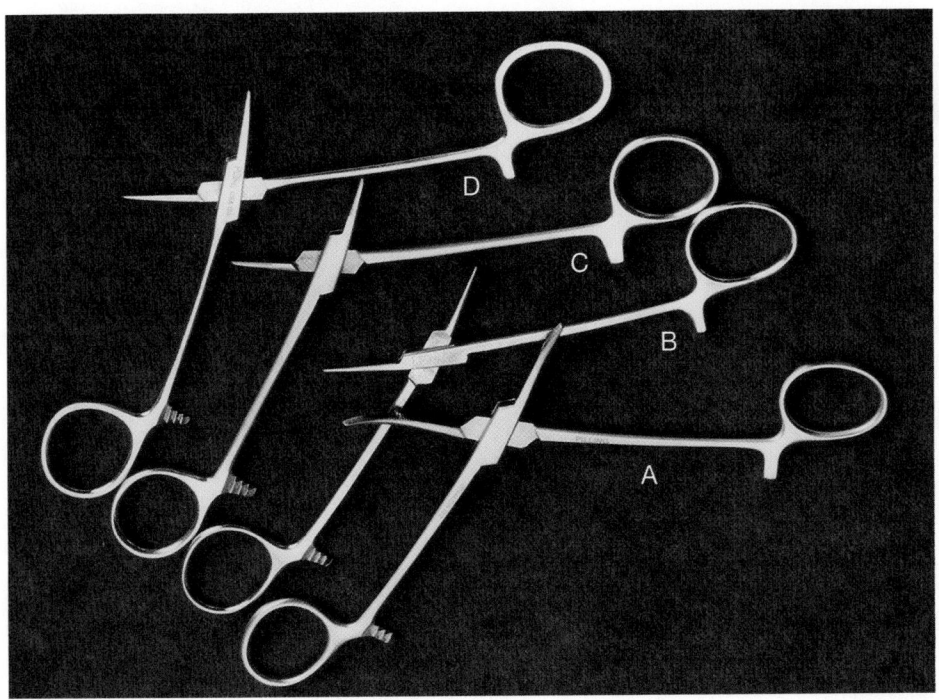

FIGURE 55-8 A, Kelly hemostat forceps. **B,** Mosquito hemostat forceps. **C,** Needle holder. **D,** Smooth-tip needle holder.

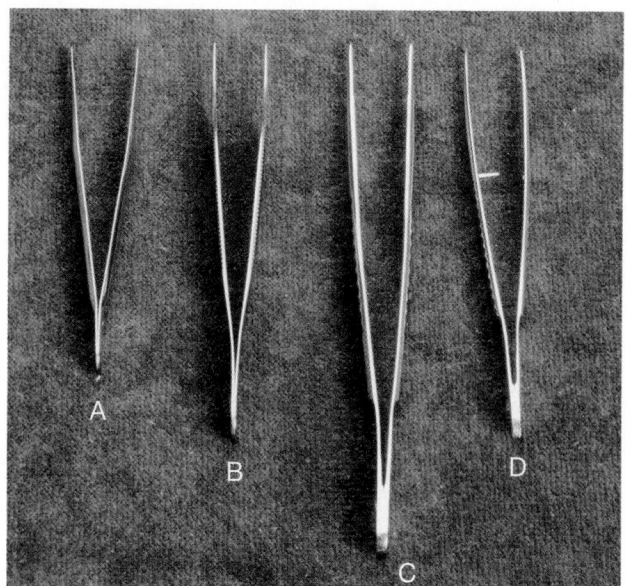

FIGURE 55-9 A, Splinter forceps. **B,** Smooth Adson forceps. **C,** Long plain-tip forceps. **D,** Short plain-tip forceps.

Towel Forceps (Towel Clamp) (Figure 55-10, *A* to *D*)
- May have sharp or atraumatic tips
- Are various lengths from 3 to 6½ inches
- Used to hold drapes in place during surgery

Allis Tissue Forceps (Figure 55-11, *A*)
- Available in different lengths and jaw widths
- Used to grasp tissue, muscle, or skin surrounding a wound

Foerster Sponge Forceps (Figure 55-11, *B*)
- Used to hold gauze squares to sponge the surgical site

Transfer Forceps (Figure 55-11, C to *E*)
- Many sizes and lengths are available
- Sterile transfer forceps may be used to arrange items on a sterile tray

Adson Thumb Forceps (Figure 55-12, *A* and *B*)
- Usually in 4-inch lengths
- Manufactured with or without teeth
- Used to grasp tissue and in suturing

Bayonet Forceps (Figure 55-12, *C* to *E*)
- Manufactured in different lengths
- Smooth tipped
- Used to insert packing into or remove objects from nose and ear

Plain-Tip Tissue Forceps (Figure 55-12, *F*)
- Manufactured in different lengths
- Atraumatic to tissue
- Used to grasp tissue, muscle, or skin surrounding a wound

Toothed Tissue Forceps (Figure 55-12, *G*)
- Manufactured in 4- to 18-inch lengths
- Pincher grip
- Used to grasp tissue, muscle, or skin surrounding a wound

Retractors

Retracting instruments hold tissue away from the surgical wound (incision). Depending on physician preference, skin hooks and Senn retractors are used to retract during most minor surgical procedures. These instruments are hand-held and are used for skin retraction.

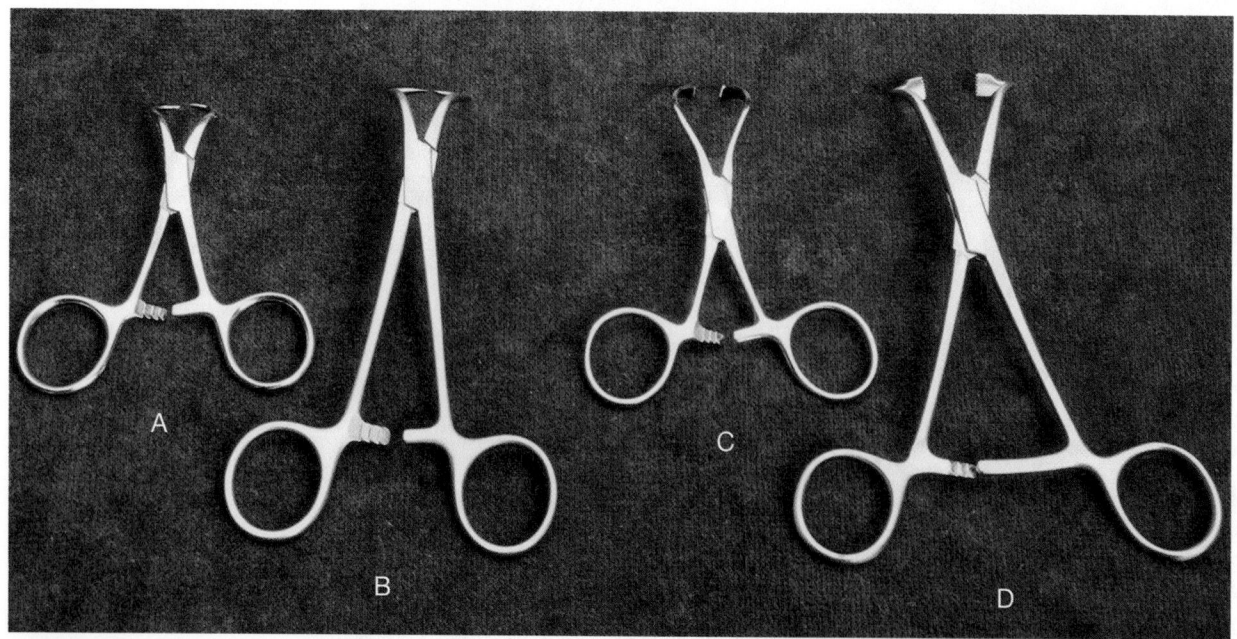

FIGURE 55-10 A, Small sharp towel forceps. **B,** Large sharp towel forceps. **C,** Small atraumatic towel forceps. **D,** Large atraumatic towel forceps.

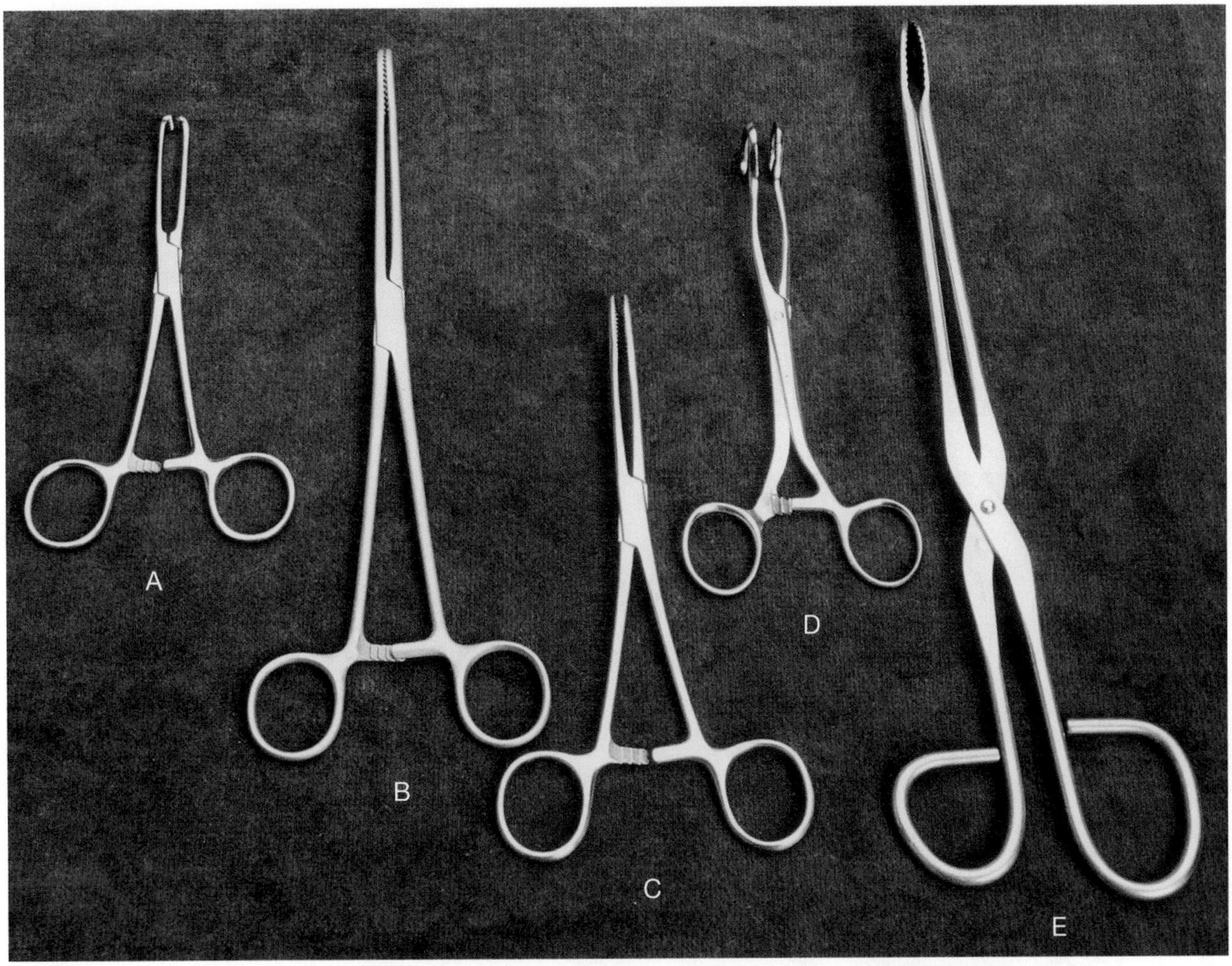

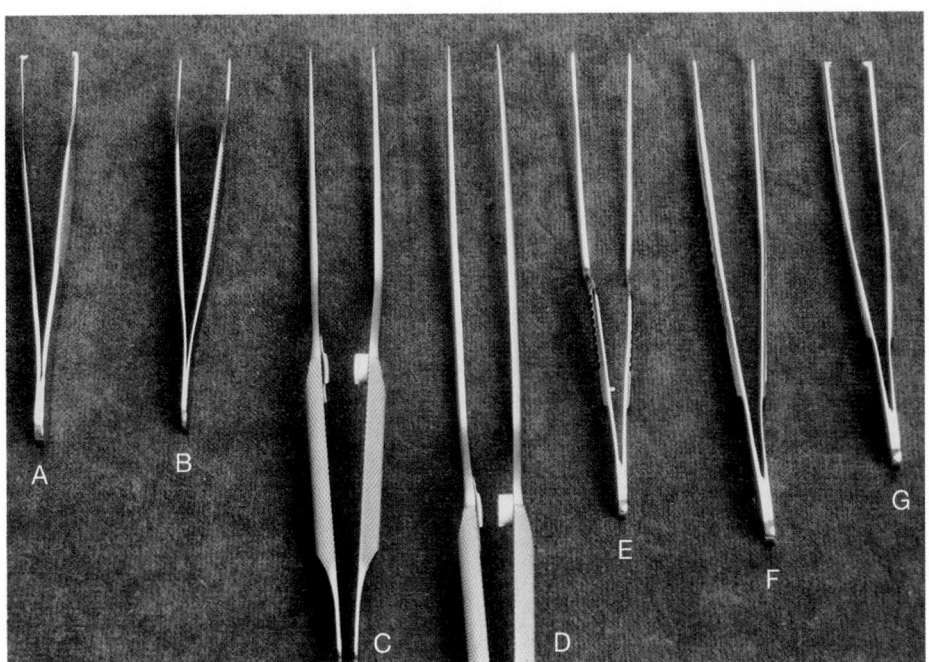

FIGURE 55-11 A, Allis forceps. **B,** Foerster sponge forceps. **C,** Straight transfer forceps. **D,** Short transfer forceps. **E,** Long transfer forceps.

FIGURE 55-12 A, Toothed Adson forceps. **B,** Smooth Adson forceps. **C,** Medium long bayonet forceps. **D,** Long bayonet forceps. **E,** Short bayonet forceps. **F,** Plain-tip tissue forceps. G, Toothed tissue forceps.

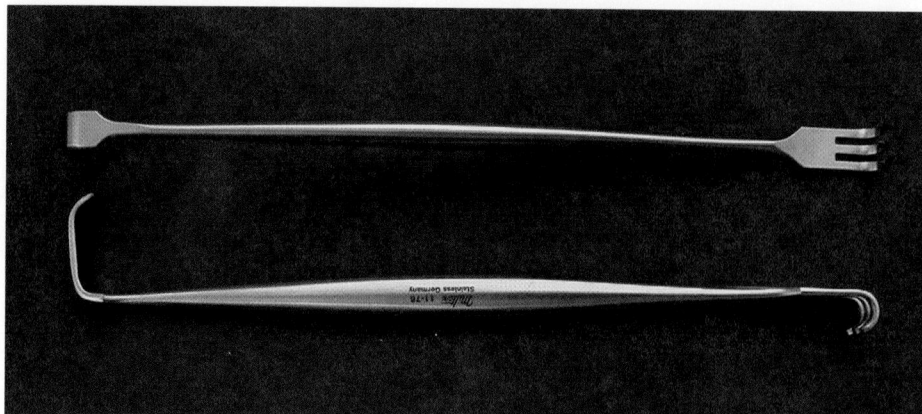

FIGURE 55-13 Senn retractor.

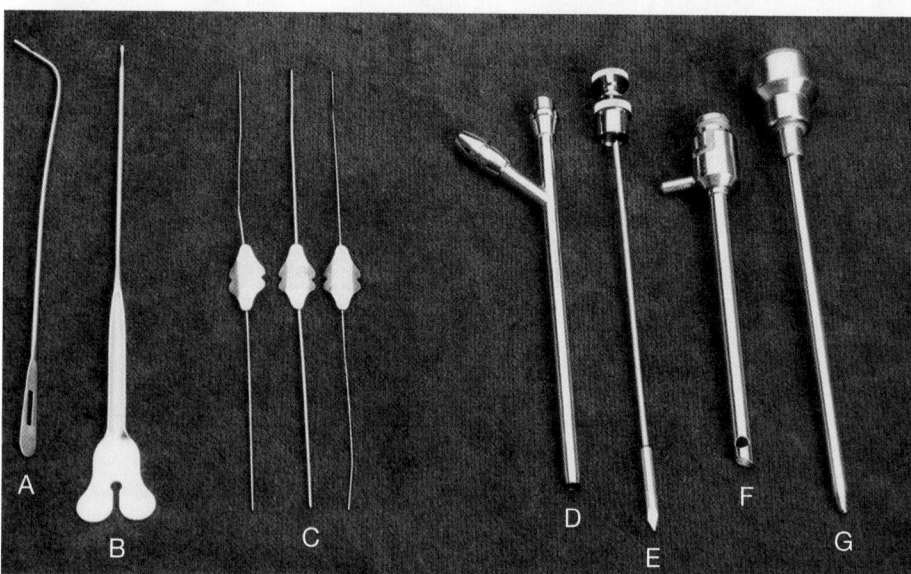

FIGURE 55-14 A, Probe. **B,** Grooved director. **C,** Lacrimal duct probes. **D,** Double-ended cannula. **E,** Sharp trocar. **F,** Cannula. **G,** Blunt-tip obturator.

Senn Retractor (Figure 55-13)

- Used to retract small incisions or to secure a skin edge for suturing
- Flat end is a blunt retractor
- Three-prong end may be sharp or dull

Probes and Dilators

These instruments are used for both surgery and examinations. Probes can be used to search for a foreign body in a wound or to enter a **fistula.** Dilators are used to stretch a cavity or opening for examination or before inserting another instrument to obtain a tissue specimen.

Probes (Figure 55-14, *A* to *C*)

- Length ranges from 4 to 12 inches; available with or without bulbous tip
- May be smooth or have a grooved director
- Used to find foreign bodies embedded in dermal tissue or muscle or to trace a wound tract

Trocars and Obturators (Figure 55-14, *D* to *G*)

- Consist of a sharply pointed stylus (obturator) contained in a cannula (outer tube)
- Available in various sizes

- Used to withdraw fluids from cavities or for draining and irrigating with a catheter

Specula (Figure 55-15, *A* to *D*)

- Most common dilator used
- Valves are spread apart, dilating the opening
- Used to open or distend a body orifice or cavity

Nasal Specula (see Figure 55-15, *A* and *B*)

- Valves can be spread to facilitate viewing
- An applicator or snare can be introduced through the valves
- Used to spread the nostrils for examination

SPECIALTY INSTRUMENTS

Although all instruments fall under the same four categories as the surgical instruments just discussed, the remaining instruments are organized into specialty groupings. Presenting the instruments in this manner makes it easy to see how the instruments relate to particular examinations. In addition to recognizing the name and use of each instrument, the medical assistant must organize and set out the instruments needed for each particular examination in what is called a *tray setup.*

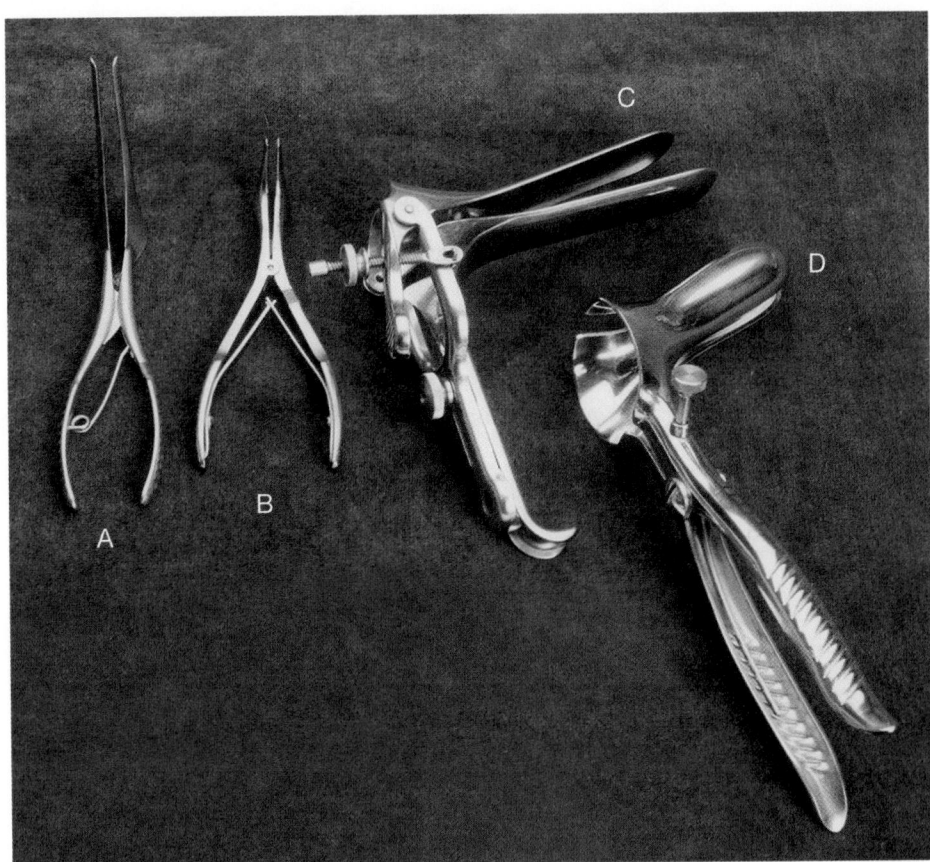

FIGURE 55-15 A, Long nasal speculum. **B,** Short nasal speculum. **C,** Graves vaginal speculum. **D,** Anal speculum, self-retaining.

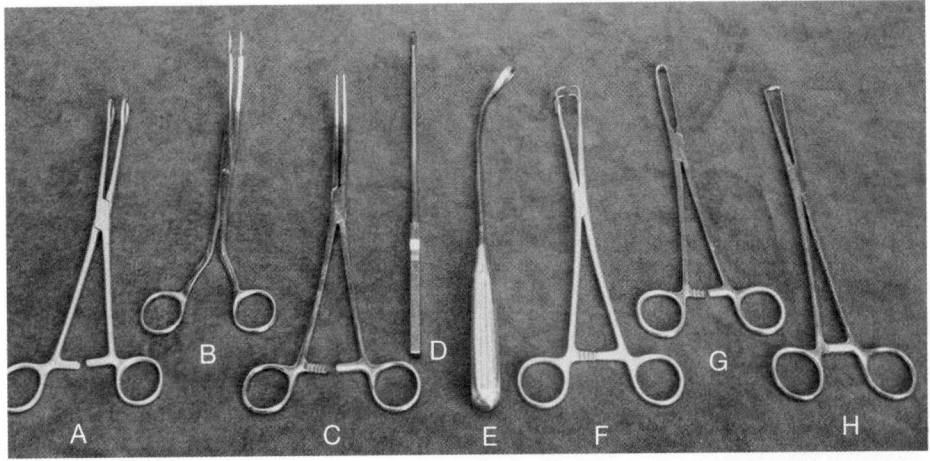

FIGURE 55-16 A, Foerster sponge forceps. **B,** Placenta forceps. **C,** Bozeman uterine dressing forceps. **D,** Endocervical curette. **E,** Sims uterine curette. **F,** Schroeder uterine vulsellum forceps. **G,** Long Allis forceps. **H,** Schroeder uterine tenaculum forceps.

Gynecologic Instruments

Foerster Sponge Forceps (Figure 55-16, *A*)
- Used in the same way as the dressing forceps
- Tips are round and serrated

Placenta Forceps (Figure 55-16, *B*)
- Used to remove tissue from the uterus

Bozeman Uterine Dressing Forceps (Figure 55-16, *C*)
- Used to swab the area or apply medication
- Designed to hold sponges or dressings
- Capable of reaching the cervix through the vagina

Endocervical Curette (Figure 55-16, *D*)
- Smaller than the uterine curette
- Used the same as the uterine curette

Sims Uterine Curette (Figure 55-16, *E*)
- Used to remove polyps, secretions, and bits of placental tissue
- Manufactured in several sizes
- Hollow and spoon shaped, used for scraping

Schroeder Uterine Vulsellum Forceps (Figure 55-16, *F*)
- Used to hold tissue (such as cervix) while obtaining a tissue specimen or to lift the cervix to view the fornix

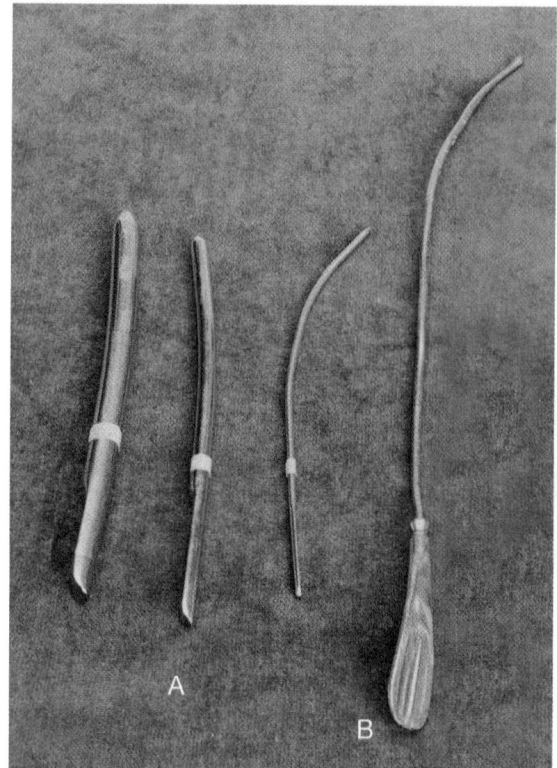

FIGURE 55-17 **A,** Uterine dilators. **B,** Sims uterine sounds.

Long Allis Forceps (Figure 55-16, *G*)
- Same as Allis forceps
- Used in deeper body cavities

Schroeder Uterine Tenaculum Forceps (Figure 55-16, *H*)
- Used in the same way as the vulsellum forceps
- Have very sharp, pointed tips

Hegar Uterine Dilators (Figure 55-17, *A*)
- Used to dilate the cervix for **dilatation** and **curettage**
- Available in sets
- Double or single ended

Sims Uterine Sounds (Figure 55-17, *B*)
- Used to check the **patency** of the cervical os or the urethral meatus

Ophthalmologic and Otolaryngologic Instruments

Krause Nasal Snare (Figure 55-18, *A*)
- Has a wire loop at the tip that can be tightened
- Used to remove **polyps** from the nares

Metal Tongue Depressor (Figure 55-18, *B*)
- Used to depress the tongue for oral examinations

Hartmann "Alligator" Ear Forceps (Figure 55-18, *C*)
- Has a $3^1/_2$-inch shaft and is made in a variety of styles
- Action of the jaw similar to that of an alligator's jaw
- Used to remove foreign bodies or polyps

Laryngeal Mirror (Figure 55-18, *D*)
- Made in various sizes
- May have a nonfogging surface
- Used for examination of the larynx and postnasal area

Ivan Laryngeal Metal Applicator (Figure 55-18, *E*)
- Holds cotton in place with its roughened end; used to swab or sponge throat or postnasal tissue
- Six to 9 inches long with curved end for use in throat or postnasal areas
- Used to remove foreign bodies imbedded in the pharynx

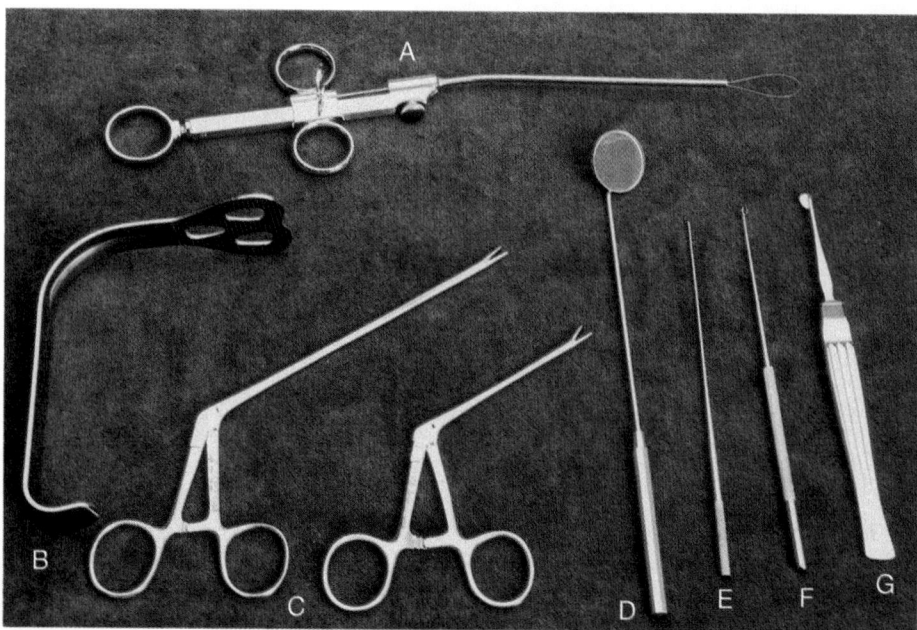

FIGURE 55-18 **A,** Krause nasal snare. **B,** Metal tongue depressor. **C,** Long and short alligator forceps. **D,** Laryngeal mirror. **E,** Ivan metal applicator. **F,** "Buck" ear curette. **G,** Sharp ear dissector.

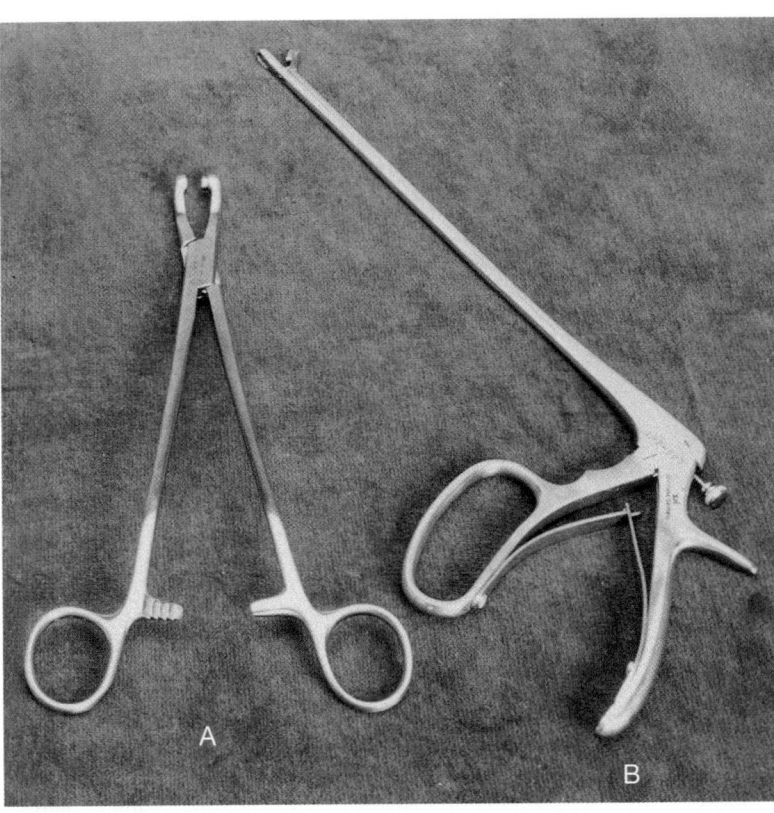

FIGURE 55-19 A, Cervical biopsy forceps. **B,** Rectal biopsy punch.

"Buck" Ear Curette (Figure 55-18, *F*)
- Made with sharp or blunt scraper ends
- Manufactured in various sizes
- Used to remove foreign matter from the ear canals

Sharp Ear Dissector (Figure 55-18, *G*)
- Used to remove debris from the ear canal

Biopsy Instruments

Cervical Biopsy Forceps (Figure 55-19, *A*)
- Available with or without teeth
- Used to obtain cervical specimens for diagnostic examination

Rectal Biopsy Punch (Figure 55-19, *B*)
- Manufactured with interchangeable stems
- Available in different lengths and styles
- Used through a proctoscope or sigmoidoscope

Silverman Biopsy Needle
- Manufactured with a split cannula
- **Stylus** is removed, and cannula is inserted to retrieve specimen
- Needle biopsy can eliminate the need for surgical incision

Genitourinary Instruments

Catheter Guide (Figure 55-20, *A*)
- Metal guide
- Used with extreme caution
- Used by the physician when it is impossible to insert a catheter by normal means

Foley Catheter with Inflated Balloon (Figure 55-20, *B*)
- Manufactured in sizes 8 to 32 French with a double rubber lining toward the tip
- After insertion, sterile solution injected into the inner lining (inflating the balloon) to hold it in the bladder
- Used as an indwelling catheter

Red Robinson Catheter (Figure 55-20, *C*)
- Soft rubber urethral catheter in sizes 8 to 32 French (each French unit is equal to 1.3 mm)
- The higher the number, the larger the **lumen**
- Inserted temporarily into the bladder for drainage or to obtain a specimen

12-mL Luer-Lok Syringe (Figure 55-20, *D*)
- Used for injecting amounts greater than 5 mL

Colorectal Procedures

Sigmoidoscope
- Used to internally view the anus, rectum, and sigmoid colon
- Used with a fiberoptic light source; may use photography or video setup

---

CRITICAL THINKING APPLICATION

Tom is preparing instrument and supply packs for specific procedures performed by Dr. Samanski. One of the packs he is preparing for the autoclave is for removal of a nasal polyp. Based on your understanding of typical and specialty instruments and supplies, what items should Tom include in the instrument pack?

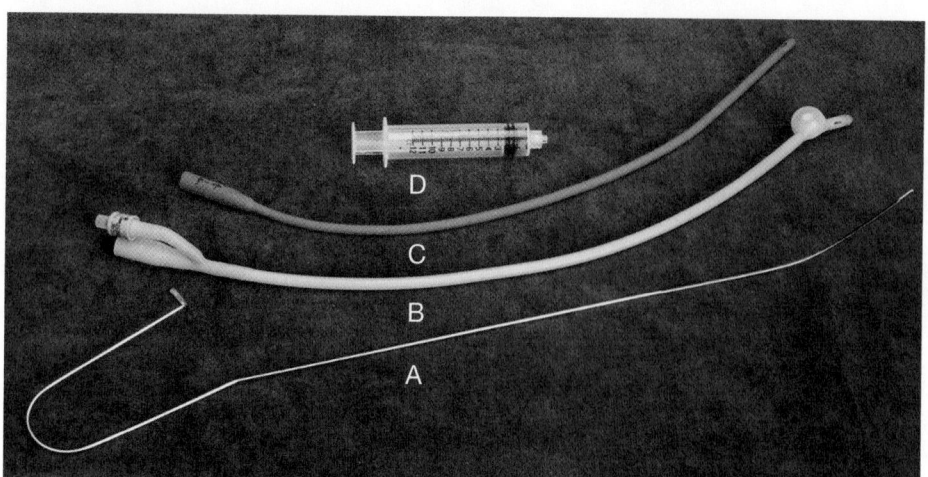

FIGURE 55-20 A, Metal catheter guide. **B,** Foley catheter with inflated balloon. **C,** Red Robinson catheter. **D,** 12-mL Luer-Lok syringe.

CARE AND HANDLING OF INSTRUMENTS

Because instruments are expensive and the physician's skill is dependent on their quality, the medical assistant must properly care for each instrument to maximize its life and ensure that every part is in safe working order.

Most instruments are made of fine-grade stainless steel. The term *stainless* is usually taken too literally. Although stainless steel does resist rust and keeps a fine edge and tip longer, even the best stainless steel may develop water spots and stains, especially if water with a high mineral content is used. Proper hardness and flexibility are important. Inexpensive instruments that are chrome plated may be too brittle or too soft. In addition, mistreatment of chrome-plated instruments can cause minute breaks in the finish, which may become a source of contamination or may tear the surgeon's gloves.

All instruments should be carefully examined when they are purchased. Scissors should be tested to see whether they shear the full length of the blades completely to the tip. If the scissors cut a piece of cloth cleanly and do not chew at any point, even at the tip, they are functioning correctly. Teeth and serrations should be checked to see whether they intermesh completely and whether the jaws are even on the sides and tip. Each instrument should be felt over its entire surface for any rough areas that may tear or snag the surgeon's gloves or act as a future source of contamination. Box-locks and hinges must work freely but should not be too loose. Thumb- and spring-handled instruments must have the correct tension and meet evenly at the tips. After inspection, instruments should be cleaned and checked again for possible faulty workmanship before sterilization.

Under no circumstances should instruments be bundled together or allowed to become entangled. Avoid mixing stainless steel instruments with others made of different metals, including chrome-plated instruments. This may cause electrolysis and result in etching. If an instrument is accidentally dropped, it may be permanently damaged. If scissors are dropped with the blades partially open, there may be a nick at the point where the blades cross. Any damaged or malfunctioning instrument must be disposed of to prevent complications during a surgical procedure.

After a surgical procedure, contaminated instruments should be placed in a basin of disinfectant solution with heavier instruments on the bottom of the basin and lighter, more delicate instruments placed on top. Always unlock each instrument before immersion in the chemical decontaminant to permit cleansing of the entire surface area. Never allow blood or other coagulable substances to dry on an instrument because they will be difficult to remove. If immediate disinfection is not possible, the instruments should be rinsed well and placed in a cold water solution with a blood solvent and mild detergent. The detergent increases the wetting ability of the water, giving the instrument surfaces better exposure to the solution. It is best to use a detergent that has a neutral pH, low suds, and the ability to be rinsed off easily. Manufacturer recommendations for the correct dilution and time of immersion of the various disinfectants and blood solvents must be strictly followed for the chemicals to be effective.

When the surgical procedure is completed, the receiving basin for instruments should be transferred from the surgical area to the disinfection and sterilization room. It is important to remove used instruments from the patient's view as soon as possible. After disinfection is completed, instruments should be thoroughly rinsed and either washed by hand or washed mechanically using an ultrasonic device.

Some delicate instruments, such as microsurgical and lensed instruments, should be washed by hand with mild, low-suds, neutral pH detergent solution and a soft brush. The instruments should be cleaned while submerged to avoid airborne spread of microorganisms. Throughout the cleaning process, the medical assistant should wear heavy utility gloves to avoid possible contaminant exposure. Instruments should then be rinsed with distilled water, dried with a lint-free cloth, and inspected for proper functioning before being packed for sterilization.

Mechanical washing, such as with an ultrasonic device, can be used for most instruments and is an especially good method for cleaning sharp instruments to avoid possible injury. An ultrasonic cleaning unit uses sound waves while instruments are immersed in a cleaning solution to clean contaminants from instrument surfaces. The unit then rinses and dries the instruments, leaving them ready for the sterilization process. However, manufacturer guidelines should be followed with rubber and plastic materials.

After disinfection and inspection, the instruments are ready for the sterilization process. This procedure is discussed in Chapter 56.

Commercially prepared disposable packs are available for most minor surgical procedures. They save time and eliminate cleaning and autoclaving reusable stainless steel instruments but may be cost prohibitive for individual practices.

CRITICAL THINKING APPLICATION

Tom is responsible for inspecting and caring for all of the surgical instruments in the minor surgical room as well as cleaning and preparing contaminated instruments for autoclaving. He is in the process of writing an addition to the office policies and procedures manual on the management of surgical instruments. Based on what you know about the care and handling of surgical instruments, what should Tom include in the policy?

DRAPES, SUTURES, AND NEEDLES

Disposable surgical drapes are available in several different materials and sizes and typically have an opening (fenestration) for the operative site (Figure 55-21). The drape is placed over the operative area using sterile technique after the patient's skin preparation has been completed. This procedure is presented in Chapter 56.

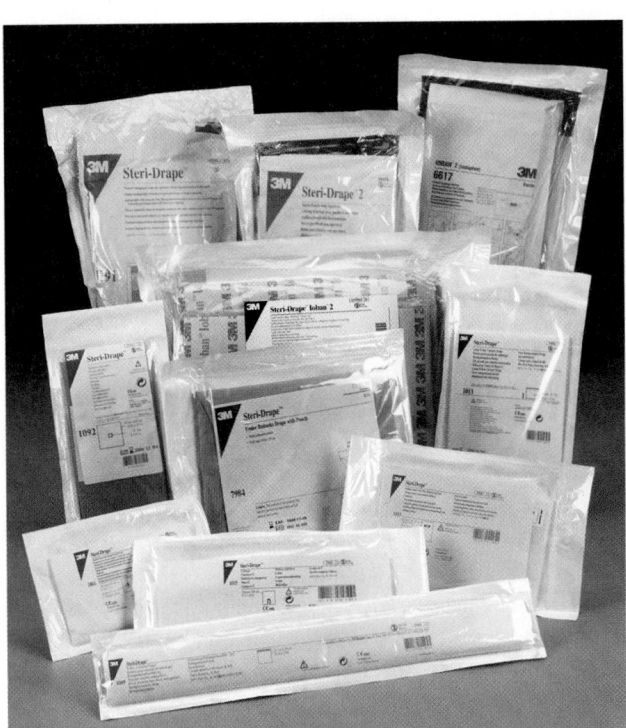

FIGURE 55-21 Sample surgical drapes. (Courtesy 3M Corp.)

Sutures

The word *suture* is used as both a noun and a verb. As a noun it refers to a surgical stitch or to the material used to close a wound. As a verb it refers to the act of stitching. Modern surgery and the use of sutures began in 1865, when Lister developed antisepsis and the disinfection of suture materials. Many kinds of materials have been used over the centuries, including precious metals, horse hair, animal tendons, and cotton and linen cord. Most of the improvements in suture materials and techniques have occurred in the past 50 years. The primary purpose of a suture is to hold the edges of a wound together until natural healing occurs.

A suture may also be used as a ligature. This is a strand of suture material used to tie off a blood vessel or to strangulate tissue. If a ligature is used to tie off an internal tubular structure, it must last permanently or long enough for the structure itself to disintegrate.

The ideal suture material has certain characteristics:

- Easy to handle and makes a secure knot
- Does not induce a localized tissue reaction and is nonallergenic
- Has adequate strength without cutting through tissue
- Can be sterilized

The physician will request a certain type of suture based on the specific properties of the suture material, the desirable rate of absorption, the size of the suture, and the type of needle the physician prefers. Both natural and synthetic suture materials are available. Sutures may be classified as either absorbable or nonabsorbable. Many different suture materials are available, each having its advantages and disadvantages. Suture materials commonly used in minor surgical procedures are described in the following paragraphs (Figure 55-22).

Absorbable Suture

The absorbable suture is dissolved by the body's enzymes during the healing process. It is used when deep incisions or lacerations require inner layers of sutures to close the wound. Absorbable suture material is also used in areas where suture removal is difficult, as in oral surgery. An example of an absorbable suture material is surgical catgut, which is obtained from sheep, cattle, or pig intestine. Plain catgut is used in tissues that heal most rapidly, such as mucous membranes and subcutaneous tissues, because it is broken down within a week. Chromic catgut is coated with chromic salts, which delays the absorption of the suture material up to 80 days.

Catgut was once the absorbable suture material of choice but has been replaced in recent years by Vicryl, a synthetic absorbable suture made of polyglactin. Other synthetic absorbable suture materials include Dexon, PDS, and Maxon. These materials remain stable longer than natural catgut, up to 11 weeks, allowing the wound to heal completely before absorption occurs.

Nonabsorbable Suture

Nonabsorbable suture material is left in the wound site until healing is complete. It is frequently used in minor surgical

FIGURE 55-22 Suture packets labeled according to size, type, length, and type of needle point and shape.

procedures performed in the medical office, because most of the suturing required is superficial, and in areas where sutures can be removed after healing has taken place. A common nonabsorbable suture material is silk because it is strong and easy to tie. It is treated with a coating to prevent tissue drag and flaking. Polyester fiber sutures, such as Dacron and Prolene, are among the strongest nonabsorbable sutures along with surgical steel. These fine filaments are braided and have great tensile strength. Nylon suture is strong and has a high degree of elasticity. It is primarily used for skin closure. Owing to its elasticity and stiffness, many knots must be used because the knots tend to untie if placed incorrectly.

Surgical staples can also be used for skin closure. They are made of stainless steel or titanium and are available in different sizes. They are applied and removed with specific staple instruments (Figure 55-23). Other techniques of wound closure include Steri-Strips, which are self-adhesive tapes that are placed over the wound, pulling the wound ends together. Steri-Strips can be used to support a wound if there is potential tension at the site or for superficial wounds such as a laceration of the forehead. Tissue adhesives, similar to glue, can also be used for superficial wounds.

Suture Sizing and Packaging

Suture material comes in a variety of diameters and lengths. The diameter of the suture strand determines its size, with the smaller gauges numbered below 0 (pronounced *aught*) and the larger gauges identified with numbers above 0. For instance, 2-0 is thinner than size 0, which is thinner than size 2. The sizes from 2-0 to 6-0 are used most frequently in the medical office. The length of the suture material may vary, with strands precut in 18-, 24-, 54-, and 60-inch lengths (Figure 55-24).

Needles

Surgical needles are chosen according to the area in which they are to be used and the depth and width of the desired suture. They are classified according to shape, which may be straight or curved (Figure 55-25). Most sutures are applied with

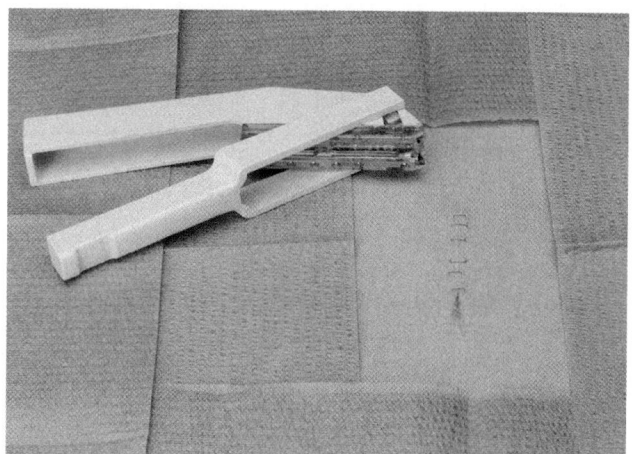

FIGURE 55-23 Disposable skin stapler.

Suture Sizes

Sutures are sized according to the United States Pharmacopoeia (USP) scale. The following sizes and diameters are available on a scale from 6-0, which is 0.07 mm in diameter, to 2, which is 0.5 mm:

6-0 = 0.07 mm
5-0 = 0.10 mm
4-0 = 0.15 mm
3-0 = 0.20 mm
2-0 = 0.30 mm
0 = 0.35 mm
1 = 0.40 mm
2 = 0.5 mm

curved needles because they allow the physician to penetrate the surface then come back up again on the other side. The sharper the curve of the needle, the deeper the surgeon can pass it into the tissue. The point of a needle can be a taper or a cutting edge. A taper is used on delicate tissues. The cutting edge needle is used on the skin. It lacerates the skin as the needle is

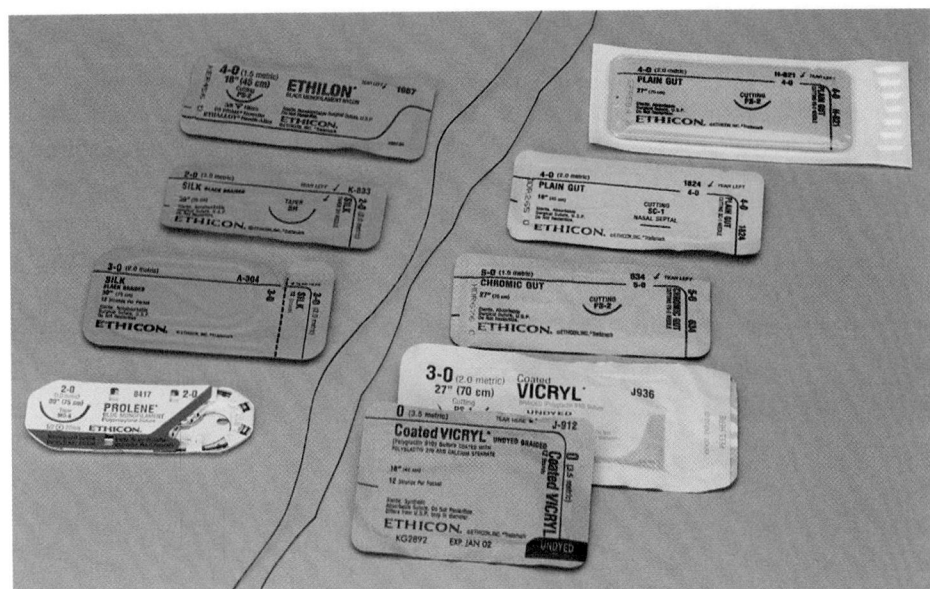

FIGURE 55-24 Suture packets (and opened suture strands) with and without needles.

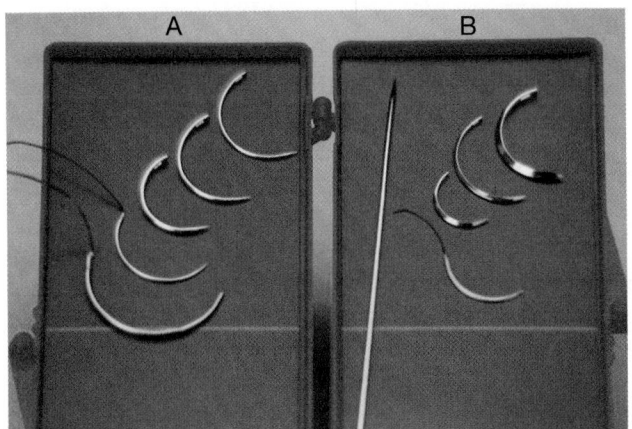

FIGURE 55-25 Surgical needle shapes. **A,** Taper point. **B,** Cutting point.

passed through. This is advantageous on tougher tissues, such as connective tissue.

Most needles are manufactured with the thread attached, or *swaged*, to the needle. These atraumatic needles do not have an eyelet and cause the least amount of tissue trauma as they are passed through the tissues. Manufacturers package the suture strands with the suture needle attached in peel-apart sterile disposable packages. These may be obtained as single, individually packed or as multipack sutures in a variety of needle types and sizes with a wide range of suture materials and lengths. The most common needle type for minor skin repair is the curved, cutting-edged, swaged needle.

CLOSING COMMENTS

Patient Education

Patients may have questions concerning the instruments the surgeon is using. The medical assistant can assist the patient by answering his or her questions to help alleviate any fears. Explaining patient preparation for the procedure, how it will be conducted, and what to expect afterward helps make the procedure easier to perform and encourages the patient to follow the physician's advice and orders.

Legal and Ethical Issues

When surgical procedures are done in the medical office, awareness of legal responsibilities is imperative. The medical assistant must know what surgery is planned and whether the patient has been informed regarding the procedure. In the surgical setting the medical assistant must realize the full extent of his or her role as the "patient's advocate" and the "physician's agent."

The medical assistant should confirm the fact that the physician has explained the surgery to the patient and that the patient fully understands all aspects of the procedure that will be performed. This means that when the patient signs the consent for surgery, he or she is fully informed. Increasing the patient's understanding ensures greater compliance with presurgical preparations, the surgical procedure, and postsurgical care.

SUMMARY OF SCENARIO

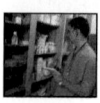

Tom has worked for Dr. Samanski for 2 years and is familiar with her preference in surgical solutions, local anesthesia, suture materials, and the typical instruments used in her practice. He also has worked hard to update the policy and procedures manual to include standards for instrument care so other medical assistants in the office will know how instruments should be sanitized, disinfected, inspected, and prepared for the autoclave. Tom realizes he needs to continue his education in surgical procedures and takes advantage of professional workshops on the topic. He and Dr. Samanski work well together in the minor surgery area of the office, and Tom consistently attempts to stay up to date on the surgical advances, medications, and instruments Dr. Samanski uses in her practice.

SUMMARY of LEARNING OBJECTIVES

1. Define, spell, and pronounce the terms listed in the vocabulary.
   - Spelling and pronouncing medical terms correctly adds credibility to the medical assistant. Knowing the definition of these terms promotes confidence in communication with patients and co-workers.
2. Describe typical solutions and medications used in minor surgical procedures.
   - The solutions used in minor surgery include sterile water for mixing with medications or rinsing instruments; sterile saline for injection or wound irrigations; antiseptic skin cleansers such as Betadine or Hibiclens for site preparations; and local anesthetics, including ethyl chloride or Fluori-Methane topical applications as well as lidocaine, Nesacaine, or Sensorcaine injectables. These local anesthetics may come packaged with or without epinephrine. The physician may also use topical silver nitrate to control local bleeding.
3. Summarize methods for identifying surgical instruments used in minor office surgery.
   - Procedure 55-1 summarizes methods for identifying surgical instruments.
4. Outline the general classifications of surgical instruments.
   - Surgical instruments are classified according to their use as cutting, grasping, retracting, probing, or dilating tools. The components of the instrument include the type of handle, the closing mechanism, and the jaws. Instrument tips may be either straight or curved and toothed or not toothed. The instruments used in minor surgical procedures depend on the type of procedure and physician preference.
5. Describe the care of surgical instruments.
   - Surgical instruments are expensive and must be cared for properly to maintain function and maximize life. Instruments must be examined when purchased for proper working order and possible faults with mechanisms. Stainless steel instruments should be kept separate from other metal types. Each instrument must be cleaned according to manufacturer guidelines, unlocked, and disinfected immediately after use. Most instruments can be cleaned with an ultrasonic washer, which helps avoid possible injury.
6. Identify types of sutures and surgical needles.
   - Suture material is available as absorbable for internal sutures or nonabsorbable for skin closures. Catgut and Vicryl are the two most popular absorbable materials; nonabsorbable sutures can be made out of silk, nylon, or staples. Suture materials range in size, with smaller gauges for finer tissues below 0 (aught) and thicker gauges above 0, and they come in various lengths. Surgical needles are either straight or curved. Most needles are manufactured with swaged suture material.

CONNECTIONS

Study Guide Connection: Go to Chapter 55 Study Guide. Read the Case Study and Workplace Applications and complete the assignments. Do online research for answers to the questions in the Internet Activities associated with surgical supplies and instruments.

CD Connection: Go to the Medical Assisting Competency Challenge CD and do the training activities under Infection Control. For a better understanding of the inflammatory response and controlling infection, view the animations for antibiotics and phagocytosis.

Evolve Connection: For more information related to surgical supplies and instruments, go to evolve.elsevier.com/kinn and visit related weblinks for Chapter 55. Click on the Medical Assisting Exam Review and do the practice questions to sharpen your test-taking skills.

Surgical Asepsis and Assisting with Surgical Procedures

56

SCENARIO

Melissa Gelbart has been a surgical medical assistant for Lakeside Surgical Associates for just over 1 month. She was hired to work as an administrative medical assistant at the front desk, but when one of the surgical assistants unexpectedly quit, the supervisor of surgery offered Melissa the position. At least she was familiar with a number of the patients, most of the staff, and the kinds of outpatient surgeries that were performed on a daily basis. Surgical asepsis and assisting with surgery were her favorite topics when she was in medical assisting school. She is very eager to get into the operating room, but they are starting her out in the supply and sterilization area. The supervisor of surgery wants her to become familiar with all of the surgical trays and instruments used daily at Lakeside Surgical Associates. It will probably be about 4 months before she gets to start working in the surgical suite. Before assisting with surgeries Melissa must prove she can set up a sterile field without contaminating the site. Melissa will also have to perform sterile dressing and bandage changes, so she must demonstrate these skills as well.

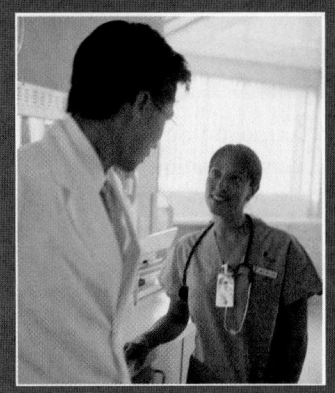

While studying this chapter, think about the following questions:

- What are the crucial steps Melissa must follow to set up and maintain a sterile field?
- How does an autoclave work and what are the important rules to remember when preparing surgical trays for the autoclave and correctly operating the machine?
- How will Melissa know if surgical trays processed in the autoclave are actually sterile?
- What techniques must Melissa follow to prepare for and assist with a surgical procedure?

- What are common surgical procedures performed in an ambulatory care facility?
- What is the medical assistant's role in preparing the patient, equipment, and room for a surgical procedure?
- Why is it important that Melissa understand and be prepared to answer patient questions about the process of wound healing?
- What bandaging techniques should Melissa be prepared to perform?

LEARNING OBJECTIVES

1. Define, spell, and pronounce the terms listed in the vocabulary.
2. Define the concepts of aseptic technique.
3. Explain the differences among sanitization, disinfection, and sterilization.
4. Demonstrate how to wrap instrument packs for autoclave sterilization.
5. Explain the types and uses of sterilization indicators.
6. Summarize the correct methods for loading, operating, and unloading an autoclave.
7. Demonstrate how to operate an autoclave.
8. Summarize common minor surgical procedures.
9. Detail the medical assistant's role in minor office surgery.
10. Perform a skin prep for surgery.
11. Perform a surgical hand scrub.

12. Outline the rules for setting up and maintaining a sterile field.
13. Open a sterile pack to create a sterile field.
14. Transfer sterile instruments and pour solutions into a sterile field.
15. Apply sterile gloves without contamination.
16. Don a sterile gown and gloves while maintaining a sterile field.
17. Demonstrate how to assist with a minor surgical procedure and suturing.
18. Summarize postoperative instructions and care of wounds.
19. Explain the process of wound healing.
20. Properly apply dressings and bandages to surgical sites.
21. Conduct patient education in aseptic technique and surgical procedures.
22. Discuss the legal and ethical concerns regarding surgical asepsis and infection control.

National Accreditation Competencies and Content

CAAHEP COMPETENCIES

Clinical
3.b.(1)(a). Perform hand washing
3.b.(1)(b). Wrap items for autoclaving
3.b.(1)(c). Perform sterilization techniques
3.b.(4)(f). Prepare patients for and assist with procedures, treatments, and minor office surgery

ABHES COMPETENCIES

Clinical Duties
4.c. Apply principles of aseptic techniques and infection control
4.o. Wrap items for autoclaving
4.p. Perform sterilization techniques
4.h. Prepare patient for and assist physician with routine and specialty examinations and treatments and minor office surgeries

VOCABULARY

antiseptic Substance that kills microorganisms.

contamination Becoming nonsterile through contact with any nonsterile material.

diseases Pathologic processes having a descriptive set of signs and symptoms.

disinfection Destruction of pathogens by physical or chemical means.

edema Swelling between layers of tissue.

infection Invasion of body tissues by microorganisms that then proliferate and damage tissues.

microorganisms Living organisms that can be seen only with a light microscope.

pathogens Disease-causing microorganisms.

permeable (pehr´-me-uh-buhl) Allowing a substance to pass or soak through.

sanitization Cleaning the environment to reduce the number of pathogenic microorganisms.

spores Thick-walled dormant form of bacteria, very resistant to disinfection measures.

sterilization Complete destruction of all forms of microbial life.

*A*sepsis means freedom from **infection** or infectious material. *Medical asepsis* is the destruction of organisms after they leave the body. The principles of medical asepsis are implemented to prevent reinfection of a patient and cross-infection of another patient or ourselves. Isolating potential **microorganisms** and **pathogens** by following standard blood and body fluid precautions and disinfecting or sterilizing objects as soon as possible after they are contaminated is required to prevent cross-contamination. As discussed in Chapter 26, medical asepsis is the process of either decreasing the number of or destruction of all pathogens, which creates a clean environment but not a sterile (microorganism free) one.

Surgical asepsis is the complete destruction of organisms on instruments or equipment that will enter the patient's body. This technique is mandatory for any procedure that invades the body's skin or tissues, such as surgery. Everything that comes in contact with the patient must be sterile including surgical gowns, drapes, and instruments as well as the gloved hands of the surgeon and surgical assistants. Any time the skin or a mucous membrane is punctured or pierced, as in venipunctures or injections, aseptic techniques must be practiced. Urinary catheterizations, biopsies, and dressing changes on open wounds are performed using sterile technique.

A medical assistant must develop an inner sense for sterile procedures. It is important that these techniques be performed on such a routine basis that they become an unbreakable habit. Conscientious attention must be given to sterilizing all items at all times. Frequent checking and rechecking of procedures helps to ensure that they are effective and are employed without any "breaks" in technique. Using single-use, disposable items is the best method of infection control and they are being used more frequently in medical offices. However, when disposable equipment is used, the assistant must be conscious of disposal guidelines and provide the office and the environment with continuous protection.

STERILIZATION

Before an instrument or piece of equipment can be used in a surgical procedure it must first be sanitized, then disinfected, and finally sterilized to remove all forms of microorganisms. **Sanitization** and **disinfection** were described in Chapter 26. It is essential that you understand these two concepts, so review them if needed before learning **sterilization** methods.

To ensure proper sterilization for surgical aseptic procedures, an area (usually a utility room) should be set aside in each office for just this purpose. The area should be divided into two sections, one dirty and one clean. The dirty section is used for receiving contaminated instruments and other materials at the conclusion of surgical procedures. This area should have a sink as well as receiving basins, proper cleaning agents, brushes, utility gloves, autoclave wrapping paper or cloth, autoclave envelopes and tape, sterilizer indicators, and disposable gloves. Designated biohazard waste containers are needed for gloves worn when handling contaminated items. The clean section should be reserved for receiving the sterile items after they are removed from the sterilizer. Clear, clean plastic bags in which to store sterile packs may be kept in the clean area. Both areas should be spotlessly clean and well organized. Sterilization can be achieved by moist heat in an autoclave, by gas, or with chemicals. Most medical offices use the autoclave method. A written sterilization procedure should be in place for each workplace.

CRITICAL THINKING APPLICATION

Melissa has spent the first few days reading the surgical supply and sterilization room procedure manual. Why is this important before she starts performing sterilization procedures? What information in this manual would be most important to Melissa as she starts this new position? Why?

Autoclave

Steam under pressure in the autoclave (Figure 56-1) is the best method of sterilization, because it kills all pathogens and **spores.** Pressurized steam is fast, convenient, and dependable. The pressure allows for heat higher than the boiling point, and when combined with moisture, these two factors create a very effective mechanism for killing all **microorganisms.** When steam is admitted into the autoclave chamber, it simultaneously heats and wets the object, coagulating the proteins present in all living organisms. When the cycle is complete and the chamber cooled, the steam condenses and explodes the cells of microorganisms, thus destroying them. To be effective the steam moisture must

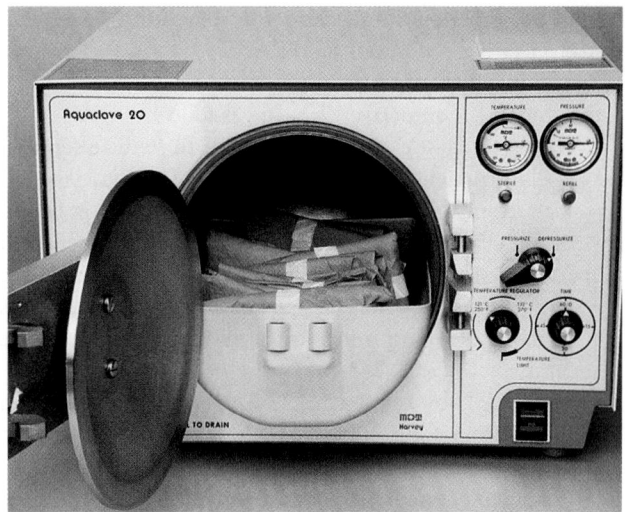

FIGURE 56-1 Steam autoclave. (Courtesy Aquaclave by MDT.)

come into contact with all surfaces to be sterilized. Steam under pressure is capable of much faster penetration of fabrics and textiles than dry heat, but its use has definite limitations if the proper techniques are not followed.

The recommended temperature for sterilization in an autoclave is 121° to 123° C (250° to 255° F). Unwrapped items should be sterilized for 20 minutes, small wrapped items for 30 minutes (Table 56-1), and large or tightly wrapped items for

TABLE 56-1 Sterilization Chart

ARTICLE	METHOD	TEMPERATURE (F)	TIME
Gauze, small, loosely packed	Autoclave	250°	30 min
Gauze, large, loosely packed	Autoclave	270°	30 min
Gauze, small, tightly packed	Autoclave	250°	40 min
Gauze, large, tightly packed	Autoclave	270°	40 min
Gauze, tightly packed	Dry heat	320°	3 hr
Gauze, loosely packed	Dry heat	320°	2 hr
Glass syringes in tubes	Autoclave	250°	30 min
Glass syringes in muslin	Dry heat	320°	1 hr
Instruments on tray, muslin under and over	Dry heat	320°	1 hr
Instruments on tray, muslin under and over	Autoclave	250°	15 min
Solutions in flasks with gauze plug	Autoclave	250°	30 min
Glassware unwrapped	Dry heat	320°	1 hr
Glassware wrapped	Autoclave	250°	30 min
Petroleum jelly, 1-oz jar	Dry heat	340°	1 hr
Petroleum jelly, 2-oz jar	Dry heat	320°	2 hr
Petroleum gauze in instrument tray	Dry heat	320°	150 min
Powder, 1-oz jar	Dry heat	320°	2 hr
Powder, small glove packs	Autoclave	250°	15 min

Remember to always place a sterilization indicator in areas where there is doubt that the steam will penetrate.
Do not measure by chamber pounds per square inch. A thermometer and sterilization indicator are the reliable methods of judging a killing temperature.

40 minutes. Processing time starts *after* the autoclave reaches normal operating conditions of 121° C (250° F) and 15 pounds per square inch (psi) pressure.

The three basic autoclave cycles are as follows:

- Gravity or "fast exhaust" cycle–Used to sterilize stainless steel instruments, glassware, and so on. The autoclave fills with steam and is held at a set temperature for a set period of time. When the cycle is completed, a valve opens and the chamber rapidly returns to atmospheric pressure. Drying time may be added to the end of the cycle. This is the cycle most often used in the physician office setting.
- Liquid or "slow exhaust" cycle–Used to prevent sterilized liquids from boiling. Steam is exhausted slowly at the end of the cycle, allowing the liquids to cool.
- Prevacuum cycle–Used for porous materials. The chamber is partially evacuated before the introduction of steam for greater steam penetration; this is not available on all machines.

Incorrect operation of an autoclave may result in superheated steam. If steam is brought to too high a temperature, it is literally dried out, and the advantage of a higher heat is diminished. Wet steam is another cause of incomplete sterilization. Wet steam results from failing to preheat the chamber, which causes excessive condensation in the interior of the chamber. Condensation is necessary, but too much prevents the sterilization process from being properly completed. It can be compared with taking a hot shower in a cold bathroom, which results in heavily steamed mirrors, walls, and towels. If fabric packs become too saturated to dry during the drying cycle, the packs will pick up and absorb bacteria from the air or any surface on which they are placed. Placing cold instruments in a hot chamber also increases condensation. Other causes of wet steam include opening the door too wide at the end of the cycle or allowing a rush of cold air into the chamber. Overfilling the water reservoir may produce this same effect.

The main cause of incomplete sterilization in the autoclave is the presence of residual air. Without the complete elimination of air, an adequately high temperature cannot be reached. Air and steam do not mix. Because air is heavier than steam, it will pool wherever possible. One tenth of 1% (0.1%) residual air trapped around an instrument will prevent complete sterilization. This is especially dangerous in older autoclaves that do not have a chamber thermometer separate from the pressure gauge. Adequate chamber pressure does not guarantee a proper chamber temperature. Table 56-2 provides tips for improving autoclave techniques.

Wrapping Materials

Maintenance of sterility depends completely on the wrapper and method of wrapping (Procedure 56-1). The wrapping material must be **permeable** to steam but impervious to contaminants. Acceptable wrapping materials for autoclaving should be made of a substance that allows the steam to

TABLE 56-2 Tips for Improving Autoclaving Techniques		
PROBLEM	**CAUSES**	**HOW TO CORRECT**
Damp linens	Clogged chamber drain Goods removed from chamber too soon after cycle Improper loading	Remove strainer; free openings of lint Allow goods to remain in sterilizer an additional 15 min with door slightly open Place packs on edge; arrange for least possible resistance to flow of steam and air
Stained linens	Dirty chamber	Clean chamber with Calgonite solution; never use strong abrasives, such as steel wool; rinse thoroughly after cleaning
Corroded instruments	Poor cleaning; residual soil Exposure to hard chemicals (e.g., iodine, salt, and acids) Inferior instruments	Improve cleaning; do not allow soil to dry on instruments; sanitize first Do not expose instruments to these chemicals; if exposure occurs, rinse immediately Use only top-quality instruments
Spotted or stained instruments	Mineral deposits on instruments Residual detergents from cleaning Mineral deposits from tap water	Wash with soft soap and detergent with good wetting properties Rinse instruments thoroughly Rinse with distilled water
Instruments that have soft hinges or joints	Corrosion or soil in joint Instrument parts out of alignment	Clean with warm, weak acid solutions (10% nitric acid solution); rinse thoroughly Have instrument realigned by qualified instrument repair professional
Ebullition, or caps that blow off solutions	Exhausting chamber too rapidly	Use slow exhaust, cool liquids, or turn autoclave off and let cool on its own; that is, let the pressure decrease at its own rate
Steam leakage	Worn gasket Door closes improperly	Replace Reopen door and shut carefully; have serviced if unable to close door properly
Chamber door does not open	Vacuum in chamber (check chamber pressure gauge)	Turn on controls to starting steam pressure; wait until equalized, then vent and open door

PROCEDURE 56-1

Wrap Items for Autoclaving: Wrap Instruments and Supplies for Sterilization in an Autoclave

<u>CAAHEP COMPETENCY:</u> 3.b.(1)(b)
<u>ABHES COMPETENCY:</u> 4.(o)

GOAL: *To place dry, checked, sanitized, and disinfected supplies and instruments inside appropriate wrapping materials for sterilization and storage without contamination.*

EQUIPMENT and SUPPLIES

- Dry, checked, sanitized, and disinfected items
- Autoclave paper or cloth wrapping material
- Autoclave tape
- Indicator tape
- A waterproof felt-tipped pen

PROCEDURAL STEPS

1. Collect and assemble already sanitized and disinfected items to be wrapped. Gloves may be worn.
2. Place the wrapping material on a clean flat surface.
3. Place the item (or items) diagonally at the approximate center of the wrapping material. Make sure the size of the square is large enough for the items (Figure 1).
    <u>PURPOSE:</u> Each of the four corners must fold over and completely cover the items, with a few extra inches of overlap for folding.
4. With the squares that are cloth fabric, use two pieces if the cloth is single layered, or follow the manufacturer's recommendation when using commercial autoclave wrapping paper.
    <u>PURPOSE:</u> To ensure sterility until the sterile item is needed for use.
5. Open any hinged instruments. If the instrument is sharp, its teeth or tip should be shielded with cotton or gauze.
    <u>PURPOSE:</u> To prevent puncture of the package or injury to the operator.

6. If the package is to contain several items, place a commercial sterilization indicator inside the package at the approximate center.
    <u>PURPOSE:</u> To ensure that the autoclave is reaching effective levels of heat and pressure.
7. Bring up the bottom corner of the wrap, and fold back a portion of it.
    <u>PURPOSE:</u> This folded-back flap is the only part of each wrapper corner that can be touched when opening a sterile package (Figure 2).

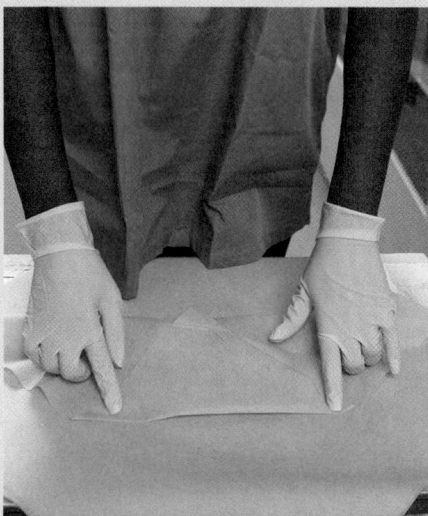

FIGURE 2

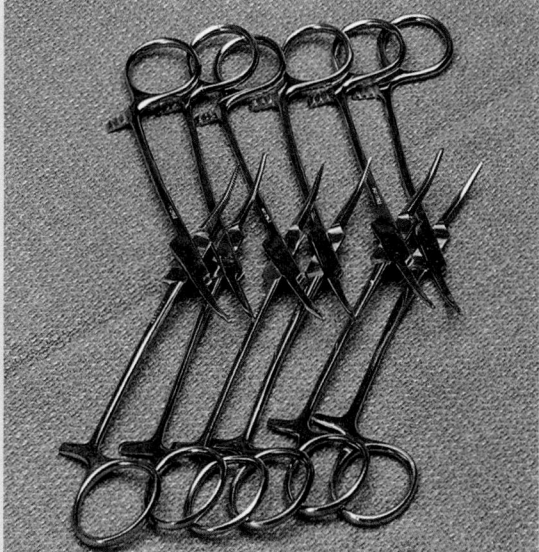

FIGURE 1

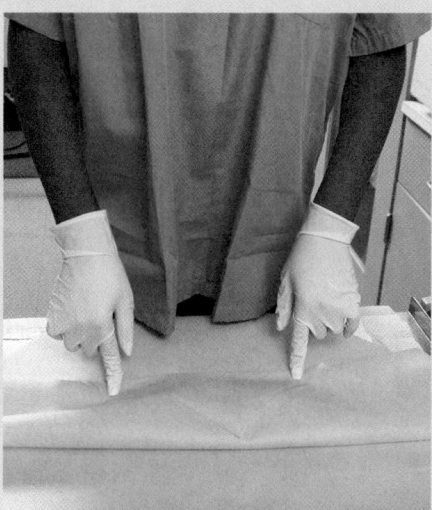

FIGURE 3

Continued

PROCEDURE 56-1—cont'd

8. Repeat the above step with each corner, making sure to turn back a portion each time (Figures 3 and 4).
9. Fold the last flap over (Figure 5).
10. Secure with autoclave tape (Figure 6).
11. Secure with autoclave tape and label package with the date including year, contents, and your initials (Figure 7).

PURPOSE: To know what is in the pack at a later date, whether the shelf life has expired (expiration date), and who performed the task. As a general rule, most office-autoclaved packs are considered sterile (usable) for up to 28 days.

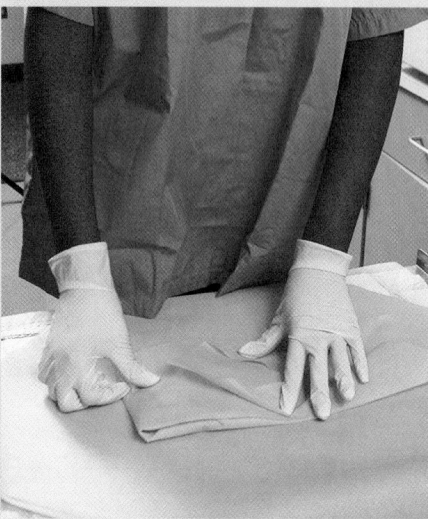

FIGURE 4

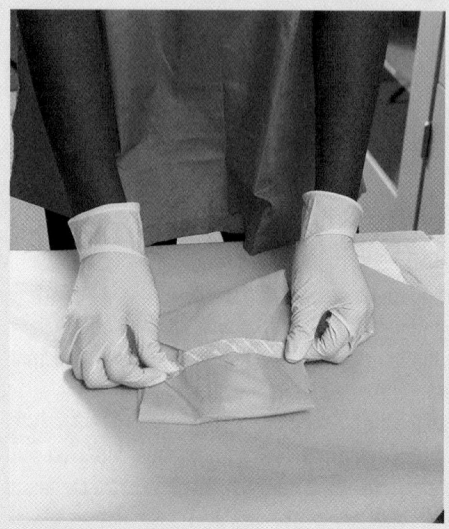

FIGURE 6

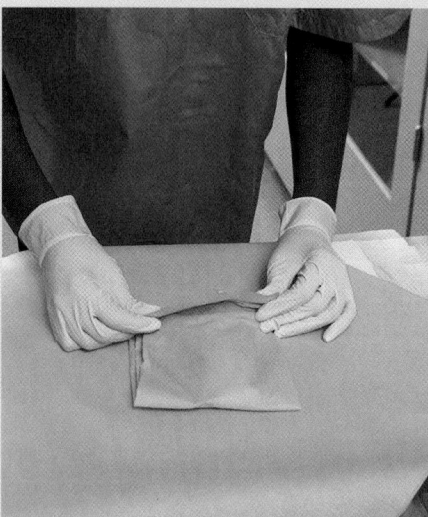

FIGURE 5

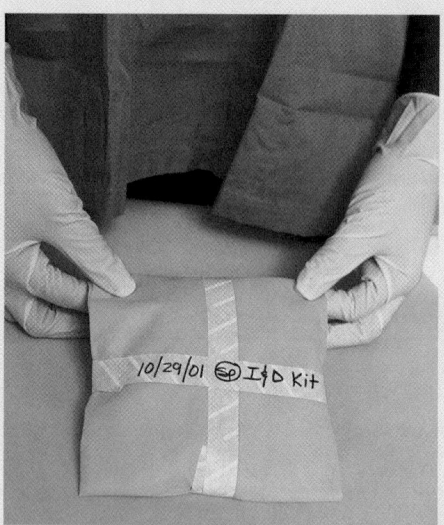

FIGURE 7

penetrate while preventing pathogens from entering during storage and handling. A wrapper should not be used if it is torn or has a hole in it. Clean muslin, disposable autoclave paper, and polypropylene bags are examples of autoclave instrument wraps (Figure 56-2).

Wrapping Instruments

The method used to wrap instruments for autoclave sterilization must allow the pack to be opened without becoming conta-minated. The rules for protecting package content include the following:

• Inspect muslin wrappers for holes before each use and discard if any holes are found.
• Wrap all hinged instruments in the open position to allow full steam penetration of the joint.
• Place a gauze sponge around the tips of sharp instruments to prevent them from piercing the wrapping material.

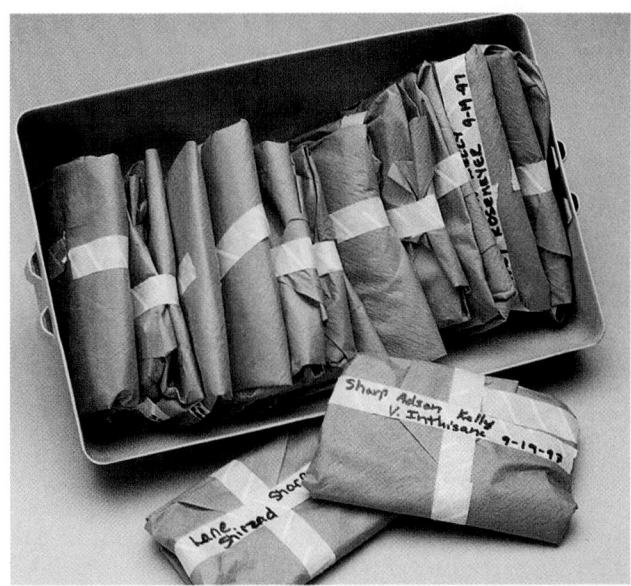

FIGURE 56-2 Autoclave paper wrap. Note chemical lines of indicator tape before autoclaving.

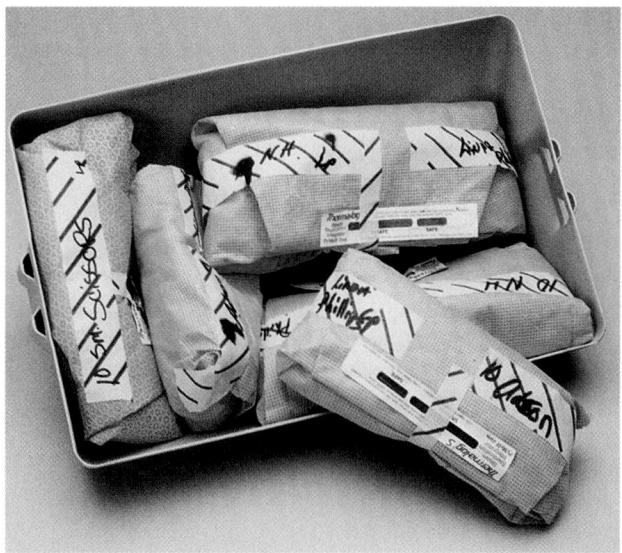

FIGURE 56-3 Wrapped autoclaved instruments with strip indicators on packages.

- If a number of instruments are to be placed on a stainless steel tray for wrapping, first place a double-folded towel on the tray, then position the instruments. This helps to protect them.
- Polypropylene is a plastic capable of withstanding autoclaving but resistant to heat transfer. Therefore materials contained in a polypropylene pan will take longer to autoclave than the same materials in a stainless steel pan.
- When using sterilizing bags, insert the jaws of the instruments first to ensure that the grasping end of the instrument can be reached easily when the bag is opened.
- Indicate on the wrapper what is in the package, or label it with a code. This code should correspond to a list of instruments that is stored with the pack after sterilization.
- Label each pack according to the instrument contents, sterilization date, and your initials. Use a permanent marker, never a ballpoint pen.
- Whether you are wrapping one item or many items together on a tray as a surgical pack, the procedure is the same; be sure the wrapper is large enough to cover the items to be sterilized.

CRITICAL THINKING APPLICATION

Melissa has now moved to processing instruments and trays. She notices one of her co-workers never inspects a muslin wrapper before wrapping a pack. What is the significance of Melissa's observation? How should she handle this situation? Why?

Sterilization Indicators

Sterilization is achieved only when steam reaches an optimal temperature for a designated length of time and has penetrated to the center of the articles. Sterilization indicators must be used routinely to determine if destruction of all microorganisms is achieved. The two basic types of sterilization indicators are chemical (autoclave tape) and biologic (bacterial spore strips).

Chemical Sterilization Indicators. Autoclave tape, a commonly used sterilization indicator, contains a chemical dye that changes color when exposed to steam (Figure 56-3). The tape is not an absolute indication that the proper sterilization time, temperature, and steam have been maintained; it merely indicates that a high temperature was reached while the article was in the autoclave. The strip must completely change color (colors vary by manufacturer) or reveal the word "autoclaved" to ensure effective operation. The main function of autoclave tape, besides holding the wrapping material together or closing a sterilization bag, is to verify that the package has been autoclaved.

Biologic Sterilization Indicators. The facility should have a policy for how frequently the autoclave is tested using biologic methods. One type, a spore strip indicator, contains a temperature-sensitive dye that changes color when the proper combination of steam, temperature, and time has been achieved. An indicator strip should be placed in the center of the largest pack that would typically be autoclaved in the facility to determine the accuracy of the autoclave and autoclave procedures. There are also test indicator kits available commercially that use ampules of *Bacillus stearothermophilus*, which is destroyed at 250° F or 121° C. On completion of the cycle, the ampule is sent to the lab for analysis of any type of microbial growth, which would indicate that the autoclave is not sterilizing properly.

Quality-Assurance Records for Office Sterilization

Every office should have specific protocols to follow for quality-assurance evaluations of the autoclave. This is done at specified intervals, depending on the volume and frequency of autoclave use. A log must be kept of the type of control test done, when it was performed, and the testing results. If the testing results indicate that sterilization was inadequate, a report must be made and filed. This report will identify the nature of the problem and how and when it was corrected. The report should also contain proof of correction by indicating the date and time of a first, subsequent, and successful sterilization run.

Loading the Autoclave

Prepare all packs and arrange the load in a way that will allow maximum circulation of steam and heat (Procedure 56-2). Articles should be resting on their edges and not crowded (see Figure 56-2). Placing the packs in stainless steel racks will prevent packing the autoclave too tightly. Jars, bottles, and trays must be wrapped and placed on their sides if they are to be used to store sterile items. Covers on jars and containers should be put to one side or left open to allow steam to penetrate. Extreme care must be taken not to contaminate jars when replacing their lids after autoclaving is complete.

Instruments may be autoclaved unwrapped if they do not need to be sterile when used later. For example, although vaginal speculums do not need to be sterilized for use (the vagina is a body cavity that is naturally open to the external environment), they must be sanitized, disinfected, and sterilized to prevent cross-contamination among patients. They can be placed unwrapped on a perforated stainless steel tray in the autoclave, then stored in a clean area for future use.

Unloading Guidelines

When the autoclave's sterilization cycle is complete, release the pressure according to the manufacturer's guidelines. Once the pressure gauge reads "0," stand back from the door and, with heat-resistant gloves, open the door approximately $1/4$ inch. Allow the load to dry for at least 15 minutes (this will vary according to the type of autoclave and the size of the load). Capillary attraction is the action that draws moisture through the surface of materials. Packs can act like a sponge, attracting outside moisture and microorganisms. Touching a wet pack allows microorganisms on your hands to penetrate the wrappings, making the contents of the pack nonsterile. Dry, wrapped packs may be removed with clean, dry hands, but it is safer to wear heat-resistant gloves to reduce the possibility of burns from the hot instruments inside the packs. If possible, allow all packs to cool in the autoclave with the door open. Place the packs on a dry, dust-free surface inside an enclosed cupboard or drawer for storage. Avoid placing the packs on cold surfaces, because hot packs may cause condensation, and moisture will contaminate the contents.

Guidelines for Unloading an Autoclave

- Stand behind the door when opening it, to prevent accidental steam burns.
- Slowly open the door only a crack, allowing the items to cool for 15-20 minutes before removing them.
- If for any reason the integrity of the sterilization process is in question, the load should be considered contaminated and reautoclaved. Reasons for concern include the following:
  - Any load that fails to convert a sterilization indicator strip
  - Any loads processed after a biologic test indicates that the autoclave is not working properly

---

Shelf-Life of Sterilized Packs. Each office will have its own guidelines regarding the shelf-life of sterile packs. Generally, muslin and autoclave paper packs are considered sterile for up to 28 days from the date of sterilization. Polypropylene autoclave bags are sterile for up to 6 months from the sterilization date. All sterile packs should be stored on dry, dust-free, covered shelves or in drawers. Fabric wrappers must be inspected for holes and laundered after each use. A damaged pack or a broken seal renders the package nonsterile; spills of any fluid onto a package will also contaminate it. When a pack is no longer sterile for any reason, including expiration date, the contents must be reprocessed as if the pack had been used for surgery. The contents must be sanitized, disinfected, wrapped, and sterilized as usual.

CRITICAL THINKING APPLICATION

Melissa discovers a number of packages of paper-wrapped sterile instruments that have no dates on them. The indicator tape shows that they have been autoclaved. What should she do with these packs? Why?

Gas Sterilization

A variety of gas sterilizers are available. Each has its own very specific operating guidelines to ensure operator safety. Because of the long processing times, very specific Occupational Safety and Health Administration (OSHA) requirements for gas ventilation, and the associated hazards of reproductive organ damage and cancer, it is unrealistic to use gas sterilization in the physician's office.

Chemical Sterilization

In the medical office, chemical sterilization is used for instruments that cannot be exposed to the high temperatures of steam sterilization. The sterilizing chemical solution must be mixed

---

Personal Protective Equipment for Autoclave Procedures

- Heat-resistant autoclave gloves for loading and unloading.
- Fluid-resistant gloves to prevent contact with contaminants.
- Lab coat or impervious gown if needed to protect against splashes.
- Face shield and/or goggles if a splash hazard is present.

Checking the Integrity of a Sterilized Package

- Check for evidence of moisture collection on the pack.
- Verify the expiration date
- Make sure the autoclave indicator tape is reactive.

PROCEDURE 56-2

Perform Sterilization Techniques: Operate the Autoclave

CAAHEP COMPETENCY: 3.b.(1)(c)
ABHES COMPETENCY: 4.(p)

GOAL: *To sterilize properly prepared supplies and instruments using the autoclave.*

EQUIPMENT and SUPPLIES

- An autoclave
- Wrapped items ready to be sterilized
- Heat-resistent gloves

PROCEDURAL STEPS

NOTE: The specific instructions for operating an autoclave may vary based on the model number and manufacturer. Refer to instructions that accompany the autoclave to be sure that the appropriate steps are followed.

1. Check the water level in the reservoir, and add distilled water as necessary.
   PURPOSE: Too much or too little water may alter the effectiveness of the equipment. Tap water will leave lime deposits in the chamber.
2. Turn the control to "fill" to allow water to flow into the chamber. The water will flow until you turn the control to its next position. Do not let the water overflow.
3. Load the chamber with wrapped items, then space them for maximum circulation and penetration.
   PURPOSE: Ensure sterilization of all items.
4. Close and seal the door.
   PURPOSE: The door must be closed, or the heated water in the chamber will evaporate.

5. Turn the control setting to "on" or "autoclave" to start the cycle.
6. Watch the gauges until the temperature gauge reaches at least 121° C (250° F) and the pressure gauge reaches 15 lb of pressure.
   PURPOSE: Proper temperature and pressure must be reached before sterilization can begin.
7. Set the timer for the desired time.
8. At the end of the timed cycle, turn the control setting to "vent."
   PURPOSE: This releases the steam and pressure. The water at the bottom of the chamber will drain back into the reservoir.
9. Wait for the pressure gauge to reach zero.
10. Carefully open the chamber door $1/4$ inch.
    PURPOSE: To allow steam to escape faster. Be careful to avoid accidental burns.
11. Leave the autoclave control at "vent" to continue releasing heat.
    PURPOSE: To dry the items faster.
12. Allow complete drying of all articles.
13. Using heat-resistant gloves or pads, remove the items from the chamber and place the sterilized packages on dry, covered shelves or open autoclave door and allow items to cool.
14. Turn the control knob to "off," and keep the door slightly ajar.
    PURPOSE: Allows the inside of the autoclave to dry completely.

---

exactly according to the instructions on the bottle. The solution must be marked with the date of preparation and expiration. Materials to be sterilized must be submerged in this chemical bath with a closed lid for 8 hours or more. Items are removed with sterile forceps and must be rinsed with sterile water to remove all traces of the chemical before the items are used on a patient. Removed items are then dried with a sterile towel. You must avoid skin contact with the sterilizing solution because it is very caustic.

SURGICAL PROCEDURES

Common surgical procedures that are routinely performed in the primary care office include suturing, cyst removal, I&D of abscesses, and collection of biopsy specimens. The medical assistant should be proficient in explaining each of these procedures to the patient, preparing the patient and the room, assisting the physician with the surgery, and applying a sterile dressing and bandage after the procedure is completed.

Each surgical procedure requires appropriate skin preparation and draping with a *fenestrated* drape, also called an *eye sheet*.

This is a surgical drape with an opening in the center. The size of the opening is dependent on the size of the surgical field. The opening is placed directly over the surgical site after the site has been suitably prepared (or "prepped," as it is called in healthcare practice). A minor surgery tray is opened, and a sterile field is created on a Mayo instrument stand. Sutures, scalpel, and any other instruments are added to the field, according to the surgeon's preference. Have a local anesthetic ready, also according to the physician's preference.

After achieving suitable local anesthesia, the physician will open the skin with an incision. If a cyst is being removed, the physician will dissect around it and usually try to "deliver" it from the wound intact. If the procedure is an incision and drainage (I&D), foul matter will start oozing out of the wound immediately after the skin is incised. The wound is drained completely and flushed out with copious amounts of sterile saline solution. A drain may be placed in the wound and left for several days. If the procedure is a biopsy, a small amount of tissue is removed and placed in a specimen container with preservative. The specimen container must be carefully labeled with the appropriate patient information, date, and specifics about the specimen type and location then sent to the laboratory, where it will be examined microscopically for changes or abnormalities.

Electrosurgery

Electrosurgery is also known as *electrocautery*. An electrosurgical unit (ESU) uses high-frequency current to cut through tissue and coagulate blood vessels. A small probe with an electric current running through it is used to *cauterize* (burn or destroy) the tissue. When the electric current comes in contact with tissue and blood cells, they are vaporized, producing carbon and steam. This process seals blood vessels, minimizing cellular oozing and bleeding. Electrosurgery may be used to destroy granulations and small polyps.

Necessary components are the ESU's power source, the grounding cable and pad, and the active electrode (a pencil-like instrument with a tip and cord). Tips are disposable and are used according to the type of procedure being performed. The two most commonly used tips are the needle and flat.

The surgeon, holding the pencil-like instrument, touches the tissue with the tip and activates the electric current with a switch on the instrument or a foot pedal. The electric current is then delivered to the tissues, and tissue is vaporized at the site of contact.

Important Tips About the Grounding Pad

- Carefully inspect the pad, cable, and skin before the procedure.
- Place the pad close to the operative site.
- The pad must be tight against the patient's skin.
- Apply the pad to a fleshy area like the thigh.
- Do not place the pad over a bony area.
- Do not place the pad over body hair.
- Do not place the pad over metal implants or a pacemaker.
- Carefully inspect the pad site on the skin after the procedure.

Laser Surgery

LASER is an acronym for Light Amplification by Stimulated Emission of Radiation. Because a laser beam is so small and precise, it can be used to safely treat specific tissue with minimal damage to surrounding tissues and limited scar formation. Lasers were first used in medicine to treat **diseases** of the retina and now are used in multiple applications including excision of lesions, cauterization of blood vessels, removal of warts or moles, and cosmetic surgical procedures.

There are several types of lasers, including the carbon dioxide, YAG (yttrium aluminum garnet), and pulsed dye lasers. Each laser has a specific use. The color of the laser light beam is directly related to the type of surgery being performed.

A medical assistant must be specially trained to operate a laser before assisting with laser surgery. Laser equipment requires very careful handling, care, and maintenance. Laser light destroys tissue and can harm the patient, the physician, and you if improperly handled. A full laser safety program should be completed before assisting in laser procedures.

Medical Assistant's Role During Laser Surgery

- Observe the surgical field through safety goggles for possible contamination, and protect the patient's eyes.
- Keep wet sponges ready.
- Remove any flammable item from the laser's path.
- Assist with suctioning of the plume to maintain a clear visual field.
- Have a basin of sterile normal saline solution and a filled irrigating syringe ready.
- Watch each application of the laser beam, anticipating needs for protective supplies, special equipment, or instruments.

Microsurgery

Microsurgery involves the use of an operating microscope to perform delicate surgical procedures. One of its major uses is in ophthalmologic surgery. It is also used in otologic, rhinologic and sinus, laryngologic, neurosurgical, microvascular, gynecologic, and genitourinary procedures. A medical assistant must acquire basic knowledge about the operation and care of a microscope before being qualified to assist in these types of procedures.

The basic components include the light source, eyepieces (also called the *oculars)*, lenses, and cord. Accessory pieces include assistant and observer lenses, cameras, video recorders, television monitors, and printers. These are all valuable for both documentation and teaching purposes. Disposable sterile drapes and handle covers are used on the microscope during surgical procedures.

Surgical microscopes are expensive, delicate instruments and require extreme care when handling and cleaning. All lenses and cords should be carefully inspected before and after each use.

Endoscopic Procedures

An endoscope is a medical device consisting of a miniature camera mounted on a flexible tube with an optical system and a light source that is used to examine within an organ or cavity. There are many types of endoscopes, and they are named according to the organs or areas they explore, such as the urinary bladder, bronchus, larynx, colon (Figure 56-4), stomach, uterus, abdomen, and various joints. Small instruments can be used to take samples of suspicious tissues through the endoscope.

Direct visualization via endoscopes is used for diagnostic purposes or to perform surgical procedures. Endoscopes may be rigid (for example laparoscope or hysteroscope), semirigid, or flexible (colonoscopes, bronchoscopes, gastroscopes). All are delicate and expensive and require extreme care in handling to be protected from damage.

Accessory equipment used with endoscopes includes a fiberoptic light cable, a light source, an irrigator for solution instillation and suction, a camera, a monitor, a printer, and a video recorder. The fiberoptic light cable consists of hundreds of glass fibers. It is important to protect it from being bent, dropped, kinked, squashed, or smashed. The light source can become very hot and must be kept out of contact with the

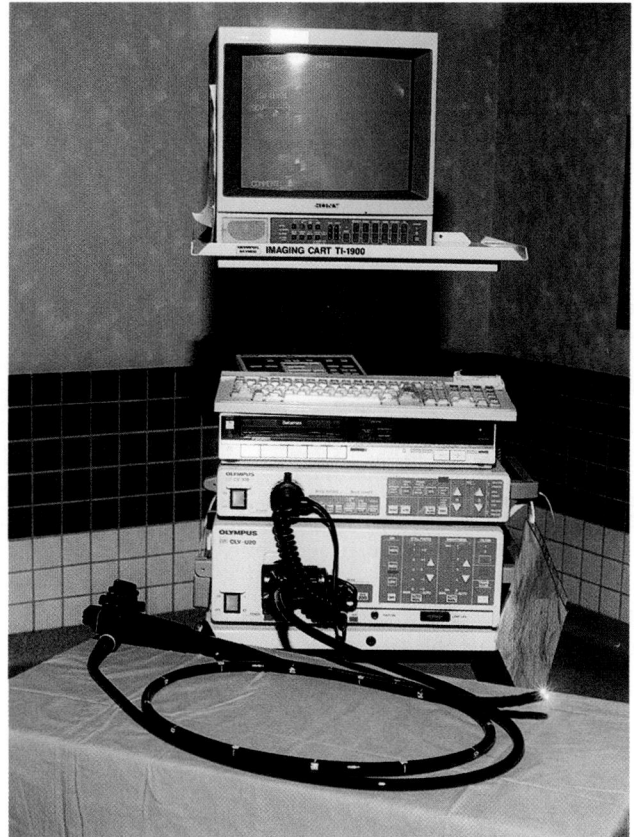

FIGURE 56-4 Flexible colonoscope with monitor and video recorder.

patient, the physician, the staff, and any flammable material, such as surgical draping. All equipment must be checked before and after use. Always follow manufacturer's recommendations for use, care, and maintenance of equipment.

Cryosurgery

In cryosurgery a very–low-temperature probe is used to destroy tissue by freezing it on contact. The probe temperature is usually below –20°C (–4°F). This cold temperature is achieved by circulating liquid nitrogen through the tip of the probe. A local anesthetic is usually administered before cryosurgery. Cryosurgery is used to treat cancers of the skin, prostate, liver, pancreas, and kidney. Cryosurgery is, in many situations, less invasive than traditional surgery and therefore generally has fewer associated complications. Cryosurgery is often performed in an office setting or in an outpatient surgery center.

ASSISTING WITH SURGICAL PROCEDURES

Surgery performed in a medical office is restricted to the management of minor problems and injuries. The medical assistant is expected to assist with preparing the patient and setting up the sterile field. The following procedures must be used without exception when assisting with minor surgery. Individual facilities may have specific guidelines for some of these procedures; however, the theory behind sterile technique is universal regardless of where you work.

Preparation of the Patient

Whether minor surgery is performed because of an unforeseen accident or is a planned, elective procedure, the patient needs both psychologic and physical support. A patient facing a surgical procedure may be concerned about pain, disfigurement, and a possible diagnosis of cancer. An injured patient may feel anxious about medical bills or possible loss of employment. Because surgery is a frightening experience, the medical assistant must take the time, both preoperatively and at the time of surgery, to help the patient deal with fears and anxieties. The best way to help is to make sure the patient understands the details about the procedure, that all questions are answered by the physician, and that the patient has the opportunity to talk about the procedure and voice any concerns.

Questions should be answered directly, but you should answer only those questions that are within your scope of experience and the policies of the office. If you cannot answer a question, assure the patient that you will relay the question to the physician before the procedure, and then be sure to do so. What may seem to be a minor or unimportant question to you may be very frightening to the patient. The minor-surgery room can look very frightening, so unless the patient is sedated, try to make conversation with the patient while you prepare for the physician's arrival.

Preoperative preparation may include blood and urine tests, completion of a consent form, and gathering of the current history concerning any recent illnesses, medications, and allergies. Patient preparations the day before surgery may include a shave prep, cleansing enemas, food intake restrictions, special bathing, and administration of a sedative medication.

On the day of surgery the patient is instructed to empty the bladder, undress and gown as requested, and vital signs are recorded in preparation for the procedure.

Preoperative Instructions

When office surgery is planned, certain procedures are followed before the appointment. These include the following:
- Having the necessary consent forms ready to sign
- Giving the patient the necessary preoperative instructions, such as medications to be used and special skin-cleansing instructions
- Telling the patient to bring a relative or friend to drive him or her home after the surgery
- Instructing the patient to leave jewelry and other valuables at home
- Calling the patient the day before the scheduled surgery to confirm any special instructions

Informed Consent

The physician must have the patient's written informed consent before beginning any surgical procedure. To sign an informed consent form permitting the physician to legally perform the surgery, the patient must understand what procedure will be performed, why it should be done, the potential risks and benefits of the surgery, alternative treatments (including no treatment), and the possible risks of any alternative treatment. This legal requirement is not met simply by having the patient sign an operative permit; a discussion must occur during which the physician provides the patient or the patient's legal representative with enough information to decide whether to proceed with the proposed surgical treatment. After this discussion, the patient either consents to or refuses the surgery. The patient then signs or refuses to sign the consent form. If the patient signs with an X, the medical assistant should write "patient's mark" beside the X, and in addition should have a family member witness the signature. The discussion must be fully documented in the patient's medical record. A copy of the signed form must also be included in the patient record. Treatment may not exceed the scope of the permit.

The patient must not be under the influence of any sedative medication at the time he or she signs the consent form. This condition must *never* be violated.

> ## CRITICAL THINKING APPLICATION
>
> Melissa is preparing a patient for a breast biopsy. The consent form was previously signed and is in the chart. When Melissa is chatting with the patient while completing the final setup for the procedure, it becomes clear that the patient thinks she is having a "cyst removed" from her breast. What action should Melissa take, if any? What is the significance of what the patient said in this situation?

Positioning

Have the patient disrobe sufficiently to completely expose the surgical site so accidental contamination does not occur during the procedure. Clothing may also act as a tourniquet or may make it difficult to apply a proper dressing or bandage. In addition, the patient's clothing may become stained from the skin prep solution or it may interfere with adequate site preparation.

The patient needs to be positioned as comfortably as possible for the procedure. An uncomfortable position can be held for only a limited time, and the patient will have to move, often in the middle of a procedure, if you have not ensured his or her comfort from the beginning. When deciding on the correct position, consider where you and the physician will stand or sit, where the instruments will be placed, and where other needed equipment will be located. If the patient has an open wound that will need irrigation during the procedure, wear nonsterile gloves to assist the patient into position. If there is active and profuse bleeding, a gown and gloves should be worn. If there is danger of blood and body fluid contamination to your face or eyes, wear goggles, mask, or face shield.

Skin Preparation

The human skin is a reservoir of bacteria but cannot be sterilized without potentially damaging cells and tissues. The goal of adequate skin preparation for a surgical procedure is to decrease the number of transient and resident microorganisms so that transference of harmful organisms at the incision site is limited. Cleansing the patient's skin before surgery with surgical soap and an **antiseptic** and shaving the area if needed is called a *skin prep*. The steps for performing this are listed in Procedure 56-3. Sometimes the patient may be instructed to repeatedly cleanse the surgical area with bacteriostatic or antiseptic soap several

days before the surgery. Disposable skin prep trays and razors are commonly used in a physician's office.

Preparation of the Room

If it is your responsibility to assist in a minor surgical procedure, study the physician's care preferences, review the procedure, and note the materials that are needed. Next, prepare the room and gather the supplies to be used (Table 56-3). Sterile supplies are opened just before the procedure. Opened materials that have been exposed longer than 1 hour, usually because of a delay, are considered nonsterile. Supplies should not be placed where they can be knocked over or dropped. Wrapped sterile supplies that fall to the floor must not be used. Once supplies are opened, the sterile field should be covered with a sterile drape, and a team member should stay in the room to monitor them.

Sterile Technique

Accurately performing surgical aseptic technique involves a degree of dexterity and vigilance that can come only with practice. It requires a great deal of concentration and planning of all movements and procedural steps. The procedures covered in this chapter are for minor surgery, but they are the same techniques used during major surgery. To develop sound knowledge of sterility and sterile technique, use the following memory aid: *Everything sterile is white and everything that is not sterile is black. There is no gray!* Sterile surfaces must *never* come into contact with nonsterile surfaces. If this occurs, the sterile surface immediately is considered contaminated or nonsterile. Constant vigilance and absolute honesty are essential for maintaining sterile techniques. If a sterile surface comes into contact with a nonsterile item, this action is called a "break" in sterility or a "break" in the sterile field. During any procedure, everything must stop at this point and the "break" must be corrected immediately—which usually means the assistant must start over again at the very beginning of the procedure. Any break could lead to serious wound contamination, postoperative infection, and even death.

Before assisting with minor surgery, the medical assistant must first perform a series of procedures to ensure surgical asepsis (Procedures 56-4 to 56-10). These skills must be learned, practiced, and followed precisely to establish and maintain the sterile environment that is required during a surgical procedure. Medical asepsis directly affects the health and well-being of the patient, physician, and office staff and must be adhered to without fail.

> ## CRITICAL THINKING APPLICATION
>
> After completing a surgical scrub before assisting with a minor surgical procedure, Melissa sneezes. She does not touch her face, but instinctively raises her hands toward her face in the "sneeze range." Can she go ahead with putting on her sterile gloves? Why or why not?

Sterile Field

A sterile field is any sterile surface on which sterile items are placed. In the office, a sterile field will most often be set up on a Mayo stand (Figure 56-5, p. 1300). In surgery a sterile field

Text continues on p. 1300

PROCEDURE 56-3

Prepare Patient for and Assist with Procedures, Treatments, and Minor Office Surgeries: Perform Skin Prep for Surgery

<u>CAAHEP COMPETENCY:</u> 3.b.(4)(f)
<u>ABHES COMPETENCY:</u> 4.(h)

GOAL: *To prepare the patient's skin and remove hair from the surgical site to reduce the risk of wound contamination.*

EQUIPMENT and SUPPLIES

- Disposal skin prep kit containing the following:
  - Gauze sponges
  - Cotton-tipped applicators
  - Antiseptic soap
  - Disposable gloves
  - Disposable razor
  - Two small bowls
  - Antiseptic
  - Sterile normal saline solution
  - Optional: cotton balls, nail pick, scrub brush
- Sterile drape
- Biohazard sharps container and waste receptacle
- Patient record

PROCEDURAL STEPS

1. Wash your hands, and dry them carefully.
   <u>PURPOSE:</u> Follow standard precautions.
2. Instruct the patient on the skin preparation procedure.
   <u>PURPOSE:</u> To ensure cooperation and keep the patient comfortable.
3. Ask the patient to remove any clothing that might interfere with exposure of the site, and provide a gown if needed.
4. Assist the patient into the proper position for site exposure. Provide a drape if necessary to protect patient privacy.
5. Expose the site. Use a light if necessary.
6. Apply gloves, and open the skin prep pack.
7. Add the surgical soap and antiseptic solutions to the two bowls.
8. Start at the incision site and begin washing with the antiseptic soap on a gauze sponge in a circular motion, moving from the center to the edges of the area to be scrubbed (Figure 1).
   <u>PURPOSE:</u> Circular motion from inside to outside drags contaminants away from the incision site.
9. After one complete wipe, discard the sponge, and begin again with a new sponge soaked in the antiseptic solution.
   <u>PURPOSE:</u> After one circular sweep, the sponge is now contaminated with skin bacteria and debris.
10. When you return to the incision site for the next circular sweep, you must use clean material.
11. Repeat the process, using sufficient friction for 5 minutes (or follow office policy for the length of time required for a particular prep).
12. If there is hair growth, the area may need to be shaved. Hold skin taut, and shave in the direction of growth (Figure 2). Use caution to avoid injury to yourself or your patient. Immediately after completion, dispose of the razor in the sharps container.
    <u>PURPOSE:</u> Follow standard precautions.
13. After shaving, scrub the skin a second time.
    <u>PURPOSE:</u> Hair should be removed before any invasive procedure, to limit the potential for infection.
14. Rinse the area with a sterile normal saline solution (Figure 3).
15. Dry the area, using the same circular technique with dry sponges. The area may be dried by blotting with a third sterile towel.
16. Paint on the antiseptic with the cotton-tipped applicators or gauze sponges, using the same circular technique and never returning to an area that has already been painted (Figure 4).

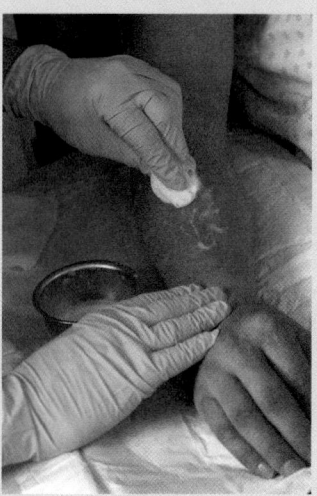

FIGURE 1

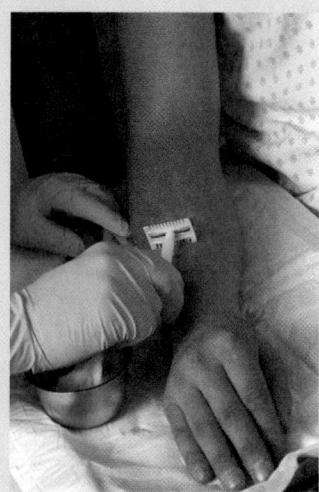

FIGURE 2

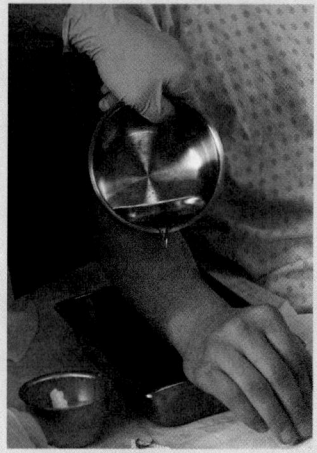

FIGURE 3

Continued

PROCEDURE 56-3—*cont'd*

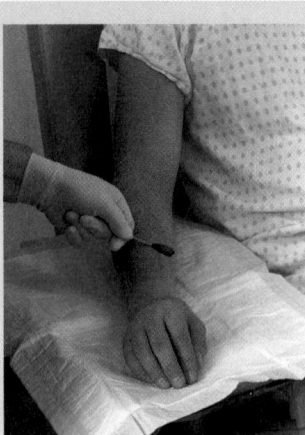

FIGURE 4

17. Place a sterile drape and/or towel over the area.
18. Answer all patient questions to relieve anxiety about the upcoming surgical procedure.
19. Document completion of the skin prep in the patient's chart.

TABLE 56-3 Single Assistant Preparation for Minor Surgery

1. Wash your hands; gather all supplies.
   Sterile side (Mayo tray): Two towel packs, skin prep pack, patient drape pack, instrument pack, miscellaneous pack(s), three glove packs, masks, goggles, aprons or gowns
   Nonsterile side (side counter): Syringes, suture material, anesthesia solutions, additional sponges, dressings, bandages, transfer forceps, waste basin, waste receptacle, nonsterile gloves, masks, goggles, aprons or gowns
2. Escort patient into the room.
3. Greet and converse with patient.
4. Position patient on table.
5. Wash your hands.
6. Open first towel pack.
7. Open skin prep pack.
8. Pour soap and antiseptic solutions.
9. Expose the site to be prepped.
10. Scrub with the surgical hand wash.
11. Glove and arrange prep items within sterile field.
12. Place sterile towels at skin scrub boundaries using sterile technique.
13. Prep the patient's skin.
14. Discard skin prep materials.
15. Discard gloves; wash your hands.
16. Open table drape pack on Mayo stand to create sterile field.
17. Open instrument pack (packs), and transfer instruments to sterile field. Add sterile syringe unit.
18. Add sterile items as requested.
19. Physician joins you and converses with the patient.
20. Open the physician's glove pack (the physician now puts on gloves).
21. Open the patient drape pack (the physician now drapes the surgical site).
22. Cleanse and hold up anesthesia vial for the physician to withdraw anesthesia with sterile syringe (the physician will now administer the anesthesia).
23. Repeat surgical hand wash; reglove with a new glove pack.
24. Arrange sterile field instruments and other materials for safety and in sequence; check instrument condition.
25. Unwind suture materials; load the first suture into the needle holder.
26. Place two gauze sponges at the site.
27. Assist with the procedure.*
    For the physician: pass instruments; maintain field; anticipate needs; cut sutures.
    For the patient: retract tissue; sponge blood from wound; apply bandage; and care for specimen.
28. Escort the patient to recovery area, and check vital signs as instructed.
29. Record and prepare specimens.
30. Clean the room; clear materials; discard gloves.
31. Chart the procedure on the medical record.
32. Help the patient to prepare to leave the office.
33. Disinfect and sterilize equipment at the first available time.

*By law, the assistant may not clamp tissues, place sutures, or alter body tissues in any way.

PROCEDURE 56-4

Perform Hand Washing: Perform a Surgical Hand Scrub

<u>CAAHEP COMPETENCY:</u> 3.b.(1)(a)
<u>ABHES COMPETENCY:</u> 4.(c)

GOAL: *To scrub your hands with surgical soap, using friction, running water, and a sterile brush to sanitize your skin before assisting with any procedure that requires surgical asepsis.*

EQUIPMENT and SUPPLIES

- Sink with foot, knee, or arm control for running water
- Surgical soap in a dispenser
- Towels
- Nail file or orange stick
- Sterile brush

PROCEDURAL STEPS

1. Remove all jewelry.
   <u>PURPOSE:</u> Jewelry harbors bacteria and is not permitted in surgical asepsis.
2. Roll long sleeves above the elbows.
3. Inspect your fingernails for length and your hands for skin breaks.
4. Turn on the faucet and regulate the water to a comfortable temperature, being careful to stand away from the sink to prevent contamination of clothing.
5. Keep your hands upright and held at or above waist level (Figure 1).
   <u>PURPOSE:</u> Water running from the unscrubbed area above the elbow down to the hands can carry bacteria back onto the

hands. All areas below the waist are considered contaminated during all surgical procedures.
6. Clean your fingernails with a file, discard it (in most situations you will drop the file into the sink and discard it later to prevent contamination by lowering your hands and/or touching a waste receptacle), and rinse your hands under the faucet without touching the faucet or the inside of the sink basin (Figure 2).
7. Allow the water to run over your hands from the fingertips to the elbows without moving the arm back and forth under the water.
   <u>PURPOSE:</u> Water running from the elbow down to the hands can carry bacteria back onto the hands.
8. Apply surgical soap from the dispenser to the sterile brush (or use a preprepared disposable brush), and start the scrub by scrubbing the palm of the hand in a circular fashion.
9. Continue from the palm to the base of the thumb, then move on to the other fingers, scrubbing from the base, along each side, and across the nail, holding fingertips upward, remembering to rub between the fingers (Figures 3 and 4). After fingers are completely scrubbed, clean the posterior surface of the hand in a circular fashion, then proceed to the wrist. The scrub process should take at least 5 minutes for each hand and arm.
   <u>PURPOSE:</u> The surfaces of the fingers have four sides.

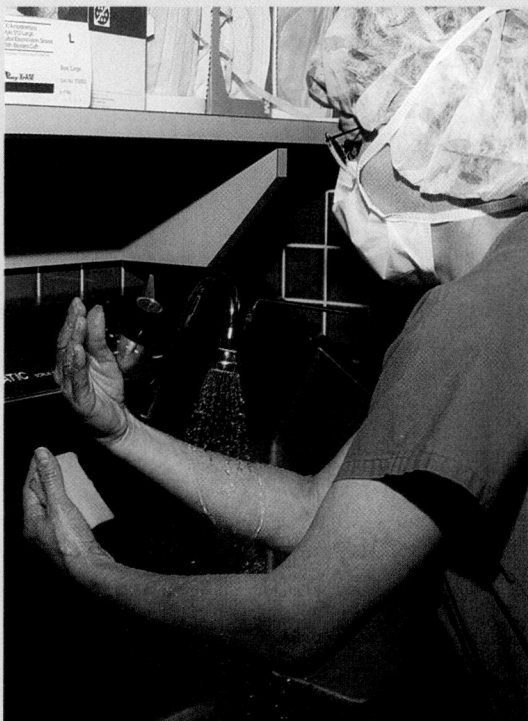

FIGURE 1

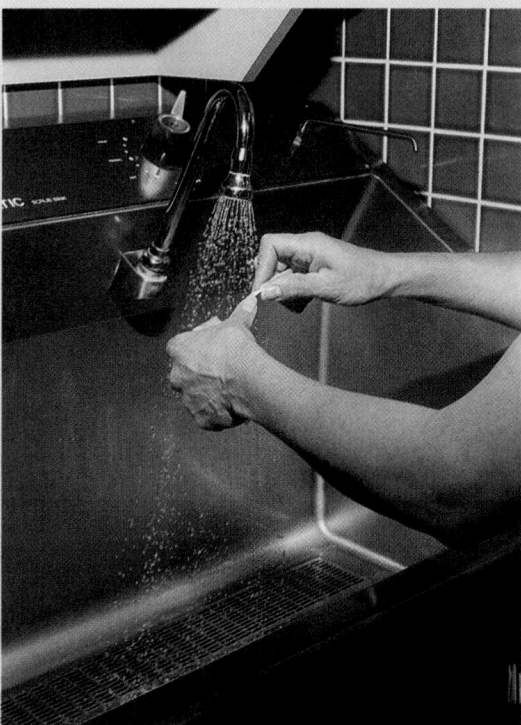

FIGURE 2

Continued

PROCEDURE 56-4—cont'd

10. Do not return to a clean area after you have moved to the next part of the hand.
PURPOSE: Once an area has been scrubbed, it is considered surgically clean, and to rub that area again will contaminate it.

11. Wash wrists and forearms in a circular fashion around the arm while holding your hands above waist level (Figure 5).

12. Rinse arms and forearms from the fingertips upward, holding the fingers up, without touching the faucet or the inside of the sink basin (Figure 6).

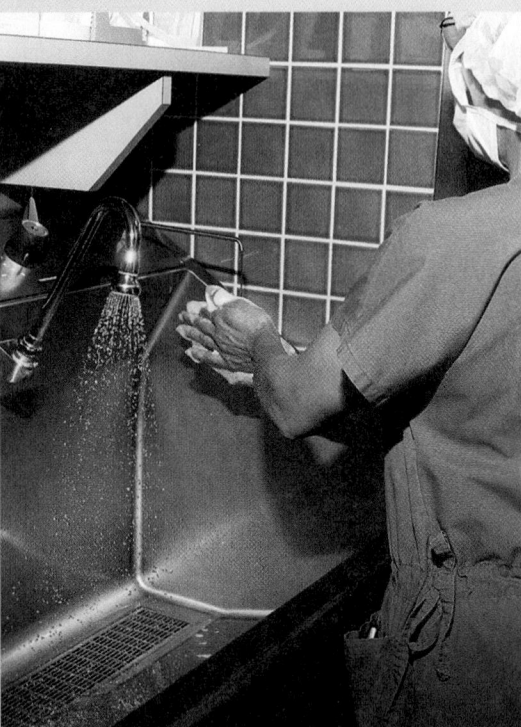

FIGURE 3

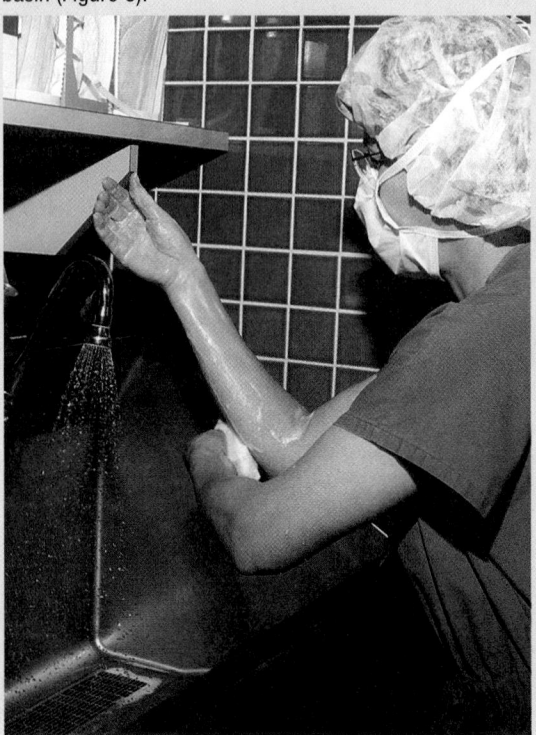

FIGURE 5

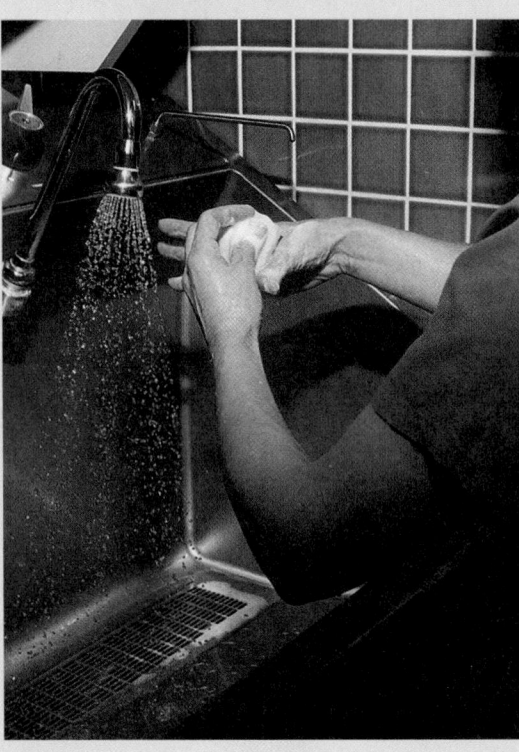

FIGURE 4

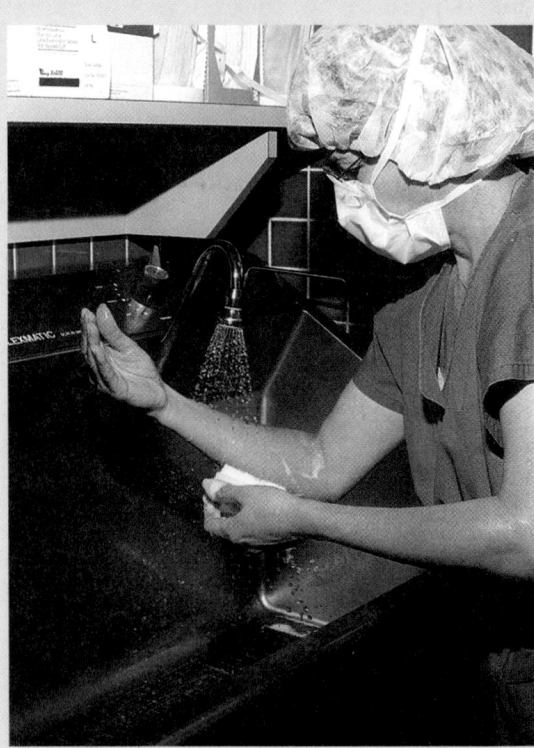

FIGURE 6

Continued

PROCEDURE 56-4—cont'd

<u>PURPOSE:</u> Keep fingers higher than the rest of the arm to prevent contamination from water running downward from the elbow. Touching the dirty faucet and/or basin will cause contamination.

13. Apply more solution without touching any dirty surface, and repeat the scrub on the other side, remembering to wash and use friction between each finger with a firm, circular motion (Figures 7 and 8).

14. Scrub all surfaces with a brush, being careful not to abrade your skin. The second hand and arm should take at least 5 minutes (Figures 9 and 10).

15. Rinse thoroughly, keeping your hands up and above waist level. Discard scrub brush without lowering arms below the waist (Figures 11 to 13).

16. Turn off the faucet with the foot, knee, or forearm lever, if available.

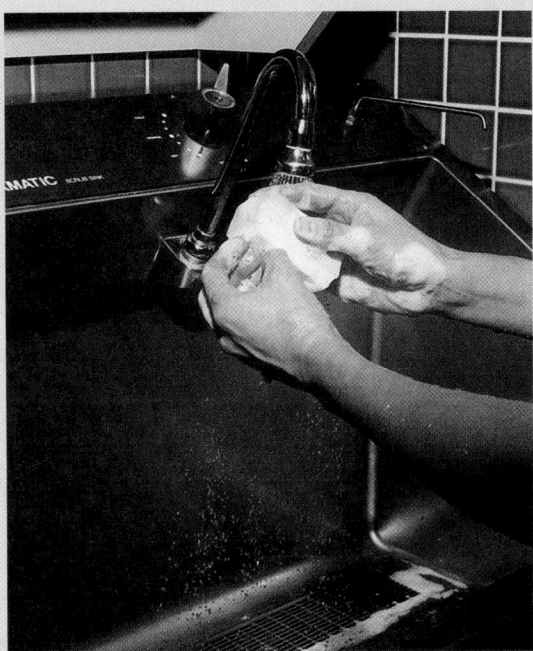

FIGURE 7

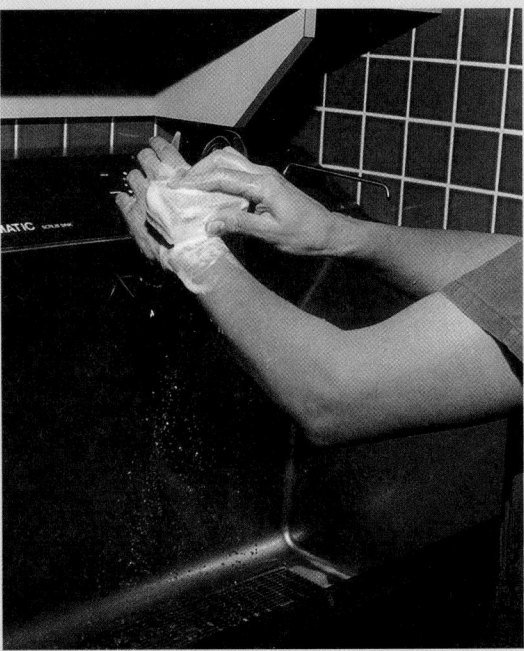

FIGURE 9

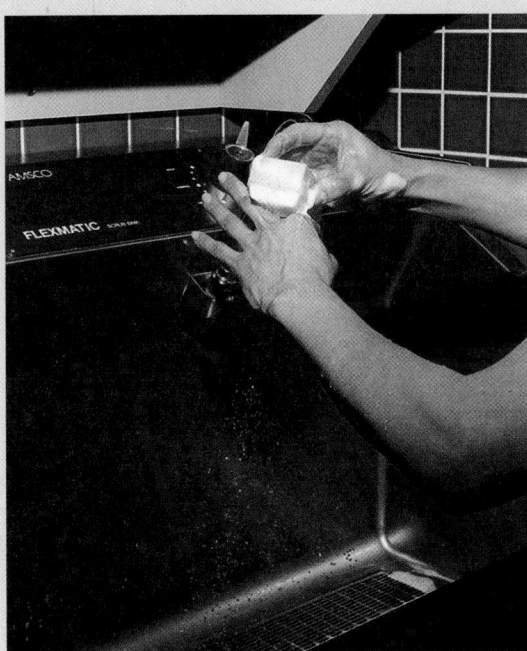

FIGURE 8

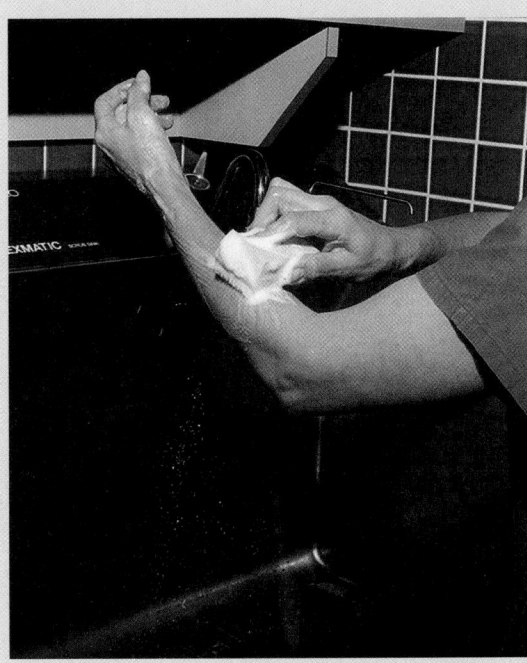

FIGURE 10

Continued

PROCEDURE 56-4—cont'd

PURPOSE: To prevent clean hands from touching the contaminated faucet handles.

17. Dry your hands with a sterile towel, being careful to keep fingers pointing upward and hands above the waist. Do not rub back and forth, dragging contaminants from the dirtier area of the upper arm down toward the hands (Figures 14 and 15). Use the opposite end of the towel for the other hand (Figures 16 and 17).

PURPOSE: To keep your clean hands from touching the part of the towel that comes into contact with your forearms, which are not as clean as your hands. If you are to gown and glove for a procedure, you will be required to use a sterile towel.

18. Using a patting motion, continue to dry the forearms (Figure 18). Discard the towel and keep your hands up and above waist level (Figures 19 and 20).

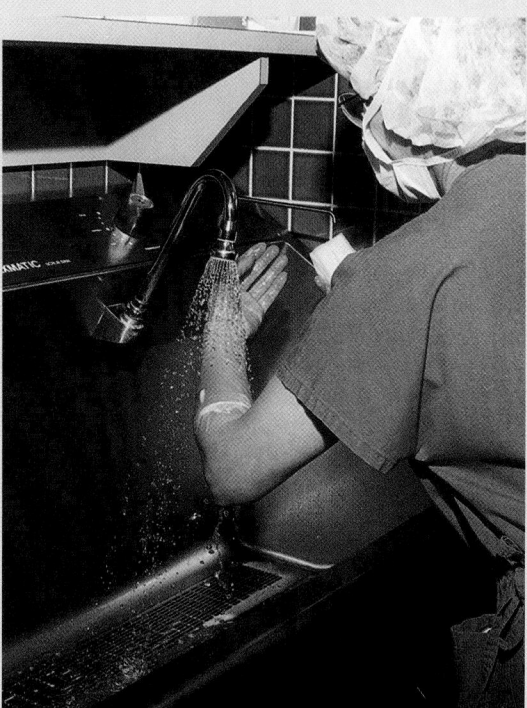

FIGURE 11

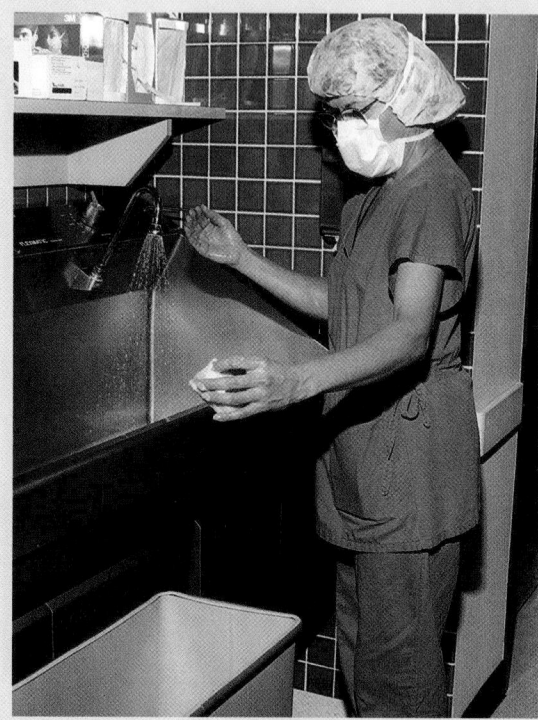

FIGURE 13

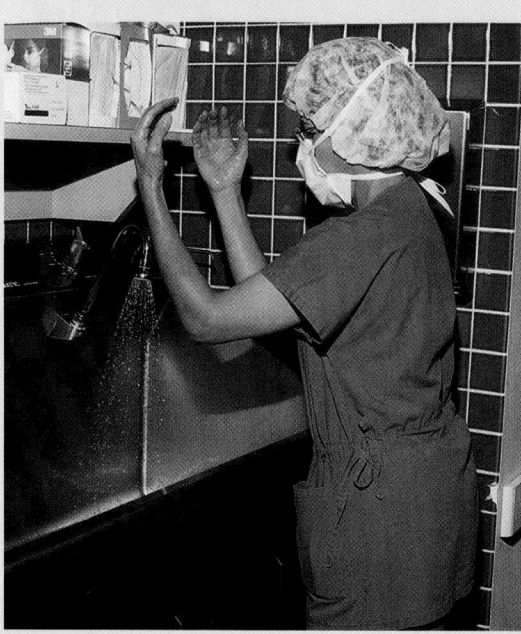

FIGURE 12

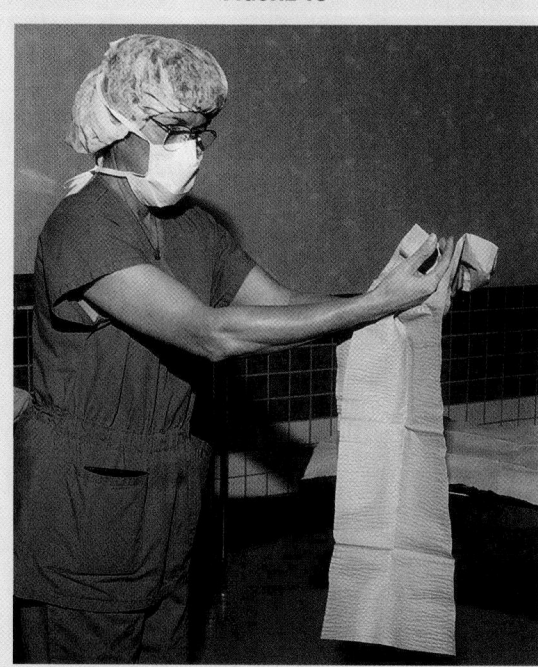

FIGURE 14

Continued

PROCEDURE 56-4—*cont'd*

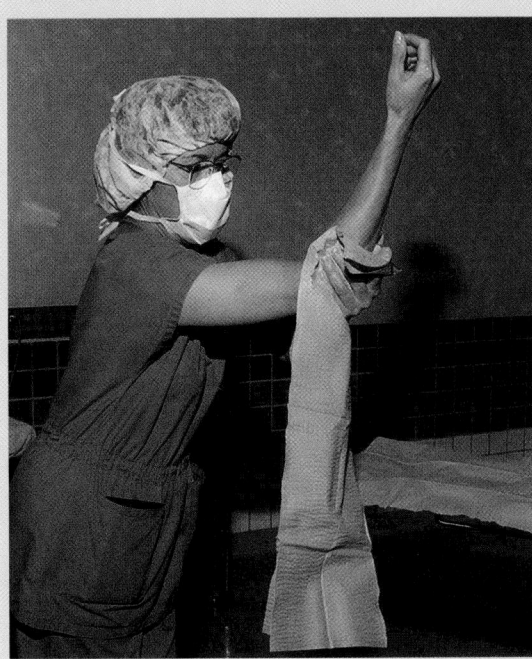

FIGURE 15

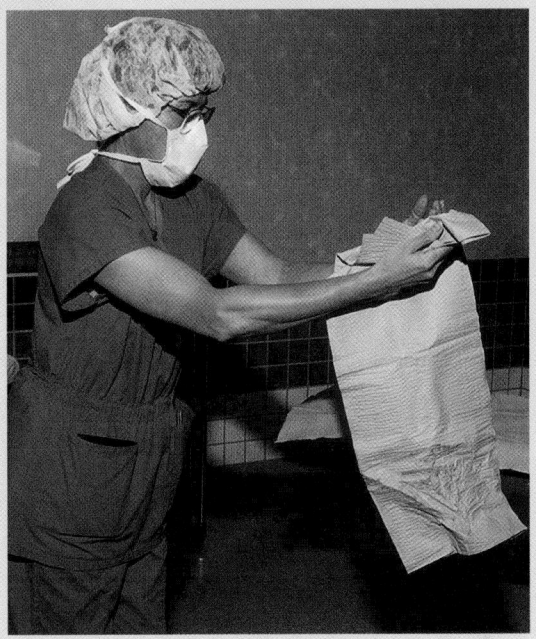

FIGURE 17

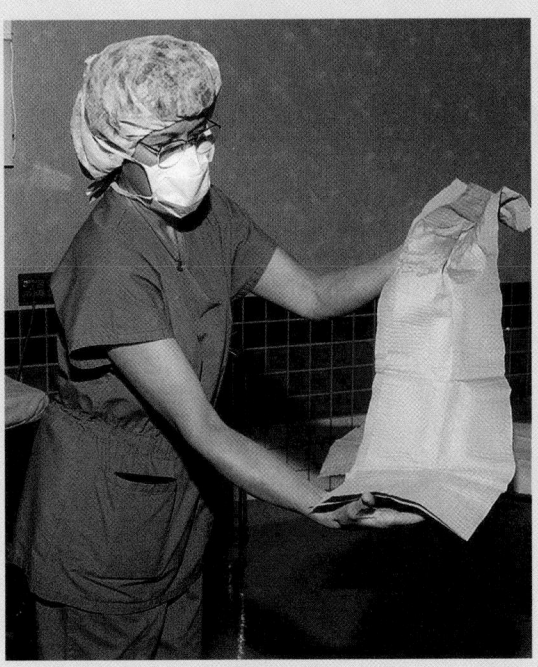

FIGURE 16

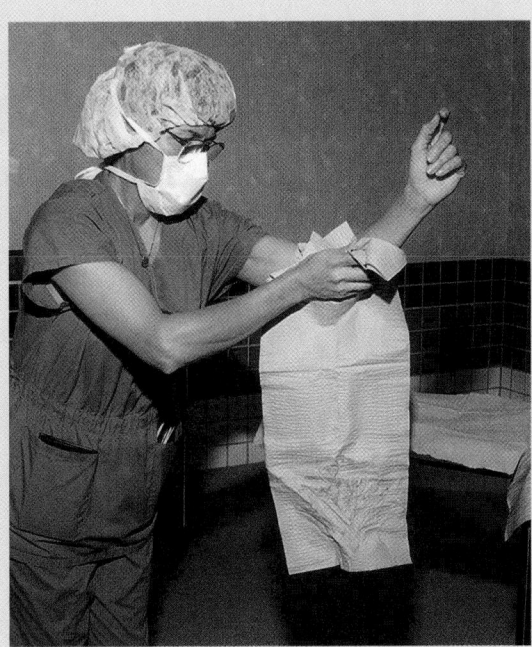

FIGURE 18

Continued

PROCEDURE 56-4—cont'd

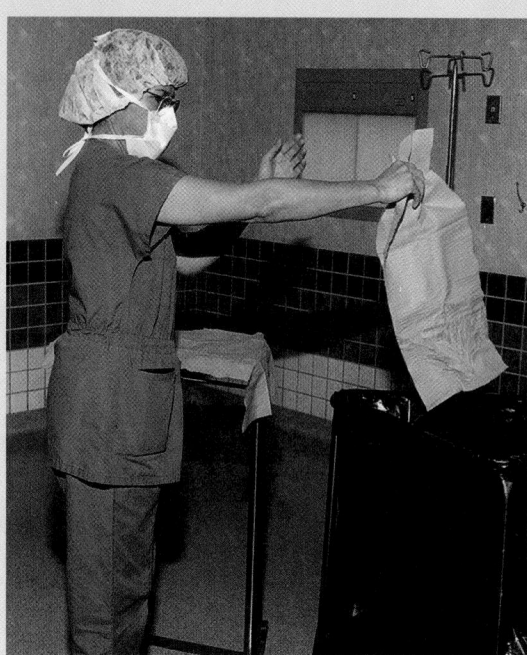

FIGURE 19

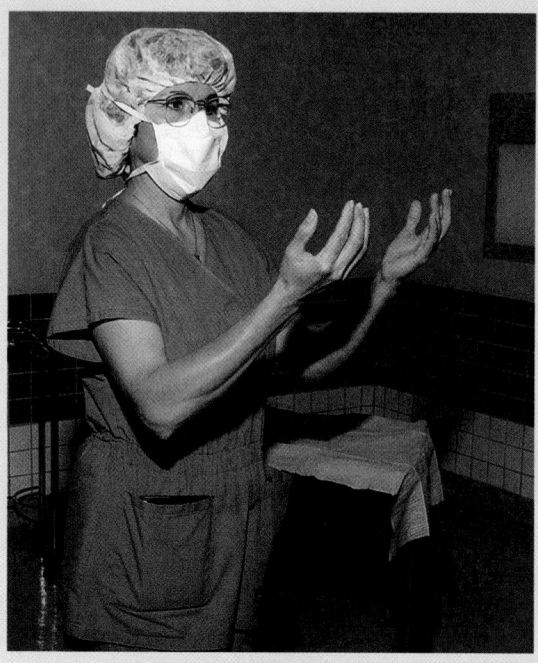

FIGURE 20

PROCEDURE 56-5

Prepare Patient for and Assist with Procedures, Treatments, and Minor Office Surgeries: Open a Sterile Pack and Create a Sterile Field

<u>CAAHEP COMPETENCY:</u> 3.b.(4)(f)
<u>ABHES COMPETENCY:</u> 4.(h)

GOAL: *To open a sterile pack that contains a table drape using correct aseptic technique*

EQUIPMENT and SUPPLIES

- A sterile pack (autoclaved linen or disposable) that will serve as a sterile table drape or field
- Mayo stand or countertop
- Disinfectant and gauze sponges

PROCEDURAL STEPS

1. Check that the Mayo stand or countertop is dust free and clean. If it is not, clean with 70% alcohol or another disinfectant, and dry carefully.
   <u>PURPOSE:</u> Although some areas cannot be sterile, steps must be taken to keep contamination to a minimum; moisture on tray will contaminate the pack.
2. Wash your hands, and dry them carefully. If you will be assisting with a surgical procedure immediately after opening the sterile pack, perform the surgical hand scrub as explained in Procedure 56-4.

<u>PURPOSE:</u> To decrease the number of transient and resident bacteria on your hands and forearms; moisture on your hands will contaminate the pack.

3. Place the sterile pack on the Mayo stand or countertop, and read the label.
   <u>PURPOSE:</u> Take care to open the required pack. Most medical offices have a limited supply of autoclaved packs. To open a wrong package could mean not having enough sterile supplies for a different procedure.
4. Check the expiration date. If using an autoclaved pack, check the indicator tape for color change.
   <u>PURPOSE:</u> An expired pack is not considered sterile. Autoclave indicator tape changes color after the sterile processing cycle.
5. Open outside cover (Figure 1). Position the package so that the outer envelope flap is at the top and facing you.
   <u>PURPOSE:</u> This positions the pack for correct opening so you do not have to cross over the sterile pack to open it.

Continued

PROCEDURE 56-5—*cont'd*

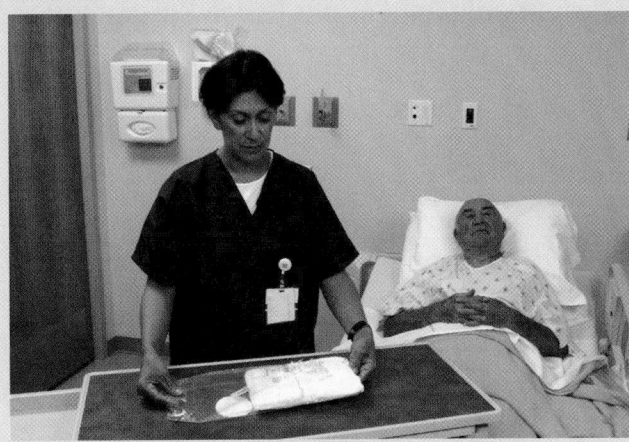

FIGURE 1

6. Open the outermost flap (Figure 2). Next open the first flap away from you. Do not cross over the pack.
7. Open the second corner, pulling to side (Figure 3).
   <u>PURPOSE:</u> Prevents contamination of the sterile field.
8. Be careful to lift the flaps by touching only the small folded-back tab and without touching or crossing over the inner surface of the pack or its contents. Open the remaining two corners of the pack. (Figures 4 and 5).
9. You now have a sterile drape as a sterile field to work from and for the distribution of additional sterile supplies and instruments.

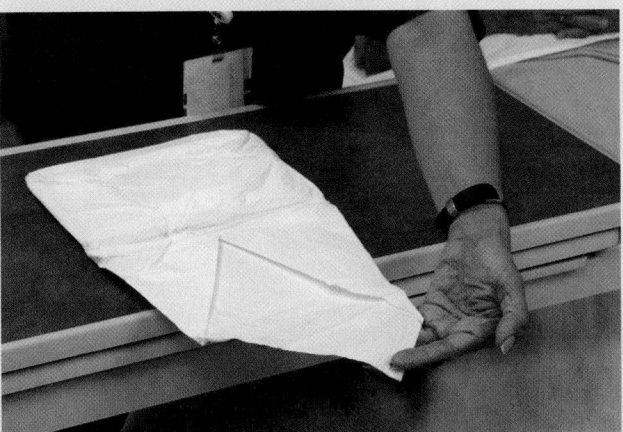

FIGURE 2

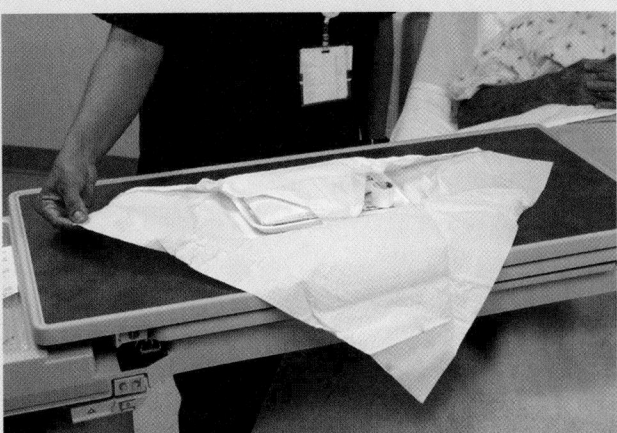

FIGURE 4

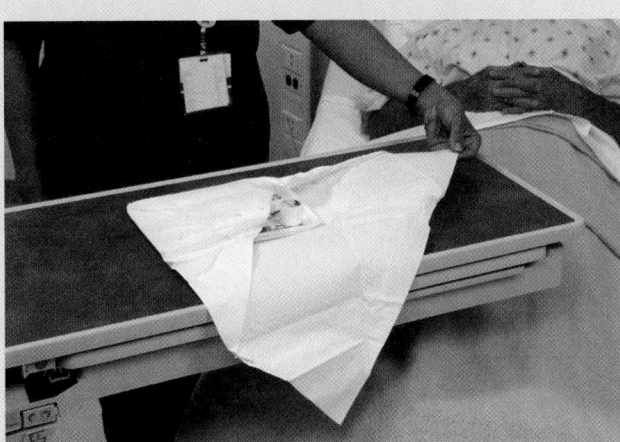

FIGURE 3

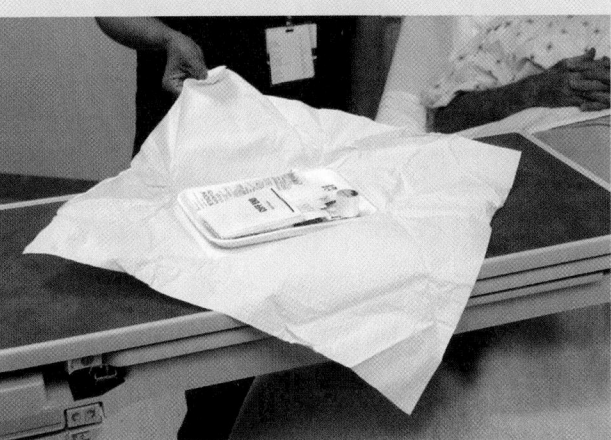

FIGURE 5

PROCEDURE 56-6

Prepare Patient for and Assist with Procedures, Treatments, and Minor Office Surgeries: Use Transfer Forceps

<u>CAAHEP COMPETENCY:</u> 3.b.(4)(f)
<u>ABHES COMPETENCY:</u> 4.(h)

GOAL: *To move sterile items on a sterile field or transfer sterile items to a gloved team member.*

EQUIPMENT and SUPPLIES

- Sterile item to move or transfer
- Sterile wrapped transfer forceps
- Mayo stand setup with a sterile field and sterile instruments

PROCEDURAL STEPS

1. Wash your hands, and dry them carefully. If you will be assisting with a surgical procedure immediately after this procedure, perform the surgical hand scrub as explained in Procedure 56-4.
   <u>PURPOSE:</u> To decrease the number of transient and resident bacteria on your hands and forearms; moisture on your hands will contaminate the pack.

2. Open a package containing a sterile transfer forceps (Figure 1).

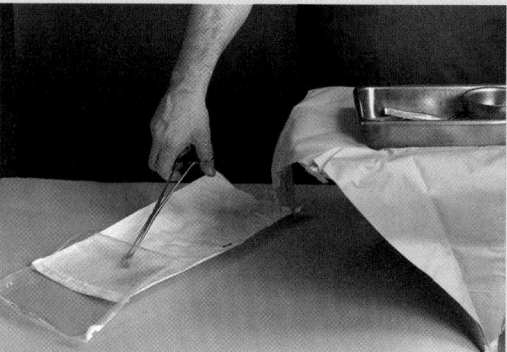

FIGURE 1

3. Using sterile technique, handle sterile forceps by ring handle only. Always point forceps tips down.
   <u>PURPOSE:</u> If the tips are turned upward, any solution encountered will run onto the nonsterile area, then back down over the sterile end when the tips are turned down again, thus contaminating the forceps.

4. Grasp an item on the sterile field with sterile forceps, points down, and move it to its proper position for the procedure, making sure not to cross the sterile field with the hand or contaminated end of the forceps (Figure 2).

5. Or, transfer an instrument from the autoclave to the sterile field.

6. Remove the transfer forceps after one-time use.

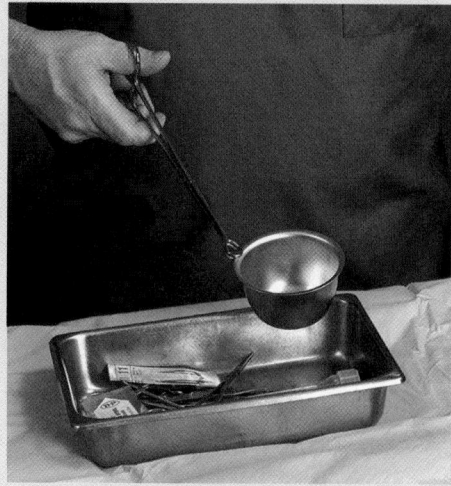

FIGURE 2

PROCEDURE 56-7

Prepare Patient for and Assist with Procedures, Treatments, and Minor Office Surgeries: Pour Sterile Solution onto a Sterile Field(s)

<u>CAAHEP COMPETENCY:</u> 3.b.(4)(f)
<u>ABHES COMPETENCY:</u> 4.(h)

GOAL: *Pour a sterile solution into a sterile stainless-steel bowl or container that is sitting at the edge of a sterile field.*

EQUIPMENT and SUPPLIES

- Bottle of sterile solution
- Sterile bowl or container
- Sterile field
- Sink or waste receptacle

NOTE: The sterile bowl should be placed near one edge of the field and the perimeter of the 1-inch barrier.

PROCEDURAL STEPS

1. Wash your hands, and dry them carefully. If you will be assisting with a surgical procedure immediately after this procedure, perform the surgical hand scrub as explained in Procedure 56-4.
   <u>PURPOSE:</u> To decrease the number of transient and resident bacteria on your hands and forearms; moisture on your hands will contaminate the pack.

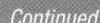

Continued

PROCEDURE 56-7—cont'd

2. Read the label of the ordered solution.
   PURPOSE: Always perform the three label checks before administering any solution or medication.
3. Place your hand over the label and lift the bottle.
   NOTE: If the container has a double cap, set the outer cap on the counter inside up, then proceed.
4. Lift the lid of the bottle straight up, then slightly to one side, and hold the lid in your nondominant hand facing downward.
   PURPOSE: Air currents carry contaminants that could settle on the inside of the lid.
5. Pour away from the label (Figure 1).
   PURPOSE: Spills down the side of the bottle stain or make the label unreadable.

6. If the container does not have a double cap, before pouring the solution into the sterile container pour off a small amount of the solution into a waste receptacle.
   PURPOSE: To rinse any contaminants off the bottle lip.
7. Pour away from the label, into the bowl, without allowing any part of the bottle to touch the bowl and without crossing over the sterile field (Figure 2).
   PURPOSE: The bottle exterior is not sterile.
8. Tilt the bottle up to stop the pouring while it is still over the bowl.
   PURPOSE: Solutions spilled on the sterile field may contaminate the field.
9. Replace the cap (or caps) off to the side, away from the sterile field.

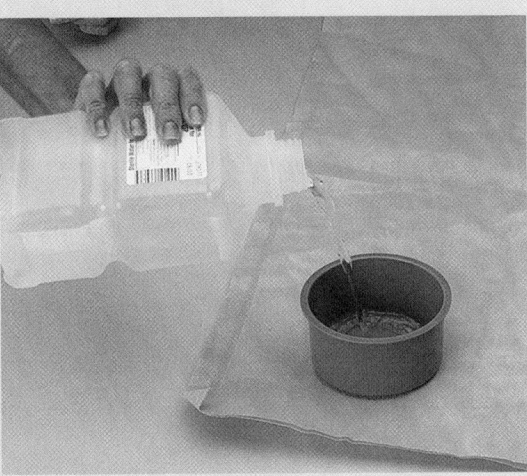

FIGURE 1

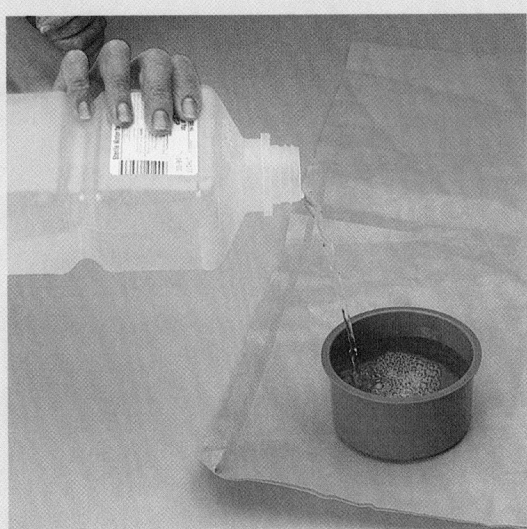

FIGURE 2

PROCEDURE 56-8

Prepare Patient for and Assist with Procedures, Treatments, and Minor Office Surgeries: Apply Sterile Gloves

CAAHEP COMPETENCY: 3.b.(4)(f)
ABHES COMPETENCY: 4.(h)

GOAL: *To apply sterile gloves before performing sterile procedures.*

EQUIPMENT and SUPPLIES

- Pair of packaged sterile gloves in your size

PROCEDURAL STEPS

1. Perform the surgical hand scrub as explained in Procedure 56-4 before applying sterile gloves.
2. Open the glove pack, being careful not to cross over the open

area in the middle of the pack. Remember, a 1-inch area around the perimeter of the glove wrapper is considered not sterile.
   PURPOSE: The open glove pack is a sterile field.
3. Glove your dominant hand first.
   PURPOSE: This will set up your dominant hand to do the more difficult step, which is to apply the second glove.
4. With your nondominant hand, pick up the glove for your dominant hand with your thumb and forefinger, grabbing the top

Continued

PROCEDURE 56-8—*cont'd*

of the folded cuff, which is the inside of the glove, being careful not to cross over the other sterile glove (Figure 1).

<u>PURPOSE:</u> The inside of the glove will be next to your skin and is considered not sterile.

5. Lift the glove up and away from the sterile package.

<u>PURPOSE:</u> To prevent accidental contamination from touching the glove on the 1-inch area around the perimeter of the glove wrapper.

6. Hold your hands up and away from your body, and slide the dominant hand into the glove (Figure 2).

7. Leave the cuff folded (Figure 3).

<u>PURPOSE:</u> You will unfold the cuff later.

8. With your gloved dominant hand, pick up the second glove by slipping your gloved fingers under the cuff, extending the thumb up and away from the glove, so that your gloved fingers touch only the outside of the second glove (Figure 4).

<u>PURPOSE:</u> Sterile surfaces must always touch sterile surfaces.

9. Slide your nondominant hand into the glove, without touching the exterior of the glove or any part of the gloved hand (Figures 5 to 7).

10. Still holding your hands away from you, unroll the cuff by slipping the fingers into the cuff and gently pulling up and out. Do not touch your bare arm or the internal surface of the glove with any part of the sterile glove (Figure 8).

11. Now, slip your gloved fingers up under the first cuff and unroll it, using the same technique (Figures 9 to 11).

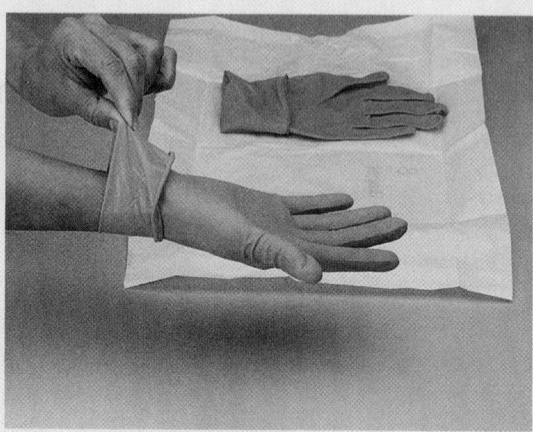

FIGURE 3

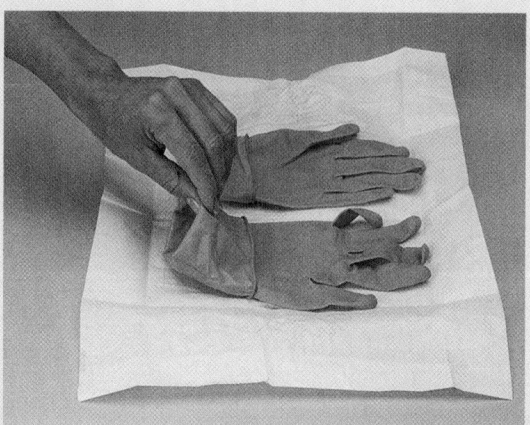

FIGURE 1

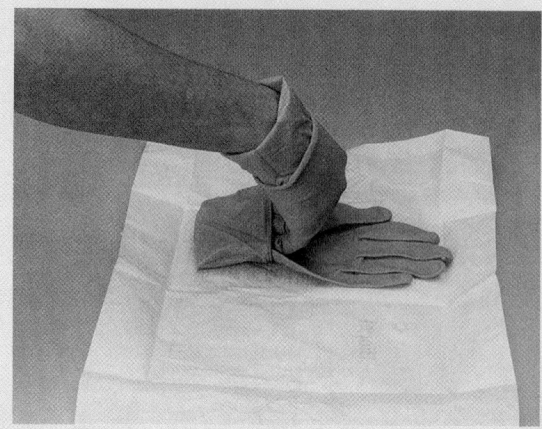

FIGURE 4

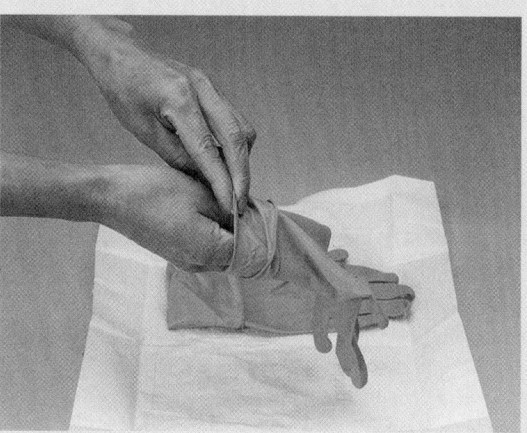

FIGURE 2

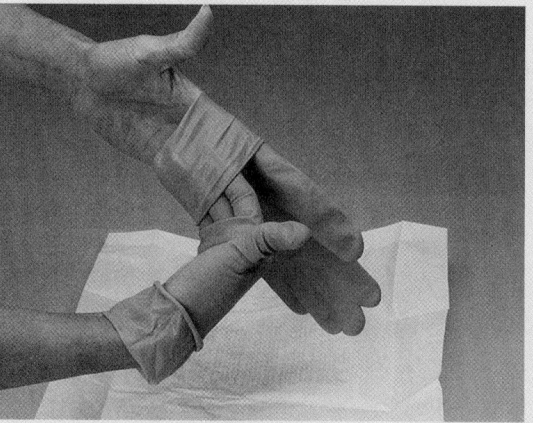

FIGURE 5

Continued

PROCEDURE 56-8—*cont'd*

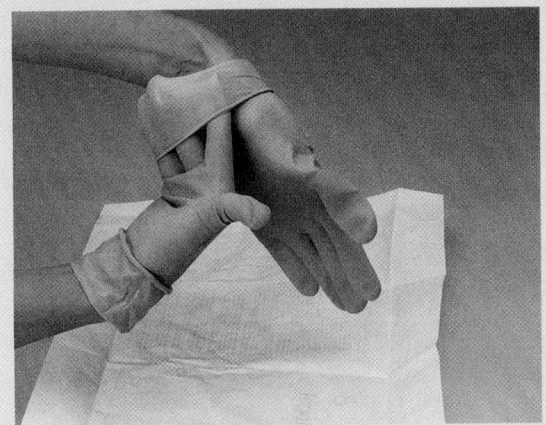

FIGURE 6

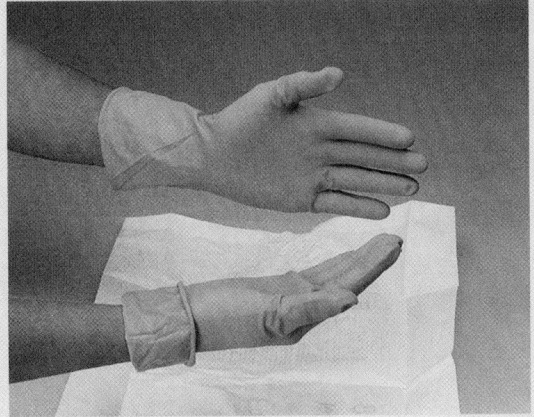

FIGURE 9

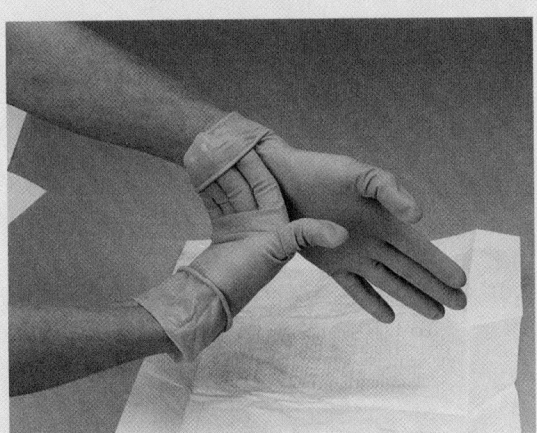

FIGURE 7

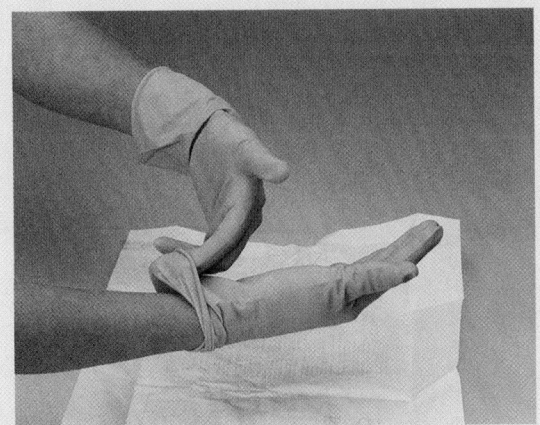

FIGURE 10

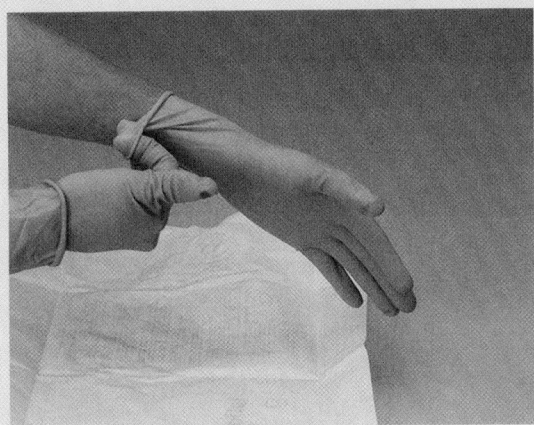

FIGURE 8

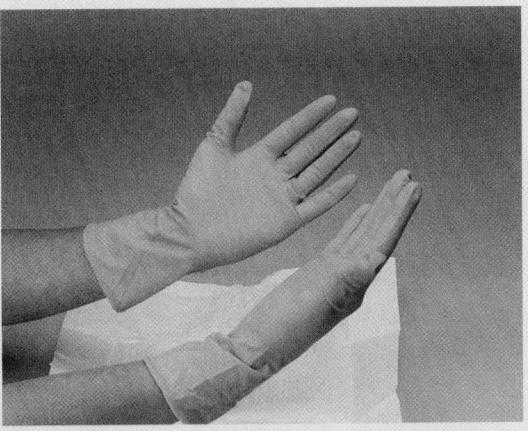

FIGURE 11

PROCEDURE 56-9

Prepare Patient for and Assist with Procedures, Treatments, and Minor Office Surgeries: Don a Sterile Gown

CAAHEP COMPETENCY: 3.b.(4)(f)
ABHES COMPETENCY: 4.(h)

GOAL: *To don a sterile gown before assisting with a surgical procedure.*

EQUIPMENT and SUPPLIES

*   Sterile gown and gloves (opened on a waist-high counter or Mayo stand, in an opened area for dressing)
NOTE: A mask, goggles, and hair cover are worn.

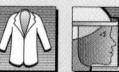

PROCEDURAL STEPS

1. Scrub, using aseptic technique (see Procedure 56-4). Remember to keep your hands up and above waist level (Figure 1).
    PURPOSE: Protect the patient from your resident bacteria.
2. Grasp the sterile gown (which is packaged with the outside of the gown on the surface) by the collar, and gently lift it from the sterile gown wrapper (Figures 2 and 3).
    PURPOSE: The sterile gown will not be contaminated by the edges of the wrapper.
3. Hold the gown away from your body. Allow it to gently unfold, grasping only the inside of the gown (Figures 4 and 5).
    PURPOSE: Only the inside of the gown touches you; the outside of the gown must remain sterile.
4. Slip your hands into the sleeve openings. Remember to touch only the inside of the gown (Figure 6).

PURPOSE: Keep the outside of the gown sterile and away from contaminants.

5. The hand and forearms are advanced only to the edge of the gown cuff.
    PURPOSE: The hands are kept covered to avoid contamination of the gown.
6. The circulating assistant touches only the inside of the gown, pulling the gown over the scrub assistant's shoulders (Figure 7).
7. The waistline and neck ties are tied (Figures 8 and 9).
    PURPOSE: The gown is fastened to prevent contamination from a flapping gown while applying sterile gloves.

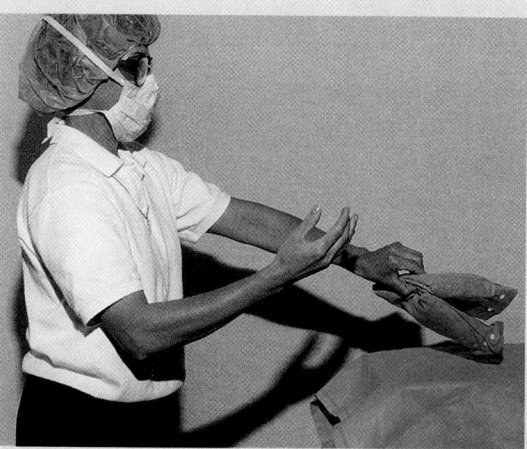

FIGURE 2

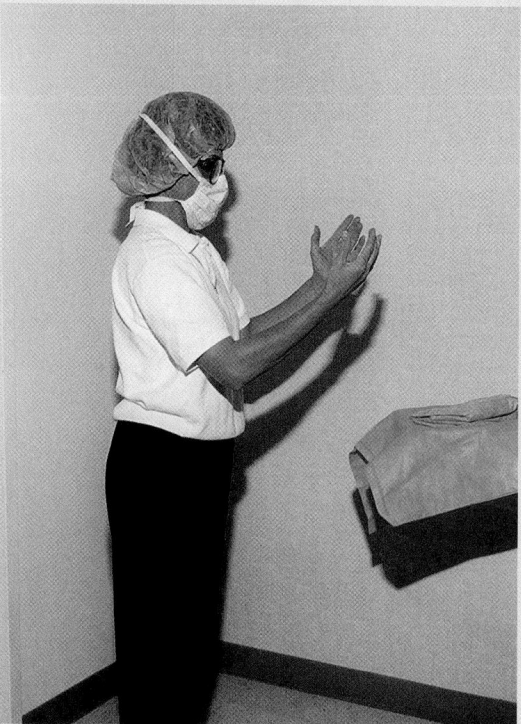

FIGURE 1

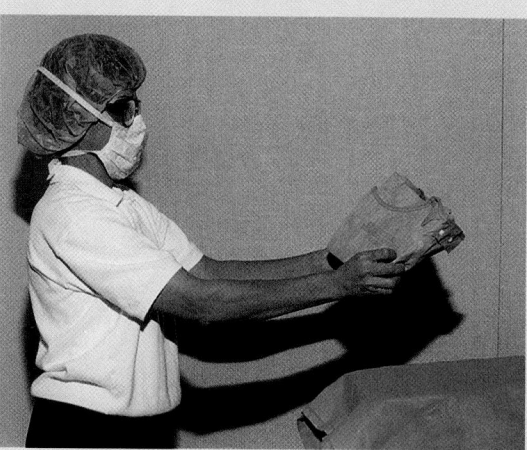

FIGURE 3

Continued

PROCEDURE 56-9—*cont'd*

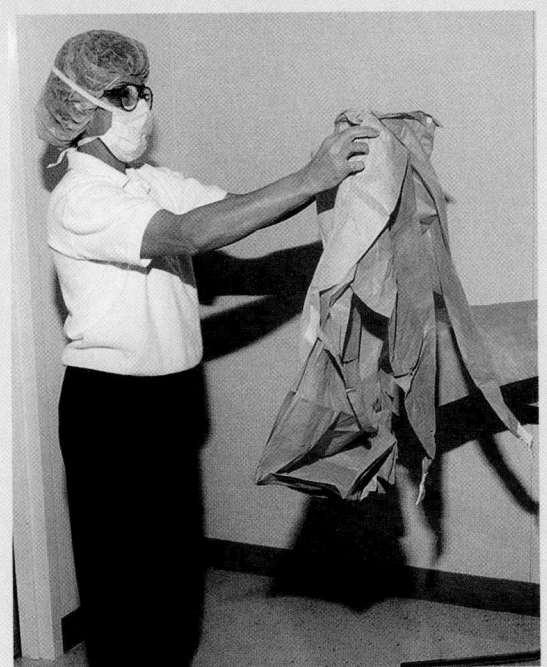

FIGURE 4

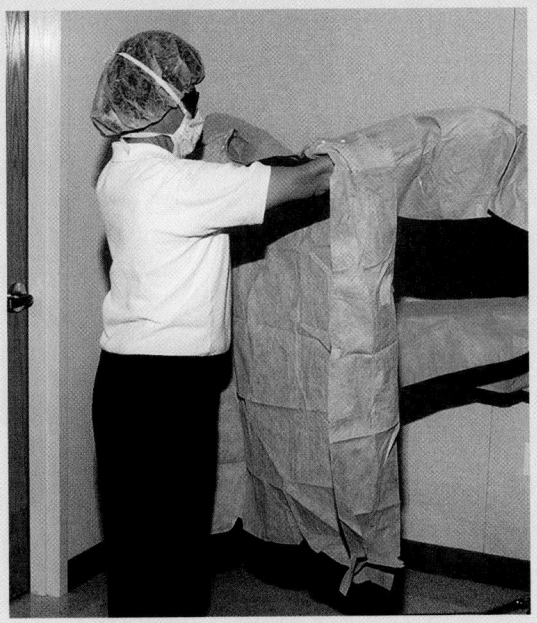

FIGURE 6

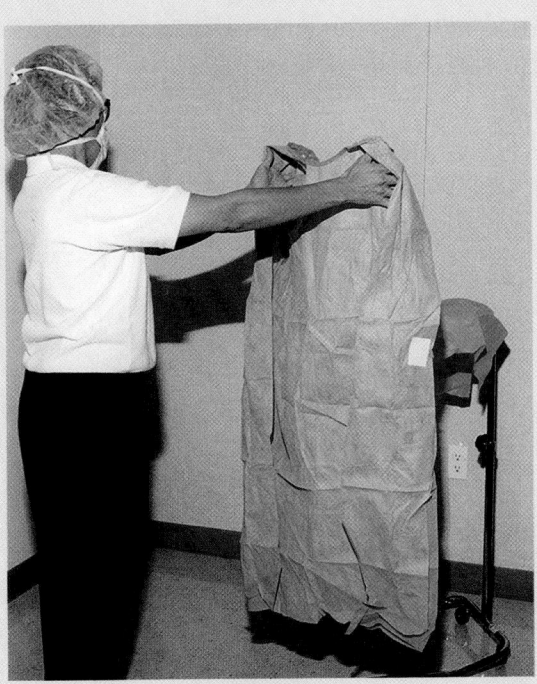

FIGURE 5

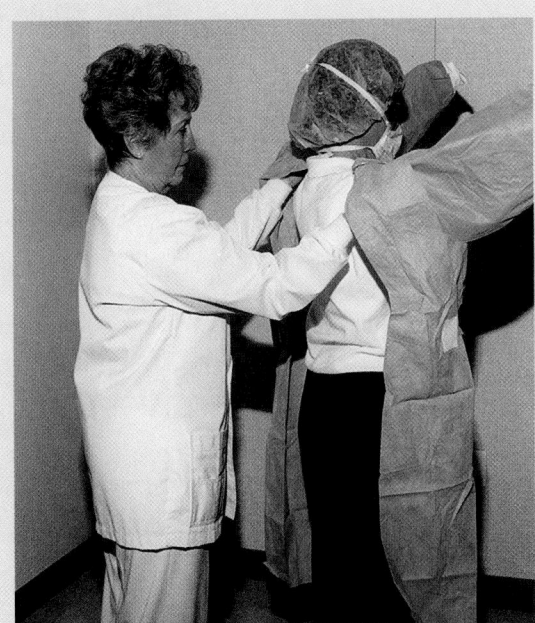

FIGURE 7

Continued

PROCEDURE 56-9—*cont'd*

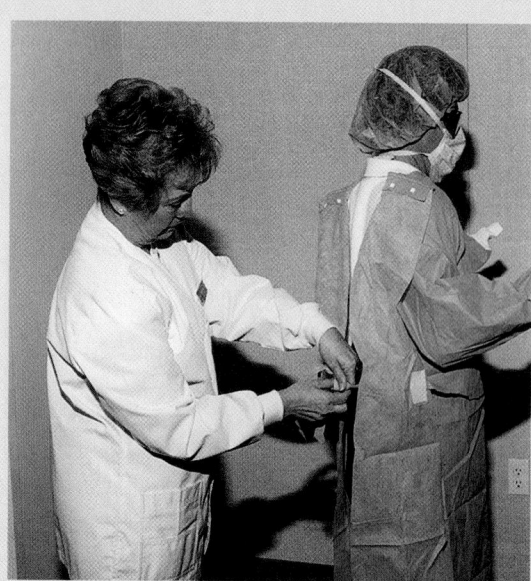

FIGURE 8

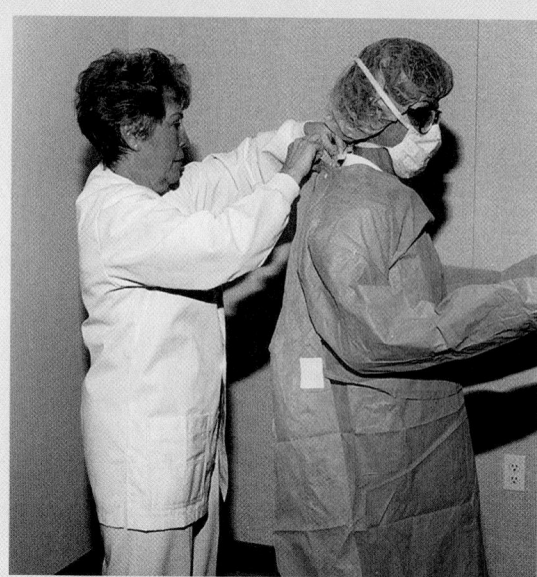

FIGURE 9

PROCEDURE 56-10

Prepare Patient for and Assist with Procedures, Treatments, and Minor Office Surgeries: Glove While Wearing a Sterile Gown

<u>CAAHEP COMPETENCY:</u> 3.b.(4)(f)
<u>ABHES COMPETENCY:</u> 4.(h)

GOAL: *To apply sterile gloves while dressed in a sterile gown before assisting with a surgical procedure.*

EQUIPMENT and SUPPLIES

- Sterile gloves, opened on a sterile field
  <u>NOTE:</u> A mask, goggles, hair cover, and a sterile gown are worn. The gloves are applied with the hands covered by the sterile gown to avoid contamination.

PROCEDURAL STEPS

1. Glove your nondominant hand first.
   <u>PURPOSE:</u> The dominant hand does the most difficult step, which is to apply the first glove.
2. Lift the glove with your major hand, and use your thumb and forefinger to grasp the top of the folded cuff (Figure 1). Remember, your hands are covered with the sterile gown sleeves.
   <u>PURPOSE:</u> Only sterile objects can touch sterile objects to prevent contamination.
3. Place the glove in the palm of your nondominant hand, with glove fingers pointing to elbows (Figure 2).
   <u>PURPOSE:</u> Your bare hand will touch only the inside of the glove as it slides into the glove.

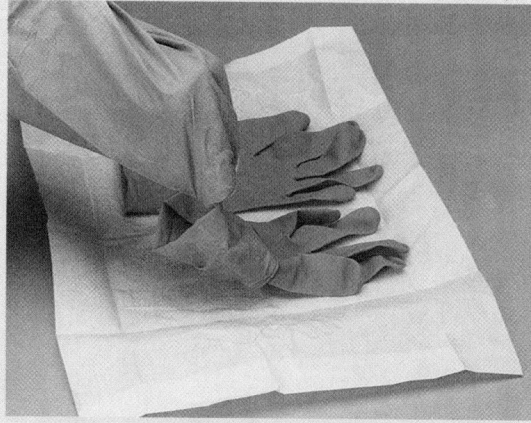

FIGURE 1

4. Grasp the inside of the cuff with your fingers, and gently stretch the glove cuff (Figure 3).
   <u>PURPOSE:</u> Sterile surfaces touch only sterile surfaces.
5. Pull the glove over your hand as you push through the gown cuff (Figures 4 to 6).
   <u>PURPOSE:</u> Your bare hand touches only the inside of the glove.

Continued

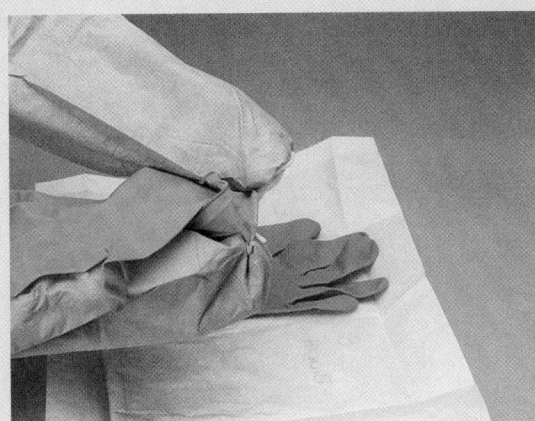

FIGURE 2

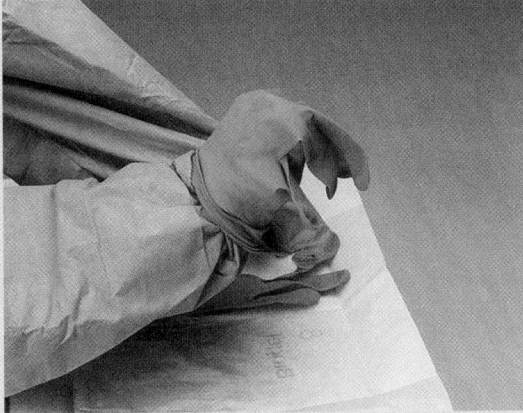

FIGURE 5

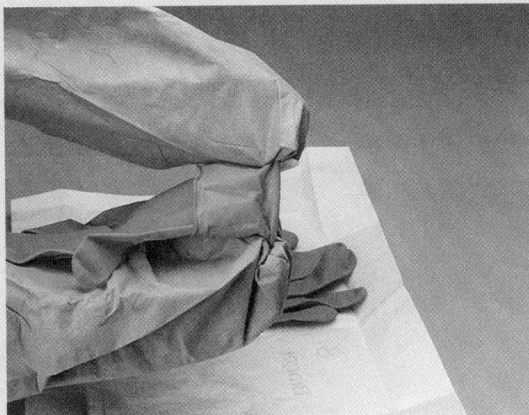

FIGURE 3

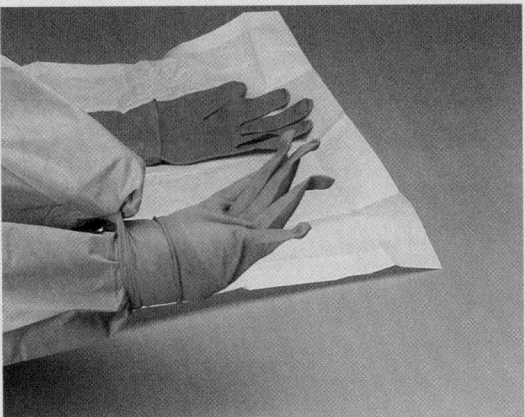

FIGURE 6

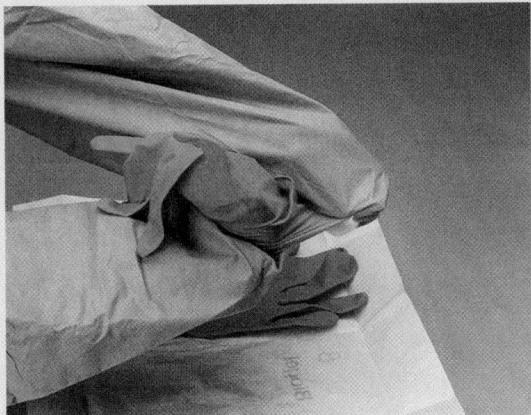

FIGURE 4

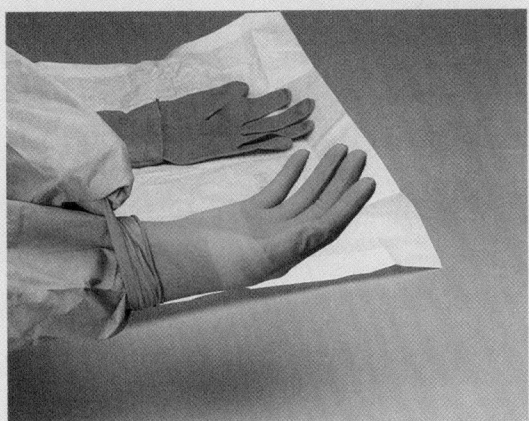

FIGURE 7

6. Gently slide your fingers in the glove (Figure 7).

7. With your minor gloved hand, slip your fingers under the cuff of the second glove (Figure 8).
   <u>PURPOSE:</u> Sterile items touch only sterile items.

8. Pull the glove over the hand as you push through the gown cuff (Figures 9 to 12).

9. The cuffs may now be adjusted (Figures 13 and 14).

10. The outside sterile gown ties may now be tied with the circulator's assistance (Figures 15 to 18).

11. The circulator grasps the red part of the tag by the corner (Figures 17 and 18).
    <u>PURPOSE:</u> This will be discarded after the scrub assistant is able to fasten the waist ties. Nonsterile areas do not touch sterile areas.

Continued

PROCEDURE 56-10—*cont'd*

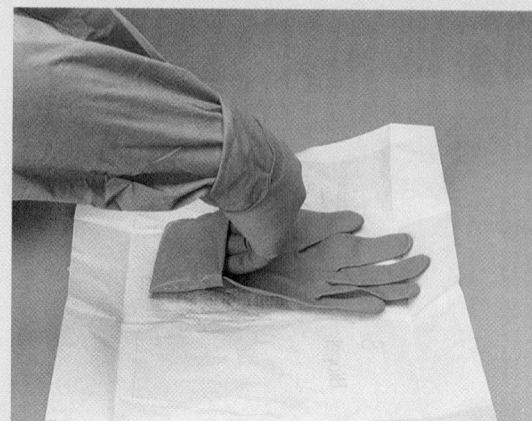
FIGURE 8

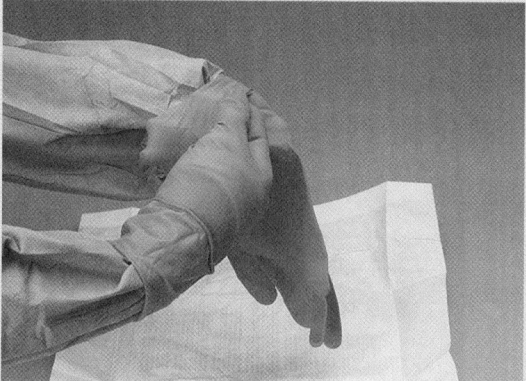
FIGURE 9

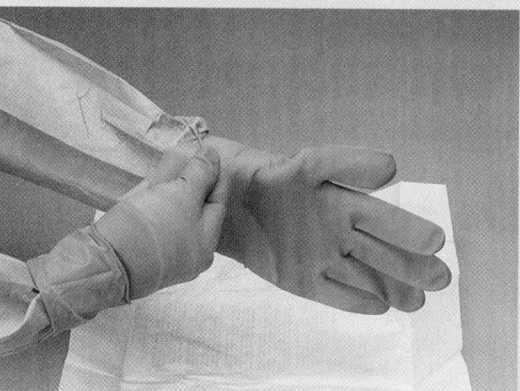
FIGURE 10

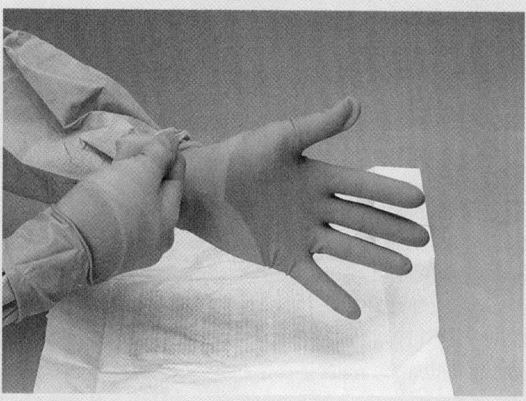
FIGURE 11

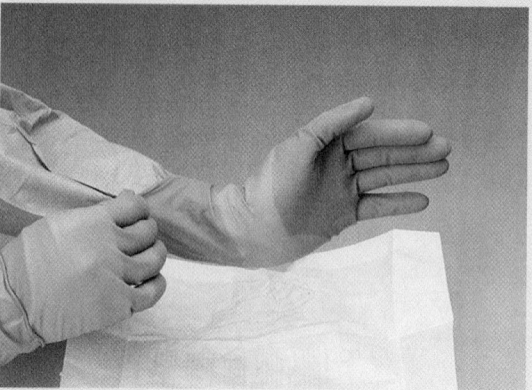
FIGURE 12

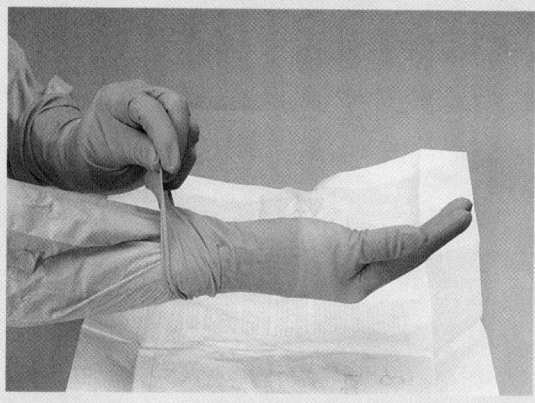
FIGURE 13

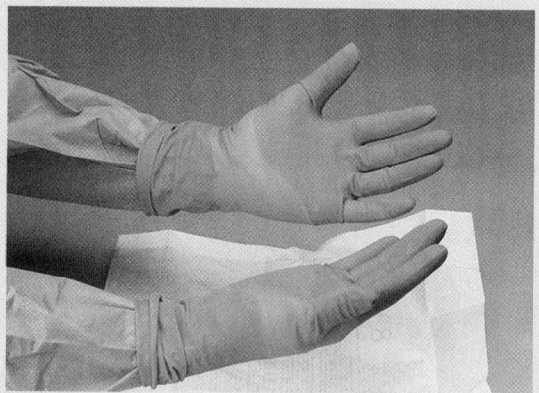
FIGURE 14

Continued

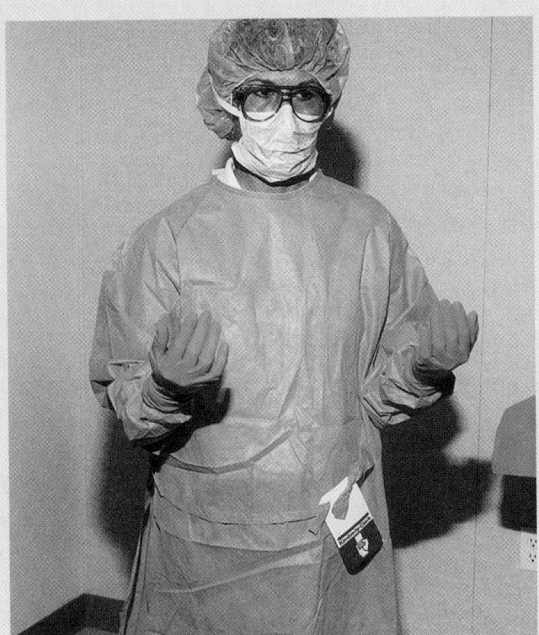

FIGURE 15

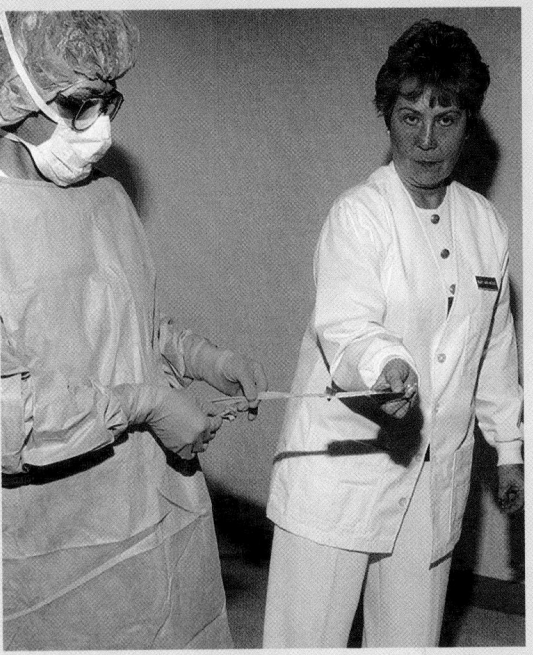

FIGURE 17

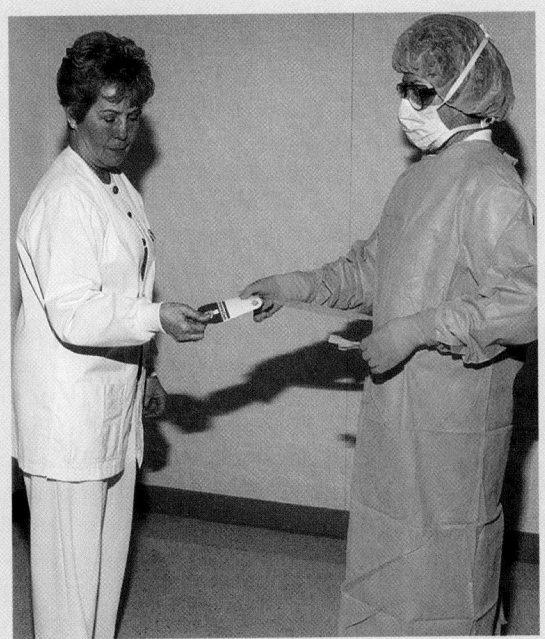

FIGURE 16

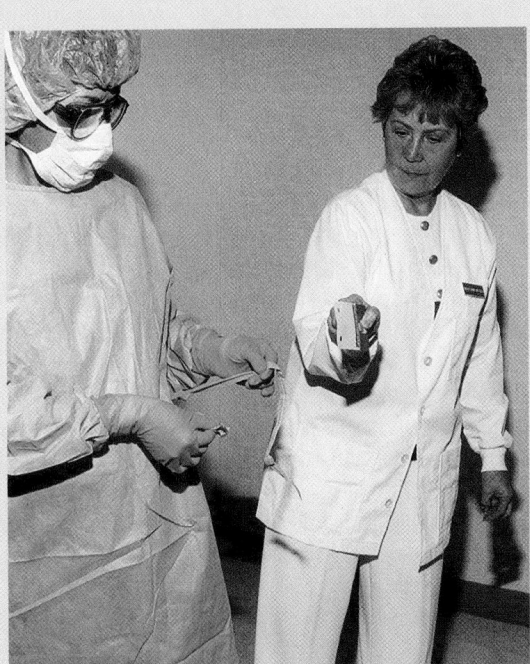

FIGURE 18

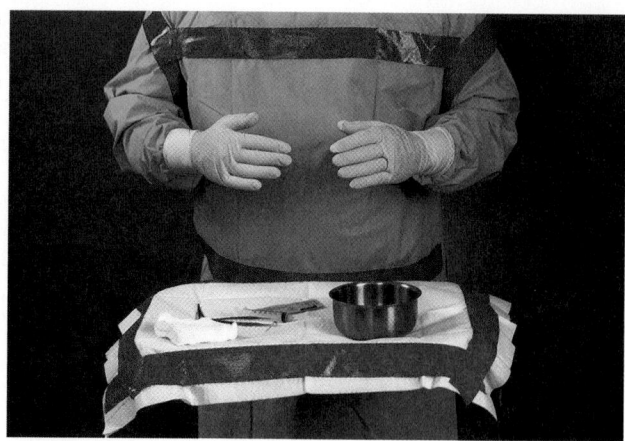

FIGURE 56-5 Sterile field (outlined in red).

is created by draping sterile towels (either disposable or from autoclaved packs) over a Mayo stand or table. The surgical site on the patient's skin is prepared, then draped with sterile towels or drapes so it also becomes a sterile field.

Hands and hair are two of the greatest sources of contamination when setting up a sterile field. With practice, you will learn to know what may be touched with your hands and what must be touched only with sterile gloved hands. Hair that falls freely over the shoulders and forward gives off a cloud of bacteria with every movement. It must always be secured back and up, not touching the shoulders.

Rules for Maintaining a Sterile Field

- Talking should be kept to a minimum because air currents carry bacteria.
- Sterile team members should always face one another.
- Always keep the sterile field in your view. If you turn your back on a sterile field or lose sight of it, it is considered contaminated.
- Nonsterile persons or items should never cross over the sterile field.
- Tables are sterile only at table level; anything that falls below the edge of the Mayo tray is considered contaminated. A 1-inch border surrounding the tray is considered contaminated, so anything placed on the tray within that 1-inch border is contaminated.
- Consider a sterile barrier contaminated if it has been wet, cut, or torn.
- Packages placed on a clean surface are contaminated on the outside, but the inside of the sterilized package may be used as a sterile field.
- Keep sterile gloved hands above waist level at all times; do not let hands drop below the waist.
- Never remove then replace any item in the field (such as using sterile forceps to cleanse a wound), or the field will be contaminated.
- The inside of a sterile package remains so if the package is peeled open properly; it should be opened the entire way, then the contents tossed onto the field without crossing over the sterile area.
- If a sterile package falls to the floor, it must be discarded
- *NOTE: If you are in doubt about the sterility of anything, consider it contaminated.*

Assisting the Physician During Surgery

The physician is ultimately responsible for the patient; however, the medical assistant is responsible for ensuring that everything the assistant and the physician will use in caring for the surgical patient is accounted for, ready for use, and prepared in a safe and sterile manner (Procedure 56-11). Every team will have preferences regarding the sequence they follow during routine minor surgery. Once a routine is established, it should be followed in every case. Sample setups for various types of minor surgery are provided in Table 56-4 (p. 1304).

The medical assistant sorts and places the scalpels, hemostats, scissors, tissue forceps, and retractors on the sterile field according to their sequence and frequency of use (Figure 56-6, p. 1304). Scalpels and sharp instruments should be conspicuously placed so that they do not accidentally harm a team member. The physician enters the room after scrubbing, then puts on gloves. The physician drapes the patient with towels or a fenestrated drape as the medical assistant hands the drapes, one at a time. Once the site is draped, the Mayo stand with the sterile field is positioned below the site and the medical assistant stands opposite the physician over the patient, ready to help as needed.

Passing Instruments

During a procedure, the medical assistant must protect the sterile field from contamination. Notify the physician if there is a break in sterile technique, dispose of soiled sponges into the biohazard waste container, and anticipate the surgeon's need for instruments. The physician may verbally request instruments or may use hand signals (Figure 56-7, p. 1305). As the team works together over time, the physician may not need to give any signals because the assistant will be able to anticipate what instrument is needed next during the procedure.

Instrumentation is logical: if the physician requests a suture, scissors will be needed next to cut the suture strand. In the case of sudden hemorrhage from a bleeding vessel, the physician will need an appropriately sized hemostat. While gaining experience the assistant watches, listens, and learns to judge what will be needed or performed next. Pass instruments with a firm and purposeful motion so that the physician will not have to look up. Wait until you feel the physician grasp the instrument so it will not drop onto the patient or to the floor, and be careful that you and the physician are protected from injury. Pass the scalpel with the blade down, and present the handle to the surgeon. Hold all instruments by their tips, and pass the handle ends into the physician's palm or fingers.

CRITICAL THINKING APPLICATION

While passing the scalpel to the surgeon when assisting with an I&D, Melissa feels the blade "slice" through her glove. She quickly and secretly looks at it and notices a "very tiny" nick in her glove. Because this is a "dirty" procedure, she decides to say nothing and continues assisting with the procedure. Is her reasoning sound here? What is the best approach to handling this situation? Why?

PROCEDURE 56-11

Prepare Patient for and Assist with Procedures, Treatments, and Minor Office Surgeries: Assist with Minor Surgery

<u>CAAHEP COMPETENCY:</u> 3.b.(4)(f)
<u>ABHES COMPETENCY:</u> 4.(h)

GOAL: *To maintain the sterile field and to pass instruments in a prescribed sequence during a surgical procedure that involves the making of a surgical incision and the removal of a growth.*

EQUIPMENT and SUPPLIES

- Open patient drape pack on the side counter
- Mayo stand covered with a sterile drape
- Packaged sterile gloves (two pairs)
- Needle and syringe for anesthesia medication
- Vial of local anesthetic medication
- Sterile drape
- Disposable scalpel with No. 15 blade
- Allis tissue forceps
- One skin retractor
- Three hemostats
- Supply of gauze sponges
- Biohazard waste receptacle
- Needle with suture material
- Specimen cup
- Lab requisitions
- Patient record

PROCEDURAL STEPS

1. Prep the patient's skin with surgical soap and antiseptic solution as explained in Procedure 56-3. Instruct the patient of prep procedure.
   <u>PURPOSE:</u> Infection control and to ensure the patient's cooperation.

2. Perform the surgical hand scrub as explained in Procedure 56-4.
3. Set up the sterile field with instruments and supplies, in the sequence to be used (Figure 1*). If it is necessary to touch sterile supplies, apply sterile gloves as explained in Procedure 56-8 or use sterile transfer forceps as shown in Procedure 56-6. After the sterile field is set up, cover it with a sterile drape.
4. Position the Mayo stand near the patient and the operative site, making sure the patient understands not to touch the sterile field (Figure 2).
   <u>PURPOSE:</u> To prevent contamination of supplies and provide easy access for the physician.
5. Apply sterile gloves, using aseptic technique.
6. Grasp the patient drape by holding one edge or corner in each hand (Figure 3).
7. Drape the surgical site without touching any part of the patient or the operating area with your gloved hands (Figure 4).

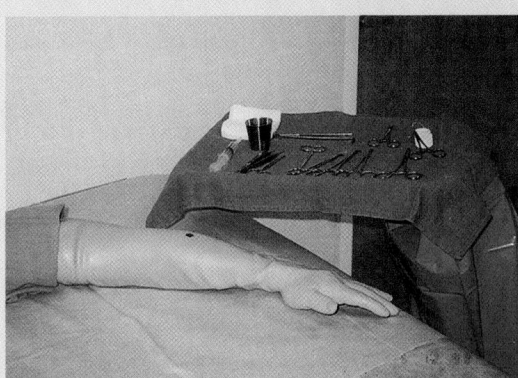

FIGURE 2

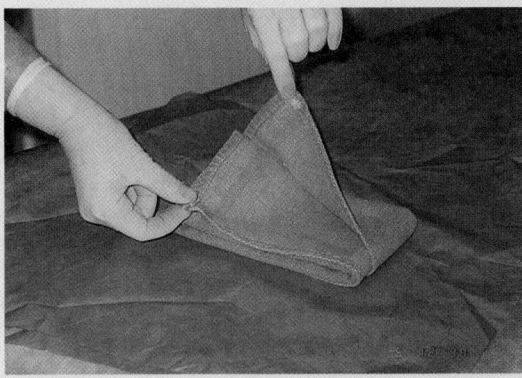

FIGURE 3

FIGURE 1

Continued

PROCEDURE 56-11—cont'd

8. If the physician requests medication such as a local anesthetic, a second circulating assistant holds the vial of local anesthetic so the physician can read the label. The physician withdraws the desired amount using sterile technique (Figure 5).
PURPOSE: The vial of local anesthetic medication must be held by the second assistant away from the sterile field to prevent crossing over the field with nonsterile item. The medication label must be checked before dispensing or administering a medication.

9. The surgeon injects the local anesthetic and waits a few minutes for it to take effect.

10. Position yourself across from the surgeon. Arrange the sterile field. Check placement location on Mayo stand (Figure 6).

11. Place two sponges on the patient, next to the wound site (Figure 7).

12. Grasp the scalpel blade with a hemostat, and mount the scalpel blade onto the scalpel handle if using nondisposable items. Keep all sharp equipment conspicuously placed on the sterile field (Figure 8).
PURPOSE: Sharp instruments that are not clearly visible may injure a team member.

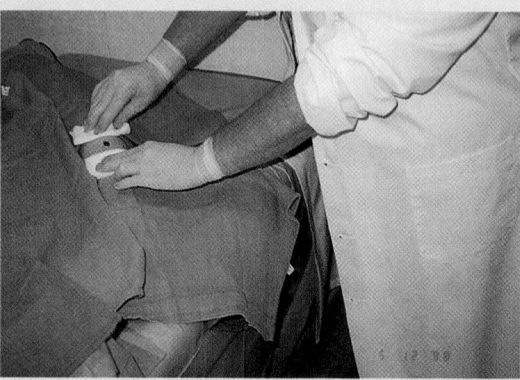

FIGURE 7

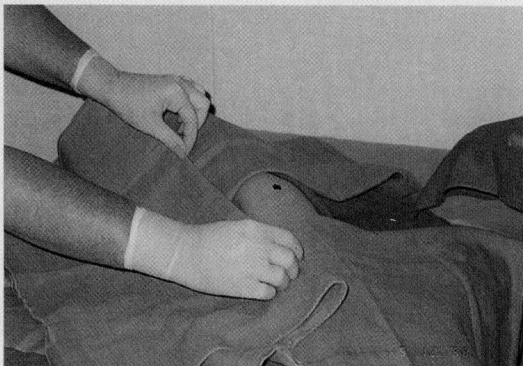

FIGURE 4

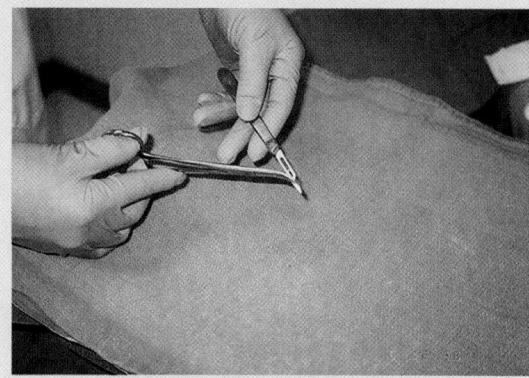

FIGURE 8

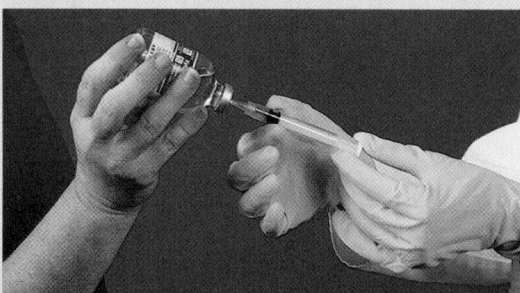

FIGURE 5

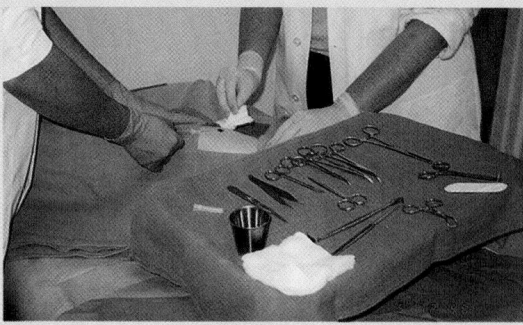

FIGURE 6

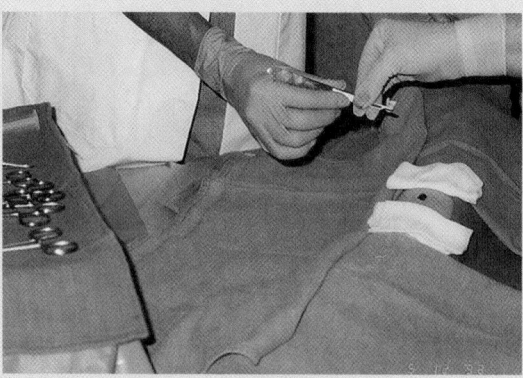

FIGURE 9

Continued

13. Pass the scalpel, blade down and handle first, to the surgeon or the surgeon will reach for it himself or herself. The surgeon will take the scalpel with the thumb and forefinger in the position ready for use (Figure 9).
    PURPOSE: To protect the surgeon and yourself from injury.

14. Grasp an Allis tissue forceps by the tips, and pass it to the surgeon to grasp a piece of the tissue to be excised (Figure 10).

15. Pass the handles into the surgeon's open palm with a firm and purposeful motion. A gentle "snap" is heard as it comes in contact with the surgeon's gloved hand.
    PURPOSE: The surgeon will not have to look up to receive the instrument.

16. Dispose of soiled sponges, using the biohazard waste receptacle, being careful to keep hands above your waist and not touching any nonsterile items.

17. Hold clean sponges in your hand, to pat or sponge the wound, as needed (Figure 11).

18. Safely position the specimen (if any) where it will not be disturbed on the sterile field (Figure 12).

19. If there is a bleeding vessel, or if a hemostat is requested, pass the hemostat in the manner described in steps 14 and 15.

20. Continue to sponge blood from the wound site.

21. Retract the wound edge, as needed, with a skin retractor.

22. Continue to monitor the sterile field and assist the surgeon as needed.

23. Pass the needle and suture material to close the wound, and apply a sterile dressing as requested (Figure 13).

24. Monitor the patient, and provide assistance as needed.

25. After the physician is finished, clean the area using aseptic technique.

26. Collect the specimen, place it into a labeled specimen cup, and send it to the lab with the proper requisitions.

27. Document the procedure, wound condition, and patient education on wound care.

*Figure from Bonewit-West K: *Clinical procedures for medical assistants*, ed 5, Philadelphia, 2000, WB Saunders.

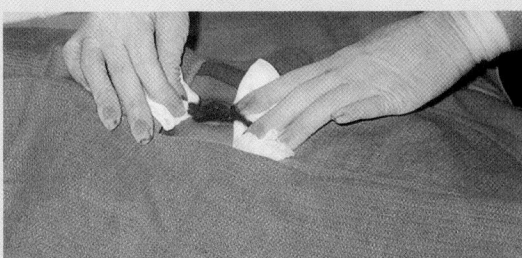

FIGURE 10

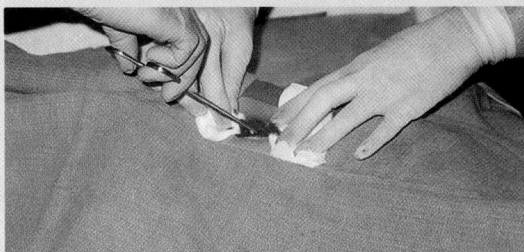

FIGURE 11

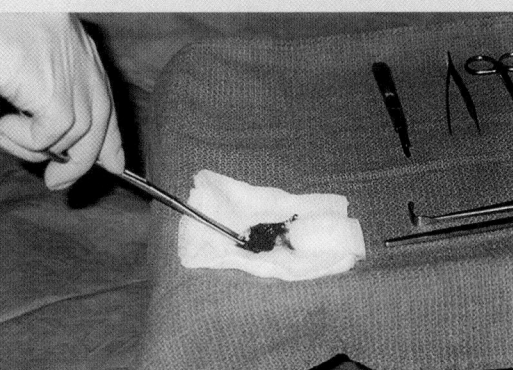

FIGURE 12

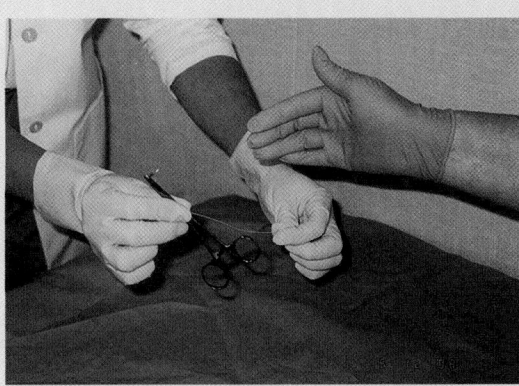

FIGURE 13

TABLE 56-4 Setups for Minor Surgeries

PROCEDURE	SIDE COUNTER	STERILE FIELD	COMMENTS	POSTOPERATIVE CARE
Suture repair	Local anesthetic, dressings and bandages, splints or guards, tape, drape, gloves, sterile normal saline solution	Syringe and needle, hemostats (three), scissors, sponges, suture material and needle, tissue forceps or skin hook, needle holder	If a patient arrives with a pressure dressing over a laceration, follow standard precautions. Do not remove the pressure dressing until the physician is ready to suture. If the patient's pressure cloth must be removed, have ample sterile dressings ready to apply immediately. Ask the patient the possible length, depth, and exact location of the laceration. Follow the physician's directions regarding cleansing of the wound.	Clean lacerations in a moderately protected area may not require a dressing. The patient is instructed to keep the area clean and dry. Some lacerations may be closed with Steri-Strips or an adhesive bond.
Needle biopsy	Specimen container with prepackaged fixative or preserving solution, laboratory form and label, local anesthetic, gloves	Biopsy needle, syringe and needle, sponges	A biopsy is the examination of tissue removed from the living body. Biopsies are usually done to determine whether a growth is malignant or benign; however, a biopsy may be done as a diagnostic aid in other diseases or infections. A needle biopsy may be done by aspiration with a needle and syringe or with a special biopsy needle. The specimen is then sent to a pathologist for either a cytologic or histologic examination.	Usually there is no special dressing required after a needle biopsy. A Band-Aid is often sufficient.
Cyst removal	Local anesthetic, disinfectant (skin prep), laboratory form, dressing (size depends on site), gloves, drape, specimen container with prepackaged fixative or preserving solution	Kelly hemostats (two straight and two curved), dressing forceps (two), suture and needle, scissors, dissector (physician's choice), skin hook, syringe and needle, disposable scalpel No. 11 or No. 15 blade, tissue forceps (two), Allis forceps, needle holder, sponges	A sebaceous cyst is a benign retention cyst of a sebaceous gland containing fatty substance from the gland. The cyst is attached to the skin and moves freely over the underlying tissue. For cosmetic reasons the physician will make the incision on the natural skin crease lines if possible.	See suture repair above, or apply a small sterile dressing depending on the size of incision.

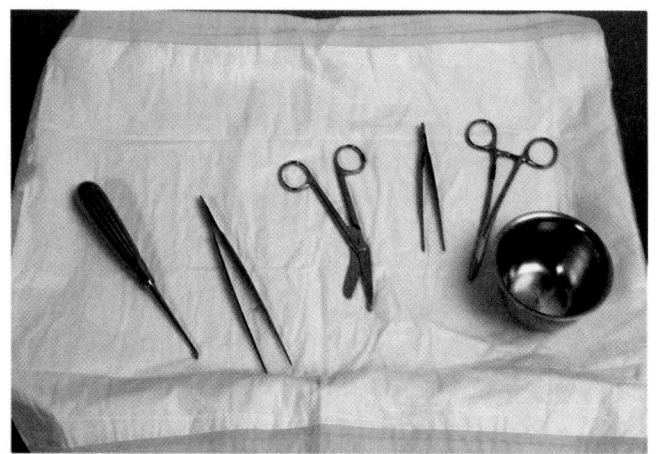

FIGURE 56-6 Mayo stand with surgical setup on sterile field.

Specimen Collection

If a specimen is collected during a procedure, it is placed in a sterile glass or basin. Do not remove the specimen from the sterile field until the physician gives the order. The surgeon may want to examine the specimen again during the surgery. After the procedure is completed, place the specimen into an appropriate container, label it, and send it to the lab for analysis.

Completing the Surgical Procedure

At the conclusion of the procedure the physician will begin wound closure (Procedure 56-12). The techniques and methods of tissue closure vary greatly, and it would be impossible to describe or illustrate all of them. The two basic methods of suturing are the continuous running suture and the interrupted suture, in which each knot is placed and tied one at a time, so

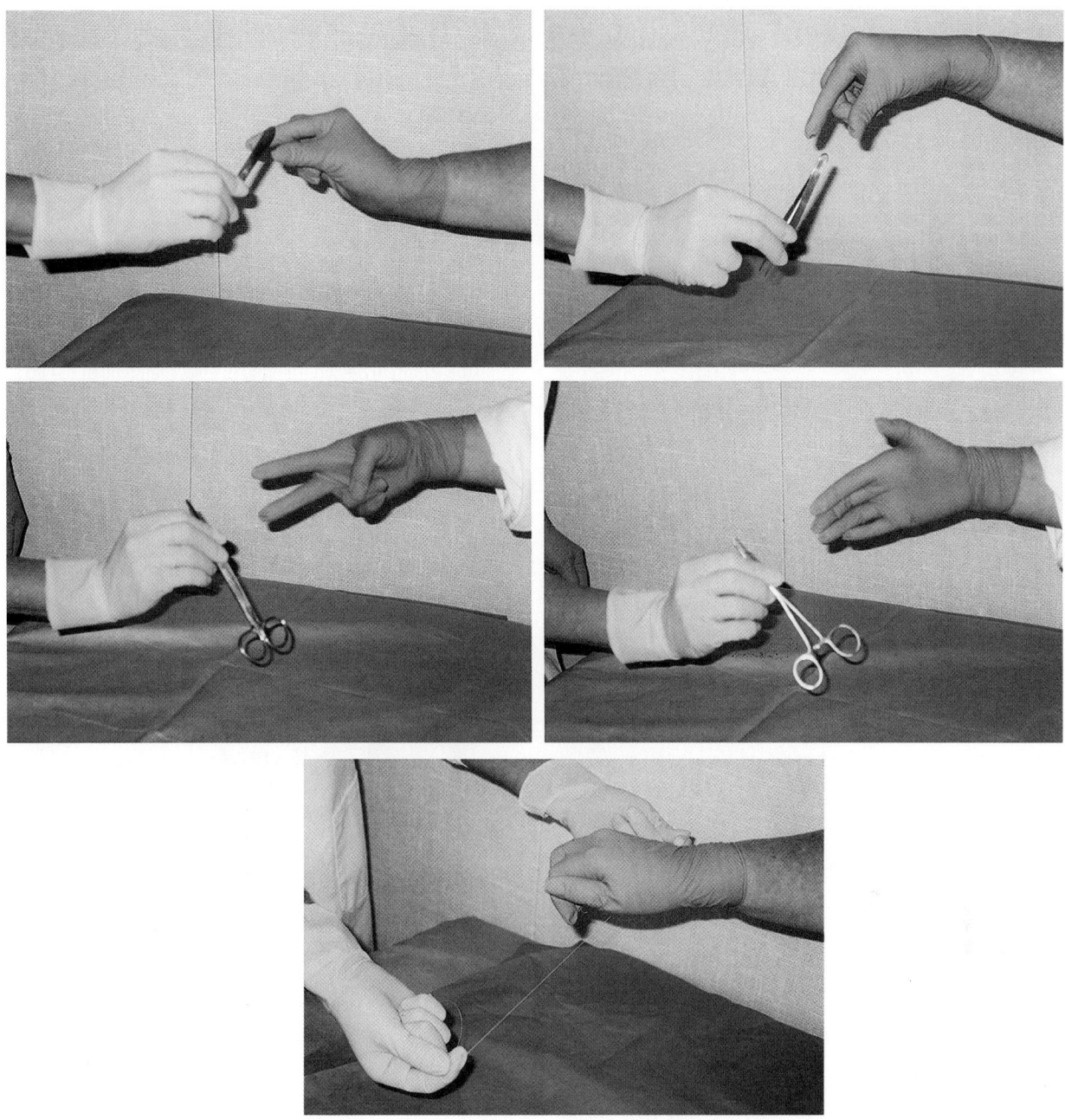

FIGURE 56-7 Passing sterile surgical instruments. **A,** Scalpel. **B,** Forceps. **C,** Scissors. **D,** Clamp. **E,** Free suture pass (free tie).

that if one breaks, the others keep the wound closure intact (Figure 56-8). For the majority of skin closures in a medical office, the interrupted technique is used.

The physician may prefer that the medical assistant place the needle into a needle holder and pass it, handle first. As the physician closes the wound, you may assist by cutting the suture and sponging the site. The physician places the first interrupted suture at the midpoint of the incision. Then each side of the first suture is mentally divided in half again, and the next two sutures are placed at each of these midpoints. The rest of the sutures are placed using the same technique until the wound edges are completely approximated.

After the skin closure, the wound site is cleaned with wet (using sterile, normal saline solution) and sterile dry sponges by the surgeon or the assistant. Care must be taken not to disturb the wound edges or sutures. Next, a sterile dressing is placed over the incision (Procedure 56-13) and a bandage is applied to support the dressing.

Postoperative Responsibilities

After caring for the patient, clear the sterile field following standard procedures. Wear disposable gloves until all contaminated materials are properly removed and handled. Place disposable equipment and supplies in biohazard waste cans and/or sharps containers. The room should be checked for any blood spills or other contamination and cleaned appropriately. After completing this process, remove the contaminated gloves and wash your hands.

PROCEDURE 56-12

Prepare Patient for and Assist with Procedures, Treatments, and Minor Office Surgeries: Assist with Suturing

<u>CAAHEP COMPETENCY:</u> 3.b.(4)(f)
<u>ABHES COMPETENCY:</u> 4.(h)

GOAL: *To assist the surgeon in wound closure, using sterile technique.*

EQUIPMENT and SUPPLIES

- Sterile field on Mayo stand
- Surgical scissors
- Suture material
- Sterile gloves
- Needle holder
- Gauze sponges
- Patient record

NOTE: This procedure may be a continuation of Procedure 56-11. If done independently, you must perform the surgical scrub and glove before beginning step 1.

PROCEDURAL STEPS

1. Hold the curved needle point in your minor hand, 4 to 5 inches over the sterile field (Figure 1).
   <u>PURPOSE:</u> Always work over a sterile field and take care not to puncture gloves with the sharp needle.

2. With the needle holder, clamp the suture needle at the upper third of its total length (Figure 2).
   <u>PURPOSE:</u> Clamping in the middle weakens and may distort the shape of the needle. Clamping too near the thread may cause the suture to detach from the needle. Clamping at the tip of the needle damages the needle point.

3. With your dominant hand, hold the needle holder halfway down its shaft with the suture needle point up.

4. With your nondominant hand, hold the suture strand, and pass the needle holder into the surgeon's hand (Figures 3 and 4).

5. Pick up the surgical scissors with your dominant hand and a gauze sponge with your nondominant hand.

6. After the surgeon places a closure suture, knots it, and holds the two strands taut, cut both suture strands in one motion.

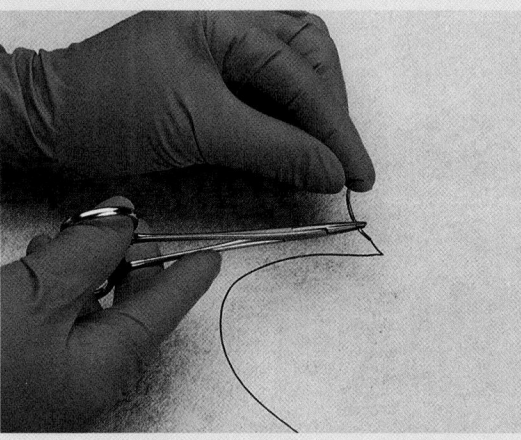

FIGURE 1

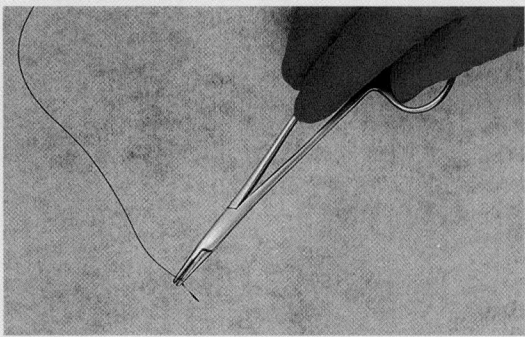

FIGURE 2

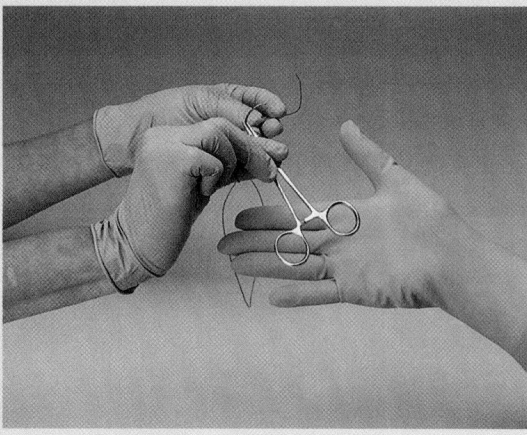

FIGURE 3

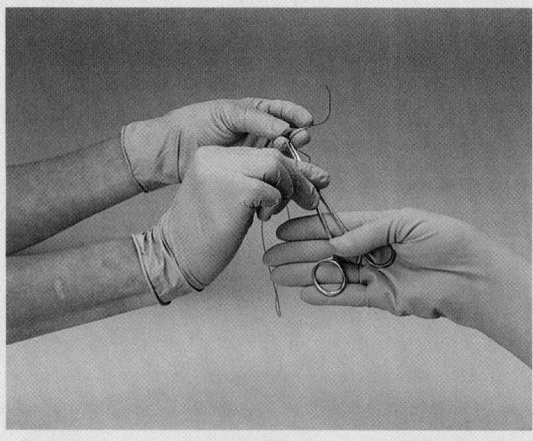

FIGURE 4

Continued

PROCEDURE 56-12—cont'd

Cut between the knot and the surgeon, at the length requested, approximately ⅛ inch.
PURPOSE: Too long a suture may irritate the patient during recovery, and too short a suture may untie during recovery.

7. Gently blot the closure once with the gauze sponge in your nondominant hand.
PURPOSE: Rubbing or friction may damage the wound edges.

8. If additional strands of suture are needed, repeat the process.

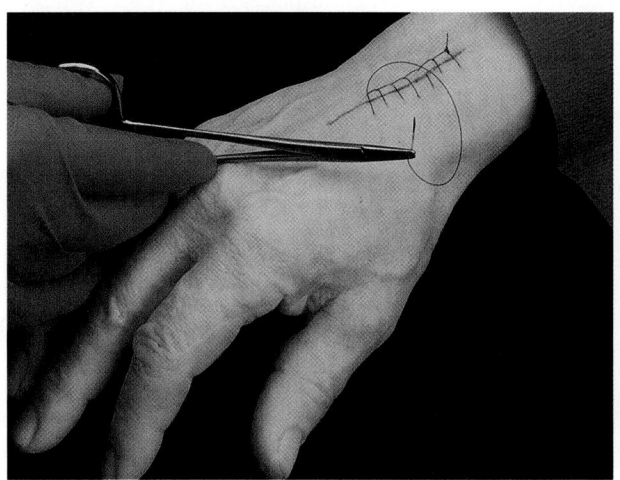
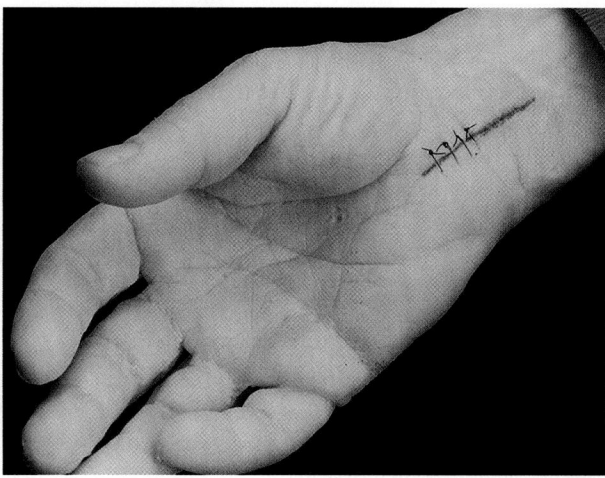

FIGURE 56-8 **A,** Continuous (running) suture placement. **B,** Interrupted suture placement.

PROCEDURE 56-13

Prepare Patient for and Assist with Procedures, Treatments, and Minor Office Surgeries: Apply or Change a Sterile Dressing

CAAHEP COMPETENCY: 3.b.(4)(f)
ABHES COMPETENCY: 4.(h)

GOAL: *To properly apply a sterile dressing at the completion of a surgical procedure.*

EQUIPMENT and SUPPLIES

- Sterile dressing material or Telfa

PROCEDURAL STEPS

1. After surgery is completed, before the sterile drape is removed, and with sterile gloves in place, the dressing is picked up from the sterile field, placed on the wound, and held.
   PURPOSE: To prevent introducing microorganisms to the wound area.

2. The drape is then removed while switching hands to hold the dressing in place.
   PURPOSE: To keep the wound as clean as possible.

3. The dressing is secured with paper tape and/or an appropriate bandage.
   PURPOSE: To keep the wound covered and protected.

4. The procedure is documented in the patient's medical record.
   PURPOSE: A procedure is not completed until it is recorded.

See Appendix D for a charting example.

Use clean gloves to disinfect the room, including the table, Mayo stand, side and back tables, any other equipment in the room, and the floor. Used instruments must be sanitized, disinfected, and resterilized for future use. The surgeon and medical assistant both document the procedure in the patient's medical record.

Postoperative Instructions and Care

The patient should be given time to rest after the surgery. If a sedative was administered, make certain that the patient is sufficiently recovered to avoid injury after the surgery or during the journey home. If the patient has been given a topical or local anesthetic, explain to the patient that the anesthesia effect will wear off and that there may be discomfort at the operative site. Check with the physician if pain medication needs to be prescribed. If medication has been prescribed, review the purpose of the medication and directions for its use with the patient and his or her companion. Before the patient leaves the office, a follow-up appointment should be made.

Postoperative care extends for the total recovery period, not just for the time of immediate care before the patient leaves the office. Most medical assistants are responsible for teaching patients to care for themselves at home after surgery. The concentration of a postoperative patient is diminished after the stress of surgery, so all instructions should be given to the patient in writing. They should be simple in style and easily understood by both the patient and caregivers. These instructions can be preprinted forms for each type of surgery, or a general form with checked boxes for particular postoperative instructions that apply specifically to the individual patient (Figure 56-9).

Warning Signs

Explain to the patient the importance of calling the office if any questions arise or changes occur that he or she is concerned about. If the patient does not call within the next 24 hours, you should call the patient. Many patients tend to "ride it out" or say they did not want to disturb you. Never allow the postoperative patient to leave the office without the physician's knowledge and approval. Tell the patient to call the office immediately if he or she notes redness around the operative site, bleeding from the wound, fever, swelling, or increasing or severe pain. The wound should be kept clean and dry, and the patient should be taught how to change the dressing if needed.

Follow-Up

If the healing process is a long one, or if the wound becomes infected, the patient may return for follow-up care. If the wound requires a new dressing, follow standard precautions; wear gloves and other protective barriers, as appropriate. If at any time you determine that the wound may be infected, stop and have the physician examine it. Generally, no bandaging material should be reused, including Ace wraps. Tape applied directly to a patient's skin is not a good dressing immobilizer. If tape is used, always keep it to a minimum. If there is tape holding a dressing in place, always remove it by pulling toward the wound. If it is adhering to a hairy area of the body, lift the outer tape edge with one hand and slowly and gently separate the underlying hair and skin from the tape with the thumb of your other hand. Peel the skin from the bandage, not the bandage from the skin. Never rapidly "rip" tape from the body-the patient's skin may be injured. If the tape is not irritating to the patient, it may be advisable to leave the tape in place until total healing has taken place. If the wound is healed the physician may ask the medical assistant to remove the patient's sutures (Procedure 56-14).

WOUND CARE

A wound can be intentional (from a surgical incision) or accidental, and may be open or closed (Figure 56-10). An open wound has an outward opening where the skin is broken, causing the underlying tissues to be exposed. A closed or nonpenetrating wound does not have an outward opening, but the underlying tissues are damaged, as in a hematoma, contusion, or bruise. Closed wounds are usually the result of some type of blunt trauma to the body. An aseptic (clean) wound is not infected with pathogens. Septic wounds are infected with pathogens.

Open wounds may be classified according to the appearance of their openings. An incised wound has a clean edge and is made with a cutting instrument. An incised wound may be the result of intentional surgery, an accident, or a knife wound. A lacerated wound has torn or mangled tissues and is made by a dull or blunt instrument. A penetrating or puncture wound is caused by a sharp, slender object, such as a needle or ice pick, and passes through the skin into the underlying tissues. A perforated wound is a penetrating wound that passes through to a body organ or cavity, such as a gunshot wound.

Wound Healing

All wounds go through a healing or repair process that has three phases. The *lag phase* occurs first when the blood vessels contract

---

POSTOP INSTRUCTIONS FOR _____

☐ Elevate your arm.
☐ Elevate your leg.
☐ Limit food intake to _____.
☐ Limit activity to _____.
☐ Do not bathe or shower.
☐ Sponge bath only.
☐ Change dressing as instructed.
☐ Call the office for fever, redness, pain, swelling, or bleeding.
☐ Take _____ every 4 hours as needed for pain.
☐ Return to school/work in _____ days.
☐ Call the office tomorrow before _____ p.m.
☐ Your next appointment is on M T W Th F S _____ at _____.

FIGURE 56-9 An example of preprinted postoperative patient instructions.

PROCEDURE 56-14

Prepare Patient for and Assist with Procedures, Treatments, and Minor Office Surgeries: Remove Sutures

CAAHEP COMPETENCY: 3.b.(4)(f)
ABHES COMPETENCY: 4.(h)

GOAL: *To remove sutures from a healed incision, using sterile technique and without injuring the closed wound.*

EQUIPMENT and SUPPLIES

- Suture removal pack containing the following:
  - Suture removal scissors
  - Gauze sponges
  - Thumb dressing forceps
  - Steri-Strips or Band-Aids
  - Skin antiseptic
- Biohazard waste container
- Sterile gloves
- Patient record

PROCEDURAL STEPS

1. Assemble necessary supplies.
2. Wash and dry your hands. Follow standard precautions.
3. Instruct patient of procedure and to lie or sit still during procedure.
   PURPOSE: To ensure cooperation during the procedure.
4. Position patient comfortably, and support the sutured area.
5. Place dry towels under the site.
6. Open the suture removal pack, and apply sterile gloves.
7. Place a sterile gauze sponge next to the wound site.
   PURPOSE: To place the removed sutures.

8. Grasp the knot of the suture with the dressing forceps, without pulling.
9. Cut the suture at skin level (Figure 1).
10. Lift, do not pull, the suture toward the incision and out with the dressing forceps (Figure 2).
11. Place the suture on the sterile gauze sponge, and check that the entire suture strand has been removed.
    PURPOSE: Suture fragments left in a wound may cause irritation and/or infection and may prolong the healing process.
12. If any bleeding occurs, blot the area with a sterile gauze sponge before continuing.
13. Continue in the same manner until all sutures have been removed.
14. Remove the gauze sponge with the sutures on it, and dispose of contaminated materials in the biohazard waste container.
15. The surgeon may apply or order that you apply Steri-Strips or a Band-Aid for added support, strength, and protection.
16. The patient is instructed to keep the wound edges clean and dry and not place excessive strain on the area.
17. Document the procedure, wound condition, and patient education on wound care.
    PURPOSE: A procedure that is not documented was not done.

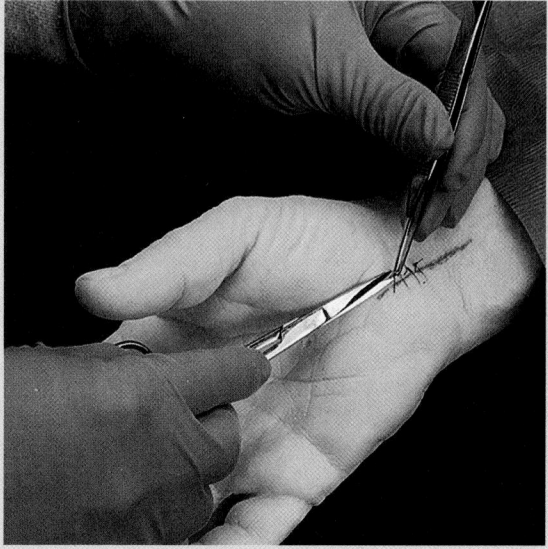

FIGURE 1

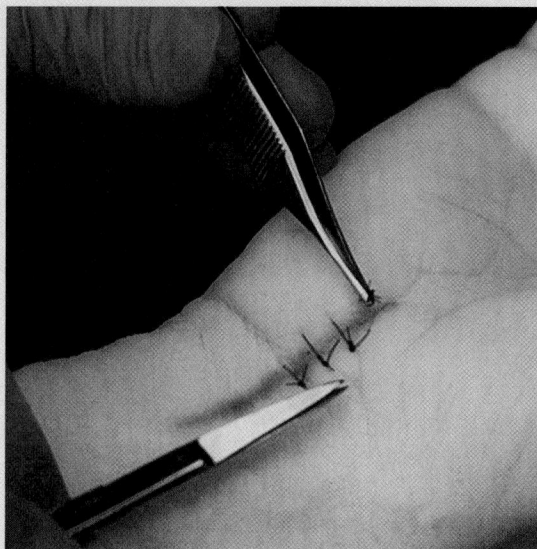

FIGURE 2

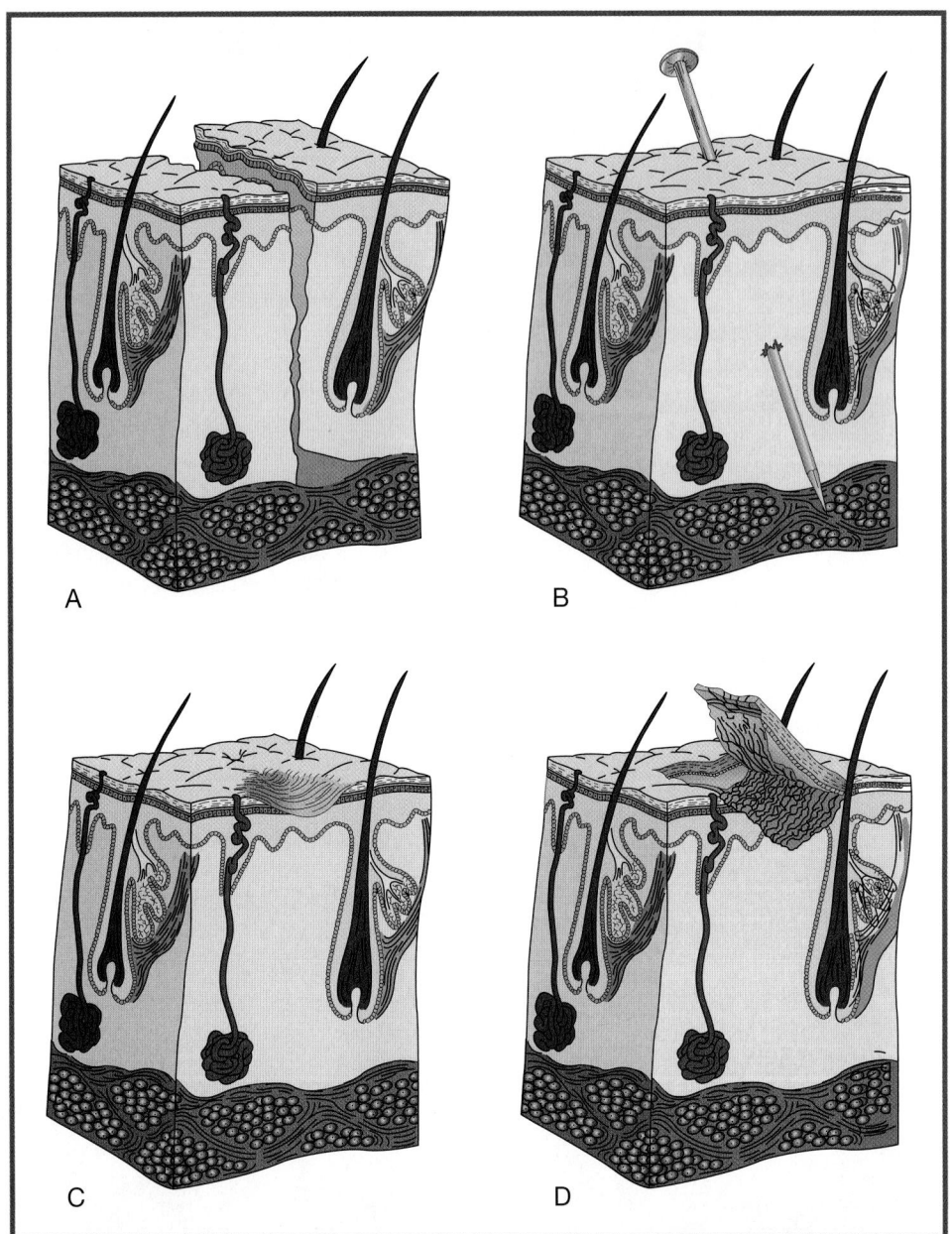

FIGURE 56-10 Types of wounds. **A,** Laceration—jagged, irregular breaking or tearing of tissues, usually caused by blunt trauma. **B,** Puncture—skin is pierced by a pointed object, such as a pin, nail, splinter, or bullet. **C,** Abrasion—superficial wound, scraping of the skin. **D,** Avulsion—tissue forcibly torn or separated, caused by accidents.

to control hemorrhage, and blood platelets form a network in the wound that acts like glue to plug the wound. After a cascade of chemical reactions, fibrin is released into the wound and clotting begins. Fibrin continues to collect red blood cells (RBCs) and the clot dries into a scab. About 12 hours later, special white blood cells (WBCs), macrophages, arrive to clear away bacteria and dead tissue. Within 1 to 4 days the fibrin threads contract and pull the edges of the wound together under the scab.

The second phase, *proliferation,* is the wound healing and new growth period, lasting from 5 to 20 days. It is during this phase

that the tissues repair themselves. New cells form and the wound continues to contract and seal. If the wound is a clean surgical incision, complete contraction usually takes place during this phase, and there is little scarring or permanent fibrous tissue *(cicatrix)* formation.

The final or *remodeling phase* occurs from the twenty-first day onward. Clean, shallow wounds may contract in the first two stages; large or mangled wounds require the time and cellular activity of this third phase to build a bridge of new tissue to close the gap of the wound. The cells produce a fibrous protein substance called collagen (connective tissue) that gives the

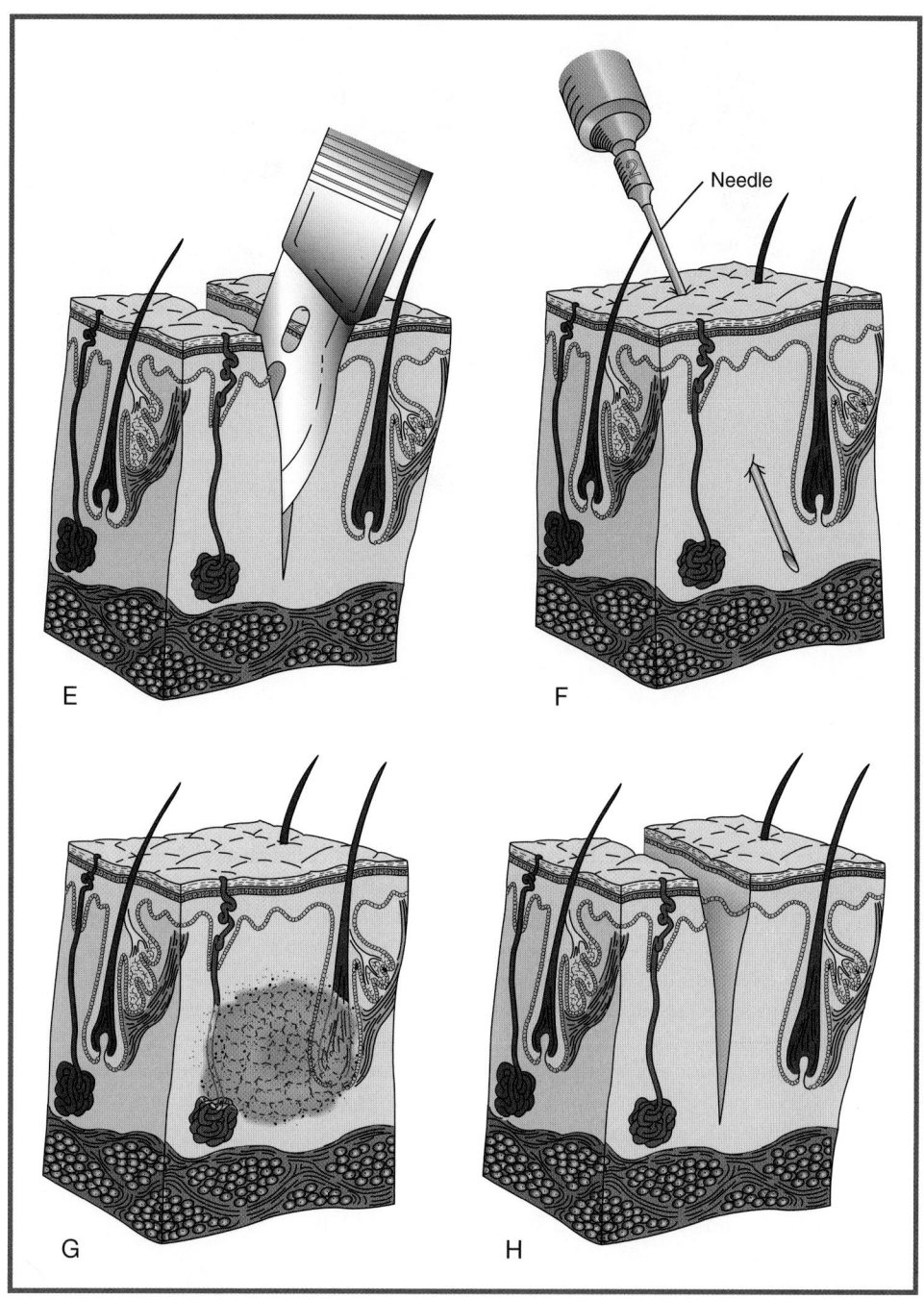

FIGURE 56-10-*cont'd* Types of wounds. **E,** Surgical incision—a neat, clean cut. **F,** Hypodermic puncture—injection under the skin. **G,** Contusion—closed nonpenetrating wound in which blood from broken vessels accumulates in tissues. **H,** Incision—neat, clean cut from sharp objects, such as glass, knives, or metal.

wounded tissues strength and forms scar tissue. Scar tissue is not true skin; it is usually very strong, but it lacks the elasticity of normal skin tissue. Scar tissue is also devoid of a normal blood supply and nerves.

Wounds are classified by the way they repair themselves. The clean, surgical wound that has been sutured closed and heals quickly without much scarring does so by *first intention*. Tissues that are severely damaged, purposely kept open, or fail to close are said to heal by *granulation* (healing from the bottom of the wound outward), which is called *second intention*.

Several factors influence the healing process. People who are young, are in good general health, and have adequate nutrition heal more rapidly. Adequate protection and rest of the injured area also enhance the healing process. Destruction or reinjury during the second phase can delay healing and increase scarring. Wounds are susceptible to infection because the normal skin barrier is broken. If there is debris in a wound as the result of the breakdown of various cellular components, this dead *(necrotic)* tissue acts as a culture medium for bacterial growth. *Suppuration* (pus) contains necrotic tissue,

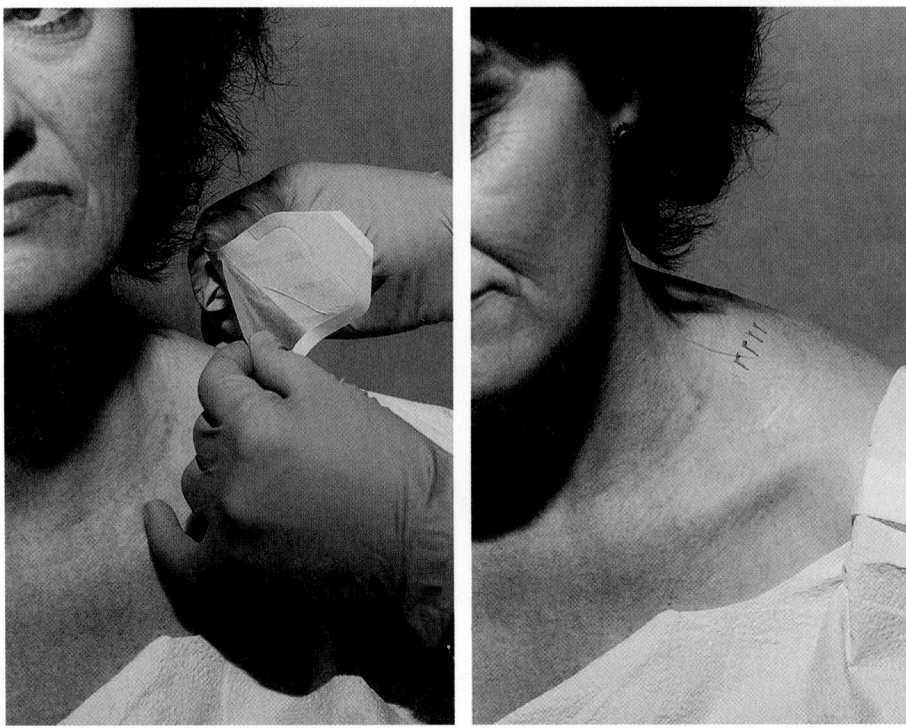

A   B

FIGURE 56-11 A, Placing a clear dressing on a sutured wound. **B,** Clear dressing in place over a sutured wound.

bacteria, dead WBCs, and other products of tissue breakdown. Necrotic tissue must be removed. Removal of debris is called *debridement,* which may occur naturally or be performed surgically.

Sometimes the physician may prefer no dressing or bandage on small wounds. This is called *open wound healing.* Some advantages to open wound healing include the following:

- It allows air to freely circulate around the wound.
- The wound is not irritated or rubbed by a dressing.
- The wound stays dry, which inhibits bacterial growth, reducing the chance of infection.
- Sutures stay dry and hold together better.
- Any preexisting infection remains localized and is not spread by the dressing or bandage.

Dressings

A dressing is a sterile covering placed over a wound to do the following:

- Protect the wound from injury and contamination
- Maintain constant pressure to minimize bleeding and swelling
- Hold the wound edges together
- Absorb drainage and secretions

A dressing usually consists of a strip of lubricated mesh gauze, a nonstick Telfa pad, or a clear dressing placed over a sutured wound (Figure 56-11). Gauze sponges may be placed over nonadhering material, depending on the physician's preference. Body cavities or wounds that need to remain open for a time are dressed with long, thin packing material that is often impregnated with an antiseptic or lubricant. This is

sometimes called *packing.* A good dressing must be effective and comfortable and must remain in place. If the dressing covers a hairless area, it may be anchored with tape, but no tape should touch the wound.

Frequently, small, clean lacerations may be closed with Steri-Strips (Figure 56-12). These strips reduce the chance of infection and do not leave suture scars. Steri-Strips are used on areas of the body that are protected from movement and stress. They are often used on the face. Because they are a suture replacement, only the physician should place them. They are placed on the wound in the same sequence and at the same intervals as interrupted sutures and are left in place until they fall off or the wound heals.

Bandages

Bandages hold dressings in place and also help maintain even pressure, support the affected part, and help protect the wound from injury and contamination. Bandages can be gauze, cloth, or elastic cloth rolls and are bound by clips, tape, or ties. Dressing and bandages frequently appear easy and simple to apply; however, special skill is required to apply a functional bandage (Procedure 56-15). Bandages that are too loose fall off, and those that are too tight may compromise circulation and further harm the patient.

Plain roller gauze is seldom used. It is difficult to handle, because it must be applied with reverse spiral turns if the area is uneven. It has no elasticity and tends to bind. It also tends to slip, because it does not adhere to itself. Wrinkled crepe-type roller bandages (e.g., Kling) are preferred, because they easily conform to various shapes of the body and adhere to themselves

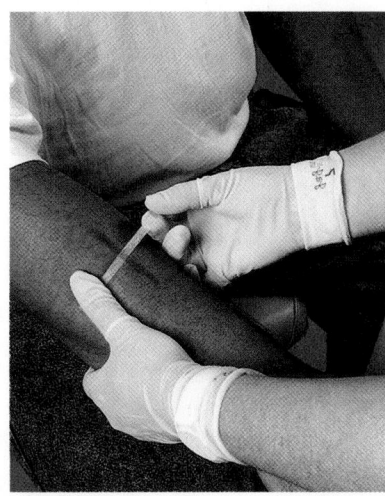

FIGURE 56-12 Steri-Strips on a wound. (From Bonewit-West K: *Clinical procedures for medical assistants*, ed 6, Philadelphia, 2003, Saunders.)

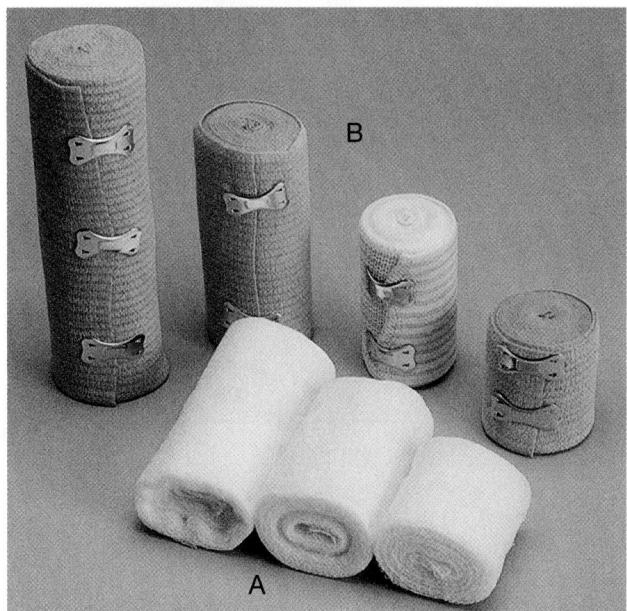

FIGURE 56-13 A, Kling bandages. **B,** Roller bandages.

(Figure 56-13, *A*). A bandage should always be applied over a sterile dressing.

Plain elastic cloth bandages (e.g., Ace) or elastic roller cloth with adhesive backing make a flexible and secure cover (Figure 56-13, *B*). When applying an Ace elastic roller bandage as a pressure bandage, especially to the lower limbs, it is essential to keep the bandage consistent in spacing and tension to ensure even pressure. Even, gentle pressure stimulates circulation and healing. Uneven pressure causes constriction points that can create pressure sores, ulcers, or **edema.** Roller bandages are usually applied from the distal to the proximal part of the area because it is more even and snug if it is wrapped from a smaller to a larger circumference. Elevate the limb while you are bandaging and work with the roller facing upward, close to the patient's skin. Elastic bandages are excellent for bandaging the

hand and wrist (Figure 56-14, p. 1316) and the foot and ankle (Figure 56-15, p. 1317).

hand and wrist (Figure 56-14, p. 1316) and the foot and ankle (Figure 56-15, p. 1317).

CRITICAL THINKING APPLICATION

Melissa applies a figure-eight elastic bandage to the hand and wrist of a patient who came into the office for suturing. She immediately sends the patient home after applying the bandage. She does not complete the chart at that time because the office is quite busy. Discuss all of your concerns regarding this situation. In what ways were office procedures ignored here? What would be a worst-case scenario for the outcome of this situation? How can this be corrected after the fact?

Seamless tubular gauze bandage, with or without elastic, is superior material for covering round narrow surfaces such as fingers or toes. It can be used as either a dressing or a bandage. A tubular gauze bandage is applied with a cagelike applicator (Figure 56-16, p. 1317). Work with the U-shaped cutting channel of the applicator toward the patient. Start in the middle of the area to be dressed, and anchor the dressing, if there is one, with a small piece of tape. Hold the applicator in the dominant hand, and control the tension flow with your fingers as the applicator is gradually rotated and the material slides off. Tubular dressing may be applied with or without slight pressure. Beyond the tip of the bandaged part, give the applicator a full half-turn, place the applicator again over the part, and repeat the process, being careful not to create a tourniquet effect when you reverse the applicator. When the desired thickness of the bandage is reached, cut the gauze and anchor the final dressing by tape or by tying at the wrist.

CLOSING COMMENTS

Patient Education

A medical assistant can help the patient in many ways. The best time to instruct your patient in aseptic techniques to be used at home is while you are performing an aseptic procedure. For example:

- While washing your hands before a procedure or examination, explain to the patient that hands should be washed before meals; after sneezing, coughing, or nose blowing; after using the bathroom; before and after changing a dressing or bandage; and after changing an infant's diaper.
- Explain to the patient how using disposable tissues to cover the nose and mouth when coughing or sneezing decreases the possibility of transmitting illness among household members.
- Discuss proper ways for disposing of used tissues, especially when one member of the household is suspected of having a communicable disease.
- Instruct the patient regarding the differences between sterile and clean dressings and bandages. Show him or her step by step how to change a dressing properly and then how to dispose of the contaminated items.

PROCEDURE 56-15

Prepare Patient for and Assist with Procedures, Treatments, and Minor Office Surgeries: Apply an Elastic Support Bandage Using a Spiral Turn

<u>CAAHEP COMPETENCY:</u> 3.b.(4)(f)
<u>ABHES COMPETENCY:</u> 4.(h)

GOAL: *To apply an elastic bandage to the forearm.*

EQUIPMENT and SUPPLIES

- One 3- or 4-inch elastic bandage

PROCEDURAL STEPS

1. Choose the proper size bandage for the size of the arm you are bandaging.
   <u>PURPOSE:</u> To provide proper support for the area.
2. Perform a circular turn at the starting point, securing a corner of the bandage as you circle the site.
   <u>PURPOSE:</u> To anchor the bandage at the starting point.
3. Hold the roll so the bandage can be rolled away from you (Figure 1).
   <u>PURPOSE:</u> To easily and securely apply the bandage.
4. Keep the roll close to the patient, and keep it facing upward (Figure 2). With each successive turn, overlap the previous bandage turn by one half.
5. Maintain even tension and spacing as you continue to apply the bandage up the forearm.
   <u>PURPOSE:</u> To maintain even, light pressure over the entire area.
6. When crossing a joint, slightly flex the joint (Figure 3).
   <u>PURPOSE:</u> To facilitate patient comfort and maintain normal circulation.
7. Fasten the end of the bandage with clips or tape (Figure 4).

8. Check the nail beds for cyanosis; ask the patient if the bandage is comfortable or feels too tight.
   <u>PURPOSE:</u> To ensure that the bandage is not acting as a tourniquet if applied too tightly.

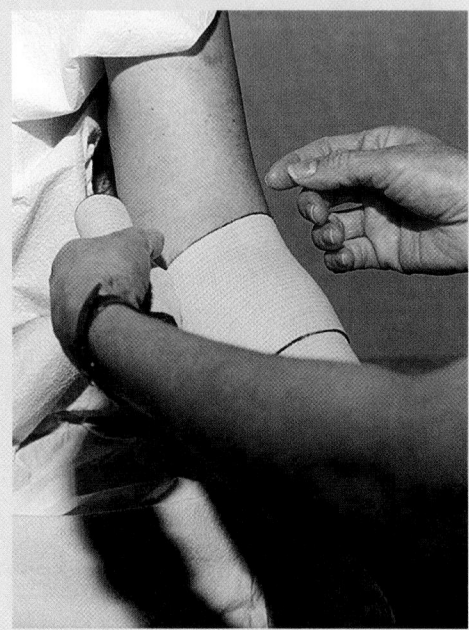

FIGURE 2

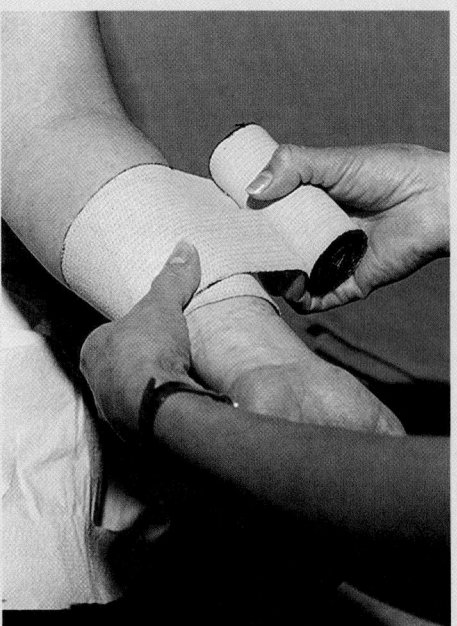

FIGURE 1

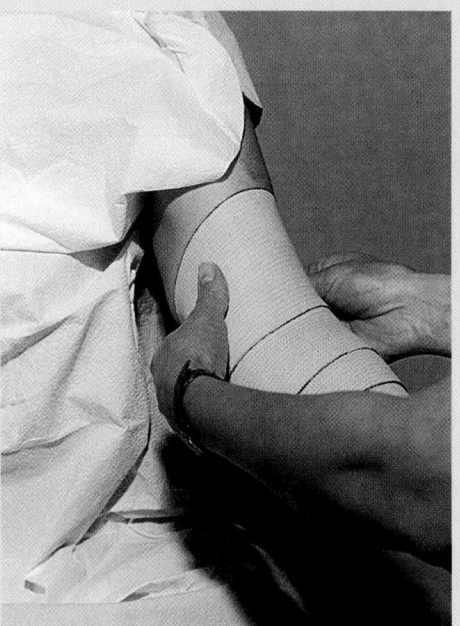

FIGURE 3

Continued

PROCEDURE 56-15—*cont'd*

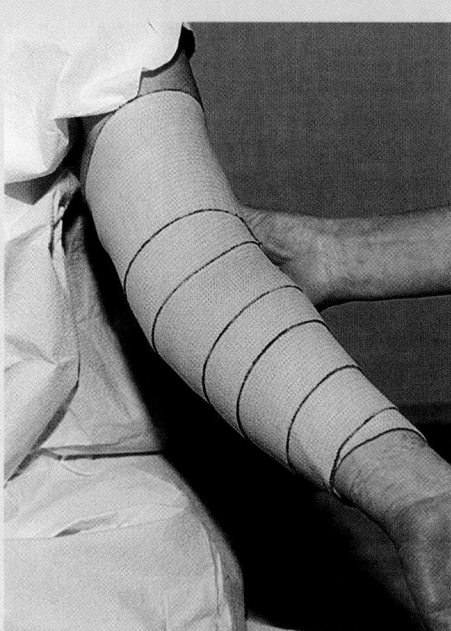

FIGURE 4

9. Check the radial pulse.
   <u>PURPOSE:</u> To ensure that the bandage is not acting as a tourniquet if applied too tightly.
10. Have the patient move his or her fingers.
   <u>PURPOSE:</u> To check that there is normal nerve function.
11. Document the procedure in the patient's medical record as well as patient instructions regarding bandage care and replacement.
   <u>PURPOSE:</u> The procedure is not completed until it is written down, dated, and signed.

See Appendix D for a charting example.

A medical assistant's duty may include calling the patient the day before surgery to confirm the scheduled surgical procedure and appointment time. Explaining the procedure and what to expect during and after surgery will prepare the patient and help to calm the patient's fears or concerns. Lying still during surgery is important, and eating a light meal the night before should be encouraged. Bathing before coming to the office will help reduce the amount of bacteria on the skin, and wearing comfortable loose clothing is recommended. Sometimes in the course of general conversation the medical assistant can pick up hints of concern that the patient may have and can direct the conversation into a discussion of these concerns.

Patients should be informed that they may need someone to accompany them home. There will be a bandage applied after surgery, and it must be kept clean and dry. There may be pain, and the physician will probably prescribe some type of analgesic. After the procedure is completed, make sure the patient makes an appointment for a return visit and examination.

Legal and Ethical Issues

Many minor surgical procedures previously performed in the hospital are now being done in a medical office, surgery center, or clinic. As insurance companies continue to recognize the cost-effectiveness of performing minor surgical procedures in these settings, the role of the medical assistant continues to expand.

Personal discipline is the primary concern in surgical asepsis. Often the assistant is alone when performing a surgical aseptic procedure; if contamination occurs, no one may know except

the medical assistant. It is the surgical assistant's responsibility to begin the procedure again with clean or sterile supplies if it is possible that contamination occurred. One of the medical assistant's main responsibilities is to carry out sanitization, disinfection, and sterilization procedures with precision and with total effectiveness. There is no room for compromise.

Patients should have absolute assurance that they are being taken care of in an aseptic atmosphere and under the most stringent aseptic conditions. This assurance is just as important for the protection of the office staff as it is for the patient. Allowing the physician to assume that the correct aseptic techniques have been employed in the preparation of equipment and allowing him or her to use contaminated equipment on a patient can result in claims of malpractice and charges of battery. Absolute, uncompromising honesty on the part of the assistant builds self-respect and contributes to professional achievement and satisfaction.

To have a good understanding of the subject, you must become familiar with the various techniques of sanitization, disinfection, and sterilization. Ignorance or carelessness can be dangerous and is inexcusable before the law.

The medical assistant must know what procedure is to be performed and whether the patient has been informed regarding the procedure. In the surgical setting the medical assistant must realize the full extent of his or her role as patient advocate and physician agent.

Confirm that the physician has explained the procedure to the patient and that the patient fully understands all aspects of the procedure that will be performed. This means that when the

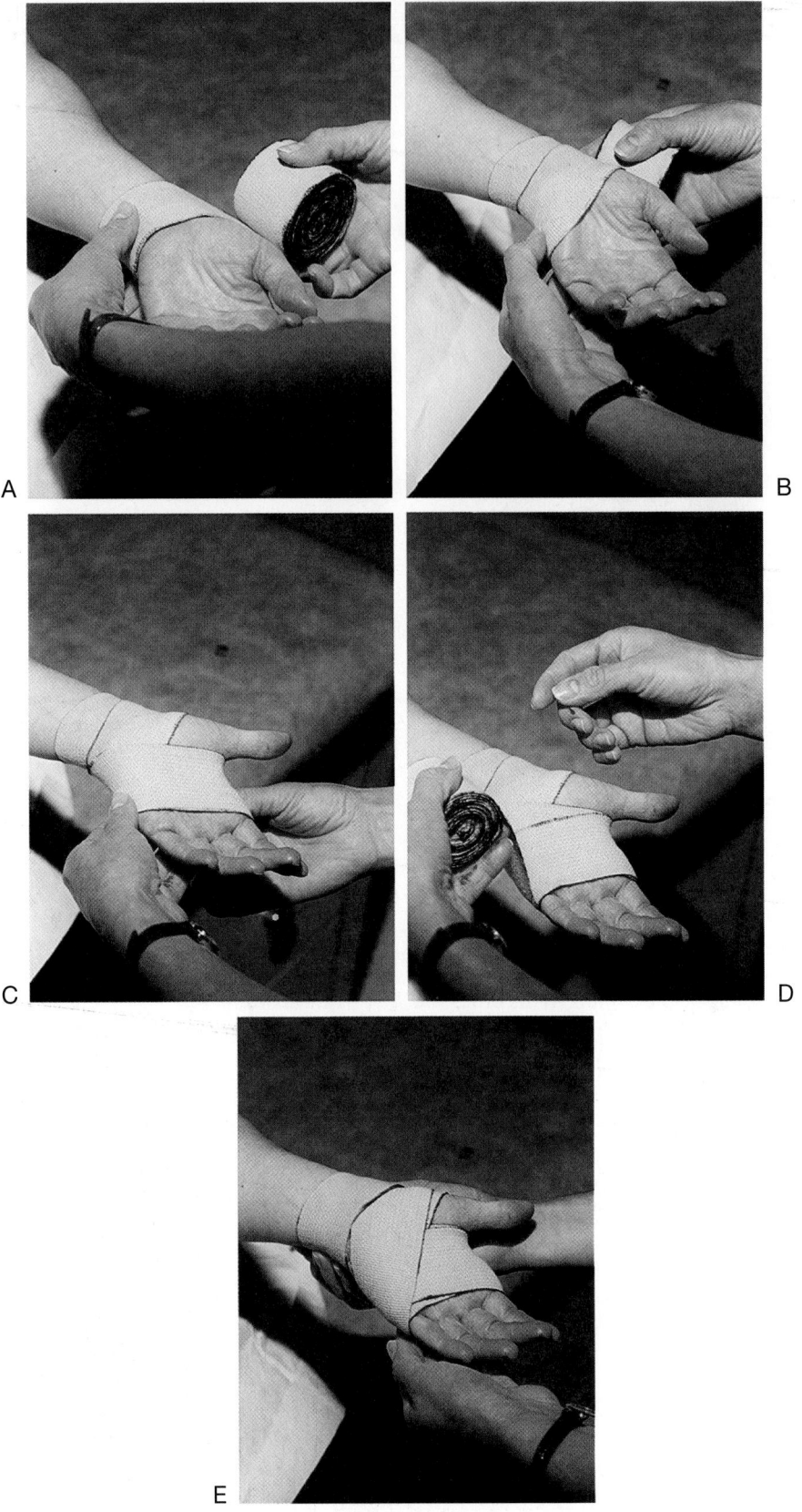

FIGURE 56-14 A, Use combination of recurrent and figure-of-eight turns for the hand. **B,** Start at wrist. **C,** Applying a roller bandage to the hand. **D,** Roller bandage applied to the hand. **E,** Maintain consistent tension while applying bandage.

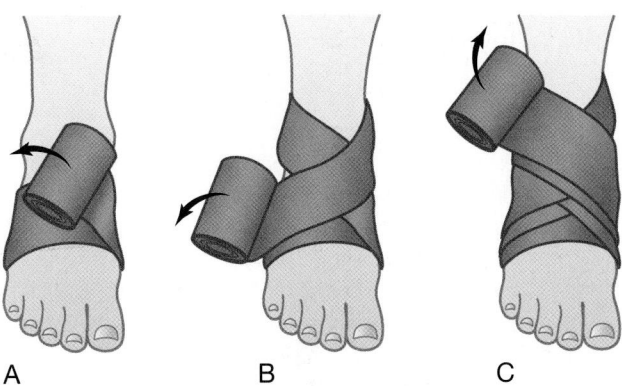

FIGURE 56-15 Use of the figure-of-eight turn for the ankle.

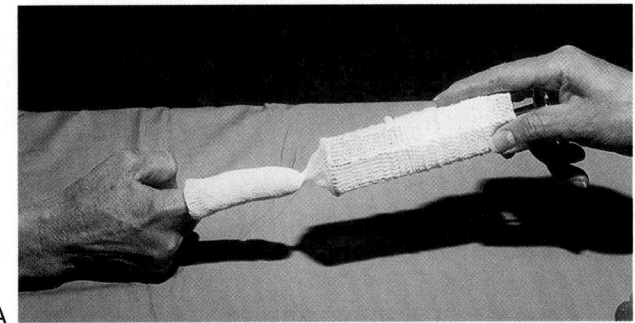

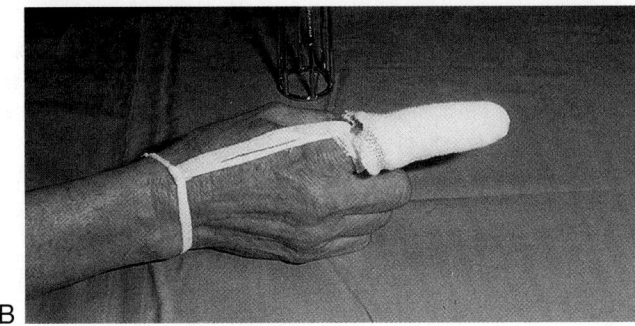

FIGURE 56-16 A, Tube gauze applied with even tension, twisting at fingertip before applying next layer. **B,** Tube gauze bandage applied and secured by tying at the wrist.

patient signs the consent for surgery, he or she is fully informed. Legal action can occur when complications arise from failure to complete procedure and consent forms. The surgical procedure is expedited when the patient is given instructions and knows what to expect. Increasing the patient's understanding ensures greater compliance with presurgical preparations, and the patient will be more likely to follow instructions and advice after surgery.

Finally, the medical assistant must practice perfect aseptic technique. A break in technique may invite infection and possible legal action. It is the medical assistant's duty to protect the patient. A major responsibility for the medical assistant is commitment to adhere strictly to aseptic technique and to immediately correct any break in technique.

SUMMARY OF SCENARIO

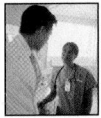

Melissa is finding her surgical medical assisting position at Lakeside Surgical Associates to be rewarding, exciting, and challenging. She enjoys coming to work every day and has learned all aspects of her position much more quickly than most of her peers. Melissa frequently reads the latest information on new developments in minor surgery practice. Her concern for her patient's well-being makes her stand out, and the clinic constantly gets positive comments on her level of professionalism.

Melissa made several mistakes during her first year as a surgical medical assistant, but she learned from each situation and has never covered up a mistake. She has communicated with her supervisor and the surgeon whenever she realized later that she did not follow procedure. This allowed errors to be discussed and corrected if possible and will most likely result in her not making similar mistakes again.

Melissa is a team player who consistently tries to anticipate the surgeon's and patient's needs both before and during surgery. Her cooperative, supportive manner is appreciated by everyone on the surgical team.

SUMMARY of LEARNING OBJECTIVES

1. Define, spell, and pronounce the terms listed in the vocabulary.
   - Spelling and pronouncing medical terms correctly adds credibility to the medical assistant. Knowing the definition of these terms promotes confidence in communication with patients and co-workers.

2. Define the concepts of aseptic technique.
   - Medical asepsis is the process of either decreasing the number of or destruction of all pathogens and surgical asepsis is the complete destruction of all organisms on instruments or equipment that will enter the patient's body. Using proper

Continued

SUMMARY of LEARNING OBJECTIVES

Continued

surgical aseptic technique is the primary means of preventing unnecessary postoperative infections in surgical patients. Everyone on the surgical team is responsible for preventing and correcting breaks in technique.

3. Explain the differences among sanitization, disinfection, and sterilization.
   - Sanitization is the cleaning of instruments and the environment to reduce the number of pathogenic microorganisms. Disinfection is the destruction of pathogens by physical or chemical means. Sterilization is the destruction of all microorganisms.

4. Demonstrate how to wrap instrument packs for autoclave sterilization.
   - Procedure 56-1 describes how to wrap instruments for sterilization.

5. Explain the types and uses of sterilization indicators.
   - Autoclave tape contains a chemical dye that changes color when exposed to steam. Biologic sterilization indicators include a spore strip indicator, which contains a temperature-sensitive dye that changes color when the proper combination of steam, temperature, and time has been achieved. An indicator strip should be placed in the center of the largest pack.

6. Summarize the correct methods for loading, operating, and unloading an autoclave.
   - Arrange the load so there is maximum circulation of steam and heat. Articles should be resting on edges; jars and bottles should be placed on their sides. When the cycle is complete, release the pressure according to the manufacturer's guidelines, stand back from the door, and, with heat-resistant gloves, open the door approximately $1/4$ inch. Allow the load to dry for at least 15 minutes before removal.

7. Demonstrate how to operate an autoclave.
   - Procedure 56-2 describes how to operate an autoclave.

8. Summarize common minor surgical procedures.
   - Typical minor surgical procedures include I&D of a cyst; electrosurgery, which uses high-frequency current to cut through tissue and coagulate blood vessels; laser surgery, which uses tiny light beams to safely treat specific tissues with minimal damage to surrounding tissues and limit scar formation; microsurgery, which involves the use of an operating microscope to perform delicate surgical procedures; endoscopic procedures, which use a fiberoptic instrument with a miniature camera mounted on a flexible tube to examine within an organ or cavity and which are named according to the organs or areas they explore; and cryosurgery, which is the use of extreme cold to destroy tissues such as warts and skin lesions.

9. Detail the medical assistant's role in minor office surgery.
   - The medical assistant is responsible for preparing the patient for surgery; performing the physician's preoperative orders; confirming the patient has signed an informed consent;

making sure that all patient questions and concerns have been addressed; assisting with positioning the patient; performing skin preparation if ordered; and preparing the room for the procedure.

10. Perform a skin prep for surgery.
    - Procedure 56-3 describes how to perform a surgical skin prep.

11. Perform a surgical hand scrub.
    - A surgical hand scrub is done to lower the number of transient and resident bacteria on practitioner hands so that the risk of wound contamination is decreased. Procedure 56-4 outlines how to perform a surgical hand scrub.

12. Outline the rules for setting up and maintaining a sterile field.
    - Sterile surfaces must never come into contact with nonsterile surfaces. If this occurs, the sterile surface immediately is considered contaminated. The rules for maintaining a sterile field include keeping talking to a minimum; maintaining sight of the sterile field; and never crossing over the sterile field. Anything that falls below the edge of the Mayo tray and within a 1-inch border surrounding the tray is considered contaminated. A sterile barrier that is wet, cut, or torn is contaminated. Keep sterile gloved hands above waist level at all times. Never remove then replace any item into the field. A sterile package should be opened the entire way and the contents tossed onto the field without crossing over the sterile area; if a sterile package falls to the floor, it must be discarded. If there is ever any doubt about sterility, consider the field contaminated and start all over again.

13. Open a sterile pack to create a sterile field.
    - Procedure 56-5 describes how to open a sterile pack to create a sterile field.

14. Transfer sterile instruments and pour solutions into a sterile field.
    - Procedures 56-6 and 56-7 outline how to use sterile transfer forceps and pour solutions into a basin on a sterile field.

15. Apply sterile gloves without contamination.
    - Procedure 56-8 describes how to apply sterile gloves.

16. Don a sterile gown and gloves while maintaining a sterile field.
    - Procedures 56-9 and 56-10 list how to don a sterile gown and sterile gloves with a gown on.

17. Demonstrate how to assist with a minor surgical procedure and suturing.
    - Procedures 56-11 and 56-12 explain the details of assisting with a minor surgical procedure and the application of sutures.

18. Summarize postoperative instructions and care of wounds.
    - If medication is prescribed, review the purpose of the medication and directions for its use with the patient and his or her companion and make a follow-up appointment. The patient should be taught to care for himself or herself at home after surgery and should receive both verbal and written instructions. Explain to the patient the importance of calling the office if there are any questions or if he or she notes redness around the operative site, bleeding from the wound, fever, swelling, or

Continued

SUMMARY of LEARNING OBJECTIVES
Continued

increasing or severe pain. If the patient does not call within the next 24 hours, you should call the patient.

19. Explain the process of wound healing.
    - All wounds go through a healing or repair process that has three phases. The lag phase occurs first when the blood vessels contract to control hemorrhage, and platelets form a fibrin network and a clot dries into a scab. Proliferation is a new growth period during which tissues repair themselves. During the final or remodeling phase a bridge of new tissue is built to close the gap of the wound. Collagen gives the wounded tissues strength and forms scar tissue. Wounds are classified by the way they repair themselves—either by first intention, with clean straight edges that heal quickly, or by granulation, with tissues that are severely damaged and are left open or fail to close, which is called second intention.

20. Properly apply dressings and bandages to surgical sites.
    - Procedures 56-13 and 56-15 describe how to apply a sterile dressing and supportive bandage to a wound.

21. Conduct patient education in aseptic technique and surgical procedures.

- The best time to instruct your patient in aseptic techniques to be used at home is while you are performing an aseptic procedure. Patient education includes the purpose and importance of hand washing; using disposable tissues to cover the nose and mouth when coughing or sneezing and properly disposing of used tissues; the differences between sterile and clean dressings and bandages and step by step instructions on how to change a dressing properly and dispose of contaminated items.

22. Discuss the legal and ethical concerns regarding surgical asepsis and infection control.
    - The medical assistant must know what procedure is to be performed and whether the patient has received and provided informed consent. The medical assistant must realize the full extent of his or her role as patient advocate and physician agent. Increasing the patient's understanding ensures greater compliance with presurgical preparations, and the patient will be more likely to follow instructions and advice after surgery. A major responsibility for the medical assistant is commitment to adhere strictly to aseptic techniques and to immediately correct any break in technique.

CONNECTIONS

 Study Guide Connection: Go to Chapter 56 Study Guide. Read the Case Study and Workplace Applications and complete the assignments. Do online research for answers to the questions in the Internet Activities associated with surgical asepsis and assisting with surgical procedures.

 CD Connection: Go to the Medical Assisting Competency Challenge CD and do the training activities under Infection Control and Patient Care. For a better understanding of the inflammatory response and controlling infection, view the animations for antibiotics and phagocytosis.

 Evolve Connection: For more information related to surgical asepsis and assisting with surgical procedures, go to evolve.elsevier.com/kinn and visit related weblinks for Chapter 56. Click on the Medical Assisting Exam Review and do the practice questions to sharpen your test-taking skills.

Career Development and Life Skills

57

SCENARIO

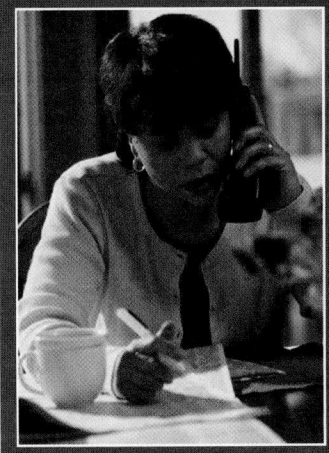

Lisa Walker is 1 month away from graduating from her medical assisting program. She has been an excellent student and is looking forward to beginning her career in the medical field. Lisa wants to begin her job search now to minimize the time during which she is not employed after her externship ends.

Lisa has participated in several volunteer activities while she has been attending school. She plans to list these experiences on her resume. She met many office managers and physicians while doing volunteer work, and she will be contacting those people in hopes of obtaining more job leads.

Lisa began saving for interview clothing when she first began school. She is on a strict budget, but she found several outfits appropriate for interviews at secondhand clothing shops and discount stores. Her best-looking suit cost only $25!

Not a person afraid to interview, Lisa looks forward to sharing her skills and experience with potential employers. She looks on each interview as a practice session for the next one, and this helps her to relax more and present a true picture of herself to the office manager. She has a great smile and projects a natural friendliness and positive attitude.

Lisa has given much thought to what she wants from her first job as a medical assistant. She knows that she may not start at a high salary, but she also realizes that there are benefits and perquisites ("perks") to working in a physician's office. She plans to commit to working for 2 years on her first job, gaining experience before looking for her next job at a higher salary and with additional benefits.

Lisa is excited about her future as a medical assistant. She is ready to put the training she received to work with actual patients. She plans to perform exceptionally well at her externship site and to go above and beyond her designated duties to impress the staff in that facility, who will become references for her first paid position. Lisa is dedicated to becoming the best medical assistant possible and becoming indispensable to her employer.

While studying this chapter, think about the following questions:

- How can the medical assistant prepare for his or her first job throughout the duration of training?
- What is meant by "writing your resume every day"?

- How can the medical assistant organize the job search?
- How can the new medical assistant employee make a positive, lasting impression on co-workers and supervisors?

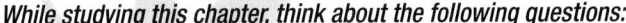

LEARNING OBJECTIVES

1. Define, spell, and pronounce the terms listed in the vocabulary.
2. Discuss the reasons that job search training is important to a medical assistant.
3. List three expectations that employers have of employees.
4. Understand the three types of employee skill strengths.
5. Explain the two best job search methods.
6. Describe some of the errors that should be avoided on a resume.
7. Explain the importance of having demographic information about former jobs before appearing for an interview.
8. List the four phases of the interview process.

9. Discuss the importance of the probationary period for a new employee.
10. List some mistakes that should be avoided by a new employee.
11. Explain why a performance appraisal's ratings are usually not perfect.
12. Prepare a resume.
13. Organize a job search.
14. Complete a job application.
15. Interview for a job.
16. Negotiate a salary.

National Accreditation Competencies and Content

CAAHEP COMPETENCIES

General

3.a.(1)(a). Schedule and manage appointments
3.c.(1)(a). Respond to and initiate written communications
3.c.(1)(b). Recognize and respond to verbal communications
3.c.(1)(c). Recognize and respond to nonverbal communications

ABHES COMPETENCIES

Professionalism

1.a. Project a positive attitude
1.g. Evidence a responsible attitude
1.i. Conduct work within scope of education, training, and ability

Communication

2.e. User proper telephone techniques
2.f. Interview effectively
2.j. Use correct grammar, spelling, and formatting techniques in written works
2.o. Fundamental writing skills
2.q. Allied health professions and credentialing

VOCABULARY

appraisals Expert judgments of the value or merit of; also, evaluations of work performance.

counteroffer Return offer made by one who has rejected an offer or job.

defaults Fails to pay financial debts, such as a student loan.

deferment Postponement, especially of a student loan.

genuineness Expressing sincerity and honest feeling.

intolerable Not tolerable or bearable.

mock Simulated; intended for imitation or practice.

networking Exchange of information or services among individuals, groups, or institutions; also, meeting and getting to know individuals in the same or similar career fields and sharing information about available opportunities.

pertinent (pur′-tuh-nent) Having a clear, decisive relevance to the matter at hand.

proofread To read and mark corrections.

ramifications Consequence; outgrowth; something produced by a cause or necessarily following from a set of conditions.

rectify (rek′-tuh-fy) To correct by removing errors.

subtle Ingenious; artful; delicate.

succinct (suhk-sinkt′) Marked by compact, precise expression without wasted words.

synopsis Condensed statement or outline.

vocation The work in which a person is regularly employed.

Each day that a person exists is a small portion of a whole—in this case, the person's entire lifetime. The events that happen during a day, no matter how small, shape the future. In the same way, the events that happen in the life of a medical assistant play a role in shaping his or her career. Every day, he or she "writes a resume"–through actions that will reveal strengths, highlight skills, and summarize accomplishments–that builds on the medical assistant's **vocation.** Each duty performed becomes a part of the medical assistant's sum of experience and is important in the overall growth of the individual. Each action taken can have an impact on the future for the medical assistant. If the actions are professional, accurate, and performed to his or her utmost ability, the resume that the medical assistant is writing through these actions will be one that will lead to greater opportunities. If the medical assistant performs poorly, the resume will be one that will not reflect trustworthiness and dependability. The small decisions that are made every day are those that greatly affect the overall impressions that the medical assistant makes in the workplace.

Approximately 85% of persons seeking employment have never had any type of formal training in the job search process. A newly graduated medical assistant should take advantage of job search training for three reasons:

- The training will decrease the amount of time spent searching for a job.
- The training will increase the chances of receiving better wages through negotiations.
- The training will help to eliminate the fears of looking for work and interviewing.

WHAT DOES THE EMPLOYER WANT?

Employers have three basic desires when they are interviewing individuals for a job:

- They want a person who has a neat appearance and looks as if he or she fits the job (Figure 57-1).
- They want an individual who is dependable and can prove that he or she has been a reliable team member in other job positions.
- They want a person with the skills to do the job.

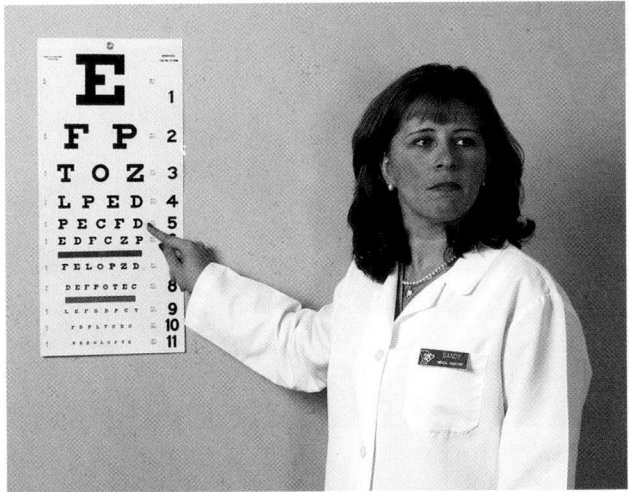

Figure 57-1 A professional appearance is mandatory in the medical office.

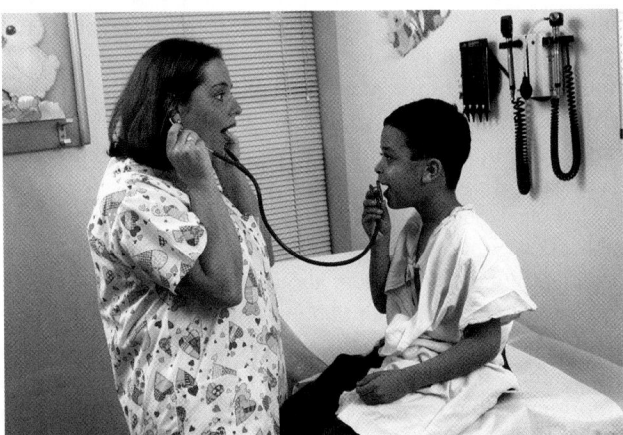

Figure 57-2 A great attitude is the best personal asset. Employers in the medical profession want medical assistants who will exhibit a positive attitude with the patients.

From the beginning of the job search process, a medical assistant's attitude is the most critical part of his or her potential success in getting a job (Figure 57-2). A good attitude is not a trait that can be developed overnight. For this reason a medical assistant must have a positive outlook in all situations, so the **genuineness** of his or her demeanor will be clear during job interviews.

CRITICAL THINKING APPLICATION

Lisa knows that attitude is of primary importance on a job. How can she prove to a potential employer in an interview that she has a good attitude? What exactly constitutes a good attitude? A bad attitude? What does it take to change an attitude from bad to good?

ASSESSING STRENGTHS

Before promoting himself or herself as a potential employee, a medical assistant must first determine the strengths that make him or her a valuable team member. There are three types of skill strengths: job skills, self-management skills, and transferable skills.

Job skills are the abilities that the medical assistant needs to perform the job. This includes such skills as performing venipuncture, billing insurance, answering the telephone, scheduling appointments, giving injections, and handling other tasks.

Self-management skills relate to the medical assistant's personality and character traits. They include such attributes as honesty, integrity, and enthusiasm.

Transferable skills can be taken from one job to another. For instance, if the medical assistant has the ability to communicate effectively, this skill can be used on every job. Leadership is a transferable skill, as are the ability to follow directions and the ability to manage people.

CRITICAL THINKING APPLICATION

Lisa expects potential employers to ask her what her strengths are. She has determined six specific strengths that she can prove with examples from past positions or her externship. What six strengths can you prove? Give examples of each of these strengths.

DEVELOPING CAREER OBJECTIVES

Each medical assistant has a reason for entering the healthcare field. This basic desire should influence decisions concerning his or her career choices. Because medical assisting is such a versatile profession, a medical assistant will have numerous options after graduation.

It is wise to take some time to think about what the medical assistant wants from his or her career. While he or she is attending school and subsequently completing an externship, ideas may surface about what specialty to enter.

When developing career objectives, the medical assistant should start by asking several questions:
- Where am I today?
- Where will I be in 5 years?
- Where will I be in 10 years?
- What additional skills do I need to get where I want to go?

Write down the questions and answers, and go into specific detail. Set realistic goals, and develop a plan as to how and when they will be reached. It is helpful to put a list of goals in a prominent place at home, where they will be seen every day. Some people use the front of the refrigerator, and some post the goals on the mirror in the area where they get dressed every day. Write goals in a visible place to keep them in mind even on the more difficult days, when they seem far from sight.

CRITICAL THINKING APPLICATION

Lisa knows that goals are important when attempting to achieve in life. She has five goals written regarding her job search and her first position as a medical assistant. What are some goals that are realistic regarding the job search? What realistic goals could be developed with regard to the first position as a medical assistant?

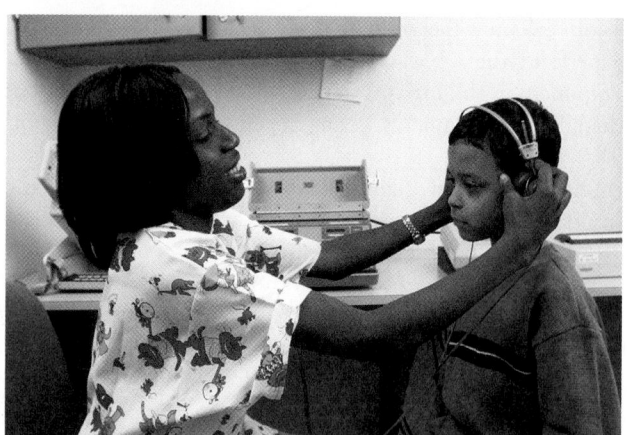

Figure 57-3 Enjoyment of the job is paramount. Medical assistants should enjoy their job and give compassionate, friendly care to all patients.

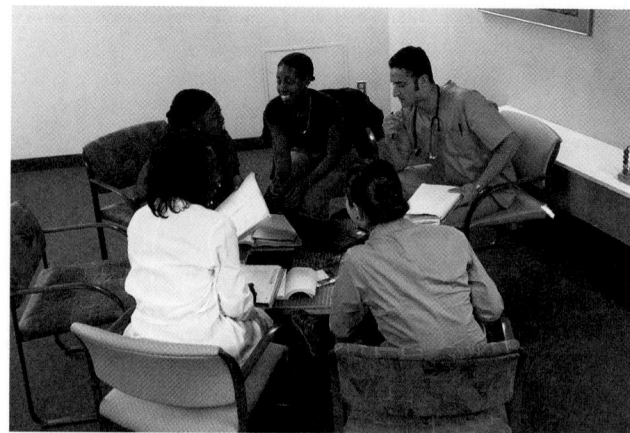

Figure 57-4 Stay in touch with classmates. Classmates are excellent networking contacts and may be able to provide job leads.

KNOWING PERSONAL NEEDS

A medical assistant must evaluate all of the needs that he or she requires in a work situation. Most people have a minimum salary that they require, as well as certain benefits. For example, if the medical assistant is a single mother, she may require a moderate salary and insist on health insurance benefits. We also have intrinsic needs, which are those internal desires that are important to us personally.

A helpful activity is to write a **synopsis** of a typical day on an ideal medical assisting job. Imagine the type of office, the job title, the daily duties, and the salary and benefits that would be a part of the ideal job (Figure 57-3). This will help to develop a focus and a goal to work toward as the medical assistant's career develops.

FINDING A JOB

Many people have misconceptions about the job market that exists today. Graduation from a medical assisting program does not guarantee that the student will obtain employment. Completion of the program will give the medical assistant the job skills needed to work, but a good attitude and positive outlook are essential for success in the job search.

Some job seekers assume that potential employers will not interact with students until they graduate. However, prospecting before graduation is a smart idea, and there are **subtle** ways of introducing oneself to a facility without bluntly asking for employment. Many also think that they must have work experience to be hired, but employers are more interested in attitude and teachability than a long resume full of experience. In fact, many physicians like hiring students fresh from school so that they can teach them how they want procedures done.

The Two Best Job Search Methods

Although there are many ways to find employment, two methods have proved to be the best and most effective. These are **networking** and direct contact with employers.

Networking is the exchange of information or services among individuals, groups, or institutions. When related to a job search, networking involves meeting and getting to know individuals in the same or similar career fields and sharing information about available opportunities. A medical assistant should begin to form a network of friends, business associates, co-workers, and acquaintances early in training, and he or she should stay in contact with these people throughout the job search effort (Figure 57-4).

How does one network? One way is by joining professional medical assisting organizations. The members that attend regular meetings often know about job leads in the area. The medical assistant should also tell his or her personal physician(s) about being in school and the approximate time of graduation. Friends and family members can be on the lookout for potential opportunities and may help by asking their personal physicians if they are aware of positions that will open for applications soon. Always keep a few resumes on hand—the opportunity to network could come at any time.

Networking is not limited to job searching, and many organizations are formed to develop networks of individuals or groups that assist one another and refer clients to one another. However, these groups are useful to the person who is looking for employment, and by attending meetings and get-togethers held for networking purposes, the medical assistant may happen onto the ideal job he or she has been looking for.

CRITICAL THINKING APPLICATION

Lisa knows that networking is a great way to secure employment. She is making a list of people with whom she can share her resume or inform that she is now ready to seek employment as a medical assistant. How many people can you think of who are good prospects for networking?

Direct contact with employers is also an effective method of job searching. Medical assistants often know of specific clinics or facilities that they would like to investigate as job possibilities. Compile a list of these places, and learn as much about them as possible. If the facility has a website, read it thoroughly. Ask for brochures about the employer. Some have an annual report that lists details about the organization. All of this information will help the medical assistant get a good basic idea of why the facility exists and what it does for the community.

Contact with employers does not necessarily begin only after the student has graduated. Students can begin networking and contacting employers from the very start of their enrollment at school. The student may wish to keep a file of potential employers. Make a list of facilities that are good prospects for employment, then begin researching them. Call to find out who supervises medical assistants in the facility. In a physician's office, this is usually the office manager. Then call the office manager and ask to make an appointment to learn about the facility. Even the busiest people are usually willing to help a student investigate healthcare facilities in the area.

Do not express to the office manager that the objective of the appointment is a job offer. The goal at this point is to learn about the facility, what it offers the community, and what roles the medical assistants in the facility perform. Suggest that the appointment be set at his or her convenience. Then treat the appointment like an actual job interview, dressing appropriately and arriving on time. Have a list of questions about the facility prepared in advance, and do not take too much of the office manager's time. Take notes about what the office manager says about the facility so that they can be referred to on graduation, during the actual job search.

After the appointment with the office manager, ask for a business card and always send a thank-you note or letter. Do not fail to remember this critical point! This helps the office manager to remember the name of the medical assistant and is a pleasant addition to the daily mail. Everyone enjoys being recognized for his or her efforts, and the office manager will appreciate the thank-you note.

Toward the time that he or she is to graduate, the medical assistant may wish to perform an externship at one of the facilities visited early in training. Check with school regulations to determine whether this is possible. Then the office manager can be approached about allowing the student to extern in the office. Be sure to follow school guidelines when investigating these possibilities. Some schools allow students to secure their own externship sites, but this must be discussed with the externship supervisor at school. Performing an externship at a medical facility is usually the first practical experience the student will have in the medical field and can be used as a reference in building a resume.

After the externship is completed, the medical assistant may wish to send a resume to all of the office managers met through the direct contact efforts made earlier in his or her training. A professional resume with a cover letter that refers to the earlier meeting will prompt the office manager to remember the student. Ask in the cover letter whether any opportunities exist in the facility. Express to the office manager that the facility and staff were impressive on the first meeting and that it would be an exciting place to begin a career. In the letter, request that if the office manager does not have any positions available at that time, the resume be kept on file or be passed along to an acquaintance who is looking for an additional staff member.

The Internet and the Job Search

The Internet opens a whole new world of opportunity when it comes to job searching. The medical assistant can find a gargantuan amount of information about writing resumes, interviewing, and follow-up methods, but perhaps most important, the Internet can provide information about who is hiring right now.

Many databases provide information about job openings. Monster, Yahoo! Jobs, and the Online Career Center are a few examples. The search can be targeted to specific geographic areas, certain career fields, or even specific job titles. Conduct a search in a selected state (or metropolitan area), then look for jobs in the medical profession, then narrow the field even more by asking for information on jobs specifically for medical assistants.

The medical assistant can also express interest in a job by perusing the company website then contacting the employer directly on the "contact us" page. Anyone looking at the website should be able to find an email address to use for gathering additional information. Express that the school encourages seeking quality businesses as potential employers, and ask for information that could be presented to a class. Most employers are happy to get the word out about their company and may give all kinds of pamphlets and "freebies" to share with a class. By sending a thank-you note and staying in touch with the company, the medical assistant creates a new lead for the job search.

Just remember, the information available to one medical assistant on the Internet is also available to every other medical assistant. The Internet is great for researching positions and companies, but networking and direct contact are still the most successful ways to obtain a job. The medical assistant's "whole package"–meaning the resume, application, interview, follow-up, attitude, appearance, and job skills–all combine to make an impression on the employer. Will that impression be favorable enough to result in a job offer?

Traditional Job Search Methods

The more traditional job search methods may be effective but are usually not as successful as networking and contacting employers directly.

Newspaper Ads

Newspaper ads normally produce a huge number of applicants and resumes for the employer. A resume or application will have to stand out in the crowd to be noticed when it arrives at the facility. Some applicants use clear envelopes, which draw attention to the resume quickly in a stack of mail.

Employment Agencies

Employment agencies usually charge a fee for their services. Even when the employer pays the fee, the medical assistant may be offered a lower wage to compensate for the fee. These agencies can be useful, however. In salary negotiation the agency will know the salary range the employer is willing to pay. This means that medical assistants can command a salary within that range and not be short-changed by asking for a salary that is much lower than the employer was willing to pay.

CRITICAL THINKING APPLICATION

Lisa keeps an eye on the local newspapers for ads that mention a need for medical assistants. What current ads in local papers are interesting and would prompt sending a resume?

Professional Societies

Joining local chapters of medical assistant organizations helps the student in many ways. Not only will valuable information be exchanged at the meetings, but the medical assistant may also hear of positions that are becoming available in various medical facilities. This is a form of networking.

Volunteering

By volunteering in medical offices or facilities, the medical assistant will meet other professionals who may be able to provide job leads. Volunteer activities should be added to the resume, because these valuable experiences can often be used in the physician's office as well. It does not matter that the position was not a paid job; experience counts, whether paid or not.

Mailing Resumes

Mailing a large number of resumes is not a very effective method of job search. Out of 100 resumes sent, one or two potential employers may respond with a request for an interview. It is much more effective to network first, then follow up with a good cover letter and resume. Resumes can be used when contacting employers directly, and this approach allows the medical assistant to meet at least one employee of the facility when the document is delivered. Be sure to ask for a business card and write down the name of the person to whom the resume was delivered. For impressive facilities, send a note of thanks to the person who accepted the resume, asking to be considered for future positions.

Cold Calling

Cold calling is contacting employers by phone and prospecting for available positions. If the medical assistant asks, "Are you hiring?" at the beginning of the conversation, he or she should expect a negative answer and has just wasted the call. This is all but useless in the job search effort. However, an assistant who calls for information about the clinic and schedules an appointment with the office manager may have more success. Never attempt to get a job over the phone. Even when interested employers call and ask questions, attempt to set up an interview to discuss your qualifications in person.

Performing Well on Externships

Performing well on externships may be one of the best ways to secure a job. If an opening exists, the medical assistant extern is already oriented to the practice and may be the perfect fit for the job. Perform duties assigned on the externship as if they were final examinations at school. Even when the office does not have a position available at that time, there may be one soon,

or the office manager or physician may know of an office that has an opening. Do the best job possible, and there may be an employment offer waiting at the conclusion of the externship. Be ready to learn from the moment the externship begins until the moment it ends.

ORGANIZING THE JOB SEARCH

Seeking a job is a full-time job. The new medical assistant must put forth effort, have stamina, and be persistent. Do not expect to get a job with the first practice that offers an interview. By keeping track of opportunities found, one will be more likely to obtain employment in a short time after graduation (Procedure 57-1).

A job lead is any information that could lead to a position, either now or in the future. Some of the most promising job leads for the newly graduated medical assistant come from the externship experience. Be friendly and meet as many people as possible while completing this part of training. Ask for business cards, and stay in contact with the medical professionals met at the externship site and nearby hospitals. Be willing to shake hands and make introductions at all times so that the circle of promising contacts for job leads continues to expand.

The medical assistant would be wise to keep a record of all job leads (Figure 57-5). The name and address of the facility, contact name, and phone numbers are all important items of information. Keep track of where the lead was obtained so that if it is provided by an individual, that person can be thanked properly, especially if the lead results in a job offer. These records are an excellent starting place when making calls to set up job interviews. Remember, the placement office at school is a resource for job leads but should not be the only source used for obtaining leads. Each medical assistant graduate must take personal responsibility for finding and following up on job opportunities.

The job lead is not the only information that should be recorded during job search efforts. Keep a record of arrangements when an interview is secured, including information such as the following:

- Day, date, and time of the interview
- Directions to the interview site
- Name of the person to interview with
- Items to bring to the interview
- Information about the company or facility

As soon as the interview is over, the medical assistant should record information about the interview itself. After several interviews, it may be difficult to remember which opportunity offered what salary, which had medical benefits, and which was closest to home. By keeping accurate records, the medical assistant can follow up in whatever way is appropriate and send a note or letter of appreciation to the person who conducted the interview (Figure 57-6).

DEVELOPING A RESUME

A resume is a fact sheet that summarizes an applicant's qualifications, education, and experience. A medical assistant must

PROCEDURE 57-1

Organize a Job Search

<u>ABHES COMPETENCY:</u> 6.f

GOAL: *To devote adequate time to and organize the job search in an efficient way so that proper follow-up can be conducted.*

EQUIPMENT and SUPPLIES

- Record of a Job Lead form
- Record of an Interview form
- Copies of resume
- List of interview questions
- Contact information for former employers and references
- Map of geographic area or printout from Internet mapping program
- Internet access
- Computer
- Job search weblinks
- Local newspapers
- Contact information for friends and family

PROCEDURAL STEPS

1. Format the resume as an accurate, up-to-date document.
   <u>PURPOSE:</u> If the resume is kept on a computer, it can be easily updated and targeted for various job opportunities.
2. Make copies of the record of job lead form and record of interview form.
3. Research job search websites and newspapers for job leads.
4. Network and contact employers directly to obtain job leads.
   <u>PURPOSE:</u> Networking and direct employer contact are the best two methods of job searching.
5. Gather information on job leads, and complete a record of Job Lead form for each one.
   <u>PURPOSE:</u> Employers are impressed when the person being

interviewed is familiar with the company; much information can be found on the company's website.

6. Prepare a targeted copy of the resume for each job lead.
   <u>PURPOSE:</u> Targeted resumes are designed to highlight the candidate's skills for a particular job, and the resume can be tailored for each specific company easily on a computer.
7. Take the resume to the facility and ask to complete an application, or....
8. Email the resume to the facility according to directions listed in the job advertisement.
9. Document all activity on each job lead.
   <u>PURPOSE:</u> The job search should be an organized process.
10. Schedule interviews for as many facilities as possible.
    <u>PURPOSE:</u> The more interviews, the better prepared the candidate will be.
11. Keep a record of job details on the record of the interview form for later reference.
    <u>PURPOSE:</u> Keeping a record of the details about each job possibility helps to keep them organized and is useful in comparing job offers.
12. Send thank-you notes to all professionals who grant an interview when the appointment is over.
    <u>PURPOSE:</u> Never fail to send a thank-you note, because this gesture may be the deciding factor in securing the job.
13. Compare opportunities when making a choice between offered positions.

---

determine what to include in the resume, remembering that he or she is "selling" himself or herself to an employer (Procedure 57-2). The resume should be developed before cover letters are written or job applications are completed so that strengths can be identified and highlighted on all job search documents.

There are many types of resumes. Three of the most common include the chronologic resume, the functional resume, and the targeted resume. A chronologic resume highlights the medical assistant's abilities in a logical order, such as most recent jobs back to the beginning of the individual's career (Figure 57-7, p. 1331). A functional resume highlights specific skill sets, emphasizing the most important abilities or the most valuable experiences that the medical assistant has performed (Figure 57-8, p. 1331). A targeted resume is perhaps the most effective: it emphasizes the skills that relate specifically to the job for which the medical assistant is applying (Figure 57-9, p. 1332).

A medical assistant should target the resume toward the specific job that he or she is applying for. This means that the job requirements should be compared with the skills on the resume, and those skills should be highlighted in the document

using action words (Figure 57-10, p. 1332). Of course, to do this effectively the medical assistant must actually know the job requirements. One can assume that clinical and administrative duties will be similar from place to place, but the ad for the position may provide further information about the scope of duties for the position. A medical assistant should read these carefully and emphasize that those are a part of his or her skill set on the resume.

Compose the resume and save it on the computer hard drive, a CD, or other storage device. Keep a copy on a flash drive so that the information is readily available if needed when away from the primary computer. Then as each job opportunity presents itself the resume can be modified to fit the job. For instance, if the resume lists back-office skills first and the job is for an administrative position, the administrative skills should be moved to the top to draw more attention to them. This is easy to accomplish when the resume is on a computer, because the medical assistant can cut and paste where necessary to make changes and save several versions of the resume. Then an original can be printed on high-quality paper for every job for which he or she applies.

Record of a Job Lead

Job Title _____ Medical Office/Facility Name _____

Phone Number_____ Fax Number _____

Contact Name _____ Contact Title _____

Contact Phone Number/Extension _____

Physician(s) _____ Office Manager _____

Office/Facility Address _____

City _____ State _____ Zip _____

Referred By _____ Phone Number _____

Date First Contacted _____ Person Spoken To _____

Information Submitted:

❏ Cover Letter   ❏   Resume   ❏   References

Date Sent _____   Date Sent _____   Date Sent _____

First Interview Scheduled: Day/Date _____   Time _____

Interviewer Name _____   Phone _____

Second Interview Scheduled: Day/Date _____   Time _____

Interviewer Name _____   Phone _____

Travel Directions _____

_____

_____

Office/Facility Information _____

_____

Basic Job Duties _____

_____

Miscellaneous Information _____

_____

_____

_____

(staple a business card to this form from the office/facility – use back for additional information)

Figure 57-5 Record of a job lead.

Record of an Interview

Job Title _____ Medical Office/Facility Name _____

Phone Number_____Fax Number _____

Contact Name _____ Contact Title _____

Contact Phone Number/Extension _____

Physician(s) _____Office Manager _____

Office/Facility Address _____

City _____ State _____ Zip _____

Interviewer Name _____ Phone _____

Travel Directions _____

_____

_____

Office/Facility Information _____

_____

Basic Job Duties _____

_____

Benefits/Salary Discussed _____

_____

Hours/Days to Work _____

General Impression of Office and Personnel _____

Questions as a result of interview _____

_____

Self-Evaluation of Interview Performance _____

_____

Thank-you sent ❑ yes ❑ no Date _____ Job Offer ❑ yes ❑ no (use back for notes)

Other Follow-up _____

_____

_____
(staple a business card to this form from the office/facility – use back for additional information)

Figure 57-6 Record of an interview.

PROCEDURE 57-2

Prepare a Resume

ABHES COMPETENCY: 2.j

GOAL: *To write an effective resume for use as a tool in gaining employment.*

EQUIPMENT and SUPPLIES

- Scratch paper
- Pen or pencil
- Former job descriptions, if available
- List of addresses of former employers and schools and names of supervisors
- Computer or word processor
- Quality stationery and envelopes

PROCEDURAL STEPS

1. Perform a self-evaluation by making notes about your strengths as a medical assistant. Consider job skills, self-management skills, and transferable skills.
   UNDERLINE PURPOSE: To determine the strongest aspects of your abilities so that they can be highlighted on the resume.

2. Explore formatting, and decide on a professional resume appearance that best highlights your skills and experience. Use the templates available in word processing software, or design your own.
   PURPOSE: To construct an attractive document.

3. Place your name, address, and two telephone numbers where you can be contacted at the top of the resume.
   PURPOSE: To make certain that potential employers have a means of contact.

4. Write a job objective that specifies your employment goals.
   PURPOSE: To give the prospective employer an idea of what you are looking for in a medical assisting position.

5. Provide details about your educational experience. List degrees and/or certifications obtained.

6. Provide details about your work experience. Include all contact information and names of supervisors. Do not include salary expectations or reasons for leaving former jobs.
   PURPOSE: No negative information should be put on the resume. Salaries should be discussed; if a certain salary is listed on the resume, it may limit the amount that the facility will offer the medical assistant.

7. Prepare a cover letter and a list of references. Send the references with the resume only when requested.

8. Type the resume carefully, and make certain that there are no errors on the document.
   PURPOSE: Resumes submitted with errors are often discarded without consideration.

9. Proofread the resume. Allow another person to read it as well and look for missed errors.
   PURPOSE: To make certain that the resume is error free.

10. Print the resume on high-quality paper. Review the resume again for errors and to assure that it looks attractive on the printed page.

11. Target each resume to a specific person or position. Do not send generic resumes to each prospective employer.
    PURPOSE: Targeted resumes get better results during the job search.

12. For all resumes that are distributed, follow up with a phone call to arrange an interview.
    PURPOSE: A resume sent without follow-up is usually ineffective.

A resume is an important job search tool, but it should never be expected to get the medical assistant a job on its own merit. It is but one of many tools that should be used when looking for employment. Developing a professional resume takes some time and effort, and it will prove to be a good investment. Give the document some thought, and follow generally accepted guidelines for its construction.

CRITICAL THINKING APPLICATION

Lisa has drafted her resume and given a copy to her placement director. She has recommended that Lisa remove the mention of her volunteer experience, because it was not in the medical field. Should Lisa do this? Why or why not?

Critical Resume Errors

The first error that should be avoided on a resume is just that—any error. There should be no errors at all on a resume;

many employers will automatically disqualify a job candidate if one is found.

One medical assistant who was having a difficult time finding a job consulted her placement director at school. The director suggested that she come in for a **mock** interview. About halfway through the interview, the placement director realized the problem. The medical assistant had worked for 2 years at a local grocery store and had misspelled the name of the store on the resume. From an employer's point of view, a person who cannot spell the name of a facility in which she worked for a length of time, even though she cashed a paycheck with the company name on it, might well make critical errors in charting or in other aspects of her duties. Within a week after this error was corrected, the medical assistant found a job.

Never list salary expectations on the resume. If the medical assistant lists a salary of $25,000 on the last job held, the future employer might not offer more than $26,000 to $27,000, realizing that this is a step up from the last salary. However, if

Ruby Dunham
9362 Caesar Creek Road
Mytown, OH 45458
(937) 555-1899
rdunham@comcast.net

Education

• 1998: A.S. in Medical Assisting, Community College, Mytown, OH

Experience:

1995–present: Medical Transcriptionist, Community Hospital, Mytown, OH

• Transcribe 55 wpm
• Specialist in medical terminology
• Excellent attendance record
• Detail oriented
• Increased personal productivity each quarter

1990–1995: Secretary, State University School of Medicine, Mytown, OH

• Coordinated schedules of four full-time professors
• Maintained office supply and assistant budget
• Created final examination scheduling guidelines for department
• Developed excellent written communication skills
• Familiar with a variety of office machines

1986–1990: Shift Manager, Burger World, Mytown, OH

• Managed 10 employees, including hiring, training, evaluating, and firing
• Developed excellent oral communication skills and team player concept
• Improved inventory supply techniques, reducing losses by 10%
• Maintained cleanliness standards highest in chain
• Developed customer-focused service goals for store

Figure 57-7 Chronologic resume.

they had been willing to pay $32,000, the medical assistant has lost an opportunity for much higher wages.

Avoid using "I" or other personal pronouns on the resume. If abbreviations are used on the resume, be sure to spell them out for clarity the first time they are used, if they are not well-known abbreviations. Never include personal information, such as height, weight, age, marital status, number of children, or any other information that is not **pertinent** to the job requirements.

Do not list dates along the left-hand side of the paper. This is distracting and draws attention away from the points that should be emphasized. A resume must be visually appealing and easy to read. The medical assistant should make good use of spacing, margins, indention, capitalization, and underlining to ensure an attractive document. **Proofread** the document several times to be sure there are no errors. It is helpful to have someone else proofread it, because many times the writer of a document misses errors when proofreading.

Never include a photograph with the resume. Photographs can be a discriminatory factor in the hiring process, and the medical assistant should be wary of any employer who requests a photograph with the resume.

One of the most senseless errors common to resumes is not having the appropriate contact information, such as an address

Max Bryan
1234 Rolling View Court
Mytown, OH 45431
(937) 555-3137
maxbryan@yahoo.com

OBJECTIVE

• An entry level position in medical assisting, with the opportunity to utilize and refine skills and training

EDUCATION

• 1998: A.S. in Medical Assisting, Community College, Mytown, OH
Dean's list senior year, cumulative GPA 3.5

STRENGTHS

• Possess excellent interpersonal and communication skills
• Demonstrate consistent positive attitude and high energy
• Caring and compassionate
• Responsible, self-motivated, precise in work
• Experienced in customer-focused service

ACCOMPLISHMENTS

• Tutored students in medical assisting and 12-lead EKG courses Received excellent evaluations and positive results
• Certified Medical Assistant, active member of local AAMA
• Experienced in MS Office programs
• Consistent "excellent" ratings in clinical externships

COMMUNITY ACTIVITIES

• 1995–present: Organized, recruited, and trained 20 others for church hand bell choir, direct weekly practices and monthly performances
• 1996–present: Teach community CPR twice yearly to high school students
• Vice-President Student Government, Community College, Mytown, OH. Recruited members, organized fund-raisers, campaigned successfully for policy changes

EMPLOYMENT

• 1996–present: Tutor, Community College, Mytown, OH
• Waiter, Scott's Place, Mytown, OH

Figure 57-8 Functional resume.

and telephone number. Two phone numbers are suggested, such as a cell phone number and a home phone number, so that there is a better chance of reaching the candidate when it is time to schedule an interview. Place an email address on the front page so that potential employers can make contact quickly. If an interview time becomes available late in the day, having access to job candidates by email may make a difference in who is scheduled and who ultimately gets the job.

The Argument about Length

Professionals disagree about the acceptable length of a resume. One page may be considered the ideal length, but a person with 20 years' experience in the job market will never get all of his or her skills on one page. A medical assistant without previous work experience may easily fit the resume on one page.

Recent trends indicate that a good rule of thumb is to allow one page for every 6 years of experience. If a person has a 20-

Roscoe Patterson
3472 Vienna Woods Lane
Mytown, OH 45449
(937) 555-8874
rpatt@aol.com

Job Target:

• A long-term medical assistant position in a busy and varied medical office

Education:

• 1992: BA in Art History, State University, Mytown, OH
• 1998: AS in Medical Assisting, Community College, Mytown, OH

Capabilities:

• Excellent interpersonal skills and caring attitude
• Detail oriented, with strong analytical and problem-solving abilities
• Utilize solid organizational and time-management abilities in coordinating multiple projects
• Self-starter, take initiative to ensure jobs get done properly and efficiently
• Upbeat, personable, and highly energetic
• Ability to communicate in Spanish and American Sign Language

Accomplishments/Achievements:

• Campaigned for and raised consistent 15% annual increase in contributions and grants, allowing expansion of exhibits and needed renovations to art museum
• Maintained museum budget with 100% accountability
• Organized annual "Art Ball" for 100 contributors under budget
• Museum employee of the year 1995
• Certificates in CPR and EKG; Certified Nursing Assistant; will sit for CMA exam this November

Work History:

• 1998–present: Certified Nursing Assistant, Friendly Nursing Home, Mytown, OH
• 1992–1998: Assistant to the Curator, Mytown Museum of Art, Mytown, OH

Figure 57-9 Targeted resume.

USEFUL ACTION WORDS

Accelerated	Manage
Actively	Motivated
Adapted	Organized
Administered	Originate
Analyze	Participated
Approve	Perform
Completed	Pinpointed
Conceived conduct	Plan
Control	Proficient
Coordinate	Program
Created	Proposed
Delegate	Proved
Demonstrate	Provide
Develop	Recommended
Direct	Reduced
Effect	Reinforced
Eliminated	Reorganized
Established	Responsibilities
Evaluate	Revamped
Expanded	Review
Expedite	Revise
Founded	Schedule
Generated	Significantly
Implemented	Simplify
Improved	Solve
Increased	Strategy
Influence	Streamline
Interpret	Structure
Launched	Successfully
Lead	Supervise
Lecture	Support
Maintain	Teach

Figure 57-10 Use action words when describing skills on the resume.

year career, the resume would be approximately three pages long. This is a general guideline; the document should be as **succinct** as possible while clearly communicating the strengths and background of the applicant. Make certain that contact information such as name, phone number, and an email address are provided on each subsequent page of the resume. The pages should also be numbered if there is more than one.

The Purpose of a Resume

The purpose of a resume is not to get the medical assistant a job, although this is a commonly held belief. The purpose of the cover letter is to get the employer to look at the resume. The purpose of the resume is to get the applicant an interview. The purpose of the interview, of course, is to get the job. Remember this, and use the resume as a tool, along with other strategies for job searching.

The medical assistant should be the person to write the resume, or at the very least should have a hand in its composition. Professional resume services may be helpful, but the person who

knows the most about the experience and education gained is the medical assistant.

CRITICAL THINKING APPLICATION

Lisa has been asked by a potential employer to email her resume. She has used an unusual font on her cover letter and the top of the resume. What concerns should Lisa have about emailing the document? How can Lisa make certain that her document arrives in a readable format when sending it electronically?

THE COVER LETTER

When sending a resume, always include a cover letter (Figure 57-11). This is the introduction to the resume and the person sending the document. A cover letter should always be sent to an individual, not to the facility or "to whom it may concern." A simple phone call will usually reveal the name of the person to whom the resume should be sent. Ask for the name of the office manager, or if this information is not obtained, address it specifically to the physician.

Brutis Walter
2345 Morrow Court
Mytown, OH 45310
(937) 555-7426

May 23, 1998

Andrea Foreman, CMA
Office Manager
Family Health, Inc.
123 Timberleaf Drive
Mytown, OH 45432

Ms. Foreman:

I will be graduating from Community College with an A.S. in Medical Assisting on June 9 and am interested in an entry-level medical assistant position in your office. I will consider part-time or temporary work to gain experience in a diverse office such as yours.

My training includes hands-on experience in pediatrics, cardiology, internal medicine, obstetrics, and geriatrics. My administrative training would allow me to fill in wherever needed in the office. I am highly motivated and have supported myself and paid my own way through college. I understand responsibility and am a true team player. Belinda Mallet, RN, a fellow church member, told me the office will be short-staffed this summer owing to vacations and a maternity leave. I believe I could help your office run smoothly this summer, and beyond.

I look forward to hearing from you. I am available Tuesday and Thursday afternoons and Friday mornings until graduation. I will call you next Tuesday to set up an appointment for an interview.
Thank you for your consideration.

Very truly yours,

Brutis Walter

Figure 57-11 Basic cover letter.

EXECUTIVE BRIEFING

Allison Aubrey, R.M.A.
3040 Wood Branch Drive
Austin, Texas 78716
512-434-9902

James Richardson, M.D.
Family Practice Clinic
5508 Lamar Blvd.
Austin, Texas 78752

Dear Dr. Richardson:

Although my attached resume will provide you with a general outline of my work history, my problem-solving abilities, and some of my achievements, it may take longer than a few moments to peruse. For your convenience, I have listed your specified requirements for the medical assistant position at the Lakewood office below, and the skills I have developed that match those specifications. I hope this briefing will allow you to quickly determine my eligibility for the position and will prompt you to contact me for an interview.

Your Requirements:	My Skills:
1. Two years' experience as a medical assistant.	1. Three years' experience as a registered medical assistant.
2. Ability to work with a larger supervisory team in planning, budgeting, and policy formulating.	2. Experience as employee council president, intricately involved in planning and budgeting.
3. Familiarity with HIPAA regulations.	3. Trained in HIPAA compliance and received three certificates for continuing education related to HIPAA compliance.
4. Ability to work with others as a team.	4. Awarded "Employee of the Quarter" honors twice during past year, and nominated for "Employee of the Year" by my coworkers.

I know that my experience and abilities will be of benefit to your organization. I look forward to discussing my qualifications and your requirements in person. I am confident that we can develop an exceptional working relationship and that I am the right individual for your organization. I will telephone you on Monday to arrange an interview to take place at your convenience.

Sincerely yours,

Allison Aubrey, R.M.A.

Figure 57-12 Executive briefing.

The purpose of the cover letter is to gain attention. Many potential employers will schedule an interview with an individual based strictly on the content of the cover letter. Some are general letters that provide basic information without targeting the requirements of one specific job. An executive briefing, as described by Martin Yate in his book *Cover Letters That Knock 'Em Dead*, is a variation on the traditional cover letter. It provides a comprehensive picture of a thorough professional, plus a personalized, fast, and easy-to-read synopsis that details exactly how the applicant meets the major job requirements. This type of cover letter is extremely effective, but the applicant must have some idea of the job requirements in advance. To produce a dynamic executive briefing, the medical assistant should choose the most important qualifications listed on the ad for the job, then explain how he or she fits those qualifications (Figure 57-12).

Remember, not all direct supervisors will be the first recipient of the resume, so the impression formed by the cover letter may make the difference in getting to the next step in the hiring process. Make it easy for screeners to find the strengths that match the job description. The cover letter should be brief and interesting. Use the same paper stock weight and color as the resume. Be sure to include contact information, such as an address and at least two phone numbers, even if these are on the attached resume. The supervisor may separate the two documents, so there must be a method of contact on each one. Never start a cover letter with the sentence, "I saw your ad in the newspaper" or a similar phrase. Be creative with the opening line, and try to capture the attention of the reader.

A cover letter should be one to three paragraphs long. The final section should include a call to action that will prompt an interview. If the document concludes with a request for a meeting, the medical assistant should state when he or she will call for a time and date.

JOB APPLICATIONS

Many facilities require a job application along with a resume (Figure 57-13). Arrive 15 minutes before the scheduled interview to allow time to fill out an application (Procedure 57-3).

Job applications can be considered a legal document if the person is hired. Therefore they should be neat and filled out correctly and completely. Always read the application before filling it out, so that directions make sense and information is not placed in the wrong area of the form. Carry a planner or address book to the interview so that former employers' and supervisors' names, addresses, and phone numbers are handy. The medical assistant should not be in a position that he or she must ask for a phone book to get an address. Have all of this information ready for when it is needed.

Applications often ask for a date that the medical assistant is available for work. Be careful with this question. If the applicant currently has a job, yet writes that he or she is "immediately available," it may indicate that the applicant intends to quit without notice. On the other hand, the current employer may be aware that the person is seeking other employment and may have granted him or her permission to quit immediately once a new job is found.

Be careful on the sections that ask the reason for leaving former positions. Think about the answers that are listed in those spaces, and try to put the information in as positive a light as possible. Ask the advice of the placement counselor if unsure what to say in these sections.

If there are sections available for listing special skills and qualifications, fill them out fully. Describe cardiopulmonary resuscitation (CPR) and first aid certifications and any professional organizations joined. If references are requested, list the name, title, employer, and a means of contact. Be sure to get permission before using someone as a reference.

One of the most common mistakes on the job application is writing "see resume." This is an indication of laziness and must be avoided. Even if the same information is found on the resume, the application must still be completed in its entirety. In addition, most job applications include a disclaimer that states that if a false or incomplete statement is made on the application, the individual can be dismissed from any position for which he or she was hired.

THE JOB INTERVIEW

A medical assistant may interview with the office manager, the physician, or both. It is possible that other staff members may be brought in for a portion of the interview. This is especially true in offices that have a cohesive team of employees.

The interview is usually the most stressful of the job search steps. Some individuals dread job interviews and become extremely nervous at the prospect of interviewing. Others are

---

PROCEDURE 57-3

Complete a Job Application

ABHES COMPETENCY: 2.j

GOAL: *To complete an accurate, detailed job application legibly in order to secure a job offer.*

EQUIPMENT and SUPPLIES

- Record of a Job Lead form
- Record of an Interview form
- Copies of resume
- Contact information for former employers and references
- Contact information for friends and family

PROCEDURAL STEPS

1. Read the entire job application before completing any portion of the document.
   PURPOSE: Reading through the entire application helps to avoid mistakes while filling out the document.
2. Gather any information that may be necessary to answer all questions on the application.
   PURPOSE: The candidate should have all information available for completing a job application.
3. Begin to complete the application legibly.
   PURPOSE: The interviewer will evaluation the candidate's handwriting to make certain that it would be legible on medical records.

4. Answer each question on the document, or write "not applicable."
5. Do not leave any space blank.
   PURPOSE: Leaving a space blank on the application may suggest that the candidate did not wish to answer a certain question or accidentally overlooked it. By writing "not applicable" on such questions, the candidate demonstrates competence and attention to detail.
6. Do not write "see resume" anywhere on the document.
   PURPOSE: Many supervisors view this practice as laziness. Always completely fill out the job application, and do not leave blank spaces.
7. Be completely honest about every fact written on the document.
8. Sign the document and date it.
9. Proofread the document and make certain that no information conflicts with the resume.
   PURPOSE: Proofreading will help the candidate to catch any errors before submitting the application.
10. Submit the application.

APPLICATION FOR POSITION / Medical or Dental Office
AN EQUAL OPPORTUNITY EMPLOYER

(In answering questions, use extra blank sheet if necessary)

No employee, applicant, or candidate for promotion, training or other advantage shall be discriminated against (or given preference) because of race, color, religion, sex, age, physical handicap, veteran status, or national origin.

PLEASE READ CAREFULLY AND WRITE OR PRINT ANSWERS TO ALL QUESTIONS. DO NOT TYPE.

Date of Application

A. PERSONAL INFORMATION

Name - Last | First | Middle | Social Security No. | Area Code/Phone No. ( )

Present Address: - Street | (Apt #) | City | State | Zip | How Long At This Address?:

Previous Address: - Street | City | State | Zip | Person to notify in case of Emergency or Accident - Name:

From: | To: | Address: | Telephone:

B. EMPLOYMENT INFORMATION

For What Position Are You Applying?: | ☐ Full-Time ☐ Part-Time ☐ Either | Date Available For Employment?: | Wage/Salary Expectations:

List Hrs./Days You Prefer To Work | List Any Hrs./Days You Are Not Available: (Except for times required for religious practices or observances) | Can You Work Overtime, If Necessary? ☐ Yes ☐ No

Are You Employed Now?: ☐ Yes ☐ No | If So, May We Inquire Of Your Present Employer?: ☐ No ☐ Yes, If Yes:
Name Of Employer: | Phone Number: ( )

Have You Ever Been Bonded? ☐ Yes ☐ No | If Required For Position, Are You Bondable? ☐ Yes ☐ No ☐ Uncertain | Have You Applied For A Position With This Office Before? ☐ No ☐ Yes If Yes, When?:

Referred By / Or Where Did You Learn Of This Job?:

Can You, Upon Employment, Submit Verification Of Your Legal Right To Work In The United States?: ☐ Yes ☐ No
Submit Proof That You Meet Legal Age Requirement For Employment? ☐ Yes ☐ No | Language(s) Applicant Speaks or Writes (If Use Of A Language Other Than English Is Relevant To The Job For Which The Applicant Is Applying:

C. EDUCATIONAL HISTORY

Name & Address Of Schools Attended (Include Current)	Dates From	Thru	Highest Grade/Level Completed	Diploma/Degree(s) Obtained/Areas of Study
High School				
College				Degree/Major
Post Graduate				Degree/Major
Other				Course/Diploma/License/Certificate

Specific Training, Education, Or Experiences Which Will Assist You In The Job For Which You Have Applied.

Future Educational Plans

D. SPECIAL SKILLS

CHECK BELOW THE KINDS OF WORK YOU HAVE DONE:

☐ MEDICAL INSURANCE FORMS ☐ RECEPTIONIST

☐ BLOOD COUNTS ☐ DENTAL ASSISTANT ☐ MEDICAL TERMINOLOGY ☐ TELEPHONES
☐ BOOKKEEPING ☐ DENTAL HYGIENIST ☐ MEDICAL TRANSCRIPTION ☐ TYPING
☐ COLLECTIONS ☐ FILING ☐ NURSING ☐ STENOGRAPHY
☐ COMPOSING LETTERS ☐ INJECTIONS ☐ PHLEBOTOMY (Draw Blood) ☐ URINALYSIS
☐ COMPUTER INPUT ☐ INSTRUMENT STERILIZATION ☐ POSTING ☐ X-RAY
OFFICE EQUIPMENT USED: ☐ COMPUTER ☐ DICTATING EQUIPMENT ☐ WORD PROCESSOR ☐ OTHER:

Other Kinds Of Tasks Performed Or Skills That May Be Applicable To Position: | Typing Speed | Shorthand Speed

ORDER # 72-110 • © 1976 BIBBERO SYSTEMS, INC. • PETALUMA, CA. • (Rev. 1/95)
TO REORDER CALL TOLL FREE: (800) BIBBERO (800-242-2376) OR FAX (800) 242-9330 MFG IN U.S.A.

(PLEASE COMPLETE OTHER SIDE)

Figure 57-13 Application for employment. (Courtesy Bibbero Systems, Petaluma Calif. 94654, (800) 242-2376, www.bibbero.com.)

E. EMPLOYMENT RECORD

LIST MOST RECENT EMPLOYMENT FIRST

May We Contact Your Previous Employer(s) For A Reference? ☐ Yes ☐ No

1) Employer

Work Performed. Be Specific:

Address   Street   City   State   Zip Code

Phone Number
(   )

Type of Business

Dates   Mo. Yr.   Mo. Yr.
From   To

Your Position

Hourly Rate/Salary
Starting   Final

Supervisor's Name

Reason For Leaving

2) Employer

Worked Performed. Be Specific:

Address   Street   City   State   Zip Code

Phone Number
(   )

Type of Business

Dates   Mo. Yr.   Mo. Yr.
From   To

Your Position

Hourly Rate/Salary
Starting   Final

Supervisor's Name

Reason For Leaving

3) Employer

Worked Performed. Be Specific:

Address   Street   City   State   Zip Code

Phone Number
(   )

Type of Business

Dates   Mo. Yr.   Mo. Yr.
From   To

Your Position

Hourly Rate/Salary
Starting   Final

Supervisor's Name

Reason For Leaving

F. REFERENCES — FRIENDS / ACQUAINTANCES NON-RELATED

(1)
Name   Address   Telephone Number   (☐ Work ☐ Home) Occupation   Years Acquainted

(1)
Name   Address   Telephone Number   (☐ Work ☐ Home) Occupation   Years Acquainted

Please Feel Free To Add Any Information Which You Feel Will Help Us Consider You For Employment

READ THE FOLLOWING CAREFULLY, THEN SIGN AND DATE THE APPLICATION

"I certify that all answers given by me on this application are true, correct and complete to the best of my knowledge. I acknowledge notice that the information contained in this application is subject to check. I agree that, if hired, my continued employment may be contingent upon the accuracy of that information. If employed, I further agree to comply with Company/Office rules and regulations."

Signature: _____   Date: _____

Figure 57-13, *cont'd* For legend see previous page.

very comfortable and consider the interview as much for their own purposes as for the employer's.

There are four phases to interviews. These are the preparation, the interview itself, the follow-up, and the negotiation.

Preparation for the Interview

When preparing for an interview, the medical assistant should learn everything possible about the employer. Look on the Internet for information about the facility. Practice answering potential interview questions. Prepare an outfit to wear to interviews. It is wise to drive to the interview site on a day preceding the interview date if the location is unfamiliar to avoid getting lost on the day of the important event. The better prepared the medical assistant is, the more comfortable he or she will be while interviewing.

The critical part of the interview is the medical assistant's ability to present himself or herself as the best candidate for the job. By preparing to answer interview questions before the interview, the medical assistant will be much more prepared. Although no one can guess exactly what questions will be asked, some standard interview questions are very common (Figure 57-14).

Review these questions thoroughly, answer them in writing, then study them before the interview. Then when the medical assistant is asked, "What are your three greatest strengths?" he or she can confidently answer, "I am professional, reliable, and honest."

When preparing on the day of the interview, be conservative with wardrobe choices. For women a skirt and blouse or business suit is appropriate. For men a business suit is the best choice. Depending on the office situation, one may be given very specific instructions on wardrobe. Some office managers or physicians will even tell the potential employee to arrive in jeans. Is this a test? The physician may be curious as to whether the medical assistant can follow directions and actually wear jeans. Obtain a hint about clothing by visiting the office before the interview, even if it is just to ask for directions. This way, the potential employee can see what the office staff members are wearing. Similar wardrobe should be sufficient for an interview. If the staff wears scrubs, then wear neatly pressed scrubs with clean shoes, avoiding the slouchy scrubs one might find in a hospital surgical suite. Conservative business suits should always be acceptable in an interview.

Be sure clothing is fresh and wrinkle free and shoes are shined. It is a good idea to carry a planner or other method of taking notes during the interview. This makes a good impression and indicates interest in the job. Always arrive 15 minutes early for the interview. Do not use heavy perfumes or colognes, do not chew gum, and avoid excessive jewelry. Never take anyone along on a job interview, especially children, even if they are older.

Pay particular attention to other aspects of appearance (Figure 57-15). Be sure that the hair is clean and styled attractively, teeth are clean, and breath is fresh. Nails are also important and should be clean and well groomed, because the medical assistant will want to give the interviewer a firm handshake. Expect to be a little nervous. Any interview can be a stressful situation. The better prepared the medical assistant is, the more of a success the interview will be.

The Interview

During the actual interview, maintain good eye contact. Many supervisors refuse to hire people who seem uncomfortable with making strong eye contact. Never take control of the interview. Allow the supervisor to ask questions at his or her own pace. Do not fidget in the chair, and observe the interviewer's body language for clues as to how interested he or she might be. Do not volunteer any negative information, be honest, and do not exaggerate experience or lengths of employment. Never speak negatively about former employers.

Remember that the interview is centered on the medical assistant, so freely discuss the skills and attributes that will be brought to the job. The better prepared the medical assistant is, the smoother the interview will be. Be able to prove the skills claimed, and explain how they meet the needs of the company or facility. Avoid a "know-it-all" attitude, which indicates overconfidence and reluctance in taking direction. Always express an interest in the employer and its projects as opposed to what the employer can do for the employee. Ask intelligent questions at the end of the interview if given the opportunity. Never let your first question be, "How much will I be paid?" Money, although important, cannot seem to be your primary concern.

Before the interview ends, the medical assistant should ask when a decision will be made and if it would be acceptable to call to follow up (Procedure 57-4, p. 1340).

CRITICAL THINKING APPLICATION

Lisa is enjoying a good interview when the supervisor, a man, asks her if she is married. When Lisa replies that she is not, he asks if she has a steady boyfriend. What might the supervisor's motive be with this line of questioning? How should Lisa respond? Are these questions inappropriate, or do they serve a purpose?

Follow-Up after the Interview

Follow-up is critical after an interview. Always send a written thank-you note or letter to the person who conducted the interview. Many employers wait to see who sends a thank-you letter before making the final hiring decision. Limit follow-up calls to no more than one or two a week. Most employers will give an indication of when the hiring decision will be made. The company should notify all those who interviewed once a decision has been made, unless specific protocols were set during the interview about follow-up. For instance, if the office manager says that a decision will be made on Friday, and the final three candidates will be called for a second interview, then the medical assistant knows if a call is not received to continue the job search. Although not all companies provide this type of notification, it is considered professional etiquette to tell the candidates who interviewed for the job if they are no longer under consideration. Never place all hope on one job—continue to prospect until an offer is made and accepted. In addition, always be on the watch for the next job opportunity.

TOP 100 INTERVIEW QUESTIONS

1. Tell me about yourself.
2. Why do you want to work for this company?
3. Why should I hire you?
4. How do you work under pressure?
5. What type of job or salary do you expect to make in 5 years?
6. How do you handle criticism?
7. What do you think your co-workers think about you?
8. What is your opinion of the company you last worked for?
9. Describe your last supervisor.
10. What is your view of management?
11. What would you like to change about yourself and how would you do it?
12. What is your best asset?
13. What adjectives would you use to describe yourself?
14. What aspects of your life are you most happy with?
15. How would you describe the perfect job?
16. Why did you leave your last job?
17. Why did you choose this type of profession?
18. What salary do you expect?
19. What are your strongest and weakest personal qualities?
20. What motivates you?
21. What have you learned from some of your previous jobs?
22. What personal characteristics are necessary for success in your chosen field?
23. What do you know about this facility and our competitors?
24. What were your major courses of study in school?
25. Do you plan to continue your education?
26. Did school meet your expectations or were you disappointed?
27. How did you pay for your education?
28. Sell this pen to me.
29. To what extent do your grades reflect how much you have learned?
30. Do you feel your education was worthwhile?
31. What were the major responsibilities of your last job?
32. What has been your most rewarding experience at work?
33. What was your single most important accomplishment for the company on your last job?
34. What was the toughest problem you have ever solved and how did you do it?
35. How do you see yourself fitting in with our company?
36. What skills did you learn on your last job that can be used here?
37. What would you do if you were fired in two years?
38. What kinds of additional education do you think you need to meet your career goals?
39. How long do you plan to stay with our company?
40. What immediate contribution could you make if you came to work for us today?
41. Do you feel that you have received good general training?
42. If you were starting school all over again, what courses would you take?
43. How much money do you hope to earn in 5 years? 10 years?
44. Do you think that your extracurricular activities were worth the time spent?
45. Are you interested in making money or do you have other reasons for entering this career field?
46. Do you prefer working with others or by yourself?
47. Can you take instructions or criticism without being upset?
48. Tell me a story.
49. What do you know about the opportunities in the field in which you are trained?
50. How long do you expect to work?
51. Have you ever had any difficulty in getting along with a co-worker, classmate, or instructor?
52. Which of your school years was most difficult?
53. Do you like routine work?
54. Define cooperation.
55. Will you fight to get ahead?
56. Do you have an analytical mind?
57. Are you willing to go where the company sends you?
58. What job in this company would you choose if you could?
59. Do you think that employers should consider grades?
60. What have you done that shows initiative and willingness to work?
61. What benefits did you receive from your last employer?
62. What has been your most important accomplishment during your school years?
63. Have you ever helped to reduce operating costs, and how?
64. Have you ever developed or helped develop any programs, and how did you do this?
65. What do you think determines a person's progress in a company?
66. What would you do if a personal problem interfered with your work?
67. What would you do if you became bored with your job?
68. What would you do if you had a personality clash with a supervisor?
69. How will you be getting to work each day?
70. Do you have reliable transportation?
71. How do you feel about working with someone who is HIV positive?
72. What person has most influenced your life?
73. What is the last book you read?
74. Who do you most admire?
75. Who is your favorite relative?
76. What will previous supervisors say about you?
77. What makes a good supervisor?
78. Why would you be successful in this job?
79. Why have you held so many jobs?
80. Can you explain this gap in your employment history?
81. Have you ever been fired from a position?
82. Do you have adequate child care arrangements that will allow you to be at work when scheduled?
83. What is your philosophy of life?
84. How many other positions are you considering?
85. Why were your grades in school so low?
86. Are you a member of any professional organizations?
87. How old were you when you began to support yourself?
88. Do you participate in continuing education activities or seminars?
89. Have you had the hepatitis B injection series?
90. Where did you perform your externship?
91. How many days of school did you miss?
92. Why did you decide to attend the college/school you attended?
93. What kind of boss do you prefer?
94. How do you usually spend your weekends?
95. Why types of people seem to rub you the wrong way?
96. What planning procedures do you use?
97. What frustrates you about your current job?
98. What is unique about you?
99. What have you done that indicates you are qualified for this job?
100. Do you have any questions?

Figure 57-14 Top 100 interview questions.

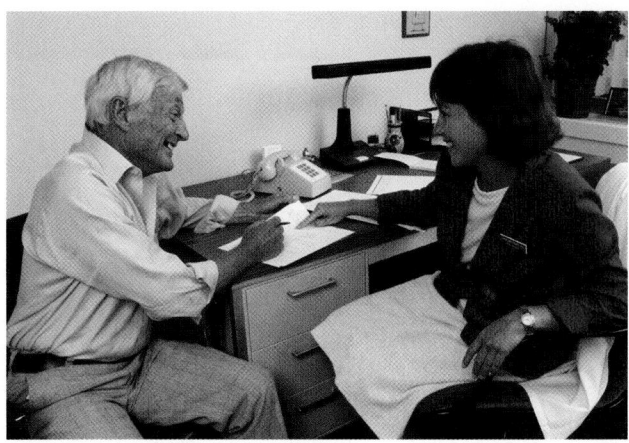

Figure 57-15 Present a professional appearance during the job interview, and be sure to smile often.

Reasons People Do Not Get Hired

Below is a ranked list of reasons that interviewers do not hire job candidates. The list is compiled from the results of a nationwide survey of 153 companies performed by North Central Technical Institute.

1. Poor personal appearance
2. Lack of interest or enthusiasm
3. Overemphasis on money
4. Poor voice, diction, grammar
5. Lack of planning
6. No purpose or goals
7. Condemnation of past employers
8. Poor eye contact
9. Limp, fishy handshake
10. Late to interview
11. Lack of tact
12. Lack of maturity
13. Lack of courtesy
14. Asking no questions
15. Overbearing "know-it-all"
16. Lack of confidence and poise
17. Failure to participate in activities
18. Making excuses, evading unfavorable factors on record
19. Indecisiveness
20. Just shopping around
21. No interest in company
22. Sloppy application form
23. Wanting a job for a short time
24. Unwillingness to relocate
25. Cynical attitude
26. Low moral standards
27. Laziness
28. Intolerance or strong prejudices
29. No sense of humor
30. Narrow interests
31. Inability to take criticism
32. No appreciation for the value of experience
33. Radical ideas
34. Too aggressive during interview

Negotiation

The negotiation stage of job acceptance can be as stressful as the actual interviews. A medical assistant should know the lowest salary he or she can afford, then should ask for a little more than that figure. Bracket salary requests: instead of asking for $12.00 per hour, ask for a salary in the "mid to high twenties." Let the employer mention a figure first, or a range of salary. Usually the person who mentions a salary range first has the disadvantage. If the medical assistant requests $12.00 per hour and the facility was willing to pay $15.00 per hour, the medical assistant will probably get $12.00.

Never say "no" to a job offer on the spot. Request at least 24 hours to consider the offer (Procedure 57-5). A medical assistant should not let the salary amount be the main factor in the decision to accept a position. Consider whether the position carries any authority, the benefits, the hours, the distance from home, and the potential for advancement before accepting or rejecting a job offer. Reasons exist for accepting a job other than the salary; remember the value of experience.

YOU GOT THE JOB!

Once the job offer has been made and accepted, a start date will be determined (Figure 57-16). Before the first day, use the computer to map several ways to get to work. Because you may be unsure of traffic flow, leave home extra early the first day so that arrival on time is guaranteed.

Most employees are placed on a 30- to 90-day probationary period, during which employment may be terminated if the employee's performance is not satisfactory. It is also an opportunity for the employer and employee to learn about each other. The medical assistant will interact with other co-workers, with patients, and with providers. A new medical assistant should volunteer to help others and efficiently complete the duties assigned. Use the probationary period as a testing ground, carefully observing ways in which the office might run in a smoother manner. However, do not make numerous suggestions for change during this period. Discover why certain methods are used, and make an effort to fit in with the rest of the team before suggesting that the routine of the office be changed. Remember, the people at the office may have been employed for substantially longer periods and may resent suggestions from a new staff member. Learn the office's rhythms, procedures, and culture first, and demonstrate a team-oriented attitude.

Common Early Mistakes

Some medical assistants make mistakes early on a new job. Never be disruptive to the office by gossiping or complaining. A medical assistant must realize that there may be different ways of performing procedures and that the way he or she was taught in school is probably not the only correct way. Be open to learning new ideas, concepts, and procedures. Although some mistakes are to be expected, be certain that once a mistake is pointed out, it is corrected. Do not make the same mistakes over and over.

Supervisors may or may not work very closely with the medical assistants. Some will be expected to carry out orders

PROCEDURE 57-4

Recognize and Respond to Verbal Communications: Interview for a Job

CAAHEP COMPETENCIES: 3.c.(1)(b), 3.c.(1)(c)
ABHES COMPETENCY: 2.f

GOAL: To project a professional appearance during a job interview and be able to express the reasons that the medical assistant is the best candidate for the position.

EQUIPMENT and SUPPLIES

- Record of a Job Lead form
- Record of an Interview form
- Job application
- Copies of resume
- Contact information for former employers and references
- Contact information for friends and family
- Sample interview questions

PROCEDURAL STEPS

1. Prepare for the interview by studying sample interview questions and researching basic information about the facility.
   PURPOSE: Employers are impressed by candidates who have researched the company and know some details about its operation.
2. Know all of the information that is contained on the resume so that it can be discussed confidently during the interview.
3. Prepare clothing that reflects a professional image for the facility in which the medical assistant is hoping to gain employment.
   PURPOSE: Most medical facilities prefer conservative dress.
4. Gather all materials that might be needed during the interview, such as copies of resumes, contact information, and copies of earned certificates.
   PURPOSE: All information must be handy and prepared in advance of the interview.

5. Arrive for the interview at least 15 minutes early.
   PURPOSE: Arrive early in case there are papers to complete in advance of the interview.
6. Stand and shake hands with the interviewer when he or she appears.
   PURPOSE: A confident, firm handshake is a positive gesture.
7. Listen intently to the interviewer as the position is described, and be ready to explain how you fit the requirements for the position.
   PURPOSE: The interviewer will evaluate how well the candidate listens and answers the questions asked.
8. Answer all interview questions confidently, smiling when appropriate, and displaying a positive attitude.
9. Ask intelligent questions after the interviewer finishes.
   PURPOSE: The questions asked at the end of an interview should indicate an interest in the position and should not focus on how the candidate would benefit from the job, but rather on what the candidate can do for the company.
10. Determine a day and time when the next contact will be made.
11. Express interest in the position.
    PURPOSE: Employers expect some type of confirmation that the candidate is interested in the job.
12. Send a thank-you note or letter to the interviewer within 24 hours of the interview.
    PURPOSE: A thank-you note is impressive and reinforces the candidate's interest in the position.
13. Follow-up as appropriate on the interview.

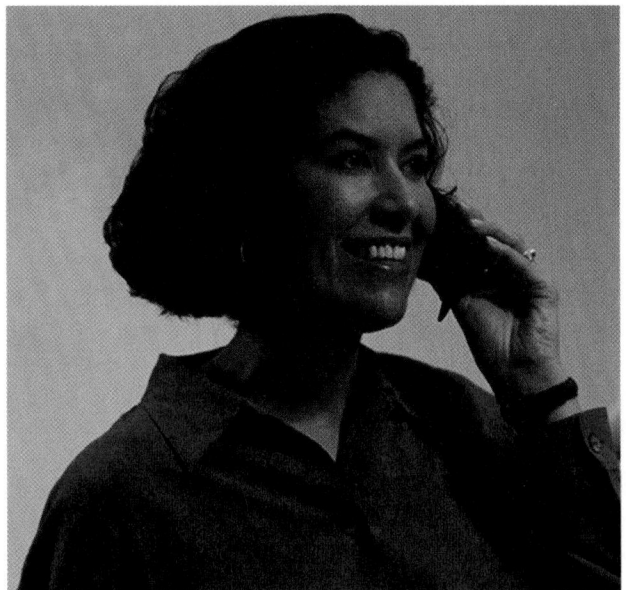

Figure 57-16 Congratulations, you're hired! The first job after school is an exciting experience for a medical assistant.

on their own. Do not make too much supervision necessary or force the office manager to constantly check the work that is done. Finish all assigned duties in a timely manner, and avoid procrastination. When problems arise, communicate them openly with the supervisor and attempt to find a quick resolution. Last, limit absences and tardy days to a minimum and miss work only when absolutely necessary—especially during the probationary period.

How to Be a Good Employee

There are several ways in which a medical assistant can be a better employee. First and foremost, arrive for the scheduled shift on time and do not leave early. Even the best medical assistant cannot benefit an office when he or she does not come to work. Be honest and demonstrate trustworthiness and professionalism. Get along with co-workers in the facility. A medical assistant should be able to resolve simple problems with others easily without involving the supervisor. Reflect a friendly attitude toward others, even if they are difficult to get along with. Arrive every single day ready to learn. The medical

PROCEDURE 57-5

Recognize and Respond to Verbal Communications: Negotiate a Salary

CAAHEP COMPETENCIES: 3.c.(1)(b), 3.c.(1)(c)
ABHES COMPETENCY: 2.i

GOAL: *To develop negotiation skills that will help the medical assistant obtain the salary and benefits that will sustain his or her family.*

EQUIPMENT and SUPPLIES

- Record of a Job Lead form
- Record of an Interview form
- Information about job offers received
- Contact name at medical facility

PROCEDURAL STEPS

1. Study the job offer at hand.
2. Determine if the offer is sufficient as it stands.
3. Make a list of what additional salary requirements and/or benefits are needed at a minimum.
   PURPOSE: Know the minimum salary and benefits that you can accept when evaluating a job offer.
4. Arrive at the second or subsequent interview appointment to discuss the job with the hiring supervisor.
5. Thank the supervisor for the offer that has been presented, and express interest in the position.

6. Express the additional salary and/or benefits desired.
   PURPOSE: The candidate should be able to express what he or she needs with regard to salary and benefits.
7. Discuss whether the facility would be willing to increase the offer to match your desires.
8. Express valid reasons that explain why the additional benefits should be offered, based on past performance, experience, or other valid factors.
9. Discuss reasonable compromises regarding the additional salary and/or benefits.
   PURPOSE: The ability to compromise is a valuable employee trait.
10. Ask what level of performance is expected for salary and/or benefits to be increased.
11. Express interest in and promise serious consideration of the position.
12. Determine the next contact time with the supervisor.
13. Weigh the offer and compromises to make a good decision about the job offer.

---

assistant's education does not end on graduation from school. The medical field is one of constant change, and those who work in it must learn and change along with the field.

A medical assistant should constantly be performing assigned duties and not expect frequent breaks in the medical office. Most offices are fast paced, and the supervisor will expect the medical assistant to keep up with the activity. Even when there are slow periods, there is always a counter to clean or filing to do. Be supportive of the leadership in the facility, and ask for more responsibility if necessary. Take initiative to perform duties that are cumbersome or repetitive, and get them done quickly.

It is vital to treat the patients with compassion. Remember that they are not always at their best when ill, so be kind and courteous to them and their families. The patients are the reason that the facility exists. Treat them with great respect and care.

CRITICAL THINKING APPLICATION

On Lisa's second day at the externship site, she clearly sees a co-worker taking and using a controlled drug from the storage area. What should Lisa do? What potential problems will this situation prompt? To whom should Lisa report this incident, if anyone?

Dealing with Supervisors

Supervisors appreciate employees who come to them when there are questions but who are able to handle minor decisions on their own. Never hesitate to approach supervisors when there is an issue at hand that needs their attention. Do not allow a situation to go unaddressed and then say, "I didn't want to bother you with that." It is the responsibility of the office manager to deal with difficult issues, and these should be handled immediately when they arise.

A medical assistant should never attempt to cover up a mistake; admitting the error is a much better approach to solving the problem. When talking with the supervisor, do not hesitate to speak and do not avoid the subject. State the problem clearly, and explain what routes are available to **rectify** the situation. Work with the supervisor to resolve issues and accept the advice given with a positive attitude.

Performance Appraisals

Performance **appraisals** are usually done after the initial probationary period and annually after that. The performance appraisal is designed to inform the employee of his or her strengths and weaknesses on the job, according to the supervisor's point of view. Most of these appraisals offer a scale to rate the employee's performance, such as 1 to 5. Do not expect to receive a perfect appraisal, because employees are seldom perfect in all aspects of their jobs. If the supervisor gives perfect scores to an employee, there is no room for growth or improvement. It is the rare employee who completes all duties without any errors. When asked to sit down with your supervisor for a performance appraisal, go into the meeting open to addressing areas that may need improvement. Ask questions and work with the supervisor to improve in the areas that may need more effort or a different approach.

If the employee strongly disagrees with any area of the performance appraisal, discuss this with the supervisor. There may have been a misunderstanding as to the duties involved. Clarify this, and strive to do better next time.

Asking for a Raise

Most facilities have some type of schedule for pay increases. Some offer a cost of living increase on an annual basis; others use a merit system, offering raises only when earned and deserved based on performance.

There may come a time when the medical assistant feels the need to ask for a raise. Before doing so, a little self-reflection should be performed to determine whether a raise is in order. Has attendance been exemplary? How many times was the medical assistant tardy? Does he or she work well with little supervision? Has he or she performed all the expected duties well and in a timely manner?

Approach the supervisor at a relatively calm part of the day, and ask how a salary raise might be earned in the near future. Do not expect a raise of more than 4% to 5% at any given time. If the supervisor is unable to grant a raise, determine whether the reasons are valid. If they are not, the medical assistant may wish to pursue other employment options. It is always easier to find a job if one already has a job, so do not quit outright unless the work environment is **intolerable.** Begin networking again, and discover the options available.

Leaving a Job Professionally

Always offer at least a 2-week notice when resigning from a job. Give the supervisor a written notice of resignation, and take this to him or her in person. Do not just leave it on a desk or place it in the interoffice mail.

It is a dangerous practice to resign from a job just to attempt to get a salary increase. Once the employer doubts the employee's loyalty, the future is usually not bright for the employee at that facility. Resign only after a final decision has been made. If the medical assistant is resigning to take another position, the current employer may be expected to make a **counteroffer.** However, be wary about accepting counteroffers. What led to looking for a new job in the first place? Has the situation been resolved? Ask these questions before agreeing to stay with the current employer.

LIFE SKILLS

To be successful in the job search, the medical assistant must have the basic entry-level skills needed to perform in the workplace. Even more important, however, he or she must develop certain life skills that are essential to excel in any profession. If these skills are not developed and refined, the medical assistant may find fewer opportunities and advancements available, as well as less impressive salaries and benefits.

The most important life skill one can possess is the willingness to change. Many employees insist on doing things the same way they have always been done, and they resist any changes in policy or procedure. However, a medical assistant who does not welcome and work hard to adjust to change is a failure waiting to happen.

Personal Growth

Personal growth is a comprehensive term that applies to many aspects of a person's mental, physical, and spiritual health. This growth is a result of goals that are set for self-improvement. Without clear goals, people rarely experience personal growth that is initiated from within. There may be growth that is a result of some outside influence, but a conscious effort toward personal growth is an innate decision.

No matter how great the training or how many opportunities are placed in front of a person, fear and doubt can sabotage efforts to improve the self-image, confidence, and future potential of an individual. Personal growth involves such traits as self-control, self-esteem, problem-solving skills, decision-making skills, and stress management.

Self-Control

Self-control is a vital trait in the medical office. Some patients may not be at their best because of their illness, and this may make them less than cordial toward the staff. Remember that this is usually a temporary situation. A medical assistant must exercise self-control and not respond in kind to patients who are disagreeable.

Self-control is important in other areas of the medical office. Never remove drugs from the storage areas without permission, and be careful when dealing with petty cash. A medical assistant must get enough rest during the work week that he or she can care for the patients in an enthusiastic manner.

Self-Esteem

Everyone has certain strengths and weaknesses. Good self-esteem is the result of knowing what those strengths are and overcoming the weaknesses. It is having a positive outlook about the self and others. A person with good self-esteem is motivated, able to express love, and capable of handling criticism. A person's self-esteem will improve if he or she has developed adaptive skills. Especially in the medical profession, one thing that is guaranteed in the workplace is change. Change can be positive or negative; this depends mostly on the way it is viewed by the individual.

A person is not doomed to live with poor self-esteem forever. With a degree of effort and open-mindedness, an individual can work toward better self-esteem, which can make a tremendous difference in the individual's future potential.

Problem-Solving Skills

For individuals to work together, they must have a degree of trust and be willing to make suggestions for the good of the group. The phrase "two heads are better than one" is still true when it comes to problem solving. Employees usually want to play a part in solving the problems in the workplace, and they appreciate knowing that their opinions make a difference. A medical assistant who can listen to the concerns of others and is willing to give and take will be an excellent problem solver.

Decision-Making Skills

People who know how to make good decisions are usually successful. Thinking through a decision requires logic, and it is best to take some time to carefully think of all of the "pros and cons." Unfortunately, a medical assistant may not always have time to consider decisions in a leisurely fashion, especially when dealing with emergencies. A good decision-maker is honest when identifying the real problems and attempts to keep personal feelings isolated from the process.

There are several steps toward making a sound decision. The problem must be specifically defined and evaluated so that the individual understands clearly what needs to happen to resolve the situation at hand. Gather as much information as possible and consider all alternatives. It is sometimes helpful to choose an alternative then consider all of the **ramifications** of making a decision using that alternative. Then, when the best alternative is determined, the decision should be made and put into action. Care should be taken to avoid making a decision simply because it is easy and comfortable, because more problems could arise later as a result of not addressing the true problem in the beginning.

CRITICAL THINKING APPLICATION

Lisa has been on several interviews and likes the prospect of working for three different physicians. If an offer is made at each office, how can Lisa decide which to accept? What will help Lisa make this decision?

Stress Management

The demands of the medical profession make it a stressful environment at times. Stress is not always bad. In fact, some stress is a positive motivator toward a goal. A stressor is a stimulus that prompts a reaction from the body. Positive stress, or eustress, includes exhilarating activities or success, which often leads to higher expectations from the person experiencing the eustress. The opposite is distress, which includes disappointment, failure, or embarrassment. Stress management is a conscious effort toward controlling the stressors and resulting reactions so that the body and mind operate evenly, even when stress is present in an individual's life.

By learning to recognize the signs of stressful overload, a medical assistant can possibly ward off the negative reactions that are so physically and mentally draining to the body. Many people notice a headache or fatigue when overly stressed. Breathing correctly is one way to reduce stress. Often an accelerated breathing pattern that is quick and shallow is a stress indicator. Breathing from the abdomen at a slower pace, inhaling through the nose, and exhaling through the mouth may help reduce tension. Taking time for relaxing activities and getting plenty of exercise are other methods of stress reduction.

Planning a Budget

A newly graduated medical assistant should formulate a simple budget and attempt to live within that budget. It is helpful to track spending with checkbook ledgers, bill stubs, receipts, and daily records for 3 months before developing a firm budget, so

that there is a realistic accounting of where money goes when it leaves the checkbook. Use that information to design a spending plan for monthly income that accounts for monthly, quarterly, and annual expenses, as well as special activities.

Even when making only a small salary, building savings is important. A medical assistant should set aside 5% to 10% of the net income in a savings account. The money in savings should not be touched except in emergencies. It is even better to establish an emergency fund, which would ideally hold 3 months' salary. This way, there is enough cash to pay bills for 3 months in case of a sudden job loss or emergency. No one can do this immediately when beginning a new job, but it can be done over a period of time if one is committed to the effort.

Avoid going into debt whenever possible. If credit cards are used, they should be used conservatively and not for impulse purchases. Instead of using credit, set spending goals and save for a purchase or use layaway programs. Make more than the minimum payment on credit cards to avoid excessive interest from accruing on the account. Everyone should work toward being debt free as soon as possible.

Limit housing and utilities to no more than 30% of the net income. Other monthly installment debt should total less than 15% of the net income. Many financial institutions figure a debt ratio when they consider loaning money to an individual. If that debt ratio is too high, the bank may not lend money, even to a person with stellar credit.

Student Loans

Student loans are extremely important and are designed to provide the opportunity to obtain a good education. They must be paid back. If an individual **defaults** on a student loan, he or she becomes ineligible for future student loans until the original loan is paid back, and amounts owed may be deducted from tax refunds involuntarily. There is never a reason to default on a student loan. The medical assistant should contact the company that services the student loan and explain any problems that are keeping him or her from repaying the debt. These companies want to work with students to clear their accounts. Often a **deferment** is available, which allows the student to postpone the payments for a period of time (Figure 57-17). Deferments may be available when the student is unemployed, attending school to continue his or her education, suffering economic hardship, completing a graduate fellowship, completing rehabilitation training, or in other situations. Contact the lender to find out whether a deferment is in order.

The Guideline Budget

Dealing with personal finances can be a stressor. Developing a realistic budget will assist a medical assistant in planning his or her spending. When careful planning is implemented, more can be accomplished with less money if a commitment has been made to staying on budget and resisting the temptation to spend.

Dangerous Habits

Some individuals practice dangerous habits related to finances. For instance, if this month's bills are arriving and last month's

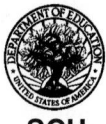

SCH

IN-SCHOOL DEFERMENT REQUEST
Federal Family Education Loan Program

OMB No. 1845-0005
Form Approved
Exp. Date 09/30/XXXX

WARNING: Any person who knowingly makes a false statement or misrepresentation on this form or on any accompanying documents shall be subject to penalties which may include fines, imprisonment or both, under the U.S. Criminal Code and 20 U.S.C. §1097.

SECTION 1: BORROWER IDENTIFICATION

Please enter or correct the following information.

SSN |___|___|___| - |___|___| - |___|___|___|___|

Name _____

Address _____

City, State, Zip _____

Telephone - Home (   ) _____

Telephone - Other (   ) _____

E-mail Address (optional) _____

SECTION 2: DEFERMENT REQUEST

Before answering any questions, carefully read the entire form, including the instructions and other information in Sections 5 and 6.

■ I meet the qualifications for the deferment checked below and request that my loan holder defer repayment of my loan(s):

❑ While I am enrolled at an eligible school as a **FULL-TIME STUDENT** . (For borrowers with a FFEL Program loan.)

❑ While I am enrolled at an eligible school as a **LESS THAN FULL-TIME BUT AT LEAST HALF-TIME STUDENT**. (For borrowers who, on the date they signed the promissory note, did not have an outstanding balance on a FFEL Program loan made **before July 1, 1987**.)

NOTE: *Your promissory note or other loan documents may state that a borrower with an outstanding balance on a FFEL Program loan made **prior to July 1, 1993**, must receive another loan in order to qualify for a half-time student deferment. This requirement was eliminated by the Higher Education Amendments of 1998. **Effective October 1, 1998**, no FFEL Program borrower who is eligible for a deferment based on enrollment as at least a half-time student is required to receive another loan in order to qualify for this deferment.*

SECTION 3: BORROWER UNDERSTANDINGS AND CERTIFICATIONS

■ **I understand that: (1)** I am not required to make payments of loan principal during my deferment. Interest will not be charged on my subsidized loan(s) during my deferment. However, interest will be charged on my unsubsidized loan(s). **(2)** I have the option of making interest payments on my unsubsidized loan(s) during my deferment. **(3)** I may choose to make interest payments by checking the box below. Interest that I do not pay during the deferment period will be capitalized by my loan holder.

❑ I wish to make interest payments on my unsubsidized loan(s) during my deferment.

(4) My deferment will begin on the date the condition that qualifies me for a deferment began, as certified by the authorized official who completes Section 4 of this form. **(5)** My deferment will end on the earlier of the date that I no longer meet the condition that qualifies me for the deferment, or the ending date of that condition as certified by the authorized official. **(6)** If my deferment does not cover all my past due payments, my loan holder may grant me a forbearance for all payments due before the begin date of my deferment or—if the period for which I am eligible for a deferment has ended—a forbearance for all payments due at the time my deferment request is processed. **(7)** If I am eligible for a post-deferment grace period on loans made before October 1, 1981, my loan holder may grant me a forbearance on my other loans for this period so that I can begin repayment of all my loans at the same time. I understand that my loan holder may capitalize the interest that accrues on my other loans during the six-month period and that this will increase the principal balance of my other loans. **(8)** My loan holder may grant me a forbearance on my loans for up to 60 days, if necessary, for the collection and processing of documentation related to my deferment request. Interest that accrues during the forbearance will not be capitalized.

■ **I certify that: (1)** The information I provided in Sections 1 and 2 above is true and correct. **(2)** I will provide additional documentation to my loan holder, as required, to support my deferment status. **(3)** I will notify my loan holder immediately when the condition(s) that qualified me for the deferment ends. **(4)** I have read, understand, and meet the eligibility criteria of the deferment for which I have applied.

Borrower's Signature _____   Date _____

SECTION 4: AUTHORIZED OFFICIAL'S CERTIFICATION

NOTE: As an alternative to completing this section, the school may attach its own enrollment certification report listing the required information.

I certify, to the best of my knowledge and belief, that the borrower named above:

(1) is/was enrolled as (check the appropriate box) ❑ a full-time student ❑ at least a half-time student

during the academic period from |___|___| - |___|___| - |___|___|___|___| to |___|___| - |___|___| - |___|___|___|___| and

(2) is reasonably expected to complete his/her program requirements on |___|___| - |___|___| - |___|___|___|___|.

Name of Institution _____   OPE-ID _____

Address _____   City, State, Zip _____

Name/Title of Authorized Officia _____   Telephone (   ) _____

Authorized Official's Signature _____   Date _____

Page 1 of 2

Figure 57-17 In-school deferment form. Do not allow yourself to default on your student loans. Contact the financial aid office at your educational institution for assistance and answers to questions about student loans.

SECTION 5: INSTRUCTIONS FOR COMPLETING THE FORM

Type or print using dark ink. Report dates as month-day-year (MM-DD-YYYY). For example, 'January 31, 2002' ='01-31-2002'. An authorized school official must either (A) complete Section 4, or (B) attach the school's own enrollment certification report listing the required information. If you need help completing this form, contact your loan holder.

Return the completed form and any required documentation to the address shown in Section 7.

SECTION 6: DEFINITIONS FOR IN-SCHOOL DEFERMENT REQUEST

■ The **Federal Family Education Loan (FFEL) Program** includes Federal Stafford Loans (both subsidized and unsubsidized), Federal Supplemental Loans for Students (SLS), Federal PLUS Loans, and Federal Consolidation Loans.

■ A **deferment** is a period during which I am entitled to postpone repayment of the principal balance of my loan(s). The federal government pays the interest that accrues during an eligible deferment for all subsidized Federal Stafford Loans and for Federal Consolidation Loans for which the Consolidation Loan application was received by my loan holder **(1)** on or after January 1, 1993, but before August 10, 1993, **(2)** on or after August 10, 1993, if it includes **only** Federal Stafford Loans that were eligible for federal interest subsidy, or **(3)** on or after November 13, 1997, for that portion of the consolidation loan that paid a subsidized FFEL Loan or a subsidized Federal Direct Loan. I am responsible for the interest that accrues during this period on all other FFEL Program loans.

■ **Forbearance** means permitting the temporary cessation of payments, allowing an extension of time for making payments, or temporarily accepting smaller payments than previously scheduled. I am responsible for the interest that accrues on my loan(s) during a forbearance. If I do not pay the interest that accrues, the interest may be capitalized.

■ The **holder** of my FFEL Program loan(s) may be a lender, guaranty agency, secondary market, or the U.S. Department of Education.

■ **Capitalization** is the addition of unpaid interest to the principal balance of my loan. This will increase the principal and the total cost of my loan.

■ An **authorized certifying official** for an In-School Deferment is an authorized official of the school where I am/was enrolled as a full-time or at least half-time student.

SECTION 7: WHERE TO SEND THE COMPLETED DEFERMENT REQUEST

RETURN THE COMPLETED DEFERMENT REQUEST AND ANY REQUIRED DOCUMENTATION TO:
(IF NO ADDRESS IS SHOWN, RETURN TO YOUR LOAN HOLDER)

SECTION 8: IMPORTANT NOTICES

Privacy Act Notice

The Privacy Act of 1974 (5 U.S.C. 552a) requires that the following notice be provided to you:

The authority for collecting the requested information from and about you is §428(b)(2)(A) et seq. of the Higher Education Act of 1965, as amended (20 U.S.C. 1078(b)(2)(A) et seq.) and the authority for collecting and using your Social Security Number (SSN) is §484(a)(4) of the HEA (20 U.S.C. 1091(a)(4)). Participating in the Federal Family Education Loan (FFEL) Program and giving us your SSN are voluntary, but you must provide the requested information, including your SSN, to participate.

The principal purposes for collecting the information on this form, including your SSN, are to verify your identity, to determine your eligibility to receive a loan or a benefit on a loan (such as a deferment, forbearance, discharge, or forgiveness) under the FFEL program, to permit the servicing of your loan(s), and, if it becomes necessary, to locate you and to collect on your loan(s) if your loan(s) become delinquent or in default. We also use your SSN as an account identifier and to permit you to access your account information electronically.

The information in your file may be disclosed to third parties as authorized under routine uses in the appropriate systems of records. The routine uses of this information include its disclosure to federal, state, or local agencies, to other federal agencies under computer matching programs, to agencies that we authorize to assist us in administering our loan programs, to private parties such as relatives, present and former employers, business and personal associates, to credit bureau organizations, to educational institutions, and to contractors in order to verify your identity, to determine your eligibility to receive a loan or a benefit on a loan, to permit the servicing or collection of your loan(s), to counsel you in repayment efforts, to enforce the terms of the loan(s), to investigate possible fraud and to verify compliance with federal student financial aid program regulations, to locate you if you become delinquent in your loan payments or if you default, to provide default rate calculations, to provide financial aid history information, to assist program administrators with tracking refunds and cancellations, or to provide a standardized method for educational institutions efficiently to submit student enrollment status.

In the event of litigation, we may send records to the Department of Justice, a court, adjudicative body, counsel, party, or witness if the disclosure is relevant and necessary to the litigation. If this information, either alone or with other information, indicates a potential violation of law, we may send it to the appropriate authority for action. We may send information to members of Congress if you ask them to help you with federal student aid questions. In circumstances involving employment complaints, grievances, or disciplinary actions, we may disclose relevant records to adjudicate or investigate the issues. If provided for by a collective bargaining agreement, we may disclose records to a labor organization recognized under 5 U.S.C. Chapter 71. Disclosures may also be made to qualified researchers under Privacy Act safeguards.

Paperwork Reduction Notice

According to the Paperwork Reduction Act of 1995, no persons are required to respond to a collection of information unless it displays a currently valid OMB control number. The valid OMB control number for this information collection is 1845-0005. The time required to complete this information collection is estimated to average 0.16 hours (10 minutes) per response, including the time to review instructions, search existing data resources, gather and maintain the data needed, and complete and review the information collection. *If you have any comments concerning the accuracy of the time estimate(s) or suggestions for improving this form, please write to:*

U.S. Department of Education, Washington, DC 20202-4651

If you have any comments or concerns regarding the status of your individual submission of this form, write directly to the address shown in Section 7.

Figure 57-17, *cont'd* For legend see previous page.

Top Ten Ways to Avoid Defaulting on a Student Loan

1. Understand your rights and responsibilities regarding your repayment obligation as well as your repayment options.
2. Borrow for college expenses only. Borrow only the amount you need and only what you can reasonably expect to be able to repay.
3. Keep all records regarding your loan. Make copies of all letters, canceled checks, and any forms you sign.
4. Notify your lender or servicer when you have a change of address, phone number, or name or if you change schools or your enrollment status.
5. Seek help as early as possible if you have any difficulty maintaining your student loan repayment arrangement.
6. If you have any questions, talk to your lender or student loan guarantor about the particular terms of your loan.
7. Keep credit card debt to a minimum or avoid credit card debt completely.
8. Create and maintain a budget that is within your monthly income.
9. Consider making nominal student loan payments while in school. This will reduce the amount you owe after graduation.
10. Make loan payments on time.

Courtesy Texas Guaranteed Student Loan Corporation. Available at: www.tgslc.org.

MONTHLY INCOME	AMOUNT
Net Income	
Spouse Net Income	
Child Support	
Other Income	

MONTHLY EXPENSES	AMOUNT
Rent	
Gas	
Electric	
Home/Renters Insurance	
Water/Sewage	
Trash	
Home Telephone	
Cell Telephone	
Pager	
Cable TV/Satellite	
Internet/DSL	
Child Care	
Lawn Care	
Clothing	
Food - Home	
Food - Work or School	
Food - Eating Out	
Laundry/Dry Cleaning	
Medical Expenses	
Dental Expenses	
Life Insurance	
Medical Insurance	
Dental Insurance	
Eyeglasses	
Prescriptions	
Automobile Payment	
Automobile Insurance	
Repairs	
Gas/Oil	
Furniture	
Beauty/Barber Shop	
Pet Expenses	
Student Loan	
Other Loans	
Credit Cards	
Church/Charities	
Birthdays	
Anniversaries	
Christmas	
Vacation Planning	
Entertainment	

Figure 57-18 The guideline budget.

have not been paid, frustration and depression may result. Some people may even avoid opening letters or bills just so they do not have to deal with seeing the balance due. Writing checks on funds that are not in the checking account is not only unwise—it is also illegal. All states have laws related to insufficient fund checks, and most legislation considers this a form of theft. It is possible to be arrested for writing "hot" checks. People headed for financial disaster also purchase daily items, such as bread and milk, with a credit card. All of these behaviors are signs of financial trouble.

A sample budget outline is shown in Figure 57-18. Take an honest look at each item listed, and determine what amount is spent monthly in each category. Compare these amounts with the monthly income and see if the current budget is positive or negative. Remember that the gross salary is the amount earned before taxes and other deductions. The net salary is the take-home pay. Adjustments may be needed to bring the budget into balance.

CLOSING COMMENTS

The period surrounding graduation will be a celebration, but also a busy time for which much planning is required. Cooperate with the school when securing externship sites, and make an effort to obtain a site that will be of the most benefit to the career desired. Do not take an externship just because it is close to home. Think about the skills that will be offered, and learn as much as possible. Then perform well, so that the staff and physicians are happy to offer a good reference to potential employers. Strive to attain goals and once they are reached, set additional goals to continue moving forward in life.

Even though the medical assistant educational experience ends, remember that there is constantly something new to learn in the medical profession. Join professional societies, and participate in as many educational seminars and continuing education classes as possible. Remain in a continual state of learning, and be determined to be the best medical assistant you can be.

Steps for Achieving Goals

- Decide what you want
- Write the goal down
- Set the date for accomplishment
- Read the goal three times daily
- Think of the goal often
- See yourself accomplishing the goal
- Develop a plan of action for reaching the goal
- Do not discuss the plan with others who might be discouraging
- Be confident
- Act successful, and you will be!

Always be completely honest when completing a job application and offering information on a resume. Most facilities stipulate that if an individual is not truthful on these documents, his or her employment can be terminated once the deception is discovered. Employers are more interested in honesty and a forthright explanation than in minor problems that affect the job performance.

If a medical assistant has had some brush with the law that requires disclosure on the job application, the best policy is to be honest and deal with the ramifications of telling the truth. Most businesses can verify whether a potential employee has any type of criminal record. A solid explanation of the facts, admission of a past mistake, and excellent, current references will often prompt an employer to have faith and make a positive decision about extending employment.

SUMMARY OF SCENARIO

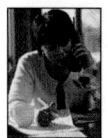

The end of medical assistant training is a time of great excitement and perhaps a small bit of apprehension. Lisa is prepared to accept the challenges ahead as she readies herself for her future in her new career. She has begun her externship and has been expanding her network of acquaintances in the medical profession for several months. Lisa has met many office managers and a few physicians and has learned a great deal about several area medical facilities. Through her research, she has decided that she would like to work with one of three local physicians who need a medical assistant. One is a pediatrician, another is a well-known neurologist, and the third is a family practitioner just out of medical school. Lisa has gathered information about all of these professionals, and each has invited her for a job interview.

Lisa knows that she will need to be at her best, so she takes care of herself and gets plenty of rest. She has a long list of interview questions and has taken the time to write out answers to the questions in preparation for her interviews. She is careful about her grooming every day that she reports to the externship, because she knows that the physician at her site is her first reference in the medical field. In addition, she knows that she may be called for an interview any day that might be scheduled just after her workday ends. Looking professional prepares her for this each day.

Lisa is comfortable during her interviews because she is well prepared. She has identified her strengths and can share them with a potential employer. She is focused on her objectives and knows what the minimum requirements will be for her to accept a position. She has a healthy self-esteem, and her good decision-making skills will help her to determine which position will be right for her. Her enthusiasm and excitement show in her eyes, and she is dedicated to making a difference in the lives of her patients and co-workers.

SUMMARY of LEARNING OBJECTIVES

1. Define, spell, and pronounce the terms listed in the vocabulary.
   - Spelling and pronouncing medical terms correctly adds credibility to the medical assistant. Knowing the definition of these terms promotes confidence in communication with patients and co-workers.
2. Discuss the reasons that job search training is important to a medical assistant.
   - Because approximately 85% of individuals do not have any formal training in job search skills, taking the time to learn the best methods will place the medical assistant at an advantage. Training decreases the time spent looking for work and increases the benefits and salary offered when using good

negotiating skills. The medical assistant will also be more comfortable during interviews and throughout the job search process.
3. List three expectations that employers have of employees.
   - Employers have three basic expectations of their medical assistant employees. They want an employee with a good appearance, who looks as if he or she fits in the medical profession. A medical assistant should also be dependable and have the skills to do the job for which he or she was hired.
4. Understand the three types of employee skill strengths.
   - There are three types of skill strengths that may be used by employees. Job skills are those used to actually perform

Continued

SUMMARY of LEARNING OBJECTIVES
Continued

a job, such as venipunctures or scheduling appointments. Self-management skills are usually a part of the medical assistant's personality; these include honesty and dependability. Transferable skills are those that can be taken from one job to another or used on any job. Examples include the ability to communicate effectively and lead and manage individuals.

5. Explain the two best job search methods.
   - Networking and contacting employers directly are the two best methods of job searching. Networking involves developing a network of individuals that can assist in finding employment. This group may include co-workers, other students, relatives, or friends who provide leads to potential employers. Contacting employers directly includes taking resumes to specific offices or setting appointments to gain knowledge about the facility, then later using that knowledge during the job search. These two methods are more effective than most traditional means of finding a job.

6. Describe some of the errors that should be avoided on a resume.
   - Any error on a resume should be avoided. Be sure that everything is spelled correctly, but do not rely on the computer's spell-check feature alone. Proofread the document, and have someone else proofread it to catch errors that may have been overlooked. Salary expectations should never be stated on the resume, and a photograph should not be included. Do not include personal information, such as height and weight.

7. Explain the importance of having demographic information about former jobs before appearing for an interview.
   - Demographic information on other employers should be taken to interviews and kept handy when filling out job applications. A medical assistant should never have to ask for a phone book to look up the address of a former employer. This demonstrates a lack of preparation and planning on the part of the potential employee.

8. List the four phases of the interview process.
   - The four phases of the interview process include the preparation, the actual interview, the follow-up, and the negotiation. The preparation includes all efforts made before the actual interview in obtaining information about the company, deciding on the wardrobe, and making sure nails are groomed and shoes are shined. The interview itself is designed to help the employer and potential employee get to know each other and discover whether they are compatible. The follow-up is perhaps the most critical stage, wherein the medical assistant should send a thank-you letter and continue to stay in touch with the facility until the job is filled. The negotiation includes discussion of the salary and benefits that will be offered to the new employee.

9. Discuss the importance of the probationary period for a new employee.
   - The probationary period is a time for the new medical assistant to become oriented to the facility. It also allows the employer to assess whether the medical assistant fits with the team and performs the duties of the job in a satisfactory way. During this time, the medical assistant should demonstrate that he or she is a productive team member with an excellent attitude. There should never be idle time; instead, look for ways to assist others when all duties are completed.

10. List some mistakes that should be avoided by a new employee.
    - A new employee in the medical office should avoid arriving late or being absent, especially during the probationary period. Never participate in office gossip, and make a good attempt to get along with every employee. A medical assistant should not make excessive supervision necessary and should be open to learning new ways of performing procedures. Fit in with the team, and the job will be more rewarding.

11. Explain why a performance appraisal's ratings are usually not perfect.
    - No employee is perfect, so performance appraisals rarely have perfect ratings. Even an employee who is doing an excellent job has room for improvement in some area. Without comments that suggest improvement, the employee may not feel that the position offers growth potential. Constructive comments will help a medical assistant to perform better and take on more responsibility.

12. Prepare a resume.
    - The resume must be accurate and error-free. The process for preparing a resume is outlined in Procedure 57-2.

13. Organize a job search.
    - Time management and organizational skills will help the medical assistant to launch an effective job search. The process for organizing a job search is outlined in Procedure 57-1.

14. Complete a job application.
    - Job applications must be competed accurately and in their entirety. The process for completing a job application is outlined in Procedure 57-3.

15. Interview for a job.
    - The interview is the job search step that most influences hiring decisions. The process for interviewing for a job is outlined in Procedure 57-4.

16. Negotiate a salary.
    - The medical assistant should develop skills in negotiating salary after he or she has determined the minimum amount in both benefits and pay that can be accepted. The process for negotiating a salary is outlined in Procedure 57-5.

CONNECTIONS

    Study Guide Connection: Go to Chapter 57 Study Guide. Read the Case Study and Workplace Applications and complete the assignments. Do online research for answers to the questions in the Internet Activities associated with career development and life skills.

    CD Connection: Go to the Medical Assisting Competency Challenge CD and do the training activities under Communication.

    Evolve Connection: For more information related to career development and life skills, go to evolve.elsevier.com/kinn and visit related weblinks for Chapter 57. Click on the Medical Assisting Exam Review and do the practice questions to sharpen your test-taking skills.

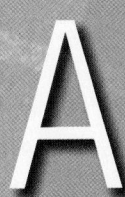
English-Spanish Phrases

Commonly Used Phrases

Are you having pain? Where?
¿Siente usted dolor? ¿Dónde?

What does the pain feel like?
¿Qué tipo de dolor es?

How long have you had problems with this?
¿Desde cuándo tiene este tipo de problemas?

When did it start?
¿Cuándo comenzó?

Does your child have a temperature?
¿Tiene fiebre su hijo?

Have you given your child any medication?
¿Le ha dado alguna medicina a su hijo?

Are you allergic to any medication?
¿Es usted alérgico a algo?

How did your child get hurt?
¿Cómo se lastimó su hijo?

What is your name?
¿Cómo se llama usted?

How old are you?
¿Qué edad tiene?

Do you take any medication regularly?
¿Toma usted alguna medicación con regularidad?

How many times have you been pregnant?
¿Cuántas veces ha estado embarazada?

How many children were born alive?
¿Cuántos niños sanos ha dado usted a luz?

Who is your closest relative?
¿Quién es su familiar más cercano?

Do you speak English?
¿Habla usted inglés?

Can someone come with you the next time who does speak English?
¿Puede acompañarle alguien que hable inglés la próxima vez?

Can you read English?
¿Sabe usted leer en inglés?

Does someone in your family read English?
¿Alguien de su familiar sabe leer en inglés?

My name is… You are…
Yo soy… Usted es…

Please put the gown on.
Por favor, póngase la bata.

Your blood pressure is…
Su presión arterial es de…

Your blood sugar is…
Su nivel de azúcar en la sangre es de…

The doctor recommends a low-fat diet.
El médico recomienda una dieta baja en grasa.

Does this hurt?
¿Le duele esto?

Do you have medical insurance?
¿Tiene usted seguro médico?

Please point to where it hurts.
Por favor, indíqueme dónde le duele.

Where do you work?
¿Dónde trabaja usted?

Have you seen blood in your urine?
¿Ha visto algo de sangre en su orina?

Do you have pain when urinating?
¿Siente algún dolor al orinar?

Please fill out this form.
Por favor, llene este formulario.

Do you have an insurance card?
¿Tiene usted una tarjeta del seguro?

Do you have a telephone? What is the number?
¿Tiene usted teléfono? ¿Cuál es el número?

Please come back to see the doctor on…
Por favor, regrese para ver al médico el…

The doctor wants you to see another doctor.
El médico quiere que la vea otro médico.

Go to the hospital.
Vaya al hospital.

Call the ambulance now.
Pida una ambulancia ahora mismo.

Take your medication as ordered.
Tómese la medicación tal como se le indicó.

These are the side effects of your medication.
Su medicación tiene algunos efectos secundarios.

Thank you.
Gracias.

You are welcome.
De nada.

Please.
Por favor.

Please come this way.
Venga por aquí, por favor.

Please come with me.
Acompáñeme, por favor.

Please wait here to see the doctor.
Por favor, espere aquí para ver al médico.

You may leave now.
Ya puede marcharse.

We need to get a blood sample.
Necesitamos una muestra de su sangre.

We need to get a urine sample.
Necesitamos una muestra de su orina.

You owe "xxx" today.
Hoy debe abonar "xxx."

Who should we call to pick you up?
¿A quién debemos contactar para que lo recojan?

Please go to the laboratory at this address.
Por favor, vaya al laboratorio que está en este lugar.

When did you last eat?
¿Cuándo comió por última vez?

Have you had nausea?
¿Ha tenido náuseas?

Have you vomited?
¿Ha vomitado?

Please sign your name here.
Por favor, firme aquí.

Take this medicine (3) times a day.
Tómese esta medicina (3) veces al día.

This paper allows us to file your insurance.
Este papel nos permite presentarle su caso al seguro.

This paper allows the insurance company to pay the doctor.
Este papel es para que el seguro le pague al médico.

The doctor will see you now.
El médico le puede ver ahora.

Good morning.
Buenos días.

Good afternoon.
Buenas tardes.

Here is information (written) about your illness.
Aquí se incluye información (escrita) sobre su enfermedad.

Please follow these directions.
Por favor, siga estas instrucciones.

It is nice to meet you.
Es un placer conocerle.

Thank you for coming.
Gracias por su visita.

Take care of yourself.
¡Cuídese!

Do you drink alcohol?
¿Toma usted alcohol?

Do you smoke? How much?
¿Fuma? ¿Cuántos cigarrillos al día?

Have you had this problem before?
¿Ha tenido antes este problema?

Days of the week

Los días de la semana

Monday
lunes

Tuesday
martes

Wednesday
miércoles

Thursday
jueves

Friday
viernes

Saturday
sábado

Sunday
domingo

Months of the year

Los meses del año

January
enero

February
febrero

March
marzo

April
abril

May
mayo

June
junio

July
julio

August
agosto

September
septiembre

October
octubre

November
noviembre

December
diciembre

Times

Horas

One o'clock
Es la una

Two o'clock
Son las dos

Three o'clock
Son las tres

Four o'clock
Son las cuatro

Five o'clock
Son las cinco

Six o'clock
Son las seis

Seven o'clock
Son las siete

Eight o'clock
Son las ocho

Nine o'clock
Son las nueve

Ten o'clock
Son las diez

Eleven o'clock
Son las once

Twelve o'clock
Son las doce

Numbers

Números

1
uno

2
dos

3
tres

4	cuatro	18	dieciocho
5	cinco	19	diecinueve
6	seis	20	veinte
7	siete	21	veintiuno
8	ocho	22	veintidos
9	nueve	23	veintitres
10	diez	24	veinticuatro
11	once	25	veinticinco
12	doce	26	veintiséis
13	trece	27	veintisiete
14	catorce	28	veintiocho
15	quince	29	veintinueve
16	dieciséis	30	treinta
17	diecisiete	31	treinta y uno

ICD-10-CM and ICD-10-PCS

The tenth revision of Volumes 1, 2, and 3 of the International Classification of Diseases (ICD) brings massive changes. There are now two separate systems: ICD-10-CM for diagnostic coding and ICD-10-PCS for procedural coding.

- ICD-10-CM (International Statistical Classifications of Diseases and Related Health Problems, Tenth Revision, Clinical Modification) is the replacement for Volumes I and II—the diagnoses, signs, symptoms, and health-related codes.
- ICD-10-PCS (International Statistical Classifications of Diseases and Related Health Problems, Tenth Revision, Procedural Coding System) replaces Volume III—the procedures generally performed within a hospital environment.

TENTH REVISION OF ICD

The World Health Organization (WHO) published the tenth revision of the ICD system in 1992 in order to:

- Expand the content, purpose, and scope of system
- Include ambulatory care services
- Increase clinical detail
- Capture risk factors in primary care
- Include emergent diseases
- Group diagnoses for epidemiologic purposes

ICD-10-CM IMPLEMENTATION

The National Center for Health Statistics (NCHS) began testing the clinical modification of ICD-10 in 1997. The American Health Information Management Association (AHIMA), in cooperation with the American Hospital Association (AHA), has begun field testing coding and records management using the ICD-10-CM. Implementation of ICD-10-CM is likely to happen no sooner than October 2007. However, the massive changes to the coding system and the huge impact on all of healthcare in implementing these changes require that planning and training in the new coding system begin now.

BENEFITS OF ICD-10-CM

- Greater specificity
- Added descriptions relevant to ambulatory care and managed care encounters
- Allows for the possibility of expansion

- Extends beyond classification of diseases and injuries to include health-related risk factors
- General terminology and disease classification have been updated to current standards

ICD-10-CM

With the release of Volume 1 of the ICD-10 in 1992 by WHO, the United States requested and was granted permission to develop an adaptation of ICD-10 for use in the United States for government purposes. Currently this clinical modification is underway and is being called *ICD-10-CM*. Other countries have already made or are developing their own modifications of ICD-10 for use within their respective countries. ICD-10-CM will replace ICD-9-CM Volumes 1 and 2 only. Like the ICD-9-CM system, this new coding system is closely related to its ICD counterpart (ICD-10). Therefore it closely follows the changes to ICD-10. It contains significantly more codes than the current ICD-9-CM. It is also alphanumeric and has up to seven digits. Please note that Volume 3 (the inpatient procedures) is not included in ICD-10-CM. A separate coding system, called *ICD-10-PCS* (procedure coding system), has been proposed as a replacement.

COMPARISON OF ICD-10-CM WITH ICD-9-CM

The advantages and benefits of ICD-10-CM are significant in both quality and usefulness of data for various healthcare settings.

- The hierarchic structure is the same for both classification systems, but ICD-10-CM codes are alphanumeric and include all letters except U, which is reserved for new diseases of uncertain etiology.
- ICD-9-CM's V and E codes have been incorporated into the main classification of ICD-10-CM.
- ICD-10-CM codes can be up to seven characters, compared with the maximum of five for ICD-9-CM.
- ICD-10-CM incorporates additional information related to ambulatory care and managed care encounters.
- Conditions that were not uniquely identified in ICD-9-CM have been assigned code numbers in ICD-10-CM.
- In ICD-10-CM, as in ICD-9-CM, some three-character categories are left vacant to allow for code revisions and future additions.
- The ICD-10-CM groups injuries first by site (arm,

shoulder, ankle), then by type (fracture, sprain), rather than just by type, as they are in the ICD-9-CM.

- The Excludes guidelines and notes have been expanded to provide guidance on hierarchy of the chapters and help clarify code assignment.
- Some conditions are listed in more appropriate chapters in the ICD-10-CM.

Some new or expanded features of the ICD-10-CM include the following:

- Combination codes are used for both symptom and diagnosis and for etiology and manifestations.
- Many codes have been expanded to include laterality (identification of a specific side of the body), a feature that was missing from ICD-9-CM.

- Classifications that indicate a patient's trimester are included in the OB chapter. In the section on diabetes, codes are included for types that require insulin therapy and types that do not.
- Codes for postoperative complications have been expanded.
- Codes have been expanded to allow for distinctions between intraoperative complications and postprocedural disorders.

For more information about ICD-10-CM and ICD-10-PCS, contact the National Center for Health Statistics (NCHS) (www.cdc.gov/nchs) or AHIMA (www.ahima.org).

Understanding Medical Terms

Medical terminology is similar to a foreign language. Many medical terms are derived from Latin and Greek sources. They often consist of two or more simple words or word elements. A word root or *combining form* may be put together with a *prefix* and a *suffix*.

Root–the basis of a word
Example: *nephr*/o/tic (degenerative changes in the kidney)
Root: nephr- (kidney)

Linking vowel–a vowel that joins the combining form to the suffix or another combining form
Example: nephr/*o/sis* (disease of the kidneys)
Linking vowel: o

Prefix–the beginning of a word
Example: *hyper*/active (excessively active)
Prefix: hyper- (excessive)

Suffix–the ending of a word
Example: nephr/itis (inflammation of the kidney)
Suffix: -itis (inflammation)

Combining form–the union of a word root with a linking vowel
Example: *hepato*/megaly (enlargement of the liver)
Combining form: hepato- (liver)

The following table provides some of the most commonly used terminology for your reference.

Common Prefixes

PREFIX	DEFINITION
a-	without
ab-	away from
abd-	abdominal
acu-	sharp
ad-	toward
adip-	fat
ad lib-	freely, as wanted
aero-	air, gas
al-	toward
ambi-	both
an-	not
ana-	up
ante-	before, in front of
anti-	against
arteri-	artery
arthro-	joint
auto-	self
bi-	two

PREFIX	DEFINITION
brady-	slow
cata-	down
chole-	bile
cili-	eyelid
circum-	around
co-	with, together
cogni-	know
colo-	colon
con-	with, together
contra-	against
crani-	skull
cut-	skin
cyt-	cell
de-	from, lack of
demi-	half
dent-	tooth
derm-	skin
dia-	through, across
diplo-	double, twofold
dis-	to free or undo
dors-	back
dur-	hard
dy-	two
dys-	bad, painful, difficult, abnormal
ec-	out, out from
ecto-	outside
em-	in
embol-	to insert
encephalo-	brain
endo-	in, within
entero-	intestine
epi-	above, upon
erythro-	red
eso-	within, inward
et-	and
eu-	good, normal
ex-	out, away from
exo-	outside
extra-	outside
faci-	face
fiss-	split, cleft
fore-	before, in front of
gastro-	stomach
glosso-	relating to the tongue

PREFIX	DEFINITION
glyco-	sugar
haplo-	simple, single
heme-	iron-based
hemi-	one half
hepat-	liver
hetero-	different
histo-	tissue
homo-	same
hydro-	wet, water
hyper-	excessive, above normal
hypo-	under, below
im-	not
in-	in, not
infra-	under, below
inter-	between
intra-	in, within
isch-	deficiency
iso-	equal, alike
lapis-	stone
lapra-	loin or flank, sometimes abdomen
latero-	side
macro-	large
mal-	bad
meato-	opening
medi-	middle
melano-	black
mesa-	middle
meso-	middle
meta-	beyond, change
micro-	small
mono-	one
morpho-	form, structure
multi-	many, much
neo-	new
nephro-	kidney
oculo-	eye
onco-	tumor
oro-	mouth
osteo-	bone
pan-	all
para-	beside, beyond
per-	through, by
peri-	around
phago-	eating
poly-	many, much
post-	after, behind
pre-	before, in front of
primi-	first
pro-	before, in front of
pseudo-	false
quadri-	four
re-	again, backward
retro-	backward, behind
rhabdo-	rod-shaped, striated
rhodo-	red
scler-	hardening

PREFIX	DEFINITION
semi-	one half
sub-	under, below
super-	above, excessive
supra-	above, excessive
stetho-	chest
sym-	together
syn-	union, together, joined
tachy-	rapid
tetra-	four
therm-	heat
trans-	through, across
tri-	three
ultra-	beyond, excess
uni-	one
vas-	vessel or duct
xantho-	yellow
xero-	dry

Common Suffixes

SUFFIX	DEFINITION
-ac	pertaining to
-agra	excessive pain
-al	pertaining to
-algia	painful condition, pain
-apheresis	removal
-ar	pertaining to
-ary	pertaining to
-ase	enzyme
-bi	two, double
-blast	developing cell
-cele	hernia, swelling, sac
-centesis	puncture of a cavity
-clasis	break, fracture
-clysis	irrigation, washing
-coccus	berry shaped
-crit	to separate
-cyte	cell
-desis	fusion, binding, fixation
-drome	to run
-dynia	pain
-ectasis	expansion, dilation
-ectomy	excision, removal of a body part
-emesis	vomiting
-emia	blood
-er	one who
-gen	forming, producing, origin
-genesis	forming, producing, origin
-genic	origin, formation
-grade	to go
-gram	the record made, mark
-graph	instrument for recording, machine
-graphy	the process, process of recording
-ia	condition
-iasis	morbid condition
-iatry	treatment, medicine
-ic/-ical	pertaining to

SUFFIX	DEFINITION	SUFFIX	DEFINITION
-icle	small, minute	-plasia	formation, growth
-ism	condition	-plasm	growth, formation
-ist	one who specializes in, specialist	-plasty	mold, shape, repair
-itis	inflammation	-plegia	paralysis
-lith	stone, calculus	-poiesis	formation, production
-logist	specialist in the study of	-ptosis	downward displacement, falling
-logy	process of study	-ptysis	spitting
-lysis	dissolution, setting free	-rrhage	bursting forth, rupture
-malacia	softening, soft	-rrhaphy	suturing in place
-megaly	enlargement	-rrhea	flow, discharge
-meter	instrument for measuring	-rrhexis	rupture
-metry	act of measuring	-scope	instrument to visually examine
-odynia	pain	-scopy	process of examining, visual
-oid	form, shape		examination
-ole	small, minute	-sepsis	infection
-ology	study or science of	-sis	state of, condition
-oma	tumor	-spasm	involuntary spasm
-opsy	to view	-stalsis	constriction
-or	one who	-stasis	control, constant level, stop
-orrhea	flow, discharge	-stenosis	narrowing, stricture
-osis	condition or state	-stomy	creation of an opening
-ous	pertaining to	-therapy	treatment
-para	to bear (offspring)	-tic	pertaining to
-paresis	partial paralysis	-tome	instrument for cutting
-pathy	disease, suffering	-tomy	process of cutting, incision
-penia	deficiency, lack of, decrease	-toxic	poison
-pexy	fixation	-tresia	opening
-phagia	eating, swallowing	-tripsy	surgical crushing
-phasia	speech	-trophy	nourishment
-philia	attraction for	-ula	small, minute
-phobia	fear	-ule	small, minute
-physis	to grow	-y	process

Procedure Charting Examples

Procedure 30-1 Obtaining an Oral Temperature Using a Digital Thermometer		
Date	Time	Note
3/27/XX	10:05 AM	T – 97.7°F orally ———————————————————— C. Ricci, CMA

Procedure 30-2 Obtaining an Aural Temperature Using the Tympanic Thermometer		
Date	Time	Note
3/30/XX	2:20 PM	T – 101.2°F (T) ———————————————————— C. Ricci, CMA

Procedure 30-3 Obtaining an Axillary Temperature		
Date	Time	Note
4/2/XX	9:30 AM	T – 98.2°F (A) ———————————————————— C. Ricci, CMA

Procedure 30-4 Obtaining an Apical Pulse		
Date	Time	Note
4/22/XX	4:10 PM	AP – 92 irregular ———————————————————— C. Ricci, CMA

Procedure 30-5 Assessing the Patient's Pulse (radial pulse)		
Date	Time	Note
5/6/XX	8:35 AM	P – 72, reg ———————————————————— C. Ricci, CMA

Procedure 30-6 Determining Respirations		
Date	Time	Note
5/12/XX	1:15 PM	R – 18 ———————————————————— C. Ricci, CMA

Procedure 30-7 Determining a Patient's Blood Pressure		
Date	Time	Note
5/19/XX	3:20 PM	BP – 120/80 Ⓛ arm ———————————————————— C. Ricci, CMA

Orthostatic Hypotension Documentation:		
Date	Time	Note
5/19/XX	3:25 PM	BP – 120/80 sitting, BP – 102/68 standing Ⓛ arm ——————— C. Ricci, CMA

Procedure 30-8   Measuring a Patient's Height and Weight

Date	Time	Note
5/26/XX	11:07 AM	Wt – 136½ lb, Ht – 64¼ in _____ C. Ricci, CMA

Procedure 34-1   Safety Measures in Preparing, Administering, and Documenting

Date	Time	Note
1/12/XX	11:22 AM	Administered 10 mcg Recombivax IM to Ⓛ deltoid. Pt informed this is the first of 3 doses.
		No side effects noted. Appointment scheduled for patient to return in 1 mo for second dose.
		_____ D. Gaston, CMA

Procedure 34-2   Maintaining Medication Records

Date	Time	Note
4/02/XX	9:30 AM	Administered Lasix 20 mg and potassium chloride 20 mEq PO without difficulty. Pt informed
		of importance of taking medications as prescribed for treatment of hypertension; warned
		she will have to urinate more frequently. No side effects noted. Appointment scheduled for
		patient to return in 1 mo for follow-up. _____ D. Gaston, CMA

Procedure 34-3   Dispensing, Administering, and Documenting Oral Medications

Date	Time	Note
6/8/XX	9:45 AM	Aldomet tab 250 mg po administered per physician order _____ Dorothy Gaston, CMA

Procedure 34-7   Giving an Intradermal Injection

Date	Time	Note
8/22/XX	9:10 AM	Administered Mantoux TB test as ordered, 0.1 ml ID, lot # MF4780D, exp date 2/xx, to Ⓡ
		anterior forearm. Pt tolerated procedure well. No questions. Appointment made to return
		8/24 for reading. _____ Dorothy Gaston, CMA

Procedure 34-8   Giving an Intradermal Injection

Date	Time	Note
6/14/XX	11:35 AM	0.5 ml Varicella virus vaccine administered SQ to Ⓡ posterior upper arm, lot # V5829K,
		exp date 9/xx. VIS form given to mother. She had no questions. Pt tolerated
		procedure well. _____ Dorothy Gaston, CMA

Procedure 34-9   Giving an Intramuscular Injection into the Deltoid

Date	Time	Note
9/8/XX	8:35 AM	300,000 U Penicillin G administered IM to Ⓡ deltoid without complication. Patient observed
		for allergic reaction and none noted. Patient had no questions. Instructed to call office if he
		experiences any problems from injection. _____ D. Gaston, CMA

Procedure 34-10	Administering a Pediatric Intramuscular Vastus Lateralis Injection	
Date	Time	Note
3/27/XX	1:30 PM	Hib lot # 98525, exp date 10/08, administered IM to Ⓛ vastus lateralis. Caregiver given Hib
		VIS, answered questions regarding follow-up care. No adverse effects noted. Appointment
		made for next immunizations in 1 month. _____ D. Gaston, CMA

Procedure 34-11	Giving a Z-Track Intramuscular Injection Into the Dorsogluteal Site	
Date	Time	Note
7/13/XX	1:25 PM	1 ml INFeD administered Z-Track IM in Ⓡ dorsogluteal site. Injection site not massaged
		after administration. No evidence of skin discoloration after administration. _____
		_____ Dorothy Gaston, CMA

Procedure 35-2	Perform Telephone Screening and Document Appropriately	
Date	Time	Note
7/12/XX	2:45 PM	Patient's mother reports child fell against a window and lacerated his arm. Bleeding is moderate
		but controlled. There are no reported signs of dyspnea or altered consciousness. Mother will
		bring child to office immediately for physician assessment. _____ C. Skurka, CMA

Procedure 35-4	Administering Oxygen	
Date	Time	Note
7/24/XX	3:05 PM	R – 28 and labored. Oxygen initiated at 4 L/min via nasal cannula per physician order. Pt
		observed for signs of dyspnea and tachypnea. _____ Cheryl Skurka, CMA

Procedure 35-5	Responding to an Adult With an Obstructed Airway	
Date	Time	Note
7/22/XX	8:35 AM	Pt in waiting room coughing forcefully but clutching throat. After confirming pt choking,
		abdominal thrusts administered until foreign body expelled. Pt breathing without difficulty;
		R – 18. Situation reported to physician. _____ Cheryl Skurka, CMA

Procedure 35-6	Caring for a Patient Who Fainted	
Date	Time	Note
7/29/XX	4:18 PM	Pt in waiting room states she feels faint. Pt lowered to floor, clothes loosened, and legs
		elevated. Physician notified. P – 88 and regular, R – 22, BP 112/66. Syncopal episode
		persisted for 90 sec, feeling of vertigo lasted 10 minutes post-syncope. Pt transferred to
		exam room via wheelchair after recovery. _____ Cheryl Skurka, CMA

Procedure 36-1	Measuring Distance Visual Acuity Using the Snellen Chart	
Date	Time	Note
8/01/XX	2:20 PM	Visual acuity exam completed c̄ Snellen eye chart. OD 20/40; OS 20-30 –1; OU 20/30 c̄
		corrective lenses. No squinting noted. _____ Kim Tau, CMA

Procedure 36-3   Irrigating a Patient's Eyes

Date	Time	Note
8/06/XX	9:00 AM	OD irrigated with 500 cc normal saline. Sclera clear post-irrigation. No c/o discomfort.
		Kim Tau, CMA

Procedure 36-4   Instilling Eye Medication

Date	Time	Note
8/8/XX	1:45 PM	Thin ribbon of Neosporin ophthalmic ung applied in lower conjunctival sac of OS. No pt
		complaints. Pt instructed on homecare application of med including washing hands before
		and after procedure and taking care not to touch eye with applicator.
		Kim Tau, CMA

Procedure 36-6   Irrigating a Patient's Ear

Date	Time	Note
8/12/XX	10:15 AM	AS irrigated with 500 cc warm saline soln. Large amt of dark brown cerumen expelled. Post-irrigation TM visible and pearly gray. No c/o discomfort. Kim Tau, CMA

Procedure 36-7   Instilling Medicated Ear Drops

Date	Time	Note
8/12/XX	3:22 PM	ii gtts Auralgan otic soln administered to AD. No c/o discomfort. Pt instructed on home use.
		Kim Tau, CMA

Procedure 36-8   Collecting a Specimen for Throat Culture

Date	Time	Note
8/14/XX	8:35 AM	Throat specimen collected via swab from tonsillar area. Sent to University Laboratories for Strep testing. Kim Tau, CMA

Procedure 39-1   Teaching Testicular Self-Examination

Date	Time	Note
8/19/XX	11:12 AM	Pt shown and successfully demonstrated testicular self-exam on model. Given pamphlet and shower card for home use. Dorothy Gaston, CMA

Procedure 40-1   Assisting With Examination of the Female Patient and Pap Smear

Date	Time	Note
8/23/XX	2:00 PM	Pap smear prepared. Slides placed for pick-up by University Laboratory for cytology.
		Betsy Davis, CMA

Procedure 40-2   Preparing the Patient for Cryosurgery

Date	Time	Note
7/22/XX	10:25 AM	Cervical cryosurgery procedure completed without incident. Pt stable, T-98.6°, BP 118/72.
		No c/o discomfort. Pt to call office if any problems noted.
		B. Davis, CMA

Procedure 41-1   Documentation of Immunizations

Date	Time	Note
4/2/XX	3:25 PM	Administered second dose of Hep B to (L) vastus lateralis. Mother given VIS form. Had no
		questions. No problems noted after injection.
		S. Kwong, CMA

Procedure 41-3   Measuring Infant Length and Weight

Date	Time	Note
8/24/XX	10:20 AM	Wt 17 lb 4 oz Length 27 in ———————————————— Susie Kwong, CMA

Procedure 41-5   Applying a Urinary Collection Device

Date	Time	Note
8/24/XX	10:45 AM	Urine specimen collected for culture. Placed for pick-up by North Hills Laboratory.
		Susie Kwong, CMA

Procedure 42-1   Assisting With Cold Application

Date	Time	Note
8/27/XX	1:45 PM	Ice pack applied to (R) knee for 20 min. No c/o of discomfort. Pt instructed to continue ice
		application q 3 hrs while awake for 24 hrs at 20 min intervals. To call physician if edema
		persists. ——————————————— Kaiwan Tillman, CMA

Procedure 42-2   Assisting With Hot Moist Heat Application in the Office

Date	Time	Note
9/2/XX	8:35 AM	Commercial hot pack applied to lumbar region for 20 min. Pt states muscle cramps relieved.
		Instructed to continue hot packs q 2 hrs for 20 min prn for relief of muscular pain. To return
		to office 9/5/XX for further evaluation. ——————— Kaiwan Tillman, CMA

Procedure 42-3   Assisting With Therapeutic Ultrasonography

Date	Time	Note
9/6/XX	4:33 PM	Ultrasound treatment applied to (R) lower back @ 3 watts X 6 minutes. No pt discomfort
		during procedure. Pt states pain relief, increased muscle relaxation.
		Kaiwan Tillman, CMA

Procedure 42-4   Assisting With Cast Application

Date	Time	Note
9/7/XX	3:17 PM	Applied short fiberglass cast to (R) leg. Skin under cast is clean and intact. Pt given written
		instructions on cast care. ——————————— Kaiwan Tillman, CMA

Procedure 42-7   Assisting the Patient With Crutch Walking

Date	Time	Note
9/8/XX	1:50 PM	Pt instructed in crutch walking using 3-point gait on steps and floor. Pt understands he is to
		be non-weight bearing on (R) leg. Demonstrated techniques without difficulty.
		Kaiwan Tillman, CMA

Procedure 43-3	Preparing the Patient For and Assisting With a Lumbar Puncture	
Date	Time	Note
9/15/XX	8:32 AM	Lumbar puncture performed by Dr. Song. 30 cc of CSF placed for pick-up by North Hills
		Laboratory. Pt to remain in prone position for at least 8 hours. Pt to be given instructions
		for home care and pain relief upon leaving the office. ——— Mai Lee, CMA

Procedure 44-1	Performing a Blood Glucose Accu-Chek Test	
Date	Time	Note
8/16/XX	1:00 PM	Glucometer screening completed as ordered. NFBS 144. Pt took routine dose of 10 U Regular
		insulin at noon. Reinforced pt ed on using control methods. No questions. ———
		——— M. Vasco, CMA

Procedure 48-1	Obtaining a 12-lead ECG	
Date	Time	Note
9/22/XX	12:45 PM	12-lead ECG recorded without incident. ——— Martha Reyes, CMA

Procedure 48-2	Applying a Holter Monitor	
Date	Time	Note
9/29/XX	3:10 PM	Holter monitor applied per physician order. Pt given instructions to leave leads in place until
		she returns to office tomorrow afternoon. Understands to record cardiac symptoms in diary,
		to use event marker if symptoms occur, and not to shower until monitor removed.
		——— Martha Reyes, CMA

Procedure 51-3	Measuring Urine Specific Gravity With a Refractometer	
Date	Time	Note
10/1/XX	9:28 AM	SG: 1.010 ——— Rosa Gonzales, CMA

Procedure 51-8	Performing a Pregnancy Test	
Date	Time	Note
10/2/XX	3:47 PM	LMP: 8/16/XX. QuickVue pregnancy test: Positive. ——— Rosa Gonzales, CMA

Procedure 52-2	Collecting a Venous Blood Sample Using the Evacuated Tube Method	
Date	Time	Note
10/5/XX	1:45 PM	Venous blood drawn from Ⓡ arm for CBC with differential and SMA 12. Placed for pick-up by
		Health Alliance Labs. ——— Leah Barney, CMA

Procedure 53-1	Performing a Microhematocrit	
Date	Time	Note
10/7/XX	11:25 AM	Hct: 44. ——— Dana Cummings, CMA

Procedure 53-3	Performing a Hemoglobin Test	
Date	Time	Note
10/9/XX	9:25 AM	Hb 15.5 g/dL. ——— Dana Cummings, CMA

Procedure 53-9 Performing a Blood Glucose Accu-Check Test		
Date	Time	Note
10/11/XX	8:30 AM	Pt last ate on 10/10 @ 12:30 AM. FBS: 92 mg/dl Dana Cummings, CMA

Procedure 56-13 Applying/Changing a Dressing		
Date	Time	Note
10/12/XX	2:15 PM	Dressing change completed to wound on Ⓛ mid-forearm. Area slightly inflamed, mod amt of
		serosanguineous drainage noted. Site cleansed and sterile dressing applied. Pt instructed on
		home wound care and to notify physician if drainage changes, inflammation increases, or fever
		occurs. ———————————————————————————— Melissa Gelbart, CMA

Procedure 56-15 Applying an Elastic Support Bandage Using a Spiral Turn		
Date	Time	Note
10/22/XX	9:35 AM	Spiral elastic bandage applied to Ⓡ forearm. Pt denies bandage too tight. Fingers warm to
		touch. ———————————————————————————— Melissa Gelbart, CMA

Glossary

abandonment To withdraw protection or support; in medicine, to discontinue medical care without proper notice after accepting a patient.

abscesses Localized collections of pus that may be under the skin or deep within the body and that cause tissue destruction.

abstract An outline or summary of the diagnostic statement and/ or procedures and services performed. In procedural coding, the outline or summary assists in ensuring that all procedures and services are included in an insurance claim submission, and that nothing was omitted or added to the encounter form or charge ticket; to abstract also means to compile this outline or summary for use in procedural coding.

academic degree A title conferred by a college, university, or professional school on completion of a program of study.

accommodation Adjustment of the eye for seeing various sizes of objects at different distances.

account A statement of transactions during a fiscal period and the resulting balance.

account balance The amount owed on an account.

accounts payable Debts incurred and not yet paid.

accounts receivable Amounts owed to the physician.

accounts receivable ledger A record of the charges and payments posted on an account.

accounts receivable trial balance A method of determining that the journal and the ledger are in balance.

accreditation The process through which an organization is recognized for adherence to a group of standards that meet or exceed expectations of the accrediting agency.

accrual basis of accounting Method of accounting in which income is recorded when earned and expenses are recorded when incurred.

acronyms Abbreviations, such as ECG for electrocardiography.

act The formal action of a legislative body; a decision or determination of a sovereign state, a legislative council, or a court of justice.

adage A saying, often in metaphoric form, that embodies a common observation.

add-on code A code that indicates additional or supplemental procedures carried out in addition to the primary procedure.

adhesions Bands of scar tissue that bind together two anatomic surfaces that are normally separate.

adnexal Pertaining to adjacent or accessory parts.

adrenocorticotropic hormone (ACTH) A hormone that stimulates the production and secretion of glucocorticoids; released by the anterior pituitary gland.

advent A coming into being or use.

advocate One who pleads the cause of another; one who defends or maintains a cause or proposal.

affable Being pleasant and at ease in talking to others; characterized by ease and friendliness.

agenda A list or outline of things to be considered or done.

aggressive Forceful or intended to dominate; hostile, injurious, or destructive, especially when referring to a behavior caused by frustration.

albuminuria Abnormal presence of albumin in the urine.

allegation A statement by a party to a legal action of what the party undertakes to prove; an assertion made without proof.

allied health fields Occupational disciplines in which professionals involved with the delivery of healthcare or related services assist physicians with the diagnosis, treatment, and care of patients in many different specialty areas.

allocating Apportioning for a specific purpose or to particular persons or things.

allopathic A word used to contrast homeopathic medicine with mainstream medicine; describes medicine supposedly characterized by an effort to counteract the symptoms of a disease by administration of treatments that produce effects that are opposite to the symptoms.

allowed charge (allowable amount) The maximum amount of money that many third-party payors allow for a specific procedure or service.

alopecia Partial or complete lack of hair.

alphabetic filing Any system that arranges names or topics according to the sequence of the letters in the alphabet.

Alphabetic Index The reference section of the CPT-4 manual that is used to help find a code or code range.

alphanumeric Of or relating to systems made up of combinations of letters and numbers.

alternative medicine A variety of therapeutic or preventative health care practices that are alternatives to mainstream medicine, such as chiropractic, homeopathy, naturopathy, and herbal medicine.

ambiguous Capable of being understood in two or more possible senses or ways; unclear.

amblyopia Reduction or dimness of vision with no apparent organic cause; often referred to as *lazy eye syndrome*.

ambulatory Able to walk about and not be bedridden.

amenity Something conducive to comfort, convenience, or enjoyment.

amiable Having qualities that make one liked and easy to deal with.

amino acids Organic compounds that form the chief constituents of protein and are used by the body to build and repair tissues.

amorphous Lacking a defined shape.

anaphylaxis Exaggerated hypersensitivity reaction that in severe cases leads to vascular collapse, bronchospasm, and shock.

anaplastic Relating to alteration in cells to a more primitive form; describes cancer-producing cells.

anastomosis The surgical joining together of two normally distinct organs.

ancillary diagnostic services Services that support patient diagnoses (e.g., laboratory or radiology services).

ancillary Subordinate; auxiliary.

ancillary therapeutic services Services that support patient treatment (specialists or surgery).

"and" In the context of ICD-9-CM, the word *and* should be interpreted as *and/or.*

anemia A condition marked by deficiency of RBCs.

angina pectoris Spasm-like pain in the chest caused by myocardial anoxia.

angiocardiography Radiography of the heart and great vessels using an iodine contrast medium.

angiography Radiography of blood vessels using an iodine contrast medium.

angioplasty Interventional technique using a catheter to open or widen a blood vessel to improve circulation.

animate To fill with life; to give spirit and support to expressions.

annotations Notes added by way of comment or explanation.

anomalies Deformities or deviations from a normal condition, resulting from faulty development of a fetus.

anorexia Lack or loss of appetite for food.

anteroposterior (AP) Frontal projection in which the patient is supine or facing the x-ray tube.

antibodies Immunoglobulins produced by the immune system in response to bacteria, viruses, or other antigenic substances.

antigen Foreign substance that causes the production of a specific antibody.

antimicrobial agents Drugs used to treat infection.

antiseptic Substances such as alcohol and povidone-iodine solution (Betadine) that inhibit the growth of microorganisms on living tissue.

aortogram Radiography of the aorta using an iodine contrast medium.

apnea Absence or cessation of breathing.

appeal A legal proceeding by which a case is brought before a higher court for review of the decision of a lower court.

appellate Having the power to review the judgment of another tribunal or body of jurisdiction, such as an appellate court.

application software Computer programs designed to perform specific tasks.

appraisal An expert judgment of the value or merit of; judgment as to quality.

arbitration The hearing and determination of a cause in controversy by a person or persons either chosen by the parties involved or appointed under statutory authority.

arbitrator A neutral person chosen to settle differences between two parties in a controversy.

archaic Of, relating to, or characteristic of an earlier or more primitive time.

archived To have filed or collected records or documents.

arrhythmia Abnormality or irregularity in the heart rhythm.

arteriography Radiography of arteries using an iodine contrast medium.

arthritis Inflammation of a joint.

arthrogram Fluoroscopic examination of the soft-tissue components of joints with direct injection of a contrast medium into the joint capsule.

arthropods Members of a class of invertebrate animals that includes the insects, crustaceans, and arachnids.

articular Pertaining to a joint.

artifacts Structures or features not normally present but visible as a result of an external agent or action, such as one seen in a microscopic specimen after fixation or in an image produced by radiology or electrocardiography.

artificial intelligence The aspect of computer science that deals with computers taking on the attributes of humans, such as mimicking human thought. One example is expert systems, which are capable of making decisions, such as software that is designed to help a physician diagnose a patient, given a set of symptoms.

ASCII codes Acronym for American Standard Code for Information Interchange; a code representing English characters as numbers, where each is given a number from 0 to 255.

ascites An abnormal collection of fluid in the peritoneal cavity that contains high levels of protein and electrolytes.

asepsis The process of removing pathogenic microorganisms or protecting against infection by such organisms.

assault An intentional, unlawful attempt of bodily injury to another by force.

assent To agree to something, especially after thoughtful consideration.

assets The entire property of a person, association, corporation, or estate applicable or subject to the payment of debts.

assignment of benefits The transfer of the patient's legal right to collect benefits for medical expenses to the provider of those services, authorizing the payment to be sent directly to the provider.

asymptomatic Without symptoms of a disease process.

asystole The absence of a heartbeat.

ataxia Failure or irregularity of muscle actions and coordination.

atria The two upper chambers of the heart.

atrioventricular (AV) node Part of the cardiac conduction system located between the atria and the ventricles.

atrophy Decrease in the size of a normally developed organ.

attenuated Weakened, or changed; refers to the virulence of a pathogenic microorganism.

audiologist An allied healthcare professional specializing in evaluation of hearing function, detection of hearing impairment, and determination of the anatomic site of impairment.

audit A formal examination of an organization's or individual's accounts or financial situation; a methodic examination and review. *Also,* A process done prior to claims submission to examine claims for accuracy and completeness. An audit can be performed manually, or, if computer billing software is used, electronically.

audit trail The path left by a transaction when it has been completed; often referred to when tracking medical services used by patients or researching claims.

augment To make greater, more numerous, larger, or more intense.

aura Peculiar sensation preceding the appearance of a more definite disturbance.

authenticated Proved; with regard to medical records, it applies to a signature, initials, or computer keystroke by the maker of the record to verify that the record is correct.

authorization A term used in managed care for an approved referral.

autoimmune Pertaining to a disturbance in the immune system in which the body reacts against its own tissue. Examples of autoimmune disorders include multiple sclerosis, rheumatoid arthritis, and systemic lupus erythematosus.

axial projections Radiographs taken with a longitudinal angulation of the x-ray beam; sometimes referred to as semiaxial projections.

azotemia Retention in the blood of excessive amounts of nitrogenous wastes.

backorder An ordered item that has not been delivered when promised or demanded but will be supplied at a later date.

backup Any type of storage of files to prevent their loss in the event of hard disk failure.

bailiff An officer of some U.S. courts usually serving as a messenger or usher, who keeps order at the request of the judge.

balance sheet A financial statement for a specific date that shows the total assets, liabilities, and capital of the business.

banners Advertisements often found on a Web page that can be animated to attract the user's attention in hopes that he or she will click on the ad, be redirected to the advertiser's home page, and purchase from the site or gain information from the site.

battery An offensive touching or use of force on a person without his or her consent.

beneficence The act of doing or producing good, especially performing acts of charity or kindness.

beneficiary Individual entitled to receive benefits from an insurance policy or program or a governmental entitlement program offering healthcare benefits. Also called a *participant, subscriber, dependent, enrollee,* or *member.*

benefits Services or payments provided under a health plan, employee plan, or some other agreement, including programs such as health insurance, pensions, retirement planning, and many other options that may be offered to employees of a company or organization.

benign Not cancerous and not recurring.

bevel Angled tip of a needle.

bifurcation The point of forking or separating into two branches.

bilirubin Orange pigment in bile that when it accumulates leads to jaundice.

bilirubinuria Presence of bilirubin in the urine.

biophysical Pertaining to the science dealing with the application of physical methods and theories to biologic problems.

birthday rule Under law, the rule stating that when an individual is covered under two insurance policies, the insurance plan of the policyholder whose birthday comes first in the calendar year (month and day, not year) becomes the primary insurance. This rule applies when there is a question as to whose insurance should be determined as primary, such as for a dependent child, and not used when the individual is the owner of one of the two policies, which would make that the primary policy.

bits The smallest units of information inside the computer, each represented by either the digit "0" or "1"; 8 bits equal 1 byte.

blatant Completely obvious, conspicuous, or obtrusive, especially in a crass or offensive manner; brazen.

blood-brain barrier An anatomic-physiologic structure made up of astrocyte glial cells that prevents or slows the transfer of chemicals into the neurons of the CNS.

bond A durable, formal paper used for documents.

bookkeeping The recording of business and accounting transactions.

bookmarking Marking a document or a specific place within a document for later retrieval; a feature supported by most browsers that allows the user to save the address (or URL) so that the document can be located when it is needed again.

bounding Describes a pulse that feels full because of increased power of cardiac contractions or as a result of increased blood volume.

bradycardia A slow heartbeat; a pulse below 60 beats per minute.

bradypnea Respirations that are regular in rhythm but slower than normal in rate.

broad-spectrum antimicrobial agents Drugs used to treat a broad range of infections.

bronchiectasis Dilation of the bronchi and bronchioles associated with secondary infection or ciliary dysfunction.

bronchoconstriction Narrowing of the bronchiole tubes.

bronchodilator A drug that relaxes contractions of the smooth muscle of the bronchioles to improve lung ventilation.

bruit Abnormal sound or murmur heard on auscultation of an organ, vessel, or gland.

bucky Moving grid device that prevents scatter radiation from fogging the film.

budget A plan for the coordination of resources and expenditures; the amount of money that is available or required for a particular purpose.

bundle of His Specialized muscle fibers that conduct electrical impulses from AV node to ventricular myocardium.

bundled codes Codes designating procedures or services that are grouped together and paid for as one procedure or service.

burnout Exhaustion of physical or emotional strength or motivation, usually as a result of prolonged stress or frustration.

bursae Fluid-filled, saclike membranes that provide for cushioning and frictionless motion between two tissues.

business associates Individuals or organizations that perform or assist a covered entity in the performance of a function or activity that involves the use or disclosure of individually identifiable health information.

byte A unit of data that contains 8 binary digits, or bits.

cache A special high-speed storage that can either be a part of the computer's main memory or can be a separate storage device. One function of a cache is to store websites visited in the computer memory for faster recall the next time the website is requested.

candidiasis Infection caused by a yeast that typically affects the vaginal mucosa and skin.

cannula Rigid tube that surrounds a blunt trocar or a sharp, pointed trocar inserted into the body; when withdrawn, fluid may escape from the body through the cannula, depending on where it is inserted.

capitation Payment method used by many managed care organizations wherein a fixed amount of money is reimbursed to the provider for patients enrolled during a specific period of time, no matter what services were received or how many visits were made.

caption A heading, title, or subtitle under which records are filed.

carcinogens Substances or agents that cause the development of or increase the incidence of cancer.

cardiac arrest Condition in which cardiac contractions completely stop.

cardiac arrhythmias Irregular heartbeats resulting from a malfunction of the electrical system of the heart.

cardioversion Use of electroshock to convert an abnormal cardiac rhythm to a normal one.

carriers As related to insurance, companies that assume the risk of an insurance policy.

cartilage Rubbery, smooth, somewhat elastic connective tissue covering the ends of bones.

case management The process of assessing and planning patient care, including referral and follow-up, to ensure continuity of care and quality management.

cash basis of accounting Method of accounting in which income is recorded when received and expenses are recorded when paid.

cash flow statement A financial summary for a specific period that shows the beginning balance on hand, the receipts and disbursements during the period, and the balance on hand at the end of the period.

casts Tubular structures found in urine composed mainly of mucoprotein secreted by certain cells of the kidney.

categorically Placed in a specific division of a system of classification.

categories Indented one level below a subsection in the CPT-4 coding manual, usually refers to a specific anatomic site or procedures and/or services.

category I code The primary procedure or service code selected when performing insurance billing or statistical research.

category II codes Special codes that can help providers track revenue and reimbursement.

category III codes Codes for a new or experimental procedure or service.

cathartics Laxative preparations.

caustic Marked by sarcasm.

CD burner A device that is capable of "writing" data onto a blank compact disk (CD) or copying data from one CD to a blank CD.

centrifuge An apparatus consisting essentially of a compartment spun about a central axis to separate contained materials of different specific gravities or to separate colloidal particles suspended in a liquid.

certification The attesting of something as being true, as represented, or as meeting a standard; the result of having been tested, usually by a third party, and awarded a certificate based on proven knowledge.

cerumen A waxy secretion in the ear canal; commonly called *ear wax*.

cervical Pertaining to the neck region which contains seven cervical vertebrae.

chain of command A series of executive positions in order of authority.

channels Means of communication or expression; courses or directions of thought.

chapters Broad sections of the ICD-9-CM coding manual grouped by disease or illness, (e.g., Chapter 10 contains diagnostic codes for diseases of the genitourinary system).

characteristics Distinguishing traits, qualities, or properties.

chief complaint The reason for the patient's seeking medical care.

chiropractic A medical discipline that focuses on the nervous system and involves manual adjustment of the vertebral column to affect the nervous system to treat various disorders and to promote patient wellness.

cholesterol Substance produced by the liver and found in plant and animal fats that can produce fatty deposits or atherosclerotic plaques in the blood vessels.

chronic bronchitis Recurrent inflammation of the membranes lining the bronchial tubes.

chronic obstructive pulmonary disease (COPD) A progressive and irreversible lung condition that results in diminished lung capacity.

chronologic order Of, relating to, or arranged in or according to the order of time.

cilia Hairlike projections that are capable of movement; in the lungs cilia waves move unwanted substances such as mucus, dust, and pus upward; cilia are destroyed by smoking.

circumvent To manage to get around, especially by ingenuity or strategy.

cirrhosis A chronic degenerative disease of the liver that interferes with normal liver function.

cited Quoted by way of example, authority, or proof or mentioned formally in commendation or praise.

Civilian Health and Medical Program of the Uniformed Services (CHAMPUS) See TRICARE.

Civilian Health and Medical Program of the Veterans Administration (CHAMPVA) A health benefits program run by the Department of Veterans Affairs (VA) that helps eligible beneficiaries pay the cost of specific healthcare services and supplies.

clarity The quality or state of being clear.

clauses Groups of words containing a subject and predicate and functioning as a member of a complex or compound sentence.

clean claims Insurance claim forms that have been completed correctly (no errors or omissions) and can be processed and paid promptly if they meets the restrictions on covered services and items.

clearinghouse A centralized facility to which insurance claims are transmitted. Clearinghouses separate, check, and redistribute claims electronically to various insurance carriers and may offer additional services to the physician.

clinical trials Research studies that test how well new medical treatments or other interventions work in the subjects, usually human beings.

clitoris Small, elongated erectile body situated above the urinary meatus at the superior point of the labia minora.

clubbing Abnormal enlargement of the distal phalanges (fingers and toes), associated with cyanotic heart disease or advanced chronic pulmonary disease.

coagulate To form into clots.

"code also" Used when more than one code is necessary to fully identify a given condition, "code also" or "use additional code" is used.

Code of Federal Regulations (CFR) A coded delineation of the rules and regulations published in the *Federal Register* by the various departments and agencies of the federal government. The CFR is divided into 50 titles that represent broad subject areas, and then chapters that provide specific detail.

coding Converting verbal or written descriptions into numeric and alphanumeric designations.

cognitive Pertaining to the operation of the mind; referring to the process by which we become aware of perceiving, thinking, and remembering.

cohesive Sticking together tightly; exhibiting or producing cohesion.

co-insurance A policy provision frequently found in medical insurance whereby the policyholder and the insurance company share the cost of covered losses in a specified ratio (e.g., 80/20 means 80% is covered by the insurer and 20% by the insured).

coitus Sexual union between male and female; also known as *intercourse.*

collagen Protein that forms the inelastic fibers of tendons, ligaments, and fascia.

collect on delivery (COD) Method of payment used when an article or item is delivered and payment is expected before it is released.

colloidal Pertaining to a gluelike substance.

colonoscopy Examination of the large intestine with a fiberoptic scope.

colony-forming units (CFU) Term used when reporting bacteriuria; one CFU represents one bacterium present in the urine sample.

colostrum Thin, yellow, milky fluid secreted by the mammary glands a few days before and after delivery.

coma An unconscious state from which the patient cannot be aroused.

comfort zone A place in the mind where an individual feels safe and confident.

commensurate Corresponding in size, amount, extent, or degree; equal in measure.

commercial insurance Plans that reimburse the insured for expenses resulting from illness or injury according to a specific fee schedule as outlined in the insurance policy and on a fee-for-service basis. Sometimes called *private insurance.*

competent Having adequate abilities or qualities; having the capacity to function or perform in a certain way.

complainant Person making a complaint against a person or organization.

compression The state of being pressed together.

computed tomography (CT) Computerized x-ray imaging modality providing axial and three-dimensional scans.

computer A machine that is designed to accept, store, process, and give out information.

concise Expressing much in brief form.

concurrently Occurring at the same time.

condescending Assuming an air of superiority.

cones Structures found in the retina that make the perception of color possible.

congruent Being in agreement, harmony, or correspondence; conforming to the circumstances or requirements of a situation.

connotation An implication; something suggested by a word or thing.

contaminated Soiled with pathogens or infectious material; nonsterile.

contamination A process by which something is made impure, unclean, or unfit for use by the introduction of unwholesome or undesirable elements.

continuation pages The second and following pages of a letter.

continuing education units (CEUs) Credits for courses, classes, or seminars related to an individual's profession, designed to promote education and to keep the professional up to date on current procedures and trends in his or her field; CEUs are often required for licensing.

continuity of care Continuation of care smoothly from one provider to another, so that the patient receives the most benefit and no interruption in care.

contraindications Factors, such as symptoms or conditions, that make a particular treatment or procedure inadvisable.

contralateral Pertaining to the opposite side of the body.

contrast media Radiopaque substances used to enhance visibility of soft tissues in imaging studies.

contributory negligence Statutes in some states that may prevent a party from recovering some damages if he or she contributed in any way to the injury or condition.

cookies Messages sent to a Web browser from a Web server that identify users and can prepare custom Web pages for them, possibly displaying their name on return to the site.

copayment A sum of money that is paid at the time of medical service; a form of co-insurance.

copulation Sexual intercourse.

coronal plane Plane that divides the body into anterior and posterior parts.

corticosteroids Antiinflammatory hormones, natural or synthetic.

costal Pertaining to the ribs.

coulombs per kilogram (C/kg) International unit of radiation exposure.

counteroffer Return offer made by one who has rejected an offer or job.

covered entity An organization that transmits information in an electronic form during a transaction, as defined by HIPAA.

creatinine Nitrogenous waste from muscle metabolism excreted in urine.

credentialing The act of extending professional or medical privileges to an individual; the process of verifying and evaluating that person's credentials.

credibility The quality or power of inspiring belief.

credit An entry on an account constituting an addition to a revenue, net worth, or liability account; the balance in a person's favor in an account.

crenate Forming notches or leaflike scalloped edges on an object.

crepitation Dry, crackling sound or sensation.

critical thinking The constant practice of considering all aspects of a situation when deciding what to believe or what to do.

cross-training Training in more than one area so that a multitude of duties may be performed by one person or so that substitutions of personnel may be made in an emergency or at other necessary times.

cryosurgery Technique of exposing tissue to extreme cold to produce a well-defined area of cell destruction.

cryptogenic Having a hidden origin.

cultivate To foster the growth of; to improve by labor, care, or study.

culture and sensitivity (C&S) A procedure performed in the microbiology laboratory in which a specimen is cultured on artificial media to detect bacterial or fungal growth, followed by appropriate screening for antibiotic sensitivity.

curettage Act of scraping a body cavity with a surgical instrument, such as a curette.

cursor A symbol appearing on the monitor that shows where the next character to be typed will appear.

curt Marked by rude or peremptory shortness.

cyanosis Blue color of the mucous membranes and body extremities caused by lack of oxygen.

cyberspace The nonphysical space of the online world of computer networks in which communication takes place.

cystoscopy A telescopic examination of the urinary bladder.

cysts Small capsule-like sacs that enclose certain organisms in their dormant or larval stage.

damages Loss or harm resulting from injury to person, property, or reputation; compensation in money imposed by law for losses or injuries.

database A collection of related files that serves as a foundation for retrieving information.

debit An entry on an account constituting an addition to an expense or asset account or a deduction from a revenue, a net worth, or a liability account.

debit cards Cards that looks like credit cards and by which money may be withdrawn or the cost of purchases paid directly from the holder's bank account without the payment of interest.

debridement Removal of foreign material and dead, damaged tissue from a wound.

decedent A legal term for a deceased person.

decodes Convert, as in a message, into intelligible form; recognizes and interprets.

decubitus ulcers Sores or ulcers over a bony prominence that are the result of ischemia from prolonged pressure; bedsores.

deductibles Specific amounts of money a patient must pay out of pocket before the insurance carrier begins paying. Usually this amount ranges from $100 to $500. This deductible amount is met on a yearly or per-incident basis.

defaults Fails to pay financial debts, such as a student loan.

defendant A person required to make answer in a legal action or suit; in criminal cases, the person accused of a crime.

defense mechanisms Psychologic methods of dealing with stressful situations that are encountered in day-to-day living.

deferment Postponement, especially of a student loan.

defibrillator Machine used to deliver an electroshock to the heart through electrodes placed on the chest wall.

deficiencies Conditions caused by a below-normal intake of a particular substance.

demeanor Behavior toward others; outward manner.

demographic The statistical characteristics of human populations (as in age or income) used especially to identify markets.

dependents The spouse, children, and sometimes domestic partner or other individuals designated by the insured who are covered under a healthcare plan.

depleted Lessened markedly in quantity, content, power, or value.

detrimental Obviously harmful or damaging.

device driver The program or commands given to a device connected to a computer that enable the device to function. For instance, a printer may come equipped with software that must be loaded onto the computer first, so that the printer will work.

diabetes mellitus type 1 A disease in which the beta cells in the pancreas no longer produce insulin. Patients must rely on daily insulin administration to use glucose for energy and prevent complications.

diabetes mellitus type 2 A disease in which the body is unable to use glucose for energy as a result of either a lack of insulin production in the pancreas or resistance to insulin on the cellular level.

diagnosis Concise technical description of the cause, nature, or manifestations of a condition or problem. *Initial:* Physician's temporary impression, sometimes called a *working diagnosis.* *Differentiated diagnosis:* Comparison of two or more diseases with similar signs and symptoms. *Final:* Conclusion physician reaches after evaluating all findings, including laboratory and other test results.

diaphoresis The profuse excretion of sweat.

diaphysis Midportion of a long bone containing the medullary cavity.

dictation The act or manner of uttering words to be transcribed.

diction The choice of words especially with regard to clearness, correctness, or effectiveness.

digestion Process of converting food into chemical substances that can be used by the body.

digital subscriber line (DSL) High-speed, sophisticated modulation scheme that operates over existing copper telephone wiring systems; often referred to as "last-mile technologies," because DSL is used for connections from a telephone switching station to a home or office, and not between switching stations.

digital video disk (DVD) An optical disk that holds approximately 28 times more information than a CD; a DVD is most commonly used to hold full-length movies. Compared with a CD, which holds approximately 600 megabytes, a DVD has the capacity to hold approximately 4.7 gigabytes. Also called a *digital versatile disk.*

dilatation and curettage The widening of the cervix and scraping of the endometrial wall of the uterus.

dilatation Opening or widening the circumference of a body orifice with a dilating instrument.

dilation The opening of the cervix through the process of labor, measured as 0 to 10 cm dilated.

direct billing A method of electronic claims submission where computer software allows a provider to submit an insurance claim directly to an insurance carrier for payment.

direct filing system A filing system in which materials can be located without consulting an intermediary source of reference.

dirty claims Claims that contain errors or omissions which must be corrected and resubmitted to an insurance carrier in order to obtain reimbursement.

disability income insurance Insurance that provides periodic payments to replace income when an insured person is unable to work as a result of illness, injury, or disease.

disbursements Funds paid out.

disbursements journal A summary of accounts paid out.

discrepancies Differences among conflicting facts, claims, or opinions.

discretion The quality of being discrete; having or showing good judgment or conduct, especially in speech.

diseases Pathologic processes having a descriptive set of signs and symptoms.

disinfectant Substance such as alcohol or povidone-iodine solution (Betadine) that inhibits the growth of microorganisms on inanimate surfaces or objects.

disk A removable device shaped like a hard plastic square with a magnetic surface that is capable of storing computer programs; also called *diskettes,* and early versions were called *floppy disks.*

disk drives Devices that load a program or data stored on a disk into the computer.

disparaging Slighting; having a negative or degrading tone.

disparities Fundamentally different and often incongruous elements; elements that are markedly distinct in quality or character.

dispense To prepare a drug for administration.

disposition The tendency of something or someone to act in a certain manner under given circumstances.

disruption An unexpected event that throws a plan into disorder; an interruption that prevents a system or process from continuing as usual or as expected.

dissect To cut or separate tissue with a cutting instrument or scissors.

dissection Separation into pieces and exposure of parts for scientific examination.

disseminate To disperse throughout.

diurnal rhythm Patterns of activity or behavior that follow day-night cycles.

diverticulosis Presence of pouchlike herniations through the muscular layer of the colon.

divulge To make known, as a confidence or secret.

docket A formal record of judicial proceedings; a list of legal cases to be tried.

domestic mail Mail that is sent within the boundaries of the United States and its territories.

dosimeter Badge for monitoring radiation exposure of personnel.

downcoding A change in code submitted for reimbursement, usually performed by the insurance company. This change generally occurs because the code submitted does not match in some way to the specifications of the insurance company.

drawee Bank or facility on which a check is drawn or written.

drawer Person who writes a check.

due diligence Also known as *due care;* the effort made by an ordinarily prudent or reasonable party to avoid harm to another party or himself; doing everything possible to prevent something from happening.

due process A fundamental constitutional guarantee that all legal proceedings will be fair; that one will be given notice of the proceedings and given an opportunity to be heard before the government acts to take away life, liberty, or property; a constitutional guarantee that a law will not be unreasonable or arbitrary.

duty Obligatory tasks, conduct, service, or functions that arise from one's position, as in life or in a group.

dysplasia An alteration in cell growth causing differences in size, shape, and appearance.

dyspnea Difficult or painful breathing.

e-banking Electronic banking via computer modem or over the Internet.

ecchymosis A hemorrhagic skin discoloration commonly called *bruising.*

e-commerce An abbreviation for electronic commerce; used to describe the sale and purchase of goods and services over the Internet; doing business over the Internet.

ectopic Originating outside of the normal tissue.

edema Abnormal accumulation of fluid in the interstitial spaces of tissues.

effacement The thinning of the cervix during labor, measured in percentages from 0% to 100% effaced.

effective date The date on which an insurance policy or plan takes effect so that benefits are payable.

elastin Essential part of elastic connective tissue that, when moist, is flexible and elastic.

electrocardiogram A graphic record of electrical conduction through the heart.

electrodesiccation Destruction of cells and tissue by means of short high-frequency electrical sparks.

electronic (or digital) signature A scanned signature or other such mark that is accepted as proof of approval of and/or responsibility for the content of an electronic document.

electronic claims Claims that are submitted to insurance processing facilities using a computerized medium, such as direct data entry, direct wire, dial-in telephone digital fax, or personal computer download or upload.

electronic data interchange (EDI) The transfer of data back and forth between two or more entities using an electronic medium.

electronic media Means of electronic transmission, including the Internet, private networks, dial-up phone lines, and fax modems; includes information moved from one place to another while stored on an electronic device.

eligibility A term which describes whether a patient's insurance coverage is in effect, and eligible for payment of insurance benefits

e-mail Communications transmitted via computer or computer network.

emancipated minor A person under legal age who is self-supporting and living apart from parents or guardian; a mature minor considered by the courts to possess a sufficient understanding of self-care and responsibility.

embezzlement Stealing from an employer; to appropriate goods, services, or funds for personal use without permission.

embolization Interventional technique using a catheter to block off a blood vessel to prevent hemorrhage.

embolus Foreign material blocking a blood vessel, frequently a blood clot that has broken away from some other part of the body.

emetic A substance that causes vomiting.

empathy Sensitivity to the individual needs and reactions of patients.

emphysema Pathologic accumulation of air in the tissues or organs; in the lungs the bronchioles become plugged with mucus and lose elasticity.

employer identification number (EIN) The number used by the Internal Revenue Service that identifies a business or individual functioning as a business entity for income tax reporting.

encodes Converts from one system of communication to another; converts a message into code.

encounter Any contact between a healthcare provider and a patient that results in treatment or evaluation of the patient's condition; not limited to in-person contact.

encroachments Actions that advance beyond the usual or proper limits.

encrypted Encoded; converted from one system of communication to another.

endemic Disease or microorganism that is specific to a particular geographic area.

endocervical curettage The scraping of cells from the wall of the uterus.

endorser Person who signs his or her name on the back of a check for the purpose of transferring title to another person.

enteric-coated Referring to an oral medication to which a coating has been added that resists the effects of stomach juices; designed so that medicine is absorbed in the small intestine.

enunciate To utter articulate sounds; the act of being very distinct in speech.

environment The state of a computer, usually determined by the programs that are running as well as hardware and software characteristics.

enzymatic reaction Chemical reaction controlled by an enzyme.

enzymes Complex proteins that are produced by cells and act as catalysts in specific biochemical reactions.

epiphysis End of a long bone.

eponyms Procedures, services, or diagnoses named after people, such as Mohs' micrographic surgery or Crohn's disease.

equities The money value of a property or of an interest in a property in excess of claims or liens against it.

erroneous Containing or characterized by error or assumption.

erythropoietin Substance released from the kidney and liver that promotes red blood cell formation.

esophageal varices Varicose veins of the esophagus occurring as a result of portal hypertension; vessels can easily hemorrhage.

essential hypertension Elevated blood pressure of unknown cause that develops for no apparent reason; sometimes called *primary hypertension.*

established patient (EP) A patient who has been seen by the same physician or same group of physicians over time. An established patient becomes a new patient if not seen by the physician or group in 3 years.

etiology The cause of the disorder; a claim may be classified according to etiology.

eukaryotes Single-celled or multicellular organisms whose cells contain a distinct membrane-bound nucleus.

euthanasia The act or practice of killing or permitting the death of hopelessly sick or injured individuals in a relatively painless way for reasons of mercy.

exacerbation An increase in the seriousness of a disease marked by greater intensity in the signs and symptoms.

"excludes" Exclusion terms are always written in italics, and the word "excludes" is often enclosed in a box to draw particular attention to these instructions. Exclusion terms may apply to a chapter, a section, a category, or a subcategory. The applicable code number usually follows the exclusion term.

exclusions Limitations on an insurance contract for which benefits are not payable.

excoriated Having undergone injury to the skin caused by scratching; abraded.

expediency A means of achieving a particular end, as in a situation requiring haste or caution.

expert witnesses People who provide testimony to a court as experts in certain fields or subjects to verify facts presented by one or both sides in a lawsuit, often compensated and used to refute or disprove the claims of one party.

explanation of benefits (EOB) A letter or statement from the insurance carrier describing what was paid, denied, or reduced in payment. It also contains information about amounts applied to the deductible, the patient's co-insurance, and the allowed amounts.

explanation of Medicare benefits (EOMB) The EOMB is the name for an explanation of benefits from Medicare. See explanation of benefits above for the definition.

external noise Sounds or factors outside the brain that interfere with the communication process.

externalization The attribution of an event or occurrence to causes outside the self.

externship or internship A training program that is part of a course of study of an educational institution and is taken in the actual business setting of that field of study; the terms are often interchanged in reference to medical assistant training.

extrinsic External to a thing, its essential nature, or its original character.

familial Occurring in or affecting members of a family more than would be expected by chance.

fascia Sheet or band of fibrous tissue located deep in the skin that covers muscles and body organs.

fastidious Requiring specialized media or growth factors to grow.

fax Abbreviation for facsimile; also, a document sent using a facsimile (fax) machine.

febrile Pertaining to an elevated body temperature.

fecalith A hard, impacted mass of feces in the colon.

fee for service An established schedule of fees set for services performed by providers and paid by the patient.

fee profile A compilation or average of physician fees over a given period of time.

fee schedule A compilation of preestablished fee allowances for given services or procedures.

feedback The transmission of evaluative or corrective information to the original or controlling source about an action, event, or process.

felony A major crime, such as murder, rape, or burglary; punishable by a more stringent sentence than that given for a misdemeanor.

fermentation An enzymatically controlled transformation of an organic compound.

fervent Exhibiting or marked by great intensity of feeling.

fibrillation Rapid, random, ineffective contractions of the heart.

fidelity Faithfulness to something to which one is bound by pledge or duty.

filtrate Fluid that remains after a liquid is passed through a membranous filter.

fine A sum imposed as punishment for an offense; a forfeiture or penalty paid to an injured party or the government in a civil or criminal action.

fiscal agent An organization under contract to the government as well as some private plans to act as financial representatives in handling insurance claims from providers of health care; also referred to as *fiscal intermediary.*

fiscal intermediary An organization that contracts with the government to handle and mediate insurance claims from medical facilities, home health agencies, or providers of medical services or supplies.

fiscal year An accounting period of 12 months during which a company determines earnings and profit; the fiscal year does not necessarily begin in January—instead, the beginning of the fiscal year is determined by the business.

fissures Narrow slits or clefts in the abdominal wall.

fistula Abnormal, tubelike passage between internal organs or from an internal organ to the body surface.

flagged Marked in some way as to remind or remember that specific action needs to be taken.

Flash Animation technology often used on the opening page of a website to draw attention, excite, and impress the user.

flash drive A small portable device that connects into the USB port that can carry 2 to 8 or more gigabytes of information.

flatus Gas expelled through the anus.

fluoroscopy Direct observation of the x-ray image in motion.

flush Directly abutting or immediately adjacent, as set even with an edge of a type page or column; having no indention.

follicle-stimulating hormone (FSH) A hormone secreted by the anterior pituitary; stimulates oogenesis and spermatogenesis.

font A design for a set of type characters; a combination of typeface, spacing, pitch, and other qualities. Fonts are named; examples include Times Roman, Arial, and Garamond.

format To magnetically create tracks on a disk where information will be stored, usually done by the manufacturer of the disk.

fovea centralis A small pit in the center of the retina that is considered the center of clearest vision.

free radicals Compounds with at least one unpaired electron that makes the compound unstable and highly reactive.

frontal projection Radiographic view in which the coronal plane of the body or body part is parallel to the film plane; AP or PA.

fundus the curved, top portion of the uterus; the fundal height can be used as a measurement of fetal growth and estimated gestation.

gait The manner or style of walking.

gametes Mature male or female germ cells, usually possessing a haploid chromosome set and capable of initiating formation of a new diploid individual; a sex cell, whether sperm or ovum.

gangrene Death of body tissue as a result of loss of nutritive supply and followed by bacteria invasion and putrefaction.

gantry Doughnut-shaped portion of a scanner that surrounds the patient and functions, at least in part, to gather imaging data.

generic Not protected by trademark.

genome The genetic material of an organism.

genuineness Expressing sincerity and honest feeling.

germicides Agents that destroy pathogenic organisms.

gigabyte Approximately 1 billion bytes; abbreviated GB.

girth A measure around a body or item.

gleaned Gathered bit by bit (e.g., information or material); picked over in search of relevant material.

glomerulonephritis Inflammation of the glomerulus of the kidney.

gluconeogenesis The formation of glucose in the liver from proteins and fats.

glycogen The sugar (starch) formed from glucose and stored mainly in the liver.

glycosuria The abnormal presence of glucose in the urine.

gold standard A paragon of excellence; the one to which all others are compared.

goniometer Instrument for measuring the degrees of motion in a joint.

government plans Entitlement programs or healthcare plans that are sponsored and/or subsidized by the state or federal government, such as Medicaid and Medicare.

gradients Changes in response with distance from a stimulus.

grammar The study of the classes of words, their inflections, and their functions and relations in the sentence; a study of what is to be preferred and what avoided in inflection and syntax.

gray (Gy) International unit of radiation dose.

grief Reaction to an unfortunate outcome; a deep distress caused by bereavement, a loss, or a perceived loss.

group policy Insurance written under a policy that covers a number of people under a single master contract issued to their employer or to an association with which they are affiliated.

growth hormone (GH) Also called *somatotropic hormone;* stimulates tissue growth and restricts tissue glucose dependence when nutrients are not available.

guarantor The person who is responsible for paying a medical bill.

guardian ad litem Legal representative for a minor.

guidelines Found at the beginning of each of the six sections of the CPT-4. The guidelines define items that are necessary to appropriately interpret and report the procedures and services found in the section.

hard copy The readable paper copy or printout of information.

hardware The physical components of the computer system, such as the CPU, monitor, and printer.

harmonious Marked by accord in sentiment or action; having the parts agreeably related.

Health Care Common Procedural Coding System (HCPCS) Level II codes created to supplement procedures and services not covered in the CPT-4.

Health Insurance Portability and Accountability Act (HIPAA) The Kassebaum-Kennedy Act, designed to improve portability and continuity of health insurance coverage; to combat waste, fraud, and abuse in health insurance and healthcare delivery; to promote the use of medical savings accounts; to improve access to long-term care services and coverage; to simplify the administration of health insurance; and to serve other purposes.

health insurance Protection in return for periodic premium payments that provides reimbursement of expenses resulting from illness or injury. Includes the following forms of insurance: accident, disability income, medical expense, and accidental death and dismemberment. Also known as *accident and health insurance* or *disability income insurance.*

health maintenance organization (HMO) An organization that provides a wide range of comprehensive healthcare services for a specified group at a fixed periodic payment. HMOs can be sponsored by the government, medical schools, hospitals, employers, labor unions, consumer groups, insurance companies, and hospital-medical plans.

healthcare providers Providers of medical or health services, individually or as organizations, that furnish, bill for, or are paid for services or products.

hematemesis Vomiting of bright red blood, indicating rapid upper gastrointestinal bleeding; associated with esophageal varices or peptic ulcer.

hematocrit The percentage by volume of packed red blood cells in a given sample of blood after centrifugation.

hematopoiesis Formation and development of blood cells in the bone marrow.

hematuria Blood in the urine.

hemoconcentration A situation in which the concentration of blood cells is increased in proportion to the plasma.

hemoglobin Protein found in erythrocytes that transports molecular oxygen in the blood.

hemolysis The destruction or dissolution of red blood cells, with subsequent release of hemoglobin.

hepatomegaly Abnormal enlargement of the liver.

hereditary Pertaining to a characteristic, condition, or disease transmitted from parent to offspring on the DNA chain.

hermetically sealed Sealed so that no air can enter.

hertz A unit of measurement used in hearing examinations; a wave frequency equal to one cycle per second.

holder Person presenting a check for payment.

holistic Related to or concerned with all of the systems of the body, rather than breaking it down into parts.

homeopathy A type of alternative medicine that attempts to stimulate the body to recover itself; a system of therapy based on the concept that disease can be treated with minute doses of drugs thought capable of producing the same symptoms in healthy people as the disease itself.

homeostasis Internal adaptation and change in response to environmental factors.

hormones Substances produced by one tissue and conveyed by the bloodstream to another to effect physiologic activity, such as growth or metabolism.

hospice A concept of care that involves health professionals and volunteers who provide medical, psychologic, and spiritual support to terminally ill patients and their loved ones.

HTML Acronym for HyperText Markup Language, which is the language used to create documents for use on the Internet.

HTTP Acronym for HyperText Transfer Protocol, which defines how messages are formatted and transmitted over the Internet. When a URL is entered into the computer, an HTTP command tells the Web server to retrieve the requested Web page.

hub A common connection point for devices in a network

containing multiple ports, often used to connect segments of a LAN.

human chorionic gonadotropin A hormone secreted by the placenta; is found in the urine of pregnant females.

hydrocephaly Enlargement of the cranium caused by abnormal accumulation of cerebrospinal fluid within the cerebral system.

hydrogenated Combined with, treated with, or exposed to hydrogen.

hypercapnia Excess levels of carbon dioxide in the bloodstream.

hypercholesterolemia Elevated blood levels of cholesterol.

hyperplasia An increase in the number of normal cells.

hyperpnea Increase in the depth of breathing.

hypertension High blood pressure (systolic pressure consistently above 140 mm Hg and diastolic pressure above 90 mm Hg).

hyperventilation Abnormally prolonged and deep breathing usually associated with acute anxiety or emotional tension.

hypotension Blood pressure that is below normal (systolic pressure below 90 mm Hg and diastolic pressure below 50 mm Hg).

icons Pictures, often on the desktop of a computer, that represent programs or objects. By clicking on an icon, the user is directed to the program.

idealism The practice of forming ideas or living under the influence of ideas.

idiopathic Pertaining to no known cause of a condition or disease.

ileostomy Surgical formation of an opening of the ileum onto the surface of the abdomen through which fecal material is emptied.

immigrant A person who comes to a country to take up permanent residence.

immunosuppressant Pertaining to a substance that suppresses or prevents an immune system response.

immunotherapy Administering repeated injections of diluted extracts of a substance that causes an allergy; also called *desensitization*.

impaired Being in a less-than-perfect or less-than-whole condition; includes having handicaps or functional defects and being under the influence of drugs, alcohol, and/or controlled substances.

impenetrable Incapable of being penetrated or pierced; not capable of being damaged or harmed.

implied consent Presumed consent, such as when a patient offers an arm for a phlebotomy procedure.

in balance State in which the total ending balances of patient ledgers equals total of accounts receivable.

in vitro Refers to conditions outside of a living body.

incentives Things that incite or spur to action; rewards or reasons for performing a task.

"includes" This term appearing under a subdivision, such as a category (three-digit code) or two-digit procedure code, indicates that the code and title include these terms. Other terms also classified to that particular code and title are listed in the Alphabetic Indexes.

incomplete claim A claim that is missing information and is returned to the provider for correction and resubmission. This is sometimes also called an invalid claim.

incur To become liable or subject to; to bring down on oneself.

indemnity plans Traditional health insurance plans that pay for all or a share of the cost of covered services, regardless of which physician, hospital, or other licensed healthcare provider is used. Policyholders of indemnity plans and their dependents choose when and where to get healthcare services.

indicators An important point or group of statistic values that, when evaluated, indicate the quality of care provided in a healthcare facility.

indicted Charged with a crime by the finding or presentment of a jury according to due process of law.

indigent Totally lacking in something of need.

indirect filing system A filing system in which an intermediary source of reference, such as a card file, must be consulted to locate specific files.

individual policy An insurance policy designed specifically for the use of one person (and his or her dependents), not associated with the amenities of a group policy, namely higher premiums. Often called *personal insurance*.

individually identifiable health information Any part of a patient's health record that is created or received by a covered entity.

induration An abnormally hard, inflamed area.

infarction Area of tissue that has died from lack of blood supply.

infection Invasion of body tissues by microorganisms that then proliferate and damage tissues.

infer To derive as a conclusion from facts and premises.

infertile Not fertile or productive; not capable of reproducing.

inflammation Tissue reaction to trauma or disease that includes redness, heat, swelling, and pain.

inflection A change in pitch or loudness of the voice.

informed consent A consent, usually written, which states understanding of what treatment is to be undertaken and of the risks involved, why it should be done, and alternative methods of treatment available (including no treatment) and their attendant risks.

infractions Breaking the law; minor offenses against the rules, usually punishable by fines.

initiative To cause or facilitate the beginning of; to initiate something into happening.

innate Existing in, belonging to, or determined by factors present in an individual since birth.

innocuous Having no effect, adverse or otherwise; harmless.

input Information entered into and used by the computer.

instigate To goad or urge forward; to provoke.

insubordination Disobedience to authority.

insured An individual or organization covered by an insurance policy according to the policy terms, usually the individual or group that pays the premiums. Blue Cross/Blue Shield refers to this person or group as the *subscriber*.

intangibles Qualities that are incapable of being perceived, especially by touch, or incapable of being precisely identified or realized by the mind.

integral Essential; being an indispensable part of a whole.

Intelligent Character Recognition (ICR) The electronic scanning of printed items as images and use of special software to recognize these images (or characters) as ASCII text for upload into a computer database.

interaction A two-way communication; mutual or reciprocal action or influence.

intercellular Between cells.

intercom A two-way communication system with a microphone and loudspeaker at each station for localized use.

interferon A protein that forms when a cell is exposed to a virus, blocking viral action on the cell and providing protection against viral invasion.

interleukin A protein produced by certain white blood cells that regulates immune responses by activating lymphocytes and initiating fever.

intermittent Coming and going at intervals; not continuous.

intermittent pulse Pulse in which beats are occasionally skipped.

internal noise Factors inside the brain that interfere with the communication process.

International Classification of Diseases, Ninth Revision, Clinical Modification (ICD-9-CM) System for classifying disease to facilitate collection of uniform and comparable health information, for statistical purposes and indexing medical records for data storage and retrieval.

international mail Mail that is sent outside the boundaries of the United States and its territories.

International Statistical Classifications of Diseases and Related Health Problems, Tenth Revision, Clinical Modification (ICD-10-CM) System containing the greatest number of changes in ICD history. To allow more specific reporting of disease and newly recognized conditions, the ICD-10-CM contains approximately 5500 more codes than ICD-9.

interval Space of time between events.

intolerable Not tolerable or bearable.

intravenous urogram (IVU) Radiographic examination of the urinary tract using intravenous injection of an iodine contrast medium.

intrinsic Belonging to the essential nature or constitution of a thing; indwelling, inward.

introspection An inward, reflective examination of one's own thoughts and feelings.

invariably Consistently; not changing or capable of change.

invasive Involving entry into the living body as by incision or insertion of an instrument.

invoice A paper describing a purchase and the amount due.

ipsilateral Pertaining to the same side of the body.

ischemia Decreased blood flow to a body part or organ, caused by constriction or plugging of the supplying artery.

jargon The technical terminology or characteristic idiom of a particular group or special activity.

jaundice Yellow discoloration of the skin and mucous membranes resulting from deposits of bile pigments because of excess bilirubin in the blood.

Java A commonly used object-oriented high-level programming language that is well suited for the Internet.

judicial Of or relating to a judgment, the function of judging, the administration of justice, or the judiciary.

jurisdiction A power constitutionally conferred on a judge or magistrate to decide cases according to law and to carry sentence into execution; jurisdiction is original when it is conferred on the court in the first instance, called *original jurisdiction;* or it is appellate when an appeal is given from the judgment of another court.

jurisprudence The science or philosophy of law; a system or body of law or the course of court decisions.

Kaposi's sarcoma A malignant tumor that begins as brown or purple papules on the feet and slowly spreads in the skin.

keloid A raised, firm scar formation caused by overgrowth of collagen at the site of a skin injury.

keratin Very hard, tough protein found in hair, nails, and epidermal tissue.

keratinocytes Any one of the skin cells that synthesizes keratin.

kilobyte Approximately 1024 bytes, abbreviated KB.

kyphotic Relating to normal convex curvature of the thoracic spine region.

lacrimation The secretion or discharge of tears.

language barrier Any type of interference that inhibits the communication process and is related to languages spoken by the people attempting to communicate.

laryngoscopy Visual examination of the voice box area through an endoscope equipped with a light and mirrors for illumination.

latent image Invisible changes in exposed film that will become an image when the film is processed.

lateral projections Radiographic views in which the sagittal plane of the body or body part is parallel to the film.

law A binding custom or practice of a community; a rule of conduct or action prescribed or formally recognized as binding or enforceable by a controlling authority.

learning style The way that an individual perceives and processes information to learn new material.

leukoderma Lack of skin pigmentation, especially in patches.

liabilities Things that are owed; debts.

liable or circumstance.

libel A written defamatory statement or representation that conveys an unjustly unfavorable impression.

ligaments Tough connective tissue bands that hold joints together by attaching to the bones on either side of a joint.

limited radiography Limited-scope radiography practice, usually in an outpatient setting, that does not require the same credentials needed for professional radiologic technology; also called *practical radiography.*

lithotripsy A procedure for eliminating a stone by crushing or dissolving it in situ through the use of high-intensity sound waves.

litigious Prone to engage in lawsuits.

loading dose A double dose administered as the first dose of a medication; usually used with antibiotic therapy so that therapeutic blood levels are reached quickly.

lordotic Relating to normal concave curvature of the cervical and lumbar spine regions.

lower gastrointestinal series Fluoroscopic examination of the colon, usually employing rectal administration of barium sulfate as a contrast medium; also called a *barium enema.*

lumbar Lower back region containing five lumbar vertebrae.

lumen Open space, such as within a blood vessel, the intestine, the inside of a needle, or an examining instrument.

luteinizing hormone (LH) Hormone produced by the anterior pituitary gland; promotes ovulation.

luxation Dislocation of a bone from its normal anatomic location.

lymphadenopathy Any disorder of the lymph nodes or lymph vessels.

lymphedema Swelling caused by the accumulation of lymph fluid in soft tissues.

macromolecules The molecules needed for metabolism: carbohydrates, lipids, proteins, and nucleic acids.

macular degeneration A progressive deterioration of the macula of the eye; causes loss of central vision.

magnetic resonance imaging (MRI) Imaging modality that uses a magnetic field and radiofrequency pulses to create computer images of both bones and soft tissues in multiple planes.

mailpiece A piece of mail.

maker In reference to a check, any individual, corporation, or legal party who signs a check or any type of negotiable instrument.

malaise Indefinite feeling of debility or lack of health, often indicative of or accompanying the onset of an illness.

malediction Speaking evil or the calling of a curse.

malignant Cancerous.

managed care plans An umbrella term for all healthcare plans that provide healthcare in return for preset monthly payments and coordinated care through a defined network of primary care physicians and hospitals.

manifestation Something that is easily understood or recognized by the mind. *Also,* the signs and symptoms of a disease.

manipulation Moving or exercising a body part via an externally applied force.

marketing The process or technique of promoting, selling, and distributing a product or service.

mastication Chewing.

matrix Something in which a thing originates, develops, takes shape, or is contained; a base on which to build.

m-banking Banking through the use of wireless devices, such as cellular phones and wireless Internet services.

media Term applied to agencies of mass communication, such as newspapers, magazines, and telecommunications.

mediastinum Space in the center of the chest under the sternum.

Medicaid A federal and state sponsored health insurance program for the medically indigent.

medical savings accounts Tax-deferred bank or savings accounts that are combined with a low-premium, high-deductible insurance policy, designed for individuals or families who choose to fund their own healthcare expenses and medical insurance.

medically indigent Able to take care of ordinary living expenses but not able to afford medical care.

Medicare A federally sponsored health insurance program for those over 65 or individuals under 65 but disabled.

Medigap A term sometimes applied to private insurance products that supplement Medicare insurance benefits.

medullary cavity Inner portion of diaphysis containing bone marrow.

megabyte Approximately 1 million bytes; abbreviated MB.

megahertz The measuring device for microprocessors, abbreviated MHz. A megahertz is 1 million cycles of electromagnetic currency alternation per second and is used as a unit of measure for the clock speed of computer microprocessors. The hertz is a unit of measure named after Heinrich Hertz, a German physicist.

meniscus The curved surface of liquids in a container.

mentors Trusted counselors or guides.

metabolic alkalosis Condition characterized by the significant loss of acid in the body or an increased amount of bicarbonate; severe levels can lead to coma and death.

metabolite The product of the metabolism of a substance such as a drug.

meticulous Marked by extreme or excessive care in the consideration or treatment of details.

microcephaly Small size of the head in relationship to the rest of the body.

microfiche A sheet of microfilm containing rows of microimages of pages of printed matter.

microfilm A film bearing a photographic record on a reduced scale of printed or other graphic matter.

micromanage To manage with great or excessive control or attention to details.

microorganisms Organisms of microscopic or submicroscopic size.

MIDI Acronym for Musical Instrument Digital Interface; a MIDI interface allows computers to record and manipulate sound.

miotic Any substance or medication that causes constriction of the pupil.

misdemeanor A minor crime, as opposed to a felony, punishable by fine or imprisonment in a city or county jail rather than in a penitentiary.

mock Simulated; intended for imitation or practice.

modem A device that allows information to be transmitted over telephone lines, at speeds measured in bits per second (bps); short for modulator-demodulator. Modem speed is generally listed somewhere on the actual unit.

modifiers Code additions that explain circumstances that alter a provided service, or provide additional clarification or detail about a procedure or service.

molecules Groups of like or different atoms held together by chemical forces.

monochromatic Having or consisting of one color or hue.

mononuclear white blood cells Leukocytes having an unsegmented nucleus; monocytes and lymphocytes in particular.

monotone A succession of syllables, words, or sentences in one unvaried key or pitch.

mons pubis Fat pad that covers the symphysis pubis.

morale The mental and emotional condition, enthusiasm, loyalty, or confidence of an individual or group with regard to the function or tasks at hand.

motivation The process of inciting a person to some action or behavior.

multimedia The presentation of graphics, animation, video, sound, and text on a computer in an integrated way, or all at once. CD-ROMs are efficient multimedia devices.

multiparous Pertaining to women who have had two or more pregnancies.

multitasking Performing multiple tasks at the same time.

municipal courts Courts that sit in some cities and larger towns and that usually have civil and criminal jurisdiction over cases arising within the municipality.

murmur Abnormal sound heard when auscultating the heart that may or may not have a pathologic origin.

myelin sheath Segmented, fatty tissue that wraps around the axon of the nerve cell and acts as an electrical insulator to speed the conduction of nerve impulses.

myelography Fluoroscopic examination of the spinal canal with spinal injection of an iodine contrast medium.

myelomeningocele A herniation of a portion of the spinal cord and its meninges that protrudes through a congenital opening in the vertebral column.

myocardial Pertaining to the heart muscle.

myocardium The muscular lining of the heart.

myoglobinuria Abnormal presence of a hemoglobin-like chemical of muscle tissue in urine that is the result of muscle deterioration.

mysticism The experience of seeming to have direct communication with God or ultimate reality.

nanometer One billionth (10^{-9}) of a meter.

National Provider Identifier (NPI) A lifetime number consisting of 10 digits that Medicare will use to replace the Provider Identification Number (PIN) and the Unique Physician Identification Number (UPIN).

naturopathy An alternative to conventional medicine in which holistic methods are used, as well as herbs and natural supplements, with the belief that the body will heal itself. Naturopathic physicians can currently be licensed in 15 states, Puerto Rico, and the Virgin Islands.

necrosis The death of cells or tissue.

negligence Failure to exercise the care that a prudent person usually exercises; implies inattention to one's duty or business; implies want of due or necessary diligence or care.

negotiable Legally transferable to another party.

networking Exchange of information or services among individuals, groups, or institutions; also, meeting and getting to know individuals in the same or similar career fields and sharing information about available opportunities.

neural tube defect Any of a group of congenital anomalies involving the brain and spinal column that are caused by failure of the neural tube to close during embryonic development.

new patient (NP) A patient who has his or her first encounter (visit) with a physician or physician group or who was an established patient with a physician or provider but has not been seen in 3 years.

nocturia Excessive urination during the night.

nodules Small lumps, lesions, or swellings felt when palpating the skin.

nomogram A graph on which variables are plotted so that a particular value can be read on the appropriate line.

nonmaleficence Refraining from the act of harming or committing evil.

nonstress tests (NSTs) Fetal monitoring used in combination with maternal reports of fetal movement to evaluate fetal heart rate response.

no-show A person who fails to keep an appointment without giving advance notice.

nosocomial infections Infections acquired during hospitalization or in a healthcare setting; often caused by *Escherichia coli*, hepatitis viruses, *Pseudomonas*, and *Staphylococcus* microorganisms.

notations Notations, also known as instructional notations, are found in both the Alphabetic Index and the Tabular Index as instructions or guides in classification assignments, defining category content or the use of subdivision codes.

NPO Nothing by mouth, from the Latin *nil per os.*

nuclear medicine Imaging modality that uses radioactive materials injected or ingested into the body to provide information about the function of organs and tissues.

numeric filing The filing of records, correspondence, or cards by number.

obesity An excessive accumulation of body fat; defined as a body mass index (BMI) of 30 or higher.

objective information Information that is gathered by watching or observation of a patient.

objectives Something toward which effort is directed; aims, goals, or ends of action.

oblique projections Radiographic views in which the body or part is rotated so that the projection is neither frontal nor lateral.

obliteration Act of making undecipherable or imperceptible by obscuring or wearing away.

obturator Metal rod with a smooth, rounded tip that is placed into hollow instruments to decrease injury to body tissues during insertion.

occlusion Complete blocking off of an opening.

Office for Civil Rights (OCR) The division of the federal government that enforces privacy standards.

Office of Inspector General (OIG) Established to protect the integrity of the Department of Health and Human Services (HHS), the office conducts audits, investigations, and inspections involving the laws that pertain to HHS.

opaque Not translucent or transparent; murky.

opinions Formal expressions of judgment or advice by an expert; formal expressions of the legal reasons and principles on which a legal decision is based.

opportunistic infections Infections caused by a normally nonpathogenic organism in a host whose resistance has been decreased.

optic disc Region at the back of the eye where the optic nerve meets the retina; considered the blind spot of the eye, because it contains only nerve fibers and no rods or cones and thus is insensitive to light.

optic nerve Second cranial nerve, which carries impulses for the sense of sight.

optimistic Inclined to put the most favorable construction on actions and events or to anticipate the best possible outcome.

ordinances Authoritative decrees or directions; laws set forth by a governmental authority—specifically, municipal regulations.

organelles Differentiated structures within a cell, such as mitochondrion, vacuoles, and chloroplasts, that perform a specific function.

orthopnea Condition in which an individual must sit or stand to breathe comfortably.

orthostatic (postural) hypotension Temporary fall in blood pressure when a person rapidly changes from a recumbent position to a standing position.

osteopathic A type of medicine based on the theory that disturbances in the musculoskeletal system affect other bodily parts, causing many disorders that can be corrected by various manipulative techniques in conjunction with conventional medical, surgical, pharmacologic, and other therapeutic procedures.

osteoporosis Loss of bone density; lack of calcium intake is a major factor in its development.

other potentially infectious materials (OPIM) Substances or materials other than blood that have the potential to carry infectious pathogens, such as body fluid, urine, semen, and others.

otitis externa Inflammation or infection of the external auditory canal.

otosclerosis Formation of spongy bone in the labyrinth of the ear, often causing the auditory ossicles to become fixed and unable to vibrate when sound enters the ears.

ototoxic A medication or substance that is capable of producing damage to the eighth cranial nerve or the organs of hearing and balance.

OUTfolder A folder used to provide space for the temporary filing of materials.

OUTguide A heavy guide that is used to replace a folder that has been temporarily moved from the filing space.

output Information that is processed by the computer and transmitted to a monitor, printer, or other device.

outreach The process of using marketing and education strategies to reach and involve diverse audiences through the use of key messages and effective programs.

outsourcing The practice of subcontracting work to an outside company.

over-the-counter (OTC) drugs Medications sold without a prescription.

packing slip A list of items that are included in a shipment.

palliative Relieving or alleviating symptoms without curing the disease.

pandemic A condition in which the majority of the people in a country, a number of countries, or a geographic area are affected.

paper claims Hard copies of insurance claims that have been completed and sent by surface mail.

papilledema Swelling of the optic disc from increased intracranial pressure.

paraphrasing To express an idea in different wording in an effort to enhance communication and clarify meaning.

parenteral Relating to injection or introduction of substances into the body through any route other than the digestive tract such as subcutaneous, intravenous, or intramuscular administration.

paresthesia Abnormal sensation of burning, prickling, or stinging.

paroxysmal Pertaining to a sudden recurrent spasm of symptoms.

participating provider (PAR) A physician or other healthcare provider who enters into a contract with a specific insurance company or program, and by doing so agrees to abide by certain rules and regulations set forth by that particular third-party payor.

parturition Act or process of giving birth to a child.

patency Open condition of a body cavity or canal.

pathogen A disease-causing microorganism.

pathophysiology Study of the biological and physical manifestations of disease as they are related to system abnormalities and physiological disturbances.

patient status (PS) The state of a patient as either new or established; appears in the Evaluation and Management section of the CPT-4.

payables Balances due to a creditor on an account.

payee Person named on a draft or check as the recipient of the amount shown.

payor Person who writes a check in favor of the payee.

peer review organization A group of medical reviewers contracted by the Centers for Medicare and Medicaid Services to ensure quality control and medical necessity of services provided by a facility.

pegboard system Also called the *write-it-once system;* a method of tracking patient accounts that allows the figures to be proved accurate through mathematic formulas.

perceiving How an individual looks at information and sees it as real.

perception Capacity for comprehension; an awareness of the elements of the environment.

periosteum The thin, highly innervated, membranous covering of a bone.

peripheral Pertaining to an area that is outside or away from an organ or structure.

peristalsis Rhythmic contraction of involuntary muscles lining the gastrointestinal tract.

peristalsis Wavelike movement by which the gastrointestinal tract moves food downward.

perjured testimony The voluntary violation of an oath or vow either by swearing to what is untrue or by omission to do what has been promised under oath; false testimony.

perks Extra advantages or benefits from working in a specific job that may or may not be commonplace in that particular profession; a shortened form of *perquisites*.

permeable Allowing a substance to pass or soak through.

persona An individual's social facade or front that reflects the role in life the individual is playing; the personality that a person projects in public.

personal health information The patient's own information that pertains to his or her health.

pertinent Having a clear, decisive relevance to the matter at hand.

petechiae Small, purplish hemorrhagic spots on the skin.

petty cash fund A fund maintained to pay small unpredictable cash expenditures.

phenylalanine Essential amino acid found in milk, eggs, and other foods.

philanthropist An individual who makes an active effort to promote human welfare.

philosopher A person who seeks wisdom or enlightenment; an expounder of a theory in a certain area of experience.

phlebitis Inflammation of a vein, with the possible complication of clot formation at the site *(thrombophlebitis)*.

phlebotomy The invasive procedure used to obtain a blood specimen for testing, experimentation, or diagnosis of disease.

phonetic Constituting an alteration of ordinary spelling that better represents the spoken language, that employs only characters of the regular alphabet, and that is used in a context of conventional spelling.

phosphors Fluorescent crystals that give off light when exposed to x-rays.

photophobia Abnormal sensitivity to light.

physical status The physical condition of the patient.

physician office laboratories (POLs) Laboratories owned by a private physician or corporation, such as the laboratory inside a physician's office or a freestanding laboratory.

physiologic noise Physiologic interferences with the communication process.

pitch The property of a sound, especially a musical tone, that is determined by the frequency of the waves producing it; the highness or lowness of sound.

place-of-service (POS) codes Codes that indicate where a procedure or service was performed.

plaintiff The person or group bringing a case or legal action to court.

plaque Abnormal accumulation of a fatty substance.

plasma The liquid portion of whole blood that contains active clotting agents.

policyholder A person who pays a premium to an insurance company and in whose name the policy is written in exchange for the insurance protection provided by a policy of insurance.

polycythemia vera A condition marked by an abnormally large number of RBCs in the circulatory system.

polydipsia Excessive thirst.

polymorphonuclear white blood cells Leukocytes having a segmented nucleus. Also known as *polymorphonuclear neutrophils* (PMNs) or *segmented neutrophils*.

polyphagia Increased appetite.

polyps Tumors on outgrowths found in the mucosal lining of the colon; considered precancerous.

polyuria Excretion of an unusually large amount of urine.

portal circulation Pathway of blood flow through the portal vein from the gastrointestinal system to the liver.

portal hypertension An increased venous pressure in the portal circulation caused by cirrhosis or compression of the hepatic vascular system.

portfolio A set of pictures, drawings, documents, or photographs either bound in book form or loose in a folder.

posteroanterior (PA) Frontal projection in which the patient is prone or facing the x-ray film or image receptor.

posting Transferring or carrying from a book of original entry to a ledger; entering figures in an accounting system.

postmortem Done, collected, or occurring after death.

power of attorney A legal statement in which a person authorizes another person to act as his or her attorney or agent. The authority may be limited to the handling of specific procedures. The person authorized to act as the agent is known as the *attorney in fact*.

preauthorization A process required by some insurance carriers where the provider obtains permission to perform certain procedures or services, or refer a patient to a specialist.

precedence To surpass in rank, dignity, or importance; to be, go, or come ahead or in front of.

precedents A person or thing that serves as a model; something done or said that may serve as an example or rule to authorize or justify a subsequent act of the same kind.

preclude To rule out in advance.

premium The periodic (monthly, quarterly, or annual) payment of a specific sum of money to an insurance company for which the insurer, in return, agrees to provide certain benefits.

preponderance A superiority or excess in number or quantity; a majority.

preponderance of the evidence Evidence that is of greater weight or more convincing than the evidence offered in opposition to it; evidence that as a whole shows that the fact sought to be proven is more probable than not.

prerequisite Something that is necessary to an end or to carry out a function.

present illness The chief complaint, written in chronologic sequence, with dates of onset.

pressboard A strong, highly glazed composition board resembling vulcanized fiber; heavy card stock.

prevalent Generally or widely accepted, practiced, or favored.

primary care provider (PCP) A general practice, or non-specialists provider or physician responsible for the care of a patient for some health maintenance organizations. Also called a gatekeeper.

primary diagnosis Initial identification of the condition or complaint that the patient expresses in the outpatient medical setting.

principal A capital sum of money due as a debt or used as a fund for which interest is either charged or paid.

privacy officer A person designated to ensure compliance with privacy standards for a covered entity.

proactive Acting in anticipation of future problems, needs, or changes.

processing How an individual internalizes new information and makes it his or her own.

procrastination Intentionally putting off doing something that should be done.

procurement To get possession of, to obtain by particular care and effort.

professional behaviors Those actions that identify the medical assistant as a member of a healthcare profession, including being dependable, performing respectful patient care, exercising initiative, demonstrating a positive attitude, and using teamwork.

professional courtesy Reduction or absence of fees to professional associates.

professionalism The conduct or qualities characterized by or conforming to the technical or ethical standards of a profession; exhibiting a courteous, conscientious, and generally businesslike manner in the workplace

proficiency Competency as a result of training or practice.

profit sharing Offer of a part of a company's profits to employees or other designated individuals or groups.

progress notes Notes used in the patient chart to track the progress and condition of the patient.

prokaryote A unicellular organism having cells that lack a membrane-bound nucleus.

prolactin (PRL) Hormone secreted by the anterior pituitary gland; stimulates the development of the mammary gland.

proofread To read and mark corrections.

prostaglandins Chemicals released from cells that cause smooth muscle contraction and pain.

prosthesis Artificial replacement for a body part.

prosthetic The surgical or dental specialty concerned with the design, construction, and fitting of prostheses, which are artificial devices that replace missing parts of the body.

protected health information (PHI) Any individually identifiable health information that is transmitted and/or maintained in electronic form.

provider Any company, individual, or group that provides medical, diagnostic, or treatment services to a patient.

Provider Identification Numbers (PINs) Numbers assigned to providers by a carrier for use in submission of claims.

provider Individual or company that provides medical care and services to a patient or the public.

provisional diagnosis A temporary diagnosis made before all test results have been received.

proxemics The study of the nature, degree, and effect of the spatial separation individuals naturally maintain.

prudent Marked by wisdom or judiciousness; shrewd in the management of practical affairs.

psoriasis Usually chronic, recurrent skin disease marked by bright red patches covered with silvery scales.

psychosocial Pertaining to a combination of psychologic and social factors.

psyllium Grain that is found in some cereal products, in certain dietary supplements, and in certain bulk fiber laxatives; a water-soluble fiber.

public domain The realm embracing property rights that belong to the community at large, are unprotected by copyright or patent, and are subject to use or appropriation by anyone.

pulmonary consolidation Process by which the lungs become solidified as they fill with exudates in pneumonia.

pulse deficit Condition in which the radial pulse is less than the apical pulse; may indicate peripheral vascular abnormality.

pulse pressure Difference between the systolic and the diastolic blood pressures (30 to 50 mm Hg is considered normal).

pure culture A bacterial or fungal culture that contains a single organism.

putrefaction Decomposition of animal matter that results in a foul smell.

pyemia The presence of pus-forming organisms in the blood.

quackery The pretense of curing disease.

quality assurance Activities designed to increase the quality of a product or service through process or system changes that increase efficiency or effectiveness.

quality control An aggregate of activities designed to ensure adequate quality, especially in manufactured products or in the service industries.

queries Requests for information from a database.

rad Conventional unit of radiation dose.

radiograph An x-ray image.

radiographer Person qualified to perform radiographic examinations.

radiography Making diagnostic images using x-rays.

radiologist Physician specialist in medical imaging or therapeutic applications of radiation.

radiolucent Describing a substance that is easily penetrated by x-rays; these substances appear dark on radiographs.

radiopaque Substance that can easily be visualized on an x-ray film.

rales Abnormal or crackling breath sounds during inspiration.

ramifications Consequence; outgrowth; something produced by a cause or necessarily following from a set of conditions.

rapport Relationship of harmony and accord between the patient and the healthcare professional.

Raynaud's phenomenon Intermittent attacks of ischemia of the extremities; results in cyanosis, numbness, tingling, and pain.

ream A quantity of paper consisting of, variously, 480, 500, or 516 sheets.

reasonable doubt Doubt based on reason and arising from evidence or lack of evidence; it is not doubt that is imagined or conjured up, but doubt that would cause reasonable persons to hesitate before acting.

receipts Amounts paid on patient accounts.

receivables Total monies received on accounts.

recipient The receiver of some thing or item.

reconciliation The process of proving that a bank statement and checkbook balance are in agreement.

recourse A turning to something or someone for help or protection.

rectify To correct by removing errors.

reduction The return to correct anatomic position, as in reduction of a fracture.

referral An insurance term used when a primary care provider wants to send a patient to a specialist. Typically, the provider must obtain authorization from the insurance carrier in advance to refer a patient.

reflection The process of considering new information and internalizing it to create new ways of examining information.

refractile Causing light to refract, thus creating a sharp boundary or image.

registered dietitian (RD) Person with a minimum of a bachelor's degree in foods and nutrition who is concerned with the maintenance and promotion of health and the treatment of diseases through diet.

rejected claims Claims returned unpaid to the provider for clarification of any question and that must be corrected before resubmission.

relapse The recurrence of the symptoms of a disease after apparent recovery.

relevant Having significant and demonstrable bearing on the matter at hand.

rem Convention unit of radiation dose equivalent.

remission The partial or complete disappearance of the clinical and subjective characteristics of a chronic or malignant disease.

remittance advice (RA) An explanation of benefits which comes from Medicaid. See explanation of benefits above for the definition.

renal thresholds Levels above which substances cannot be reabsorbed by the renal tubules and are therefore excreted in the urine.

reparations Amends, acts of atonement, or satisfaction given as a result of a wrong or injury.

reprimands Criticisms for a fault; severe or formal reproofs.

reproach An expression of rebuke or disapproval; a cause or occasion of blame, discredit, or disgrace.

requisites Entities considered essential or necessary.

resource-based relative value scale (RBRVS) A fee schedule designed to provide national uniform payment of Medicare benefits after being adjusted to reflect the differences in practice costs across geographic areas.

respondent The person required to make answer in a civil legal action or suit; similar to a defendant in a criminal trial.

retention The act of keeping in possession or use; keeping in one's pay or service.

retention schedule A method or plan for retaining or keeping medical records, and their movement from active, to inactive, to closed filing.

rhinitis Inflammation of the mucous membranes of the nose.

rhinorrhea Discharge of nasal drainage.

rhonchi Abnormal rumbling sounds on expiration that indicate airway obstruction by thick secretions or spasms.

rider A special provision or group of provisions that may be added to a policy to expand or limit the benefits otherwise payable. It may increase or decrease benefits, waive a condition or coverage, or in any other way amend the original contract.

robotics Technology dealing with the design, construction, and operation of robots in automation.

rods Structures located in the retina of the eye and forming the light-sensitive elements.

roentgen (R) Conventional unit of radiation exposure.

router A device used to connect any number of LANs, which communicate with other routers and determine the best route between any two hosts.

sagittal plane Plane that divides the body into right and left parts.

salutation An expression of greeting, goodwill, or courtesy by words or gestures.

sanitization Cleaning the environment to reduce the number of pathogenic microorganisms.

sarcasm A sharp and often satirical response or ironic utterance designed to cut or give pain.

scanner Device that reads text or illustrations on a printed page and can translate the information on that page into a form that the computer can understand.

sclera White part of the eye that forms the orbit.

sclerotherapy Injection of sclerosing solutions in the treatment of hemorrhoids, varicose veins, or esophageal varices.

scoliosis Abnormal lateral curvature of the spine.

scored Slashed; for example, describes a tablet that is manufactured with an indentation for division through the center.

screen Something that shields, protects, or hides; to select or eliminate through a screening process.

search engines Programs that search documents for keywords and return a list of documents containing those words.

seborrhea Excessive discharge of sebum from the sebaceous glands forming greasy scales or cheesy plugs on the body.

secondary hypertension Elevated blood pressure resulting from another condition.

section The main divisions of the CPT-4 manual.

"see" A direction given to the coder to look in another place. This term must always be followed and is found in the Alphabetic Index, Volumes 2 and 3.

"see also" A direction given to the coder to look elsewhere if the main term or subterm (or subterms) for that entry are not sufficient for coding the information. If a code number follows, "see also" is enclosed in parentheses. If there is no code number, "see also" is preceded by a dash.

"see category" A direction given to the coder to see a specific category (three-digit code). This must always be followed.

self-insured plan An insurance plan funded by an organization having a large enough employee base that it can afford to fund its own insurance program.

self-referral The act of a patient or insured individual who refers himself or herself to a specialist without requesting the referral from the primary provider, such as a woman seeking an annual gynecologic examination. Managed care guidelines may require the patient to report the self-referral.

sentinel events Unexpected occurrences involving death or serious physical or psychologic injury, or the risk thereof.

sequentially Of, relating to, or arranged in a sequence.

serous Thin, watery, serum-like drainage.

serum The liquid portion of whole blood that remains after the blood has clotted.

server A computer or device on a network that manages shared network resources.

service benefit plans Plans that provide benefits in the form of certain surgical and medical services rendered, rather than cash. A service benefit plan is not restricted to a fee schedule.

shelf filing A system that uses open shelves rather than cabinets for storing records.

shingling A method of filing whereby one report is laid on top of the older report, resembling the shingles of a roof.

Sievert (Sv) International unit of radiation dose equivalent.

sinoatrial (SA) node Pacemaker of the heart, located in the right atrium.

sinus arrhythmia Irregular heartbeat originating in the sinoatrial node (pacemaker).

socioeconomic Relating to a combination of social and economic factors.

sociologic Oriented or directed toward social needs and problems.

sonography Imaging modality that uses sound waves to produce images of soft tissues; also called *diagnostic ultrasound.*

sound card Device that allows a computer to output sound through speakers that are connected to the main circuitry board, or motherboard.

specific gravity Weight of urine compared with an equal volume of water.

specimen A sample, as of tissue, blood, or urine, used for analysis and diagnosis.

spermicide A chemical substance that kills sperms cells.

spirometer Instrument that measures the volume of inhaled and exhaled air.

spores Thick-walled dormant form of bacteria, very resistant to disinfection measures.

staff privileges Allowance of a healthcare professional to practice within a specific facility.

standards Models or examples established by authority, custom, or general consent; something set up and established by authority as a rule for the measure of quantity, weight, extent, value, or quality.

stat With no delay; at once.

statement A request for payment.

statement of income and expense A summary of all income and expenses for a given period.

stationers Sellers of stationery.

statutes Laws enacted by the legislative branch of a government.

stereotactic An x-ray procedure to guide the insertion of a needle into a specific area of the breast.

stereotype Something conforming to a fixed or general pattern; a standardized mental picture that is held in common by many and represents an oversimplified opinion, prejudiced attitude, or uncritical judgment.

sterile Free of all microorganisms, pathogenic and nonpathogenic.

sterilization Complete destruction of all forms of microbial life.

stertorous Describes a strenuous respiratory effort that has a snoring sound.

stipulate To specify as a condition or requirement of an agreement or offer; to make an agreement or covenant to do or forbear from doing something.

stock options Offers of stocks for purchase to a certain group of individuals or certain groups, such as employees of a for-profit hospital.

stressors Stimuli that cause stress.

stridor Shrill, harsh respiratory sound heard during inhalation in the presence of a laryngeal obstruction.

stylus Metal probe that is inserted into or passed through a catheter, needle, or tube used for clearing purposes or to facilitate passage into a body orifice.

subcategory Indented one level below a category, usually a procedure or service unique to a specific category.

subjective information Information that is gained by questioning the patient or taken from a form.

subluxation Incomplete dislocation of a bone from its normal anatomic location.

subordinate Submissive to or controlled by authority; placed in or occupying a lower class, rank, or position.

subpoena A writ or document commanding a person to appear in court under a penalty for failure to appear.

subpoena duces tecum A legally binding request to appear in court and provide records or documents that pertain to a particular case.

subsection Indented one level below a section, a subsection usually describes an anatomic site or organ system—e.g., integumentary system or cardiology.

substance number A number based on the weight of a ream of paper containing 500 sheets.

subtle Difficult to understand or perceive; having or marked by keen insight and ability to penetrate deeply and thoroughly.

succinct Marked by compact, precise expression without wasted words.

superfluous Exceeding what is sufficient or necessary.

suppurative Characterized by formation and/or discharge of pus.

supravital Of, relating to, or capable of staining living cells after their removal from a living or recently dead organism.

surface area The total area of the body exposed to the outside environment.

surrogate A substitute; to put in place of another.

switch In networks, a device that filters information between LAN segments and decreases overall network traffic and increases speed and bandwidth usage efficiency.

syncope Fainting; a brief lapse in consciousness.

synopsis Condensed statement or outline.

synovial fluid Clear fluid found in joint cavities that facilitates smooth movements and nourishes joint structures.

system software The operating system and all utility programs that allow the computer to function and perform operations.

tachycardia Rapid but regular heart rate exceeding 100 beats per minute.

tachypnea Respirations that are rapid and shallow; hyperventilation.

tactful Having a keen sense of what to do or say to maintain good relations with others or to avoid offense.

tangible Capable of being appraised at an actual or approximate value; capable of being precisely identified or realized by the mind.

target market A specific group of individuals toward whom the marketing plan is focused.

targeted Directed or used toward a target; directed toward a specific desire or position.

TCP/IP Acronym for Transmission Control Protocol/ Internet Protocol; a suite of communications protocols used to connect users or hosts to the Internet.

tedious Tiresome because of length or dullness

telecommunications The science and technology of communication by transmission of information from one location to another via telephone, television, telegraph, or satellite.

telemedicine The use of telecommunications in the practice of medicine, in which great distances can exist among healthcare professionals, colleagues, patients, and students.

teleradiology The use of telecommunications devices to enhance and improve the results of radiologic procedures.

tendons Tough bands of connective tissue connecting muscle to bone.

terabyte Approximately 1 trillion bytes, abbreviated TB.

teratogen Any substance that interferes with normal prenatal development.

testimony A solemn declaration usually made orally by a witness under oath in response to interrogation by a lawyer or authorized public official.

thanatology The study of the phenomena of death and of psychologic methods of coping with death.

therapeutic range Blood concentration of a drug that produces the desired effect without toxicity.

third-party administrator An organization that processes claims and performs other business-related functions for a health plan.

third-party payor Someone other than the patient, spouse, or parent who is responsible for paying all or part of the patient's medical costs.

thixotropic gel A material that appears to be a solid until subjected to a disturbance, such as centrifugation, upon which it becomes a liquid.

thready Describes a pulse that is scarcely perceptible.

thrombolytics Agents that dissolve blood clots.

thrombus Blood clot.

thyroid-stimulating hormone (TSH) A hormone secreted by the anterior pituitary gland that stimulates the secretion of hormones produced by the thyroid gland.

tickler file A chronologic file used as a reminder that something must be taken care of on a certain date.

tinea Any fungal skin disease that results in scaling, itching, and inflammation.

tissue culture The technique or process of keeping tissue alive and growing in a culture medium.

toxemia An abnormal condition of pregnancy characterized by hypertension, edema, and protein in the urine.

tracers Radioactive substances administered to patients for nuclear medicine imaging procedures.

tracheostomy Surgical opening through the neck into the trachea for breathing.

transaction An exchange or transfer of goods, services, or funds. *Also,* As defined by HIPAA, transmissions of information between two parties to carry out financial or administrative activities related to healthcare.

transcription To make a written copy of, either in longhand or by machine.

transducer Part of the sonography machine that is in contact with the patient; the transducer sends high-frequency sound waves and receives the sound echoes that return from the patient's body.

transection Cross-section; division made by cutting across.

transient ischemic attack Temporary neurologic symptoms caused by a gradual or partial occlusion of a cerebral blood vessel.

transillumination Inspection of a cavity or organ by passing light through its walls.

transport medium A medium used to keep an organism alive during transport to the laboratory.

transposed Altered in sequence; interchanged.

transverse plane Plane that divides the body into superior and inferior parts.

trauma Physical injury or wound caused by an external force or violence.

treatises Systematic expositions or arguments in writing including a methodic discussion of the facts and principles involved and the conclusions reached.

triage Process of evaluating the urgency of medical need and prioritizing treatment.

trial balance A method of checking the accuracy of accounts.

TRICARE A government-sponsored program wherein authorized dependents of military personnel receive medical care. This program was originally called *CHAMPUS.*

triglyceride Fatty acid and glycerol compound that combines with a protein molecule to form high- or low-density lipoprotein.

tubercle A nodule produced by the tuberculosis bacillus.

turgor Resistance of the skin to being grasped between the fingers and released; refers to normal skin tension; is decreased in dehydration and increased with edema.

type and cross-match Tests performed to assess the compatibility of blood to be transfused.

unbundled codes Codes in which the components of a procedure are separated and reported separately.

Uniform Commercial Code (UCC) A unified set of rules covering many business transactions; it has been adopted in all 50 states, the District of Columbia, and most U.S. territories. It regulates the fields of sales of goods; commercial paper, such as checks; secured transactions in personal property; and particular aspects of banking, letters of credit, warehouse receipts, bills of lading, and investment securities.

unique provider identification number (UPIN) A number assigned by fiscal intermediaries to identify providers on claims for services.

unit dose Method of preparing individual doses of medications by the pharmacy.

universal claim form The form developed by the Health Care Financing Administration (HCFA) (now known as the Centers for Medicare and Medicaid Services [CMS]) and approved by the AMA for use in submitting all government-sponsored claims. Also known as the CMS-1500 form.

upcoding A deliberate increase in a CPT-4 code, despite the lack of documentation, to the next highest reimbursable code in order to receive higher reimbursements.

upper gastrointestinal (UGI) series Fluoroscopic examination of the esophagus, stomach, and duodenum using oral administration of barium sulfate as a contrast medium.

urea The major nitrogenous end product of protein metabolism and the chief nitrogenous component of the urine.

urease An enzyme that catalyzes the hydrolysis of urea to form ammonium carbonate.

urgency Sudden, compelling desire to urinate and the inability to control the release of urine.

URL Acronym for Uniform Resource Locator; specifies the global address of documents or information on the Internet. The URL provides the IP address and the domain name for the Web page, such as microsoft.com.

urticaria A skin eruption creating inflamed wheals; hives.

"use additional code" This term appears only in Volume 1 in those subdivisions in which the user should add further information by means of an additional code to give a more complete picture of the diagnosis. In some cases you will find "if desired" following the term. For the purpose of coding, the "if desired" phrase will not be used. When the term "use additional code…if desired" appears, disregard "if desired" and assign the appropriate additional code.

utilization review A review of individual cases by a committee to make sure that services are medically necessary and to study how providers use medical care resources.

Valsalva's maneuver Occurs when one strains to defecate and urinate, uses the arms and upper trunk muscles to move up in bed, or strains during laughing, coughing, or vomiting; causes a trapping of blood in the great veins, preventing it from entering the chest and right atrium, and may cause heart attack and death.

vasoconstriction Contraction of the muscles lining blood vessels that results in decreased lumen size.

vasodilation Increase in the diameter of a blood vessel.

vectors Animals or insects (e.g., ticks) that transmit the causative organisms of disease.

vehemently In a manner marked by forceful energy; intensely emotionally.

ventricles The two lower chambers of the heart.

veracity A devotion to or conformity with the truth.

verbiage A manner of expressing oneself in words.

verdict The finding or decision of a jury on a matter submitted to it in trial.

versatile Embracing a variety of subjects, fields or skills; having a wide range of abilities.

vertigo Dizziness; a sensation of faintness or an inability to maintain normal balance.

vested Granted or endowed with a particular authority, right, or property; to have a special interest in.

viable Capable of living, developing, or germinating under favorable conditions.

virtual reality An artificial environment presented to a computer user that feels as if it were a real environment, often involving use of special gloves, earphones, and goggles to enhance the experience.

virulent Exceedingly pathogenic, noxious, or deadly.

viscosity The quality of being thick and of lacking the capability of easy movement.

vocation The work in which a person is regularly employed.

voided Urinated.

volatile Easily aroused; tending to erupt in violence.

volatile Capable of vaporizing at a low temperature; describes an explosive substance.

vulva The external female genitalia, which begins at the mons pubis and terminates at the anus.

wasting syndrome Physical deterioration resulting in profound weight loss, fatigue, anorexia, and mental confusion.

watermark A marking in paper resulting from differences in thickness usually produced by the pressure of a projecting design in the mold or on a processing roll and visible when the paper is held up to the light.

wet mount A slide preparation in which a drop of liquid specimen or the like is covered with a coverslip and observed with a microscope.

wheal Localized area of edema or a raised lesion.

"with" In the context of ICD-9-CM, the terms "with," "with mention of," and "associated with" in a title dictate that both parts of the title be present in the statement of the diagnosis order to assign the particular code.

workers' compensation Insurance against liability imposed on certain employers to pay benefits and furnish care to employees who are injured and to pay benefits to dependents of employees killed in the course of or arising out of their employment.

zip drive A small, portable disk drive that is primarily used for backing up information and archiving computer files. A 100-megabyte Zip disk will hold the equivalent of approximately 70 floppy disks.

Index

Page numbers followed by *t* indicate tables; *f*, figures.

Strengthen your medical assisting skills and boost your confidence

with these interactive review and clinical preparation products!

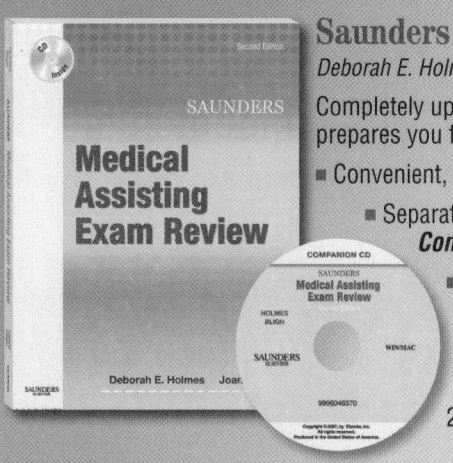

Saunders Medical Assisting Exam Review, 2nd Edition

Deborah E. Holmes, RN, MLT, CMA-C and Joanna Bligh, MEd, RT(R) (Ret.), CMA

Completely updated to meet the current standards of the AAMA and the AMT, this essential resource prepares you for the CMA and RMA exams.

■ Convenient, **easy-to-read outline format** streamlines key information for at-a-glance review.

  ■ Separate **general, administrative, and clinical pre-tests** in the text and on the *Companion CD* test your knowledge of important concepts.

    ■ **Practice tests** provide a realistic testing experience and include **clear rationales** to help you identify areas where more study is needed.

    ■ **Test-taking tips and study techniques** offer helpful suggestions on improving your retention and recall.

2007 • 288 pp., 120 illus. • **ISBN: 978-1-4160-2440-8**

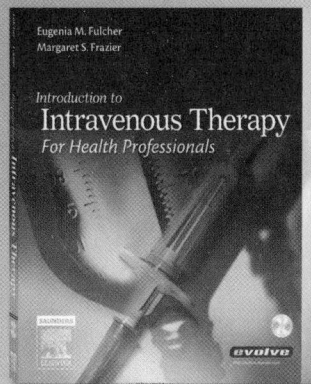

Introduction to Intravenous Therapy for Health Professionals

Eugenia M. Fulcher, RN, BSN, MEd, EdD, CMA and Margaret S. Frazier, RN, CMA, BS

This comprehensive guide teaches you the principles and techniques necessary to administer basic IV fluids and medications safely and effectively.

■ Basic overviews of **anatomy and physiology, IV equipment and supplies, and pharmacology** issues prepare you for practice.

■ A variety of exercises help you master complex skills, such as **IV calculations and patient teaching**.

■ **Multiple-choice chapter review questions** test and reinforce your understanding of key concepts.

■ *Competency Check Sheets* allow you to compare your performance to standards for proficiency, as well as competency-based education requirements.

2007 • 176 pp., illustd. • **ISBN: 978-1-4160-3399-8**

Virtual Medical Office

Elsevier's **Virtual Medical Office** learning system combines this textbook with a study guide and interactive software that let you practice key medical assisting skills before you start working in the real world.

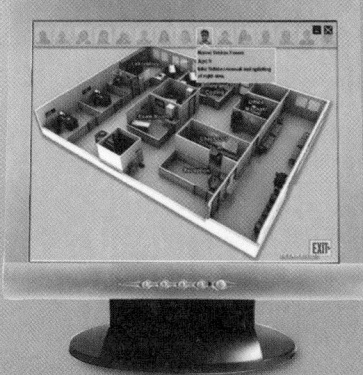

■ **Realistic simulations** provide valuable patient care experience and illustrate how **national curriculum competencies** come into play in the workplace.

■ Tasks such as handling a difficult patient, setting up the exam room, and troubleshooting rejected insurance claims help you develop the **critical thinking and decision-making skills** you will need to succeed on the job.

■ **Performance summaries** allow you to compare your decisions to those of an expert and evaluate any differences between the two.

■ More than two hours of video clips highlight **communication and professionalism aspects of patient care**.

2007 • **ISBN: 978-1-4160-4189-4**

Get your copies today!

Order securely at	Call toll-free	Visit your	
www.elsevierhealth.com	**1-800-545-2522**	**local bookstore**	**SAUNDERS** ELSEVIER

P-06677

The American Association of Medical Assistants and Commission on Accreditation of Allied Health Education Programs

Essentials/Standards initially adopted in l969; Revised in 1971, 1977, 1984, 1991, 1999, 2003

The Entry-Level Competencies for the medical assistant include, but are not limited to:

3.a. Administrative Competencies:

(1) Perform Clerical Functions
- (a) Schedule and manage appointments
- (b) Schedule inpatient and outpatient admissions and procedures
- (c) Organize a patient's medical record
- (d) File medical records

(2) Perform Bookkeeping Procedures
- (a) Prepare a bank deposit
- (b) Post entries on a daysheet
- (c) Perform accounts receivable procedures
- (d) Perform billing and collection procedures
- (e) Post adjustments
- (f) Process a credit balance
- (g) Process refunds
- (h) Post non-sufficient fund (NSF) checks
- (i) Post collection agency payments

(3) Process Insurance Claims
- (a) Apply managed care policies and procedures
- (b) Apply third party guidelines
- (c) Perform procedural coding
- (d) Perform diagnostic coding
- (e) Complete insurance claim forms

3.b. Clinical Competencies:

(1) Fundamental Procedures
- (a) Perform handwashing
- (b) Wrap items for autoclaving
- (c) Perform sterilization techniques
- (d) Dispose of biohazardous materials
- (e) Practice Standard Precautions

(2) Specimen Collection
- (a) Perform venipuncture
- (b) Perform capillary puncture
- (c) Obtain specimens for microbiological testing
- (d) Instruct patients in the collection of a clean-catch, mid-stream urine specimen
- (e) Instruct patients in the collection of a fecal specimen

(3) Diagnostic Testing
- (a) Perform electrocardiography
- (b) Perform respiratory testing
- (c) CLIA Waived Tests:
  - (i) Perform urinalysis
  - (ii) Perform hematology testing
  - (iii) Perform chemistry testing
  - (iv) Perform immunology testing
  - (v) Perform microbiology testing

(4) Patient Care
- (a) Perform telephone and in-person screening
- (b) Obtain vital signs
- (c) Obtain and record patient history
- (d) Prepare and maintain examination and treatment areas
- (e) Prepare patient for and assist with routine and specialty examinations
- (f) Prepare patient for and assist with procedures, treatments, and minor office surgeries
- (g) Apply pharmacology principles to prepare and administer oral and parenteral (excluding IV) medications
- (h) Maintain medication and immunization records
- (i) Screen and follow-up test results

3.c. General Competencies

(1) Professional Communications
- (a) Respond to and initiate written communications
- (b) Recognize and respond to verbal communications
- (c) Recognize and respond to nonverbal communications
- (d) Demonstrate telephone techniques

(2) Legal Concepts
- (a) Identify and respond to issues of confidentiality
- (b) Perform within legal and ethical boundaries
- (c) Establish and maintain the medical record
- (d) Document appropriately
- (e) Demonstrate knowledge of federal and state health care legislation and regulations

(3) Patient Instruction
- (a) Explain general office policies
- (b) Instruct individuals according to their needs
- (c) Provide instruction for health maintenance and disease prevention
- (d) Identify community resources

(4) Operational Functions
- (a) Perform an inventory of supplies and equipment
- (b) Perform routine maintenance of administrative and clinical equipment
- (c) Utilize computer software to maintain office systems
- (d) Use methods of quality control

General Competencies may be addressed in clinical, administrative, or both areas.